W9-BIT-190

ENDOCRINOLOGY

VOLUME 3

ENDOCRINOLOGY

THIRD EDITION

Edited by

LESLIE J. DeGROOT

MICHAEL BESSER
HENRY G. BURGER
J. LARRY JAMESON
D. LYNN LORIAUX
JOHN C. MARSHALL
WILLIAM D. ODELL
JOHN T. POTTS, Jr.
ARTHUR H. RUBENSTEIN

Consulting Editors

GEORGE F. CAHILL, Jr.
LUCIANO MARTINI
DON H. NELSON

W.B. SAUNDERS COMPANY

A Division of Harcourt Brace & Company

PHILADELPHIA   LONDON   TORONTO   MONTREAL   SYDNEY   TOKYO

W.B. SAUNDERS COMPANY
A Division of
Harcourt Brace & Company

The Curtis Center
Independence Square West
Philadelphia, Pennsylvania 19106

Library of Congress Cataloging-in-Publication Data

Endocrinology / edited by Leslie J. DeGroot . . . [et al.] ; consulting editors, George F. Cahill, Jr., Luciano Martini, Don H. Nelson.—3rd ed.

p.   cm.

Includes bibliographical references and index.

ISBN 0–7216–4262–4 (set). ISBN 0–7216–4263–2 (v.1).—ISBN 0–7216–4264–0 (v.2).—ISBN 0–7216–4265–9 (v. 3)

1. Endocrine glands—Diseases.   2. Endocrinology.   I. DeGroot, Leslie J.
   [DNLM: 1. Endocrine Diseases.   2. Endocrine Glands.   3. Hormones.   WK 100 E5345 1995]
RC648.E458   1995

616.4—dc20

DNLM/DLC
                                           93–8208

ENDOCRINOLOGY

                     Set ISBN 0–7216–4262–4
        Volume 1 ISBN 0–7216–4263–2
        Volume 2 ISBN 0–7216–4264–0
        Volume 3 ISBN 0–7216–4265–9

Last digit is the print number: 9   8   7   6   5   4   3   2   1

Contributors

NOBUYUKI AMINO, M.D.
Professor of Medicine, Department of Laboratory Medicine, Osaka University Medical School, Staff Physician, Osaka University Hospital, Osaka, Japan.
Autoimmune Thyroid Disease/Thyroiditis

JOSEPHINE ARENDT, Ph.D.
Professor of Endocrinology, School of Biological Sciences, University of Surrey, Surrey, England.
The Pineal Gland: Basic Physiology and Clinical Implications

ANDREW ARNOLD, M.D.
Associate Professor of Medicine, Harvard Medical School. Chief, Laboratory of Endocrine Oncology, Massachusetts General Hospital, Boston, Massachusetts.
Hyperparathyroidism; Hypoparathyroidism

LOUIS V. AVIOLI, M.D.
Schoenberg Professor of Medicine and Director, Division of Bone and Mineral Diseases, Washington University School of Medicine. Director, Division of Endocrinology and Metabolism, The Jewish Hospital of St. Louis, St. Louis, Missouri.
Disorders of Calcification: Osteomalacia and Rickets

SAMI T. AZAR, M.D.
Formerly Instructor in Medicine, Boston University School of Medicine. Presently Assistant Professor in Medicine, American University in Beirut, Beirut, Lebanon.
Hypoaldosteronism and Mineralocorticoid Resistance

DAVID T. BAIRD, M.B., D.Sc.
M.R.C. Clinical Research Professor, University of Edinburgh. Consultant Gynaecologist, Royal Infirmary, Edinburgh, Scotland.
Amenorrhea, Anovulation, and Dysfunctional Uterine Bleeding

H. W. GORDON BAKER, M.D., B.S., Ph.D., FRACP
Senior Research Fellow, Department of Obstetrics and Gynaecology, University of Melbourne. Andrologist, The Royal Women's Hospital and Austin Hospital; Senior Research Associate, Prince Henry's Institute of Medical Research, Monash Medical Centre, Clayton, Victoria, Australia.
Male Infertility

RANDALL B. BARNES, M.D.
Associate Professor, Department of Obstetrics and Gynecology, University of Chicago Pritzker School of Medicine. Attending Physician, Chicago Lying-in Hospital, Chicago, Illinois.
Hyperandrogenism, Hirsutism, and the Polycystic Ovary Syndrome

GEORGE B. BARTLEY, M.D.
Associate Professor of Ophthalmology, Mayo Medical School. Chair, Department of Ophthalmology, Mayo Clinic, Rochester, Minnesota.
Ophthalmopathy

ETIENNE-EMILE BAULIEU, M.D., Ph.D.
Professor, Collège de France. Chef de Service de Biochimie Hormonale, Hôpital de Bicêtre, Bicêtre, France.
Nuclear Receptor Superfamily

PETER H. BAYLIS, B.Sc., M.D., FRCP
Professor, The Medical School, University of Newcastle-Upon-Tyne. Consultant Physician, Royal Victoria Infirmary, Newcastle-Upon-Tyne, England.
Vasopressin and Its Neurophysin

GREGORY P. BECKS, M.D., FRCPC
Assistant Professor, Department of Medicine, Division of Endocrinology and Metabolism, University of Western Ontario. Attending Staff, Department of Medicine, Endocrine Division, St. Joseph's Health Centre of London, London, Ontario, Canada.
Diagnosis and Treatment of Thyroid Disease During Pregnancy

GRAEME I. BELL, Ph.D.
Professor of Biochemistry and Molecular Biology, and Medicine, University of Chicago Pritzker School of Medicine, Chicago, Illinois.
Chemistry and Biosynthesis of the Islet Hormones: Insulin, Islet Amyloid Polypeptide (Amylin), Glucagon, Somatostatin, and Pancreatic Polypeptide

RICHARD M. BERGENSTAL, M.D.
Clinical Associate Professor, University of Minnesota Medical School. Senior Vice President, International Diabetes Center, and Chairman, Endocrinology, Park Nicollet Medical Center, Minneapolis, Minnesota.
Diabetes Mellitus: Therapy

MICHAEL BESSER, M.D., D.Sc., FRCP
Professor of Medicine and Endocrinology, and Head, Departments of Medicine and Endocrinology, Medical College of St. Bartholomew's Hospital, University of London. Honourary Consultant Physician in Charge, Department of Endocrinology, St. Bartholomew's Hospital, London, England
Tests of Pituitary Function

DENNIS M. BIER, M.D.
Professor of Pediatrics, Baylor College of Medicine. Director, Children's Nutrition Research Center; Attending Physician, Texas Children's Hospital, Houston, Texas.
Metabolic Aspects of Fuel Homeostasis in the Fetus and the Neonate

HÅKAN BILLIG, M.D., Ph.D.
Assistant Professor, Department of Physiology, Göteborg University, Göteborg, Sweden.
Ovarian Hormone Synthesis and Mechanism of Action

MARC R. BLACKMAN, M.D.
Associate Professor of Medicine, Johns Hopkins University School of Medicine. Chief, Division of Endocrinology and Metabolism, and Associate Program Director, General Clinical Research Center, Francis Scott Key Medical Center, Baltimore, Maryland.
Endocrinology and Aging

STEPHEN R. BLOOM, M.A., M.D., D.Sc., FRCP
Professor of Endocrinology, Royal Postgraduate Medical School, Hammersmith Hospital, London, England.
Hormones of the Gastrointestinal Tract

GEORGE A. BRAY, M.D.
Professor of Medicine, Louisiana State University School of Medicine. Executive Director, Pennington Biomedical Research Institute, Baton Rouge, Louisiana.
The Syndromes of Obesity: An Endocrine Approach

H. BRYAN BREWER, Jr., M.D.
Chief, Molecular Disease Branch, National Heart, Lung, and Blood Institute, National Institutes of Health, Bethesda, Maryland.
Disorders of Lipoprotein Metabolism

F. RICHARD BRINGHURST, M.D.
Associate Professor of Medicine, Harvard Medical School. Associate Physician, Massachusetts General Hospital, Boston, Massachusetts.
Parathyroid Hormone: Physiology, Chemistry, Biosynthesis, Secretion, Metabolism, and Mode of Action; Calcium and Phosphate Distribution, Turnover, and Metabolic Actions

ARTHUR E. BROADUS, M.D., Ph.D.
Professor and Chairman, Division of Endocrinology, Yale University School of Medicine. Staff Physician, Yale-New Haven Hospital, New Haven, Connecticut
Malignancy-Associated Hypercalcemia

HENRY G. BURGER, M.D., FRACP, FCP(SA), FRACOG
Honorary Professor of Medicine, Monash University. Director, Prince Henry's Institute of Medical Research, and Director, Endocrine Unit, Monash Medical Centre, Clayton, Victoria, Australia.
Gonadal Regulatory Peptides

GERARD N. BURROW, M.D.
Dean and Professor of Internal Medicine, Yale University School of Medicine. Attending Physician, Department of Internal Medicine, Yale-New Haven Hospital, New Haven, Connecticut.
Diagnosis and Treatment of Thyroid Disease During Pregnancy

ROBERT K. CAMPBELL, Ph.D.
Executive Research Director, Ares Advanced Technology, Randolph, Massachusetts.
Gonadotropins

ERNESTO CANALIS, M.D.
Professor of Medicine and Orthopedics, University of Connecticut School of Medicine. Director of Research, St. Francis Hospital and Medical Center, Hartford, Connecticut.
Metabolic Bone Disease: Introduction and Classification

JOSÉ F. CARA, M.D.
Assistant Professor, University of Chicago Pritzker School of Medicine. Attending Physician, Wyler Children's Hospital, Chicago, Illinois.
Somatic Growth and Maturation

DON H. CATLIN, M.D.
Associate Professor, Departments of Medicine and of Molecular and Medical Pharmacology, University of California Los Angeles School of Medicine. Attending Physician, UCLA Hospital and Clinics, Los Angeles, California.
Anabolic Steroids

WILLIAM W. CHIN, M.D.
Professor of Medicine, Harvard Medical School. Investigator, Howard Hughes Medical Institute; Chief, Division of Genetics, and Senior Physician, Brigham and Women's Hospital, Boston, Massachusetts.
Hormonal Regulation of Gene Expression

JACK W. COBURN, M.D.
Adjunct Professor of Medicine, University of California Los Angeles School of Medicine. Staff Physician, Veterans Affairs Hospital, Los Angeles, California.
The Renal Osteodystrophies

NANCY E. COOKE, M.D.
Associate Professor of Medicine and Genetics, University of Pennsylvania School of Medicine. Staff Physician, Hospital of the University of Pennsylvania, Philadelphia, Pennsylvania.
Prolactin: Basic Physiology

ELIZABETH ANNE COWDEN, B.Sc.(Hons), M.B.Ch.B., FRCP (Glasgow), M.D. (Hons)
Acting Head, University Section of Endocrinology and Metabolism, University of Manitoba. Head, Section of Endocrinology and Metabolism, St. Boniface General Hospital, Winnipeg, Manitoba.
Endocrinology of Lactation and Nursing: Disorders of Lactation

MICHAEL J. CRONIN, Ph.D.
Visiting Associate Professor of Physiology, University of Virginia. Adjunct Professor of Physiology, University of Southern California, San Francisco, California.
Growth Hormone–Releasing Hormone: Basic Physiology and Clinical Implications

WILLIAM F. CROWLEY, Jr., M.D.
Professor of Medicine, Harvard Medical School. Chief, Reproductive Endocrine Sciences Center and National Center for Infertility Research, Massachusetts General Hospital, Boston, Massachusetts.
Gonadotropins and the Gonad: Normal Physiology and Their Disturbances in Clinical Endocrine Diseases

PHILIP E. CRYER, M.D.
Professor of Medicine and Director, Division of Endocrinology, Diabetes and Metabolism, Washington University School of Medicine. Physician, Barnes Hospital, St. Louis, Missouri.
Orthostatic (Postural) Hypotension

GARY C. CURHAN, M.D., M.S.
Instructor in Medicine, Harvard Medical School. Chief, Clinical Nephrology, Brockton/West Roxbury Veterans Administration Medical Center, West Roxbury, Massachusetts.
Calcium Nephrolithiasis

GORDON B. CUTLER, Jr., M.D.
Chief, Section on Developmental Endocrinology, Developmental Endocrinology Branch, National Institute of Child Health and Human Development, and Senior Staff Physician, Warren Grant Magnuson Clinical Center, National Institutes of Health, Bethesda, Maryland.
Cushing's Syndrome

DAVID L. DANIELS, M.D.
Professor of Radiology, Medical College of Wisconsin. Neuroradiologist, Froedtert Memorial Lutheran Hospital, Consultant in Radiology, Veterans Administration Medical Center, Milwaukee, Wisconsin.
Radiographic Evaluation of the Pituitary and Anterior Hypothalamus

DOMINIQUE DARMAUN, M.D., Ph.D.
Visiting Associate Professor of Pediatrics, University of Florida/Health Sciences Center. Attending Physician, Nemours Children's Clinic, Jacksonville, Florida.
Metabolic Aspects of Fuel Homeostasis in the Fetus and the Neonate

WILLIAM H. DAUGHADAY, M.D.
Irene M. and Michael E. Karl Professor Emeritus of Medicine, Washington University School of Medicine. Physician, Barnes Hospital, St. Louis Jewish Hospital, St. Louis, Missouri.
Growth Hormone, Insulin-Like Growth Factors, and Acromegaly

VAL DAVAJAN, M.D.†
Professor, Department of Obstetrics and Gynecology, Los Angeles County/University of Southern California Medical Center, Los Angeles, California.
Infertility: Causes, Evaluation, and Treatment

RALPH A. DeFRONZO, M.D.
Professor of Medicine and Chief, Diabetes Division, University of Texas Health Science Center, San Antonio, Texas.
Regulation of Intermediary Metabolism During Fasting and Feeding

LESLIE J. DeGROOT
Professor of Medicine, University of Chicago Pritzker School of Medicine. Staff Physician, University of Chicago Medical Center, Chicago, Illinois.
Mechanisms of Thyroid Hormone Action; Thyroid Neoplasia; Congenital Defects in Thyroid Hormone Formation and Action

---

†Deceased 7/13/93.

DAVID M. de KRETSER
Professor and Director, Institute of Reproduction and Development, Monash University. Consultant, Reproductive Biology Unit, Monash Medical Centre, Clayton, Victoria, Australia.
Basic Endocrinology of the Testis

MARIE B. DEMAY, M.D.
Assistant Professor of Medicine, Harvard Medical School. Assistant in Medicine, Massachusetts General Hospital, Boston, Massachusetts.
Hereditary Defects in Vitamin D Metabolism and Vitamin D Receptor Defects

ROBERTO Di LAURO, M.D.
Professor of Genetics, Dipartimento Di Scienze e Biotecnologie Mediche, Universita di Udine. Head, Laboratory of Biochemistry and Molecular Biology, Stazione Zoologica Anton Dohrn, Naples, Italy.
Biosynthesis and Secretion of Thyroid Hormones

JOHN L. DOPPMAN, M.D.
Director of Radiology, Department of Radiology, National Institutes of Health, Bethesda, Maryland.
Adrenal Imaging

J. E. DUMONT, M.D., Ph.D.
Professor of Biochemistry, School of Medicine and School of Sciences, University of Brussels. Consultant in Endocrinology, University Hospital Erasme, Brussels, Belgium.
Thyroid Regulation

CHRISTOPHER R. W. EDWARDS, M.D.
Professor of Clinical Medicine, Department of Medicine, University of Edinburgh. Honourary Consultant Physician, Western General Hospital, Edinburgh, Scotland.
Primary Mineralocorticoid Excess Syndromes

EDWARD N. EHRLICH, M.D.
Professor Emeritus, Section of Endocrinology and Metabolism, Department of Medicine, University of Wisconsin Medical School. Attending Physician, University of Wisconsin Hospital and Clinics, Madison, Wisconsin.
Hormonal Regulation of Electrolyte and Water Metabolism

DAVID A. EHRMANN, M.D.
Assistant Professor, Section of Endocrinology, Department of Medicine, University of Chicago Pritzker School of Medicine. Attending Physician, University of Chicago Hospitals, Chicago, Illinois.
Hyperandrogenism, Hirsutism, and the Polycystic Ovary Syndrome

RAGNAR EKHOLM, M.D., Ph.D.
Professor Emeritus of Anatomy, Department of Anatomy, University of Göteborg, Göteborg, Sweden.
Thyroid Gland: Anatomy and Development

DARIUSH ELAHI, Ph.D.
Associate Professor of Medicine, Department of Medicine, University of Maryland School of Medicine Veterans Affairs Medical Center, Geriatrics and Guest Researcher, NIH/NIA, Laboratory of Clinical Physiology, Baltimore, Maryland.
Endocrinology and Aging

ERIC A. ESPINER, M.B., M.D., FRACP, FRSNZ
Professor in Medicine, Christchurch School of Medicine, University of Otago. Head, Department of Endocrinology, Christchurch Hospital, Christchurch, New Zealand.
Hormones of the Cardiovascular System

STEFAN S. FAJANS, M.D.
Professor Emeritus (Active) of Internal Medicine, Division of Endocrinology and Metabolism, University of Michigan Medical School, Ann Arbor, Michigan.
Diabetes Mellitus: Definition, Classification, Tests

ELEUTERIO FERRANNINI, M.D.
Chief, Metabolic Branch, CNR Institute of Physiology, Pisa, Italy.
Regulation of Intermediary Metabolism During Fasting and Feeding

DELBERT A. FISHER, M.D.
Professor Emeritus, Pediatrics and Medicine, University of California Los Angeles School of Medicine. Senior Scientist, Research and Education Institute, Harbor-UCLA Medical Center, Torrance, California.
Thyroid Disease in the Fetus, Neonate, and Child; Fetal and Neonatal Endocrinology

LORRAINE A. FITZPATRICK, M.D.
Associate Professor of Medicine, Mayo Graduate School of Medicine, Mayo Clinic and Mayo Foundation. Consultant in Endocrinology, Mayo Clinic, St. Mary's Hospital, Rochester Methodist Hospital, Rochester, Minnesota.
Hypoparathyroidism

JEFFREY S. FLIER, M.D.
Professor of Medicine, Harvard Medical School. Chief, Division of Endocrinology, Beth Israel Hospital, Boston, Massachusetts.
Syndromes of Insulin Resistance and Mutant Insulin

MAGUELONE G. FOREST, M.D.
Director of Research, INSERM. Hôpital Debrousse, Lyons, France.
Diagnosis and Treatment of Disorders of Sexual Development

DANIEL W. FOSTER, M.D.
Donald W. Seldin Distinguished Chair and Chairman, Department of Internal Medicine, University of Texas Southwestern Medical School, Dallas, Texas.
Diabetes Mellitus: Acute Complications, Ketoacidosis, Hyperosmolar Coma, Lactic Acidosis

AARON L. FRIEDMAN, M.D.
Professor, Nephrology Section, Department of Pediatrics, University of Wisconsin Medical School. Attending Physician, University of Wisconsin Hospital and Clinics, Madison, Wisconsin.
Hormonal Regulation of Electrolyte and Water Metabolism

ELI A. FRIEDMAN, M.D.
Distinguished Teaching Professor of Medicine, State University of New York Health Science Center at Brooklyn. Attending Physician and Director, Division of Renal Disease, University Hospital of Brooklyn and Kings County Hospital Center, Brooklyn, New York.
Diabetes Mellitus: Late Complications, Nephropathy

HENRY G. FRIESEN, M.D.
President, Medical Research Council of Canada, Ottawa, Ontario, Canada.
Endocrinology of Lactation and Nursing: Disorders of Lactation

JOHN W. FUNDER, M.D.
Director, Baker Medical Research Institute, Prahran, Victoria, Australia.
Aldosterone Action: Biochemistry

MATS E. GÅFVELS, M.D., Ph.D.
Visiting Assistant Professor, Department of Obstetrics and Gynecology, University of Pennsylvania School of Medicine, Philadelphia, Pennsylvania.
Placental Hormones

ROBERT F. GAGEL, M.D.
Professor of Medicine, University of Texas M.D. Anderson Cancer Center; Associate Professor of Medicine, Baylor College of Medicine, Houston, Texas.
Multiple Endocrine Neoplasia Type 2

HENRIK GALBO, M.D., D.M.Sc.
Professor, Exercise Physiology, Department of Medical Physiology, University of Copenhagen. Chief Physician, Internal Medicine and Rheumatology, University Hospital, Copenhagen, Denmark.
Integrated Endocrine Responses and Exercise

STEEN GAMMELTOFT, M.D.
Professor, University of Copenhagen. Medical Director, Glostrup Hospital, Copenhagen, Denmark.
Hormone Signaling via Membrane Receptors

THOMAS GARDELLA, Ph.D.
Assistant Professor of Medicine, Harvard Medical School. Assistant Professor in Biochemistry, Massachusetts General Hospital, Boston, Massachusetts.
Parathyroid Hormone: Physiology, Chemistry, Biosynthesis, Secretion, Metabolism, and Mode of Action

EDWARD P. GELMANN, M.D.
Professor of Medicine, Georgetown University School of Medicine. Chief, Division of Medical Oncology, Vincent T. Lombardi Cancer Research Center, Washington, D.C.
Endocrine Management of Malignant Disease

FABRIZIO GENTILE, M.D., Ph.D.
Investigator, Centro di Endocrinologia e Oncologia Sperimentale del Consiglio Nazionale delle Ricerche, Naples, Italy.
Biosynthesis and Secretion of Thyroid Hormones

HANS GERBER, M.D.
Privatdozent, University of Bern School of Medicine. Head of Division, Department of Clinical Chemistry, University Hospital, Inselspital, Bern, Switzerland.
Multinodular Goiter

MARVIN C. GERSHENGORN, MD.
Abby Rockefeller Mauze Distinguished Professor of Endocrinology in Medicine, and Chief, Division of Molecular Medicine; Cornell University Medical College. Attending Physician, The New York Hospital, New York, New York.
Second Messenger Signaling Pathways: Phosphatidylinositol and Calcium

MOHAMMAD A. GHATEI, Ph.D.
Lecturer, Division of Endocrinology and Metabolism, Royal Postgraduate Medical School, Hammersmith Hospital, London, England.
Hormones of the Gastrointestinal Tract

STEVEN R. GOLDRING, M.D
Associate Professor of Medicine, Harvard Medical School. Chief of Rheumatology, New England Deaconess Hospital; Clinical Associate, Massachusetts General Hospital, Boston, Massachusetts
Disorders of Calcification: Osteomalacia and Rickets

LOUIS J. G. GOOREN, M.D., Ph.D.
Professor of Medicine, Free University, Amsterdam. Head of Division of Andrology, Department of Endocrinology, Free University Hospital, Amsterdam, The Netherlands.
Normal and Abnormal Sexual Behavior

COLUM A. GORMAN, M.B., B.Ch., Ph.D.
Professor of Medicine, Mayo Medical School. Consultant, Mayo Clinic, Rochester, Minnesota.
Ophthalmopathy

NICHOLAS M. GOUGH, Ph.D.
Head, Molecular Hematology Laboratory, The Walter and Eliza Hall Institute of Medical Research, Royal Melbourne Hospital, Melbourne, Australia.
Hormones and Blood Cell Production

ANDREW J. GREEN, M.D.
Medical Director, Diabetes Center of Excellence, Overland Park Regional Medical Center, Overland Park, Kansas.
The Neuropathies of Diabetes

ASHLEY GROSSMAN, B.A., B.Sc., M.D., FRCP
Professor of Neuroendocrinology, St. Bartholomew's Hospital Medical College, University of London. Honourary Consultant Physician, St. Bartholomew's Hospital, London, England.
Corticotropin-Releasing Hormone: Basic Physiology and Clinical Applications

JOEL F. HABENER, M.D.
Professor of Medicine, Harvard Medical School. Investigator, Howard Hughes Medical Institute; Chief, Laboratory of Molecular Endocrinology, and Associate Physician, Massachusetts General Hospital, Boston, Massachusetts.
Cyclic AMP Second Messenger Signaling Pathway; Hyperparathyroidism

JANET E. HALL, M.D.
Assistant Professor in Medicine, Harvard Medical School. Assistant in Medicine, Massachusetts General Hospital, Boston, Massachusetts.
Gonadotropins and the Gonad: Normal Physiology and Their Disturbances in Clinical Endocrine Diseases

REGINALD HALL, B.Sc., M.D., FRCP, OBE
Professor Emeritus of Medicine, University of Wales College of Medicine, Cardiff, Wales.
Thyrotropin-Releasing Hormone: Basic and Clinical Aspects

DAVID J. HANDELSMAN, M.B., B.S., Ph.D., FRACP
Associate Professor, Departments of Obstetrics and Gynaecology and of Medicine, University of Sydney. Director, Andrology Unit and Department of Endocrinology, Royal Prince Alfred Hospital, Sydney, Australia.
Testosterone and Other Androgens: Physiology, Pharmacology, and Therapeutic Use; Contraception in the Male

HISATO HARA, M.D.
Visiting Research Associate, University of Chicago Hospitals, Chicago, Illinois.
Developmental Abnormalities of the Thyroid; Surgery of the Thyroid

S. MITCHELL HARMAN, M.D., Ph.D.
Associate Professor, Department of Medicine, Johns Hopkins University School of Medicine. Section Chief, Endocrinology Section, Gerontology Research Center, National Institute on Aging, National Institutes of Health. Attending Physician, Francis Scott Key Medical Center, Baltimore, Maryland.
Endocrinology and Aging

VICTOR M. HAUGHTON, M.D.
Professor of Radiology and Director of MRI Research, Medical College of Wisconsin. Radiologist, Milwaukee County Medical Complex, Froedtert Memorial Lutheran Hospital; Consultant in Radiology, Veterans Administration Medical Center, Milwaukee, Wisconsin.
Radiographic Evaluation of the Pituitary and Anterior Hypothalamus

MOREY W. HAYMOND, M.D.
Professor of Pediatrics, Mayo Medical School. Medical Director, Nemours Children's Clinic, Jacksonville, Florida.
Metabolic Aspects of Fuel Homeostasis in the Fetus and the Neonate

DAVID HEBER, M.D., Ph.D.
Professor of Medicine and Chief, Division of Clinical Nutrition, Department of Medicine, University of California Los Angeles School of Medicine. Director, Clinical Nutrition Research Unit, University of California Los Angeles, Los Angeles, California.
Endocrine Responses to Starvation, Malnutrition, and Illness

KEVAN C. HEROLD, M.D.
Assistant Professor, Department of Medicine, University of Chicago Pritzker School of Medicine. Attending Physician, Chicago Children's Diabetes Center and LaRabida Children's Hospital, Chicago, Illinois.
Immunological Mechanisms Causing Autoimmune Endocrine Disease

ARMIN E. HEUFELDER, M.D.
Instructor in Internal Medicine and Endocrinology, and Molecular Thyroid Research Laboratory Director, Medizinische Klinik, Klinikum Innenstadt, Ludwig-Maximilians-University, Munich, Germany.
Ophthalmopathy

RICHARD A. HIIPAKKA, Ph.D.
Senior Research Associate, Ben May Institute, University of Chicago, Chicago, Illinois.
Androgen Receptors and Action

GARY D. HODGEN, Ph.D.
Professor and President, The Jones Institute for Reproductive Medicine, Department of Obstetrics and Gynecology, Eastern Virginia Medical School, Norfolk, Virginia
Ovarian Follicular Maturation, Ovulation, and Ovulation Induction

JEFFREY M. HOEG, M.D.
Head, Section of Cell Biology, Molecular Disease Branch, National Heart, Lung, and Blood Institute, National Institutes of Health, Bethesda, Maryland.
Disorders of Lipoprotein Metabolism

J. J. HOET, M.D.
Professor of Medicine, University of Louvain, Louvain, Belgium.
Anatomy, Developmental Biology, and Pathology of the Pancreatic Islets

MICHAEL F. HOLICK, Ph.D., M.D.
Professor of Medicine, Physiology and Dermatology, Boston University School of Medicine. Chief, Endocrinology, Diabetes, and Metabolism Section, Boston University Medical Center and Boston City Hospital and Veterans Administration Hospital; Director, General Clinical Research Center, and Director, Vitamin D, Skin, and Bone Research Laboratory, Boston University School of Medicine, Boston, Massachusetts
Vitamin D: Photobiology, Metabolism, and Clinical Applications

EVA HORVATH, Ph.D.
Associate Professor of Pathology, University of Toronto. Research Associate, St. Michael's Hospital, Toronto, Ontario, Canada.
Anatomy and Histology of the Normal and Abnormal Pituitary Gland

AARON J. W. HSUEH, Ph.D.
Professor, Division of Reproductive Biology, Stanford University Medical Center, Stanford, California
Ovarian Hormone Synthesis and Mechanism of Action

HIROO IMURA, M.D.
President, Kyoto University, Kyoto, Japan.
Adrenocorticotropic Hormone

KARL L. INSOGNA, M.D.
Associate Professor, Endocrinology, Yale University School of Medicine. Attending Physician, Yale-New Haven Hospital, New Haven, Connecticut.
Malignancy-Associated Hypercalcemia

ROBERT ISRAEL, M.D.
Professor, University of Southern California School of Medicine, Los Angeles. Attending Physician, Women's Hospital; Hospital of the Good Samaritan, Los Angeles, California.
Infertility: Causes, Evaluation, and Treatment

KOICHI ITO, M.D.
Visiting Research Associate, University of Chicago Hospitals, Chicago, Illinois.
Developmental Abnormalities of the Thyroid; Surgery of the Thyroid

J. LARRY JAMESON, M.D., Ph.D.
Charles F. Kettering Professor of Medicine; Chief, Division of Endocrinology, Metabolism, and Molecular Medicine, Northwestern University Medical School. Chief, Section of Endocrinology and Metabolism, Northwestern Memorial Hospital, Chicago, Illinois.
Applications of Molecular Biology in Endocrinology; Mechanisms of Thyroid Hormone Action

JONATHAN B. JASPAN, M.D.
Tullis-Tulane Alumni Chair in Diabetes, and Professor of Medicine, Tulane University Medical Center School of Medicine. Attending Physician, Endocrinology and General Internal Medicine, Tulane University Medical Center and Clinics; Medical Center of Louisiana; and Veterans Administration Medical Center, New Orleans, Louisiana.
The Neuropathics of Diabetes

NATHALIE JOSSO, M.D.
Research Director, Institut de la Santé et de la Recherche Médicale, Ecole Normale Supérieure. Hôpital Saint-Vincent de Paul, Paris, France.
Anatomy and Endocrinology of Fetal Sex Differentiation

C. RONALD KAHN, M.D.
Mary K. Iacocca Professor of Medicine, Harvard Medical School. Research Director, Elliott P. Joslin Research Laboratory, Joslin Diabetes Center, Boston, Massachusetts.
Hormone Signaling via Membrane Receptors; the Molecular Mechanism of Insulin Action

EDWIN L. KAPLAN, M.D.
Professor of Surgery, University of Chicago Pritzker School of Medicine and University of Chicago Hospitals, Chicago, Illinois.
Developmental Abnormalities of the Thyroid; Surgery of the Thyroid

JOSEPHINE Z. KASA-VUBU, M.D.
Assistant Professor of Pediatrics, University of Michigan Medical School. Assistant Professor of Pediatrics, University of Michigan Medical Center, Ann Arbor, Michigan.
Precocious and Delayed Puberty: Diagnosis and Treatment

HARRY R. KEISER, M.D.
Clinical Professor of Medicine, Georgetown University School of Medicine, Washington, D.C. Clinical Director, National Heart, Lung, and Blood Institute, National Institutes of Health, Bethesda, Maryland.
Pheochromocytoma and Related Tumors

ROBERT P. KELCH, M.D.
Professor of Pediatrics, Department of Pediatrics, University of Michigan Medical School. Chairman, Department of Pediatrics, University of Michigan Medical Center, and Physician-in-Chief, C.S. Mott Children's Hospital, Ann Arbor, Michigan.
Precocious and Delayed Puberty: Diagnosis and Treatment

DANIEL KENIGSBERG, M.D.
Clinical Associate Professor, State University of New York at Stony Brook. Chief, Section of Reproductive Endocrinology, John T. Mather Memorial Hospital, Fort Jefferson, New York.
Ovarian Follicular Maturation, Ovulation, and Ovulation Induction

JEFFREY B. KERR, Ph.D.
Associate Professor, Department of Anatomy, Monash University, Clayton, Victoria, Australia.
Basic Endocrinology of the Testis

BARRY F. KING, Ph.D.
Professor of Cell Biology and Human Anatomy, University of California School of Medicine, Davis, California.
Placental Hormones

RONALD KLEIN, M.D., M.P.H.
Professor, Department of Ophthalmology and Visual Sciences, University of Wisconsin Medical School. Attending Physician, University of Wisconsin Hospitals and Clinics, Madison, Wisconsin.
Diabetes Mellitus: Late Complications, Oculopathy

STANLEY G. KORENMAN, M.D.
Professor of Medicine and Associate Dean, University of California Los Angeles. Chief of Endocrinology, Center for the Health Sciences; Attending Physician, University of California Los Angeles Medical Center, Los Angeles, California.
Male Impotence

KALMAN KOVACS, M.D., Ph.D.
Professor of Pathology, University of Toronto. Pathologist, St. Michael's Hospital, Toronto, Ontario, Canada.
Anatomy and Histology of the Normal and Abnormal Pituitary Gland

STEPHEN M. KRANE, M.D.
Persis, Cyrus and Marlow B. Harrison Professor of Medicine, Harvard Medical School. Physician and Chief of Arthritis Unit, Massachusetts General Hospital, Boston, Massachusetts
Metabolic Bone Disease: Introduction and Classification; Disorders of Calcification: Osteomalacia and Rickets

HENRY KRONENBERG, M.D.
Professor of Medicine, Harvard Medical School. Chief, Endocrine Unit, Massachusetts General Hospital, Boston, Massachusetts.
Parathyroid Hormone: Physiology, Chemistry, Biosynthesis, Secretion, Metabolism, and Mode of Action

A. H. LAUBER, M.D.
Laboratory of Neurobiology and Behavior, The Rockefeller University, New York, New York.
Hypothalamus and Hormone–Regulated Behaviors

VALERIANO LEITE, M.D.
Post-doctoral Fellow, Department of Physiology, University of Manitoba, Winnipeg, Canada. Endocrinologist, Department of Endocrinology, Portuguese Cancer Institute, Lisbon, Portugal.
Endocrinology of Lactation and Nursing: Disorders of Lactation

ÅKE LERNMARK, Ph.D.
Professor in Experimental Endocrinology, and Chairman, Department of Endocrinology and Clinical Genetics, Karolinska Institute, Stockholm, Sweden.
Insulin-Dependent (Type I) Diabetes: Etiology, Pathogenesis, and Natural History

MICHAEL A. LEVINE, M.D.
Professor of Medicine and Pathology, Johns Hopkins University School of Medicine. Physician, Johns Hopkins Hospital, Baltimore, Maryland.
Pseudohypoparathyroidism

SHUTSUNG LIAO, Ph.D.
Professor, Ben May Institute and the Department of Biochemistry and Molecular Biology, University of Chicago.
Androgen Receptors and Action

GRAHAM C. LIGGINS, M.D., Ph.D.
Professor Emeritus, University of Auckland. Director, Research Centre in Reproductive Medicine, National Women's Hospital, Auckland, New Zealand.
Endocrinology of Parturition

DENNIS W. LINCOLN, D.Sc.
Director, MRC Reproductive Biology Unit, Edinburgh, Scotland.
Gonadotropin-Releasing Hormone (GnRH): Basic Physiology

MARC E. LIPPMAN, M.D.
Professor of Medicine and Pharmacology, Georgetown University School of Medicine. Director, Vincent T. Lombardi Cancer Research Center, Washington, D.C.
Endocrine Management of Malignant Disease

JONATHAN S. LoPRESTI, M.D., Ph.D.
Assistant Professor of Medicine, University of Southern California School of Medicine. Attending Physician, Los Angeles County/USC Medical Center, Los Angeles, California.
Nonthyroidal Illnesses

D. LYNN LORIAUX, M.D.
Professor of Medicine, University of Oregon School of Medicine. Head, Division of Endocrinology, Oregon Health Sciences University, Portland, Oregon.
An Introduction to Endocrinology; Adrenal Insufficiency

IAIN MacINTYRE, M.D., D.Sc., FRCP
Associate Director, The William Harvey Research Institute, St. Bartholomew's Hospital Medical College, London, England.
Calcitonin: Physiology, Biosynthesis, Secretion, Metabolism, and Mode of Action

NOEL K. MACLAREN, M.D.
Professor and Chairman, Department of Pathology and Laboratory Medicine, University of Florida College of Medicine. Attending Physician, Shands Hospital, Gainesville, Florida.
Polyglandular Failure Syndromes

WILLY J. MALAISSE, M.D., Ph.D.
Professor of Chemical Pathology and Director of the Laboratory of Experimental Medicine, Brussels Free University, Brussels, Belgium.
Insulin Secretion and Beta Cell Metabolism

CARL D. MALCHOFF, M.D., Ph.D.
Associate Professor of Surgery and Medicine, University of Connecticut Health Center. Associate Professor of Surgery and Medicine, John Dempsey Hospital, Farmington, Connecticut.
Glucocorticoid Resistance

DIANA M. MALCHOFF, Ph.D.
Assistant Professor of Surgery and Medicine, University of Connecticut Health Center, Farmington, Connecticut
Glucocorticoid Resistance

LEIGHTON P. MARK, M.D.
Associate Professor of Radiology, Medical College of Wisconsin. Neuroradiologist, Froedtert Memorial Lutheran Hospital, Consultant in Radiology, Veterans Administration Medical Center, Milwaukee, Wisconsin.
Radiographic Evaluation of the Pituitary and Anterior Hypothalamus

JOHN C. MARSHALL, M.D., Ph.D.
Professor and Chair, Department of Internal Medicine, University of Virginia School of Medicine. Physician in Chief, University of Virginia Hospitals, University of Virginia Health Sciences Center, Charlottesville, Virginia.
Regulation of Gonadotropin Secretion; Hormonal Regulation of the Menstrual Cycle and Mechanisms of Anovulation

JOSEPH B. MARTIN, M.D., Ph.D.
Professor of Neurology, University of California San Francisco School of Medicine, San Francisco, California.
Functional Anatomy of the Hypothalamic–Anterior Pituitary Complex

T. J. MARTIN, M.D., D.Sc., FRACP
Professor of Medicine, Department of Medicine, University of Melbourne. Director, St. Vincent's Institute of Medical Research, St. Vincent's Hospital, Melbourne, Australia.
Parathyroid Hormone–Related Protein

DIANA MARVER, M.D.
Associate Professor of Internal Medicine, Division of Nephrology, Department of Internal Medicine, University of Texas Southwestern Medical Center, Dallas, Texas.
Aldosterone Action: Biochemistry

WALTER J. McDONALD, M.D.
Associate Dean for Education; Oregon Health Sciences University. Active Staff, University Hospital, Portland, Oregon.
Adrenal Insufficiency

J. DENIS McGARRY, Ph.D.
Professor of Internal Medicine and Biochemistry, University of Texas Southwestern Medical School, Dallas, Texas.
Diabetes Mellitus: Acute Complications, Ketoacidosis, Hyperosmolar Coma, Lactic Acidosis

J. MAXWELL McKENZIE, M.D.
Kathleen and Stanley Glaser Professor and Chairman, Department of Medicine; Professor, Department of Physiology and Biophysics, University of Miami School of Medicine. Chief, Medical Services, Jackson Memorial Hospital; Staff Physician, University of Miami Hospital and Clinics, Miami, Florida.
Hyperthyroidism

GERALDO MEDEIROS-NETO, M.D.
Associate Professor of Endocrinology, University of São Paulo Medical School. Chief, Thyroid Laboratory, Division of Endocrinology, Department of Medicine, Hospital das Clinicas, São Paulo, Brazil.
Iodide Deficiency Disorders

CHRISTOPH A. MEIER, M.D.
Instructor, University Hospital. Research Associate, Thyroid Unit, Department of Endocrinology, University Hospital, Geneva, Switzerland.
Thyroid-Stimulating Hormone in Health and Disease

A. WAYNE MEIKLE, M.D.
Professor of Medicine, Division of Endocrinology, University of Utah School of Medicine. University of Utah Hospital, and Associated Regional and University Pathologists, Director of Endocrine Testing, Salt Lake City, Utah.
Endocrinology of the Prostate and of Benign Prostatic Hyperplasia

JAMES C. MELBY, M.D.
Professor of Medicine, Boston University School of Medicine, Boston, Massachusetts.
Hypoaldosteronism and Mineralocorticoid Resistance

SHLOMO MELMED, M.D.
Professor of Medicine, University of California Los Angeles School of Medicine. Director, Cedars-Sinai Medical Center Research Institute, Los Angeles, California.
Tumor Mass Effects of Lesions in the Hypothalamus and Pituitary; General Aspects of the Management of Pituitary Tumors by Surgery or Radiation Therapy

JAN MESTER, M.D.
Unité de Recherches sur les Peptides, Neurodigestifs et le Diabète, Institut Nationel de la Santé et de la Recherche Médicale, Paris, France.
Nuclear Receptor Superfamily

DONALD METCALF, M.D.
Research Professor of Cancer Biology, The Walter and Eliza Hall Institute of Medical Research, Royal Melbourne Hospital, Melbourne, Australia.
Hormones and Blood Cell Production

BOYD E. METZGER, M.D.
Professor of Medicine, Division of Endocrinology and Metabolism, Northwestern University Medical School. Attending Physician, Northwestern Memorial Hospital, Chicago, Illinois.
Diabetes Mellitus and Pregnancy

ROGER L. MIESFELD, Ph.D.
Associate Professor of Biochemistry, University of Arizona, Arizona Cancer Center, Tucson, Arizona.
Glucocorticoid Action: Biochemistry

DANIEL R. MISHELL, Jr., M.D.
Lyle T. McNeile Professor and Chairman, Department of Obstetrics and Gynecology, University of Southern California School of Medicine. Chief of Professional Services, Los Angeles County/University of Southern California Medical Center, Women's Hospital, Los Angeles, California.
Contraception

MARK E. MOLITCH, M.D.
Professor of Medicine, Center for Endocrinology, Metabolism and Molecular Medicine, Northwestern University Medical School. Attending Physician, Northwestern Memorial Hospital; Consultant, Lakeside Veterans Administration Hospital, Chicago, Illinois.
Pitfalls in Endocrine Tests and Testing in Pregnancy

JOHN MONEY, M.D.
Professor Emeritus of Medical Psychology and Professor Emeritus of Pediatrics, Johns Hopkins University and Johns Hopkins University School of Medicine. Director, Psychohormonal Research Unit, Johns Hopkins Hospital, Baltimore, Maryland
Normal and Abnormal Sexual Behavior

THOMAS J. MOORE, M.D.
Associate Professor of Medicine, Harvard Medical School. Director, Ambulatory Clinical Center, and Director, Cardiac Risk Reduction Center, Brigham and Women's Hospital, Boston, Massachusetts.
Hormonal Aspects of Hypertension

RICHARD M. MORTENSEN, M.D., Ph.D.
Assistant Professor of Medicine, Harvard Medical School. Associate Physician, Brigham and Women's Hospital, Boston, Massachusetts.
Aldosterone Action: Physiology

J. M. MOSELEY, Ph.D.
Senior Research Fellow, University of Melbourne. Department of Medicine, St. Vincent's Hospital, Melbourne, Australia.
Parathyroid Hormone–Related Protein

WILLIAM R. MOYLE, Ph.D.
Professor of Obstetrics and Gynecology, University of Medicine and Dentistry of New Jersey–Robert Wood Johnson Medical School, Piscataway, New Jersey.
Gonadotropins

ANDREW MUIR, M.D.
Assistant Professor, Department of Pathology and Laboratory Medicine, Department of Pediatrics, University of Florida College of Medicine. Attending Physician, Shands Hospital, Gainesville, Florida.
Polyglandular Failure Syndromes

EUGENIO E. MÜLLER, M.D.
Professor and Chairman, Department of Pharmacology, School of Medicine, University of Milan. Professor of Pharmacology, University of Milan, Milan, Italy.
Role of Neurotransmitters and Neuromodulators in the Control of Anterior Pituitary Hormone Secretion

ALLAN MUNCK, Ph.D.
Third Century Professor of Physiology, Dartmouth Medical School, Lebanon, New Hampshire.
Glucocorticoid Action: Physiology

ANIKÓ NÁRAY-FEJES-TÓTH, M.D.
Associate Professor of Physiology, Dartmouth Medical School, Lebanon, New Hampshire.
Glucocorticoid Action: Physiology

ROBERT M. NEER, M.D.
Associate Professor of Medicine, Harvard Medical School. Director, Osteoporosis Center, Massachusetts General Hospital, Boston, Massachusetts.
Medical Management of Hyperparathyroidism and Hypercalcemia; Osteoporosis

DON H. NELSON, M.D.
Professor Emeritus of Medicine, University of Utah Medical School. Attending Physician, University Hospital, Salt Lake City, Utah.
A Historical Overview of the Adrenal Cortex

MARIA I. NEW, M.D.
Professor and Chairman, Department of Pediatrics, Cornell University Medical College. Chairman, Department of Pediatrics, The New York Hospital, New York, New York.
Congenital Adrenal Hyperplasia

NICOS A. NICOLA, Ph.D.
Head, Laboratory for Molecular Regulators, The Walter and Eliza Hall Institute of Medical Research, Royal Melbourne Hospital, Melbourne, Australia.
Hormones and Blood Cell Production

JOHN T. NICOLOFF, M.D.
Professor of Medicine, University of Southern California School of Medicine. Attending Physician, Los Angeles County/USC Medical Center, Los Angeles, California.
Thyroid Hormone Transport and Metabolism; Nonthyroidal Illnesses

LYNNETTE K. NIEMAN, M.D.
Chief, Unit on Reproductive Medicine, Developmental Endocrinology Branch, and Senior Staff Physician, National Institute of Child Health and Human Development, National Institutes of Health, Bethesda, Maryland.
Cushing's Syndrome

JEFFREY A. NORTON, M.D.
Professor of Surgery, Chief of Endocrine and Oncologic Surgery, Washington University School of Medicine. Attending Surgeon, Barnes Hospital, St. Louis, Missouri.
Surgical Management of Hyperparathyroidism

SAMUEL R. NUSSBAUM, M.D.
Associate Professor of Medicine, Harvard Medical School. Director, Endocrine Associates, Massachusetts General Hospital, Boston, Massachusetts.
Parathyroid Hormone: Physiology, Chemistry, Biosynthesis, Secretion, Metabolism, and Mode of Action; Medical Management of Hyperparathyroidism and Hypercalcemia

WILLIAM D. ODELL, M.D., Ph.D.
Professor of Medicine and Physiology, University of Utah School of Medicine. Chairman, Department of Internal Medicine, University of Utah, Salt Lake City, Utah.
Genetic Basis of Sexual Differentiation; Endocrinology of Sexual Maturation; The Menopause and Hormonal Replacement

JERROLD M. OLEFSKY, M.D.
Professor of Medicine and Chief, Endocrinology and Metabolism Section, University of California San Diego School of Medicine, La Jolla. Attending Physician, University Hospital, and Veterans Administration Medical Center, San Diego, California.
Diabetes Mellitus (Type II): Etiology and Pathogenesis

NIALL M. O'MEARA, M.D.
Consultant Physician/Endocrinologist, Department of Diabetes and Endocrinology, Mater Misericordiae Hospital, Dublin, Ireland.
Secretion and Metabolism of Insulin, Proinsulin, and C-Peptide

LELIO ORCI, M.D.
Professor, Histology and Cell Biology, Department of Morphology, University of Geneva Medical School, Geneva, Switzerland.
Glucagon Secretion, Alpha Cell Metabolism, and Glucagon Action

LAWRENCE N. PARKER, M.D.
Professor of Medicine, University of California at Irvine College of Medicine. Assistant Chief of Endocrinology, Veterans Administration Medical Center, Long Beach, California.
Adrenal Androgens

JEFFREY H. PERLMAN, M.D.
Senior Fellow in Medicine, Cornell University Medical College. Clinical Fellow, New York Hospital, and Memorial Sloan-Kettering Cancer Center, New York, New York.
Second Messenger Signaling Pathways: Phosphatidylinositol and Calcium

D. W. PFAFF, M.D.
Professor of Neurobiology and Behavior, The Rockefeller University, New York, New York.
Hypothalamus and Hormone-Regulated Behaviors

RICHARD L. PHELPS, M.D.
Assistant Clinical Professor of Medicine, Northwestern University Medical School. Attending Physician, Northwestern Memorial Hospital, Chicago, Illinois.
Diabetes Mellitus and Pregnancy

BRIAN T. PICKERING, B.Sc, Ph.D, D.Sc.
Professor of Anatomy, University of Bristol, Bristol, England.
Oxytocin

DANIEL H. POLK, M.D.
Associate Professor, Department of Pediatrics, University of California Los Angeles School of Medicine, Los Angeles, California. Physician Specialist, Harbor-UCLA Medical Center, Torrance, California.
Thyroid Disease in the Fetus, Neonate, and Child; Fetal and Neonatal Endocrinology

KENNETH S. POLONSKY, M.D.
Professor of Medicine and Chief, Section of Endocrinology. Director, Diabetes Research and Training Center, University of Chicago Pritzker School of Medicine, Chicago, Illinois.
Secretion and Metabolism of Insulin, Proinsulin, and C-Peptide

JOHN T. POTTS, Jr., M.D.
The Jackson Professor of Clinical Medicine, Harvard Medical School. Physician-in-Chief, Massachusetts General Hospital, Boston, Massachusetts.
Parathyroids: Introduction; Parathyroid Hormone: Physiology, Chemistry, Biosynthesis, Secretion, Metabolism, and Mode of Action; Hyperparathyroidism; Differential Diagnosis of Hypercalcemia; Medical Management of Hyperparathyroidism and Hypercalcemia

EDWIN L. PRIEN, Jr., M.D.
Instructor in Medicine, Harvard Medical School. Assistant Physician, Massachusetts General Hospital, Boston, Massachusetts.
Calcium Nephrolithiasis

LISA P. PURDY, M.D., C.M., FRCP(C)
Fellow in Endocrinology, Northwestern University Medical School, Chicago, Illinois.
Diabetes Mellitus and Pregnancy

JOSÉ QUINTANS, M.D., Ph.D.
Professor, Department of Pathlogy, Committee on Immunology and the College, University of Chicago and University of Chicago Cancer Center, Chicago, Illinois.
Immunological Mechanisms Causing Autoimmune Endocrine Disease

JORGE A. RAMIREZ, M.D.
Assistant Director, Medical Education, Arnold Palmer Hospital for Women and Children, Orlando, Florida.
The Renal Osteodystrophies

MICHAEL B. RANKE, M.D.
Professor of Pediatrics, University of Tübingen. Head, Department of Endocrinology, Children's Hospital, University of Tübingen, Tübingen, Germany.
Growth Hormone Insufficiency: Clinical Features, Diagnosis, and Therapy

SAMUEL REFETOFF, M.D.
Professor of Medicine and Pediatrics, University of Chicago Pritzker School of Medicine. Attending Physician, University of Chicago Hospitals, Chicago, Illinois.
Thyroid Hormone Transport and Metabolism; Thyroid Function Tests

SEYMOUR REICHLIN, M.D., Ph.D.
Professor of Medicine, Tufts University School of Medicine. Senior Endocrinologist, New England Medical Center, Boston, Massachusetts.
Endocrine-Immune Interaction

CLAUDE REMACLE, Ph.D.
Professor of Biology, University of Louvain, Louvain, Belgium.
Anatomy, Developmental Biology, and Pathology of the Pancreatic Islets

IVANA PAVLIC RENAR, M.D.
Institute Vuk Vrhovac, Zagreb, Croatia
Neuroendocrine Tumors of Carcinoid Variety

B. REUSENS, Ph.D.
Department of Biology, University of Louvain, Louvain, Belgium.
Anatomy, Developmental Biology, and Pathology of the Pancreatic Islets

GAIL P. RISBRIDGER, Ph.D.
NH and MRC Senior Research Fellow, Institute of Reproduction and Development, Monash University, Melbourne, Australia.
Basic Endocrinology of the Testis

PETER N. RISKIND, M.D., Ph.D.
Assistant Professor of Neurology, Harvard Medical School. Assistant Neurologist, Massachusetts General Hospital, and Spaulding Rehabilitation Hospital, Boston, Massachusetts.
Functional Anatomy of the Hypothalamic–Anterior Pituitary Complex

ROBERT L. ROSENFIELD, M.D.
Professor of Pediatrics and Medicine, University of Chicago Pritzker School of Medicine. Head, Section of Pediatric Endocrinology, Wyler Children's Hospital, Chicago, Illinois.
Hyperandrogenism, Hirsutism, and the Polycystic Ovary Syndrome; Somatic Growth and Maturation

ZEV ROSENWAKS, M.D.
Professor, Department of Obstetrics and Gynecology, Cornell University Medical College. Director, The Center for Reproductive Medicine and Infertility, The New York Hospital-Cornell Medical Center, New York, New York.
Ovarian Follicular Maturation, Ovulation, and Ovulation Induction

ARTHUR H. RUBENSTEIN, M.D.
Professor and Chairman, Department of Medicine, University of Chicago Pritzker School of Medicine, Chicago, Illinois.
Chemistry and Biosynthesis of the Islet Hormones: Insulin, Islet Amyloid Polypeptide (Amylia), Glucagon, Somatostatin, and Pancreatic Polypeptide; Diabetes Mellitus: Therapy

WILLIAM E. RUSSELL, M.D.
Associate Professor of Pediatrics and Cell Biology, Vanderbilt University. Attending Physician, Vanderbilt Children's Hospital, Nashville, Tennessee.
Peptide Growth Factors

ISIDRO B. SALUSKY, M.D.
Professor of Pediatrics, University of California Los Angeles School of Medicine. Director, Pediatric Dialysis Program, and Program Director, General Clinical Research Center, UCLA Medical Center, Los Angeles, California.
The Renal Osteodystrophies

GAETANO SALVATORE, M.D.
Full Professor, Dipartimento di Biologia e Patologia Cellulare e Molecolare, Universita di Napoli Federico II. Dean, Medical School, Universita di Napoli Federico II. President, Stazione Zoologica Anton Dohrn, Naples, Italy.
Biosynthesis and Secretion of Thyroid Hormones

SALVIA SANTAMARINA-FOJO, M.D.
Head, Section of Molecular Biology, National Heart, Lung, and Blood Institute, National Institutes of Health, Bethesda, Maryland.
Disorders of Lipoprotein Metabolism

RICHARD J. SANTEN, M.D.
Professor of Medicine, and Chairman, Department of Internal Medicine, Wayne State University School of Medicine. Physician-in-Chief, Detroit Medical Center, Detroit, Michigan.
Gynecomastia

DAVID H. SARNE, M.D.
Associate Professor of Medicine, University of Illinois at Chicago. Physician, University of Illinois at Chicago Medical Center, Veterans Administration Center–Westside, Chicago, Illinois.
Thyroid Function Tests

MAURICE F. SCANLON, B.Sc., M.D., FRCP
Professor of Endocrinology, University of Wales College of Medicine. Consultant Physician, University Hospital of Wales, Cardiff, Wales.
Thyrotropin-Releasing Hormone: Basic and Clinical Aspects

DESMOND A. SCHATZ, M.D.
Associate Professor, Department of Pediatrics, University of Florida College of Medicine. Attending Physician, Shands Hospital, Gainesville, Florida.
Polyglandular Failure Syndromes

ALAN L. SCHILLER, M.D.
Irene Heinz Given and John LaPorte Given Professor of Medicine, Mount Sinai School of Medicine. Chairman of Pathology, Mount Sinai Medical Center and Mount Sinai Hospital, New York, New York.
Metabolic Bone Disease: Introduction and Classification

ROBERT E. SCULLY, M.D.
Professor Emeritus of Pathology, Harvard Medical School. Pathologist, Massachusetts General Hospital, Boston, Massachusetts.
Ovarian Tumors with Endocrine Manifestations; Testicular Tumors with Endocrine Manifestations

GINO V. SEGRE, M.D.
Associate Professor of Medicine, Harvard Medical School. Associate Physician and Director, Endocrine Clinical Laboratory, Massachusetts General Hospital, Boston, Massachusetts.
Parathyroid Hormone: Physiology, Chemistry, Biosynthesis, Secretion, Metabolism, and Mode of Action; Differential Diagnosis of Hypercalcemia

F. JOHN SERVICE, M.D., Ph.D.
Professor of Medicine, Mayo Medical School. Consultant in Endocrinology and Metabolism, Mayo Clinic, Rochester, Minnesota.
Hypoglycemia, Including Hypoglycemia in Neonates and Children

YORAM SHENKER, M.D.
Associate Professor, Section of Endocrinology and Metabolism, Department of Medicine, University of Wisconsin Medical School. Attending Physician, William S. Middleton Memorial Veterans Administration Hospital and University of Wisconsin Hospital and Clinics, Madison, Wisconsin.
Hormonal Regulation of Electrolyte and Water Metabolism

LOUIS M. SHERWOOD, M.D.
Adjunct Professor of Medicine, University of Pennsylvania School of Medicine. Visiting Professor of Medicine, Albert Einstein College of Medicine. Senior Vice President, Medical and Scientific Affairs, U.S. Human Health Division, Merck & Co., West Point, Pennsylvania. Attending Physician, Montefiore Medical Center, Bronx Municipal Hospital Center, Bronx, New York.
Paraneoplastic Endocrine Disorders (Ectopic Hormone Syndromes)

MANAN SHUKLA, M.D.
Visiting Research Associate, University of Chicago Hospitals, Chicago, Illinois.
Developmental Abnormalities of the Thyroid; Surgery of the Thyroid

EVAN R. SIMPSON, Ph.D.
Professor of Obstetrics/Gynecology and Biochemistry, The University of Texas Southwestern Medical Center, Dallas, Texas.
Steroid Hormone Biosynthesis in the Adrenal Cortex and its Regulation by Adrenocorticotropin

FREDERICK R. SINGER, M.D.
Clinical Professor of Medicine, University of California Los Angeles School of Medicine. Medical Director, Osteoporosis/Metabolic Bone Disease Program, St. John's Hospital and Health Center, Santa Monica, California.
Paget's Disease of Bone

PETER J. SNYDER, M.D.
Professor of Medicine, University of Pennsylvania School of Medicine. Attending Physician, Hospital of the University of Pennsylvania, Philadelphia, Pennsylvania.
Gonadotroph Adenomas

ALLEN M. SPIEGEL, M.D.
Chief, Molecular Pathophysiology Branch, National Institute of Diabetes and Digestive and Kidney Diseases, National Institutes of Health, Bethesda, Maryland.
Pseudohypoparathyroidism

DONALD F. STEINER, M.D.
Professor of Biochemistry and Molecular Biology and Medicine, University of Chicago Pritzker School of Medicine, Chicago, Illinois.
Chemistry and Biosynthesis of the Islet Hormones: Insulin, Islet Amyloid Polypeptide (Amylin), Glucagon, Somatostatin, and Pancreatic Polypeptide

ANDREW F. STEWART, M.D.
Professor of Medicine and Endocrinology, Yale University School of Medicine. Chief, Endocrinology, West Haven Veterans Administration Medical Center; Attending Physician, Yale-New Haven Hospital, New Haven, Connecticut.
Malignancy-Associated Hyercalcemia

JEROME F. STRAUSS III, M.D., Ph.D.
Luigi Mastroianni, Jr. Professor, and Director, Center for Research in Women's Health and Reproduction and Associate Chairman, Department of Obstetric and Gynecology, University of Pennsylvania School of Medicine. Attending Physician, Hospital of the University of Pennsylvania, Philadelphia, Pennsylvania.
Placental Hormones

HUGO STUDER, M.D.
Full Professor of Medicine, University of Bern. Head, Department of Medicine, University Hospital, Inselspital, Bern, Switzerland.
Multinodular Goiter

SONIA L. SUGG, M.D.
Medical Staff Fellow, Surgery Branch, National Cancer Institute, National Institutes of Health, Bethesda, Maryland.
Surgical Management of Hyperparathyroidism

HISATO TADA, M.D.
Research Associate, Department of Laboratory Medicine, Osaka University Medical School. Staff Physician, Osaka University Hospital, Osaka, Japan.
Autoimmune Thyroid Disease/Thyroiditis

HOWARD S. TAGER, Ph.D.
Professor of Biochemistry and Molecular Biology and Medicine, University of Chicago Pritzker School of Medicine, Chicago, Illinois.
Chemistry and Biosynthesis of the Islet Hormones: Insulin, Islet Amyloid Polypeptide (Amylin), Glucagon, Somatostatin, and Pancreatic Polypeptide

RAJESH V. THAKKER, M.A., FRCP
M.R.C. Clinical Scientist and Senior Lecturer, Royal Postgraduate Medical School. Honourary Consultant Physician and Endocrinologist, The Hammersmith Hospital, London, England.
Multiple Endocrine Neoplasia Type 1

MICHAEL O. THORNER, M.B., B.S., D.Sc., FRCP
Kenneth R. Crispell Professor of Medicine; Chief, Division of Endocrinology and Metabolism, University of Virginia Health Sciences Center, Charlottesville, Virginia.
Growth Hormone–Releasing Hormone: Basic Physiology and Clinical Implications; Prolactin: Hyperprolactinemic Syndromes and Management

FRED W. TUREK, Ph.D.
Professor and Chairman, Department of Neurobiology and Physiology, Northwestern University Medical School, Chicago, Illinois.
Endocrine and Other Biological Rhythms

ROGER H. UNGER, M.D.
Touchstone/West Distinguished Chair in Diabetes Research and Professor of Internal Medicine, University of Texas Southwestern Medical School. Senior Medical Investigator, Veterans Administration Medical Center; Director, Center for Diabetes Research, University of Texas Southwestern Medical Center, Dallas, Texas.
Glucagon Secretion, Alpha Cell Metabolism, and Glucagon Action

ROBERT D. UTIGER, M.D.
Clinical Professor of Medicine, Harvard Medical School. Attending Physician, Brigham and Woman's Hospital, Boston, Massachusetts.
Hypothyroidism

EVE VAN CAUTER, Ph.D.
Research Associate (Professor); University of Chicago Pritzker School of Medicine, Chicago, Illinois.
Endocrine and Other Biological Rhythms

JUDSON J. VAN WYK, M.D.
Kenan Professor of Pediatrics, University of North Carolina School of Medicine. Attending Pediatrician, University of North Carolina Children's Hospital, Chapel Hill, North Carolina.
Peptide Growth Factors

MARY LEE VANCE, M.D.
Associate Professor of Medicine, University of Virginia School of Medicine. Staff Physician, University of Virginia Hospital, Charlottesville, Virginia.
Prolactin: Hyperprolactinemic Syndromes and Management

G. VASSART, M.D., Ph.D.
Professor of Medical Genetics, Free University of Brussels, Faculty of Medicine. Director, Department of Medical Genetics, Erasme Hospital, Brussels, Belgium.
Thyroid Regulation

AARON VINIK, M.D.
Professor of Internal Medicine and Anatomy/Neurobiology and Director, Diabetes Research Institute, Eastern Virginia Medical School, Norfolk, Virginia.
Neuroendocrine Tumors of Carcinoid Variety

ROBERT VOLPÉ, M.D., FRCP(C), FACP, FRCP (Edin)
Professor Emeritus, Division of Endocrinology and Metabolism, Department of Medicine, University of Toronto. Active Staff and Director of Endocrinology Research Laboratory, The Wellesley Hospital; Consultant, Department of Medicine, Princess Margaret Hospital (Ontario Cancer Institute), Toronto, Ontario, Canada.
Subacute and Sclerosing Thyroiditis

MICHELLE P. WARREN, M.D.
Associate Professor of Clinical Obstetrics and Gynecology and Clinical Medicine, Columbia College of Physicians and Surgeons. Head, Reproductive Endocrinology, Roosevelt Site, St. Luke's–Roosevelt Hospital Center, New York, New York.
Anorexia Nervosa

JOHN A. H. WASS, M.D., FRCP
Professor of Clinical Endocrinology, St. Bartholomew's Hospital Medical College. Honourary Consultant Physician, St. Bartholomew's Hospital, London, England.
Somatostatin; Tests of Pituitary Function

MICHAEL R. WATERMAN, Ph.D.
Professor and Chairman, Department of Biochemistry, Vanderbilt University School of Medicine, Nashville, Tennessee.
Steroid Hormone Biosynthesis in the Adrenal Cortex and its Regulation by Adrenocorticotropin

BRUCE D. WEINTRAUB, M.D.
Director, NIH Interinstitute Endocrinology Training Program. Chief, Molecular and Cellular Endocrinology Branch, National Institute of Diabetes and Digestive and Kidney Diseases, National Institutes of Health, Bethesda, Maryland.
Thyroid-Stimulating Hormone in Health and Disease

MORRIS F. WHITE, Ph.D.
Associate Professor of Biological Chemistry, Department of Medicine, Harvard Medical School. Investigator, Elliott P. Joslin Research Laboratory, Joslin Diabetes Center, Boston, Massachusetts.
Molecular Mechanism of Insulin Action

JOHN F. WILBER, M.D.
Professor of Medicine, University of Maryland School of Medicine. Staff Physician, University of Maryland Systems, Baltimore, Maryland.
Control of Thyroid Function: The Hypothalamic-Pituitary-Thyroid Axis

JOHN P. H. WILDING, B.M., MRCP
Senior Registrar, Division of Endocrinology and Metabolism, Hammersmith Hospital, London, England.
Hormones of the Gastrointestinal Tract

E. DILLWYN WILLIAMS, M.D.
Professor of Histopathology, University of Cambridge. Consultant Histopathologist, Addenbrookes Hospital, Cambridge, England.
Medullary Carcinoma of the Thyroid

GORDON H. WILLIAMS, M.D.
Professor of Medicine, Harvard Medical School. Senior Physician and Chief, Endocrine-Hypertension Service, Brigham and Women's Hospital, Boston, Massachusetts.
Aldosterone Action: Physiology; Hormonal Aspects of Hypertension

STEPHEN J. WINTERS, M.D.
Professor of Medicine, University of Pittsburgh School of Medicine, Pittsburgh, Pennsylvania.
Clinical Disorders of the Testis

ROBERT J. WITTE, M.D.
Assistant Professor, University of Nebraska School of Medicine. Radiologist, University of Nebraska Medical Center, Omaha, Nebraska
Radiographic Evaluation of the Pituitary and Anterior Hypothalamus

FREDRIC E. WONDISFORD, M.D.
Assistant Professor of Medicine, Harvard Medical School. Chief, Thyroid Unit, Division of Endocrinology and Metabolism, Beth Israel Hospital, Boston, Massachusetts.
Thyroid-Stimulating Hormone in Health and Disease

MARGITA ZAKARIJA, M.D.
Professor, Department of Medicine and Department of Microbiology and Immunology, University of Miami School of Medicine. Staff Physician, University of Miami Hospital and Clinics, and Jackson Memorial Hospital, Miami, Florida.
Hyperthyroidism

Preface

One of the most awe-inspiring experiences in medicine occurs on meeting each new patient. In the course of an hour an individual, previously quite unknown, allows the physician total access to his innermost problems, fears, and secrets, and to his body. A good physician must accept this gift with humility and respond with candor, empathy, and responsibility. The opportunity presented to help a fellow human suffering from illness provides the most fundamental satisfaction in being a physician. The physician must bring to bear on the problem his knowledge of pathophysiology, presented with an understanding of human interactions.

To prepare for this task, doctors subject themselves to a demanding education and a long apprenticeship. They then must almost totally relearn their art and science every decade in order to stay abreast of advances. Endocrinology shares in this development of knowledge, perhaps even leads in the change, as the constant stream of new clinical and laboratory observations forces us to update our prior ideas. It is the challenge to encompass this evolving field of endocrinology—and bring it to clinicians and researchers in a useful manner—that we address in the third edition of ENDOCRINOLOGY.

Our goals remain as stated in the first edition:

- To review basic knowledge of endocrine physiology and biochemistry in a complete and up-to-date manner
- To provide a thorough clinical discussion of each topic
- To integrate the basic and clinical material around human endocrinology
- To make clear the integration of the endocrine system in a gland-by-gland manner, as well as the important multi-hormonal integration in relation to physiological functions
- To have our presentations made by the most accomplished endocrinologists throughout the world.

Reflecting these goals, our book is divided into three complementary sections. The first six chapters provide a foundation for understanding contemporary molecular endocrinology, emphasizing the function of cell membrane and nuclear receptors, and "second messengers". The second section provides a traditional gland-oriented presentation of basic endocrine physiology and clinical problems. The third section integrates contemporary knowledge around important physiological or pathological functions, such as feeding, obesity, rhythms, and polyglandular autoimmunity.

Our book is in every sense the product of a joint effort by eight distinguished co-editors. They have taken the responsibility for organizing each of the sections, which are in a real sense equal to whole books in themselves. In keeping with our plan to bring the most current concepts to our readers, we have the privilege of introducing three new section editors for this edition. Dr. Lynn Loriaux now edits the chapters on Adrenal Disease, Dr. Larry Jameson has organized the introductory chapters and "Integrated Endocrinology," and in an acknowledgment of the "One World" of endocrinology, Dr. Henry Burger of Melbourne has taken responsibility for the section on Male Reproduction.

We are blessed by having experts from around the world write our chapters, and even to submit them more or less promptly. Readers will note many totally new chapters including those on the application of molecular biological techniques to endocrine disease, the molecular basis of insulin action, adrenal imaging, adrenal androgens, glucocorticoid resistance, gonadal regulatory peptides, endocrine testing in pregnancy, male contraception, multiple endocrine neoplasias, hormones of the cardiovascular system, and endocrine hypertension, to name a few. And the rest of the chapters have been largely rewritten as well.

It is with a sense of accomplishment and excitement that we bring this edition to the endocrine community. We believe it will provide students, fellows, clinical endocrinologists, academicians, and researchers around the world with a complete source to which they can turn to find answers to their questions. The chief editor is continually awed by the brilliance displayed by the authors in each section. To these distinguished scientists and clinicians, I express my great respect and most sincere thanks. It is their knowledge and hard work that make this volume possible and unique in its scope and contribution.

LESLIE J. DEGROOT, M.D.

Contents

PART III   THYROID GLAND

VOLUME 2

PART IV PARATHYROIDS

PART VI   ADRENAL CORTEX

PART VII SEXUAL DIFFERENTIATION AND PUBERTY

VOLUME 3

PART VIII FEMALE REPRODUCTION

PART IX ENDOCRINOLOGY OF PREGNANCY

PART X MALE REPRODUCTION

†Deceased.

PART XI   INTEGRATED ENDOCRINE SYSTEMS

PART VIII

FEMALE REPRODUCTION

113

Regulation of Gonadotropin Secretion

JOHN C. MARSHALL

HYPOTHALAMIC-PITUITARY-OVARIAN AXIS

The major hormones involved in the regulation of reproductive function in women are shown in Figure 113–1.

Gonadotropin-releasing hormone (GnRH, or luteinizing hormone–releasing hormone [LHRH]) is a decapeptide secreted by hypothalamic neurons. It stimulates the synthesis and secretion of both luteinizing hormone (LH) and follicle-stimulating hormone (FSH) by the pituitary gonadotroph cells. Hypothalamic secretion of GnRH is influenced by other hypothalamic neurotransmitters, and in general, the catecholamines norepinephrine and epinephrine increase GnRH release, whereas endogenous opioid peptides, such as β-endorphin, inhibit GnRH secretion. LH and FSH are glycoprotein hormones composed of two subunits designated alpha and beta. The α subunit is identical in both LH and FSH, whereas the β subunit is structurally dissimilar and conveys specificity to the hormones. Both LH and FSH are secreted by the same gonadotroph cells, and gonadotrophs constitute 7 to 10 per cent of cells in the anterior pituitary gland. Metabolic clearance rates of the two hormones are different so that the plasma half-life of LH (about 60 to 90 minutes) is shorter than that of FSH (about 180 to 200 minutes). FSH and LH act in concert to produce ovarian follicular maturation, ovulation, and secretion of estradiol and progesterone. Prolactin is an important regulator of ovarian function in rodents, but in humans this action does not appear to be physiologically significant and the exact role of prolactin remains uncertain. The inhibins are proteins that consist of a common α subunit linked to either a β_A subunit (inhibin A) or β_B subunit (inhibin B). The activin group of compounds are homodimers or heterodimers of the β subunits activin A (β_A,β_A) and activin B (β_A,β_B). Activin B (β_B,β_B) has not yet been isolated, but recombinant material has been shown to be as effective as activin A. Follistatin is an unrelated single-chain protein that has been cloned, and all three compounds, originally obtained from gonadal extracts, have been found to be widely distributed in different tissues. The proteins have been shown to exert multiple actions in other systems (inhibin and activin are related to the transforming growth factor β compounds), but in relation to gonadotropins, inhibin and follistatin reduce FSH secretion, whereas activin increases FSH synthesis and secretion (see Ch. 114). The exact mechanisms of action of these compounds in regulating FSH secretion remain unclear. They are active in both sexes, with effects being more marked in females and immature males. Plasma inhibin is inversely related to plasma FSH, indicating an endocrine role for inhibin of ovarian origin. The exact roles of activin and follistatin are less clear, and because both compounds are also present in the pituitary, they may have paracrine or autocrine mechanisms of action.

Considerable evidence exists from animal studies that the extrahypothalamic CNS (shown as suprahypothalamic in Fig. 113–1) can exert a major influence on reproductive function. In rodents, odors from a male mouse can coordinate the timing of estrous cycles in female mice housed in colonies (Whitten effect). These effects are mediated by pheromones, and their action has been reviewed by Bronson.[1] Other observations suggest that similar mechanisms may be involved in primates. If vaginal secretions from a female rhesus monkey at midcycle are placed on the perineum of a castrate female, male monkeys are attracted to the castrate animal. Human vaginal secretions have similar effects when applied to castrate female monkeys.[2] Exposure to light, and in particular duration of light exposure, is also an important factor in some species. The effects of light vary with the species. Regulation of light exposure (constant day-night length) can regularize the estrous cycle of rats, and constant light can result in earlier puberty in female rats. The duration of light exposure appears to be a major factor in the regulation of reproductive function in species that are seasonal breeders. Extensive studies have been performed in female sheep,[3] and during summer (long days) LH secretion is inhibited. With the advent of the fall, gonadotropin secretion increases and cyclical estrous function continues during the winter breeding season (short days). The transition from anestrus (summer) to the breeding season is associated with an increase in the frequency of pulsatile LH secretion,[4] suggesting that the duration of light exposure can regulate secretion of GnRH. The exact mechanisms by which these effects are mediated remain uncertain, and little evidence is available to indicate that similar factors play any role in reproductive function in women. Higher CNS regulation of reproductive function probably exists, however, and may be important in the cause of anovulation and amenorrhea seen in some women under conditions of stress or after weight loss or intensive exercise (see Ch. 117).

GnRH is the major hormone that controls the secretion of LH and FSH and the only hypothalamic hormone known to consistently stimulate release of pituitary gonadotropins. Thus, in this summary of regulation of gonadotropin secretion, we review the secretion of GnRH and also examine the factors that regulate the action of GnRH at the level of the pituitary gland.

GnRH SECRETION AND THE MECHANISMS OF GnRH ACTION

Patterns of GnRH Secretion

Early studies of the patterns of LH secretion in humans revealed that LH was released into the circulation in a series of pulses[5, 6] and that similar secretory patterns are present in all species. These data suggested that each LH pulse resulted from the pulsatile release of GnRH by the hypothalamus. This assumption cannot be tested in humans because the measurement of GnRH in hypothalamic-portal blood is impractical, but data from sheep, rodents, and primates support this view. Simultaneous measurement of GnRH in portal blood and LH in jugular venous blood[7] has shown good concordance between GnRH and LH pulses (Fig. 113–2), and this suggests that the patterns of GnRH secretion can be inferred from the measurement of LH pulses in peripheral plasma. FSH is also secreted in a pulsatile manner, but FSH peaks often are obscured because the long half-life of FSH often exceeds the interval between pulses.

Pulsatile secretion of GnRH appears to be essential for the maintenance of normal gonadotropin synthesis and secretion. The crucial importance of a pulsatile GnRH stimulus was initially observed in castrate monkeys rendered GnRH-deficient by the placement of hypothalamic lesions.[8] When GnRH was administered by continuous infusion, initial release of LH and FSH was seen, but serum gonadotropins subsequently fell despite continuing the GnRH infusion. In contrast, if GnRH is given in a pulsatile manner to lesioned monkeys, LH and FSH secretion could be maintained for prolonged periods, whereas a subsequent continuous GnRH infusion again produced a decline in serum LH and FSH (Fig. 113–3).

These observations have been confirmed in humans, and pulsatile administration of GnRH to patients with isolated GnRH deficiency can stimulate gonadotropin secretion

HYPOTHALAMIC-PITUITARY-OVARIAN AXIS

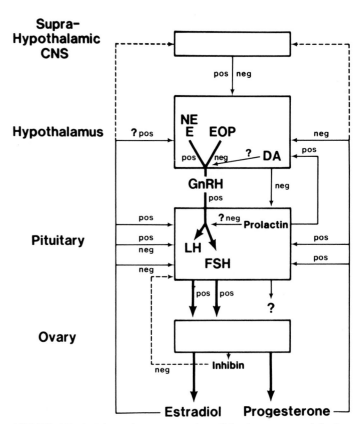

FIGURE 113–1. Schematic representation of the hormones and feedback control mechanisms in the hypothalamic-pituitary-ovarian axis. Solid lines indicate established and dotted lines putative regulatory pathways. Pos shows stimulatory and neg shows inhibitory regulation. NE, norepinephrine; E, epinephrine; EOP, endogenous opioid peptides; DA, dopamine.

and induce pubertal maturation,[9–11] reproduce the hormonal changes seen during the menstrual cycle,[12, 13] and induce ovulation.[14]

The frequency of the pulsatile GnRH stimulus is also important in determining gonadotropin secretion. Increasing the frequency of GnRH pulses from one per hour to two or three per hour reduces plasma gonadotropins in hypothalamic-lesioned monkeys,[15] and this effect is reversed by returning to an hourly frequency. Similarly, slow frequencies of GnRH stimulation (one pulse every three to four hours) do not maintain serum LH concentrations, and together these data indicate that a narrow range of GnRH pulse frequency is required to maintain pituitary responsiveness and normal gonadotropin secretion. Additional evidence suggests that the frequency of GnRH stimulation may regulate release of LH or FSH by the pituitary gonadotrophs. GnRH pulse frequencies of one per hour induce release of both LH and FSH in monkeys, sheep, and humans. Slower frequencies, one pulse every three to four hours, produce an increase in serum FSH concentrations but LH declines. The fall in LH may be explained by the short half-life of LH, but the rise in FSH suggests that a slow frequency of GnRH stimulation may favor FSH release by the pituitary.[15, 16] Similar observations have been made in rats, and a GnRH pulse frequency of every 30

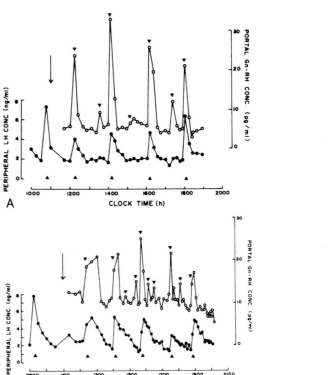

FIGURE 113–2. Patterns of gonadotropin-releasing hormone (GnRH) in hypothalamic-portal blood and LH in jugular venous blood in ovariectomized ewes. Good concordance between GnRH and LH pulses is present. (From Clark IJ, Cummins JT: The temporal relationship between gonadotropin-releasing hormone [GnRH] and luteinizing hormone [LH] secretion in ovariectomized ewes. Endocrinology 111:1737–1739, © by The Endocrine Society, 1982.)

HYPOTHALAMIC LESIONED MONKEYS:
SERUM LH AND FSH AFTER PULSATILE OR CONTINUOUS GnRH

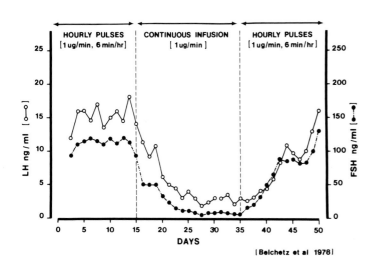

[Belchetz et al 1978]

FIGURE 113–3. The effects of pulsatile or continuous administration of GnRH to ovariectomized monkeys rendered GnRH-deficient by placement of a lesion in the hypothalamus. Gonadotropin secretion was restored by hourly GnRH pulses, reduced during a continuous GnRH infusion, and again increased after reinstitution of pulsatile GnRH administration. (From Belchetz PE, et al: Hypophysial responses to continuous and intermittent delivery of hypothalamic gonadotropin-releasing hormone. Science 202:631–633, Copyright 1978 by the American Association for the Advancement of Science.)

minutes was required to maintain LH responsiveness, whereas FSH release was seen after pulses given every 60 to 120 minutes.[17] GnRH pulse frequency may also determine the amount of LH released in response to a GnRH pulse. The amplitude of LH release is small when GnRH pulse frequency is high, and amplitude increases when a slower frequency of GnRH stimulation is used.[16] This may in part explain the differences in LH pulsatile release seen during the follicular phase of the menstrual cycle (low amplitude and fast frequency) and the luteal phase (high amplitude and slow frequency).[18, 19]

The evidence presented above clearly demonstrates the critical importance of a pulsatile GnRH stimulus in the maintenance of normal pituitary gonadotropin secretion. The exact frequencies and amount of GnRH required to produce optimal gonadotroph stimulation vary in different species, but all share a requirement for an intermittent stimulus. The full effects of variation of the patterns of GnRH stimulation on pituitary responsiveness remain to be elucidated, but evidence suggests that these are crucial aspects in the regulation of gonadotropin secretion.

Mechanisms of GnRH Action

GnRH acts on pituitary gonadotrophs to stimulate the acute release and synthesis of both LH and FSH. The mechanisms involved in GnRH action are shown in Figure 113–4 and have been reviewed.[20–22]

The initial step in GnRH action is binding to a receptor on the gonadotroph plasma membrane, and GnRH agonist analogues have been extensively used to quantitate GnRH receptors.[23] The number of GnRH receptors vary in different physiological situations, such as during sexual maturation and during the estrous cycle.[24] GnRH receptors are highest when responsiveness to GnRH is maximal, suggesting that the number of receptors plays a role in modulating

GnRH ACTION ON THE GONADOTROPH

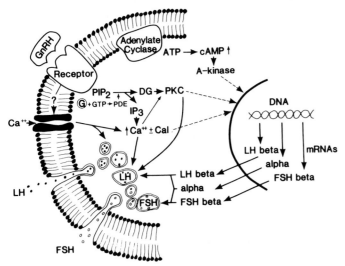

FIGURE 113–4. Mechanisms involved in GnRH action on the gonadotroph. Dashed lines indicate pathways where the mechanisms are unknown. PIP₂, phosphatidylinositol (4,5) phosphate; DG, diacylglycerol; PKC, protein kinase C; IP₃, inositol triphosphate; G, G protein; PDE, phosphodiesterase (phospholipase C); cal, calmodulin.

GnRH action. GnRH itself has been shown to be the main factor regulating GnRH receptor concentration. GnRH receptors are increased in situations where endogenous GnRH secretion is increased, such as after castration, and GnRH administration can increase the number of GnRH receptors.[25, 26] Thus the number of pituitary GnRH receptors appears to reflect endogenous GnRH secretion, but the manner of GnRH secretion is also important in determining the receptor response. In rats, GnRH pulses given every 30 minutes produce a maximum increase in receptor concentration,[17] and faster or slower frequencies of GnRH stimulation result in smaller responses.

After the initiation of GnRH action by binding to the membrane receptor, multiple steps appear to be involved in GnRH-stimulated LH and FSH secretion and subunit gene expression. GnRH stimulates a phospholipase C enzyme in the plasma membrane, a step that involves a guanosine triphosphate–binding protein. Phosphatidylinositol 4,5 diphosphate is hydrolyzed to inositol triphosphate (IP₃) and diacylglycerol (DG).[27] The increase in IP₃ releases calcium from intracellular stores by way of a specific IP₃ receptor, and this transient calcium increase appears to be responsible for the initial burst of LH release lasting from 1 to 1½ minutes. Both the elevated intracellular calcium and DG probably induce the translocation of protein kinase C (PKC) subspecies from the cytosol to the membrane. The activated PKC phosphorylates proteins that are involved in initiating the secretory reactions leading to LH and FSH release. GnRH receptor binding also initiates the influx of extracellular calcium by way of calcium channels, leading to a further increase in intracellular calcium, which appears necessary, together with effects of PKCs, to maintain the sustained phase (over several minutes) of gonadotropin secretion. GnRH also induces the production of arachidonic acid and lipoxygenase and/or epoxygenase products of the fatty acid, which appear to be involved in exocytosis.

Several reports have shown that intracellular cAMP is increased three to four hours after GnRH stimulation,[28] but the mechanisms are unclear because GnRH does not stimulate adenylate cyclase activity. Because cAMP response elements are present on the α subunit gene, this mechanism may be involved in regulating α subunit gene expression. The mechanisms involved in stimulating expression of the two β subunit genes are also unclear. GnRH is critical for initiating transcription (see below), and LH β mRNA has been shown to increase after stimulation of PKC pathways. GnRH is less effective in PKC-depleted cells,[29] suggesting that PKC pathways are important in β subunit expression.

Self-Priming Action of GnRH

In addition to stimulating the release of LH and FSH, GnRH enhances pituitary responsiveness to subsequent stimulation by GnRH. When a second injection of GnRH is given within one to two hours of the first injection, increased secretion of LH occurs in response to the second stimulus.[30] This action of GnRH is termed a self-priming effect and depends on protein synthesis because it is blocked by inhibitors such as cycloheximide. The self-priming effect of GnRH is enhanced in the presence of estradiol, and data are shown in Figure 113–5. LH responses to

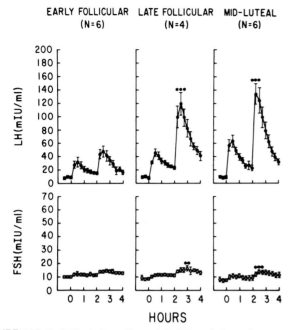

EARLY FOLLICULAR (N=6) LATE FOLLICULAR (N=4) MID-LUTEAL (N=6)

HOURS

FIGURE 113–5. Self-priming effect of GnRH and the enhancement of this effect in the presence of estradiol. The response to a second GnRH pulse injection is increased during the late follicular and midluteal stages of the menstrual cycle when plasma estradiol concentrations are elevated. (From Wang CF, et al: The functional changes of the pituitary gonadotrophs during the menstrual cycle. J Clin Endocrinol Metab 42:718–728, © by The Endocrine Society, 1976.)

the second and subsequent injections of GnRH are increased at times when plasma estradiol is elevated, such as during the late follicular and midluteal phases of the menstrual cycle.[31] The self-priming action of GnRH is one component of the positive feedback effect of estradiol in enhancing pituitary responses to GnRH (see below).

Cyclic AMP and progesterone also augment responses to subsequent GnRH stimulation, and these effects are blocked by the progesterone receptor antagonist RU486. This suggests that GnRH activation of protein kinase A may interact with the progesterone receptor and that GnRH self-priming may be mediated by way of this mechanism. Studies have supported this view, and in pituitary cells transfected with a progesterone response element linked to a reporter gene, GnRH has been shown to increase reporter gene activity. These data suggest the possibility that GnRH self-priming may result from GnRH-stimulated intracellular mechanisms (? cAMP) acting by way of the progesterone receptor to enhance responsiveness to subsequent GnRH stimuli.[32]

Effect of GnRH on Prolactin Secretion

Studies have indicated that GnRH may also stimulate secretion of prolactin in some circumstances. Administration of GnRH results in acute release of prolactin in addition to LH and FSH in normal cycling women.[33] In addition, simultaneous spontaneous secretion of prolactin and LH has been noted during the menstrual cycle,[18] and concordance of LH and prolactin pulses is most notable during the luteal phase[34] and in hypogonadal women.[35] The mechanisms of GnRH-induced prolactin release are uncertain. Some evidence suggests that GnRH acts at the pitui-

tary level,[36] but in rodents GnRH antagonists block LH pulses, whereas prolactin pulse release continues.[37] This suggests that prolactin pulses may result from release of a prolactin-releasing factor, the secretion of which is loosely coupled to the secretion of GnRH.

EXPRESSION OF THE GONADOTROPIN SUBUNIT GENES

The cDNAs and genes for the common α and the specific LH β and FSH β subunits have been isolated and characterized in several species.[38] For α, a single gene is composed of four exons and three introns, and cAMP response elements have been identified in the 5′ flanking region. The LH β gene is smaller, with three exons and two introns, and a putative estrogen response element has been demonstrated.[39] The FSH β subunit is also coded by a single gene, which differs from other glycoprotein hormone β genes in having a long 3′ untranslated region. This region contains sequences that in other genes have been shown to be important in determining RNA stability.[40] Data are not available concerning the presence of regulatory elements in the 5′ region of the FSH β gene. The availability of the cDNA's has allowed quantitation of subunit mRNA's, which together with measurements of transcription rates, has allowed insights into the mechanisms that regulate the expression of the three gonadotropin subunit genes.

Gonadal Steroids and Peptides

Gonadectomy in male and female rats has revealed evidence of differential expression of the gonadotropin subunit genes.[38, 41, 42] In females serum LH and α and LH β subunit mRNA's do not increase until several days after ovariectomy, whereas serum FSH and FSH β mRNA increase within hours. In male rats all three subunit mRNA concentrations are increased within 24 hours, although the increase in FSH β is less marked than in females.

Replacement of estradiol (E_2) and progesterone (P) at the time of ovariectomy prevents the increase in α and LH β mRNA, but the increase in FSH β mRNA was not suppressed. Similar changes occur in the presence of a GnRH antagonist, suggesting that the increase in α and LH β mRNA depend on GnRH, but that of FSH β mRNA is independent of GnRH.[43] Current data suggest that the increase in FSH β depends on loss of ovarian inhibin in female animals,[42] and in vitro inhibin rapidly reduces FSH β mRNA in cultured pituitary cells.[44]

In male rats testosterone replacement at castration prevents the increase in all three subunit mRNA's, and when given to castrate animals, it suppresses α and LH β, although FSH β mRNA remains elevated. Studies have shown that testosterone can selectively increase FSH mRNA in the absence of GnRH, and the half-life of FSH β mRNA appears to be prolonged in the presence of testosterone.[45]

The gonadal peptides activin and follistatin also appear to regulate FSH β mRNA by modifying mRNA stability. Both compounds are active in vitro, and their mRNAs are present in the pituitary as well as in other tissues. These observations have led to the suggestion that activin may

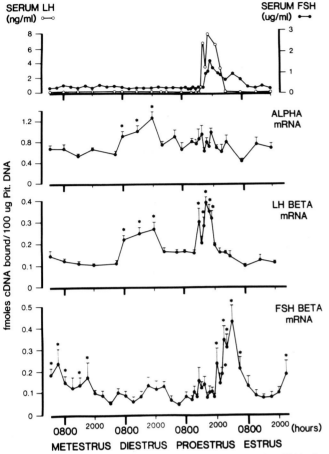

FIGURE 113–6. Serum LH, FSH, and gonadotropin subunit mRNAs during the four-day estrous cycle in rats. *P < .05 versus basal values. (From Marshall JC, Dalkin AC, Haisenleder DJ et al: Gonadotropin releasing hormone pulses: Regulators of gonadotropin synthesis and ovulatory cycles. Recent Prog Horm Res 47:155–189,1991.)

normally stabilize FSH β mRNA in the pituitary and that this action can be modified by the presence of inhibin or follistatin (see below).

Estrous Cycle

During the four-day cycle in female rats, the concentrations of serum LH and FSH and of the subunit mRNA's in the pituitary change in both a coordinate and a differential manner.[43] On metestrus FSH β mRNA alone is increased, whereas on diestrus α and LH β mRNA expression increases and FSH β remains unchanged. During the proestrus gonadotropin surge, α mRNA is unchanged, LH β mRNA is increased, and FSH β mRNA increases several hours later (Fig. 113–6). The increase in β subunit mRNA's at the time of increased gonadotropin secretion suggests that they depend on increased GnRH secretion, which occurs at the time of the surge. The increase in FSH β mRNA on metestrus is seen at the time when GnRH secretion is low, suggesting that it may be consequent on a reduction in the actions of ovarian inhibin.[46]

These physiological data during the ovulatory cycle in rats indicate that complex mechanisms are involved in the differential expression of gonadotropin subunit gene expression. Although the exact interrelations remain un-

certain, studies have concentrated on the role of altered GnRH secretion in regulating subunit mRNA expression.

Role of GnRH Pulses

A pulsatile GnRH stimulus is as important in increasing subunit gene expression as it is in maintaining hormone release. GnRH appears essential for subunit gene expression, and the administration of GnRH antagonists reduces the elevated mRNA levels seen in castrate animals. Similarly, if long-acting GnRH agonists are used to desensitize the gonadotroph, β mRNA expression is not increased, although α mRNA concentrations rise. This suggests that α mRNA expression may not be as sensitive to intermittent GnRH stimuli as that of the two β subunits. Studies in GnRH-deficient sheep and rodent models have shown that the administration of GnRH pulses can increase subunit mRNA concentrations, and further studies have suggested that both the amplitude and the frequency of GnRH stimuli may be important in differential gene expression.

GnRH Pulse Amplitude

GnRH pulses given at intervals of every 30 minutes (to mimic the frequency of pulsatile GnRH secretion in cas-

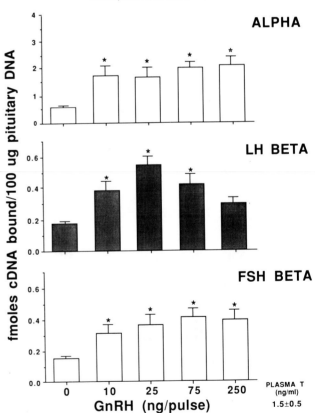

FIGURE 113–7. Effects of GnRH pulse amplitude on expression of gonadotropin subunit mRNAs in male rats. Castrate testosterone-replaced rats were given GnRH pulses every 30 minutes for 48 hours. Pulse amplitude (ng/pulse) is shown. *P < .05 versus 0 ng GnRH (saline controls). (From Marshall JC, Dalkin AC, Haisenleder DJ et al: Gonadotropin releasing hormone pulses: Regulators of gonadotropin synthesis and ovulatory cycles. Recent Prog Horm Res 47:155–189,1991.)

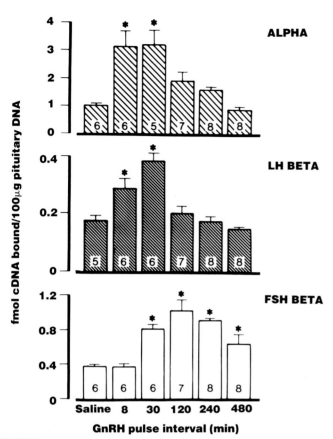

FIGURE 113–8. Effect of GnRH pulse frequency on expression of gonadotropin subunit mRNAs in castrate testosterone-replaced male rats. The dose-pulse of GnRH was constant (25 ng) and the pulse intervals are shown. *$P < .05$ versus saline. (From Dalkin AC, Haisenleder DJ, Ortolano GA, et al: The frequency of gonadotropin-releasing hormone stimulation differentially regulates gonadotropin subunit mRNA expression. Endocrinology 125:917–924, © by The Endocrine Society, 1989.)

trate rats) increased α and FSH β mRNA three- to four-fold over a wide range of pulse amplitudes (Fig. 113–7). In contrast, LH β mRNA concentrations were maximal after GnRH pulses that produced physiological concentrations of GnRH (about 200 pg/ml), and higher doses were less effective.[43] FSH β mRNA is expressed more rapidly than α, and significant increases in LH β are seen only after 24 or more hours of GnRH stimulation.

GnRH Pulse Frequency

When a constant amplitude of GnRH stimulus is given, the frequency of GnRH administration also appears important in determining which gonadotropin mRNA is expressed.[47] Faster frequencies (every 30 minutes or faster) increase α and LH β subunit mRNA's but do not alter the concentration of FSH β mRNA. In contrast, slower frequency pulses (every two hours or slower) only increase expression of FSH β mRNA (Fig. 113–8). These effects of GnRH pulse frequency appear to be exerted at the level of subunit gene transcription.[48, 49] Fast-frequency GnRH pulses increased α transcription, only 30-minute pulses increased LH β transcription, and the transcription rate of FSH β was increased only by slower (every two hours) pulses.

Overall, these data suggest that alterations in the frequency and amplitude of pulsatile GnRH secretion may be

one mechanism whereby a single GnRH can differentially exert expression of the three gonadotropin subunit genes. This in turn imparts physiological import to the observed changes in GnRH pulse frequency shown to occur during ovulatory cycles in several species.

REGULATION OF GnRH SECRETION AND FACTORS THAT MODULATE GONADOTROPH RESPONSES TO GnRH

Regulation of GnRH Secretion

GnRH is released in a pulsatile manner from isolated hypothalami in vitro, and evidence suggests that the GnRH neurons possess the intrinsic ability to secrete GnRH in an intermittent manner.[50] This inherent pattern of secretion can be modified by gonadal steroids and other neural signals. The most important neurotransmitters involved in this action are norepinephrine (NE), epinephrine (E), and endogenous opioid peptides. Concepts of the neural mechanisms involved in the regulation of GnRH secretion are predominantly based on studies performed in rodents and have been thoroughly reviewed by Kalra,[51] who proposed the model system shown in Figure 113–9.

The essential features of the system include a modulatory mechanism consisting of opioid peptide- and catecholamine-secreting neurons that are interposed between the suprahypothalamic "neural clock" and the GnRH secretory neurons. These mechanisms regulate the function of the GnRH neurons, the "pattern generator."

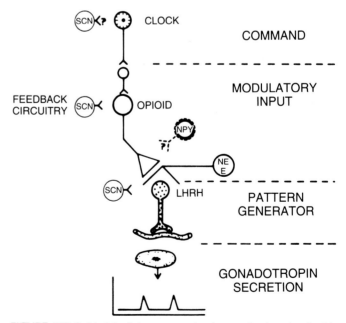

FIGURE 113–9. Model of the neuroendocrine mechanisms involved in the regulation of GnRH secretion. The neurons depicted on the left (feedback circuitry) indicate the proposed sites of gonadal steroid hormonal feedback, which may be positive or negative and may be exerted at different levels of the regulatory system. NE and E represent norepinephrine- and epinephrine-secreting neurons. NPY, neuropeptide Y. (From Kalra SP: In Ganong W, Martini L [eds]: Frontiers in Neuroendocrinology [ed 9]. New York, Raven Press, 1986, pp 31–75.)

Catecholamines

Norepinephrine can exert both inhibitory and stimulatory effects on LH secretion. In ovariectomized rats NE inhibits LH release, whereas it stimulates LH secretion by way of increased GnRH release in intact or steroid-replaced castrate rats. In the latter model, the administration of pulses of NE by way of the cerebral ventricles produces synchronous pulsatile LH release.[52] Thus the effects of NE appear to depend on the presence of ovarian steroids, particularly estradiol. In contrast, E does not alter LH secretion in ovariectomized animals but is more potent than NE in stimulating GnRH and LH release in steroid-primed rats. This suggests that E may be important in the steroid-related increase in GnRH secretion that occurs at the time of the ovulatory LH surge. The role of dopamine (DA) in the regulation of GnRH secretion is less clear. DA has been shown to stimulate a small increase in GnRH release from hypothalami in vitro, but many in vivo studies have shown inconsistent or little effect of DA on LH secretion in rats.

The majority of evidence regarding catecholamine regulation of GnRH release has been obtained in rodents, and the role of this mechanism in women is less clear. α-Adrenergic receptor blocking drugs, such as phentolamine, can abolish pulsatile LH release in monkeys and reduce serum LH levels in postmenopausal women. DA infusions inhibit LH secretion in women, and this probably reflects reduced GnRH release. Thus, although data are incomplete, evidence suggests that catecholamines regulate GnRH secretion in primates, but the exact nature of the mechanisms involved remain uncertain.

Neuropeptide Y, Galanin, and N-Methyl-D-Aspartic Acid

Neuropeptide Y (NPY) is a 36-amino-acid peptide of the pancreatic polypeptide family. It is present throughout the brain and in high concentrations in the hypothalamus and certain brain stem nuclei. Intracerebroventricular administration of NPY stimulates LH release, and immunoneutralization of NPY blocks LH surges on proestrus. A series of studies have indicated that NPY exerts actions to stimulate GnRH secretion in the presence of ovarian steroids,[51] and in general, the actions of NPY are similar to those of E. In some conditions NPY can directly cause LH release from pituitary cells in culture and augment LH release in response to GnRH.[53, 54] Data suggest that NPY concentrations in the median eminence change in parallel to GnRH. NPY is also increased in portal blood coincident with the proestrus rise in GnRH. NPY binding sites have been identified in the anterior pituitary, and the peptide can also enhance binding of GnRH to anterior pituitary receptors.[55] Taken together these data suggest that NPY plays an important role in augmenting GnRH secretion and GnRH action in releasing LH—both sites of action requiring the presence of ovarian steroids.

Galanin is a peptide of 29 amino acids, initially isolated from intestine but also widely distributed in the brain, particularly in the hypothalamus and median eminence of the rodent. Studies have shown that galanin can stimulate GnRH release from the median eminence in vitro, an action that appears to be mediated through α-adrenergic mechanisms.[56] Galanin is secreted in a pulsatile manner into portal blood, and pulses coincide with GnRH pulses. Galanin has been co-localized with GnRH in hypothalamic neurons, particularly in female rodents, suggesting that galanin and GnRH may be co-secreted.[57, 58] In vitro galanin has also been shown to stimulate LH release from isolated pituitary cells and to augment GnRH action in stimulating LH release, actions that are enhanced in the presence of ovarian steroids. These data suggest that both NPY and galanin play a role in production of the marked increase in LH secretion during the LH surge by actions at both the hypothalamic and the pituitary level.

N-Methyl-D-aspartic acid (NMDA) is an excitatory amino acid that is known to stimulate LH secretion in both rodents and primates. NMDA stimulates release of GnRH from hypothalamic neurons and has proved a useful tool in assessing the effects of stimulated endogenous GnRH secretion. NMDA receptor antagonists markedly attenuate the proestrus LH surge,[59] suggesting that NMDA and analogues may play a role in initiating the LH surge, but its exact role in normal physiology remains uncertain.

Endogenous Opioid Peptides

Early studies demonstrated that morphine could inhibit LH secretion and suppress the proestrus LH surge and ovulation in rats. These observations suggested that the endogenous opioid peptides—endorphin, enkephalin, and dynorphin—may regulate GnRH secretion, and considerable evidence is now available to show that opioid peptides exert a major inhibitory influence on GnRH secretion. β-Endorphin and long-acting enkephalin analogues inhibit both the amplitude and the frequency of LH secretion in rats, and naloxone (an opiate receptor blocker) stimulates LH release. Opioid peptides also inhibit GnRH secretion in humans and primates. Long-acting enkephalin analogues inhibit LH secretion, and naloxone stimulates LH release in women.[60] Naloxone appears to act by increasing the frequency of GnRH secretion because naloxone infusions increase the frequency of LH pulses. This action is most prominent during the late follicular and luteal phases of the menstrual cycle,[61] suggesting that endogenous opioid peptides are involved in steroid hormone regulation of GnRH secretion. Inhibition of GnRH secretion by opioid peptides is enhanced in the presence of ovarian steroids, and naloxone is ineffective in increasing LH release in postmenopausal women.[62] Other evidence indicates that ovarian steroid inhibition of GnRH secretion is exerted by way of increased hypothalamic opioid activity. β-Endorphin concentrations in hypophysioportal blood are increased during the luteal phase of the menstrual cycle, and replacement of estradiol and progesterone to ovariectomized monkeys increases β-endorphin in portal blood.[63] Furthermore, opiate receptor blockers prevent the inhibition of pulsatile LH release that occurs after intravenous infusion of estradiol.[64] Thus strong evidence indicates that endogenous opioids exert an inhibitory influence on GnRH secretion and are involved in the steroid regulation of GnRH release in women.

Ovarian Steroids

Earlier studies in animals and humans showed that plasma gonadotropin levels were elevated after ovariectomy and were suppressed after the administration of estrogens and progestogens. These data indicated that the ovarian steroids exerted an inhibitory influence on LH and FSH secretion. Subsequent experiments have shown that both estradiol and progesterone could also stimulate secretion of pituitary gonadotropins. The inhibitory and stimulatory effects of ovarian steroids involve regulation of both GnRH secretion and pituitary responses to GnRH. The effects on GnRH secretion are considered here, and steroid action on pituitary responses to GnRH are discussed in the subsequent section.

ESTRADIOL. The inhibitory action of estradiol on GnRH secretion is supported by observations that the concentration of GnRH in hypophysioportal blood is increased after ovariectomy.[65, 66] In addition, the frequency of pulsatile LH release is increased in ovariectomized rats and primates, suggesting that estradiol inhibits GnRH secretion by slowing its frequency. Other evidence casts some doubt on this interpretation. Some investigators have not found elevated GnRH concentrations after ovariectomy,[67] and estradiol did not reduce the frequency of LH pulses in castrate sheep (Fig. 113–10). Other studies have shown that estra-

diol can stimulate GnRH secretion. The concentration of GnRH in hypothalamic-portal blood is increased at the time of the LH surge,[67, 68] which coincides with an elevation of the plasma estradiol level. In addition, the frequency of pulsatile LH secretion is increased during the late follicular phase of the menstrual cycle (when plasma estradiol concentrations are rising[18, 19]), and GnRH pulses increase in frequency at this time.[69] These data suggest that estradiol can stimulate the frequency of GnRH secretion, and this action may depend on crucial time-dose relations of hypothalamic exposure to estradiol. Studies have confirmed this in sheep. Estradiol injection was initially followed by reduced GnRH pulse amplitude (for about eight hours), followed by an increase in pulse frequency and a marked increase in mean GnRH (and LH) concentrations.[70, 71] The chronic inhibitory actions of estradiol on GnRH secretion remain uncertain, and the decline in plasma gonadotropins after the administration of estradiol probably results from inhibition of pituitary responses to GnRH (see below).

PROGESTERONE. Progesterone inhibits GnRH secretion, and this action is exerted by a decrease in the frequency of GnRH secretion.[72] The effects of the administration of progesterone to ovariectomized ewes are shown in Figure 113–10.

In normal women this effect of progesterone is seen as reduced LH pulse frequency during the luteal phase of the menstrual cycle.[18, 19] Confirmation that the slow luteal LH pulse frequency is due to the effects of progesterone is found in the results of studies during the follicular phase,[73] when the administration of progesterone results in a slowing of the frequency of LH pulses (see Fig. 117–5). Progesterone may exert this action by increasing the activity of hypothalamic opioid peptides because the administration of naloxone during the luteal phase of the menstrual cycle increases LH pulse frequency in normal women.[74]

In certain circumstances progesterone can also increase LH secretion, and the administration of progesterone to estrogen-replaced postmenopausal women or ovariectomized animals is followed by a surge of LH a few hours later.[75] This positive effect of progesterone requires the presence of estradiol and is mediated in part by enhanced pituitary responses to GnRH (see below). Increased GnRH secretion may also be involved because progesterone has been shown to stimulate GnRH release from hypothalamic tissue in vitro.[76]

Prolactin

Luteinizing hormone secretion is suppressed in postpartum women and suckling female rats. In these physiological situations where serum prolactin concentrations are elevated, pituitary responsiveness to GnRH usually is maintained. This suggests that the elevated prolactin level inhibits GnRH secretion. This effect is profound in suckling mothers, and pulsatile release of LH is not seen.[77] Hyperprolactinemia may act to suppress the amount of GnRH secreted, but the frequency of pulsatile GnRH release also appears to be reduced. In rats that are ovariectomized during suckling, a slower frequency of LH pulses is observed compared with nonsuckling controls. Prolactin appears to exert similar effects in humans, and irregular patterns of slow frequency LH release are consistently seen in women with anovulation due to hyperprolactinemia (see Ch. 117). Suppression of serum prolactin by the adminis-

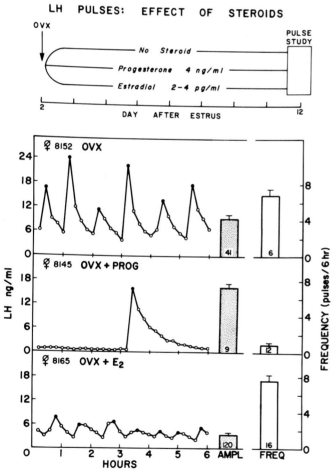

FIGURE 113–10. Effects of progesterone and estradiol on pulsatile LH secretion in ovariectomized ewes. Progesterone reduced LH pulse frequency and estradiol decreased LH pulse amplitude. LH responses to GnRH were reduced in estradiol-replaced ewes, indicating that estradiol was acting on the gonadotroph to suppress responsiveness to GnRH. (From Goodman RL, Karsch FJ: The estradiol induced surge of GnRH in the ewe. Endocrinology 127:1375–1384, © by The Endocrine Society, 1990.)

tration of bromocriptine is associated with an increase in the frequency of LH pulses and resumption of ovulatory menstrual cycles.[78, 79] The mechanisms of inhibition of GnRH secretion by prolactin are uncertain. Hypothalamic DA turnover is increased in hyperprolactinemic animals, and DA may inhibit GnRH release. Alternatively, an increase in hypothalamic opioid activity may be involved because infusions of naloxone increase LH pulsatility in hyperprolactinemic women.[80]

Hyperprolactinemia exerts a profound effect in inhibiting secretion of GnRH and may act as a natural contraceptive. The elevated serum prolactin level present during suckling inhibits ovulation and thus spares the mother the additional stress of pregnancy when she is feeding the existing offspring.

Factors That Modulate Gonadotroph Responses to GnRH

Gonadotropin-releasing hormone stimulation of LH and FSH release can be modified by other hormones. These interactions may enhance or inhibit gonadotroph responses to GnRH. Evidence points to estradiol and progesterone as the most important hormones involved in the regulation of gonadotroph responsiveness. Other ovarian compounds such as inhibin, pituitary hormones such as prolactin, and adrenal steroids may also play a role in modulating responses to GnRH.

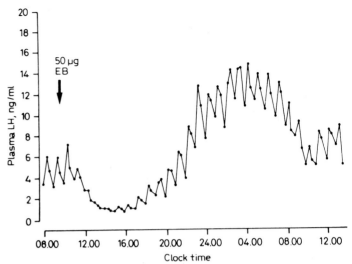

FIGURE 113–12. Inhibitory and stimulatory effects of estradiol on LH responsiveness to GnRH. Ovariectomized ewes, with surgical disconnection of the hypothalamus from the pituitary, were given GnRH pulse injections (500 ng every hour). LH responses to each GnRH pulse were measured after injection of 50 μg of estradiol benzoate (EB). LH responses were diminished between 12 noon and 1600 hours and subsequently augmented between 2000 and 0900 hours. (From Clarke IJ, Cummins JT: Direct pituitary effects of estrogen and progesterone on gonadotropin secretion in the ovariectomized ewe. Neuroendocrinology 39:267–274, 1984.)

Estradiol

The administration of estradiol to women or female animals is followed by an initial suppression of plasma LH and FSH, but both gonadotropins, particularly LH, are subsequently increased.[81] These observations have been confirmed in numerous studies, and estradiol consistently exerts a biphasic effect on gonadotropin secretion. The time course of the biphasic action depends on the species and the dose of estradiol used. In women the inhibitory effects persist two to three days and are followed by augmentation of LH secretion—"positive feedback" (Fig. 113–11).

Studies using single or multiple injections of GnRH have shown that both the inhibitory and the stimulatory effects of estradiol are exerted on the pituitary gonadotroph. After estradiol administration to normal women, LH responses to GnRH are suppressed during the first 36 hours[82] but are augmented after 48 hours, and the enhanced responses persist for several days.[82, 83] As noted, the time course of the negative and positive feedback effects of estradiol depend on both the species studied and the dose of estradiol used. The temporal relations in sheep, together with the pituitary site of estradiol action, are shown in Figure 113–12.[84]

As seen in Figure 113–12, estradiol initially inhibits LH release to each GnRH pulse, but subsequently LH responses are augmented and mean plasma LH concentrations increase. This positive action of estradiol accounts for the variation in pituitary responsiveness to GnRH that occurs during the menstrual cycle. LH responses to GnRH are augmented during the late follicular and midluteal phases of the cycle, when plasma estradiol concentrations are elevated. Confirmation that the positive effect of estradiol is exerted directly on the gonadotroph is found in

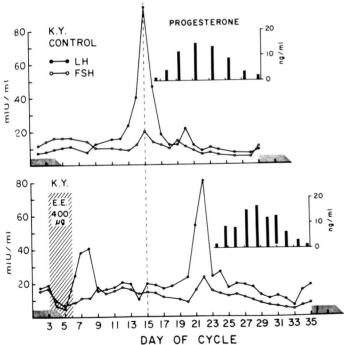

FIGURE 113–11. Effects of administration of ethinyl estradiol during the early follicular phase of the menstrual cycle on plasma gonadotropins (*lower panel*). Both LH and FSH were initially suppressed by estradiol, but plasma LH increased during the last day of estradiol and remained elevated for three days. Administration of estradiol delayed the midcycle LH surge (compared to the control cycle, *upper panel*), which reflects the reduction in FSH and consequent delay of ovarian follicular maturation. (From Tsai CC, Yen SSC: The effect of ethinyl estradiol administration during the early follicular phase of the cycle on gonadotropin levels and ovarian function. J Clin Endocrinol Metab 33:917–923, © by The Endocrine Society, 1971.)

studies that have examined the effects of estradiol on cultured pituitary cells.[85] When rat pituitary cells are incubated with estradiol, LH responses to GnRH are augmented after 12 hours of exposure to the steroid. The exact mechanisms of this estradiol effect are uncertain but may involve alteration of the number of cells that release LH as well as an increase in the amount of LH released by each cell. Smith et al.[86] have shown that GnRH stimulates release of LH from twice as many cells from proestrous rats (high estradiol) as compared with cells from diestrous animals (low estradiol).

In contrast to the effects on LH, estradiol exerts a predominantly inhibitory action on FSH release. The differential effects of estradiol on pituitary LH and FSH secretion are seen in studies in which GnRH pulses are given to women with isolated GnRH deficiency (Kallmann's syndrome). Pretreatment of these patients with estradiol abolishes FSH responses to GnRH, but LH responsiveness is maintained.[87] As shown in Figure 113–13, the inhibitory effect of estradiol on FSH release is evident when plasma estradiol values exceed 50 to 75 pg/ml.

Experiments using pituitary cells in culture have shown that estradiol inhibition of FSH responses to GnRH involves inhibition of FSH synthesis. Synthesis of FSH is decreased after six to eight hours of gonadotroph exposure to estradiol.[88]

Progesterone

Progesterone can also augment gonadotropin responses to GnRH, but this action is seen only after previous exposure to estradiol. LH responses to GnRH are inhibited when progesterone alone is added to rat pituitary cells in culture. In contrast, the addition of progesterone after prior incubation with estradiol results in a transient (12- to 16-hour) augmentation of LH release and a more prolonged enhancement of FSH responsiveness to GnRH.[89] This transient augmentation of pituitary responsiveness to GnRH also occurs in vivo, and data are shown in Figure 113–14.

Thus progesterone acts synergistically with estrogen to augment gonadotroph responsiveness to GnRH. The combined effects of these steroids are crucial in the production of the mid-cycle LH and FSH surge (see Ch. 117), and progesterone augments and prolongs the positive feedback effects of estradiol.[90, 91]

Prolactin

The major effects of prolactin on LH and FSH secretion appear to be exerted by inhibiting secretion of GnRH. Prolactin may, however, also exert a direct effect on the gonadotroph. GnRH-stimulated LH release from cultured pituitary cells is impaired in the presence of elevated prolactin concentrations, and this is reversed by bromocriptine.[92] Similar results have been observed in vivo and in bromocriptine-enhanced responses to GnRH pulses in hyperprolactinemic rats.[93, 94] Thus prolactin may also inhibit pituitary responses to GnRH and contribute to the low gonadotropin levels seen in hyperprolactinemic states.

Inhibin, Activin, and Follistatin

The concept that ovarian follicular fluid contains substances in addition to steroid hormones that may play a role in the regulation of gonadotropin secretion has existed for more than half a century. Despite many investigations the nature of these substances, shown to be proteins and to selectively inhibit FSH secretion in vivo and in vitro, remained obscure. Recent studies have cast major light in this area, and the inhibins, activins, and follistatin are compounds now known to be active in regulating gonadotropin

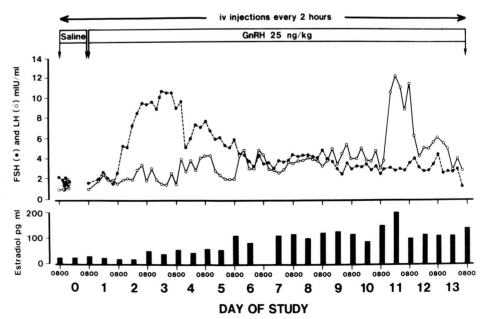

**ISOLATED GONADOTROPIN DEFICIENCY
– "PHYSIOLOGICAL" GnRH INJECTIONS FOR 13 DAYS**

FIGURE 113–13. Differential effects of estradiol on LH and FSH responsiveness to GnRH. GnRH pulses (25 ng/kg/pulse) were given every two hours for 13 days to a woman with isolated GnRH deficiency. Hormone values shown are those obtained immediately before a GnRH pulse injection. The initial predominance of FSH secretion declined as plasma estradiol rose (days 3 to 6). In addition, the preovulatory increase in estradiol (day 11) was associated with augmented LH, but not FSH, responsiveness to GnRH. (Redrawn from Valk TW, et al: Simulation of the follicular phase of the menstrual cycle by intravenous administration of low dose pulsatile gonadotropin releasing hormone. Am J Obstet Gynecol 141:842–843, 1981.)

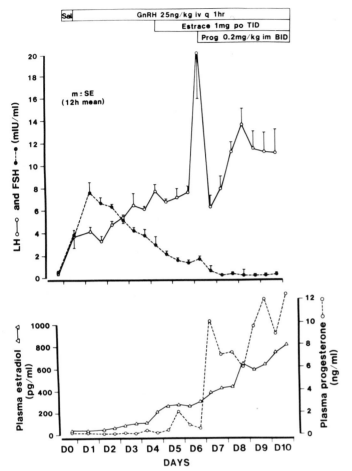

ISOLATED GONADOTROPIN DEFICIENCY: RESPONSES TO PULSATILE GnRH GIVEN HOURLY - EFFECTS OF ESTRADIOL AND PROGESTERONE

FIGURE 113–14. Effects of estradiol and progesterone on gonadotropin responses to GnRH. GnRH pulses (25 ng/kg/pulse) were given hourly for 10 days to a woman with isolated GnRH deficiency. The effects of addition of estrogen alone (Estrace on days 4 to 6) and estrogen together with progesterone (days 6 to 10) on plasma LH and FSH are shown. Plasma LH and FSH (mean values over four hours from samples obtained before GnRH pulses) are shown in the upper panel, and ovarian steroids, in the lower panel. The rapid and transient augmentation of LH and, to a lesser extent, FSH responses to GnRH are evident soon after addition of progesterone on day 6. (Redrawn from Nippoldt TB, et al: Gonadotropin responses to GnRH pulses in hypogonadotropic hypogonadism: LH responsiveness is maintained in the presence of luteal phase concentrations of estrogen and progesterone. Clin Endocrinol 26:293–301, 1987.)

synthesis and secretion.[95] All three compounds were originally isolated from gonadal tissue, but either the protein or mRNAs for all three compounds are widely distributed. Of interest, inhibin, activin, and follistatin have all been shown to be present in the pituitary in addition to the CNS and other tissues.

Inhibin circulates in plasma being secreted by the ovarian granulosa cells during the follicular phase (under the control of FSH), but it is also secreted during the luteal phase under the control of LH.[96] In vitro studies showed that inhibin predominantly reduced FSH release from the gonadotroph. Together these data suggest that inhibin may regulate the reduction in plasma FSH in the late follicular phase and the low levels of FSH present in the luteal phase of the menstrual cycle. The availability of recombi-

nant inhibin has allowed further study. In rats the injection of inhibin caused dose-related decreases in mean plasma FSH with little effect on LH. Similarly, inhibin decreased the evening proestrus FSH surge and abolished the secondary FSH surge on the subsequent morning.[97] These effects are exerted directly on the gonadotroph because inhibin lowers plasma FSH in animals pretreated with a GnRH antagonist and is also active on gonadotrophs in vitro. The exact mechanisms of inhibin's actions in suppressing FSH secretion remain uncertain, but in part they are exerted on FSH β mRNA concentrations. In vitro inhibin rapidly reduces FSH β mRNA,[44] and in vivo administration of anti-inhibin sera results in a marked increase in FSH β mRNA concentrations during the proestrus surge in rats.[98]

Activins were discovered during the characterization of inhibin and found to be homodimers or heterodimers of the inhibin β subunits. Activin was shown to increase secretion of FSH by pituitary cells in vitro, and studies using recombinant material has shown that similar effects are present in vivo. Activin increases plasma FSH in female rats, and FSH β mRNA is also increased.[99, 100] It is unclear whether activin from the ovary acts in an endocrine manner to selectively increase FSH synthesis and secretion. The observation that activin subunits are present in the pituitary suggests an alternative whereby activin exerts paracrine and autocrine mechanisms in normal physiology. The availability of sensitive assays to detect activin in plasma will allow these issues to be addressed.

Follistatin bears no structural relation to inhibins and activins but exhibits potent and specific inhibition of pituitary FSH secretion in vitro. Its effects are similar to those of inhibin but appear to persist longer in vivo.[101] It is not known whether follistatin acts in an endocrine manner, but it also is present in the pituitary.

The mechanism and site of activin, inhibin, and follistatin action remain unclear, as do the relative contributions of circulating hormone versus intrapituitary compounds. The α and $β_B$ subunits have been shown to be present in gonadotrophs and thus may act directly on FSH mRNA expression. Antisera to activin B inhibited FSH β mRNA accumulation in vitro, supporting a direct role for the $β_B$ subunit. Of interest, an activin-binding protein purified from pituitary tissue was shown to be identical to follistatin. Follistatin binds to both activin and inhibin through the common β subunit.[102] The presence of $β_B$ subunit mRNA in the gonadotroph suggests the possibility that activin may act within the cell to regulate mRNA expression, presumably by increasing FSH β mRNA stability.[103] These actions of activin may be locally modulated by inhibin or by follistatin binding to the β subunit of activin. The availability of sensitive to specific assays for the three compounds will clarify the endocrine versus paracrine and autocrine roles, but evidence suggests that these compounds exert a large part of their action by modifying the stability of the FSH β mRNA.

CLOMIPHENE CITRATE

Clomiphene citrate (Clomid) is a nonsteroidal compound with either antiestrogenic or estrogenic actions, depending on the target tissue.[104] It is widely used to induce ovulation and is effective in women with polycystic ovarian syndrome and in those with anovulation caused by abnormalities of hypothalamic function. Clomiphene acts by binding to estradiol receptors in the hypothalamus and anterior pituitary (antiestrogenic effect) to prevent estradiol negative feedback on gonadotropin secretion.[105] Clomiphene may also act in an estrogen-like manner on the gonadotroph to enhance responses to GnRH, but not all studies have confirmed this action.

The administration of clomiphene to women for five to seven days increases LH and FSH secretion, which initiates maturation of ovarian follicular development and estradiol secretion. Thus clomiphene initiates hormonal changes that are similar to those seen during the follicular phase of the normal menstrual cycle. Clomiphene induces ovulation in 65 to 75 per cent of women with polycystic ovarian syndrome or hypothalamic anovulation, but the pregnancy rate is considerably lower, being in the range of 30 to 40 per cent. Multiple factors may be involved in this discrepancy, but in many clomiphene-induced cycles the luteal phase is short and implantation of the fertilized ovum may be impaired. The inadequate luteal phase may relate to the fact that clomiphene stimulates the secretion of LH more than that of FSH. Thus FSH stimulation of the ovarian follicles often is suboptimal, which may account for subsequent abnormal function of the corpus luteum with reduced progesterone secretion and early menses (see Ch. 117). As noted, clomiphene is not effective in inducing ovulation in all women and does not always stimulate gonadotropin secretion. Examples of gonadotropin and estradiol responses after clomiphene administration are shown in Figure 113–15.

A normal response to clomiphene consists of elevation of plasma gonadotropins and estradiol. The rise in estradiol exerts a positive action at both the hypothalamic and the pituitary level to induce an LH surge. In some women plasma estradiol is increased after clomiphene but an LH surge does not ensue (absent positive feedback). These patients can be identified by their failure to increase plasma LH after an injection of estradiol,[106] and good correlation exists between the absence of an LH response to estradiol and the absence of an LH surge after clomiphene.[107] The ability to respond to clomiphene has been related to the plasma estradiol concentration, but estradiol itself is probably not directly involved in determining clomiphene responsiveness. In many women with hypothalamic amenorrhea consequent to exercise or weight loss, the frequency of pulsatile GnRH secretion is reduced and LH pulses occur infrequently (see Ch. 117). The degree of inhibition of GnRH pulse frequency is variable, and this may be an important factor in determining clomiphene responsiveness. If GnRH secretion is absent, clomiphene will be ineffective. When GnRH pulse frequency is moderately reduced, clomiphene may increase gonadotropin secretion, but the frequency of endogenous GnRH pulses may not be sufficient to allow full expression of estradiol positive feedback and an LH surge does not ensue. In women with less impairment of pulsatile GnRH activity, endogenous GnRH pulse frequency is adequate to allow estradiol positive feedback, and an LH surge and ovulation follow the administration of clomiphene.

REFERENCES

1. Bronson FH: Pherohormonal influences on mammalian reproduction. *In* Diamond N. (ed): Perspectives in Reproduction and Sexual Behavior. Bloomington, Indiana University Press, 1968.
2. Michael RP: Hormone steroids and sexual communication in primates. J Steroid Biochem 6:161–168, 1975.
3. Karsch FJ: Seasonal reproduction—a saga of reversible fertility. Physiologist 23:29–38, 1981.
4. Jackson GL, Davies SL: Comparison of luteinizing hormone and prolactin levels in cycling and anestrous ewes. Neuroendocrinology 28:256–263, 1979.
5. Midgley AR, Jaffe RB: Regulation of human gonadotropins—episodic fluctuation of LH during the menstrual cycle. J Clin Endocrinol Metab 33:962–969, 1971.
6. Santen RJ, Bardin CW: Episodic luteinizing hormone secretion in man. J Clin Invest 52:2617–2628, 1973.
7. Clarke IJ, Cummins JT: The temporal relationship between gonadotropin releasing hormone (GnRH) and luteinizing hormone (LH) secretion in ovariectomized ewes. Endocrinology 111:1737–1739, 1982.
8. Belchetz PE, Plant TM, Nakai Y, et al: Hypophysial responses to continuous and intermittent delivery of hypothalamic gonadotropin-releasing hormone. Science 202:631–633, 1978.
9. Marshall JC, Kelch RP: Low dose pulsatile gonadotropin-releasing hormone in anorexia nervosa—a model of human pubertal development. J Clin Endocrinol Metab 49:712–718, 1979.
10. Valk TW, Corley KP, Kelch RP, Marshall JC: Hypogonadotropic hypogonadism hormonal responses to low dose pulsatile administration of gonadotropin-releasing hormone. J Clin Endocrinol Metab 51:730–738, 1980.
11. Hoffman AR, Crowley WF: Induction of puberty in men by long term pulsatile administration of low dose gonadotropin-releasing hormone. N Engl J Med 307:1237–1241, 1982.
12. Valk TW, Marshall JC, Kelch RP: Simulation of the follicular phase of the menstrual cycle by intravenous administration of low dose

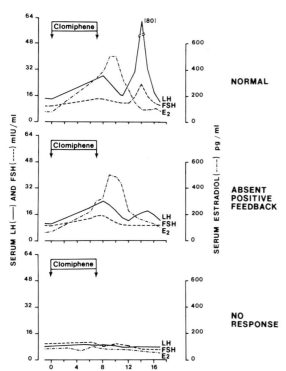

HYPOTHALAMIC AMENORRHEA - RESPONSES TO CLOMIPHENE CITRATE

FIGURE 113–15. Patterns of LH, FSH, and estradiol responses to clomiphene citrate in women with hypothalamic anovulation and amenorrhea. The normal response is shown in the upper panel, stimulation of estradiol secretion without an LH surge in the middle panel (absent positive feedback), and absence of response in the lower panel.

pulsatile gonadotropin-releasing hormone. Am J Obstet Gynecol 141:842–843, 1981.

13. Crowley WF, McArthur JW: Simulation of the normal menstrual cycle in Kallmann's syndrome by pulsatile administration of LHRH. J Clin Endocrinol Metab 51:173–175, 1980.

14. Leyendecker G, Wildt L, Hansmen M: Pregnancies following chronic intermittent pulsatile administration of GnRH. J Clin Endocrinol Metab 51:1214–1216, 1980.

15. Wildt L, Hausler A, Marshall JC, et al: Frequency and amplitude of gonadotropin-releasing hormone stimulation and gonadotropin secretion in the rhesus monkey. Endocrinology 109:376–385, 1981.

16. Clarke IJ, Cummins JT, Findlay JK, et al: Effects on plasma LH and FSH of varying frequency and amplitude of gonadotropin-releasing hormone pulses in ovariectomized ewes with hypothalamic-pituitary disconnection. Neuroendocrinology 39:214–221, 1984.

17. Katt JA, Duncan JA, Herbon L, et al: The frequency of gonadotropin-releasing hormone stimulation determines the number of pituitary gonadotropin-releasing hormone receptors. Endocrinology 116:2113–2116, 1985.

18. Backstrom CT, McNeilly AS, Leask RM, Baird DT: Pulsatile secretion of LH, FSH prolactin, estradiol and progesterone during the human menstrual cycle. Clin Endocrinol (Oxf) 17:29–38, 1982.

19. Reame N, Sauder SE, Kelch RP, Marshall JC: Pulsatile gonadotropin secretion during the human menstrual cycle—evidence for altered frequency of gonadotropin-releasing hormone secretion. J Clin Endocrinol Metab 59:328–337, 1984.

20. Hazum E, Conn PM: Molecular mechanisms of gonadotropin releasing hormone (GnRH) action. I: The GnRH receptor. Endocr Rev 9:379–386, 1988.

21. Huckle WR, Conn PM: Molecular mechanisms of gonadotropin releasing hormone action. II: The effector system. Endocr Rev 9:387–395, 1988.

22. Naor Z: Signal transductor mechanisms of Ca^{2+} mobilizing hormones: The case of gonadotropin releasing hormone. Endocr Rev 11:326–353, 1990.

23. Clayton RN, Shakespear RA, Duncan JA, Marshall JC: Radioiodinated nondegradable gonadotropin-releasing hormone analogues—new probes for the investigation of pituitary GnRH receptors. Endocrinology 60:1369–1377, 1979.

24. Savoy-Moore RT, Schwartz NB, Duncan JA, Marshall JC: Pituitary gonadotropin releasing hormone receptors during the estrous cycle. Science 209:942–945, 1980.

25. Frager MS, Pieper DR, Tonetta SA, et al: Pituitary gonadotropin releasing hormone (GnRH) receptors—effects of castration, steroid replacement and the role of GnRH in modulating receptors in the rat. J Clin Invest 67:615–623, 1981.

26. Clayton RN, Katt KJ: Gonadotropin-releasing hormone receptors—characterization, physiological regulation, and relationship to reproductive function. Endocr Rev 2:186–209, 1981.

27. Andrews WV, Conn PM: Gonadotropin-releasing hormone stimulates mass changes in phosphoinositides and diacylglycerol accumulation in purified gonadotrope cell cultures. Endocrinology 118:1148–1158, 1986.

28. Borgeat P, Chavancy G, Dupont A, et al: Stimulation of adenosine 3,5-monophosphate accumulation in anterior pituitary gland in vitro by synthetic LHRH. Proc Natl Acad Sci USA 69:2677–2679, 1972.

29. Andrews WV, Conn PM: Stimulation of rat luteinizing hormone beta mRNA levels by gonadotropin releasing hormone. J Biol Chem 263:13755–13758, 1988.

30. Aiyer MS, Chiappa SA, Fink G: A priming effect of luteinizing hormone-releasing factor on the anterior pituitary gland in the female rat. J Endocrinol 62:573–588, 1974.

31. Wang CF, Lasley BL, Lein A, Yen SSC: The functional changes of the pituitary gonadotrophs during the menstrual cycle. J Clin Endocrinol Metab 42:718–728, 1976.

32. Turgeon JL, Waring DW: Activation of the progesterone receptor in gonadotropes by GnRH and cAMP. 74th Annual Meeting of the Endocrine Society, San Antonio, June 1992, Abstr 517.

33. Casper RF, Yen SSC: Simultaneous pulsatile release of prolactin and luteinizing hormone induced by luteinizing hormone-releasing factor agonist. J Clin Endocrinol Metab 52:934–939, 1981.

34. Braund W, Roeger DC, Judd SJ: Synchronous secretion of luteinizing hormone and prolactin in the human luteal phase—neuroendocrine mechanisms. J Clin Endocrinol Metab 58:293–297, 1984.

35. Cetel NS, Yen SSC: Concomitant pulsatile release of prolactin and luteinizing hormone in hypogonadal women. J Clin Endocrinol Metab 56:1313–1315, 1983.

36. Denef C, Andries M: Evidence for paracrine interaction between gonadotrophs and lactotrophs in pituitary cell aggregates. Endocrinology 112:813–822, 1983.

37. Pohl CR, Weiner RI, Smith MS: Relation between luteinizing hormone and prolactin pulses in ovariectomized rats with or without dopamine inhibition. Endocrinology 123:1591–1597, 1988.

38. Gharib SD, Wierman ME, Shupnik MA, Chin WW: Molecular biology of the pituitary gonadotropins. Endocr Rev 11:177–199, 1990.

39. Shupnik MA, Weinmann CM, Notides AC, Chin WW: An upstream region of the rat luteinizing hormone beta gene binds estrogen receptor and confers estrogen responsiveness. J Biol Chem 264:80–84, 1989.

40. Shaw G, Kamen R: A conceived AU sequence from the 3′ untranslated region of GM-CSF mRNA mediates selective mRNA degradation. Cell 46:659–663, 1980.

41. Papavasiliou SS, Zmeili S, Herbon L, et al: α and LH beta mRNA of male and female rats after castration: Quantitation using an optimized RNA dot blot hybridization assay. Endocrinology 119:691–698, 1986.

42. Dalkin AC, Haisenleder DJ, Ortolano GA, et al: Gonadal regulation of gonadotropin subunit gene expression: Evidence for regulation of FSH beta mRNA by non-steroidal hormones in female rats. Endocrinology 127:798–806, 1990.

43. Marshall JC, Dalkin AC, Haisenleder DJ, et al: Gonadotropin releasing hormone pulses: Regulators of gonadotropin synthesis and ovulatory cycles. Recent Prog Horm Res 47:155–189, 1991.

44. Carroll RS, Corrigan AZ, Gharib SD, et al: Inhibin, activin and follistatin: Follicle-stimulating hormone messenger ribonucleic acid levels. Mol Endocrinol 3:1969–1976, 1989.

45. Paul SJ, Ortolano GA, Haisenleder DJ, et al: Gonadotropin subunit mRNA concentrations after blockade of GnRH action: Testosterone selectively increases FSH beta subunit mRNA by posttranscriptional mechanisms. Mol Endocrinol 4:1943–1955, 1990.

46. Haisenleder DJ, Ortolano GA, Jolly D, et al: Inhibin secretion during the rat estrous cycle: Relationships to FSH secretion and FSH beta subunit mRNA concentrations. Life Sci 47:1769–1773, 1990.

47. Dalkin AC, Haisenleder DJ, Ortolano GA, et al: The frequency of gonadotropin-releasing hormone (GnRH) stimulation differentially regulates gonadotropin subunit mRNA expression. Endocrinology 125:917–924, 1989.

48. Haisenleder DJ, Dalkin AC, Ortolano GA, et al: A pulsatile GnRH stimulus is required to increase transcription of the gonadotropin subunit genes: Evidence for differential regulation of transcription by pulse frequency in vivo. Endocrinology 128:509–517, 1991.

49. Shupnik MA: GnRH effects on rat gonadotropin subunit gene transcription in vitro: Requirement for pulsatile administration for LH beta gene stimulation. Mol Endocrinol 4:1444–1450, 1990.

50. Estes KS, Simpkins JW, Kalra SP: Resumption with clonidine of pulsatile LH release following acute norepinephrine depletion in ovariectomized rats. Neuroendocrinology 35:56–64, 1982.

51. Kalra SP: Neural circuitry involved in the control of LHRH secretion: A model for preovulation LH release. In Ganong W, Martini L (eds): Frontiers in Neuroendocrinology (ed 9). New York, Raven Press, 1986, pp 31–75.

52. Kalra SP, Gallo RV: Effects of intraventricular catecholamines on luteinizing hormone release in morphine treated rats. Endocrinology 113:23–28, 1983.

53. Sutton SW, Toyama TT, Otto S, Plotsky PM: Evidence that neuropeptide Y (NPY) released into the hypophysial-portal circulation participates in priming gonadotropes to the effects of GnRH. Endocrinology 123:1208–1210, 1988.

54. Bauer-Dantoin A, McDonald JK, Levine JE: Neuropeptide Y potentiates LH-RH stimulated LH surges in pentobarbital-blocked proestrous rats. Endocrinology 129:402–408, 1991.

55. Parker SL, Kalra SP, Crowley WR: Neuropeptide Y modulates the binding of a GnRH analog to anterior pituitary GnRH receptor sites. Endocrinology 128:2309–2316, 1991.

56. Lopez FJ, Negro-Vilar A: Galanin stimulates LH-RH secretion from arcuate nucleus–median eminence fragments in vitro: Involvement of an α-adrenergic mechanism. Endocrinology 127:2431–2436, 1990.

57. Lopez FJ, Merchenthaler I, Ching M, et al: Galanin: A hypothalamic-hypophysiotropic hormone modulating reproductive functions. Proc Natl Acad Sci USA 88:4508–4512, 1991.

58. Merchenthaler I, Lopez FJ, Lennard DE, Negro-Vilar A: Sexual differences in the distribution of neurons coexpressing galanin and LH-RH in the rat brain. Endocrinology 129:1977–1986, 1991.

59. Brann DW, Mahesh VB: Endogenous excitatory amino acid involvement in the preovulatory and steroid-induced surge of gonadotropins in the female rat. Endocrinology 128:1541–1547, 1991.

60. Grossman A, Moult PJA, Gaillard RC, et al: The opioid control of LH and FSH release—effects of a met-enkephalin analogue and naloxone. Clin Endocrinol (Oxf) 14:41–47, 1981.

61. Quigley ME, Yen SSC: The role of endogenous opiates on LH secretion during the menstrual cycle. J Clin Endocrinol Metab 51:179–181, 1980.

62. Reid RL, Quigley ME, Yen SSC: The disappearance of opioidergic regulation of gonadotropin secretion in post-menopausal women. J Clin Endocrinol Metab 57:1107–1110, 1983.

63. Wardlaw SL, Wehrenberg WB, Ferin M, et al: Effect of sex steroids on beta-endorphin in hypophysial-portal blood. J Clin Endocrinol Metab 55:877–881, 1982.

64. Veldhuis JD, Rogol AD, Samojlik E, Ertel NH: Role of endogenous opiates in the expression of negative feedback actions of androgens and estrogen on pulsatile properties of luteinizing hormone secretion in man. J Clin Invest 74:47–55, 1984.

65. Neill JD, Patton JM, Daily RA, et al: Luteinizing hormone releasing hormone (LHRH) in pituitary stalk blood of rhesus monkeys—relationship to level of LH release. Endocrinology 101:430–434, 1977.

66. Sarkar DK, Fink G: Luteinizing hormone-releasing factor in pituitary stalk plasma from long term ovariectomized rats—effects of steroids. J Endocrinol 86:511–524, 1980.

67. Levine JE, Ramirez VD: Luteinizing hormone-releasing hormone release during the rat estrous cycle and after ovariectomy as estimated with push-pull cannulae. Endocrinology 111:1439–1448, 1982.

68. Sarkar DK, Chiappa SA, Fink G, Sherwood NM: Gonadotropin-releasing hormone surge in proestrous rats. Nature 264:461–463, 1975.

69. Moenter SM, Caraty A, Locatelli A, Karsch FJ: Pattern of GnRH secretion leading up to ovulation in the ewe—existence of a preovulatory GnRH surge. Endocrinology 129:1175–1182, 1991.

70. Caraty A, Locatelli A, Martin GB: Biphasic response to GnRH in ovariectomized ewes treated with estradiol. J Endocrinol 123:375–382, 1989.

71. Moenter SM, Caraty A, Karsch FJ: The estradiol induced surge of GnRH in the ewe. Endocrinology 127:1375–1384, 1990.

72. Goodman RL, Karsch FJ: Pulsatile secretion of luteinizing hormone—differential suppression by ovarian steroids. Endocrinology 107:1286–1292, 1980.

73. Soules MR, Steiner RA, Clifton DK, et al: Progesterone modulation of pulsatile luteinizing secretion in normal women. J Clin Endocrinol Metab 58:378–383, 1984.

74. Van Vugt DA, Lam NY, Ferin M: Reduced frequency of pulsatile luteinizing hormone secretion in the luteal phase of the rhesus monkey—involvement of endogenous opiates. Endocrinology 115:1095–1101, 1984.

75. Odell WD, Swerdloff RS: Progesterone induced luteinizing and follicle-stimulating hormone surge in post-menopausal women—a simulated ovulatory peak. Proc Natl Acad Sci USA 61:529–536, 1968.

76. Kim K, Ramirez VD: In vitro progesterone stimulates the release of luteinizing hormone-releasing hormone from superfused hypothalamic tissue from ovariectomized estradiol-primed prepuberal rats. Endocrinology 111:750–757, 1982.

77. Fox SR, Smith SM: The suppression of pulsatile leutinizing hormone secretion during lactation in the rat. Endocrinology 115:2045–2051, 1984.

78. Sauder SE, Frager M, Case GD, et al: Abnormal patterns of pulsatile luteinizing hormone secretion in women with hyperprolactinemia and amenorrhea—responses to bromocriptine. J Clin Endocrinol Metab 59:941–948, 1984.

79. Klibanski A, Beitins IZ, Merriam GR, et al: Gonadotropin and prolactin pulsations in hyperprolactinemic women before and during bromocriptine therapy. J Clin Endocrinol Metab 58:1141–1147, 1984.

80. Cook CB, Nippoldt TB, Kletter GB, et al: Naloxone increases the frequency of LH (GnRH) pulsatile secretion in hyperprolactinemia. J Clin Endocrinol Metab 73:1099–1105, 1991.

81. Tsai CC, Yen SSC: The effect of ethinyl estradiol administration during the early follicular phase of the cycle on gonadotropin levels and ovarian function. J Clin Endocrinol Metab 31:917–923, 1971.

82. Shaw RW, Butt WR, London DR: The effect of estrogen pretreatment on subsequent response to luteinizing hormone-releasing hormone in normal women. Clin Endocrinol (Oxf) 4:297–304, 1975.

83. Jaffe RB, Keyes WR: Estradiol augmentation of pituitary responsiveness to gonadotropin-releasing hormone in women. J Clin Endocrinol Metab 39:850–856, 1974.

84. Clarke IJ, Cummins JT: Direct pituitary effects of estrogen and progesterone on gonadotropin secretion in the ovariectomized ewe. Neuroendocrinology 39:267–274, 1984.

85. Drouin J, Lagace L, Labrie F: Estradiol induced increase of LH responsiveness to LH-releasing hormone (LHRH) in rat anterior pituitary cells in culture. Endocrinology 99:1477–1481, 1976.

86. Smith PF, Frawley LS, Neill JD: Detection of LH release from individual pituitary cells by the reverse hemolytic plaque assay—estrogen increases the fraction of gonadotropes responding to GnRH. Endocrinology 115:2484–2486, 1984.

87. Marshall JC, Case GD, Valk TW, et al: Selective inhibition of follicle-stimulating hormone secretion by estradiol—a mechanism for modulation of gonadotropin responses to low dose pulses of gonadotropin-releasing hormone. J Clin Invest 71:248–257, 1983.

88. Miller WL, Knight MM, Grimek HJ, Gorski J: Estrogen regulation of follicle-stimulating hormone in cell cultures of sheep pituitaries. Endocrinology 100:1306–1316, 1977.

89. Lagace L, Massicotte J, Labrie F: Acute stimulatory effects of progesterone on luteinizing hormone and follicle-stimulating hormone release in rat anterior pituitary cells in culture. Endocrinology 106:684–692, 1980.

90. Nippoldt TB, Khoury S, Barkan A, et al: Gonadotropin responses to GnRH pulses in hypogonadotropic hypogonadism: LH responsiveness is maintained in the presence of luteal phase concentrations of estrogen and progesterone. Clin Endocrinol 26:293–301, 1987.

91. Liu JH, Yen SSC: Induction of the mid-cycle gonadotropin surge by ovarian steroids in women. A critical evaluation. J Clin Endocrinol Metab 57:797–802, 1983.

92. Cheung CY: Prolactin suppresses luteinizing hormone secretion and pituitary responses to LHRH by a direct action at the anterior pituitary. Endocrinology 113:632–638, 1983.

93. Garcia A, Herbon L, Barkan A, et al: Hyperprolactinemia inhibits gonadotropin-releasing hormone (GnRH) stimulation of the number of pituitary GnRH receptors. Endocrinology 117:954–959, 1985.

94. Duncan JA, Barkan A, Herbon L, Marshall JC: Regulation of pituitary GnRH receptors by pulsatile GnRH in female rats: Effects of estradiol and prolactin. Endocrinology 118:320–327, 1986.

95. Ying SY: Inhibins, activins, and follistatins: Gonadal proteins modulating the secretion of follicle-stimulating hormone. Endocr Rev 9:267–293, 1988.

96. McLachlan RI, Robertson DM, Healy DL, et al: Circulating immunoreactive inhibin levels during the normal human menstrual cycle. J Clin Endocrinol Metab 65:954–961, 1987.

97. Rivier C, Schwall R, Mason A, et al: Effect of recombinant inhibin on gonadotropin secretion during proestrus and estrus in the rat. Endocrinology 128:2223–2228, 1991.

98. Attardi B, Vaughan J, Vale W: Regulation of FSH beta mRNA levels in the rat by endogenous inhibin. Endocrinology 129:2802–2804, 1991.

99. Rivier C, Vale W: Effect of recombinant activin-A on gonadotropin secretion in the female rat. Endocrinology 129:2463–2465, 1991.

100. Carroll RS, Kowash PM, Lofgren JA, et al: In vivo regulation of FSH synthesis by inhibin and activin. Endocrinology 129:3299–3304, 1991.

101. Inouye S, Guo Y, DePaolo L, et al: Recombinant expression of human follistatin with 315 and 288 amino acids: Chemical and biological comparison with native porcine follistatin. Endocrinology 129:815–822, 1991.

102. Shimonaka M, Inouye S, Shimasaki S, Ling N: Follistatin binds to both activin and inhibin through the common beta subunit. Endocrinology 128:3313–3315, 1991.

103. Carroll RS, Corrigan AZ, Vale W, Chin WW: Activin stabilizes FSH-beta mRNA levels. Endocrinology 129:1721–1726, 1991.

104. Lunan CB, Klopper A: Antiestrogens—a review. Clin Endocrinol (Oxf) 4:551–572, 1975.

105. Kato J, Kobayashi T, Villee CA: Effect of clomiphene on the uptake of estradiol by the anterior hypothalamus and hypophysis. Endocrinology 82:1049–1052, 1968.

106. Shaw RW, Butt WR, London DR, Marshall JC: The estrogen provocation test—a method for assessing the hypothalamo-pituitary axis in patients with amenorrhea. Clin Endocrinol (Oxf) 4:267–276, 1975.

107. Shaw RW, Butt WR, London DR: Pathological mechanisms to explain some cases of amenorrhea without organic disease. Br J Obstet Gynecol 82:337–340, 1975.

114

Gonadal Regulatory Peptides

HENRY G. BURGER

The term *gonadal regulatory peptides* encompasses a group of proteins and peptides, primarily of gonadal origin, involved in endocrine (long-loop feedback), paracrine, and autocrine regulation of reproductive function. This chapter focuses particularly on three members of this family—inhibin, activin, and follistatin (also known as follicle-stimulating hormone [FSH]–suppressing protein [FSP])—emphasizing their endocrine roles in women. Historically, the notion that a nonsteroidal factor was involved in the regulation of pituitary gonadotropin secretion originated from studies of male reproductive function and the demonstration by McCullagh[1] that an aqueous testicular extract was capable of preventing the appearance of castration cells in the pituitaries of male rats. The active principle, inhibin, eluded isolation until 1985, when it was first purified from bovine follicular fluid,[2] it having been recognized that a specific inhibitor of pituitary FSH was present in follicular fluid[3] as well as in testicular extracts.[4] Inhibin is characterized by its ability to inhibit the secretion of FSH and has been shown to circulate, with a substantial body of evidence indicating that it is involved in the physiological regulation of FSH secretion in a number of species (reviewed in refs. 5–10). The isolation of activin, a dimeric peptide that stimulates rather than inhibits FSH, followed shortly on the isolation of inhibin.[11, 12] Although it has subsequently been shown that activin has various physiological properties,[10] it has not yet been shown to circulate, and its physiological role in the regulation of reproductive function remains to be fully elucidated. Follistatin was also isolated initially from ovarian follicular fluid[13, 14] and has been demonstrated to have FSH-suppressing properties similar to those of inhibin, but only limited studies of its physiology, particularly its endocrine physiology, have so far been published.[15, 16, 16a]

STRUCTURE–FUNCTION RELATIONS

Inhibin

The structure–function relations of inhibin have been extensively reviewed,[5–10] and only the major features are summarized here. Inhibin is a glycoprotein hormone made up of an α subunit of varying molecular size linked to one of two types of β subunit (β_A or β_B) by disulfide bonds. Three separate genes code for the precursors of these subunits; the subunits are cleaved from the C-terminal ends of these precursors. The α subunit precursor has four segments, including a signal peptide, a pro-sequence (pro), together with N-terminal (αN) and C-terminal (αC) peptides. Inhibin as initially isolated from bovine follicular fluid had a molecular mass of 58 kDa, incorporating a 43-kDa α subunit (αN-αC) and the 15-kDa β subunit. Inhibin of about 31 to 32 kDa subsequently was isolated in several species and has αC as its α subunit. Analysis of bovine follicular fluid in particular indicates the presence of a large number of inhibin forms, ranging as high as 120 kDa in molecular weight. The free pro-αN-αC together with αN and pro-αC (the α subunit precursor with αN cleaved out) have all been isolated from follicular fluid, as has the β_A free subunit.[17–19] There is 85 per cent homology in the sequence of the α chain among human, bovine, porcine, murine, and ovine inhibins and 100 per cent homology in the β_A subunit sequences among human, bovine, porcine, and murine, with one amino acid substitution in the ovine β_A subunit. Similarly, there is 95 per cent sequence homology among the β_B subunits of the various species. The major structural features of inhibin and activin are shown in Figure 114–1.

The inhibin β subunit sequences in particular are homologous with a number of other biologically active peptides. These include transforming growth factor-β, which affects the proliferation and/or differentiation of a number of cell lines in vitro; müllerian inhibiting substance, which is responsible for müllerian duct regression during male sexual differentiation; the gene product of the decapentaplegic complex, which affects morphogenesis in *Drosophila,* an mRNA product in *Xenopus* involved in the differentiation of the frog embryo (subsequently shown to be activin); the bone morphogenetic proteins, which can induce cartilage and bone formation; and the product of the growth differentiation factor I (GDF-I) gene, which may mediate cell differentiation events during embryonic development.

Activin

Activin is the name given to the group of dimers of the inhibin β subunits. Activin A is a dimer of β_A; activin AB, a dimer of $\beta_A\beta_B$; and activin B, a dimer of β_B. All three species have been isolated from porcine follicular fluid,[11, 12, 19a] whereas the β_B dimer has not been isolated under natural conditions, although it has been produced using recombinant methodology. The β_A subunit monomer is calculated to be present at 25 to 60 per cent of the level of the dimer in bovine follicular fluid and resembles the dimer in both biological and immunological activity.[19] The erythroid differentiation factor isolated from the culture medium of a human leukemia cell line has been shown to be activin A and shares its biological activity.[20] The activins may play fundamental roles in embryonic differentiation, specifically in mesoderm induction.[21, 22] The exposure of animal pole cells of the *Xenopus* embryo to

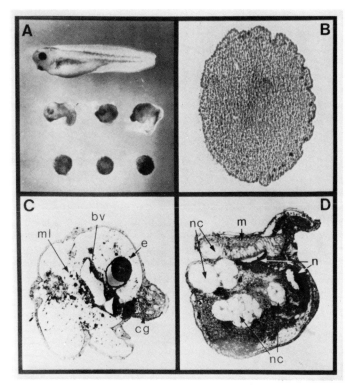

FIGURE 114–2. **Activin induces anterior and dorsal tissues.** *A,* Upper: Normal tadpole. Middle: Two-day-old animal caps treated with activin A. Note the presence of a small head with eyes and cement gland and rudimentary anteroposterior polarity. Lower: Untreated control animal caps that form balls of ciliated epidermis. *B* through *D,* Histological sections of an untreated two-day-old animal cap (*B*) and those treated with activin A (*C* and *D*). Note the presence of an eye (e), melocytes (ml), notochord (nc), neural tissue (n), muscle (m), cement gland (cg), and cavity resembling brain ventricle (bv). Animal caps were cut from stage 8 blastulae and exposed to 50 pM porcine activin A as described in experimental procedures. (From Thomsen G, et al: Activins are expressed early in *Xenopus* embryogenesis and can induce axial mesoderm and anterior structures. Cell 63:486, 1990, © 1990 Cell Press.)

activin A or activin B leads to the formation of a miniature embryo, complete with head and rudimentary trunk (as shown in Fig. 114–2). Activin B is transcribed very early in embryonic development, at the blastula stage, several hours before activin A.[21] Related studies in the chick embryo have shown that activins can induce the formation of organized axial structures from epiblasts and that activin B is expressed in the hypoblast, which normally induces axial differentiation in the epiblast.[22] Other diverse effects of activin include the stimulation of insulin secretion by rat pancreatic islets and of glucose production in isolated rat adipocytes. The effects on pituitary cells other than gonadotrophs have included reduction in growth hormone–releasing factor–mediated growth hormone release and thyrotropin-releasing hormone–mediated prolactin release, together with inhibition of somatotroph growth and growth hormone biosynthesis and secretion (reviewed in ref. 10).

Follistatin

An FSP with properties similar to those of inhibin has been isolated from both bovine and porcine follicular fluids.[13, 14] It is a single-chain protein that ranges in molec-

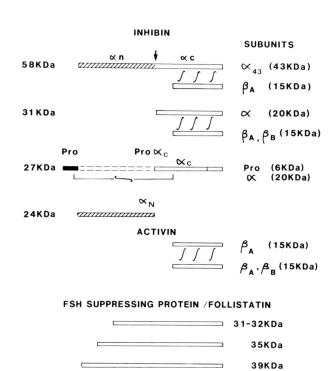

FIGURE 114–1. Schema of the structures of inhibin, the α subunit containing peptide Pro-αC, αN, activin, and FSH-suppressing protein, or follistatin. Note that 31-kDa inhibin is derived from the 58-kDa form by proteolytic cleavage of αN from the α_{43} subunit.

ular mass from 31 to 45 kDa, has no sequence homology with the α or β subunits of inhibin, but has 5 to 33 per cent of inhibin's potency in suppressing pituitary FSH in vitro. Molecular cloning and sequence analysis of follistatin cDNA's from porcine, ovine, murine, and human species indicate that it is coded by a single gene with a high degree of conservation of primary structure. Two types of follistatin precursor are generated by alternative splicing, FS 344 and FS 317. The ultimate products are FS 300 and FS 288, with various forms resulting from varying degrees of glycosylation. It has been shown that recombinant human follistatin of 288 amino acids is similar to inhibin A in its in vitro FSH-suppressing properties and is more potent than inhibin A when administered in vivo.[23] Follistatin shares structural features with a human pancreatic trypsin inhibitor and with epidermal growth factor and has been demonstrated to be capable of binding activin.[24] It might thus act at the pituitary level by direct effects on FSH synthesis and/or release or by inhibiting the stimulatory effects of activin.

SITES OF PRODUCTION

Inhibin

The fact that circulating concentrations of inhibin, whether measured by bioassay or radioimmunoassay, fall to undetectable levels after gonadectomy and that inhibin is also undetectable in most normal postmenopausal women indicates that in females, the ovary is the major source of the circulating molecule.[25–27] The main source of inhibin during the follicular phase of the reproductive cycle is the granulosa cell. Inhibin biological and immunological activities were detected in media in which rat, bovine, porcine, or human granulosa cells had been cultured.[28–31] Using antibodies generated against either 32-kDa inhibin or the inhibin α subunit, immunoreactivity was localized in ovarian granulosa cells in various species, including the human.[32] The mRNA's for α, β_A, and β_B subunits were detectable in rat granulosa cells by in situ hybridization[33, 34] and have also been demonstrated in bovine and primate ovaries, although β_B subunit mRNA is not present in the bovine ovary. Weak β_B subunit immunoreactivity was detectable in the granulosa cells of some primary follicles in midgestation human fetal ovaries, but all three subunits were demonstrable in the granulosa cells of primary and secondary follicles late in gestation in the rhesus monkey fetal ovary.[35] In the adult human ovary, preantral and early antral follicular granulosa cells showed positive immunostaining for β_A and β_B subunits, whereas medium-sized healthy antral follicles and preovulatory follicles were positive for α, β_A, and β_B.[36]

In primates the corpus luteum is also a site of inhibin production. Tsonis et al.[37] demonstrated the production of inhibin in vitro by luteinized human granulosa cells, and cells from isolated human corpora lutea were shown to be capable of producing inhibin in vitro under basal conditions, responding to human chorionic gonadotropin (hCG) with an increase in inhibin production when isolated from the early to mid luteal phase corpus luteum.[38] The subunit genes for inhibin α and β_A subunits were demonstrable in the human and the monkey corpus luteum.[39, 40] Immunocytochemical studies with α subunit antiserum have shown localization in human luteal cells.[41] In contrast to the situation in the human and primate, there is substantial evidence that the corpus luteum of the cow and sheep does not produce inhibin α or β_A subunits; the situation in the rat remains uncertain, with some groups demonstrating inhibin α subunit gene expression.

Inhibin subunit mRNA's have also been demonstrated in the placenta[42] and the decidua[43] as well as in both fetal and adult adrenals.[44] Inhibin α mRNA is present in extracts of early pregnancy placenta and is much more abundant than β_A mRNA, with β_B mRNA being detected at low levels only in term placenta.[45] Inhibin α subunit was demonstrable in the cytotrophoblast and β_B, in the syncytial layer of the villi; β_A was widely distributed. A discussion of the testicular production of inhibin and its subunits is beyond the scope of this chapter. In brief there is evidence for the production of inhibin, particularly by the Sertoli cells of the testis[46] but also by the interstitial cells.[47]

Recent evidence indicates that the pituitary is another potential site of inhibin production. In the rat, gonadotrophs have been shown to contain immunoreactive inhibin α and β_B subunits and their mRNA's.[48] In male monkeys inhibin-like immunoreactivity was noted in clusters of chromophobe cells, frequently lying close to gonadotrophs,[49] suggesting a possible paracrine role for inhibin in the regulation of gonadotropin production. It has, however, not been possible to detect inhibin bioactivity or immunoreactivity in culture medium from cultured rat anterior pituitary cells, and the incubation of such cells in medium that contains anti-inhibin antiserum does not alter basal FSH secretion. Thus the possible role of any inhibin that might be secreted by pituitary cells remains unclear. That activin, locally produced in the pituitary, may have a role in the regulation of FSH secretion is suggested by the report that the administration of an anti–activin B monoclonal antibody dose dependently suppressed serum FSH 12 hours after removal of the ovaries in hypophysectomized rats bearing renal pituitary allografts.[50] Similarly, the administration of this antibody on the evening of proestrus attenuated the serum FSH rise that normally occurs early on the day of estrus in rats.

Activin

Little progress has been made in the development of specific assays for activin,[19, 51] and the major conclusions regarding its sites of production are based on immunohistochemical and in situ hybridization evidence. Activin activity has been isolated from porcine and bovine follicular fluids,[11, 12, 19] and in the rat the highest activin A immunoreactivity has been found in the ovary.[51] It is not known whether activin circulates and how the circulating concentrations are regulated.

The demonstration of inhibin β subunits in the absence of demonstrable α subunit has been taken as implicit evidence for the production of activin rather than inhibin. Small antral follicular granulosa cells express β_B inhibin mRNA, as demonstrated by in situ hybridization in the monkey ovary,[40] and weak β_B subunit immunoreactivity has also been detected in granulosa cells in midgestation human fetal ovaries.[35] Both β_A and β_B, but not α, were demonstrable in preantral granulosa cells in women.[36] The demonstration of activin A and activin B in the embryo has been referred to above. β Subunit has also been demonstrated immunohistochemically in a cell group centered in the nucleus of the solitary tract with a fiber distribution consistent with known projections of that tract, involving particularly the regulation of oxytocin secretion.[52] Several forms of activin receptor have been expression-cloned from AtT20 mouse corticotropic cells, and the binding of ^{125}I activin A to Cos cell transfections can be completed by activin A, activin B, and inhibin A.[53]

Follistatin

Various tissues express the follistatin gene, with Northern analyses indicating that the ovary contains the most abundant mRNA.[54, 55] Using the techniques of in situ hybridization and immunohistochemistry, it has been demonstrated that follistatin mRNA and protein are present in granulosa and luteal cells but not in other ovarian cell types.[56] mRNA and protein production by granulosa cells are regulated by gonadotropin, specifically FSH, in the immature rat ovary, with FSH stimulation being inhibited by epidermal growth factor.[54, 57] Various other tissues have been shown to contain follistatin mRNA,[55] including the pituitary gonadotroph, where it may be involved in the local regulation of activin action.[50, 58]

ASSAYS

Inhibin

Bioassays

Although the original bioassays for inhibin were based on its administration to intact or castrate animals, all recent advances, particularly the progress in the isolation and characterization of inhibin, have been based on in vitro bioassays, using dispersed cultured rat anterior pituitary cells and measuring basal FSH release, cell content, or gonadotropin-releasing hormone (GnRH)-stimulated release.[5] Control of specificity has been achieved by attention to indices of cellular toxicity and/or the simultaneous measurement of luteinizing hormone (LH), which is little affected by inhibin in the dose range that produces FSH suppression.[5] Bioassays using dispersed ovine pituitary cells have been of sufficient sensitivity for application to physiological studies of inhibin regulation.[59] These bioassays have a place in the validation of newly developed radioimmunoassay systems and were crucial in the identification of substances such as activin and follistatin. In vivo bioassays based on suppression of circulating FSH levels in castrate or intact rats and sheep have been of value in the characterization of inhibin and related molecules, synthesized by recombinant techniques.[60–62]

Radioimmunoassays

A number of radioimmunoassays for human inhibin have been developed, the majority being based on the strong immunological cross-reactivity that is observed between bovine or porcine and human inhibin.[27, 63, 64, 64a] In initial studies these assays appeared to be highly specific because there was negligible cross-reactivity with a wide range of potentially related peptides. The α subunit precursor, pro-αC, which has been isolated from follicular fluid,[17, 18] together with other α subunit–related peptides that are present in peripheral blood,[65] has shown significant cross-reactivity in the assay, casting doubt on the specificity of measurements reported to date. It has, however, been shown that biological inhibin activity corresponds with immunological inhibin activity during the follicular phase of the human menstrual cycle,[66] and it thus appears probable that measurements made under such circumstances, in the absence of the corpus luteum, are representative of the concentrations of biologically active inhibin dimer. The major findings with respect to inhibin physiology in humans, using such radioimmunoassays, are in accord with a physiological role for inhibin as a component of the closed-loop feedback regulating system involved in the control of FSH secretion.[10] It seems probable that during the luteal phase of the menstrual cycle, when immunoreactive inhibin concentrations are at their peak, α subunit peptides may also be measured, since the ratio of biological to immunological activity is only about half of that seen during the follicular phase.[66] Alternative explanations would include the presence of activin or follistatin, which would modify biological as compared with immunological inhibin activity, since activin and follistatin do not cross-react in the radioimmunoassay. Although the assay appears to represent biologically active inhibin in the follicular phase of the cycle and in the absence of a corpus luteum, the situation is far more complex in men. A detailed discussion is beyond the scope of this chapter, but it is clear that in men, for instance, immunoreactive inhibin levels are normal or even elevated in patients with severe seminiferous tubule damage, including men with Klinefelter's syndrome.[67] No evidence has been found for the postulated inverse relation between immunoreactive inhibin and serum FSH in men with testicular disorders, despite the initial observation that bioassayable inhibin in seminal plasma was inversely related to serum FSH.[68] There is a clear need for the development of new assays that will measure specifically the inhibin dimer without measuring cross-reacting α subunit–related peptides. Two reports of immunoradiometric assays[69, 70] give evidence of some progress in this direction, although no detailed studies of inhibin physiology in humans have been reported with them. A potential problem in the application of such assays, with both serum and follicular fluid, is the demonstration of circulating and follicular fluid binding proteins, such as α_2-macroglobulin and follistatin (so far presented only in abstract form).[71, 72]

Activin

Some progress has been made toward the establishment of an activin radioimmunoassay,[19, 51] but its presence in the circulation in humans has not been reported. The bioassay on which the isolation of activin was based has been referred to. The major difficulty encountered in the establishment of an activin immunoassay applicable to serum is potential interference caused by circulating binding proteins, particularly follistatin,[71, 72] as well as the high probability of cross-reactivity with the β subunit of the inhibin dimer, which may be present in substantially higher concentrations than activin.

Follistatin

Follistatin was recognized and isolated on the basis of its biological activity in dispersed cultured rat anterior pituitary cells. Two specific radioimmunoassays[15, 16] and an affinity gel assay[73] have been developed, and some studies of its production in vivo and in vitro have been reported. Follistatin is secreted by cultured rat[73] and bovine[16] granulosa cells, whereas cultured theca interna tissue does not produce the hormone.[16] One report of follistatin measurements in women has indicated a two-fold increase in its levels after ovarian hyperstimulation with gonadotropins.[15] There was a direct positive relation between follistatin and estradiol levels. Corresponding data have been obtained in vitro in the bovine, in which FSH stimulates granulosa cell follistatin secretion.[16]

PHYSIOLOGY

With the exception of the report of follistatin stimulation by gonadotropins in women undergoing ovarian hyperstimulation,[15] there are no reports of the physiology of the gonadal regulatory peptides in women other than those concerning inhibin. Their role in other species with particular emphasis on their paracrine and autocrine roles has been reviewed.[74] A discussion of immunoreactive inhibin concentrations in the male is beyond the scope of this chapter; the reader is referred to Chapter 130 for more detail.

Fetus

Although it has been demonstrated that the fetal gonad in the sheep secretes immunoassayable inhibin when FSH is administered in a pulsatile manner,[75] and that porcine follicular fluid treated with charcoal leads to decreased circulating FSH but not LH levels in ovine fetuses,[76] there are no data regarding the secretion of inhibin or activin by the human or primate fetal gonad. Rabinovici et al.[35] showed weak immunostaining for the β_A subunit in some of the follicles that had formed at midgestation (16 to 23 weeks) but were unable to demonstrate α or β_B subunit staining. In late-gestation fetal rhesus monkey ovaries, granulosa cells surrounding oocytes showed positive immunostaining for all three inhibin subunits. Inhibin levels were undetectable in media from cultures of midgestation human ovaries, and no studies were reported on rhesus monkey fetal ovary cultures. In the fetal bovine ovary both inhibin bioactivity and immunoactivity have been detected, as has follistatin.[77]

Early Postnatal Period

Immunoreactive inhibin may participate in the regulation of the pituitary gonadal axis during the period of activation that occurs in the first few months of life in both sexes.[78] In a study of girls aged two months to two years, inhibin levels were found to be in the low follicular phase range of adults in the youngest girls, with FSH levels elevated at times into the postmenopausal range and LH in the early follicular phase range. Estradiol was in the mid-follicular range in the youngest girls studied, but beyond age one year all four hormones were at extremely low concentrations. In contrast, in boys of a similar age FSH levels were around the lower limit of adult values, whereas inhibin levels were in the adult midrange. Inhibin might in part contribute to the differing FSH levels seen in young girls and young boys, with the higher inhibin levels of the latter playing a role in maintaining substantially lower FSH levels than in girls. Similar observations were made in the postnatal male rhesus monkey,[79] but no data are available for very young female monkeys.

Puberty

Serum immunoreactive inhibin concentrations in girls were low before the onset of puberty and rose in parallel with levels of FSH, LH, and estradiol.[80] The values were lower than those seen in boys at equivalent stages. A wide range of values was seen at different stages of puberty, but the increase in mean concentrations with increasing maturation was highly significant. The only report of inhibin levels during disturbances of pubertal development describes concentrations in children treated with cytotoxic therapy for childhood leukemia.[81] Such children undergo puberty at a significantly earlier age than normal, and in these patients there was a relatively high frequency of undetectable inhibin concentrations, presumably reflecting the ovarian damage caused by chemotherapy.

Menstrual Cycle

The initial report of immunoreactive serum inhibin levels throughout the menstrual cycle was in 1987,[63] when it was shown that levels remained relatively constant throughout most of the follicular phase, rose immediately before the midcycle gonadotropin surge, fell transiently, and rose again to reach their highest levels during the midluteal phase. These findings have been confirmed and expanded in subsequent reports (Fig. 114–3).[82–84] A detailed study of the hormonal relations, particularly around midcycle,[83] showed that although estradiol levels began to fall 18 hours before the LH peak, inhibin continued to rise, peaking 6 hours before the LH peak (Fig. 114–4). Inhibin levels were positively correlated with those of LH and FSH for 24 hours before and after the LH peak, respectively. Estradiol was negatively correlated with the gonadotropins and inhibin from 24 hours before the LH peak until the peak itself. From 24 hours before the peak until the peak itself and from 48 to 60 hours afterward inhibin was correlated positively with progesterone, but there was an inverse correlation for the first 48 hours after the peak. It thus appears that the maturing follicle secretes inhibin and estradiol in parallel until 18 hours before the midcycle LH surge, when luteinization is initiated. Estradiol falls but inhibin continues to rise, indicating that there is differential regulation

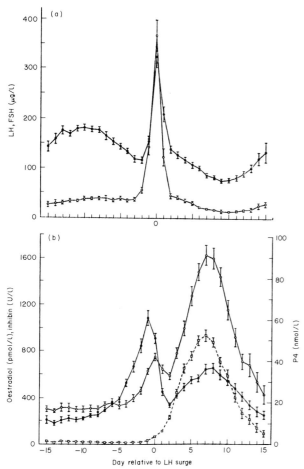

FIGURE 114-3. Daily mean (± SEM) serum levels of (a) LH (○), FSH (●), (b) inhibin (○), estradiol (●), and progesterone (□) during the menstrual cycle are shown for 33 normal women. Data have been normalized around the day of the LH surge (day 0). (From McLachlan RI, et al: Serum inhibin levels during the periovulatory interval in normal women: Relationships with sex steroid and gonadotrophin levels. Clin Endocrinol 32:43, 1990.)

strongly suggest that the corpus luteum is the major source. Both α and β subunit gene expression together with bioactive and immunoreactive inhibin have been demonstrated in the corpus luteum.[39] Immunocytochemical localization of α, β_A, and β_B subunits has been demonstrated in this tissue,[41, 87] and luteectomy in the cynomolgus monkey during the midluteal phase results in a major fall in serum inhibin levels.[88] Whether the fall in immunoreactive inhibin that occurs late in the luteal phase is important in the reciprocal rise of FSH in particular remains unclear, since FSH levels are also clearly inversely related to estradiol and progesterone at that time.[89]

Different regulatory mechanisms appear to be involved in the control of inhibin secretion during the follicular and luteal phases. During the follicular phase, inhibin appears to be predominantly under FSH control. Urinary gonadotropin preparations that contain both FSH and LH given for the purpose of ovarian hyperstimulation[90] or biologically purified FSH given to women with polycystic ovarian disease undergoing ovulation induction[91] leads to rises in circulating immunoreactive inhibin and estradiol. A dose-response relation between serum immunoreactive in-

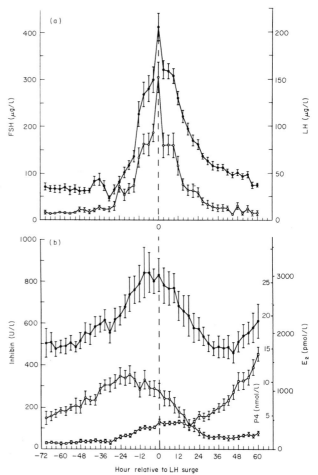

FIGURE 114-4. Mean (± SEM) serum levels of (a) LH (○), FSH (●), (b) inhibin (●), estradiol (○), and progesterone (□) between −69 hours and +60 hours relative to the peak LH value are shown for the seven normal women who had blood samples drawn every 3 hours around midcycle (each point consists of data from at least six women). (From McLachlan RI, et al: Serum inhibin levels during the periovulatory interval in normal women: Relationships with sex steroid and gonadotrophin levels. Clin Endocrinol 32:44, 1990.)

of the secretion of the two hormones from the maturing follicle. Because of the close correlation between inhibin and gonadotropin levels at midcycle, it appears that the latter may stimulate inhibin at that time, with any negative feedback effects of inhibin on FSH being overcome. During the middle to late follicular phase, inhibin is inversely related to serum FSH as measured by radioimmunoassay, although no correlation was seen with biologically active FSH.[82] Plasma estradiol was negatively correlated with bioactive FSH during the late follicular phase, suggesting that estradiol may be more important than inhibin in FSH regulation at that time. During the luteal phase, inhibin is correlated positively with serum progesterone and inversely with FSH.[63] Although it seemed likely that the dominant follicle was the source of follicular phase inhibin secretion, a recent study failed to show any difference in ovarian vein inhibin levels between the ovary containing the dominant follicle and that on the contralateral side,[85] despite the fact that follicular fluid inhibin bioactivity was related to the degree of follicular maturity.[86] It is possible that inhibin has an important ovarian paracrine role during the follicular phase.

The pattern of immunoreactive inhibin secretion during the luteal phase and its parallelism with progesterone hibin and 100 and 200 units of FSH given as single injections in the early follicular phase of the menstrual cycle was demonstrated recently.[91a] During the luteal phase, LH appears to be the major regulatory gonadotropin. Human granulosa lutein cells in long-term culture responded to LH and testosterone with increased inhibin production,[37] and a GnRH antagonist given to normal women in the midluteal phase caused a fall in circulating inhibin levels that could be prevented or reversed by hCG but not FSH administration.[92] Confirmatory evidence has been obtained in the luteal phase of the macaque monkey treated with a GnRH antagonist, with hCG but not FSH reversing the inhibitory effects of the antagonist on inhibin levels.[93] The possible role of inhibin in the phenomenon of twinning has been examined in one study,[94] in which elevated early follicular phase levels of FSH and LH were accompanied by raised inhibin concentrations, suggesting a hypothalamic-pituitary cause for the increased gonadotropin concentrations.

Pregnancy and Lactation

The circulating levels of both bioactive and immunoreactive inhibin rise throughout normal pregnancy,[95–97] an early rise being originally noted in the studies of McLachlan et al.,[98] who observed parallel increasing concentrations of inhibin and hCG in women who became pregnant after embryo transfer in an in vitro fertilization program. Levels rose from the midluteal phase to peak at about week 11 of gestation, with a subsequent decline to a plateau from 14 to 25 weeks and a further slow rise to peak concentrations at 41 weeks, the levels then being up to four times those of the midluteal phase. The levels subsequently fell in a biexponential manner after delivery.[99] A rise in inhibin was noted relatively early in pregnancy in women without endogenous ovarian function,[100] suggesting that the ovary was not essential to the early inhibin rise of pregnancy. The rise in such women was quantitatively less than that observed in women with intact ovarian function,[97] and one report has suggested that women who lack a corpus luteum do not appear to secret inhibin until at least eight weeks of gestation, indicating that a luteal source of immunoreactive inhibin is normal early in pregnancy.[101] In that study detectable and similar immunoreactive concentrations were found in women without corpora lutea at two to three weeks and four to six weeks of pregnancy, lower than those in normals. Placental content of both bioactive and immunoreactive inhibin has been reported, with hCG having been shown capable of stimulating inhibin secretion from cultured placental cells.[102] Physiological doses of hCG given to normal women during the midluteal phase result in increases of both progesterone and inhibin, compatible with the corpus luteum as a significant source of inhibin early in pregnancy.[103] Another possible source of inhibin during pregnancy is the decidua, as α, β_A, and β_B inhibin subunits have been demonstrated in decidual tissue.[43] Unpublished observations (Burger HG, 1992) indicate that inhibin levels remain low throughout lactational amenorrhea and rise at the time of re-initiation of ovarian activity.

Reproductive Aging and the Menopausal Transition

Studies have shown that serum FSH levels increase in women over age 40 who continue to have regular menstrual cycles.[104, 105] Lenton et al.[106] found a significant increase in serum FSH in a group of women aged 40 to 41 with a further gradual rise throughout their 40's. LH became significantly elevated in the 48-to-49-year age group. When related to the time of the menopause, the increase in FSH was seen five to six years earlier, whereas the LH increase occurred three to four years earlier. This group further reported that follicular phase inhibin concentrations in cycles from older women (mean age 44.2 years) were lower than those of younger women (mean age 27.4 years) in cycles in which pregnancy did not occur but were similar to those of a group of mean age 29.7, sampled during a conception cycle.[84] When estradiol and progesterone levels were measured as a function of increasing age, no change was seen.[105] In a cross-sectional study of 37 women aged 20 to 49 years sampled in the early follicular phase of their regular menstrual cycles, mean follicular phase levels of inhibin were significantly lower in the 45-to-49-year age group than in all younger age groups, with FSH levels being significantly elevated.[107] Serum inhibin and FSH were negatively correlated, as were estradiol and FSH. A significant negative relation was found between inhibin and age, with inhibin showing a steady decline with increasing age at a rate of 49.3 units/L for every 10-year increase in age across the population studied. FSH levels appeared to be constant up to age 43 and then rose progressively, whereas estradiol levels were constant until age 38 and then fell progressively. It thus appears probable that decreasing levels of both estradiol and inhibin may contribute to the increasing concentrations of FSH seen as a function of reproductive aging, although the question of whether estradiol levels change with increasing reproductive age remains controversial. There is some evidence for differential secretion of inhibin and estradiol by the aging granulosa cell. Although parallel changes in estradiol and inhibin were observed during ovarian hyperstimulation for the purposes of in vitro fertilization,[64, 90] an age-related reduction in inhibin but not in estradiol response in women over age 35 was noted.[108] Serum inhibin may provide a sensitive and early index of declining ovarian function with advancing age. Further data in support of this concept have come from a study of women with "incipient" ovarian failure, presenting for the investigation of infertility but having regular menstrual cycles. In these subjects early follicular phase FSH levels were elevated, whereas serum inhibin levels were lower than normal with estradiol being in the normal range.[109] After the menopause, inhibin levels usually are undetectable by the currently available immunoassays.

CLINICAL USES OF INHIBIN ASSAYS

The relatively recent development of inhibin radioimmunoassays, their restricted availability, and the doubts about assay specificity have limited the widespread applicability of the assays to clinical problems. The major area of diagnostic promise is in the monitoring of patients with

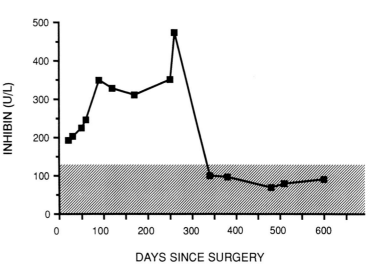

FIGURE 114–5. Serum inhibin concentrations in an 80-year-old patient with stage 2 granulosa cell tumor of the right ovary. Despite apparent clinical remission, serum inhibin levels rose steadily for nine months after cytoreductive surgery. Second-look laparotomy 272 days after primary surgery confirmed residual granulosa cell tumor, which was successfully removed, after which the patient remained clinically disease-free. The serum inhibin range seen in functionally agonadal postmenopausal women is shown as a shaded band.

stromal and epithelial tumors of the ovary. An initial report indicated that circulating inhibin concentrations were markedly elevated in patients with granulosa cell tumor of the ovary[110] (Fig. 114–5), and that at least in some patients rising inhibin levels were observed up to 20 months before clinical evidence of tumor recurrence was obtained. Inhibin assays are clearly of greatest value in patients who have previously undergone bilateral oophorectomy or in those who are postmenopausal, both situations in which endogenous inhibin levels are expected to be undetectable. Observations from my laboratory also indicate that serum inhibin concentrations are elevated in most postmenopausal women with mucinous cystadenocarcinoma of the ovary and in about 15 per cent of patients with nonmucinous epithelial cancers. Successful surgical removal of such tumors leads to a rapid fall in serum inhibin to nonsignificant levels by one week postoperatively (unpublished observations, 1992–3). In postmenopausal women with proven ovarian cancer, serum inhibin is inversely correlated with FSH and positively correlated with estradiol and progesterone, particularly in those with granulosa cell tumors. In women with mucinous tumors the inverse correlation with FSH is lost, one possible explanation for which is that mucinous tumors may secrete α subunit–related peptides.

One report indicates that inhibin levels may be of diagnostic value in patients with hydatidiform mole.[111] Levels were elevated in patients with this tumor and fell much more rapidly after evacuation than did the levels of the traditional marker, hCG. Failure to remove all diseased tissue led to a fall in inhibin but not into the normal range, whereas complete evacuation restored inhibin levels to normal.

Because inhibin is a product of the corpus luteum, it might be predicted that it could provide a useful marker of luteal insufficiency. Published reports to date are conflicting in this regard, with one group reporting that women with an inadequate luteal phase had lowered serum inhibin concentrations during that time,[112] whereas another group reported that women with luteal phases of normal length but markedly decreased progesterone concentrations had normal concentrations of inhibin and estradiol.[84]

The normal pattern of inhibin secretion has been established during pregnancy, and there is a recent preliminary report about its diagnostic use in suspected abnormalities.[113]

The observation that inhibin levels rise in parallel with estradiol during ovarian hyperstimulation makes it possible in theory to use inhibin measurements as an alternative to estradiol in the assessment of the ovarian response.[64, 90] No prognostic significance for circulating inhibin concentrations has been demonstrated.[108] It is clearly important that assays specific for the inhibin dimer as well as assays for activin be developed to allow exploration of the full diagnostic potential of the inhibin assay.

REFERENCES

1. McCullagh DR: Dual endocrine activity of the testis. Science 76:19–20, 1932.
2. Robertson DM, Foulds LM, Leversha L, et al: Isolation of inhibin from bovine follicular fluid. Biochem Biophys Res Commun 126:220–226, 1985.
3. de Jong FH, Sharpe RM: Evidence for inhibin-like activity in bovine follicular fluid. Nature 263:71–72, 1976.
4. Keogh EJ, Lee VWK, Rennie GC, et al: Selective suppression of FSH by testicular extracts. Endocrinology 98:997–1002, 1976.
5. McLachlan RI, Robertson DM, de Kretser DM, Burger HG: Advances in the physiology of inhibin and inhibin-related peptides. Clin Endocrinol 29:77–114, 1988.
6. de Jong FH: Inhibin. Physiol Rev 68:555–607, 1988.
7. Ying SY: Inhibins, activins and follistatins: Gonadal proteins modulating the secretion of follicle-stimulating hormone. Endocr Rev 9:267–293, 1988.
8. Vale W, Rivier C, Hsueh A, et al: Chemical and biological characterization of the inhibin family of protein hormones. Recent Prog Horm Res 44:1–34, 1988.
9. de Kretser DM, Robertson DM: The isolation and physiology of inhibin and related proteins. Biol Reprod 40:33–47, 1989.
10. Burger HG: Inhibin. Reprod Med Rev 1:1–20, 1992.
11. Ling N, Ying SY, Ueno N, et al: Pituitary FSH is released by a heterodimer of the subunits of the two forms of inhibin. Nature 321:779–782, 1986.
12. Vale W, Rivier J, Vaughan J, et al: Purification and characterization of an FSH releasing protein from porcine follicular fluid. Nature 321:776–779, 1986.
13. Robertson DM, Klein R, de Vos FL, et al: The isolation of polypeptides with FSH suppressing activity from bovine follicular fluid which are structurally different from inhibin. Biochem Biophys Res Commun 149:744–749, 1987.
14. Ueno N, Ling N, Ying SY, et al: Isolation and partial characterization of follistatin: A single chain Mr 35000 monomeric protein that inhibits the release of follicle stimulating hormone. Proc Natl Acad Sci USA 84:8282–8286, 1987.

15. Sugawara S, DePaolo L, Nakatani A, et al: Radioimmunoassay of follistatin: Application for *in vitro* fertilization procedures. J Clin Endocrinol Metab 71:1672–1674, 1990.

16. Klein R, Robertson DM, Shukovski L, et al: The radioimmunoassay of follicle stimulating hormone (FSH)-suppressing protein (FSP); stimulation of bovine granulosa cell FSP secretion by FSH. Endocrinology 128:1048–1056, 1991.

16a. Klein R, Findlay JK, Clarke IJ, et al: Radioimmunoassay of FSH-suppressing protein in the ewe:concentrations during the oestrous cycle and following ovariectomy. J Endocrinol 137:433–443, 1993.

17. Robertson DM, Giacometti M, Foulds LM, et al: Isolation of inhibin α-subunit precursor proteins from bovine follicular fluid. Endocrinology 125:2141–2149, 1989.

18. Sugino K, Nakamura T, Takio N, et al: Inhibin α-subunit monomer is present in follicular fluid. Biochem Biophys Res Commun 159:1323–1329, 1989.

19. Robertson DM, Foulds LM, Prisk M, Hedger MP: Inhibin/activin β subunit monomer: Isolation and characterisation. Endocrinology 130:1680–1687, 1992.

19a. Nakamura T, Asashima M, Eto Y, et al: Isolation and characterization of native activin B. J Biol Chem 267:16385–16389, 1992.

20. Eto Y, Takazawa M, Takano S, et al: Purification and characterization of erythroid differentiation factor (EDF) isolated from human leukemia cell line THP-1. Biochem Biophys Res Commun 142:1095–1103, 1987.

21. Thomsen G, Woolf T, Whitman M, et al: Activins are expressed early in *Xenopus* embryogenesis and can induce axial mesoderm and anterior structures. Cell 63:485–493, 1990.

22. Mitrani E, Ziv T, Thomsen G, et al: Activin can induce the formation of axial structures and is expressed in the hypoblast of the chick. Cell 63:495–501, 1990.

23. Inouye S, Guo Y, DePaolo L, et al: Recombinant expression of human follistatin with 315 and 288 amino acids: Chemical and biological comparison with native porcine follistatin. Endocrinology 129:815–822, 1991.

24. Nakamura T, Takio K, Eto Y, et al: Activin-binding protein from rat ovary is follistatin. Science 247:836–838, 1989.

25. Lee VWK, McMaster J, Quigg H, Leversha L: Ovarian and circulating inhibin levels in immature female rats treated with gonadotropin and after castration. Endocrinology 111:1849–1854, 1982.

26. Robertson DM, Hayward S, Irby D, et al: Radioimmunoassay of rat serum inhibin: Changes after PMSG stimulation and gonadectomy. Mol Cell Endocrinol 58:1–8, 1988.

27. McLachlan RI, Robertson DM, Burger HG, de Kretser DM: The radioimmunoassay of bovine and human follicular fluid and serum inhibin. Mol Cell Endocrinol 46:175–185, 1986.

28. Erickson GF, Hsueh AJW: Secretion of "inhibin" by rat granulosa cells in vitro. Endocrinology 103:1960–1961, 1978.

29. Henderson KM, Franchimont P: Inhibin production by bovine ovarian tissues in vitro and its regulation by androgens. J Reprod Fertil 67:291–298, 1983.

30. Channing CP, Hoover DJ, Anderson LD, Tanabe K: Control of follicular secretion of inhibin *in vitro* and *in vivo*. Adv Biosci 34:41–55, 1982.

31. Channing CP, Tanabe K, Chacon M, Tildon JT: Stimulatory effects of follicle-stimulating hormone and luteinizing hormone upon secretion of progesterone and estradiol activity by cultured infant human ovarian granulosa cells. Fertil Steril 42:598–605, 1984.

32. Merchenthaler I, Culler MD, Petrusz P, Negro-Vilar A: Immunocytochemical localization of inhibin in rat and human reproductive tissues. Mol Cell Endocrinol 54:239–243, 1987.

33. Meunier H, Rivier C, Evans RM, Vale W: Gonadal and extragonadal expression of inhibin α, β_A and β_B subunits in various tissues predicts diverse functions. Proc Natl Acad Sci USA 85:247–251, 1988.

34. Woodruff TK, D'Agostino J, Schwartz NB, Mayo KE: Dynamic changes in inhibin messenger RNAs in rat ovarian follicles during the reproductive cycle. Science 239:1296–1299, 1988.

35. Rabinovici J, Goldsmith PC, Roberts VJ, et al: Localization and secretion of inhibin/activin subunits in the human and subhuman primate fetal gonads. J Clin Endocrinol Metab 73:1141–1149, 1991.

36. Yamoto M, Minami S, Nakano R, Kobayashi M: Immunohistochemical localization of inhibin/activin subunits in human ovarian follicles during the menstrual cycle. J Clin Endocrinol Metab 74:989–993, 1992.

37. Tsonis CG, Hillier SG, Baird DT: Production of inhibin bioactivity by human granulosa-lutein cells; stimulation by LH and testosterone *in vitro*. J Endocrinol 112:R11–R14, 1987.

38. Wang H-Z, Lu S-H, Han X-J, et al: Control of inhibin production by dispersed human luteal cells in vitro. Reprod Fertil Dev 4:67–75, 1992.

39. Davis SR, Krozowski Z, McLachlan RI, Burger HG: Inhibin gene expression in the human corpus luteum. J Endocrinol 115:R21–R23, 1987.

40. Schwall RH, Mason AJ, Wilcox JN, et al: Localization of inhibin/activin subunit mRNAs within the primate ovary. Mol Endocrinol 4:75–79, 1990.

41. Smith KB, Millar MR, McNeilly AS, et al: Immunocytochemical localization of inhibin α-subunit in the human corpus luteum. J Endocrinol 129:155–160, 1991.

42. Mayo KE, Cerelli GM, Spiess J, et al: Inhibin-A subunit cDNAs from porcine ovary and human placenta. Proc Natl Acad Sci USA 83:5849–5853, 1986.

43. Petraglia F, Calza L, Garuti GC, et al: Presence and synthesis of inhibin subunits in human decidua. J Clin Endocrinol Metab 71:487–492, 1990.

44. Voutilainen R, Eramaa M, Ritvos O: Hormonally regulated inhibin gene expression in human fetal and adult adrenals. J Clin Endocrinol Metab 73:1026–1030, 1991.

45. Petraglia F, Garuti GC, Calza L, et al: Inhibin subunits in human placenta: Localization and messenger ribonucleic acid levels during pregnancy. Am J Obstet Gynecol 165:750–758, 1991.

46. Steinberger A, Steinberger E: Secretion of an FSH-inhibiting factor by cultured Sertoli cells. Endocrinology 99:918–921, 1976.

47. Risbridger G, Clements J, Robertson DM, et al: Imuno- and bioactive and inhibin α-subunit expression in rat Leydig cell cultures. Mol Cell Endocrinol 66:119–122, 1989.

48. Roberts V, Meunier H, Vaughan J, et al: Production and regulation of inhibin subunits in pituitary gonadotropes. Endocrinology 124:552–554, 1989.

49. Schlatt S, Weinbauer GF, Nieschlag E: Inhibin-like and gonadotropin-like immunoreactivity in pituitary cells of male monkeys (*Macaca fascicularis, Macaca mulatta*). Cell Tissue Res 265:203–209, 1991.

50. DePaolo LV, Bald LN, Fendly BM: Passive immunoneutralization with a monoclonal antibody reveals a role for endogenous activin-B in mediating FSH hypersecretion during estrus and following ovariectomy of hypophysectomized, pituitary-grafted rats. Endocrinology 130:1741–1743, 1992.

51. Shintani Y, Takada Y, Yamasaki R, Saito S: Radioimmunoassay for activin A/EDF: Method and measurement of immunoreactive activin A/EDF levels in various biological materials. J Immunol Methods 137:267–274, 1991.

52. Sawchenko PE, Plotsky PM, Pfeiffer SW, et al: Inhibin β in central neural pathways involved in the control of oxytocin secretion. Nature 334:615–617, 1988.

53. Matthews LS, Vale WW: Expression cloning of an activin receptor, a predicted transmembrane serine kinase. Cell 65:973–982, 1991.

54. Shimasaki S, Koga M, Buscaglia ML, et al: Follistatin gene expression in the ovary and extragonadal tissues. Mol Endocrinol 3:651–659, 1989.

55. Michel U, Albiston A, Findlay JK: Rat follistatin: Gonadal and extragonadal expression and evidence for alternative splicing. Biochem Biophys Res Commun 173:401–407, 1990.

56. Nakatani A, Shimasaki S, DePaolo LV, et al: Cyclic changes in follistatin messenger ribonucleic acid and its protein in the rat ovary during the estrous cycle. Endocrinology 129:603–611, 1991.

57. Michel U, McMaster JW, Findlay JK: Regulation of steady-state follistatin mRNA levels in rat granulosa cells *in vitro*. J Mol Endocrinol 9:147–156, 1992.

58. Kaiser UB, Lee BL, Carroll RS, et al: Follistatin gene expression in the pituitary: Localization in gonadotropes and folliculostellate cells in diestrous rats. Endocrinology 130:3048–3056, 1992.

59. Tsonis CG, McNeilly AS, Baird DT: Measurement of exogenous and endogenous inhibin in sheep serum using a new and extremely sensitive bioassay for inhibin based on inhibition of ovine pituitary FSH secretion *in vitro*. J Endocrinol 110:341–352, 1986.

60. Tierney ML, Goss NH, Tomkins SM, et al: Physiochemical and biological characterization of recombinant human inhibin A. Endocrinology 126:3268–3270, 1990.

61. DePaolo LV, Shimonaka M, Schwall RH, Ling N: *In vivo* comparison of the follicle-stimulating hormone-suppressing activity of follistatin and inhibin in ovariectomized rats. Endocrinology 128:668–674, 1991.

62. Rivier C, Schwall R, Mason A, et al: Effect of recombinant inhibin on luteinizing hormone and follicle-stimulating hormone secretion in the rat. Endocrinology 128:1548–1554, 1991.

63. McLachlan RI, Robertson DM, Healy DL, et al: Circulating immuno-

reactive inhibin levels during the normal human menstrual cycle. J Clin Endocrinol Metab 65:954–961, 1987.

64. Tsuchiya K, Hasegawa Y, Seki M, et al: Correlation of serum inhibin concentrations with results in an ovarian hyperstimulation program. Fertil Steril 52:88–94, 1989.

64a. Burger HG: Clinical review—clinical utility of inhibin measurements. J Clin Endocrinol Metab 76:1391–1396, 1993.

65. Schneyer AL, Mason AJ, Burton LE, et al: Immunoreactive inhibin α-subunit in human serum: Implications for radioimmunoassay. J Clin Endocrinol Metab 70:1208–1212, 1990.

66. Robertson DM, Tsonis CG, McLachlan RI: Comparison of inhibin immunological and in vitro biological activities in human serum. J Clin Endocrinol Metab 67:438–443, 1988.

67. de Kretser DM, McLachlan RI, Robertson DM, Burger HG: Serum inhibin levels in normal men and men with testicular disorders. J Endocrinol 120:517–523, 1989.

68. Scott RS, Burger HG: An inverse relationship exists between seminal plasma inhibin and serum FSH in man. J Clin Endocrinol Metab 52:796–803, 1981.

69. Knight PG, Groome N, Beard AJ: Development of a two-site immunoradiometric assay for dimeric inhibin using antibodies against chemically synthesized fragments of the α and β subunit. J Endocrinol 129:R9–R12, 1991.

70. Betteridge A, Craven RP: A two-site enzyme-linked immunosorbent assay for inhibin. Biol Reprod 45:748–754, 1991.

71. Schneyer AL, O'Neil DA, Crowley WF: Activin-binding proteins in human serum and follicular fluid. J Clin Endocrinol Metab 71:1320–1324, 1992.

72. Krummen LA, Woodruff TK, DeGuzman G: Identification and characterization of binding proteins for inhibin and activin in human serum and follicular fluids. Endocrinology 132:431–443, 1993.

73. Saito S, Nakamura T, Titani K, Sugino H: Production of activin-binding protein by rat granulosa cells in vitro. Biochem Biophys Res Commun 176:413–422, 1991.

74. Findlay JK, Xiao Sai, Shukovski L, Michel U: Novel peptides in ovarian physiology. In Adashi EY, Leung PCK (eds): The Ovary. New York, Raven Press, 1993, pp 413–432.

75. Albers N, Bettendorf M, Hart CS, et al: Hormone ontogeny in the ovine fetus. XXIII. Pulsatile administration of follicle-stimulating hormone stimulates inhibin production and decreases testosterone synthesis in the ovine fetal gonad. Endocrinology 124:3089–3094, 1989.

76. Albers N, Hart CS, Kaplan SL, Grumbach MM: Hormone ontogeny in the ovine fetus. XXIV. Porcine follicular fluid "inhibins" selectively suppress plasma follicle-stimulating hormone in the ovine fetus. Endocrinology 125:675–678, 1989.

77. Torney AH, Robertson DM, de Kretser DM: Characterization of inhibin and related proteins in bovine fetal testicular and ovarian extracts: Evidence for the presence of inhibin subunit products and FSH-suppressing protein. J Endocrinol 133:111–120, 1992.

78. Burger HG, Yamada Y, Bangah ML, et al: Serum gonadotropin, sex steroid and immunoreactive inhibin levels in the first two years of life. J Clin Endocrinol Metab 72:682–686, 1991.

79. Abeyawardene SA, Vale WW, Marshall GR, Plant TM: Circulating inhibin α concentrations in infant, prepubertal, and adult male rhesus monkeys (Macaca mulatta) and in juvenile males during premature initiation of puberty with pulsatile gonadotropin-releasing hormone treatment. Endocrinology 125:250–256, 1989.

80. Burger HG, McLachlan RI, Bangah ML, et al: Serum inhibin concentrations rise throughout normal male and female puberty. J Clin Endocrinol Metab 67:689–694, 1988.

81. Quigley C, Cowell C, Jimenez M, et al: Normal or early development of puberty despite gonadal damage in children treated for acute lymphoblastic leukemia. N Engl J Med 321:143–151, 1989.

82. Reddi K, Wickings EJ, McNeilly AS, et al: Circulating bioactive follicle stimulating hormone and immunoreactive inhibin levels during the normal human menstrual cycle. Clin Endocrinol 33:547–557, 1990.

83. McLachlan RI, Cohen NL, Dahl KD, et al: Serum inhibin levels during the periovulatory interval in normal women: Relationships with sex steroid and gonadotrophin levels. Clin Endocrinol 32:39–48, 1990.

84. Lenton LA, de Kretser DM, Woodward AJ, Robertson DM: Inhibin concentrations throughout the menstrual cycles of normal, infertile, and older women compared with those during spontaneous conception cycles. J Clin Endocrinol 73:1180–1190, 1991.

85. Illingworth PJ, Reddi K, Smith KB, Baird DT: The source of inhibin secretion during the human menstrual cycle. J Clin Endocrinol Metab 73:667–673, 1991.

86. Marrs RP, Lobo R, Campeau JD, et al: Correlation of human follicu-

87. Yamoto M, Minami S, Nakano R: Immunohistochemical localization of inhibin subunits in human corpora lutea during menstrual cycle and pregnancy. J Clin Endocrinol Metab 73:470–477, 1991.

88. Basseti SG, Winters SJ, Keeping HS, Zeleznik AJ: Serum immunoreactive inhibin levels before and after luteectomy in the cynomolgus monkey (Macaca fascicularis). J Clin Endocrinol Metab 70:590–594, 1990.

89. Roseff SJ, Bangah ML, Kettel LM: Dynamic changes in circulating inhibin levels during the luteal-follicular transition of the human menstrual cycle. J Clin Endocrinol Metab 69:1033–1039, 1989.

90. McLachlan RI, Robertson DM, Healy DL, et al: Plasma inhibin levels during gonadotrophin-induced ovarian hyperstimulation for IVF: A new index of follicular function? Lancet 1:1233–1234, 1986.

91. Buckler HM, Healy DL, Burger HG: Purified FSH stimulates inhibin production from the human ovary. J Endocrinol 122:279–285, 1989.

91a. Hee J, MacNaughton J, Bangah M, et al: FSH induces dose-dependent stimulation of immunoreactive inhibin secretion during the follicular phase of the human menstrual cycle. J Clin Endocrinol Metab 76:1340–1343, 1993.

92. McLachlan RI, Cohen NL, Vale WW, et al: The importance of LH in the control of inhibin and progesterone secretion by the human corpus luteum. J Clin Endocrinol Metab 68:1078–1085, 1989.

93. Smith KB, Fraser HM: Control of progesterone and inhibin secretion during the luteal phase in the macaque. J Endocrinol 128:107–113, 1991.

94. Martin NG, Robertson DM, Chenevix-Trench G, et al: Elevation of follicular phase inhibin and luteinizing hormone levels in mothers of dizygotic twins suggests nonovarian control of human multiple ovulation. Fertil Steril 56:469–474, 1991.

95. Qu J, Vankrieken L, Brulet C, Thomas K: Circulating bioactive inhibin levels during human pregnancy. J Clin Endocrinol Metab 72:862–866, 1991.

96. Abe Y, Hasegawa Y, Miyamoto K, et al: High concentrations of plasma immunoreactive inhibin during normal pregnancy in women. J Clin Endocrinol Metab 71:133–137, 1990.

97. Yohkaichiya T, Polson D, O'Connor A, et al: Concentrations of immunoactive inhibin in serum during human pregnancy: Evidence for an ovarian contribution. Reprod Fertil Dev 3:671–678, 1991.

98. McLachlan RI, Healy DL, Robertson DM, et al: Circulating immunoreactive inhibin in the luteal phase and early gestation of women undergoing ovulation induction. Fertil Steril 48:1001–1005, 1987.

99. Kettel LM, Roseff SJ, Bangah ML, et al: Circulating levels of inhibin in pregnant women at term: Simultaneous disappearance with estradiol and progesterone after delivery. Clin Endocrinol 34:19–23, 1991.

100. McLachlan RI, Healy DL, Lutjen PJ, et al: The maternal ovary is not the source of circulating inhibin levels during human pregnancy. Clin Endocrinol 27:663–668, 1987.

101. Santoro N, Schneyer AL, Ibrahim J, Schmidt CL: Gonadotropin and inhibin concentrations in early pregnancy in women with and without corpora lutea. Obstet Gynecol 79:579–585, 1992.

102. Petraglia F, Sawchenko P, Lim ATW, et al: Localization, secretion, and action of inhibin in human placenta. Science 237:187–189, 1987.

103. Illingworth PJ, Reddi K, Smith K, Baird DT: Pharmacological "rescue" of the corpus luteum results in increased inhibin production. Clin Endocrinol 33:323–332, 1990.

104. Sherman BM, West JH, Korenman SG: The menopausal transition: Analysis of LH, FSH, estradiol, and progesterone concentrations during menstrual cycles of older women. J Clin Endocrinol Metab 42:629–636, 1976.

105. Lee SJ, Lenton EA, Sexton L, Cooke ID: The effect of age on the cyclical patterns of plasma LH, FSH, oestradiol and progesterone in women with regular menstrual cycles. Hum Reprod 3:851–855, 1988.

106. Lenton EA, Sexton L, Lee S, Cooke ID: Progressive changes in LH and FSH and LH: FSH ratio in women throughout reproductive life. Maturitas 10:35–43, 1988.

107. MacNaughton J, Bangah M, McCloud P, et al: Age related changes in follicle stimulating hormone, luteinizing hormone, oestradiol and immunoreactive inhibin in women of reproductive age. Clin Endocrinol 36:339–345, 1992.

108. Hughes EG, Robertson DM, Handelsman DJ, et al: Inhibin and estradiol responses to ovarian hyperstimulation: Effects of age and predictive value for in vitro fertilization outcome. J Clin Endocrinol Metab 70:358–364, 1990.

109. Buckler HM, Evans CA, Mamtora H, et al: Gonadotropin, steroid

and inhibin levels in women with incipient ovarian failure during anovulatory and ovulatory rebound cycles. J Clin Endocrinol Metab 72:116–124, 1991.

110. Lappohn R, Burger H, Bouma J, et al: Inhibin as a marker for granulosa-cell tumors. N Engl J Med 321:790–793, 1989.

111. Yohkaichiya T, Fukaya T, Hoshiai H, et al: Inhibin a new circulating marker of hydatidiform mole. Br Med J 298:1684–1686, 1989.

112. Soules MR, McLachlan RI, Marit EK, et al: Luteal phase deficiency: Characterization of reproductive hormones over the menstrual cycle. J Clin Endocrinol Metab 69:804–812, 1989.

113. de Kretser DM, Yohkaichiya T, Healy DL, et al: Patterns of secretion of inhibin and related proteins during pregnancy and its disorders. Hormones in Gynaecological Endocrinology. *In* Genazzani AR, Petraglia F (eds): Carnforth, Parthenon Publishing Group, 1992, pp 261–267.

Ovarian Hormone Synthesis and Mechanism of Action

AARON J. W. HSUEH
HÅKAN BILLIG

The basic functional unit of the mammalian ovary is the follicle, each of which consists of an outer layer of theca interna cells that encircle inner layers of granulosa cells. Stratified granulosa cells in turn surround the innermost oocyte–cumulus cell complex. The maturation of these follicles, subsequent release of oocytes from the follicles, and the eventual transformation of follicles into corpora lutea are cyclic events controlled by a diversity of hormones. Pituitary gonadotropins, follicle-stimulating hormone (FSH) and luteinizing hormone (LH), stimulate follicular maturation and estrogen biosynthesis during the early part of the menstrual cycle. Hormonal interactions at the hypothalamic, pituitary, and ovarian levels lead to a pre-ovulatory elevation of serum estrogens that in turn trigger the ovulatory gonadotropin surge (see Ch. 17). After the climactic increases in serum gonadotropins, the dominant graafian follicle releases its mature oocyte and transforms into a LH-dependent corpus luteum. The luteal secretion of progesterone and estrogens during the second half of the menstrual cycle ensures adequate uterine development for implantation of fertilized eggs. In the absence of blastocyst implantation, the corpus luteum regresses and progesterone secretion declines before menses.

Ovarian steroid production depends on the de novo biosynthesis of cholesterol as well as the provision of serum cholesterol carried by circulating lipoproteins. In response to cyclic pituitary gonadotropin secretion, various follicular compartments interact in a highly integrated manner to convert cholesterol into steroids that are readily secreted. In addition, ovarian cells produce peptide hormones and other factors to regulate pituitary FSH release, oocyte maturation, steroidogenesis, and the ovulatory process.

Not all follicles in a given ovary respond to the pituitary hormones. At menarche in the human female about 400,000 oocytes are found within primordial follicles.[1] Most of these follicles never develop to preovulatory graafian follicles, and only around 400 "selected" follicles ovulate during the female life span. Most ovarian follicles undergo atresia, which is characterized by apoptotic cell death of follicle cells.[2, 3] The selection of the dominant follicles as well as the atresia of the remaining follicles is under the control of intra-ovarian hormones, such as gonadal steroids and peptides, as well as neurotransmitters.

Although the ovaries are the major site of estrogen biosynthesis, nonovarian production of these steroids by peripheral aromatization of adrenal androgens is also important. After secretion ovarian steroids are bound by serum-binding proteins and transported to target tissues that contain steroid hormone receptors. Interaction between steroids and their specific receptors results in the transformation of the receptor molecule, which is capable of binding to specific chromatin sites and initiates genomic events leading to the synthesis of new mRNA and proteins. The principal action of ovarian steroids is the stimulation of growth of the female reproductive organs, in particular the uterus, vagina, and mammary glands. The steroid-induced events are also responsible for the differentiation of secondary sex characteristics (pelvic enlargement and fat deposition), development of sexual behavior, nidation of fertilized ovum, maintenance of pregnancy, and feedback control of the hypothalamic-pituitary-ovarian axis.

BIOSYNTHESIS AND METABOLISM OF PROGESTINS, ANDROGENS, AND ESTROGENS

The general steps in the steroid biosynthetic pathway and the subcellular localization of the major steroid enzymes are similar in all steroid-producing glands, including the ovary, testis, placenta, and adrenal (Fig. 115–1). In the ovary the theca interna cells possess all the enzymes necessary for androgen biosynthesis, and the granulosa cells are capable of producing progestins and aromatizing androgens to estrogens. The luteal cells, which are derived from both granulosa and theca cells, contain enzymes necessary for both progestin and estrogen biosynthesis.

De Novo Cholesterol Synthesis and Role of Lipoproteins

In vitro studies using radioactive acetate as the precursor have demonstrated that the ovarian steroid-producing cells are capable of carrying out de novo synthesis of acetylcoenzyme A, leading to the formation of cholesterol (see Fig. 115–1, step B). The rate-limiting enzyme involved in cholesterol biosynthesis is the cytoplasmic 3-hydroxy-3-methylglutaryl coenzyme A reductase (HMG-CoA reductase), which catalyzes the formation of mevalonate from β-hydroxy-β-methylglutaryl CoA. The 6-carbon mevalonate is further converted to the 27-carbon cholesterol through phosphorylation, condensation of isomers, and cyclization. Cellular cholesterol is stored in the form of cholesterol ester in the lipid granules. After the activation of cholesterol esterase by gonadotropins, stored cholesterol can be mobilized (see Fig. 115–1, step D).[4]

Cellular cholesterol may also be derived from plasma lipoproteins (see Fig. 115–1, step A).[5] Lipoproteins are complex macromolecules that carry plasmid lipids, including cholesterol and its esters. Each lipoprotein particle consists of a lipid core surrounded by a protein coat composed of specific apoproteins. The lipoproteins are classified according to their lipid-protein ratio (densities). In humans a low-density lipoprotein (LDL) is the predominant form that provides cholesterol to steroidogenic tissues.

In organ culture of human corpus luteum, treatment with LDL enhances progesterone biosynthesis.[6] LDL particles bind to specific plasma membrane receptors and enter the cell by receptor-mediated endocytosis.[7] The internalized vesicles fuse with lysosomes; the protein component of LDL is then cleaved to amino acids, and the cholesterol ester component is hydrolyzed to free fatty acids and unesterified cholesterol. The rise in cellular unesterified cholesterol suppresses HMG-CoA reductase activities and activates the enzyme acyl CoA:cholesterol acyl transferase, which re-esterifies cholesterol (see Fig. 115–1, step C). The cholesterol esters are stored in lipid granules within the cells for steroid biosynthesis. Increases in cellular cholesterol content also lead to a suppression of the synthesis of plasma membrane LDL receptors, resulting in decreased LDL uptake.

Lipoprotein dependence varies with the stages of the menstrual cycle. Owing to its high molecular weight, only low concentrations of LDL are found in human follicular fluid.[8] Because granulosa cells in the avascular compartment of the follicle do not have ready access to LDL in the systemic circulation, de novo cholesterol biosynthesis is essential for steroidogenesis. After ovulation, extensive neovascularization of the follicles takes place, exposing the granulosa cells to circulating LDL. This increased access of LDL to the luteinized granulosa cells is correlated with substantial increases in progesterone biosynthesis during the luteal phase of the menstrual cycle. Furthermore, the number of LDL binding sites in the corpus luteum increases during the midluteal phase,[6] and treatment of cultured human granulosa–luteal cells with human chorionic gonadotropin (hCG) increases their LDL receptor mRNA content.[9] Genetic defects of the LDL receptor molecule and its internalization mechanism have been found in patients with altered lipoprotein metabolism.[10] Possible changes in ovarian steroidogenesis in affected patients remain to be elucidated.

Conversion of Cholesterol to Ovarian Steroids

The molecular structure and enzymatic steps involved in the conversion of cholesterol to ovarian steroids are shown in Figure 115–2.

Although the availability of cellular cholesterol is under stringent control, hormonal regulation of steroid biosynthesis is primarily exerted at the level of the cholesterol side chain cleavage enzyme, which removes the 6-carbon isocaproic acid from cholesterol, resulting in the formation of pregnenolone. This process requires the cofactor nicotinamide adenine dinucleotide phosphate, reduced form (NADPH), and molecular oxygen and involves a complex of three enzymes: cytochrome P-450scc, a flavoprotein

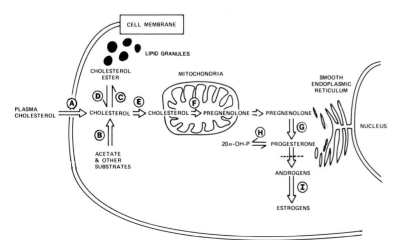

FIGURE 115–1. Diagrammatic representation of cellular organelles and key enzymes involved in ovarian steroid biosynthesis. Dashed line between progesterone and androgens emphasizes the deficiency of 17β-hydroxylase and 17, 20-desmolase in granulosa cells. A, lipoprotein receptors; B, 3-hydroxy-3-methylglutaryl coenzyme A reductase (HMG-CoA reductase); C, acyl-coenzyme A: cholesterol acyl transferase; D, cholesterol esterase; E, cholesterol transport to the mitochondria; F, cholesterol side-chain cleavage enzymes (phospholipid membrane environment and enzyme levels); G, 3β-hydroxysteroid dehydrogenase (3β-HSD); H, 20α-hydroxysteroid dehydrogenase (20α-HSD); I, aromatases.

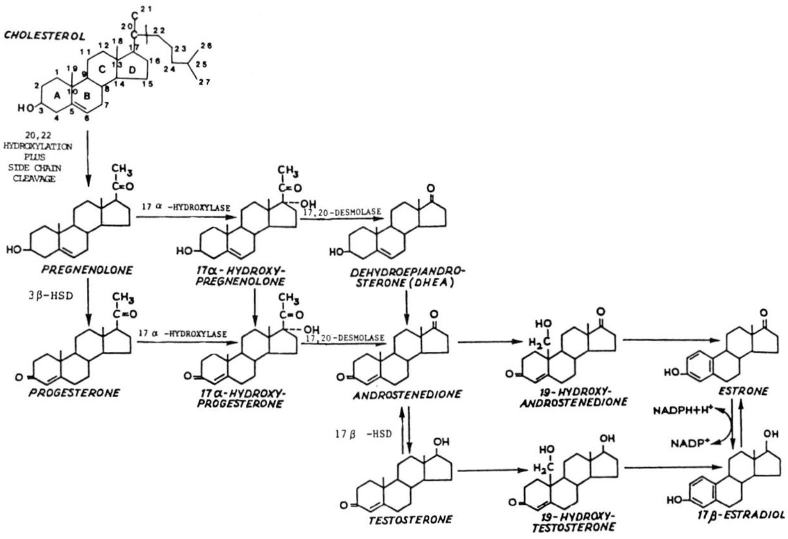

FIGURE 115–2. Steroidogenic pathways involved in the formation of progestins, androgens, and estrogens from cholesterol.

(NADPH: adrenodoxin reductase), and an iron-sulfur protein, adrenodoxin.[11] The cDNA's for all three enzymes have been cloned.[12] A multistep reaction occurs without release of intermediates during the formation of pregnenolone. At least three steps in the cholesterol side chain cleavage reaction may be under hormonal control (see Fig. 115–1, steps E and F): (1) transfer of cholesterol into mitochondria by sterol carrier protein,[13] (2) availability of phospholipids important for the formation of complexes between cholesterol and the cytochrome P-450 enzyme,[14] and (3) modulation of the mitochondria cytochrome P-450 levels. Clinically useful drugs such as aminoglutethimide have been synthesized to inhibit the cholesterol side chain cleavage activity.[15]

Pregnenolone was thought to be converted to progesterone by a complex of two tightly linked enzymes, 3β-hydroxysteroid dehydrogenase (3β-HSD) and Δ^5,Δ^4-isomerase. Recent molecular biology analysis, however, indicates that one gene confers both enzyme activities.[16] Although this enzyme is mainly localized in the smooth endoplasmic reticulum of steroidogenic cells (see Fig. 115–1, step G), its presence in the mitochondria has also been reported. Because isomerase activity appears to be in excess, the production of progesterone from pregnenolone is regulated by 3β-HSD. Steroid oxidation requires the cofactor nicotinamide adenine dinucleotide (NAD), and this reaction is followed by the shift of the double bond from the Δ^5 to the Δ^4 position. The conversion of pregnenolone to progesterone is rate-limiting and can be inhibited by cyanoketone. Progesterone is secreted by granulosa or luteal cells and used as a substrate for further enzymatic reactions leading to androgens and estrogens. Progesterone may also be metabolized to its inactive metabolite, 20α-hydroxypregn-4-en-3-one (20α-OH-P) by 20α-HSD (see Fig. 115–1, step H). The elevation of 20α-HSD activity is associated with luteolysis.

The conversion of progesterone to C_{19} androgens is catalyzed by an enzyme complex in the endoplasmic reticulum composed of a specific form of cytochrome P-450, P-$450_{17\alpha}$, and the flavoprotein NADPH-cytochrome P-450 reductase. Although two separate enzymes, 17α-hydroxylase and $C_{17,20}$-lyase, have been designated for the conversion of progesterone to 17α-hydroxyprogesterone and 17α-hydrox-

yprogesterone to androstenedione, respectively, molecular biology studies have attributed both activities to the same P-$450_{17\alpha}$. Activities of 17,20-lyase (also known as 17,20-desmolase) can be demonstrated in nonsteroidogenic cells transfected with cDNA clone for the P-$450_{17\alpha}$ enzyme.[17, 18] Because 17α-hydroxyprogesterone is secreted by the ovary but not by the placenta, it serves as a marker for ovarian secretion during pregnancy.

Pregnenolone can also be converted by the 17α-hydroxylase enzyme complexes to form 17α-hydroxypregnenolone and dehydroepiandrosterone (DHEA). This offers an alternative route (the Δ^5 pathway) for androgen formation. DHEA is in turn converted by 3β-HSD and isomerase to androstenedione. The major androgen secreted by the ovary is androstenedione, which is much less potent than testosterone.

Estrone and estradiol are formed from androstenedione and testosterone, respectively. This reaction takes place in the smooth endoplasmic reticulum and requires enzyme complexes referred to as aromatases (see Fig. 115–1, step I). Aromatization involves the loss of the angular C-19 methyl group and the steroid-specific elimination of the 1-β and 2-β hydrogens from the androgens.[19, 20] This process includes three enzymatic hydroxylations using 3 mol of O_2 and NADPH per mole of estrogen formed. The irreversible reaction requires the participation of both a specific cytochrome P-450 enzyme (P-450 aromatase) and the NADPH-cytochrome c reductase. The former enzyme has been cloned from human placenta.[21] Several aromatase inhibitors, such as androstene-3,6,17-trione, have been found to be clinically useful in suppressing estrogen biosynthesis in patients with steroid-dependent breast tumor.[22]

Although androstenedione is the most abundant androgen secreted by the ovary, estradiol is the major ovarian estrogen released. The conversion of androstenedione to testosterone, or estrone to estradiol, is mediated by 17β-HSD.[23] The participation of both aromatase and 17β-HSD leads to optimal estradiol biosynthesis.

The essential role of steroidogenic enzymes in female reproductive performance is exemplified in patients with 17α-hydroxylase deficiency. This congenital enzyme defect results in altered adrenal and gonadal steroidogenesis with decreases in glucocorticoids, androgens, and estrogens.[24]

Cloning of the enzyme has made it possible to demonstrate the molecular defect of this disease, including point mutation, insertion, and deletion of the gene.[25] The clinical syndrome of these patients includes sexual immaturity and primary amenorrhea associated with failure of follicle growth.[26]

GONADOTROPIN CONTROL OF OVARIAN STEROIDOGENESIS AND DIFFERENTIATION

Follicle-stimulating hormone is the prime inducer of ovarian follicle maturation[27] and responsible for the development of granulosa cell responsiveness to LH and prolactin.[28, 29] Because FSH receptors are present exclusively on the granulosa cells, various ovarian effects of FSH are believed to be mediated through granulosa cells. In contrast, theca interna cells contain LH but not FSH receptors, and androgen production by these cells is regulated by LH. The binding of gonadotropins to their respective plasma membrane receptors enhances receptor interaction with a stimulatory guanine nucleotide binding protein (G$_s$ protein; see Ch. 4). This coupling protein activates the adenyl cyclase, resulting in increased intracellular cAMP levels. The binding of cAMP to protein kinases augments the phosphorylation of a family of CREBP's (cAMP response element binding proteins), leading to the active transcription of different steroidogenic enzymes.

Recent cloning of the cDNA's for FSH[30-32] and LH/hCG[33-35] receptors demonstrates their structural similarity to a superfamily of G protein–coupled receptors. This group of receptors is characterized functionally by their interaction with G proteins and structurally by seven hydrophobic transmembrane domains. The gonadotropin receptors, constituting a receptor subfamily together with the thyroid-stimulating hormone receptor, have a large extracellular domain at the amino terminus, which is responsible for ligand binding.

Both FSH and LH are required for estrogen biosynthesis by immature hypophysectomized rats.[36, 37] In a classic study of Falck,[38] autotransplantation of both theca interna and granulosa cells to the anterior chamber of the eye of the rat showed that both cell types are needed for estrogen biosynthesis. The hypothesis that androgen precursors leave theca cells before aromatization by granulosa cells is documented by the ability of infused testosterone antiserum to decrease follicular estrogen secretion in the sheep ovary.[39] Studies of monkey follicles further demonstrate that granulosa cells are the major site of estrogen production because scraping of these cells in situ abolishes the secretion of estrogens into the ovarian vein.[40]

A two-cell, two-gonadotropin hypothesis for ovarian estrogen biosynthesis has been proposed (Fig. 115–3). According to this model, LH stimulates the biosynthesis of androstenedione from cholesterol in the theca interna. Androgens diffuse across the lamina basalis and are converted to estrogens by granulosa cells. The aromatase activity in the granulosa cells is regulated by FSH in immature follicles and by both FSH and LH in mature graafian follicles. Furthermore, granulosa cell progesterone may diffuse into theca cells to serve as a substrate for androgen biosynthesis.[41] Theca cells mainly produce androstenedione, and

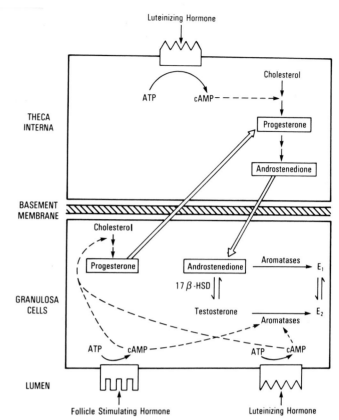

FIGURE 115–3. Gonadotropin control of ovarian estrogen biosynthesis: A two-cell, two-gonadotropin hypothesis. (Adapted from Hsueh AJH, et al: Hormonal regulation of the differentiation of cultured ovarian granulosa cells. Endocr Rev 5:76–127, 1984.)

the participation of granulosa cell 17β-HSD is necessary for optimal estradiol biosynthesis.

LH is the most important hormone involved in the breakdown of the follicular wall, which results in ovum release. The ovulatory event is associated with increases in proteolytic activity, including plasminogen activators and collagenase to allow disaggregation of basement membrane and stromal tissues and the physical release of the oocyte-cumulus complex. Furthermore, the LH stimulus signals the resumption of meiotic maturation of the oocyte. After ovulation both granulosa and theca cells undergo luteinization and form epithelial-like luteal cells that contain large numbers of lipid droplets. During luteinization granulosa cell size increases and the cells appear to gain surface microvilli. This is correlated with a substantial increase in LH receptor number as well as LH-induced cAMP production. Concurrently, FSH receptor number and FSH responsiveness decrease. Extensive neovascularization of the follicle also takes place during luteinization, leading to increases in new blood vessel formation in the corpus luteum.[42]

Progesterone is the main steroid secreted by the LH-dependent corpus luteum during the second half of the menstrual cycle. The functional life span of the human corpus luteum is 14 ± 2 days, after which it spontaneously regresses. If pregnancy occurs, hCG secreted by the fetal trophoblast prolongs progesterone secretion and maintains early pregnancy.[43] In addition, the human corpus luteum secretes estrogens.

Follicle growth depends on optimal stimulation by both

FSH and LH. Polycystic ovarian syndrome is characterized by an increased ratio of serum LH to FSH, leading to excess theca androgen production and stunted follicle growth. Defective ovarian responsiveness to gonadotropins occurs in patients with "resistant ovary" syndrome. Despite elevated levels of FSH and LH, the ovaries of these amenorrheic patients are small and contain many primordial follicles that show no evidence of maturation.[44] Studies have indicated that deglycosylated gonadotropins are capable of binding to ovarian receptors without eliciting steroidogenesis, thus serving as potential gonadotropin antagonists.[45, 45a] It is unclear whether defective carbohydrate content of the gonadotropins contributes to abnormal gonadal responsiveness. One also cannot rule out the existence of abnormal gonadotropin receptors or circulating receptor antibodies in "resistant ovary" syndrome. Furthermore, patients with genetically defective G proteins for cAMP production have been identified.[46] Although the syndrome is named pseudohypoparathyroidism because of the decreases in cAMP production stimulated by parathyroid hormone, the defect in G protein affects all tissues and results in decreased ovarian responsiveness to gonadotropins.

In addition to LH, prolactin modulates luteal steroidogenesis. In rodents and sheep, prolactin is an indispensable part of the luteotrophic complex. Physiological levels of prolactin may also be important in the maintenance of human ovarian steroidogenesis, but prolonged hyperprolactinemia is associated with suppression of ovarian steroidogenesis.[47] A direct inhibitory effect of high concentrations of prolactin on ovarian aromatase activity has been demonstrated in rats.[48]

BIOSYNTHESIS OF PEPTIDE HORMONES AND FOLLICULAR CONSTITUENTS

Ovarian follicles and corpora lutea also secrete peptide hormones (e.g., inhibin, activin, relaxin, and oxytocin), prostaglandins, regulatory proteins (e.g., plasminogen activators), growth factors, and mucopolysaccharides. Some of these secretory products have endocrine roles by acting outside the ovary; others exert intraovarian regulatory functions in the control of ovulation and oocyte maturation.

The presence of a nonsteroidal testis inhibitor of FSH secretion was proposed as early as 1932 by McCullagh.[49] An ovarian inhibin-like factor that specifically suppresses FSH secretion in castrated male and female rats has been found in ovarian extracts and follicular fluid.[50] Studies using cultured cells have shown that the granulosa cells secrete inhibin and the pituitary gonadotrophs are a site of action of this peptide.[51] FSH production is suppressed by inhibin, and inhibin production by the developing granulosa cells is stimulated by FSH and LH, thus forming a closed-loop feedback system.[52] Isolation and cloning studies indicate that inhibins are heterodimers with dissimilar α and β subunits covalently linked by disulfide bonds.[53] The β subunits have sequence homology with transforming growth factor-β and müllerian duct inhibition factor. Although the αβ dimers suppress FSH secretion, the ββ dimers (see Ch. 114) have been shown to stimulate FSH release. In addition to its well-known endocrine action at the anterior

pituitary gland, inhibin has been shown to exert paracrine effects at the ovary level by enhancing LH-stimulated androgen biosynthesis by theca interna cells.[54] In vivo studies also suggest a role for activin in inducing atresia.[55] Although deletion of inhibin-α gene in mice using homologous recombination resulted in the formation of gonadal tumors,[55a] the exact role of inhibin-α as a cancer-suppressor gene with gonadal specificity is still unclear in humans. Relaxin, a peptide hormone structurally related to insulin and insulin-like growth factors, has been purified from the corpus luteum. Relaxin has been demonstrated to inhibit myometrial activity and increase connective tissue remodeling of the cervix through its collagenolytic effect.[56, 57] Human corpora lutea of pregnancy, but not of the menstrual cycle, produce relaxin when treated with hCG in vitro.[58] The exact physiological importance of relaxin in the ovarian control mechanism is unclear. The presence of mRNA and immunoreactive relaxin has been demonstrated in theca cells and in nonpregnant corpora lutea.

Although oxytocin has been shown to be secreted by human luteal cells,[59] its suspected role in ovarian steroidogenesis and uterine activity remains to be elucidated. During ovulation, rupture of the follicular wall for oocyte release depends on the actions of several follicular secretory products. Based on the observation that inhibitors of prostaglandin biosynthesis prevent ovulation, it is believed that prostaglandins are involved in the ovulatory event.[60] Prostaglandins also modulate follicular and luteal steroidogenesis. In nonprimate studies prostaglandin E_2 (PGE_2) has been shown to increase cAMP and steroidogenesis by the ovarian cells, whereas $PGF_2\alpha$ of uterine origin is essential for suppressing progesterone biosynthesis during luteolysis.[61]

Oocyte release from the graafian follicle during ovulation requires extensive proteolysis.[62] Breakdown of collagen fibers in the ovarian capsule involves the activation of collagenase and the decrease of its inhibitors controlled by the pre-ovulatory surge of gonadotropins. In addition, identification of a protease plasminogen activator, its substrate (plasminogen), and its product (plasmin) in the follicular fluid supports the concept that a fibrinolytic system similar to those found in blood clot dissolution is operating in the ovary.[63] Both FSH and LH stimulate the production of tissue plasminogen activator (TPA) by cultured granulosa cells.[64] The secreted activator converts plasminogen to the active protease, plasmin, which may in turn initiate proteolytic events and activate collagenase to promote ovulation. Intrabursal injection of antibodies to TPA or α_2-antiplasmin blocks gonadotropin induction of ovulation in rats.[65]

INTRA-OVARIAN CONTROL MECHANISMS

Autocrine and Paracrine Actions of Ovarian Steroids

In addition to their presence in peripheral plasma, ovarian steroids are found in high concentrations inside the developing follicles. The human follicular fluid content of estrogens and androgens closely reflects the developing or atretic status of a given follicle.[66] The estrogen-androgen ratio is high in healthy dominant follicles, whereas a high androgen-estrogen ratio is invariably associated with atretic follicles.

Multiple evidence suggests autocrine and paracrine actions of the ovarian steroids at the follicle level.[29] Estrogen treatment increases granulosa cell proliferation and estrogen receptor content in laboratory animals. Furthermore, estrogen enhances FSH-induced ovarian weight increase as well as FSH-stimulated cAMP production and LH receptor formation in rat granulosa cells.[28, 29] Although estrogens also augment gonadotropin-stimulated estrogen biosynthesis[67] in rat granulosa cells, the exact intra-ovarian action of estrogens in women is still unclear. Treatment of hypogonadotropic women with recombinant FSH induces the growth of pre-ovulatory follicles in the absence of significant follicle estrogen production.[68]

In contrast to estrogen, ovarian androgens induce atretic events inside the follicles.[69] Treatment with androgens stimulates follicular atresia, and this effect is accompanied by apoptosis of granulosa cells and ovum death.[69a] The counteracting actions of estrogens and androgens inside a given follicle are important in determining the ultimate fate of that follicle.

Ovarian progesterone may also modulate intra-ovarian events. Unilateral ovarian implants of progesterone in monkeys directly inhibit follicular growth without affecting the function of the contralateral ovary.[70] Follicular growth begins immediately after luteectomy, suggesting that a locally high concentration of progesterone may inhibit folliculogenesis. In contrast, local luteal progesterone may facilitate progesterone biosynthesis by way of an autocrine positive feedback mechanism.[71] It is clear that intra-ovarian hormonal milieu determines the maturation and development of individual follicles and corpora lutea.

Role of Growth Factors and Neurohormones

Studies using cultured granulosa cells suggest important intra-ovarian regulatory roles of several peptide growth factors, including epidermal growth factor (EGF),[72] insulin-like growth factors (IGF-I),[73–75] gonadotropin-releasing hormone,[76] and transforming growth factor-β.[77] In addition, oxytocin is produced by the luteal cells.[78] Because secretion, specific receptor, and biological action of several growth factors have been demonstrated in the ovary, they are believed to play autocrine or paracrine roles.

Of the growth factors studied, IGF-I is perhaps the most well characterized as an intra-ovarian regulator with production, reception, and action within the ovary.[75, 79] In addition, synthesis of IGF binding proteins (IGFBP)[80] has been demonstrated in follicles at different stages of development and atresia. In rodents, IGF-I is produced in granulosa cells and secreted into the follicular fluid. Of all the tissues studied, the levels of ovarian IGF-I gene expression is exceeded only by the liver and uterus.[81] Ovarian IGF-I production is gonadotropin-regulated,[79] and the expression of IGF-I depends on the cyclic variations of gonadotropins.[82] As in most tissues, IGF-I is stimulated by growth hormone.[83] After stimulation by gonadotropins and growth hormone, ovarian IGF-I augments gonadotropin action, including steroid production and LH receptor induction. Unlike in rodents, IGF-II is the predominant IGF type pro-

duced by human granulosa cells. All but one (IGFBP-1) of the six known IGFBP's[80] are expressed in the ovary.[84, 85] These high-affinity binders are believed to block the actions of endogenous IGF-I and IGF-II. Indeed, high levels of IGFBP's are found in atretic follicles in normal women and cystic follicles in PCO patients.[85a] IGFBP's may also serve as a transport protein and prolong the half-life of the growth factor.[86]

EGF has been demonstrated in human follicular fluid[87] and corpora lutea.[88] In the rat the cellular localization of transforming growth factor-α (TGFα), a structural and functional analogue of EGF,[89] has been localized to the theca-interstitial cells and is stimulated by FSH.[90] EGF/TGF-α stimulates proliferation and inhibits differentiation of granulosa cells. The stimulatory effect of FSH on DNA synthesis in hamster follicles is blocked by neutralizing antibodies against EGF, suggesting that FSH stimulates the follicle cells to increase ovarian levels of EGF, which in turn enhances cell division.[91]

In cells of mesodermal and neuroectodermal origin, basic fibroblast growth factor (bFGF) is a potent mitogen. In the ovary bFGF has been isolated from corpora lutea and is also produced by granulosa cells. Like EGF, bFGF stimulates proliferation and inhibits differentiation of granulosa cells in several species. bFGF, being a potent angiogenic stimulator, has been suggested to be involved in the rapid neovascularization during corpus luteum formation.[92] In addition to their effects on granulosa cell proliferation, both EGF and bFGF have been shown to inhibit apoptotic granulosa cell death.[93]

Although gonadotropins are the major regulators of follicular development, only one dominant preovulatory follicle is selected during a given menstrual cycle. The selected follicle, by way of its estrogen production, reduces systemic and intrafollicular FSH levels, thereby impeding the maturation of other follicles[94]; however, the selected follicle continues to mature in the face of declining FSH levels because intrafollicular growth factors enhance the action of FSH to stimulate vascularity in the selected follicle. The exact growth factors involved in the maintenance of the dominant follicle is unclear, but studies suggest an endothelial cell growth factor as a potential candidate.[95]

Adrenergic nerves are found in proximity to ovarian vessels and perifollicular musculature. Adrenergic control mechanisms may be important in intraovarian vasomotor activity and ovulation.[96] Also, many nerve fibers appear to be in proximity to ovarian follicles and corpora lutea.[97] A potential role of catecholamines in the regulation of steroid biosynthesis is suggested by the finding of β₂-adrenergic receptors in rat granulosa and luteal cells and the stimulation of progesterone biosynthesis by adrenergic agents.[29] Treatment of neonatal rats with antiserum against nerve growth factor (NGF) resulted in abnormal ovarian development. In addition, both NGF and NGF receptors are found in the ovary, suggesting a potential role of this neurohormone.[98]

SECRETION AND METABOLISM OF OVARIAN STEROIDS

Unlike protein and peptide hormones, most of the steroid hormones are not stored and are secreted immediately after biosynthesis. The secretion of ovarian steroids has been directly estimated by the measurement of hormones in peripheral and ovarian veins. Higher concentrations in the venous effluent indicate steroid secretion, and the concentration gradient multiplied by ovarian blood flow gives a direct estimate of secretion rate.

The "production rate" of a given steroid is defined as the amount of hormone entering the circulation per unit of time from all sources, including the ovary, adrenal, and peripheral nonglandular tissue. When the steroid is secreted only by the ovary, the production rate equals the ovarian secretion rate. If a steroid is secreted by more than one gland, it is necessary to suppress the secretion of a given gland and measure the residual production rate to estimate the contribution of the gland. The production rate of a hormone can be calculated by multiplying its concentration in blood by its metabolic clearance rate (MCR). The MCR is defined as the volume of blood or plasma from which a substance is cleared per unit of time.[99] This parameter is independent of transfer among body compartments and metabolism and can be measured by infusing labeled steroid until equilibrium is attained. Because the rate of infusion of labeled steroid is known and the rate of removal at equilibrium equals the infusion rate, the MCR equals the rate of infusion divided by the concentration of the labeled steroid in blood.

If the MCR is not altered, changes in the concentration of a hormone in circulation directly reflects changes in its production rate. Furthermore, the absolute value of the MCR is informative about the site of metabolism. If the value is much greater than hepatic blood flow (1500 L/d), then extrahepatic clearance must be substantial.[100, 101] In general, the binding of steroids to high-affinity serum binders (e.g., sex steroid–binding globulin) decreases their MCR. The plasma concentration of various ovarian steroids as well as their metabolic clearance, production, and secretion rates are shown in Table 115–1.

The circulating half-lives of ovarian steroids are extremely short (within minutes). These steroids are hydroxylated and/or conjugated to form steroid glucuronide or sulfate. The steroid metabolites are less active but more soluble for renal clearance. Estrogens are hydroxylated at the C-2 and C-16 positions to form 2-methoxyestrone and estriol, respectively. Estriol is the most abundant estrogen

in urine, mainly as the result of nonovarian metabolism of estradiol and estrone. The chief route of progesterone metabolism is the formation of pregnanediol after hydroxylation at the C-3 and C-20 positions. Urinary pregnanediol levels give an adequate index of corpus luteum function.

SERUM STEROID BINDING AND TRANSPORT

More than 95 per cent of the steroids secreted into systemic circulation are bound by serum-binding proteins (Fig. 115–4, step 1). Binding of steroids primarily occurs to albumin and to two other well-characterized binding proteins. Albumin has a high capacity but low affinity for ovarian steroids, whereas sex hormone–binding globulin (SHBG) and corticosteroid-binding globulin (CBG) bind steroids with high affinities but much lower capacity.[102–104] Both SHBG and CBG are of hepatic origin, and their primary structures have been determined.[105, 106]

SHBG, also known as testosterone-estrogen–binding globulin, is capable of binding estradiol, testosterone, and dihydrotestosterone.[107] This serum β-globulin is homologous to androgen-binding protein secreted by the testis Sertoli cells and is transcribed from the same gene.[108] Because of its higher affinity for SHBG, tritiated dihydrotestosterone has been used as the ligand for the measurement of SHBG binding. Treatment with estrogens and thyroid hormone increases serum SHBG concentrations, whereas androgen administration decreases serum SHBG concentrations. The circulating concentration of SHBG is higher in women than in men, and SHBG is elevated during pregnancy, in hyperthyroidism, and in male hypogonadism. Conversely, SHBG levels are lowered after menopause and in patients with hypothyroidism.

CBG, also known as transcortin, binds progesterone and cortisol with equal affinity.[104] Serum CBG levels are elevated during pregnancy, and the administration of estrogens to men or nonpregnant women raises serum CBG levels to concentrations similar to those found during pregnancy. Increases in the CBG level may explain the failure of pregnant women to develop Cushing-like symptoms, despite their markedly elevated plasma cortisol levels. CBG is structurally unrelated to SHBG but resembles thyroxine-

TABLE 115–1. Plasma Concentrations, Metabolic Clearance Rates, Production Rates, and Ovarian Secretion Rates of Ovarian Steroid Hormones

STEROID	MCR (L/d)	PHASE OF MENSTRUAL CYCLE	PLASMA CONCENTRATION (ng/100ml)	PRODUCTION RATE (mg/d)	SECRETION RATE (mg/d)
Estradiol	1350	Early follicular	6	0.08	0.07
		Late follicular	33–70	0.5–1.0	0.4–0.8
		Midluteal	20	0.27	0.25
Estrone	2210	Early follicular	5	0.11	0.08
		Late follicular	15–30	0.3–0.7	0.25–0.50
		Midluteal	11	0.24	0.16
Progesterone	2200	Follicular	50–100	2.1	1.5
		Luteal	1000–1500	25.0	24.0
17α-hydroxyprogesterone	2000	Early follicular	30	0.6	0.2
		Late follicular	200	4.0	3–4
		Midluteal	200	4.0	3–4
Androstenedione	2010		130–160	3.2	0.8–1.6
Testosterone	690		38	0.3	—

Adapted from Lipsett MB: Steroid hormone. In Yen SSC, Jaffe RB (eds): Reproductive Endocrinology. Philadelphia, WB Saunders Co, 1978, pp 80–92.

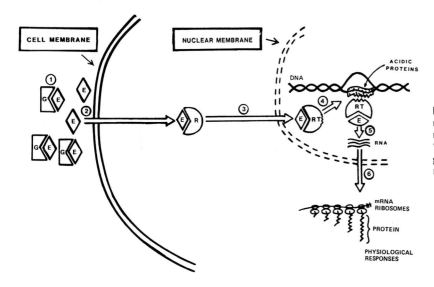

FIGURE 115–4. Molecular mechanism of estrogen action in target tissues. Nuclear membrane is depicted as dashed lines to denote the uncertain cellular localization of the unbound "free" receptors. E, estrogen; G, serum steroid-binding globulin; R, receptor; RT, transformed receptor; SRE, steroid-responsive element.

binding globulin and several other members of the serine protease inhibitor superfamily. The existence of membrane-bound receptors for both CBG[109] and SHBG[110] has been demonstrated, but the physiological function of these receptors remains unclear.

There is no unified concept regarding the physiological role of serum binders. It is clear that the abundant serum albumin prevents the rapid degradation of circulating sex steroids, resulting in a prolonged half-life and decreased MCR. The major role of steroid-binding globulins appears to be the provision of a reservoir of bound hormone that effectively dampens wide fluctuations in the free steroid concentration. Because only the unbound steroids are capable of interacting with specific target tissue receptors, the presence of serum binders maintains a dynamic equilibrium between serum binding and target cell activation. This is followed by the dissociation of steroids into the "free" pool before binding to target cell receptors.

Although the serum binders may reduce the metabolism of steroids and provide the "buffering" mechanism, they do not play an obligatory role in steroid action. Patients with SHBG deficiency are not infertile,[111] and potent synthetic steroids with minimum binding affinity to serum binders are powerful drugs in modulating reproductive functions. The lack of an essential role of serum binders is also demonstrated by the action of various steroids in serum-free culture systems.

MECHANISM OF STEROID HORMONE ACTION

Role of Steroid Hormone Receptors

Sex steroids diffuse into cells within seconds through the plasma membrane lipid bilayer (see Fig. 115–4, step 2). Carrier-mediated transport may occur but plays no apparent regulatory function. Although steroid hormones enter all cells of the body, steroid-modulated physiological responses occur only in selective tissues that contain specific receptor molecules. Except in target tissues, steroids exit from cells at the same rate as plasma concentrations decrease, and the retention of hormones is a hallmark of target cells. Jensen and Jacobson synthesized tritiated estra-

diol and showed that estrogen target tissues, such as the uterus, retain significant quantities of the hormone, whereas nontarget tissues, such as the diaphragm, do not.[112]

Steroid receptors are proteins of high molecular weight and are present in low concentrations (about 100,000 binding sites per cell). Because the physiological concentration of steroid hormones in the blood ranges from 10^{-8} to 10^{-10} M, the high affinity (Kd:10^{-10} M) of the receptors for steroid hormones allows optimal binding. Furthermore, receptors display characteristic binding stereospecificity for each class of hormones. Specific receptors are present only in steroid-responsive target cells. The presence of steroid receptors is a necessary (but not sufficient) step in hormone action. That receptors are essential for hormone action is best demonstrated by the defective tissue responsiveness found in androgen-resistant pseudohermaphroditic male patients with normal androgen production but apparent female phenotype.[113]

It is clear that the primary role of steroid hormones is to act as an allosteric effector that unmasks a DNA binding site on the receptor protein. Sex steroids, as well as other steroid hormones and several vitamins, appear to function by way of the two-step model involving the transformation of the intracellular steroid receptors (see Fig. 115–4, step 3). The "free" receptor exists in an inactive form sequestered with a complex of proteins, including heat shock proteins.[114] Binding of the hormone ligand results in a conformational change of the receptor to an active form capable of binding to specific DNA sequences. The transformation process takes 5 to 30 minutes after hormone exposure and is temperature- and hormone-dependent.[115] This process also involves dissociation of receptor-associated proteins[114] as well as dimerization[116] and phosphorylation of receptors.[117]

Although earlier studies using harsh tissue homogenization conditions suggest a steroid-induced transformation of the inactive receptor into DNA-binding form as well as the translocation of the "cytoplasmic" form of the "free" receptor to the nucleus, immunocytochemical studies using estrogen receptor antibodies demonstrate that the "free" receptors are present in the nucleus.[118] Likewise, cell fractionation using gentler conditions indicates that the estrogen receptors are mainly present in the nucleus.[119] It is now believed that both forms of receptors for sex steroids are always located in the nucleus.

Activation of Genomic Events

Cloning of the receptors for glucocorticoid,[120] estrogen,[121] progesterone,[122] and androgen[123, 124] has shown that these intracellular proteins are structurally related, constituting a family of nuclear transcription factors.[125] The structural homology between the steroid receptors provides important insight on the role of the transformed receptors in their interaction with DNA enhancer elements (steroid response elements [SRE]) of steroid-dependent genes, leading to increased transcription (see Fig. 115–4, step 4). Consensus sequences in the receptor genes indicate the presence of two separate domains responsible for hormone binding and enhancer DNA interaction, respectively. The hormone-binding domain is specific for each steroid, whereas the DNA-binding domain is highly conserved with homology to the oncogene erb A and contains 20 invariant amino acids constituting two regions named zinc-finger domains. The DNA-binding specificity of different steroid receptors to respective SRE is determined by three amino acids at the base of the first zinc-finger domain.[126] Binding of steroids to the hormone-binding domain increases affinity of the receptor protein with the SRE and enhances the binding of additional transcription factors,[127] whereas deletion of the binding domain allows the receptor to act as constitutive transcription factors. In addition, the product of the cellular erb A oncogene has been shown to bind thyroxine and represents the cellular thyroid receptor.[128, 129] It is apparent that receptors for steroid hormones, thyroid hormones, and vitamins A and D, together with several "orphan" receptors with unknown ligands, are members of a superfamily of genes important for transcriptional regulation.[125] During evolution, transcriptional factors with zinc-finger domains acquire ligand-binding ability and become steroid-regulated receptor proteins.

The transformed receptors initiate genomic events leading to increased (and, in some cases, decreased) transcription of specific genes. The classes of new mRNA produced in response to a given steroid are cell-specific, and their utilization in the production of new proteins leads to characteristic tissue responses. The transformed receptors bind to specific nuclear sites. The DNA sequence for the SRE of the different hormones comprise complete or partial palindromic DNA structures (see Fig. 115–4, step 4). Genetic manipulation of glucocorticoid-induced expression of a mammary tumor virus demonstrated the essential role of enhancer DNA sequences in the recognition of transformed receptors.[130] The insertion of foreign genes "downstream" from these DNA sequences enables the induction of new gene products by glucocorticoid, whereas deletion of the regulatory DNA sequences abolishes glucocorticoid responsiveness.

Transcriptional events induced by the ligand-bound steroid receptors include increases of RNA polymerase and binding of multiple general transcription factors like TFIIA, TFIIB, TFIID, TFIIE, and TFIIF to the TATA promoter, followed by the synthesis of heterogeneous nuclear RNA and specific proteins (see Fig.115–4, step 6). Synergistic interaction with other transcription factors to modulate gene expression induced by steroids has also been demonstrated.[127] Depending on the target tissue, steroid hormones may induce structural proteins involved in the formation of new subcellular organelles, modulatory proteins for fine tuning of cell functions, or regulatory proteins that amplify the initial responses leading to tissue growth or cell division.

Although the essential role of intracellular receptors in the mediation of steroid action is well accepted, alternative mechanisms cannot be excluded. The observation that a soluble macromolecular progesterone agonist, which does not enter cells, induces Xenopus oocyte maturation suggests that the progesterone action may be mediated by cell membrane–associated recognition sites.[131] Indeed, progesterone is ineffective if injected into the oocyte, and an oocyte maturation-promoting factor can be induced in enucleated cells. Similarly, estrogen-induced changes in neuronal electrical activity can be detected within seconds and is unlikely to be mediated by the classic intercellular receptors. Furthermore, it was demonstrated that certain steroid receptors can be activated in the absence of their steroid ligands. Binding of dopamine to its membrane receptor activates several steroid receptors, including the receptor for estrogen and progesterone.[132]

Modulation of Receptor Content and Action of Hormone Analogues

Tissue concentrations of steroid receptors vary widely during different physiological conditions. Because changes in steroid receptor content are correlated with alterations in hormonal responsiveness of the target cells, tissue receptor concentration provides a useful parameter for understanding hormonal actions. In the uterus, estrogen treatment increases both estrogen and progesterone receptor content. Conversely, progesterone treatment decreases these receptors.[133] These findings are consistent with the priming effect of estrogen required for optimal estrogen and progesterone action in the endometrium, as well as the antagonistic properties of progesterone on estrogen-induced responses. Variations of human endometrial steroid receptor concentration during the menstrual cycle reinforces the important role of ovarian steroids in the regulation of target cell receptor content and tissue responsiveness.[134]

Because the likelihood that mammary tumor cells will respond to various endocrine therapies (such as ovarian ablation or treatment with estrogen antagonists) is correlated with the presence of tissue estrogen receptors in individual patients, the measurement of estrogen receptor content in mammary tumors provides a useful diagnostic tool for predicting the success of endocrine therapies.[135] To rule out possible postreceptor defects in some estrogen receptor–positive tumors, the estrogen-induced progesterone receptor content is used as an additional parameter. Similar diagnostic procedures have also been applied for endometrial cancers.

Studies on the mechanism of action of steroid hormones provide the opportunity to design potent hormone analogues based on their high intrinsic affinity to tissue receptors. The analogues usually have prolonged serum half-lives because of lower metabolic breakdown and do not interact with serum-binding proteins. The agonists are more effective than the native hormones in eliciting various physiological responses, whereas the antagonists are capable of blocking the action of endogenous hormones by occupying the receptors without eliciting physiological responses.

Representative synthetic steroid agonists include diethylstilbestrol (an estrogen), R5020 (a progestin), methyltrienolone (an androgen), and dexamethasone (a glucocorticoid). Various synthetic agonists of estrogens and progestins are effective contraceptives because they inhibit pituitary secretion of gonadotropins. Synthetic progestins, such as medroxyprogesterone acetate, also cause remission of endometrial and renal carcinomas. Conversely, various steroid antagonists may act by way of formation of inactive antagonist receptor complexes or facilitation of the dissociation of native steroids from their receptors.[136] Trans-tamoxifen, a potent estrogen antagonist, is used in the treatment of mammary tumors, whereas clomiphene citrate, a mixed estrogen agonist-antagonist, induces ovulation in anovulatory women.[137] Although clomiphene citrate is one of the most effective fertility drugs, the effectiveness of using tamoxifen to prevent breast cancer in healthy women[137a] is still controversial because of the potential non–receptor-mediated action of tamoxifen. In syndromes with excess androgens, antiandrogens, such as flutamide and cyproterone acetate, have also gained clinical usage. The compound RU 486 binds to both progesterone and glucocorticoid receptors and acts as an antiprogestin[138] and an antiglucocorticoid.[139] In combination with prostaglandin $F_{2\alpha}$ this drug is effective in terminating early pregnancies. RU 486 acts by antagonizing the action of circulating progesterone at the endometrium to prevent implantation.

REFERENCES

1. Baker TG: A quantitative and cytological study of germ cells in human ovaries. Proc R Soc Lond [Biol] 158:417–433, 1963.
2. Tilly JL, Kowalski KI, Johnson AL, Hsueh AJW: Involvement of apoptosis in ovarian follicular atresia and postovulatory regression. Endocrinology 129:2799–2801, 1991.
3. Hughes FM Jr, Gorospe WC: Biochemical identification of apoptosis (programmed cell death) in granulosa cells: Evidence for a potential mechanism underlying follicular atresia. Endocrinology 129:2415–2422, 1991.
4. Behrman HR, Armstrong DT: Cholesterol esterase stimulation by luteinizing hormone in luteinized rat ovaries. Endocrinology 85:474–480, 1969.
5. Brown MS, Goldstein JL: Receptor-mediated control of cholesterol metabolism. Science 191:150–154, 1976.
6. Carr BR, MacDonald PC, Simpson ER: The role of lipoproteins in the regulation of progesterone secretion by the human corpus luteum. Fertil Steril 38:303–311, 1982.
7. Gwynne JT, Strauss JF III: The role of lipoproteins in steroidogenesis and cholesterol metabolism in steroidogenic glands. Endocr Rev 3:299–329, 1982.
8. Simpson ER, Rochelle DB, Carr BR, MacDonald PC: Plasma lipoproteins in follicular fluid of human ovaries. J Clin Endocrinol Metab 38:394–400, 1974.
9. Golos TG, Strauss JF III: Regulation of low density lipoprotein receptor gene expression in cultured human granulosa cells: Role of human chorionic gonadotropin 8-bromo 3′,5′-cyclic adenosine monophosphate and protein synthesis. Mol Cell Endocrinol 1:321–326, 1987.
10. Goldstein JL, Brown MS: Binding and degradation of low density lipoproteins by cultured human fibroblast. Comparison of cells from a normal subject and from a patient with homozygous familial hypercholesterolemia. J Biol Chem 249:5153–5162, 1974.
11. Waterman MR, Simpson ER: Regulation of the biosynthesis of cyto-chrome P–450 involved in steroid hormone synthesis. Mol Cell Endocrinol 39:81–89, 1985.
12. Simpson E, Lauber M, Demeter M, et al: Regulation of the genes encoding steroidogenic enzymes in the ovary. J Steroid Biochem Molec Biol 41:409–413, 1992.
13. Rennert H, Amsterdam A, Billheimer JT, Strauss JF III: Regulated expression of sterol carrier protein 2 in the ovary: A key role for cyclic AMP. Biochemistry 30:11280–11285, 1991.
14. Leaven HA, Boyd GS: Control of steroidogenesis in rat corpus luteum: The rate of access of cholesterol to the active site of the cholesterol side-chain cleavage enzyme. J Endocrinol 91:123–133, 1981.
15. Dexter RW, Fishman LM, Ney RL, Liddle GW: Inhibition of adrenal corticosteroid by aminoglutethimide: Studies on the mechanism of action. J Clin Endocrinol Metab 27:473–480, 1967.
16. Zhao HZ, Labrie C, Simard J, et al: Characterization of rat 3β-hydroxysteroid dehydrogenase/delta5-delta4 isomerase cDNA and different tissue-specific expression of the corresponding mRNA in steroidogenic and peripheral tissues. J Biol Chem 266:583–593, 1991.
17. Zuber MX, Simpson ER, Waterman MR: Expression of bovine 17α-hydroxylase cytochrome P-450 CDNA in nonsteroidogenic (COS1) cells. Science 234:1258–1261, 1986.
18. Chung BC, Picado-Leonard J, Maniu M, et al: Cytochrome P-450c17: Cloning of human adrenal and testis cDNAs indicates the same gene is expressed in both tissues. Proc Natl Acad Sci USA 84:407–411, 1987.
19. Fishman J: Biochemical mechanisms of aromatization. Cancer Res 42:3277S–3280S, 1982.
20. Thompson EA Jr, Siiteri PK: Partial resolution of the placental microsomal aromatase complex. J Steroid Biochem 7:635–639, 1976.
21. Evans GT, Ledesma DB, Schultz TZ, et al: Isolation and characterization of a complementary DNA specific for human aromatase system cytochrome P–450 mRNA. Proc Natl Acad Sci USA 83:6387–6391, 1986.
22. Brodie A: Aromatase and its inhibitors—an overview. J Steroid Biochem Molec Biol 40:255–261, 1991.
23. Bjersing L: On the morphology and endocrine function of granulosa cells in ovarian follicles and corpora lutea. Acta Endocrinol 125:1–23, 1967.
24. Biglieri EG, Herron MA, Brust N: 17α-hydroxylation deficiency in men. J Clin Invest 45:1946–1954, 1966.
25. Yanase T, Simpson ER, Waterman MR: 17α-hydroxylase/17,20-lyase deficiency: From clinical investigation to molecular definition. Endocr Rev 12:91–108, 1991.
26. Goldsmith O, Solomon DH, Morton R: Hypogonadism and mineralocorticoid excess: The 17α-hydroxylase syndrome. N Engl J Med 277:673–677, 1967.
27. Dorrington JH, Armstrong DT: Effect of FSH on gonadal function. Recent Prog Horm Res 35:301–342, 1979.
28. Richards JS: Hormonal control of ovarian follicular development: 1978 perspective. Recent Prog Horm Res 35:343–373, 1979.
29. Hsueh AJW, Adashi EY, Jones PBC, Welsh TH Jr: Hormonal regulation of the differentiation of cultured ovarian granulosa cells. Endocr Rev 5:76–127, 1984.
30. Sprengel R, Braun T, Nikolics K, et al: The testicular receptor for follicle stimulating hormone: structure and functional expression of cloned cDNA. Mol Endocrinol 4:525–530, 1990.
31. Minegish T, Nakamura K, Takakura Y, et al: Cloning and sequencing of human FSH receptor cDNA. Biochem Biophys Res Commun 175:1125–1130, 1991.
32. Tilly JL, Aihara T, Nishimori K, et al: Expression of recombinant human follicle-stimulating hormone receptor: Species-specific ligand binding, signal transduction, and identification of multiple ovarian messenger ribonucleic acid transcripts. Endocrinology 131:799–806, 1992.
33. Loosfelt H, Misrahi M, Atger M, et al: Cloning and sequencing of porcine LH-hCG receptor cDNA: Variants lacking transmembrane domain. Science 245:525–527, 1989.
34. McFarland KC, Sprengel R, Phillips HS, et al: Lutropin-choriogonadotropin receptor: An unusual member of the G protein-coupled family. Science 245:494–499, 1989.
35. Minegish T, Nakamura K, Takakura Y, et al: Cloning and sequencing of human LH/hCG receptor cDNA. Biochem Biophys Res Commun 172:1049–1054, 1990.
36. Fevoid HL: Synergism of follicle stimulating and luteinizing hormone in producing estrogen secretion. Endocrinology 28:33–36, 1941.
37. Greep RO, VanDyke HB, Chow BF: Gonadotropins of the swine

pituitary. I. Various biological effects of purified thylakenstrin (FSH) and pure metakentrin (ICSH). Endocrinology 30:635–649, 1942.

38. Falck B: Site of production of oestrogen in rat ovary s studied in microtransplants. Acta Physiol Scand 163(Suppl 47):1–101, 1959.

39. Baird DT: Evidence in vivo for the two-cell hypothesis of oestrogen biosynthesis by the sheep graafian follicle. J Reprod Fertil 50:183–185, 1977.

40. Marut EL, Huang S-C, Hodgen GD: Distinguishing the steroidogenic roles of granulosa and theca cells of the dominant ovarian follicle and corpus luteum. J Clin Endocrinol Metab 57:925–930, 1983.

41. Liu YX, Hsueh AJW: Synergism between granulosa and theca-interstitial cells on estrogen biosynthesis by gonadotropin-treated rat ovaries: Studies on the two-cell, two-gonadotropin hypothesis using steroid antisera. Biol Reprod 35:27–36, 1986.

42. Reynolds PL, Killilea D, Redmer DA: Angiogenesis in the female reproductive system. FASEB J 6:886–892, 1992.

43. Yoshimi TC, Strott C, Marshall J, Lipsett M: Corpus luteum function in early pregnancy. J Clin Endocrinol Metab 29:225–230, 1969.

44. Seegar-Jones G, De Moraes-Ruehsen M: A new syndrome of amenorrhea in association with hypergonadotropism and apparently normal ovarian follicular apparatus. Am J Obstet Gynecol 104:597–600, 1969.

45. Sairam MR, Bharagavi, GN: A role for glycosylation of the α subunit in transduction of biological signal in glycoprotein hormones. Science 229:65–67, 1985.

45a. Dunkel L, Jia XC, Nishimori K, et al: Deglycosylated human chorionic gonadotropin antagonizes hCG stimulation of cyclic AMP accumulation through a non-competitive interaction with recombinant human LH receptors. Endocrinology 32:763–769, 1993.

46. Farfel Z, Brickman AS, Kaslow HR, et al: Defect of receptor-cyclase coupling protein in pseudohypoparathyroidism. N Engl J Med 303:337–342, 1980.

47. McNeilly AS, Glasier A, Jonassen J, Howie PW: Evidence for a direct inhibition of ovarian function by prolactin. J Reprod Fertil 66:559–569, 1982.

48. Wang C, Hsueh AJW, Erickson GF: Prolactin inhibition of estrogen production by cultured rat granulosa cells. Mol Cell Endocrinol 20:135–144, 1980.

49. McCullagh GR: Dual endocrine activity of the testes. Science 76:19–20, 1932.

50. Grady RR, Charlesworth MC, Schwartz NB: Characterization of the FSH-suppressing activity in follicular fluid. Recent Prog Horm Res 38:409–456, 1982.

51. Erickson GF, Hsueh AJW: Secretion of "inhibin" by rat granulosa cells in vitro. Endocrinology 103:1960–1963, 1978.

52. Bicsak TA, Tucker EM, Cappel S, et al: Hormonal regulation of granulosa cell inhibin biosynthesis. Endocrinology 119:2711–2719, 1986.

53. Mason AJ, Hayflick JS, Ling N, et al: Complementary DNA sequences of ovarian follicular fluid inhibin show precursor structure and homolog with transforming growth factor-β. Nature 318:659–661, 1985.

54. Hsueh AJW, Dahl KD, Vaughan J, et al: Hetero- and homo-dimers of inhibin subunits have different paracrine actions in the modulation of LH-stimulated androgen biosynthesis. Proc Natl Acad Sci USA 84:5082–5086, 1987.

55. Woodruff TK, Lyon RJ, Hansen SE, et al: Inhibin and activin locally regulate ovarian folliculogenesis. Endocrinology 127:3196–3205, 1990.

55a. Matzuk M, Feingold M, Su J-GJ, et al: Alpha-Inhibin is a tumour-suppressor gene with gonadal specificity in mice. Nature 360:313–319, 1992.

56. Schwabe C, Steinetz B, Weiss G, et al: Relaxin. Recent Prog Horm Res 34:123–211, 1982.

57. Bryant-Greenwood, GD: The human relaxins: Consensus and dissent. Mol Cell Endocrinol 79:C125–C132, 1991.

58. Weiss G: The physiology of human relaxin. Contrib Gynecol Obstet 18:130–146, 1991.

59. Scaeffer JM, Lia J, Hsueh AJW, Yen SSC: Presence of oxytocin and arginine vasopressin in human ovary, oviduct and follicular fluid. J Clin Endocrinol Metab 59:970–973, 1984.

60. Behrman HR: Prostaglandins in hypothalamo-pituitary and ovarian function. Ann Rev Physiol 41:685–700, 1979.

61. Challis JRG: Prostaglandins. In Austin CR, Short RV (eds): Reproduction in Mammals. Book 7. London, Cambridge University Press, 1977, pp 81–116.

62. Espey LL: Ovulation as an inflammatory reaction—a hypothesis. Biol Reprod 22:73–106, 1980.

63. Beers WH: Follicular plasminogen and plasminogen activator and the effect of plasmin on ovarian follicle wall. Cell 6:379–386, 1975.

64. Ny T, Bjersing L, Hsueh AJW, Loskutoff DJ: Cultured granulosa cells produce two plasminogen activators and an antiactivator, each regulated by gonadotropins. Endocrinology 116:1666–1668, 1985.

65. Tsafriri A, Bicsak TA, Cajander SB, et al: Suppression of ovulation rate by antibodies to tissue-type plasminogen activator and alpha 2-antiplasmin. Endocrinology 124:415–421, 1989.

66. McNatty KP, Baird DT, Balton H, et al: Concentration of estrogens and androgens in human follicular fluid throughout the menstrual cycle. J Endocrinol 71:77–85, 1976.

67. Adashi EY, Hsueh AJW: Estrogens augment the stimulation of ovarian aromatase activity by follicle-stimulating hormone in cultured rat granulosa cells. J Biol Chem 257:6077–6083, 1982.

68. Schoot DC, Bennink HJTC, Mannaerts BMJL, et al: Human recombinant follicle-stimulating hormone induces growth of preovulatory follicles without concomitant increase in androgens and estrogen biosynthesis in a woman with isolated gonadotropin deficiency. J Clin Endocrinol Metab 74:1471–1473, 1992.

69. Harman SM, Louvet J-P, Ross GT: Interaction of estrogen and gonadotropins on follicular atresia. Endocrinology 96:1145–1152, 1975.

69a. Billig H, Furuta I, Hsueh AJW: Estrogens inhibit and androgens enhance ovarian granulosa cell apoptotic cell death. Endocrinology, in press.

70. Goodman A, Hodgen G: Between-ovary interaction in the regulation of follicle growth: Corpus luteum function and gonadotropin secretion in the primate ovarian cycle. II. Effects of luteoectomy and hemiovariectomy during the luteal phase in cynomolgus monkeys. Endocrinology 104:1310–1316, 1979.

71. Rothchild I: The regulation of the mammalian corpus luteum. Recent Prog Horm Res 37:183–298, 1981.

72. Mondschein HS, Schomberg DW: Growth factors modulate gonadotropin receptor induction in granulosa cell cultures. Science 211:1179–1180, 1981.

73. Adashi EY, Resnick CE, Svoboda ME, Van Wyk JJ: A novel role for somatomedin-C in the cytodifferentiation of the ovarian granulosa cell. Endocrinology 115:1127–1129, 1984.

74. Davoren JB, Hsueh AJW: Growth hormone increases ovarian levels of immunoreactive somatomedin C/insulin-like growth factor I in vivo. Endocrinology 118:880–890, 1986.

75. Adashi EY, Resnick CE, D'Ercole AJ, et al: Insulin-like growth factor as intraovarian regulators of granulosa cell growth and function. Endocr Rev 6:400–420, 1985.

76. Hsueh AJW, Jones PBC: Gonadotropin-releasing hormone: Extrapituitary actions and paracrine control mechanisms. Ann Rev Physiol 45:83–94, 1983.

77. Skinner MK, Keski-Oja J, Osteen KG, Moses HL: Ovarian thecal cells produce transforming growth factor-β which can regulate granulosa cell growth. Endocrinology 121:786–792, 1987.

78. Wathes DC: Possible actions of gonadal oxytocin and vasopressin. J Reprod Fertil 71:315–345, 1984.

79. Adashi EY, Resnick CE, Hurwitz A, et al: Insulin-like growth factors: The ovarian connection. Hum Reprod 6:1213–1219, 1991.

80. Shimasaki S, Ling N: Identification and molecular characterization of insulin-like growth factor binding proteins (IGFBP-1, -2, -3, -4, -5, -6). Prog Growth Factor Res 3:243–266, 1991.

81. Murphy LJ, Bell GI, Friesen HG: Tissue distribution of insulin-like growth factor I and II messenger ribonucleic acid in the adult rat. Endocrinology 120:1279–1282, 1987.

82. Carlsson B, Carlsson L, Billig H: Estrus cycle-dependent co-variation of insulin-like growth factor I (IGF-I) messenger ribonucleic acid and protein in the rat ovary. Mol Cell Endocrinol 64:271–275, 1989.

83. Davoren JB, Hsueh AJW: Growth hormone increases ovarian levels of immunoreactive somatomedin C/insulin-like growth factor I in vivo. Endocrinology 118:880–890, 1986.

84. Nakatani A, Shimasaki S, Erickson GF, Ling N: Tissue-specific expression of four insulin-like growth factor-binding proteins (1, 2, 3 and 4) in the rat ovary. Endocrinology 129:1521–1529, 1991.

85. Erickson GF, Nakatani A, Ling N, Shimasaki S: Localization of insulin-like growth factor-binding protein-5 messenger ribonucleic acid in rat ovaries during the estrous cycle. Endocrinology 130:1867–1878, 1992.

85a. Giudice LC: Insulin-like growth factors in ovarian follicular development. Endocr Rev 13:641–669, 1992.

86. Baxter RC, Martin JL: Binding proteins for the insulin-like growth factors. Prog Growth Factor Res 1:49–68, 1989.

87. Westergaard LG, Andersen CY: Epidermal growth factor (EGF) in human preovulatory follicles. Hum Reprod 4:257–260, 1989.

88. Khan-Dawood FS: Human corpus luteum: immunocytochemical localization of epidermal growth factor. Fertil Steril 47:916–919, 1987.

89. Massague J: Epidermal growth factor-like transforming growth factor. II. Interaction with epidermal growth factor receptor in human placenta membranes and A431 cells. J Biochem 258:13614–13620, 1983.

90. Kudlow JE, Kobrin MS, Purchio AF, et al: Ovarian transforming growth factor-α gene expression: Immunohistochemical localization to the theca-interstitial cells. Endocrinology 121:1577–1579, 1987.

91. Roy SK, Greenwald GS: Mediation of follicle-stimulating hormone action on follicular deoxyribonucleic acid synthesis by epidermal growth factor. Endocrinology 129:1903–1908, 1991.

92. Gospadarowicz D, Ferrara N, Schweigerer L, Neufeld G: Structural characterization and biological function of fibroblast growth factor. Endocr Rev 8:95–114, 1987.

93. Tilly JL, Billig H, Kowalski KI, Hsueh AJW: Epidermal growth factor and basic fibroblast growth factor suppress the spontaneous onset of apoptosis in cultured rat ovarian granulosa cells and follicles by tyrosine kinase-dependent mechanism. Mol Endocrinol 6:1942–1950, 1992.

94. Hillier SG, Zeleznik AJ, Knazek RA, Ross GT: Hormonal regulation of preovulatory follicle maturation in the rat. J Reprod Fertil 60:219–229, 1980.

95. Phillips HS, Hains J, Leung DW, Ferrara N: Vascular endothelial growth factor is expressed in rat corpus luteum. Endocrinology 127:965–967, 1990.

96. Espey LL: Ovarian contractility and its relationship to ovulation: A review. Biol Reprod 19:540–551, 1978.

97. Owman CH, Rosengren E, Sjoberg N-O: Adrenergic innervation of the human female reproductive organs: A histochemical and chemical investigation. Obstet Gynecol 30:763–773, 1967.

98. Dissen GA, Hill DF, Costa ME, et al: Nerve growth factor receptors in the peripubertal rat ovary. Mol Endocrinol 5:1642–1650, 1991.

99. Tait JF: The use of isotopic steroids for the measurement of production rates in vivo. J Clin Endocrinol Metab 23:1285–1297, 1963.

100. Gurpide E: Tracer Methods in Hormone Research. Berlin, Springer-Verlag, 1975.

101. Baird DT, Horton R, Longcope C, Tait JF: Steroid dynamics under steady state conditions. Recent Prog Horm Res 25:611–664, 1969.

102. Westphal U: Steroid-Protein Interactions. Berlin, Springer-Verlag, 1971.

103. Anderson DC: Sex-hormone-binding globulin. Clin Endocrinol 2:69–96, 1974.

104. Rosner W: Plasma steroid-binding proteins. Endocrinol Metab Clin North Am 20:697–720, 1991.

105. Walsh KA, Titani K, Takio K, et al: Amino acid sequence of the sex steroid binding protein of human blood plasma. Biochemistry 25:7584–7590, 1986.

106. Hammond GL, Smith CL, Goping IS, et al: Primary structure of corticosteroid binding globulin, deduced from hepatic and pulmonary cDNAs, exhibits homology with serine protease inhibitors. Proc Natl Acad Sci USA 84:5153–5157, 1987.

107. Rosenbaum W, Christy NP, Kelly W: Electrophoretic evidence for the presence of estrogen-binding β-globulins in human plasma. J Clin Endocrinol Metab 26:1399–1403, 1966.

108. Hammond GL, Underhill DA, Rykse HM, et al: The human sex hormone-binding globulin gene contains exons for androgen-binding protein and two other testicular messenger RNAs. Mol Endocrinol 3:1869–1876, 1989.

109. Hryb DJ, Khan MS, Romas NA, et al: Specific binding of human corticosteroid globulin to cell membranes. Proc Natl Acad Sci USA 83:3253, 1986.

110. Strel'chyonok OA, Avvakumov GV, Survilo LI: A recognition system for sex-hormone–binding protein-estradiol complex in human decidual endometrium plasma membranes. Biochem Biophys Acta 802:459–466, 1984.

111. Ahrentsen OD, Jensen HK, Johnson SG: Sex-hormone-binding globulin deficiency. Lancet 2:377, 1982.

112. Jensen EV, Jacobson HI: Fate of steroid estrogens in target tissues. *In* Puncus G, Vollmer EP (eds): Biological Activities of Steroids in Relation to Cancer. New York, Academic Press, 1960, p 161.

113. Griffin JE, Leshin M, Wilson JD: Androgen resistance syndrome. Am J Physiol 243:E81–E87, 1982.

114. Smith DF, Toft DO: Steroid receptors and their associated proteins. Mol Endocrinol 7:4–11, 1993.

115. Shymala G, Goski J: Estrogen receptors in the rat uterus: Studies on the interaction of cytosol and nuclear binding sites. J Biol Chem 244:1097–1103, 1969.

116. Tsai SY, Carlstedt-Duke J, Weigel NL, et al: Molecular interactions of steroid hormone receptor with its enhancer element: Evidence for dimer formation. Cell 55:361–369, 1988.

117. Takimoto GS, Tasset DM, Eppert EC, Horwitz KB: Hormone induced progesterone receptor phosphorylation consists of sequential DNA-independent and DNA-dependent stages. Analysis with zinc-finger mutants and the progesterone antagonist ZK-98299. Proc Natl Acad Sci USA 89:3050–3052, 1992.

118. King WJ, Greene GL: Monoclonal antibodies localize oestrogen receptor in the nuclei of target cells. Nature 307:745–747, 1984.

119. Welshons WV, Lieberman ME, Gorski J: Nuclear localization of unoccupied oestrogen receptors. Nature 307:747–749, 1984.

120. Hollenberg SM, Weinberger C, Ong ES, et al: Primary structure and expression of a functional human glucocorticoid receptor cDNA. Nature 318:635–641, 1985.

121. Walter P, Green S, Greene G: Cloning of the human estrogen receptor cDNA. Proc Natl Acad Sci USA 82:7889–7893, 1985.

122. Misrahi M, Atger M, d'Auriol L, et al: Complete amino acid sequence of the human progesterone receptor deduced from cloned cDNA. Biochem Biophys Res Commun 143:740–748, 1987.

123. Chang C, Kokontis J, Liao S: Molecular cloning of human and rat complementary DNA encoding androgen receptors. Science 240:324–326, 1988.

124. Lubahn DB, Joseph DR, Sullivan PM, et al: Cloning of human androgen receptor complementary DNA and localization to the X chromosome. Science 240:327–330, 1988.

125. O'Malley B: The steroid receptor super family: More excitement predicted for the future. Mol Endocrinol 4:363–369, 1990.

126. Forman BM, Samuels HH: Interactions among a subfamily of nuclear receptors: The regulatory zipper model. Mol Endocrinol 9:1293–1301, 1990.

127. Bagchi MK, Tsai M-J, O'Malley BW, Tsai SY: Analysis of the mechanism of steroid hormone-dependent gene activation in cell-free system. Endocr Rev 13:525–535, 1992.

128. Sap J, Munoz A, Damm K, et al: The c-erb-A protein is a high affinity receptor for thyroid hormone. Nature 324:635–640, 1986.

129. Weinbeger C, Thompson CC, Ong ES, et al: The c-erb-A gene encodes a thyroid hormone receptor. Nature 324:641–646, 1986.

130. Ringold GM, Dobson DE, Grove JR, et al: Glucocorticoid regulation of gene expression: Mouse mammary tumor virus as a model system. Recent Prog Horm Res 39:387–421, 1983.

131. Baulieu E-E: Cell membrane, a target for steroid hormones. Mol Cell Endocrinol 12:247–254, 1978.

132. Power RF, Mani SK, Connely OM, O'Malley BW: Dopaminergic and ligand-independent activation of steroid receptors. Science 254:1636–1639, 1992.

133. Hsueh AJW, Peck EJ, Clark JH: Progesterone antagonism of the estrogen receptor and estrogen-induced uterine growth. Nature 254:337–339, 1975.

134. Bayard F, Damiliano S, Robel P, Baulieu E-E: Cytoplasmic and nuclear estradiol and progesterone receptors in human endometrium. J Clin Endocrinol Metab 46:635–648, 1978.

135. McGuire WL, Osborne CK, Clark GM, Knight WA III: Steroid hormone receptors and carcinoma of the breast. Am J Physiol 243:E99–E102, 1982.

136. Gronmeyer H, Benhamou, Berry M, et al: Mechanisms of antihormone action. J Steroid Biochem Molec Biol 41:217–221, 1992.

137. Ross GT, Cargille CM, Lipsett MB, et al: Pituitary and gonadal hormones in women during spontaneous and induced ovulatory cycles. Recent Prog Horm Res 267:1–62, 1970.

137a. Henderson BE, Ross RK, Pike MC: Hormonal chemoprevention of cancer in women. Science 259:633–638, 1993.

138. Baulieu E-E: Contragestation and other clinical application of RU 486, an antiprogesterone at the receptor. Science 245:1351–1357, 1989.

139. Bertagna X, Bertagna C, Luton JP, et al: The new steroid analog RU 486 inhibits glucocorticoid action in man. J Clin Endocrinol Metab 59:25–28, 1984.

116

Ovarian Follicular Maturation, Ovulation, and Ovulation Induction

DANIEL KENIGSBERG
ZEV ROSENWAKS
GARY D. HODGEN

The human ovarian follicle is a paradox of timeless and timely biological functions—the former because it can "sleep away" up to three decades before giving way to the latter, a fortnightly burst of growth and cell proliferation in preparation for ovulation.

Neither of these fates is likely for any given ovarian follicle. Indeed, from a maximum of about 6 million ovarian follicles in the two gonads at the seventh month of intrauterine life, only about 2 million survive to reach neonatal life. By the time of menarche, this number has been depleted to only about 400,000 viable follicles. If a healthy woman who never becomes pregnant ovulates 13 times per year between ages 15 and 50, fewer than 500 of the original 6 million ovarian follicles ever achieve ovulation. Thus, quantitatively and in terms of the probable fate of a given follicle, there is much to say about the process of follicular atresia.[1]

There are two intervals in the life cycle of an oocyte that can be termed folliculogenesis. Embryologically, this term refers to the migration of the germ cell and the organization of the surrounding stroma. Functionally, when one considers fertility, folliculogenesis is that phenomenon that occurs cyclicly and results in ovulation. In considering reproductive functions as they relate to ovulation induction, there are now two broad categories of experience and demand for ovarian stimulation: endocrinologically normal women undergoing ovarian stimulation for in vitro fertilization (IVF) and women with intrinsic defects of cyclic ovarian function who require exogenous therapy to achieve ovulation. After a review of basic embryology of the ovary and the mechanics of follicular growth, follicular atresia and enhancement of the ovarian cycle for either ovulation induction or assisted reproductive technologies are discussed.

Embryology

Peters[2] defines folliculogenesis as the transformation of oocytes, lying in cell nests, to small follicles. Embryologically, the germ cells arise on the yolk sac and migrate to an area known as the gonadal ridge. Here the interplay between the contact of the germ cell and stromal cell and the expression of the underlying chromosomal composition in that part of the embryo, sex chromosome positive or negative, determines the formation of an ovary or a testis, respectively.

In the female the germ cells first reside in the developing gonad in a stage known as the *cell syncytium,* in which cytoplasmic boundaries between nuclei are indistinct (nonexistent). As the nucleus reaches the diplotene stage of the first meiotic division, the plasma membrane around separate nuclei closes and gives the appearance of a "naked oocyte." Closure of the cell membrane over multiple nuclei or nuclear fragments results in the occasional occurrence of polynuclear ova.[3] The final stage in embryonic folliculogenesis continues into the first few months of postnatal life and results in the *small follicle,* also known as the primordial follicle. This structure consists of the oocyte with nucleus arrested in the diplotene stage and a basement membrane that separates the germ cell from the single layer of surrounding stromal cells, the granulosa. Until gonadotropic stimulation occurs, there is little change in this structure, but the potential for dynamic interaction between the oocyte and the granulosa cell can be seen in the close relation between the oocyte microvilli and granulosa cell projections (Fig. 116–1). Furthermore, oocytes that do not become encapsulated degenerate. The envelopment of more than one oocyte by a stromal ring results in a polyovular follicle, known to be common in histological preparations of the ovary and recognized clinically by both sonography and oocyte aspiration during IVF (Fig. 116–2).[4] "Seeding" of the gonadal ridge is insufficient for stimulating the development of ovaries, as shown by several investigators.[5–7] This has been demonstrated in the case of fetuses with XO gonadal dysgenesis, in which some primordial germ cells arrive at the gonad but fail to develop follicles. Hormonal input is obligatory for embryological development of ovarian follicles, as indicated by the failure of gonadal development in the anencephalic human fetus[8] and the decreased number of oocytes after fetal hypophysectomy in monkeys (Fig. 116–3). Factors

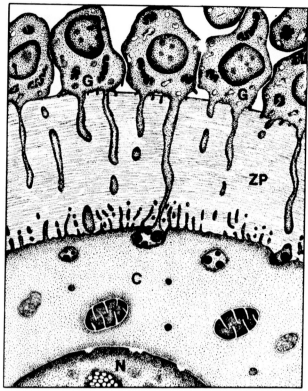

FIGURE 116–1. **Structure of a fully formed zona pellucida (ZP) around an oocyte in graafian (secondary) follicle.** Microvilli arising from the oocyte interdigitate with processes from granulosa cells (G). These processes penetrate into the cytoplasm of the oocyte (C) and may provide nutrients and maternal protein. N, oocyte nucleus. (From Baker TG: Oocytesis and ovulation. *In* Austin CR, Short RV (eds): Germ Cells and Fertilization. Cambridge, Cambridge University Press, 1972, p 25.)

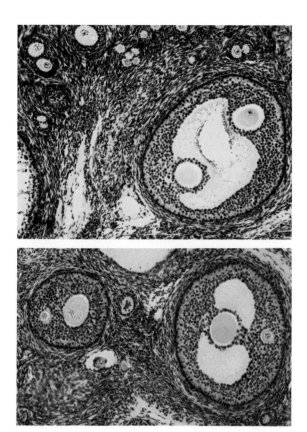

FIGURE 116–2. **Section through the cortex of an ovary (2203L) showing numerous polyovular follicles.** In these follicles the oocytes are of similar size and stage of development (× 100). (From Koering MJ et al: Preantral follicle development during the menstrual cycle in the *Macaca mulatta* ovary. Am J Anat 166:429, 1983.)

apart from the hypothalamic-pituitary axis influence ovarian development. In monkeys, fetal thymectomy reduced ovarian size and the number of follicles.[9, 10]

Prepubertal Phase

During juvenile life, plasma gonadotropins are low and the ovaries are relatively quiescent in terms of hormone production. In normal children there is histological evidence of early follicular development to the preantral stage (see below) seemingly independent of follicle-stimulating hormone (FSH) or luteinizing hormone (LH) secretion. The significance of this gonadotropin-independent phase of follicular growth is unknown, but germ cell depletion occurs, reducing the number of oocytes from 5 million to 7 million during fetal life to only approximately 400,000 at menarche. Atresia may not be a necessary concomitant in those follicles that manifest prepubertal gonadotropin-independent growth, since some enter a secondary growth arrest until gonadotropin-dependent recruitment and maturation occurs in adolescent or adult life.

Folliculogenesis

When considering folliculogenesis in the ovarian cycle, one must anticipate the probable existence of unidentified factors in the regulation of this process. For example, in

humans, as opposed to litter-bearing mammals, the normal ovulatory quota is one. We may ask, Why is there almost exclusively only one ovulation in the human ovarian cycle? How is the selection process regulated? What functional

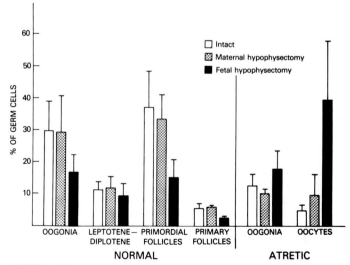

FIGURE 116–3. Graphic presentation of the differential germ cell count in the ovaries of three groups of term infant monkeys. Results expressed as mean ± S.E. (From Gulyas BJ et al: Effects of fetal or maternal hypophysectomy on endocrine organs and body weight in infant rhesus monkeys (*Macaca mulatta*) with particular emphasis on oogenesis. Biol Reprod 16:216, 1977.)

characteristics of the follicle destined to ovulate enable it to thrive in a milieu where other growing follicles undergo atresia? Why do most others remain inactive (at rest) throughout the same cycle? Which processes act through the hypothalamic-pituitary-ovarian axis, whereas others depend on intra-ovarian factors? When exogenous gonadotropin therapy is used, how are the events of the ovarian cycle changed? The list of important questions seems endless.

The ovary performs dual roles as an organ of gametogenesis and as a gland of steroid and peptide secretion. To distinguish the regulation of these ovarian activities, we shall characterize the gametogenic activity as *folliculogenesis* and the secretory activity as *hormonogenesis*.[11] Some ovarian secretions may act locally within the ovary in a paracrine—perhaps even in an autocrine—manner and, therefore, are not always, in the strictest sense, endocrine. Also, because some ovarian hormones secreted into the circulation may be nonsteroidal (inhibin and gonadotropin surge–inhibiting factor), steroidogenesis is too restrictive; accordingly, the term hormonogenesis encompasses all such ovarian secretions.

The anatomy of maturational follicular progression correlates with the physiology of gametogenesis and hormonogenesis (Fig. 116–4). The primordial follicle is the structure composed of the dictyate oocyte, a single granulosa layer, and a surrounding basement membrane. Growth of the *primordial follicle* to a *primary follicle* entails enlargement of the oocyte from about 15 to 100 μm, with the appearance of a zona pellucida and investment by at least two layers of granulosa cells. Specialized gap junctions between granulosa cells and oocytes appear at this time and are thought to be important in cell-to-cell communications and transport. These changes are examples of gonadotropin-independent follicle growth.[12]

The distinguishing feature of the follicle is its development of a fluid-filled cavity or antrum. This accumulation of fluids is the result of both the secretion of mucopolysaccharides by granulosa cells and the transudation of plasma

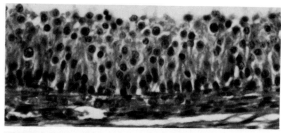

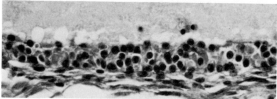

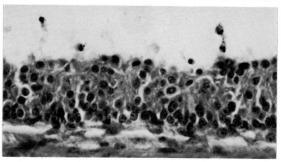

FIGURE 116–5. **Sections from the walls of a dominant follicle** *(top and middle)* **and an early atretic follicle** *(bottom)* **12 days after the initiation of new follicle growth.** The dominant follicle with its accompanying elevated estrogen levels shows variation in the structures of its walls. The major portion of the wall is several cell layers in thickness *(top)*, but in certain areas some of the luminal granulosa cells have pyknotic nuclei *(middle)*. The early atretic follicle has more granulosa cells with pyknotic nuclei lining its lumen *(bottom)* (× 425). (From Koering MJ et al: Granulosa cell pyknosis in the dominant follicle of monkeys. Fertil Steril 37:837, 1982.)

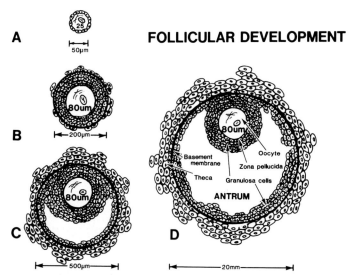

FIGURE 116–4. **Follicular development.** *A,* Primordial follicle. *B,* Preantral follicle. *C,* Antral follicle. *D,* Pre-ovulatory follicle. (From Fritz MA, Speroff L: The endocrinology of the menstrual cycle: The interaction of folliculogenesis and neuroendocrine mechanisms. Fertil Steril 38:509, 1982.)

proteins from the newly acquired theca layer with its vasculature. The overt connection of this follicular apparatus to the peripheral bloodstream is coincident with the onset of gonadotropin-dependent follicular growth. At the stage of the secondary follicle recruitment occurs and, subsequently, selection of the dominant follicle (see below), typically with atresia of all other gonadotropin-dependent follicles. The preovulatory dominant follicle then becomes increasingly vascularized and increasingly richer in LH receptors as ovulation approaches.[13, 14] Simultaneously, among the follicles not selected, the first signs of atresia are foretold by the prevalence of granulosa cell nuclear pyknosis, which usually precedes oocyte degeneration (Fig. 116–5).[15]

During each ovarian-menstrual cycle, primordial follicles depart the resting pool and begin a well-characterized pattern of growth and development. Groups of (quasi-)synchronously growing follicles are called cohorts. In a given cycle a few (or at least one) members of the follicular cohort continue to develop and escape atresia, until one becomes the preovulatory (graafian) follicle, ultimately providing the species-characteristic ovulatory quota of eggs—usually one in a woman.

The term *recruitment* indicates that a follicle has entered this gonadotropin-dependent, rapid-growth phase. Recruitment includes the entry of primordial follicles and the re-entry of slightly more advanced follicles that may have been transiently at rest. Once the recruitment phase has been attained, the follicle must achieve ovulation or become atretic within a single cycle. Specifically, Pederson's[16] studies in mice have been interpreted to mean that once a follicle leaves the resting primordial pool, it must continue to mature or succumb to atresia; it does not again rest. Whether this viewpoint is true for primates is not fully established, although published data are agreeable.[11] Because follicles at various preantral stages of development are observed in the ovaries of hypophysectomized subjects and of patients with hypogonadotropic hypogonadism (Kallmann's syndrome), the recruitment of primordial follicles may not be exclusively dependent on gonadotropins but strikingly enhanced by these hormones.[17] Growing follicles are vulnerable to atresia, which may occur at any point. Thus, although an obligatory step, recruitment does not guarantee ovulation. This is particularly important when attempting to stimulate the ovarian cycle as discussed below.

The term *selection* indicates the final decrease of the cohort size down to the species-characteristic ovulatory quota. When the number of healthy follicles (i.e., with ovulatory potential) in the cohort equals the size of the ovulatory quota, then selection is complete. Selection, then, involves the simultaneous emergence of a follicle or follicles destined to ovulate and the atresia of the others. Implicit in this definition is the notion that the cohort may be the regulated variable rather than the fate of an individual follicle. Which particular follicles are culled from the cohort may be due to a random process that continues until cohort size matches the ovulatory quota, in contrast to a deterministic process in which specific follicles are individually chosen according to some unknown criteria. What is certain, however, is that the process operates with great precision. In humans a spontaneous multiple ovulation is atypical, although not a rarity. Like recruitment, selection does not guarantee ovulation, but given its greater temporal proximity to ovulation, selection secures ovulation in an ovarian or menstrual cycle. Primate models have been used to demonstrate that selection is begun and completed only during the cycle in which ovulation occurs.[18, 19] In contrast, the time of initiation of recruitment is not conclusively known; its tenure lasts until the dominate follicle is selected.[11]

The *dominant follicle* is the sole follicle destined to ovulate, and somehow it continues to thrive in a milieu it has helped to make inhospitable for other follicles. An operational definition of dominance is the time and condition at which one particular follicle orchestrates the remaining events of the entire ovarian cycle. The achievement of dominance occurs between days 5 and 7 of the idealized 28-day ovarian-menstrual cycle. Before this interval one or more other recruited follicles retain the potential to ovulate.

The selected follicle plays a key role in regulating the size of the ovulatory quota. Indeed, the follicle, once selected for ovulation, is functionally (not merely morphologically) dominant; it inhibits the development of other competing follicles on both ovaries. It is unknown whether this capacity to thrive results from a unique ability of the dominant follicle that is newly acquired or from a preexisting ability originally shared by the entire cohort but only retained by the dominant follicle. Whichever is the case, the dominant follicle maintains its eminence for the

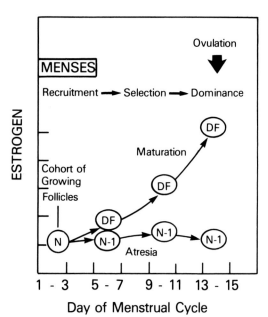

FIGURE 116–6. Time course for recruitment, selection, and ovulation of the dominant ovarian follicle (DF) with onset of atresia among other follicles of the cohort (N1). (From Hodgen GD: The dominant ovarian follicle. Fertil Steril 38:281, 1982.)

remainder of the follicular phase, but it is unresolved whether the mechanism by which the follicle attains dominance is the same by which the follicle maintains dominance (Fig. 116–6).

Mechanism of Ovulation

Once growth of the dominant follicle has achieved the necessary level and systemic hormonal effects are adequate, a cascade of events begins both centrally and within the ovary that results in ovum release. Because ovarian activity and ovulation can occur in the absence of the uterus and fallopian tubes in women and primates, we look to ovarian and hypothalamic-pituitary function as the temporal determinants of the physical act of extrusion of the oocyte.

The most prominent marker for impending ovulation is the midcycle LH surge, which is preceded by an accelerated rise in serum estradiol. Ovulation often occurs within 10 to 12 hours after the peak and 40 hours after the onset of the LH surge.[20, 21] As described below, LH has specific effects on the oocyte and follicle. Recognizing that the LH surge is promoted by rising estrogen secretion, it is regulated by an "ovarian clock."

Ovulation

Primate experiments have shown that in gonadotropin-releasing hormone (GnRH)-deficient monkeys, ovarian stimulation was achieved by administering GnRH in a fixed-dose pulsatile regimen, resulting in timely LH-FSH surges and ovulation.[22] This is the most compelling evidence of an ovarian pacemaker that dictates the timing of these peri-ovulatory events.

Several specific biochemical and biophysical phenomena occur at the time of ovulation; most of them are associated with the LH surge and its metabolic effects (Fig. 116–7). Until the LH surge the oocyte remains in the dictyate stage of meiosis I. At this time the resumption of meiosis occurs, the first polar body is extruded, and the oocyte becomes "mature" (i.e., ready for fertilization); these changes are both nuclear and cytoplasmic. This process can be stimulated in vitro by the addition of cAMP, which suggests a classic second-messenger mechanism with LH as the stimulus. However, it is known that the mere removal of the oocyte from the follicular milieu and subsequent incubation in culture media can result in oocyte maturation. The latter phenomenon has led to a purported intrafollicular regulatory factor known as oocyte maturation inhibitor (OMI).[23, 24]

At the time of the LH surge the granulosa cells surrounding the follicle begin to become transformed or luteinized. These cells enlarge and, along with a decrease in rough endoplasmic reticulum and increased lipid content, become more specialized toward synthesis and secretion of progesterone and estrogen instead of the predominantly estrogenic and peptide products of the follicular phase. Luteinization is also associated with an increase in cAMP within these cells. When granulosa cells obtained from large follicles are cultured, spontaneous luteinization oc-

curs, whereas granulosa cells from small follicles fail to undergo this change. This has led to other hypothesized regulators of follicular maturation, either a luteinizing stimulator (LS) that is produced during follicle growth or a luteinizing inhibitor (LI) that is overcome near the time of ovulation.[25] These putative regulators (OMI, LS, LI) are appealing concepts in explaining the differential behavior of neighboring follicles from cycle to cycle. It is remarkable that adjacent ovarian stromal cells can respond or not respond to ambient conditions in proximity.

Prostaglandins of the F and E series have been implicated in the mechanism of ovum release. Prostaglandin concentrations are increased in follicular fluid at the time of ovulation and can be further enhanced by LH or human chorionic gonadotropin (hCG). Also, prostaglandins have stimulatory effects on smooth muscle fibers found in the theca externa. In animals a degree of ovulation inhibition has been achieved by the administration of antiprostaglandins, which can be overcome by the addition of prostaglandin F_2 (PGF_2).[26]

Concurrent with these biochemical events of the periovulatory interval are characteristic architectural changes in follicular structure. Immediately preceding ovulation the biophysical properties of the follicular wall are altered. With a rapidly increasing antral volume, a coincident increase of intrafollicular pressure does not occur, suggesting an increased distensibility of the follicle.[27] Both progesterone, a potent smooth muscle relaxant, and proteolytic enzymes such as plasmin and collagenase are contained in follicular fluid; they have been implicated in this phenomenon.[28, 29] Before follicular rupture the antrum remains avascular; during and after release of the ovum, transient hemorrhage and neovascular development are prominent preludes to formation of the corpus luteum. Recent studies have demonstrated angiogenic activity in follicular fluid of animals and women (Fig. 116–7).[30, 31]

Luteal Function as a Sequel to Folliculogenesis

During typical normal menstrual cycles in which pregnancy is not initiated, the life span of the corpus luteum is limited to 12 to 16 days. Corpus luteum function is established after ovulation, when the newly ruptured follicle completes luteinization. Throughout the luteal phase progesterone and estradiol are the principal steroidal secretory products of the corpus luteum, although other hormones, such as relaxin, are also secreted. Supplementation of agonadal patients with only progesterone and estradiol is sufficient for the establishment and maintenance of pregnancy.[32, 33] In the nonfertile menstrual cycle this transient endocrine milieu is truncated by spontaneous regression of the corpus luteum, marked by cessation of progesterone secretion and menstruation. In a fertile cycle hCG from the placenta induces prolongation of the luteal phase by extension of corpus luteum function. Although the role of luteal progesterone in the support of gestation is incompletely understood, its requirement for nidation and maintenance of intrauterine early pregnancy is well established.[34] Indeed, deficiencies in either the duration of progesterone secretion or the amount secreted during the postovulatory phase of the menstrual cycle have been

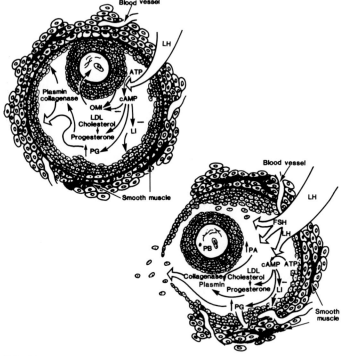

FIGURE 116–7. Mechanism of ovulation. (1) Rising LH levels stimulate an increase in cAMP. (2) cAMP mediates luteinization and resumption of meiosis, overcoming the action of local inhibitors, luteinization inhibitor (LI), and oocyte maturation inhibitor (OMI). (3) As luteinization proceeds, progesterone levels rise, enhancing the activity of proteolytic enzymes and increasing follicle wall distensibility. (4) Prostaglandin (PG) levels increase and, together with plasmin and collagenase, may serve to digest the follicle wall. (5) The midcycle LH surge brings about completion of reduction division and formation of the first polar body (PB). (6) Midcycle FSH stimulates expansion of the cumulus and production of plasminogen activator (PA). (7) Continued enzymatic digestion results in follicle wall rupture. (8) PG's may stimulate contraction of smooth muscle in the theca externa, causing oocyte expulsion. (9) Branching vessels penetrate the luteinized granulosa. (From Fritz MA, Speroff L: The endocrinology of the menstrual cycle: The interaction of folliculogenesis and neuroendocrine mechanisms. Fertil Steril 38:509, 1982.)

widely correlated with reproductive failure. Whether extra-uterine pregnancy requires progestational support is unknown.

Deficiencies in progesterone secretion by the corpus luteum lead to inappropriate (delayed) endometrial development such that normal nidation is impaired or prevented. As originally reported, the *short luteal phase* defect in women was defined as a duration of eight days or less from ovulation to menses.[35, 36] A second luteal phase abnormality has been termed the *inadequate luteal phase,* in which the interval from ovulation to menses is normal but progesterone output is subnormal.[37, 38]

Inappropriate patterns of circulating pituitary gonadotropins lead to abnormalities in the developing dominant follicle and, in turn, the corpus luteum. For example, relative FSH deficiency results in decreased estrogen secretion in the proliferative phase and decreased progesterone secretion in the secretory phase. From the initial defect in FSH action, estradiol is not maximally secreted; these two hormones within the microenvironment of the follicle are then at suboptimal levels for both FSH and, later, LH receptor induction on the granulosa cells as well as proliferation of the granulosa cells. Consequently, the uterine end-organ is understimulated. Therefore, pituitary and ovarian derangements during folliculogenesis are likely to limit luteal function and fertility.

The first morphological signs of luteinization begin concurrently with the preovulatory LH surge. Thus ovulation transforms the dominant structure of the ovarian cycle from primarily an estrogen source (before ovulation) to an equally transient endocrine tissue that principally secretes progesterone after ovulation. The main sites of progesterone synthesis and secretion are the granulosa-luteal cells, but their metabolic capabilities are surely linked with those of the thecal compartment, especially in the preovulatory interval.[39]

Studies of human follicles and antral fluid have suggested that at least three criteria need to be fulfilled before the rupturing follicle can be transformed into an appropriately functional corpus luteum: (1) there must be sufficient numbers of granulosa cells in the follicle before ovulation because thereafter granulosa-luteal cells cease proliferation; (2) the follicle must contain granulosa cells with the capacity to secrete sufficient progesterone after ovulation; and (3) the granulosa cells, as well as the theca cells, must be responsive to trophic stimuli, especially LH and/or hCG.[40] In culture, granulosa cells undergo the highest rate of mitosis when they are harvested from follicles that contain elevated levels of FSH in the antral fluid.[41–43] Conversely, in follicles with lower FSH concentrations, little estradiol was present in the antral fluid regardless of the number of granulosa cells present. Evidence derived in vitro suggests that the FSH delays degeneration of granulosa cells. Granulosa cells from antral follicles grown in a culture medium devoid of FSH undergo atresia. In contrast, when FSH is present the cells remain viable longer and retain steroidogenic responsiveness to trophic stimuli. Thus, without adequate FSH support, the dominant follicle cannot develop normally for its sequel, the functioning corpus luteum.[44–46] However, the capacity of FSH to extend follicular viability is finite; atresia eventually occurs despite continued FSH therapy.

Foremost among the functional characteristics of luteal phase deficiency is the frequent inability of the corpus luteum to adequately respond to hCG, thereby precluding one of the earliest events in maternal recognition of pregnancy. Even among normal corpora lutea, the decline of luteal function in the late luteal phase is associated with a decrease in responsiveness of the luteal cells to hCG. The progressive inability of the corpus luteum to respond to LH or hCG in the late luteal phase may be associated with the loss of receptors. In instances of luteal phase defects, luteal cells are likely to be deficient in LH or hCG receptors and/or the intracellular apparatus needed to mediate progesterone secretion. FSH, augmented by estrogen, induces expression of LH receptors during folliculogenesis. It follows that appropriate gonadotropin secretion in the antecedent follicular phase is the principal determinant of the normalcy of subsequent corpus luteum function.

Luteolysis describes the declining capacity of the corpus luteum to produce progesterone and estradiol. Is the demise of the corpus luteum an active process, or merely a passive response secondary to a relative gonadotropin deficiency, that is, tonic LH in the nonfertile cycle and hCG in the fertile menstrual cycle? In cycles of conception hCG is secreted at increased levels that are detectable as early as 8 to 10 days post ovulation[47]; this defines the beginning of the "window" through which the corpus luteum may be "rescued" from luteolysis. Interestingly, it has been demonstrated that the corpus luteum can be revived by hourly GnRH pulse therapy during both the postpartum nursing interval[48] and the subsequent early follicular phase after a nonfertile menstrual cycle.

Alternatively, luteolysis may be an active process; rising estrogen levels in the midluteal phase can decrease progesterone secretion. This mechanism may act through suppression of LH secretion or by decreasing intra-ovarian LH actions. The process can be reversed by prostaglandin synthesis inhibitors, which implicates a role for these substances. The intra-ovarian production of PGF_2 increases in the late luteal phase, and PGF_2 can directly inhibit progesterone synthesis.[49] Another nonsteroidal ovarian factor, LH receptor binding inhibitor, has been identified in rats and shown to increase throughout the luteal phase.[25]

Lastly, there is an event known as the luteal-placental shift, when the maintenance of pregnancy can be totally subsumed by hormones derived from the conceptus, indeed, in the absence of ovaries. Human studies in which the corpus luteum was eliminated suggest that the ovaries are dispensable after the seventh to eighth week of pregnancy.[34] Castration of luteectomy before this interval is associated with high abortion rates; thus progesterone supplementation in early pregnancy aids the maintenance of gestation until the conceptus has achieved autonomy from ovarian support.

Follicular Atresia

Most developing follicles degenerate; only about 200 ovulate during reproductive life in macaques and about 400 in the human. Although the atretic process is characterized morphologically by cell death, the theca interna of some atretic follicles may become involved in folliculogenesis. In these atretic follicles the theca interna hypertrophies and forms interstitial gland tissue. This tissue is abundant during ovulation in macaque ovaries, late in

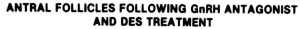

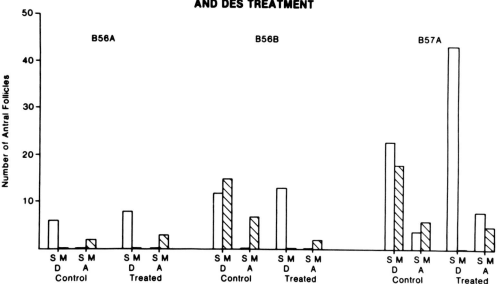

FIGURE 116–8. Status of the number of small (S) (< 0.5 mm) and medium (M)-sized (0.5 to 1.0 mm) developing (D) and early-atretic (A) antral follicles in the left (control) ovary before and in the right (treated) ovary after GnRH antagonist and diethylstilbestrol treatment in three juvenile monkeys. (From Koering M et al: Early folliculogenesis in primate ovaries: Testing the role of estrogen. Biol Reprod 45:890–897, 1991.

pregnancy in the human and in some new-world monkeys, and may have secretory activity.[50]

To recognize atresia certain morphological criteria have been established, even though it is likely that the initial cellular stages of degeneration have already occurred at the molecular level. For preantral follicles the best indicator is degenerative changes in the oocyte, since the granulosa cells appear normal. In the rhesus monkey preantral follicle atresia is minimal. In antral follicles the best evidence for regression is the presence of pyknotic nuclei in granulosa cells lining the lumen. Such a nuclear change has been used to identify cellular degeneration in other tissues. It has been shown, however, that larger developing follicles can have a small percentage of granulosa cells with pyknotic nuclei in both the human and the monkey. With advancing regression the number of degenerating granulosa cells increases. The basement (glassy) membrane thickens as the follicle collapses. Finally, the glassy membrane is the only visual remnant of atretic follicles.

In macaque ovaries early atresia is most prevalent in medium-sized (0.5 to 1.0 mm) antral follicles. Similarly, atretic follicles are most common in an equivalent size range in the human. After selection of the dominant follicle in the monkey, the percentage of medium-sized follicles increases, which suggests that the competing follicles can no longer survive in the new microenvironment where the dominant follicle has taken control.[50]

The process of apoptosis has been studied to elucidate the mechanism that programs cell death in ovarian follicles.[51]

In both the adult cycling monkey and the human, specific stimulation of certain primordial follicles and their development into antral follicles are required. After attaining about 1 mm in diameter in the monkey and 4 to 5 mm in diameter in the human, these follicles degenerate if not adequately supported by FSH.[52] The same growth pattern is clearly seen in ovaries from immature rhesus monkeys, where the hypothalamic-pituitary axis is still juvenile and plasma gonadotropins are low. This suggests that the growth of follicles from primordial into the medium-sized

category in these primates does not rely strictly on gonadotropic stimulation. The hormonal regulation of this process remains unknown.

The data obtained on preantral follicles in primate ovaries differ from observations in the immature hypophysectomized rat, in which preantral follicle development proliferated in the presence of diethylstilbestrol or estradiol treatment. In addition, in the rat there is an increased responsiveness to FSH, which results in the enhancement of antrum formation and seems to be mediated by way of the theca interna. In contrast, antrum formation in the monkey occurs in an environment devoid of FSH (Fig. 116–8). Developing antral follicles can attain diameters up to 1 mm before becoming sensitive to FSH, as seen both in immature monkeys studied here and in adult monkeys. Similarly, developing antral follicles characterize the ovary of human infants.[52]

OVULATION INDUCTION FOR ASSISTED REPRODUCTIVE TECHNOLOGIES

Controlled Ovarian Hyperstimulation

In vitro fertilization with embryo transfer (IVF-ET) is now a widespread and well-accepted therapy for infertility secondary to fallopian tube obstruction. It is also being applied for problems of oligospermia, severe endometriosis, and cervical factor infertility. In these settings the female patient usually is endocrinologically normal with regular cyclic ovarian function. The steps of IVF are, briefly, as follows: (1) ovarian stimulation to achieve multiple follicular development; (2) recovery of oocytes by needle aspiration, usually at ultrasonography; (3) inspection, incubation, and grading of oocytes for maturity and suitability for fertilization; (4) addition of washed sperm; (5) incubation and inspection for fertilization and cleavage of the embryo; and then (6) transcervical transfer of the embryo to the uterus.

Before the era of IVF much of the information on the

physiology of the human menstrual cycle was based on peripheral blood hormone measurements and focused on ovarian hormonogenesis and its interactions with the central nervous system–hypothalamic–pituitary axis. The ability to examine follicular fluids and oocytes obtained by aspiration during the natural cycle or after a defined stimulation protocol has provided a technique by which ovarian hormonogenesis can be correlated with gametogenesis, fertilizability of the gamete, and even viability of the early conceptus.

Early experience with monitoring the "natural cycle" provided important information on the variability of the temporal relations of prostaglandin E_2 (PGE_2), LH, and ovulation during the menstrual cycle. For example, the estradiol peak in the periovulatory interval may occur for 24 to 72 hours before the onset of the LH surge in both animals and humans.[20, 21, 53] It was also observed that ovulation occurred about 28 hours after the onset of the ascending limb of the LH surge.

The first IVF birth was accomplished without ovarian stimulation—in the natural cycle. Further experience confirmed that there were problems related to timing the follicular aspiration because of variability in the temporal relation of the estradiol peak to the LH surge. In addition to measurement timing, the overall pregnancy rates of IVF with the natural cycle were low. Methods to promote multiple follicular development have proved superior to the natural cycle not only in terms of increased oocyte yield but also in allowing more controlled protocols of ovarian stimulation. This control, achieved by the administration of exogenous agents that override the natural cycle, has resulted in increased pregnancy rates in IVF programs worldwide. Stimulation of endocrinologically normal menstruating females with exogenous gonadotropins also offers new insight into basic feedback mechanisms and increases our understanding of gonadotropin–granulosa cell–oocyte interaction.

Stimulation of the Natural Cycle

A number of treatment methods have been used to obtain multiple follicle development and increased oocyte retrieval.[54, 55] Minor variations exist between clinics, but these methods are as follows.

1. *Gonadotropins plus hCG.* By administering exogenous FSH, with or without LH, multiple follicular stimulation can be reliably achieved. At this level of ovarian stimulation, spontaneous LH surges occur infrequently, and therefore, hCG must be added to complete intrafollicular oocyte development. This method is discussed in detail below as a paradigm example of ovarian stimulation in the endocrinologically normal patient.

2. *Clomiphene citrate alone.* This strategy most resembles the natural cycle and relies on an endogenous LH surge. Because of the resultant increase in gonadotropins that is promoted by this anti-estrogen, there often is multiple follicular development. The problems of timing inherent with awaiting a spontaneous LH surge have made this approach less popular for IVF.

3. *Clomiphene citrate plus hCG.* Here a pharmacological "LH surge" is provided when parameters of follicle development, ultrasonography, and/or peripheral estradiol lev-

els reach a critical level indicative of impending maturity. Consequently, the problems of timing oocyte recovery are diminished by predetermining the "LH surge" and, thus, the retrieval at optimal times after that surge.

4. *Clomiphene citrate, gonadotropin, and hCG.* The combination of all three agents has provided another reliable method of ovarian stimulation practiced in many IVF programs. The addition of gonadotropins, usually after or concurrent with the clomiphene, extends the increased follicular growth initiated by clomiphene citrate.

Gonadotropin Stimulation for Assisted Reproductive Technologies

Although various centers have used gonadotropins in different regimens with success, here we discuss a gonadotropin-only protocol used at the Howard and Georgeanna Jones Institute for Reproductive Medicine in Norfolk, Virginia, to provide a basis for presentation and discussion. This gonadotropin-plus-hCG protocol has been successfully executed with pure FSH preparations and equal combinations of FSH and LH, the latter constituting the usual urinary preparation of human menopausal gonadotropins (hMG).

Two to four ampules (150 to 300 IU of FSH and LH) usually are administered beginning about day 3 of the menstrual cycle. The hMG is administered at 1600 hours. Rapid serum estrogen assays are performed daily in the morning along with ultrasonography. Sonographic examinations are performed beginning on day 6 of the cycle. hMG therapy usually is discontinued when the largest follicular diameter on sonography approaches 17 mm. Decisions to discontinue hMG injections are based on a combination of ovarian sonography, serum estradiol levels above 300 pg/ml, and estrogenic manifestations in cervical mucus. hCG most often is administered as a single 10,000-IU injection about 50 hours after gonadotropic stimulation is discontinued. Follicular aspiration is performed about 35 hours after hCG administration to avoid spontaneous ovulations, which frequently begin to occur 36 hours after hCG administration.

Changes in the FSH-LH ratio during the first two days of treatment have been found to influence the number of follicles developed. Increasing the amount of FSH administered during days 3 and 4 by adding 150 IU of pure FSH to the previously administered hMG (usually 150 IU of FSH and LH) increased the number of large follicles obtained and the yield of fertilized oocytes per cycle. This is shown in Table 116–1,[56] in which the number of oocytes obtained and the number of concepti transferred are compared using more versus less FSH therapy.

This is especially important, since a person's response to a given regimen is repetitive (Fig. 116–9). The response can be influenced by changing the first two days of treatment, during which more FSH promotes a greater response.

The tendency toward repetitive patterns exists in measurements of peripheral estradiol levels in response to a fixed hMG stimulation protocol. Relative to the time a clinical shift toward an estrogen milieu is detected (thinning of cervical mucus), these response patterns have been arbitrarily characterized as low for patients whose serum

TABLE 116–1. IVF RESULTS USING DIFFERENT COMBINATIONS OF GONADOTROPIN THERAPY IN RELATION TO STIMULATION ON DAYS 3 AND 4 OF CYCLE

STIMULATION	DAILY GONADOTROPIN REGIMENS		
	2 hMG/hCG	2 FSH/2 hMG/hCG	4 FSH/hCG
Pre-ov/laparoscopy	1.59	3.04	3.09
Pre-ov/total no. oocytes	41%	49%	53%
Pre-ov/cycle with transfer	1.63	2.86	2.7
Total oocytes transferred/transfer cycle	2.1	3.93	3.90
Pregnancy rate/transfer	23.8%	27%	23%

Each ampule of hMG contains 75 IU FSH and 75 IU LH; each ampule of FSH contains 75 IU without LH. The hCG was administered as a 10,000-IU single injection. (From Bernardus R et al: The significance of the ratio in follicle-stimulating hormone and leuteinizing hormone in induction of multiple follicular growth. Fertil Steril 43:373–378, 1985.)

estradiol levels remain below 300 pg/ml, intermediate for patients with circulating estradiol of 300 to 600 pg/ml, and high for patients with estradiol levels greater than 600 pg/ml (Fig. 116–10).[57]

Among these endocrinologically normal ovulating women, treatment with hMG almost always results in inhibition of the estrogen-induced LH surge. In intermediate normal and high responders serum levels of estradiol equal to or greater than those found nearing ovulation in spontaneous cycles (Fig. 116–10) usually do not bring a spontaneous LH surge competent for ovulation.

It has been suggested that this inhibition of positive estrogen feedback in patients with a presumably normally

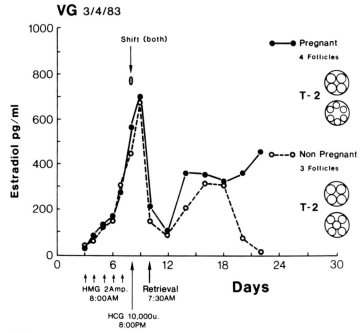

FIGURE 116–9. The pattern of estradiol response, given the same stimulation, is remarkably repetitive from cycle to cycle in the same patient 0 shift refers to the time of the thinning of the cervical mucus. Oocyte retrieval occurred on day 9. (From Jones GS: Update on *in vitro* fertilization. Endocr Rev 5:62, 1984.)

responsive hypothalamic-pituitary axis is due to a putative inhibitory substance called gonadotropin surge-inhibiting factor produced by supraphysiological ovarian stimulation.[58] In monkeys similarly stimulated with exogenous gonadotropins, removal of the ovaries rapidly reverses this pituitary refractoriness. The observation that endogenous gonadotropin secretion is inhibited during exogenous gonadotropin administration may contribute to the repetitiveness of individual response to a given stimulation protocol and permit the correlation of a given stimulation with granulosa cell response and, ultimately, pregnancy outcome. Indeed, the pregnancy rate and quality of oocytes retrieved are correlated with secretory characteristics of PGE_2 from the ovaries.

A surprising finding during the stimulation of endocrinologically normal monkeys was the brisk serum estradiol response pattern using "pure" FSH that is devoid of any discernible LH bioactivity.[59] The responses of women undergoing IVF-ET therapy are similar.

"Pure" FSH stimulation was initiated as an adjunct in an effort to increase the number of follicles in patients who exhibited an insufficient follicular recruitment in response to the standard hMG regimen described above. FSH alone has also been administered in similar dosage and manner as described above for hMG. Here 300 IU of "pure" FSH is given intramuscularly on days 3 and 4 of the cycle followed by 150 IU daily after day 5 until estradiol levels of 300 to 600 pg/ml are reached and the largest follicular diameter is increased to about 14 mm by ultrasonography. The low endogenous LH levels are sufficient to sustain follicle growth stimulated by exogenous pure FSH.

Apparently owing to inhibitory feedback by ovarian factors, endogenous gonadotropin secretions are significantly reduced. Follicular development proceeds with an increased number of large follicles, increased oocyte recovery, and more oocytes fertilized. Preliminary findings with this FSH-rich protocol indicate a higher pregnancy rate in these patients.[60, 61] Therefore, estrogen synthesis as well as oocyte maturation may proceed normally in the absence of exogenous LH. These findings agree with previous observations in monkeys. In monkeys a model for "medical hypophysectomy" by way of a GnRH antagonist causes low or undetectable endogenous serum levels of pituitary gonadotropins. Follicular development and estrogen steroidogenesis with "pure" FSH stimulation are equal to that induced by the FSH-LH combination in hMG. Furthermore, GnRH antagonist plus "pure" FSH induce follicles that achieve ovulation of fertilizable oocytes after hCG treatment. These human and nonhuman primate data raise questions as to the relative importance of FSH versus LH in the follicular phase of the primate menstrual cycle. Indeed, FSH may be of far greater significance than LH until the peri-ovulatory interval.

Oocyte Morphology

Follicular development is a reflection of granulosa and theca cell proliferation, with an increasing steroidogenic capacity by these cells. Maturation of follicles is accompanied by increased follicular volume and enhanced synthesis of various follicular fluid constituents, both steroidal and nonsteroidal. Aspiration at about 34 hours after hCG administration reveals that most preovulatory (mature) oocytes are derived from larger follicles (average volume greater than 2.5 ml per follicle). When aspirate volumes of 1 ml or less are obtained, the incidence of immature and degenerate oocytes is strikingly higher.[62, 63]

After aspiration, oocytes are classified as preovulatory (mature), immature, or atretic on the basis of nuclear morphology and the appearance of the associated granulosa cell mass. A mature oocyte has an expanded cumulus mass with a radiant corona, germinal vesicle breakdown, and an extruded first polar body. The granulosa cells of mature oocytes are spread out as opposed to being clumped. Individually, these cells are large, plump, and without dark lipid-filled cytoplasm (Fig. 116–11A). In contrast, immature oocytes have a small unexpanded cumulus, a tight corona, and no polar bodies, and a germinal vesicle often is still present in the ooplasm (Fig. 116–11B). These small granulosa cells have little cytoplasm and often are found in clumps. Thus during egg maturation the cumulus cells that surround the oocyte undergo a synchronous transformation with the oocyte from a compact mass to a dispersed and mucified structure. Mucification involves the deposition of a hyaluronic acid matrix, the synthesis of which is thought to be stimulated by FSH.[64] Follicular fluid from mature oocyte cumulus cells contained higher FSH concentrations than that from follicles containing an immature oocyte.[65] Oocytes and cumulus cells derived from cycles of "pure" FSH therapy often display more asynchronous oocyte granulosa development than after hMG. The oocyte may still contain the germinal vesicle, whereas the cumulus is fully expanded. This suggests that oocyte maturation may be a more LH-dependent phenomenon, whereas granulosa cell development may be primarily FSH-dependent. Most degenerate or atretic oocytes have no cumulus mass. The naked egg typically has dark ooplasm

pulled away from the zona with distortion. If present, the associated granulosa cells are dark and clumped to one another.

Abnormalities of the zona pellucida may be characterized by fractures, especially prevalent among postmature eggs. These may be seen as a small defect, a poorly defined zona, or fragments of zona. Such abnormalities of the gamete occasionally are associated with mature, normal-appearing granulosa cells. Follicular fluid volumes associated with oocytes that have damaged zona pellucidae often are similar to the volume obtained from follicles with a preovulatory oocyte. This is consistent with an interpretation of postmaturity among such inferior eggs.

Oocyte development, as reflected by morphological criteria, can be predicted in part from estradiol response patterns. High and intermediate responders have a greater proportion of preovulatory (mature) oocytes than do the low-estradiol responders.[66] That more favorable development has occurred is reflected by the fact that 90 per cent of aspirated preovulatory oocytes fertilize, whereas only 65 per cent of the immature oocytes do so, despite being allowed to mature in vitro before insemination.

Microenvironment, Steroidogenesis, and Oocyte Maturity

Studies of follicular fluids and aspirated granulosa cells have allowed assessment of the follicular microenvironment and its relation to oocyte maturity, the potential for fertilization, and the ultimate success of the conceptus. Several investigators have noted that follicular status and oocyte viability correlate with high concentrations of estrogens and low concentrations of androgens in follicular fluid. Presumably, estrogen is required to sustain granulosa

FIGURE 116–10. Serum LH and 17β-estradiol (E₂) in hMG/hCG stimulated cycles, normalized to the time of hCG administration (day 0). The three E₂ responses are represented. All cycles resulted in aspiration of preovulatory oocytes. (From Ferraretti AP, et al: Serum LH during ovulation induction with human menopausal gonadotropin for *in vitro* fertilization in normally menstruating women. Fertil Steril 40:742, 1983.)

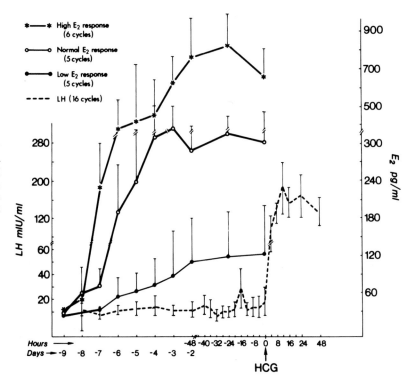

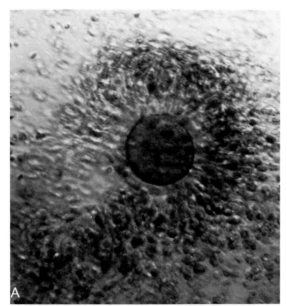

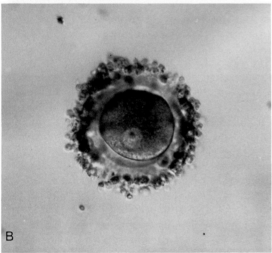

FIGURE 116–11. *A*, Preovulatory (mature) oocyte. Note the expanded cumulus mass, radiant corona, and absence of germinal vesicle. The first polar body is not visualized. *B*, Immature oocyte. Note the germinal vesicle, unexpanded cumulus, and tight corona. No polar bodies are seen. (Photographs courtesy of Lucinda Veeck.)

cell mitosis, whereas FSH is necessary to permit the granulosa and theca cells to aromatize androgens to estrogens. Fluid obtained at aspiration for IVF therapy from follicles that contain mature oocytes has a higher progesterone concentration than fluid aspirated from follicles that contain immature oocytes.[62] Furthermore, granulosa cells isolated from preovulatory follicles secrete large quantities of progesterone, compared with granulosa cells from follicles that contain immature oocytes. This ability to synthesize progesterone may reflect the degree of luteinization of the granulosa cells, which is the culmination of previous exposure to FSH and estrogens, induction by FSH or LH receptors, and, therefore, subsequent responsiveness to hCG when it is presented to the follicle. Indeed, the hallmark of granulosa cell maturity, and perhaps that of theca cell maturity too, is the conversion to a luteinized progesterone-secreting unit in temporal concert with the periovulatory cascade.[67] One must bear in mind that the principal difference between ovarian stimulation for IVF-ET and true ovulation induction for anovulatory states is that in IVF, all the oocytes used are aspirated within the same hour, whereas in true ovulation induction, eggs are released for as long as four to five days after hCG treatment; thus disparity of oocyte maturity may be greater in IVF therapy.

OVULATION INDUCTION FOR ANOVULATORY STATES

Axiomatic Considerations

In achieving ovulation induction in anovulatory conditions, the objective is to modify the pathophysiological condition toward replication of the temporal, quantitative, and qualitative events of the natural fertile menstrual cycle. Any treatment regimen undertaken requires both ovarian follicles that can respond to endogenous or exogenous gonadotropins and a milieu within the reproductive tract that is conducive to intrauterine conception. Because defects of the ovarian cycle are the primary cause in 15 to 20 per cent of infertile couples, the need to more fully understand the origins and mechanisms of this ovarian pathophysiology continues.

Whereas some anovulatory infertility is almost absolute, other forms manifest sporadic intervals of spontaneous ovulation. Oligoovulation may have occult abnormalities so subtle that they defy detection. Indeed, the degree of derangement within the hypothalamic-pituitary-ovarian-uterine axis is a primary factor in choosing an appropriate therapeutic course. The pretreatment evaluation usually is critical in determining the opportunity for success of ovulation induction. When the overall health status of the patient is understood, then reversal of pathophysiology is the first objective. Not uncommonly some patients in evaluation spontaneously ovulate and become pregnant before therapeutic intervention. When the infertility has persisted for two or more years, attainment of successful pregnancy seldom occurs without medical or surgical treatment.

Anovulation most often results from either a relative or an absolute gonadotropin deficiency or imbalance. Accordingly, the next consideration is the method of elevating or correcting biologically active gonadotropin levels in circulation. This may be achieved by enhancement of endogenous pituitary gonadotropin secretion or by administration of gonadotropins of pituitary or urinary origin. Recent developments foretell the availability of FSH, LH, and hCG synthesized by recombinant DNA technology in the near future.

Whatever the method used for ovulation induction, the follicular phase conditions must allow progressive maturation of one or more ovarian follicles with concurrent proliferation of the uterine endometrium. If a timely LH surge does not occur spontaneously, its effects may be mimicked by an injection of hCG, which acts as a surrogate LH surge. Further, the oocyte or egg released by rupture of a mature ovarian follicle will have resumed first meiosis in response to the preovulatory LH surge or hCG treatment. Thus the haploid nucleus and its surrounding investments are rendered competent for fertilization.

In the luteal phase both the secretory endometrium and the normalcy of the corpus luteum are primary determinants of successful ovulation induction. Not uncommonly the iatrogenic effects of the therapeutic course contribute to failure in treatment. Forcing an oocyte out of the ovary is not sufficient to suppose a good opportunity of achieving pregnancy. Indeed, both the gametogenic and the hormonogenic factors must act in concert during ovulation induction, as they do in the spontaneous fertile menstrual cycle.

Means for Intervention

OVARIAN WEDGE RESECTION. Even before medical therapies for ovulation induction were available, the elimination of one third to one half of the ovarian mass from patients presenting with polycystic ovarian disease often induced ovulation, ovarian cyclicity lasting for a few months to years. The means by which this disease prevents ovulation is not fully understood; it is clear, however, that the wedge resection often accommodates a disinhibition involving a relative FSH deficiency and an LH excess. FSH levels usually rise after wedge resection, either because steroid effects centrally and/or locally are diminished or in part because of the reduction of purported inhibin levels secreted in excess by ovarian cells of the woman with polycystic ovaries. Liabilities of the wedge resection include adhesive disease, limited efficacy, and operative risks. Accordingly, it is now infrequently applied.[68, 69]

BROMOCRIPTINE. Central defects that result in hyperprolactinemia can cause an associated deficiency of gonadotropin secretion. Administration of the ergot alkaloid bromocriptine, a dopamine agonist, frequently can inhibit pituitary prolactin release concurrent with resumption of the ovarian cycle and ovulation in patients presenting with overt hyperprolactinemia. The primacy of prolactin in mediating the anovulation has yet to be conclusively demonstrated. As the level of prolactin in circulation declines into the normal range, pituitary gonadotropin secretion rises, often promoting the resumption of fertile menstrual cycles almost immediately.[70] Bromocriptine has been shown to have efficacy in some normoprolactinemic anovulatory patients.[71]

CLOMIPHENE CITRATE. The indications favoring use of this nonsteroidal weak estrogen are paradoxical yet convincing. The best results occur in patients who are already near the threshold for spontaneous ovulation. Indeed, significant extant pituitary and ovarian function is essential to any clomiphene citrate regimen. Sufficient endogenous estrogen to a level allowing withdrawal bleeding after a progesterone challenge indicates an appropriate patient for this form of ovulation induction therapy. Despite more than 20 years of its broad application, the real mechanism by which clomiphene citrate promotes ovulation is only partially deciphered.[72] In part, administration of clomiphene citrate in the midfollicular phase causes transient small elevations of gonadotropin secretion. Both quantitative changes in FSH and/or LH and enhanced responsiveness of ovarian follicles to prevailing gonadotropin levels may contribute to the promotion of fertile ovulations. The previously discussed mechanism for selection of one dominant follicle can be overcome, and it is not uncommon for patients who receive clomiphene citrate to mature up to three follicles during a cycle of therapy. Importantly, a hyperstimulation syndrome (see below) is infrequently observed with this agent. When clomiphene citrate is given from days 5 to 9 of the "cycle," a spontaneous LH surge usually develops by days 15 to 17; if it does not, hCG may be used to accomplish ovulation (Fig. 116–12). Other regimens that use this agent are also effective, especially if given earlier in the follicular phase, before selection of the spontaneous dominant follicle or in combination with gonadotropin therapy.[73–76]

EXOGENOUS GONADOTROPINS. Among anovulatory patients, those most deficient in pituitary gonadotropin and estrogen secretion—that is, hypopituitary-hypogonadal women—often are appropriate candidates for administration of gonadotropins. This is particularly true when pituitary response to GnRH is diminished or the pituitary is absent. The primary advantage to ovulation induction by direct injection of gonadotropin preparations is the high rate of ovarian response to the supraphysiological levels of FSH and/or LH provided. Several follicles usually mature quasi-synchronously, with spontaneous LH surges often absent (Fig. 116–13). Accordingly, the injection of hCG as the surrogate LH surge frequently leads to multiple ovulations, with a significant rate of multiple pregnancies if the stimulation is excessive. Hyperstimulation syndrome, which can result in a massive third-space fluid shift into the peritoneal cavity and even ovarian rupture, is a very real potential adverse effect. The use of daily rapid estrogen assays, along with ovarian sonographic monitoring, greatly diminishes the risks of this problem.[77–79]

A supraphysiological FSH-LH milieu created during gon-

CLOMIPHENE THERAPY
(CONVENTIONAL)

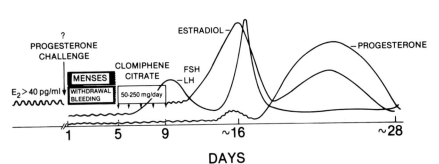

FIGURE 116–12. Conceptual illustration of a conventional regimen of clomiphene citrate for ovulation induction. Note that initial circulating estradiol (E_2) levels (best results at or above 40 pg/ml) must be high enough to augment the transient elevation of serum FSH and LH derived from clomiphene treatment. Spontaneous menses or previous progesterone withdrawal bleeding indicates sufficient estrogen for endometrial proliferation and ovulation induction.

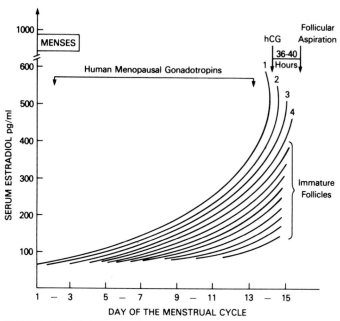

INDUCED FOLLICULAR MATURATION
hMG/hCG

FIGURE 116–13. hMG-stimulated follicular maturation overrides selection of a single dominant follicle in the natural cycle. Note that only a few follicles can be regarded to be developing quasi-synchronously. If hCG is given too late, the most advanced follicles may yield postmature eggs of low potential viability. (From Hodgen GD: Hormonal stimulation of the natural ovarian cycle and oocyte transfer for fertilization in vivo. In Crosignini P and Rubin BL (eds): Proceedings from the Serono Symposium of In Vitro Fertilization and Embryo Transfer. New York, Academic Press, 1983, p 239.)

adotropin administration prevents the selection of a single dominant follicle, as in the natural cycle. Further, maturation of the most advanced follicle is hastened such that maturity often is achieved by day 7 to day 10 of the treatment regimen, compared with about 14 days in the normal menstrual cycle. Thus the "ovarian clock" can be accelerated by supraphysiological levels of gonadotropins. FSH is paramount in ovulation induction until the need for an LH surge effect for follicular rupture and oocyte nuclear and ooplasmic maturation.[59]

PULSATILE GnRH. The elucidation of the importance of pulse amplitude and frequency in the regulation of pituitary gonadotropin secretion has brought a new solution to ovulation induction when the causative factor is a lesion of

hypothalamic function. That is, the absence of appropriate pulsatile stimulation of the pituitary by GnRH (Kallmann's syndrome, hypogonadotropic hypogonadism, or olfacto-genital dysplasia) can be efficaciously treated by the use of "mechanical hypothalamus." The patient typically wears a belt or strap that holds a small pulse pump programmed to inject GnRH, 1 to 20 μg per pulse, at intervals of about 60 to 120 minutes, mimicking the natural overt GnRH pulse frequency in the normal follicular phase (Fig. 116–14). Interestingly, even with an unvarying intermittent pulse schedule and a wide dose range, both subcutaneously and intravenously, the temporal and endocrine characteristics of cycles induced by GnRH pulse therapy are similar to those of the spontaneous menstrual cycle if the dose is within certain limits. Spontaneous LH surges normally occur when there is maturation of one dominant follicle. Some evidence suggests that high-amplitude GnRH pulses may promote multiple follicular development,[80] but this may only be a reflection of asynchronous pituitary discharges during the early stages of exposure to the administered GnRH. Indeed, the risk of multiple ovulations and multiple pregnancies with pulsatile GnRH may be increased either early in the course of therapy or if the dose is too high. In patients without sufficient endogenous LH, the corpus luteum depends on continued GnRH pulse therapy throughout the luteal phase, although the dose, frequency, and amplitude may change from that of the follicular phase. Alternatively, hCG can be substituted as a means of corpus luteum support.

Recent findings persuade us that the infusion interval is a key factor in determining dose–response patterns. Similarly, intravenous versus subcutaneous administration may radially affect efficacy, patient tolerance, and the multiple pregnancy rate.

Because of the ability of differential dose frequencies to change FSH-LH ratios, it is likely that GnRH pulse pump therapy will also be applicable to the treatment of polycystic ovarian disease in certain patients who require only a minimal increase of FSH secretion to resume ovulatory menstrual cycles.[81–84]

SUMMARY AND FUTURE

Throughout the 1980's ovarian physiologists have increasingly recognized the need to understand ovarian folliculogenesis at the paracrine and autocrine levels of cellu-

FIGURE 116–14. Ovulation can be induced by pulsatile administration of GnRH for treatment of secondary amenorrhea and anovulatory infertility in primates. A mechanical pump delivered GnRH pulse (6 μg per pulse, IV) once every 90 minutes. Note the elevation of circulating estrogen levels emanating from the dominant follicle before ovulation followed by normal serum progesterone levels in the luteal phase with continued GnRH therapy. In these monkeys with secondary amenorrhea (greater than eight months), only three weeks of GnRH therapy were required to induce ovulation. (From Sopelak VM et al: A mechanical "hypothalamus" for ovulation induction therapy. JAMA 251:1477, copyright 1984, the American Medical Association.)

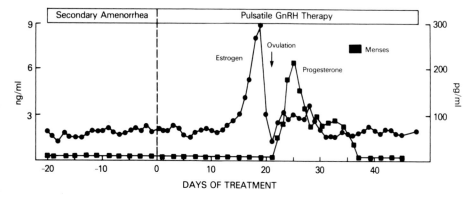

lar regulation, in addition to the more traditional endocrine approaches. Clearly, elucidation of the roles of growth factors that regulate theca, granulosa, and germ cell responses to the stimulation of gonadotropin receptors, and clarification of neovascular events will soon explain some of the mysteries, while raising new questions.[85] The important issue as to whether apoptosis among these cell populations is causal or reflective of follicular atresia may soon be elucidated.[51]

REFERENCES

1. Irianni F, Hodgen GD: Mechanism of ovulation. Endocrinol Metab Clin North Am 21:19–38, 1992.
2. Peters H: Folliculogenesis in mammals. In Jones RE (ed): The Vertebrate Ovary. New York, Plenum Press, 1978, pp 121–140.
3. Brambell FWR: Ovarian changes. In Parkes AS (ed): Marshall's Physiology of Reproduction. New York, Longman, 1956, p 397.
4. Sandow BA, Veeck LL, Acosta AA, Garcia JE: Asynchronous oocyte maturation in polyovular follicles aspirated for in vitro fertilization. Fertil Steril 39:424, 1983.
5. Singh RP, Carr DH: The anatomy and histology of XO human embryos and fetuses. Anat Rec 155:369, 1966.
6. Marishiena F, Grumbach MM: The interrelationship of sex chromosome constitution and phenotype in the syndrome of gonadal dysgenesis and its variants. Ann NY Acad Sci 155:695, 1968.
7. Weiss L: Additional evidence of gradual loss of germ cells in the pathogenesis of streak ovaries in Turner's syndrome. J Med Genet 8:540, 1971.
8. Kaplan SL, Grumbach MM, Aubert ML: The ontogenesis of pituitary hormones and hypothalamic factors in the human fetus: Maturation of the central nervous system regulation of anterior pituitary function. Recent Prog Horm Res 32:161, 1976.
9. Gulyas BJ, Hodgen GD, Tullner WW, Ross GT: Effects of fetal or maternal hypophysectomy on endocrine organs and body weight in infant rhesus monkeys (Macaca mulatta) with particular emphasis on oogenesis. Biol Reprod 16:216, 1977.
10. Healy DL, Bacher J, Hodgen GD: Thymic regulation of primate fetal ovarian-adrenal differentiation. Biol Reprod 32:1127–1133, 1985.
11. Goodman AL, Hodgen GD: The ovarian triad of the primate menstrual cycle. Recent Prog Horm Res 39:1, 1983.
12. Ericson GF: Normal ovarian function. Clin Obstet Gynecol 21:31, 1978.
13. Zelznik AJ, Schuler HM, Reichert LE: Gonadotropin-binding sites in the rhesus monkey ovary: Role of the vasculature in the selective distribution of human chorionic gonadotropin to the preovulatory follicle. Endocrinology 109:356, 1981.
14. diZerega GS, Hodgen GD: Fluorescence localization of luteinizing hormone/human chorionic gonadotropin uptake in the primate ovary. II. Changing distribution during selection of the dominant follicle. J Clin Endocrinol Metab 51:903, 1980.
15. Koering MJ, Baehler EA, Goodman AL, Hodgen GD: Developing morphological asymmetry of ovarian follicular maturation in monkeys. Biol Reprod 27:989, 1982.
16. Pedersen T: Follicle kinetics in the ovary of cyclic mouse. Acta Endocrinol 64:304–323, 1970.
17. Lunenfeld B, Kraiem Z, Eshkol A: Structure and functions of the growing follicle. Clin Obstet Gynecol 3:27, 1976.
18. Goodman AL, Hodgen GD: Between-ovary interaction in the regulation of follicle growth, corpus luteum function, and gonadotropin secretion in the primate ovarian cycle. I. Effects of follicle cautery and hemiovariectomy during the follicular phase in cynomolgus monkeys. Endocrinology 104:1304, 1979.
19. Goodman AL, Hodgen GD: Between-ovary interaction in the regulation of follicle growth, corpus luteum function, and gonadotropin secretion in the primate ovarian cycle. II. Effects of luteectomy and hemiovariectomy during the luteal phase in cynomolgus monkeys. Endocrinology 104:1310, 1979.
20. Pauerstein CJ, Eddy CA, Croxatto HD, et al: Temporal relationship of estrogen, progesterone, and luteinizing hormone levels to ovulation in women and infrahuman primates. Am J Obstet Gynecol 130:876, 1978.
21. Garcia JE, Jones GS, Wright GL: Prediction of time of ovulation. Fertil Steril 36:308, 1981.
22. Knobil E: The neuroendocrine control of the menstrual cycle. Recent Prog Horm Res 36:53, 1980.
23. Pincus G, Enzmann EV: The comparative behaviors of mammalian eggs in vivo and in vitro. J Exp Med 62:655, 1935.
24. Tsafriri A, Dekel N, Bar-Ami S: The role of oocyte maturation inhibitor in follicular regulation of oocyte maturation. J Reprod Fertil 64:541, 1982.
25. Channing CP, Schaerf FW, Anderson LD, Tsafrir A: Ovarian follicular and luteal physiology. In Greep RO (ed): International Review of Physiology, Vol 22. Baltimore, University Park Press, 1980, p 117.
26. Wallach EE, Wright KH, Hamada Y: Investigation of mammalian ovulation with an in vitro perfused rabbit ovary preparation. Am J Obstet Gynecol 132:728, 1978.
27. Lipner H: Mechanism of mammalian ovulation. In Greep RO (ed): Handbook of Physiology, Vol 2, Sec 7. Washington, DC, American Physiological Society, 1973, p 409.
28. Stickland S, Beers WH: Studies on the role of plasminogen activator in ovulation: In vitro response of granulosa cells to gonadotropins, cycle nucleotides, and prostaglandins. J Biol Chem 251:5694, 1976.
29. Espey LI: Ovarian proteolytic enzymes and ovulation. Biol Reprod 10:216, 1974.
30. Koos R, LeMaire W: Evidence for angiogenic factor from rat follicles. In Greenwals GS, Terranova PF (eds): Factors Regulating Ovarian Function. New York, Raven Press, 1983, pp 191–195.
31. Frederick JL, Shimanuki T, diZerega GS: Initiation of angiogenesis by human follicular fluid. Science 224:389, 1984.
32. Hodgen GD: Surrogate embryo transfer combined with estrogen-progesterone therapy in monkeys: Implantation, gestation, and delivery without ovaries. JAMA 250:2167, 1983.
33. Lutjen P, Trounson A, Leeton J, et al: The establishment and maintenance of pregnancy using in vitro fertilization and embryo domination in a patient with primary ovarian failure. Nature 307:174, 1984.
34. Csapo AI, Pulkkinen MO, Ruttner B, et al: The significance of the human corpus luteum in pregnancy maintenance. Am J Obstet Gynecol 11:1061, 1972.
35. Strott CA, Cargille CM, Ross GT, Lipsett MB: The short luteal phase. J Clin Endocrinol Metab 30:246, 1970.
36. Sherman BM, Korenman SG: Measurement of plasma LH, FSH, estradiol, and progesterone in disorders of the human menstrual cycle: The short luteal phase. J Clin Endocrinol Metab 38:89, 1974.
37. Wentz AC: Physiologic and clinical considerations in luteal phase defects. Clin Obstet Gynecol 22:169, 1979.
38. Moszkowski E, Woodruff JD, Jones GS: The inadequate luteal phase. Am J Obstet Gynecol 83:363, 1962.
39. Murut EL, Huang S-C, Hodgen GD: Distinguishing the steroidogenic roles of granulosa and theca cells of the dominant ovarian follicle and corpus luteum. J Clin Endocrinol Metab 57:925, 1983.
40. McNatty KP, Sawyers RS: Relationship between the endocrine environment within the graafian follicle and the subsequent rated progesterone secretion by human granulosa cells in vitro. J Endocrinol 66:391, 1975.
41. McNatty KP: Cyclic changes in antral fluid hormone concentration in humans. Clin Endocrinol 7:577, 1979.
42. Moon YS, Tsang BK, Simpson C, Armstrong DT: Estradiol biosynthesis in cultured granulosa and theca cells of human ovarian follicles: Stimulation by follicle-stimulating hormone. J Clin Endocrinol Metab 47:1331, 1978.
43. McNatty KP, Smith DM, Makris A, et al: The micro-environment of the human antral follicle: Interrelationships among the steroid levels in antral fluid, the population of granulosa cells, and the status of the oocyte in vivo and in vitro. J Clin Endocrinol Metab 49:851, 1979.
44. diZerega GS, Hodgen GD: Luteal phase dysfunction infertility: A sequel to aberrant folliculogenesis. Fertil Steril 35:489, 1981.
45. Bomsel-Helmreich O, Gougeon A, Thebault A, et al: Healthy and atretic human follicle in the preovulatory phase: Differences in evolution of follicular morphology and steroid contents of follicular fluid. J Clin Endocrinol Metab 48:686, 1979.
46. Sanval MK, Berger MJ, Thompson IE, et al: Development of graafian follicles in adult human ovary. I. Correlation of estrogen and progesterone concentration in antral fluid with growth of follicle. J Clin Endocrinol Metab 38:828, 1974.
47. Catt KJ, Dufau L, Vaitukaitis JL: Appearance of hCG in pregnancy plasma following the initiation of implantation of the blastocyst. J Clin Endocrinol Metab 40:537, 1975.
48. Aso T, Williams RF: Lactational amenorrhea with failure of pulsatile GnRH to induce ovulation: Synergistic actions of LH and prolactin to rejuvenate the corpus luteum of pregnancy. 7th International Congress of Endocrinology, July 1–7, 1984, Quebec City, Canada, Abstr 181.

49. Fritz MA, Speroff L: The endocrinology of the menstrual cycle: The interaction of folliculogenesis and neuroendocrine mechanism. Fertil Steril 38:509, 1982.

50. Koering MJ: Follicle maturation and atresia. In Stouffer RL (ed): The Primate Ovary. New York, Plenum Press, 1987, pp 3–23.

51. Schomberg DW, Tilly JL, Kowalski KI: Down-regulation of luteinizing hormone (LH) receptor messenger RNA during apoptosis in atretic porcine ovarian follicles. 7th Annual Meeting of the Endocrine Society, June 24–27, 1992, San Antonio, Texas, Abstr 26.

52. Koering MJ, Danforth DR, Hodgen GD: Early folliculogenesis in primate ovaries: Testing the role of estrogen. Biol Reprod 45:890–897, 1991.

53. Korenman SG, Sherman BM: Further studies of gonadotropins and estradiol secretion during the preovulatory phase of the human menstrual cycle. J Clin Endocrinol Metab 36:1205, 1981.

54. Trounson A, Wood C: Extracorporeal fertilization and embryo transfer. Clin Obstet Gynecol 8:681, 1981.

55. Jones GS: Update on in vitro fertilization. Endocr Rev 5:62–75, 1984.

56. Bernardus RE, Jones GS, Acosta AA, et al: The significance of the ratio in follicle-stimulating hormone and luteinizing hormone in induction of multiple follicular growth. Fertil Steril 43:373–378, 1985.

57. Ferraretti AP, Garcia JE, Acosta AA, Jones GS: Serum LH during ovulation induction for in vitro fertilization in normally menstruating women. Fertil Steril 40:742, 1983.

58. Schenken RS, Hodgen GD: FSH-induced ovarian hyperstimulation in monkeys: Blockade of the LH surge. J Clin Endocrinol Metab 57:50, 1983.

59. Kenigsberg D, Littman BA, Williams RF, Hodgen GD: Medical hypophysectomy. II. Variability of ovarian response to gonadotropin therapy. Fertil Steril 42:116, 1984.

60. Jones GS, Garcia JE, Rosenwaks Z: The role of pituitary gonadotropins in follicular stimulation and oocyte maturation in the human. J Clin Endocrinol Metab 59:178–180, 1984.

61. Jones GS, Acosta AA, Garcia JE, et al: The effect of FSH without additional LH on follicular stimulation and oocyte development in normal ovulatory women. Fertil Steril 43:696–702, 1985.

62. Simonetti S, Veeck LL, Jones HW: Correlation of follicular fluid volume with oocyte morphology from follicles stimulated by human menopausal gonadotropin. Fertil Steril 44:177–180, 1985.

63. Acosta AA, Jones GS, Garcia JE, et al: Correlation of hMG, hCG stimulation and oocyte quality in an in vitro fertilization program. Fertil Steril 111:196, 1984.

64. Eppig JJ: Regulation of cumulus oophorus expansion by gonadotropins in vivo and in vitro. Biol Reprod 23:545, 1980.

65. Laufer N, Botero-Ruiz W, DeCherney AH, et al: Gonadotropin and prolactin levels in follicular fluid of human ova successfully fertilized in vitro. J Clin Endocrinol Metab 58:430, 1984.

66. Laufer N, DeCherney AM, Haseltine F, Behrman H: Steroid secretion by the human-egg-corona-cumulus complex in culture. J Clin Endocrinol Metab 58:1153, 1984.

67. Veldius JD, Klase PA, Sandow B, Kolp CA: Progesterone secretion by highly differentiated human granulosa cells isolated from preovulatory graafian follicles induced by exogenous gonadotropins and human chorionic gonadotropin. J Clin Endocrinol Metab 57:87–93, 1983.

68. Lunde O: Polycystic ovarian syndrome: A retrospective study of the therapeutic effect of ovarian wedge resection after unsuccessful treatment with clomiphene citrate. Ann Chir Gynaecol 71:330, 1982.

69. Jones HW: Polycystic ovarian syndrome: A retrospective study on the therapeutic effect of ovarian wedge resection after unsuccessful treatment with clomiphene citrate (editorial). Obstet Gynecol Surv 38:483, 1983.

70. Pepperel RJ, McBain JC, Healy DL: Ovulation induction with bromocriptine in patients with hyperprolactinemia. Aust NZ J Obstet Gynaecol 17:181, 1977.

71. Ben-David M, Schenker JG: Transient hyperprolactinemia: A correctable cause of idiopathic female infertility. J Clin Endocrinol Metab 57:442, 1983.

72. Adashi EY: Clomiphene citrate, mechanism(s) and site(s) of action—a hypothesis revisited. Fertil Steril 42:331, 1984.

73. Talbert LM: Clomiphene citrate induction of ovulation. Fertil Steril 39:742, 1983.

74. Kase N, Crouch A, Olsen LE: Clomid therapy for anovulatory infertility. Am J Obstet Gynecol 98:1057, 1967.

75. Ross GT, Cargille CM, Lipsett MB, et al: Pituitary and gonadal hormones in women during spontaneous and induced ovulatory cycles. Recent Prog Horm Res 26:1, 1970.

76. March CM, Tredway DR, Mishell DR: Effect of clomiphene citrate upon amount and duration of human menopausal gonadotropin therapy. Am J Obstet Gynecol 125: 699, 1976.

77. Schwartz M, Jewelewitz R: The use of gonadotropins for reduction of ovulation. Fertil Steril 35:3, 1981.

78. Gemzell C: Induction of ovulation with human gonadotropins. Recent Prog Horm Res 21:179, 1965.

79. Ben-Rafae Z, Dor J, Mashiach S, et al: Abortion rates in pregnancies following ovulation induced by human menopausal gonadotropin/human chorionic gonadotropin. Fertil Steril 39:157, 1983.

80. Liu JH, Durfee R, Muse K, Yen SSC: Induction of multiple ovulation by pulsatile administration of gonadotropin-releasing hormone. Fertil Steril 40:18, 1983.

81. Crowley WF, MacArthur JW: Stimulation of the normal menstrual cycle in Kallman's syndrome by pulsatile administration of luteinizing hormone-releasing hormone (LHRH). J Clin Endocrinol Metab 51:173, 1980.

82. Leyendecker G, Wildt L, Hansmann M: Pregnancies following chronic intermittent (pulsatile) administration of GnRH by means of a portable pump ("Zyklomat")—a new approach to the treatment of infertility in hypothalamic amenorrhea. J Clin Endocrinol Metab 51:1214, 1980.

83. Shoemaker J, Simons AHM, van Osnabrugge GJC, et al: Pregnancy after prolonged pulsatile administration of luteinizing hormone-releasing hormone in patients with clomiphene-resistant secondary amenorrhea. J Clin Endocrinol Metab 52:882, 1981.

84. Hurley DM, Brian R, Outch K, et al: Induction of ovulation and fertility in amenorrheic women by pulsatile low-dose gonadotropin-releasing hormone. N Engl J Med 310:1069, 1984.

85. Hernandez ER, Hurwitz A, Vera A, et al: Expression of the genes encoding the insulin-like growth factors and their receptors in the human ovary. J Clin Endocrinol Metab 74:419–426, 1992.

117

Hormonal Regulation of the Menstrual Cycle and Mechanisms of Anovulation

JOHN C. MARSHALL

In women and female primates reproductive function follows a cyclical pattern between menarche and the menopause that is termed the menstrual cycle. Cyclical function is recognized clinically by menstrual bleeding, and by convention the first day of bleeding is designated day 1 of the cycle. In women, during the 12 to 18 months after menarche cycles often are anovulatory and cycle length is irregular. Regular menses occur the next 20 to 25 years, and cycle length usually is between 25 and 30 days. Before the menopause, irregular cycles of longer duration are again seen. Early studies of vaginal and endometrial histology together with measurement of urinary steroids had indicated different hormonal activity during the cycle that was divided into two parts; the follicular phase and the luteal phase, separated by ovulation. The follicular phase persists for 12 to 16 days and is the stage of growth and maturation of ovarian follicles, one of which is destined to become the ovulatory follicle. Conventionally, the follicular phase begins on the first day of menstrual bleeding, but follicular maturation begins during the latter part of the preceding luteal phase. After ovulation the luteal phase persists for 10 to 16 days and is associated with the presence of a corpus luteum in the ovary. Estradiol and progesterone secreted by the corpus luteum induce proliferation and secretory changes in the endometrial glands. In the absence of a fertilized ovum the corpus luteum regresses 9 to 11 days after ovulation, and the decline in estradiol and progesterone results in shedding of the endometrium as the menstrual flow.

HORMONAL CHANGES DURING THE MENSTRUAL CYCLE

The dynamic relationship between pituitary gonadotropin and ovarian steroid secretion has been recognized for several decades, but detailed understanding of the nature of these interactions has occurred only in recent years. The development of radioligand assays provided methods of sufficient sensitivity and specificity to measure pituitary gonadotropin and ovarian steroid and peptide hormones in small volumes of blood. This in turn allowed delineation of the temporal and causal relations between luteinizing hormone (LH), follicle-stimulating hormone (FSH), estradiol, progesterone, and inhibin, initially on a day-to-day and more recently on a minute-to-minute basis. These studies have resulted in our current understanding of the control mechanisms that regulate the menstrual cycle. The day-to-day changes of hormones in plasma during a typical menstrual cycle are shown in Figure 117–1 and are based on studies using radioimmunoassays.[1–5]

The early follicular phase is characterized by plasma levels of FSH that are relatively high and by low levels of LH, estradiol, progesterone, and inhibin. The initial predominance of FSH stimulation of the ovary is critical for the recruitment and maturation of a cohort of ovarian follicles, one of which is destined to ovulate.[6–9] FSH stimulates follicular growth, induces the appearance of LH receptors on granulosa cells, and stimulates the activity of aromatase enzymes in granulosa cells that are required to convert androstenedione (from the theca cells) to estradiol (see Chs. 115 and 116). The combined effects of FSH and LH stimulate secretion of estradiol, which by the middle to late follicular phase is secreted predominantly by the follicle destined to ovulate, the dominant follicle. The exact mechanisms whereby one follicle achieves dominance while many others become atretic are not fully understood, but FSH appears to be important in primates. Suppression of plasma FSH by exogenous estradiol during the early follicular phase delays the development of the dominant follicle[10] and prolongs the follicular phase in both monkeys and humans. Large doses of FSH administered to women or animals stimulate more than one follicle—often several—to develop. If an antiestrogen is given to hypophysectomized rats, along with FSH, this FSH-stimulated folliculogenesis is prevented. Thus estrogens acting locally within the ovary are involved in follicular maturation initiated by FSH. In addition, regulatory proteins that are secreted by granulosa cells and that inhibit follicle growth have been identified. These have been termed follicle regulatory proteins, or oocyte maturation inhibitor.[11] It is pos-

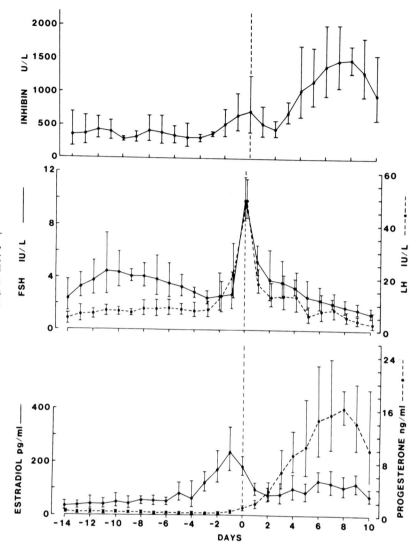

FIGURE 117–1. Plasma concentrations of pituitary gonadotropins (LH, FSH, *middle panel*) and ovarian steroids (estradiol, progesterone, *lower panel*) and inhibin (*upper panel*) during the menstrual cycle. Data from ovulatory cycles in six normal women are normalized around the LH surge (day 0). (From McLachlan RI et al: Circulating immunoreactive inhibin levels during the normal human menstrual cycle. J Clin Endocrinol Metab 65:954–961, © by the Endocrine Society, 1987.)

tulated that these materials assist the dominant follicle to be selected, producing atresia and failure to survive in smaller follicles. Just as an adequate FSH stimulus is important in initiating follicle development, it also may be important for determining subsequent function of the corpus luteum; women with short luteal phases have lower levels of serum FSH during the follicular phase of the cycle.

During the middle of the follicular phase, serum estradiol increases rapidly and suppresses secretion of FSH by a selective action on the pituitary.[12] Plasma inhibin also increases at this time[5] and may play a role in suppressing FSH release. This reduction in FSH may be causally related to atresia of the nondominant follicles. The increase in estradiol in the late follicular phase is important in the development of the midcycle LH surge. Estradiol exerts a positive feedback effect and enhances LH responsiveness to gonadotropin-releasing hormone (GnRH). Plasma progesterone is also rising and similarly can augment LH responses to GnRH[13]; thus the combined effects of estradiol and progesterone result in markedly enhanced LH release, which produces the midcycle LH surge (see Ch. 113). GnRH secretion is also increased in sheep and monkeys, and estradiol can increase secretion of GnRH.[14] In essence, this ovarian estradiol-progesterone signal system produced by the mature follicle induces the GnRH–LH–FSH ovula-

tory surge.[11] The LH surge persists for 40 to 48 hours and induces rupture of the mature follicle and subsequent release of the ovum, which occurs 16 to 24 hours after the initiation of the LH surge. Concomitant with the abrupt rise in LH, serum estradiol falls precipitously and progesterone secretion increases, reflecting the altered function of the luteinized follicle. The transient fall in estradiol may allow FSH release to produce the smaller midcycle FSH peak. After ovulation the luteinized follicle responds to LH by secreting progesterone, 17-hydroxyprogesterone, estradiol, and estrone, and plasma concentrations of these hormones increase during the 7 to 8 days after ovulation (see Fig. 117–1). The elevated plasma estradiol, probably acting synergistically with inhibin, which is also secreted by the corpus luteum, inhibits FSH secretion, and FSH remains low during the luteal phase. LH appears to be essential for normal function of the corpus luteum. The nature of other factors that dictate the duration of corpus luteum function is uncertain, but in many species, prostaglandins of ovarian or uterine origin appear to be involved.[15] If the ovum is fertilized, corpus luteum function is maintained by human chorionic gonadotropin (hCG), but in the absence of conception, plasma levels of estradiol and progesterone decline during the final days of the cycle. The fall in ovarian hormones allows an increase in plasma gonadotropins, particularly FSH, which initiates the recruitment and maturation of ovarian follicles for the next cycle.

MECHANISMS THAT REGULATE HORMONE SECRETION

The exact nature of the mechanisms involved in the interaction of the hypothalamic-pituitary-ovarian axis to produce the orderly sequential hormonal changes seen during the normal cycle remains uncertain. Studies have focused on the detailed examination of hormonal changes in blood samples obtained every 10 to 20 minutes during the cycle. These studies have revealed differences in the patterns of LH and FSH secretion that suggest that alterations in pulsatile hypothalamic GnRH secretion are important for the maintenance of normal cyclicity. In human subjects estimation of GnRH secretion has to be indirect, and changes in GnRH secretion are inferred from the patterns of LH and FSH seen in plasma. Studies in animals have shown that GnRH is secreted in an intermittent manner, and each episode of GnRH release from the hypothal-

amus is followed by an acute increase in plasma LH. Thus the frequency and/or amplitude of LH pulses in peripheral blood can be used as an indirect measurement of GnRH secretion. FSH is less helpful in this regard because the long half-life of FSH (about three hours) obscures pulsatile patterns. The frequency of LH pulses varies during different stages of the cycle.[16–19] In the early follicular phase, LH pulses are of of constant amplitude and occur at a frequency of every one to two hours. Slower frequencies of LH pulses (every two to six hours) are present during the luteal phase, and the amplitude of LH pulses is much more variable. The patterns of plasma LH and FSH during cycles in two normal women are shown in Figure 117–2.

Follicular Phase and the Midcycle Gonadotropin Surge

During the early follicular phase (days 3 to 4), plasma concentrations of LH and FSH are similar and LH pulses are of constant amplitude and occur every 90 to 100 min-

PULSATILE LH AND FSH SECRETION DURING A NORMAL MENSTRUAL CYCLE

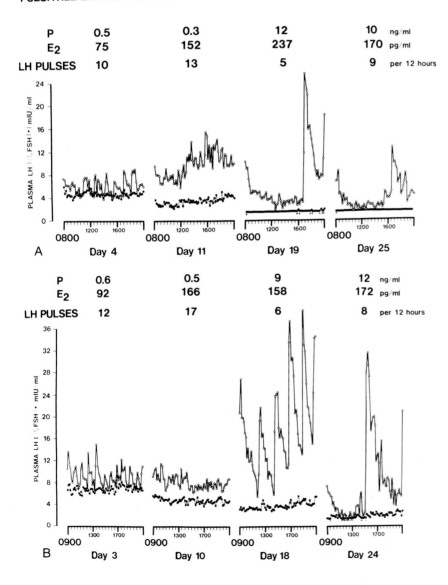

FIGURE 117–2. Pulsatile LH and FSH secretion in two women during ovulatory menstrual cycles. Blood samples were obtained at 10-minute intervals during the early and late stages of both the follicular and the luteal phases of the cycle. Mean values for ovarian steroids are shown. The number of LH pulses per 12 hours is shown for each day. P, progesterone; E_2, estradiol. (From Reame N et al: Pulsatile gonadotropin secretion during the human menstrual cycle: Evidence for altered frequency of gonadotropin-releasing hormone secretion. J Clin Endocrinol Metab 59:328–337, © by the Endocrine Society, 1984.)

utes. In the late follicular phase, estradiol levels are increased and FSH falls, whereas LH is stable or increased. The reduction in plasma FSH probably reflects selective inhibition of FSH release by estradiol.[9] The ovarian peptides inhibin and follistatin can also suppress FSH secretion, and plasma inhibin tends to be elevated during the late follicular phase. The exact role of inhibin remains uncertain because it is not increased in the midfollicular stage when FSH begins to fall. Data on follistatin in plasma are not yet available. Administration of exogenous estradiol at this stage of the cycle reduces plasma FSH,[6] suggesting that estradiol feedback is more important in reducing FSH secretion. LH pulse frequency increases to about one pulse per hour during the late follicular phase and probably stimulates increased estradiol secretion by the maturing follicle.[20, 21] The mechanisms involved in increasing the frequency of LH pulses in humans are unclear, but similar changes have been observed in sheep and appear to be consequent on the rise in estradiol.[22, 23] Direct measurement of portal blood GnRH in sheep after estradiol has shown that GnRH pulse frequency and amplitude increase and estradiol induces a massive increase in GnRH secretion.[14, 22] The pulsatile release of GnRH is obscured, and GnRH levels are continuously elevated and remain elevated throughout the LH surge. Ovulatory midcycle LH surges have been induced by the administration of constant-amplitude GnRH pulses to GnRH-deficient monkeys and humans,[24, 25] but the magnitude of LH secretion usually is less than occurs spontaneously. The data suggest that an increase in GnRH secretion is not an absolute requirement to produce an LH surge, but these studies used supraphysiological doses of GnRH, and the amount of GnRH delivered to the pituitary may have been similar to concentrations of endogenous GnRH, which are present only during a midcycle surge in vivo. In addition to the increase in GnRH secretion, ovarian steroids enhance LH responsiveness to GnRH. Both estradiol and progesterone enhance LH responses. Plasma estradiol is maximal, and progesterone and 17α-hydroxyprogesterone concentrations rise immediately before the LH surge[26] (Fig. 117–3). Thus the increase in estradiol is probably the primary signal that triggers increased GnRH secretion and enhanced LH responsiveness to GnRH. The latter is augmented by the rise in progesterone, resulting in the ovulatory LH surge.[27]

During the LH surge, progesterone concentrations continue to rise but estradiol falls rapidly. These changes reflect the LH-induced luteinization of granulosa cells and an acute change in steroidogenesis to favor progesterone secretion.[28] The duration of the LH surge is probably limited by a combination of factors. The fall in estradiol results in loss of enhanced LH responses to GnRH, and progesterone is not effective in maintaining LH responsiveness in the absence of estradiol. GnRH secretion continues to be elevated during the declining part of the surge.[23] Thus the reduced amplitude of LH pulsatile secretion may also reflect a degree of gonadotrope desensitization after the prolonged rapid frequency or even continuous stimulation by GnRH.

Luteal Phase and Initiation of the Next Wave of Follicular Recruitment

During the three to four days after ovulation, LH pulse frequency falls, and by the midluteal stage, LH pulses occur

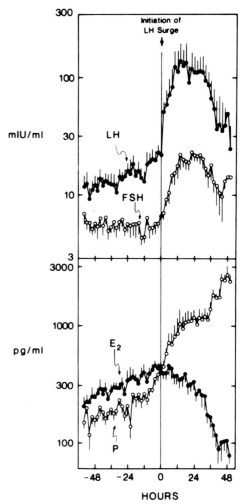

FIGURE 117–3. Plasma LH, FSH, estradiol, and progesterone concentrations in samples obtained at two-hour intervals for five days at midcycle during seven cycles. Zero time represents initiation of the gonadotropin surge. Data are plotted on a logarithmic scale. (From Hoff JD et al: Hormonal dynamics at mid cycle: A reevaluation. J Clin Endocrinol Metab 57:792–796, © by the Endocrine Society, 1983.)

every three to five hours. In addition, the pattern of LH pulses varies through the luteal phase. In the early luteal phase, LH pulses occur regularly and are of large amplitude, whereas irregularity of both amplitude and frequency is seen in the midluteal to late luteal phase (see Fig. 117–2). The variable LH secretory patterns reflect altered hypothalamic GnRH secretion because LH responsiveness to GnRH is not impaired during the luteal phase.[29] The elevation in progesterone concentrations appears to be the main factor that reduces GnRH secretion in the luteal phase. The administration of progesterone during the follicular phase results in LH secretory patterns that resemble those of the normal luteal phase,[30] and the effects of progesterone on LH secretion are shown in Figure 117–4. Similar effects of progesterone in slowing LH pulse frequency have been observed in castrate estrogen-replaced ewes.[31]

The mechanism of progesterone action in altering GnRH secretion involves an increase in hypothalamic opioid activity. β-Endorphin concentrations in hypothalamic portal blood are increased in the luteal phase, and the administration of naloxone, an opiate receptor

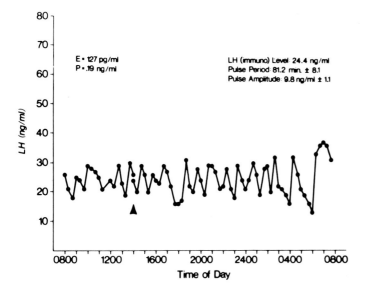

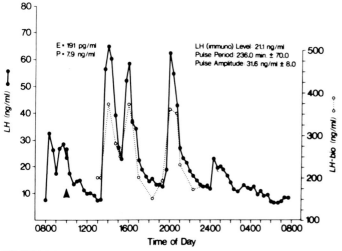

FIGURE 117–4. Patterns of plasma LH in samples obtained at 20-minute intervals during the late follicular phase (*upper panel*) and during the late follicular phase after administration of progesterone for eight days (*lower panel*) in a normally cycling woman. The dotted lines in the lower panel represent serum LH measured by bioassay. (From Soules MR et al: Progesterone modulation of pulsatile luteinizing hormone secretion in normal women. J Clin Endocrinol Metab 58:378–383, © by the Endocrine Society, 1984.)

blocker, increases LH pulse frequency during the luteal phase in both women and monkeys.[32, 33] Naloxone is ineffective during the follicular phase. The slowing of GnRH pulsatile secretion during the luteal phase may have important consequences for the life span of the corpus luteum. The factors that regulate the life span of the corpus luteum are uncertain, but LH is required for normal luteal function in primates. In the absence of LH secretion, the corpus luteum life span is shortened; in the presence of large doses of exogenous LH or the secretion of hCG (an LH-like hormone) in normal pregnancy, the corpus luteum life span is lengthened.[34] Studies have shown that in the early luteal phase, before LH pulse frequency has decreased, serum progesterone is stable and only minor fluctuations occur. During the midluteal to late luteal phase, progesterone secretion only occurs coincident with LH pulses.[18, 35] Thus the alteration in the pattern of the LH stimulus may be important for corpus luteum function,

and the reduced LH pulse frequency may play a role in the demise of the corpus luteum. The slower frequency of GnRH pulses may also affect gonadotropin synthesis in the luteal phase. GnRH is known to be required for gonadotropin synthesis, and in rodents faster-frequency GnRH pulses favor LH synthesis, and slower pulses, FSH synthesis.[36] The slow irregular luteal GnRH stimulus would thus be expected to maintain FSH synthesis but may not be optimal for maintaining LH synthesis. This, together with LH release, would result in depletion of pituitary LH stores during the luteal phase.

Plasma FSH remains low during the luteal phase (see Fig. 117–2), which again reflects inhibition of release by estradiol and inhibin. With the demise of the corpus luteum, serum estradiol, progesterone, and inhibin levels fall and LH pulse frequency and plasma FSH levels increase during the last two to three days of the cycle. Detailed studies of the late luteal–early follicular phase transition in individual patients suggest that the fall in progesterone allows an increase in GnRH pulse frequency (Fig. 117–5). The increase in GnRH stimulation of the pituitary results in predominant FSH release because the selective inhibition by estradiol and inhibin is no longer present and LH stores have been depleted. FSH release and the long half-life of FSH contribute to a selective increase in plasma FSH. Thus the critically important increase in plasma FSH that initiates recruitment of ovarian follicles for the next cycle occurs during the late luteal phase and results from increased GnRH stimulation of a pituitary that is primed to release FSH.

Role of Altered GnRH Secretion in Cycle Regulation

As outlined above, regulation of the normal menstrual cycle consists of a complex series of interactions between the hypothalamus, pituitary, and ovaries. Changes in the pattern of GnRH secretion appear to play an important role, and the presumed patterns of GnRH secretion during a normal cycle are shown in Figure 117–6.

Follicular recruitment and maturation is initiated by FSH, which is secreted in response to the late luteal increase in GnRH pulse frequency in the presence of low levels of estradiol and inhibin. Estradiol secreted by the maturing follicle selectively inhibits FSH secretion and stimulates the increase in GnRH pulse frequency during the late follicular phase. This in turn increases plasma LH, which stimulates estradiol secretion by the dominant follicle. The midcycle LH surge results from increased frequency and amplitude of GnRH secretion and from estradiol and progesterone augmentation of LH responses to GnRH. After ovulation and luteinization of the ruptured follicle, progesterone from the corpus luteum increases hypothalamic opioid activity, which in turn reduces the frequency of GnRH secretion, and GnRH pulse amplitude is variable. GnRH pulses do not release FSH (inhibited by high plasma estradiol and inhibin levels), and pituitary FSH stores are maintained. The fall in progesterone allows an increase in GnRH pulse frequency, which now affects FSH secretion because estradiol and inhibin levels are low.

This synopsis of the role of GnRH secretion is based on data from women and several animal species, and the pat-

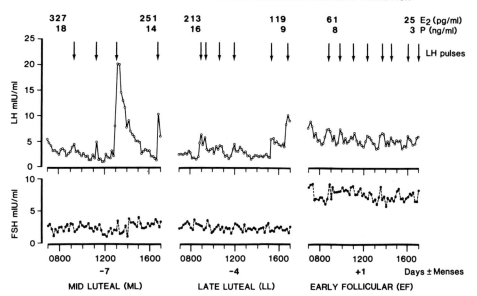

FIGURE 117–5. Gonadotropin secretion and gonadal steroids during the intercycle period of an ovulatory cycle. The transition of hormone secretion from the midluteal to the early follicular phase is shown. Arrows indicate LH (GnRH) pulses. (From Marshall JC et al: Gonadotropin-releasing hormone pulses: Regulators of gonadotropin synthesis and ovulatory cycles. Recent Prog Horm Res 47:155–189, 1991.)

terns of hormone secretion have been consistently observed. The importance of changes in GnRH secretion remains uncertain because the administration of a fixed dose of GnRH at a fixed frequency has been shown to induce ovulation both in women with GnRH deficiency and in GnRH-deficient monkeys (induced by hypothalamic lesions).[24, 25, 37–39] This apparent contradiction may reflect the manner of GnRH administration. In most cycles where ovulation has been induced with exogenous GnRH, the dose of GnRH used was supraphysiological, and this may override the need to change the frequency of the GnRH stimulus. Additionally, few studies have examined the efficacy of exogenous GnRH in the stimulation of ovulatory

cycles over prolonged periods, and the ability to alter GnRH frequency may be important in the continued maintenance of normal cyclicity. Slowing of pulse frequency in the luteal phase appears to be important in this regard. The administration of GnRH at rapid frequencies in the luteal phase has led to deficient follicular development and corpus luteum function in subsequent cycles, perhaps a consequence of inadequate late luteal FSH secretion.[40, 41] The fact that GnRH pulse frequency varies during the cycle appears well established, but the exact role and the requirement for altered frequency to maintain cyclicity await the results of future studies.[42]

The changes in the pattern of GnRH secretion during

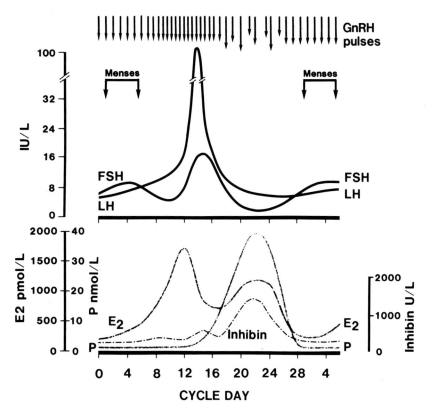

FIGURE 117–6. Schematic representation of alterations in gonadotropin-releasing hormone (GnRH) secretion and the relation to gonadotropin and ovarian hormone secretion during the normal menstrual cycle. The arrows represent pulses of GnRH release. The length of an arrow indicates the amount of GnRH secreted and the distance between arrows represents pulse intervals. For estradiol (E_2) ÷ 3.7 to pg/ml; for progesterone (P) ÷ 3.2 to ng/ml. (From Marshall JC et al: Gonadotropin-releasing hormone pulses: Regulators of gonadotropin synthesis and ovulatory cycles. Recent Prog Horm Res 47:155–189, 1991.)

the cycle—an increase in frequency during the follicular phase with slowing in the luteal phase—are similar to the changes in GnRH secretion that occur during pubertal maturation. In prepubertal girls LH (by inference GnRH) pulse amplitude is low and pulses occur infrequently, every three to four hours, with a minor augmentation during sleep.[43] Pubertal maturation is initiated by a marked amplification of the sleep-entrained secretion of GnRH. Over time increased GnRH pulsatile secretion persists throughout the day, and thus the transition from prepubertal to pubertal secretory patterns is consequent on increases in the amplitude and frequency of endogenous GnRH secretion. Gonadotropin responses to GnRH also change during pubertal maturation from a predominant FSH secretory response in prepubertal girls to the adult pattern of dominant LH release. Thus the increased frequency of GnRH secretion occurring in pubertal girls over that in prepubertal girls is a mechanism similar to the increase in frequency that occurs during progression from the luteal phase to the follicular phase in ovulatory cycles. In concert, FSH responses to GnRH predominate in the late luteal–early follicular phase but diminish as LH responsiveness increases in the late follicular phase. The ability to secrete GnRH at a rapid frequency (one pulse per hour) is reacquired at puberty (data suggest that fast-frequency secretion is present in utero), and this is a necessary event in the development of ovulatory cycles. A fast frequency of GnRH secretion is needed to allow estradiol augmentation of LH responses to GnRH, an important event in the genesis of the LH surge. The luteal phase could then be viewed as a time when the ovarian steroids inhibit GnRH release to a pattern that is not optimal for LH secretion but allows ongoing FSH synthesis to stimulate the next wave of follicular development.[36]

MECHANISMS OF ANOVULATION

In view of the complex nature of the interrelations between the hypothalamus-pituitary and the ovary that are required for normal cyclical function, it is not surprising that disorders of any part of this axis can result in anovulation and amenorrhea. In many instances, however, anovulation occurs in the absence of recognized pathological abnormalities. Anovulatory cycles frequently occur during the year after menarche, and because regular cycles subsequently ensue, this suggests that the hormonal interrelations are established over time. Specifically, the ability of estradiol to induce a positive feedback effect to increase LH release is absent in immature girls,[44] and this may in part account for the anovulatory cycles that occur soon after menarche.

In several instances anovulation in the absence of pathological abnormality has been shown to be associated with abnormal patterns of LH (GnRH) pulsatile secretion, and these are discussed below.

Hypothalamic Amenorrhea

Hypothalamic amenorrhea, the most common form of amenorrhea, is a diagnosis made only after exclusion of pituitary and ovarian abnormalities. Conditions that often precede anovulation include marked weight loss, strenuous exercise such as gymnastics or competitive running, psychological stress, and, occasionally, the prior use of combination oral contraceptive preparations.[45] In most women (about 70 per cent) the removal of these antecedent conditions results in the return of ovulatory menses within 12 months, but in the remainder anovulation and amenorrhea persist. Basal hormone measurements show that plasma LH, FSH, and estradiol levels often are normal or low, prolactin is not elevated, and LH and FSH responsiveness to GnRH usually is preserved. Daily hormone measurements have shown that cyclical changes do not occur, and abnormalities of estrogen and progesterone feedback, with failure of positive feedback, have been described.[46–49] Studies from several groups have shown that the frequency

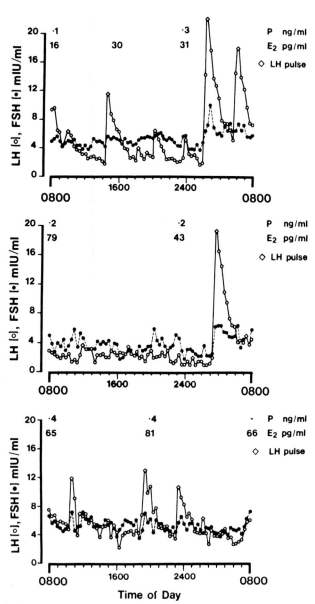

FIGURE 117–7. Patterns of pulsatile LH secretion over 24 hours in women with hypothalamic amenorrhea. Plasma estradiol (E_2) and progesterone (P) levels are also shown. From top to bottom panels, patients showed 4, 3.5, and 5 pulses per 12 hours, respectively. (From Reame NE et al: Pulsatile gonadotropin secretion in women with hypothalamic amenorrhea—evidence for reduced frequency of GnRH secretion. J Clin Endocrinol Metab 61:851–858, © by the Endocrine Society, 1985.)

of GnRH pulsatile secretion is markedly reduced in most women with hypothalamic amenorrhea[50–52] (Fig. 117–7). GnRH pulse frequency (one pulse every three to four hours) and the irregular amplitude of LH pulses resemble the patterns seen during the luteal phase of ovulatory cycles. This similarity led to the suggestion that the disorder may reflect abnormal suppression of GnRH pulse frequency by increased hypothalamic opioid activity. The administration of the opiate receptor blocker naloxone results in rapid (within one to two hours) restoration of normal-frequency GnRH secretion in some 60 to 70 per cent of women with hypothalamic amenorrhea[53–55] (Fig. 117–8). This suggests that most women with this disorder have anovulation on the basis of a persistent slow frequency of pulsatile GnRH secretion that is inadequate to maintain the level of LH synthesis and secretion required for the production of an ovulatory LH surge. Support for this view is found in studies in which administration of GnRH pulses at a slow frequency (every three hours) to GnRH-deficient primates did not maintain plasma LH concentrations.[56]

The observation that patterns of GnRH secretion are variable but of slower than normal pulse frequency would also explain observations that some women with hypothalamic amenorrhea ovulate after administration of clomiphene citrate (Clomid) and others do not (see Ch. 113). If pulse frequency were markedly impaired, clomiphene would not be able to enhance GnRH and gonadotropin secretion to the levels required for an LH surge. On the other hand, lesser degrees of GnRH slowing may be overcome by clomiphene, allowing follicular maturation and ovulation.

As noted above, not all women with hypothalamic amenorrhea have slow-frequency GnRH pulses at the time of study, and not all those who do have slow-frequency pulses respond to opiate blockade. The mechanisms of amenorrhea in these women are uncertain, but some data have suggested that abnormalities of the hypothalamic-pituitary-adrenal axis may be involved. Stress can elevate corticotropin-releasing hormone (CRH), and CRH can directly inhibit GnRH secretion and reproductive function in animal studies. Some women with hypothalamic amenorrhea have elevated plasma cortisol levels and blunted responses to CRH, suggesting stress-induced abnormalities of CRH secretion.[57] These issues remain unproven, and evidence suggests that most women with hypothalamic amenorrhea are anovulatory on the basis of slow-frequency GnRH secretion caused by enhanced hypothalamic opioid activity. Naltrexone (an orally active opiate receptor blocker) has been given to these patients for two to three weeks, and in a small number of studies it has been shown to be effective in inducing ovulation.[58]

Hyperprolactinemia

Amenorrhea and anovulation commonly occur when serum prolactin is elevated. This may follow the administration of medications that block dopamine action or reduce hypothalamic dopamine secretion or reflect the presence of a prolactinoma of the pituitary gland. Initial studies revealed slow, irregular patterns of GnRH secretion, which were restored to normal follicular phase patterns after suppression of serum prolactin by the dopamine agonist bromocriptine[59, 60] (Fig. 117–9).

Of interest, the mechanisms of reduced GnRH pulsatile secretion in hyperprolactinemic patients also appear to involve a final common pathway of excess hypothalamic opioid activity. The administration of naloxone to hyperprolactinemic women (serum prolactin remains elevated) results in a rapid increase of pulsatile GnRH secretion in a manner similar to that seen in women with hypothalamic amenorrhea.[61, 62] This suggests that an elevated prolactin level enhances hypothalamic opioid activity, which in turn

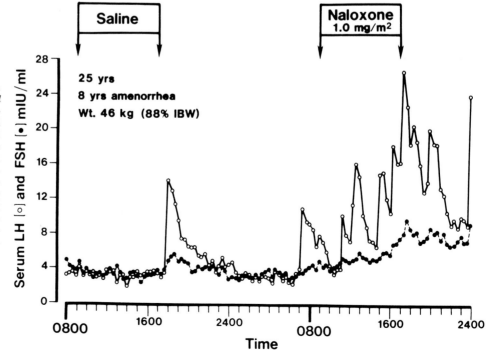

FIGURE 117–8. Effects of naloxone on pulsatile LH (*open circles*) and FSH (*closed circles*) secretion in a woman with hypothalamic amenorrhea. The 25-year-old woman had a history of weight loss and amenorrhea for eight years and, despite regaining weight to 90 per cent of ideal one year ago, had remained amenorrheic. (Data from Khoury SA et al: Diurnal patterns of pulsatile luteinizing hormone secretion in hypothalamic amenorrhea: Reproducibility and responses to opiate blockade and in α_2-adrenergic agonist. J Clin Endocrinol Metab 64:755–762, © by the Endocrine Society, 1987.)

LH PULSES IN A WOMAN WITH HYPERPROLACTINEMIA

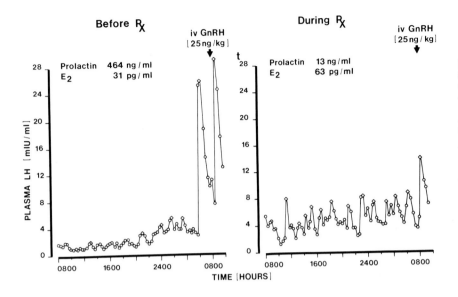

FIGURE 117–9. Patterns of pulsatile LH secretion before and after administration of bromocriptine in a woman with hyperprolactinemia. Note the initial irregular amplitude and infrequent LH pulses (6/24 hours) (*left panel*), which return to a more regular pulsatile pattern similar to that of follicular phase (12 pulses/24 hours) after administration of bromocriptine and reduction of serum prolactin (*right panel*). ◇, LH pulses. E₂, plasma estradiol. (From Sauder SE et al: Abnormal patterns of pulsatile luteinizing hormone secretion in women with hyperprolactinemia and amenorrhea—responses to bromocriptine. J Clin Endocrinol Metab 59:941–948, © by the Endocrine Society, 1984.)

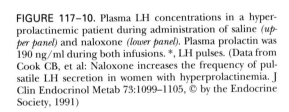

FIGURE 117–10. Plasma LH concentrations in a hyperprolactinemic patient during administration of saline *(upper panel)* and naloxone *(lower panel)*. Plasma prolactin was 190 ng/ml during both infusions. *, LH pulses. (Data from Cook CB, et al: Naloxone increases the frequency of pulsatile LH secretion in women with hyperprolactinemia. J Clin Endocrinol Metab 73:1099–1105, © by the Endocrine Society, 1991)

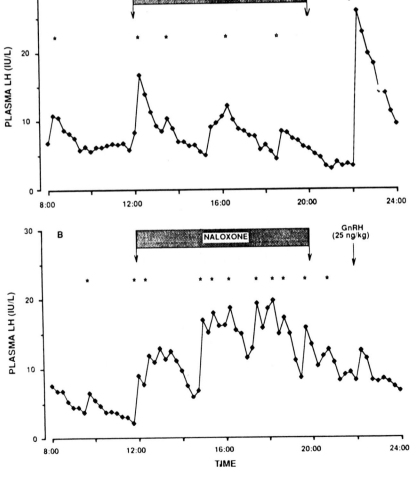

reduces GnRH secretion, particularly by reducing pulse frequency (Fig. 117–10).

These data suggest that both hypothalamic amenorrhea and hyperprolactinemia produce ovulation consequent on a slow frequency of endogenous GnRH secretion. This results in persistent GnRH stimuli similar to those present in the normal luteal phase. The inability to increase pulsatile GnRH secretion results in a failure of follicular maturation and failure of estradiol and progesterone to augment LH release (the latter would not occur in the absence of an adequate GnRH stimulus). In addition, data show that the abnormalities of GnRH secretion may be variable[55] and not consistently present on a week-to-week basis. This may account for why some women with apparent hypothalamic amenorrhea have "normal" LH pulse frequencies during some studies. If an underlying mechanism such as stress acting through increased hypothalamic opioid activity were the underlying mechanism, this may be variable in both degree and duration. If the mechanism was present for long enough to affect the hypothalamic mechanisms involved in normal follicular maturation and ovulation, anovulation would be expected to ensue.

Polycystic Ovarian Syndrome

Polycystic ovarian (PCO) syndrome is a disorder of unknown cause associated with anovulation, hirsutism, obe-sity, and multiple cysts in the ovaries. The excess androgen secretion in PCO has been shown to be predominantly of ovarian origin, but adrenal abnormalities exist, and it is probable that the syndrome encompasses several disorders. An ovarian abnormality, including abnormal ovarian steroidogenesis or follicular maturation, may be the primary cause of excess androgen secretion in some patients.[63] In a majority, however, the syndrome is associated with increased LH secretion, and some 75 per cent of patients with PCO have elevated mean serum LH levels. Blockade of LH secretion by desensitization using a long-acting GnRH agonist is followed by reduced androgen secretion, confirming the importance of LH stimulation of the ovary.[64] Studies have demonstrated that the frequency and amplitude of LH pulses usually are increased in patients with PCO.[65, 66] This suggests the possibility that a persistent rapid frequency of GnRH secretion causes the excess LH synthesis and secretion, which in turn produces enhanced androgen production by the ovary and failure of follicular maturation. Some authorities view the abnormal GnRH secretion as secondary to abnormal secretion from the ovary, but evidence to support this view is lacking. An alternative view is that the abnormal pulsatile GnRH secretion is the underlying abnormality in PCO. In normal cycles estradiol and progesterone inhibit pulse frequency in the luteal phase, and if a relative inability of these steroids to reduce GnRH secretion were present, this would be expected to result in persistent increased GnRH and LH secretion. Many patients with PCO had an onset of symp-

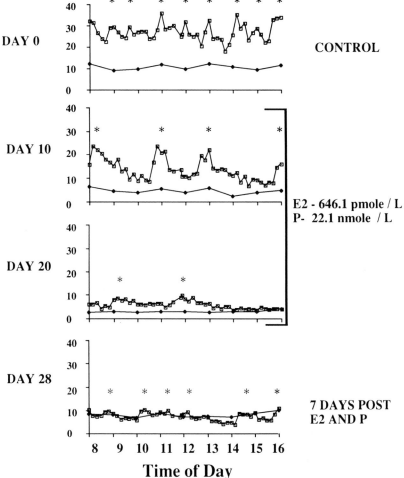

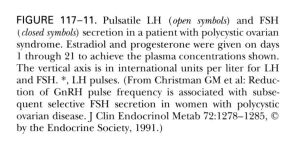

FIGURE 117–11. Pulsatile LH (*open symbols*) and FSH (*closed symbols*) secretion in a patient with polycystic ovarian syndrome. Estradiol and progesterone were given on days 1 through 21 to achieve the plasma concentrations shown. The vertical axis is in international units per liter for LH and FSH. *, LH pulses. (From Christman GM et al: Reduction of GnRH pulse frequency is associated with subsequent selective FSH secretion in women with polycystic ovarian disease. J Clin Endocrinol Metab 72:1278–1285, © by the Endocrine Society, 1991.)

toms soon after pubertal maturation, a time when the ability to secrete GnRH at a fast frequency is achieved. Thus, if women destined to develop PCO were relatively resistant to the effects of estradiol and progesterone in slowing GnRH, the normal slowing of the luteal phase may not occur. This would be expected to result in a relative deficiency in selective FSH secretion, with abnormalities of follicular maturation and irregular infrequent ovulation. Over time increased GnRH pulse frequency and LH secretion would increase ovarian androgen production and cause hirsutism and cyst formation in the ovaries. These views extend existing data, but some evidence suggests that these events may occur. In half of the adolescent girls with anovulation studied, LH pulse amplitude and frequency were increased, and this was associated with elevated plasma estradiol and progesterone.[67, 68] It is uncertain whether these adolescents will later develop changes consistent with PCO.

To explore these causative possibilities, studies have assessed the ability of physiological luteal concentrations of estradiol and progesterone to suppress the rapid frequency of GnRH secretion in women with PCO.[69] The data in Figure 117–11 show that the administration of estrogen and progesterone initially slowed the frequency of GnRH

secretion (day 10), with later persistent slowing and marked reduction in LH pulse amplitude. Withdrawal of ovarian steroids was associated with increased GnRH pulse frequency and a selective increase in FSH, which increased more rapidly than LH. This relative increase in FSH after steroids were discontinued and normalization of the LH-FSH ratio are seen in Figure 117–12. The enhanced FSH secretion resulted in follicular maturation in all patients studied and ovulation in some.

The observation that most patients with PCO have increased frequency and amplitude of pulsatile LH secretion appears well established, and the results in Figures 117–11 and 117–12 are consistent with a relative inability to slow GnRH pulsatile secretion in the manner that normally occurs in the luteal phase. Proof of these suggestions awaits further study, but the data suggest a potential line of therapy, at least for the subset of women with PCO who have elevated plasma LH levels and rapid-frequency GnRH secretion.

These observations in anovulatory patients indicate that some disorders resulting in anovulation are associated with abnormalities of GnRH secretory patterns. Both slow frequency with inability to increase GnRH pulse frequency and persistence of rapid GnRH frequencies have been recognized. This suggests that the ability to change the pattern of GnRH secretion in normal cycles is an important part of the cyclical process of repeated ovulation. Moreover, these data suggest new approaches to therapy whereby the administration of opioid receptor antagonists in hypothalamic amenorrhea or of exogenous hormones to slow GnRH frequency in PCO may be efficacious in restoring normal pulsatile GnRH secretion and ovulatory cycles.

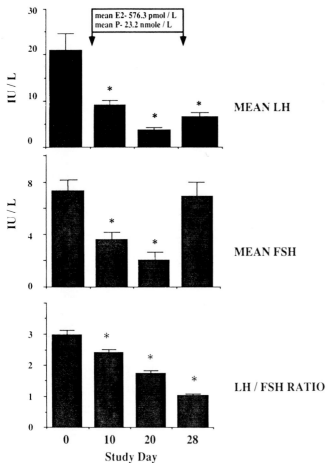

FIGURE 117–12. Mean plasma concentrations of LH and FSH and LH-FSH ratios in six women with polycystic ovarian syndrome given estradiol and progesterone on days 1 through 21. *$P < .001$ compared to day 0. (From Christman GM et al: Reduction of GnRH pulse frequency is associated with subsequent selective FSH secretion in women with polycystic ovarian disease. J Clin Endocrinol Metab 72:1278–1285, © by the Endocrine Society, 1991.)

REFERENCES

1. Cargille CM, Ross GT, Yoshimi TJ: Daily variations in plasma follicle-stimulating hormone, luteinizing hormone and progesterone in a normal menstrual cycle. J Clin Endocrinol Metab 29:12–16, 1969.
2. Abraham GE, Odell WD, Swerdloff RS, et al: Simultaneous radioimmunoassay of plasma FSH, LH, progesterone, 17-hydroxyprogesterone and estradiol-17 during the menstrual cycle. J Clin Endocrinol Metab 34:312–318, 1972.
3. Speroff L, Vande Weile L: Regulation of the human menstrual cycle. Am J Obstet Gynecol 109:234–237, 1971.
4. Baird DT, Fraser HM, Hillier SG, et al: Production and secretion of ovarian inhibin in women. In Yen SSC, Vale WW (eds): Neuroendocrine Regulation of Reproduction. Norwell, MA, Serono Symposia USA, 1990, pp. 195–206.
5. McLachlin RI, Robertson DM, Healy DL, et al: Circulating immunoreactive inhibin levels during the normal human menstrual cycle. J Clin Endocrinol Metab 65:954–961, 1987.
6. DiZerega GS, Hodgen GD: Folliculogenesis in the primate ovarian cycle. Endocr Rev 2:27–49, 1981.
7. Baird DT: Factors regulating the growth of the pre-ovulatory follicle in the sheep and human. J Reprod Fertil 69:343–352, 1983.
8. Tonetta SA, DiZerega GS: Intragonadal regulation of follicular maturation. Endocr Rev 10:205–229, 1989.
9. Adashi EY: The potential revelance of cytokines to ovarian physiology: The emerging role of ovarian cells of the white blood cell series. Endocr Rev 11:454–464, 1990.
10. Zeleznik AJ: Premature elevation of systemic estradiol reduces serum FSH and lengthens the follicular phase of the menstrual cycle in rhesus monkeys. Endocrinology 109:352–355, 1981.
11. Hsueh AJW, Adashi EY, Jones PBC, Welsh TH Jr: Hormonal regulation of the differentiation of cultured ovarian granulosa cells. Endocr Rev 5:76–127, 1984.
12. Marshall JC, Case GD, Valk TW, et al: Selective inhibition of follicle-

stimulating hormone secretion by estradiol. Mechanism for modulation of gonadotropin responses to low dose pulses of gonadotropin-releasing hormone. J Clin Invest 71:248–258, 1983.

13. Odell WD, Swerdloff RS: Progesterone induced luteinizing and follicle-stimulating hormone surge in postmenopausal women—a stimulated ovulatory peak. Proc Natl Acad Sci USA 61:629–631, 1968.

14. Moenter SM, Caraty A, Karsch FJ: The estradiol induced surge of GnRH in the ewe. Endocrinology 127:1375–1384, 1990.

15. Auletta FJ, Flint ADF: Mechanisms controlling corpus luteum function in sheep, cows, nonhuman primates and women especially in relation to the time of luteolysis. Endocr Rev 9:88–105, 1988.

16. Yen SSC, Tsai CC, Naftolin F, et al: Pulsatile patterns of gonadotropin release in subjects with and without ovarian function. J Clin Endocrinol Metab 34:671–676, 1972.

17. Santen RJ, Bardin CW: Episodic luteinizing hormone secretion in man. J Clin Invest 52:2617–2628, 1973.

18. Backstrom CT, McNeilly AS, Leask RM, Baird DT: Pulsatile secretion of LH, FSH, prolactin, estradiol and progesterone during the human menstrual cycle. Clin Endocrinol (Oxf) 17:29–40, 1982.

19. Reame N, Sauder SE, Kelch RP, Marshall JC: Pulsatile gonadotropin secretion during the human menstrual cycle: Evidence for altered frequency of gonadotropin-releasing hormone secretion. J Clin Endocrinol Metab 59:328–337, 1984.

20. Baird DT: Pulsatile secretion of LH and ovarian estradiol in the follicular phase of the sheep estrous cycle. Biol Reprod 18:359–364, 1978.

21. Djahanbakhch O, Warner P, McNeilly AS, Baird DT: Pulsatile release of LH and estradiol during the periovulatory period in normal women. Clin Endocrinol (Oxf) 20:579–589, 1984.

22. Karsch FJ, Foster DL, Bittman EL, Goodman RL: A role for estradiol in enhancing LH pulse frequency during the follicular phase of the estrous cycle of sheep. Endocrinology 113:1333–1339, 1983.

23. Moenter SM, Caraty A, Locatelli A, Karsch FJ: Pattern of GnRH secretion leading up to ovulation in the ewe: Existence of a preovulatory GnRH surge. Endocrinology 129:1175–1182, 1991.

24. Knobil E, Plant TM, Wildt L, et al: Control of the rhesus monkey menstrual cycle: Permissive role of hypothalamic gonadotropin-releasing hormone. Science 207:1371–1374, 1980.

25. Leyendecker G, Wildt L, Hansmann M: Pregnancies following chronic intermittent (pulsatile) administration of GnRH by means of a pulsatile pump (zyklomat)—a new approach to the treatment of infertility in hypothalamic amenorrhea. J Clin Endocrinol Metab 51:1214–1216, 1980.

26. Hoff JD, Quigley ME, Yen SSC: Hormonal dynamics at mid cycle: A reevaluation. J Clin Endocrinol Metab 57:792–796, 1983.

27. Liu JH, Yen SSC: Induction of the mid cycle gonadotropin surge by ovarian steroids in women—a critical evaluation. J Clin Endocrinol Metab 57:797–802, 1983.

28. McNatty KP, Makras A, DeGrazia C, et al: The production of progesterone, androgens and estrogens by human granulosa cells, thecal tissue and stromal tissue from human ovaries in vitro. J Clin Endocrinol Metab 49:687–694, 1979.

29. Nippoldt TB, Khoury S, Barkan A, et al: Gonadotropin responses to GnRH pulses in hypogonadotropic hypogonadism: LH responsiveness is maintained in the presence of luteal phase concentrations of estrogen and progesterone. Clin Endocrinol 26:293–301, 1987.

30. Soules MR, Steiner RA, Clifton DK, et al: Progesterone modulation of pulsatile luteinizing hormone secretion in normal women. J Clin Endocrinol Metab 58:378–383, 1984.

31. Goodman RL, Bittman EL, Foster DL, Karsch FJ: The endocrine basis of the synergistic suppression of luteinizing hormone by estradiol and progesterone. Endocrinology 109:1414–1417, 1981.

32. Ropert JF, Quigley ME, Yen SSC: Endogenous opiates modulate pulsatile luteinizing hormone release in humans. J Clin Endocrinol Metab 52:583–588, 1981.

33. Van Vugt DA, Lam NY, Ferin M: Reduced frequency of pulsatile luteinizing hormone secretion in the luteal phase of the rhesus monkey: Involvement of endogenous opiates. Endocrinology 115:1095–1101, 1984.

34. Vande Wiele RL, Bogumil J, Dyrenfurth I, et al: Mechanisms regulating the menstrual cycle in women. Recent Prog Horm Res 26:63–103, 1970.

35. Filicori M, Butler JP, Crowley WF: Neuroendocrine regulation of the corpus luteum in the human—evidence for pulsatile progesterone secretion. J Clin Invest 73:1638–1647, 1984.

36. Marshall JC, Dalkin AC, Haisenleder DJ, et al: Gonadotropin-releasing hormone pulses: Regulators of gonadotropin synthesis and ovulatory cycles. Recent Prog Horm Res 47:155–189, 1991.

37. Crowley WF, MacArthur JW: Simulation of the normal menstrual cycle

38. Valk TW, Marshall JC, Kelch RP: Simulation of the follicular phase of the menstrual cycle by intravenous administration of low dose pulsatile gonadotropin-releasing hormone. Am J Obstet Gynecol 141:842–844, 1981.

39. Filicori M, Flamigni C, Merriggiola MC, et al: Ovulation induction with pulsatile gonadotropin-releasing hormone: Technical modalities and clinical perspectives. Fertil Steril 56:1–13, 1991.

40. Lam NY, Ferin M: Is the decrease in the hypophysiotropic signal frequency normally observed during the luteal phase important for menstrual cyclicity in the primate? Endocrinology 120:2044–2050, 1987.

41. Soules MR, Clifton DK, Bremner WJ, Steiner RA: Corpus luteum insufficiency induced by a rapid gonadotropin-releasing hormone-induced gonadotropin secretion pattern in the follicular phase. J Clin Endocrinol Metab 65:457–464, 1987.

42. Marshall JC, Kelch RP: Gonadotropin-releasing hormone: Role of pulsatile secretion in the regulation of reproduction. N Engl J Med 315:1459–1468, 1986.

43. Hale PM, Khoury S, Foster CM, Beitins IZ, et al: Increased luteinizing hormone pulse frequency during sleep in early to midpubertal boys: Effects of testosterone infusion. J Clin Endocrinol Metab 66:785–791, 1988.

44. Reiter EO, Kulin HE, Hamwood SM: The absence of positive feedback between estrogen and luteinizing hormone in sexually immature girls. Pediatric Res 8:740–745, 1974.

45. Schwartz B, Cumming DC, Riordan E, et al: Exercise-associated amenorrhea: A distinct entity? Am J Obstet Gynecol 141:662–668, 1981.

46. Santen RJ, Friend JN, Trojanowski D, et al: Prolonged negative feedback suppression after estradiol administration: Proposed mechanism of eugonadal secondary amenorrhea. J Clin Endocrinol Metab 47:1220–1229, 1978.

47. Shaw RW, Butt WR, London DR, Marshall JC: The estrogen provocation test—a method for assessing the hypothalamic-pituitary axis in patients with amenorrhea. Clin Endocrinol (Oxf) 4:267–276, 1975.

48. Shaw RW, Butt WR, London DR: Pathological mechanisms to explain some cases of amenorrhea without organic disease. Br J Obstet Gynaecol 82:337–340, 1975.

49. Rakoff JS, Rigg LA, Yen SSC: The impairment of progesterone induced pituitary release of prolactin and gonadotropin in patients with hypothalamic chronic anovulation. Am J Obstet Gynecol 130:807–812, 1978.

50. Reame NE, Sauder SE, Kelch RP, et al: Pulsatile gonadotropin secretion in women with hypothalamic amenorrhea—evidence for reduced frequency of GnRH secretion. J Clin Endocrinol Metab 61:851–858, 1985.

51. Veldhuis JD, Evans WS, Demers LM, et al: Altered neuroendocrine regulation of gonadotropin secretion in women distance runners. J Clin Endocrinol Metab 61:557–563, 1985.

52. Crowley WF, Filicori M, Spratt DI, Santoro NF: The physiology of GnRH secretion in men and women. Recent Prog Horm Res 41:473–531, 1985.

53. Quigley ME, Sheehan KL, Casper RF, Yen SSC: Evidence for increased dopaminergic and opiate activity in patients with hypothalamic hypogonadotropic amenorrhea. J Clin Endocrinol Metab 50:949–954, 1980.

54. Sauder SE, Case GD, Hopwood NJ, et al: The effects of opiate antagonism on gonadotropin secretion in children and in women with hypothalamic amenorrhea. Pediatr Res 18:322–328, 1984.

55. Khoury SA, Reame NE, Kelch RP, Marshall JC: Diurnal patterns of pulsatile luteinizing hormone secretion in hypothalamic amenorrhea: Reproducibility and responses to opiate blockade and in α_2-adrenergic agonist. J Clin Endocrinol Metab 64:755–762, 1987.

56. Pohl CR, Richardson DW, Hutchison JS, et al: Hypophysiotropic signal frequency and the functioning of the pituitary-ovarian axis in the rhesus monkey. Endocrinology 112:2076–2080, 1983.

57. Biller BMK, Federoff HJ, Koenig JI, Klibanski A: Abnormal cortisol secretion and responses to corticotropin-releasing hormone in women with hypothalamic amenorrhea. J Clin Endocrinol Metab 70:311–317, 1990.

58. Wildt L, Leyendecker G: Induction of ovulation by the chronic administration of naltrexone in hypothalamic amenorrhea. J Clin Endocrinol Metab 64:1334–1335, 1987.

59. Klibanski A, Beitins IZ, Merriam GR, et al: Gonadotropin and prolactin pulsations in hyperprolactinemic women before and during bromocriptine therapy. J Clin Endocrinol Metab 58:1141–1147, 1984.

60. Sauder SE, Frager M, Case GD, et al: Abnormal patterns of pulsatile luteinizing hormone secretion in women with hyperprolactinemia and amenorrhea—responses to bromocriptine. J Clin Endocrinol Metab 59:941–948, 1984.

61. Grossman A, Moult PJA, McIntyre H, et al: Opiate mediation of amenorrhea in hyperprolactinemia and in weight loss related amenorrhea. Clin Endocrinol (Oxf) 17:379–388, 1982.

62. Cook CB, Nippoldt TB, Kletter GB, et al: Naloxone increases the frequency of pulsatile LH secretion in women with hyperprolactinemia. J Clin Endocrinol Metab 73:1099–1105, 1991.

63. Ehrmann DA, Rosenfield RL, Barnes RB, et al: Detection of functional ovarian hyperandrogenism in women with androgen excess. N Engl J Med 327:157–162, 1992.

64. Chang RJ, Laufer LR, Meldrum DR, Judd HL: Steroid secretion in polycystic ovarian disease after ovarian suppression by a long acting GnRH agonist. J Clin Endocrinol Metab 56:897–903, 1983.

65. Kazer RR, Kessel B, Yen SSC: LH pulse frequency in women with PCO. J Clin Endocrinol Metab 65:223–226, 1987.

66. Waldstreicher J, Santoro NF, Hall JE, et al: Hyperfunction of the hypothalamic pituitary axis in women with PCO. J Clin Endocrinol Metab 66:165–172, 1988.

67. Porcu E, Venturoli S, Magini O, et al: Circadian variations of luteinizing hormones can have two different profiles in adolescent anovulation. J Clin Endocrinol Metab 65:488–494, 1987.

68. Zumoff B, Freeman R, Coupey S, et al: A chronobiologic abnormality in luteinizing hormone secretion in teenage girls with polycystic ovary syndrome. N Engl J Med 309:1206–1209, 1983.

69. Christman GM, Randolph J, Kelch RP, Marshall JC: Reduction of GnRH pulse frequency is associated with subsequent selective FSH secretion in women with polycystic ovarian disease. J Clin Endocrinol Metab 72:1278–1285, 1991.

Amenorrhea, Anovulation, and Dysfunctional Uterine Bleeding

DAVID T. BAIRD

Regular menstrual cycles are the most obvious manifestation of cyclical ovarian activity, which depends on a carefully regulated feedback system that involves the hypothalamus, anterior pituitary, and ovary (Chs. 113 and 116). Hence a disturbance in the pattern of menstruation usually is the most obvious symptom of a disorder of ovarian activity and is the most common reason women in the reproductive age (15 to 50 years) consult a physician.[1, 2] Yet the almost universal expectation of the menstrual cycle as the norm among women is a relatively new phenomenon, a product of the decline in fertility rates in modern Western society.[3] For most of humankind's existence most women were amenorrheic, either because they were pregnant or because they were lactating. Hence the problems associated with menstrual cycles have reached epidemic proportions in the latter half of the 20th century. Although most cases of amenorrhea are due to a defect in ovarian function, developmental and acquired abnormalities of the genital tract may present with similar symptoms. In particular, before it can be assumed that disturbance in the pattern of menstruation is due to an endocrine cause, local intrauterine pathology must be excluded. Although this chapter concentrates on the endocrine causes of a disturbance in the pattern of menstruation, the variety of organic abnormalities is included for the sake of completeness. It is usual to classify amenorrhea into primary and secondary, depending on whether or not the subject has ever menstruated. Although this distinction has some clinical usefulness in focusing on the likely causes, the overlap is wide, and I prefer to consider the conditions based on their underlying pathology.

NORMAL OVARIAN AND MENSTRUAL CYCLES

The developmental changes in neuroendocrine function that occur throughout puberty are discussed in detail in Chapters 111 and 113 and are referred to only briefly here. In response to increased activity of the hypothalamic neurons responsible for secreting gonadotropin-releasing hormone (GnRH), there is a progressive rise in the secretion of follicle-stimulating hormone (FSH) and luteinizing hormone (LH) beginning many years before the physical manifestations of puberty. In association with a change in the sensitivity of the hypothalamic-pituitary unit to the feedback effects of ovarian steroids, there is cyclical growth of ovarian follicles and secretion of estradiol, which stimulates the uterine endometrium. The first menstrual period often is due to estrogen withdrawal, and it is not until some months after the menarche that ovulatory cycles become established.[4, 5] Maturation of the positive feedback system that involves both the hypothalamus and the anterior pituitary may be delayed for years and result in a period of irregular menstruation in late puberty.[6] As soon as regular ovulatory cycles have become established, the pattern of menstrual cycles for each person is remarkably constant (Fig. 118–1).[7, 8] In the years between ages 20 and 40, there is a slight but significant decrease in the mean length of the menstrual cycle owing to a shorter follicular phase. The variability in the length of the cycle increases markedly in the decade before the menopause, reflecting a gradual decline in ovarian function before complete failure. Hence

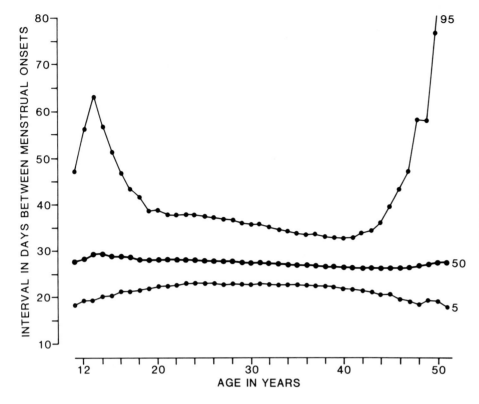

FIGURE 118–1. **Menstrual cycle length in relation to age.** The median and 5th and 95th centiles are indicated. Note the marked variation in the length of the menstrual cycle at the extremes of reproductive life. (Redrawn from Treloar AE, et al: Variation of the human menstrual cycle through reproductive life. Int J Fertil 12:77–126, 1967.)

disorders in the pattern of menstruation are much commoner at the extremes of reproductive life in association with establishment and demise of ovarian function.

MECHANISM OF MENSTRUATION

Although the relation between ovarian function and menstruation has been known for centuries, it was not until the discovery and isolation of estradiol and progesterone earlier this century that the mechanism by which steroid withdrawal induced bleeding was investigated.[9, 10] After priming with estrogen, bleeding from the endometrium occurs in response to withdrawal of either estradiol or progesterone, although the levels of both steroids drop at luteal regression before the onset of menstruation. It seems likely that prostaglandins are involved in the vascular changes that accompany endometrial shedding, and that priming with both estradiol and progesterone is necessary for optimal synthesis of prostaglandin $F_{2\alpha}$ and prostaglandin E_2.[11, 12] Hence any alteration in the sequence of hormonal priming with estradiol followed by progesterone, which is characteristic of the normal ovarian cycle, disturbs the synthesis of prostaglandins by the endometrium and, therefore, produces an abnormality in menstrual pattern.

ASSESSMENT OF PITUITARY OVARIAN FUNCTION

History and Clinical Examination

Because uterine bleeding occurs in response to the withdrawal of sex steroids, it is clear that a careful menstrual history is of great importance in assessing ovarian activity.

In the absence of exogenous hormone medication, the presence of even scanty bleeding indicates that the ovaries are secreting sufficient estrogen to stimulate proliferation of the endometrium. Thus it can be assumed that in women with a history of oligomenorrhea, some ovarian activity is present. If complete amenorrhea is present, it is important to establish whether it is primary or secondary and, if the latter, whether it was followed by hot flushes, indicating primary ovarian failure. If primary amenorrhea is due to ovarian agenesis, hot flushes do not occur, unless the woman has been previously treated with exogenous estrogens. A careful dietary history and weight record should be sought in all women who complain of amenorrhea. The most common clinical feature of women who present with this symptom is a history of weight loss, usually caused by voluntary dietary restriction.[13] Psychological stress owing to such factors as bereavement and separation may coincide with cessation of menstruation. Various psychotropic drugs may interfere with normal hypothalamic function either by depleting the amounts of catecholamines (e.g., reserpine) or by blocking dopamine receptors (e.g., phenothiazines). A number of clinical signs are useful indices of ovarian activity on physical examination. The development of secondary sex characteristics, including female contours and breasts, is mainly due to the increased secretion of estradiol by the ovary at puberty. Adequate breast development, therefore, indicates that at some time the ovaries (or, rarely, the testes) have secreted adequate quantities of estrogen. A more sensitive clinical index of current estrogenic status is the thickness of the vaginal epithelium and the quality of cervical mucus. Under the influence of unopposed estrogen, the walls of the vagina become well vascularized and thicken owing to hypertrophy and cornification of the squamous epithelial cells. There is an increased secretion of cervical mucus that becomes watery because of changes in the content of water, electrolytes, and mucopolysaccharides.[14] These estrogen-induced changes in consistency are responsible for the change in physical properties that allow the mucus to be stretched out for several centimeters before breaking—spinnbarkeit. Estrogen production can be confirmed either by the finding of a proliferative endometrium on biopsy or by menstrual bleeding in response to a progestogen challenge.

Diagnostic Tests

An additional investigation that can be useful in the management of women with oligomenorrhea or amenorrhea is a pelvic ultrasound examination. The ovaries, uterus, endometrium, and vagina can all be visualized with either an abdominal or a vaginal probe.[15] The resolution of modern real-time scanning is such that follicles as small as 2 mm in diameter can be identified in the ovary. The shape and size of the uterus and measurement of uterine thickness are helpful in assessing estrogenic status.

Although various elaborate diagnostic tests of the hypothalamic-hypophyseal-ovarian axis have been described, they are mainly of use for research purposes and have little practical importance in planning the management of the individual patient. In the vast majority of patients it should be possible to make a diagnosis sufficient to plan therapy after history, physical examination, and basic investigations.[16]

Basic Diagnostic Investigation

At the initial consultation blood should be withdrawn for the measurement of FSH, LH, prolactin, estradiol, and thyroxine and/or thyroid-stimulating hormone (TSH). Any spontaneous ovarian activity can be monitored by serial measurements once or twice weekly of the concentration in plasma of estradiol and progesterone or their metabolites in urine. I prefer to measure sex steroids directly rather than rely solely on the progesterone challenge test for assessment of ovarian activity. In all women with amenorrhea a right lateral and anteroposterior radiograph of the skull should be taken to outline the sella turcica. These basic investigations should allow classification of the patients into a number of diagnostic categories that correspond to the basic endocrine defect and are useful when planning therapy.

Dynamic Tests of Pituitary-Ovarian Activity

As indicated above, dynamic tests of pituitary-ovarian activity have limited place in routine clinical practice.[17, 18] The responsiveness of the pituitary to GnRH can be tested by single or repeated injections of GnRH in doses ranging from 100 to 5 μg.[19, 20] The injection of a large supraphysiological dose of GnRH (100 μg) tests the responsiveness and gives some index of the capacity of the pituitary to secrete gonadotropins.[21] The response is closely correlated with the basal level of gonadotropins, and it may be helpful in establishing the degree of gonadotropin deficiency. A single injection, however, cannot determine the total functional capacity of the anterior pituitary (i.e., the pituitary

reserve), a better index of which can be obtained by measuring the response to repeated injections of "physiological" amounts of GnRH (5 to 10 μg) at intervals of two to three hours. This test of secretory capacity correlates better with the degree of spontaneous secretion as measured by the amplitude and frequency of LH pulses. Estradiol plays a key role in regulating the secretion of gonadotropins by the hypothalamus. The negative and positive feedback response to estrogen can be tested by various provocation tests. Exogenous estrogen is administered either by injection as estradiol benzoate (1 to 3 mg) or by ingestion of ethinyl estradiol (100 μg/d for three days).[17, 22] In normal women after initial suppression (negative feedback), a surge of LH and FSH occurs within 72 to 96 hours (positive feedback). Alterations in both negative and positive feedback occur in various conditions, resulting in amenorrhea or anovulatory cycles.

The negative feedback system can be indirectly tested using anti-estrogens such as clomiphene citrate or tamoxifen.[23, 24] By antagonizing the biological effect of endogenous estrogen, administration of these compounds results in an elevation in both FSH and LH. When the levels of endogenous estrogen are very low (e.g., in prepubertal children or hypogonadotropic amenorrhea), however, they act as weak agonists, resulting in suppression of gonadotropins.[25]

The response of the ovaries to gonadotropins can be indirectly assessed by measuring the level of estradiol after elevation of gonadotropins induced by GnRH or anti-estrogen. Alternatively, exogenous gonadotropins can be injected and the rise in estradiol concentration and/or the growth of ovarian follicles monitored by serial ultrasound measurements.[26] Either purified FSH or human chorionic gonadotropin (hCG) can be used to test the response to FSH or LH, respectively.

AMENORRHEA

Abnormalities in ovarian activity may be indicated by various changes in the menstrual pattern, ranging from amenorrhea to continuous menstrual bleeding. A normal menstrual cycle occurs at intervals of between 21 and 35 days and lasts no longer than 7 days. By convention, *amenorrhea* is defined as absence of menstrual bleeding for six months; *oligomenorrhea*, as bleeding that occurs at intervals of between 35 days and 6 months.

Physiological Causes

Pregnancy and lactation are two common physiological causes of amenorrhea. The early signs of pregnancy are easy to overlook, and all women in the reproductive age group who have missed a period should be assumed to be pregnant until it has been proved otherwise. Ovulation and pregnancy can occur without resumption of menstruation after lactation or after recovery from hypothalamic suppression associated with weight loss. The physician should never omit a full physical examination, including a pelvic examination, before ordering further investigations. The measurement of hCG in blood or urine excludes pregnancy.

Local Genital Causes

Malformation or absence of the lower genital tract is a relatively common congenital abnormality.[27] The presenting clinical symptoms depend on the degree of maldevelopment. Imperforate hymen or incompletely canalized vagina results in primary amenorrhea with normal secondary sex characteristics and cyclical abdominal pain during puberty. The diagnosis can be easily made from the history and presence of a pelvic swelling and bulging septum at the introitus. It is important to make the diagnosis promptly because unless surgically corrected, the distention of the uterus and tubes with retrograde menstruation may produce permanent damage and sterility. Complete failure of the müllerian duct system to develop results in primary amenorrhea in association with absence of the uterus, fallopian tubes, and upper vagina.

Because, embryologically, the genital and urinary tracts are derived from common structures, it is hardly surprising that abnormalities of the urinary tract often are found in association with absence of the uterus and/or vagina. Intravenous pyelography may reveal duplex ureters or the absence of one kidney and collecting duct system.

The diagnosis of absence of the uterus can easily be made clinically by the presence of normal secondary sex characteristics in the absence of a palpable uterus or cervix. The presence of normal axillary and pubic hair excludes testicular feminization. The diagnosis can be confirmed by normal female karyotype and, if necessary, inspection of the pelvic organs by ultrasonography and/or laparoscopy.

If the cervix or upper vagina is absent but the uterus is present, retrograde menstruation into the pelvic cavity will result in cyclical lower abdominal pain. Endometriosis may develop in the pelvic peritoneum with subsequent fibrosis and adhesions. Examination under anesthesia, and laparoscopy are necessary to confirm the diagnosis.

Secondary amenorrhea owing to a uterine cause may also occur because of the development of endometrial synechiae after repeated curettage of the uterus, abortion, myomectomy, or cesarean section, or the destruction of the endometrium after tuberculous infection (Asherman's syndrome). In developed countries with good medical services, these causes are becoming fairly rare; hysterectomy is a much more common iatrogenic cause of amenorrhea.

Disorders of Sexual Differentiation

Because the acquisition of the male genitalia and sexual characteristics depends on the secretion of the fetal testis, any defect in the synthesis of testosterone results in varying degrees of female phenotype.[28–30] Congenital disorders owing to the absence or reduction in five key enzymes required in the synthesis of testosterone are dealt with in Chapter 109 (20,22-cholesterol desmolase, 3β-hydroxy-Δ^5-steroid dehydrogenase, 17-keto-reductase, 17α-hydroxylase, and 17,20-desmolase). In these genetic males, incomplete masculinization of the urogenital sinus and external genitalia may result in male pseudohermaphroditism. If unrecognized at birth, these people may be raised as girls and present with primary amenorrhea at the time of expected puberty. The diagnosis can be made by the presence of normal XY karyotype and by the measurement of raised levels of precursor steroids, reflecting the defects in steroid enzymes.

Testicular Feminization (Androgen Insensitivity)

Another inherited disorder that results in male pseudohermaphroditism is insensitivity of the peripheral tissues to the action of androgens.[31, 32] Deficiency in the androgen receptor and/or the enzyme responsible for the conversion of testosterone to 5α-dihydrotestosterone (5α-reductase) results in lack of androgenization to varying degrees.[33] Several mutations in the gene coding for the androgen receptor have been described and may explain the variability in clinical phenotype.[34] In the complete testicular feminization syndrome, the phenotype is fully female, although the uterus and upper vagina are absent because of the production of müllerian duct inhibitory factor by the fetal testes. The testes also secrete the normal male amounts of testosterone and estradiol, although the former is ineffective in producing androgenization. The testes, therefore, fail to descend into the scrotum and are retained within the abdominal cavity or inguinal canal. Because of the secretion of estradiol, there is good breast development and the normal female contours. Axillary and pubic hair are scanty or absent. The diagnosis is easily made from the family history, absence of body hair, XY karyotype, and the male levels of testosterone in plasma. The intra-abdominal testes are more likely to develop tumors and should be surgically removed as soon as growth and breast development are complete. The so-called incomplete testicular feminization is associated with some evidence of masculinization of the external genitalia at birth (e.g., partial fusion of the labia) but absence of the penis and scrotum. Partial virilization often occurs at puberty owing to increased secretion of testosterone. Pubic hair develops, and there is absence of breast development. Some of these people have deficiency of 5α-reductase enzyme, which converts testosterone to dihydrotestosterone. Because this conversion is required for the action of testosterone on the genital tubercle (but not on other target organs), the external genitalia are incompletely androgenized.

DISORDERS OF HYPOTHALAMIC-PITUITARY-OVARIAN AXIS

Because normal functioning of the ovaries depends on a feedback system that involves the anterior pituitary and the hypothalamus, a defect or malfunctioning in any one component leads to a breakdown in cyclicity and a disturbance in the pattern of menstruation. A classification of amenorrhea based on the basic defect in the hypothalamic-pituitary-ovarian (HPO) system is shown in Table 118–1 (Fig. 118–2). The degree of failure may range from total (e.g., amenorrhea in association with ovarian failure or hypopituitarism) to minor deficiencies in gonadotropin secretion, resulting in slight upsets in ovarian cycles. Defects in the HPO system may present with primary or secondary amenorrhea, although the latter is much more common.

The HPO system is composed of both positive and negative feedback loops. Although the positive feedback loop

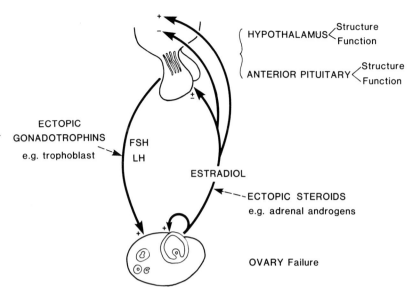

FIGURE 118–2. **Defects in the hypothalamic-pituitary-ovarian axis.** Estradiol feeds back at the level of both the anterior pituitary and the hypothalamus to regulate the secretion of gonadotropins. Ovarian failure results in elevated levels of FSH and LH; steroids and gonadotropins from extraovarian sources lead to a disturbance in the normal feedback mechanism; structural or functional disease of the hypothalamic and/or pituitary leads to hypogonadotropic hypogonadism. (Adapted from Baird D [ed]: Abnormalities of gonadotropin secretion in women. Clin Obstet Gynaecol 3, 1976.)

Ovarian Failure

Unlike the testis, an ovary without gametes (oocytes) cannot function as an endocrine gland. The gonad may fail to develop normally and be present in adulthood merely as a streak.[35] The cause of gonadal agenesis in either sex is unknown but results in a similar clinical presentation (i.e., primary amenorrhea with sexual infantilism) (Fig. 118–3). A normal uterus, fallopian tubes, and vagina are present. The testis-determining gene (Tdy) is situated on the short arm of the Y chromosome and that responsible for the H-Y antigen, on the long arm.[36] Thus in XY gonadal dysgenesis, the testis may fail to develop due to the loss or mutation of the Tdy.[37] Because the levels of estrogen are very low, the concentration of FSH is elevated into the castrate range. If the karyotype reveals 46XY, the gonadal streaks should be removed because there is a risk of malignant transformation. Replacement therapy with cyclical estrogen and progestogen should be started to induce secondary sex characteristics and prevent premature demineralization of skeletal bone.

Gonadal dysgenesis usually also occurs in Turner's syndrome—perhaps the most common sex chromosomal abnormality in neonates (1 in 2500 girls).[38] The incidence in spontaneous abortion is much higher, suggesting that less

than 10 per cent of XO fetuses reach viability.[39] The classic syndrome associated with 45XO chromosomes is short stature, shield chest and web-shaped neck, short fourth metacarpal, and congenital heart disease.[40, 41] A range of phenotypes may be found with varying mosaic karyotypes 45XO/46XX. Oocytes are formed in fetal life in the ovaries of women with Turner's syndrome, but atresia occurs at an accelerated rate, so that by the time of expected puberty, the ovary usually is devoid of oocytes. In some women, however, sufficient oocytes apparently survive to adoles-

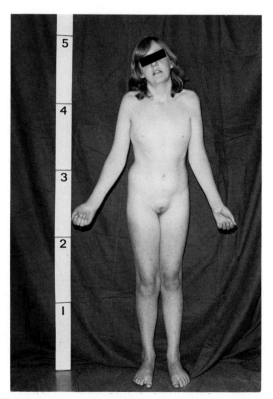

FIGURE 118–3. **Subject with gonadal agenesis.** This phenotype girl presented at 14½ years with primary amenorrhea and sexual infantilism. Karyotype of peripheral leukocytes and skin and gonadal tissue revealed 46XY. "Streak" gonads were removed at laparotomy when the presence of normal uterus and tubes was confirmed.

TABLE 118–1. DISTURBANCES IN THE HYPOTHALAMIC-PITUITARY-OVARIAN AXIS

DISTURBANCES OF THE NEGATIVE FEEDBACK LOOP
Ovarian failure
Failure of the hypothalamus and/or anterior pituitary

INTERFERENCE WITH THE FEEDBACK LOOP OWING TO "ECTOPIC" STEROIDS OR GONADOTROPINS

DISTURBANCE OF THE POSITIVE FEEDBACK LOOP
Adolescent and perimenopausal anovulatory cycles

cence, so that a few ovarian cycles may occur before premature menopause occurs. A few well-documented cases of pregnancy have even been reported.[42]

Premature Ovarian Failure

By the time of the menopause (median age, 50 years), few oocytes remain in the ovary. The factors that determine the age of menopause are largely unknown, although there is a genetic element. If ovarian failure occurs spontaneously before age 40, premature menopause is said to have occurred. A gradual decline in ovarian activity often occurs, with periods of ovarian activity associated with menstruation alternating with several months of ovarian failure, when the gonadotropin levels rise.[43, 44] It is thought that when the population of oocytes falls below a certain number (probably 10,000 to 20,000), there are an insufficient number to ensure that at least one survives the process of atresia to develop as a large graafian follicle each month.

Ovarian failure can occur in association with autoantibodies to ovarian tissue (Fig. 118–4).[45, 46] These antibodies occur much more frequently in patients with other evidence of autoimmune disease. Of 105 patients with idiopathic Addison's disease, 57 had antibodies to adrenal cortex and 13, to ovarian or testicular cells. In contrast, antibodies to ovary and adrenal were absent in all of 35 cases of Addison's disease owing to tuberculosis. Virtually all the 10 female patients of reproductive age had premature ovarian failure. These studies strongly suggest that the development of autoantibodies to antigens present in theca and granulosa cells can lead to destruction of the ovary and premature menopause. The tests for detecting autoantibodies to ovarian antigens are complex and relatively nonspecific, which probably accounts for the inconsistency in the prevalance of positive results in published series.[47]

In most cases of premature ovarian failure, no identifying cause can be found. Previous treatment with x-rays or cytotoxic drugs for malignant disease (e.g., Hodgkin's lymphoma) deplete the ovaries of oocytes. Minor autosomal abnormalities in chromosomes have been reported in 25 per cent of cases.[48] Ovarian failure after pelvic surgery for endometriosis or infection is probably due to interference with ovarian blood supply.

In most cases it is unnecessary to confirm the absence of oocytes by ovarian biopsy. However, if there is concern about future fertility, biopsy should be recommended to exclude the condition of "resistant ovary," a syndrome in which the ovaries contain primordial follicles that are apparently resistant to gonadotropins.[49, 50] Suppression of the elevated gonadotropin values for several months by exogenous estrogen may subsequently result in spontaneous ovarian cycles. There is not good evidence that suppression of gonadotropins with analogues of GnRH, steroids, or treatment with gonadotropins significantly enhances the chance of pregnancy.[51–53] Studies that involve the measurement of LH and FSH receptors in ovarian tissue in this condition would be of great interest.

In summary, with the exception of the rare resistant ovary syndrome, if the level of FSH is grossly elevated, it can be assumed that the ovaries are virtually devoid of oocytes and that irreversible ovarian failure has occurred. Restoration of fertility is impossible, although it is possible

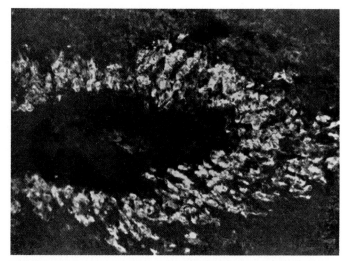

FIGURE 118–4. Immunofluorescent photomicrograph of antibodies to granulosa cells in the serum of a patient with premature ovarian failure. Note that the immunofluorescence is localized in granulosa cells of the follicle ($\times$ 144). (From Irvine WJ: Autoimmune ovarian failure. *In* Irvine WJ, Loraine JA [eds]: Reproductive Endocrinology. Edinburgh, Churchill Livingstone, 1970, pp 106–114.)

to achieve pregnancies after hormone replacement therapy and the transfer of donor embryos into the uterus.[54, 55] In any case, replacement therapy with cyclical estrogen and progestogen is indicated.

Hypothalamic-Pituitary Failure

Failure of the hypothalamus and/or anterior pituitary is a much more common cause of amenorrhea than ovarian failure[56] (Table 118–2). A disturbance in ovarian function also occurs if the feedback loops are interrupted by steroids or gonadotropins extrinsic to the HPO axis. In the absence of clearly localized destruction, injury, or disease (e.g., pituitary infarction, as in Sheehan's syndrome), it often is difficult to distinguish between disorders of the hypothalamus and the anterior pituitary. Because normal functioning of the anterior pituitary depends on continued pulsatile stimulation by GnRH, even in hypothalamic disease, it may be impossible to demonstrate the potential function of the anterior pituitary without priming the pituitary for several days with GnRH. In clinical practice, therefore, it often is convenient to regard the hypothalamic-pituitary system as a single unit and to classify the conditions accordingly.

TABLE 118–2. CAUSES OF GONADOTROPIN FAILURE

STRUCTURAL
Craniopharyngioma
Kallmann's syndrome
Panhypopituitarism (e.g., Sheehan's syndrome)
Pituitary adenomas

FUNCTIONAL
Weight loss, including anorexia nervosa
Exercise
Debilitating disease (e.g., regional ileitis)
Drugs (e.g., reserpine, phenothiazine)
Psychological stress

The common feature of amenorrhea owing to hypothalamic-pituitary failure is a reduction in the pulsatile secretion of LH.[57-60] Although the basal levels of LH and FSH may be within the range of the normal follicular phase of the cycle, careful analysis of the pattern of pulsatile secretion of gonadotropins demonstrates a reduction in the frequency of pulses of LH and FSH (Fig. 118–5). These changes represent a continuum ranging from a hypogonadotropic state resembling infancy to minor abnormalities of cycle control, as represented by the formation of an inadequate corpus luteum. Although the degree of inactivity of the hypothalamic-pituitary unit can be tested directly by measuring the pattern of gonadotropin secretion, in practice it often is more convenient to assess the estrogenic status. In the absence of adequate gonadotropic stimulation, the ovaries secrete minimal quantities of estradiol, the levels of which are very low (less than 50 pg/ml) in peripheral blood. Because the endometrium remains unstimulated, administration of progesterone fails to induce a withdrawal hemorrhage. Assessment of estrogenic status by progestogen challenge is of diagnostic value in determining the degree of hypogonadism and in selecting the most appropriate therapy (see below).

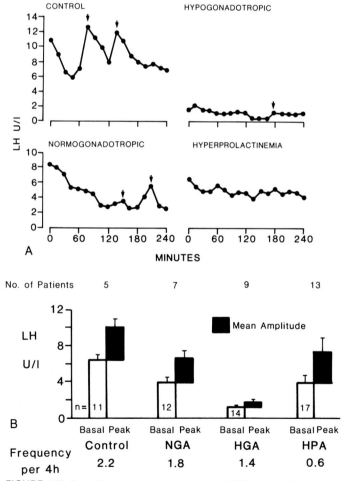

FIGURE 118–5. *A*, Patterns of concentration of LH in serum in patients with secondary amenorrhea. Note the absence of pulsatile release of LH in hyperprolactinemic patients, although the basal level is within the normal range. *B*, The mean basal level and pulse amplitude and frequency in women with amenorrhea. NGA, normogonadotropic; HGA, hypogonadotropic; HPA, hyperprolactinemic. (Courtesy of CW Vaughan Williams and DT Baird.)

TABLE 118–3. ETIOLOGY OF SECONDARY AMENORRHEA IN PATIENTS ATTENDING THE REPRODUCTIVE ENDOCRINE CLINIC, ROYAL INFIRMARY, EDINBURGH (1974–1978)

CAUSE	NO. OF PATIENTS (%)
Hyperprolactinemia (PRL >360 mU/L; PRL >20 ng/ml)	34 (23)
Normal gonadotropins	47 (31)
Low gonadotropins	70 (46)
Total	151

Secondary Amenorrhea

It is useful to divide women with secondary amenorrhea into three groups, depending on the basal levels of prolactin, FSH, LH, and estradiol:[2, 16, 61] (1) hyperprolactinemia, (2) normogonadotropic hypogonadism, and (3) hypogonadotropic hypogonadism (Table 118–3). Although a history of weight loss of greater than 10 per cent of body weight is common in the normoprolactinemic groups, it occurs in less than 10 per cent of those with hyperprolactinemia (Table 118–4). There are no clear features in the history to distinguish between the groups, although the finding of galactorrhea suggests a raised level of prolactin. This classification is useful not only because most patients with pituitary tumors have raised levels of prolactin but also because effective treatment can be chosen earlier.

Hyperprolactinemia

About 15 to 20 per cent of women with secondary amenorrhea have prolactin concentrations that are persistently elevated above the normal range (greater than 20 ng/ml Friesen Standard; 360 mU/L International Standard).[13, 62] Prolactin is an important component of the complex of hormones responsible for lactation, although in only about 50 per cent of amenorrheic women with hyperprolactinemia is it possible to demonstrate galactorrhea. The relation between galactorrhea and the secretion of prolactin is complex; only about one half the women who present with galactorrhea have raised levels of prolactin.[63] Galactorrhea occurs in some hypothyroid women who have normal levels of prolactin, and it is likely that other factors in addition to thyroxine affect the sensitivity of the breast to prolactin.

The association of amenorrhea and galactorrhea has been described under a number of eponyms (e.g., Chiari-Frommel [postpartum], Argonz-Del Costello [without rela-

TABLE 118–4. CLINICAL FEATURES OF 151 PATIENTS WITH SECONDARY AMENORRHEA (1974–1978)

	PERCENTAGE OF EACH GROUP		
	Hyperprolactinemia (N = 34)	*Normal Gonadotropins (N = 47)*	*Low Gonadotropins (N = 70)*
Weight loss>10%	9	30	43
Following pill	24	32	37
History of pill	9	19	10
Psychological	12	17	14
Pregnancy	6	0	3
Drugs	9	2	6

TABLE 118–5. CAUSES OF HYPERPROLACTINEMIA

Prolactin-secreting tumors (e.g., chromophobe, eosinophilic, or basophilic)
Interference with pituitary stalk (e.g., trauma, tumor)
Drugs that interfere with dopamine activity
   Receptor blockade (e.g., phenothiazine, metoclopramide, sulpiride, haloperidol)
   Depletors of catecholamines (e.g., reserpine or methyldopa)
Disease of central nervous system (e.g., craniopharyngioma, encephalitis, sarcoidosis)
Hyperplasia of lactotrophs (e.g., postpartum, hypothyroidism)
Neural stimulation (e.g., chest wall thoracotomy, herpes zoster, burns, nipple stimulation, pseudocyesis)

tion to pregnancy], and Forbes-Albright [galactorrhea with pituitary tumor]) but are now considered in relation to the cause.[64, 65] Various conditions result in hyperprolactinemia (Table 118–5), but in the absence of thyroid disease or drugs, a prolactin-secreting tumor of the pituitary should be suspected. The development of sensitive radioimmunoassays for the measurement of prolactin has permitted the identification of most women with amenorrhea who are likely to harbor a pituitary tumor. With modern methods of computed tomography (CT) and magnetic resonance imaging of the sella turcica, tumors can be identified in about 50 per cent of women with hyperprolactinemia (see Ch. 34). In the remainder it is assumed that either the tumor is too small to be identified even with the most sophisticated CT scanner or there is some defect in the hypothalamic production of dopamine leading to hypertrophy of the lactotrophs. The latter occurs physiologically during pregnancy and is important in maintaining the increased secretion of prolactin during lactation. In hypothyroidism excessive secretion of thyrotropic-releasing hormone has been suggested as responsible for the increased secretion of prolactin from the lactotrophs, but this is unproven. Not all hypothyroid women are hyperprolactinemic.[66] In some hyperprolactinemic states, including lactation, the levels of estradiol are much lower than one would expect in relation to the concentration of LH and FSH, suggesting that prolactin may directly inhibit follicular development and ovarian secretion of estradiol. Follicular development and ovulation can be induced in hyperprolactinemic amenorrhea by pulsatile administration of gonadotropins or GnRH.[59]

The clinical features and detailed investigations of patients with pituitary tumors are dealt with elsewhere (Chs. 31 and 32). The degree of hypogonadism in hyperprolactinemic women can vary from gross evidence of estrogenic deficiency to minor disturbance in the regulation of ovarian function. Many women with amenorrhea associated with hyperprolactinemia complain of dyspareunia associated with vaginal dryness and estrogen deficiency. Although the single basal levels of gonadotropins are within the normal range, the concentration of estradiol may be less than 50 pg/ml, and there is no bleeding in response to a progestogen challenge. This suppression of ovarian activity is due to an absence or marked reduction in the frequency of LH pulses (see Fig. 118–5).[67–69] In others there may be spontaneous episodes of vaginal bleeding, reflecting estrogen levels in the range 50 to 200 pg/ml in association with follicular activity. In these women LH pulses are present, although with a reduced frequency. The

inactivity of the hypothalamic neurons that secrete GnRH results in a secondary decrease in the secreting capacity of the anterior pituitary. In contrast to the apparently normal release of LH in response to a single injection of GnRH, the secretory capacity is markedly impaired when tested by repeated injections at two-hour intervals. As in most severely hypogonadotropic states, the positive feedback response to estrogen usually is markedly impaired or absent (Fig. 118–6).[70, 71]

The mechanism by which hyperprolactinemia produces hypogonadotropism is incompletely understood. Some authors have reported that administration of naloxone is followed by an immediate increase in the frequency of LH pulses, suggesting in these hyperprolactinemic states that endogenous opioids may play a role in inhibiting hypothalamic GnRH-secreting neurones.[72, 73] This is not a consistent finding even in those women in whom there is no evidence of a prolactin-secreting adenoma and the hyperprolactinemia is thought to be due to a functional abnormality in the hypothalamus (Fig. 118–7). The fact that selective enucleation of a prolactin-secreting tumor results in restoration of normal secretion of gonadotropins and of cyclical ovarian activity suggests that prolactin may have a direct effect on hypothalamic activity.

The management of the hyperprolactinemic woman with amenorrhea depends on whether she wants to become pregnant, the presence or absence of a pituitary tumor and its size, and her estrogenic status. If she is com-

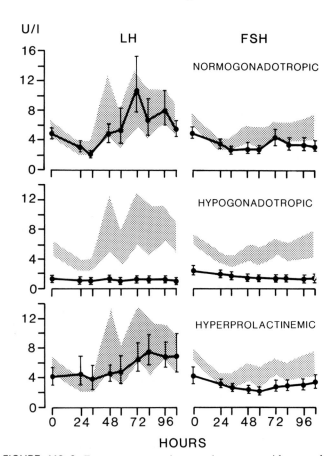

FIGURE 118–6. Estrogen provocation test in women with secondary amenorrhea. The range of normal control women in the early follicular phase of the cycle is indicated by the shaded area. Note the absence of a secondary rise of LH concentration in the hypogonadotropic women. (Courtesy of CW Vaughan Williams, AS McNeilly, and DT Baird.)

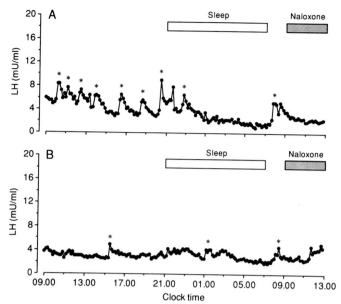

FIGURE 118–7. Twenty-four-hour secretory pattern of LH in two women with amenorrhea caused by hyperprolactinemia and during four-hour infusions with naloxone (1.6 μg/h). Statistically significant LH pulses are indicated by *. Note the reduced number of LH pulses in both women. (From Tay CCK, Glasier AF, Illingworth PJI, et al: Abnormal 24-hr pattern of pulsatile hormone secretion and the response to naloxone in women with hyperprolactinemic amenorrhea. Clin Endocrinol, in press.)

plaining of infertility, it is important to identify the size of any pituitary tumor and its possible suprasellar extension. Modern CT scanning has made air encephalography an obsolete investigation for all but rare cases of empty sella syndrome. If the tumor diameter exceeds 1 cm, it should be surgically removed or reduced in size by medical treatment before the patient becomes pregnant.[74] If untreated, there is a small but definite risk of further enlargement of the tumor during pregnancy, with pressure on the optic chiasma. For this reason it has been suggested that women contemplating pregnancy should have radiotherapy to the pituitary. This does not reduce the risk of enlargement during pregnancy completely, and if large macroadenomas are treated surgically, the subsequent pregnancies usually are uneventful. Many of these tumors may be safely enucleated by the transsphenoidal route with minimal morbidity and preservation of function of the anterior pituitary.[75] The operation is not totally without risk, however, and is curative in only about 70 per cent of patients.[76] Moreover, it has been suggested that the development of prolactinomas is secondary to an intrinsic defect in the catecholamine-secreting neurons of the tubero-infundibular system, implying that surgical removal is unlikely to result in a permanent cure.[77]

For most women with infertility due to hyperprolactinemia, whether functional or resulting from a prolactinoma, the treatment of choice is bromocriptine or another dopamine agonist, such as pergolide or lisuride.[78–80] These drugs interact with the dopamine receptors of the lactotrophs and inhibit the secretion of prolactin. At a dosage ranging from 2.5 to 15.0 mg/d bromocriptine reduces the levels of prolactin and produces a coincidental rise in the frequency of LH pulses. Although menses usually return within three months, the first few cycles may be anovulatory or have a short and/or inadequate luteal phase. Normal ovarian cycl-

icity is restored within six months in most cases, and the fertility rates are satisfactory.

It usually is recommended that bromocriptine be stopped as soon as pregnancy has been diagnosed, although there is no evidence that it can be teratogenic. During pregnancy there is a small but definite risk of further enlargement of a pituitary adenoma, which rarely may cause symptoms because of pressure on the optic nerve.[74] In these circumstances, bromocriptine can be restarted safely during pregnancy and usually results in prompt shrinkage of the tumor with relief of symptoms.

The treatment of hyperprolactinemic women who do not want to conceive is more controversial. It would seem reasonable to treat those with large pituitary tumors or with symptoms of estrogen deficiency with bromocriptine.[80] Some authorities recommend that all hyperprolactinemic women should be treated with bromocriptine to prevent any growth of a pituitary adenoma and to reduce the premature demineralization of bone owing to estrogen deficiency.[81] However, although the natural history of prolactinemia is not yet known, about 10 per cent of hyperprolactinemic women have a spontaneous remission.[80a] If bromocriptine is given to those who are sexually active, it is necessary to provide some form of contraception (avoiding the combined pill) to prevent unwanted pregnancy. Moreover, not all hyperprolactinemic women are deficient in estrogen, and restoration of cyclical ovarian function may provoke menstrual symptoms that require treatment. The long-term consequences of repeated ovarian cycles (breast and endometrial cancer) may well outweigh the risks of osteoporosis. The relative health risks and benefits of treatment versus no treatment must be carefully weighed in each case. Whatever the choice, the woman should be informed of the possible long-term risks and followed-up at intervals of 6 to 12 months.

Normal Gonadotropins

Most patients in the second group have some evidence of estrogen secretion as well as having basal levels of LH and FSH within the normal range. The concentration of estradiol usually is between 50 and 100 pg/ml, and bleeding occurs in response to a progestogen challenge.[58, 61] LH pulses are of normal amplitude but of slightly reduced frequency when compared with the follicular phase of the cycle, and estrogen provocation produces an LH surge (positive feedback) (see Figs. 118–5 and 118–6). With all the components of the HPO axis intact and responding appropriately to dynamic stimuli, it is difficult to understand why these women remain acyclic. It may be that they have reverted to a state that is equivalent to early puberty, when the hypothalamus remains so sensitive to the inhibitory effects of ovarian steroids that follicular development is inhibited shortly after its initiation.

Induction of ovulation and restoration of fertility can be achieved relatively easily by the administration of an antiestrogen, such as clomiphene citrate or tamoxifen (see Ch. 113).[82] Antiestrogens bind to the estrogen receptor but initiate little stimulation of new receptor. Clomiphene is a mixture of two isomers of which only one (trans or en) is an antiestrogen and the cis or zu isomer is a weak estrogen.[83] It is now clear that the ovulatory properties of clomiphene (and tamoxifen) are due solely to the trans (zu) isomer (Fig. 118–8). Whether the *cis* isomer has any beneficial therapeutic role remains to be established. Both isomers have an extremely long half-life, and traces of the *cis* isomer can be detected in body fluid for up to 30 days after a single treatment.[84] It is usual to start clomiphene in a dosage of 50 mg/d for five days on the third day of progesterone-induced menstrual bleeding. During the treatment there is a rise of both FSH and LH, which stimulates follicular development, and an increased secretion of estradiol, which induces a surge of LH by means of the positive feedback mechanism. Thus clomiphene is effective in inducing ovulation only when both negative and positive feedback mechanisms are intact. The timing of ovulation after treatment with clomiphene varies between 7 and 14 days after starting therapy. It is wise to monitor the response at least during the first few cycles by measuring the concentration of progesterone on day 21. If there is no response to 50 mg, the dosage may be increased in subsequent cycles up to 150 mg/d.

In some women follicular development is stimulated in response to clomiphene, but ovulation fails to occur, presumably because of a failure of the positive feedback system. Ovulation may be induced by administration of hCG (5000 to 10,000 units), although the injection must be

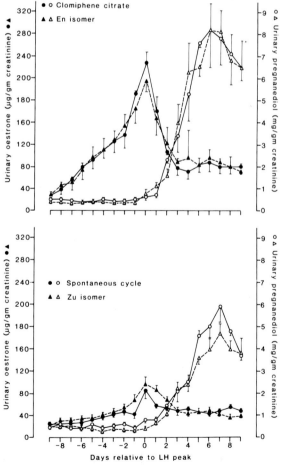

FIGURE 118–8. Mean excretion of estrone and pregnanediol glucuronide in women taking isomers of clomiphene from day 2 to day 6 of the cycle. *A*, Clomiphene citrate (100 mg/d) and En (trans) isomer (50 mg/d) n = 10. *B*, Spontaneous cycle and Zu (cis) isomer (50 mg/d). (From Glasier AF et al: A comparison of the effects on follicular development between clomiphene citrate, its two separate isomers and spontaneous cycles. Hum Reprod 4:252–256, 1989.)

timed to coincide with maximum follicular development as assessed by ultrasonography and/or estrogen levels. Although an ovulation rate of more than 70 per cent may be achieved if patients for antiestrogen therapy are properly selected, the pregnancy rate is disappointingly low.[85] In some cases luteinization of the follicle without rupture may occur; in others it has been suggested that the suppression of cervical mucus production by the antiestrogen prevents the sperm from ascending the cervix into the uterus and tubes.[61] It has been claimed that the administration of estrogen (e.g., ethinyl estradiol, 100 μg/d) for three to four days after the clomiphene treatment improves the pregnancy rate, although this treatment has never been subjected to critical trial.[14]

Many amenorrheic patients with normal levels of gonadotropins display some or all of the features of polycystic ovary syndrome (PCO) (i.e., obesity, hirsutism, anovulation associated with enlarged microcystic ovaries).[86, 87] The levels of LH are elevated because of frequent high-amplitude pulses, whereas those of FSH are normal or suppressed. It is considered that this syndrome is the end result of a number of conditions that lead to chronic anovulation in the absence of hypogonadotropism.[88] There is increased secretion of androstenedione and testosterone from the ovaries and/or adrenal glands, with resulting clinical evidence of hyperandrogenization, including hirsutism (Ch. 119). It is now evident that many women with PCO display abnormalities in peripheral resistance to insulin that may play a role in the pathogenesis.[89] It is relevant to note that the extraglandular production of estrogen from androgen precursors is raised in PCO and interferes with the normal feedback mechanisms.[90] The relatively constant production of estrogen suppresses FSH and at the same time increases the amount of LH produced from the anterior pituitary in response to GnRH. The high-amplitude LH pulses stimulate androgen production from the theca and stromal tissue and, hence, further perpetuate the endocrine abnormality. The normal sequence of follicular development is prevented by the low levels of FSH. Thus the persistent anovulation in PCO is due to the production of feedback signals (estrogen) "ectopic" to the main HPO axis.[2]

Ovulation can be induced in women with amenorrhea caused by PCO by the administration of clomiphene or FSH. About 25 per cent of women with PCO fail to ovulate in response to clomiphene or tamoxifen. If there is evidence of excessive secretion of adrenal androgens, treatment with corticosteroids (e.g., 0.5 mg of dexamethasone per day) may restore cyclical ovarian activity or make them responsive to clomiphene. The traditional treatment of wedge resection is probably effective by reducing the mass of ovarian tissue and, hence, the secretion of excessive androgens.[91] This treatment results in restoration of ovulation in about 70 per cent of women but fell into disrepute because its effect usually is temporary (about 6 to 12 months) and runs a significant risk of postoperative adhesions, which may impair tubal function. More recently there have been reports that destruction of ovarian follicles by laser or diathermy through the laparoscope gives similar results to ovarian wedge resection.[92, 93] If these preliminary studies are confirmed, then this less invasive form of surgical treatment may be useful in those women who fail to become pregnant after clomiphene.

The alternative treatment for women with PCO who are resistant to clomiphene is human menopausal gonadotropin (hMG) or purified FSH. Women with PCO are sensitive to FSH, and it often is extremely difficult to restrict the number of ovulatory follicles (see later).

Low Gonadotropins

If hypothalamic activity is minimal or there is pituitary disease, basal levels of gonadotropins are below the normal female range, reflecting a markedly reduced frequency of GnRH pulses. The ovaries receive minimal stimulation, and hence the secretion of estradiol is markedly reduced. There may be clinical signs of estrogen deficiency (e.g., atrophy of the breast and vaginal epithelium). The serum estradiol level usually is less than 20 pg/ml, and there is no bleeding in response to progestogen.

In Kallmann's syndrome the hypogonadotropic hypogonadism is associated with a congenital maldevelopment of the olfactory tissues and lack of GnRH secretion.[94] It originally was thought that there was deficiency of pituitary gonadotropins, but injection with GnRH produces some rise in the concentration of LH in most cases, and full reproductive function can be restored by prolonged pulsatile administration.[95] Most females with this condition present with primary amenorrhea and lack of development of secondary sex characteristics.

The hypothalamus may be destroyed owing to such tumors as craniopharyngiomas or gliomas, or it may be infiltrated by such conditions as tuberculosis, sarcoidosis, or Hand-Schüller-Christian disease. The clinical features are similar to those of Kallmann's syndrome, but the sense of smell remains intact.

Unlike hypogonadism owing to hypothalamic disease, pituitary conditions are unresponsive to treatment with GnRH. Pituitary infarction may occur at any age but most often follows severe postpartum hemorrhage (Sheehan's syndrome).[96] The initial clinical sign is a failure of lactation followed in subsequent months by signs of panhypopituitarism (i.e., fatigue, lethargy, and loss of pubic and axillary hair). Destruction owing to a tumor or in association with empty sella syndrome is a much more common pituitary cause of gonadotropin deficiency. Hemorrhage into a chromophobe adenoma may precipitate an acute emergency owing to a rise in intracranial pressure and pituitary failure. Many pituitary tumors secrete prolactin and may present as amenorrhea-galactorrhea syndrome.

In most subjects with hypogonadotropic hypogonadism, no organic structural abnormality is identified. A functional cessation of the activity of the hypothalamic neurons responsible for secretion of GnRH leads to a marked reduction in the secretion of gonadotropins and ovarian steroids (hypothalamic amenorrhea).[97–99] Under minimal stimulation by GnRH, the pituitary secretion of LH is reduced to a relatively greater extent than FSH. The response to acute stimulation by GnRH is markedly impaired. Although various factors may lead to a suppression of gonadotropin secretion, by far the most common in Western society is weight loss associated with dieting or anorexia nervosa. The mechanism underlying the change in hypothalamic function that occurs in association with weight loss is unknown, although it is assumed to be a disturbance in the synthesis of catecholamines and other neural transmitters.

It is hardly surprising, therefore, that even when the hypothalamus and anterior pituitary are structurally intact, there is no response to antiestrogens or bromocriptine. In those women in whom the amenorrhea is due to severe weight loss (e.g., anorexia nervosa), appropriate counseling aimed at correcting the dietary deficiency and restoring normal weight should be started (Fig. 118–9). If strenuous exercise is the precipitating factor, a reduction in weekly running schedules may be advised if restoration of cyclic ovarian activity is desired. In those who wish pregnancy, it may be necessary to use pharmacological means. Until recently the treatment of choice for all hypogonadotropic patients was exogenous gonadotropins prepared from either human pituitary glands (hPG) or human menopausal urine (hMG).[26, 100–103]

It is necessary to use human material because preparations of gonadotropins of animal origin either are ineffective or rapidly induce production of antibodies. The treatment introduced in 1958 by Carl Gemzell and Paul Roos involved daily injections of hPG to induce follicular development followed by administration of hCG to induce ovulation. Although hPG has now been replaced by hMG, the original schedule of daily injections is still probably the most effective and safest way to induce ovulation with gonadotropins (Fig. 118–10). It has proved extremely difficult, however, to simulate the normal ovarian cycle in which a single dominant follicle is selected for ovulation. The fact that during treatment with gonadotropins, stimulation of multiple follicles almost always occurs no matter how carefully the dose is adjusted is hardly surprising because the therapy overrides the normal feedback system. Severe hyperstimulation syndrome can be avoided by with-

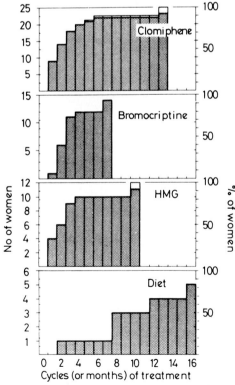

FIGURE 118–9. Conceptions after treatment of amenorrheic women with clomiphene, hMG, bromocriptine, or diet. Selection of therapy was based on the cause of the amenorrhea. (From Hull MGR et al: Investigation and treatment of amenorrhea resulting in normal fertility. Br Med J 1:1257–1261, 1979.)

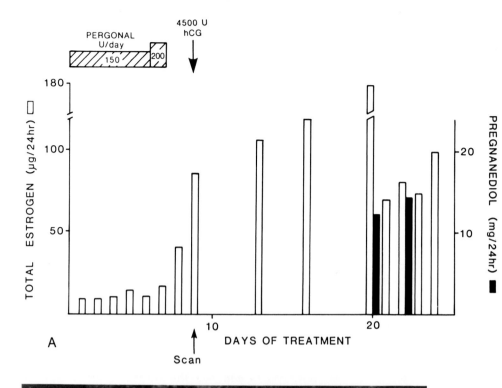

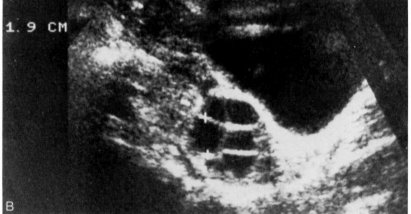

FIGURE 118–10. *A,* Induction of ovulation in a woman with secondary amenorrhea caused by hypogonadotropic hypogonadism. hMG (Pergonal) was given by intramuscular injection every day, the dose being adjusted in relation to the total estrogen excretion. Although the hCG was given when the total estrogen excretion was optimal (50 to 150 μg/24 h), superovulation was induced as demonstrated by ultrasound scan. *B,* Five fetuses were aborted at 19 weeks' gestation.

holding hCG if estrogen levels and ultrasound measurements indicate excessive stimulation of the ovary. Even in the best centers, the multiple-pregnancy rate may be as high as 30 per cent with subsequent increase in abortion and perinatal mortality.[103] The cumulative pregnancy rate in women treated with gonadotropins is more than 90 per cent after five cycles and is similar to that in normal fertile couples if hypogonadotropism is the sole cause of infertility (see Fig. 118–9).

Because the primary cause of amenorrhea in most patients with hypogonadotropism is a defect in the synthesis of GnRH by the hypothalamus, replacement with GnRH is the logical therapy.[104, 105] After the demonstration in the rhesus monkey that pulsatile administration of GnRH was important to stimulate the anterior pituitary, this knowledge was quickly applied to amenorrheic women.[106] Follicular development and ovulation can be induced in most hypogonadotropic women by the administration of GnRH in a pulsatile manner by means of a portable infusion pump programmed to deliver a pulse of GnRH (5 to 20 μg) every 60 to 120 minutes (Fig. 118–11). Most patients respond to subcutaneous administration, although a few may require the pulses to be given intravenously.

The optimum regimen is one pulse every 60 minutes, which stimulates the pulse frequency observed during the late follicular phase of the cylce.[107] Although a spontaneous LH surge occurs in most women, it may be more convenient to induce ovulation by the injection of 5000 to 10,000 units of hCG when at least one follicle has reached a diameter of 18 mm. Intercourse can then be timed 36 to 48 hours later and the pump removed. If pulsatile GnRH is withheld during the luteal phase, it will be necessary to provide luteotropic support by injection of a "booster" dose of hCG four and eight days after ovulation. Because the feedback system between the ovary and the anterior pituitary remain intact during pulsatile GnRH therapy, stimulation of multiple follicular development is rare and the risk of multiple births markedly reduced compared with treatment with gonadotrophins. Moreover, intense daily monitoring of ovarian response by serial measurements of estradiol concentration and follicular diameter by ultrasonography is unnecessary. Many large series have

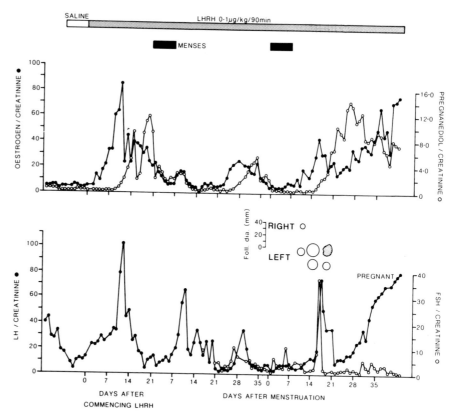

FIGURE 118–11. Induction of ovulation with pulsatile GnRH therapy in women with hypogonadotropic hypogonadism. GnRH (LHRH) was administered subcutaneously by way of a portable pump in a 40-μl bolus at a dosage of 0.1 μg/kg every 90 minutes. Note the occurrence of an LH surge without a change in the frequency of GnRH pulses. Pregnancy occurred during the third cycle. (Courtesy of AF Glasier, AS McNeilly, and DT Baird.)

demonstrated that the cumulative pregnancy rate of this form of treatment in properly selected women with hypogonadotropic hypogonadism is similar to that in normal women but without the risk of multiple births.[107–110]

In contrast to women with hypogonadotropic hypogonadism, induction of ovulation with pulsatile GnRH or gonadotropins is much more difficult in normogonadotropic women who are unresponsive to clomiphene.[107] The ovulation rate with pulsatile GnRH is low, although encouraging results have been reported with this form of treatment used after a period of down-regulation with GnRH analogues. As mentioned earlier, women with PCO are extremely sensitive to gonadotropins, and it is difficult to avoid stimulation of multiple follicles. In addition, premature discharge of an LH surge may result in luteinization of follicles before they have reached preovulatory maturity. Even if ovulation and pregnancy occur, there is about a 30 to 40 per cent chance of miscarriage. The causes of the increased abortion rate in women with PCO is only partially related to the high incidence of multiple births. It has also been suggested that high levels of LH in the follicular phase of the cycle in some way compromise the orderly maturation of the oocyte such that the completion of the meiotic divisions before fertilization is impaired.[111, 112]

Various therapeutic approaches have been tried to improve the pregnancy rate and reduce the incidence of multiple births in these women. The daily dose of FSH should be gradually increased from the initial low dose (37 IU) by no more than 30 per cent only when there has been no ovarian response after 7 to 10 days.[113] The aim should be to inject no more than the threshold amount of FSH necessary to induce the development of a single large follicle. Initial reports are encouraging that a low incidence of multiple births can be achieved using this regimen, although the "take home baby" rate per cycle is disappointing. Moreover, the requirement for multiple biochemical and ultrasound measurements makes the method expensive and tedious for the patient.

Another approach has been to stimulate follicular development after a period of down-regulation with GnRH agonists for two to four weeks.[114] When the levels of LH, FSH, and estradiol have reached basal levels, follicular development is induced with hMG or FSH in the same way as in women with hypogonadotropic hypogonadism. Although some authors have claimed cumulative pregnancy rates approaching normal using this regimen, others have reported a high rate of miscarriage and multiple pregnancy.[115, 116]

A second approach has involved the use of down-regulation with analogues of GnRH followed by pulsatile GnRH therapy.[106] Not surprisingly, treatment with pulsatile GnRH is unsuccessful in women with PCO in view of the high frequency of pulses of endogenous LH (and presumably GnRH). If, however, after suppression of the endogenous level of LH by prolonged treatment with a GnRH agonist, it is possible to override the endogenous GnRH and induce ovulation in a high percentage of cycles. Disappointingly, the abortion rate of pregnancies remains high.

EXTRAOVARIAN DISEASES

Disturbances of ovarian cyclicity occur in other diseases that interfere with the normal feedback loops of the HPO axis.

Thyroid Disease

In thyroid disease the disturbance in menstrual pattern may range from amenorrhea to dysfunctional uterine bleeding.[117]

In hyperthyroidism the concentration of sex hormone–binding globulin (SHBG) increases, and hence the concentrations of both estradiol and testosterone are increased.[118] The metabolic clearance rate of both steroids is reduced, and an increased extraglandular production of estrogens from androgens occurs, as in the PCO syndrome.

In hypothyroidism, estradiol is preferentially metabolized in favor of estriol, which has weak intrinsic biological activity.[119] The concentration of prolactin may be elevated because of stimulation with thyrotropin-releasing hormone. Treatment with thyroxine causes reduction of TSH and prolactin with disappearance of galactorrhea. Because the concentration of SHBG is reduced, the amount of unbound estradiol is increased, although the total concentration is reduced owing to an increased metabolic clearance rate.

Adrenal Disease

The normal adrenal secretes large quantities of androgens (androstenedione, testosterone, and dehydroepiandrosterone and its sulfate) but little estrogen. Androstenedione is an important precursor for estrogen that is produced in the liver, skin, and fatty tissue. Although adrenal androgens may modulate the sensitivity of the HPO axis, they are not essential for ovarian cyclicity, which apparently occurs normally in their absence in Addison's disease or after bilateral adrenalectomy. Any condition that leads to excessive secretion of sex steroids from the adrenal will lead to amenorrhea. The secretion of gonadotropins may be directly suppressed by androgens or by the estrogens produced in excess quantities by extraglandular production.[120] The suppression of ovarian activity that occurs with congenital adrenal hyperplasia has been mentioned in an earlier section. When the secretion of adrenal androgens is sufficiently high in Cushing's syndrome to cause androgenization, amenorrhea usually occurs. As adrenal carcinoma may selectively secrete testosterone or estradiol, gross disturbances in ovarian cyclicity usually occur.

DYSFUNCTIONAL UTERINE BLEEDING

Any abnormality in the HPO axis short of total acyclicity usually presents clinically as a disturbance in the pattern of menstruation. Dysfunctional uterine bleeding is defined as heavy and/or irregular periods that occur in the absence of recognizable pregnancy, pelvic pathology, or general bleeding disorder.[121] The menstrual blood loss is extremely variable from one woman to another, with a mean of 35 ml per period and an upper limit of normal between 60 and 80 ml. Throughout most of their reproductive life women have a highly reproducible pattern of menstrual cycle bleeding that occurs for 3 to 7 days at intervals of 25 to 35 days. The mean length of the menstrual cycle declines slightly with age because of a shortening by one or two days of the length of the follicular phase (see Fig. 118–1). Although the length of the luteal phase remains relatively constant within individuals, a short or insufficient luteal phase occurs in about 10 per cent of cycles in otherwise apparently healthy women.

Because dysfunctional uterine bleeding is a symptom of a disturbance in the HPO axis, it is hardly surprising that it is much more common at the extremes of reproductive life (i.e., in adolescence and in premenopausal transition). The range in the length of menstrual cycles that occurs at these times is due to a various abnormalities in ovarian activity, which can be classified as follows:

1. Anovulatory
   a. Inadequate signal (e.g., inadequate follicular development in PCO syndrome or premenopausally)
   b. Impaired positive feedback
2. Ovulatory
   a. Inadequate or insufficient luteal phase
   b. Idiopathic bleeding

Anovulatory Dysfunctional Uterine Bleeding

Although an occasional anovulatory cycle may occur in otherwise normal women with little change in the pattern of menses, chronic anovulation usually is associated with an irregular and unpredictable pattern of bleeding ranging from short cycles with scanty bleeding to prolonged periods of irregular heavy loss. Normal menstruation occurs in response to withdrawal of both progesterone and estradiol after a period of priming with estradiol followed by both steroids. If the sequence or length of the priming process deviates from normal, the pattern of synthesis of steroid receptors, prostaglandins, and other locally active endometrial products is deficient, and an abnormal pattern of bleeding may result.[12] The common feature of anovulatory dysfunctional uterine bleeding is that bleeding occurs from an endometrium that has been exposed to estrogen unopposed by progesterone and, hence, is proliferative or hyperplastic. The exact mechanism of estrogen withdrawal bleeding is not known, but characteristically it is painless and of irregular amount.[122] Recent evidence suggests that persistent proliferative or hyperplastic endometrium has a reduced capacity to synthesize prostaglandin $F_{2\alpha}$ ($PGF_{2\alpha}$), whereas the production of PGE_2 and PGD_2 is enhanced.[123] Thus there is a relative reduction in the synthesis of those prostaglandins that cause vasoconstriction and myometrial contraction in favor of those with vasodilatory properties (PGE_2 and PGI_2). The absence of dysmenorrhea in anovulatory bleeding is probably an index of the lack of high-amplitude uterine contractions, which are associated with the production of $PGF_{2\alpha}$.

Because of the irregular and unpredictable pattern of menstruation, the diagnosis of anovulation often is difficult to confirm. Serial measurements of estradiol and progesterone over a period of several weeks may be necessary to establish the pattern of ovarian activity in relation to menstrual bleeding.[1] The occurrence of cystic glandular hyperplasia of the endometrium in a premenstrual biopsy may confirm prolonged unopposed estrogen and indicate chronic anovulation.

Ovulation occurs in response to the midcycle surge of LH induced by rising levels of estradiol. Only a mature large follicle with a full complement of granulosa cells secretes sufficient estrogen to induce positive feedback. This mechanism ensures that by the time of ovulation, the oocyte is competent to permit fertilization and that a fully functional corpus luteum will be formed. Thus, if for any reason the development of the follicle is deficient so that the secretion of estradiol is insufficient to provoke an LH surge, ovulation does not occur.

Inadequate Signal

PCO syndrome is one of the most common conditions in which the failure to ovulate is due not to any intrinsic defect in the positive feedback system but to a failure of normal follicular development. Details of the cause and pathogenesis of this condition are dealt with above and in detail in Chapter 119 and are only summarized here.[87] When tested, both FSH and LH respond normally to estrogen by both negative and positive feedback. Although there is no spontaneous midcycle surge, the basal levels of LH are elevated owing to frequent LH pulses of high amplitude. There is good evidence that the raised levels of LH are responsible for stimulating the increased ovarian secretion of testosterone and androstenedione characteristic of this condition. By interacting with its receptor, LH stimulates not only increased secretion of androgens but also hypertrophy of the theca and stromal cells. In contrast, the secretion of FSH is too low to maintain development of healthy large antral follicles, and hence the ovarian secretion of estradiol is low.

Despite the reduced secretion of estradiol by the ovaries, women with PCO syndrome show no evidence of estrogen deficiency. There is copious production of cervical mucus and good breast development, and the endometrium is proliferative or hyperplastic. The excretion of total estrogen is within the range of the follicular phase of the cycle. Most estrogen in women with PCO syndrome is derived from aromatization of androgen precursors (mainly androstenedione) in peripheral tissues, such as the fat and skin.[90] Not only is there an abundant source of precursor owing to excessive secretion of androstenedione from both the ovary and the adrenals, but the obesity that may be present enhances the sites of aromatization. Because most of the estrogen in peripheral blood is derived from androstenedione, the concentration of estrone exceeds that of estradiol.[88] The chronically raised estrogen levels sensitize the anterior pituitary to GnRH and probably account for the increased amplitude of LH pulses. The levels of FSH are low because its secretion is more sensitive to the negative feedback effect of estrogen and/or the increased production of inhibin from the ovaries. Because of the low levels of FSH, granulosa cells do not develop normal aromatase activity, and hence the follicles are unable to convert the increased amounts of androgens to estrogens.[124] The high local concentration of androgens within the ovary may further aggravate the situation by inhibiting aromatase and inducing atresia.

The treatment of women with PCO syndrome depends on the primary complaint. If infertility is a problem, normal follicular development and ovulation can be readily restored by the administration of exogenous FSH or by raising the endogenous levels by administration of an antiestrogen, such as clomiphene citrate.

The most effective treatment of hirsutism is a combination of cyproterone acetate and estrogen.[125] Being a strong gestogen as well as a potent antiandrogen, in combination with estrogen, cyproterone acetate suppresses the secretion of LH to very low levels. Whether as a combined pill (2 mg of cyproterone acetate for 21 days) or in the reverse sequential manner (100 mg of cyproterone acetate for 10 days), it must be used in combination with ethinyl estradiol (30 to 50 µg/d for 21 days) to control menstrual bleeding and inhibit ovulation.[126] Cyproterone acetate, being an anti-androgen, can feminize a male fetus so that reliable contraception is essential. Other treatments that include spironolactone and cimetidine are not as effective but may be useful alternatives in those countries in which cyproterone acetate is not available.[127]

Even if hirsutism is not a problem, some form of hormonal therapy is desirable to avoid hypertrophy of the endometrium. In addition to the inconvenience of irregular bleeding, those women run an increased risk of developing carcinoma of the endometrium owing to the action of unopposed estrogen.[128] If contraception is required, a combined estrogen-gestogen preparation usually gives good cycle control. If no contraceptive is required, cyclical administration of an orally active gestogen (e.g., norethindrone 5 mg/d) for 7 to 10 days each month induces regular bleeding within a few days of stopping therapy and prevents hyperplasia of the endometrium.

Follicular development insufficient to provide an adequate estrogen signal to induce an LH surge is one of the more common reasons for the irregularities in menstrual cycle pattern in premenopausal women.[129, 130] As the stock of oocytes in the ovaries declines, there are intervals of apparent ovarian inactivity associated with low levels of estrogens ranging from a few days to several weeks, followed by some evidence of follicular development. Characteristically, the secretion of FSH and LH rises during the time when the feedback of ovarian steroids (and inhibin) is minimal and declines slowly as the follicles develop. During this time the secretion of estradiol may never reach a level sufficient to induce positive feedback, although an LH surge can be induced by the administration of exogenous estrogen. The exact pathogenesis of the impaired follicular development in these women is unknown, although it may be due to the exposure of the antral follicles at a crucial stage in their development to inappropriate levels and/or ratio of gonadotropins.

Although the levels of estradiol may never exceed 200 pg/ml, cystic hyperplasia may develop owing to the chronic exposure of the uterus to unopposed estrogen over a prolonged period. Hence the pattern of bleeding is irregular and unpredictable. Bleeding of this type in perimenopausal women always requires full gynecological investigation. If local pelvic pathology has been excluded by curettage of the uterus and/or hysteroscopy, then cycle control usually can be obtained by cyclical administration of gestogens (e.g., norethindrone 10 mg/d) for 10 days each month. If there are troublesome hot flushes, estrogen should be given in combination with cyclical gestogens.

Impaired Positive Feedback

Less commonly older women may experience persistent anovulatory cycles and irregular bleeding in association

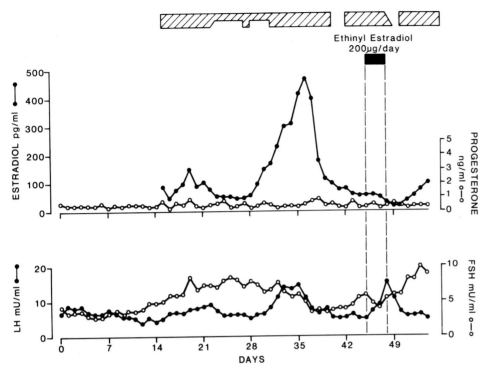

FIGURE 118–12. Ovarian hormone and gonadotropin levels in women aged 37 years with dysfunctional bleeding because of recurrent anovulatory cycles. Hatched bar at top indicates menses. (From Van Look PFA et al: Hypothalamic-pituitary-ovarian function in perimenopausal women. Clin Endocrinol 7:13–31, 1977.)

with cystic hyperplasia of the endometrium (Fig. 118–12). In a normal cycle, ovulation occurs in response to the midcycle surge of LH provoked by the secretion of estradiol secreted by the mature graafian follicle. In prepubertal girls the positive feedback mechanism is absent, and it may take some time after menarche for it to mature.[25] Hence the first few menstrual cycles usually are anovulatory and the bleeding scanty and painless. If anovulatory cycles persist for more than a few months, the pattern of bleeding may become totally irregular. There typically is a period of amenorrhea lasting for a few months during which time the endometrium thickens and becomes hyperplastic (Fig. 118–13). The hyperplastic endometrium eventually becomes necrotic and breaks down, resulting in several weeks of prolonged and often heavy bleeding.[122]

Recent studies have thrown light on the endocrine basis

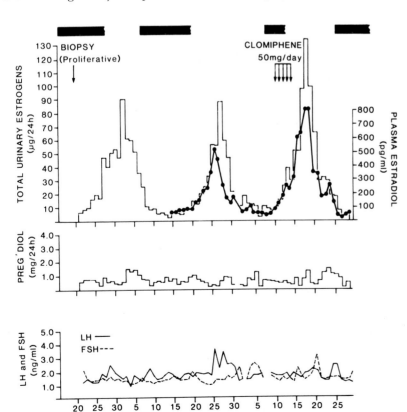

FIGURE 118–13. Steroid and gonadotropin levels in a girl with persistent anovulatory dysfunctional uterine bleeding. Note the absence of a preovulatory LH surge despite the raised levels of estrogen. Solid bar at top indicates menses. (From Fraser IS et al: Pituitary gonadotropins and ovarian function in adolescent dysfunctional uterine bleeding. J Clin Endocrinol Metab 37:407–414, © by the Endocrine Society, 1973.)

of this condition.[131] There appear to be waves of coordinated follicular development, as indicated by the fluctuating levels of estradiol.[6, 130, 131] In contrast to a normal cycle, a single dominant follicle fails to establish itself with the result that the ovary becomes multicystic. Despite the raised levels of estradiol, an LH surge does not occur because of an absence of the positive feedback mechanism (Fig. 118–14).[130] There is some evidence that the secretion of FSH is slightly more resistant than normal to the negative feedback effects of estrogen and may account for the persistence of more than one large antral follicle. It is not known whether the failure of positive feedback is due to a defect in the hypothalamus or the anterior pituitary. The fact that the frequency of LH pulses is similar to that found in the early follicular phase of the cycle suggests that hypothalamic activity is normal, at least at the initiation of the cycle.[131, 132]

The morbidity associated with chronic anovulatory cycles is considerable.[122] In addition to anemia associated with excessive bleeding, a proportion of women develop a form of PCO syndrome, infertility, or cancer of the endometrium.[133] An attempt should be made to suppress ovarian activity with the combined estrogen-gestogen pill and, hence, impose a regimen of exogenous steroids on the endometrium. In older women, if contraception is not required, cyclical gestogen therapy should be given to prevent hyperplasia of the endometrium.

Ovulatory Dysfunctional Uterine Bleeding

Insufficient or Inadequate Luteal Phase

In most ovarian cycles the luteal phase lasts for at least 10 days, during which time the concentration of progesterone exceeds 5 ng/ml on at least one day. A luteal phase that falls below these limits is deemed to be inadequate, although the precise values incompatible with the maintenance of pregnancy are unknown.[134] The diagnosis of inadequate luteal phase depends on accurate detection of ovulation and frequent measurements of plasma progesterone in the luteal phase. In practice the rise in basal body temperature usually is taken to time ovulation, and two or three samples of blood are collected in the next 10 days. The fact that the concentration of progesterone varies considerably from minute to minute may add to the difficulties of confirming a diagnosis.

Short luteal phases are thought to arise from inadequate development of the follicle[135] and can be reproduced experimentally in rhesus monkeys if the rise in the secretion of FSH in the early follicular phase of the cycle is prevented by the injection of porcine follicular fluid. The concentration of FSH in the early follicular phase of the cycle is lower in women with short luteal phases as compared with normal. Although some authorities claim that an inadequate luteal phase is an important cause of infertility,[136] 10 per cent of cycles in otherwise healthy women have a short luteal phase.[137] Short luteal phases commonly occur during the resumption of ovarian activity after weaning and after treatment of hyperprolactinemic amenorrhea with bromocriptine.[138] These physiological states of infertility are associated with an abnormality in the pattern of LH pulses, and it seems likely, therefore, that follicular development is abnormal. In some cases the follicle may luteinize in response to LH without rupture (luteinized unruptured follicle syndrome), and the levels of progesterone may be lower than normal.[139]

Although a wide variety of treatments have been used in inadequate luteal phase, none has conclusively improved fertility.[140] Treatment with hCG to stimulate increased secretion of progesterone by the corpus luteum and administration of exogenous progesterone both produce a lengthening of the luteal phase. Treatment during the early follicular phase with clomiphene or hMG restores the pattern of ovarian steroids to normal but does not increase the pregnancy rate. All these therapies, by increasing the level of progesterone during the luteal phase, may alleviate the breakthrough bleeding that may occur in this condition.

Idiopathic Bleeding

In most women who present with excessively heavy menses, no abnormality in ovarian activity can be identified.[141]

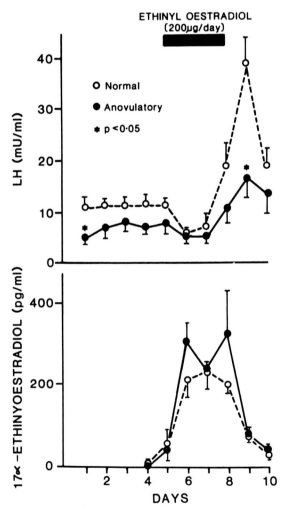

FIGURE 118–14. Estrogen provocation test in young women with anovulatory dysfunctional uterine bleeding. In normal women in the early follicular phase of the cycle after administration of ethinyl estradiol, the level of LH is initially suppressed (negative feedback). A discharge of LH commences on the third day of estrogen treatment (positive feedback). In adolescent girls with dysfunctional uterine bleeding, the positive feedback response to estrogen is absent or impaired. (From Van Look PFA et al: Impaired estrogen-induced luteinizing hormone release in young women with anovulatory dysfunctional uterine bleeding. J Clin Endocrinol Metab 46:816–823, © by The Endocrine Society, 1978.)

It is likely that there is some defect locally in the mechanism by which the endometrium is "programmed" for menstruation. When incubated in vitro, the endometriums of women with excessive menstrual blood loss synthesize more prostaglandins than those of women with normal loss.[142-144] Moreover, more PGE_2 and PGI_2, prostaglandins that induce vasodilation and inhibition of platelet aggregation, are produced relative to $PGF_{2\alpha}$, a vasoconstrictor.[145] The biochemical mechanism responsible for the change in biosynthesis of prostaglandins is unknown, but it gives some rational reason for the reduction in blood observed after treatment with inhibitors of prostaglandin biosynthesis.[146] Mefenamic acid (1.5 g/d in three divided doses) started on day 1 for the duration of bleeding results in a reduction of menstrual blood loss by one third. Similar results can be obtained with inhibitors of fibrinolysis (e.g., tranexamic acid), but because of their general affects on the vascular system, they are not widely used. Gestogen therapy is ineffective in ovulatory dysfunctional uterine bleeding in contrast to anovulatory conditions. Danazol in amounts insufficient to suppress ovarian function (200 mg/d) has been demonstrated to result in a significant reduction in blood loss. The mechanism is unknown, although through its mild androgenic properties it may reduce proliferation of the endometrium. In larger dosages (800 mg/d) danazol induces amenorrhea by suppressing FSH and LH. At this dosage the adverse effects of weight gain, hirsutism, and other manifestations of androgenization may preclude its use.

Two recent developments are likely to be of value in the medical management of women with excessive menstrual blood loss. As mentioned earlier, amenorrhea can be induced by suppression of the pituitary-ovarian axis by analogues of GnRH.[147-150] After an initial period of stimulation, receptors for GnRH in the pituitary are downregulated and a hypogonadotropic state and amenorrhea result. GnRH analogues may be given by nasal sniff, daily subcutaneous injection, or, more conveniently, biodegradable depot lasting up to three months.[149] Although amenorrhea is produced almost universally, the prolonged low levels of estrogen produce symptoms of estrogen deficiency such as flushes and vaginal dryness. In the long term the accelerated loss of calcium from the skeleton may lead to premature menopause and the lack of estrogen, to increased risk of heart disease.[148] It is possible to combine GnRH analogue treatment with estrogen and/or gestogen replacement therapy.[151-153] The blood loss that follows the cyclical withdrawal of progestogen is much less and more predictable than in spontaneous cycles.

Analogues of GnRH have already had widespread application in the treatment of benign gynecological conditions (e.g., endometriosis, uterine fibromyomata, premenstrual syndrome) as well as hormone-dependent cancers (e.g., uterus, breast, and prostate). Their widespread use in association with gonadotropins has facilitated stimulation of multiple follicular development for in vitro fertilization and other techniques of assisted conception. By allowing manipulation of the hormonal environment with exogenous agents after suppression of ovarian activity, analogues of GnRH have raised the possibility of medical management of many disorders of the reproductive system that hitherto could only be treated surgically.

REFERENCES

1. Brown JB, Matthew GD: The application of urinary estrogen measurements to problems in gynecology. Recent Prog Horm Res 18:337–373, 1962.
2. Baird D (ed): Abnormalities of gonadotrophin secretion in women. Clin Obstet Gynaecol 3, 1976.
3. Short RV: The evolution of human reproduction. Proc R Soc Lond 195:3–24, 1976.
4. Apter D, Viinikka L, Vihko R: Hormonal pattern of adolescent menstrual cycles. J Clin Endocrinol Metab 47:944–954, 1978.
5. Metcalf MG, McKenzie JA: Incidence of ovulation in young women. J Biosoc Sci 12:345–352, 1980.
6. Venturoli S, Porcu E, Fabbri R, et al: Longitudinal evaluation of the different gonadotropin pulsatile patterns in anovulatory cycles of young girls. J Clin Endocrinol Metab 74:836–841, 1992.
7. Treloar AE, Boynton RE, Behn BG, Brown BW: Variation of the human menstrual cycle through reproductive life. Int J Fertil 12:77–126, 1967.
8. Sherman BM, Wallace RB: Menstrual patterns: Menarche through menopause. In Baird DT, Michie EA (eds): Mechanism of Menstrual Bleeding. New York, Raven Press, 1985, pp 157–163.
9. Heape W: Menstruation and ovulation of Macacus rhesus with observations on the changes undergone by the discharged follicles. Philos Trans R Soc Lond [Biol] 188:135–166, 1987.
10. Corner GW: Our knowledge of the menstrual cycle, 1910–1950. Lancet 1:919–923, 1951.
11. Abel MH: Prostanoids and menstruation. In Baird DT, Michie EA (eds): Mechanism of Menstrual Bleeding. New York, Raven Press, 1985, pp 139–156.
12. Baird DT, Abel MH, Kelly RW, Smith SK: Endocrinology of dysfunctional uterine bleeding: The role of endometrial prostaglandins. In Crosignani PG, Rubin BL (eds): Endocrinology of Human Infertility: New Aspects. New York, Academic Press, 1981, pp 399–417.
13. Jacobs HS: Failures of the components of the negative feedback system. Clin Obstet Gynaecol 3:515–534, 1976.
14. Insler V, Zakut H, Serr DM: Cycle patterns and pregnancy rate following combined clomiphene-estrogen therapy. Obstet Gynecol 41:602–607, 1973.
15. Adams J, Mason PW, Tucker M, et al: Ultrasound assessment of changes in the ovary and uterus during LHRH therapy. Upsala J Med Sci 89:39–41, 1984.
16. Baird DT: Endocrinology of female infertility. Br Med Bull 35:193–198, 1979.
17. Shaw RW: Tests of the hypothalamic-pituitary-ovarian axis. Clin Obstet Gynaecol 3:485–503, 1976.
18. Baird DT, Fraser IS: Disorders of the hypothalamic-pituitary-ovarian axis. Clin Endocrinol Metab 2:469–488, 1973.
19. Yen SSC, Van den Berg G, Rebar R, Ehara Y: Variation of pituitary responsiveness of synthetic LRF during different phases of the menstrual cycle. J Clin Endocrinol Metab 35:931–934, 1972.
20. Nillius SJ, Wide L: The LH-releasing hormone test in 31 women with secondary amenorrhoea. Br J Obstet Gynaecol 79:874–882, 1972.
21. Yen SSC, Rebar R, Van den Berg G, et al: Pituitary gonadotrophin responsiveness to synthetic LRF in subjects with normal and abnormal hypothalamic-pituitary-ovarian axis. J Reprod Fertil 20:137–161, 1973.
22. Van Look PFA: Failure of positive feedback. Clin Obstet Gynaecol 3:555–578, 1976.
23. Newton J, Dixon P: Site of action of clomiphene and its use as a test of pituitary function. Br J Obstet Gynaecol 78:812–821, 1971.
24. Van den Berg G, Yen SSC: Effect of anti-estrogenic action of clomiphene during the menstrual cycle: Evidence for a change in the feedback sensitivity. J Clin Endocrinol Metab 37:356–365, 1973.
25. Kulin HE, Grumbach MM, Kaplan SL: Gonadal-hypothalamic interaction in prepubertal and pubertal man: Effect of clomiphene citrate on urinary follicle stimulating hormone and luteinizing hormone and plasma testosterone. Pediatr Res 6:162–171, 1972.
26. Gemzell C: Induction of ovulation with human gonadotropins. Recent Prog Horm Res 21:179–198, 1965.
27. Leduc B, Van Campenhout J, Simard R: Congenital absence of the vagina: Observations on 25 cases. Am J Obstet Gynecol 100:512–520, 1968.
28. Jost A, Vigier B, Prepin J, Perchellet JP: Studies on sex differentiation in mammals. Recent Prog Horm Res 29:1–41, 1973.

29. Wilson JD, Griffin JE, George FW, Leshin M: Studies on the endocrine control of male phenotype development. *In* Serio M, Motta M, Zanisi M, Martini L (eds): Sexual Differentiation: Basic and Clinical Aspects. New York, Raven Press, 1984, pp 223–224.

30. Serio M, Motta M, Zanisis N, Martini L (eds): Sexual Differentiation: Basic and Clinic Aspects. New York, Raven Press, 1984.

31. Morris JM: The syndrome of testicular feminization in male pseudohermaphrodites. Am J Obstet Gynecol 65:1192–1211, 1953.

32. Bardin CW, Bullock LP, Sherins RJ, et al: Androgen metabolism and mechanism of action in male pseudohermaphroditism: A study of testicular feminization. Recent Prog Horm Res 29:65–109, 1973.

33. Imparato-McGinley J, Guerrero L, Gautier T, et al: Steroid 5α-reductase deficiency in man: An inherited form of pseudohermaphroditism. Science 186:1213–1215, 1974.

34. French FS, Lubahn DB, Brown TR, et al: Molecular basis of androgen insensitivity. Recent Prog Horm Res 46:1–42, 1990.

35. Sohval AR: The syndrome of pure gonadal dysgenesis. Am J Med 38:615–625, 1965.

36. Muller J, Schwartz M, Skakkebaek NE: Analysis of the sex-determining region of the Y chromosome (SRY) in sex reversed patients: Point mutation in SRY causing sex reversion in 46XY female. J Clin Endocrinol Metab 75:(1)331–333, 1992.

37. McLaren A: Somatic and germ-cell sex in mammals. Philos Trans R Soc Lond [Biol] B322:3–9, 1988.

38. MacLean N, Harnden DG, Courtbrown WM, et al: Sex-chromosome abnormalities in newborn babies. Lancet 1:286–290, 1964.

39. Carr DH: Chromosomes and abortions. Adv Hum Genet 2:201–257, 1971.

40. Turner HH: A syndrome of infantilism, congenital webbed neck and cubitus valgus. Endocrinology 23:566–574, 1938.

41. Ferguson-Smith MA: Review article: Karyotype-phenotype correlations in gonadal dysgenesis and their bearing on the pathogenesis of malformations. J Med Genet 2:93–98, 1965.

42. Bahner F, Schwarz G, Hienz HA, Walter K: Turner-syndrome mit voll ausgebildeten sekundaren Geschlechsmerkmalen und Fertilitat. Acta Endocrinol 35:397–404, 1960.

43. Sherman BM, Korenman SG: Hormonal characteristics of the human menstrual cycle throughout reproductive life. J Clin Invest 55:699–706, 1975.

44. Metcalf MG, Donald RA, Livesey JH: Pituitary-ovarian function before, during and after the menopause: A longitudinal study. Clin Endocrinol 17:489–494, 1982.

45. Irvine WJ, Chan MMW, Scarth L, et al: Immunological aspects of premature ovarian failure associated with idiopathic Addison's disease. Lancet 2:883–887, 1968.

46. Irvine WJ: Autoimmune ovarian failure. *In* Irvine WJ, Loraine JA (eds): Reproductive Endocrinology. Edinburgh, Churchill Livingstone, 1970, pp 106–114.

47. Rabinowe SL, George KL, Ravnikar VA, et al: Premature menopause: Monoclonal antibody defined T lymphocyte abnormalities and antiovarian antibodies. Fertil Steril 51:450–459, 1989.

48. Rolland R, Kirkels VGHJ: Gonadal disorders of genetic origin. *In* Crosignani PG, Rubin BL (eds): Endocrinology of Human Infertility: New Aspects. London, Academic Press, 1981, pp 359–375.

49. Jones SG, de Moraea-Ruehsen M: A new syndrome of amenorrhoea in association with hypergonadism and apparently normal ovarian follicular apparatus. Am J Obstet Gynecol 104:597–600, 1969.

50. Starup J, Sele V, Henriksen B: Amenorrhoea associated with increased production of gonadotrophins and a morphologically normal ovarian follicular apparatus. Acta Endocrinol 66:248–256, 1971.

51. Ledger WL, Thomas EJ, Browning D, et al: Suppression of gonadotropin secretion does not reverse premature ovarian failure. Br J Obstet Gynaecol 96:196–199, 1989.

52. Nelson LM, Kimzey LM, White BJ, Merrian GR: Gonadotropin suppression for the treatment of karyotypically normal spontaneous premature ovarian failure: A controlled trial. Fertil Steril 57:50–55, 1992.

53. Evers JLH, Rolland R: The gonadotrophin resistant ovary syndrome: A curable disease? Clin Endocrinol 14:99–103, 1981.

54. Lutjen P, Trounson A, Leeton J, et al: The establishment and maintenance of pregnancy using in vitro fertilization and embryo donation in a patient with primary ovarian failure. Nature 307:174–175, 1984.

55. Saver MV, Partsson RJ: Oocyte donation to women with ovarian failure. Contemp Obstet Gynecol 34:125–135, 1989.

56. Speroff L, Glass RH, Kase NG (eds): Clinical Gynecologic Endocrinology and Infertility (ed 4). Baltimore, Williams & Wilkins, 1989, p 165.

57. Lachelin GCL, Yen SSC: Hypothalamic chronic anovulation. Am J Obstet Gynecol 130:825–831, 1978.

58. Letsky OA, Davajan V, Nakamura RM, Mishell DR Jr: Classification of secondary amenorrhoea based on distinct hormonal patterns. J Clin Endocrinol Metab 41:660–668, 1975.

59. Leyendecker G, Wildt L: Induction of ovulation with chronic intermittent (pulsatile) administration of Gn-RH in women with hypothalamic amenorrhoea. J Reprod Fertil 69:397–409, 1983.

60. Crowley WF, Filicori M, Spratt DI, Santoro NF: The physiology of gonadotropin-releasing hormone (GnRH) secretion in man and women. Recent Prog Horm Res 41:473–477, 1985.

61. Lunenfeld B, Insler V: Classification of amenorrhoeic states and their treatment by ovulation induction. Clin Endocrinol 3:223–237, 1974.

62. Jacobs HS, Franks S, Murray MAF, et al: Clinical and endocrine features of hyperprolactinemic amenorrhoea. Clin Endocrinol 5:439–454, 1976.

63. Kleinberg DL, Noel GL, Frantz AG: Galactorrhea: A study of 235 cases including 48 with pituitary tumors. N Engl J Med 296:589–600, 1977.

64. Argonz J, del Castillo EB: A syndrome characterized by estrogen deficiency, galactorrhea and gonadotropin secretion. J Clin Endocrinol Metab 13:79–87, 1953.

65. Forbes AP, Hennemann PH, Griswold GC, Albright F: Syndrome characterized by galactorrhea, amenorrhea and low urinary FSH: Comparison with acromegaly and normal lactation. J Clin Endocrinol Metab 14:265–271, 1974.

66. Honbo KS, Van Kellett KA: Serum prolactin levels in untreated primary hypothyroidism. Am J Med 64:782–787, 1978.

67. Bohnet HG, Dahlen HG, Wuttke W, Schneider HPG: Hyperprolactinemic anovulatory syndrome. J Clin Endocrinol Metab 42:132–143, 1976.

68. Lachelin GCL, Abu-Fadil S, Yen SSC: Functional delineation of hyperprolactinemic amenorrhoea. J Clin Endocrinol Metab 44:1163–1174, 1977.

69. Vaughan Williams CA, McNeilly AS, Baird DT: The effects of chronic treatment with LHRH on gonadotrophin secretion and pituitary responsiveness to LHRH in women with secondary hypogonadism. Clin Endocrinol 19:9–19, 1983.

70. Aono T, Miyake A, Shioji T, et al: Impaired LH release following exogenous estrogen administration in patients with amenorrhea-galactorrhea syndrome. J Clin Endocrinol Metab 42:696–702, 1976.

71. Glass MR, Shaw RW, Butt WR, et al: An abnormality of oestrogen feedback in amenorrhoea-galactorrhea. Br Med J 3:274–275, 1975.

72. Ropert JF, Quigley ME, Yen SSC: Endogenous opiates modulate pulsatile luteinizing hormone release in humans. J Clin Endocrinol Metab 52:583–585, 1981.

73. Grossman A, Moult PJA, McIntyre H, et al: Opiate mediation of amenorrhoea in hyperprolactinaemia and in weight loss related amenorrhoea. Clin Endocrinol 17:379–388, 1982.

74. Gemzell C, Wang CF: Outcome of pregnancy in women with pituitary adenoma. Fertil Steril 31:363–372, 1979.

75. Hardy T: Transsphenoidal surgery of hypersecreting tumours. *In* Kohler PO, Ross GT (eds): Diagnosis and Treatment of Pituitary Tumors. Amsterdam, Excerpta Medica, 1973, pp 179–185.

76. Serri O, Rajio E, Beauregard H, et al: Recurrence of hyperprolactinemia after selective transsphenoidal adenectomy in women with prolactinoma. N Engl J Med 309:280–283, 1983.

77. Van Loon GR: A defect in catecholamine neurons in patients with prolactin-secreting pituitary adenoma. Lancet 2:868–871, 1978.

78. Thorner MO, McNeilly AS, Hagen C, Besser GM: Long-term treatment of galactorrhoea and hypogonadism and bromocriptine. Br Med J 2:419–422, 1974.

79. Nillius SJ: Medical therapy of prolactin-secreting pituitary tumours. *In* L'Hermite M, Judd SL (eds): Advances in Prolactin. Progress in Reproductive Biology, Vol 6. Basel, Karger, 1980, pp 194–221.

80. Molitch ME, Elton RL, Blackwell RE, et al: Bromocriptine as primary therapy for prolactin-secreting adenomas: Results of a prospective multicentre study. J Clin Endocrinol Metab 60:698–705, 1985.

80a. Glasier AF, Hendry RA, Seth T, et al: Does treatment with bromocriptine influence the chance of hyperprolactinemia? 5:359–366, 1987.

81. Trends in the management of prolactinomas. Br Med J 281:338–339, 1980.

82. Greenblatt RB, Zarate A, Mahesh VB: Stimulation of gonadal function by clomiphene citrate. *In* Astwood EB, Cassidy CE (eds): Clinical Endocrinology II. New York, Grune & Stratton, 1969, pp 630–642.

83. Glasier AF, Irvine DS, Wickings EJ, et al: A comparison of the effects of follicular development between clomiphene citrate, its two separate isomers and spontaneous cycles. Hum Reprod 4:252–256, 1989.

84. Mikkelson TJ, Kroboth PD, Cameron WJ, et al: Single-dose pharmacokinetics of clomiphene citrate in normal volunteers. Fertil Steril 46:392–396, 1986.

85. Macgregor AH, Johnson JE, Bunde CA: Further clinical experience with clomiphene citrate. Fertil Steril 19:616–622, 1968.

86. Stein IF, Leventhal ML: Amenorrhoea associated with bilateral polycystic ovaries. Am J Obstet Gynecol 29:181–191, 1935.

87. Yen SSC: The polycystic ovary syndrome. Clin Endocrinol 12:177–208, 1980.

88. Baird DT, Corker CS, Davidson DW, et al: Pituitary-ovarian relationships in polycystic ovary syndrome. J Clin Endocrinol Metab 45:798–809, 1977.

89. Dunaif A, Segal KR, Futterweit W, Dobrjansky A: Profound peripheral insulin resistance independent of obesity, in polycystic ovary syndrome. Diabetes 38:1165–1174, 1989.

90. Siiteri PK, Macdonald PC: Role of extraglandular estrogen in human endocrinology. In Field J (ed): Handbook of Physiology, Vol II, Sec 7. Baltimore, Williams & Wilkins, 1973, pp 615–629.

91. Adashi EY, Rock JA, Guzick D, et al: Fertility following bilateral ovarian wedge resection: A critical analysis of 90 consecutive cases of polycystic ovary syndrome. Fertil Steril 36:320–325, 1981.

92. Vaughan Williams CA: Ovarian electrocautery or hormone therapy in PCOS. Clin Endocrinol 33:569–572, 1990.

93. Aakavaag A, Gjonnaess H: Hormonal response to electrocautery of the ovary in patients with polycystic ovarian disease. Br J Obstet Gynaecol 92:1258–1264, 1985.

94. Kallman FJ, Schoefield WA, Barrera SE: The genetic aspects of primary eunuchoidism. Am J Ment Defic 48:203–236, 1944.

95. Valk TW, Corley KP, Kelch RP, Marshall JC: Hypogonadotropic hypogonadism—hormonal responses to low dose pulsatile administration of gonadotrophin-releasing hormone. J Clin Endocrinol Metab 51:730–738, 1980.

96. Sheehan HL: Simmond's disease due to post partum necrosis of the anterior pituitary. Q J Med 8:277–309, 1939.

97. Yen SSC, Rebar R, Van den Berg G, Judd H: Hypothalamic amenorrhea and hypogonadotropism: Responses to synthetic LRF. J Clin Endocrinol Metab 36:811–816, 1973.

98. Santen RJ, Friend JN, Trujanowski D, et al: Prolonged negative feedback suppression after estradiol administration: Proposed mechanism of eugonadal secondary amenorrhea. J Clin Endocrinol Metab 47:1220–1229, 1978.

99. Vigersky RA, Loriaux DL, Anderson AE, et al: Delayed pituitary hormone response to LRF and TRF in patients with anorexia nervosa and with secondary amenorrhea associated with simple weight loss. J Clin Endocrinol Metab 43:893–900, 1976.

100. Hull MGR, Savage PE, Jacobs HS: Investigation and treatment of amenorrhoea resulting in normal fertility. Br Med J 1:1257–1261, 1979.

101. Brown JB, Evans JH, Adey FD, et al: Factors involved in the induction of fertile ovulation with human gonadotrophins. Br J Obstet Gynaecol 76:289–307, 1969.

102. Lunenfeld B, Insler V: Diagnosis and Treatment of Functional Infertility. Berlin, Gross Verlag, 1978.

103. West CP, Baird DT: Induction of ovulation with gonadotrophins–a ten year review. Scott Med J 29:212–217, 1984.

104. Yoshimoto Y, Moridera K, Imura H: Restoration of normal pituitary gonadotropic reserve by administration of luteinizing hormone-releasing hormone in patients with hypogonadotropic hypogonadism. N Engl J Med 292:242–245, 1975.

105. Leyendecker G, Wildt L, Hansmann M: Pregnancies following chronic intermittent (pulsatile) administration of Gn-RH by means of a portable pump ("Zyklomat")—a new approach to the treatment of infertility in hypothalamic amenorrhea. J Clin Endocrinol Metab 51:1214–1216, 1980.

106. Belchetz PE, Plant TM, Nakai Y, et al: Hypophyseal responses to continuous and intermittent delivery of hypothalamic gonadotrophin-releasing hormone. Science 202:631–633, 1978.

107. Filicori M, Falmigni C, Meriggiola MC, et al: Endocrine response determines the clinical outcome of pulsatile gonadotropin-releasing hormone ovulation induction in different disorders. J Clin Endocrinol Metab 72:965–972, 1991.

108. Homburg R, Eshel A, Armar NA, et al: One hundred pregnancies after treatment with pulsatile luteinising hormone releasing hormone to induce ovulation. Br Med J 298:809–812, 1989.

109. Mason P, Adams J, Morris DV, et al: Induction of ovulation with pulsatile luteinising hormone releasing hormone. Br Med J 288:181–185, 1984.

110. Braat DDM, Boghelman D, Coelingh Bennink HJT, et al: The outcome of pregnancies established in GnRH induced cycles with special reference to the multiple pregnancies in 5 Dutch centres. In Coelingh Bennink HJT, Dogterom AA, Lapphon RE, et al (eds): Pulsatile GnRH. Haarten, Feming, 1986, pp 207–211.

111. Regan L, Owen EJ, Jacobs HS: Hypersecretion of LH, infertility and miscarriage. Lancet 336:1141–1144, 1990.

112. Homburg R, Armar NA, Eshel A, et al: Influence of serum luteinising hormone concentrations on ovulation, conception and early pregnancy loss in polycystic ovary syndrome. Br Med J 297:1024–1026, 1988.

113. Hamilton-Fairley D, Kiddy D, Watson H, et al: Low-dose gonadotrophin therapy for induction of ovulation in 100 women with polycystic ovary syndrome. Hum Reprod 6:1095–1099, 1991.

114. Fleming R, Coutts JRT: Induction of multiple follicular growth in normally menstruating women with endogenous gonadotropin suppression. Fertil Steril 45:226–230, 1986.

115. Fleming R, Coutts JT: LHRH analogues for ovulation induction with particular reference to polycystic ovarian syndrome. Baillieres Clin Obstet Gynaecol 2:677–687, 1988.

116. Homburg R, Eshel A, Kilborn J, et al: Combined luteinising hormone releasing hormone analogue and exogenous gonadotrophins for the treatment of infertility associated with polycystic ovaries. Hum Reprod 5:32–35, 1990.

117. Goldsmith RE, Sturgis SH, Lerman J, Stanbury JB: The menstrual pattern in thyroid disease. J Clin Endocrinol Metab 12:846–855, 1952.

118. Ridgway EC, Longcope C, Malouf F: Metabolic clearance and blood production rates of estradiol in hyperthyroidism. J Clin Endocrinol Metab 41:491–497, 1975.

119. Rishman J, Hellman L, Zumoff B, Gallacher TF: Influence of thyroid hormone on estrogen metabolism in man. J Clin Endocrinol Metab 22:389–392, 1961.

120. Goldzieher JW: Oestrogens in congenital adrenal hyperplasia. Acta Endocrinol 54:51–62, 1967.

121. Wallach EE: Symposium on dysfunctional uterine bleeding. Clin Obstet Gynecol 13:363–488, 1970.

122. Southam AL, Richart RM: The prognosis for adolescents with menstrual abnormalities. Am J Obstet Gynecol 94:637–643, 1966.

123. Smith SK, Abel MH, Kelly RW, Baird DT: The synthesis of prostaglandins from persistent proliferative endometrium. J Clin Endocrinol Metab 55:284–289, 1982.

124. Erickson GF, Hsueh AJW, Quigley ME, et al: Functional studies of aromatase activity in human granulosa cells from normal and polycystic ovaries. J Clin Endocrinol Metab 49:514–519, 1979.

125. Hammerstein J, Meekies J, Leo-Rossberg I, et al: Use of cyproterone acetate (CPA) in the treatment of acne, hirsutism, and virilism. J Steroid Biochem 6:827–836, 1975.

126. McKenna TJ: The use of anti-androgens in the treatment of hirsutism. Clin Endocrinol 35:1–3, 1991.

127. Barth JH, Cherry CA, Wojnarowska F, Dawber RPR: Spironolactone is an effective and well tolerated systemic anti androgen therapy for hirsute women. J Clin Endocrinol Metab 68:966–970, 1989.

128. Coulam CB, Annegers JF, Kranz JS: Chronic anovulation syndrome and associated neoplasia. Obstet Gynecol 61:403–407, 1983.

129. Metcalf MG, Donald RA, Livesey JH: Classification of menstrual cycles in pre- and perimenopausal women. J Endocrinol 91:1–10, 1981.

130. Van Look PFA, Lothian H, Hunter WM, et al: Hypothalamic-pituitary-ovarian function in perimenopausal women. Clin Endocrinol 7:13–31, 1977.

131. Baird DT: Anovulatory dysfunctional uterine bleeding in adolescence. In Flamigni C, Venturoli S, Givens JR (eds): Adolescence in Females. Chicago, Year Book Medical Publishers, 1985, pp 273–285.

132. Fraser IS, Michie EA, Wide L, Baird DT: Pituitary gonadotropins and ovarian function in adolescent dysfunctional uterine bleeding. J Clin Endocrinol Metab 37:407–414, 1973.

133. Fraser IS, Baird DT: Endometrial cystic glandular hyperplasia in adolescent girls. Br J Obstet Gynaecol 79:1009–1015, 1972.

134. Coutts JRT: The abnormal luteal phase. In Jeffcoate SL (ed): The Luteal Phase. New York, John Wiley & Sons, 1985, pp 101–114.

135. Strott CA, Cargille CM, Ross GT, Lipsett MB: The short luteal phase. J Clin Endocrinol Metab 30:246–251, 1970.

136. Jones GES: Some newer aspects of the management of infertility. JAMA 141:1123–1128, 1949.

137. Lenton EA, Landeren BM: The normal menstrual cycle. In Shearman RP (ed): Clinical Reproductive Endocrinology. Edinburgh, Churchill Livingstone, 1985, pp 81–108.

138. McNeilly AS: Prolactin and the control of gonadotrophin secretion in the female. J Reprod Fertil 58:537–549, 1980.

139. Koninckx PR, De Moor P, Brosens IA: Diagnosis of the luteinized unruptured follicle syndrome by steroid hormone assays in peritoneal fluid. Br J Obstet Gynaecol 87:929–934, 1980.
140. Macnaughton MC: Treatment of the defective luteal phase. In Jacobs HS (ed): Advances in Gynaecological Endocrinology. London, Royal College of Obstetricians and Gynaecologists, 1978, pp 92–101.
141. Haynes PJ, Anderson ABM, Turnbull AC: Patterns of menstrual blood loss in menorrhagia. Res Clin Forums 1:73–78, 1979.
142. Drife JO: Dysfunctional uterine bleeding and menorrhagia. Baillieres Clin Obstet Gynaecol 3 (No. 2), 1989.
143. Willman EA, Collins WP, Clayton SG: Studies on the involvement of prostaglandins in uterine symptomatology and pathology. Br J Obstet Gynaecol 83:337–341, 1976.
144. Smith SK, Abel MH, Kelly RW, Baird DT: Prostaglandin synthesis in the endometrium of women with ovular dysfunctional uterine bleeding. Br J Obstet Gynaecol 88:434–442, 1981.
145. Smith SK, Abel MH, Kelly RW, Baird DT: A role for prostacyclin (PGI$_2$) in excessive menstrual bleeding. Lancet 1:522–524, 1981.
146. Cameron IT: Dysfunctional uterine bleeding. Baillieres Clin Obstet Gynaecol 3:315–327, 1989.
147. Meldrum DR, Chang RJ, Lu J, et al: "Medical oophorectomy" using a long-acting GnRH agonist—a possible new approach to the treatment of endometriosis. J Clin Endocrinol Metab 54:1081–1083, 1982.
148. Fraser HM, Baird DT: Clinical applications of LHRH analogues. Clin Endocrinol Metab 1:43–70, 1987.
149. West CP, Baird DT: Suppression of ovarian activity by Zoladex depot (ICI 118630), a long acting LHRH agonist analogue. Clin Endocrinol 26:213–220, 1987.
150. Shaw RW, Fraser HM: Use of a superactive luteinizing hormone releasing hormone (LHRH) agonist in the treatment of menorrhagia. Br J Obstet Gynaecol 91:913–916, 1984.
151. Maheux R, Lemay A, Blanchet P, et al: Maintained reduction of uterine leiomyomata following addition of hormone replacement therapy to a monthly luteinising hormone-releasing hormone agonist implant: A pilot study. Hum Reprod 6:500–505, 1991.
152. West CP, Lumsden M-A, Hillier H, et al: Potential role for medroxyprogesterone acetate as an adjunct to goserelin (Zoladex) in the medical management of fibroids. Hum Reprod 7:328–332, 1992.
153. Friedman AJ: Treatment of leiomyota uteri with short-term leuprolide followed by oestrogen-progestin hormone replacement therapy for two years: A pilot study. Fertil Steril 51:526–528, 1989.
154. Tay CCK, Glasier AF, Illingworth PJI, et al: Abnormal 24 hour pattern of pulsatile hormone secretion and the response to naloxone in women with hyperprolactinaemic amenorrhoea. Clin Endocrinol, in press.

119

Infertility: Causes, Evaluation, and Treatment

VAL DAVAJAN†
ROBERT ISRAEL

Approximately 10 to 15 per cent of all married couples (2.5 million women) in the United States are childless.[1] The diagnosis of infertility is usually made when conception has not occurred after one year of unprotected sexual exposure in a couple trying to achieve a pregnancy. The term *primary infertility* is used when no conception has ever taken place. In contrast, secondary infertility implies that at least one previous conception has been either hormonally or histologically documented. The diagnosis of sterility by ultrasonography should be made only when the cause of infertility is such that no conception is possible without therapy. Fecundity is defined by rate of conception occurring in a population in a given time interval, usually one month. The normal fertile population fecundity rate is approximately 20 per cent per cycle. This rate steadily decreases in each subsequent month, with conception rates being 50 per cent after three months of trying to conceive, 75 per cent at the end of six months, and approximately 90 per cent at the end of one year. Following the first year, those couples who have not conceived can be subdivided into two groups. The first group includes those who are sterile and cannot conceive without specific therapy (for example, bilateral tubal occlusion). The second group includes those with relative infertility (for example, oligospermia) or those with idiopathic infertility. It has been stated that in the latter group approximately two thirds can be expected to conceive spontaneously within the following two years.

The causes of infertility can be divided into four major categories: (1) the female factor, (2) the male factor, (3) combined factors, and (4) infertility of undetermined cause. It is difficult to assign exact percentages to each of these categories. Approximately 40 per cent of the infertility cases are due to a female factor and 40 per cent to a male factor, and in 2 to 15 per cent no diagnosis can be made after a complete investigation.[2] It has also been reported that in as many as 35 per cent of patients, the infertility may be of multiple origins.[3]

Various surveys in the United States have listed the following prevalence of infertility among women in the different age groups: 8 per cent in the 20- to 29-year-old category, 15 per cent in ages 30 to 34, 22 per cent from ages 35 to 39, and 29 per cent from ages 40 to 44. The decline appears to begin after women reach age 31. Using artificial insemination data, it can be stated that after age 35 pregnancy rates are only about half those of women under age 31 and by age 40 only about one third. Therefore, the two major factors determining fecundity rates appear to be (1) length of time during which the couple has been attempting to conceive and (2) the age of the woman.

The diagnostic approach to infertility should be systematic and as rapid as possible. At the initial interview the total diagnostic and therapeutic plan should be explained to the infertile couple. The therapy for each causative factor should be discussed, as well as the expected prognosis. Patients should be told that in a significant number of instances no diagnosis can be made after completing the work-up. The incidence of spontaneous conception in couples with unexplained infertility is stated to be only 3 per cent.[4] An honest assessment of the problems of infertility

†Deceased.

does help to reduce the frustrations experienced by both physicians and patients.

The following scheme for evaluating the infertile couple is the method used in the Los Angeles County/University of Southern California Endocrine-Infertility Clinic.

INVESTIGATION OF THE INFERTILE COUPLE

Investigation of infertility should be complete, and all couples should have a complete history and physical examination. Routine laboratory tests include complete blood counts, urinalysis, Venereal Disease Research Laboratory (VDRL) test for syphilis, and a fasting and two-hour postprandial blood sugar. A sexual history should be obtained with special emphasis on the frequency and timing of intercourse and the use of lubricants during intercourse. Not infrequently an infertile couple abstains from intercourse and has only one "timed" exposure in the middle of the cycle. There is no evidence that "storing up" sperm increases the chances of conception. In fact, decreasing the number of exposures per week seems to be related to infertility. Intercourse should be advised for at least two to three days after the rise in basal body temperature (BBT). With the introduction of the urinary luteinizing hormone (LH) detection kits for home use, it is now possible to accurately time intercourse based on the LH surge rather than relying on the BBT alone. Unless the male partner is found to have oligospermia, no abstinence should be recommended. The use of lubricants should be avoided and the couple advised to use small amounts of warm water if lack of lubrication is a problem. Male impotence that seems to be related to the demand for "timed" intercourse is not uncommon. If this problem is encountered, the couple should be instructed to have intercourse as often as possible, without any specific instructions as to the exact days or time for intercourse. The exact positioning and technique of intercourse should be pursued only if the postcoital test reveals no sperm in the cervical canal or vaginal vault.

The investigation of infertility should be initiated in the following manner: (1) documentation of ovulation (presumptive), (2) semen analysis, (3) postcoital test, and (4) investigation of the female upper genital tract. If these tests are normal, the following additional tests can be performed: (5) immunological test, (6) bacterial cultures of cervical mucus and semen, (7) endometrial biopsy and serum progestin to establish the diagnosis of inadequate luteal phase, and (8) serum thyroid-stimulating hormone (TSH) to rule out hypothyroidism (see Ch. 45).

Documentation of Ovulation (Presumptive)

A woman who gives the history of having regular monthly menstrual cycles is probably ovulating. Nevertheless, ovulation should be documented in the work-up of infertile patients. There are five methods available to make the presumptive diagnosis of ovulation: (1) serum progesterone, (2) BBT, (3) endometrial biopsy, (4) ultrasonographic detection of follicle maturation, and (5) detection of urinary LH surge by the use of monoclonal antibody kits developed for home use.

SERUM PROGESTERONE. A single serum progesterone value obtained between days 20 and 24 of the menstrual cycle that is greater than 3 ng/ml can be considered indicative of ovulation.[5] If the sample is obtained too early or too late in the luteal phase, a false-negative result may be obtained because of the rise and fall of serum progesterone in a normal cycle. Although serum progesterone values of 3 to 5 ng/ml are sufficient to cause secretory changes in the endometrium, it has been reported that in all cycles in which a pregnancy occurred the serum progesterone values were found to be above 10 ng/ml. Because of this finding we have treated infertile patients who have serum progesterone values of less than 10 ng/ml with clomiphene citrate.

BASAL BODY TEMPERATURE. Because of the thermogenic properties of progesterone, the BBT shifts to a higher temperature in the luteal phase of the cycle. A mean increase of at least 0.4°F over the proliferative phase temperature is considered a normal biphasic shift. The patient should be instructed to take her temperature orally each morning before getting out of bed. The length of the luteal phase should be greater than 11 days. Ovulation usually takes place following the nadir of the BBT and the early rise of the temperature.

ENDOMETRIAL BIOPSY. A biopsy obtained between days 20 and 22 of the cycle should reveal histological evidence of ovulation by the presence of secretory changes in the endometrial glands. The biopsy should be obtained with a single swipe of the endometrium high on the anterior wall of the uterine fundus. (Endometrial biopsy for documentation of "inadequate" luteal phase is done later in the luteal phase and is discussed later in this chapter).

ULTRASONOGRAPHY. Serial ultrasonographic evaluations of ovarian follicular growth now have been used with success in establishing whether or not ovulation is taking place.[6]

DETECTION OF LH SURGE BY HOME URINARY MONITORING. In recent years several kits have become available to detect the increase in urinary LH at the time of the midcycle LH surge. Most kits use an anti-LH antiserum linked to an enzyme system as a dipstick. Increased amounts of LH in the urine bind to the antiserum, which triggers the enzyme system to produce a color change that can be read by the patient.

After presumptive documentation of ovulation, the investigation should proceed to the next step as outlined. However, if the patient is not ovulating, an endocrine work-up should be instituted to determine the cause of anovulation.

Diagnosis and Treatment of Anovulation

Some 10 to 15 per cent of all infertile women are anovulatory.[2] These patients are categorized into three groups according to their menstrual patterns: (1) primary amenorrhea, (2) secondary amenorrhea, and (3) oligomenorrhea.

The correct diagnosis in these patients is not difficult to make, and in-depth discussion of these patients is covered in Chapters 31, 118, and 120. If the diagnosis does not preclude the possibility of pregnancy, the patient should be treated. Many patients with primary amenorrhea have a normal karyotype and normal development of secondary sex characteristics. These patients and those with secondary amenorrhea or oligomenorrhea should be given an intramuscular injection of 100 to 200 mg of progesterone in oil. Approximately two thirds of such patients have uterine bleeding after this challenge test. These patients should be treated with clomiphene citrate.[7, 8]

All patients treated with ovulation-inducing drugs should be given an informed consent form stating the incidence of multiple pregnancies, development of ovarian cysts, and incidence of fetal anomalies. The incidences from this clinic are listed in Table 119–1.

Clomiphene therapy is started on the fifth day of the cycle at 50 mg/d for five days. Semen analysis should be obtained before instituting therapy. If the patient fails to ovulate at this dose, the dose is increased to 100 mg/d and, if necessary, to 150, 200, and, finally, 250 mg/d for five days. At the 150-mg dose, 10,000 units of human chorionic gonadotropin (hCG) can be given seven days after the last dose of clomiphene or when a dominant follicle as seen by ultrasonography reaches a diameter of 20 to 22 mm. If this dose fails to induce ovulation, eight days of 250 mg/d of clomiphene should be administered. If the patient fails to ovulate at this dose, she is then treated with gonadotropins (Pergonal) or gonadotropin-releasing hormone (GnRH) via a pump designed for pulsatile intravenous or subcutaneous administration of the drug.

With an intact hypothalamic-pituitary axis and intact ovaries, clomiphene has been successful in more than 90 per cent of cases.[7, 8] The ovulatory rate with Pergonal therapy is close to 100 per cent. Documentation of ovulation by either a BBT record, a serum progesterone, urinary LH kits, or serial ultrasonography should be obtained in each treatment cycle. Patients receiving clomiphene should have a pelvic examination at monthly intervals before taking the next dose. The exact mode of administration of Pergonal with steroid monitoring is discussed in Chapter 116.

The couple should try to achieve pregnancy for at least three ovulatory cycles before instituting further diagnostic procedures. Eighty per cent of patients treated with clomiphene who get pregnant do so within three cycles of therapy. If no conception occurs after three ovulatory cycles, the postcoital test and hysterosalpingography should be performed. If these tests are normal, the patient should be allowed at least six ovulatory cycles before undergoing a laparoscopy. If the patient successfully ovulates with clomiphene and if no other factors for infertility can be found, the patient should be continued on this drug for as long as

TABLE 119–1. Side Effects of Clomiphene and Pergonal Therapy

	Clomid (%)	Pergonal (%)
Multiple pregnancies	5	8–22
Ovarian cysts	5–10	6–15
Fetal anomalies	2–3	2–3
Ovulation	60–92	85–100
Term pregnancies	70–80	65–70
Abortions	20–25	30–35

Data from the Los Angeles County/University of Southern California Endocrine-Infertility Clinic.

TABLE 119–2. Normal Semen Analysis

Volume	3–5 ml
Count*	>20 million/ml
Motility	50–60%
Normal morphology	50–60%
Cytology	<5 WBC/HPF
Viscosity	Total liquefaction within 20 min

Data from Los Angeles County/University of Southern California Clinic.
*Lower counts/ml can be found in men with proven fertility in any one sample and therefore one low sperm count may not be definitive evidence of oligospermia.

she desires. One patient in this clinic was treated for 29 ovulatory cycles before conception occurred.[9] It is now common to try the new technology methods much more quickly if pregnancy does not occur.

If the amenorrheic or oligomenorrheic patient shows clinical evidence of excess cortisol production, she should be evaluated for possible Cushing's syndrome (see Ch. 100) before considering anovulatory therapy. The same principle applies to the amenorrheic patient who has clinical findings compatible with excess androgen production. The ovarian and adrenal evaluation for this condition is discussed in Chapters 100 and 120. Finally, if the patient has galactorrhea or is found to have hyperprolactinemia, an appropriate evaluation should be instituted before the patient is treated with bromocriptine in order to induce ovulation (see Ch. 31).

THE EXAMINATION OF SEMEN

The examination of semen is an integral part of the clinical investigation of infertility. It should be one of the first steps in the investigation of the infertile couple. It is beyond the scope of this chapter to discuss male infertility in detail (see Ch. 136), but a portion of the male factor is discussed under "In Vivo Fractional Postcoital Test."

Briefly, the semen should be collected in a clean glass container. Interval of abstinence should be determined by the frequency of intercourse routinely practiced by the couple. In areas where the weather is mild, the specimen need not be kept warm when transporting it to the laboratory. Because most of the spermatozoa are found in the first 1 ml of the ejaculate, the patient should be instructed to take extreme precautions not to spill any portion of the specimen. Examination of the semen should be performed within the first hour after collection (Table 119–2). More recently, the hamster egg (zona pellucida–free) human sperm penetration test has become popular in the evaluation of male infertility. This test assesses sperm penetration, but its exact role in the investigation of infertile men is uncertain at present.

ABNORMAL CERVICAL MUCUS–SPERMATOZOON INTERACTION (CERVICAL FACTOR)

The exact incidence of infertility secondary to abnormal midcycle cervical mucus–spermatozoon interaction is unknown, but it has been reported to be between 10 and 30 per cent.[10] The existence of this factor is based on the finding that in certain infertile couples, the microscopic examination of midcycle postcoital cervical mucus contains few or no sperm or in some cases only immobilized sperm.

In the evaluation of infertility the postcoital test (PCT) is the only routinely performed in vivo test that brings together both partners in a testing system.

In Vivo Fractional Postcoital Test

The cervical mucus is aspirated with a large syringe attached to a polyethylene suction catheter. Catheters, size 8 to 14 French, can be used, depending on the diameter of the external os.[9,10] The tubing is grasped 2.5 cm from the distal end with an atraumatic cervical clamp or a large Allis clamp. The aspiration must be initiated just as the tip of the catheter is inserted into the external os. A constant negative pressure is maintained with the syringe as the catheter is advanced to the internal os level (2.5 cm). The catheter is then gently withdrawn and the trailing mucus cut away with scissors in order to prevent the sample from being pulled out of the catheter. The catheter segment containing the mucus is then cut into four segments. The mucus in the segment from the tip of the catheter contains mucus collected from the internal os level and the segment most proximal (closest to the clamp) represents mucus from the level of the external os. A smear of the posterior vaginal fornix should always be obtained to make sure that spermatozoa were deposited into the vaginal vault. The PCT should be performed after two days of abstinence and within two hours of coitus. It has been reported that at 2 to 2½ hours, maximum numbers of sperm are present in the cervical canal.[10-14] The day of examination should be scheduled for one or two days before the expected rise and one day after the rise of the BBT. A test considered normal should show at least five motile sperm per high-power field at the internal os level.[10-14] The spinnbarkeit measured in the same mucus sample should be no less than 6 cm (Table 119–3).

Differential Diagnosis and Treatment of the Cervical Factor

The possible cervical factors involved may be categorized as (a) anatomical defects, (b) abnormal quality and quantity of cervical mucus, and (c) abnormal postcoital test with normal cervical mucus.

Anatomical Defects of the Cervix

CERVICAL STENOSIS. Less than 10 per cent of patients with cervical factors have anatomical defects. Conization of the cervix is still the most common cause of cervical stenosis. The diagnosis is made by history when there is resis-

TABLE 119–3. NORMAL POSTCOITAL TEST

Days of abstinence	2
Days of examination	BBT rise-2
Hours from coitus to examination	2–2.5
Number of sperm/HPF (internal os level)	5 or more
Spinnbarkeit (internal os level)	>6 cm

tance in attempting to pass a catheter into the endocervical canal. Neither estrogen therapy nor attempts to recanalize the endocervix with dilators or cryosurgery have been successful. The use of small lamineria has been suggested, but little success has been reported. Intrauterine insemination using washed sperm has given encouraging results.[15] This technique is now used throughout the world in dealing with all aspects of infertility due to the cervical or the male factor.

VARICOSITIES OF HYPOPLASTIC ENDOCERVICAL CANAL. In some patients any attempt to collect cervical mucus leads to immediate bleeding. These patients have poorly developed columnar epithelium with prominent superficial varicosities. They are best treated with the intrauterine insemination technique. Care must be taken not to do the insemination if the patient has infectious cervicitis.

Abnormal Cervical Mucus

Some 50 to 60 per cent of patients with cervical factor problems have an abnormality of cervical mucus. In approximately 40 per cent of the patients (excluding the anatomical defects) there is an abnormal postcoital test with normal cervical mucus. Of the patients with abnormal cervical mucus, 45 per cent have poor quality and 55 per cent have inadequate quantity of mucus. Both types of patients can be treated with daily doses of 0.1 mg of diethylstilbestrol (DES) given on days 5 through 15 of a 28-day menstrual cycle. If the patient shows no improvement, the DES dose should be increased to 0.2 mg. If no improvement is noted after the increased dose of DES, intrauterine insemination should be utilized. In fact, most infertility specialists are now treating patients with abnormal cervical mucus with the latter technique rather than DES therapy.

Abnormal Postcoital Test with Normal Cervical Mucus

FAULTY COITAL TECHNIQUE. In some infertile patients no spermatozoa can be seen in the cervical mucus or in the vagina after intercourse. Microscopic examination of samples taken from the labia may reveal spermatozoa. In such patients where penetration or intravaginal ejaculation failed to take place, careful review of coital technique is all that is necessary to make a diagnosis and institute proper therapy.

"VAGINAL FACTOR." If no sperm or only immobilized sperm are seen in the cervical mucus and the male has a normal semen analysis, intrauterine washed sperm insemination can be used to bypass the so-called vaginal factor. If intrauterine insemination is not available, a cervical cup insemination followed in one hour by a PCT should be performed. The procedure is performed by placing a specially designed cup on the cervix. Semen is then introduced through the stem and allowed to be exposed to the cervix for one hour. The cup is removed, the portio vaginalis cleansed, and an in vivo PCT performed. If motile sperm are seen at the internal os level, the procedure can be instituted as therapy in the ensuing cycles. Pregnancy has occurred in approximately one third of such cases. The exact cause of the "vaginal factor" has not yet been established.

OLIGOSPERMIA. If the abnormal PCT is secondary to oligospermia (counts of less than 20 million per milliliter), the same cervical cup therapy as outlined above should be attempted. If an improvement is noted on the postcup PCT, the cup insemination should be used for therapy. Using this technique, in selected cases of oligospermia, a pregnancy rate of 30 per cent has been achieved in this clinic. Currently at our institution all such patients are treated with intrauterine insemination, with pregnancy rates of 30 to 40 per cent.

LACK OF SPERM PENETRATION OWING TO LOW VOLUME OF SEMEN OR OLIGOSPERMIA OWING TO HYPERVOLUME. The lack of sperm penetration into the cervical canal may be due to an abnormally low (less than 2 ml) or an abnormally high volume of semen (more than 8 ml). If the semen specimens are found to be consistently less than 2 ml or more than 8 ml, a cervical cup insemination or intrauterine washed sperm insemination should be tried as therapy.

IMMOBILIZATION OF SPERM IN THE ENDOCERVICAL CANAL. Not infrequently the PCT is abnormal owing to sperm immobilization. In such cases immunological tests should be obtained (see "Other Factors"), although most of these patients have a low correlation between a positive immunological test and immobilization in the cervical canal. Mycoplasma or other infections in both the man and woman may play a role in this finding. Both the immunological factor and mycoplasma infections are discussed below. If the immunological tests and bacterial cultures are both negative, a cup insemination or intrauterine insemination should be attempted. A technique whereby motile sperm are allowed to "swim-up" and thus separate from immobilized sperm is now being evaluated, but the preliminary results have not been very encouraging.

PELVIC FACTOR

Along with the male factor, pelvic abnormalities (tubal occlusion, adhesions, and endometriosis) account for the majority of cases of infertility. In most clinics 30 to 40 per cent of infertility can be attributed to the pelvic factor. With indigent populations, tubal disease is much more prevalent than endometriosis. Although the diagnosis of tubal or pelvic disease is relatively straightforward, the various therapeutic modalities do not yield especially satisfying results.

Tubal Disease

The diagnostic techniques for evaluating tubal function and the pelvis in general have become more sophisticated. However, they still indicate only patency, obstruction, or distortion and fail to indicate the degree of physiological impairment that exists; the capability for reproductive function remains unmeasured.

Hysterosalpingography (HSG)

A radiologic study of the fallopian tubes involves transuterine dye instillation under radiographic visualization. The study is performed in the follicular phase of the cycle before ovulation. Exactness and care are essential. If a ra-

diologist is going to perform the HSG, the gynecologist should be in attendance or, at the very least, review the radiographs. Preferably the dye instillation should be set up and administered by the gynecologist. Image intensification fluoroscopy adds to the interpretation of the final radiographs and should be part of the procedure. However, it must be carried out by a radiologist skilled in the technique. If one minute of fluoroscopy is used during HSG, the patient receives a radiation dose equal to one conventional film. The predominant contrast media used today are water-soluble. Siegler outlines the HSG complications in detail.[16] In patients with a history of pelvic inflammatory disease (PID), the HSG should be deferred until the white blood cell count and erythrocyte sedimentation rate have returned to normal. Antibiotic coverage before and after HSG provides additional protection. A flare-up of PID after HSG is a poor prognostic sign regarding the success of any subsequent reparative surgery. If even attempted, the latter should be deferred at least three months.

HSG is extremely valuable in the work-up of the infertile patient. In a population prone to PID, an HSG should be obtained relatively early in the infertility investigation. The discovery of extensive tubal disease may alter and certainly speed up the other infertility studies. Multifactor infertility does not have a good prognosis, and an abnormal HSG hastens laparoscopy and possibly brings the investigation to an early end. In some conditions, the HSG can be the definitive study, and, as noted by Klein and colleagues, the HSG in tuberculosis is diagnostic.[17]

To the infertility surgeon the HSG must be illuminated in the operating room at the time of surgery. Although, in some series, discrepancies between HSG and definitive laparoscopy occur as often as 25 per cent of the time, it is still a valuable study.[18] A radiographic technique does have technical problems that endoscopy can overcome. For example, a unilateral tubal block visualized on HSG occasionally can be overcome at laparoscopy by occluding the patent tube at the uterine cornu with a probe while continuing to instill the dye transcervically. If several months have elapsed between the HSG and surgery, advancing disease or a reaction to the HSG may explain tubal occlusion found at laparoscopy and not present on an earlier HSG. On occasion, mechanical problems with laparoscopic chromopertubation can occur, and the illuminated HSG can be quite comforting. In summary, if the HSG is obtained as the "final" evaluation in the infertility work-up or only for its "therapeutic" benefit, then its continuing value must be questioned. However, as an adjuvant study to those of the laparoscopist and the infertility surgeon, the HSG can be of significant benefit.

Laparoscopy

Laparoscopy has added a significant tool to the gynecologist's diagnostic and therapeutic armamentarium.[19] The panoramic view of the pelvis provided by the laparoscope is unsurpassed. In addition to its usefulness in pelvic pain syndromes and tubal sterilization, the laparoscope has become an integral part of the infertility investigation.

The ovulatory infertile patient with a normal PCT and semen analysis undergoes HSG. If the latter is abnormal, laparoscopy should follow in the next cycle. However, if the HSG is entirely normal, three months should elapse before laparoscopy is undertaken. Although the therapeutic value of HSG is debatable, reports by Horbach and co-workers[20] and Kletzky and Halbracht[21] indicate that a patient should be given some time to conceive after tubal flushing. If an abnormal parameter is found during the infertility work-up (for example, a poor PCT), that abnormality should be treated. However, an HSG should be obtained so that the pelvic status is somewhat illuminated before extensive time and therapy are devoted to correcting a cervical problem.

The anovulatory infertile patient should be evaluated and therapeutically ovulated before an extensive infertility work-up is undertaken. Although a PCT should be deferred until ovulatory cycles have been achieved, an early semen analysis and HSG rule out or rule in other significant pathology. If more than one factor exists to account for the infertility, pregnancy becomes even more difficult, and the entire situation should be reviewed. On the other hand, if all studies have been normal and clomiphene-induced ovulatory cycles have been achieved for at least six months, laparoscopy should be undertaken to eliminate the possibility of unsuspected pelvic pathology. Even in the asymptomatic patient with unexplained infertility, the laparoscope can reveal significant disease.

In addition to its value in diagnosing unsuspected pelvic pathology, laparoscopy is an essential primary step when conservative infertility surgery is contemplated. The laparoscope can reveal a normal pelvis, thus eliminating the need for further surgery. With the laparoscope the infertility surgeon can begin to define and categorize the degree of pelvic disease and distortion. In some instances surgery can be deferred and the medical work-up and/or therapy continued on a more solid basis with the accurate laparoscopic view of the pelvis. In other cases laparoscopy can reveal such extensive pelvic destruction that a laparotomy is avoided and the patient can be advised to abandon further infertility studies and consider in vitro fertilization (see Ch. 116) and/or adoption. In view of its importance in determining the degree of pelvic pathology and the necessity for conservative infertility surgery, laparoscopy in the infertile patient should be carried out only by a gynecological surgeon who is prepared to make endoscopic judgments and perform the required surgery.

As with any study of tubal function, laparoscopy should be performed in the follicular phase of the menstrual cycle. A thorough examination of the pelvis must be carried out, using the accessory probe to lift, move, and feel all areas of the pelvis. Because the manipulations are extensive and adhesive disease is often encountered, a double-puncture technique under general endotracheal anesthesia is preferred. Prior pelvic surgery is usually not a deterrent to an adequate laparoscopic examination. During laparoscopy, chromopertubation (transuterine tubal dye instillation) is carried out with a dilute indigo carmine solution.

The decision to proceed with conservative infertility surgery is made at the time of laparoscopy and, in many instances of minimal or moderate adhesive disease, laparoscopy alone can be used to carry out reconstructive pelvic surgery. Therefore, before laparoscopy, all possible pelvic findings and surgical risks are explained to the patient and her partner. If pelvic pathology is confirmed or unsuspected pathology is found, the patient is prepared to undergo definitive tubal or pelvic surgery by laparoscopy or by immediate laparotomy using the same anesthetic. In skilled hands, the laparoscope has become a primary surgical tool in infertility. If pelvic/tubal pathology is extensive, only a laparotomy may provide the needed space and exposure to properly perform the job. According to Israel and March,[18] the presence or absence of additional infertility factors plays a prognostic role when combined with the laparoscopic findings. When laparoscopy reveals a normal pelvis, the presence of an infertility factor that has responded to treatment is an encouraging sign. Continuing to treat the problem in the light of a normal pelvis results in a number of pregnancies. On the other hand, the patient who has minimal or unilateral disease at laparoscopy has a more favorable outlook for pregnancy if the pelvic pathology is not compounded by an additional infertility factor. In view of the generally poor results achieved with conservative tubal surgery, the laparoscope must be used critically in order to select the best candidates for reparative operations.

Surgical Correction

After the laparoscopic decision to perform conservative surgery, the surgeon and the patient are faced with end results that leave much to be desired. In most instances subsequent pregnancy rates do not exceed 50 per cent and include abortions and ectopic pregnancies as well as term gestations. With tubal closure, surgery can achieve patency in the majority of cases. However, a postoperative patent tube is not a guarantee of pregnancy. Prior involvement of the endosalpinx or its distortion by the surgery itself may disturb the reproductive physiology of the fallopian tube to such an extent that pregnancy never occurs.

Four basic operative procedures are used in conservative tubal surgery: (1) lysis of peritubal adhesions (salpingolysis), (2) opening of the occluded distal tube (salpingostomy), (3) correction of midsegment occlusions (end-to-end anastomosis), and (4) repair of interstitial occlusions.

SALPINGOLYSIS. The most successful type of tubal surgery involves the lysis of peritubal and/or pelvic adhesions and does not involve primary tubal surgery. In most instances, this form of surgery can be carried out laparoscopically. Ovum pick-up is impeded by adhesions that isolate the tubes and ovaries. The tubes may spill dye into isolated pockets of adhesions, but the fimbriated ends are open and the endosalpinx is intact. Ultimate success depends on the extent and type of adhesions encountered and whether they re-form postoperatively. In reported series the overall pregnancy rate varies from 40 to 70 per cent, with 70 to 90 per cent of the pregnancies going to term.

SALPINGOSTOMY. Opening distal tubal occlusions is the least successful type of tubal surgery. A hydrosalpinx is the end stage of generalized tubal disease. Although the surgeon may be able to open the tube and have it remain open, anatomical and physiological damage to the remainder of the tube only rarely supports the numerous normal reproductive processes necessary to achieve an intrauterine pregnancy. The fimbria are often gone, the endosalpinx is partially or totally denuded, the tubal musculature is nonfunctional, and various degrees of tubal dilation may be present. In addition, distal tubal closure is usually associated with pelvic adhesions varying from minimal and filmy to extensive and thick.

To compound the salpingostomy problem, some surgeons include lesser degrees of fimbrial pathology in this surgical category. Fimbrial "agglutination" and "phimosis" are two of the favorites. Teasing apart filmy strands between the fimbria or "dilating" the fimbriated end of the tube with small bougies does not represent salpingostomy surgery. If these two methods can be considered "indicated" forms of conservative infertility surgery, they should be classified in a subcategory under salpingolysis.

Cuff salpingostomy by laparoscopy or laparotomy yields overall pregnancy rates of 10 to 40 per cent. As noted, the ultimate result depends on the condition of the remainder of the tube rather than on the operative method used. If tubal patency were the only consideration, the operation would be a success. The percentage of patent tubes after salpingostomy varies between 60 and 90 per cent. The surgeon can open the pipeline in most instances, but proper function cannot be restored. The increased incidence of ectopic pregnancies in post-salpingostomy tubes reinforces the concept that tubal closure is not the only problem in such cases.[18]

END-TO-END ANASTOMOSIS. If there is a place for magnification in any area of tubal reparative surgery, end-to-end anastomosis would seem to be the logical choice. Using improved binocular telescopic eye pieces or the operating microscope, the most successful primary tubal surgery is correction of tubal occlusion secondary to previous tubal sterilization. The remainder of the tube, proximally and distally, is normal and the pelvis is free of adhesions. However, as tubal sterilization often destroys a significant amount of tissue, especially with prior laparoscopic fulguration, reapproximation of all remaining viable tissue is extremely important and often difficult without the aid of magnification. As has been stressed with any form of conservative surgery, prelaparotomy laparoscopy should be used to confirm the normal status of the pelvis and to decide that adequate tubal segments exist for anastomosis. Ideally, for end-to-end reconstruction, the prior tubal sterilization should have been a small segmental resection in the midisthmic portion of the tube. If an intact ampullary-isthmic junction is present, and the anastomosis can be performed in the isthmus, the chance of success should be extremely high. In a young woman undergoing sterilization, segmental isthmic resection, banding, or clipping should be considered, so that if the future brings a change of mind, reanastomosis success could be a reality. The pregnancy rate after end-to-end anastomosis ranges from 60 to 80 per cent with high term pregnancy rates (70 to 90 per cent).

INTERSTITIAL OCCLUSION REPAIR. Proximal (interstitial) tubal occlusion is the least common form of tubal pathology. Clinically, the patient usually has a history of "uterine invasion" (that is, D and C, pregnancy with sepsis, or intrauterine device insertion). In many instances these events were not accompanied by any clinical evidence of pelvic sepsis, yet the end result is a bilateral interstitial block. As the interstitial portion of the tube is important in reproduction and impossible to duplicate surgically, it is fortunate that a nonsurgical corrective procedure has been developed which should be tried before the more complex surgical repairs of either implantation or anastomosis are attempted. Although instrumentation, technique, and acceptance are still undergoing revision and debate, transcervical cannulation of the proximal tube can be done by

fluoroscopy or hysteroscopy. Cannulation not only confirms or refutes whether interstitial obstruction exists, but, if it is present, a coaxial wire or balloon can be used to eliminate the occlusion. Obviously, if the tube(s) is distally obstructed as well, correcting the proximal block is worthless and should not be attempted. Tubes with both proximal and distal blocks have too much abnormality for correction. These patients are candidates for assisted reproductive technologies such as in vitro fertilization.

Following successful transcervical tubal cannulation and elimination of the obstruction(s), preliminary results indicate that one third of the patients conceive, one third remain with tubal patency, and the other third reobstruct. If desired, the latter group could undergo proximal (interstitial) tubal surgical repair by implantation or anastomosis, with anticipated pregnancy rates ranging from 35 to 50 per cent, including term pregnancy rates of 60 to 80 per cent.

Endometriosis

In 1921 Sampson described endometriosis as "the presence of ectopic tissue which possesses the histological structure and function of the uterine mucosa."[22] Although the occurrence of aberrant endometrium had been described by various authors in the nineteenth century, it was not until the classic contribution of J. A. Sampson that there was any appreciation of the frequency, pathology, and clinical characteristics of this enigmatic gynecological disorder.

Histogenesis

As Ridley noted in 1968, there are at least 11 published theories regarding the histogenesis of endometriosis.[23] They can be divided into three broad categories: transportation, in situ development, and a combination of the two.

TRANSPORTATION. *Retrograde Menstruation (Sampson's Theory) by Means of the Fallopian Tubes.* Red blood cells, leukocytes, endometrial cells, and amorphous material can traverse the tubes in an antiperistaltic, anticilial manner. In a series of experiments in monkeys, TeLinde and Scott demonstrated that transported endometrial cells are viable and can implant.[24] Subsequently, Ridley and others confirmed the viability of human endometrial cells after tubal transport.

Mechanical. Direct dissemination of endometrial tissue occurs at surgery. For example, endometriosis subsequently develops at the incision site after cesarean section or hysterotomy.

Lymphatic and Venous Metastasis. The presence of endometrial tissue in distant, unusual sites must be attributed to venous or lymphatic transportation.

IN SITU DEVELOPMENT: COELOMIC METAPLASIA. This theory is based on the fact that certain cells under certain stimuli can change their character and physiological function. However, if this theory explains the origin of endometriosis, the condition should occur as frequently in the thoracic cavity as it does in the peritoneal cavity. Obviously this does not occur, although the coelomic membrane contributes to the thoracic lining as well as to the peritoneal lining. In addition, if coelomic metaplasia contributes to endometriosis, the condition should be found in men.

COMBINATION OF TRANSPORTATION AND IN SITU DEVEL-

OPMENT. Although this theory includes the ability of the endometrium to reproduce itself, it relies on direct extension or vascular system metastasis to explain endometrial movement. This theory is unacceptable to the coelomic metaplasia "purists."

Clinical Characteristics

Because endometriosis depends on ovarian steroids for its existence and proliferation, its occurrence and clinical importance are generally confined to the reproductive years. The peak incidence is in the fourth decade of life. The "typical" patient with endometriosis is a nulliparous patient in her late 20s or early 30s.

Whether the emergence and widespread use of steroidal contraceptives over the past 30 years has reduced the incidence of endometriosis by reducing menstrual flow, thereby preventing tubal reflux, remains an unanswered question. However, if operative statistics from predominantly private practice hospitals are used, endometriosis continues to be a significant gynecological entity.

Thirty to 40 per cent of patients with endometriosis have concomitant infertility,[25] although in many instances the endometriosis does not appear to be interfering with normal reproductive processes. Sperm ascension, ovulation, and ovum pick-up and transport can all take place. A multifactorial concept for the cause of infertility in the presence of mild endometriosis has been postulated.[26] However, it may well be that persistent infertility is the reason that endometriosis develops and not the other way around.

The most frequent pelvic locations for endometriosis are the ovaries, uterine ligaments (round, broad, uterosacral), pelvic peritoneum, and rectovaginal septum. Other sites include the umbilicus, laparotomy scars, hernial sacs, appendix, small intestine, rectum, sigmoid colon, bladder, ureters, vulva-vagina-cervix, lymph nodes, extremities, pleural cavity, and lungs. The multiplicity and widespread distribution of these sites make acceptance of any one histogenetic theory difficult.

Pathology

Like everything else connected with endometriosis, the one characteristic of the gross pathology is its variability. Until Acosta and associates proposed a classification in 1973,[27] the extent of pelvic endometriosis was described by individual cases. With mild involvement, the adnexa are free of adhesions and a variable number of reddish blue (raspberry) or brown fibrin-like implants are present on the ovaries and/or peritoneal surfaces. With progressive disease the older implants coalesce and "burn out," leaving scarred, retracted areas that may involve peritoneal surfaces only or include peritubal and periovarian involvement and fixation. Not all endometriotic areas are pigmented. Whitish plaques, cribriform spaces, and other areas of noncolor, when biopsied, may turn out to be endometriosis.[28] More significant ovarian involvement means the formation of single or multiple, unilateral or bilateral endometrial cysts (endometriomas, "chocolate" cysts). As the endometrium grows into the ovary during formation of these cysts, menstrual reaction occurs and the cysts become hemorrhagic. With deeper penetration, the cyst content darkens, resembling thick chocolate syrup. Even when quite small the cysts show a strong tendency to perforate, with escape of menstrual blood and subsequent ovarian adherence to any adjacent structure, usually the posterior surface of the broad ligament or uterus. If early perforation does not occur, larger endometriomas form with thicker walls and few surrounding adhesions. When the uterine ligaments are involved, especially the uterosacrals, endometriotic nodules form that can often be palpated on bimanual or rectovaginal examination. Endometrial islands may occur on any part of the pelvic peritoneum, involving the serosal surface of any pelvic structure. Occasionally invasion and penetration occur in the sigmoid colon so that progressive submucosal scarring results in luminal constriction. Mucosal involvement with associated rectal bleeding is a late phenomenon in bowel endometriosis.

Definitive diagnosis requires microscopic demonstration of endometrial tissue, preferably both glands and stroma. However, a wide range of histological appearances may occur. Some specimens reveal endometrium that histologically and functionally cannot be distinguished from normal uterine epithelium. In others the endometrium has been completely denuded owing to repeated menstrual bleeding and desquamation. Hemorrhage and pigment-laden macrophages may be the only microscopic clues. According to the Gynecologic Pathology Laboratory at The Johns Hopkins Hospital, no specific pathological diagnosis can be made definitely in one third of clinically typical endometriosis cases.[29]

Diagnosis

The symptomatology associated with endometriosis is also extremely variable. Dysmenorrhea, dyspareunia, and dyschezia may be present as a symptom complex or individually. However, even with extensive endometriosis, pain may not be a significant clinical entity. Unless rupture occurs, ovarian endometriomas can painlessly expand. On the other hand, incapacitating dysmenorrhea and pelvic pain may be associated with minimal amounts of active peritoneal surface endometriosis.[30] Thus, the degree of endometriotic involvement and spread bears no constant relationship to the presence or absence of subjective discomfort. More than 50 per cent of patients complain of dysmenorrhea. Usually it is the secondary or acquired variety, although, on occasion, primary dysmenorrhea worsens. The dysmenorrhea can be attributed to secretory changes in the endometriotic islands, with subsequent miniature menstruation and bleeding in areas encapsulated by fibrous tissue. With involvement of the rectovaginal septum or uterosacral ligaments, the dysmenorrhea is often referred to the rectum or the lower sacrococcygeal area, and dyspareunia is a common complaint. Dyschezia results from endometriotic bleeding in the rectosigmoid muscularis or serosa with subsequent fibrosis. Abnormal uterine bleeding (such as premenstrual spotting) may occur. Anovulation is not uncommon.

Although the diagnosis may be suggested by the history, it cannot be made with any certainty on symptoms alone. Even a pelvic examination, which, at times, can be quite distinctive, cannot be considered pathognomonic. Tender, nodular uterosacral ligaments combined with a fixed, retroverted uterus are findings highly suggestive of endometriosis, but inflammation and cancer cannot be ruled out by a bimanual examination. For definitive diagnosis, laparoscopic visualization of the pelvis must be carried out and the extent of the endometriosis staged according to the classification (minimal, mild, moderate, severe) established by the American Fertility Society.[31] When lesions are identified and the examiner still remains in doubt, confirmatory endoscopic biopsy should be performed. Double-puncture laparoscopy should be used so that a careful, complete pelvic inspection can be carried out. In addition, one of several available instruments for uterine manipulation must be placed in the cervical canal. It should have a central cannula for transuterine tubal dye instillation. The palpating probe, placed through the accessory trocar, should be used as an examining finger running over various structures (for example, the uterosacral ligaments) to detect subperitoneal implants. Each ovary must be lifted up to visualize the undersurface adjoining the broad ligament. The serosa of any bowel in the pelvis should be carefully inspected for any endometriotic implants, as should the appendix.

Therapy

Although controversy continues in the areas of histogenesis, symptomatology, and detection, more uniformity of thinking exists with regard to the therapy of endometriosis in the infertile patient. Hormonal suppression and/or conservative surgery constitute the available therapeutic modalities. Diagnosis and stage (minimal, mild, moderate, severe) are established by laparoscopy and become the basis for selection of subsequent therapy.

MINIMAL/MILD/MODERATE ENDOMETRIOSIS. Satisfactory pregnancy rates (40 to 75 per cent) have been reported with laparoscopic observation only, laparoscopic laser or electrocoagulation only, or medical therapy alone. When laparoscopy diagnoses endometriosis, minimal, mild, and many degrees of moderate endometriosis should be treated at the same time with either laparoscopic electrocoagulation or laser therapy.[32] Even if therapy does not improve fertility, it does serve to suppress the lesions of a progressive gynecological entity. Postoperative medical therapy only suppresses ovulation, thus further postponing any conception attempt, and it does not increase future fertility chances. As both danazol and continuous oral contraceptive therapy have been shown to have post-use pregnancy rates of 20 to 50 per cent, neither form of medical therapy should be used in the treatment of infertility. Even with moderate endometriosis consisting of small endometriosis and accessible adhesions, the diagnosing laparoscope can be used as a therapeutic agent without preoperative or postoperative hormonal suppression. Because complication rates rise with "endoscopic gymnastics," extensive laparoscopic surgical manipulations are contraindicated for all but the most experienced endoscopists.

With the laparoscope, the uterus and adnexa must be mobilized and carefully inspected. This may require triple, or even quadruple, puncture sites. The serosa of the large and small bowel either in or contiguous to the pelvis, including the appendix, must be visualized for any endometriotic involvement. All endometriotic areas should be electrocoagulated, vaporized, or excised.

The ovaries must be carefully palpated and cystic areas punctured or incised so that small endometriomas are not missed. Ovarian endometriomas should be excised or drained and the lining completely destroyed. Although a major portion of one or both ovaries may have to be sacrificed, pregnancy can still occur after unilateral oophorectomy and resection of three quarters of the contralateral ovary.

If secondary dysmenorrhea is part of the symptomatology, presacral neurectomy and resection of the uterosacral ligaments at their uterine insertion are indicated. If the uterus is not anterior and/or the cul-de-sac is scarred, a uterine suspension should be performed. Although these procedures can be performed by the highly skilled endoscopist, laparotomy is the standard approach.

Prophylactic antibiotic treatment started preoperatively and Interceed (Johnson & Johnson, New Brunswick, NJ), a biodegradable barrier left in the pelvis at the conclusion of surgery, may be of benefit.

SEVERE ENDOMETRIOSIS. With extensive pathology attributable to endometriosis, the postsurgical pregnancy outlook is 25 to 30 per cent at best. In addition to massive pelvic adhesions, the fallopian tubes can be involved to the point of closure. Reconstructive or ablative surgery for severe degrees of endometriosis can be the most difficult gynecological surgery encountered, even more difficult than end-stage salpingitis or oncology operations.

In the presence of extensive and/or deep-seated rectovaginal septum endometriosis, preoperative therapy with a GnRH agonist for two to three months may enhance the surgery by reducing and/or softening the active areas of endometriosis. Whether this therapy improves the pregnancy rate remains to be proved. In any case, after conservative surgery, endometriosis recurs in 5 to 25 per cent of patients.

OTHER FACTORS

In approximately 2 to 15 per cent of couples no abnormalities can be found after establishing the fact that ovulation is occurring, obtaining a semen analysis, performing a PCT, and investigating the upper female genital tract with an HSG and laparoscopy. Because a large percentage of couples do end up in this category of "unexplained" infertility, the following additional factors may be considered in an effort to reduce the percentage of unexplained infertility: (1) infertility secondary to immunological factors, (2) genital mycoplasma as a cause of infertility, (3) inadequate luteal phase, and (4) TSH as a test for primary hypothyroidism.

Infertility Secondary to Immunological Factors

Immunological incompatibility may be the cause of infertility in some couples. The exact incidence of this phenomenon is not known. The fact that antibodies can be induced in laboratory animals by injecting semen has been known for more than 75 years.[33–35] In the human, two different immune systems have been implicated as the possible cause of infertility: (1) autoimmunity in men and (2) the presence of circulating sperm-agglutinating and -immobilizing antibodies in women.

AUTOIMMUNITY IN MEN. The first report of autoimmunity in men as a cause of infertility was reported by Wilson.[36, 37] In 1959 Rumke and Hellinga reported this finding in 3 per cent of 2000 infertile couples.[38] The titer that appeared to be significant was stated to be 1:32. Some of these men also showed spontaneous agglutination of spermatozoa in their own seminal plasma. A significant number of these men had a history of genital tract infection, surgery, or trauma.

In 1968, Fjallbrant and Obrant not only demonstrated the presence of autoantibodies in 400 infertile men but also related this finding to the decreased ability of sperm from these men to penetrate normal cervical mucus.[39] A correlation between autoimmunity and infertility is present in a certain percentage of infertile couples, although it should be noted that the presence of sperm-agglutinating antibodies does not always interfere with fertility. No successful therapy has yet been found, although some investigators have recommended high doses of cortisone therapy.[40] Artificial insemination using donor semen may be the only treatment.

SPERM-AGGLUTINATING AND -IMMOBILIZING ANTIBODIES IN WOMEN. Agglutination of the man's sperm by the woman's serum has been reported to be a possible factor in infertility. Franklin and Dukes[41] in 1964 first published their observations on the relationship of circulating sperm agglutinins to infertility of unknown cause and reported an incidence of 72 per cent, compared with the control group, who had a 5.7 per cent incidence of sperm agglutinins. Sexual abstinence or the use of condoms for two to six months has been recommended in order to lower the antibody titer. In the first report this therapy was found to be extremely successful. However, by 1968 the same authors reported that the incidence of sperm-agglutinating antibody in infertile women was only 48 per cent, with a control group showing an incidence of 13 per cent. Again, some 57 per cent of their patients became pregnant after using the recommended condom therapy. Of the 20 couples who refused condom therapy, only 2 (10 per cent) became pregnant. Other authors have not found the incidence of sperm-agglutinating antibodies in infertile women to be as high as in the original report by Franklin and Dukes. Schwimmer and colleagues[42, 43] reported a 33.5 per cent incidence of sperm-agglutinating antibodies in women with primary unexplained infertility. Glass and Vaidya[44] reported a 20 per cent incidence of sperm agglutination in a group of 122 women with unexplained infertility. None of their 24 patients had become pregnant after condom therapy.

Currently, therefore, the only statement that can be made concerning sperm-agglutination antibodies in the serum of women as a cause of infertility is that the phenomenon appears to exist in a small percentage of infertile couples and that if it is a cause of infertility, it is probably titer dependent.

Another test for identifying the existence of sperm-agglutinating antibodies in the female serum is the Kibrick test.[45] The incidence of positive tests using this technique has varied between 5 and 20 per cent.

Isojima and colleagues[46] reported a complement-dependent serum-sperm immobilization technique. Their incidence of positive tests has varied between 12 and 19 per cent, with a 0 per cent incidence in controls.

The incidence of positive tests in our medical center for the agglutination test using both the Franklin-Dukes test and the Kibrick test is approximately 5 per cent. Only 12 per cent of these patients have become pregnant using condom therapy, compared with an 8 per cent pregnancy rate in patients who either refused therapy or voluntarily discontinued it. The incidence of positive Isojima tests has been 3 per cent, and no pregnancy has been achieved using condom therapy. More recently an immunobead technique has been developed to identify specific sperm surface antigens. Proponents of this technique claim that this is a more precise and accurate test. However, at present controlled studies comparing this test with older methods are not available.

Until the role of immune reactions as a cause of infertility is totally disproved for a couple, the immunobead test should be performed if all other tests previously outlined prove to be negative. If an immunological test is positive at 1:4 titer, condom therapy can be recommended for three months or the couple put through intrauterine inseminations.

Genital Mycoplasma and Its Role in Infertility

The isolation of the mycoplasma has been reported to be a possible factor in patients with undiagnosed infertility, and the T mycoplasma appears to be the significant organism.[47–50] Both the cervical mucus and the semen should be cultured for this organism.[51] The treatment recommended has been doxycycline, 200 mg the first day, starting on the seventh day of the cycle, followed by 100 mg/d for 9 days. Both partners should be treated for two to three cycles.[52, 53] If the cultures remain positive, the dose should be doubled and treatment continued for another two months. A pregnancy rate after antibiotic therapy of 42 per cent after three months and 84 per cent after one year has been reported.[53] Both published[54] and unpublished studies have shown little or no relationship between the incidence of T mycoplasma infection and infertility. However, until further results are published, T mycoplasma cultures should be obtained in couples with infertility, and if the cultures are positive, treatment should be instituted.

The Inadequate Luteal Phase

The inadequate luteal phase is a histological diagnosis made in a small number of infertile women in whom the endometrial biopsy shows a lag of two or more days in two menstrual cycles.[55] The inappropriate maturation of the endometrium may be due to inadequate production of progesterone from the corpus luteum (see Ch. 116). It is assumed that with poorly developed endometrium implantation of the fertilized ovum is unsuccessful.

It is important to differentiate between the inadequate luteal phase and the short luteal phase. In the short luteal phase the interval between the luteinizing hormone peak and the onset of menses is less than 10 days.[56] The inadequate luteal phase must be documented in two cycles. Normal infertile women may, on occasion, have out-of-phase endometrial biopsies. A BBT chart cannot be used in making this diagnosis. The daily progesterone values obtained in the luteal phase of these women appear to be somewhat lower than those of normal women; however, the differences in the absolute values are debatable.[55]

The therapy for this condition has been 25 mg of progesterone as a vaginal suppository inserted twice daily in the luteal phase, or a daily dose of 12.5 mg of progesterone-in-oil intramuscularly starting with the rise of BBT until the onset of menses.[55] If the patient becomes pregnant, it has been recommended that the therapy at a higher dosage be continued until the second trimester. The use of hCG (2500 to 5000 IU given intramuscularly every other day during the luteal phase) has also been suggested. In addition, as it has been postulated that the inadequate luteal phase may be secondary to a "poor" follicular development in these ovulatory patients, clomiphene citrate therapy has been suggested in order to develop a "better" follicle and thus a "better" corpus luteum. All three modes of therapy may be beneficial, and currently no single method of treatment has definitely proved to be the best.

Thyroid-Stimulating Hormone as Test for Hypothyroidism

In a rare instance the only finding after instituting an extensive infertility work-up is an abnormal serum TSH value, indicating a "subclinical" hypothyroid state. The incidence at our medical center appears to be between 1:500 and 1:1000. In some of these patients the serum T_4 levels have been in the normal range. If the infertile patient has an elevated serum TSH level, we recommend instituting throxine therapy.

THE NEW TECHNOLOGY: ASSISTED REPRODUCTIVE TECHNOLOGY

It is beyond the scope of this chapter to discuss in any great detail the assisted reproductive techniques being offered to patients with various infertility problems. The in vitro fertilization (IVF) technique, which was first successful in producing a viable human pregnancy in 1978, was at first performed only in patients with nonfunctioning fallopian tubes. IVF is now being offered to most infertile couples who do not achieve a pregnancy through other less involved treatment methods. The essential steps in an IVF cycle include (1) hyperstimulation of the ovaries, (2) retrieval (follicle aspiration) of ova, (3) sperm preparation, (4) in vitro fertilization and embryo culture, and (5) embryo transfer into the uterine cavity.

Hyperstimulation of the Ovaries

The increased rate of successful pregnancies is associated with multiple embryo transfer into the uterine cavity. In order to achieve this, most centers use human menopausal gonadotropin (hMG) or follicle-stimulating hormone (FSH). Combination clomiphene citrate (cc) and hMG is the third most commonly used regimen. All these treatment methods result in increased follicle recruitment. In order to better control the follicular hyperstimulation, in 1988 most IVF programs began using pituitary "downregulation" by gonadotropin-releasing hormone-agonist (GnRH-a) prior to starting the hyperstimulation protocols. This method is more costly but has resulted in increased numbers of oocytes becoming available for aspiration. When the cost factor makes the use of these drugs impossible, unstimulated cycles for IVF have been advocated. All methods use transvaginal ultrasonography to follow follicular size and serum estradiol (E_2) measurements in order to follow the cycle and determine when ovulation should be induced with the administration of 2500 to 10,000 IU of human chorionic gonadotropin (hCG) given intramuscularly.

Egg Retrieval (Follicle Aspiration)

The oocytes are recovered 34 to 36 hours after the intramuscular administration of hCG. Both laparoscopic aspiration and ultrasonography-directed transvaginal aspirations are being used for egg retrieval. The latter procedures can be performed in an operating suite or in a room in the clinic specifically designed for the procedure. Light inhalation anesthesia, intravenous sedation, or both are used to make the procedure tolerable. Oral prophylactic antibiotics are used commonly to minimize the risk of pelvic infection. Under direct ultrasonographic visualization, the needle is inserted into the ovary and each follicle greater than 14 mm is aspirated into a separate sterile tube by means of gentle suction. The test tubes with culture media are placed in a controlled environment chamber at 37°C. Using a dissecting microscope, the oocytes are identified and placed in culture medium. Complication rates are very low, and successful ovum retrieval rates are extremely high. At the present time most centers are using the transvaginal approach to ovum retrieval rather than the laparoscopic approach unless there is added clinical reason to evaluate the pelvic organs.

Sperm Preparation

The spermatozoa are separated from the seminal plasma by various techniques. One of the simplest methods is mixing the semen with Ham's F-10 solution and placing the mixture in a centrifuge at 300 g for 5 to 10 minutes. The supernatant is then discarded and the pellet again mixed with Ham's F-10 and centrifuged for 3 to 10 minutes at 300 g. The pellet is then incubated in the same solution and in some cases the patient's own serum is added to the mixture. The incubation takes place at 37°C and the sperm contained within the pellet "swim up" out of the pellet into the solution. The sperm concentration is then measured and a predetermined number of sperm are prepared for introduction into the fertilization dishes containing one ovum each.

Another commonly used method of separating the sperm from the seminal plasma is the Percoll-column method. This technique uses a density gradient principle to select out the motile sperm from immobilized and defective sperm, white cells, and other seminal debris. The Percoll solution is an inert biological preparation made up into various concentration, layered on top of each other.

The semen is placed on top of the column and the entire preparation centrifuged for 20 minutes at 300 g. The 80 per cent fraction is used for recovery of the "normal" sperm. The pellet is resuspended in culture medium and used to fertilize the retrieved ova.

In Vitro Fertilization

The harvested oocytes are placed in modified Ham's F-10 physiological solution or commercially available human tubal fluid (HTF)–like solution. The medium is almost always supplemented with the patient's serum or serum albumin. The concentration of sperm used in each culture dish varies from program to program; as few as 2500 spermatozoa have been used successfully during a gamete intrafallopian transfer (GIFT) cycle. The most common concentration of sperm used in IVF centers varies between 50,000 and 500,000 motile sperm per milliliter of culture medium. The maintenance of physiological temperature and pH is extremely important. The culture dishes are incubated at 37°C in an atmosphere containing 5 per cent carbon dioxide and with a pH of 7.4. The spermatozoa are usually added to the ova six hours after the eggs have been aspirated. The eggs are examined at regular intervals, usually 16 to 20 hours after insemination, for the presence of pronuclei, the indicator that fertilization has taken place. The fertilized eggs are then transferred to fresh medium supplemented with maternal serum and cultured for an additional 24 hours.

Embryo Transfer

The developing embryos are transferred at any stage of development from two pronuclei to blastocyst stage. Most transfers occur after about 48 hours following oocyte aspiration. Most embryos have undergone at least one mitotic division and are at least at the two-cell stage. The endometrial cavity is sounded and the length documented accurately prior to the transfer cycle in order to avoid unnecessary trauma. Antibiotic prophylaxis is given prior to transfer. Mild sedation is used prior to placement of the embryos into the endometrial cavity via a special semi-rigid catheter. The catheter is examined microscopically after placement to make sure that a successful transfer was accomplished. The patient is kept in Trendelenburg position for three hours.

Hormonal Support of the Luteal Phase after Embryo Transfer

Most failures of IVF occur after embryo transfer, and much of the research being performed at the present time is directed toward possible correction of this problem. The altered endometrial receptivity seems to be the major hindrance to successful embryo implantation. When embryos are transferred to unstimulated endometrium, the results for implantation are markedly improved. The luteal inadequacy may be the result of ovarian hyperstimulation prior to follicle aspiration or possibly due to mechanical trauma to the follicles and removal of granulosa cells with resulting

decrease in progesterone secretion. Empirical progesterone therapy during the luteal phase is now commonly practiced. The serum β-hCG levels are measured, usually on days 11 and 16 following follicle aspiration. The progesterone therapy is usually discontinued after ultrasound confirmation of presence of a fetal heart beat. According to a report published by the Society for Assisted Reproductive Technology (SART), clinical pregnancy rates of 16 per cent per retrieval and 19 per cent per embryo transfer were achieved nationally. Although multiple embryos are transferred during most IVF cycles, multiple gestations occur in only 20 to 25 per cent of deliveries. Extrauterine pregnancy rates of 5 to 7 per cent have been reported, although the embryos are placed directly in the uterine cavity.

Because only three or four embryos are transferred into the uterine cavity per cycle, the extra embryos are stored by means of cryopreservation for use in subsequent cycles. The first successful human pregnancy after cryopreservation was reported in 1983. In 1988 the national registry reported 73 deliveries in the United States resulting from cryopreservation.

Gamete Intrafallopian Transfer (GIFT)

This procedure was first described in 1984 and is now used throughout the world. The procedure is identical to the IVF procedure in techniques of stimulating multiple follicle development by use of clomiphene-hMG-hCG in various combinations. After the ova are retrieved, the ova and prepared spermatozoa are placed into each fallopian tube by means of catheters placed through the abdominal wall as observed through a laparoscope. Usually two embryos and 100,000 sperm are placed in the ampullary portion of each fallopian tube. Live birth pregnancy rates of 25 to 30 per cent per attempt were reported in 1991.

Superovulation and Intrauterine Insemination (IUI)

This technique uses clomiphene both alone and in combination with hMG therapy to superovulate the patient. Based on ultrasound findings, intramuscular hCG is used to trigger ovulation. Thirty-six hours following the hCG injection, the semen is prepared by means of either Ham's F-10 wash or Percoll-column separation. The prepared spermatozoa are then placed into the uterine cavity. Pregnancy rates of 20 to 25 per cent per cycle have been reported by the use of this technique.

Other Techniques

Modification of IVF and GIFT procedures have been reported. A procedure using pronuclear-stage ova, fertilized by IVF procedure and placed into the ampullary portion of the fallopian tube analogous to the GIFT procedure, is known as the PROST technique. Transfer of a zygote obtained by IVF procedure into the fallopian tube via laparoscopy is known as the ZIFT procedure. Transfer of an embryo into the fallopian tube is known as the TET procedure. A newer technique of placing fertilized ova into the fallopian tube via a transcervical approach through the endometrial cavity into the tube appears to be promising. This latter technique has the advantage of avoiding the laparoscopic procedure.

Two new techniques under extensive investigation for use with abnormal semen are transcervical intratubal insemination and injection of sperm into the perivitelline space by microscopically cutting a slit in the zona pellucida. Microscopic injection of one sperm directly into the ovum has resulted in fertilization in animals but has not been successful in humans. The future of such micromanipulation techniques appears very promising, but clinical applications at the present time need further investigative work.

REFERENCES

1. Romeny S, Gray MJ, Little B, et al: The Health Care of Women in Gynecology and Obstetrics. New York, McGraw-Hill, 1975, p 345.
2. Speroff L, Glass RH, Kase NG: Clinical Gynecologic Endocrinology and Infertility. Baltimore, Williams & Wilkins, 1983, p 173.
3. Behrman SJ, Kistner RW: Progress in Infertility (ed 2). Boston, Little, Brown & Company, 1974, p 4.
4. Warner MP: Results of 25 year study of 1553 infertile couples. NY State J Med 62:2663, 1962.
5. Israel R, Mishell DR Jr, Stone SC, et al: Single luteal phase serum progesterone assay as an indicator of ovulation. Am J Obstet Gynecol 112:1043, 1972.
6. Marrs RP, Vargyas JM, March CM: Correlation of ultrasonic measurements in human menopausal gonadotropin therapy. Am J Obstet Gynecol 145:417, 1983.
7. Adams R, Mishell DR Jr, Israel R: Treatment of refractory anovulation with increased dosage and prolonged duration of cyclic clomiphene citrate. Obstet Gynecol 39:562, 1972.
8. Rust LA, Israel R, Mishell DR Jr: An individualized therapeutic regimen for clomiphene citrate. Am J Obstet Gynecol 129:785, 1974.
9. March CM, Israel R, Mishell DR Jr: Pregnancy following 29 cycles of clomiphene citrate therapy: A case report. Am J Obstet Gynecol 124:209, 1976.
10. Davajan V, Kunitake GM: Fractional in-vivo and in-vitro examination of post-coital cervical mucus in the human. Fertil Steril 20:197, 1967.
11. Davajan V, Nakamura RM, Kharma K: Spermatozoa transport in cervical mucus. Obstet Gynecol Surv 25:1, 1970.
12. Davajan V, Nakamura RM, Mishell DR Jr: A simplified technique for evaluation of the biophysical properties of cervical mucus. Am J Obstet Gynecol 109:1042, 1971.
13. Tredway DR, Settlage DSF, Nakamura RM, et al: The significance of timing for the post-coital evaluation of cervical mucus. Am J Obstet Gynecol 121:387, 1975.
14. Tredway DR: The interpretation and significance of the fractional post-coital test. Am J Obstet Gynecol 124:352, 1976.
15. Davajan V, Vargyas JM, Kletzky OA, et al: Intrauterine insemination with washed sperm to treat infertility. Abstracts of the American Fertility Society. Fertil Steril 40:419, 1983.
16. Siegler AM: Hysterosalpingography. Fertil Steril 40:139, 1983.
17. Klein TA, Richmond JA, Mishell DR Jr: Pelvic tuberculosis in an infertility clinic. Obstet Gynecol 48:99, 1976.
18. Israel R, March CM: Diagnostic laparoscopy: A prognostic aid in the surgical management of infertility. Am J Obstet Gynecol 124:969, 1976.
19. Cohen MR: Laparoscopy, Culdoscopy and Gynecology. Philadelphia, WB Saunders, 1970.
20. Horbach JGM, Maathuis JB, Van Hall EV: Factors influencing the pregnancy rate following hysterosalpingography and their prognostic significance. Fertil Steril 24:15, 1973.
21. Kletzky OH, Halbracht JG: Hydrotubation in the treatment of the tubal factor. Acta Eur Fertil 2:31, 1970.
22. Sampson JA: Perforating hemorrhagic (chocolate) cysts of the ovary. Arch Surg 3:245, 1921.
23. Ridley JH: The histogenesis of endometriosis. Obstet Gynecol Surv 23:1, 1968.
24. TeLinde RW, Scott RB: Experimental endometriosis. Am J Obstet Gynecol 60:1147, 1950.
25. Schenken RS: Endometriosis. Contemporary Concepts in Clinical Management. Philadelphia, JB Lippincott, 1989.
26. Muse KN, Wilson EA: How does mild endometriosis cause infertility? Fertil Steril 38:145, 1982.
27. Acosta AA, Buttram VC Jr, Besch PK, et al: A proposed classification of endometriosis. Obstet Gynecol 42:19, 1973.
28. Jansen RPS, Russell P: Nonpigmented endometriosis: Clinical, laparoscopic, and pathologic definition. Am J Obstet Gynecol 155:1154, 1986.
29. Spangler DB, Jones GS, Jones HW Jr: Infertility due to endometriosis. Conservative surgical therapy. Am J Obstet Gynecol 109:850, 1971.
30. Koninckx PR, Meuleman C, Demeyere S, et al: Suggestive evidence that pelvic endometriosis is a progressive disease, whereas deeply infiltrating endometriosis is associated with pelvic pain. Fertil Steril 55:759, 1991.
31. American Fertility Society: Classification of endometriosis. Fertil Steril 32:633, 1979 (revised 1985).
32. Cook AS, Rock JA: The role of laparoscopy in the treatment of endometriosis. Fertil Steril 55:663, 1991.
33. Landsteiner K: Kur Kenntnis der spezifich aufblutkorperehen winkenden Sera. Zentralbl Parasitent 25:546, 1899.
34. Metalnifoff S: Etudes sur la spermotorine. Ann Inst Pasteur 14:577, 1900.
35. Meknifoff E: Etudes sur la resorption des cellules. Ann Inst Pasteur 13:737, 1899.
36. Wilson L: Sperm agglutinins in human semen and blood. Proc Soc Exp Biol Med 85:652, 1954.
37. Wilson L: Sperm agglutination due to autoantibodies: A new cause of sterility. Fertil Steril 7:262, 1956.
38. Rumke P, Hellinga G: Autoantibodies against spermatozoa in sterile men. Am J Clin Pathol 32:357, 1959.
39. Fjallbrant B, Obrant O: Clinical and seminal findings in men with sperm antibodies. Acta Obstet Gynecol Scand 47(Suppl 4):451, 1968.
40. Shulman S, Harlin B, Davis P, Reyniak JV: Immune infertility and new approaches to treatment. Fertil Steril 29:309, 1978.
41. Franklin RR, Dukes CDL: Antispermatozoal antibodies and unexplained infertility. Am J Obstet Gynecol 89:6, 1964.
42. Schwimmer WB, Ustay KA, Behrman SJ: An evaluation of immunological factors of fertility. Fertil Steril 18:167, 1967.
43. Schwimmer WB, Ustay KA, Behrman SJ: Sperm agglutinating antibodies and decreased fertility in prostitutes. Obstet Gynecol Surv 23:195, 1968.
44. Glass RH, Vaidya RA: Sperm-agglutinating antibodies in infertile women. Fertil Steril 21:657, 1970.
45. Kibrick S, Relding D, Merrill B: Methods for the detection of antibodies against mammalian spermatozoa II. A gelatin agglutination test. Fertil Steril 3:430, 1952.
46. Isojima S, Li TS, Ashitaka Y: Immunologic analysis of sperm immobilizing factor found in sera of women with unexplained infertility. Am J Obstet Gynecol 101:677, 1968.
47. Horne HW Jr, Hertig AW, Kundsin RB, et al: Subclinical endometrial inflammation and T-mycoplasma: A possible case of human reproductive failure. Int J Fertil 18:226, 1973.
48. Horne HW Jr, Kundsin RB, Kosasa TS: The role of mycoplasma infection in human reproduction failure. Fertil Steril 25:380, 1974.
49. McCormack WM, Braun P, Lee YH, et al: The genital mycoplasmas. N Engl J Med 288:78, 1973.
50. O'Leary WM, Frick J: The correlation of human male infertility with the presence of mycoplasma T-strain. Andrologia 7:309, 1975.
51. Gnarpe H, Griberg J: Mycoplasma and human reproductive failure. The occurrence of different mycoplasma in couples with reproductive failures. Am J Obstet Gynecol 114:727, 1972.
52. Gnarpe H, Friberg J: T-mycoplasma on spermatozoa and infertility. Nature 245:97, 1973.
53. Friberg J, Gnarpe H: Mycoplasma and human reproductive failure. III. Pregnancies in infertile couples treated with doxycycline for T-mycoplasma. Am J Obstet Gynecol 116:23, 1973.
54. de Louvous J, Blades M, Harrison RF, et al: Frequency of mycoplasma in fertile and infertile couples. Lancet 1:1073, 1974.
55. Jones GS, Aksel S, Wentz AC: Serum progesterone values in the luteal phase defects. Obstet Gynecol 44:26, 1974.
56. Strott CA, Cargille CM, Ross GT, Lipsett MB: The short luteal phase. J Clin Endocrinol 30:246, 1970.

Hyperandrogenism, Hirsutism, and the Polycystic Ovary Syndrome

DAVID A. EHRMANN
RANDALL B. BARNES
ROBERT L. ROSENFIELD

Recent insights into the physiology and pathophysiology of androgen biosynthesis and action have fostered improved diagnostic and therapeutic measures for disorders that cause androgen excess in women. In this chapter we first review what is known about androgen biosynthesis, regulation, and action. The clinical manifestations and differential diagnosis of androgen excess and an approach to diagnostic and therapeutic strategies follow.

ANDROGEN PHYSIOLOGY AND PATHOPHYSIOLOGY

Androgen Biosynthesis

The core pathway for the biosynthesis of all steroid hormones begins with the rate-limiting conversion of cholesterol to pregnenolone by the side-chain cleavage enzyme (P450scc) (Fig. 120–1).[1] Thereafter, pregnenolone undergoes a two-step conversion to the 17-ketosteroid (17-KS) dehydroepiandrosterone (DHA) along the Δ^5-steroid pathway. This conversion is accomplished by way of cytochrome P450c17, an enzyme with both 17-hydroxylase and 17,20-lyase activities.[2, 3] Progesterone undergoes a parallel transformation to androstenedione (AD) in the Δ^4-steroid path. In humans it is not established whether the Δ^4-17,20-lyase activity is due to P450c17.[4] The metabolism of Δ^5- to Δ^4-intermediates is accomplished by Δ^5-isomerase-3β-hydroxysteroid dehydrogenase (3β-HSD). A single gene appears

to code for the type II 3β-HSD isozyme, which accounts for the vast majority of the 3β-HSD activity of the human ovary and adrenal.[5] In the adrenal, 17-hydroxyprogesterone (17-PROG) is the branch point at which cortisol and sex hormone synthesis diverge (by way of 21-hydroxylase and 17,20-lyase, respectively). In the ovary, AD is the branch point at which testosterone and estrogen synthesis diverge (by way of 17β-reductase and aromatase, respectively). Viewed from another perspective, androgens (AD and testosterone) are obligate intermediates in the biosynthesis of estrogens (estrone and estradiol, respectively). Testosterone alternatively can be converted by 5α-reductase to the more potent androgen dihydrotestosterone (DHT).

Regulation of Androgen Production

Androgens are secreted by both the adrenal glands and the ovaries in response to the respective tropic hormones ACTH and luteinizing hormone (LH). Because of this they undergo about two-fold episodic, diurnal, and cyclic variation. Because they are by-products of estradiol and cortisol secretion, androgens in women are not specifically under negative feedback control via these pituitary hormones. The regulation of adrenal and ovarian androgen production is summarized below.

Adrenal Glands

Adrenal 17-KS secretion gradually begins in midchildhood as a result of adrenarche, a ''puberty'' of the adrenal

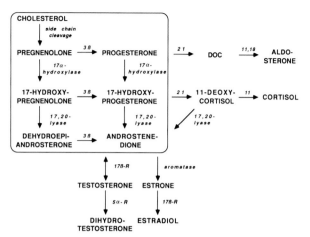

FIGURE 120–1. Outline of the major steroid biosynthetic pathways. The enclosed area contains the core steroidogenic pathway used by the gonads and adrenal glands; the Δ^5-path is in the left-hand column, the Δ^4-path is in the right-hand column. The steroidogenic enzymes are italicized. Cytochrome P450 enzyme steps are side-chain cleavage; 17α-hydroxylase/17,20-lyase; 21-hydroxylase (21); 11β-hydroxylase/18-hydroxylase-dehydrogenase (11, 18); and aromatase. Non-P450 enzyme steps are Δ^5-isomerase-3β-hydroxysteroid dehydrogenase (3β), 17-ketosteroid 17β-reductase (17β-R), and 5α-reductase (5α-R). DOC, deoxycorticosterone. (Modified from Ehrmann DA, Rosenfield RL: An endocrinologic approach to the patient with hirsutism. J Clin Endocrinol Metab 71:1–4. © The Endocrine Society, 1990.)

gland during which the adrenal cortex develops the ability to secrete 17-KS's in response to ACTH.[6] During adrenarche, DHA sulfate (DHAS) becomes as prominent an adrenocortical secretion as cortisol. Adrenarche represents a change in the pattern of adrenal secretory response to ACTH: There are striking increases in 17-hydroxypregnenolone and DHA responsiveness to ACTH. The cause of the changes that underlie adrenarche is unclear. Both in vivo and in vitro data are consistent with maturational increases in 17-hydroxylase and 17,20-lyase activities. These changes seem to be related in part to the development of the zona reticularis of the adrenal cortex. This zone produces large amounts of DHA and DHAS.

The existence and nature of an "adrenarche factor" has been the subject of considerable controversy. It has been postulated to be a pituitary hormone, since adrenal androgen production is more depressed than is cortisol production in hypopituitarism and after glucocorticoid administration.[7, 8] A portion of the joining peptide of proopiomelanocortin is the leading candidate for a glucocorticoid-suppressible pituitary adrenarche factor.[9] Whether an adrenarche factor is an adrenocortical androgen-stimulating hormone, as postulated by some,[9] remains to be determined. The fact that the adrenarchal secretion pattern represents a change in the pattern of steroidogenic response to ACTH suggests, alternatively, that an adrenarche factor may control the growth and differentiation of the zona reticularis or regulate steroidogenic enzymes, such as by increasing the 17,20-lyase activity of P450c17 (see below).

Ovary

Normal ovarian function depends on the combined action of LH on theca-interstitial-stromal (thecal) cells and follicle-stimulating hormone (FSH) on granulosa cells. Ac-

cording to the two-cell model of ovarian steroidogenesis[10, 11] (Fig. 120–2), the thecal cell compartment secretes AD in response to LH, and the AD formed by the thecal cells is converted within granulosa cells to estrogen by aromatase under the influence of FSH. In actuality, this model represents an oversimplification because estradiol can be formed by thecal cells in response to LH both very early and very late (luteinized follicle) in the follicular phase of the menstrual cycle.[12] In any case, as a dominant follicle emerges, increased amounts of both AD and estradiol are secreted, but estradiol normally predominates. The normal female pattern of response to gonadotropin-releasing hormone (GnRH) is one of relative FSH predominance over LH, favoring estrogen over androgen secretion.[13]

Intraovarian modulation of androgen synthesis in response to LH seems to be a crucial aspect of the regulation of androgen biosynthesis, since LH secretion (and, therefore, androgen secretion) is not very sensitive to long-loop feedback by the modest changes in plasma estradiol or testosterone levels that occur during the normal menstrual cycle.[4, 14–19] A crucial aspect of this intraovarian modulation of the response to LH appears to occur at the level of 17-hydroxylase/17,20-lyase. These activities seem to be regulated so as to coordinate thecal androgen synthesis with estrogen secretion and thus prevent both hyperandrogenism and hyperestrogenism. Stimulation of 17-hydroxylase/17,20-lyase by LH seems augmented by specific autocrine/intracrine, paracrine, and hormonal factors such as those shown in Figure 120–2. The processes up-regulating 17-hydroxylase/17,20-lyase activities are counterbalanced by processes of desensitization to LH. Desensitization of

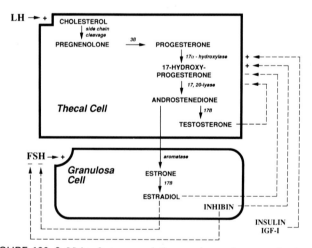

FIGURE 120–2. Major factors regulating ovarian androgen and estrogen biosynthesis. LH stimulates androgen formation within theca-interstitial-stromal (thecal) cells by way of the steroidogenic pathway common to the gonads and adrenal glands. FSH regulates estradiol biosynthesis from androgen by granulosa cells according to the two-gonadotropin, two-cell model of ovarian steroidogenesis.[10] Long-loop negative feedback of estradiol on gonadotropin secretion does not suppress LH at physiological levels of estradiol. Androgen formation in response to LH appears to be modulated by intra-ovarian feedback at the levels of 17-hydroxylase and 17,20-lyase, both of which may be activities of cytochrome P450c17. Androgen, by way of DHT (not shown), and estradiol inhibit (minus signs) and inhibin, insulin, and insulin-like growth factor 1 (IGF 1) stimulate (plus signs) 17-hydroxylase and 17,20-lyase activities. 3β,Δ^5-isomerase-3β-hydroxysteroid dehydrogenase; 17β,17-β-reductase. (Modified from Ehrmann DA et al: Detection of functional ovarian hyperandrogenism in women with androgen excess. By permission of The New England Journal of Medicine [327:157–162, 1992].)

LH to itself (homologous desensitization) sets in as LH stimulation increases and involves in part down-regulation of 17-hydroxylase/17,20-lyase activities by other intraovarian factors, some of which are shown in Figure 120–2.

DHT is synthesized from testosterone by both thecal and granulosa cells.[20] Negative autocrine/intracrine feedback by androgen on testosterone secretion appears to be receptor-mediated in testicular interstitial cells.[21] Androgen receptors have been identified in monkey thecal and granulosa cells.[22] These data are compatible with androgen directly affecting thecal AD secretion, but this remains to be demonstrated. The role of the estrogen receptor in estrogen action in the primate ovary is controversial.[23] Estradiol inhibits thecal secretion of androgen rapidly (half-life 10 min) in the rat, an observation that is compatible with a direct, post-translational inhibitory effect of estradiol on steroidogenesis.[10]

All the elements of the insulin-like growth factor (IGF) system are present in the ovary[24]: IGF production, receptors, and action. Both IGF-I and insulin are synergistic in augmenting LH-stimulated androgen production.[25-27] They act in the rat by increasing thecal levels of P450scc mRNA and augment the ability of LH to increase P450c17 mRNA levels.[28] In addition, IGF-I receptors appear to be up-regulated by insulin.[29] Insulin may affect ovarian androgen production through diverse mechanisms.[30] Insulin may act through its own receptor, through alternatively spliced insulin receptors,[30a] through the homologous type I IGF receptor,[31] or through a hybrid receptor that contains a combination of α- and β-subunits of both receptors.[32] It has also been postulated that by lowering levels of IGF binding protein 1, insulin may raise the fraction of IGF-I that is bioavailable.[32, 33] IGF-II, however, may prove to be the major member of the IGF family within the human ovary.[33a]

Various other ovarian peptides are potentially capable of modulating thecal androgen synthesis. Stimulators include inhibin, prostaglandin, and angiotensin.[4, 27, 34, 35] Inhibitors include activin, transforming growth factor β, epidermal growth factor (EGF), tumor necrosis factor, and cytokines.[36-41]

Granulosa cell proliferation is an important determinant of ovarian androgen production. Immature follicles (less than or equal to 4 mm in diameter) produce low amounts of all the sex hormones. Mature follicles (greater than or equal to 8 mm in diameter) have high numbers of granulosa cells with high aromatase activity; they predominantly convert AD to estradiol[20, 42, 43] (Fig. 120–3). On the other hand, aromatase activity is low in atretic or cystic follicles, so such follicles become relatively androgenic. What factors determine the proliferation and health of the granulosa cell population? FSH is necessary for granulosa cell proliferation and is concentrated by the emerging dominant follicle. In addition, IGF's appear to be important regulators of granulosa cell function.[44] In synergy with FSH, IGF-I and insulin (usually in greater concentrations) stimulate progesterone and estradiol production in a dose-dependent manner in cultured rat granulosa cells.[45] A similar effect of IGF-I has been demonstrated in human granulosa cells.[46] In addition, the 53-kD subunit of IGF binding protein 3 inhibits FSH bioactivity.[47, 48] EGF appears to inhibit FSH-induced estradiol production by human granulosa cells in culture.[49] Androgens, in low concentration, promote gonadotropin-stimulated granulosa cell aromatase activity.[50, 51] In high concentration, however, DHT acts as a

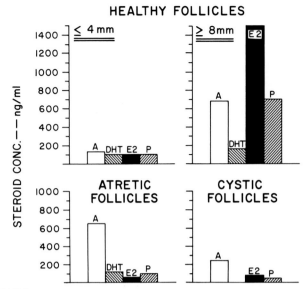

FIGURE 120–3. **Human follicular fluid steroid concentrations.** As healthy follicles grow, the androstenedione they produce is predominantly metabolized to estradiol. In atretic or cystic follicles, little estradiol is formed. Testosterone concentrations are only about one third those of dihydrotestosterone. A, androstenedione; DHT, dihydrotestosterone; E2, estradiol; P, progesterone. (From Barnes R, Rosenfield RL: The polycystic ovary syndrome: Pathogenesis and treatment. Ann Intern Med 110:386–399, 1989.)

competitive inhibitor of aromatase activity in the granulosa cell.[51, 52]

Peripheral Conversion of Secreted Precursors

Despite their great abundance, the 17-KS's are proandrogens: peripheral conversion to the 17β-hydroxysteroids testosterone and DHT is required for biological activity. Testosterone is the most important circulating androgen because of its relative potency and free plasma concentration. About one half of plasma testosterone is derived from the peripheral conversion of secreted AD. The remainder is derived equally from direct ovarian and adrenal secretion. The major clinically important sites of peripheral conversion are liver, adipose tissue, and target organs.[6, 53] The factors that control these conversions are poorly understood.

Plasma DHT arises virtually entirely from peripheral formation from secreted precursors. Plasma AD is the major precursor of DHT in women, accounting for more than 60 per cent of circulating levels; testosterone accounts for only 15 per cent, and the remaining 25 per cent is accounted for by DHA and Δ5-androstenediol.[54-56]

Blood Levels and Transport

More than 96 per cent of 17β-hydroxysteroids circulate bound to the carrier proteins albumin and sex hormone–binding globulin (SHBG). Because of its high binding affinity, the SHBG concentration is the major determinant of the distribution of 17β-hydroxysteroids to the plasma albumin and free fractions.[57, 58] A number of physiological and pathological states impact on the SHBG concentration: It is increased by estrogens and thyroid hormone excess; it is decreased primarily by insulin, with androgen, glucocorticoid, and growth hormone seemingly playing lesser roles.[58-60] Although there has been interest in the possibility that albumin-bound testosterone is bioactive, most evidence suggests that it is the free steroid intermediate that is bioavailable.[61-63] Consequently, plasma free testosterone appears to be the most important single hormonal factor in the pathogenesis of hirsutism.

Mechanism of Androgen Action

Androgens, like other steroid hormones, exert their biological activity by freely crossing the cell membrane and entering the cell nucleus. The biological activity of testosterone is affected in large part by its conversion to DHT by 5α-reductase.[57] In turn, 5α-reductase activity is enhanced by DHT.[64] The 5α-reductase and androgen receptor of skin are localized primarily in sebaceous glands, dermal papilla cells, and sweat glands, to a greater extent than in hair or dermis.[6, 65] 3α-Androstanediol glucuronide, a metabolite of DHT, has been promulgated by some,[66, 67] but not all,[68, 69] to be a marker of hypersensitivity of the hair follicle to androgen, particularly in women with idiopathic hirsutism. Because this metabolite is also formed from secreted precursors,[70, 70a] serum levels may not accurately reflect changes at the level of the hair follicle.

DHT is more potent than testosterone primarily because of its higher affinity for and slower dissociation from the androgen receptor. DHT and testosterone bind to their specific nuclear receptor, thereby activating gene transcription.[71, 72] The androgen receptor gene resides on the X chromosome. Androgen binding to the hormone-binding domain of the receptor causes conformational changes that permit the DNA-binding domain of the androgen receptor complex to bind to the hormone response element of genomic DNA and relieve transcription inhibition. The androgen receptor shares a high degree of sequence conservation in its DNA and hormone-binding domains with other members of the steroid hormone receptor subfamily of nuclear receptors, particularly the progesterone and corticoid receptors.

MANIFESTATIONS OF ANDROGEN EXCESS

Cutaneous Manifestations

Androgens are a prerequisite for sexual hair and sebaceous gland development.[57] In conjunction with other regulatory factors, including induction factors elaborated by the dermal papilla, androgens cause the prepubertal pilosebaceous unit (PSU) in androgen-dependent areas to differentiate into either a sexual hair follicle, in which the vellus hair transforms into a terminal hair, or a sebaceous follicle, in which the sebaceous component proliferates and the hair remains vellus[6, 57] (Fig. 120–4). Terminal hairs are long, wide, pigmented, and medullated; vellus hairs are not. Hair follicles cyclically pass through anagen (growth), catagen (transitional), and telogen (resting) phases. The growth cycle of sexual hairs lasts about three months. Seasonal changes occur, with beard growth maximal in the

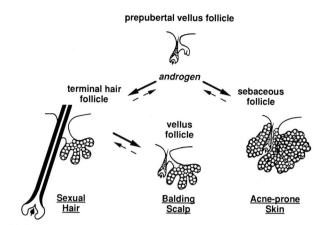

FIGURE 120–4. **Role of androgen in the development of the pilosebaceous unit.** *Solid lines* indicate effects of androgens; *dotted lines*, those of anti-androgens. Hairs are depicted only in the anagen phase of the growth cycle. In conjunction with other regulatory factors, androgens cause the prepubertal pilosebaceous unit in androgen-dependent areas to differentiate into either a sexual hair follicle, in which the vellus hair transforms into a terminal hair, or into a sebaceous follicle, in which the sebaceous component proliferates and the hair remains vellus. (Modified from Rosenfield RL, Lucky AW: Acne, hirsutism and alopecia in adolescent girls: Clinical expressions of androgen excess. Clin Endocrinol Metab 22:507, 1993.)

summer.[73] Ambisexual hair development occurs equally in both sexes in sites (e.g., pubis) where relatively low levels of androgen are necessary for PSU differentiation. Male-pattern sexual hair development occurs in sites (e.g., abdomen) where higher levels of androgen are necessary for PSU differentiation. The greater density of sexual hairs in the androgen-sensitive areas of men than of women is accounted for by a greater proportion of PSU's with terminal rather than vellus hairs. Male-pattern baldness involves conversion of terminal to vellus hair follicles.

Hirsutism, acne, and balding are variably expressed manifestations of androgen excess.[74] Some hyperandrogenic women have hirsutism, some acne, some both, and some neither. Balding alone, in a diffuse pattern commencing on the crown (rather than in the vertex and bifrontal areas, as in men), may be the sole manifestation.[6] It is normal for women to have a few sexual hairs in most of the "male" areas. Hirsutism is defined as excessive male-pattern hair growth in women. One half of the cases of mild hirsutism are associated with elevated plasma free testosterone levels, and moderately severe hirsutism is even more likely to be hyperandrogenic. Conversely, about one third of women with modest (up to two-fold) elevations of plasma free testosterone have no evidence of hirsutism.

Hyperandrogenism is an incitant of acne vulgaris, along with a combination of luminal hyperkeratinization, sebocyte hyperplasia, and secondary infection. When the onset of inflammatory acne is prepubertal, persists into or begins in the third decade, or is resistant to dermatological therapy, underlying hyperandrogenism should be suspected.[6] An increased plasma free testosterone is found in one third of the cases of even persistent comedonal acne,[74] whereas cystic acne usually is hyperandrogenic.[75]

The amount of sexual hair and sebaceous gland development thus seems to depend as much on the biological factors that determine sensitivity of the PSU to androgens as on the plasma androgen level.[57] At one end of the spectrum are women whose PSU's seem hypersensitive to normal blood androgen levels; this seems to account for idiopathic hirsutism and acne. At the other end of the spectrum are women whose PSU's are relatively insensitive to androgen; this seems to account for cryptic hyperandrogenism (hyperandrogenemia without skin manifestations).

Acanthosis nigricans has been reported in anywhere from 5 to 50 per cent of hyperandrogenic women.[76] The lesion appears hyperpigmented and velvety and usually is found over the nape of the neck, in the axillae, or beneath the breasts. Histologically, it is characterized by epidermal papillomatosis and hyperkeratosis and often is present on biopsy when it is not evident on clinical skin examination.[76] Its presence has been used as a marker of insulin resistance in general and the syndrome of hyperandrogenism, insulin resistance, and acanthosis nigricans ("HAIR-AN") in particular.[77] The best biochemical correlate of histological acanthosis nigricans appears to be decreased insulin action, rather than elevated insulin or androgen levels per se.[76]

Ovarian Manifestations

Any disorder that causes high intraovarian androgen concentrations causes follicular maturation arrest, atresia, and anovulation,[13] the clinical correlates of which are oligoamenorrhea, dysfunctional uterine bleeding, and infertility (see below).

In the face of excessive intraovarian androgen concentrations, viable follicles seldom develop beyond about the 6-mm stage.[78] Androgen-induced follicular atresia is thought to be mediated by the androgen receptor complex that activates cell death in the granulosa cells of preantral follicles.[79, 80] The atretogenic effect of LH is mediated by increased intraovarian androgen production, as indicated by the fact that it is antagonized by antiandrogen.[81] Studies in the rat also suggest that androgen-induced atresia is related to antagonism of granulosa cell proliferation and development by estradiol.[82]

Follicular atresia is self-perpetuating in part because the atretic follicle becomes an androgenic follicle by a "default" mechanism: Because aromatase activity is low in atretic follicles, AD is preferentially metabolized to testosterone and then to DHT[20, 42, 43] (see Fig. 120–3). Structurally, follicular atresia is characterized by the attrition of granulosa cells, whereas thecal cells remain in the stroma. This results in an increasingly large stromal compartment of hypertrophic "interstitial gland cells" that retain LH responsiveness and continue to secrete androgen.[10]

Frankly masculinizing plasma concentrations of androgens seem capable of inducing histopathological changes in the ovary (pseudoluteinization of theca and thickening of the ovarian capsule), as documented during the induction of virilization of transsexuals,[83, 84] and thecal hyperandrogenism, as reported in classic congenital adrenal hyperplasia (CAH).[85] In addition, injection of testosterone into a single ovary results in local follicular and oocyte degeneration, whereas the opposite ovary and gonadotropins remain unaffected.[86]

HYPERANDROGENIC DISORDERS

The causes of androgen excess in women are listed in Table 120–1 and discussed in detail below.

Functional Adrenal Hyperandrogenism

Premature Adrenarche

The appearance of sexual pubic hair before 8.5 years of age (premature pubarche) usually is due to premature adrenarche.[87] That is, most girls with the precocious onset of pubic hair development have undergone early maturation of adrenal androgen secretion. Less often, premature pubarche represents inordinate sensitivity of sexual hair follicles to normal adrenal androgen levels. The best hormonal indicator of adrenarche is a plasma level of DHAS over 40 μg/dl with concomitant plasma testosterone levels that are in the midpubertal range at most. Clinically, the androgen excess is so subtle that the only other sign of increased androgen production may be a few microcomedones. No evidence of virilization is found: There is no clitoromegaly, no growth spurt, no excessive bone maturation. The responses of steroid intermediates to ACTH are between the prepubertal and adult range in more than 90 per cent of children with premature adrenarche (Fig. 120–5).

Considerable controversy surrounds the distinction of premature adrenarche from mild virilizing CAH.[6] Some have estimated the incidence of nonclassic 21-hydroxylase deficiency CAH to be as high as 40 per cent in children with premature pubarche.[88] This estimate probably is skewed by the high prevalence in such studies of certain ethnic groups, such as Ashkenazic Jews and Hispanics, that have a high incidence of nonclassic CAH. Some also make the controversial claim that 3β-HSD deficiency is a common cause of premature adrenarche.[88] Such investigators have designated Δ5-steroid responses greater than those of Tanner stage II to III controls as 3β-HSD deficiency. However, our interpretation and that of many others is that 3β-HSD deficiency is rare.[6] We only make the diagnosis of 3β-HSD deficiency when there is evidence of virilization, including abnormal advancement of bone age, and when the responses to ACTH of the Δ5-steroids, 17-hydroxypregnenolone and DHA, are much greater than those of normal adults. As additional criteria for this diagnosis, we also require a subnormal acute rise in Δ4-steroids (17-PROG and AD). There will continue to be controversy in this field

TABLE 120–1. CAUSES OF ANDROGEN EXCESS IN WOMEN

Functional Adrenal Hyperandrogenism
  Premature adrenarche
  Dysregulation/exaggerated adrenarche
  Congenital adrenal hyperplasia
  Cushing's syndrome
  Hyperprolactinemia
  Abnormal cortisol action/metabolism
Functional Gonadal Hyperandrogenism
  Functional ovarian hyperandrogenism/polycystic ovary syndrome
    Follicular atresia and maturation arrest
    Extraovarian androgen excess
    Ovarian steroidogenic blocks
    Dysregulation of 17-hydroxylase/17,20-lyase
      LH excess
      Syndromes of insulin resistance
  True hermaphroditism
  Chorionic gonadotropin–related hyperandrogenism
Peripheral Androgen Overproduction
  Obesity
  Idiopathic
Tumoral Hyperandrogenism

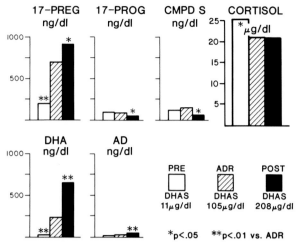

FIGURE 120–5. **Changing pattern of adrenal steroidogenic response to ACTH with maturation.** Shown are plasma steroid levels 30 minutes post ACTH (10 μg per m²) in prepubertal children (PRE), children with premature adrenarche as an isolated phenomenon (ADR), and postadrenarchal follicular phase adult females (POST). The layout is organized according to the biosynthetic pathway (see Fig. 120–1). Note that 17-hydroxypregnenolone (17-PREG) and dehydroepiandrosterone (DHA) responses of children with premature adrenarche are intermediate between the prepubertal and adult responses. 17-PROG, 17-hydroxyprogesterone; CMPD S, 11-deoxycortisol, AD, androstenedione. (From Rosenfield RL: The ovary and female sexual maturation. *In* Kaplan SA (ed): Clinical Pediatric and Adolescent Endocrinology. (ed 2). Philadelphia, WB Saunders, 1990, pp 259–324.)

until hormonal and molecular genetic data are compared. Normal ranges for plasma androgens and intermediates at baseline and in response to ACTH for preadrenarchal, prematurely adrenarchal, and postadrenarchal subjects are shown in Tables 120–2 and 120–3.

Exaggerated Adrenarche

One half of hyperandrogenic women with 17-KS hyperresponsiveness to ACTH have a pattern of steroid intermediates that resembles an exaggeration of adrenarche.[91] That is, they have moderately excessive DHA, 17-hydroxypregnenolone, and AD hyperresponsiveness to ACTH. This is the single most common adrenal secretory abnormality in hyperandrogenic women. Menses are more often normal in these women than in women with functional ovarian hyperandrogenism (FOH).[11]

Some investigators have considered patients with excessive DHA and 17-hydroxypregnenolone responses to ACTH to have mild 3β-HSD deficiency.[92] This appears unlikely, since many of these patients have greater than aver-

age AD responses to ACTH stimulation, which suggests that they, too, have exaggerated adrenarche. In addition, GnRH agonist testing in such cases typically shows a pattern of ovarian steroid response that is different from that encountered in 3β-HSD deficiency.[93] Symptomatic heterozygosity for 21-hydroxylase deficiency, on the other hand, is an alternative possibility. A slightly elevated 17-PROG response often is found in women with an otherwise typical exaggerated adrenarche steroid pattern.[94]

The cause of exaggerated adrenarche is unknown. We favor the possibility that it may be due to abnormal regulation of adrenal P450c17 activity of the same sort that seems to co-exist in one half of the cases of FOH.[93] Alternatively, it may represent hyperplasia of the zona reticularis. Whether it is related to premature adrenarche is unknown. Although the menstrual cycle usually is normal in those women with isolated exaggerated adrenarche, some would consider this an adrenal variant of polycystic ovary syndrome (PCOS)[95, 96] (see below).

Congenital Adrenal Hyperplasia

Congenital adrenal hyperplasia results from deficient activity of one of the enzymes necessary for the biosynthesis of cortisol, thus leading to excessive 17-KS (and hence testosterone) production. Classic CAH occurs in people homozygous for two alleles that together code for a severe enzymatic defect; nonclassic (late-onset) CAH results from mild allelic variations of the classic form.[97]

Deficiency of 21-hydroxylase accounts for more than 90 per cent of classic CAH[98]; 21-hydroxylase deficiency CAH accounts for between 2.5[11] and 6.0 per cent[99] of hirsutism in women. The incidence is higher in Hispanic, Ashkenazic Jewish, and Yupik Eskimo populations. Women with nonclassic deficiency of this enzyme may present with premature pubarche or peripubertal or postpubertal hirsutism, acne, or amenorrhea. On the other hand, it may be "cryptic," without manifestations of androgen excess.[100] Cryptic disease has been shown to be due to distinct 21-hydroxylase gene mutations that cause only mild enzyme deficiencies.[101] Women with classic and nonclassic 21-hydroxylase deficiency CAH may have polycystic ovaries and elevated levels of serum LH.[85, 102–104] Thus, in the absence of specific testing of ovarian function, women with nonclassic 21-hydroxylase deficiency CAH may be clinically indistinguishable from women with ovarian hyperandrogenism.[105]

It has been well demonstrated that the 17-PROG response to a rapid ACTH test distinguishes the various forms of 21-hydroxylase deficiency from normal better than does a baseline measurement.[101] The degree of clini-

TABLE 120–2. TYPICAL NORMAL RANGES FOR PLASMA ANDROGENS AND INTERMEDIATES*

	17-HYDROXY-PREGNENOLONE (ng/dl)	17-HYDROXY-PROGESTERONE (ng/dl)	11-DEOXY-CORTISOL (ng/dl)	CORTISOL (μg/dl)	DHA (ng/dl)	ANDRO-STENE-DIONE (ng/dl)	TESTOS-TERONE (ng/dl)	DHAS (μg/dl)
Prepubertal, 2–8 yr	<25–235	<25–65	<25–160	5–25	<25–120	<25–50	<15	<40
Adrenarchal†	<25–355	<25–95	<25–120	5–25	100–420	30–75	10–<45	40–400
Adult female	40–360	30–130‡	30–220	5–25	100–1000	55–200	20–75	100–400

*Normal range may differ slightly among laboratories.
†Children with premature adrenarche.
‡17-Hydroxyprogesterone rises in the preovulatory phase to a peak as high as 360 ng/dl in the luteal phase of the cycle.
From Rosenfield RL, Lucky AW: Acne, hirsutism, and alopecia in adolescent girls: Clinical expressions of androgen excess. Clin Endocrinol Metab 22:507, 1993.

TABLE 120–3. TYPICAL NORMAL RANGE OF STEROID LEVELS POST-ACTH*

	17-HYDROXY-PREGNENOLONE (ng/dl)	17-HYDROXY-PROGESTERONE (ng/dl)	11-DEOXY-CORTISOL (ng/dl)	CORTISOL (µg/dl)	DHA (ng/dl)	ANDROSTENE-DIONE (ng/dl)
Prepubertal, 2–8 yr	130–340	80–180	<25–350	13–50	45–120	<25–80
Adrenarche†	240–1100	40–190	40–300	13–50	285–495	55–140
Adult female	150–1070	35–130‡	40–200	13–50	225–1470	55–185

*Thirty minutes post-ACTH 10 µg/m² as I.V. bolus. Values 60 minutes after 250 µg of ACTH are slightly greater.[89]
†Children with premature adrenarche.
‡17-Hydroxyprogesterone rises in the preovulatory phase to a peak as high as 360 ng/dl in the luteal phase of the cycle.
From Rosenfield RL, Lucky AW: Acne, hirsutism, and alopecia in adolescent girls: Clinical expressions of androgen excess. Clin Endocrinol Metab 22:507, 1993.

cal severity is correlated with the degree of 21-hydroxylase deficiency as reflected by the 17-PROG response to ACTH. The response of 17-PROG to ACTH usually distinguishes carriers from noncarriers, but molecular genetic analysis is most discriminating for this purpose.[106]

Deficiency of 11β-hydroxylase accounts for 5 to 8 per cent of cases of classic CAH.[98] A large proportion of these cases have been reported in Moroccan Jews.[92] About two thirds of patients with classic 11β-hydroxylase deficiency have hypertension as a result of concomitant 11-deoxycorticosterone excess,[98, 107] although in its milder forms, hypertension may not be present. Moderate hyper-responsiveness of 11-deoxycortisol to ACTH administration occasionally is found in subjects with nonclassic 21-hydroxylase deficiency; this has been attributed to secondary inhibition of 11β-hydroxylase by elevated intra-adrenal androgens.[92] Because there are no independent direct enzymatic measurements or genetic studies for 11β-hydroxylase deficiency, precise diagnostic criteria for nonclassic deficiency of this enzyme are lacking.

Although the classic form of 3β-HSD deficiency is rare, late-onset 3β-HSD deficiency often has been hypothesized to be a common cause of the adrenal hyperandrogenism of hirsute women.[92, 108, 109] Based on elevation of various Δ⁵-steroids in response to ACTH, investigators report that as many as 10 to 40 per cent of hirsute women have 3β-HSD deficiency.[92, 108, 109] Firm diagnostic criteria for late-onset 3β-HSD deficiency have not been established.[110] In most cases there is concomitant hyper-responsiveness of Δ⁴-steroids, consonant with exaggerated adrenarche (see above). In our recent study of 40 consecutive hyperandrogenic, hirsute women undergoing evaluation of adrenal steroidogenic responses to ACTH, 8 had Δ⁵-steroid hyper-responsiveness suggestive of 3β-HSD deficiency.[93] If this were the diagnosis, stimulation of ovarian steroidogenesis with the GnRH agonist nafarelin would be predicted to have resulted in an elevated Δ⁵:Δ⁴ steroid ratio. This was not the case in any of these women. Rather, their ovarian steroidogenic response frequently was characterized by an increase in Δ⁴-steroids, consistent with abnormal regulation of ovarian 17,20-lyase activity[11, 94] (see below). Thus much of what has been labeled 3β-HSD deficiency may be due to abnormal regulation of adrenal 17-KS secretion.

Other

A number of other causes of functional adrenal hyperandrogenism are known but are relatively rare. Cushing's disease typically is accompanied by DHAS levels that are relatively less elevated than AD levels.[111] Cortisol resistance

may cause adult-onset hirsutism.[112, 113] In these patients a functional abnormality of the glucocorticoid receptor leads to compensatory hypersecretion of ACTH and hypercortisolemia without other clinical or biochemical findings of Cushing's syndrome. The clinical manifestations are due to overproduction of nonglucocorticoid adrenal steroids. Consequently, hypertension with hypokalemia may accompany the syndrome. Congenitally excessive cortisol metabolism caused by 11-ketoreductase deficiency resembles cortisol resistance and may present as hirsutism and amenorrhea.[114, 115]

Women with hyperprolactinemia may present with hirsutism and acne,[116] polycystic ovaries,[117] and LH hyperresponsiveness to GnRH.[117, 118] Galactorrhea occurs in only about one half of cases. Elevation of plasma free testosterone, sometimes accompanied by elevated plasma DHAS concentrations, is characteristic. These elevations result from the multiple effects of hyperprolactinemia on steroid metabolism.[116, 119–121] The hyperandrogenemia typically is suppressible by glucocorticoid administration. Adrenal androgenic hyperfunction has also been reported in acromegaly.[122]

Functional Gonadal Hyperandrogenism

Most women with androgen excess have ovarian hyperandrogenism, as demonstrated by the results of ovarian vein catheterization,[123] dexamethasone suppression testing,[11, 123–125] long-term administration of GnRH agonists,[70, 126] and, most recently, the acute ovarian steroidogenic response to the administration of a GnRH agonist.[11, 127] The causes of gonadal androgen excess in women are listed in Table 120–1, the most common of which is FOH/PCOS.

Functional Ovarian Hyperandrogenism and Polycystic Ovary Syndrome

In 1935, Stein and Leventhal reported the association of polycystic ovaries with amenorrhea, hirsutism, and obesity.[128] Later, increased serum LH concentrations or an increase in the ratio of LH to FSH were shown to be characteristic[129] and became common diagnostic criteria in lieu of biopsy evidence of polycystic ovaries. More recently, hyperandrogenemia was shown to be typical,[124] and improvements in ultrasonographic techniques have made it possible to noninvasively demonstrate polycystic ovaries.[130]

Hyperandrogenism in association with either an increased serum concentration of LH or LH:FSH ratio[131] or polycystic ovaries on ultrasonography currently are the usual diagnostic criteria for what is termed PCOS.[132] Some women without polycystic ovaries or gonadotropin abnormalities, however, have been considered to have the syndrome.[125, 126, 133–136] Indeed, some investigators have required only the presence of oligomenorrhea and hirsutism to make the diagnosis.[137] Furthermore, women with as well as those without the characteristic histological[135] or sonographic[11] changes of the ovaries have evidence of similar ovarian dysfunction. Ovarian vein catheterization has also suggested that excessive ovarian androgen production occurs not only with but also without polycystic ovaries.[123, 138] It is our thesis that PCOS is a form of FOH and, conversely, that FOH occurs without the LH or ultrasonographic criteria for PCOS.

CLINICAL CHARACTERISTICS. Women with PCOS in its full-blown state present with symptoms of anovulation, hyperandrogenemia, and obesity.[128, 129, 139] The anovulation typically is expressed as oligoamenorrhea or infertility and the hyperandrogenism, as hirsutism. Structurally, classic polycystic ovaries are two- to five-fold enlarged with a thickened tunica albuginea, thecal hyperplasia, and 20 or more subcapsular follicles about 1 to 15 mm in diameter.

The disorder often presents difficulties in diagnosis. First, not all patients have the typical clinical syndrome: The anovulation may result in dysfunctional uterine bleeding or may be undetected because of cyclic menses; the hyperandrogenism may present as acne rather than as hirsutism or be cryptic with no cutaneous manifestations; and obesity is present in only 40 per cent of patients.[139] Second, women with PCOS may be clinically indistinguishable from those with other disorders that cause androgen excess, such as nonclassic CAH, as already discussed. Finally, patients with the hyperthecosis form of PCOS, considered to be the most severe form of the syndrome, do not have LH excess, seem to "burn out" their follicles, and do not have polycystic ovaries.[133, 136]

Symptoms of ovarian hyperandrogenism typically begin at about the time of menarche, and the disorder can be diagnosed during adolescence.[140–142] The incidence of PCOS is about 3 per cent in both the adolescent and the adult populations.[142, 143]

PATHOGENESIS. There is abundant evidence to suggest that PCOS may be caused by congenital disorders of ovarian function that first appear in adolescence. PCOS has been documented in concordantly affected monozygotic twins.[144] Both autosomal[145] and X-linked[146] modes of inheritance have been proposed, and human leukocyte antigen abnormalities may be linked.[147] Furthermore, congenital type A insulin resistance (see below) can cause PCOS. All this suggests a genetic basis for the syndrome, although in the vast majority of cases there is no clear family history of the disorder.

The most widely promulgated hypothesis regarding the pathogenesis of PCOS has been termed the "estrone hypothesis," according to which PCOS results from a complex vicious cycle whereby AD, which originates in part from the adrenal glands, is aromatized peripherally to estrone.[96] The elevation in estrone is postulated to sensitize the pituitary to secrete excess LH, which initiates or maintains excessive ovarian AD secretion. The observation that antiestrogens such as clomiphene citrate beneficially alter the abnormal gonadotropin secretion in women with PCOS is cited as evidence that this is the result of estrone

excess. Recent evidence, however, casts doubt on the tenets of this hypothesis.[13] Estrone is a weak estrogen, and attempts to alter gonadotropin secretion by altering estrone levels have not supported the hypothesis. In addition, the estrone hypothesis does not account for the occurrence of ovarian hyperandrogenism in women with normal levels of LH.

We have proposed a new model for the pathogenesis of PCOS as FOH.[13] The central abnormality in FOH appears to be an elevated intraovarian androgen concentration. This is responsible, on the one hand, for the cutaneous and anovulatory manifestations discussed above. On the other hand, FOH appears to be the end-point of several heterogeneous but interrelated processes,[13] including follicular atresia, extraovarian androgen excess, ovarian steroidogenic blocks, abnormal regulation (dysregulation) of steroidogenesis,[11, 13, 94] excessive LH stimulation, and insulin resistance syndromes (Fig. 120–6). The salient features of this model follow.

Follicular Atresia and Maturation Arrest. Attenuation of follicular development, primarily at the level of selection of a dominant preovulatory follicle, is characteristic in women with PCOS[148] and evidenced by the presence of an increased number of small, immature follicles within PCOS ovaries.[149] Graafian follicles from women with PCOS have fewer granulosa cells, suggesting that their capacity to proliferate may be reduced.[150] The reduction in granulosa cell proliferation is associated with an abundance of polysomes and the lack of gap junctions between granulosa cells that could lead to altered responsiveness to regulatory factors[150] with follicles committing to atresia before reaching a stage at which healthy oocytes can be sustained.

Because FSH is necessary for granulosa cell proliferation, a reduction of its serum levels, a decrease in its biological activity, or inhibition of its activity could account for the lesser number of granulosa cells in PCOS. The correction of ovarian function in PCOS by the repetitive administration of very low doses of FSH in vivo lowers serum androgen levels, increases serum estradiol, and results in ovulation.[151–153] The biological activity of FSH in women with PCOS appears to be normal as assessed by a rat granulosa cell assay, however.[154] This suggests inhibition of FSH ac-

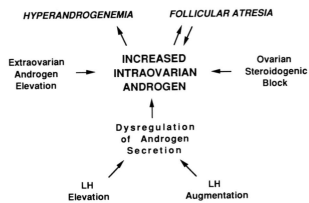

FIGURE 120–6. Model of pathogenesis of functional ovarian hyperandrogenism. An increased intraovarian androgen concentration can both induce and result from follicular atresia. Additional causes of increased intraovarian androgen levels include extraovarian androgen excess, ovarian steroidogenic blocks, and dysregulation of androgen secretion. The latter may occur from LH excess or by augmentation of LH action.

tion at the level of the granulosa cell, perhaps by IGF-binding proteins[47, 48] and/or EGF.[38]

Extraovarian Androgen Excess. Frankly virilizing levels of androgen appear to boost the intraovarian concentration of androgen sufficiently to initiate the anatomical and functional ovarian changes typical of PCOS, as discussed above. Very high plasma concentrations of androgen seem to be required for this effect ordinarily because it is unlikely that modest elevations of plasma androgens interfere with ovarian function by causing follicular atresia or inhibiting gonadotropins. In particular, mild adrenal androgen excess does not seem likely to account for ovarian dysfunction. Women with mild adrenal hyperandrogenemia typically are eumenorrheic,[15] and those with nonclassic 21-hydroxylase deficiency, with mild plasma androgen elevations, can be fertile.[100, 155] Furthermore, the characteristic ovarian steroidogenic defect of women with PCOS does not appear to be due to increased adrenal androgen secretion or to occur in nonclassic CAH.[11]

These studies are compatible with the concept that any disorder that causes very high intraovarian androgen levels—such as poorly controlled classic CAH—causes follicular maturation arrest, atresia, polycystic ovaries, and anovulation.[83–86] Enzymatic defects that interfere with the synthesis of estradiol from androgen within the ovary can bring about this result (see below).

Ovarian Steroidogenic Blocks. Primary defects in ovarian biosynthesis of estrogen from androgen result in increased intra-ovarian androgen concentrations. This makes for a particularly potent atretogenic environment and, not surprisingly, has been shown to cause PCOS. Deficiencies of 3β-HSD, 17-KS oxidoreductase, and aromatase have all been reported in association with PCOS. However, in a prospective study of 40 consecutive women with androgen excess, there was no evidence of ovarian enzyme deficiency in any subject.[11]

3β-HSD Deficiency. Concomitant ovarian and adrenal 3β-HSD deficiency as a cause of PCOS has been reported.[127, 156–158] Loss of heterozygosity for the single gene coding for the main 3β-HSD isozyme within the human ovary and adrenal[5] would seem to be responsible. The type I 3β-HSD isozyme found in skin and placenta would seem to account for the peripheral formation of Δ^4-3-ketosteroids from Δ^5-3β-hydroxysteroid precursors that occurs in 3β-HSD deficiency syndrome.

Ovarian 3β-HSD deficiency appears to be rare. The responses to nafarelin testing in a patient with PCOS known to be secondary to partial deficiency of 3β-HSD contrasted with those in typical PCOS.[127] Her block in ovarian steroidogenesis was evident in plasma levels of Δ^5-3β-hydroxysteroids increasing markedly, whereas responses of the Δ^4-3-ketosteroids immediately beyond the block, 17-PROG and AD, and those of estrone were low.

17-Ketosteroid Reductase Deficiency. 17-KS reductase (17β-R, see Fig. 120–1) converts AD to testosterone and estrone to estradiol. A diagnosis of ovarian 17-KS reductase deficiency has been made when plasma levels of AD and estrone are elevated and the ratio of estrone to estradiol is increased.[159, 160] The ratio of AD to testosterone usually is normal because there appears to be normal peripheral conversion of AD to testosterone.[159] This enzymatic defect has been associated with PCOS in three patients reported to date.[159, 160] Direct evidence of deficiency of this enzyme in the ovary has not been obtained.

Aromatase Deficiency. Examination of polycystic ovary follicular fluid reveals high levels of AD with an elevated ratio of AD to estradiol, suggesting a defect in aromatization.[150] Whatever deficiency of aromatase there may be in polycystic ovary granulosa cells appears to be reversed by the administration of FSH.[38, 78, 161] This suggests that whatever aromatase deficit may be present in typical PCOS is secondary to the gonadotropin abnormalities of the syndrome and is not intrinsic to the disorder.

Dysregulation of Steroidogenesis. Women with typical PCOS have a characteristic ovarian steroidogenic response to the endogenous gonadotropin secretion induced by the administration of the GnRH agonist nafarelin.[127] Like men, they had significantly greater plasma 17-PROG ($P < .01$), AD ($P < .05$), and testosterone responses to endogenous LH and FSH secretion than normal women in the early follicular phase of the menstrual cycle (Fig. 120–7).[127, 141] There was evidence of oversecretion of all steroids on the pathway between progesterone and estradiol, without evidence of a steroidogenic block. This characteristic PCOS type of response suggested a newly recognized abnormality of steroidogenesis: abnormal regulation (dysregulation) of 17-hydroxylase and 17,20-lyase activities. This abnormality accounts for about 80 per cent of FOH identified by the dexamethasone suppression test.[11] The high correlation between the results of these two tests indicates that poor suppression of plasma free testosterone by dexamethasone and the 17-PROG hyper-responsiveness to nafarelin reflect related aspects of ovarian androgenic function (Fig. 120–8).

Subsequent clinical research has indicated that PCOS gonads, while overproducing androgen, appear to be producing it less efficiently than testes.[127, 141] Analysis of the apparent efficiency of ovarian androgen biosynthesis also has suggested that women with FOH have high, yet relatively inefficient 17,20-lyase activity concomitant with in-

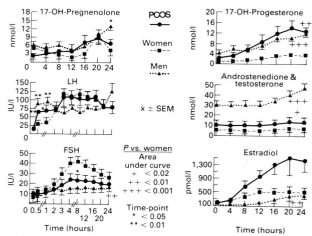

FIGURE 120–7. Responses to nafarelin of normal men (n = 5) and women with PCOS (n = 5) compared with normal follicular phase women (n = 9). Nafarelin was administered at 0 min. Statistics at time points are shown only when areas under the response curve are not significantly different. P values are two-tailed. (Modified from Rosenfield RL et al: Ovarian steroidogenic abnormalities in polycystic ovary syndrome: Evidence for abnormal coordinate regulation of androgen and estrogen secretion. *In* Dunaif A et al [eds]: Current Issues in Endocrinology and Metabolism: Polycystic Ovary Syndrome. Cambridge, MA: Blackwell Scientific, 1992, pp 83–110. By permission of Blackwell Scientific Publications, Inc.)

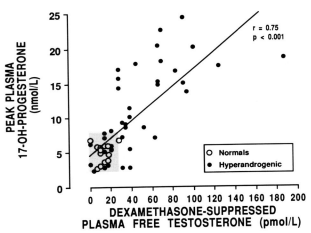

FIGURE 120–8. Relationship between plasma free testosterone concentration after administration of dexamethasone for four days and the peak plasma 17-hydroxyprogesterone concentration in response to nafarelin in a consecutive series of 40 hyperandrogenic women. The peak plasma 17-PROG response to nafarelin correlates well with the plasma free testosterone concentration after dexamethasone suppression of adrenal function ($P < .001$). The shaded area depicts the mean ± 2 SD response of normal women. (Modified from Ehrmann DA et al: Detection of functional ovarian hyperandrogenism in women with androgen excess. N Engl J Med 327:157–162, 1992.)

creased 17-hydroxylase activity compared with normal women.[4] Although basal levels of 17-PROG and AD were both increased in FOH relative to normals, in response to nafarelin the 17-PROG response was excessive ($P<.001$), but AD rose relatively less in FOH than in normals. Indexes of 17,20-lyase activity in the Δ^4-pathway were significantly less than normal ($P <.02$). There was no evidence of hindered estrogen secretion or abnormality at any of the other enzyme steps on the steroidogenic pathway.

The data suggest an abnormality in the dose-response between LH and estrogen precursors. LH-estradiol dose-response curves are normal. However, women with PCOS/FOH have higher baseline ovarian 17-PROG production and respond to a given increase of LH with a greater rise in 17-PROG than normal. Women with PCOS/FOH also have elevated baseline ovarian AD production, but in response to a given increase in LH they have a normal rise of AD. The basis of the abnormalities seems to lie in abnormal down-regulation of 17-hydroxylase and 17,20-lyase activities.

The dose-response curves for LH as opposed to the 17-hydroxylase and 17,20-lyase activities of rat P450c17 are modeled in Figure 120–9.[4] Because the Km of 17-hydroxylase is about one half as great, and V_{max} twice as great, as that of 17,20-lyase, P450c17 forms more 17-PROG than AD in the absence of LH stimulation. LH at low doses stimulates both 17α-hydroxylase and 17,20-lyase activities. Because of down-regulation as LH concentrations increase, 17,20-lyase is initially not stimulated as much as 17-hydroxylase. High doses of LH cease to stimulate P450c17 activities.

Although the enzyme kinetics of the underlying reactions are poorly understood in humans, we favor the interpretation that PCOS/FOH results primarily from partial escape from down-regulation rather than from operating on the right limb of the dose-response curves. The data are compatible with increased activity of the insulin/IGF sys-

tem or decreased activity of the sex steroid system for modulating androgen formation in response to LH stimulation. Insulin and IGF may left-shift the curves and raise the maximal androgen synthesis; they have been shown to increase production of P450c17 mRNA. Sex steroids, on the other hand, appear to mediate LH-induced down-regulation of these activities, depressing the dose-response curves; interference with the process would be expected to increase their slopes and maximal androgen secretion. However, the predominance of ovarian AD over 17-PROG production at baseline in PCOS makes it difficult to interpret with certainty the available clinical research data in terms of P450c17 activities.

In essence, dysregulation represents a flaw in the coordinate regulation of ovarian androgen and estrogen secretion at the level of 17-hydroxylase/17,20-lyase (see Fig. 120–2).[141] It appears to result from imbalance among LH and the heterogeneous intra-ovarian and endocrine factors that modulate LH stimulation of ovarian androgen secretion. About one half of patients with FOH have evidence of LH excess, but one half do not.

LH Excess. Not only is the serum LH concentration or LH:FSH ratio increased in women with classic PCOS, but they have a pattern of gonadotropin secretion similar to that of men in response to GnRH agonist testing, with greater early LH and lesser, although substantial, FSH responses.[127] LH abnormalities have been postulated to result from primary hypothalamic or pituitary abnormalities. Some women with PCOS appear to have an increase in LH pulse amplitude and frequency when compared with follicular phase controls.[131, 162, 163] The increase in LH pulse frequency implies an increased GnRH pulse frequency, which has been corroborated using free α-subunit measurements as a marker of GnRH secretion.[164, 165] A primary CNS abnormality is also suggested by the abnormal diurnal pattern of LH secretion in both postmenarcheal teenagers[166, 167] and adults[168] with PCOS. These people have a morning rise in LH that is distinctly different from the nocturnal rise char-

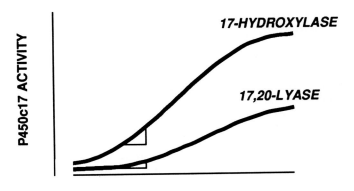

FIGURE 120–9. Hypothetical dose-response curve of relationship between LH and 17-hydroxylase/17,20-lyase activities of P450c17. In response to low doses of LH, 17,20-lyase activity at first rises less than 17-hydroxylase activity because of its lower Km. At higher doses of LH, as in PCOS, down-regulation of 17,20-lyase seems to increasingly set in, with decreasing stimulation at LH doses, which up-regulate 17-hydroxylase. FOH patients with dysregulation and normal LH levels behave as if they have left-shifted dose-response curves. (From Rosenfield RL et al: Gonadotropin releasing hormone agonist as a probe for the pathogenesis and diagnosis of ovarian hyperandrogenism. Ann NY Acad Sci 687:162–181, 1993.)

acteristic of normal premenarcheal pubertal girls[169] and anovulatory adolescents without the syndrome.[167, 170] The possibility that neuroendocrine abnormalities are due to elevated levels of estrone or abnormal secretion of neurotransmitters has not been consistently supported by the data to date.[13]

Could the gonadotropin abnormalities be secondary to an effect of androgens at the level of the hypothalamus and/or pituitary? Taken together, the data suggest that if androgens have a direct stimulatory effect on LH secretion, the effect must be relatively subtle.[13] Although the data are inconsistent, the various studies are compatible with the possibility that moderate elevations of plasma testosterone stimulate an increase in the ratio of serum LH to FSH, whereas greater elevations inhibit gonadotropins. Such an outcome might be explicable by the action of androgen on higher CNS centers. Recent evidence indicates that androgens have complex, potentially counterbalancing effects on hypothalamic GnRH turnover. These effects include the ability to increase GnRH neuron pulse frequency in vitro.

Our preliminary data in CAH patients suggest that perinatal exposure of the neuroendocrine axis to excess levels of androgen may program the neuroendocrine system to secrete excessive LH at the time of puberty, thus stimulating excessive ovarian thecal androgen secretion at that time;[103] this "masculinization" of gonadotropin secretion in women appears to depend on the duration and intensity of perinatal androgen exposure.

The secretion of an LH molecule with enhanced bioactivity has been postulated to account for the subset of women with ovarian androgen excess and normal immunoreactive levels of LH.[154, 171] Abnormal modulation of ovarian androgen responsiveness to LH by autocrine, paracrine, and endocrine factors seems to be a more attractive explanation for ovarian hyperandrogenism in the presence of normal LH levels.

Syndromes of Insulin Resistance. Hyperinsulinemia is a contributing factor to ovarian hyperandrogenism,[77, 172, 173] independent of LH excess, as demonstrated in women with generalized insulin resistance. In fact, every form of severe insulin resistance has been associated with PCOS. These include insulin receptor gene mutations,[174–179] auto-antibodies to the insulin receptor,[180] and postreceptor defects.[181–183]

Women with PCOS are, as a group, insulin-resistant. Barbieri and Ryan were the first to recognize the frequent association of hyperandrogenism, insulin resistance, and acanthosis nigricans, dubbing it the "HAIR-AN" syndrome.[77] This resistance to insulin is independent of obesity; women with PCOS are more hyperinsulinemic than weight-matched controls.[184, 185]

Some investigators[173, 186] have reported an increase in vivo in serum concentrations of AD, testosterone, and/or DHAS in response to endogenous or exogenous hyperinsulinemia, independent of changes in gonadotropin or adrenocorticotropin levels.[173, 187] The putative effects of insulin on androgen secretion have not been confirmed in other studies.[188, 189] The mechanism by which insulin might augment LH stimulation of androgen secretion in insulin-resistant states is unclear. Although it is tempting to speculate that insulin acts through IGF-I receptors, it has less than 1 per cent the affinity of IGF-I for the IGF-I receptor. The possibility exists that insulin acts by binding to hybrid receptors or indirectly by lowering IGF binding protein 1

levels, thereby raising free IGF-I levels.[32] The acromegaloid features that occasionally are found seem to represent a phenotypical expression of an IGF action of insulin and present a therapeutic challenge.[190, 190a]

True Hermaphroditism

Subjects with true hermaphroditism are characterized by the presence of functional testicular and ovarian tissue. This tissue may be separate, or it may be combined in the same gonad, in which case it is referred to as an ovotestis. Most true hermaphrodites have an XX karyotype,[191] although the use of Y-specific probes has detected Y-specific material on an X chromosome in some patients.[192] True hermaphrodites occasionally present as menstruating, phenotypical females with signs of androgen excess.[193]

Human Chorionic Gonadotropin–Related Hyperandrogenism

Virilization during pregnancy may be due to androgen hypersecretion by a luteoma or hyperreactio luteinalis. These conditions represent benign hyperplastic thecal luteinization of the ovary, solid and cystic, respectively, which spontaneously regress postpartum. Luteomas appear not to be associated with excessive levels of human chorionic gonadotropin (hCG); in contrast, hyperreactio luteinalis is almost always associated with hCG excess. Maternal virilization occurs in 10 to 50 per cent of women with luteomas and in 25 per cent of those with hyperreactio luteinalis.[194] Fetal virilization is rare because of the placental aromatization of androgen to estrogen.[194]

Peripheral Androgen Overproduction

About 10 per cent of women have idiopathic hyperandrogenism.[11] That is, a specific abnormality of androgen secretion cannot be demonstrated after extensive endocrinological evaluation. The failure to delineate a source of androgen excess may be a function of the insensitivity of available tests. The increased mass of adipose tissue of obese women is conceivably the sole source of androgen excess on occasion, since weight reduction normalizes androgen levels in some cases.[195–197] The source of androgen excess in many of these patients is unclear. We postulate that genetically increased peripheral conversion of precursors secreted by both the adrenal glands and the ovaries underlies such cases.

Tumoral Hyperandrogenism

Adrenocortical tumors, particularly carcinoma, are characterized by very high DHAS levels. Some degree of ACTH or gonadotropin dependency may be found in adrenal or ovarian virilizing tumors.[124, 198]

The most common virilizing ovarian tumor is arrhenoblastoma. Ovarian lipid cell tumors typically are gonadotropin-responsive and are dependent in part on ACTH as well.[199] Ovarian virilizing tumors typically secrete predominantly AD and are thus characterized by a disproportionate elevation of plasma AD relative to testosterone. Mild elevation of urinary 17-KS secretion characteristically results.

DIAGNOSIS OF HYPERANDROGENIC STATES

Evaluation of the woman with androgen excess includes an assessment of the pattern and quantity of hair growth. Hypertrichosis must be differentiated from hirsutism: The former is the term reserved to describe androgen-independent growth of hair that is vellus, prominent in nonsexual areas, and most commonly congenital or caused by metabolic disorders (e.g., hypothyroidism, anorexia nervosa, porphyria cutanea tarda) or medications (e.g., phenytoin, minoxidil, cyclosporine).

The degree of hirsutism may be scored, although imperfectly, by the method of Ferriman and Gallwey (Fig. 120–10) in which the body areas that possess androgen-sensitive PSU's are graded and summed. A total score of 8 or more is seen in only 5 per cent of premenopausal white women; these women, by definition, are hirsute. Acne vulgaris may be clinically scored as outlined in Table 120–4.

We recommend screening for hyperandrogenemia by measuring blood levels of total and free testosterone, and DHAS. A normal plasma total testosterone does not exclude an important hyperandrogenic disorder, such as virilizing CAH or FOH. A random value may be misleadingly normal in part because of the variation in secretion of androgens and in part because a depressed SHBG level may lower the total testosterone while an abnormally great fraction of the total testosterone is free and bioavailable. LH, FSH, AD, and prolactin may also be obtained at the time of initial evaluation.[1] A baseline plasma testosterone level in the male range (over 350 ng/dl; 12 nM) indicates a virilizing tumor, and a level over 200 ng/dl (7 nM) is suggestive. A basal DHAS level over 800 μg/dl (18.5 μM) suggests an adrenal tumor. Ultrasonography, computed tomography, or magnetic resonance imaging usually demonstrates the mass.

It is both costly and impractical to measure many steroids on multiple occasions; a strategy must be used to derive maximal diagnostic information from limited sampling. This may be accomplished by dexamethasone suppression testing (Fig. 120–11).[1]

The dexamethasone androgen-suppression test is performed by obtaining a blood sample before and after ad-

TABLE 120–4. GRADING OF ACNE LESIONS

SEVERITY	PAPULES/PUSTULES	NODULES
Microcomedonal (<1 mm)	None	None
Comedonal (≥1 mm)	None	None
Mild inflammation	Few to several	None
Moderate inflammation	Several to many	Few to several
Severe inflammation	Numerous and/or excessive*	Many

*Persistent draining, sinus tracks, ongoing scarring.
From Rosenfield RL, Lucky AW: Acne, hirsutism, and alopecia in adolescent girls: Clinical expressions of androgen excess. Clin Endocrinol Metab 22:507, 1993.

ministering a "low dose" of dexamethasone: 2 mg daily in divided doses by mouth for four days (or longer in patients who are very obese or who have relatively high DHAS levels). The pattern of response of plasma free testosterone, DHAS, and cortisol segregates patients diagnostically. Normal suppression of androgens is most specifically indicated by a reduction of the plasma free testosterone into the normal range for *dexamethasone-suppressed, nonhirsute* women. In our laboratory, dexamethasone suppressibility is considered normal in a perimenarchal or postmenarchal female if the plasma free testosterone is less than 8 pg/ml (27 pmol/L).[11] Normal adrenal suppression is indicated by a reduction of both DHAS and cortisol levels below the normal range for adult controls (less than 70 and less than 3 μg/dl, respectively, in our laboratory). Inadequate cortisol suppression indicates Cushing's syndrome or noncompliance. Subnormal suppressibility of free testosterone with normal adrenal suppression usually is due to FOH. If cortisol is suppressed, the only other considerations are virilizing tumor, true hermaphroditism, and, in pregnancy, hCG-related disorders.

An elevated serum LH level may be a useful corroborative test. However, elevation of serum LH is not specific for FOH, and about one half of women with FOH have levels that are normal.[11] Suppression of plasma free testosterone after a therapeutic trial of estrogen-progestin may also be

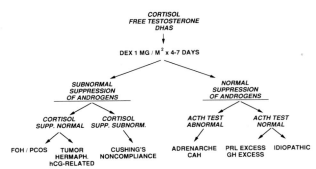

FIGURE 120–11. Algorithm for the differential diagnosis of hyperandrogenemia. The response of the plasma free testosterone, DHAS, and cortisol to DEX for four or more days is evaluated. Subnormal suppression of androgens by DEX points toward FOH/PCOS (if both DHAS and cortisol suppress normally), tumor, true hermaphroditism, or hCG-related androgen excess (if only cortisol suppresses normally), or Cushing's syndrome or noncompliance (if cortisol does not suppress normally). CAH, congenital adrenal hyperplasia; DEX, dexamethasone; FOH, functional ovarian hyperandrogenism; GH, growth hormone; HERMAPH, true hermaphroditism; PCOS, polycystic ovary syndrome; PRL, prolactin. (Modified from Ehrmann DA, Rosenfield RL: An endocrinologic approach to the patient with hirsutism. J Clin Endocrinol Metab 71:1–4. © The Endocrine Society, 1990.)

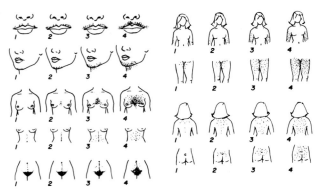

FIGURE 120–10. **Hirsutism scoring scale of Ferriman and Gallwey.** The nine body areas that possess androgen-sensitive PSU's are graded from 0 (no terminal hair) to 4 (frankly virile) and then summed. Normal hirsutism score is less than 8. (From Ehrmann DA, Rosenfield RL: An endocrinologic approach to the patient with hirsutism. J Clin Endocrinol Metab 71:1–4. © The Endocrine Society, 1990.)

confirmatory. However, gonadotropin dependence occasionally has been reported with virilizing ovarian[124] and adrenal[201] tumors.

Ovaries from women with FOH are sonographically normal in about one half of cases.[11] Conversely, polycystic ovaries may be found on ultrasound examination of women without FOH. Therefore, polycystic ovaries are not only relatively insensitive but also nonspecific for the diagnosis of ovarian hyperandrogenism. The best ultrasound correlate of ovarian steroidogenic function in hyperandrogenic women is stromal area rather than ovarian area, cyst area, or cyst number.[4, 202]

GnRH agonist testing is a promising means of making a specific diagnosis of FOH. Our data suggest that a peak 17-PROG level more than 259 ng/dl (7.8 nmol/L) after the administration of 100 μg of nafarelin subcutaneously is virtually diagnostic.[11] The results of nafarelin testing are highly concordant (85 per cent) with dexamethasone suppression testing.

TREATMENT OF HYPERANDROGENISM

Hirsutism and Acne

The pharmacological therapy of androgen excess is directed at interrupting one or more of the steps in the pathway leading to its expression: (1) suppression of adrenal and/or ovarian androgen production, (2) alteration of binding of androgens to their plasma binding proteins, (3) impairment of the peripheral conversion of androgen precursors to active androgen, and (4) inhibition of androgen action at the target tissue level.

Combination estrogen-progestin therapy in the form of an oral contraceptive is the first-line endocrine treatment for hirsutism and acne after cosmetic and dermatological management. The estrogenic component of most oral contraceptives currently in use is either ethinyl estradiol or mestranol. The estrogenic component in particular is responsible for the suppression of LH and, thus, serum androgen levels[203] and also results in a dose-related increase in SHBG,[204] thus lowering the fraction of plasma testosterone that is unbound. Combination therapy has also been demonstrated to decrease DHAS levels, perhaps by reducing ACTH levels.[205, 206] Estrogens also have a direct, dose-dependent suppressive effect on sebaceous cell function, with a uniform effect on acne at a dose of 100 μg of mestranol.[207]

The choice of a specific oral contraceptive should be predicated on the progestational component because each progestin has a variably suppressive effect on SHBG levels as well as some androgenic potential. Ethynodiol diacetate has a relatively low androgenic potential, whereas progestins such as norethindrone, norethindrone acetate, norgestrel, and levonorgestrel are particularly androgenic,[208] as can be judged from their attenuation of the estrogen-induced increase in SHBG.[209]

Assessment of adequacy of ovarian suppression can be made at the end of the third week after starting treatment; by this time ovarian androgen suppression is complete.[203] The effect on acne can be expected to be maximal in one to two months. In contrast, the effect on hair growth may not be evident for 6 months, and the maximum effect

requires 9 to 12 months because of the length of the hair growth cycle. In most trials estrogen-progestin therapy alone improves the extent of acne by 50 to 70 per cent.[210] Although similar claims have been made for hirsutism,[211] it is our experience that this treatment typically does little more than arrest progression of hair growth.

GnRH agonists have been reported to be effective in the treatment of hirsutism.[212–214] Their chronic administration suppresses pituitary-ovarian function, thus inhibiting both ovarian androgen and estrogen secretion. The addition of dexamethasone (0.5 mg/day) to leuprolide has been reported to further improve the response of some women with PCOS.[70] Because of the concomitant reduction of serum estrogen levels and the attendant, albeit apparently reversible, reductions in bone mineral density observed when GnRH agonists are used alone,[215, 216] it appears unwise to use these agents for longer than six months. It has been suggested that "add back" therapy in which combination estrogen and progestin is prescribed in conjunction with a GnRH agonist may be effective in treating androgen excess without the adverse effects of hypoestrogenemia.[217]

Adrenal androgens are more sensitive than cortisol to the suppressive effects of glucocorticoids.[7] Therefore, glucocorticoids are the mainstay of treatment of the adrenal androgen excess of CAH but appear to be less effective in other forms of functional adrenal androgen excess.[218, 219] It has been claimed, however, that menstrual irregularities are corrected in about 50 per cent of patients with PCOS by prednisone treatment.[220]

Prednisone in doses of 5 to 10 mg at bedtime usually is effective in suppressing adrenal androgens while posing minimal risk of the sequelae of glucocorticoid excess. We do not advocate the use of dexamethasone because it is difficult to prevent cushingoid striae even with dosages as low as 0.5 mg daily. DHAS levels are used to indicate the degree of adrenal suppression; the target is a level of about 70 μg/dl. It has been suggested by some that anti-androgen therapy in the form of cyproterone acetate[221] or spironolactone[219] is at least as effective as glucocorticoid for the treatment of hirsutism caused by adrenal androgen excess (see below).

Ketoconazole, a synthetic imidazole antifungal agent, inhibits multiple steps in the biosynthesis of testosterone but acts primarily to inhibit 17-hydroxylase/17,20-lyase and 11β-hydroxylase activities.[222, 223] In dosages of 400 mg/day for six months, it has been demonstrated to have a moderate salutary effect on acne and hirsutism, although adverse effects are relatively frequent and include nausea, dry skin, pruritus, and transaminase elevation.[224]

Cyproterone acetate is the prototypical antiandrogen. It acts mainly by competitive inhibition of the binding of testosterone and DHT to the androgen receptor.[225] In addition, it may act to enhance the metabolic clearance of testosterone by inducing hepatic enzymes. Although not available for use in the United States, cyproterone acetate is an effective treatment for hirsutism and acne[226, 227] and is used throughout Canada, Mexico, and Europe. Because of its potent progestational activity and its prolonged half-time, it is administered in a "reverse sequential" manner: cyproterone acetate 50 to 100 mg/day from day 5 to day 15 of the cycle with ethinyl estradiol in a dosage of 35 to 50 μg/day from day 5 to day 26 of the cycle.[226] The dose of cyproterone acetate may be reduced incrementally at six-month intervals. Diane (2 mg of cyproterone acetate with

50 μg of ethinyl estradiol) may be effective in maintaining improvement in milder cases of hirsutism. The adverse effects of cyproterone acetate include irregular uterine bleeding, nausea, headache, fatigue, weight gain, and decreased libido.

Spironolactone appears to be as effective an anti-androgen as cyproterone acetate in dosages of 100 to 200 mg daily.[228, 229] It is a potent antimineralocorticoid that was developed as a progestational analogue and has diverse effects on steroid metabolism.[230–233] Although there has been concern about possible toxicity, its adverse effects are remarkably few; however, patients must be monitored for hyperkalemia and hypotension. Its major adverse effect is menstrual irregularity when used alone. Estrogen-progestin should be given in conjunction with spironolactone[234, 235] not only for this reason but to prevent pregnancy because of the danger of feminization of a male fetus.

Flutamide is a potent nonsteroidal antiandrogen without progestational, estrogenic, corticoid, antigonadotropic, or androgenic activity.[236] Preliminary data indicate that it may be efficacious in the treatment of hirsutism. In a seven-month trial of flutamide (250 mg twice daily) in conjunction with an estrogen-progestin, marked improvement in acne, seborrhea, and hirsutism was reported.[237] Concerns about the induction of hepatocellular dysfunction have limited its use.

Finasteride, a 4-aza steroid, is a competitive inhibitor of 5α-reductase that does not compete with DHT for binding to the androgen receptor.[238] Although only recently approved for the treatment of benign prostatic hyperplasia, this compound holds potential for the therapy of hirsutism, acne, and male-pattern baldness.

Finally, administration of a long-acting somatostatin analogue has been reported to lower serum androgen concentrations in women with PCOS.[239]

Anovulatory Symptoms

Progestin alone is useful in the management of anovulatory symptoms in patients who present without hirsutism or acne. Progestins are ineffective in correcting androgen levels when used alone, however.[240] Progestin-induced withdrawal bleeding is indicated in the attempt to reduce the increased risk of endometrial cancer[241] imparted by unopposed estrogen stimulation. A common regimen is to give 10 mg of medroxyprogesterone acetate daily for 10 days each month.

Ovulation induction usually can be accomplished by medical maneuvers that improve the LH:FSH ratio. The standard therapy for ovulation induction in PCOS is clomiphene citrate. This causes an increase in both pulsatile LH and FSH secretion[242] and an overall improvement (decrease) in the LH:FSH ratio, allowing for recruitment and selection of a dominant follicle. Using a graduated regimen of 50 to 250 mg daily for five days, ovulation can be induced in about 80 per cent of women with PCOS, of whom about one half conceive.[243, 244] If ovulation does not occur, combined therapy with dexamethasone and clomiphene often is successful in those patients in whom adrenal androgens are significantly elevated.[245]

Failure to achieve pregnancy in women made ovulatory with clomiphene most commonly is a result of associated tubal disease, poor cervical mucus, or male infertility.[243, 244] Both an antiestrogenic effect on cervical mucus production and an inadequate luteal phase have been proposed as treatment-related factors that limit conception after ovulation induction with clomiphene therapy.[244] Poor cervical mucus on an appropriately timed postcoital test during an ovulatory clomiphene cycle can be successfully treated with intrauterine insemination[246] or with the administration of estrogen during a clomiphene cycle.[244] An inadequate luteal phase is best treated by increasing the clomiphene dose.[244, 247, 248] Luteal-phase progesterone supplementation may also be effective.[248]

Patients who fail to ovulate or to become pregnant using clomiphene therapy present a challenging management problem. Advances in therapy with human menopausal gonadotropin (hMG), purified FSH, pulsatile GnRH, and GnRH agonist pretreatment have greatly expanded treatment options.

hMG is effective in ovulation induction in PCOS.[249, 250] Despite the equal amounts of LH and FSH administered, the LH:FSH ratio is corrected because of the longer serum half-life of FSH, and ovulation occurs. The pregnancy rate is about 60 per cent after two or three treatment cycles. Indeed, the challenge with hMG is to prevent ovarian hyperstimulation, which is frequent in this syndrome. During hMG therapy, follicular development should be monitored by frequent ultrasound measurement of follicular diameter and frequent estradiol levels. hCG is given to induce ovulation when the largest follicle has a mean diameter of 16 to 18 mm. To prevent hyperstimulation, hCG should not be given if estradiol is greater than 2000 pg/ml (7500 pmol/L). Purified human FSH has been approved to induce ovulation in PCOS. The pregnancy rate and incidence of ovarian hyperstimulation appear to be similar with hMG or purified FSH.[251]

Because conventional doses of gonadotropins of 150 IU/day often cause ovarian hyperstimulation in PCOS, several groups have attempted to induce ovulation using lower doses. Therapy usually is begun with 75 IU/day of purified FSH or hMG. Patients remain on this dose for 7 to 14 days, and the dose is then increased by one-half ampul (37.5 IU) at seven-day intervals if no significant follicle growth occurs.[252–255] Compared with conventional doses of gonadotropins, low-dose protocols result in significant decreases in the number of developing follicles, estradiol on the day of hCG, and risk of ovarian hyperstimulation.[252, 253, 255] In a prospective, randomized trial, low-dose hMG was as effective as low-dose purified FSH in ovulation induction in PCOS. There was no difference between the two gonadotropin preparations in the number of ampuls required, number of follicles recruited, estradiol level on the day of hCG, pregnancy rate, or spontaneous abortion rate.[254]

Another therapeutic approach to normalize the LH:FSH ratio and induce ovulation is pulsatile administration of exogenous GnRH. When GnRH is given to patients as intravenous pulses every 90 to 120 minutes, it appears to override the endogenous pattern of GnRH secretion and normalize the LH:FSH ratio. LH levels may become normal, and ovulation may occur with less chance of ovarian hyperstimulation.[256, 257] Ovulation is not always achieved in patients with PCOS, and ovulation and pregnancy rates are much lower than for women with hypogonadotropic amenorrhea similarly treated.[258, 259]

Inhibition of pituitary gonadotropin production by prolonged daily administration of GnRH agonists before administration of hMG, purified FSH, or pulsatile GnRH has also been attempted in women with PCOS in whom pregnancy has not occurred with the latter agents alone. The rationale for this regimen is that conversion of the pituitary-ovarian axis from a high-LH, hyperandrogenic, prematurely luteinized to a hypogonadotropic, hypogonadal state may favor ovum maturation and fertilizability.[260–263]

In a prospective, randomized trial GnRH agonist treatment before and during hMG administration eliminated premature luteinization as determined by levels of LH and progesterone on the day of hCG administration.[264] Cycle fecundity was almost doubled in the GnRH agonist–treated group, but the groups were not large enough for the difference to reach statistical significance. The incidence of hyperstimulation was unchanged. The persistent occurrence of hyperstimulation despite elimination of excessive LH secretion by the GnRH agonist is compatible with the concept that PCOS may be caused by intrinsic ovarian abnormalities. GnRH agonist treatment may also reduce the high incidence of recurrent spontaneous abortion found in PCOS.[264a–c]

GnRH agonist pretreatment may also improve PCOS response to pulsatile GnRH. GnRH agonist pretreatment for two months about doubles both ovulatory and pregnancy rates compared with untreated cycles.[258, 263] GnRH agonist pretreatment was particularly successful in the nonobese patients with PCOS.

Because of the difficulty of medically inducing ovulation in many patients with PCOS, there has been a revival of interest in surgical therapies. For many years the mainstay of ovulation induction in PCOS was ovarian wedge resection, which resulted in pregnancy in about 65 per cent of patients.[265] Wedge resection fell out of favor with the development of medical means of ovulation induction and because of concern about postsurgical tubo-ovarian adhesion formation worsening infertility.[265] Recent authors have described laparoscopic techniques using either the laser or the electrocautery to burn multiple small, shallow holes in the ovarian cortex.[266, 267] About 80 per cent of patients ovulate spontaneously after surgery, and many of those remaining respond to clomiphene. Pregnancy rates vary from 45 to 70 per cent with 6 to 12 months of follow-up. Although the risk of severe postoperative adhesion formation is not great, these laparoscopic techniques should be limited to patients who are unresponsive to medical induction of ovulation.[267–269]

REFERENCES

1. Ehrmann DA, Rosenfield RL: An endocrinologic approach to the patient with hirsutism. J Clin Endocrinol Metab 71:1–4, 1990.
2. Miller WL: Molecular biology of steroid hormone synthesis. Endocrinol Rev 9:295–318, 1988.
3. Fevold HR, Lorence MC, McCarthy JL, et al: Rat P450c17α from testis: Characterization of a full-length cDNA encoding a unique steroid hydroxylase capable of catalyzing both Δ4- and Δ5-steroid-17,20-lyase reactions. Mol Endocrinol 3:968–973, 1989.
4. Rosenfield RL, Ehrmann DA, Barnes RB, Sheikh Z: Gonadotropin releasing hormone agonist as a probe for the pathogenesis and diagnosis of ovarian hyperandrogenism. Ann NY Acad Sci 687:162–181, 1993.
5. Rheaume E, Lachance Y, Zhao H-F, et al: Structure and expression of a new complementary DNA encoding the almost exclusive 3β-hydroxysteroid dehydrogenase/Δ5-Δ4-isomerase in human adrenals and gonads. Mol Endocrinol 5:1147–1157, 1991.
6. Rosenfield RL, Lucky AW: Acne, hirsutism and alopecia in adolescent girls: Clinical expressions of androgen excess. Clin Endocrinol Metab 22:507, 1993.
7. Rittmaster RS, Loriaux DL, Cutler GB: Sensitivity of cortisol and adrenal androgens to dexamethasone suppression in hirsute women. J Clin Endocrinol Metab 61:462–466, 1985.
8. Cutler GB, Davis ES, Johnsonbaugh RE, Loriaux DL: Dissociation of cortisol and adrenal androgen secretion in patients with secondary adrenal insufficiency. J Clin Endocrinol Metab 49:604–609, 1979.
9. Parker LN: Adrenarche. Endocrinol Metab Clin North Am 20:71–83, 1991.
10. Erickson GF, Magoffin DA, Dyer CA, Hofeditz C: The ovarian androgen producing cells: A review of structure/function relationships. Endocrinol Rev 6:371–399, 1985.
11. Ehrmann DA, Rosenfield RL, Barnes RB, et al: Detection of functional ovarian hyperandrogenism in women with androgen excess. N Engl J Med 327:157–162, 1992.
12. Inkster SE, Brodie AMH: Expression of aromatase cytochrome P-450 in premenopausal and postmenopausal human ovaries: An immunocytochemical study. J Clin Endocrinol Metab 73:717–726, 1991.
13. Barnes R, Rosenfield RL: The polycystic ovary syndrome: Pathogenesis and treatment. Ann Intern Med 110:386–399, 1989.
14. Ross GT, Cargille CM, Lipsett MB, et al: Pituitary and gonadal hormones in women during spontaneous and induced ovulatory cycles. Recent Prog Horm Res 26:1–62, 1970.
15. Rosenfield RL, Ehrlich EN, Cleary RE: Adrenal and ovarian contributions to the elevated free plasma androgen levels in hirsute women. J Clin Endocrinol 34:92–98, 1972.
16. Abraham GE: Ovarian and adrenal contributions to peripheral androgens during the menstrual cycle. J Clin Endocrinol Metab 39:340–346, 1974.
17. Dunaif A: Do androgens directly regulate gonadotropin secretion in the polycystic ovary syndrome? J Clin Endocrinol Metab 63:215–221, 1986.
18. Serafini P, Silva PD, Paulson RJ, et al: Acute modulation of the hypothalamic-pituitary axis by intravenous testosterone in normal women. Am J Obstet Gynecol 155:1288–1292, 1986.
19. Rosenfield RL: The ovary and female sexual maturation. In Kaplan SA (ed): Clinical Pediatric and Adolescent Endocrinology (ed 2). Philadelphia, WB Saunders, 1990, pp 259–324.
20. McNatty KP, Makris A, Reinhold VN, et al: Metabolism of androstenedione by human ovarian tissues in vitro with particular reference to 5α-reductase and aromatase activity. Steroids 34:429–434, 1979.
21. Adashi EY, Hsueh AJW: Autoregulation of androgen production in a primary culture of rat testicular cells. Nature 293:737–738, 1981.
22. Hild-Petito S, West NB, Brenner RM, Stouffer RL: Localization of androgen receptor in the follicle and corpus luteum of the primate ovary during the menstrual cycle. Biol Reprod 44:561–567, 1991.
23. Billiar RB, Loukides JA, Miller MM: Evidence for the presence of the estrogen receptor in the ovary of the baboon (Papio anubis). J Clin Endocrinol Metab 75:1159–1165, 1992.
24. Hernandez ER, Hurwitz A, Vera A, et al: Expression of the genes encoding the insulin-like growth factors and their receptors in the human ovary. J Clin Endocrinol Metab 74:419–425, 1992.
25. Cara JF, Rosenfield RL: Insulin-like growth factor-I and insulin potentiate luteinizing hormone-induced androgen synthesis by rat ovarian theca-interstitial cells. Endocrinology 123:733–739, 1988.
26. Hernandez ER, Resnick CE, Svoboda ME, et al: Somatomedin-C/insulin-like growth factor I as an enhancer of androgen biosynthesis by cultured rat ovarian cells. Endocrinology 122:1603–1612, 1988.
27. Hillier SG, Yong EL, Illingworth PJ, et al: Effect of recombinant inhibin on androgen synthesis in cultured human thecal cells. Mol Cell Endocrinol 75:R1–R6, 1991.
28. Magoffin DA, Kurtz KM, Erickson GF: Insulin-like growth factor-I selectively stimulates cholesterol side-chain cleavage expression in ovarian theca-interstitial cells. Mol Endocrinol 4:489–496, 1990.
29. Poretsky L, Glover B, Laumas V, et al: The effects of experimental hyperinsulinemia on steroid secretion, ovarian [125I]insulin binding, and ovarian [125I]insulin-like growth-factor I binding in the rat. Endocrinology 122:581–585, 1988.
30. Barbieri RL, Smith S, Ryan KJ: The role of hyperinsulinemia in the pathogenesis of ovarian hyperandrogenism. Fertil Steril 50:197–212, 1988.
30a. Prager D, Melmed S: Insulin and insulin-like growth factor I recep-

tors: Are there functional distinctions? Endocrinology 132:1419–1420, 1993.

31. Poretsky L: On the paradox of insulin-induced hyperandrogenism in insulin-resistant states. Endocrinol Rev 12:3–13, 1991.

32. Nobels F, Dewailly D: Puberty and polycystic ovarian syndrome: The insulin/insulin-like growth factor I hypothesis. Fertil Steril (in press).

33. Yen SSC: Interface between extra- and intra-ovarian factors in PCOS. Ann NY Acad Sci 687:98–111, 1993.

33a. Bondy C, Zhou J: Insulin-like growth factor system gene expression in the postpubertal human ovary. Ann NY Acad Sci 687:65–76, 1993.

34. Rainey S: Prostaglandin E₂ is a positive regulator of adrenocorticotropin receptor, 3β-hydroxysteroid dehydrogenase, and 17α-hydroxylase expression in bovine adrenocortical cells. Endocrinology 129:1333–1339, 1991.

35. Palumbo A, Carcangiu ML, Roa L, et al: The ovarian renin-angiotensin system in polycystic ovarian syndrome. Ann NY Acad Sci 687:39–45, 1993.

36. Adashi EY: The potential relevance of cytokines to ovarian physiology: The emerging role of resident ovarian cells of the white blood cell series. Endocrinol Rev 11:454–464, 1990.

37. Hernandez ER, Hurwitz A, Payne DW, et al: Transforming growth factor-β1 inhibits ovarian androgen production: Gene expression, cellular localization, mechanism(s) and site(s) of action. Endocrinology 127:2804–2811, 1990.

38. Franks S, Mason HD: Polycystic ovary syndrome: Interaction of follicle stimulating hormone and polypeptide growth factors in oestradiol production by human granulosa cells. J Steroid Biochem Molec Biol 40:405–409, 1991.

39. Hillier SG, Yong EL, Illingworth PJ, et al: Effect of recombinant activin on androgen synthesis in cultured human thecal cells. J Clin Endocrinol Metab 72:1206–1211, 1991.

40. Jaattela M, Ilvesmaki V, Voutilainen R, et al: Tumor necrosis factor as a potent inhibitor of adrenocorticotropin-induced cortisol production and steroidogenic P450 enzyme gene expression in cultured human fetal adrenal cells. Endocrinology 128:623–629, 1991.

41. Hurwitz A, Payne DW, Packman JN, et al: Cytokine-mediated regulation of ovarian function: Interleukin-1 inhibits gonadotropin-induced androgen biosynthesis. Endocrinology 129:1250–1256, 1991.

42. McNatty KP, Baird DT: Relationship between follicle stimulating hormone, androstenedione and estradiol in human follicular fluid. J Endocrinol 76:527–531, 1978.

43. McNatty KP, Smith DM, Makris A, et al: The microenvironment of the human antral follicle: Interrelationships among the steroid levels in antral fluid, the population of granulosa cells, and the status of the oocyte in vivo and in vitro. J Clin Endocrinol Metab 49:851–860, 1979.

44. Mondschein JS, Canning SF, Miller DQ, Hammond JM: Insulin-like growth factors (IGFs) as autocrine/paracrine regulators of granulosa cell differentiation and growth: Studies with a neutralizing monoclonal antibody to IGF-I. Biol Reprod 40:79–85, 1989.

45. Adashi EY, Resnick CE, D'Ercole AJ, et al: Insulin-like growth factors as intraovarian regulators of granulosa cell growth and function. Endocrinol Rev 6:400–420, 1985.

46. Bergh C, Carlsson B, Olsson J-H, et al: Effects of insulin-like growth factor and growth hormone in cultured human granulosa cells. Ann NY Acad Sci 626:169–176, 1991.

47. Shimasaki S, Shimonaka M, Ui M, et al: Structural characterization of a follicle-stimulating hormone action inhibitor in porcine ovarian follicular fluid. J Biol Chem 265:2198–2202, 1990.

48. Bicsak TA, Shimonaka M, Malkowski M, Ling N: Insulin-like growth factor-binding protein (IGF-BP) inhibition of granulosa cell function. Endocrinology 126:2184–2189, 1990.

49. Mason HD, Margara R, Winston RML, et al: Inhibition of oestradiol production by epidermal growth factor in human granulosa cells of normal and polycystic ovaries. Clin Endocrinol 33:511–517, 1990.

50. Hillier SG, van den Boogard AJM, Reichart LE Jr, van Hall EV: Alterations in granulosa cell aromatase activity accompanying preovulatory follicular development in the rat ovary with evidence that 5α-reduced C19 steroids inhibit the aromatase reaction in vitro. J Endocrinol 84:409–419, 1980.

51. Harlow CR, Shaw HJ, Hillier SG, Hodges JK: Factors influencing follicle-stimulating hormone-responsive steroidogenesis in marmoset granulosa cells: Effects of androgens and the stage of follicular maturity. Endocrinology 122:2780–2786, 1988.

52. Brailly S, Gougeon A, Milgrom E, et al: Androgens and progestins in the human ovarian follicle: Differences in the evolution of preovulatory, healthy nonovulatory and atretic follicles. J Clin Endocrinol Metab 53:128–134, 1981.

53. Bleau G, Roberts KD, Chapdelaine A: The in vitro and in vivo uptake and metabolism of steroids in human adipose tissue. J Clin Endocrinol Metab 39:236–246, 1974.

54. Kirschner MA, Bardin CW: Androgen production and metabolism in normal and virilized women. Metabolism 21:667–688, 1972.

55. Vermeulen A, Ando S: Metabolic clearance rate and interconversion of androgens and influence of the free androgen fraction. J Clin Endocrinol Metab 48:320–325, 1979.

56. Mauvais-Jarvis P: Regulation of androgen receptor and 5α-reductase in the skin of normal and hirsute women. Clin Endocrinol Metab 15:307–317, 1986.

57. Rosenfield RL: Pilosebaceous physiology in relation to hirsutism and acne. Clin Endocrinol Metab 15:341–362, 1986.

58. Rosenfield RL, Moll GW Jr: The role of proteins in the distribution of plasma androgens and estradiol. *In* Molinatti G, Martini L, James VHT (eds): Androgenization in Women. New York, Raven Press, 1989, pp 25–45.

59. Nestler JE, Powers LP, Matt DW, et al: A direct effect of hyperinsulinemia on serum sex hormone–binding globulin levels in obese women with the polycystic ovary syndrome. J Clin Endocrinol Metab 72:83–89, 1991.

60. Rosner W: Plasma steroid–binding proteins. Endocrinol Metab Clin North Am 20:697–720, 1991.

61. Moll GW Jr, Rosenfield RL: Estradiol inhibition of pituitary luteinizing hormone release is antagonized by serum proteins. J Steroid Biochem 25:309–314, 1986.

62. Mendel CM: The free hormone hypothesis: A physiologically based mathematical model. Endocrinol Rev 10:232–274, 1989.

63. Ekins R: Measurement of free hormones in blood. Endocrinol Rev 11:5–46, 1990.

64. Mowszowicz I, Melanitou E, Kirchoffer MD, Mauvais-Jarvis P: Dihydrotestosterone stimulates 5α-reductase activity in pubic skin fibroblasts. J Clin Endocrinol Metab 79:29–34, 1978.

65. Itami S, Kurata S, Sonoda T, Takayasu S: Characterization of 5α-reductase in cultured human dermal papilla cells from beard and occipital scalp hair. J Invest Dermatol 96:57–62, 1991.

66. Lobo RA, Goebelsman U, Horton R: Evidence for the importance of peripheral tissue events in the development of hirsutism in polycystic ovary syndrome. J Clin Endocrinol Metab 57:393–397, 1983.

67. Lobo RA, Paul WL, Gentzschein E, et al: Production of 3α-androstanediol glucuronide in human genital skin. J Clin Endocrinol Metab 65:711–714, 1987.

68. Scanlon MJ, Whorwood CB, Franks S, et al: Serum androstanediol glucuronide concentrations in normal and hirsute women and patients with thyroid dysfunction. Clin Endocrinol 29:529–538, 1988.

69. Pang S, Wang M, Jeffries S, et al: Normal and elevated 3α-androstanediol glucuronide concentrations in women with various causes of hirsutism and its correlation with degree of hirsutism and androgen levels. J Clin Endocrinol Metab 75:243–248, 1992.

70. Rittmaster RS, Thompson DI: Effect of leuprolide and dexamethasone on hair growth and hormone levels in hirsute women: The relative importance of the ovary and the adrenal in the pathogenesis of hirsutism. J Clin Endocrinol Metab 70:1096–1102, 1990.

70a. Rittmaster R, Zwicker H, Thompson DL, et al: Androstanediol glucuronide production in human liver, prostate, and skin. J Clin Endocrinol Metab 76:977–982, 1993.

71. French FS, Lubahn DB, Brown TR, et al: Molecular basis of androgen insensitivity. Rec Prog Horm Res 46:1–20, 1990.

72. Bagchi MK, Tsai MJ, O'Malley BW, Tsai SY: Analysis of the mechanism of steroid hormone receptor-dependent gene activation in cell-free systems. Endocrinol Rev 13:525–535, 1992.

73. Randall VA, Ebling FVG: Seasonal changes in human hair growth. Br J Dermatol 124:146–151, 1991.

74. Reingold SB, Rosenfield RL: The relationship of mild hirsutism or acne in women to androgens. Arch Dermatol 123:209–212, 1987.

75. Marynick SP, Chakmakjian ZH, McCaffree DL, et al: Androgen excess in cystic acne. N Engl J Med 308:981–984, 1983.

76. Dunaif A, Green G, Phelps RG, et al: Acanthosis nigricans, insulin action, and hyperandrogenism: Clinical, histological, and biochemical findings. J Clin Endocrinol Metab 73:590–595, 1991.

77. Barbieri RL, Ryan KJ: Hyperandrogenism, insulin resistance and acanthosis nigricans syndrome: A common endocrinopathy with distinct pathophysiologic features. Am J Obstet Gynecol 147:90–101, 1983.

78. Erickson GF, Hsueh AJ, Quigley ME, et al: Functional studies of aromatase activity in human granulosa cells from normal and polycystic ovaries. J Clin Endocrinol Metab 49:514–519, 1979.

79. Schreiber JR, Reed R, Ross GT: A receptor-like testosterone-binding

protein in ovaries from estrogen-stimulated hypophysectomized immature female rats. Endocrinology 98:1206–1213, 1976.
80. Uilenbrock JTJ, Woutersen PJA, Van der Schoot P: Atresia in preovulatory follicles: Gonadotropin binding and steroidogenic activity. Biol Reprod 23:219–229, 1980.
81. Louvet JP, Harman SM, Schreiber JR, Ross GT: Evidence for a role of androgens in follicular maturation. Endocrinology 97:366–372, 1975.
82. Hillier S, Ross GT: Effects of exogenous testosterone on ovarian weight, follicular morphology and intraovarian progesterone concentration in estrogen-primed hypophysectomized immature female rats. Biol Reprod 20:261–268, 1979.
83. Futterweit W, Deligdisch L: Histopathological effects of exogenously administered testosterone in 19 female to male transsexuals. J Clin Endocrinol Metab 62:16–21, 1986.
84. Spinder T, Spijkstra JJ, Van Den Tweel JG, et al: The effects of long term testosterone administration on pulsatile luteinizing hormone secretion and on ovarian histology in eugonadal female to male transsexual subjects. J Clin Endocrinol Metab 69:151–157, 1989.
85. Erickson GF, Magoffin DA, Jones KL: Theca function in polycystic ovaries of a patient with virilizing congenital adrenal hyperplasia. Fertil Steril 51:173–176, 1989.
86. Hoffman F, Meger C: On the action of intraovarian injection of androgen on follicle and corpus luteum maturation in women. Geburtshilfe Frauenheilkd 25:1132–1137, 1965.
87. Rosenfield RL, Rich BH, Lucky AW: Adrenarche as a cause of benign pseudopuberty in boys. J Pediatr 101:1005–1009, 1982.
88. Oberfield SE, Mayes DM, Levine L: Adrenal steroidogenic function in a black and Hispanic population with precocious pubarche. J Clin Endocrinol Metab 70:76–82, 1990.
89. Lashansky G, Saenger P, Fishman K, et al: Normative data for adrenal steroidogenesis in a healthy pediatric population: Age- and sex-related changes after adrenocorticotropin stimulation. J Clin Endocrinol Metab 73:674–686, 1991.
90. Rich BH, Rosenfield RL, Lucky AW, et al: Adrenarche: Changing adrenal response to ACTH. J Clin Endocrinol Metab 52:1129–1136, 1981.
91. Lucky AW, Rosenfield RL, McGuire J, et al: Adrenal androgen hyperresponsiveness to ACTH in women with acne and/or hirsutism: Adrenal enzyme defects and exaggerated adrenarche. J Clin Endocrinol Metab 62:840–848, 1986.
92. Eldar-Geva T, Hurwitz A, Vecsei P, et al: Secondary biosynthetic defects in women with late-onset congenital adrenal hyperplasia. N Engl J Med 323:855–863, 1990.
93. Barnes RB, Ehrmann DA, Brigell DF, Rosenfield RL: Ovarian steroidogenic responses to gonadotropin-releasing hormone agonist testing with nafarelin in hirsute women with adrenal responses to ACTH suggestive of 3β-hydroxy-Δ⁵-steroid dehydrogenase deficiency. J Clin Endocrinol Metab 76:450–455, 1993.
94. Rosenfield RL, Barnes RB, Cara JF, Lucky AW: Dysregulation of cytochrome P450c17α as the cause of polycystic ovary syndrome. Fertil Steril 53:785–791, 1990.
95. Lobo RA: The role of the adrenal in polycystic ovary syndrome. Reprod Endocrinol 2:251–264, 1984.
96. McKenna TJ: Current concepts: Pathogenesis and treatment of polycystic ovary syndrome. N Engl J Med 318:558–562, 1988.
97. Miller WL, Levine LS: Molecular and clinical advances in congenital adrenal hyperplasia. J Pediatr 111:1–17, 1987.
98. White PC, New MI, Dupont B: Congenital adrenal hyperplasia. N Engl J Med 316:1519–1524, 1580–1586, 1987.
99. Kuttenn F, Couillin P, Girard P, et al: Late-onset adrenal hyperplasia in hirsutism. N Engl J Med 313:224–231, 1985.
100. Levine LS, Dupont B, Lorenzen F, et al: Genetic and hormonal characterization of cryptic 21-hydroxylase deficiency. J Clin Endocrinol Metab 53:1193–1198, 1981.
101. New MI, Lorenzen F, Lerner AJ, et al: Genotyping steroid 21-hydroxylase deficiency: Hormonal reference data. J Clin Endocrinol Metab 57:320–326, 1983.
102. Dewailly D, Vantyghem-Haudiquet MC, Sainsard C, et al: Clinical and biological phenotypes in late-onset 21-hydroxylase deficiency. J Clin Endocrinol Metab 63:418–423, 1986.
103. Barnes RB, Rosenfield RL: Masculinization of the human pituitary-ovarian axis by perinatal androgen exposure: Polycystic ovary syndrome (PCOS) in congenital adrenal virilizing disease (CAVD). 73rd Annual Meeting of the Endocrine Society, Washington, DC, June 19–22, 1991.
104. Levin JH, Carmina E, Lobo RA: Is the inappropriate gonadotropin secretion of patients with polycystic ovary syndrome similar to that of patients with adult-onset congenital adrenal hyperplasia? Fertil Steril 56:635–640, 1991.
105. Chrousos GP, Loriaux DL, Mann DL, Cutler GB Jr: Late-onset 21-hydroxylase deficiency mimicking idiopathic hirsutism or polycystic ovarian disease. Ann Intern Med 96:143–148, 1982.
106. Speiser PW, Dupont J, Zhu D, et al: Disease expression and molecular genotype in congenital adrenal hyperplasia due to 21-hydroxylase deficiency. J Clin Invest 90:584–595, 1992.
107. Rosler A, Weshler N, Lieberman E, et al: 11β-hydroxylased deficiency congenital adrenal hyperplasia: Update of prenatal diagnosis. J Clin Endocrinol Metab 66:830–838, 1988.
108. Siegel SF, Finegold DN, Lanes R, Lee PA: ACTH stimulation tests and plasma dehydroepiandrosterone sulfate levels in women with hirsutism. N Engl J Med 323:849–854, 1990.
109. Schram P, Zerah M, Mani P, Jewelewicz R, et al: Nonclassical 3β-hydroxysteroid dehydrogenase deficiency: A review of our experience with 25 female patients. Fertil Steril 58:129–136, 1992.
110. Mathieson J, Couzinet B, Wekstein-Noel S, et al: The incidence of late-onset congenital adrenal hyperplasia due to 3β-hydroxysteroid dehydrogenase deficiency among hirsute women. Clin Endocrinol 36:383–388, 1992.
111. Hauffa BP, Kaplan SL, Grumbach MM: Dissociation between plasma adrenal androgens and cortisol in Cushing's disease and ectopic ACTH-producing tumour: Relation to adrenarche. Lancet 1:1373–1375, 1984.
112. Malchoff CD, Javier EC, Malchoff DM, et al: Primary cortisol resistance presenting as isosexual precocity. J Clin Endocrinol Metab 70:503–507, 1990.
113. Lamberts SWJ, Koper JW, Biemond P, et al: Cortisol receptor resistance: The variability of its clinical presentation and response to treatment. J Clin Endocrinol Metab 74:313–321, 1992.
114. Taylor NF, Bartlett WA, Dawson DJ, Enoch BA: Cortisone reductase deficiency: Evidence for a new inborn error in metabolism of cortisone to cortisol. J Endocrinol 102S:90–96, 1984.
115. Phillipou G, Higgins BA: A new defect in the peripheral metabolism of cortisone to cortisol. J Steroid Biochem 22:435–436, 1985.
116. Glickman SP, Rosenfield RL, Bergenstal RM, Helke J: Multiple androgenic abnormalities, including elevated free testosterone in hyperprolactinemic women. J Clin Endocrinol Metab 55:251–257, 1982.
117. Futterweit W, Krieger DT: Pituitary tumors associated with hyperprolactinemia and polycystic ovary disease. Fertil Steril 31:608–613, 1979.
118. Monroe SE, Levine L, Chang J, et al: Prolactin-secreting pituitary adenomas. V. Increased gonadotroph responsivity in hyperprolactinemic women with pituitary adenomas. J Clin Endocrinol Metab 52:1171–1178, 1981.
119. Vermeulen A, Ando S, Verdonck L: Prolactinomas, testosterone binding globulin, and androgen metabolism. J Clin Endocrinol Metab 54:409–412, 1982.
120. Higuchi K, Nawata H, Maki T, et al: Prolactin has a direct effect on adrenal androgen secretion. J Clin Endocrinol Metab 59:714–718, 1984.
121. Schiebinger RJ, Chrousos GP, Cutler GB, Loriaux DL: The effect of serum prolactin on plasma adrenal androgens and the production and metabolic clearance rate of dehydroepiandrosterone sulfate in normal and hyperprolactinemic subjects. J Clin Endocrinol Metab 62:202–209, 1986.
122. Lim NY, Dingman JF: Androgenic adrenal hyperfunction in acromegaly. N Engl J Med 271:1189–1194, 1964.
123. Kirschner MA, Zucker IR, Jesperson D: Idiopathic hirsutism—an ovarian abnormality. N Engl J Med 294:637–640, 1976.
124. Hatch R, Rosenfield RL, Kim MH, Tredway D: Hirsutism: Implications, etiology, and management. Am J Obstet Gynecol 140:815–830, 1981.
125. Abraham GE, Maroulis GB, Buster JE, et al: Effect of dexamethasone on serum cortisol and androgen levels in hirsute patients. Obstet Gynecol 47:395–402, 1976.
126. Chang RJ, Laufer LR, Meldrum DR, et al: Steroid secretion in polycystic ovary disease after ovarian suppression by a long-acting gonadotropin-releasing hormone agonist. J Clin Endocrinol Metab 56:897–903, 1983.
127. Barnes RB, Rosenfield RL, Burstein S, Ehrmann DA: Pituitary-ovarian responses to nafarelin testing in the polycystic ovary syndrome. N Engl J Med 320:559–565, 1989.
128. Stein IF, Leventhal ML: Amenorrhea associated with bilateral polycystic ovaries. Am J Obstet Gynecol 29:181–191, 1935.
129. Yen SSC: The polycystic ovary syndrome. Clin Endocrinol 12:177–208, 1980.

130. Conway GS, Honour JW, Jacobs HS: Heterogeneity of the polycystic ovary syndrome: Clinical, endocrine and ultrasound features in 556 patients. Clin Endocrinol 30:459–470, 1989.
131. Waldstreicher J, Santoro NF, Hall JE, et al: Hyperfunction of the hypothalamic-pituitary axis in women with polycystic ovarian disease: Indirect evidence for partial gonadotroph desensitization. J Clin Endocrinol Metab 66:165–172, 1988.
132. Franks S: Polycystic ovary syndrome: A changing perspective. Clin Endocrinol 31:87–120, 1989.
133. Judd HL, Scully RE, Herbst Al, et al: Familial hyperthecosis: Comparison of endocrinologic and histologic findings with polycystic ovarian disease. Am J Obstet Gynecol 117:976–982, 1973.
134. Berger MJ, Taymor ML, Patton WC: Gonadotropin levels and secretory patterns in patients with typical and atypical polycystic ovarian disease. Fertil Steril 26:619–626, 1975.
135. Kim MH, Rosenfield RL, Hosseinian AH, Schneir HG: Ovarian hyperandrogenism with normal and abnormal histologic findings of the ovaries. Am J Obstet Gynecol 134:445–452, 1979.
136. Nagamani M, Lingold JC, Gomez LG, Garza JR: Clinical and hormonal studies in hyperthecosis of the ovaries. Fertil Steril 36:326–332, 1981.
137. Chang RJ, Nakamura RM, Judd HL, Kaplan SA: Insulin resistance in nonobese patients with polycystic ovary syndrome. J Clin Endocrinol Metab 57:356–359, 1983.
138. Wajchenberg BL, Achando A, Okada H, et al: Determination of the source(s) of androgen overproduction in hirsutism associated with polycystic ovary syndrome by simultaneous adrenal and ovarian venous catheterization. Comparison with the dexamethasone suppression test. J Clin Endocrinol Metab 636:1204–1210, 1986.
139. Goldzieher MW, Green JA: The polycystic ovary. I. Clinical and histologic features. J Clin Endocrinol Metab 22:325–338, 1962.
140. Emans SJ, Grace E, Woods ER, et al: Treatment with dexamethasone of androgen excess in adolescent patients. J Pediatr 112:821–826, 1988.
141. Rosenfield RL, Ehrmann DA, Barnes RB, et al: Ovarian steroidogenic abnormalities in polycystic ovary syndrome: Evidence for abnormal coordinate regulation of androgen and estrogen secretion. In Dunaif A, Givens J, Haseltine F, Merriam G (eds): Current Issues in Endocrinology and Metabolism: Polycystic Ovary Syndrome. Cambridge, MA, Blackwell Scientific, 1992, pp 39–48.
142. Moll GW Jr, Rosenfield RL: Plasma free testosterone in the diagnosis of adolescent polycystic ovary syndrome. J Pediatr 102:461–464, 1983.
143. Declercq JA, van de Calseyde JF: Polycystic ovarian disease: Diagnosis, frequency and symptoms in a general gynecological practice. Br J Obstet Gynaecol 84:380–385, 1977.
144. McDonough PG, Mahesh VB, Ellegood JO: Steroid, follicle-stimulating hormone and luteinizing hormone profiles in identical twins with polycystic ovaries. Am J Obstet Gynecol 113:1072–1076, 1972.
145. Cooper HE, Spellacy WN, Prem KA, Cohen WD: Hereditary factors in the Stein-Leventhal syndrome. Am J Obstet Gynecol 100:371–387, 1968.
146. Wilroy RS, Givens JR, Wiser WL, et al: Hyperthecosis: An inheritable form of polycystic ovarian disease. Birth Defects 11:81–85, 1975.
147. Hague WM, Adams J, Algar V, et al: HLA associations in patients with polycystic ovaries and in patients with congenital adrenal hyperplasia caused by 21-hydroxylase deficiency. Clin Endocrinol 32:407–415, 1990.
148. Erickson GF, Yen SSC: New data on follicle cells in polycystic ovaries: A proposed mechanism for the genesis of cystic follicles. Semin Reprod Endocrinol 2:231–243, 1984.
149. Hughesdon PE: Morphology and morphogenesis of the Stein-Leventhal ovary and of so-called "hyperthecosis." Obstet Gynecol Surv 37:59–77, 1982.
150. Erickson GF: Folliculogenesis in polycystic ovary syndrome. In Dunaif A, Givens J, Haseltine F, Merriam G (eds): Current Issues in Endocrinology and Metabolism: Polycystic ovary syndrome. Cambridge, MA, Blackwell Scientific, 1992, pp 111–128.
151. Kamrava MM, Seibel MM, Berger MJ, et al: Reversal of persistent anovulation in polycystic ovarian disease by administration of chronic low dose follicle-stimulating hormone. Fertil Steril 37:520–523, 1982.
152. Polson DW, Mason HD, Saldahna MBY, Franks S: Ovulation of a single dominant follicle during treatment with low-dose pulsatile follicle stimulating hormone in women with polycystic ovary syndrome. Clin Endocrinol 26:205–212, 1987.
153. Polson DW, Mason HD, Kiddy DS, et al: Low-dose follicle-stimulating hormone in the treatment of polycystic ovary syndrome: A comparison of pulsatile subcutaneous with daily intramuscular therapy. Br J Obstet Gynaecol 96:746–748, 1989.
154. Fauser BCJM, Pache TD, Lamberts SWJ, et al: Serum bioactive and immunoreactive luteinizing hormone and follicle-stimulating hormone levels in women with cycle abnormalities, with or without polycystic ovarian disease. J Clin Endocrinol Metab 73:811–817, 1991.
155. Feldman S, Billaud L, Thalabard J-C, et al: Fertility in women with late-onset adrenal hyperplasia due to 21-hydroxylase deficiency. J Clin Endocrinol Metab 74:635–639, 1992.
156. Axelrod LR, Goldzieher JW: The polycystic ovary. III. Steroid biosynthesis in normal and polycystic ovarian tissue. J Clin Endocrinol 22:431–440, 1962.
157. Rosenfield RL, Rich BH, Wolfsdorf JE, et al: Pubertal presentation of congenital Δ⁵-3β-hydroxysterone dehydrogenase deficiency. J Clin Endocrinol Metab 51:345–353, 1980.
158. Pang S, Levine LS, Stoner E, et al: Non-salt losing congenital adrenal hyperplasia due to 3β-hydroxysteroid dehydrogenase deficiency with normal glomerulosa function. J Clin Endocrinol Metab 56:808–818, 1983.
159. Pang S, Softness B, Sweeney W, New MI: Hirsutism, polycystic ovarian disease, and ovarian 17-ketosteroid reductase deficiency. N Engl J Med 316:1295–1301, 1987.
160. Toscano V, Balducci R, Bianchi P, et al: Ovarian 17-ketosteroid reductase deficiency as a possible cause of polycystic ovarian disease. J Clin Endocrinol Metab 71:288–292, 1990.
161. Erickson GF, Magoffin DA, Cragun JR, Chang RJ: The effects of insulin and insulin-like growth factors I and II on estradiol production by granulosa cells of polycystic ovaries. J Clin Endocrinol Metab 70:894–902, 1990.
162. Burger CW, Korsen T, van Kessel H, et al: Pulsatile luteinizing hormone patterns in the follicular phase of the menstrual cycle, polycystic ovarian disease (PCOD) and non-PCOD secondary amenorrhea. J Clin Endocrinol Metab 61:1126–1132, 1985.
163. Filicori M, Campaniello E, Michelacci L, et al: Gonadotropin-releasing hormone (GnRH) analog suppression renders polycystic ovarian disease patients more susceptible to ovulation induction with pulsatile GnRH. J Clin Endocrinol Metab 66:327–333, 1988.
164. Hall JE, Whitcomb RW, Rivier JE, et al: Differential regulation of luteinizing hormone, follicle-stimulating hormone, and free α-subunit secretion from the gonadotrope by gonadotropin-releasing hormone (GnRH): Evidence from the use of two GnRH antagonists. J Clin Endocrinol Metab 70:328–335, 1990.
165. Hall JE, Taylor AE, Martin KA, Crowley WF Jr: Neuroendocrine investigation of polycystic ovary syndrome: New approaches. In Dunaif A, Givens J, Haseltine F, Merriam G (eds): Current Issues in Endocrinology and Metabolism: Polycystic Ovary Syndrome. Cambridge, MA, Blackwell Scientific, 1992, pp 39–56.
166. Zumoff B, Freeman R, Coupey S, et al: A chronobiologic abnormality in luteinizing hormone secretion in teenage girls with the polycystic-ovary syndrome. N Engl J Med 309:1206–1209, 1983.
167. Porcu E, Venturoli S, Magrini O, et al: Circadian variations of luteinizing hormone can have two different profiles in adolescent anovulation. J Clin Endocrinol Metab 65:488–493, 1987.
168. Moll GW Jr, Rosenfield RL, van Cauter E, Burstein S: Origin of episodic fluctuations of plasma testosterone in women: Adrenal, ovarian, and TeBG contributions. In Crowley WF Jr, Hofler JG (eds): The Episodic Secretion of Hormones. New York, John Wiley/Churchill Livingstone, 1987, pp 403–414.
169. Boyar R, Finkelstein J, Roffwarg H, et al: Synchronization of augmented luteinizing hormone secretion with sleep during puberty. N Engl J Med 287:582–586, 1982.
170. Venturoli S, Porcu E, Fabbri R, et al: Longitudinal evaluation of the different gonadotropin pulsatile patterns in anovulatory cycles of young girls. J Clin Endocrinol Metab 74:836–841, 1992.
171. Imse V, Holzapfel G, Hinney B, et al: Comparison of luteinizing hormone pulsatility in the serum of women suffering from polycystic ovarian disease using a bioassay and five different immunoassays. J Clin Endocrinol Metab 74:1053–1061, 1992.
172. Nestler JE, Clore JN, Blackard WG: Effects of insulin on steroidogenesis in vivo. In Dunaif A, Givens J, Haseltine F, Merriam G (eds): Current Issues in Endocrinology and Metabolism: Polycystic Ovary Syndrome. Cambridge, MA, Blackwell Scientific, 1992, pp 265–278.
173. Stuart DA, Nagamani M: Acute augmentation of plasma androstenedione and dehydroepiandrosterone by euglycemic insulin infusion: Evidence for a direct effect of insulin on ovarian steroidogenesis. In Dunaif A, Givens J, Haseltine F, Merriam G (eds): Current Issues in Endocrinology and Metabolism: Polycystic Ovary Syndrome. Cambridge, MA, Blackwell Scientific, 1992, pp 279–288.
174. Kahn CR, Flier JS, Bar RS, et al: The syndromes of insulin resistance and acanthosis nigricans. N Engl J Med 294:739–742, 1976.

175. Yoshimasa Y, Seino S, Whittaker J, et al: Insulin-resistant diabetes due to a point mutation that prevents insulin proreceptor processing. Science 240:784–787, 1988.

176. Moller DE, Flier JS: Detection of an alteration in the insulin-receptor gene in a patient with insulin resistance, acanthosis nigricans, and the polycystic ovary syndrome (type A insulin resistance). N Engl J Med 319:1526–1529, 1988.

177. Kadawaki T, Berins C, Cama A: Two mutant alleles of the insulin receptor gene in a patient with extreme insulin resistance. Science 240:787–790, 1988.

178. Accili D, Frapier C, Mosthat L, et al: A mutation in the insulin receptor gene that impairs transport of the receptor to the plasma membrane and causes insulin-resistant diabetes. EMBO J 8:2509–2517, 1989.

179. Taylor SI, Cama A, Accili D, et al: Mutations in the insulin receptor gene. Endocrinol Rev 13:566–595, 1992.

180. Taylor SI, Dons RF, Hernandez E, et al: Insulin resistance associated with androgen excess in women with autoantibodies to the insulin receptor. Ann Intern Med 97:851–855, 1982.

181. Bar RS, Muggeo M, Roth J, et al: Insulin resistance, acanthosis nigricans, and normal insulin receptors in a young woman: Evidence for a postreceptor defect. J Clin Endocrinol Metab 47:620–625, 1978.

182. Harrison LC, Dean B, Peluso I, et al: Insulin resistance, acanthosis nigricans, and polycystic ovaries associated with a circulating inhibitor of postbinding insulin action. J Clin Endocrinol Metab 60:1047–1052, 1985.

183. Dunaif A, Segal KR, Shelley DR, et al: Evidence for distinctive and intrinsic defects in insulin action in polycystic ovary syndrome. Diabetes 41:1257–1266, 1992.

184. Dunaif A, Graf M, Mandeli J, et al: Characterization of groups of hyperandrogenic women with acanthosis nigricans, impaired glucose tolerance and/or hyperinsulinemia. J Clin Endocrinol Metab 65:499–507, 1987.

185. O'Meara N, Blackman JD, Ehrmann DA, et al: Defects in beta cell function in functional ovarian hyperandrogenism. J Clin Endocrinol Metab 76:1241–1247, 1993.

186. Micic D, Popovic V, Nesovic M, et al: Androgen levels during sequential insulin euglycemic clamp studies in patients with polycystic ovary disease. J Steroid Biochem 31:995–999, 1988.

187. Dunaif A, Segal KR, Futterweit W, Dobrjansky A: Profound peripheral insulin resistance, independent of obesity, in polycystic ovary syndrome. Diabetes 38:1165–1174, 1989.

188. Burghen GA, Givens JR, Kitabchi AE: Correlation of hyperandrogenism with hyperinsulinemia in polycystic ovarian disease. J Clin Endocrinol Metab 50:113–116, 1980.

189. Nestler JE, Clore JN, Strauss JF III, Blackard WG: The effects of hyperinsulinemia on serum testosterone, progesterone, dehydroepiandrosterone sulfate, and cortisol levels in normal women and in a woman with hyperandrogenism, insulin resistance, and acanthosis nigricans. J Clin Endocrinol Metab 64:180–184, 1987.

190. Flier JS: Lilly lecture: Syndromes of insulin resistance. Diabetes 41:1207–1219, 1992.

190a. Flier JS, Moller DE, Moses AC, et al: Insulin-mediated pseudoacromegaly: Clinical and biochemical characterization of a syndrome of selective insulin resistance. J Clin Endocrinol Metab 76:1533–1541, 1993.

191. Van Niekerk WA: True hermaphroditism—analytic review with a report of 3 new cases. Am J Obstet Gynecol 126:890–907, 1976.

192. Vergnaud G, Page DC, Simmler MC, et al: A deletion map of the human Y chromosome based on DNA hybridization. Am J Hum Genet 38:109–124, 1986.

193. Talerman A, Jarabak J, Amarose AP: Gonadoblastoma and dysgerminoma in a true hermaphrodite with a 46,XX karyotype. Am J Obstet Gynecol 140:475–477, 1981.

194. Hensleigh PA, Woodruff JD: Differential maternal-fetal response to androgenizing luteoma or hyperreactio luteinalis. Obstet Gynecol Surv 33:262–271, 1978.

195. Kopelman PG, White N, Pilkington FRE, et al: The effect of weight loss on sex steroid secretion and binding in massively obese women. Clin Endocrinol 14:113–118, 1981.

196. Bates GW, Whitworth NS: Effect of body weight reduction on plasma androgens in obese, infertile women. Fertil Steril 38:406–409, 1982.

197. Pasquali R, Antenucci D, Casimirri F, et al: Clinical and hormonal characteristics of obese amenorrheic hyperandrogenic women before and after weight loss. J Clin Endocrinol Metab 68:173–179, 1989.

198. Rosenfield RL: Congenital adrenal hyperplasia and reproductive function in females. In Flamigni C, Venturoli S, Givens J (eds): Adolescence in Females. Chicago, Year Book Medical Publishers, 1985, pp 373–387.

199. Rosenfield RL, Cohen RM, Talerman A: Lipid cell tumor of the ovary in reference to adult-onset congenital adrenal hyperplasia and polycystic ovary syndrome. J Reprod Med 32:363–367, 1987.

200. Pochi PE, Shalita AR, Strauss JS, Webster SB: Report of the consensus conference on acne classification. J Am Acad Dermatol 24:495–501, 1991.

201. Werk EE, Sholiton LJ, Kalejs L: Testosterone-secreting adenoma under gonadotropin control. N Engl J Med 289:767–770, 1973.

202. Dewailly D, Robert Y, Helin I, et al: Interrelationship between ultrasonography and biology in the diagnosis of polycystic ovarian syndrome. Ann NY Acad Sci 687:206–216, 1993.

203. Givens JR, Andersen RN, Wiser WL, et al: Dynamics of suppression and recovery of plasma FSH, LH, androstenedione and testosterone in polycystic ovarian disease using an oral contraceptive. J Clin Endocrinol Metab 38:727–735, 1974.

204. Mandel FP, Geola FL, Lu JKH, et al: Biological effects of various doses of ethinyl estradiol in postmenopausal women. Obstet Gynecol 58:673–679, 1982.

205. Carr BR, Parker CR, Madden JD, et al: Plasma levels of adrenocorticotropin and cortisol in women receiving oral contraceptive steroid treatment. J Clin Endocrinol Metab 49:346–349, 1979.

206. Wild RA, Umstot ES, Andersen RN, Givens JR: Adrenal function in hirsutism. II. Effect of an oral contraceptive. J Clin Endocrinol Metab 54:676–681, 1982.

207. Palitz LL: Estrogen-progestin in the control of acne in girls. Clin Med 75:43–54, 1968.

208. Brotherton J: Animal biological assessment. In Brotherton J (ed): Sex Hormone Pharmacology. London, Academic Press, 1976, pp 43–78.

209. Thijssen JHH: Hormonal and nonhormonal factors affecting sex hormone–binding globulin levels in blood. Ann NY Acad Sci 538:280–286, 1988.

210. Lemay A, Dewailly SD, Grenier R, Huard J: Attenuation of mild hyperandrogenic activity in postpubertal acne by a triphasic oral contraceptive containing low doses of ethynyl estradiol and d,l-norgestrel. J Clin Endocrinol Metab 71:8–14, 1990.

211. Hancock KW, Levell MJ: The use of oestrogen/progestogen preparations in the treatment of hirsutism in the female. J Obstet Gynaecol Br Commonweal 81:804–811, 1974.

212. Andreyko JL, Monroe SE, Jaffe RB: Treatment of hirsutism with a gonadotropin-releasing hormone agonist (nafarelin). J Clin Endocrinol Metab 63:854–859, 1986.

213. Steingold K, DeZiegler C, Cedars M, et al: Clinical and hormonal effects of chronic gonadotropin-releasing hormone agonist treatment in polycystic ovarian disease. J Clin Endocrinol Metab 65:773–778, 1987.

214. Rittmaster RS: Differential suppression of testosterone and estradiol in hirsute women with the superactive gonadotropin-releasing hormone agonist leuprolide. J Clin Endocrinol Metab 67:651–655, 1988.

215. Sidenius-Johansen J, Juel-Riis B, Hassager C, et al: The effect of a gonadotropin-releasing hormone agonist analog (nafarelin) on bone metabolism. J Clin Endocrinol Metab 67:701–706, 1988.

216. Matta WH, Shaw RW, Hesp R, Evans R: Reversible trabecular bone density loss following induced hypooestrogenism with the GnRH analogue buserelin in premenopausal women. Clin Endocrinol 29:45–51, 1988.

217. Adashi EY: Potential utility of gonadotropin-releasing hormone agonists in the management of ovarian hyperandrogenism. Fertil Steril 53:765–779, 1990.

218. Rittmaster RS, Givner ML: Effect of daily and alternate day low dose prednisone on serum cortisol and adrenal androgens in hirsute women. J Clin Endocrinol Metab 67:400–403, 1988.

219. Carmina E, Lobo RA: Peripheral androgen blockade versus glandular androgen suppression in the treatment of hirsutism. Obstet Gynecol 78:845–849, 1991.

220. Steinberger E, Rodriguez-Rigau LJ, Petak SM, et al: Glucocorticoid therapy in hyperandrogenism. Ballieres Clin Obstet Gynaecol 4:457–471, 1990.

221. Spritzer P, Billaud L, Thalabard J-C, et al: Cyproterone acetate versus hydrocortisone treatment in late-onset adrenal hyperplasia. J Clin Endocrinol Metab 70:642–646, 1990.

222. Rajfer J, Sikka SC, River F, Handelsman DJ: Mechanism of inhibition of human testicular steroidogenesis by oral ketoconazole. J Clin Endocrinol Metab 63:1193–1198, 1986.

223. Couch RM, Muller J, Perry YS, Winter JSD: Kinetic analysis of human adrenal steroidogenesis by ketoconazole. J Clin Endocrinol Metab 65:551–555, 1987.

224. Venturoli A, Fabri R, Dal Prato L, et al: Ketoconazole therapy for women with acne and/or hirsutism. J Clin Endocrinol Metab 71:335–339, 1990.

225. Mowszowicz I, Wright F, Vincens M, et al: Androgen metabolism in hirsute patients treated with cyproterone acetate. J Steroid Biochem 20:757–761, 1984.

226. Miller JA, Jacobs HS: Treatment of hirsutism and acne with cyproterone acetate. Clin Endocrinol Metab 15:373–389, 1986.

227. Miller J, Wojnarowska F, Dowd P, et al: Antiandrogen treatment in women with acne: A controlled trial. Br J Dermatol 114:705–716, 1986.

228. Barth JH, Cherry CA, Wojnarowska F, Dawber RPR: Spironolactone is an effective and well tolerated systemic antiandrogen therapy for hirsute women. J Clin Endocrinol Metab 68:966–970, 1989.

229. O'Brien RC, Cooper ME, Murray RML, et al: Comparison of sequential cyproterone acetate versus spironolactone/oral contraceptive in the treatment of hirsutism. J Clin Endocrinol Metab 72:1008–1013, 1991.

230. Edgren RA, Elton RL: Estrogen antagonisms: Effects of several steroidal spironolactones on estrogen-induced uterine growth in mice. Proc Soc Exp Biol Med 104:664–665, 1960.

231. Camino-Torres R, Ma L, Snyder PJ: Gynecomastia and semen abnormalities induced by spironolactone in normal men. J Endocrinol Metab 45:255–260, 1977.

232. Serafini P, Lobo RA: The effects of spironolactone on adrenal steroidogenesis in hirsute women. Fertil Steril 44:595–599, 1985.

233. Serafini P, Catalino J, Lobo RA: The effect of spironolactone on genital skin 5α-reductase activity. J Steroid Biochem 23:191–194, 1985.

234. Givens JR: Treatment of hirsutism with spironolactone. Fertil Steril 43:841–843, 1985.

235. Crosby PDA, Rittmaster RS: Predictors of clinical response in hirsute women treated with spironolactone. Fertil Steril 55:1076–1081, 1991.

236. Neri RO, Monahan M: Effects of a novel nonsteroidal antiandrogen on canine prostatic hyperplasia. Invest Urol 10:123–130, 1972.

237. Cusan L, Dupont A, Belanger A, et al: Treatment of hirsutism with the pure antiandrogen flutamide. J Am Acad Dermatol 23:462–469, 1990.

238. Liang T, Rasmusson GH, Brooks JR: Biochemical and biological studies with 4-aza-steroidal 5α-reductase inhibitors. J Steroid Biochem 19:385–390, 1983.

239. Prelevic GM, Wurzburger MI, Balint-Peric L, Nesic JS: Inhibitory effect of sandostatin on secretion of luteinising hormone and ovarian steroids in polycystic ovary syndrome. Lancet 336:900–903, 1990.

240. Venturoli S, Porcu E, Gammi L, et al: Different gonadotropin pulsatile fashions in anovulatory cycles of young girls indicate different maturational pathways in adolescence. J Clin Endocrinol Metab 65:785–791, 1987.

241. Jafari K, Tavaheri C, Ruiz G: Endometrial adenocarcinoma and the Stein-Leventhal syndrome. Obstet Gynecol 51:97–100, 1978.

242. Kerin JF, Liu JH, Phillipou G, Yen SSC: Evidence for a hypothalamic site of action of clomiphene citrate in women. J Clin Endocrinol Metab 61:265–268, 1985.

243. Gysler M, March CM, Mishell DR Jr, Bailery EJ: A decade's experience with an individualized clomiphene treatment regimen including its effect on the postcoital test. Fertil Steril 37:161–167, 1982.

244. Hammond MG, Halme JK, Talbert LM: Factors affecting the pregnancy rate in clomiphene citrate induction of ovulation. Obstet Gynecol 62:196–202, 1983.

245. Lobo RA, Paul W, March CM, et al: Clomiphene and dexamethasone in women unresponsive to clomiphene alone. Obstet Gynecol 60:497–501, 1982.

246. Allen NC, Herbert CM, Maxson WS, et al: Intrauterine insemination: A critical review. Fertil Steril 44:569–580, 1985.

247. Garcia J, Jones GS, Wentz AC: The use of clomiphene citrate. Fertil Steril 28:707–717, 1977.

248. Huang KE: The primary treatment of luteal phase inadequacy: Progesterone versus clomiphene citrate. Am J Obstet Gynecol 155:824–828, 1986.

249. Wang CF, Gemzell C: The use of human gonadotropins for the induction of ovulation in women with polycystic ovarian disease. Fertil Steril 33:479–486, 1980.

250. Kemmann E, Tavakoli F, Shelden RM, Jones JR: Induction of ovulation with menotropins in women with polycystic ovary syndrome. Am J Obstet Gynecol 141:58–64, 1981.

251. Seibel MM, McArdle C, Smith D, Taymor ML: Ovulation induction in polycystic ovary syndrome with urinary follicle-stimulating hormone or human menopausal gonadotropin. Fertil Steril 43:703–708, 1985.

252. Buvat J, Buvat-Herbaut M, Marcolin G, et al: Purified follicle-stimulating hormone in polycystic ovary syndrome: Slow administration is safer and more effective. Fertil Steril 52:553–559, 1989.

253. Shoham Z, Patel A, Jacobs HS: Polycystic ovarian syndrome: Safety and effectiveness of stepwise and low-dose administration of purified follicle-stimulating hormone. Fertil Steril 55:1051–1056, 1991.

254. Sagle A, Hamilton-Fairley D, Kiddy DS, Franks S: A comparative, randomized study of low-dose human menopausal gonadotropin and follicle-stimulating hormone in women with polycystic ovarian syndrome. Fertil Steril 55:56–60, 1991.

255. Mizunuma H, Takagi T, Yamada K, et al: Ovulation induction by step-down administration of purified urinary follicle-stimulating hormone in patients with polycystic ovarian syndrome. Fertil Steril 55:1195–1196, 1991.

256. Burger CW, van Kessel H, Schoemaker J: Induction of ovulation by prolonged pulsatile administration of luteinizing hormone releasing hormone (LRH) in patients with clomiphene resistant polycystic ovary-like disease. Acta Endocrinol 104:357–364, 1983.

257. Burger CW, Korsen T, Hompes PG, et al: Ovulation induction with pulsatile luteinizing releasing hormone in women with clomiphene citrate resistant polycystic ovary-like disease: Clinical results. Fertil Steril 46:1045–1054, 1986.

258. Jansen RP, Handelsman DJ, Boylan LM, et al: Pulsatile intravenous gonadotropin-releasing hormone for ovulation-induction in infertile women. I. Safety and effectiveness with outpatient therapy. Fertil Steril 48:33–38, 1987.

259. Filicori M, Flamigni C, Meriggiola MC, et al: Ovulation induction with pulsatile gonadotropin-releasing hormone: Technical modalities and clinical perspectives. Fertil Steril 56:1–13, 1991.

260. Fleming R, Haxton MJ, Hamilton MP, et al: Successful treatment of infertile women with oligomenorrhoea using a combination of an LHRH agonist and exogenous gonadotrophins. Br J Obstet Gynaecol 92:369–373, 1985.

261. Dodson WC, Hughes CL, Whitesides DB, Haney AF: The effect of leuprolide acetate on ovulation induction with human menopausal gonadotropins in polycystic ovary syndrome. J Clin Endocrinol Metab 65:95–100, 1987.

262. Lanzone A, Fulghesu AM, Spina MA, et al: Successful induction of ovulation and conception with combined gonadotropin-releasing hormone agonist plus highly purified follicle-stimulating hormone in patients with polycystic ovarian disease. J Clin Endocrinol Metab 65:1253–1258, 1987.

263. Filicori M, Flamigni C, Meriggiola MC, et al: Endocrine response determines the clinical outcome of pulsatile gonadotropin-releasing hormone ovulation induction in different ovulatory disorders. J Clin Endocrinol Metab 72:965–972, 1991.

264. Dodson WC, Hughes CL Jr, Yancy SE, Haney AF: Clinical characteristics of ovulation induction with human menopausal gonadotropins with and without leuprolide acetate in polycystic ovary syndrome. Fertil Steril 52:915–918, 1989.

264a. Sagle M, Bishop K, Ridley N, et al: Recurrent early miscarriage and polycystic ovaries. Br Med J 297:1027–1028, 1988.

264b. Regan L, Owen EJ, Jacobs HS: Hypersecretion of luteinising hormone, infertility, and miscarriage. Lancet 336:1141–1144, 1990.

264c. Homburg R, Feldberg D, Levy T, et al: Gonadotropin-releasing hormone agonist reduces the miscarriage rate for pregnancies achieved in women with polycystic ovarian syndrome. Fertil Steril 59:527–531, 1993.

265. Goldzieher JW: Polycystic ovarian disease. Fertil Steril 35:371–394, 1981.

266. Gjönnaess H: Polycystic ovarian syndrome treated by ovarian electrocautery through the laparoscope. Fertil Steril 41:20–25, 1984.

267. Casper RF, Greenblatt EM: Laparoscopic ovarian cautery for induction of ovulation in women with polycystic ovarian disease. Semin Reprod Endocrinol 8:208–212, 1990.

268. Dabirashrafi H, Mohamad K, Behjatnia Y, Moghadami-Tabrizi N: Adhesion formation after ovarian electrocauterization on patients with polycystic ovarian syndrome. Fertil Steril 55:1201–1203, 1991.

269. Gurgan T, Urman B, Aksu T, et al: The effect of short-interval laparoscopic lysis of adhesions on pregnancy rates following Nd-YAG laser photocoagulation of polycystic ovaries. Obstet Gynecol 80:45–47, 1992.

Ovarian Tumors with Endocrine Manifestations

ROBERT E. SCULLY

"Ovarian Tumors with Endocrine Manifestations" is a more appropriate title for this chapter than "Functioning Ovarian Tumors" because steroid hormones produced by these neoplasms may be converted to other steroid hormones elsewhere in the body, and the latter, rather than the ovarian hormones themselves, may be responsible for associated endocrine abnormalities. Ovarian tumors with overt endocrine manifestations account for less than 5 per cent of all ovarian neoplasms, and those that are malignant for less than 10 per cent of all ovarian cancers. The frequency of ovarian tumors that produce hormones at a subclinical level is probably considerably higher in view of evidence afforded by various laboratory data. For example, more than one third of ovarian cancers in postmenopausal women have been reported to be associated with increased maturation of vaginal epithelial cells in cytological smears, suggesting an increased estrogen level.[1] Even more compelling is the finding that 50 per cent of postmenopausal women with surface epithelial-stromal tumors (tumors derived from the surface epithelium and adjacent stroma of the ovary), which usually are considered to be nonfunctioning, have abnormally high levels of total urinary estrogens.[2] The appearance of the stroma of many ovarian tumors, including those of the surface epithelial-stromal type, suggest that it is largely responsible for the production of steroid hormones in these cases.[3]

Most ovarian tumors with endocrine manifestations are associated with changes in end-organs and clinical syndromes related to overproduction of steroid hormones, most often estrogens, but androgens and exceptionally progesterone or corticosteroids occasionally are produced. Rare tumors secrete chorionic gonadotropin (hCG), which stimulates the stroma of the neoplasm or uninvolved ovarian tissue to produce steroid hormones. Highly specialized cells within ovarian tumors, such as thyroid epithelial cells, argentaffin cells, or pituitary cells, occasionally elaborate their specific secretory products. Finally, sometimes cancers of the ovary, such as those that arise elsewhere in the body, are associated with ectopic hormone production of various types.

A classification of ovarian tumors with endocrine manifestations, based on the World Health Organization histological typing of ovarian tumors,[3] is presented in Table 121–1. Non-neoplastic processes associated with clinical or laboratory manifestations that closely simulate those of hormone-secreting ovarian tumors are included in the classification.

CLINICAL MANIFESTATIONS OF STEROID HORMONE ABNORMALITIES

Estrogenic Manifestations

Estrogen secretion by an ovarian tumor in infancy and childhood produces isosexual pseudoprecocity (see Ch. 111).[4] This syndrome may develop any time from early infancy to the onset of true puberty, with most cases encountered before the age of five years. Enlargement of the breasts is the most common initial manifestation, followed

TABLE 121–1. CLASSIFICATION OF OVARIAN TUMORS WITH ENDOCRINE MANIFESTATIONS

I. Steroid hormone–secreting tumors
  A. Sex cord–stromal tumors
    1. Granulosa–stromal cell tumors
      a. Granulosa cell tumor
      b. Tumors in thecoma-fibroma group
        i. Thecoma
        ii. Fibroma*
        iii. Sclerosing stromal tumor
    2. Sertoli–stromal cell tumors (androblastomas)
    3. Sex cord tumor with annular tubules
    4. Gynandroblastoma
  B. Steroid (lipid; lipoid) cell tumors
  C. Gonadoblastoma
  D. Tumors with functioning stroma
II. Gonadotropin-secreting tumors
  A. Choriocarcinoma
  B. Embryonal carcinoma
  C. Polyembryoma
  D. Dysgerminoma with syncytiotrophoblastic cells
  E. Mixed primitive germ cell tumors
  F. Ovarian carcinomas with ectopic chorionic gonadotropin production
III. Highly specialized teratomas with hormone production
  A. Struma
  B. Carcinoid
  C. Strumal carcinoid
  D. Pituitary adenomas in teratomas
IV. Tumors with ectopic hormone production
V. Tumor-like conditions
  A. Solitary follicle cyst
  B. Multiple follicle cysts (polycystic ovaries)
  C. Hyperplasia of ovarian stroma and stromal hyperthecosis
  D. Massive edema
  E. Fibromatosis
  F. Pregnancy luteoma
  G. Hyperreactio luteinalis
  H. Large solitary luteinized follicle cyst of pregnancy and puerperium†
  I. Autoimmune oophoritis

*Nonfunctioning but included to maintain integrity of classification.
†Hormone secretion not yet proved.

by the development of pubic and axillary hair, enlargement of the external and internal secondary sex organs, irregular uterine bleeding, and a white vaginal discharge, which originates in the stimulated endocervix. Bone growth often is accelerated, and if the tumor is not removed, premature closure of the epiphyses and short stature may result. Vaginal cytology reveals maturation of squamous epithelial cells, and elevated levels of estrogens may be demonstrated in the blood and urine. Although gonadotropin levels might be expected to be depressed by the excess of estrogens in the circulation, values have been elevated in some cases. Palpation of a mass on abdominal examination is almost diagnostic of an ovarian tumor as the cause of the sexual precocity, but if unilateral or bilateral adnexal masses are detectable only on rectal examination, ovarian enlargement by cystic follicles and/or corpora lutea is more likely. Central precocity, which usually is constitutional (idiopathic), accounts for 85 to 90 per cent of cases of sexual precocity in females and has been designated true precocity because the hypothalamic-pituitary axis is prematurely activated, with the release of follicle-stimulating hormone (FSH) and luteinizing hormone (LH) and the possibility of ovulation (see Ch. 111). Ultrasound examination may be of great value in distinguishing follicle cysts from ovarian tumors in sexually precocious girls.[5]

In women of reproductive age, estrogen secretion by an ovarian tumor inhibits ovulation and cyclic progesterone secretion by means of the hypothalamic-pituitary feedback mechanism, resulting in continuous, unopposed estrogenic stimulation of the endometrium (see Ch. 118). The latter is manifested morphologically by cystic hyperplasia, often accompanied by varying degrees of precancerous atypicality and occasionally by the development of endometrial carcinoma, which typically is low grade.[6] The clinical expression of the endometrial stimulation may be excessive, irregular uterine bleeding (metropathia hemorrhagica), but a period of amenorrhea lasting for months to years often precedes the onset of abnormal bleeding or is the only menstrual disorder at the time of diagnosis. A patient with an estrogenic ovarian tumor occasionally presents with swelling of the breasts, which may be accompanied by pain and tenderness. Estrogenic changes should be evident in cytological smears of the vagina, and elevated estrogen levels have been demonstrated in the plasma and urine.

After the menopause, estrogen production by an ovarian tumor rejuvenates the endometrium, producing morphological changes similar to those described in younger women. Postmenopausal bleeding is the typical presenting symptom of endocrine origin, but occasionally bleeding from the stimulated endometrium has not occurred by the time of recognition of the tumor. Associated carcinoma of the endometrium is more common in postmenopausal women than in younger women. In one large series of granulosa cell tumors and thecomas,[6] endometrial carcinoma was found in 24 per cent of the postmenopausal women but in only 12.5 per cent of those in the reproductive age group. These figures apply only to those women whose endometrial tissue was available for microscopic examination. A review of several large series of unselected cases in the literature indicates that less than 5 per cent of all women with granulosa cell tumors or thecomas have endometrial cancer. Symptoms of mammary stimulation may also develop after the menopause. Laboratory parameters of hyperestrogenism are helpful diagnostic aids, particularly elevation of plasma or urinary estrogen levels and maturation of vaginal epithelial cells, which is strikingly different from the expected atrophy in this age group.

A mass usually is palpable, at least on pelvic examination, in patients with estrogenic ovarian tumors, but in about 12 per cent of affected adults the tumor is a surprise finding at the time of hysterectomy for abnormal uterine bleeding caused by endometrial hyperplasia or carcinoma.[7]

Androgenic Manifestations

Rarely, androgen secretion by an ovarian tumor before puberty seldom results in heterosexual precocity, with virilizing manifestations superimposed on accelerated somatic growth.[8] During the reproductive-age period the typical picture is one of oligomenorrhea followed by amenorrhea, defeminization (atrophy of breasts and loss of female body contours), and progressive virilization (see Ch. 120). The latter is characterized by acne, hirsutism, temporal balding, enlargement of the clitoris, deepening of the voice, and muscular development. Excessive, irregular uterine bleeding occasionally precedes the onset of diminished menstruation. This phenomenon may reflect an initial plasma elevation of androgens that inhibits ovulation by means of the hypothalamic-pituitary feedback mechanism but allows gonadotropic stimulation of the ovarian follicles and estrogen secretion to continue. Sometimes an androgenic ovarian tumor results in a more insidious onset of menstrual disturbances and virilization, and rarely androgen levels may not be high enough to interfere with ovulation. A postmenopausal woman occasionally becomes masculinized by an ovarian tumor or has a history of long-standing mild virilism that began during her reproductive years.

Although urinary 17-ketosteroid (17-KS) levels usually are normal, their measurement may be helpful in the diagnosis of an androgenic ovarian tumor. An elevation depends not only on the amount but also on the type of androgens being secreted. Testosterone, a potent androgen, is not significantly metabolized to 17-KS, and elevations of this hormone commonly cause masculinization without a detectable abnormality in the 17-KS level. Weaker androgens, such as androstenedione and dehydroepiandrosterone, are 17-KS's but must be present in large amounts to virilize a patient; as a result, an increase in 17-KS's is detectable in the urine when these hormones alone are responsible for virilization, or when they are secreted in significant amounts in addition to testosterone. Elevation of various androgens, free and protein-bound—particularly the former—in the plasma is the most sensitive and accurate laboratory index of a high androgen state (see Ch. 120). An elevation of testosterone is most characteristic of virilizing ovarian tumors and non-neoplastic disorders but can also occur in association with adrenal hyperplasia and neoplasia (see Ch. 105).[9] Androstenedione and dehydroepiandrosterone may be secreted by tumors and other pathological processes originating in either the ovary or the adrenal cortex. The results of stimulation by tropic hormones (hCG and ACTH) and of suppression by sex hormones and corticosteroids are not decisive in distinguishing ovarian from adrenal virilism in view of many exceptions to the results expected on theoretical grounds.[10] Measurements of hormone levels in ovarian and adrenal vein blood may be of diagnostic value, detecting ovarian tumors as small as 0.6 cm in diameter,[11-13] but they can be misleading as a result of technical errors.

A testosterone level of 2 ng/ml (7 nmol/L) has been proposed as a diagnostic dividing line between androgen-secreting tumors and non-neoplastic lesions such as polycystic ovarian disease and stromal hyperthecosis.[12] Friedman et al.,[14] however, found that the latter disorders often are associated with levels over 2 ng (7 nmol), and that such levels in the absence of an adnexal mass or rapidly progressive virilism do not warrant the use of invasive diagnostic approaches, including surgical exploration.

Manifestations of Other Types of Steroid Hormone Excess

Combinations of estrogenic and androgenic phenomena, such as virilization and cystic hyperplasia of the endometrium, seldom have been observed in patients with ovarian tumors. Likewise, histological evidence of progesterone stimulation is present in exceptional cases of estrogen or androgen excess. Thus a patient with an estrogenic ovarian tumor may have secretory changes superimposed on hyperplasia of the endometrium, and a rare patient has decidual transformation of the endometrium.[3] It has not been clear in most of these unusual cases which hormones have been produced directly by the tumor and which have resulted from peripheral conversion of its secretory products.

Virilizing ovarian tumors often have been accompanied by one or more clinical or laboratory findings suggestive of Cushing's syndrome (see Ch. 100).[13] These include erythrocytosis, which can be a manifestation of androgen excess alone, and obesity, hypertension, and diabetes, all of which are common disorders that may be unrelated to the hormones secreted by the tumor. Very rarely a virilizing ovarian tumor is associated with true Cushing's syndrome, with elevation of free cortisol in both the peripheral and the ovarian vein blood.[15]

OVARIAN TUMORS ASSOCIATED WITH STEROID HORMONE ABNORMALITIES

Sex Cord–Stromal Tumors

The category of sex cord–stromal tumors includes all neoplasms that contain granulosa cells, theca cells, Sertoli cells, Leydig cells, and stromal fibroblasts singly or in any combination and in various degrees of differentiation.[3] A number of terms have been assigned to these tumors, reflecting differing views of gonadal embryology. These designations include "mesenchymomas," "sex cord–mesenchyme tumors," and "gonadal stromal tumors." The term *sex cord–stromal tumors* is a compromise between the latter two designations, recognizing the presence in these neoplasms of derivatives of two of the morphological components of the developing gonad:[5] groups of cells arranged in epithelial configurations and referred to as sex cords, and mesenchyme or stroma. Granulosa cells and Sertoli cells are the offspring of the sex cords, whereas theca cells, Leydig cells, and fibroblasts develop from the mesenchyme or stroma. Most tumors in the sex cord–stromal category are composed of ovarian cell types, but some contain those of testicular-type Sertoli cells, Leydig cells, or both; rarely cells and patterns of growth characteristic of both gonads are present within a single neoplasm. If the relatively common endocrinologically inactive ovarian fibroma is excluded from consideration, most tumors in the sex cord–stromal category are associated with clinically apparent endocrine disturbances. It is not possible on the basis of microscopic examination alone to distinguish these tumors from those that are not functioning at a clinical level.

Granulosa–Stromal Cell Tumors

The category of granulosa–stromal cell tumors includes all ovarian tumors composed of granulosa cells and cells of ovarian stromal derivation (theca cells and fibroblasts) singly or in various combinations.

GRANULOSA CELL TUMOR. The granulosa cell tumor may be composed exclusively of granulosa cells, or it may contain a significant component of them in association with theca cells, fibroblasts, or both.[3, 16, 17] The granulosa cell tumor is the most common form of clinically manifest estrogenic tumor of the ovary, accounting for 1 to 2 per cent of all ovarian tumors and 5 to 10 per cent of all ovarian cancers. Five per cent of granulosa cell tumors occur before the onset of true puberty, and about three fourths of these tumors are associated with isosexual pseudoprecocity, accounting for 3 to 10 per cent of all cases of sexual precocity.[4, 5] The remaining granulosa cell tumors are encountered after the menarche, more often in postmenopausal than in premenopausal women. The tumors range in size from small nodules that cannot be felt on pelvic examination but may be demonstrable on ultrasound examination to huge masses that distend the abdomen.

Among estrogenic ovarian tumors, granulosa cell tumors may be associated with distinctive clinical and laboratory features seldom shared by other neoplasms in this category. Those granulosa cell tumors that occur in the first two decades of life (juvenile granulosa cell tumors) have been a component of Ollier's disease (enchondromatosis) or Maffucci's syndrome (enchondromatosis and hemangiomatosis) in at least 10 reported cases.[18] From a laboratory viewpoint, in addition to being associated with elevated estrogen values, granulosa cell tumors may be accompanied by high plasma levels of inhibin[19, 19a] and follicle-regulatory protein.[20]

Abdominal exploration in cases of granulosa cell tumor reveals solid or cystic ovarian enlargements, which are unilateral in more than 95 per cent of cases. Sectioning a solid granulosa cell tumor discloses a gray or yellow color, depending on the cellularity and the amount of intracellular lipid, and a soft or firm consistency, depending on the relative proportions of cells and fibrothecomatous stroma. Foci of yellow, often partly necrotic tissue and red hemorrhagic tissue are frequent and characteristic findings. A more common gross expression of a granulosa cell tumor is in the form of a predominantly cystic mass in which numerous compartments, usually filled with fluid or clotted blood, are separated by bridges of solid yellow tissue. An interesting clinical corollary of necrosis and hemorrhage in these tumors is their presentation in almost 10 per cent of the cases, not in the form of overt endocrine disturbances but with abdominal pain that results from rupture of the tumor with hemoperitoneum. A rare granulosa cell tumor has a gross appearance simulating that of a serous cystadenoma—a large mass composed of one or more thin-walled cysts that contain watery fluid.

On microscopic examination the granulosa cells are observed to grow in a wide variety of patterns. Well-differentiated forms may be characterized by microfollicular, macrofollicular, trabecular, insular, solid tubular, gyriform, and watered-silk (moiré) patterns or a combination thereof. The less well-differentiated form of granulosa cell tumor has been designated diffuse, or sarcomatoid, and appears as a monotonous cellular growth resembling a round cell sarcoma. Because various patterns of granulosa cell tumors may be simulated by ovarian carcinomas, sometimes the latter are misdiagnosed as granulosa cell tumors. If the clinical course of the patient is atypical for a granulosa cell tumor, the possibility of such an error must be considered. The single best criterion for the microscopic diagnosis of a granulosa cell tumor is the appearance of its nuclei, which typically are pale and commonly grooved.

Most granulosa cell tumors contain theca cells in varying quantities, and several histochemical reactions characteristic of steroid hormone–producing cells are positive more often in these cells than in the neoplastic granulosa cells. Also, when a granulosa cell tumor recurs outside the ovary, theca cells often are poorly developed or absent and clinical evidence of estrogen secretion is lacking.[21] These observations have led to the conclusions[5] that the theca cells are the steroid hormone producers in most granulosa cell tumors, with the granulosa cells merely aromatizing androgens of theca cell origin to estrogens, and that the theca cells may not be truly neoplastic but reactive cells developing from the ovarian stroma in response to the proliferating granulosa cells. In some cases histochemical and other evidence has suggested that the granulosa cells themselves are entirely responsible for the estrogen production.

Either the granulosa cells or the theca cells or both occasionally assume the appearance of lutein cells (i.e., cells that resemble those of the corpus luteum), containing abundant cytoplasm, which may be dense and eosinophilic or spongy, reflecting a rich lipid content; in such cases the term "luteinized granulosa cell tumor" is appropriate. The formation of irregularly shaped follicles of medium size, which typically contain mucin, nuclear hyperchromatism, and pleomorphism, and an abundance of cytoplasm are so characteristic of granulosa cell tumors encountered in the first two decades that the designation "juvenile granulosa cell tumor" has been applied to tumors with these morphological features.[4]

Most granulosa cell tumors are estrogenic; it is impossible to give an accurate figure for the frequency of function because in many cases the endometrium is not available for microscopic examination to evaluate the presence or absence of estrogenic changes. After the removal of a functioning granulosa cell tumor from a young woman whose uterus has been conserved, estrogen withdrawal bleeding typically occurs in one to two days, and regular menses ensue shortly thereafter. Exceptional granulosa cell tumors have been associated with virilization rather than estrogenic manifestations.[8] Enigmatically, about 40 per cent of these tumors have been of the huge, thin-walled, oligolocular or unilocular cystic variety on gross examination, a rare appearance for granulosa cell tumors in general. Ten per cent of granulosa cell tumors have extended beyond the ovary, usually into the pelvis, by the time of exploration, and stage I tumors often recur, typically in the pelvis and lower abdomen, after apparently successful operative removal; distant metastases, although rare, have been reported in numerous sites. Some recurrences appear within five years, but many are not evident until a longer postoperative interval has elapsed, and numerous cases have been reported in which the tumor has reappeared two or even three or more decades after its removal. Juvenile granulosa cell tumors are clinically benign in about 90 per cent of cases, but unlike their adult counterparts, they tend to have a rapid course when they are malignant, with death usually occurring within two years postoperatively.[4]

Optimal treatment of stage I granulosa cell tumors in menopausal and postmenopausal women is total hysterectomy with bilateral salpingo-oophorectomy. In young women and children, in whom the preservation of fertility is an important consideration, removal of the involved ovary alone is justifiable if extra-ovarian spread is not demonstrable and the contralateral ovary is uninvolved. Sometimes recurrences have been successfully treated by reoperation, radiation therapy, or a combination thereof.[22]

Relatively few data are available on the results of chemotherapy of granulosa cell tumors to permit evaluation of the comparative merits of various agents, but several of them have been used with varying degrees of success.[22] Hormone-related therapy, such as the administration of a progestin, tamoxifen, or a gonadotropin-releasing hormone agonist, has been tried in sporadic cases with promising results.[22] Most of the reported 10-year survival figures for patients with granulosa cell tumors are in the 80 to 90 per cent range, but a progressive decline in survival has been documented after longer follow-up periods.[16, 17] The stage of the tumor is the most important indicator of prognosis; in stage I cases the occurrence of rupture and a high degree of nuclear atypicality are unfavorable prognostic features.[16]

TUMORS IN THE THECOMA-FIBROMA GROUP. These tumors are composed exclusively—or almost exclusively—of theca cells, fibroblasts of ovarian stromal origin, or both types of cells; rarely, a few nests of granulosa cells are present.[3, 23] Fibromas, which are composed of fibroblasts, contain little or no lipid and are not associated with biochemical or clinical evidence of estrogen production. Tumors that have larger quantities of lipid and are accompanied by equivocal evidence of estrogen production belong in an unclassified category. Thecomas typically contain abundant lipid and are characteristically accompanied by estrogenic manifestations. They are only one third as common as granulosa cell tumors, occur at an older average age (59 years) than the latter, and are rare before puberty. Thecomas range in size from small tumors that are not palpable on pelvic examination to large solid masses that have a fibrous consistency, and are yellow or predominantly white and flecked with yellow. On microscopic examination two types of thecoma are encountered: The more common, the typical thecoma, is characterized by ill-defined masses of rounded vacuolated cells laden with lipid; the second type, a luteinized thecoma, has the basic appearance of a fibroma or a typical thecoma but also contains lutein cells singly or in nests.[24] Typical thecomas are almost always estrogenic; the luteinized forms are estrogenic in one half the cases but virilizing in about 10 per cent of the cases.[23]

The thecoma is bilateral in only 3 per cent of the cases[23] and is almost never malignant. Several tumors purported to be malignant thecomas have appeared in the literature, but most of them are better interpreted as endocrinologically inactive fibrosarcomas or diffuse granulosa cell tumors.[25]

In cases in which the preservation of fertility is important, a thecoma can be treated adequately by unilateral oophorectomy.

A rare benign tumor in the thecoma-fibroma group is the sclerosing stromal tumor, characterized by an admixture of lipid-laden cells and fibroblasts with prominent sclerosis.[26] More than 80 per cent of these tumors occur in the first three decades of life, and occasional examples have been associated with evidence of estrogen or androgen secretion.[27]

Sertoli–Stromal Cell Tumors (Androblastomas)

Sertoli–stromal cell tumors contain Sertoli cells, Leydig cells, indifferent stromal cells, or all three in varying proportions and varying degrees of differentiation.[3, 28–30]

Sertoli–stromal cell tumors are about one fifth as frequent as granulosa cell tumors; they occur at all ages but are most often encountered in women in the early reproductive-age period, with an average age at diagnosis of 25 years.[28] Virilization occurs in more than one third of cases. Plasma testosterone levels are always elevated in the virilized patients, ranging from 1.2 to 7.0 ng/ml (4.2 to 24.2 nmol/L)[12]; weaker androgens and other steroid hormones may also be increased to varying extents.[12, 31] 17-KS values usually are normal or only slightly elevated, although an occasional high level has been recorded. One small, well-differentiated Sertoli-Leydig cell tumor secreted inhibin into the circulation.[32] More than 20 Sertoli–stromal cell tumors have been associated with elevated plasma levels of α-fetoprotein, which may be demonstrated immunohistochemically in various tumor cell types, but the levels typically are not as high as those associated with ovarian yolk sac tumors.[33] At operation the tumor varies in size from a small nodule that was not palpable preoperatively to a huge mass that distends the abdomen. The wide variety of gross appearances that have been described for granulosa cell tumors can be duplicated by Sertoli–stromal cell tumors.

The microscopic patterns of these tumors vary more widely than those of any other ovarian neoplasms with the exception of teratomas. Most of the specimens contain mixtures of Sertoli and Leydig cells and have been subdivided into well-differentiated forms, tumors of intermediate differentiation, poorly differentiated (sarcomatoid) tumors, a heterogenous group identified by a content of one or more heterologous elements, and a retiform type. The well-differentiated Sertoli–stromal cell tumor[30] is characterized by solid or hollow tubules filled with or lined by cells best interpreted as Sertoli cells and separated by well-developed Leydig cells; the latter occasionally contain crystals of Reinke, the specific cytoplasmic inclusions of testicular Leydig cells. In the intermediate form, well-defined islands and cords or ill-defined masses of immature Sertoli cells alternate with cellular tissue of stromal derivation, which typically contains islands of well-differentiated Leydig cells. In the poorly differentiated Sertoli–stromal cell tumor the appearance may be that of fibrosarcoma, poorly differentiated carcinoma, or a combination of the two; in such cases identification of mature elements compatible with Sertoli cells and Leydig cells permits a specific diagnosis. The heterologous tumor, in addition to containing intermediate or poorly differentiated elements, is characterized by the presence of unexpected heterologous tissues, the genesis of which is difficult to explain.[34, 35] These tissues include mucinous glands and cysts, the epithelium of which often contains argentaffin cells, foci of carcinoid tumor, rhabdomyoblasts, and cartilage. Although a teratomatous origin has been postulated to account for the presence of these foreign elements, more characteristic components of teratomas are not encountered in heterologous Sertoli–stromal cell tumors, and ovarian tumors clearly recognizable as teratomas have never been reported to contain gonadal tissue. The occurrence of heterologous elements in these tumors is better explained by neometaplasia (alteration of neoplastic cells into cells of a type not normally found in the tissue of origin of the tumor). Retiform Sertoli–stromal cell tumors have a prominent component that simulates morphologically the rete testis.

Instead of containing both testicular cell types, neoplasms in the Sertoli–stromal cell category may be composed exclusively, or almost exclusively, of either Sertoli cells or Leydig cells in various degrees of differentiation. Pure Sertoli cell tumors may contain lipid in varying amounts and may be associated with estrogenic manifestations.[29] One distinctive form of estrogenic ovarian tumor, which originally was designated *folliculome lipidique* (lipid-rich granulosa cell tumor), has been reinterpreted as a Sertoli cell tumor with lipid storage because of its basic tubular architecture.[29] Tumors composed exclusively of Leydig cells may not have the same histogenesis as other tumors in the Sertoli–stromal cell category, arising in many cases directly from the hilus cells (hilar Leydig cells), which can be found in the ovarian hilus of more than 80 per cent of adult women on careful microscopic sampling.[36] Hilus cell tumors are discussed in greater detail below, in the section on steroid cell tumors.

Although Leydig cells and their morphological variants are the obvious producers of androgens in Sertoli–stromal cell tumors, it is more difficult to pinpoint the source of the estrogen excess that is associated with occasional tumors in this category. In view of the well-established existence of pure Sertoli cell tumors that are estrogenic in canine and human testes (see Ch. 136) and ovaries,[29] it is reasonable to conclude that the Sertoli cell component of Sertoli–stromal cell tumors may secrete estrogens as well. In a similar vein, the knowledge that testicular Leydig cell tumors are capable of estradiol production[37] (see Ch. 136) suggests that Leydig cells within ovarian tumors may also secrete estrogens. A final possibility in some cases is the conversion of androgens produced by neoplastic Leydig cells into estrogens by the Sertoli cells in the tumor or peripherally.

After removal of a virilizing Sertoli–stromal cell tumor, normal menses characteristically resume in about four weeks. In most cases the hirsutism improves but often incompletely. Clitoromegaly and particularly deepening of the voice are less apt to regress.

The overall five-year survival rate of patients with Sertoli–stromal cell tumors is about 80 per cent, but the prognosis varies widely, depending on the stage and degree of differentiation of the tumor.[28] Almost all the tumors are stage I. Well-differentiated Sertoli–Leydig cell tumors are benign, whereas the poorly differentiated forms typically have a rapidly malignant course, with only a 41 per cent survival rate. Tumors of intermediate differentiation are associated with a survival rate of 89 per cent, and those with heterologous elements, 81 per cent. Almost all the malignant tumors in the latter category contain sarcoma with islands of cartilage or rhabdomyosarcoma. Recurrences usually are recognized within the first postoperative year and are rare after five years. Pelvic and intra-abdominal spread is much more common that distant metastasis.

Because Sertoli–stromal cell tumors predominantly occur in young women and are bilateral in less than 2 per cent of cases, unilateral oophorectomy or salpingo-oophorectomy is justifiable if the preservation of fertility is an important consideration and there is no evidence of extension beyond the involved ovary. The role of radiation therapy and chemotherapy in the treatment of these tumors after they have spread beyond surgical control is uncertain, but these approaches have been effective in some cases.[22, 28]

Sex Cord Tumor with Annular Tubules

The sex cord tumor with annular tubules is composed of simple and complex ring-like solid tubular structures whose appearance is intermediate between that of tubules filled by Sertoli cells and islands of granulosa cells.[38] Tavassoli and Norris[39] have shown that some cells of the annular tubules contain Charcot-Bottcher bundles of filaments, apparently specific inclusions of Sertoli cells; focal differentiation into granulosa cells may be observed as well. When sex cord tumors with annular tubules grow in the form of multiple tumorlets with a prominent tendency to undergo calcification, they are almost always associated with the Peutz-Jeghers syndrome (gastrointestinal polyposis, mucocutaneous pigmentation, and, occasionally, adenoma malignum of the cervix). When they occur in the absence of the syndrome, they typically form large solitary ovarian masses, are commonly estrogenic and frequently secrete progesterone, and often metastasize to lymph nodes. In one remarkable case[40] a woman had repeated lymph node recurrences of this type of tumor over a 22-year period. The recurrences were associated with striking elevations in müllerian-inhibiting substance in the plasma; inhibin and progesterone were also present in high levels.

Gynandroblastoma

An extremely rare tumor, the gynandroblastoma should be diagnosed only if clearly recognizable, well-differentiated ovarian and testicular cellular elements co-exist, each forming a significant component of the neoplasm.[3, 41] The presence of occasional foci of ovarian cell types in an otherwise typical Sertoli–stromal cell tumor or of testicular cell types in a granulosa–stromal cell tumor is insufficient evidence for the diagnosis. The gynandroblastoma is a morphological curiosity rather than a clinicopathological entity and has been overdiagnosed as shown in the literature. The coexistence of estrogenic and androgenic clinical manifestations alone does not warrant a diagnosis of gynandroblastoma, and indeed, the true gynandroblastoma is not typically associated with this combination of clinical findings.

Steroid Cell Tumors

These rare tumors are composed exclusively of cells that have the morphological features of typical steroid hormone–producing cells (lutein cells, Leydig cells, and adrenal cortical cells).[3, 42] The patient is virilized in almost one half the cases, but endocrine manifestations often are absent and, rarely, estrogenic changes or Cushing's syndrome is associated. The tumors appear as red-brown, yellow, or orange masses that vary greatly in size and may be too small to be palpable on pelvic examination or even recognizable before bisection of the involved ovary at operation. Steroid cell tumors can be conveniently divided into three categories according to their cell of origin, known or unknown (Table 121–2).

About two thirds of these tumors have been designated "not otherwise specified" (NOS) because of their uncertain cellular lineage.[42] Such tumors have also been referred to as lipoid cell tumors, lipid cell tumors, adrenal rest

TABLE 121–2. CLASSIFICATION OF STEROID CELL TUMORS

1. Not otherwise specified (lipid cell tumor; lipoid cell tumor)
2. Stromal luteoma
3. Leydig cell tumors
   a. Hilus cell tumor
   b. Leydig cell tumor, nonhilar type

tumors, adrenal-like tumors, masculinovoblastomas, luteomas, and hypernephromas. The first two terms, which are in wide usage, are inappropriate because of their lack of specificity and the paucity or absence of fat in about one fourth of tumors in this category.[42] Steroid cell tumors NOS occur in patients of all ages, but most of them are encountered during the reproductive period, in patients with an average age of 43 years. When they are masculinizing, they are much more often associated with high levels of weak androgens in the plasma and elevated levels of 17-KS's in the urine than are Sertoli–stromal cell tumors; however, because of overlaps in results, these two types of tumor cannot be reliably distinguished by hormone assays in individual patients. A wide variety of other steroid hormones, including testosterone, androgen precursors, and estrogens, have also been reported to be elevated in the plasma of patients with these tumors.[12, 42, 43]

The presence of some of the features of Cushing's syndrome and the finding of high levels of 17-KS's in the urine have led to the speculation that at least some steroid cell tumors originate in adrenal cortical rests, which have been identified in the broad ligament near the ovary in about one fourth of hysterectomy specimens.[44] Only rarely, however, has convincing evidence of corticosteroid production by a steroid cell tumor been reported. In one unusual case[45] a six-year-old girl had a unilateral adrenalectomy after a diagnosis of adrenogenital syndrome had been made but did not experience a regression of masculinization until an ovarian steroid cell tumor, which arose in the hilar or medullary area, was removed two years later. Preoperative elevated urinary levels of 17-KS's, 17-ketogenic steroids, and pregnanetriol and the demonstration of cortisol and corticosterone production by the tumor in vitro favored neoplasia of cells of adrenal cortical rather than gonadal type. Marieb et al.[46] described the case of a metastasizing steroid cell tumor accompanied by evidence of androgen excess and Cushing's syndrome; the level of free cortisol in the peripheral blood was elevated, and its level in the ovarian vein draining the tumor was significantly higher. We have seen two additional cases of metastasizing ovarian steroid cell tumor with hirsutism, Cushing's syndrome, and elevated values for free cortisol in the peripheral blood[15] and one case of an apparently benign steroid cell tumor with hypercortisolemia and Cushing's syndrome in a child.[42] An additional case of steroid cell tumor in a child with isosexual precocity and Cushing's syndrome has been described.[47] Although the occurrence of the aforementioned tumors, which functioned like adrenal cortex, suggests an origin from adrenal cortical rests, all the tumors appeared to be situated within the ovary, where such rests are exceedingly rare and have not been observed except in fetuses. The intraovarian location of the tumors is more suggestive of ectopic adrenocortical function on the part of neoplastic cells of gonadal origin. Virilizing tumor-like hyperplastic nodules of adrenal rest cells have been observed within the mesosalpinx and mesovarium in a case of Nelson's syndrome[48] (see Ch. 100); testosterone production by these lesions was demonstrated to be dependent on the high ACTH level characteristic of this disorder.

If a steroid cell tumor is small and situated within the ovarian stroma, an origin from lutein cells of the ovarian stroma appears almost certain. Tumors in this category have been designated stromal luteomas[3, 49, 50] and account for almost one fourth of steroid cell tumors. These tumors are benign, resulting in estrogenic manifestations and, occasionally, virilization and are almost always associated with underlying stromal hyperthecosis. An unknown number of unclassified steroid cell tumors probably are stromal luteomas that have grown to a large size and obliterated evidence of their site of origin.

Steroid cell tumors that contain crystals of Reinke in the cytoplasm of some of their cells are appropriately designated Leydig cell tumors and account for more than 10 per cent of all steroid cell tumors. Many of these neoplasms are situated in the hilus of the ovary, where cells that have the morphological features of Leydig cells have been demonstrated in more than 80 per cent of adult women.[36] Leydig cell tumors in this location are referred to as hilus cell tumors.[36, 36a, 36b] Other Leydig cell tumors appear to arise directly from the ovarian stroma.[51] With few exceptions, a diagnosis of Leydig cell tumor is uncertain unless the presence of crystals of Reinke is clearly documented. Conversely, it is probable that many and perhaps most ovarian Leydig cell tumors cannot be identified as such and remain within the NOS category of steroid cell tumors in view of the absence of crystals of Reinke in up to 60 per cent of Leydig cell tumors of the testis (see Ch. 136).[52]

Recognizable Leydig cell tumors of the ovary occur in an older age group than do steroid cell tumors NOS, are typically virilizing, and are characterized by high levels of testosterone rather than by the weaker androgens that often are the predominant products of the latter group of tumors. However, a variety of androgens and their precursors[53–55] have been identified in the ovarian veins that drain Leydig cell tumors.

Almost one half of steroid cell tumors NOS are malignant, with occasional recurrences many years after removal of the primary tumor. Cancer has not been reported in childhood and is more common in postmenopausal than premenopausal women. The most reliable pathological correlates of cancer are two or more mitotic figures per 10 high-power fields (92 per cent malignant), necrosis (86 per cent malignant), a diameter of 7 cm or greater (78 per cent malignant), hemorrhage (77 per cent malignant), and grade 2 or 3 nuclear atypia (64 per cent malignant).[42] No tumor recognizable as a stromal luteoma has been reported to be malignant, and with possible rare exceptions,[56] Leydig cell tumors have also been uniformly benign.

Gonadoblastoma

A complex tumor, the gonadoblastoma is composed of germ cells, sex cord derivatives, and, in two thirds of cases, stromal derivatives.[57, 58] The germ cells, which resemble those of the ovarian dysgerminoma and the testicular seminoma, and the sex cord elements, which have the appearance of immature Sertoli or granulosa cells, characteristically grow within circumscribed nests. The stromal derivatives resemble lutein cells and Leydig cells; they have not been reported to contain crystals of Reinke. Foci of calcification are present in the germ cell–sex cord component in most of cases and may become confluent. The calcification often is so extensive that it can be observed on an x-ray film of the pelvis. In about one half of cases of gonadoblastoma, the germ cells transgress the limits of the circumscribed nests and invade the stroma to form a germinoma (dysgerminoma or seminoma). A more highly malignant form of germ cell tumor, such as yolk sac tumor, embryonal carcinoma, or choriocarcinoma, occasionally develops in association with a gonadoblastoma.[57, 58] The gonadoblastoma may be of microscopic dimensions or may form a large mass, which can be soft and fleshy if there is significant germinomatous overgrowth, totally calcified, or of mixed consistency.

Almost all gonadoblastomas arise in people with abnormal gonads (see Ch. 109), although a rare example has been observed in an otherwise normal male or female. Many of the smaller tumors can be demonstrated to originate in streak gonads or dysgenetic testes, but it usually is impossible to determine the nature of the underlying gonad because the tumor has replaced it. The sexual disorders that are most commonly associated with gonadoblastomas are 46,XY pure gonadal dysgenesis and mixed gonadal dysgenesis, but an occasional patient has had Turner's syndrome, or true hermaphroditism.[58] The great majority of patients have been chromatin-negative, and the most common karyotypes have been 46,XY and 45,X / 46,XY. Other types of mosaicism have also been recorded, and a rare patient has been 46,XX. The tumor may be detected in childhood or during adult life. Four fifths of the patients are phenotypic females, who usually are masculinized to some extent. Although it often is difficult to determine whether endocrine abnormalities in a patient with a gonadoblastoma are related to the tumor or to the underlying gonadal abnormality, both clinical and biochemical evidence, including in vitro studies of tumor tissue, indicate that the Leydig-like cells of the tumor are capable of androgen production, which may result in virilization. In vitro evidence of estrogen production has also been reported, and a few patients have experienced hot flashes after the removal of a gonadoblastoma.[57]

Although the gonadoblastoma unassociated with an invasive germ cell tumor has not been demonstrated to exhibit a malignant behavior and can be regarded as an in situ germ cell cancer, the common complication of invasive germinoma and the occasional association with a more malignant type of germ cell tumor indicate that a gonad containing a gonadoblastoma is hazardous and should be removed. Because the tumor is bilateral in more than one third of cases and arises almost invariably in patients with abnormal gonads, the removal of the contralateral gonad is also indicated in almost all cases. Because many gonadoblastomas are of microscopic dimensions and are incidental findings in biopsy specimens of gonads obtained to establish the nature of a sexual disorder, and because 25 per cent of patients with gonadal dysgenesis and a Y chromosome have been reported to have gonadoblastomas or other malignant germ cell tumors, routine gonadectomy is recommended for patients with this disorder. A 100 per cent survival can be expected after the removal of gonads that harbor one or more gonadoblastomas if significant germ cell infiltration of the stroma has not occurred. A germinoma that arises within a gonadoblastoma is capable of metastatic spread, and the yolk sac tumor, embryonal carcinoma, and choriocarcinoma that occasionally are associated with gonadoblastomas can be expected to have the same poor prognosis that has been established for these tumors when they occur in pure form.

Tumors with Functioning Stroma

In tumors with functioning stroma the neoplastic cells stimulate the tumor stroma or the adjacent ovarian stroma to differentiate into cells that are capable of secreting androgens, estrogens, or progesterone, or a combination of these hormones[3, 59–68]; in rare cases hilus cells are stimulated to proliferate along the hilar margin of the tumor.[66] These tumors may be benign or malignant and primary or metastatic. Many forms of ovarian neoplasia have been reported to be associated with a functioning stroma, which is unique in the ovary among all the endocrine glands. The evidence for the existence of tumors with functioning stroma is the appearance of an endocrine disorder that regresses after removal of the tumor; abnormal preoperative results of steroid assays that revert to normal after removal of the tumor; the presence of cells that resemble steroid hormone–secreting cells in the stroma of the tumor, in a rim of adjacent ovarian stroma or in the ovarian hilus[66]; histochemical and immunohistochemical reactions in these cells that are characteristic of steroid hormone–secreting cells; the recovery of various steroids from the neoplastic tissue; and the demonstration in vitro of an ability of the tumor to synthesize steroid hormones from precursors.

In some cases hCG appears to be a factor in stimulating the stroma to develop into steroid hormone–secreting tissue. A number of ovarian tumors with functioning stroma have virilized pregnant women,[59–63] and it is possible that other tumors with a similar stroma secrete estrogens, which would not cause clinical manifestations during pregnancy. The relation of the stromal stimulation and androgen production to the hCG level of pregnancy is strongly suggested by various findings in individual reported cases of this type. In several patients the virilizing tumor was a benign neoplasm that had probably been present before the onset of pregnancy, at a time when virilism was absent. In one case of a masculinizing Krukenberg tumor that occurred during pregnancy,[61] a similar tumor that had been found in the contralateral ovary before the onset of the pregnancy had not masculinized the patient; in addition, regression of the virilism and a decline in androgen levels occurred after the termination of the pregnancy but before the removal of the tumor; finally, the postpartum administration of hCG caused an increase in plasma androgens and urinary 17-KS's. In still another case[62] a Brenner tumor that virilized a pregnant woman was unable to produce testosterone in vitro unless hCG was added to the incubate.[63] In one case of an ovarian tumor with functioning stroma that occurred in the absence of pregnancy,[64] hCG, secreted by a dysgerminoma containing syncytiotrophoblast cells, stimulated the stroma in and around the tumor to luteinize and produce androgens, resulting in virilization; in another case of a morphologically similar tumor[65] the associated clinical syndrome was isosexual pseudoprecocity.

In most cases of ovarian tumors with functioning stroma that occur in nonpregnant patients, there is no obvious explanation of why the stroma has been stimulated to secrete steroid hormones. However, the findings that carcinomas of diverse origin, including those arising in the ovary, may be associated with elevated levels of hCG in the serum[69] and that the epithelial components of many carcinomas of the ovary are positive for hCG by immunohistochemical staining[70] suggest that this hormone may be a pathogenetic factor in stromal stimulation in at least some cases. Finally, Quinn et al.[67] have shown that a mucinous cystadenoma of borderline cancer that secreted various steroid hormones increased its production after an intramuscular injection of hCG.

The phenomenon of functioning stroma of an ovarian tumor is only occasionally evident clinically, but it adequately explains the abnormal maturation of squamous cells in the vaginal smear that is observed in many patients with ovarian cancer[1] as well as the elevated urinary levels of estrogens that are found in about 50 per cent of women with surface epithelial tumors and metastatic carcinomas of the ovary.[2] MacDonald et al.[68] have shown that a mucinous cystadenocarcinoma with functioning stroma that was associated with endometrial hyperplasia produced androstenedione, which was converted elsewhere to estrone, the hormone directly responsible for the estrogenic manifestation; Brennecke et al.[71] made a similar observation in a case of an estrogenic metastatic cecal adenocarcinoma. Heinonen et al.[72] have demonstrated, however, that surface epithelial-stromal tumors, particularly mucinous tumors, may secrete estrogens and progesterone as well androgens directly, based on measurements of these hormones in ovarian vein blood.

Evidence based on culture of ovarian cancer cells suggests that the tumor cells themselves may also have a role in steroid hormone secretion.[73]

GONADOTROPIN-SECRETING TUMORS

Choriocarcinoma

Choriocarcinoma is composed of cytotrophoblast and syncytiotrophoblast growing in intimate association with each other. In the ovary, choriocarcinomas are only rarely of germ cell origin, and most of these tumors are admixed with other forms of malignant germ cell tumor, most often immature teratoma.[3, 74–77] Ovarian choriocarcinomas are more often metastatic from other sites in the genital tract or arise from the trophoblast of a primary ovarian pregnancy.[74] The germ cell origin of a choriocarcinoma is acceptable only if the tumor has developed before puberty or is associated with another type of germ cell cancer. Most of the tumors of germ cell derivation described in the literature have occurred in the first two decades. Isosexual pseudoprecocity has been reported in about one half the prepubertal patients, and heterosexual precocity has been present on rare occasions.[3] In older patients irregular menstrual bleeding and rapid enlargement of the breasts, occasionally with colostrum secretion, may be observed. Levels of hCG, placental lactogen, estrogens, and androgens may be elevated. The higher frequency of estrogenic than

androgenic effects may be related to the ability of the tumor cells, like normal trophoblast, to aromatize circulating androgens to estrogens. The tumor has almost always been fatal within a period of several weeks to one year, with spread throughout the abdomen and often to the lungs. Rare patients have survived for many years after simple removal of the tumor.[75] Chemotherapy, such as the combination of methotrexate, dactinomycin, and chlorambucil, has produced prolonged remission in several patients with ovarian choriocarcinoma of germ cell origin.[77]

Embryonal Carcinoma

The rare embryonal carcinoma of the ovary, which resembles morphologically that of the testis, often contains syncytiotrophoblastic cells and is associated with endocrine manifestations similar to those of the choriocarcinoma.[78]

Polyembryoma

An exceptionally rare tumor, the polyembryoma is a teratoma, most or all of which is composed of myriad embryoid bodies. Enough trophoblast may be present in these structures to produce clinically significant quantities of hCG.[79]

Dysgerminoma with Syncytiotrophoblastic Cells

The dysgerminoma with syncytiotrophoblastic cells is a typical dysgerminoma except for the presence of widely scattered syncytiotrophoblastic cells, which grow adjacent to dilated vascular sinusoids and stain immunohistochemically for hCG.[64, 65, 80] This type of tumor is discussed earlier in the section on tumors with functioning stroma.

Mixed Primitive Germ Cell Tumors

Less than 10 per cent of primitive germ cell tumors of the ovary are composed of mixtures of the various forms described above. The clinical manifestations, prognosis, and therapy of these tumors depend on the nature and, possibly, the quantity of their various components.[76, 77]

Ovarian Carcinomas with Ectopic Chorionic Gonadotropin Production

This subject is discussed in the sections on tumors with functioning stroma and tumors with ectopic hormone production.

HIGHLY SPECIALIZED TERATOMAS WITH HORMONE PRODUCTION

Struma Ovarii

Struma ovarii is a type of teratoma in which thyroid tissue is present exclusively or forms a grossly recognizable component of a more complex neoplasm.[3] The peak age of incidence is in the fifth decade; occasional examples have been encountered in postmenopausal women and rare cases before puberty. On gross examination most strumas appear to be composed entirely of thyroid tissue; others are associated with dermoid cysts, and occasional examples with mucinous or serous cystadenomas. The thyroid tissue is brown or green-brown; it may be solid but often is partly or almost entirely cystic with a content of gelatinous fluid. The contralateral ovary occasionally contains a dermoid cyst and, rarely, another struma. On microscopic examination the thyroid-type tissue is unencapsulated and typically resembles a thyroid adenoma, which may be predominantly macrofollicular, microfollicular, or embryonal. Occasionally vascular invasion and rarely a papillary pattern are observed. Less than 5 per cent of strumas have had a malignant clinical course, with metastases having been reported in the lungs, bones, liver, and brain[3, 81, 82]; evidence of recurrent disease may appear one to two decades after the removal of the primary tumor. Rarely histologically mature implants of thyroid tissue are found on the peritoneum; this process, which has been termed benign strumosis, has been associated with a long survival.

The frequency of function of ovarian strumas is unknown. In occasional cases there has been strong clinical evidence that a struma was responsible for the development of thyrotoxicosis, but such cases have appeared mostly in the older literature, before the advent of sophisticated assays of thyroid function. Likewise, enlargement of the thyroid gland has been reported in about 15 per cent of cases of struma ovarii, and the role of the thyroid gland itself in the pathogenesis of the associated thyrotoxicosis was not evaluated in some of the cases in which this disorder was ascribed solely to a struma. Scanning after the administration of radioactive iodine has been advocated as an aid in the diagnosis of struma ovarii, but at least one false-positive result has been reported.[83]

Most strumas are adequately treated by oophorectomy. If the tumor is greater than 5 cm in diameter or has solid foci on microscopic examination, x-ray examination of the lungs and bones and scanning with [131]iodine are indicated to detect possible metastases. Treatment of malignant struma ovarii should follow the same principles that dictate the management of carcinoma of the thyroid gland (see Ch. 50).

Carcinoid

Six types of ovarian carcinoid have been observed, five of which are primary and the sixth metastatic, usually from the ileum.[3, 34, 84–86] The primary forms include the insular, or midgut, variety; the trabecular, or foregut-hindgut, variety; the strumal carcinoid, in which the carcinoid grows in association with a struma; the goblet cell carcinoid (adenocarcinoid); and a very rare type that arises as a heterologous element within a Sertoli–Leydig cell tumor. Only the primary insular and metastatic insular forms have been reported to be accompanied by the carcinoid syndrome, with the exception of one case of strumal carcinoid.[87] The carcinoids of various types have occurred exclusively in adults, with the youngest patient in the third decade and the oldest in the ninth.

All the reported primary carcinoids have been unilateral, although another type of tumor, usually a dermoid cyst, may be present in the contralateral ovary. The carcinoid may form a small, firm, tan to yellow nodule that protrudes into the lumen of a dermoid cyst, diffusely thickens the wall of the cyst, lies within a predominantly solid mature teratoma, or forms a large, solid homogeneous mass in which teratomatous elements may be found on microscopic examination. The insular carcinoid is characterized by discrete islands of argentaffin cells that may be perforated, particularly at the periphery of the nests, by numerous small, round glandular spaces. Argentaffin granules usually are visible in hematoxylin-eosin sections and are almost always identifiable after argentaffin, argyrophil, or chromogranin-immunohistochemical staining. The trabecular carcinoid is characterized by a ribbon-like pattern of the tumor cells; argentaffin granules are observed much less often than in the insular carcinoid. The rare cases of carcinoid that have been found in Sertoli–Leydig cell tumors have been of the insular or goblet cell type.[34] Metastatic carcinoids usually are insular but occasionally are of the trabecular type.

One third of the reported cases of primary insular carcinoid have been associated with manifestations of the carcinoid syndrome (flushing, sometimes misinterpreted as menopausal; diarrhea; pulmonary stenosis, tricuspid insufficiency, or both; and peripheral edema) (see Ch. 150). Because the effluent of the tumor is routed through the ovarian vein into the inferior vena cava and not into the portal circulation with hepatic inactivation of carcinoid hormones, an ovarian carcinoid can produce the characteristic syndrome in the absence of hepatic and extraportal metastases. Furthermore, because only a rare ovarian carcinoid is malignant, the associated syndrome has almost always been cured by removal of the tumor. In exceptional cases cardiac valvular damage has progressed despite the restoration of the hormone values to normal levels, or the tumor has recurred with or without a return of the carcinoid syndrome.

The primary insular carcinoid of the ovary must be distinguished from the metastatic form, the other type that often is associated with the carcinoid syndrome.[85] Such a distinction may be difficult for the pathologist at the time of operation because a primary carcinoid of the bowel may be small and escape detection. Clues to the differential diagnosis are as follows: metastatic carcinoids commonly are bilateral, in contrast to primary forms; metastases to the ovaries usually are associated with metastases elsewhere, particularly on the peritoneum and in the liver; other teratomatous elements usually can be detected either grossly or microscopically in specimens of primary carcinoid; postoperatively, the urinary level of 5-hydroxyindoleacetic acid can be expected to return to normal in the case of a functioning primary ovarian carcinoid but usually remains elevated or rises again within several months if the ovarian tumors are metastatic because residual disease typically is present elsewhere in the abdomen.

Primary ovarian carcinoids are adequately treated by unilateral oophorectomy in a young woman, but total hysterectomy and bilateral salpingo-oophorectomy usually is performed when preservation of fertility is not a problem. Only 5 of about 70 reported cases of primary insular carcinoid have had a malignant behavior.

Strumal Carcinoid

The strumal carcinoid contains struma and carcinoid, usually intimately admixed with each other.[3, 86, 87] In most cases this tumor is associated with a dermoid cyst or a solid mature teratoma, but it may be present in pure or almost pure form. Almost all reported patients have been between the ages of 30 and 60 years, with a range of 21 to 77 years. At operation the tumor varies considerably in appearance, depending on whether the strumal, carcinoid, or another teratomatous component predominates. All reported cases have been unilateral, although another type of tumor, usually a dermoid cyst, occasionally has been present in the contralateral ovary.

Microscopic examination reveals struma associated with a carcinoid, which has a predominantly trabecular pattern. Although the two components occasionally appear to collide with each other, much more often they are intimately admixed, with argyrophil cells lining follicles filled with colloid. Although carcinoids have not been reported in the thyroid gland itself, medullary carcinomas of the thyroid with amyloid stroma may bear a morphological resemblance to the strumal carcinoid, may contain argentaffin granules, and have been associated rarely with the carcinoid syndrome. Immunohistochemical staining of strumal carcinoids for calcitonin and the identification of amyloid in their stroma in several cases heighten their resemblance to the medullary carcinoma.[5, 88]

Only one case of strumal carcinoid has been associated with the carcinoid syndrome.[87] In a few cases preoperative or postoperative findings have suggested the possibility of hyperfunction of the thyroid component of the tumor, but unequivocal hyperthyroidism has not been reported. Although the strumal carcinoid often has been referred to in the older literature as malignant struma, only rarely does it spread beyond the ovary.

Teratoma Containing Pituitary Adenoma

Rarely pituitary tissue is found in an ovarian teratoma. Two cases have been reported of pituitary adenomas within teratomas that secreted ACTH and caused Cushing's syndrome.[89] We have seen another case in which a prolactin-secreting adenoma arose in the wall of a dermoid cyst and caused hyperprolactinemia that disappeared after removal of the tumor.[90]

TUMORS WITH ECTOPIC HORMONE PRODUCTION

A hypercalcemic state simulating hyperparathyroidism and reversed by removal of the tumor has been reported in association with a variety of ovarian cancers (see Ch. 62).[91–93] The most common of these are the small cell carcinoma and the clear cell carcinoma. The former is a rare, highly malignant ovarian tumor with an epithelial growth pattern. It occurs almost exclusively in patients in their second, third, and fourth decades, with an average age of 24 years. The nature of the neoplastic cells and that of the hypercalcemic factor it produces are unknown; the tumor is not of neuroendocrine type, differing in many respects from small cell carcinoma of the type encountered most often in the lung. Cushing's syndrome caused by ectopic ACTH production has been recorded in association with a "poorly differentiated adenocarcinoma," a malignant Sertoli cell tumor, and a presumably primary small cell carcinoma of the ovary that resembled an oat cell carcinoma of the lung; the last tumor also resulted in the carcinoid syndrome. Ectopic production of hCG, as mentioned earlier in the section on tumors with functioning stroma, is common in cases of ovarian carcinoma of surface epithelial origin. One patient with an elevated level of hCG in the urine had marked luteinization of the stroma of the contralateral ovary and a decidual reaction in the endometrium; the tumor contained syncytial giant cells that resembled syncytiotrophoblast and were positive on immunofluorescence staining for hCG. Five ovarian tumors (a serous cystadenocarcinoma, a dysgerminoma, a fibroma, a schwannoma, and a carcinoid tumor) have been associated with hypoglycemia, which disappeared after the removal of the tumor in two of the cases. Ten cases of the Zollinger-Ellison syndrome (see Ch. 153) caused by gastrin secretion by benign, borderline, and malignant mucinous cystic tumors of the ovary have been reported. (These cases are not examples of ectopic hormone production in the strict sense of the term, since mucinous cystic tumors as well as other varieties of ovarian neoplasm may contain endocrine cells of gastrointestinal and pancreatic type and produce a variety of peptide hormones, including gastrin, as well as serotonin.[94])

Six ovarian tumors, most of them in the sex cord–stromal or steroid cell category have secreted renin ectopically, resulting in secondary hyperaldosteronism and hypertension (see Ch. 96).[95, 96] Three other tumors have produced aldosterone with resultant hypertension; suppression of the plasma renin level was demonstrated in one of these cases.

TUMOR-LIKE CONDITIONS WITH ENDOCRINE MANIFESTATIONS

Solitary Follicle Cyst and Corpus Luteum Cyst

The solitary follicle cyst and the corpus luteum cyst may develop at any time during the reproductive age period. They seldom exceed 8 to 10 cm in diameter; although commonly asymptomatic, they may rupture, with intra-abdominal hemorrhage and pain, and may be associated with abnormal uterine bleeding. If what appears to be a follicle cyst does not involute spontaneously within a month to six weeks, an abdominal exploration may be necessary to exclude a neoplasm. The administration of steroid contraceptives has proved helpful diagnostically by hastening the involution of the cyst.[97] A follicle cyst occasionally forms several years after the clinical onset of the menopause; in such cases it may result in endometrial stimulation and postmenopausal bleeding.[98]

Rarely, a single follicle cyst or several of them develop autonomously before puberty and cause abdominal pain or isosexual pseudoprecocity. The latter may regress as a result of spontaneous involution of the cyst, puncture or resection of the cyst, or oophorectomy (see Ch. 111).[5] Follicle cyst formation with sexual precocity in the McCune-Albright syndrome (polyostotic fibrous dysplasia, cutaneous melanin pigmentation, and endocrine abnormalities, the most common of which is sexual precocity) is likewise almost always independent of premature release of gonadotropins from the pituitary gland.[99]

Multiple Follicle Cysts (Polycystic Ovaries)

Polycystic ovaries, commonly associated with the Stein-Leventhal syndrome (infrequent, anovulatory uterine bleeding and sterility, often accompanied by hirsutism), is characterized by the bilateral presence of multiple follicle cysts, usually accompanied by ovarian enlargement, collagenization of the outermost portion of the cortex (often erroneously designated "thickening of the capsule"), follicular hyperthecosis (proliferation and excessive luteinization of the theca interna layer of the follicles), an absence or rarity of stigmata of ovulation, and a variable amount of medullary stromal hyperplasia, sometimes accompanied by slight degrees of stromal hyperthecosis (the presence of lutein cells in the stroma) (see Ch. 120).[3, 100, 101] The syndrome typically begins in the early postmenarchal years but occasionally follows a pregnancy or the withdrawal of oral contraceptive medication.[102] It lacks the more or less abrupt onset of amenorrhea and progressive virilization associated with most androgen-secreting ovarian tumors. The differential diagnosis of polycystic ovaries and virilizing ovarian tumors is discussed further in Chapter 120.

Some patients with polycystic ovaries have endometrial hyperplasia with varying degrees of atypicality and, rarely, adenocarcinoma, which typically is low grade and develops on the basis of unopposed estrogenic stimulation. The estrogenic state may result from the peripheral conversion of excess circulating androstenedione to estrone. Some of the adenocarcinomas have apparently been cured by curettage and therapy directed at restoring progesterone stimulation to the endometrium.[103] This unexpected result has led some observers to regard the endometrial lesion as being a reversible atypical hyperplasia that mimics carcinoma.

The polycystic ovarian syndrome is not a sharply defined clinicopathological entity, since polycystic ovaries may also be seen in women with irregular cycles without hirsutism and in hirsute women with regular cycles. At the other end of the spectrum there is clinical and pathological overlap between polycystic ovaries and stromal hyperthecosis (described later) in premenopausal women.

Stromal Hyperplasia and Hyperthecosis

Stromal hyperplasia is characterized by a bilateral nodular or diffuse proliferation of stromal cells that involves primarily the ovarian medulla but may involve the cortex as well. It occurs predominantly in perimenopausal women but may be seen at any age after puberty. Stromal hyperthecosis, which has also been called thecosis, thecomatosis, and diffuse luteinization of the ovarian stroma, refers to the presence of lutein cells lying singly or in clusters usually within hyperplastic stroma.[3, 36b, 104] These two disorders are closely related and have not always been clearly distinguished in the literature. Also, in premenopausal women with stromal hyperplasia with or without hyperthecosis, varying numbers of follicle cysts with luteinization of their theca interna layers usually are present as well, creating a transitional zone between these disorders and polycystic ovarian disease and making precise classification difficult.[105, 106]

Stromal hyperthecosis in a young woman often is associated with the clinical picture of the Stein-Leventhal syndrome but occasionally is accompanied by a more profound disorder characterized by virilism, obesity (which may be of the central type), hypertension, and a disturbance in glucose tolerance. Sometimes hyperplasia and even adenocarcinoma of the endometrium have developed, as in cases of polycystic ovarian disease. Stromal hyperplasia without obvious hyperthecosis has been observed in association with similar clinical findings, but significantly virilized patients usually have considerable numbers of lutein cells in the hyperplastic ovarian stroma.

The association of masculinization with stromal hyperactivity is consistent with in vitro evidence that the stromal compartment of the ovary produces mainly androgens.[107] The occasional complication of endometrial hyperplasia or carcinoma may reflect estrogen production by the hyperplastic stroma in some cases and peripheral conversion of excess androgens to estrogens in others. The virilization associated with ovarian hyperthecosis typically is more insidious in onset than that produced by androgen-secreting ovarian tumors, but on occasion it may appear relatively abruptly. The association of stromal hyperthecosis with insulin resistance, sometimes accompanied by diabetes, and acanthosis nigricans has been receiving increasing attention (see Ch. 91).[108]

In cases of stromal hyperplasia and hyperthecosis the ovaries may not be perceptibly enlarged or may attain diameters as great as 7 cm. Sectioning reveals replacement of the entire ovaries or their central portions by solid tissue with a yellow hue. In younger women multiple follicle cysts and a white collagenization of the outer cortex are also typically observed. In contrast to virilizing ovarian tumors, which are almost always unilateral, stromal hyperplasia and hyperthecosis are almost invariably bilateral; however, we have seen two exceptional cases of unilateral virilizing hyperthecosis in which elevated androgen levels returned to normal after the removal of the involved ovary.

Wedge resections usually have been ineffective in the treatment of patients with stromal hyperthecosis accompanied by severe endocrine changes. Bilateral oophorectomy has caused considerable regression of virilism in some cases.[104, 109] Other cases in which oophorectomy has not been successful have suggested associated hyperactivity of the adrenal cortex.

According to Wiebe and Morris,[110] secretion of androstenedione exceeds that of testosterone in cases of polycystic ovarian disease and, to a lesser degree, in cases of stromal hyperthecosis, whereas the reverse is typically true in patients with Sertoli–Leydig or Leydig cell tumors.

Massive Edema and Fibromatosis

Rarely children and young women have unilateral or bilateral large ovarian masses composed of markedly edematous stroma, in which follicles and their derivatives are entrapped.[111] The inclusion of these structures indicates that the process is stromal proliferation and edema, and not neoplasia, which typically destroys or displaces follicles and their derivatives. Although most patients with massive edema present with nonspecific symptoms similar to those associated with ovarian tumors, in some cases the lesions have contained scattered lutein cells and have been accompanied by a clinical picture similar to that of the Stein-Leventhal syndrome, by virilization, or, rarely, by estrogenic manifestations. Two theories exist about the pathogenesis of this disorder. One is that repeated subclinical torsion of one or both ovaries results in lymphatic obstruction and subsequent edema; the edema is thought to stimulate proliferation of the ovarian stroma and, in some cases, its differentiation into lutein cells. The alternate theory is that the primary process is stromal hyperplasia or hyperthecosis, which enlarges the ovary, predisposing to secondary torsion and edema. Therapy should be directed toward resection of the edematous tissue with restoration of the ovary or ovaries to normal size and ovarian suspension[111] rather than oophorectomy. Young and Scully[112] have described an ovarian lesion characterized by replacement of one or both ovaries by dense fibromatous rather than loose edematous tissue. This disorder, designated fibromatosis, has many clinical and pathological features in common with massive edema, and the two processes may be variants of each other.

Pregnancy Luteoma, Hyperreactio Luteinalis, and Large Solitary Luteinized Follicle Cyst of Pregnancy and Puerperium

The pregnancy luteoma is characterized by the presence of one or more tumor-like nodules of lutein cell hyperplasia, usually encountered incidentally during a cesarean section in the last trimester of pregnancy.[113] About 80 per cent of the patients have been black. More than one fifth of them have been virilized, and when the offspring has been female, her external genitalia usually have been masculinized as well.[114] At operation the nodules, which may be more than 20 cm in diameter, are multiple in as many as one half the cases and bilateral in more than one third of them. Sectioning reveals solid, red-brown to brown-gray, well-circumscribed masses. Microscopic examination discloses a diffuse proliferation of large lutein cells, which are intermediate in size between normal granulosa lutein and theca lutein cells. The absence or paucity of intracellular lipid and the presence of numerous mitotic figures in some cases, as well as the common multiplicity of the lesions, are helpful clues in differentiating these lesions from tumors in the steroid cell category. There is evidence from postpartum morphological and biochemical findings in some cases that pregnancy luteomas are not true tumors but rather hyperplastic nodules that depend on stimulation by hCG for their structural and functional integrity.

Although hyperreactio luteinalis[113, 115, 116] also appears to depend on stimulation by hCG, it differs from the pregnancy luteoma in other respects. It is characterized by the presence of multiple lutein cysts, stromal congestion, and stromal edema, all of which may cause marked ovarian enlargement during any trimester of pregnancy. The process usually is bilateral. The lesion most often is seen in patients with trophoblastic disease but may develop during a normal twin or singleton pregnancy; it occasionally is associated with fetal hydrops. It may also be iatrogenic, complicating the administration of clomiphene citrate or, more often, gonadotropins for the induction of ovulation (ovarian hyperstimulation syndrome).[117, 118] In such cases there additionally may be multiple corpora lutea, ascites, and hydrothorax (acute Meigs' syndrome). Hyperreactio luteinalis has been reported to be associated with virilization of the mother but not of her female offspring.[113] On rare occasions pregnancy luteomas and hyperreactio luteinalis co-exist.

When the diagnosis of pregnancy luteoma is suspected at operation, removal of one of the nodules is appropriate to confirm the diagnosis. It is not necessary to remove one or both ovaries because spontaneous involution of the lesion can be expected with the decline in hCG after the termination of the pregnancy. Hemorrhage or torsion with infarction occasionally requires surgical intervention in cases of hyperreactio luteinalis, but in the great majority of the cases the process involutes spontaneously. Aspiration of ascitic fluid under ultrasound guidance has been used to relieve symptoms in cases of the ovarian hyperstimulation syndrome,[118] and aspiration of follicle cysts has been used to prevent its development.

Clement and Scully[119] have described eight cases of solitary luteinized follicle cysts discovered during pregnancy or at the time of the first postpartum visit. These cysts have ranged in size up to 26 cm in diameter. Microscopic examination has revealed a characteristic focal nuclear pleomorphism of the luteal cells lining the cyst. To date, no associated endocrine manifestations have been reported and no hormonal assays have been performed.

Autoimmune Oophoritis

Autoimmune oophoritis is a rare cause of premature ovarian failure and typically is associated with other autoimmune disorders, including endocrine diseases such as Addison's disease (see Chs. 159 and 160). Developing follicles as well as degenerating follicles are infiltrated by round cells, sometimes accompanied by granulomas; antibodies to steroid hormone–secreting cells can be demonstrated in the serum. Occasionally, presumably as a result of elevated pituitary gonadotropin levels, one or both ovaries may be enlarged by cystic dilatation of the follicles, resulting in masses up to 8 cm in diameter.[120]

REFERENCES

1. Rubin DK, Frost JK: The cytologic detection of ovarian cancer. Acta Cytol 7:191–195, 1963.
2. Rome RM, Fortune DW, Quinn MA, Brown JB: Functioning ovarian tumors in postmenopausal women. Obstet Gynecol 57:705–710, 1981.
3. Scully RE: Tumors of the Ovary and Maldeveloped Gonads. Atlas of Tumor Pathology, Second Series, Fasc. 16. Washington, D.C., Armed Forces Institute of Pathology, 1979.
4. Young RH, Dickersin GR, Scully RE: Juvenile granulosa cell tumor of the ovary. A clinicopathologic analysis of 125 cases. Am J Surg Pathol 8:575–596, 1984.
5. Liapi C, Evain-Brion D: Diagnosis of ovarian follicular cysts from birth to puberty: A report of twenty cases. Acta Paediatr Scand 76:91–96, 1987.
6. Gusberg SB, Kardon P: Proliferative endometrial response to theca-granulosa cell tumors. Am J Obstet Gynecol III:633–643, 1971.
7. Fathalla MF: The occurrence of granulosa and theca tumors in clinically normal ovaries. A study of 25 cases. J Obstet Gynaecol Br Commonw 74:279–282, 1967.
8. Nakashima N, Young RH, Scully RE: Androgenic granulosa cell tumors of the ovary. A clinicopathological analysis of seventeen cases and review of the literature. Arch Pathol Lab Med 108:786–791, 1984.
9. Aguirre P, Scully RE: Testosterone-secreting adrenal ganglioneuroma containing Leydig cells. Am J Surg Pathol 7:699–705, 1983.
10. Haning RV Jr, Loughlin J, Shapiro SS: Diagnosis and resection of an oral contraceptive–suppressible Sertoli-Leydig cell tumor with pres-

ervation of fertility and a 7-year follow-up. Obstet Gynecol 73:901–905, 1989.

11. Barkan AL, Cassorla F, Loriaux DL, et al: Steroid and gonadotropin secretion in a patient with a 30-year history of virilization due to lipoid-cell ovarian tumor. Obstet Gynecol 64:287–295, 1984.

12. Meldrum DR, Abraham GE: Peripheral and ovarian venous concentration of various steroid hormones in virilizing ovarian tumors. Obstet Gynecol 53:36–43, 1979.

13. Moltz L, Pickartz H, Sorensen R, et al: Ovarian and adrenal vein steroids in seven patients with androgen-secreting ovarian neoplasms: Selective catheterization findings. Fertil Steril 42:585–593, 1984.

14. Friedman CI, Schmidt GE, Kim MH, Powell J: Serum testosterone concentration in the evaluation of androgen-producing tumors. Am J Obstet Gynecol 153:44–49, 1985.

15. Young RH, Scully RE: Ovarian steroid cell tumors associated with Cushing's syndrome: A report of three cases. Int J Gynecol Pathol 6:40–48, 1987.

16. Bjorkholm E, Silfversward C: Prognostic factors in granulosa cell tumors. Gynecol Oncol II:261–274, 1981.

17. Stenwig JT, Hazekamp JT, Beecham JB: Granulosa cell tumors of the ovary. A clinicopathological study of 118 cases with long term follow-up. Gynecol Oncol 7:136–152, 1979.

18. Tanaka Y, Sasaki Y, Nishihira H, et al: Ovarian juvenile granulosa cell tumor associated with Maffucci's syndrome. Am J Clin Pathol 97:523–527, 1992.

19. Lappöhn RE, Burger HG, Bouma J, et al: Inhibin as a marker for granulosa-cell tumors. N Engl J Med 321:790–793, 1989.

19a. Nishida M, Jimi S, Haji M, et al: Juvenile granulosa cell tumor in association with a high serum inhibin level. Gynecol Oncol 40:90–94, 1991.

20. Rodgers KE, Marks JF, Ellefson DD, et al: Follicle regulatory protein: A novel marker for granulosa cell cancer patients. Gynecol Oncol 37:381–387, 1990.

21. Fathalla MF: The role of the ovarian stroma in hormone production by ovarian tumours. J Obstet Gynaecol Br Commonw 75:78–83, 1968.

22. Gershenson DM: Ovarian germ cell and stromal tumors. In Greer BE, Berek JS (eds): Gynecologic Oncology. Treatment Rationale and Techniques. New York, Elsevier, 1991, pp 167–184.

23. Bjorkholm E, Silfversward C: Theca-cell tumors. Clinical features and prognosis. Acta Radiol Oncol Rad Phys Biol 19:241–244, 1980.

24. Zhang J, Young RH, Arseneau J, Scully RE: Ovarian stromal tumors containing lutein or Leydig cells (luteinized thecomas and stromal Leydig cell tumors). A clinicopathological analysis of fifty cases. Int J Gynecol Pathol I:270–285, 1982.

25. Waxman M, Vuletin JC, Urcuyo R, Belling CG: Ovarian low grade stromal sarcoma with thecomatous features. A critical reappraisal of the so-called "malignant thecoma." Cancer 44:2206–2217, 1979.

26. Chalvardjian A, Scully RE: Sclerosing stromal tumors of the ovary. Cancer 31:664–670, 1973.

27. Cashell AW, Cohen ML: Masculinizing sclerosing stromal tumor of the ovary during pregnancy. Gynecol Oncol 43:281–285, 1991.

28. Young RH, Scully RE: Ovarian Sertoli-Leydig cell tumors. A clinicopathologic analysis of 207 cases. Am J Surg Pathol 9:543–569, 1985.

29. Young RH, Scully RE: Ovarian Sertoli cell tumors. A report of ten cases. Int J Gynecol Pathol 2:349–363, 1984.

30. Young RH, Scully RE: Well-differentiated ovarian Sertoli-Leydig cell tumor. A clinicopathologic analysis of 23 cases. Int J Gynecol Pathol 3:277–290, 1984.

31. Munermura M, Nakamura T, Matsuura K, et al: Endocrine profile of an ovarian androblastoma. Obstet Gynecol 15:100S–104S, 1982.

32. Ohashi M, Hasagawa Y, Haji M, et al: Production of immunoreactive inhibin by virilizing ovarian tumour. Clin Endocrinol 33:613–618, 1990.

33. Gagnon S, Teta B, Silva EG, McCaughey WTE: Frequency of α-fetoprotein production by Sertoli-Leydig cell tumors of the ovary: An immunohistochemical study of eight cases. Mod Pathol 2:63–67, 1989.

34. Young RH, Prat J, Scully RE: Ovarian Sertoli-Leydig cell tumors with heterologous elements. I. Gastrointestinal epithelium and carcinoid—a clinicopathologic analysis of thirty-six cases. Cancer 50:2448–2456, 1982.

35. Prat J, Young RH, Scully RE: Ovarian Sertoli-Leydig cell tumors with heterologous elements. II. Cartilage and skeletal muscle—a clinicopathologic analysis of twelve cases. Cancer 50:2465–2475, 1982.

36. Sternberg WH:The morphology, endocrine function, hyperplasia and tumors of the human ovarian hilus cells. Am J Pathol 25:493–521, 1949.

36a. Paraskevas M, Scully RE: Hilus cell tumors of the ovary. A clinicopathologic analysis of 12 Reinke crystal-positive and nine crystal-negative cases. Int J Gynecol Pathol 8:299–310, 1989.

36b. Honoré LH, Chari R, Mueller HD, et al: Postmenopausal hyperandrogenism of ovarian origin. A clinicopathologic study of four cases. Gynecol Obstet Invest 34:52–56, 1992.

37. Gabrilove JL, Nicolis GL, Mitty HA, Sohval AR: Feminizing interstitial cell tumor of the testis. Personal observations and a review of the literature. Cancer 35:1184–1202, 1975.

38. Young RH, Welch WR, Dickersin GR, Scully RE: Ovarian sex cord tumor with annular tubules. Cancer 50:1384–1402, 1982.

39. Tavassoli FA, Norris HJ: Sertoli tumors of the ovary. A clinicopathologic study of 28 cases with ultrastructural observations. Cancer 46:2282–2297, 1980.

40. Gustafson ML, Lee MM, Scully RE, et al: Mullerian inhibiting substance as a marker for ovarian sex cord tumor. N Engl J Med 326:466–471, 1992.

41. Jaworski RC, Fryatt JJ, Turner TB, Osborn, RA: Gynandroblastoma of the ovary. Pathology 18:348–351, 1986.

42. Hayes MC, Scully RE: Ovarian steroid cell tumors, not otherwise specified. A report of 63 cases. Am J Surg Pathol 11:835–845, 1987.

43. Shenker Y, Malazowski SN, Ayers J, et al: Steroid secretion by a virilizing lipoid cell ovarian tumor: Origins of dehydroepiandrosterone sulfate. Obstet Gynecol 74:502–506, 1989.

44. Falls JL: Accessory adrenal cortex in the broad ligament. Incidence and functional significance. Cancer 8:143–150, 1955.

45. Motlik K, Starka L: Adrenocortical tumour of the ovary. A case report with particular stress upon morphological and biochemical findings. Neoplasma 20:97–110, 1973.

46. Marieb NJ, Spangler S, Kashgarian M, et al: Cushing's syndrome secondary to ectopic cortisol production by an ovarian carcinoma. J Clin Endocrinol Metab 57:737–740, 1983.

47. Adeyemi SB, Grange AO, Giwa-Osajre OF, Elesha SO: Adrenal rest tumour of the ovary associated with isosexual pseudopuberty and cushingoid features. Eur J Pediatr 145:236–238, 1986.

48. Baranetsky NG, Zysser RD, Goebelsmann U, et al: Adrenocorticotropin-dependent virilizing parovarian tumors in Nelson's syndrome. J Clin Endocrinol Metab 49:381–386, 1979.

49. Givens JR, Kerber IJ, Wiser WL, et al: Remission of acanthosis nigricans associated with polycystic ovarian disease and a stromal luteoma. J Clin Endocrinol Metab 38:347–355, 1974.

50. Hayes MC, Scully RE: Stromal luteoma of the ovary: A clinicopathological analysis of 25 cases. Int J Gynecol Pathol 6:313–321, 1987.

51. Sternberg WH, Roth LM: Ovarian stromal tumors containing Leydig cells. I. Stromal Leydig cell tumor and non-neoplastic transformation of ovarian stroma to Leydig cells. Cancer 32:940–951, 1973.

52. Kim I, Young RH, Scully RE: Leydig cell tumors of the testis. A clinicopathological analysis of 40 cases and review of the literature. Am J Surg Pathol 9:177–192, 1985.

53. Janson PO, Hamberger L, Dambers J-E, et al: Steroid production in vitro of a hilus cell tumor of the human ovary. Obstet Gynecol 55:662–664, 1980.

54. Namamani M, Gonzales-Vitale JC: Steroid secretion patterns of a hilus cell tumor of the ovary. Obstet Gynecol 58:521–527, 1981.

55. Baramki TA, Leddy AL, Woodruff JD: Bilateral hilus cell tumors of the ovary. Obstet Gynecol 62:128–131, 1983.

56. Echt CR, Hadd HE: Androgen excretion patterns in a patient with a metastatic hilus cell tumor of the ovary. Am J Obstet Gynecol 100:1055–1061, 1968.

57. Scully RE: Gonadoblastoma. A review of 74 cases. Cancer 25:1340–1356, 1970.

58. Scully RE: Neoplasia associated with anomalous sexual development. Pediatr Adolesc Endocr 8:203–217, 1981.

59. Scully RE: Ovarian tumours with functioning stroma. In Fox H (ed): Haines and Taylor Obstetrical and Gynaecological Pathology (ed 3). Edinburgh, Churchill Livingstone, 1987, pp 724–736.

60. Verhoeven ATM, Mastboom JL, Van Leusden HAIM, Van Der Velden WHM: Virilization in pregnancy coexisting with an (ovarian) mucinous cystadenoma: A case report and review of virilizing ovarian tumors in pregnancy. Obstet Gynecol Surv 28:597–622, 1973.

61. Connor TB, Ganis FM, Levin HS, et al: Gonadotropin-independent Krukenberg tumor causing virilization during pregnancy. J Clin Endocrinol 28:198–412, 1968.

62. Hamwi GJ, Byron RC, Besch PK, et al: Testosterone synthesis by a Brenner tumor. I. Clinical evidence of masculinization during pregnancy. Am J Obstet Gynecol 86:1015–1020, 1963.

63. Besch PK, Byron RC, Barry RD, et al: Testosterone synthesis by a Brenner tumor. II. In vitro biosynthetic steroid conversion of a Brenner tumor. Am J Obstet Gynecol 86:1021–1026, 1963.

64. Case Records of the Massachusetts General Hospital: Case II-1972. N Engl J Med 286:594–600, 1972.
65. Ueda G, Hamanaka N, Hayakawa K, et al: Clinical, histochemical, and biochemical studies of an ovarian dysgerminoma with trophoblasts and Leydig cells. Am J Obstet Gynecol 114:748–754, 1972.
66. Rutgers JL, Scully RE: Functioning ovarian tumors with peripheral steroid cell proliferation: A report of twenty-four cases. Int J Gynecol Pathol 5:319–337, 1986.
67. Quinn MA, Baker HWG, Rome R, et al: Response of a mucinous ovarian tumor of borderline malignancy to human chorionic gonadotropin. Obstet Gynecol 61:121–126, 1983.
68. MacDonald PC, Grodin JM, Edman CD, et al: Origin of estrogen in a postmenopausal woman with a non-endocrine tumor of the ovary and endometrial hyperplasia. Obstet Gynecol 47:644–650, 1976.
69. Mählck CG, Grankvist K, Kjellgren O, Bäckström T: Human chorionic gonadotropin, follicle-stimulating hormone, and luteinizing hormone in patients with epithelial ovarian carcinoma. Gynecol Oncol 36:219–225, 1990.
70. Matias-Guiu X, Prat J: Ovarian tumors with functioning stroma. An immunohistochemical study of 100 cases with human chorionic gonadotropin monoclonal and polyclonal antibodies. Cancer 65:2001–2005, 1990.
71. Brennecke SP, McEvoy MI, Seymour AE, et al: Caecal adenocarcinoma metastatic to ovary inducing increased oestrogen production and postmenopausal bleeding. Aust NZ J Obstet Gynecol 26:158–161, 1986.
72. Heinonen PK, Koivulo T, Rajaniemi H, Pystynen P: Peripheral and ovarian venous concentrations of steroid and gonadotropin hormones in postmenopausal women with epithelial ovarian tumors. Gynecol Oncol 25:1–10, 1986.
73. Meehan D, Cavallo C: Human epithelial cancer cell steroid secretion and its control by gonadotropins. Gynecol Oncol 41:56–63, 1991.
74. Jacobs AS, Newland JR, Green RK: Pure choriocarcinoma of the ovary. Obstet Gynecol Surv 37:603–609, 1982.
75. Axe SR, Klein VR, Woodruff JD: Choriocarcinoma of the ovary. Obstet Gynecol 66:111–114, 1985.
76. Kurman RJ, Norris HJ: Malignant mixed germ cell tumors of the ovary. Obstet Gynecol 48:579–589, 1976.
77. Gershenson DM, Del Junco G, Copeland LJ, Rutledge FN: Mixed germ cell tumors of the ovary. Obstet Gynecol 64:200–206, 1984.
78. Kurman RJ, Norris HJ: Embryonal carcinoma of the ovary. A clinicopathologic entity distinct from endodermal sinus tumor resembling embryonal carcinoma of the adult testis. Cancer 38:2420–2433, 1976.
79. Takeda A, Ishizuka T, Goto T, et al: Polyembryoma of ovary producing alpha-fetoprotein and HCG: Immunoperoxidase and electron microscopic study. Cancer 49:1878–1889, 1982.
80. Zaloudek C, Tavassoli FA, Norris HJ: Dysgerminoma with syncytiotrophoblastic giant cells. A histologically and clinically distinctive subtype of dysgerminoma. Am J Surg Pathol 5:361–367, 1981.
81. Willemse PHB, Oosterhius JW, Aalders JG, et al: Malignant struma ovarii treated by ovariectomy, thyroidectomy, and 131-I administration. Cancer 60:178–182, 1987.
82. Rosenblum NG, LiVolsi VA, Edmonds PR, Mikuta JJ: Malignant struma ovarii. Gynecol Oncol 32:224–227, 1989.
83. Nodine JH, Maldia G: Pseudostruma ovarii. Obstet Gynecol 17:460–463, 1961.
84. Robboy SJ, Norris HJ, Scully RE: Insular carcinoid primary in the ovary: A clinicopathologic analysis of 48 cases. Cancer 36:404–418, 1975.
85. Robboy SJ, Scully RE, Norris HJ: Carcinoid metastatic to the ovary. A clinicopathologic analysis of 35 cases. Cancer 33:798–811, 1974.
86. Robboy SJ, Scully RE: Strumal carcinoid of the ovary: An analysis of 50 cases of a distinctive tumor composed of thyroid tissue and carcinoid. Cancer 46:2019–2034, 1980.
87. Ulbright TM, Roth LM, Ehrlich CE: Ovarian strumal carcinoid: An immunocytochemical and ultrastructural study of two cases. Am J Clin Pathol 77:622–631, 1982.
88. Dayal Y, Tashjian AH, Wolfe JH: Immunocytochemical localization of calcitonin producing cells in a strumal carcinoid with amyloid stroma. Cancer 43:1331–1338, 1979.
89. Axiotis CA, Lippes HA, Merino MJ, et al: Corticotroph cell pituitary adenoma within an ovarian teratoma. Am J Surg Pathol 11:218–224, 1987.
90. Palmer PE, Bogojavlensky S, Bhan AK, Scully RE: Prolactinoma in wall of ovarian dermoid cyst with hyperprolactinemia. Report of a case. Obstet Gynecol 75:540–543, 1990.
91. Clement PB, Young RH, Scully RE: Clinical syndromes associated with tumors of the female genital tract. Semin Diagn Pathol 8:204–233, 1991.
92. Dickersin GR, Kline IW, Scully RE: Small cell carcinoma of the ovary with hypercalcemia. A report of eleven cases. Cancer 49:188–197, 1982.
93. Scully RE: Small cell carcinoma of hypercalcemic type. Int J Gynecol Pathol 12:148–152, 1993.
94. Scully RE, Aguirre P, DeLellis RA: Argyrophilia, serotonin and peptide hormones in the female genital tract and its tumors. Int J Gynecol Pathol 3:51–70, 1984.
95. Korzets A, Nourial H, Steiner Z, et al: Resistant hypertension associated with a renin-producing ovarian Sertoli cell tumor. Am J Clin Pathol 85:242–247, 1986.
96. Jackson B, Valentine R, Wagner G: Primary aldosteronism due to a malignant ovarian tumor. Aust NZ J Med 16:69–71, 1986.
97. Spanos WJ: Preoperative hormonal therapy of cystic adnexal masses. Am J Obstet Gynecol 116:551–554, 1973.
98. Strickler RC, Kelly RW, Askin FB: Postmenopausal ovarian follicle cyst: An unusual cause of estrogen excess. Int J Gynecol Pathol 3:318–322, 1984.
99. Mauras N, Blizzard RM: The McCune-Albright syndrome. Acta Endocrinol 113 (Suppl 279):207–217, 1986.
100. Franks S: Review. Polycystic ovary syndrome: A changing perspective. Endocrinology 3:87–120, 1989.
101. Milewicz A, Silber D, Mielecki T: The origin of androgen synthesis in polycystic ovary syndrome. Obstet Gynecol 62:601–604, 1983.
102. Beaconsfield P, Dick R, Ginsburg J, Lewis P: Amenorrhea and infertility after the use of oral contraceptives. Surg Gynecol Obstet 138:571–575, 1974.
103. Fechner RE, Kaufman RH: Endometrial adenocarcinoma in Stein-Leventhal syndrome. Cancer 34:444–452, 1974.
104. Case Records of the Massachusetts General Hospital: Case 12–1974. N Engl J Med 290:730–736, 1974.
105. Judd HL, Scully RE, Herbst AL, et al: Familial hyperthecosis: Comparison of endocrinologic and histologic findings with polycystic ovarian disease. Am J Obstet Gynecol 117:976–982, 1973.
106. Scully RE: Correspondence. Am J Obstet Gynecol 119:864, 1974.
107. Dennefors BL, Janson PO, Knutson F, Hanberger L: Steroid production and responsiveness to gonadotropin in isolated stromal tissue of human postmenopausal ovaries. Am J Obstet Gynecol 136:997–1002, 1980.
108. Dunaif A, Hoffman AR, Scully RE, et al: The clinical, biochemical and ovarian morphologic features in women with acanthosis nigricans and masculinization. Obstet Gynecol 66:545–552, 1985.
109. Bardin CW, Lipsett MB, Edgcomb JH, et al: Studies of testosterone metabolism in a patient with masculinization due to stromal hyperthecosis. N Engl J Med 277:399–402, 1967.
110. Wiebe RH, Morris CV: Testosterone/androstenedione ratio in the evaluation of women with ovarian androgen excess. Obstet Gynecol 61:279–284, 1983.
111. Thorp JM Jr, Wells SR, Droegemueller W: Ovarian suspension in massive ovarian edema. Obstet Gynecol 76:912–914, 1990.
112. Young RH, Scully RE: Fibromatosis and massive edema of the ovary, possibly related entities. A report of 14 cases of fibromatosis and 11 cases of massive edema. Int J Gynecol Pathol 3:153–178, 1984.
113. Young RH, Scully RE: Non-neoplastic disorders of the ovary. In Fox H (ed): Haines and Taylor Obstetrical and Gynaecological Pathology (ed 3). Edinburgh, Churchill Livingstone, 1987, pp 519–541.
114. Hensleigh PA, Woodruff JD: Differential maternal-fetal response to androgenizing luteoma or hyperreactio luteinalis. Obstet Gynecol Surv 33:262–271, 1978.
115. Monty FJ, Schlaerth JB, Morrow CP: The natural history of theca lutein cysts. Obstet Gynecol 72:247–251, 1988.
116. Wajda KJ, Lucas JG, Marsh WL Jr: Hyperreactio luteinalis. Benign disorder masquerading as an ovarian neoplasm. Arch Pathol Lab Med 113:921–925, 1989.
117. Borenstein R, Elhalah U, Lunenfeld B, et al: Severe ovarian hyperstimulation syndrome: A reevaluated therapeutic approach. Fertil Steril 51:791–795, 1989.
118. Aboulghar MA, Mansour RT, Serour GI, et al: Ultrasonically guided vaginal aspiration of ascites in the treatment of severe ovarian hyperstimulation syndrome. Fertil Steril 53:933–935, 1990.
119. Clement PB, Scully RE: Large solitary luteinized follicle cyst of pregnancy and puerperium. A clinicopathological analysis of eight cases. Am J Surg Pathol 4:431–438, 1980.
120. Biscotti CV, Hart WR, Lucas JG: Cystic ovarian enlargement resulting from autoimmune oophoritis. Obstet Gynecol 74:492, 1989.

122

The Menopause and Hormonal Replacement

WILLIAM D. ODELL

In the human female, mitosis of oogonia is confined to embryonic life. From a peak number of about 7 million in the embryonic ovary, the number of germ cells decreases to about 2 million at birth and to 300,000 at menarche. Thus about 94 per cent of the oogonia cease to exist before menarche. These oogonia disappear from the ovary in a poorly understood selection process termed *atresia*. Even after menarche, during each menstrual cycle of the reproductive years, some 6 to 10 follicles that contain ova begin development, but only one is selected to reach maturity and be receptive to fertilization. Even after menarche, more than 99 per cent of oogonia disappear from the ovary by some process other than ovulation, and throughout a woman's life 99.99 per cent of oogonia or ova disappear by this process. Even the oogonia or ova contained within the selected dominant follicle during reproductive life are not equally susceptible to ovulation, as is evidenced by declining fertility with age when studied under controlled conditions. Figure 122–1 shows the cumulative conception rates of women of various ages undergoing artificial insemination with sperm from young healthy men. Conception was similar in women under age 30. In women aged 31 to 35 the frequency of conception decreased; in women over age 36 the frequency of conception was even lower. In these years of waning fertility and in later years decreased ovulation before cessation of menses is termed the *climacteric;* this lasts about 20 years. At menopause few or no follicles exist in the ovary,[2] and ovarian steroid production decreases to physiologically insignificant levels.[3] The age of menopause was determined in United States women in a prospective study of 561 women followed from before age 25 to menopause by Whelan et al.[4] Natural menopause ranged from ages 44 to 56 with a mean age of 50.5 years (Fig. 122–2). Interestingly, women with shorter menstrual cycle length (less than or equal to 26 days) at a young age had a mean menopause 2.2 years earlier than did women with a long menstrual cycle length (greater than or equal to 33 days) (Fig. 122–3). Furthermore, women who were nulliparous had an earlier menopause than women who

had at least one live birth. In contrast to age at menarche, which has decreased, age at menopause appears to be relatively constant over the past several hundred years.[5, 6] Because age of death has steadily climbed, it is evident that the proportion of living women who are menopausal has greatly increased, and currently about 30 per cent of living women are postmenopausal. Therefore, for the physician, knowledge of the physiology of the menopause, as well as the pros and cons of estrogen replacement therapy, is of major importance.

ENDOCRINOLOGY OF THE MENOPAUSE

Luteinizing and Follicle-Stimulating Hormone Secretion

As discussed in the previous paragraphs, the number of follicles that contain oogonia steadily decreases during reproductive life. Those undergoing development early appear more sensitive to the actions of follicle-stimulating hormone (FSH) than those in later reproductive life. In 1971, Adamopoulos et al.[7] reported that urinary FSH excretion was considerably greater in perimenopausal women who still had regular menses than in women in the early reproductive portion of life (Table 122–1). Later, in 1975, using radioimmunoassays for both FSH and luteinizing hormone (LH) and measuring samples daily throughout menstrual cycles, Sherman and Korenman[8] reported that serum LH concentrations measured throughout the menstrual cycle were indistinguishable in young women and in older women with regular cycles just before the age of menopause. However, FSH concentrations during the early follicular phase, when follicle development is stimulated, were considerably greater in the older women than in the young women. Figure 122–4 shows these data. After menopause, as ovarian estrogen production falls strikingly, LH and FSH concentrations increase further to castrated or postmenopausal levels. Table 122–2 shows such data. Kwek-

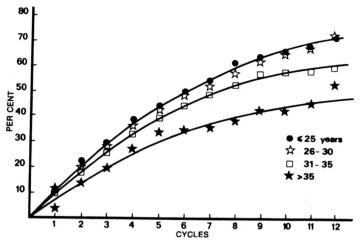

FIGURE 122–1. Theoretical cumulative success rates of artificial insemination in various age groups. The four curves differ significantly ($P <$ .01). Because the curves of the two younger groups were similar, they are represented by a single tracing. These curves differ significantly from those of the two older groups ($P <$ .03 for those 30 to 35 and $P <$ .001 for those over 35). There were 371 women in the <25 group, 1079 in the 26-to-30 group, 599 in the 31-to-35 group, and 144 in the >35 group. (From Schwartz D, Mayaux MJ: Female fecundity as a function of age. N Engl J Med 306:404–406, 1982. Reprinted by permission of the New England Journal of Medicine.)

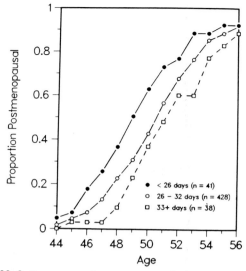

FIGURE 122–3. Percentage of postmenopausal women by median menstrual cycle length at ages 20 to 35 (Kaplan-Meier estimates), Menstruation and Reproductive History Study, 1935–1980. (From Whelan EA et al: Menstrual and reproductive characteristics and age at natural menopause. Am J Epidemiol 131:625–632, 1990.)

keboom et al.[9] have reported LH, FSH, free α-subunit, and selected steroid concentrations in 697 well-characterized postmenopausal women. These workers[9] reported that mean serum LH, FSH, and α-subunit concentrations decline slightly but significantly as postmenopausal women age further between ages 55 and 75. Table 122–3 shows mean values in postmenopausal women calculated from univarate regression analysis at ages 55, 65, and 75.

Notice that after menopause, FSH concentrations increase to a greater extent than LH concentrations when stated either as (a) relative to average follicular or luteal phase concentrations or (b) in terms of the International Reference Preparation (IRP-HMG No. 2). Thus the ratio of serum FSH to LH in postmenopausal women is greater than 1, whereas during the ovulatory FSH-LH surge, it is considerably less than 1. Furthermore, administration of

gonadotropin-releasing hormone (GnRH) to postmenopausal women increases LH secretion to a much greater extent than FSH (i.e., the ratio of FSH to LH is less than 1). These data suggest that the sustained hypersecretion of FSH and LH in the postmenopausal state is due not to hypersecretion of GnRH but to a decreased effect of circulating steroids directly on the pituitary.

At any rate, after menopause a new sustained feedback equilibrium is reached with chronic increased levels of FSH, LH, and α-subunit held in balance with the reduced steroid production from the ovary and the steroids produced by the adrenals. In addition, the short loop in autoregulatory feedback of LH on LH and FSH on FSH secretion may constitute part of this regulatory system.[10–12] In addition to the gonadotropins LH and FSH, the pituitary gland secretes small amounts of human chorionic gonadotropin (hCG).[13, 14] In postmenopausal women this pituitary hCG is secreted in greater amounts than in women in their reproductive years. Figure 122–5 shows the pulsatile secretion of hCG in parallel with that of LH in a postmenopausal woman.

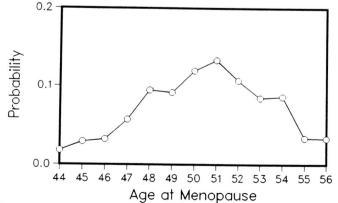

FIGURE 122–2. Probability distribution for age at natural menopause. Menstruation and Reproductive History Study, 1935–1980. (From Whelan EA et al: Menstrual and reproductive characteristics and age at natural menopause. Am J Epidemiol 131:625–632, 1990.)

TABLE 122–1. FSH AND LH EXCRETION

REPRODUCTIVE STAGE	NO. OF SUBJECTS	AGE RANGE (yr)	FSH EXCRETION* (IU/24 h)	LH EXCRETION† (IU/24 h)
Early reproductive	6	19–25	7.3 ± 0.7‡	11.1 ± 1.1†
Premenopausal	6	37–42	20.7 ± 4.6	79.4 ± 20.7
Perimenopausal	6	40–51	18.6 ± 4.6	87.1 ± 13.5
Postmenopausal	5	50–63	69.7 ± 28.0	80.1 ± 27.7

*Ovarian weight augmentation assay.
†Ovarian ascorbic acid depletion assay.
‡Mean ± SEM.
From Adamopoulos DA et al: Endocrinological studies in women approaching the menopause. J Obstet Gynaecol Br Commow 78:62–79, 1971. Used by permission of Blackwell Scientific Publishers, Ltd.

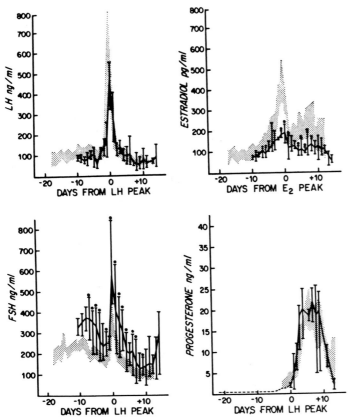

FIGURE 122–4. Mean and range of serum LH, FSH, estradiol, and progesterone in six premenopausal women (lines and brackets) with regular menses compared with mean ± 2 SEM in 10 cycles (shaded area) in women aged 18 to 30. Asterisk indicates statistically significant difference between the two groups. (From Sherman BM, Korenman SG: Hormonal characteristics of the human menstrual cycle throughout reproductive life. Reproduced from the Journal of Clinical Investigation, 1975, Vol. 55, p. 699, by copyright permission of the American Society for Clinical Investigation.)

Steroid Secretion by the Ovary in Postmenopausal Women

The postmenopausal ovary is not totally devoid of the ability to secrete steroids. Mattingly and Huang[15] demonstrated that postmenopausal ovarian slices incubated in vitro with 7-³H-pregnenolone produced dehydroepiandros-

TABLE 122–2. MEAN SERUM LH AND FSH CONCENTRATIONS IN PREMENOPAUSAL AND POSTMENOPAUSAL WOMEN

| | PREMENOPAUSAL | | POSTMENOPAUSAL |
	Follicular Phase	Luteal Phase	
LH	5.9 ± 1.7 (N = 69)	3.2 ± 2.0 (N = 125)	22.6 ± 1.6 (N = 52)
FSH	5.2 ± 1.4 (N = 66)	3.4 ± 1.5 (N = 140)	55.7 ± 1.5 (N = 57)

Mean ± SD of serum LH and FSH concentrations in women with regular menstrual cycles and in postmenopausal women. The number of subjects in each group is given in parentheses. Data were normally distributed on a log scale, and mean and SD were calculated from log distribution. Hormone concentrations were determined by chemical luminescent-sandwich–type IRMA assay at Nichols Institute, San Juan Capistrano, California.

TABLE 122–3. MEAN LH, FSH, AND FREE α-SUBUNIT IN POSTMENOPAUSAL WOMEN AT THREE AGES

	AGE 55	AGE 65	AGE 75
FSH (IU/L)	72.1	66.8	61.6
LH (IU/L)	47.1	39.8	32.4
α-subunit (μg/L)	2.6	2.2	1.9

From Kwekkeboom DJ et al: Serum gonadotropins and α-subunit decline in aging normal postmenopausal women. J Clin Endocrinol Metab 70:944–950, © 1990 by the Endocrine Society.

terone, androstenedione, and testosterone. They reported that the ovarian stroma was unable to aromatize androgens to estrogens. Judd et al.[3] measured the concentrations of testosterone, androstenedione, estradiol, and estrone in peripheral and ovarian venous blood. A higher ovarian venous concentration was found for all four steroids, but the differences for the estrogens were small (Table 122–4). Although the postmenopausal ovary has the capacity to secrete testosterone and androstenedione, blood flow through the ovary is a factor in determining these steroid production rates, and Siiteri[16] suggests that the postmenopausal ovarian contribution to blood concentrations of androstenedione and testosterone is exceedingly small. Nagamani et al.,[17] however, have reported that the ovarian stroma from postmenopausal women with endometrial cancer produces more androstenedione, testosterone, and dehydroepiandrosterone than the stroma of women without cancer when studied in vitro. The addition of LH stimulated production of all three steroids further, whereas the addition of insulin stimulated steroid production only from the stroma of women with cancer. These studies suggest that ovarian androgen production may contribute to the formation of endometrial carcinoma.

Adrenal Secretion of Androgens and Estrogens

In menopausal women the major circulating estrogen is estrone. This is formed almost exclusively by aromatization

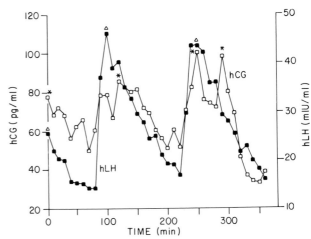

FIGURE 122–5. Chorionic gonadotropin and LH determined by specific 2 monoclonal-antibody assays at 10-minute intervals in a postmenopausal woman. (From Odell WD, Griffin J: Pulsatile secretion of human chorionic gonadotropin. N Engl J Med 317:1686–1691, 1987. Reprinted by permission of the New England Journal of Medicine.)

TABLE 122–4. CONCENTRATIONS OF STEROIDS IN OVARIAN AND PERIPHERAL BLOOD

VEIN	TESTOSTERONE (pg/ml)	ANDROSTENEDIONE (pg/ml)	ESTRADIOL (pg/ml)	ESTRONE (pg/ml)
Ovarian	3033 ± 1046	3455 ± 1330	31.1 ± 6.3	71.5 ± 133
Peripheral	198 ± 27	754 ± 174	14.6 ± 2.9	30.3 ± 3.4

Data from Judd HL et al: Endocrine function of the postmenopause ovary: Concentrations of androgens and estrogens in ovarian and peripheral vein blood. J Clin Endocrinol Metab 39:1020–1024, © by the Endocrine Society, 1974.

of androstenedione in peripheral tissues, principally adipose tissue and muscle. The daily production rate of androstenedione is 2 to 4 mg, and more than 95 per cent of this is secreted by the adrenals. Siiteri and MacDonald[16, 18] and Hemsell et al.[19] have shown that about 1 to 2 per cent of the 2 to 4 mg of androstenedione (20 to 80 μg) is converted to estrone in this manner. The result of this process (plus any small direct adrenal and ovarian secretion of estrone) is a production rate of estrone that averages 35 to 40 μg/d. Both age and obesity (the latter is the more important) increase the conversion of androstenedione to estrone; very obese women may produce 150 to 200 μg/d with a conversion ratio of about 11 per cent (Fig. 122–6). This is believed to be the explanation for the increased incidence of endometrial carcinoma in obese postmenopausal women.[18, 19] The conversion of androstenedione to estrone is also increased in women with cirrhosis. Thus the major circulating estrogen of the postmenopausal state is estrone, whereas the major circulating estrogen of the premenopausal state is estradiol (Fig. 122–7).

SYMPTOMATOLOGY OF THE MENOPAUSE

During the same years that the menopause is occurring, many women in Western countries are undergoing significant alterations in their personal lives. If a woman has not developed a career, in addition to being a housewife and mother, this often is the time when the husband is occupied most deeply in his job; promotion, responsibility, and many other aspects of the employed male partner may draw his attention and time away from the family and home. Concomitantly, the children the mother has raised usually are grown and have begun their own families, careers, and activities. Time and evaluation of life may weigh heavily on some women. In this setting the woman with pre-existing psychiatric or emotional problems may become increasingly uncomfortable. Often the complaints

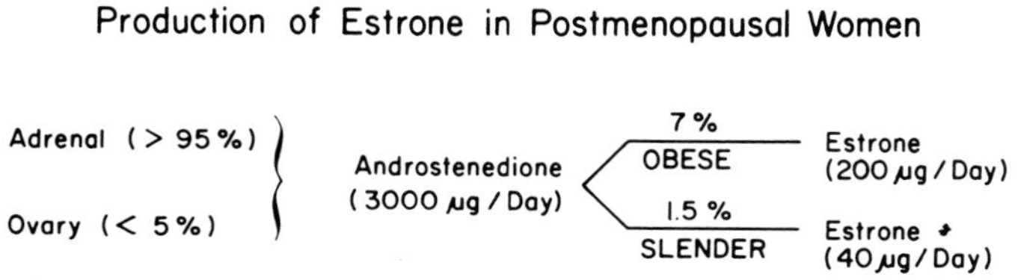

she carries to her physician are quickly attributed to the "menopause."

On the other hand, menopause (or castration) is associated with distinct symptomatology. In carefully done studies Lauritzen[21] noted that surgical castration in women resulted in characteristic hot flashes beginning four to six days later. These initially occurred three to five times daily, increased in frequency, and began to occur at night by 8 to 12 days. Serum LH and FSH levels first increased *after the onset* of flashes; for FSH the increase occurred on days 6 to 8 and for LH, on days 8 to 10 postcastration. Within three weeks FSH had increased about three-fold and LH about two-fold over baseline precastration levels.

The hot flash is an intriguing and uncomfortable symptom. Meldrum et al.[22] showed that the hot flash is a generalized body phenomenon, with the most striking rises of skin temperature and vasodilation occurring over the fingers and toes. Many women, however, perceive that the changes are limited to the upper trunk, neck, and face, a perception that appears to be incorrect. Continuous measurement of finger temperature can be used as a marker of the hot flash if subjects are studied in a cool environment.[21] Perspiration, a second prominent symptom during the flash, is most pronounced over the upper body. This symptom may be monitored by measuring skin resistance over the upper chest.[23] If these parameters are monitored, along with serial determination at 5- to 10-minute intervals of LH and FSH, there is a remarkable correlation with pulsatile release of LH.[24] Figure 122–8 shows such data reproduced

Production of Estrone in Postmenopausal Women

Adrenal (> 95 %)
Ovary (< 5 %)
Androstenedione (3000 μg / Day)
7 % OBESE → Estrone (200 μg / Day)
1.5 % SLENDER → Estrone (40 μg / Day)

FIGURE 122–6. Production of estrone from androstenedione in obese and slender postmenopausal women. Androstenedione is predominantly secreted by the adrenal, and an average of 3000 μg is produced per day. Conversion occurs in peripheral tissues; adipose tissue is active in aromatization. Thus the conversion is greater in obese than in slender women.

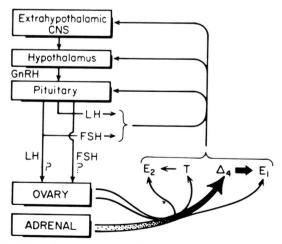

FIGURE 122–7. Hypothalamic-pituitary-adrenal-ovarian system in postmenopausal women. Control of LH and FSH secretion is by way of a short-loop feedback system (LH and FSH acting on hypothalamus and/or pituitary to control LH and FSH) and by way of steroid modulation. The latter is believed to originate predominantly from adrenal androstenedione (Δ_4). E_2, estradiol; T, testosterone; E_1, estrone.

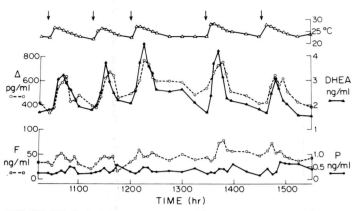

FIGURE 122–8. Serial measurements of finger temperature and serum dehydroepiandrosterone (DHEA), androstenedione (Δ), cortisol (F), and progesterone (P) levels in an individual subject. Arrows mark the onset of the temperature rises. (From Meldrum DR et al: Gonadotropins, estrogens and adrenal steroids during the menopausal hot flush. J Clin Endocrinol Metab 50:685–689, © 1980 by The Endocrine Society.)

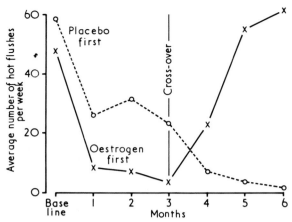

FIGURE 122–9. Results of a double-blind cross-over study of the effects of estrogen or placebo on the incidence of hot flashes. Placebo treatment produced a significant fall in incidence of hot flashes if administered initially. This was followed by total cessation of flashes when placebo was switched to estrogen. This placebo effect is an easily identifiable parameter in the treatment of postmenopausal women and must be controlled for in well-designed studies. (From Lauritzen C: The management of the premenopausal and the postmenopausal patient. In VanKeep PA, Lauritzen C [eds]: Ageing and Estrogens. Vol 2. New York, Karger, 1973, pp 2–21.)

from the publication of Meldrum et al.[25] However, women with hypopituitarism and extremely low LH and FSH secretion and men with similar very low LH and FSH secretion produced by long-acting GnRH agonist treatment have hot flashes. These data indicate that the LH pulse per se is not the cause of the flash but an associated phenomenon. The severity and frequency of hot flashes vary greatly, and this variation probably relates directly to the degree of estrogen deficiency. As shown in Figure 122–6, extraglandular production of estrone and other estrogens varies with body weight. Erlik et al.[26] have shown that women with frequent hot flashes have both lower circulating estrogen levels (estradiol) and lower body weight than do women with infrequent hot flashes.

The incidence and age of onset of hot flashes is of interest. Jaszmann et al.,[27] studying Dutch women aged 42 to 62, reported that 17 per cent with regular cycles were already having hot flashes. This increased to 40 per cent in women with irregular cycles and was 65 per cent 1 to 2 years after menopause and 35 per cent 5 to 10 years after menopause. Several studies have concluded that the hot flash is the only characteristic feature of the menopause.

Hot flashes are abolished by treatment with either estrogens or androgens. Objective study of this "best understood" symptom associated with the menopause illustrates the difficulty of interpreting most studies of treatment of menopausal symptoms. Figure 122–9[21] shows a double-blind cross-over study of treatment of two groups of postmenopausal women with either estrogen or placebo. Placebo treatment decreased the number of hot flashes that occurred but did not abolish them. When estrogen was substituted for the placebo, the frequency of hot flashes decreased further. In contrast, the group receiving estrogens first had a more dramatic fall in frequency of flashes but showed an increase under placebo treatment. This "placebo effect" appears to result in 30 to 50 per cent improvement in hot flashes and makes interpretation of treatment of less well quantifiable symptoms often attributed to the menopause (such as depression or loss of energy) even more difficult to study. Table 122–5 lists additional symptoms often associated with menopause. Even with these reservations some data suggest that estrogens

improve mood in menopausal and geriatric women when compared with placebo treatment.[28–31] The placebo effects are many, and caution in interpretation is necessary. Other studies not using blind placebo control populations probably are valueless.

ESTROGEN REPLACEMENT: INDICATIONS, DOSAGE, AND BENEFITS

Menopausal symptoms or disorders are effectively treated with oral or systemic estrogen replacement. The physician often is asked why a given woman does not have symptoms abolished on oral estrogen therapy when she has some benefits from parenteral therapy given in the physician's office. In such women the "symptoms" invariably

TABLE 122–5. MANIFESTATIONS OF THE GRADUAL DECREASE AND FINAL CESSATION OF THE OVARIAN FUNCTION IN THE CLIMACTERIC AND POSTMENOPAUSAL PERIODS

MAIN GROUPS OF SYMPTOMS	COMMON MANIFESTATIONS
Endocrine symptoms	Bleeding irregularities "Menopausal syndrome" (principally vasomotor disturbances) Local regressive changes in the urogenital tract
Nervous system disturbances	Insomnia Nervousness Headache Irritability Fluctuation in mood Depression
Metabolic changes	Osteoporosis Altered lipid and carbohydrate metabolism Atherosclerosis

Reproduced with permission from Zador G: The pathophysiology and methods of treatment of climacteric disorders. Acta Obstet Gynecol Scand [Suppl] 65:19–26, 1977.

fall into the "Nervous System Disturbances" category shown in Table 122–5, in which significant placebo effects are observed. Assuming that the appropriate dosage is used, there are no data to show that estrogens of the correct form are not effective orally. In fact, when therapy is considered for women with past breast cancer or with metabolic lipid disorders that involve triglyceride production, estrogens are well absorbed when administered intravaginally, transcutaneously, sublingually, or orally. Estradiol per se is ineffective orally because it is metabolized in the liver to inactive products. Effective estrogens include conjugated estrogens, mestranol, ethinyl estradiol, once-weekly quinestrol, and estradiol dermal patches. Dosages are discussed later. Oral administration is associated with four to five times higher concentration of the administered estrogen in the portal circulation than in the general circulation. This enhances hepatic effects such as increasing triglyceride synthesis and triglyceride blood concentrations, increasing blood high-density lipoprotein (HDL) concentrations, and decreasing cholesterol production and blood concentrations. Such changes in lipid metabolism produced by oral estrogens may be of major importance in decreasing the incidence of cardiovascular disease and are not seen when estrogen is administered transdermally. Table 122–6 shows the effects of orally administered conjugated estrogens and transdermally administered estradiol on plasma lipids.[32] Note that oral estrogens decreased total cholesterol and low-density lipoprotein (LDL) cholesterol and raised HDL cholesterol but that transdermal estradiol had no effects on these parameters. Walsh et al.[33] published a randomized double-blind crossover study comparing placebo with oral micronized estradiol (2 mg/d) and transdermal estradiol (0.1 mg twice weekly). In this study also oral, but not transdermal, estrogens favorably altered LDL and HDL levels.

In women with intact uterus present, estrogens usually are administered in a cyclic manner days 1 through 25 each month with a progestogen added days 13 through 25 each month. On cessation of treatment on day 25, menses results. As discussed later, this regimen decreases the incidence of endometrial carcinoma when compared with continuous unopposed estrogen use. A recent regimen appears more desirable and consists of continuous combined treatment with oral conjugated equine estrogen, 0.625 mg/d, or estradiol valerate, 0.2 mg/d, and a low-dose progestogen, such as medroxyprogesterone acetate, 2.5 to 5.0 mg/d, or norethindrone, 0.35 to 2.0 mg/d. These continuous regimens consistently produce amenorrhea with inactive (low mitotic index) endometrium while alleviating menopausal symptoms.[34] This treatment is attractive, since monthly menses are not experienced, and based on endometrial histology it appears that no increase in incidence of endometrial carcinoma is seen. Long-term studies of the incidence of endometrial cancer, breast cancer, and cardiovascular disease in women treated with this continuous regimen are not available.

Indications

The indications for estrogen therapy include the abolition of hot flashes, cosmetic effects, prevention of osteoporosis, decreased cardiovascular morbidity and mortality, and, possibly, decreased CNS symptoms. There is a possible biochemical explanation for estrogen modification of emotions and mood. Estradiol is metabolized in two major pathways: about two thirds by 16-α-hydroxylation and about one third by 2-hydroxylation to form 2-hydroxy-estradiol.[35, 36] The compound 2-hydroxyestradiol is a "catechol estrogen" and is further metabolized by catecholamine-o-methyl transferase, a metabolic pathway for the metabolism of centrally active catecholamines important as neurotransmitters. It is attractive to postulate, therefore, that rapid changes in estrogen concentrations in blood might produce mood or emotional alterations by means of alterations in catechol estrogen concentrations.

Cosmetic Effects

Estrogens assist in maintaining breast tissue mass, vaginal secretions, and some aspects of skin structure. Men and women deprived of gonadal steroid effects for several years develop characteristic "hypogonadal facies," characterized by fine-radiating lines around the mouth and eyes. Such changes appear to be prevented or delayed by estrogen therapy. Cigarette smoking produces facial fissuring and lining different from these subtle hypogonadal facies. These cosmetic effects have not been objectively studied and constitute only a relative indication for estrogen therapy. The exception to this statement is the effect on vaginal secretions; dyspareunia is common in estrogen-deprived women.

Osteoporosis

The process of bone growth, maturation, and maintenance is a complex one and is discussed in further detail in Chapters 71, 72, and 73. Briefly, the skeleton can be divided into two compartments or types of bone: cortical bone and trabecular bone. Cortical bone exists mainly in the shafts of long bones or in the so-called *peripheral skeleton*, which constitutes some 80 per cent of skeletal mass. Cortical bone is composed of compact plates or lamellae organized about central nutrient canals. Trabecular bone exists in the central or axial skeleton (vertebral bodies, pelvis, and proximal femur) and consists of honeycombs of vertical and horizontal bars filled with red marrow and fat cells. The metaphyseal ends of long bones also contain

TABLE 122–6. EFFECTS OF TRANSDERMAL AND ORAL ESTROGENS ON PLASMA LIPIDS

	BASELINE	TRANSDERMAL*	ORAL†
Total cholesterol	201 mg/dl	198	189‡
HDL cholesterol	63 mg/dl	62	71‡
LDL cholesterol	124	118	106‡
Triglycerides	96	97	100

*100 µg/24 h estradiol.
†1.25 mg conjugated estrogen.
‡P = <.05

Reprinted with permission from Chetkowski RJ et al: Biologic effects of transdermal estradiol. N Engl J Med 314:1615–1620, 1986. Reprinted by permission of the New England Journal of Medicine.

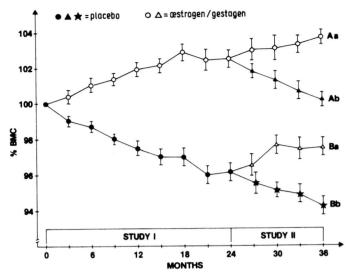

FIGURE 122–10. Bone mineral content as a function of time and treatment in women soon after menopause. In study I women were divided into two treatment groups, (A) estrogen-progestogen–treated and (B) placebo-treated, and followed for two years. In study II each group was further divided into two groups and followed an additional year: Aa continued hormone therapy; Ab were switched to placebo; Ba were switched to hormone therapy; and Bb continued placebo. (From Christiansen C et al: Bone mass in postmenopausal women after withdrawal of estrogen/progestogen replacement therapy. Lancet 1:459–461, 1981.)

trabecular bone. The greatly increased surface area of trabecular bone explains why alterations in bone formation and resorption are seen to a greater degree in the axial skeleton.

Skeletal maintenance in the adult is a dynamic process with continuous resorption and new bone formation occurring throughout life. In each unit of the skeleton, termed a "bone remodeling unit," about 90 per cent of the bone surfaces are at rest. In a small percentage of each bone remodeling unit bone resorption continuously occurs, initiated and modified by hormonal and physical signals. Bone formation is coupled to bone resorption probably through local cytokines. Thus at each unit this continuous slow process of resorption linked to formation leads to continuous remodeling of bone probably with continuous correction of microfractures or fatigue microdamage to maintain a healthy skeleton. In the adult human, however, bone remodeling does not completely restore each bone unit to its previous state, and each cycle of resorption and formation is associated with a small loss or deficit in bone. The consequence is a steady, small, age-related loss of bone in both men and women. A number of hormonal and physical factors appear to modify this age-related bone mass, including calcium and vitamin D intake, exercise, weight bearing, body weight, cigarette smoking, as well as the concentrations of hormones (glucocorticoids, gonadal steroids, and thyroid hormones). Thus excess cortisol (Cushing's syndrome), thyrotoxicosis, and long-standing estrogen or androgen deficiency are associated with increased bone resorption relative to formation and, ultimately, osteoporosis. In men and women who do not have functioning gonads at puberty (e.g., vanishing testes syndrome in men and gonadal dysgenesis or Turner's syndrome in women), osteoporosis is almost universal by age 30 if these patients are untreated. At time of menopause

the abrupt decrease in ovarian estrogen production leads to a dramatic increase in bone resorption with acceleration of the decrease in bone density, and early development of osteoporosis.

Riggs et al.[37] in 1972 showed that estrogens in high doses given to postmenopausal women with osteoporosis decreased the bone resorption rate to normal within one to four weeks, thus dramatically affecting the principal cause of the disease. Subsequently, Lindsay et al.[38] showed that relatively small dosages of estrogens (25 μg/day of mestranol) given to normal women at the time of oophorectomy prevented the decrease in bone density seen in untreated oophorectomized women. Figure 122–10 shows striking data published by Christiansen et al.[39] In this study, women of menopausal age were divided into two groups: one was treated with placebo and the other, with oral estrogen-progestogen. After 24 months the percentage of change in bone mineral content had strikingly decreased in the placebo group and had *increased* in the estrogen-progestogen group. At 24 months each group was subdivided into two groups (total four groups) of placebo or estrogen-progestogen treatment. Note the efficacy of estrogen-progestogen treatment, even though initiated at 24 months. A 10-year *prospective* study by Nachtigall et al.[40] is shown in Figure 122–11. In this study, postmenopausal

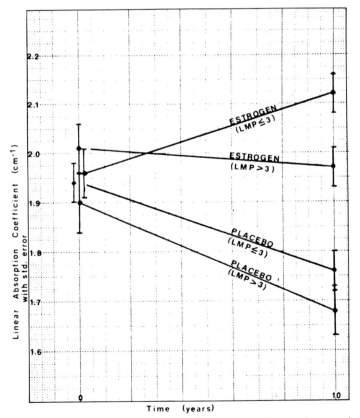

FIGURE 122–11. Densitometric linear absorption co-efficients in treated patients with last menstrual period (LMP) < three years, treated patients with LMP > three years, control patients with LMP < three years, and control patients with LMP > three years. (From Nachtigall LE et al: Estrogen replacement therapy. I. A 10-year prospective study in the relationship to osteoporosis. Obstet Gynecol 53:277–281, 1979. Reprinted with permission from The American College of Obstetricians and Gynecologists.)

women were divided into four groups: (1) a group receiving estrogen started less than three years after menopause, (2) a group receiving estrogen started more than three years after menopause, and (3 and 4) two groups receiving placebo. Again, note the striking difference in bone density at 10 years' follow-up in this prospective study.

In addition to lowering bone resorption rates to normal, estrogens act by enhancing calcium absorption. Ireland and Fordtran[41] have shown that on a given calcium intake, older subjects absorbed less calcium from the intestine than did younger subjects. Despite the decreased calcium absorption, the older subjects had higher urinary excretion of calcium than the younger subjects. Heaney et al.[42] showed that estrogen treatment of postmenopausal women produced increased calcium absorption at a given intake; net calcium balance was achieved at a lower calcium intake. The mechanism of this effect of estrogens is not certain but may involve increased production of free (non–protein-bound) 1,25-dihydroxyvitamin D.[43]

A large number of studies have verified these beneficial effects of estrogen replacement on preventing loss of bone density. In addition, use of estrogens decreases the incidence of fractures. For example, the Framingham study, published in 1987,[44] showed a decrease in relative risk of hip fracture in postmenopausal women receiving estrogen. In a prospective study Quigley et al.[45] showed that the beneficial effects of estrogen replacement continue indefinitely. Figure 122–12 shows differences in bone density in women receiving estrogens versus those receiving no estrogens grouped into three age groups: (1) 51 to 60 years, (2) 61 to 70 years, and (3) 71 to 80 years.

In addition to estrogen therapy, other factors assist in preventing osteoporosis. These probably have a more modest effect on retarding bone loss than does estrogen therapy and include increased calcium intake, weight-bearing

exercises, and augmented vitamin D intake, in addition to adverse effects of cigarette smoking, heavy alcohol intake, and immobility. More potent adverse effects are seen in thyrotoxicosis (iatrogenic or disease) and glucocorticoid therapy. Although the influence of calcium intake on osteoporosis is controversial,[46–49] most studies indicate that calcium supplementation has some value. Dawson-Hughes et al.[49] showed that healthy older postmenopausal women with a daily calcium intake of less than 400 mg can significantly reduce bone loss by increasing calcium intake to 800 mg/day. Interestingly, some forms of calcium carbonate appear to be compacted too firmly, and breakup of the tablet in the gut and absorption can be poor. In the study of Dawson-Hughes et al.,[49] calcium citrate malate was more effective than calcium carbonate. It is recommended that calcium intake be increased to at least 1 g/day to achieve calcium balance in estrogen-treated women for prevention of osteoporosis. To treat established osteoporosis, a higher calcium intake of 1.5 to 2.0 g daily is recommended. In addition, augmented vitamin D intake may be helpful. Gallagher et al.[50] have shown that physiological doses of 1,25-dihydroxyvitamin D had a better than 50 per cent reduction in the number of new vertebral fractures, as compared with placebo. Because estrogens increase 1-hydroxylation of 25-hydroxyvitamin D, we recommend supplementation of estrogen treatment with 400 to 800 IU of vitamin D, rather than 1,25-dihydroxyvitamin D.

Estrogens and Cardiovascular Disease

In the dosages used, estrogen treatment of postmenopausal women does not appear to increase the incidence of thromboembolic phenomena or stroke. The influence of estrogens on cardiovascular disease has been evaluated in 18 publications to date: three studies[51–53] reported estrogen replacement was associated with increased risk; three studies[54–56] reported no effect of estrogens on cardiovascular disease, and 12 studies[57–68] reported a decreased incidence of cardiovascular disease in estrogen-treated postmenopausal women. The Framingham studies[48, 53] are the most striking to report on the adverse effects of estrogens. Even in these studies the increased risk was not significant if women with angina were omitted. A subsequent re-analysis of the Framingham data showed a nonsignificant protective effect among younger women, with a nonsignificant adverse effect among older women.[69] Seven of the reports that indicated estrogen replacement is associated with decreased cardiovascular mortality have appeared since 1985, with two published in 1991. Barrett-Connor[70] reported that there may be a bias in selection in some studies, in that women who take estrogens may be more likely than those who do not take estrogens to have access to medical care, to be health conscious and diet conscious, and perhaps to exercise regularly. Thus perhaps not all the decrease in cardiovascular mortality is due to estrogen use. Nevertheless, the decrease in cardiovascular incidence and mortality associated with estrogen use appears to be real and probably to extend even to women in their 70's.[68]

Stampfer et al.[68] reported that the relative risk of cardiovascular mortality in women with any estrogen use after adjustment for other risk factors was 0.72 (95 per cent interval 0.55 to 0.95). Stampfer et al.[68] reported no effect

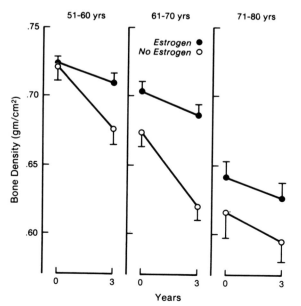

FIGURE 122–12. Mean (± SEM) bone density readings (g/cm²) in postmenopausal women subdivided by 10-year age increments (51 to 60, 61 to 70, and 71 to 80 years) treated with either estrogen (●——●, Estrace, 1 mg, or Premarin, 0.625 mg) or no estrogen (○——○) during a three-year interval. (From Quigley MET et al: Estrogen therapy arrests bone loss in elderly women. Am J Obstet Gynecol 156:1516–1523, 1987.)

on total strokes or ischemic strokes and subarachnoid hemorrhage. As discussed in previous sections of this chapter, the mechanisms of these protective effects of estrogens are attributed to their effects on serum lipids. These effects, however, are seen only with *oral* estrogens and not with estrogens administered transdermally or in micronized injected form. Further studies need to be performed to determine whether estrogens administered by other than oral routes are associated with decreased cardiovascular mortality. An intriguing report by Pines et al.[71] indicates that estrogen may beneficially affect cardiovascular function by directly affecting the heart. In a controlled prospective study of 2.5 months' duration 24 estrogen-treated women had significantly greater aortic blood peak flow velocity, increased mean blood acceleration, and increased cardiac ejection time compared with 19 non–estrogen-treated controls. Whatever the mechanisms, these reports of the beneficial effects of estrogen replacement on cardiovascular disease are important in consideration of whether to treat women, since cardiovascular disease is a common cause of death and morbidity, and other diseases to be discussed shortly, such as endometrial and breast cancers, have lower incidences.

POTENTIAL OR ACTUAL ADVERSE EFFECTS OF ESTROGEN REPLACEMENT

Endometrial Carcinoma

A normal function of estrogens is to stimulate mitotic growth of the endometrium. A large number of studies have demonstrated that unopposed estrogen action over prolonged periods leads to abnormal cystic and adenomatous endometrial hyperplasia, histological atypia, and, ultimately, carcinoma.[72–81] The odds-risk ratio of endometrial cancer ranges from three to five times greater in unopposed (no progestogen) estrogen-treated postmenopausal women versus non–estrogen-treated women. This increased risk can be reduced or eliminated by adding a progestational agent to the estrogen.[81–85] This protective effect of progestogens increases with the number of days' exposure when estrogens and progestogens are used in the usual manner (estrogens administered days 1 through 25 each month, with progestogens added at the end of the 25-day period). Although there are limited data on the optimal duration of progestogen use each month,[83, 86] these data suggest that at least 10 and possibly 12 days of progestogen treatment each month are required to abolish the stimulatory effect of estrogens on the endometrial mitotic rate. The previously discussed continuous administration of *both* estrogen and progestogen, which produces an inactive endometrium and amenorrhea, appears to be a satisfactory alternative.[36]

Breast Cancer

Although the subject is not without some controversy, it is accepted that oral contraceptive use in eugonadal women is not associated with an increased risk of breast cancer.[87] However, women of reproductive age taking oral contraceptives, especially with the newer low-estrogen–

dose contraceptives, change from fairly high exposure to endogenous estrogens to low-dose exogenous exposure. In contrast, the *postmenopausal woman* receiving estrogens is changed from an *estrogen-deprived state* to an estrogen-replete state. Thus the effect of exposure of breast tissue to estrogens in postmenopausal women over many years may be a different problem. The studies are somewhat conflicting, some indicating no risk[88–104] and others indicating some increased risk.[105–115] The increased risk in a number of these studies was frequently confined to some subgroup of the women studied, such as women who underwent premenopausal bilateral oophorectomy,[111, 112] women who had a natural menopause,[108–110] or women who received higher doses of estrogens or received estrogens for longer periods.[107, 109–114] A meta-analysis of the effect of estrogen replacement therapy on the risk of breast cancer has been published by Steinberg et al.[116] This analysis of all statistically acceptable published studies of women with any type of menopause demonstrated a small but significant increase in breast cancer with long estrogen use. This increased risk was not apparent until after at least 5 years of estrogen use, and the odds-risk ratio was 1.3:1 (95 per cent confidence 1.2 to 1.6) after 15 years of estrogen use. In women with a positive family history of breast cancer the risk was greater. These data are summarized in Table 122–7.

Hypertension

Estrogens in adequately high doses increase the concentrations of many circulating proteins produced by the liver (e.g., cortisol-binding globulin, thyroxine-binding globulin, renin substrate, transferin, and sex hormone–binding globulin). As discussed earlier, in the usual doses used for postmenopausal women, these changes are seen with oral estrogens and not with transdermal or micronized injected estrogens. A subset of women receiving oral estrogens developed hypertension, which is at times reversible on discontinuation of the estrogens.[117, 118] The hypertension has been attributed to increases in renin substrate. However, a very large fraction of (probably most) women receiving oral estrogens develop increased renin substrate levels without developing hypertension. Estrogens also cause an increase in blood volume and cardiac output in most women.[71, 119, 120] The incidence of estrogen-induced hypertension is low, probably about less than or equal to 1 per cent of postmenopausal estrogen-treated women. Nevertheless, because it is reversible in some women, it is important to keep in mind. The mechanisms remain uncertain, since the alterations in renin substrate and the hemody-

TABLE 122–7. EFFECT OF ESTROGEN REPLACEMENT THERAPY ON BREAST CANCER IS GREATER IN WOMEN WITH A FAMILY HISTORY OF BREAST CANCER

FAMILY HISTORY	MEAN RISK
Yes	3.4 (2.0–6.0)
No	1.5 (1.2–1.7)

From Steinberg KK et al: A meta-analysis of the effect of estrogen replacement therapy on the risk of breast cancer. JAMA 265:1985–1990, copyright 1991, the American Medical Association.

namic changes occur in most estrogen-treated women, and so few develop hypertension.

Hyperlipidemia

Mild increases in the levels of triglycerides are observed in most postmenopausal women who receive oral estrogens, but triglyceride concentrations usually remain within normal limits. On rare occasions estrogen treatment of postmenopausal women can produce massive hypertriglyceridemia (i.e., to several thousand milligrams per cent). Patients who develop such elevated triglycerides have a previous underlying metabolic lipid disorder, usually a mild combined triglyceride-cholesterol disorder.[121] Complications of massive triglyceridemia include fatigue, weakness, cardiac ischemia, a predisposition to pancreatitis, and fatty deposits in skin. When estrogen therapy is discontinued, the triglycerides fall over 4 to 12 weeks to a baseline slightly above normal and representative of the underlying lipid disorder.[121] Cholesterol concentrations may also become elevated to 500 to 1000 μg/dl in such patients and fall with the same time course as the triglyceride concentrations.[121] In addition to the underlying lipid disorder, other factors that can augment these adverse estrogen effects include obesity and therapy with glucocorticoids or thiazides. These adverse effects are uncommon, and as indicated earlier, as a group, postmenopausal women who receive estrogen therapy have a lower incidence of ischemic heart disease and overall mortality.

Gallbladder Disease

Bile cholesterol concentrations are increased by estrogen therapy, as well as by other parameters, such as obesity.[122] This effect of estrogens accounts for the increased incidence of cholelithiasis and cholecystitis in obese women as well as in estrogen-treated women. This, as other estrogen effects, is presumably a dose-related phenomenon. However, in women who are overweight or have past symptoms of cholecystitis, estrogen replacement should be used with caution. The relative risk for surgically confirmed gallbladder disease occurring in otherwise healthy postmenopausal women who received estrogens compared with those who did not was 2.5:1, as estimated by the Boston Collaborative Drug Surveillance Program.[123]

SUMMARY

The prolonged estrogen-deprived state seen in postmenopausal women is unusual in nature. Menses occur to very old age in higher primates other than humans, and estrus cycles occur in very old nonprimate mammals. An excellent case can be made that, with the exception of women with specific contraindications or those who are obese, estrogen replacement therapy should be offered to all women at menopause. Massively obese women produce greatly increased quantities of *endogenous* estrogens in adipose tissue and are at decreased risk for osteoporosis. In such patients periodic treatment with a progestogen only assists in decreasing the risk of endometrial carcinoma.

Contraindications to estrogen replacement include breast cancer either in the patient or in a relative. In otherwise healthy, slender women the advantages of estrogen treatment, which include decreased osteoporosis and its associated morbidity and mortality, decreased incidence of cardiovascular disease, beneficial effects on vasomotor symptoms, and beneficial effects on estrogen-sensitive tissues, appear to outweigh potential or real adverse effects.

REFERENCES

1. Tokarz RR: Oogonia, proliferation, oogenesis and folliculogenesis in nonmammalian vertebrates. *In* Jones RE (ed): The Vertebrate Ovary. New York, Plenum Press, 1978, pp 145–179.
2. Richardson SJ, Senikas V, Nelson JF: Follicular depletion during the menopausal transition: Evidence for accelerated loss and ultimate exhaustion. J Clin Endocrinol Metab 65:1231–1237, 1987.
3. Judd HL, Judd GE, Lucas WE, et al: Endocrine function of the postmenopausal ovary: Concentrations of androgens and estrogens in ovarian and peripheral vein blood. J Clin Endocrinol Metab 39:1020–1024, 1974.
4. Whelan EA, Sandler DP, McConnaughey DR, Weinberg CR: Menstrual and reproductive characteristics and age at natural menopause. Am J Epidemiol 131:625–632, 1990.
5. Beard RJ: The menopause. Br J Hosp Med 13:631–637, 1975.
6. Amundsen DW, Diers CJ: The age of menopause in medieval Europe. Hum Biol 45:605–612, 1973.
7. Adamopoulos DA, Loraine JA, Dove GA: Endocrinological studies in women approaching the menopause. J Obstet Gynaecol Br Commonw 78:62–79, 1971.
8. Sherman BM, Korenman SG: Hormonal characteristics of the human menstrual cycle throughout reproductive life. J Clin Invest 55:699–706, 1975.
9. Kwekkeboom DJ, deJong FH, Van Hemert AM, et al: Serum gonadotropins and alpha-subunit decline in aging normal postmenopausal women. J Clin Endocrinol Metab 70:944–950, 1990.
10. Patritti-Laborde N, Wolfsen AR, Heber D, Odell WD: Pituitary gland: Site of short loop feedback for luteinizing hormone in the rabbit. J Clin Invest 64:1066–1069, 1979.
11. Patritti-Laborde N, Wolfsen AR, Odell WD: Shortloop feedback system for the control of follicle stimulating hormone in the rabbit. Endocrinology 108:72–75, 1981.
12. Patritti-Laborde N, Odell WD: Shortloop feedback of LH: Dose-response relations and specificity. Fertil Steril 30:456–460, 1978.
13. Odell WD, Griffin J: Pulsatile secretion of human chorionic gonadotropin in normal adults. N Engl J Med 317:1688–1691, 1987.
14. Odell WD, Griffin J: Pulsatile secretion of chorionic gonadotropin during the normal menstrual cycle. J Clin Endocrinol Metab 69:528–532, 1989.
15. Mattingly RF, Huang WY: Steroidogenesis of the menopausal and postmenopausal ovary. Am J Obstet Gynecol 103:679–693, 1969.
16. Siiteri PK: Postmenopausal-estrogen production. *In* VanKeep PA, Lauritzen C (eds): Ageing and Estrogens, vol 3. New York, Karger, 1973, pp 40–44.
17. Nagamani M, Stuart CA, Doherty MG: Increased steroid production by the ovarian stromal tissue of postmenopausal women with endometrial cancer. J Clin Endocrinol Metab 74:172–176, 1992.
18. MacDonald PC, Siiteri PK: The relationship between the extraglandular production of estrone and the occurrence of endometrial neoplasia. Gynecol Oncol 2:259–263, 1974.
19. Hemsell DL, Grodin JM, Brenner PF, et al: Plasma precursors of estrogen. II. Correlation of the extent of conversion of plasma androstenedione to estrone with age. J Clin Endocrinol Metab 38:476–479, 1974.
20. Zador G: The pathophysiology and methods of treatment of climacteric disorders. Acta Obstet Gynecol Scand [Suppl] 65:19–26, 1977.
21. Lauritzen C: The management of the premenopausal and the postmenopausal patient. *In* VanKeep PA, Lauritzen C (eds): Ageing and Estrogens, vol 2. New York, Karger, 1973, pp 2–21.
22. Meldrum DR, Shamonki IM, Frumar AM, et al: Elevations in skin temperature of the finger as an objective index of postmenopausal hot flashes: Standardization of the technique. Am J Obstet Gynecol 135:713–717, 1979.

23. Tataryn IV, Lomax P, Meldrum DR, et al: Objective techniques for the assessment of postmenopausal hot flashes. Obstet Gynecol 57:340–344, 1981.
24. Casper RF, Yen SSC, Wilkes MM: Menopausal flushes: A neuroendocrine link with pulsatile luteinizing hormone secretion. Science 205:823–825, 1979.
25. Meldrum DR, Tataryn IV, Frumar AM, et al: Gonadotropins, estrogens and adrenal steroids during the menopausal hot flash. J Clin Endocrinol Metab 50:685–689, 1980.
26. Erlik Y, Meldrum DR, Judd HL: Estrogen levels in postmenopausal women with hot flashes. Obstet Gynecol 59:403–407, 1982.
27. Jaszmann L, Van Lith ND, Zaat JCA: The perimenopausal symptoms. Med Gynecol Sociol 4:268–277, 1969.
28. Winokur G: Depression in the menopause. Am J Psychiatry 130:92–93, 1973.
29. Sheffery JB, Wilson TA, Walsh JC: Double-blind, cross-over study comparing chlordiazepoxide, conjugated estrogens, combined chlordiazepoxide and conjugated estrogens, and placebo in treatment of the menopause. Med Ann Dist Columbia 38:433–436, 1969.
30. Utian WH: The mental tonic effect of oestrogens administered to oophorectomized females. South Afr Med J 46:1079–1082, 1972.
31. Kantor HI, Michael CM, Shore H: Estrogen for older women. A three-year study. Am J Obstet Gynecol 116:115–118, 1973.
32. Chetkowski RJ, Meldrum DR, Steingold KA, et al: Biologic effects of transdermal estradiol. N Engl J Med 314:1615–1620, 1986.
33. Walsh BW, Schiff I, Rosner B, et al: Effects of postmenopausal estrogen replacement on the concentrations and metabolism of plasma lipoproteins. N Engl J Med 325:1196–1204, 1991.
34. Sporrong T, Hellgren M, Samsioe G, Mattsson LA: Comparison of four continuously administered progestogen plus oestradiol combinations for climacteric complaints. Br J Obstet Gynaecol 95:1042–1048, 1988.
35. Yoshizawa I, Fishman J: Radioimmunoassay of 2-hydroxyestrone in human plasma. J Clin Endocrinol Metab 32:3–6, 1971.
36. Fishman J, Guzik H, Hellman L: Aromatic ring hydroxylation of estradiol in man. Biochemistry 9:1593–1598, 1970.
37. Riggs BL, Jowsey J, Goldsmith RS, et al: Short- and long-term effects of estrogen and synthetic anabolic hormone in postmenopausal osteoporosis. J Clin Invest 51:1659–1663, 1972.
38. Lindsay R, Aitken JM, Anderson JB, et al: Long-term prevention of postmenopausal osteoporosis by oestrogen. Lancet 1:1038–1040, 1976.
39. Christiansen C, Christiansen MS, Transbol I: Bone mass in postmenopausal women after withdrawal of estrogen/gestogen replacement therapy. Lancet 1:459–461, 1981.
40. Nachtigall LE, Nachtigall RH, Nachtigall RD, Beckman EM: Estrogen replacement therapy. I. A 10-year prospective study in the relationship to osteoporosis. Obstet Gynecol 53:277–281, 1979.
41. Ireland P, Fordtran JS: Effect of dietary calcium and age on jejunal calcium absorption in humans studied by intestinal perfusion. J Clin Invest 52:2672–2681, 1973.
42. Heaney RP, Recker RR, Saville PD: Menopausal changes in calcium balance performance. J Lab Clin Med 92:953–963, 1978.
43. Cheema C, Grant BF, Marcus R: Effects of estrogen on circulating "free" and total 1,25-dihydroxyvitamin D and on the parathyroid-vitamin D axis in postmenopausal women. J Clin Invest 83:537–542, 1989.
44. Kiel DP, Felson DT, Anderson JJ, et al: Hip fracture and the use of estrogens in postmenopausal women. N Engl J Med 317:1169–1174, 1987.
45. Quigley MET, Martin PL, Burnier AM, Brooks P: Estrogen therapy arrests bone loss in elderly women. Am J Obstet Gynecol 156:1516–1523, 1987.
46. Riis B, Thomsen K, Christiansen C: Does calcium supplementation prevent postmenopausal bone loss? A double-blind, controlled clinical study. N Engl J Med 316:173–177, 1987.
47. Riggs BL, Wahner HW, Melton LJ III, et al: Dietary calcium intake and rates of bone loss in women. J Clin Invest 80:979–982, 1987.
48. Baran D, Sorensen A, Grimes J, et al: Dietary modification with dairy products for preventing vertebral bone loss in premenopausal women: A three-year prospective study. J Clin Endocrinol Metab 70:264–270, 1990.
49. Dawson-Hughes B, Dallal GE, Krall EA, et al: A controlled trial of the effect of calcium supplementation on bone density in postmenopausal women. N Engl J Med 323:878–883, 1990.
50. Gallagher JC, Riggs BL, Recker RR, Goldgar D: The effect of calcitriol on patients with postmenopausal osteoporosis with special reference to fracture frequency. Proc Soc Exp Biol Med 191:287–292, 1989.
51. Gordon T, Kannel WB, Hjortland MC, McNamara PM: Menopause and coronary heart disease: The Framingham Study. Ann Intern Med 89:157–161, 1978.
52. Jick H, Dinan B, Rothman KJ: Noncontraceptive estrogens and nonfatal myocardial infarction. JAMA 239:1407–1408, 1978.
53. Wilson PWF, Garrison RJ, Castelli WP: Postmenopausal estrogen use, cigarette smoking, and cardiovascular morbidity in women over 50: The Framingham Study. N Engl J Med 313:1038–1043, 1985.
54. Rosenberg L, Armstrong B, Jick H: Myocardial infarction and estrogen therapy in post-menopausal women. N Engl J Med 294:1256–1259, 1976.
55. Petitti DB, Wingerd J, Pellegrin F, Ramcharan S: Risk of vascular disease in women: Smoking, oral contraceptives, noncontraceptive estrogens, and other factors. JAMA 242:1150–1154, 1979.
56. Rosenberg L, Slone D, Shapiro S, et al: Noncontraceptive estrogens and myocardial infarction in young women. JAMA 244:339–342, 1980.
57. Pfeffer RI, Whipple GH, Kurosaki TT, Chapman JM: Coronary risk and estrogen use in postmenopausal women. Am J Epidemiol 107:479–487, 1978.
58. Ross RK, Paganini-Hill A, Mack TM, et al: Menopausal oestrogen therapy and protection from death from ischaemic heart disease. Lancet 1:858–860, 1981.
59. Bain C, Willett W, Hennekens CH, et al: Use of postmenopausal hormones and risk of myocardial infarction. Circulation 64:42–46, 1981.
60. Adam S, Williams V, Vessey MP: Cardiovascular disease and hormone replacement treatment: A pilot case-control study. Br Med J 282:1277–1278, 1981.
61. Szklo M, Tonascia J, Gordis L, Bloom I: Estrogen use and myocardial infarction risk: A case-control study. Prev Med 13:510–516, 1984.
62. Stampfer MJ, Willett WC, Colditz GA, et al: A prospective study of postmenopausal estrogen therapy and coronary heart disease. N Engl J Med 313:1044–1049, 1985.
63. Colditz GA, Willett WC, Stampfer MJ, et al: Menopause and the risk of coronary heart disease in women. N Engl J Med 316:1105–1110, 1987.
64. Bush TL, Barrett-Connor E, Cowan LD, et al: Cardiovascular mortality and noncontraceptive use of estrogen in women: Results from the Lipid Research Clinics Program Follow-up Study. Circulation 75:1102–1109, 1987.
65. Criqui MH, Suarez L, Barrett-Connor E, et al: Postmenopausal estrogen use and mortality: Results from a prospective study in a defined, homogeneous community. Am J Epidemiol 128:606–614, 1988.
66. Henderson BE, Paganini-Hill A, Ross RK: Estrogen replacement therapy and protection from acute myocardial infarction. Am J Obstet Gynecol 159:312–317, 1988.
67. Wolf PH, Madans JH, Finucane FF, et al: Reduction of cardiovascular disease-related mortality among postmenopausal women who use hormones: Evidence from a national cohort. Am J Obstet Gynecol 164:489–494, 1991.
68. Stampfer MJ, Colditz GA, Willett WC, et al: Postmenopausal estrogen therapy and cardiovascular disease. N Engl J Med 325:756–762, 1991.
69. Eaker ED, Castelli WP: Coronary heart disease and its risk factors among women in the Framingham Study. In Eaker E, Packard B, Winger NK, et al (eds): Coronary Heart in Women. New York, Maymarket Doyma, 1987, pp 122–132.
70. Barrett-Connor E: Postmenopausal estrogen and prevention bias. Ann Intern Med 115:455–456, 1991.
71. Pines A, Fisman EZ, Levo Y, et al: The effects of hormone replacement therapy in normal postmenopausal women: Measurement of Doppler-derived parameters of aortic flow. Am J Obstet Gynecol 164:806–812, 1991.
72. Smith DC, Prentice R, Thompson DJ, Herrmann WL: Association of exogenous estrogen and endometrial carcinoma. N Engl J Med 293:1164–1167, 1975.
73. Ziel HK, Finkle WD: Increased risk of endometrial carcinoma among users of conjugated estrogens. N Engl J Med 293:1167–1170, 1975.
74. Mack TM, Pike MC, Henderson BE, et al: Estrogens and endometrial cancer in a retirement community. N Engl J Med 294:1262–1267, 1976.
75. McDonald TW, Annegers JR, O'Fallon WM, et al: Exogenous estrogen and endometrial carcinoma: Case-control and incidence study. Am J Obstet Gynecol 127:572–580, 1977.
76. Gray LA Sr, Christopherson WM, Hoover RN: Estrogens and endometrial cancer. Obstet Gynecol 49:385–389, 1977.
77. Antunes CMF, Stolley PD, Rosenshen NB: Endometrial cancer and estrogen use: Report of a large case-control study. N Engl J Med 300:9–13, 1979.

78. Shapiro S, Kaufman DW, Slone D, et al: Recent and past use of conjugated estrogens in relation to adenocarcinoma of the endometrium. N Engl J Med 303:485–489, 1980.
79. Hammond CB, Jelovsek FR, Lee KC, et al: Effects of long-term estrogen replacement therapy. II. Neoplasia. J Obstet Gynecol 133:537–547, 1979.
80. Shapiro S, Kelly JP, Rosenberg L, et al: Risk of localized and widespread endometrial cancer in relation to recent discontinued use of conjugated estrogens. N Engl J Med 313:969–972, 1985.
81. Paganini-Hill A, Ross RK, Henderson BE: Endometrial cancer and patterns of use of oestrogen replacement therapy: A cohort study. Br J Cancer 59:445–447, 1989.
82. Thom MH, White PJ, Williams RM, et al: Prevention and treatment of endometrial disease in climacteric women receiving oestrogen therapy. Lancet 2:455–457, 1979.
83. Whitehead MI, Townsend PT, Pryse-Davies J, et al: Effects of estrogens and progestin on the biochemistry and morphology of the postmenopausal endometrium. N Engl J Med 305:1599–1605, 1981.
84. Gambrell RD, Bagnell CA, Greenblatt RB: Role of estrogens and progesterone in the etiology and prevention of endometrial cancer: Review. Am J Obstet Gynecol 146:696–707, 1983.
85. Persson I, Adami H-O, Bergkvist L, et al: Risk of endometrial cancer after treatment with oestrogens alone or in conjunction with progestogens: Results of a prospective study. Br Med J 298:147–151, 1989.
86. Varma TR: Effect of long-term therapy with estrogen and progesterone on the endometrium of post-menopausal women. Acta Obstet Gynecol Scand 64:41–46, 1985.
87. Oral-contraceptive use and the risk of breast cancer—The Cancer and Steroid Hormone Study of the Centers for Disease Control and the National Institute of Child Health and Human Development. N Engl J Med 315:405–411, 1986.
88. Wallach S, Henneman PH: Prolonged estrogen therapy in postmenopausal woman. JAMA 171:1637–1642, 1959.
89. Wilson RA: The roles of estrogen and progesterone in breast and genital cancer. JAMA 182:327–331, 1962.
90. Casagrande J, Gerkins V, Mack T, et al: Brief communication: Exogenous estrogens and breast cancer in women with natural menopause. J Natl Cancer Inst 56:839–841, 1976.
91. Sartwell PE, Arthes FG, Tonascia JA: Exogenous hormones, reproductive history, and breast cancer. J Natl Cancer Inst 59:1589–1592, 1977.
92. Wynder EL, MacCornack FA, Stellman SD: The epidemiology of breast cancer in 785 United States Caucasian women. Cancer 41:2341–2354, 1978.
93. Ravinhar BA, Seigel DG, Lindtner J: An epidemiologic study of breast cancer and benign breast neoplasias in relation to the oral contraceptive and estrogen use. Eur J Cancer 15:395–405, 1979.
94. Nachtigall LE, Nachtigall RH, Nachtigall RD, Beckman EF: Estrogen replacement therapy. II. A prospective study in the relationship to carcinoma and cardiovascular and metabolic problems. Obstet Gynecol 54:74–79, 1979.
95. Hammond CB, Jelocsek FR, Lee KL, et al: Effects of long-term estrogen replacement therapy. II. Neoplasia. Am J Obstet Gynecol 133:537–547, 1979.
96. Bland KI, Buchanan JB, Weisberg BF, et al: The effects of exogenous estrogen replacement therapy on the breast: Breast cancer risk and mammographic parenchymal patterns. Cancer 45:3027–3033, 1980.
97. Kelsey JL, Fischer DB, Holford TR, et al: Exogenous estrogens and other factors in the epidemiology of breast cancer. J Natl Cancer Inst 67:327–333, 1981.
98. Sherman B, Wallace R, Bean J: Estrogen use and breast cancer. Cancer 51:1527–1531, 1983.
99. Gambrell RD Jr, Maier RC, Sanders BI: Decreased incidence of breast cancer in postmenopausal estrogen-progestogen users. Obstet Gynecol 62:435–443, 1983.
100. Horwitz RI, Stewart KR: Effects of clinical features on the association of estrogens and breast cancer. Am J Med 6:192–198, 1984.
101. Kaufman DW, Miller DR, Rosenberg L, et al: Noncontraceptive estrogen use and risk of breast cancer. JAMA 252:63–67, 1984.
102. McDonald JA, Weiss NS, Daling JR, et al: Menopausal estrogen use and the risk of breast cancer. Breast Cancer Res Treat 7:193–199, 1986.
103. Buring JE, Hennekens CH, Lipnick RJ, et al: A prospective cohort study of postmenopausal hormone use and risk of breast cancer in U.S. women. Am J Epidemiol 125:939–947, 1987.
104. DuPont WD, Page DL, Rogers LW, Parl FF: Influence of exogenous estrogens, proliferative breast disease, and other variables on breast cancer risk. Cancer 63:948–957, 1989.
105. Hulka BS, Chambless LE, Duebner DC, Wilkinson WE: Breast cancer and estrogen replacement therapy. Am J Obstet Gynecol 143:638–644, 1982.
106. Nomura AMY, Kolonel LN, Hirohata T, Lee J: The association of replacement estrogens with breast cancer. Int J Cancer 37:49–53, 1986.
107. Brinton LA, Hoover R, Fraumeni JF Jr: Menopausal oestrogens and breast cancer risk: An expanded case-control study. Br J Cancer 54:825–832, 1986.
108. Jick H, Walker AM, Watkins RN, et al: Replacement estrogens and breast cancer. Am J Epidemiol 112:586–594, 1980.
109. Hoover R, Glass A, Finkle WD, et al: Conjugated estrogens and breast cancer risk in women. J Natl Cancer Inst 67:815–820, 1981.
110. Ross RK, Paganini-Hill A, Gerkins VR, et al: A case-control study of menopausal estrogen therapy and breast cancer. JAMA 243:1635–1639, 1980.
111. Wingo PA, Layde PM, Lee NC, et al: The risk of breast cancer in postmenopausal women who have used estrogen replacement therapy. JAMA 257:209–215, 1987.
112. Hiatt RA, Bawol R, Friedman GD, Hoover R: Exogenous estrogen and breast cancer after bilateral oophorectomy. Cancer 4:139–144, 1984.
113. Hoover R, Gray LA, Cole P, MacMahon B: Menopausal estrogens and breast cancer. N Engl J Med 295:401–405, 1976.
114. Bergkvist L, Adami HO, Persson I, et al: The risk of breast cancer after estrogen and estrogen-progestin replacement. N Engl J Med 321:293–297, 1989.
115. LaVecchia C, DeCarli A, Parazihni F, et al: Noncontraceptive oestrogens and the risk of breast cancer in women. Int J Cancer 38:853–858, 1986.
116. Steinberg KK, Thacker SB, Smith SJ, et al: A meta-analysis of the effect of estrogen replacement therapy on the risk of breast cancer. JAMA 265:1985–1990, 1991.
117. Royal College of General Practitioners: Oral Contraceptives and Health, an Interim Report from the Oral Contraception Study of the Royal College of General Practitioners. New York, Pitman Publishing, 1974, pp 37–42.
118. Laragh JH, Sealey JE, Ledingham JGG, Newton MA: Oral contraceptives: Renin, aldosterone, and high blood pressure. JAMA 201:918–922, 1967.
119. Walters WAW: Haemodynamic changes in women taking oral contraceptives. J Obstet Gynaecol Br Commonw 77:1007–1012, 1970.
120. Lehtovirta P: Haemodynamic effects of combined oestrogen/progestogen oral contraceptives. J Obstet Gynaecol Br Commonw 81:517–525, 1974.
121. Molitch ME, Oill P, Odell WD: Massive hyperlipidemia during oral contraceptive and postmenopausal estrogen therapy. JAMA 227:522–526, 1974.
122. Bennion LJ, Grundy SM: Risk factors for the development of cholelithiasis in man. N Engl J Med 299:1221–1226, 1978.
123. Surgically confirmed gallbladder disease, venous thromboembolism, and breast tumors in relation to postmenopausal estrogen therapy. A report from the Boston Collaborative Drug Surveillance Program, Boston University Medical Center. N Engl J Med 290:15–19, 1974.

123

Contraception

DANIEL R. MISHELL, Jr.

CONTRACEPTIVE USE AND EFFECTIVENESS

An ideal method of contraception for all individuals is not now available and probably will never be developed. A variety of effective methods of contraception are available, each with certain advantages and disadvantages. Therefore, when giving advice about contraception, the clinician should explain to the couple the advantages and disadvantages of each method, so that they will be fully informed and can rationally choose the method most suitable for them. Because no contraceptive method other than the condom has been developed for use by the male, the contraceptive provider counsels the female partner and should inform her if there are medical reasons that contraindicate the use of certain methods and offer her alternatives.

Contraceptive Use in the United States

The last government survey in the United States was performed in 1988.[1] Data from this survey revealed that about one third of the 57.9 million women in the reproductive age group (15 to 44), or 19.2 million women, were not exposed to unwanted pregnancy. Of the remaining 38.7 million women who were exposed to the risk of pregnancy, all but 3.8 million (9.7 per cent) used a method of contraception.

The remaining 35 million women were using a method of contraception with technique. Sterilization was the most common. A total of 13.7 million women, 35 per cent of those exposed to unwanted pregnancy, used sterilization of one member of the couple, 17 per cent women and 7 per cent men, to prevent pregnancy. Use of sterilization among married women in the United States has increased dramatically in the past 25 years from one fourth of these women practicing contraception in 1977 to more than one half in 1988.

Of the nonsurgical, reversible methods of contraception, oral contraceptives (OC's) were most popular, being used by 10.7 million women, and were followed in frequency of use by the condom, periodic abstinence, withdrawal, diaphragm, intrauterine device (IUD), and spermicides alone (Table 123–1). More women using reversible contraceptive methods used OC's, 50.4 per cent, than all the other methods combined.

Between 1982 and 1988 OC and condom use increased, IUD use decreased, and the use of the other techniques remained relatively stable.

TABLE 123–1. CONTRACEPTIVE USE OF 57.9 MILLION U.S. WOMEN 15 TO 44 YEARS OLD (1988 NATIONAL SURVEY OF FAMILY GROWTH)

EXPOSURE AND CONTRACEPTIVE METHOD	NO. (MILLIONS)	PERCENTAGE OF EXPOSED WOMEN	PERCENTAGE OF ALL WOMEN AGED 15–44
Exposed users	34.7	90.0	60.3
Sterilization	13.7	35.5	23.6
Female	9.6	24.9	16.6
Male	4.1	10.6	7.0
Oral contraceptives	10.7	27.7	18.5
Condom	5.1	13.2	8.8
Spermicides	0.3	0.7	0.6
Withdrawal	0.8	2.1	1.3
Diaphragm	2.0	5.2	3.5
Periodic abstinence	0.8	2.1	1.4
IUD	0.7	1.8	1.2
Douche	0.05	0.1	0.1
Exposed nonusers	3.8	9.8	6.5
Not exposed	19.2	49.6	33.2
TOTAL	57.9		

From Mosher WD, Pratt WF: Contraceptive use in the United States. Patient Educ Couns 16:163, 1990.

Contraceptive Effectiveness

It is difficult to determine the actual effectiveness of various methods of contraception because of a large number of factors that affect contraceptive failure. The terms *method effectiveness* and *use effectiveness* (or *method failure* and *patient failure*) have been used to differentiate whether conception occurred while the contraceptive method was being used correctly or incorrectly. In general, methods used at the time of coitus, such as the diaphragm, condom, spermicides, and withdrawal, have a much greater method effectiveness than use effectiveness. With the use of methods in which coitus-related activities are not needed, such as the OC's and IUD, there is less difference between method and use effectiveness, and thus their overall effec-

tiveness is greater than that of the coitus-related methods (Table 123–2).

The overall value of a contraceptive method as used by a couple (correctly or incorrectly) is determined by calculating actual effectiveness as well as the continuation rate. To determine these rates, actuarial methods such as the log-rank life table method should be used instead of the less accurate Pearl index.

Several factors influence contraceptive failure rates. One of the most important is motivation of the couple. Contraceptive failure is more likely to occur in couples seeking to delay a wanted birth than in couples seeking to prevent any more births, especially for coitus-related methods. The woman's age has a strong negative correlation with the failure of a contraceptive method, as does the socioeconomic class and level of education. Thus one must consider many variables when evaluating the effectiveness of any method of contraception for an individual patient. In addition, failure rates of prospective studies are consistently lower than those of retrospective interview studies. Finally, for all methods, failure rates are greater during the first year of use than in subsequent years, yet most studies report only first-year use failure rates. Thus many variables must be considered when evaluating the effectiveness of any method of contraception for an individual woman.

In 1990 Trussell et al[2] published an estimate of first-year failure rates based on recently reported data. OC's, the IUD, and Norplant had the lowest method and use failure rates (Table 123–3).

Continuation rates for the various contraceptive methods are highest for the IUD and subdermal implants, which necessitate a visit to a health care facility to discontinue use, and lowest for the diaphragm, condom, and spermicide.

TABLE 123–2. CONTRACEPTIVE FAILURES WITH VARIOUS METHODS (OXFORD FAMILY PLANNING ASSOCIATION CONTRACEPTIVE STUDY)

METHOD	FAILURE RATE (PER 100 WOMAN-YEARS)
Sterilization	
Male	0.02
Female	0.13
Oral contraceptives	
<50 µg estrogen	0.27
50 µg estrogen	0.16
>50 µg estrogen	0.32
Progesterone only	1.2
IUD	
Copper T	1.2
Copper 7	1.5
Dalkon Shield	2.4
Loop A	6.8
Loop B	1.8
Loop C	1.4
Loop D	1.3
Saf-T-Coil	1.3
Not known	1.8
Diaphragm	1.9
Condom	3.6
Withdrawal	6.7
Spermicides	11.9
Rhythm	15.5

From Vessey M, et al: Efficacy of different contraceptive methods. Lancet 1:841, 1982.

Spermicides: Intravaginal Sponge, Foams, Creams, and Suppositories

All spermicidal agents contain a surfactant, usually non-oxynol-9, which immobilizes or kills sperm on contact.

TABLE 123–3. LOWEST EXPECTED, TYPICAL, AND LOWEST REPORTED FAILURE RATES DURING FIRST YEAR OF USE OF CONTRACEPTIVE METHOD

METHOD	PERCENTAGE OF WOMEN EXPERIENCING ACCIDENTAL PREGNANCY IN FIRST YEAR OF USE		
	Lowest Expected[1]	Typical[2]	Lowest Reported[3,4]
Chance[5]	85	85	43.1
Spermicides[6]	3	21	0.0
Periodic abstinence		20	
Calendar method	9		14.4[7]
Ovulation method	3		10.5[7]
Symptothermal[8] method	2		12.6
Postovulation	1		2.0[7]
Withdrawal	4	18	6.7[7]
Cap[9]	6	18	8.0
Sponge			
Parous women	9	28	27.7
Nulliparous women	6	18	13.9
Diaphragm[9]	6	18	2.1
Condom[10]	2	12	4.2
IUD		3	
Progestasert	2.0		1.9
Copper T 380A	0.8		0.5
Oral contraceptives	3		75
Combined	0.1		0.0
Progestin only	0.5		1.1
Injectable progestin			
DMPA	0.3	0.3	0.0
NET	0.4	0.4	0.0
Implants			
Norplant (6 capsules)	0.04	0.04	0.0
Female sterilization	0.2	0.4	0.0
Male sterilization	0.1	0.15	0.0

Modified from Trussell J, et al: Contraceptive failure in the United States: An update. Stud Fam Plann 21:51, 1990.

[1]Among couples who initiate use of a method (not necessarily for the first time) and who use it *perfectly* (both consistently and correctly), the authors' best guess of the percentage expected to experience an accidental pregnancy during the first year if they do not stop use for any other reason. [2]Among *typical* couples who initiate use of a method (not necessarily for the first time), the percentage who experience an accidental pregnancy during the first year if they do not stop use for any other reason. [3]In the literature on contraceptive failure, the *lowest* reported percentage who experienced an accidental pregnancy during the first year following initiation of use (not necessarily for the first time) if they did not stop use for any other reason. However, see note 8. [4]Among couples attempting to avoid pregnancy, the percentage who continue to use a method for one year, under the alternative assumptions that no one becomes pregnant (column 4) and that the proportion becoming pregnant is given by column 1 (column 5). [5]The lowest expected and typical percents are based on data from populations where contraception is not practiced and from women who cease practicing contraception in order to become pregnant. These represent our best guess of the percentage who would conceive among women now relying on reversible methods of contraception if they abandoned contraception altogether. The lowest reported percent is based on U.S. women who practice no contraception even though they do not wish to become pregnant. This group is selected for low fecundity or low coital frequency, and some fraction may use an unreported variant of periodic abstinence. [6]Foams and vaginal suppositories. [7]Too low, because rate is based on more than one year of exposure. See J. Trussell and K. Kost, "Contraceptive failure in the United States: A critical review of the literature," *Studies in Family Planning* 18 (1987):237–283. [8]Cervical mucus (ovulation) method supplemented by calendar in the pre-ovulatory and basal body temperature in the post-ovulatory phases. [9]With spermicidal cream or jelly. [10]Without spermicides.

They also provide a mechanical barrier and need to be placed into the vagina before each coital act. The effectiveness of these agents, except for the sponge, increases with increasing age of the woman and is similar to that of the diaphragm in all age and income groups.

The most popular spermicide is a contraceptive sponge, which is a cylindrical piece of soft polyurethane that has been impregnated with 1 mg of nonoxynol-9. In contrast to other spermicidal methods, the sponge does not have to be inserted into the vagina before each act of intercourse and is effective for 24 hours. In large clinical trials the one-year failure rate for the sponge was slightly but significantly higher than that for the diaphragm, about 15 per cent.[3,4]

The incidence of toxic shock syndrome appears to be slightly increased in users of the sponge, especially if it is used during the menses or the puerperium or if it is left in place for more than 24 hours. Each of these risk factors are contraindications for use of the sponge. The overall incidence of toxic shock syndrome in users of the sponge is low, estimated at one infection per 2 million sponges.[5]

Although a few early studies linked the use of a spermicide at the time of conception with an increased risk of some congenital malformations, these studies were probably flawed by recall bias. Recent studies have shown no increased risk of congenital malformation in the neonates or karyotypical abnormalities in the spontaneous abortuses of women who conceived while using spermicides.[6–8]

Diaphragm

A diaphragm must be carefully fitted by the physician or nursing personnel. The largest size that does not cause discomfort or undue pressure on the vaginal mucosa should be used. After the fitting the patient should remove the diaphragm and re-insert it herself. She should then be examined to make sure the diaphragm is covering the cervix. The diaphragm should be used with contraceptive cream or jelly and be left in place for at least eight hours after coitus. If repeated intercourse takes place or coitus occurs more than eight hours after insertion of the diaphragm, additional contraceptive cream or jelly should be used. The number of urinary tract infections in women who use diaphragms is significantly higher than in nonusers, probably because of the mechanical obstruction of the outflow of urine by the diaphragm.[9]

Diaphragm users should also be cautioned not to leave the device in place for more than 24 hours because ulceration of the vaginal epithelium may occur with prolonged usage.

Cervical Cap

The cervical cap, a cup-shaped plastic or rubber device that fits around the cervix, can be left in place longer than the diaphragm and is more comfortable. Each type of device is manufactured in different sizes and should be fitted to the cervix by a clinician. The cervical cap should not be left in place for more than 72 hours because of the possibility of ulceration, unpleasant odor, and infection.

The Prentif cavity-rim cervical cap was approved in 1988 for general use in the United States. Product labeling stipulates that the cap should be left on the cervix for no more than 48 hours and that a spermicide should always be placed inside the cap before use. The cap is manufactured in four sizes and requires more training, both for the provider in fitting it and for the user in placing it correctly, than the diaphragm. Failure rates are similar to those observed with the diaphragm.[10–12]

Condom

Use of the condom by individuals with multiple sex partners should be encouraged. It is the contraceptive method most effective in preventing transmission of sexually transmitted diseases. The condom should not be applied tightly. The tip should extend beyond the end of the penis by about 1/2 inch to collect the ejaculate.

Barrier Techniques and Sexually Transmitted Diseases

Barrier methods have the advantage of reducing the rate of transmission of sexually transmitted diseases. Several epidemiologic studies have shown that spermicides reduce the frequency of clinical infection with sexually transmitted diseases, both bacterial and viral.[13–16] In vitro studies have demonstrated that condoms prevent the transmission of viruses, specifically the herpes virus and the human immunodeficiency virus as well as *Chlamydia trachomatis*, a frequent cause of salpingitis.[17] Several epidemiologic studies, both case control and cohort, indicate that the use of the condom or diaphragm protects both men and women from clinically apparent gonorrheal infection.[18, 19] The incidence of cervical neoplasia is also markedly diminished among women in couples using condoms or diaphragms, probably because of the decreased transmission of human papillomavirus.[20] This antiviral action may be the reason women who use spermicides are only one third as likely to have cervical cancer as members of a control group. Certain strains of this virus have been causally linked to the later development of cervical neoplasia. The failure rates of users of the diaphragm or condom are highest for people younger than age 25, those most likely to become infected with a sexually transmitted disease. Therefore, to prevent the transmission of these diseases as well as unwanted pregnancy in this age group, the use of a barrier technique together with the most effective reversible method, the oral contraceptive, is advisable.

Periodic Abstinence

The avoidance of sexual intercourse during the days of the menstrual cycle when the ovum can be fertilized is used by many highly motivated couples as a means of preventing pregnancy. There are four techniques of periodic abstinence. The oldest of these is the calendar rhythm method. With this method the period of abstinence is determined solely by calculating the length of the individual woman's previous menstrual cycle. The rationale for the rhythm method is based on three assumptions: (1) the human ovum is capable of being fertilized for only about 24 hours after ovulation; (2) spermatozoa retain their fertilizing ability for only about 48 hours after coitus; and (3) ovulation usually occurs 12 to 16 days (14 ± 2 days) before the onset of the subsequent menses. According to these assumptions, after the woman records the length of her cycles for several months, she establishes her fertile period by subtracting 18 days from the length of her previous shortest cycle and 11 days from her previous longest cycle. Then, in each subse-

quent cycle, the couple abstains from coitus during this calculated fertile period.

This method requires abstinence by most women with regular menstrual cycles for nearly one half the days of each cycle and cannot be used by women with irregular menstrual cycles. Although calendar rhythm is the most widely used technique of periodic abstinence, pregnancy rates are high, ranging from 14.4 to 47 per 100 woman-years, mainly because most couples fail to abstain for the relatively long periods required. The use of the calendar rhythm method by itself is not advocated or taught to couples who are interested in practicing periodic abstinence.[21]

New techniques have been developed whereby women rely on physiological changes during each cycle to determine the fertile period. The term "natural family planning" has been used instead of "rhythm" to describe these new techniques. They include the temperature method, the cervical mucus method, and the symptothermal method. Each of these techniques requires a great amount of motivation as well as training. In most reports of use of these methods pregnancy rates are relatively high and continuation rates are low.

The temperature method relies on measuring basal body temperature daily. The woman is required to abstain from intercourse from the onset of the menses until the third consecutive day of elevated basal temperature. Because abstinence is required for the entire preovulatory period in ovulatory cycles and for the entire cycle in anovulatory cycles, the temperature method alone is no longer commonly used.[22]

The cervical mucus method requires that the woman be taught to recognize and interpret cyclic changes in the presence and consistency of cervical mucus; these changes occur in response to changing estrogen and progesterone levels. Abstinence is required during the menses and every other day after the menses ends—because of the possibility of confusing semen with ovulatory mucus—until the first day that copious, slippery mucus is observed to be present. Abstinence is required every day thereafter until four days after the last day when the characteristic mucus is present, called the "peak mucus day." In two well-designed randomized clinical trials the pregnancy rates for new users of this method in the first year after they completed a three-to-five-month training period were 20 and 24 per cent, with the discontinuation rates between 72 and 74 per cent.[23, 24] In a five-country study of 725 highly motivated couples, sponsored by the World Health Organization (WHO), the use failure rate during the first year after the completion of three cycles of training was 19.6 per cent, with a method failure rate of 3.5 per cent.[25] Most of the pregnancies (15.4 of the 19.6 per cent) resulted from conscious deviation from the rules of the method. The mean length of the fertile period in this study was 9.6 days, and abstinence was therefore required for about 17 days in each cycle.[26] In this study the continuation rate after one year was high, 64.4 per cent.

The symptothermal method, rather than relying on a single physiological index, uses several indices to determine the fertile period, most commonly calendar calculations and changes in the cervical mucus to estimate the onset of the fertile period and changes in mucus or basal temperature to estimate its end. Because several indices need to be monitored, this method is more difficult to learn than the single-index methods, but it is more effective than the cervical mucus method alone. In two large randomized studies comparing these methods, the pregnancy rates at the end of one year of use, after training phase, were 10.9 and 19.8 per cent with the symptothermal method compared with 20 and 24 per cent for the cervical mucus method.[23, 24] In addition, the continuation rate among the women who used the symptothermal method in these studies was higher after one year, about 50 per cent in each study, than that among the women who used the cervical mucus method (26 and 40 per cent).

The major reason for the lack of acceptance of natural family planning as well as the relatively high pregnancy rates among users of these methods is the need to avoid having sexual intercourse for a large number of days during each menstrual cycle. To overcome this problem, many women use barrier methods or spermicides during the fertile period.

Because the use of any method of contraception other than abstinence is unacceptable to many couples, simple, self-administered tests to detect hormonal changes have been developed to reduce the number of days of abstinence required in each cycle to a maximum of seven. Enzyme immunoassays for urinary estrogen and pregnanediol glucuronide have been developed that can easily be used at home at minimal cost and require minimal time to perform.[27] Such tests have to be performed by the woman about 12 days each month, but they should reduce the number of days of abstinence required. It remains to be determined to what extent this aid to natural family planning will be used when it becomes generally available.

ORAL STEROID CONTRACEPTIVES

Since the initial use in 1960, many OC formulations have been developed and marketed with steadily decreasing doses of both the estrogen and the progestin component. All the formulations initially marketed after 1975 contain less than 50 μg of ethinyl estradiol and 1 mg or less of several progestins. The use of these agents is associated with very low pregnancy rates, similar to those for formulations with higher doses of steroid, and a significantly lower incidence of adverse metabolic effects.

The use of formulations that contain less than 50 μg of estrogen has steadily increased in the United States since they were first marketed in 1973 to 87 per cent in 1988. Formulations with greater than 50 μg of estrogen are no longer marketed for contraceptive use in the United States, Canada, and Great Britain.

Pharmacology

There are three major types of oral steroid contraceptive formulations: fixed-dose combination, combination phasic, and daily progestin. The combination formulations are the most widely used and most effective. They consist of tablets that contain both an estrogen and a progestin given continuously for three weeks. The combination phasic formulations contain two or three different amounts of the same estrogen and progestin. Each of the tablets containing one of these various doses is given for intervals varying from 5 to 11 days during the 21-day medication period. These

formulations have been described as biphasic or triphasic and are referred to as multiphasic. The rationale for this type of formulation is that a lower total dose of steroid is administered without increasing the incidence of breakthrough bleeding. In the usual regimen for combination OC's no medication is given for one week out of four to allow withdrawal bleeding to occur. The third type of contraceptive formulation, consisting of tablets that contain a progestin without any estrogen, is designed to be taken daily without a steroid-free interval.

The OC's currently being used are formulated from synthetic steroids and contain no natural estrogens or progestins. There are two major types of synthetic progestins: (1) derivatives of 19-nortestosterone and (2) derivatives of 17 α-acetoxyprogesterone. The latter group are C21 progestins, consisting of such steroids as medroxyprogesterone acetate and megestrol acetate. In contrast to the 19-nortestosterone derivatives, when high doses of the C21 progestins were given to female beagle dogs, the animals developed an increased incidence of mammary cancer. Because of this carcinogenic effect, contraceptives that contain these progestins are no longer being made.

All OC formulations now available in the United States consist of varying doses of one of the following six 19-nortestosterone progestins: norethindrone, norethindrone acetate, ethynodiol diacetate, norgestrel, norgestimate and desogestrel (Fig. 123–1). The parent compound of d,l-norgestrel consists of two isomers, only one of which is biologically active. Currently formulations that contain only the active isomer of d,l-norgestrel, levonorgestrel, are being produced primarily. In Europe, formulations that contain three additional progestins, desogestrel, gestodene, and norgestimate, which have greater progestational activity but are less androgenic than the currently used progestins, have been marketed for several years (Fig. 123–2). Clinical testing with these formulations in the United States has been completed, and compounds containing norgestimate and desogestrel have been approved for use in the United States since 1992.

With the exception of two daily progestin-only formulations, the progestins are combined with varying doses of

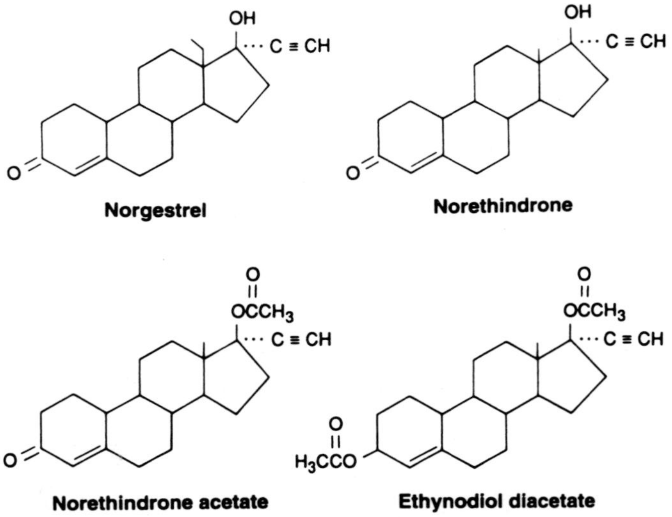

FIGURE 123–1. Structural formulas of the four progestins in oral contraceptives manufactured in the United States in 1990.

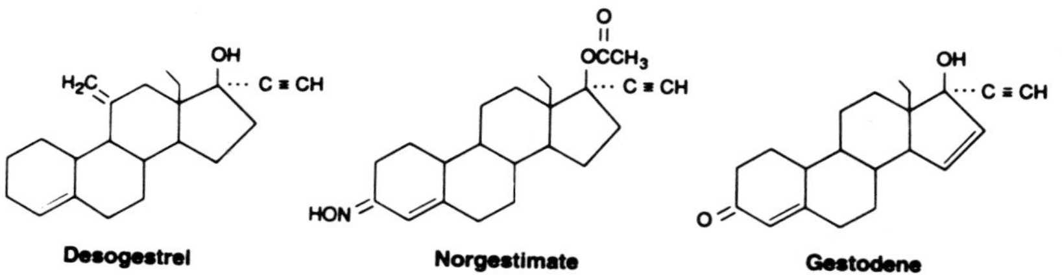

FIGURE 123–2. Structural formulas of three new progestins used in oral contraceptive formulations.

two estrogens, ethinyl estradiol and ethinyl estradiol 3-methyl ether, also known as mestranol (Fig. 123–3). All the older, higher-dose formulations contained mestranol, and this steroid is still present in some 50-μg formulations. All formulations with less than 50 μg of estrogen contain the parent compound ethinyl estradiol. All the synthetic estrogens and progestins in OC's have an ethinyl group at position 17. The presence of this ethinyl group enhances the oral activity of these agents because their essential functional groups are not as rapidly hydroxylated and then conjugated as they initially pass through the liver by way of the portal system, in contrast with what occurs when natural sex steroids are ingested orally. The synthetic steroids thus have greater oral potency per unit of weight than the natural steroids.

The various modifications in chemical structure of the different synthetic progestins and estrogens also affect their biological activity. Thus one cannot judge the pharmacological activity of the progestin or estrogen in a particular contraceptive steroid formulation only by the amount of steroid present. The biological activity of each steroid also has to be considered. Using established tests for progestational activity in animals as well as in humans, it has been found that norgestrel is several times more potent than the same weight of norethindrone.[28] Norethindrone acetate and ethynodiol diacetate are metabolized in the body to norethindrone. These three progestins have about equal potency per unit of weight, whereas levonorgestrel is 10 to 20 times as potent. The three new derivatives of levonorgestrel are as potent or more potent than the parent compound, with gestadene having the greater potency. When considering which contraceptive to prescribe, the physician needs to consider both the dose and the potency of each steroid. The currently marketed triphasic contraceptive formulations with levonorgestrel contain about 10 per cent as much progestin as triphasic formulations that contain norethindrone and have similar effects on lipid and carbohydrate metabolism. Several fixed-dose monophasic formulations currently marketed in the United States have a lower total dose of norethindrone per treatment cycle than the triphasic formulations that contain norethindrone.

The two estrogenic compounds used in OC's, ethinyl

estradiol and mestranol, also have different biological activity in women. Ethinyl estradiol is about 1.7 times as potent as the same weight of mestranol.[29] Thus it is important to evaluate the biological activity as well as the quantity of both steroid components when comparing potency of the various formulations.

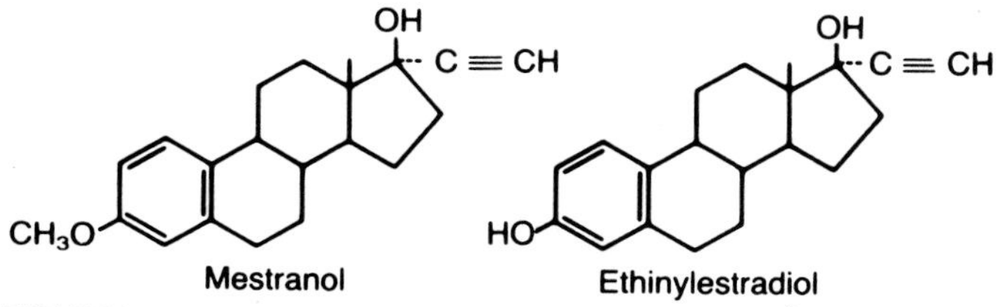

Using radioimmunoassay of levonorgestrel, it was found that substantial amounts of the chemical remained in the serum for at least the first three to four days after the last pill of the cycle was ingested.[30] These levels of steroid were sufficient to suppress gonadotropin release, and thus follicle maturation, as evidenced by rising estradiol levels, does not occur during the pill-free interval. From these data it seems reasonable to conclude that accidental pregnancies during OC therapy probably do not occur because of failure to ingest one or two pills more than a few days after treatment is initiated, but because initiation of the next cycle of medication is delayed for a few days. Therefore, it is important that the pill-free interval is limited to no more than seven days. This is best accomplished by administering either a placebo or an iron pill daily during the steroid-free interval (the so-called 28-day package). Alternatively, treatment may be started on the first Sunday after menses begins instead of the fifth day of the cycle. It is easier to remember to start the next cycle on a Sunday. Patients should be warned that the most important pill not to forget to ingest is the first pill.

Mechanism of Action

The estrogen–progestin combination is the most effective type of OC formulation because these preparations consistently inhibit the midcycle gonadotropin surge, and thus prevent ovulation. Such formulations also act on other aspects of the reproductive process. They alter the cervical mucus, making it thick, viscid, and scanty, which retards sperm penetration. They also alter motility of the uterus and oviduct, impairing transport of both ova and sperm. Furthermore, they alter the endometrium, so that its glandular production of glycogen is diminished and less energy is available for the blastocyst to survive in the uterine cavity. Finally, they may alter ovarian responsiveness to gonadotropin stimulation. Nevertheless, neither gonadotropin production nor ovarian steroidogenesis is completely abolished, and levels of endogenous estradiol in the peripheral blood during ingestion of combination OC's are similar to those found in the early follicular phase of the normal cycle.[31]

Contraceptive steroids prevent ovulation mainly by interfering with release of gonadotropin-releasing hormone (GnRH) from the hypothalamus. In rats and in a few studies in humans this inhibitory action of the contraceptive steroids could be overcome by the administration of GnRH.[32, 33] In most other human studies most women who

FIGURE 123–3. Structural formulas of the two estrogens used in combination oral contraceptives.

had been ingesting combination OC's had suppression of the release of luteinizing hormone (LH) and follicle-stimulating hormone (FSH) after infusion of GnRH, indicating that the steroids had a direct inhibitory effect on the pituitary as well as the hypothalamus.[34-36]

It is possible that when hypothalamic inhibition is prolonged, the mechanism for synthesis and release of gonadotropins may become refractory to the normal amount of GnRH stimulation. In a few OC users studied, after serial daily administration of GnRH, there was still a refractory response to a GnRH infusion. Thus the combination contraceptive steroids probably do have a direct inhibitory effect on the gonadotropin-producing cells of the pituitary, in addition to affecting the hypothalamus. This effect occurs in about 80 per cent of women who ingest combination OC steroids. It is unrelated to the age of the patient or the duration of steroid use, but it is related to the potency of the preparations. The effect is more pronounced with formulations that contain a more potent progestin and with those that contain 50 μg or more of estrogen than with 30- to 35-μg formulations. It has not been demonstrated that the amount of pituitary suppression is related to the occurrence of postpill amenorrhea, but if there is a relation, the lower-dose formulations should be associated with a lower frequency of this condition. The delay in the resumption of ovulation after discontinuation of OC use is shorter in women who ingest preparations that contain less than 50 μg of estrogen than in those who ingest formulations that contain 50 μg of estrogen or more.[37]

The daily progestin-only preparations do not consistently inhibit ovulation. They exert their contraceptive action by way of the other mechanisms listed above, but because of the inconsistent ovulation inhibition, their effectiveness is significantly less than that of the combined type. Because a lower dose of progestin is used, it is important that they be consistently taken at the same time of day to ensure that blood levels do not fall below the effective contraceptive level.

No significant difference in clinical effectiveness has been demonstrated among the various combination formulations currently available in the United States (Table 123–4). Provided no tablets are omitted, the pregnancy rate is less than 0.2 per cent at the end of one year with all combination formulations.

Metabolic Effects

Oral contraceptives have metabolic effects in addition to the effects on the reproductive axis. The estrogenic component and progestin component have different and sometimes opposite metabolic effects (Table 123–5). These metabolic effects can produce both the more common, less serious adverse effects as well as the rare, potentially serious complications. The magnitude of these effects is directly related to the dose and potency of the steroids in the formulations. In most instances the more common adverse effects are relatively mild. The most frequent symptoms produced by the estrogenic component include nausea (a CNS effect), breast tenderness, and fluid retention, which usually does not exceed three to four lb of body weight, due to decreased sodium excretion. Minor, clinically insig-

nificant changes in circulating vitamin levels also occur after ingestion of the higher-dose OC's. These changes are a decrease in levels of the B complex vitamins and ascorbic acid and an increase in levels of vitamin A. Even with the use of high doses of the steroid agents, dietary vitamin supplementation was not necessary because the changes in circulating vitamin levels were small and clinically insignificant. Estrogen can also cause chloasma, pigmentation of the malar eminences, to develop. Chloasma is accentuated by sunlight and usually takes a long time to disappear after OC's are discontinued. The incidence of all these estrogenic adverse effects is much lower now than occurred previously because the formulations in use today contain only one fifth as much estrogen as the formulations used in the 1960's. The estrogen component of OC agents also accelerates the development of symptoms of gallbladder disease in young women but does not increase the overall incidence of cholelithiasis. In a very large, retrospective cohort study the risk ratio for gallbladder disease in OC users was only 1.14, which barely achieved statistical significance.[38] Among women using formulations with less than 50 μg of estrogen, the risk ratio for gallbladder disease was 0.97.

It was previously postulated that high doses of synthetic estrogens could also produce changes in mood and depression brought about by diversion of tryptophan metabolism from its minor pathway in the brain to its major pathway in the liver.[39] The end product of tryptophan metabolism, serotonin, is thus decreased in the CNS, and it was postulated that the resultant lowering of serotonin could produce depression in some women and sleepiness and mood changes in others. Data from studies of postmenopausal women receiving estrogen therapy alone as well as estrogen-progestin sequential therapy indicate that estrogen alone improves the mood of women,[40] whereas the addition of a progestin increases depression, irritability, tension, and fatigue.[41] These studies indicate that the progestin component of the agents may be the major cause of the adverse mood changes and tiredness observed in some women after ingestion of OC's, but it has not been definitely established which of the steroid components is the major factor in producing adverse mood changes. Possibly both are involved.

The progestins, because they are structurally related to testosterone, also produce certain adverse androgenic effects. These include weight gain, acne, and a symptom perceived by some women as nervousness. Some women gain a considerable amount of weight when they take OC's, and this weight gain is produced by the anabolic effect of the progestin component. Although estrogens decrease sebum production, progestins increase sebum production and can cause acne to develop or worsen. Thus patients who have acne should be given a formulation with a low progestin-estrogen ratio. The final symptom produced by the progestin component is failure of withdrawal bleeding or amenorrhea. Because the progestins decrease the synthesis of estrogen receptors in the endometrium, endometrial growth is decreased, and some women have failure of withdrawal bleeding. Although this symptom is not important medically, since bleeding serves as a signal that the woman is not pregnant, it is desirable to have some amount of periodic withdrawal bleeding during the days she is not taking these steroids. Both steroid components can act together to produce irregular bleeding. Breakthrough bleed-

TABLE 123–4. ESTROGEN AND PROGESTIN COMPONENTS OF ORAL CONTRACEPTIVES

MANUFACTURER/ PRODUCT		TYPE*	PROGESTIN	ESTROGEN
Berlex Laboratories, Inc.				
Levlen		Comb.	0.15 mg levonorgestrel	30 μg ethinyl estradiol
Tri-Levlen 6/		Comb.-triphasic	0.05 mg levonorgestrel	30 μg ethinyl estradiol
5/			0.075 mg levonorgestrel	40 μg ethinyl estradiol
10/			0.125 mg levonorgestrel	30 μg ethinyl estradiol
GynoPharma, Inc.				
Norcept-E 1/35		Comb.	1 mg norethindrone	35 μg ethinyl estradiol
Mead Johnson Laboratories				
Ovcon-35		Comb.	0.4 mg norethindrone	35 μg ethinyl estradiol
Ovcon-50		Comb.	1.0 mg norethindrone	50 μg ethinyl estradiol
Ortho Pharmaceutical Corp.				
Micronor		Prog.	0.35 mg norethindrone	
Modicon		Comb.	0.5 mg norethindrone	35 μg ethinyl estradiol
Ortho-Novum 1/35		Comb.	1.0 mg norethindrone	35 μg ethinyl estradiol
Ortho-Novum 1/50		Comb.	1.0 mg norethindrone	50 μg mestranol
Ortho-Novum 7/7/7	7/	Comb.-triphasic	0.5 mg norethindrone	35 μg ethinyl estradiol
	7/		0.75 mg norethindrone	35 μg ethinyl estradiol
	7/		1.0 mg norethindrone	35 μg ethinyl estradiol
Ortho-Novum 10/11	10/	Comb.-biphasic	0.5 mg norethindrone	35 μg ethinyl estradiol
	11/		1.0 mg norethindrone	35 μg ethinyl estradiol
Parke-Davis				
Loestrin 1/20		Comb.	1.0 mg norethindrone acetate	20 μg ethinyl estradiol
Loestrin 1.5/30		Comb.	1.5 mg norethindrone acetate	30 μg ethinyl estradiol
Norlestrin 1/50		Comb.	1.0 mg norethindrone acetate	50 μg ethinyl estradiol
Norlestrin 2.5/50		Comb.	2.5 mg norethindrone acetate	50 μg ethinyl estradiol
Rugby Laboratories, Inc.				
Genora 1/35		Comb.	1 mg norethindrone	35 μg ethinyl estradiol
Genora 1/50		Comb.	1 mg norethindrone	50 μg ethinyl estradiol
Genora 0.5/35		Comb.	5 mg norethindrone	35 μg ethinyl estradiol
Schiapparelli Searle				
Norethin 1/35E		Comb.	1 mg norethindrone	35 μg ethinyl estradiol
Norethin 1/50M		Comb.	1 mg norethindrone	50 μg ethinyl estradiol
Searle Laboratories				
Dermulen 1/35		Comb.	1.0 mg ethynodiol diacetate	35 μg ethinyl estradiol
Demulen 1/50		Comb.	1.0 mg ethynodiol diacetate	50 μg ethinyl estradiol
Syntex Laboratories, Inc.				
Brevicon		Comb.	0.5 mg norethindrone	35 μg ethinyl estradiol
Norinyl 1 + 35		Comb.	1.0 mg norethindrone	35 μg ethinyl estradiol
Norinyl 1 + 50		Comb.	1.0 mg norethindrone	50 μg mestranol
Nor-Q D		Prog.	0.35 mg norethindrone	
Tri-Norinyl 7/		Comb.-triphasic	0.5 mg norethindrone	35 μg ethinyl estradiol
9/			1 mg norethindrone	35 μg ethinyl estradiol
5/			0.5 mg norethindrone	35 μg ethinyl estradiol
Wyeth-Ayerst Laboratories				
Lo/Ovral		Comb.	0.3 mg norgestrel	30 μg ethinyl estradiol
Nordette		Comb.	0.15 mg levonorgestrel	30 μg ethinyl estradiol
Ovral		Comb.	0.5 mg norgestrel	50 μg ethinyl estradiol
Ovrette		Prog.	75 μg norgestrel	
Triphasil 6/		Comb.-triphasic	50 μg levonorgestrel	40 μg ethinyl estradiol
5/			75 μg levonorgestrel	40 μg ethinyl estradiol
10/			125 μg levonorgestrel	30 μg ethinyl estradiol

*Comb., combination; Prog., progestin only.

ing (which usually is produced by insufficient estrogen, too much progestin, or a combination of both) as well as failure of withdrawal bleeding can be alleviated by increasing the amount of estrogen in the formulation or by switching to a more estrogenic formulation. Many women who take OC's complain of an increased frequency of headaches. It has not been determined what is the exact relation, if any, between OC use and the occurrence of headaches.

Proteins

The synthetic estrogens used in OC's cause an increase in the hepatic production of several globulins, some of which are involved in the coagulation process[42]; another,

angiotensinogen, may be converted to angiotensin and increases blood pressure in some users. The circulating levels of each of these globulins are directly correlated with the amount of estrogen in the OC formulation[42] (Table 123–6). Epidemiologic studies have shown that the incidence of both venous and arterial thrombosis is also directly related to the dose of estrogen (Table 123–7)[5, 16, 43, 44] and that users of low-estrogen-dose OC's do not have an increased risk of venous thromboembolism.

Angiotensinogen levels are lower in women who ingest formulations with 30 to 35 μg of ethinyl estradiol than in those who ingest formulations with 50 μg. However, a significant increase in blood pressure in women who receive the lower dose has been reported.[45] Thus blood pressure

TABLE 123–5. METABOLIC EFFECTS OF CONTRACEPTIVE STEROIDS

	EFFECTS	
	Chemical	Clinical
Estrogen—ethinyl estradiol		
Proteins		
Albumin	↓	None
Amino acids	↓	None
Globulins	↑	
Angiotensinogen		↑ Blood pressure
Factors VII and X		Hypercoagulability
Carrier proteins (CBG, TBG, transferrin, ceruloplasmin)		
Carbohydrate		
Plasma insulin	None	None
Glucose tolerance	None	None
Lipid		
Cholesterol	None	None
Triglyceride	↑	None
HDL cholesterol	↑	None
LDL cholesterol	↓	None
Electrolytes		
Sodium excretion	↓	Fluid retention
		Edema
Vitamins		
B complex	↓	None
Ascorbic acid	↓	None
Vitamin A	↑	None
Target tissues		
Breast	↑	Breast tenderness
Endometrial receptors	↑	Hyperplasia
Skin	↓	Sebum production
	↑	Facial pigmentation
Progestins—19-nortestosterone derivatives		
Proteins	None	None
Carbohydrate		
Plasma insulin	↑	None
Glucose tolerance	↓	None
Lipids†		
Cholesterol	↓	None
Triglyceride	↓	None
HDL cholesterol	↓ }	? ↑ Cardiovascular disease
LDL cholesterol	↑ }	
Nitrogen retention	↑	↑ Body weight
Skin—sebum production	↑	↑ Acne
Central nervous system effects	↑	Nervousness, fatigue, depression
Endometrial receptors	↓	Amenorrhea

CBG, corticosteroid-binding globulin; TBG, thyroxine-binding globulin; HDL, high-density lipoprotein; LDL, low-density lipoprotein.

should be monitored in all users of OC's. There is some indirect evidence that the progestin component may also affect blood pressure; however, women who receive progestins without estrogen do not have an increase in blood pressure over time, indicating that the estrogen component is the major factor in causing elevated blood pressure in certain users of OC's.

TABLE 123–6. MEAN FACTOR VII AND FIBRINOGEN LEVELS* IN RELATION TO ORAL CONTRACEPTIVE USE AND ESTROGEN DOSE

	NOT TAKING OCs	OC ESTROGEN DOSE	
		30 μg	50 μg
No. of patients	243	15	65
Factor VII (%)	83.0	96.6	121.1
Fibrinogen (g/L)	2.52	2.84	2.89

From Meade TW: Oral contraceptives, clotting factors, and thrombosis. Am J Obstet Gynecol 142:758, 1982.
*Age-adjusted values.

Carbohydrates

When formulations with a high dose of progestin are administered, 4 to 16 per cent of women (depending on their age) have an abnormal response on the glucose tolerance test.[46, 47] The incidence of abnormal test results is related to the dose and potency of the progestin, since estrogen does not affect carbohydrate metabolism.[48] Some studies have shown that formulations with a low dose of progestin (even one that contains levonorgestrel) do not significantly alter levels of glucose, insulin, or glucagon after a glucose load in healthy women[49] or in those with a history of gestational diabetes.[50] Other studies indicate that the multiphasic formulations with norgestrel, but not those with norethindrone,[51] produce some deterioration of glucose tolerance in normal women as well as in those with a history of gestational diabetes.[52]

When prescribing OC's for women with a history of glucose intolerance or those with diabetes mellitus, one should choose formulations with a low dose of a norethin-

TABLE 123–7. RATIO OF OBSERVED TO EXPECTED EMBOLISM AND THROMBOSIS IN RELATION TO TYPE AND DOSE OF ESTROGEN IN COMBINED ORAL CONTRACEPTIVES

| | ESTROGEN | | | | | |
| | Mestranol Dose (μg) | | | | Ethinyl Estradiol Dose (μg) | |
	150	100	75–80	50	100	50
Fatal pulmonary embolism*	2.8	1.5	0.9	0.6	1.0	0.5
Nonfatal pulmonary embolism†	2.3	1.2	0.9	1.0	1.8	0.7
Cerebral thrombosis‡	3.2	1.2	0.7	0.5	—	0.8
Coronary thrombosis*	2.6	1.2	0.3	1.1	1.8	0.9

Modified from Mann JI: Progestogens in cardiovascular disease: An introduction to the epidemiologic data. Am J Obstet Gynecol 142:752, 1982.
*Linear trend test: $P < .05$.
†Linear trend test: $P < .01$.
‡Linear trend test: $P < .001$.

drone-type progestin and monitor glucose tolerance periodically. Data from 20 years' experience of use of mainly high-dose formulations in the large Royal College of General Practitioners (RCGP) study reveal no increased risk of developing diabetes mellitus among current OC users (RR 0.80) or former OC users (RR 0.82) even among those women who had used OC's for 10 years or longer.[53] A recent study indicated that use of a low-progestin-dose OC did not cause deterioration of glucose tolerance among a group of women with gestational diabetes.[54]

Lipids

Adverse alterations in high-density lipoprotein (HDL) cholesterol and low-density lipoprotein (LDL) cholesterol are produced by all the progestins used in OC's available in the United States, and the degree of change is related to the amount and potency of the progestin. Estrogen has an opposite, beneficial effect on these lipid factors. Because of the balance of estrogen and progestin in the formulations, most currently marketed OC's, including the phasic formulations, do not significantly alter these lipid fractions. Triglycerides are elevated by all OC formulations that contain estrogen.

Cardiovascular Diseases

Although one must be concerned about the adverse changes in lipid levels produced by the progestin component of certain high-progestin-dose OC formulation, the cause of the increased incidence of both venous and arterial cardiovascular disease, including myocardial infarction (MI), in users of OC's appears to be thrombosis and not atherosclerosis.

Neither epidemiological studies of humans nor experimental studies with subhuman primates have observed an acceleration of atherosclerosis with the ingestion of OC's. There is no increased risk of MI among former users of OC's, according to several epidemiological studies.[55–57] The incidence of cardiovascular disease is also not correlated with the duration of OC use. A study with cynomolgus macaque monkeys found that the ingestion of an OC that contained high doses of norgestrel and ethinyl estradiol lowered HDL cholesterol levels significantly. After two years of ingesting this formulation and being fed an atherogenic diet, the animals had a significantly smaller area of coronary artery atherosclerosis than a control group of female monkeys fed the same diet.[57] Another group of monkeys that received levonorgestrel without estrogen also had lowered HDL cholesterol levels. In this group the extent of coronary atherosclerosis was significantly increased compared with that of the controls. The results of this study have since been confirmed in a larger study with two high-dose estrogen-progestin formulations.[58] In this study the mean coronary artery plaque extent of the high-risk control group of female animals was more than 3 times greater than that found in animals ingesting a high-dose norgestrel compound and more than 10 times greater than those ingesting a high-dose norethindrone compound. Both of these compounds lowered HDL cholesterol levels by one half and tripled the cholesterol-HDL ratio. These studies suggest that the estrogen component of OC's may have a protective effect on coronary atherosclerosis that would otherwise be accelerated by decreased levels of HDL cholesterol.

The epidemiological studies that reported an increased incidence of MI in older users of OC's were published in the late 1970s and thus used as a data base women who only ingested formulations with 50 μg or more of estrogen. In these case-control and cohort studies a significantly increased incidence of MI was found mainly among older users who had risk factors that caused arterial narrowing, such as smoking, pre-existing hypercholesterolemia, hypertension, and diabetes mellitus.

Data accumulated during the first 10 years of the RCGP study, 1968 through 1978, in which most users ingested formulations with more than 50 μg of estrogen and high doses of progestin, showed that a significantly increased relative risk of death from circulatory disease occurred only among women over age 35 who also smoked.[59] A more recent analysis of data obtained during the first 20 years of this study, 1968 through 1988, revealed that there was no significant increased relative risk of acute MI among current or former users of OC's who did not smoke any cigarettes[60] (Table 123–8). Even though most of the women in this study used high-dose formulations, a significantly increased risk of MI occurred only among both mild (less than 15 cigarettes per day) and heavy cigarette smokers, with the latter group having a greater relative risk than the former. In this and other studies cigarette smoking was an independent risk factor for MI, but the use of OC's by cigarette smokers greatly enhanced their risk of developing an MI, the two factors acting synergistically.

The mechanism whereby cigarette smoking increases the

TABLE 123–8. RELATIVE RISK OF MYOCARDIAL INFARCTION IN RELATION TO SMOKING AND ORAL CONTRACEPTIVE USE (RCGP STUDY, 1968–1987) (n = 158)

	ORAL CONTRACEPTIVE USE		
SMOKING	Never (CL)	Previously (CL)	Current (CL)
Never	1.0	1.1 (0.6–2.2)	0.9 (0.3–2.7)
<15/day	2.0 (1.0–3.9)	1.3 (0.6–2.8)	3.5 (1.3–9.5)
≥15/day	3.3 (1.6–6.7)	4.3 (2.3–8.0)	20.8 (5.2–83.1)

Modified from Croft P, Hannaford PC: Risk factors for acute myocardial infarction in women: Evidence from the Royal College of General Practitioners' oral contraceptive study. Br Med J 298:165, 1989.
CL, confidence limits.

risk of arterial thrombosis in OC users appears to be due to the effect of nicotine on the coagulation process. Although OC's increase the concentration of factors involved in producing blood coagulation, they also affect the activity of factors that inhibit coagulation. Smokers who ingested low-dose OC's had a significantly greater decrease in levels of endogenous coagulation inhibitors, mainly antithrombin III, than did OC users who did not smoke. Platelet aggregation was increased only among OC users who also smoked and not among women who smoked and did not use OC's.[61] This thrombotic effect was probably related to prostacyclin inhibition because prostacyclin formation was reduced only among the women in the study who smoked and used OC's. The usual balance of prostacyclin and thromboxane is thus altered when OC users smoke, producing a relative excess of thromboxane. The results of this study, therefore, suggest that the synergistic effects of OC's and smoking on arterial thrombosis, are produced by activation of the thromboxane A_2–mediated mechanism of platelet aggregation brought about by reduction of prostacyclin.

Although epidemiological data from studies performed in the 1970's indicated that there was possibly a causal relation between ingestion of high-dose OC formulations and stroke, the data were conflicting. Furthermore, as occurred with MI, the studies that did show a significantly increased risk of stroke in OC users indicated that the increased risk was mainly limited to older women who also smoked and/or were hypertensive.

Data from the epidemiological studies of OC use and cardiovascular disease performed in the 1960's and 1970's are not relevant to their current use because the dose of both steroid components in the formulations now being marketed is markedly less, and women with cardiovascular risk factors such as hypertension are no longer receiving these agents. Furthermore, since 1982 OC's are not prescribed to women over 35 who also smoke. All the epidemiological studies performed during the past 10 years have shown no significantly increased risk of arterial vascular events, such as MI and stroke, in OC users.[62–64]

The results of these studies indicate that the use of low-dose OC formulations by nonsmoking women without risk factors for cardiovascular disease is not associated with an increased incidence of MI or stroke. There is also no evidence showing that the risk of venous thrombosis is increased in this group of OC users.

Reproductive Effects

The magnitude and duration of the delay in the return of fertility are greater for women discontinuing use of OC's with 50 μg of estrogen or more than for women discontinuing OC's that contain lower doses of estrogen. Use of the low-dose formulations still results in a reduction in conception rates for at least the first six cycles after discontinuation but does not cause permanent infertility.[65]

Neither the rate of spontaneous abortion nor the incidence of chromosomal abnormalities in abortuses is increased in women who conceive in the first or subsequent months after ceasing to use OC's.

Several cohort and case control studies of large numbers of babies born to women who stopped using OC's have been undertaken.[66–68] These studies indicate that these infants have no greater chance of being born with any type of birth defect than infants born to women in the general population, even if conception occurred in the first month after the medication was discontinued. If these steroids are ingested during the first few months of pregnancy, a recent review of all the prospective epidemiologic studies with a control group of women not using OC's reported that there was no increased risk of congenital malformations overall or of any particular defect among the offspring of OC users.[69] A statement warning of a possible teratogenic effect of ingestion of OC's during pregnancy has been deleted from current product labeling for OC's.

Neoplastic Effects

Oral contraceptives have been extensively used for more than 30 years, and numerous epidemiologic studies of both cohort and case control design have been performed to determine the relation between use of these agents and the development of all types of neoplasm. Because no elderly women used OC's during their early reproductive years, the studies thus far published usually restrict the analysis to women under age 60.

Breast Cancer

No study has reported a significant increase or decrease in the risk of developing breast cancer among the entire population of OC users. A meta-analysis of the combined risk estimate of the 16 case control studies and four cohort studies in 1987 was 1.0.[70] In a review of 17 studies in which the risk of developing breast cancer in women under age 60 was compared with the duration of OC use, no overall dose-response was found to exist and long-term use did not increase the risk of developing breast cancer.[71]

The issue of latency, time since first use of OC's, and risk of breast cancer has also been studied. In groups of women who used OC's for more than 10 years no changes in risk of breast cancer were found with increasing duration of time since first use. Thus there is no evidence to support a long-term latent effect. The preponderance of data in studies estimating the risk of breast cancer in women under age 60 by duration of OC use before their first term pregnancy also failed to show an increased risk or a dose response. Analysis of the studies that estimated the relative risk of developing breast cancer in women under age 45 suggested that there was a trend of increasing risk with increasing duration of overall use as well as increasing duration of use before first term pregnancy, with the increased risk in both groups becoming most evident after eight years of use.[72, 73]

Three large studies suggested that prolonged use of OC's might increase the risk of developing breast cancer but only when initially diagnosed at an early age.[72, 74, 75]

The Cancer and Steroidal Hormone (CASH) study investigators found no overall change in the risk of developing premenopausal breast cancer under age 55 with increasing duration of OC use. They also found that the risk of developing breast cancer in women aged 45 to 55 was decreased in OC users.[76]

These data are consistent with the belief that long-term use of high-dose OC's could have promoted the age at which breast cancer was diagnosed clinically among susceptible nulliparous women. This promotional effect was transient, not persistent, and thus had no appreciable effect on the aggregate lifetime risk of developing breast cancer in the population, despite the widespread use of OC's.

Because low-dose estrogen formulations have only been used by the majority of women ingesting OC's since 1983, the effect of these agents, if any, on early development of breast cancer cannot be determined until several years from now. The latest review of this data by the Food and Drug Administration (FDA) resulted in a statement that no change in OC use or prescribing practice was warranted. Finally, there have been several studies of OC use and breast cancer risk in women at increased risk of developing the disease, those with a family history of breast cancer, and those with existing benign breast disease.[77] The results of these studies indicate that OC use by each of these high-risk groups is not associated with any increased risk of developing breast cancer.

Cervical Cancer

The epidemiological data obtained thus far indicate that long-term use of OC's is associated with an increased risk of preinvasive cervical neoplasia as well as both epidermoid and adenocarcinoma of the cervix, when compared with matched control groups.[70, 71] Confounding factors such as the woman's age at first sexual intercourse, the number of sexual partners, exposure to human papillomavirus (possibly greater among users of OC's), cytological screening (more frequent among OC users), and the use of barrier contraceptives or spermicides (primarily by women in the control group) as well as cigarette smoking (an independent risk factor for this disease) could have influenced these results. In most of these studies statistical corrections were made for these confounding factors, and in many of them the control group did not use barrier methods of contraception.

Data results suggest an approximate doubling of risk of development of carcinoma in situ with the use of OC's for more than one year. The data for invasive cervical cancer suggest no increased risk with less than 5 years of OC use but a gradually increasing risk after 5 years' use that results in a two-fold increase with 10 years of use. Thus, although it is uncertain whether OC's themselves increase the risk of cervical cancer, act as a co-carcinogen, or have no effect, users of OC's as a group are at high risk for cervical neo-

plasia and require at least annual screening of cervical cytology, especially if they have used OC's for more than five years.

Endometrial Cancer

Numerous studies have been published on the relation between OC's and endometrial cancer, and nearly all have indicated that the use of these agents has a protective effect against endometrial cancer, the third most common cancer among United States women.[70, 71, 78] Women who use OC's for at least one year have an age-adjusted relative risk of 0.5 of developing endometrial cancer between ages 40 and 55 compared with nonusers. This protective effect is related to duration of use, increasing from a 20 per cent reduction in risk with one year of use to a 40 per cent reduction with two years of use to 60 per cent reduction with four years of use. This protective effect appears within 10 years of initial use and persists for at least 15 years after stopping use of OC's. The greatest protective effect is in nulliparous women (relative risk 0.2) or women of low parity, who have the greatest risk of acquiring this disease.

Ovarian Cancer

Also numerous studies have related the use of OC's with subsequent development of ovarian cancer, and each of these shows a reduction in risk, specifically of the most common type, epithelial ovarian cancers.[70, 71, 79, 80] OC's reduce the risk of the four main histological types of epithelial ovarian cancer: serous, mucinous, endometrioid, and clear cell. The relative risk of ovarian cancer is 0.6 for women who use OC's for three or more years, and as little as six months of use provides protection. The magnitude of the decrease in risk is directly related to the duration of use, increasing from a 50 per cent reduction with four years' use to a 60 to 80 per cent reduction with seven or more years' use. The protective effect begins within 10 years of first use and continues for at least 15 years after the use of OC's ends. As with endometrial cancer, the protective effect occurs only in women of low parity (less than or equal to four), who are at greatest risk for this type of cancer.

Liver Adenoma and Cancer

The development of a benign hepatocellular adenoma is a rare occurrence in long-term users of OC's, and the increased risk of this tumor was associated with prolonged use of high-dose formulations, particularly those that contain mestranol. The rate of death from this disease has remained unchanged in the United States over the past 25 years, a period when millions of women have used these agents. Data from a large multicenter epidemiologic study coordinated by the WHO found no increased risk of liver cancer associated with OC users in countries with a high prevalence rate of this neoplasm.[81] This study found no change in risk with increasing duration of use or time since first or last use.

Pituitary Adenoma

OC's mask the predominant symptoms produced by prolactinoma, amenorrhea, and galactorrhea. When OC use is discontinued these symptoms occur, suggesting a causal relation. Data from several studies, however, indicate that the incidence of pituitary adenoma among users of OC's is not higher than that among matched controls.[82]

Malignant Melanoma

Several epidemiological studies have been undertaken to assess the relation of OC use and the development of malignant melanoma. The results are conflicting, since an increased risk, a decreased risk, and no effect have all been reported. In the review by Prentice and Thomas the summary relative risk for eight case control studies was 1.0 and for three cohort studies 1.4, an insignificant increase.[70] Thus there is no convincing evidence that OC use increases the risk of developing malignant melanoma.

OC Use and Overall Mortality

In 1989 Vessey et al.[83] reported the cause of mortality through 1987 among OC users and nonusers in a British study. The overall risk of death among OC users was 0.9 (C.L. 0.7 to 1.2) compared with women of similar age and socioeconomic status using a diaphragm or condom for contraception. The risk of death from breast cancer in OC users was 0.9 (0.5 to 1.4), from cervical cancer 3.3 (0.9 to 17.9), and from ovarian cancer 0.4 (0.1 to 1.2). These cancer mortality rates are consistent with the other epidemiologic data reported above. The death rate for circulatory disease was 1.5 (0.7 to 3.0), and nearly all these deaths in OC users occurred in women who were also smokers. Thus the risk of death from circulatory disease was less than that reported for the first 10 years of the RCGP study when higher-dose formulations were used and women with cardiovascular risk factors were using OC's. It thus appears that OC use has no appreciable effect on overall mortality. With exclusive use of low-dose formulations given to women without cardiovascular risk factors who have frequent cervical cytological screening, an overall beneficial effect on mortality with OC use may be expected.

Contraindications to OC Use

Oral contraceptives can be prescribed for most women of reproductive age because these women are young and generally healthy; however, there are certain absolute contraindications. These include a history of vascular disease, including thromboembolism, thrombophlebitis, atherosclerosis, and stroke, or systemic disease that may affect the vascular system, such as lupus erythematosus or hemoglobin SS disease. Cigarette smoking by users over 35, hypertension, diabetes mellitus with vascular disease, and hyperlipidemia are also contraindications because high-dose OC use in women with these disorders was reported to increase the risk of stroke or MI. One of the contraindications listed by the FDA is cancer of the breast or endometrium, although there are no data indicating that OC's are harmful to women with these diseases.

Patients with functional heart disease should not use OC's because the fluid retention they produce could result in congestive heart failure. There is no evidence, however,

that women with an asymptomatic prolapsed mitral valve should not use OC's. Patients with active liver disease should not take OC's because the steroids are metabolized in the liver. However, women who have recovered from liver disease such as viral hepatitis and whose liver function tests have returned to normal can safely take OC's.

Relative contraindications to OC use include heavy cigarette smoking under age 35, migraine headaches, depression, and amenorrhea of unknown cause. Migraine headaches can be worsened by OC use, and patients who develop strokes have been reported to have an increased incidence of headaches of the migraine type, fainting, temporary loss of vision or speech, or paresthesias before the stroke. If any of these symptoms develop in an OC user, OC's should be stopped.

Patients who are amenorrheic for a cause other than polycystic ovary syndrome should probably not take OC's because a pituitary microadenoma may be present. Because OC use may mask the symptoms produced by a prolactin-secreting adenoma, amenorrhea, and galactorrhea, amenorrheic patients should not receive OC's until the diagnosis for this symptom is established. If galactorrhea develops during OC use, they should be discontinued and after two weeks a serum prolactin level should be measured. If elevated, further diagnostic evaluation is indicated. Patients with gestational diabetes can take low-dose OC formulations because these agents do not affect glucose tolerance or accelerate the development of diabetes mellitus. Women with insulin-dependent diabetes without vascular disease can take OC's because the low-dose OC's do not affect glucose tolerance.

Starting OC's

Adolescents

In deciding whether a sexually active pubertal girl should use OC's for contraception, the clinician should be more concerned about compliance with the regimen than about possible physiological harm. Provided she has demonstrated maturity of the hypothalamic-pituitary-ovarian axis with at least three regular, presumably ovulatory menstrual cycles, it is safe to prescribe OC's without concern that permanent damage to the reproductive process will result. It is probably best not to prescribe OC's for women of any age with oligomenorrhea, except those with polycystic ovary syndrome, because of their increased likelihood of developing postpill amenorrhea. Oligomenorrhea is more frequent in adolescence than later in life. Postpill amenorrhea that lasts more than six months is not produced by OC's but becomes manifest after discontinuing OC's because OC's mask the development of the symptoms of amenorrhea. It is not necessary to be concerned about accelerating epiphyseal closure in the postmenarcheal female. Endogenous estrogens have already initiated the process a few years before menarche, and the contraceptive steroids will not hasten it.

After Pregnancy

There is a difference in the relation of the return of ovulation and bleeding in the postabortal woman and one who has had a term delivery. The first episode of menstrual bleeding in the postabortal woman usually is preceded by ovulation. After a term delivery the first episode of bleeding usually is anovulatory. Ovulation occurs sooner after an abortion, usually between two and four weeks, than after a term delivery, when ovulation usually is delayed beyond six weeks but may occur as early as four weeks in a woman who is not breastfeeding.[84]

Thus after spontaneous or induced abortion of a fetus of less than 12 weeks' gestation, OC's should be started immediately to prevent conception after the first ovulation. For patients who deliver after 28 weeks and are not nursing, the combination pills should be initiated 2 to 3 weeks after delivery. If the termination of pregnancy occurs between 21 and 28 weeks, contraceptive steroids should be started 1 week later. The reason for delay in the latter instances is that the normally increased risk of thromoembolism that occurs postpartum may be further enhanced by the hypercoagulable state associated with contraceptive steroid ingestion. Because the first ovulation is delayed for at least four weeks after a term delivery, there is no need to expose the patient to this increased risk.

Because estrogen inhibits the action of prolactin in breast tissue receptors, the use of combination OC's (those that contain both estrogen and progestin) diminishes the amount of milk produced by OC users who breastfeed their babies.[85] Although the diminution of milk production is directly related to the amount of estrogen in the contraceptive formulation, only one study has been published in which the amount of breast milk was measured by breast pump in women using formulations with less than 50 μg of estrogen. In this study the use of this low dose of estrogen reduced the amount of breast milk.[86] Thus it is probably best for women who are nursing and not using supplementary feeding to not use combination OC's.

Women who are breastfeeding every four hours, including at night, do not ovulate until at least 10 weeks after delivery and thus do not need contraception before that time. Because only a small percentage of full breastfeeding women ovulate as long as they continue full nursing and remain amenorrheic, either a barrier method or progestin-only OC can be used. The latter does not diminish the amount of breast milk and is effective in this group of women. Once supplemental feeding is introduced, ovulation can resume promptly and effective contraception is then needed, so combination OC's can be started.

All Patients

At the initial visit, after a history and physical examination have determined that there are no medical contraindications for OC's, the patient should be informed about the benefits and risks. For medicolegal reasons it is best to note on the patient's medical record that the benefits and risks have been explained to her.

Type of Formulation

In determining which formulation to use, it is best to initially prescribe a formulation with 20 to 35 μg of ethinyl estradiol because these agents are associated with less cardiovascular risk as well as less estrogenic adverse effects. It would also appear reasonable to use formulations with the lowest dose of a particular progestin because there would

be less progestogenic metabolic and clinical adverse effects associated with their use. The development of multiphasic formulations has allowed the total dose of progestin to be reduced compared with some monophasic formulations without increasing the incidence of breakthrough bleeding. However, several monophasic formulations have a lower total dose of progestin per cycle than the multiphasic formulations.

The FDA has stated that the product prescribed should be one that contains the least amount of estrogen and progestin that is compatible with a low failure rate and the needs of the individual patient. Because few randomized studies have been performed comparing the different marketed formulations, until large-scale comparative studies are performed, clinicians must decide which formulation to use based on which formulations have the least adverse effects among patients in their practice. If estrogenic or progestogenic adverse effects occur with one formulation, a different agent with less estrogenic or progestogenic activity can be given.

The contraceptive formulations that contain progestins without estrogen have a lower incidence of adverse metabolic effects than the combination formulations. Because the factors that predispose to thromboembolism are caused by the estrogen component, the incidence of thromboembolism in women who ingest these compounds is probably not increased. Furthermore, blood pressure is not affected, nausea and breast tenderness are eliminated, and milk production and quality are unchanged. Despite these advantages, these agents have the disadvantages of a high frequency of intermenstrual and other abnormal bleeding patterns, including amenorrhea, and a lower rate of effectiveness. The use failure rate of these preparations is higher than with the combined formulations, and a relatively high percentage of the pregnancies that do occur are ectopic.[87] Because nursing mothers have reduced fertility and are amenorrheic, the major disadvantages of these preparations are minimized for these patients. Furthermore, because milk production and quality are unaffected in contrast to the changes produced by combination pills, the formulations with only a progestin may be offered to these women while they are nursing. However, a small portion of these synthetic steroids has been detected in breast milk. The long-term effects, if any, of these progestins on the infant are not known, but none have been detected to date. A long-term follow-up study of breastfed children whose mothers ingested 50 μg estrogen in combined OC's while they were lactating revealed no difference in weight gain or height increase up to age 8 compared with breastfed children whose mothers did not ingest OC's.[88] There was also no difference on occurrence of disease or intellectual or psychological behavior between the two groups.

Follow-up

If the patient has no contraindications to OC use and is healthy, no routine laboratory tests are indicated except cervical cytology. At the end of three months the patient should be seen again; at this time a nondirected history should be obtained and the blood pressure measured. After this visit the patient should be seen annually, at which time a nondirected history should again be taken, blood pressure and body weight measured, and a physical examination (including breast, abdominal, and pelvic examination with cervical cytology) performed. It is important to perform annual cervical cytological examinations on OC users because they are a relatively high-risk group for development of cervical neoplasia. The routine use of other laboratory tests is not indicated unless the patient has a family history of diabetes or vascular disease. The routine use of these tests in women is not indicated because the incidence of positive results is extremely low. If the patient has a family history of vascular disease, such as MI, occurring in family members under age 50, it would be advisable to obtain a lipid panel before OC use is started because hypertriglyceridemia may be present and OC use will further raise triglycerides. Because the low-dose formulations do not alter the lipid profile except for triglycerides, it is not necessary to measure lipids, other than the routine, every five years cholesterol screening, in women without cardiovascular risk factors even if they are over age 35. If the patient has a family history of diabetes or evidence of diabetes during pregnancy, a two-hour postprandial blood glucose test should be performed before OC's are started, and if elevated, a glucose tolerance test should be performed. If the patient has a past history of liver disease, a liver panel should be obtained to make certain that liver function is normal before OC's are started.

Drug Interactions

Although synthetic sex steroids can retard the biotransformation of certain drugs (e.g., phenazone and meperidine) as a result of substrate competition, such interference is not important clinically.[89] OC use has not been shown to inhibit the action of other drugs. Some drugs, however, can clinically interfere with the action of OC's by inducing liver enzymes that convert the steroids to more polar and less biologically active metabolites. Certain drugs have been shown to accelerate the biotransformation of steroids in the human. These include barbiturates, sulfonamides, cyclophosphamide, and rifampin.[90] There is a high incidence of OC failure in women who ingest rifampin, and these two agents should not be given concurrently. The clinical data concerning OC failure in users of other antibiotics (e.g., penicillin, ampicillin, and sulfonamides), analgesics (e.g., phenytoin), and barbiturates are less clear. A few anecdotal studies have appeared in the literature, but there is no reliable evidence for a clinical inhibitory effect of these drugs, such as occurs with rifampin. Until controlled studies are performed, it would appear prudent when both agents are given simultaneously to suggest use of a barrier method in addition to the OC's because of possible interference with OC action by the action of the antibiotic on the gut flora. In addition, women with epilepsy who require medication possibly should be treated with 50 μg of estrogen formulations because a higher incidence of abnormal bleeding has been reported in these women with the use of lower-dose estrogen formulations.[91]

Noncontraceptive Health Benefits

In addition to being the most effective method of contraception, OC's provide many other health benefits. Some

are due to the fact that the combination OC's contain a potent, orally active progestin as well as an orally active estrogen, and there is no time when the estrogenic target tissues are stimulated by estrogens without a gestagen (unopposed estrogen).

Both natural progesterone and the synthetic progestins inhibit the proliferative effect of estrogen, the so-called anti-estrogenic effect. Estrogens increase the synthesis of both estrogen and progesterone receptors, whereas progesterone decreases their synthesis. Thus one mechanism whereby progesterone exerts its anti-estrogenic effects is by decreasing the synthesis of estrogen receptors. Relatively little progestin is needed to do this, and the amount present in OC's is sufficient. Another way progesterone produces its anti-estrogenic action is by stimulating the activity of the enzyme estradiol-17-β-dehydrogenase within the endometrial cell. This enzyme converts the more potent estradiol to the less potent estrone, reducing estrogenic action within the cell.

Benefits from Antiestrogenic Action of Progestins

As a result of the antiestrogenic action of the progestins in OC's, the height of the endometrium is less than in an ovulatory cycle, and there is less proliferation of the glandular epithelium. These changes produce several substantial benefits for the OC user. One is a reduction in the amount of blood lost at the time of endometrial shedding. In an ovulatory cycle the mean blood loss during menstruation is about 35 ml, compared with 20 ml for women who ingest OC's.[92] This decreased blood loss makes the development of iron deficiency anemia less likely. Data from the RCGP study showed that OC users were about half as likely to develop iron deficiency anemia as were the controls.[93] Moreover, the beneficial effect persisted to a similar degree in women who had previously used OC's and then stopped them, probably because of an increase in the iron stores that remained for several years after the drug was discontinued.

Because the OC's produce regular withdrawal bleeding, it would be expected that OC users would have fewer menstrual disorders than do controls. The results of the RCGP study confirmed the fact that OC users were significantly less likely to develop menorrhagia, irregular menstruation, or intermenstrual bleeding.[93] Because these disorders frequently are treated by curettage and/or hysterectomy, OC users require these procedures less frequently.

Because progestins inhibit the proliferative effect of estrogens on the endometrium, as mentioned earlier, women who use OC's have been found to be significantly less likely to develop adenocarcinoma of the endometrium.[78]

Estrogen exerts a proliferative effect on breast tissue, which also contains estrogen receptors. Progestins probably inhibit the synthesis of estrogen receptors in this organ as well, exerting an antiestrogenic action on the breast. Several studies have shown that OC's reduce the incidence of benign breast disease, and two prospective studies have indicated that this reduction is directly related to the amount of progestin in the compounds.[94]

Data from the Oxford study indicate that current users of OC's have an 85 per cent reduction in the incidence of fibroadenomas and 50 per cent reductions in chronic cystic disease and nonbiopsied breast lumps, compared with controls using IUD's or diaphragms.[94] The risk of developing these three diseases decreased with increased duration of OC use and persisted for about one year after discontinuation of OC's, after which no reduction in risk was observed.

Benefits from Inhibition of Ovulation

Other, noncontraceptive medical benefits of OC's result from their main action—inhibition of ovulation. Some disorders, such as dysmenorrhea and premenstrual tension, occur much more frequently in ovulatory than in anovulatory cycles. The RCGP study showed that OC users had 63 per cent less dysmenorrhea and 29 per cent less premenstrual tension than did controls.[93] Another study indicated that OC users were less likely to have variation in the degree of feeling of well-being throughout the cycle than non-OC users.[95]

Another serious adverse effect of ovulatory menstrual cycles is the development of functional ovarian cysts—specifically follicular and luteal cysts—that frequently require laparotomy because of enlargement, rupture, or hemorrhage. When ovulation is inhibited, functional cysts do not usually develop. In a survey performed in Boston less than 2 per cent of women with a discharge diagnosis of functional ovarian cysts were taking OC's, in contrast to 20 per cent of controls. However, 20 per cent of women with nonfunctional cysts were taking OC's, an incidence similar to that observed in the controls.[96] Although authors of one small case series postulated that the formation of functional ovarian cysts may be increased in users of multiphasic OC's, the rate of hospitalization for ovarian cysts in the United States has remained unchanged after the widespread use of multiphasic formulations.[97]

Another disorder linked to incessant ovulation is ovarian cancer, and as mentioned earlier, the development of ovarian cancer is significantly reduced in OC users with a duration-dependent decrease in risk.[80]

Other Benefits

Several studies, have shown that the risk of developing rheumatoid arthritis in OC users was only about one half that in controls.[98] Another benefit is protection against salpingitis, commonly referred to as pelvic inflammatory disease (PID). The relative risk of developing PID among OC users in most studies is about 0.5.[19] Only about one half as many women infected with gonorrhea (8.8 per cent) who use OC's developed PID, compared with non-OC users infected with gonorrhea (15 per cent).[99] Although the incidence of cervical infection with C. trachomatis is increased in OC users, compared with controls, the incidence of chlamydial salpingitis in OC users is only one half that in controls.[100] This protection may be related to the decreased duration of menstrual flow, which permits a smaller number of organisms to ascend to the upper genital tract and allows the body's defenses to eliminate them more easily. One sequela of PID is ectopic pregnancy, an entity that has tripled in incidence in the past decade. OC's reduce the risk of ectopic pregnancy by more than 90 per cent in current users and may reduce the incidence in former users by decreasing their chance of developing salpingitis.

Most of this information is based on data obtained with higher-dose OC formulations. Because the lower-dose agents contain a progestin that inhibits estrogenic mitotic activity and also inhibits ovulation, the scope and magnitude of beneficial effects should be similar with all combination formulations currently marketed. It is unfortunate that the infrequent adverse effects of OC's have received widespread publicity, whereas the more common noncontraceptive health benefits have attracted little attention.

LONG-ACTING CONTRACEPTIVE STEROIDS

Injectable Suspensions

Three types of injectable steroid formulations currently are in use for contraception throughout the world. These include (1) depomedroxyprogesterone acetate (DMPA), given in a dosage of 150 mg every three months; (2) norethindrone enanthate (NET-EN), given in a dosage of 200 mg every two months; and (3) several once-a-month injections of combinations of different progestins and estrogens. About 5 million women are using injectable steroid formulations, twice the number who used them in 1985.

Depo-Medroxyprogesterone Acetate

Depo-medroxyprogesterone acetate (DMPA) is the most widely used injectable contraceptive and also the most widely studied. More than 15 million women have used DMPA since it was first made available for contraceptive use in the mid-1960's, and currently there are about 3.5 million users in the world. More than 1000 scientific articles have been written about DMPA. It is approved for use as a contraceptive in more than 90 countries, including Sweden, France, Germany, and the United Kingdom, and since 1992 it has also been approved in the United States.

DMPA is extremely effective. The failure rates in various studies range from 0.0 to 1.2 per 100 woman-years. In a large WHO multiclinic study of 1587 users of DMPA, the failure rate at the end of one year was only 0.1 per cent and at the end of two years, 0.4 per cent.[101]

DMPA is formulated as a crystalline suspension. It should be given by injection in the upper outer quadrant of the gluteal region. The area should not be massaged, so that the drug is released slowly into the circulation. Administering the drug by this method should result in a very low failure rate.

For a few days after the injection, MPA levels in the serum range from 1.5 to 3 ng/ml and gradually decline thereafter, reaching 0.2 ng/ml during the sixth month, and become undetectable about 7½ to 9 months after administration.[102]

Serum estradiol levels remain at early follicular phase levels for four to six months after the DMPA injection. When serum levels of MPA fall below 0.5 ng/ml, estradiol rises to preovulatory levels. Ovulation, however, as evidenced by elevated serum progesterone levels, does not occur, apparently because the LH peak is suppressed by inhibition of the positive feedback of estrogen on its release. When serum MPA levels fall below 0.1 ng/ml, about seven to nine months after the injection, cyclic ovulatory ovarian function resumed. Thus the delay in ovulation after receiving injections of DMPA is due to prolonged MPA release and persists until serum levels of MPA become very low. The time required for the drug to disappear from the circulation after the last of several injections should be about the same as that after a single injection because MPA is rapidly cleared from the bloodstream. The prolonged presence in serum is related to the slow release from the injection site.

MPA acts by inhibiting the midcycle gonadotropin surge. Levels of LH and FSH remain in the follicular-phase range and are not completely suppressed. Mean estradiol levels remain relatively constant, about 40 pg/ml, for up to five years of treatment.[103] These estradiol levels are higher than menopausal levels, and patients receiving DMPA do not develop signs or symptoms of estrogen deficiency, such as vaginal atrophy, hot flashes, or decreased bone density. As a result of the high progestin and low estrogen levels, the endometrium becomes low-lying and atrophic. The glands are narrow and widely spaced with deciduoid stroma. With this atrophic type of endometrium, most women treated with DMPA develop amenorrhea.

The major adverse effect of DMPA is complete disruption of the menstrual cycle. In the first three months after the first injection, about 30 per cent of the women are amenorrheic and another 30 per cent have irregular bleeding and spotting occurring more than 11 days per month. As duration of therapy increases, the incidence of frequent bleeding steadily declines and the incidence of amenorrhea steadily increases, so that at the end of two years about 70 per cent of the women treated with DMPA are amenorrheic (Fig. 123–4).[104]

After treatment with DMPA is discontinued, about one half the women resume a regular cyclic menstrual pattern within six months and about three fourths have regular menses within one year. When bleeding does resume after the effect of the last injection is dissipated, it is initially regular in about one half the women and irregular in the remainder.

Additional adverse effects include slight weight gain, and

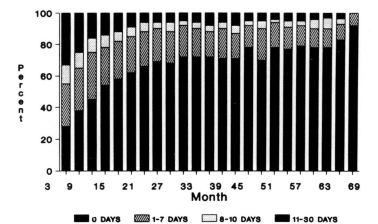

FIGURE 123–4. Percentage of patients with bleeding or spotting on days 0, 1 to 7, 8 to 10, or 11 to 30 per 30-day cycle while receiving injectable DMPA, 150 mg, every three months. (From Schwallie PC, Assenzo JR: Contraceptive use—efficacy study utilizing medroxyprogesterone acetate administered as an intramuscular injection once every 90 days. Fertil Steril 24:331, 1973.)

because of the long duration of action of the drug, there is a delay in return of fertility.

Fertility rates have been calculated for fertile couples who discontinue various methods of contraception other than DMPA to conceive. At the end of three months about 50 per cent of these women are pregnant; at the end of a year about 90 per cent are pregnant. For DMPA users the curve is shifted to the right, so the 50 per cent pregnancy rate does not occur until about one year, a delay of about nine months compared with women who discontinue barrier methods.[105]

The use of DMPA does not cause sterility but causes a temporary period of infertility. A major benefit of the prolonged effect of the drug is that when patients do not return for their scheduled injection on time but delay for one or two months, pregnancy rates remain very low. The incidence of failure to conceive as well as the interval to conception after stopping DMPA were similar among women who had used DMPA for various periods and received many or few injections of the drug.

Because DMPA does not increase liver globulin production, as does the estrogen component or OC's (ethinyl estradiol), no alteration in blood-clotting factors or angiotensinogen levels is associated with its use. Thus, unlike OC's, DMPA has not been associated with increases in hypertension or thromboembolism.

When glucose tolerance tests were performed on long-term DMPA users, a slight statistically but clinically insignificant impairment in glucose tolerance was observed when compared with a control group of women.

Long-term DMPA users have altered levels of serum lipids. Levels of triglycerides and HDL cholesterol, but not total cholesterol, were significantly lower in long-term users compared with controls of similar age. There was no significant difference in LDL cholesterol levels.[106]

Concern has also been raised that DMPA may be associated with an increased incidence of abnormal cervical cytology. In a multinational case control study conducted by WHO the adjusted relative risk for cervical cancer among women who had ever used DMPA compared with users of no contraception was 1.11, with confidence intervals of 0.96 to 1.29.[107] This insignificantly increased risk showed no trend of increasing with increasing duration of use of DMPA, as has been observed in several studies of the relation of OC use and cervical neoplasia. Thus the increased incidence of abnormal cervical cytology reported among DMPA users appears to be related to confounding factors, such as failure to use a diaphragm or many sexual partners, because there is no evidence that the drug itself causes an increase in cervical dysplasia or carcinoma.

DMPA has been associated with an increased incidence of two types of carcinoma in animals but not in humans. When given in high doses to beagle dogs it is associated with an increase in mammary cancer; however, the beagle is a poor model for study of steroid action in the human because progestins are metabolized differently in the two species. Beagles develop a high incidence of breast carcinoma after receiving various types of progestins. After 25 years of study with this agent in humans there is no evidence of an increased incidence of breast carcinoma. In a large WHO study the relative risk of developing breast cancer among ever users of DMPA was 1.2.[108]

In long-term monkey studies two monkeys developed adenocarcinoma of the endometrium when treated with

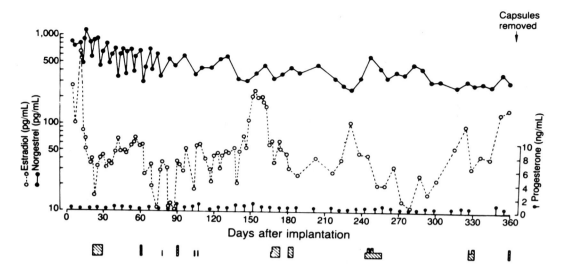

FIGURE 123–5. Serum levels of estradiol, progesterone, and *d*-norgestrel in a subject with six polysiloxane capsules, each containing 33.9 mg of *d*-norgestrel, implanted on day 0. Hatched bars represent uterine bleeding. (From Moore DE, et al: Bleeding and serum d-norgestrel, estradiol, and progesterone patterns in women using d-norgestrel subdermal polysiloxane capsules for contraception. Contraception 17:315, 1978.)

high doses of DMPA for 10 years; however, there is no evidence that DMPA produces endometrial cancer in humans. DMPA produces an atrophic endometrium and actually is used to treat metastatic endometrial carcinoma.[109] In the WHO study the relative risk of developing endometrial cancer was 0.21 (95 per cent confidence interval 0.06 to 0.79). As a result of these data an FDA advisory committee has recommended that this agent be approved for contraceptive use in the United States. Possible benefits of DMPA, in addition to its extreme effectiveness, include a reduction in menstrual blood loss, and thus anemia, and a probable decreased incidence of developing salpingitis (because most users are amenorrheic) as well as a decreased risk of developing endometrial and ovarian cancer because DMPA is progestational and inhibits ovulation.

Subdermal Implants

Subdermal implants of capsules made of polydimethylsiloxane (Silastic) that contain levonorgestrel have been developed and patented by the Population Council as Norplant. Clinical trials of this long-acting, effective, reversible method of contraception were initiated in 1975. To date Norplant has been used by more than 500,000 women in 45 countries and was approved for use in the United States in 1991. As with all steroid-containing Silastic devices, the rate of steroid delivery is directly proportional to the surface area of the capsules, and duration of action depends on the amount of steroid within the capsules. To produce effective blood levels of norgestrel, it was necessary to use six capsules filled with crystalline levonorgestrel. The cylindrical capsules are 3.4 cm long and 2.4 mm in outer diameter with the ends sealed with Silastic medical adhesive. Each capsule contains 36 mg of crystalline levonorgestrel for a total amount of 216 mg in each six-capsule set.

Insertion is performed in an outpatient area, and the entire procedure takes about five minutes. After infiltration of the skin with local anesthesia, a small (3-mm) incision is made with a scalpel, usually in the upper arm, although the lower arm and the inguinal and gluteal regions have also been used. The capsules are implanted into the subcutaneous tissue in a radial pattern through a large (10- to

12-gauge) trocar, and the incision is closed with adhesive. Stitches are not necessary. Because polydimethylsiloxane is not biodegradable, the capsules have to be removed through another incision when desired by the user or at the end of five years, which is the duration of maximal contraceptive effectiveness.

After the capsules are inserted blood levels of levonorgestrel rise rapidly to reach levels between 400 and 500 pg/ml in 24 hours.[110] The serum levels remain relatively constant during the first year of use, with a mean of about 400 pg/ml, which usually is sufficient to inhibit ovulation (Fig. 123–5). When the amount of steroid was measured in capsules removed from patients after various times, it was found that the rate of release was fairly constant during the first year of use, averaging about 50 μg of levonorgestrel per day from the six-capsule set. From about the end of the first year of use until eight years of use, daily release rates declined to about 30 μg per day but remained constant during this interval. Mean serum levels of levonorgestrel also decline slightly beyond the third year of use and average about 300 pg/ml.

With this low level of levonorgestrel, gonadotropin levels are not completely suppressed, and follicular activity results in periodic peaks of estradiol. Because the level of circulating levonorgestrel usually is sufficient to inhibit the positive feedback effect of these estradiol peaks on LH release, LH levels are lower, even in Norplant users with regular cycles, and ovulation occurs infrequently.[111]

It is difficult to determine the exact incidence of ovulatory cycles in Norplant users because different investigators have used different minimum levels of serum progesterone as a definition of presumptive ovulation and serum samples that have been obtained at various time intervals in different studies. Daily ultrasonographic scanning of ovaries of Norplant users with regular cycles and elevated luteal-phase progesterone levels revealed that only about one third of these cycles had ovarian morphological changes consistent with a normal ovulatory pattern.[112] Because only about one half the cycles of Norplant users have a fairly regular pattern, probably less than 20 per cent of the cycles are ovulatory, and a high percentage of these have deficient progesterone production.

Thus inhibition of ovulation is one of the major mechanisms of action of this method of contraception. The consistently elevated levels of norgestrel also prevent the normal midcycle thinning of the cervical mucus from occurring. The cervical mucus remains scanty and viscid, and normal sperm penetration does not take place, as demonstrated by both in vivo and in vitro studies.[113] These two mechanisms of action result in a very high level of contraceptive effectiveness. Because pregnancy rates are higher in the sixth and seventh year of use, a new set of capsules should be inserted after five years.

Annual pregnancy rates for the first five years of use in large trials are 0.2, 0.2, 0.9, 0.5, and 1.1 per 100 woman-years in the first five years, respectively.[114] All the first-year pregnancies in both trials occurred before insertion of the implants. The pregnancy rates after the second year of Norplant use were inversely related to the women's body weight, remaining at 0.2 in women who weighed less than 50 kg and increasing to more than 6.0 after three years in women who weighed more than 70 kg. In these studies the Norplant capsules were made of a denser type of tubing than is now being used and serum levels of norgestrel were slightly lower than occur with the currently used less dense tubing. In ovulatory cycles of Norplant users mean serum norgestrel levels are lower than in anovulatory cycles. Thus the higher serum levels of norgestrel associated with the less dense tubing should result in a lower incidence of ovulation and greater efficacy.

In studies performed to date the gross cumulative pregnancy rate at the end of five years in a group of women using Norplant made of the less dense tubing was only 1.1.[114] Furthermore, there was no relation between the incidence of pregnancy and the body weight of the user as the pregnancy rate was not increased in women weighing more than 70 kg. Thus, with the less dense tubing, annual pregnancy rates for the first five years of use are about 0.2 per 100 women, making Norplant one of the most effective methods of reversible contraception available. As with all progestin-only methods of contraception, when pregnancies occur with Norplant a high percentage, about 20 per cent, are ectopic. However, because of its high rate of effectiveness, the overall rate of ectopic pregnancies in Norplant users, 0.28 per 1000 woman-years of use, is reduced compared with ectopic pregnancy rates in the entire U.S. population of women of reproductive age, 1.5 per 1000 women annually.

Mean estradiol levels in Norplant users, whether or not they are ovulatory or anovulatory, are about the same as in women with regular ovulatory cycles who used IUD's. After a fall in estradiol, endometrial sloughing and uterine bleeding or spotting usually occurs. Because the peaks and declines in estradiol levels occur at irregular intervals, uterine bleeding also occurs at irregular intervals in most Norplant users.

The major adverse effect of Norplant use is the irregular pattern of uterine bleeding. Other alterations in uterine blood flow involve changes in duration and volume, with most bleeding episodes being scanty in amount. About one half the bleeding episodes can be characterized as fairly regular, with the interval between bleeding episodes ranging between 21 and 35 days, about 40 per cent irregular with intervals outside this range, and about 10 per cent as amenorrheic with no bleeding for more than a three-month interval. Because of the high incidence of bleeding irregularities, potential Norplant users must be thoroughly counseled about this potential problem before insertion. Bleeding episodes are more prolonged and irregular during the first year of use, after which there is greater frequency of a more regular pattern. The mean number of days of bleeding also declines steadily with time from 54.3 days in the first year to 44.1 days in the fifth year.[114] Mean total blood loss in Norplant users is about 25 ml per month, slightly less than the average monthly blood loss of normally cycling women. Several clinical studies have shown that the mean hemoglobin concentration in the first three years of Norplant use rises slightly. Even women who stop using the method because of bleeding problems have been found to have an increase in mean hemoglobin levels. When pregnancies occur in Norplant users they nearly always occur in women with a recent history of regular cyclic uterine bleeding.[115] Thus women who are amenorrheic or have infrequent episodes of uterine bleeding do not need to be monitored by periodic pregnancy tests.

Other problems associated with this method of contraception include infection, local irritation, or painful reaction at the insertion site. Expulsion of a capsule occasionally occurs, usually in association with infection. The incidence of insertion site infection is less than 1 per cent. Headache is the single most frequent medical problem that causes removal of the implants, accounting for about 30 per cent of the medical reasons for removal.[114] Weight gain was a common reason for medical removal in U.S. studies, whereas weight loss was more common in the Dominican Republic. Other medical problems among Norplant users include acne, mastalgia, and mood changes, including anxiety, depression, and nervousness. Because ovarian follicular development without subsequent ovulation is common among Norplant users, adnexal enlargement caused by persistent unruptured follicles has been noted during routine bimanual pelvic examination on many Norplant users. These enlarged follicles, which may reach 5 to 7 cm in diameter, usually regress spontaneously in one to two months without therapy.

Many metabolic studies have been performed among Norplant users in various population groups. Studies of carbohydrate metabolism, serum chemistries, liver function, serum cortisol levels, thyroid function, and blood coagulation have revealed only minimal changes that remain within the normal range. Several studies have been performed in different countries in which lipoproteins were measured before and after Norplant insertion. In most of these studies levels of triglycerides, total cholesterol, and LDL cholesterol declined, whereas HDL cholesterol declined slightly or increased. There was little change in the cholesterol–HDL cholesterol ratio, indicating that Norplant should not enhance the development of atherosclerosis.[116]

The removal process is, like the insertion procedure, performed in the clinic area, using local anesthesia and a small skin incision. The removal of Norplant is more difficult than its insertion because fibrous tissue develops around the capsule and must be cut before removing the capsule. It is important that the capsules be inserted superficially to enhance the ease of removal. Deeply implanted capsules are more difficult to remove.

After removal the incision is closed without stitches, and a pressure dressing is applied for about 24 hours after removal of the capsule set. If the woman wants to continue use, another set can be inserted through the same incision or in the opposite arm. If another set of Norplant is not inserted after removal, the steroid is rapidly cleared from the circulation and serum levels of norgestrel fall rapidly, reaching nearly undetectable levels in 96 hours. If pregnancy is desired, return of ovulation is prompt and similar to that in women who discontinue other, nonhormonal methods of reversible contraception, reaching 50 per cent at three months and 86 per cent at one year.[114]

Continuation rates with the Norplant method of contraception are high, ranging from 76 to 99 per cent at one year in different countries and from 33 to 78 per cent at five years. These high continuation rates are similar to those observed with IUD's and are due in large part to the fact that to discontinue use, these methods require the user to return to the clinic. This is the main reason Norplant implants and the IUD have the highest continuation rates of any methods of contraception in use today.

Postcoital Contraception

Various estrogenic compounds have been used for postcoital contraception (PCC), or what commonly is referred to as the "morning-after pill." The estrogen compounds that have been most commonly used for this purpose include diethylstilbestrol (DES), 25 to 50 mg/d; ethinyl estradiol, 5 mg/d; and conjugated estrogens, 30 mg/d. Treatment is continued for five days. If it is begun within 72 hours after an isolated midcycle act of coitus, its effectiveness is very good. If more than one episode of coitus has occurred or if treatment is initiated later than 72 hours after coitus, the method is much less effective.

A literature review reported that pregnancy rates among women treated with ethinyl estradiol were 0.6 per cent; with DES, 0.7 per cent; and with conjugated estrogen, 1.6 per cent[117] (Table 123–9). None of these rates were significantly different from the overall mean failure rate of 0.7 per cent. None of the trials included a control group, but the clinical pregnancy rate after midcycle coitus is about 7 per cent. Thus high-dose estrogen is an effective method of PCC.

Adverse effects associated with this high-dose estrogen therapy are common and severe. They include nausea, vomiting, breast soreness, and menstrual irregularities, which reduce compliance. If treatment is begun two days after coitus, the pregnancy rate is 1.7 times greater than if it was begun the day after coitus. Thus it appears best to start treatment within 24 hours of coitus.

Because the adverse effects of high-dose estrogens cause many women to fail to complete the five-day treatment

course, a regimen of four tablets of an ethinyl estradiol, 0.05 mg, and dl-norgestrel, 0.5 mg, combination OC (Ovral), given in doses of two tablets 12 hours apart, was initially tested in Canada. This regimen was found to be effective, with a shorter duration of adverse symptoms.

Results from studies with this treatment regimen involving 3802 women found that failure rates varied widely, from a low of 0.2 per cent in a Canadian study to a high of 7.4 per cent in an Italian study. The total pregnancy rate in the 11 studies was 1.8 per cent. In one large Canadian study 30 per cent of the subjects treated with this regimen reported having nausea without vomiting and another 20 per cent had nausea with vomiting.[117]

Thus the effectiveness of this method appears to be slightly less than that of higher dosages of estrogen alone, but a lower incidence of abnormal bleeding and delayed menses as well as the gastrointestinal effects occur with this regimen than with the high-dose estrogen. Also, because of the one-day treatment regimen, patient compliance is greater with this technique. Thus this method is more widely used than the high-dose estrogens.

Another method of PCC, the administration of danazol, 400 to 600 mg in two doses separated by 12 hours, has been tried by two groups of investigators. A total of 998 women were treated in these trials and the pregnancy rate, 2 per cent, was similar to that of the two doses of combined OC's.[117] The incidence of adverse effects, particularly nausea, was less with danazol, and thus patient acceptability was high. If the patient has a continuing need for contraception after the cycle in which either of these techniques is used, one of the conventional methods should be prescribed.

Several authors have advocated that intra-uterine insertion of a copper IUD within 5 to 10 days of midcycle coitus is an effective method to prevent continuation of the pregnancy. Only one pregnancy occurred after a copper IUD was inserted in 876 women.[117] The insertion of a copper IUD as well as high-dose estrogens are the most effective methods of PCC, but adverse effects limit acceptance of the latter technique, and cost and concern about introducing pathogens into the upper genital tract with IUD insertion limit its widespread use.

Antiprogestins

A few years ago Baulieu synthesized a progestogenic steroid compound that had weak progestational activity but marked affinity for progesterone receptors in the endometrium. This compound, called RU 486, or mefisterone (Fig.

TABLE 123–9. OBSERVED AND EXPECTED PREGNANCIES ACCORDING TO VARIOUS METHODS OF POSTCOITAL CONTRACEPTION

TREATMENT	NUMBER OF STUDIES	TOTAL NUMBER OF PATIENTS CONSIDERED	NUMBER OF OBSERVED PREGNANCIES	PREGNANCY RATE (%)
Ethinyl estradiol—high dosage	4	3168	19	0.6
Other estrogens—high dosage	2	975	11	1.1
Ethinyl estradiol plus *dl*-norgestrel	11	3802	69	1.8
Danazol	3	998	20	2.0
IUD	9	879	1	0.1

From Fasoli M et al: Post-coital contraception: An overview of published studies. Contraception 39:459, 1989.
$X\chi^2$ for heterogeneity = 35.31; $P < .001$.

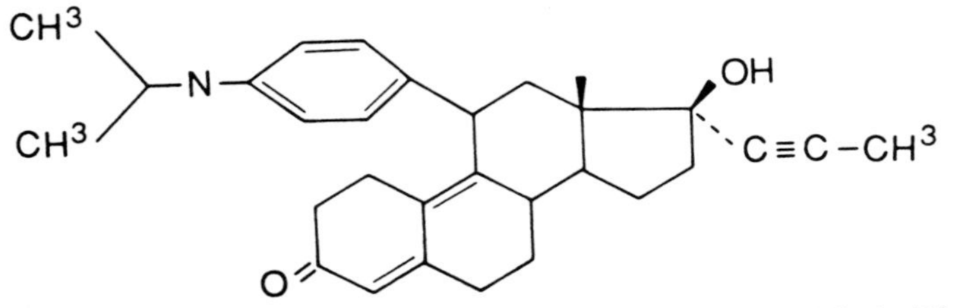

FIGURE 123–6. Molecular structure of RU 486. Molecular weight is 430, and empirical formula is $C_{29}H_{35}NO_2$. (From Healy DL, et al: Induction of menstruation by an antiprogesterone steroid [RU 486] in primates; sites of action, dose-response relationships, and hormonal effects. Fertil Steril 40:253, 1983.)

123–6), because of its high receptor affinity, prevented progesterone from binding to its receptors and thus had an antiprogesterone action.[118] In clinical trials it was found that if a single 600-mg dose of RU 486 was administered orally early in pregnancy, before six weeks after the onset of the last menses, about 85 per cent of the pregnancies spontaneously terminated.[119] When this treatment was combined with administration of a prostaglandin 36 to 48 hours later, the efficacy of pregnancy termination increases to 96 per cent.[120]

Adverse effects of RU 486 include nausea, vomiting, and abdominal pain. The main disadvantage of this method is prolonged and sometimes heavy vaginal bleeding that on occasion can cause anemia, necessitating a blood transfusion and, possibly, curettage. The mean duration of bleeding after administration of this drug is about 12 days when administered alone and 9 days when used with a prostaglandin. Distribution of this drug currently is limited to a few European countries. Compounds with similar activity or steroid enzymatic inhibitors that prevent progesterone synthesis are also being studied.

INTRAUTERINE DEVICES

The main benefits of IUD's are (1) a high level of effectiveness, (2) a lack of associated systemic metabolic effects, and (3) the need for only a single act of motivation for long-term use. In contrast to other types of contraception, there is no need for frequent motivation to ingest a pill daily or to use a coitus-related method consistently. These characteristics, as well as the necessity for a visit to a health care facility to discontinue the method, account for the fact that IUD's have the highest continuation rate of all available reversible methods of contraception. It is desirable for all women to make at least annual visits to a health care facility, but in some areas of the world this is not possible.

Unlike other contraceptives, such as the barrier methods, which rely on frequent use by the individual for effectiveness and therefore have higher use failure rates than method failure rates, the IUD has similar method effectiveness and use effectiveness rates. First-year failure rates with copper-bearing IUD's have been reported to range from less than 1 per cent to 3.7 per cent.[2] Pregnancy rates are related to the skill of the clinician inserting the device. With experience, correct high-fundal insertion occurs more frequently, and there is a lower incidence of partial or complete expulsion, with resultant lower pregnancy rates. Furthermore, the annual incidence of accidental pregnancy decreases steadily after the first year of IUD use. The incidence of all major adverse events with IUD's, including pregnancy, expulsion, or removal for bleeding and/or pain, also steadily decreases with increasing age.[121] Thus the IUD is especially suited for older parous women who want to prevent further pregnancies.

Mechanism of Action

The IUD's main mechanism of contraceptive action in the human is spermicidal, produced by a local sterile inflammatory reaction caused by the presence of the foreign body in the uterus. There is a nearly 1000 per cent increase in the number of leukocytes in washings of the human endometrial cavity 18 weeks after the insertion of an IUD, compared with washings obtained before insertion.[122] Tissue breakdown products of these leukocytes are toxic to all cells, including sperm and the blastocyst. Small IUD's do not produce as great an inflammatory reaction as larger ones. Therefore, pregnancy rates are higher with smaller IUD's than with larger devices of the same design. The addition of copper increases the inflammatory reaction. Sperm transport from the cervix to the oviduct in the first 24 hours after coitus is markedly impaired in women wearing IUD's.[123] Because of the spermicidal action of IUD's, few, if any, sperm reach the oviducts, and the ovum usually does not become fertilized.

Further evidence for this spermicidal action of IUD's was reported by investigators who performed oviductal flushing in 56 women with IUD's and in 45 who used no method of contraception, who were sterilized by salpingectomy soon after ovulation and also had unprotected sexual intercourse shortly before ovulation. Normally cleaving, fertilized ova were found in the tubal flushings of about one half of the women not wearing IUD's, whereas no eggs that had the microscopic appearance of a normally fertilized and developing preimplantation embryo were found in the oviducts of the women wearing IUD's.[124]

In rabbits the sterile inflammatory reaction changes the receptiveness of the endometrium to the nidation of the blastocyst, preventing implantation. The same effect is believed to occur in humans if fertilization does take place. The presence of copper ions increases in locally released prostaglandins, and enzymatic changes within the endometrial cavity probably also act to prevent the normal process of implantation.

On removal of both copper-bearing and non–copper-bearing IUD's, the inflammatory reaction rapidly disappears. Resumption of fertility after IUD removal is not delayed and occurs at the same rate as resumption of fertility after discontinuation of mechanical methods of contraception, such as the condom and diaphragm.[125]

Types of IUD's

In the past 25 years many types of IUD's have been designed and used clinically. The devices developed and initially used in the 1960's were made of a plastic, polyethylene that was impregnated with barium sulfate to make them radiographic. In the 1970's smaller plastic devices covered with copper wire, such as the Copper T, were developed and widely used. In the 1980's devices bearing a larger amount of copper, including sleeves on the horizontal arm, such as the copper T 380A and the copper T 220C, were developed. These devices had a longer duration of high effectiveness and thus had to be re-inserted at less frequent intervals than the devices bearing a smaller amount of copper. Although many of all the types of IUD's developed are still available for use in Europe, Canada, and elsewhere, only the copper T 380A and a progesterone-releasing IUD are being marketed in the United States (Fig. 123–7). Although the barium-impregnated plastic loop and the copper-bearing copper 7 and copper T 200B are still approved by the FDA for use in the United States, they are no longer being sold. Production and distribution of the shield device with a multifilament tail were discontinued in 1974. Because of the increased risk of infection reported with shield IUD's, if any are still in place, they should be removed. All IUD's now approved for distribution by the FDA have monofilament tails.

The T- and 7-shaped plastic devices are smaller than most non–copper-bearing types of IUD's. When T-shaped devices without copper underwent clinical trials, they were found to have a much higher pregnancy rate than the larger loops and coils. With the addition of copper wire, the effectiveness of these IUD's was increased by the mechanism described above and was comparable or higher than that of the nonmedicated IUD's.

Because of the constant dissolution of copper, which amounts daily to less than that ingested in the normal diet, all copper IUD's have to be replaced periodically. The copper T 380A is approved for use in the United States for eight years. At the scheduled time of removal the device can be removed and another inserted during the same office visit.

Adding a reservoir of progesterone to the vertical arm also increases the effectiveness of the T-shaped devices. The progesterone IUD releases 65 mg of progesterone daily. This amount is sufficient to prevent pregnancy by local action within the endometrial cavity, but it is not enough to cause a measurable increase in peripheral serum progesterone levels. The progesterone-releasing IUD needs to be replaced annually because the reservoir

of progesterone becomes depleted after about 18 months of use.

A T-shaped device containing a reservoir of levonorgestrel on the vertical arm has been developed, undergone extensive clinical testing, and been approved for use in Finland. A large comparative trial of the Cu T 380A and the levonorgestrel-releasing IUD has found that the effectiveness and complication rates of both devices were similar.[126] Because of the slower rate of release of levonorgestrel than progesterone, the levonorgestrel-releasing IUD has an estimated duration of use of at least five years.

Unlike the medicated IUD's, there is no need to change a nonmedicated plastic IUD unless the patient develops increased bleeding after it has been in place for more than one year. Calcium salts are deposited on the plastic over time, and their roughness can cause ulceration and bleeding of the endometrium. If increased bleeding develops after a non–copper-bearing IUD has been in the uterus for one or more years, the old IUD should be removed and a new device inserted.

Time of Insertion

Although it is widely believed that the optimal time for insertion of an IUD is during the menses, data indicate that if a woman is not pregnant, the IUD can safely be inserted on any day of the cycle.[127]

It has also been recommended that IUD's not be inserted until more than two to three months have elapsed after completing a term pregnancy. One- and two-year event rates among women who had copper T IUD's inserted between four and eight weeks postpartum and more than eight weeks postpartum were similar for the two groups, indicating that copper T IUD's can safely be inserted at the time of the routine postpartum visit.[128]

Although one report suggested that the perforation rate may be higher if the IUD is inserted when a woman is lactating, this finding has not been confirmed in other studies. The effect of breastfeeding on performance of the copper T 380A IUD was evaluated in a large multicenter clinical trial in which the device was inserted into 559 breastfeeding women and 590 non-breastfeeding women.[129] Significantly less pain and bleeding problems occurred at insertion in the breastfeeding group. The expulsion rate, which was low, and continuation rate, which was high, were smaller in the breastfeeding and non-breastfeeding groups six months after insertion.

Adverse Effects

Incidence

In the first year of use most IUD's have about a 1 per cent pregnancy rate, a 10 per cent expulsion rate, and a 15 per cent rate of removal for medical reasons, mainly bleeding and pain. The incidence of each of these events, especially expulsion, diminishes steadily in subsequent years.[121]

The copper T 380A IUD, which has copper on the horizontal as well as the vertical arm, has a higher rate of effectiveness, with a pregnancy rate of 0.5 per cent after one year of use. In an ongoing WHO study of this device,

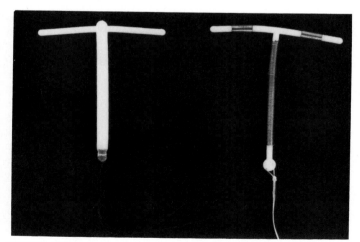

FIGURE 123–7. Intrauterine devices marketed in the United States (*left,* progesterone-releasing IUD; *right,* copper T 380A).

TABLE 123–10. CUMULATIVE DISCONTINUATION RATE FOR
COPPER T 380A IUD

EVENT	YEARS SINCE INSERTION		
	3	5	7
Pregnancies	1.0	1.4	1.6
Expulsions	7.0	8.2	8.6
Medical removals	14.6	20.8	25.8
Nonmedical removals	13.8	25.6	34.4
Loss to follow-up	10.2	15.5	22.1
All discontinuations	32.2	46.7	56.3
Woman-months	38,571	56,010	67,885

Modified from World Health Organization: Contraception 42:141, 1990.

termination rates for adverse effects continued to decline annually after the first year after insertion for each of the seven years in which sufficient data have accumulated to date.[122] In this study the cumulative discontinuation rate for pregnancy, bleeding and pain, and expulsion at the end of seven years was 1.6, 22.7, and 8.6, respectively (Table 123–10).

Uterine Bleeding

Most women who discontinue this method of contraception do so for medical reasons. Nearly all the medical reasons accounting for IUD removal involve one or more types of abnormal bleeding: heavy and/or prolonged menses or intermenstrual bleeding. The IUD does not affect the pattern or level of circulating gonadotropins and steroid hormones during the menstrual cycle. The IUD, however, does exert a local effect on the endometrium, causing menses to being about two days earlier than normal, when steroid levels are higher than in control cycles. It is possible that this early onset of menses may be produced by a premature and increased rate of local release of prostaglandins, brought about by the presence of the intrauterine foreign body. The stimulation of uterine contractions by excessive levels of prostaglandins may prolong the duration of the menstrual flow, which is significantly longer in women who wear IUD's.[130]

The amount of blood loss in each menstrual cycle is significantly greater in women wearing inert as well as copper-bearing IUD's than in nonwearers. In a normal menstrual cycle the mean amount of menstrual blood loss (MBL) is about 35 ml. After insertion of a loop IUD the mean MBL increases to 70 to 80 ml.[131, 132] The increase is less with copper-bearing devices. With the copper 7 IUD the mean MBL has been found to vary from 50 to 55 ml,[131-133] whereas with the copper T 200 the mean MBL varies from 50 to 60 ml.[134] In contrast, with the progesterone-releasing IUD the amount of blood loss is significantly reduced to about 25 ml per cycle.[135]

After the insertion of both copper and inert IUD's a greater percentage of women have MBL in excess of 80 ml, an amount that has been shown to produce severe iron deficiency than before insertion.[131] In women who use the copper 7 or copper T 200 there was no significant change in mean values for hemoglobin concentration, serum iron, and total iron-binding capacity 6 and 12 months after IUD insertion when compared with mean values before insertion.[121, 122] Blood loss studies with the Cu T 380A have not been published to date.

A sensitive indicator of tissue iron stores is the serum ferritin level. Both copper-bearing IUD's and nonmedicated plastic IUD's are associated with significant decreases in serum ferritin levels overall as well as with an increase in the percentage of women with extremely low ferritin levels (less than 16 mg/L), indicative of an absence of iron in bone marrow.[136-138] Low serum ferritin levels are a good predictor of the development of anemia. Therefore, ideally, both ferritin and hemoglobin levels should be measured annually in all women who wear nonsteroid-releasing IUD's. If either level decreases significantly, supplemental iron should be administered.

Excessive bleeding in the first few months after IUD insertion should be treated with reassurance and supplemental oral iron. The bleeding may diminish with time as the uterus adjusts to the presence of the foreign body. Excessive bleeding that continues or develops several months or more after IUD insertion may be treated by systemic administration of one of the prostaglandin synthetase inhibitors.

Mefenamic acid ingested in a dosage of 500 mg three times a day during the days of menstruation has been shown to reduce MBL significantly in IUD users.[139] If excessive bleeding continues despite this treatment, the device should be removed. After a one-month interval another type of device may be inserted if the patient still wants to use an IUD for contraception. Consideration should be given to using a progesterone-releasing IUD because this device is associated with less blood loss than a copper-bearing IUD.

Perforation

Although uncommon, one of the potentially serious complications associated with the use of the IUD is perforation of the uterine fundus. Perforation initially occurs at insertion. It can be prevented by straightening the uterine axis with a tenaculum and then probing the cavity with a uterine sound before IUD insertion. Sometimes only the distal portion of the IUD penetrates the uterine muscle at insertion. Then uterine contractions over the next few months force the IUD into the peritoneal cavity. IUD's that are correctly inserted entirely within the endometrial cavity do not wander through the uterine muscle into the peritoneal cavity. The incidence of perforation is related to the shape of the device and/or the amount of force used during its insertion as well as to the experience of the clinician performing the insertion.

Perforation rates for the copper 7 and the copper T 200 were found to be about 1 per 1000 insertions.[140] The clinician should always suspect perforation if a patient says that she cannot feel the appendage but did not notice that the device was expelled. One should not assume that an unnoticed expulsion has occurred when the appendage is not visualized. Sometimes the IUD is still in its correct position in the uterine cavity but the appendage has been withdrawn into the cavity as the position of the IUD within the cavity has changed. In this situation, after pelvic examination has been performed and the possibility of pregnancy excluded, the uterine cavity should be probed.

If the device cannot be felt with a uterine sound or biopsy instrument, pelvic ultrasonography or radiography should be performed. If the device is not visualized with pelvic ultrasonography, radiography visualizing the entire abdominal cavity should be performed because IUD's that have been pushed through the uterus may be located anywhere in the peritoneal cavity, even in the subdiaphragmatic area.

Any type of IUD found to be outside the uterus, even if asymptomatic, should be removed from the peritoneal cavity because complications such as adhesions and bowel obstruction have been reported. Both the copper IUD's and the shields have been found to produce severe peritoneal reactions. Therefore, it is best to remove these devices as soon as possible after the diagnosis of perforation is made. Unless severe adhesions have developed, most intraperitoneal IUD's can be removed by means of laparoscopy, avoiding the need for laparotomy.

Perforation of the cervix has also been reported with devices that have a straight vertical arm, such as the copper T or 7. Cervical perforation is not a major problem, but devices that have perforated downward should be removed through the endocervical canal with uterine packing forceps. Their downward displacement is associated with reduced contraceptive effectiveness.

Complications Related to Pregnancy

Congenital Anomalies

When pregnancy occurs with an IUD in place, implantation takes place away from the device itself, so the device is always extra-amniotic. Although there is a paucity of published data, so far there is no evidence of an increased incidence of congenital anomalies in infants born with an IUD in utero.

There is no evidence to indicate that the presence of a copper IUD in the uterus exerts a deleterious effect on fetal development.[141, 142] Although relatively few infants have been born with a progesterone-releasing IUD in the uterus, careful examination of these infants has revealed no increased incidence of cardiac or other anomalies.

Spontaneous Abortion

In all reported series of pregnancies with any type of IUD in situ, the incidence of fetal death was not significantly increased; however, if a patient conceives while wearing an IUD that is not subsequently removed, the incidence of spontaneous abortion is about 55 per cent, about three times greater than would occur without an IUD.[141–143]

After conception, if the IUD is spontaneously expelled or if the appendage is visible and the IUD is removed by traction, the incidence of spontaneous abortion is significantly reduced. Of women who conceived with copper T devices in place, the incidence of spontaneous abortion was only 20.3 per cent if the device was removed or spontaneously expelled.[141] Thus, if a woman conceives with an IUD in place and wants to continue the pregnancy, the IUD should be removed if the appendage is visible. This significantly reduces the chance of spontaneous abortion if the appendage is not visible. Probing of the uterine cavity may increase the chance of abortion as well as sepsis. Several recent reports indicate that with careful ultrasonography and meticulous techniques, it is possible to remove intrauterine IUD's without a visible appendage during pregnancy and have a normal outcome of gestation.

Septic Abortion

If the IUD cannot be easily removed, there is some evidence that suggests that the risk of septic abortion may be increased if the IUD remains in place. Most of the evidence is based on data from women who conceived while wearing the shield type of IUD with its multifilament tail, which allowed bacteria to enter the spaces between the filaments of the tail underneath the sheath.[144] During pregnancy, when the shield was drawn upward into the uterus as gestation advanced, the bacteria in the tail had the potential for causing a severe and sometimes fatal uterine infection, usually in the second trimester.

Although theoretical and actual evidence suggest an increased risk of septic abortion if a patient conceives with a shield IUD in place, no conclusive evidence shows an increased risk if a patient conceives with a device other than the shield in place. However, about 2 per cent of all spontaneous abortions are septic, and IUD's increase the rate of spontaneous abortion.

The patient should be informed of the possibility of a greater chance of sepsis and, if she wants to continue the pregnancy, of the need to report symptoms of infection promptly. If an intrauterine infection does occur during pregnancy with an IUD in place, treatment should proceed in the same manner as if the IUD were absent. In such a situation, the endometrial cavity should be evacuated after a short interval of appropriate antibiotic treatment.

Ectopic Pregnancy

As stated above, the IUD's main mechanism of contraceptive action is the production of a continuous sterile inflammatory reaction in the uterine cavity caused by foreign body presence. Because more inflammatory reaction is present in the endometrial cavity than in the oviducts, the IUD prevents intrauterine pregnancy more effectively than it prevents ectopic pregnancy.

Several epidemiological studies have confirmed the fact that if pregnancy occurs with an IUD in place, it is more likely to be ectopic than if pregnancy occurs in the absence of an IUD. Despite the increased incidence of ectopic pregnancy in women who conceive with an IUD in place overall, the IUD reduces the incidence of ectopic pregnancy. Women who use IUD's have only about 40 per cent as great a chance of developing ectopic pregnancy as women who use no method of contraception.

If a patient conceives with an IUD in place, her chances of having an ectopic pregnancy range from 3 to 9 per cent. This incidence is about 10 times greater than the reported ectopic pregnancy frequency of 0.3 to 0.7 per cent of total births in similar populations.[142] In two large Population Council studies the ectopic pregnancy rate in IUD wearers was about 1.0 to 1.2 per 1000 woman-years. There appears to be a higher frequency of ectopic pregnancy with the progesterone-releasing IUD.

Thus, if a patient conceives with an IUD in place, ectopic pregnancy should be suspected, and patients who conceive while wearing any IUD device should have ultrasonography performed early in gestation.[145]

The effect of the IUD on increased development of ectopic pregnancy while it is in place appears to be temporary and does not persist after removal of the IUD.

Prematurity

Several studies indicate that the rate of preterm delivery is higher if an IUD remains in the uterus throughout gestation.[141, 142, 146] If a pregnant patient has an IUD in place and the device cannot be removed but the patient wants to continue her gestation, she should be warned of the increased risk of prematurity as well as that of spontaneous abortion and ectopic pregnancy. She should also be informed of the possible increased risk of septic abortion and advised to promptly report the first signs of pelvic pain or fever. There is no evidence that pregnancies with IUD's in utero are associated with an increased incidence of other obstetrical complications. There is also no evidence that prior use of an IUD results in a greater incidence of complications in pregnancies that occur after its removal.

Infection in the Nonpregnant IUD User

In the 1960's, despite great concern among clinicians that use of the IUD would markedly increase the incidence of salpingitis, or PID, there was little evidence that such an increase did occur. During that decade the IUD was inserted mainly into parous women, and the incidence of sexually transmitted disease was not as high as occurred subsequently. Aerobic and anaerobic cultures of homogenates of endometrial tissue were obtained transfundally from uteri removed by vaginal hysterectomy at various intervals after insertion of the loop IUD. During the first 24 hours the normally sterile endometrial cavity was consistently infected with bacteria. Nevertheless, in 80 per cent of cases, the women's natural defenses destroyed these bacteria within the next 24 hours. In a bacteriological study the endometrial cavity, the IUD, and the portion of the thread within the cavity were consistently found to be sterile when transfundal cultures were obtained more than 30 days after insertion.[147] These findings support the belief that the development of PID more than one month after insertion of the loop IUD is due to infection with a sexually transmitted pathogen and is unrelated to the presence of the device.

These findings agree with the incidence of clinically diagnosed PID found in a group of 23,977 mainly parous women who were wearing non–copper-bearing IUD's.[121] When PID rates were computed according to the duration of IUD use, the rates were highest in the first three weeks after insertion and then steadily diminished. The rates after the first month were in the range of 1 to 2.5 per 100 woman-years.[148]

The results of both these studies indicate that an IUD should not be inserted into a patient who may have recently been infected with gonococci or *Chlamydia*. The insertion of the device will transport these pathogens into the upper genital tract. If there is clinical suspicion of infectious endocervicitis, cultures should be obtained and the IUD insertion delayed until the results reveal that no pathogenic organisms are present. It does not appear to be cost-effective to administer systemic antibiotics routinely with every IUD insertion, but the insertion procedure should be as aseptic as possible.

After the introduction and widespread use of the shield device, particularly among nulliparous women (in whom IUD's were previously inserted only occasionally), several studies published in the late 1970's suggested that IUD use increased the relative risk of PID from three- to sevenfold.[149–153]

There are several problems with these studies. One is that uniform guidelines were not used for the diagnosis of PID (or salpingitis). Differences in diagnostic criteria may have increased the frequency of the diagnosis among IUD users. Patients with lower abdominal pain and only minimal or no elevation in temperature may have been given the diagnosis of PID more often when an IUD was in the uterus.

A second problem is the evidence that the use of OC's, condoms, and diaphragms provides protection against development of PID. The data from numerous studies indicate that the incidence of both febrile and nonfebrile PID is about one half as much in women using OC's and barrier methods as in women using no method of contraception.[154] Most sexually active women use contraception, mainly OC's, barriers, or the IUD. The increased risk of infection reported with the IUD is due in large part to the protective effect of the other contraceptives.

A third problem is that in most of the studies performed in the 1970's, a high percentage of IUD wearers were using the shield. This device was more likely than other types to have a causal relation to PID. Examination of the sheaths of the appendages of both new shields in their sterile packages and shields removed from patients showed that 9 per cent of the new shields and 34 per cent of the used shields had breaks in the sheath around the knot attaching it to the device. These breaks could allow bacteria to have continuous access from the vagina to the endometrial cavity, and thus increase the risk of upper genital tract infection.

Finally, none of these studies differentiated between episodes of PID developing in the first few months after IUD insertion (previously shown to be related to the insertion itself) and episodes developing later. In 1987 CDC (Centers for Disease Control) investigators reported results from a multicenter case control study of the relation of the IUD and PID. They found the overall risk of PID in IUD users versus noncontraceptive users to be 1.9.[155] The risk in shield users was 8.3; in other IUD users it was only 1.6. When the risk of PID in IUD users (other than shield users) was correlated with duration of use, it was found that a significantly increased risk of PID with the loop and copper 7 was present only during the first four months after insertion. Beyond four months of use there was no significantly increased risk in IUD users other than those with shields. These data provide additional evidence that aside from the insertion process, the IUD with monofilament tail strings does not itself alter the incidence of PID. Additional support for this statement is provided by results of a large WHO study of PID incidence in copper IUD users for seven years after insertion.[148] The risk of PID was increased only, the first three weeks after insertion, after which it remained constant (Fig. 123–8).[148] It was also reported that nulliparous women with a single sexual partner who had previously used an IUD had no increased risk of tubal infertility, whereas nulliparous women with multiple sexual partners who used an IUD did have an increased risk of tubal infertility.[156]

PID that occurs more than a few months after the inser-

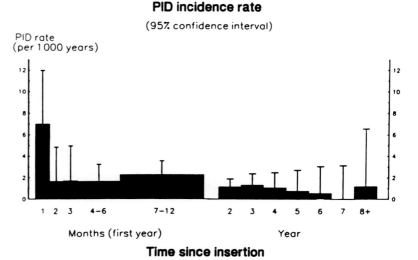

PID incidence rate

(95% confidence interval)

PID rate
(per 1000 years)

Months (first year)   Year

Time since insertion

FIGURE 123–8. Incidence rate was estimated by the number of PID cases and years of exposure in each time interval. Ninety-five per cent confidence intervals were calculated from the Poisson distribution. (From Farley MM, et al: Intrauterine devices and pelvic inflammatory disease: An international perspective. Lancet 339:785, 1992.)

tion of loop or copper devices is caused by a sexually transmitted disease and not related to the IUD.

The populations at high risk for PID include those with a prior history of PID, nulliparous women under age 25, and women with multiple sexual partners. The FDA has recommended that women with these characteristics be especially advised about the risk of developing PID during IUD use and the possibility of subsequent loss of fertility. They should be told to watch for the early symptoms of PID, so that treatment can be started before complications occur. These data, as well as those of two epidemiological studies showing an increased risk of tubal causes of infertility in nulliparous women who had used an IUD, indicate that the clinician should avoid using IUD's in nulliparous women who may want to conceive in the future. The increased risk of impairment of future fertility from PID in the first few months after IUD insertion as well as the possibility of ectopic pregnancy must be considered when deciding whether to use an IUD in a nulliparous woman.

Symptomatic PID usually can be successfully treated with antibiotics without removing the IUD until the patient becomes symptom-free. In patients with clinical evidence of a tubo-ovarian abscess or with a shield in place, the IUD should be removed only after a therapeutic serum level of appropriate parenteral antibiotics has been reached and preferably after a clinical response has been observed. An alternative method of contraception should be substituted in patients who develop PID with an IUD in place (or in those with a past history of PID).

There is evidence that IUD users may have an increased risk for colonizing actinomycosis organisms in the upper genital tract.[157] The relation of actinomycosis to PID is unclear because many women without IUD's have actinomycosis in their vaginas. If these organisms are identified on a routine annual cytological smear of IUD users, their existence should be confirmed by culture, since cytological diagnosis of actinomycosis is not precise. If the culture confirms their presence in the cervix, appropriate antimicrobial therapy should be used to eradicate the organisms, but the IUD does not have to be removed.

Overall Safety

Several long-term studies have indicated that the IUD is not associated with an increased incidence of endometrial or cervical carcinoma. Nevertheless, the IUD does produce morbidity that may result in hospitalization. The main causes of hospitalization among IUD users are complications of pregnancy, uterine perforation, and hemorrhage, as well as pelvic infection.[158] Despite the increased morbidity with IUD's, the incidence of these problems is low. IUD's are not being inserted in women at risk for developing PID, and physicians are aware of the potential complications associated with IUD's in pregnancy. The IUD is a particularly useful method of contraception for women who have completed their families and do not want permanent sterilization and have contraindications to or do not want to use OC's.[159]

REFERENCES

1. Mosher WD, Pratt WF: Contraceptive use in the United States, 1973–1988. Patient Educ Couns 16:163, 1990.
2. Trussell J, Hatcher RA, Cates W Jr, et al: Contraceptive failure in the United States: An update. Stud Fam Plann 21:51, 1990.
3. McIntyre SL, Higgins JE: Parity and use-effectiveness with the contraceptive sponge. Am J Obstet Gynecol 155:796, 1986.
4. Edelman DA, North BB: Updated pregnancy rates for the Today contraceptive sponge. Am J Obstet Gynecol 157:1164, 1987.
5. Faich G, Pearson K, Fleming D, et al: Toxic shock syndrome and the vaginal contraceptive sponge. JAMA 255:216–218, 1986.
6. Mills JL, Harley EE, Reed GF, et al: Are spermicides teratogenic? JAMA 248:2148, 1982.
7. Linn S, Schoenbaum SC, Monson RR, et al: Lack of association between contraceptive usage and congenital malformations in offspring. Am J Obstet Gynecol 147:923, 1983.
8. Louik C, Mitchell AA, Werler MM, et al: Maternal exposure to spermicides in relation to certain birth defects. N Engl J Med 317:474, 1987.
9. Fihn SD, Latham RH, Roberts P, et al: Association between diaphragm use and urinary tract infection. JAMA 254:240, 1986.
10. Cagen R: The cervical cap as a barrier contraceptive. Contraception 33:487, 1986.

11. Klitsch M: FDA approval ends cervical cap's marathon. Fam Plann Perspect 20:137, 1988.
12. Powell MG, Mears BJ, Deber RB, et al: Contraception with the cervical cap: Effectiveness, safety, continuity of use, and user satisfaction. Contraception 33:215, 1986.
13. Austin H, Louv WC, Alexander WJ: A case-control study of spermicides and gonorrhea. JAMA 251:2822–2824, 1984.
14. Jick H, Hanna MT, Stergachis A, et al: Vaginal spermicides and gonorrhea. JAMA 248:1619–1621, 1982.
15. Rosenberg MJ, Rojanapithayakron W, Feldblum PJ, Higgins JE: Effect of the contraceptive sponge on chlamydial infection, gonorrhea, and candidiasis. JAMA 257:2308–2312, 1987.
16. Hicks DR, Martin LS, Getchell JP, et al: Inactivation of HTLV-III/LAV-infected cultures of normal human lymphocytes by nonoxynol-9 in vitro. Lancet 2:1422–1423, 1985.
17. Conant MA, Spicer DW, Smith CD: Herpes simplex virus transmission: Condom studies. Sex Transm Dis 11:94, 1984.
18. Stone KM, Grimes DA, Magdar LA: Personal protection against sexually transmitted disease. Am J Obstet Gynecol 155:180, 1986.
19. Sennayake P, Kramer DG: Contraception and the etiology of pelvic inflammatory disease: New perspective. Am J Obstet Gynecol 138:852, 1980.
20. Celentano DD, Klassen AC, Weisman CS, Rosenshein NB: The role of contraceptive use in cervical cancer: The Maryland cervical cancer case-control study. Am J Epidemiol 126:592–604, 1987.
21. Klaus H: Natural family planning: A review. Obstet Gynecol Surv 37:128–150, 1982.
22. Liskin L, Fox G: Periodic abstinence: How well do new approaches work? Popul Rep [I] 9:33–71, 1981.
23. Medina JE, Cifuentes A, Abernathy JR, et al: Comparative evaluation of two methods of natural family planning in Columbia. Am J Obstet Gynecol 138:1142–1147, 1980.
24. Wade ME, McCarthy P, Abernathy JR, et al: A randomized prospective study of the use-effectiveness of two methods of natural family planning. Presented at the International Federation for Family Life Promotion Second International Congress, Navan, Ireland, September 24–October 1, 1980.
25. World Health Organization: A prospective multicentre trial of the ovulation method of natural family planning. II. The effectiveness phase. Fertil Steril 36:591–598, 1981.
26. World Health Organization: A prospective multicentre trial of the ovulation method of natural family planning. III. Characteristics of the menstrual cycle and of the fertile phase. Fertil Steril 40:773–778, 1983.
27. Brown JB, Blackwell LF, Billings JJ, et al: Natural family planning. Am J Obstet Gynecol 157:1082–1089, 1987.
28. Dorflinger LJ: Relative potency of progestins used in oral contraceptives. Contraception 31:557–570, 1985.
29. Delforge JP, Ferin J: Histometric study of two estrogens: Ethinylestradiol and its 3-methyl-ether derivative (mestranol); their comparative effect upon the growth of the human endometrium. Contraception 1:57, 1970.
30. Brenner PF, Mishell DR Jr, Stanczyk FX, et al: Serum levels of d-norgestrel, luteinizing hormone, follicle-stimulating hormone, estradiol, and progesterone in women during and following ingestion of combination oral contraceptives containing dl-norgestrel. Am J Obstet Gynecol 129:133, 1977.
31. Mishell DR Jr, Thorneycroft IH, Nakamura RM, et al: Serum estradiol levels in women receiving combination oral contraceptive steroids. Am J Obstet Gynecol 114:923, 1972.
32. Kastin AJ, Schally AV, Gaul C, et al: Administration of LH-releasing hormone to selected subjects. Am J Obstet Gynecol 108:177, 1970.
33. Thomas K, Donnez J, Ferin J: LH and FSH releasing potency of the synthetic decapeptide p-Glu-His-Trp-Ser-Tyr-Gly-Seu-Arg-Pro-Gly-NH$_2$ in human beings. Contraception 6:55, 1972.
34. Robyn C, Schondorf H, Jurgensen O, et al: Oral contraception can decrease the pituitary capacity to release gonadotropins in response to synthetic LH-releasing hormone. Arch Gynecol 216:73, 1974.
35. Becker H, Kleissel HP, Reuter A, et al: Die beeinflussbarkeit der gonadotropinabsonderung durch den synthesisierten LH-preleasingfaktor unter der mekikation eines ovulations-blockers. Klin Wochenschr 51:759, 1973.
36. Krog W, Aktories K, Jurgenson O, et al: Contrasting effects of combined and sequential oral contraceptives on LH-RH-stimulated release, of LH and FSH as compared to minipills. Acta Endocrinol 192S:21, 1975.
37. Bracken MB, Vita K: Frequency of non-hormonal contraception around conception and association with congenital malformations in offspring. Am J Epidemiol 117:281, 1983.
38. Strom BL, Tamragouri RN, Morse ML, et al: Oral contraceptives and other risk factors for gallbladder disease. Clin Pharmacol Ther 39:335–341, 1986.
39. Rose DP, Adams PW: Oral contraceptives and tryptophan metabolism: Effects of oestrogen in low dose combined with a progestagen and of a low-dose progestagen (megestrol acetate) given alone. J Clin Pathol 25:252, 1972.
40. Ditkoff EC, Crary WG, Cristo M, Lobo RA: Estrogen improves psychological function in asymptomatic postmenopausal women. Obstet Gynecol 78:991, 1991.
41. Myers LA, Dixen J, Morrissette D, et al: Effects of estrogen, androgen, and progestin on sexual psychophysiology and behavior in postmenopausal women. J Clin Endocrin Metab 70:1124–1131, 1990.
42. Meade TW: Oral contraceptives, clotting factors, and thrombosis. Am J Obstet Gynecol 142:758, 1982.
43. Meade TW, Greenberg G, Thompson SG: Progestogens and cardiovascular reactions associated with oral contraceptives and a comparison of the safety of 50- and 30-µg estrogen preparations. Br Med J 280:1157–1161, 1980.
44. Mann JI: Progestogens in cardiovascular disease: An introduction to the epidemiologic data. Am J Obstet Gynecol 142:752–757, 1982.
45. Wilson ESB, Cruickshank J, McMaster M, et al: A prospective controlled study of the effect on blood pressure of contraceptive preparations containing different types and dosages of progestogen. Br J Obstet Gynaecol 91:1254, 1984.
46. Kalkhoff RK: Relative sensitivity of postpartum gestational diabetic women to oral contraceptive agents and other metabolic stress. Diabetes Care 3:421–424, 1985.
47. Perlman JA, Russell-Briefel R, Ezzati T, Lieberknecht G: Oral glucose tolerance and the potency of contraceptive progestins. J Chronic Dis 38:857–864, 1985.
48. Spellacy W: Carbohydrate metabolism during treatment with estrogen, progestogen, and low-dose oral contraceptives. Am J Obstet Gynecol 142:732–734, 1982.
49. Van der Vange N, Kloosterboer HJ, Haspels AA: Effect of seven low-dose combined oral contraceptive preparations on carbohydrate metabolism. Am J Obstet Gynecol 156:918–922, 1987.
50. Kung AW, Ma JT, Wong VC, et al: Glucose and lipid metabolism with triphasic oral contraceptives in women with history of gestational diabetes. Contraception 35:257–269, 1987.
51. Luyckx AS, Gaspard UJ, Romus MA, et al: Carbohydrate metabolism in women with history of gestational diabetes who used oral contraceptives. Fertil Steril 45:635, 1986.
52. Skouby SO, Kuh C, Misted-Pedersen L, et al: Triphasic oral contraception: Metabolic effects in normal women and those with previous gestational diabetes. Am J Obstet Gynecol 153:495–500, 1985.
53. Hannaford PC, Kay CR (Royal College of General Practitioners): Oral contraceptives and diabetes mellitus. Br Med J 299:1315–1316, 1989.
54. Kjos SL, Shoupe D, Douham S, et al: Effect of low-dose oral contraceptives on carbohydrate and lipid metabolism in women with recurrent gestational diabetes: Results of a controlled randomized prospective study. Am J Obstet Gynecol 163:1822, 1990.
55. Layde PM, Ory HW, Schlesselman JJ: The risk of myocardial infarction in former users of oral contraceptives. Fam Plann Perspect 14:78, 1982.
56. Stampfer MJ, Willett WC, Colditz GA, et al: A prospective study of past use of oral contraceptive agents and risk of cardiovascular diseases. N Engl J M Med 3329:1313, 1988.
57. Adams MR, Clarkson TB, Koritnik DR, Nash HA: Contraceptive steroids and coronary artery atherosclerosis in cynomolgus macaques. Fertil Steril 47:1010, 1987.
58. Clarkson TB, Shively CA, Morgan TM, et al: Oral contraceptives and coronary artery atherosclerosis of cynomolgus monkeys. Obstet Gynecol 47:1010, 1990.
59. Royal College of General Practitioners' Oral Contraceptive Study: Further analysis of mortality in oral contraceptive users: Royal College of General Practitioners' Oral Contraception Study. Lancet 1:541–546, 1981.
60. Croft P, Hannaford PC: Risk factors for acute myocardial infarction in women: Evidence from the Royal College of General Practitioners' oral contraceptive study. Br Med J 298:165, 1989.
61. Mileikowsky GN, Nadler JL, Huey F, et al: Evidence that smoking alters prostacyclin formation and platelet aggregation in women who use oral contraceptives. Am J Obstet Gynecol 159:1547, 1988.
62. Thorogood M, Mann J, Murphy M, Vessey M: Is oral contraceptive use still associated with an increased risk of fatal myocardial infarction? Report of a case-control study. Br J Obstet Gynaecol 98:1245–1253, 1991.

63. Porter JB, Hunter JR, Jick H, et al: Oral contraceptives and nonfatal vascular disease. Obstet Gynecol 66:1, 1985.
64. Rosenberg L, Palmer JR, Lesko SM, et al: Oral contraceptives use and the risk of myocardial infarction. Am J Epidemiol 131:1009, 1990.
65. Bracken MB, Hellenbrand KG, Holford TR: Conception delay after oral contraceptive use: The effect of estrogen dose. Fertil Steril 53:21, 1990.
66. Rothman KJ, Luik C: Oral contraceptives and birth defects. N Engl J Med 299:522, 1978.
67. Royal College of General Practitioners' Oral Contraceptive Study: The outcome of pregnancy in former oral contraceptive users. Br J Obstet Gynaecol 83:608, 1976.
68. Vessey MP, Meisler L, Flavel R, et al: Outcome of pregnancy in women using different methods of contraception. Br J Obstet Gynaecol 86:548, 1979.
69. Bracken MB: Oral contraception and congenital malformations of offspring: A review and meta-analysis of the prospective studies. Obstet Gynecol 76:552–557, 1990.
70. Prentice RL, Thomas DB: On the epidemiology of oral contraceptives and disease. Adv Cancer Res 49:285, 1987.
71. Schlesselman JJ: Cancer of the breast and reproductive tract in relation to use of oral contraceptives. Contraception 40:1, 1989.
72. Stadel BV, Lai S, Schlesselmann JJ, et al: Oral contraceptives and premenopausal breast cancer in nulliparous women. Contraception 38:287, 1988.
73. Stadel BV, Schlesselmann JJ, Murray PA: Oral contraceptives and breast cancer. Lancet 1:1257, 1989.
74. Kay CR, Hannaford PC: Breast cancer and the pill—a further report from the Royal College of General Practitioners' Oral Contraception Study. Br J Cancer 58:676, 1988.
75. UK National Case Control Study Group: Oral contraceptive use and breast cancer risk in young women. Lancet 1:973, 1989.
76. Wingo PA, Lee NC, Ory HW, et al: Age-specific differences in the relationship between oral contraceptive use and breast cancer. Obstet Gynecol 78:161–170, 1991.
77. Centers for Disease Control: Long-term oral contraceptive use and the risk of breast cancer. JAMA 249:1591–1595, 1983.
78. Centers for Disease Control: Combination oral contraceptive use and risk of endometrial cancer. JAMA 257:796–800, 1987.
79. The Cancer and Steroid Hormone Study of the Centers for Disease Control and the National Institute of Child Health and Human Development: The reduction in risk of ovarian cancer associated with oral-contraceptive use. N Engl J Med 316:650–655, 1987.
80. Vessey M, Metcalfe A, Wells C, et al: Ovarian neoplasma, functional ovarian cysts, and oral contraceptives. Br Med J 294:1518–1520, 1987.
81. World Health Organization: Combined oral contraceptives and liver cancer. Int J Cancer 43:254, 1989.
82. Pituitary Adenoma Study Group: Pituitary adenomas and oral contraceptives: A multicenter case-control study. Fertil Steril 39:753–760, 1983.
83. Vessey MP, Villard-Mackintosh L, McPheson K, et al: Mortality among oral contraceptive users: 20 year follow up to women in a cohort study. Br Med J 299:1487, 1989.
84. Perez A, Vela P, Masnick GS, et al: First ovulation after childbirth: The effect of breast-feeding. Am J Obstet Gynecol 114:1041, 1972.
85. World Health Organization Task Force on Oral Contraceptives: Effects of hormonal contraceptives on milk volume and infant growth. Contraception 30:505, 1984.
86. Lonnerdel B, Forsum E, Hambraeus L: Effect of oral contraceptives on composition and volume of breast milk. Am J Clin Nutr 33:816, 1980.
87. World Health Organization Task Force on Oral Contraceptives: A randomized double-blind study of two combined and two progestogen-only oral contraceptives. Contraception 25:243, 1982.
88. Nilsson S, Mellbin T, Hofvander Y, et al: Long-term follow-up of children breast-fed by mothers using oral contraceptives. Contraception 34:443, 1986.
89. Field B, Cherry L, Hepner G: Inhibition of hepatic drug metabolism by norethisterone. Clin Pharmacol Ther 25:196, 1979.
90. Back DJ, Breckenridge AM, Crawford FE, et al: The effects of rifampicin on the pharmacokinetics of ethinylestradiol in women. Contraception 21:134, 1980.
91. Diamond MP, Greene JW, Thompson JM, et al: Interaction of anticonvulsants and oral contraceptives in epileptic adolescents. Contraception 31:623–632, 1985.
92. Hefnawi F, Saleh AA, Kandil O, et al: Blood loss with IUDs. In Hefnawi F, Segal SJ (eds): Analysis of Intrauterine Contraception. Amsterdam, Elsevier, 1975, p 373.
93. Oral Contraceptives and Health: An Interim Report from the Oral Contraceptive Study of the Royal College of General Practitioners. New York: Pitman Publishing, 1974.
94. Brinton LA, Vessey MP, Flavel R, et al: Risk factors for benign breast disease. Am J Epidemiol 113:203, 1981.
95. Warner P, Bancroft J: Mood, sexuality, oral contraceptives and the menstrual cycle. J Psychosom Res 32:417, 1988.
96. Ory HW: Functional ovarian cysts and oral contraceptives. JAMA 228:68, 1974.
97. Grimes DA, Hughes JM: Use of multiphasic oral contraceptives and hospitalizations of women with functional ovarian cysts in the United States. Obstet Gynecol 73:1037, 1989.
98. Hazes JMW, Dijkmans BAC, Vandenbroucke JP, et al: Reduction of the risk of rheumatoid arthritis among women who take oral contraceptives. Arthritis Rheum 33:173–179, 1990.
99. Ryden G, Fahraeus L, Molin L, et al: Do contraceptives influence the incidence of acute pelvic inflammatory disease in women with gonorrhea? Contraception 20:1459, 1979.
100. Wolner-Hanssen P, Svensson L, Mardh P-A, et al: Laparoscopic findings and contraceptive use in women with signs and symptoms suggestive of acute salpingitis. Obstet Gynecol 66:233, 1985.
101. World Health Organization Expanded Programme of Research, Development and Research Training in Human Reproduction Task Force on Long-Acting Systemic Agents for the Regulation of Fertility: Multinational comparative clinical evaluation of two long-acting injectable contraceptive steroids: Norethisterone enanthate and medroxyprogesterone acetate. I. Use-effectiveness. Contraception 15:513–533, 1977.
102. Ortiz A, Hiroi M, Stanczyk FZ, et al: Serum medroxyprogesterone acetate (MPA) concentrations and ovarian function following intramuscular injection of depo-MPA. J Clin Endocrinol Metab 44:32, 1977.
103. Mishell DR Jr, Kharma KM, Thorneycroft IH, et al: Estrogenic activity in women receiving an injectable progestagen for contraception. Am J Obstet Gynecol 113:372, 1972.
104. Schwallie PC, Assenzo JR: Contraceptive use—efficacy study utilizing medroxyprogesterone acetate administered as an intramuscular injection once every 90 days. Fertil Steril 24:331, 1973.
105. Schwallie PC, Assenzo JR: The effect of depomedroxyprogesterone acetate on pituitary and ovarian function, and the return of fertility following its discontinuation: A review. Contraception 10:181, 1974.
106. Deslypere JP, Thiery M, Vermeulen A: Effect of long-term hormonal contraception on plasma lipids. Contraception 31:633, 1985.
107. The WHO Collaborative Study of Neoplasia and Steroid Contraceptives: Depot-medroxyprogesterone acetate (DMPA) and risk of invasive squamous cell cervical cancer. Contraception 45:299–312, 1992.
108. WHO Collaborative Study of Neoplasia and Steroid Contraceptives: Breast cancer and depot-medroxyprogesterone acetate: A multinational study. Lancet 338:833–838, 1991.
109. Rosenfield A, Maine D, Rochat R, et al: The Food and Drug Administration and medroxyprogesterone acetate. JAMA 249:2922, 1983.
110. Moore DE, Ropyu S, Stanczyk FZ, et al: Bleeding and serum d-norgestrel, estradiol, and progesterone patterns in women using d-norgestrel subdermal polysiloxane capsules for contraception. Contraception 17:315, 1978.
111. Brache V, Alvarez-Sanchez F, Faundes A, et al: Ovarian endocrine function through 5 years of continuous treatment with Norplant ± subdermal contraceptive implants. Contraception 41:169, 1990.
112. Shoupe D, Horenstein J, Mishell DR Jr, et al: Characteristics of ovarian follicular development in Norplant users. Fertil Steril 55:766–770, 1991.
113. Brache V, Faundes A, Johansson E, et al: Anovulation, inadequate luteal phase and poor sperm penetration in cervical mucus during prolonged use of Norplant® implants. Contraception 31:261, 1985.
114. Sivin I: International experience with Norplant® and Norplant®-2. Stud Fam Plann 19:81, 1988.
115. Shoupe D, Mishell DR Jr, Bopp BL, Fielding M: The significance of bleeding patterns in Norplant implant users. Obstet Gynecol 77:256–260, 1991.
116. Darney PD, Atkinson E, Tanner S, et al: Acceptance and perceptions of Norplant® among users in San Francisco, USA. Stud Fam Plann 21:152–160, 1990.
117. Fasoli M, Parazzini F, Cecchetti G, et al: Post-coital contraception: An overview of published studies. Contraception 39:459, 1989.
118. Healy DL, Bauilieu EE, Hodgen GD: Induction of menstruation by an antiprogesterone steroid (RU 486) in primates; site of action, dose-response relationships, and hormonal effects. Fertil Steril 40:253, 1983.

119. Grimes DA, Mishell DR Jr, Shoupe D, Lacarra M: Early abortion with a single dose of the antiprogestin RU 486. Am J Obstet Gynecol 158:1307–1312, 1988.

120. Couzinet B, LeStrat N, Ulmann A, et al: Termination of early pregnancy by the progesterone antagonist RU 486 (mifepristone). N Engl J Med 315:1565, 1986.

121. Tietze C, Lewit S: Evaluation of intrauterine devices: Ninth progress report of the Cooperative Statistical Program. Stud Fam Plann 1:55, 1970.

122. Moyer DL, Mishell DR Jr: Reactions of human endometrium to the intrauterine foreign body. II. Long-term effects on the endometrial histology and cytology. Am J Obstet Gynecol 111:66, 1971.

123. Tredway DR, Umezaki CU, Mishell DR Jr: Effect of intrauterine devices on sperm transport in the human being: Preliminary report. Am J Obstet Gynecol 123:734, 1975.

124. Alvarez F, Guiloff E, Brache V, et al: New insights on the mode of action of intrauterine contraceptive devices in women. Fertil Steril 49:768, 1988.

125. Vessey M, Lawless M, McPherson K: Fertility after stopping use of intrauterine contraceptive device. Br Med J 286:106, 1983.

126. Sivin I, Mahgoub SE, McCarthy T, et al: Long-term contraception with the levorgestrel 20 mcg/day and the copper T 380Ag intrauterine devices; a five-year randomized study. Contraception 42:361, 1990.

127. White MK, Ory HW, Rooks JB, et al: Intrauterine device termination rates and the menstrual cycle day of insertion. Obstet Gynecol 55:220, 1980.

128. Mishell DR Jr, Roy S: Copper intrauterine contraceptive device event rates following insertion 4 to 8 weeks postpartum. Am J Obstet Gynecol 142:29, 1982.

129. Chi I-C, Potts M, Wilkins LR, et al: Performance of the copper T-380A intrauterine device in breastfeeding women. Contraception 39:603, 1989.

130. Guillebaud J, Bonnard J, Morehead J, et al: Longer though lighter menstrual and intermenstrual bleeding with copper as compared to inert intrauterine devices. Br J Obstet Gynaecol 85:707, 1978.

131. Guillebaud J, Bonnar J, Morehead J, et al: Menstrual blood-loss with intrauterine devices. Lancet 1:387, 1975.

132. Hefnawi F, Askalani H, Zaki KL: Menstrual blood loss with copper intrauterine devices. Contraception 9:133, 1976.

133. Larsson B, Hamberger L, Rybo G: Influence of copper intrauterine devices (Cu-7-IUD) on the menstrual blood-loss. Acta Obstet Gynecol Scand 54:315, 1975.

134. Liedholm P, Rybo G, Sjoberg N-O, et al: Copper IUD—influence on menstrual blood loss and iron deficiency. Contraception 12:317, 1975.

135. Rybo G: The IUD and endometrial bleeding. J Reprod Med 20:175, 1978.

136. Guillebaud J, Barnett MD, Gordon YB: Plasma ferritin levels as an index of iron deficiency in women using intrauterine devices. Br J Obstet Gynaecol 86:51, 1979.

137. Heikkila M, Nylander P, Luukkainen T: Body iron stores and patterns of bleeding after insertion of a levonorgestrel- or a copper-releasing intrauterine contraceptive device. Contraception 26:465, 1982.

138. Piedras J, Corcova MS, Perez-Toral MC, et al: Predictive value of serum ferritin in anemia development after insertion of T Cu 220 intrauterine device. Contraception 27:289, 1983.

139. Anderson ABM, Haynes PJ, Guillebaud J, et al: Reduction of menstrual blood loss by prostaglandin synthetase inhibitors. Lancet 1:774, 1976.

140. Mishell Dr Jr: Current concepts in contraception. Clin Obstet Gynecol 17:35, 1974.

141. Tatum HJ, Schmidt FH, Jain AK: Management and outcome of pregnancies associated with the copper T intrauterine contraceptive device. Am J Obstet Gynecol 126:869, 1976.

142. Vessey MP, Johnson B, Doll R, et al: Outcome of pregnancy in women using an intrauterine device. Lancet 1:495, 1974.

143. Lewit SL: Outcome of pregnancies with intrauterine devices. Contraception 2:47, 1970.

144. Christian CD: Maternal deaths associated with an intrauterine device. Am J Obstet Gynecol 119:441, 1974.

145. Sivin I: Copper T IUD use and ectopic pregnancy rates in the United States. Contraception 19:151, 1974.

146. Alvior GT Jr: Pregnancy outcome with removal of intrauterine device. Obstet Gynecol 41:894, 1973.

147. Mishell DR Jr, Bell JH, Good RG, et al: The intrauterine device: A bacteriologic study of the endometrial cavity. Am J Obstet Gynecol 96:119, 1966.

148. Farley TMM, Rosenberg MJ, Rowe PJ, et al: Intrauterine devices and pelvic inflammatory disease: An international perspective. Lancet 339:785–788, 1992.

149. Vessey MP, Yeates D, Flavel R, et al: Pelvic inflammatory disease and the intrauterine device: Findings in a large cohort study. Br Med J 282:855, 1981.

150. Faulkner WL, Ory HW: Intrauterine devices and acute pelvic inflammatory disease. JAMA 235:1851, 1976.

151. Westrom L, Bengtsson LP, Mordh PA: The risk of pelvic inflammatory disease in women using intrauterine contraceptive devices as compared to non-users. Lancet 2:21, 1976.

152. Ory HW: A review of the association between intrauterine devices and acute pelvic inflammatory disease. J Reprod Med 20:200, 1978.

153. Eschenbach DA, Harnisch JP, Holmes KK: Pathogenesis of acute pelvic inflammatory disease: Role of contraception and other risk factors. Am J Obstet Gynecol 128:838, 1977.

154. Senanayake P, Kramer DG: Contraception and the etiology of pelvic inflammatory disease: New perspectives. Am J Obstet Gynecol 138:852, 1980.

155. Lee NC, Rubin GL, Ory HW, Burkman RT: Type of intrauterine device and the risk of pelvic inflammatory disease. Obstet Gynecol 62:1, 1983.

156. Cramer DW, Goldman MB, Schiff I, et al: The relationship of tubal infertility to barrier method and oral contraceptive use. JAMA 257:2446, 1987.

157. Mishell DR Jr: Assessing the intrauterine device. Fam Plann Perspect 7:103, 1975.

158. Kahn HS, Tyler CW, Jr: IUD-related hospitalizations: United States and Puerto Rico, 1973. JAMA 234:53, 1975.

159. Jain AK: Safety and effectiveness of intrauterine devices. Contraception 11:243, 1975.

PART IX

ENDOCRINOLOGY OF PREGNANCY

124

Placental Hormones

JEROME F. STRAUSS, III
MATS GÅFVELS
BARRY F. KING

The human placenta and the fetal membranes have a remarkably diverse secretory repertoire, surpassing that of any of the other endocrine glands. These extra-embryonic tissues elaborate protein, glycoprotein, and steroid hormones, growth factors, and cytokines that control the local environment of the fetus and regulate metabolic activities of maternal and fetal tissues. The endometrium also assumes important endocrine functions during gestation. Its secretory products include hormones (e.g., prolactin, relaxin), cytokines (e.g., colony-stimulating factor I), growth factors (e.g., insulin-like growth factor I [IGF-I]), epidermal growth factor (EGF) and fibroblast growth factor (FGF), and growth factor binding proteins (e.g., IGF-binding proteins). Thus the endocrine changes that take place in the maternal organism, intra-uterine compartment, and

fetus reflect, in part, the influence of substances derived from the uterus, placenta, and fetal membranes.

Many of the hormones that the placenta produces are identical or similar to hormones of the pituitary, hypothalamus, and gonads. The placenta synthesizes the hypothalamic hormones, gonadotropin-releasing hormone (GnRH), corticotropin-releasing hormone (CRH), growth hormone–releasing hormone (GRH), a thyrotropin-releasing hormone, somatostatin, and neuropeptide Y. It also produces chorionic gonadotropin (CG), which is structurally and functionally related to luteinizing hormone (LH) and several somatotropin-like hormones, including chorionic somatomammotropin (CS) and variant growth hormones. Secretion of proopiomelanocortin-derived peptides by placental cells and a placental thyrotropin distinct from CG have been reported. The gonadal steroid and protein hormones, estrogen, progesterone, and inhibin/activin, respectively, are also synthesized by the placenta.

Receptors for many of the hormones that the placenta produces are present on trophoblast cells. Hence placental hormones are likely to have key roles in controlling the growth and function of the placenta, as well as affecting maternal organs and the fetus proper.

A detailed review of all the hormones and factors that the human placenta produces is well beyond the scope of this chapter. As noted above, many of these hormones are produced by other organs. We have selected for discussion those hormones that are unique to the trophoblast or whose synthesis and/or regulation in the placenta are novel.

FORMATION AND STRUCTURE OF THE HUMAN PLACENTA

The human zygote undergoes a series of cell divisions as it passes down the oviduct, eventually forming a cluster of cells (the morula) still surrounded by the zona pellucida.[1] It is probably as a morula that the developing embryo enters the uterus, about 7.5 days after ovulation. While in the uterus the morula undergoes transformation into the blastocyst. This involves the flattening of the outer layer of cells and the accumulation of fluid in the blastocyst cavity. The outer layer of the blastocyst is a single layer of epithelial cells, the trophoblast. Internal to the trophoblast layer is an eccentrically placed small cluster of cells, the inner (or embryonic) cell mass. Generally speaking, the trophoblast becomes the main functional tissue of the placenta, whereas the inner cell mass gives rise to the embryo proper.

Implantation

The process of implantation involves the adherence of the blastocyst to the uterine luminal epithelium, the penetration of the epithelium, and invasion into the underlying uterine stroma.[2] At the time of blastocyst formation the embryo is still surrounded by the zona pellucida. The zona is soon lost, however, allowing the trophoblast to come in contact with and adhere to the uterine epithelium. This probably occurs about seven to nine days after ovulation. Initially, the trophoblast is a layer of mononucleated cytotrophoblast, but at about the time of attachment to the uterine lining some of these cytotrophoblast cells fuse to form syncytiotrophoblast. The syncytiotrophoblast rapidly penetrates between cells of the uterine epithelium and both cytotrophoblast and syncytiotrophoblast invade deeper into the endometrium. At these early stages there is relatively little destruction of maternal tissues by the trophoblast.[3, 4] Our understanding of many of these early events in human implantation is hampered by the lack of suitable material for study. One of the earliest human implantation sites available for morphological study is estimated to be about 7.5 days after ovulation. In this specimen a large mass of syncytiotrophoblast has already invaded the uterine stroma.

As the trophoblast invades the endometrium it encoun-

ters and surrounds uterine capillaries, and the capillary endothelium is lost (Fig. 124–1). Spaces, or lacunae, form within the trophoblast, and soon the confluence of the invaded vessels with the lacunae gives rise to a system of blood-filled spaces lined by syncytiotrophoblast. The embryo invades deeper and the endometrium grows over the entire conceptus. The endometrial stroma that surrounds the conceptus is referred to as decidua; that which grows over the invaded blastocyst is referred to as the decidua capsularis; and that beneath the conceptus is called the decidua basalis.

Formation of the Placental Villi

The next important stage of placental development involves the formation of placental villi.[2] In the stage described earlier, irregular blood-filled lacunae are lined by syncytiotrophoblast. Beneath the syncytium is a layer of cytotrophoblast that in turn comes to be associated with a layer of extra-mbryonic mesoderm. Trophoblast and its associated mesoderm are referred to as chorion, and with the formation of this layer sometimes the blastocyst is referred to as the chorionic vesicle. At about 12 days of gestation certain areas of cytotrophoblast begin to proliferate rapidly, giving rise to columns of cells that radiate outward around the conceptus (see Fig. 124–1). These columns, covered by a layer of syncytiotrophoblast, are termed primary villi. This is followed shortly by the invasion of extraembryonic mesenchyme into the column of cytotrophoblast; development of a stromal core converts the primary villi to secondary villi. Almost immediately embryonic capillaries form in the mesenchyme, after which the villi are called *tertiary villi*. Although this is an important developmental process, it is well to remember that essentially all villi of the definitive placenta are vascularized and, therefore, are tertiary villi. With development of villi the blood-filled lacunae are transformed into the intervillous

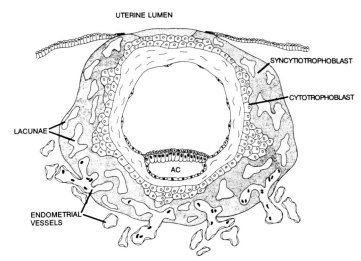

FIGURE 124–1. Human implantation site at about 12 days of gestation showing the blastocyst embedded in the endometrium. Syncytiotrophoblast (*stippled*) has invaded and surrounded some endometrial capillaries, and there is continuity between some capillaries and lacunae. Columns of cytotrophoblast have begun to grow outwardly in a few areas (primary villi). AC, amniotic cavity.

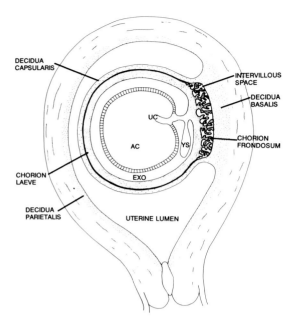

FIGURE 124–2. Diagram of the placenta and fetal membranes in early gestation. The villi adjacent to the decidua basalis are well developed (chorion frondosum), whereas elsewhere the villi have regressed (chorion laeve). The chorion laeve is made up of trophoblast *(black)* and mesoderm *(stippled)*; at this stage it is covered by the decidua capsularis but has not yet fused with the decidua parietalis. AC, amniotic cavity; UC, umbilical cord; YS, yolk sac; EXO, exocoelom.

spaces. As these changes are occurring in the villous core, continued cytotrophoblastic proliferation and migration eventually break through the peripheral syncytiotrophoblast, and these cells spread along the endometrium to form the cytotrophoblastic shell.[1, 3] The shell surrounds the developing conceptus, interrupted only where maternal blood enters or exits the developing placenta. Initially, villi develop around the entire circumference of the chorionic vesicle. As the conceptus grows and protrudes into the uterine cavity the distribution of villi begins to change. Those villi adjacent to the well-developed blood supply of the decidua basalis thrive and arborize; sometimes this region is referred to as the chorion frondosum, or leafy chorion (Fig. 124–2). It becomes discoidal in shape and forms the definitive placenta. Those villi that are associated with the decidua capsularis experience an increasingly restrictive maternal blood supply and become atrophic. This region thus evolves into the nonvillous chorion (smooth chorion), or chorion laeve. Although this layer becomes avascular, as the name indicates, it still contains trophoblast (mostly cytotrophoblast) and mesoderm (see Fig. 124–2).

From this stage onward a number of major landmarks of the placenta can be identified. The fetal-facing boundary of the placenta is called the chorionic plate. It consists of a trophoblastic lining next to the intervillous space and a thick layer of connective tissue in which course branches of the umbilical vessels. Stem villi arise from the chorionic plate. They are of large diameter and contain considerable connective tissue as well as branches of arteries and veins. Those villi that maintain their connection to the trophoblastic shell and endometrium are referred to as anchoring villi. During early gestation the peripheral extensions of

the anchoring villi, consisting of solid cytotrophoblastic cores (i.e., not invaded by fetal mesenchyme), are referred to as the cell columns. During later gestation the region of contact of trophoblast with the endometrium commonly is called the basal plate. Between the stem villi arising from the chorionic plate and the anchoring villi inserting into the basal plate, the villi undergo repeated branching to give rise eventually to numerous, small free or terminal villi.[5] These trophoblast-covered projections contain fetal capillaries and are surrounded by maternal blood in the intervillous space. Because of their numbers and size, they are considered to be of primary importance in placental function.

Structure of the Placental Villi

The terminal villi of the definitive placenta are thought to be the major site of maternal-fetal transport activities as well as the site of synthesis of many hormones.[5, 6] Therefore, we briefly describe the major components. The outermost covering of the terminal villi, bordering the intervillous space, is the syncytiotrophoblast (Fig. 124–3).[3, 4] This is a multinucleated polarized epithelium, and because it is a syncytium, it has apical and basal cell membranes but no lateral cell membranes. The surface area of the syncytiotrophoblast is enormous. The villous surface area near term is estimated to be more than 12 m²; this is further amplified many-fold by the presence of microvilli (brush border) on its apical surface. The ultrastructural features of syncytiotrophoblast include abundant cisternae of rough

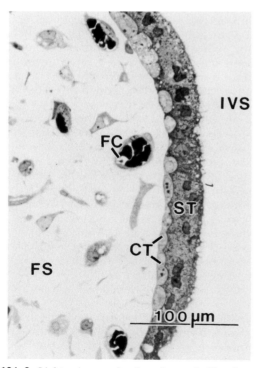

FIGURE 124–3. Light micrograph of a placental villus from the first trimester showing outer layer of syncytiotrophoblast (ST) bordering the intervillous space (IVS); a nearly complete layer of cytotrophoblast (CT) lies beneath the ST. The villous core contains fetal stroma (FS) and capillaries (FC).

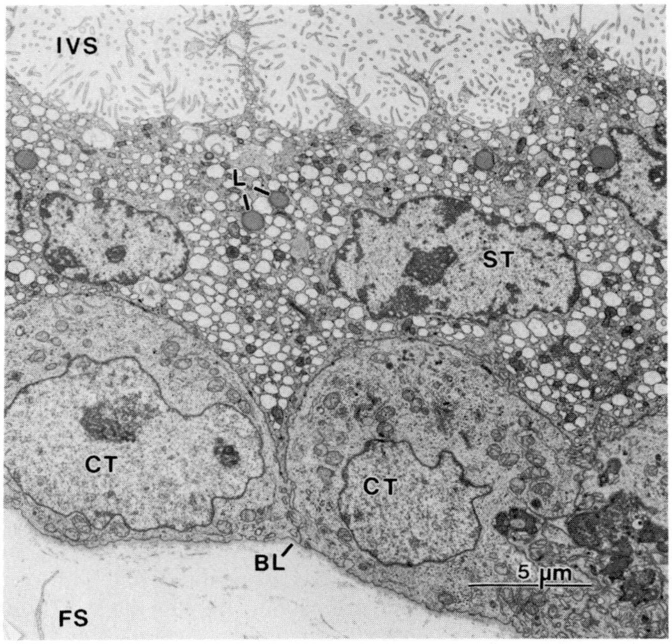

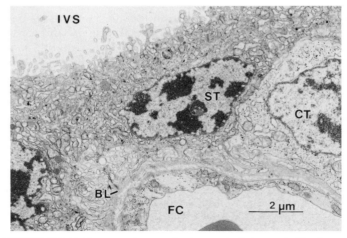

FIGURE 124–4. Electron micrograph of a first-trimester placental villus. The syncytiotrophoblast (ST) has a brush border adjacent to the intervillous space (IVS). The ST cytoplasm contains abundant rough endoplasmic reticulum and some lipid droplets (L). Underlying cytotrophoblast cells (CT) are less electron-dense and contain less endoplasmic reticulum and a few mitochondria. Trophoblast is separated from the underlying fetal stroma (FS) by a basal lamina (BL).

endoplasmic reticulum, a well-developed Golgi apparatus, and numerous mitochondria (Figs. 124–4 and 124–5).[7, 8] These are typical characteristics of cells that are engaged in the synthesis of proteins and glycoproteins. Other ultrastructural features include the presence of coated pits and vesicles and multivesicular bodies; these are undoubtedly related to the endocytic activities of syncytiotrophoblast.

Beneath the villous syncytiotrophoblast is a layer of mononuclear cytotrophoblast (Langhans' cells). This layer is nearly continuous in first-trimester villi (see Fig. 124–3) but reduced to scattered cells in the term placenta (see Fig. 124–5). Despite this apparent reduction in number, millions of cytotrophoblast cells can be isolated from term placentas and in fact are the starting material for many in vitro studies of trophoblast function. Syncytiotrophoblast and cytotrophoblast adhere to each other by means of desmosomes and the cell adhesion molecule E-cadherin.[9]

The cytotrophoblasts show varying degrees of cytoplasmic differentiation, ranging from a simple cytoplasm that contains few mitochondria, sparse endoplasmic reticulum, and numerous polyribosomes that are characteristic of proliferating immature cytotrophoblasts to cytoplasmic features similar to those of syncytiotrophoblast.[3, 4, 7, 8, 10] The latter cells are ready to fuse into the overlying syncytium. Thus the differentiation of cytotrophoblasts in the villi appears to be a continuum, with the cells progressing toward the terminal state of morphological and functional differentiation, syncytiotrophoblast formation. The factors that control this differentiation process have not been elucidated. It appears, however, that cAMP plays a key role, in that many of the genes expressed in the syncytiotrophoblast that encode hormones or hormone-synthesizing enzymes can be induced in cytotrophoblast by agents that stimulate adenylyl cyclase or cAMP analogues.[11]

The trophoblast cells of the villi are adherent to a basement membrane that also serves to separate the trophoblast from the elements of the stromal core (see Figs. 124–4 and 124–5). The basement membrane contains typical constituents, including type IV collagen and laminin.[2] Unlike some other basement membranes, it is apparently permeable to relatively large molecules (e.g., IgG). The villous stroma contains various cell types, the most important of which are the fibroblast-like mesenchymal cells, the fetal macrophages (Hofbauer cells), and the endothelial cells of the fetal vessels (see Fig. 124–3). Many of the functions of these cells remain to be elucidated. The mesenchymal cells undoubtedly produce many of the extracellular matrix components of the villous core. The latter include many types of collagen, laminin, fibronectin, and glycosaminoglycans. Hofbauer cells have numerous macrophage-associated functions, including phagocytosis and secretory activities. Endothelial cells may have some role in limiting placental permeability. The villous stroma lacks nerves and lymphatics.

Extravillous Trophoblast

Some trophoblast does not become involved in the formation of placental villi but migrates to various other locations. These populations are referred to as extravillous trophoblast. One population of these is the trophoblast associated with the cell columns and trophoblastic shell. Cells in the proximal columns (near the fetal mesenchyme) appear relatively undifferentiated, but as they migrate distally they acquire abundant glycogen stores, rough endoplasmic reticulum, and a prominent Golgi apparatus. As the cells migrate distally they begin to surround themselves with extracellular "fibrinoid." Although the composition of this substance is being investigated, it appears that some of this extracellular matrix consists in part of type IV

FIGURE 124–5. Electron micrograph of a terminal placental villus from a term placenta. Cytoplasm of the syncytiotrophoblast (ST) contains abundant endoplasmic reticulum, mitochondria, and other organelles. A brush border is adjacent to the intervillous space (IVS), and the trophoblast is adherent to an underlying basal lamina (BL). A part of a less-differentiated cytotrophoblast cell (CT) is also shown. FC, fetal capillary.

collagen, laminin, and fibronectin.[2] Changes in matrix proteins that interact with integrin receptors of the trophoblast cells undoubtedly influence cell differentiation, migration, and function.[12, 13]

Some trophoblast cells migrate deeply into the endometrium, even reaching the myometrium. Sometimes these cells are referred to as interstitial trophoblast, intermediate trophoblast, or X cells, being distinguished from villous cytotrophoblast by certain histological features, including a larger and more hypochromatic nucleus and more abundant cytoplasm.[14] Multinucleated cells, or giant wandering cells, are also found invading the endometrium. The invasion process appears to occur in two waves: one during the first trimester and a subsequent wave in the second trimester.

Trophoblast and Development of Placental Blood Supply

The maternal blood supply to the placenta is established soon after implantation begins when the trophoblast "taps" the subepithelial uterine capillaries. As gestation proceeds another population of extravillous trophoblast cells migrates intravascularly into the spiral arteries that supply the placenta.[15–18] These cells, in combination with interstitial trophoblast cells that invade the perivascular layer, proceed to modify the walls of the spiral arteries. This results in the replacement of muscular and elastic elements of the wall by trophoblast cells and fibrinoid. These changes even extend into the myometrial segments of the arteries. The remodeling of the arteries is thought to accommodate the vessels to the high-flow, low-pressure blood supply required by the developing placenta.

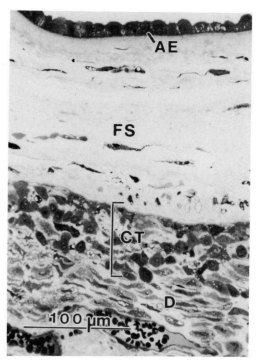

FIGURE 124–7. Light micrograph of the chorioamnion and decidua parietalis from a term placenta. Amniotic epithelium (AE) lines the amniotic cavity *(top)*. Cytotrophoblast (CT) of the chorion laeve is of irregular thickness and separated from the amniotic epithelium by a thick layer of fetal stroma (FS). Note the maternal blood vessel in the decidua parietalis (D).

Chorion Laeve

The chorionic structures that contact the decidua capsularis that lies over the implanted conceptus ultimately form the chorion laeve, an avascular membrane that consists of a layer of cuboidal cytotrophoblasts, fetal mesoderm, and the remains of degenerated villi.[3, 19] The chorion laeve is separated from the amnion by the exocoelomic cavity up until the end of the third month of pregnancy (see Fig. 124–2). After this time the chorion and amnion are in close apposition and eventually make contact with the decidua parietalis (Figs. 124–6 and 124–7). The secretory products of the cytotrophoblasts of the chorion laeve and the amnion act in a paracrine mode on the adjacent decidua and amnion, and possibly on the fetus through transfer of substances into the amniotic fluid.[19]

Placental Growth

The rate of growth of the human placenta is most rapid during the first trimester (Fig. 124–8). The placenta continues to increase in weight until term, at which time this discoid organ weighs about 500 to 600 g and measures 15 to 20 cm in diameter and 2 to 3 cm in thickness.[3, 20]

Placental growth is believed to be driven by factors produced by the trophoblast that work locally in concert with growth factors and growth factor binding proteins produced by the endometrium. The expression of the cellular oncogene c-*myc* correlates with proliferative potential of the cytotrophoblasts.[21, 22] Thus, c-*myc* presumably is involved

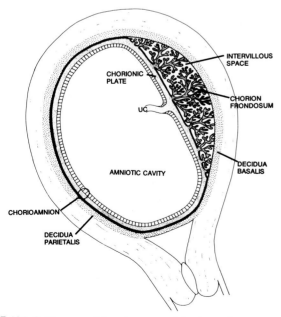

FIGURE 124–6. Diagram of the placenta and fetal membranes near term. The chorion frondosum and decidua basalis have the same relation as in Figure 124–2; however, the chorion laeve and amnion have fused (chorioamnion) and the decidua capsularis has degenerated. Thus the chorioamnion becomes apposed to the decidua parietalis, obliterating the uterine lumen. UC, umbilical cord.

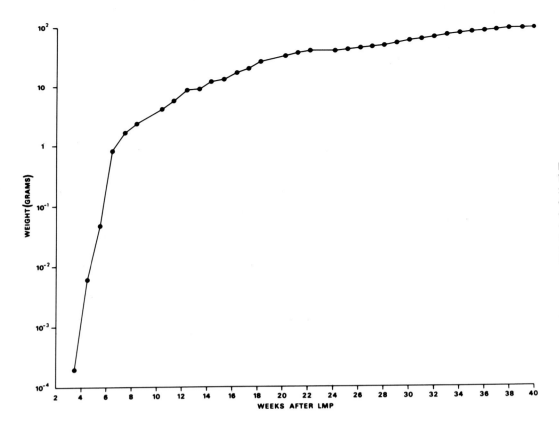

FIGURE 124–8. Estimated trophoblastic mass in grams throughout normal pregnancy. (From Braunstein GD et al: Interrelationships of human chorionic gonadotropin, human placental lactogen, and pregnancy-specific β₁-glycoprotein throughout normal human gestation. Am J Obstet Gynecol 138:1205, 1980.)

in the signal transduction pathway through which growth factors stimulate trophoblast replication.

Several growth factors have been implicated in trophoblast proliferation, including insulin-like growth factor II (IGF-II), platelet-derived growth factors (PDGF), and transforming growth factor β1 (TGFβ1).[23] These growth factors also regulate trophoblast endocrine function.[23a] The IGF-II gene is highly expressed in trophoblast cells once implantation is initiated.[24] The spatial distribution of the IGF type 1 and type 2 receptors is essentially reciprocal to that of IGF-II. Moreover, IGF-II stimulates human trophoblast cell proliferation in vitro, and deletion of the mouse IGF-II gene through homologous recombination results in reduced placental size of offspring heterozygous for the gene "knockout." These observations substantiate the role of IGF-II in trophoblast cell replication. IGF binding proteins (types 1 and 2) are produced by the decidua and placenta (type 3).[25, 26] These binding proteins may either constrain or facilitate the actions of IGF's of trophoblast or endometrial origin.

The PDGF-A and -B genes and the β-PDGF receptor are expressed by proliferating cytotrophoblast.[23, 27] Notably, the PDGF-A gene is highly expressed in cytotrophoblast cells at the base of cell columns, whereas the PDGF-B gene is expressed in the cytotrophoblast shell. TGFβ1 is co-expressed with IGF-II and PDGF-B in the cytotrophoblast shell. PDGF has been shown to induce TGFβ1 in placental cells, and TGFβ1 reportedly synergizes with IGF-II in promoting replication of cultured human trophoblast cells. TGFβ1 can also suppress trophoblast cell replication under certain conditions.[27a] These observations suggest an interactive cascade of growth factors in which IGF-II action is modified through PDGF induction of a modulating factor (TGFβ1)

that can either enhance or inhibit cell replication, depending on the local conditions. PDGF's also probably function to promote development of the villous fetal capillary endothelium. Both sets of the PDGF ligand and receptor genes are expressed at high levels in the endothelial cells of the developing fetal capillaries.[27]

EGF and colony-stimulating factor 1 (CSF-1), produced by the endometrium as well as by the trophoblast, are also postulated to have roles in trophoblast growth and differentiation early in pregnancy.[22, 28, 29] EGF and its receptor have been detected in the villous cytotrophoblast cells at four to five weeks of pregnancy. By 6 to 12 weeks EGF receptor is localized to the syncytiotrophoblast.[22, 28, 29] In vitro studies have shown that EGF stimulates cytotrophoblast differentiation and CG secretion.[30]

CSF-1 is present in the endometrium and cytotrophoblast in the first trimester and later in pregnancy in the villous mesenchyme.[31] By term, immunoreactive CSF-1 is detected only in the villous mesenchymal cells. The CSF-1 receptor, encoded by the c-fms oncogene, is found in the villi of the first-trimester placenta and the intermediate trophoblast cells of villous sprouts, but as pregnancy progresses it becomes restricted to the syncytiotrophoblast.[32] CSF-1 may affect endocrine activity of trophoblast cells, including stimulation of CG and CS secretion.[33]

These descriptive observations suggest paracrine and autocrine roles for EGF and CSF-1 in trophoblast differentiation. The ways in which they act in a temporal and spatial pattern with IGF's, PDGF, and TGFβ1 to orchestrate differentiation of the trophoblasts remain to be clarified.

The proliferative potential of cytotrophoblast cells and the pathways of differentiation once they exit from the cell cycle are also regulated by environmental factors. It is evident that the extracellular matrix has a significant impact on the morphology and function of trophoblast cells studied in vitro.[34, 35] Thus the basal lamina of the villi and factors produced by the villous mesenchymal core and overlying syncytiotrophoblast may control the structure and function of villous cytotrophoblast, causing these cells to develop features that differ from those of the extravillous trophoblast, which are exposed to a different extracellular and paracrine environment.

Oxygen tension may be another factor that regulates cytotrophoblast cell proliferation. In vitro studies have suggested that hypoxia promotes cytotrophoblast replication.[10, 36] A prominent feature of placentae of pregnancies complicated by diabetes mellitus, hypertension, maternal anemia, and Rh sensitization is an increased number of villous cytotrophoblast cells.[10, 37] The aforementioned changes in placental structure associated with disease during pregnancy are believed to be the consequence of hypoxia and would seem to be an adaptive response to compromised placental function. Kaufmann has proposed that P_{O_2} may be one of the key factors that controls trophoblast proliferation and differentiation, with cytotrophoblast replication occurring in regions of low P_{O_2} and differentiation to syncytiotrophoblast taking place in domains of higher oxygen tension.[10, 37] Although this is an attractive notion, the mechanisms by which P_{O_2} modulates the cell cycle of the cytotrophoblast have not been elucidated.

OVERVIEW OF THE ENDOCRINE FUNCTIONS OF TROPHOBLAST CELLS

Each of the morphological forms of trophoblast cells in the chorionic villi and in extravillous sites has a distinctive endocrine profile that has been elucidated by immunohistochemistry and in situ hybridization studies.[3, 14, 38, 39] A summary of some of the immunocytochemical phenotypes of the various trophoblast forms is presented in Table 124–1. Note that the function of a given morphological form of trophoblast varies during gestation. Thus the βCG subunit is produced initially by cytotrophoblast of the pre-implantation blastocyst,[40, 41] and in high levels, by the syncytiotrophoblast of the first-trimester placenta,[42] but that βCG

expression by syncytiotrophoblast is markedly reduced by term. These patterns of endocrine activity reflect the stage of differentiation of the trophoblast cells, environmental factors (e.g., extracellular matrix), and hormones, growth factors, and cytokines that function as autocrine or paracrine regulators as well as in a traditional endocrine manner. It commonly has been assumed that the functional (i.e., endocrine activity) of trophoblast cells is linked to morphological differentiation (e.g., transition from cytotrophoblast to syncytiotrophoblast). There is clear evidence from in vitro studies, however, that endocrine and morphological differentiation can be dissociated.[43, 44]

The presence of a number of hypothalamic hormones, such as GnRH and somatostatin, in villous cytotrophoblast and pituitary-like hormones (e.g., CG, CS, growth hormone [GH]-V) in the syncytiotrophoblast and the ability of the "hypothalamic" polypeptides to stimulate or inhibit secretion of their respective pituitary-like hormones by placental tissue in vitro have led to the notion that cytotrophoblast regulate the secretory function of syncytiotrophoblast through a paracrine interaction that mimics the hypothalamic-hypophyseal system (Fig. 124–9).[45, 46] Trophoblast cells, however, are distinguished from the cells of the anterior pituitary gland in that they do not have large storage granules in which preformed hormone accumulates, ready for acute release in response to a secretagogue.[46a, 46b] Placental hormones appear to be synthesized and rapidly secreted, possibly through a constitutive pathway. Therefore, many of the factors that have been shown to influence trophoblast hormone production in vitro probably act primarily at the level of hormone synthesis or perhaps control trophoblast cell differentiation, rather than primarily stimulating exocytosis of granules that contain stored hormone.

The syncytiotrophoblast is in direct contact with the maternal blood, facilitating the release of secretory products from these polarized cells into the maternal circulation. To reach the fetal circulation, syncytiotrophoblast products must cross several barriers, including a continuous layer of cytotrophoblast in the first trimester, a basement membrane, the mesenchymal stroma of the villous core, and the fetal capillary endothelium. These structural features explain in part why most placental proteins and other hor-

TABLE 124–1. REACTION OF VARIOUS TROPHOBLAST FORMS WITH ANTIBODIES TO HISTOCOMPATABILITY ANTIGENS AND PLACENTAL PROTEINS

	HLA-A,-B,-C	HLA-DR	HLA-G	αCG	βCG	CS	PSG	PP19
Villous								
Cytotrophoblast	−	−	−	− *	−	−	−	−
Syncytiotrophoblast	−	−	−	+ +†	+ +	+ +	+ +	+
Cell Column								
Mononucleate trophoblast	−	−	−	+ +	+ +	+ +	+ +	−
Syncytiotrophoblast	+	−	−	−	−	−	− −	−
Extravillous								
Mononucleate trophoblast	+	−	+	+	+‡	+	+	+
Syncytiotrophoblast	+	−	+	−	−	+	−	+

Modified from Ringler GE, Strauss JF III: In vitro systems for the study of human placental endocrine function. Endocr Rev 11:105–123, copyright © 1990 by the Endocrine Society.

αCG, α-subunit of chorionic gonadotropin; βCG, β-subunit of chorionic gonadotropin; CS, chorionic somatomammotropin; PSG, pregnancy-specific β₁-glycoprotein; PP19, pregnancy protein 19; −, negative; +, positive; + +, strongly positive.

*Some intermediate trophoblast cells in villi stain positively.

†Frequency of positive reaction declines in second trimester.

‡Positive reaction limited to mononucleate trophoblastic cells in superficial decidua of early pregnancy.

2178 / PART IX—ENDOCRINOLOGY OF PREGNANCY

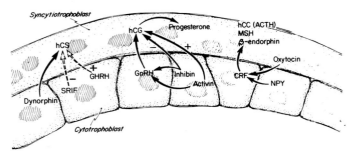

FIGURE 124–9. Model for paracrine interactions between cytotrophoblast and syncytiotrophoblast in the control of CS, CG, and proopiomelanocortin polypeptide secretion. CRF, corticotropin-releasing factor; hCS, human chorionic somatomammotropin; hCC, human chorionic corticotropin; hCG, human chorionic gonadotropin; NPY, neuropeptide Y; ACTH, adrenocorticotropic hormone; GHRH, growth hormone–releasing hormone; SRIF, somatostatin (somatotropin release-inhibiting factor); GnRH, gonadotropin-releasing hormone; MSH, melanocyte-stimulating hormone. (From Jaffe RB. *In* Yen SSC, Jaffe RB [eds]: Reproductive Endocrinology [ed 3]. Philadelphia, WB Saunders Co, 1991.)

mones are secreted almost exclusively into the maternal compartment.

Hormones in Amniotic Fluid

The placenta has three circulations: two that are active (maternal and fetal) and the amniotic fluid, which is more or less static. Many of the placental, chorion laeve, decidual, and fetal hormones accumulate in amniotic fluid.[19, 46c] The concentrations of these hormones are determined by the rates of secretion and removal, metabolism of the hormones in situ, and changes in amniotic fluid volume. Some of the hormones are inactive catabolites; other potentially act on the fetal membranes or on the fetus proper (e.g., actions on fetal lung as a consequence of lavage by amniotic fluid).

Placental-Specific Gene Expression

A number of the placental hormones and secreted proteins are synthesized only by trophoblast or a limited number of other cell types.[47, 47a] The genetic elements that determine the trophoblast-specific pattern of expression of these genes have yet to be fully elucidated. The mechanisms may include methylation of key regulatory sequences of genes in extraplacental tissues, the presence of placenta-specific trans-acting factors that regulate unique cis-acting elements in specific genes, or the absence of silencing transacting factors binding to other cis-acting elements.

Studies of the α subunit gene, which is expressed normally in primate pituitary gonadotrophs and thyrotrophs and in trophoblast, have provided some important insights regarding trophoblast-specific gene expression.[48] The presence of tandem cAMP response elements (CRE) and an upstream regulatory sequence governs the trophoblastic expression of the α-subunit gene. The CRE's bind cAMP response element binding protein (CREB), a trans-acting factor that is phosphorylated by cAMP-dependent protein kinase as well as by protein kinase C. The regulatory element upstream of the CRE's appears to bind other trans-

acting factors.[11, 47] Mutations in the CRE or deviations from the consensus CRE sequence prevent α subunit gene expression in trophoblast cells.

Nachtigall et al.[49] have identified novel nucleotide sequences in the genes of four members of the placentally expressed CS-GH family that are not present in the pituitary-expressed GH gene (GH-N). When introduced into the GH-N, these unique sequences repress promoter activity of the GH-N gene in transfected pituitary cells in an orientation-dependent manner. The DNA sequences specifically bind a protein (presumed transfactor) in gel shift assays. These observations suggest that the expression of the placenta-specific genes may be silenced in nontrophoblast tissues by transfactors acting on these novel sequences.

CHORIONIC GONADOTROPIN

Genes and Structure

Chorionic gonadotropin is the first hormone elaborated in significant quantities by the conceptus.[40, 41, 50] This glycoprotein hormone is a heterodimer consisting of two noncovalently bound subunits: the 92–amino acid α subunit, which is derived from a single gene on chromosome 6q 21.1–23 that is common to pituitary gonadotropins and thyrotropin, and a distinctive β subunit.[51, 52] There is a cluster of seven β subunit genes on chromosome 19 that includes the β-subunit of LH (six βCG genes and one βLH gene) (Fig. 124–10).[53–59] Gene 5 is expressed predominantly; genes 3 and 8 are also expressed, whereas genes 7, 1, and 2 are expressed at very low levels. Genes 1 and 2 are similar in structure and differ from genes 5, 3, 7, and 8 in that they both lack consensus donor splice sites in the first intron and have a repetitive sequence in the first exon.

The βCG subunit is structurally similar (greater than 80 per cent sequence identity) to the 121–amino acid β subunit of LH. The major difference between the β subunit of LH and the βCG subunit is a 24–amino acid carboxy-terminus extension in βCG that results from a 1-bp deletion and a 2-bp insertion that removes a termination codon, yielding an extended open reading frame. The carboxylterminal peptide of βCG contains four serine-linked (O-linked) oligosaccharide chains (Fig. 124–11). This domain of βCG does not have a major effect on biological activity in vitro, but it markedly increases the half-life of holoCG in vivo.[60]

Site-specific mutagenesis and gene transfer studies have elucidated the roles of N-linked oligosaccharide chains of the α and β subunits (see Fig. 124–11).[61–63] The absence of Asn[52] in the α subunit has no effect on secretion, but the

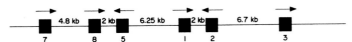

FIGURE 124–10. Structure of the CGβ locus on chromosome 19. The locus encompasses 36.5 kb of DNA. The numbers below each gene indicated by the boxes represent the number designation of each gene. The arrows above each gene denote the transcriptional orientation. Each gene is about 1.5 kb and contains two introns. (From Knoll BJ: Gene expression in the human placental trophoblast: A model for developmental gene regulation. Placenta 13:311–327, 1992.)

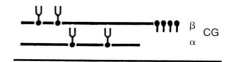

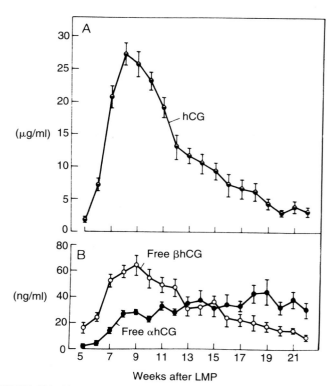

FIGURE 124–11. Glycosylation of CG. N-linked glycosylation sites at Asn[13] and Asn[30] and four O-linked sites in the carboxy terminus of the β-subunit and N-linked sites at Asn[52] and Asn[78] on the α-subunit are indicated. (Modified from Baenziger J: In Chin WW, Boime I [eds]: Glycoprotein Hormones. Norwell, MA, Serono Symposia, 1990, pp 11–26.)

lack of asparagine-linked (N-linked) oligosaccharides at this position greatly alters combination with βCG. The absence of Asn at position 78 lowers α subunit secretion, but the mutant α combines with βCG and is secreted as an assembled heterodimer. On the β subunit, the absence of the Asn[30] oligosaccharides but not Asn[13] slows secretion but not assembly. The absence of both the Asn[30] and Asn[13] oligosaccharides retards both secretion and dimer formation.

The lack of asparagine-linked oligosaccharides on the α, β, or both subunits has little effect on the binding of the mutant hormones to the LH-CG receptor. The absence of N-linked oligosaccharides from the β subunit and Asn[78] of α has no effect on the ability of the hormone to stimulate cAMP formation and steroidogenesis. In the absence of oligosaccharides on Asn[52] on the α subunit, functional activity of the hormone is markedly reduced. Thus the Asn[52] oligosaccharides are critical to signal transduction.

CG Secretion During Pregnancy

Chorionic gonadotropin is detected in maternal serum within eight days after ovulation in a fertile cycle (Fig. 124–12).[64, 65] Human oocytes fertilized in vitro secrete measurable amounts of CG within 64 hours, when they have reached the late morula stage.[40, 50] In situ hybridization has confirmed that the CG genes are expressed in the trophectoderm of the human pre-implantation embryo.[41] Later, as the trophoblast organizes into chorionic villi during the first trimester, CG production becomes localized to the syncytiotrophoblast of the villi.[66, 67] Whereas α subunit gene expression sometimes is detected in cytotrophoblast cells, βCG transcripts are essentially restricted to villous syncytiotrophoblast in the villi after six weeks of pregnancy.[42]

CG levels in maternal blood increase progressively during the first 60 to 90 days of pregnancy, with levels estimated to double every 1.3 to 2.3 days (see Fig. 124–12).[65, 68, 69] This increase can be resolved into two phases: an initial fast phase followed by a slower phase.[65, 70] Peak CG levels are reached in maternal serum at 7 to 10 weeks of pregnancy, at which time the placenta is producing 26 mg of CG/d.[71] CG secretion then declines, falling to comparatively low levels by term.

CG levels in maternal blood are higher in multiple pregnancies.[72, 73] There is no correlation between CG levels

early in pregnancy and fetal sex or birth weight. However, higher CG levels are found in pregnancies complicated by chromosomal abnormalities.[74, 75] Late in pregnancy CG levels appear to be higher in association with a female fetus.[76]

The majority of CG produced by the placenta is secreted into the maternal circulation. In the first trimester some authors have found episodic fluctuations in maternal CG levels, with a nadir at 1900 hours followed by a progressive rise to peak levels at 0700 hours.[77] These pulses and nyctohemeral variations in CG reflect pulsatile secretion as well as changes in volumes of distribution or random time-to-time fluctuations that have been reported to range from 5 to 15 per cent.[78]

High levels of CG are found in extra-embryonic coelomic fluid early in pregnancy (7 to 12 weeks), and some CG is found in fetal blood.[79] CG in the fetal circulation may be derived from the placenta or fetal organs because there is evidence that the fetal kidney and, possibly, other fetal tissues, such as the adrenals, are capable of synthesizing CG.[80, 81]

Free CG α and β-subunits are found in the circulation during pregnancy (see Fig. 124–12).[82-84] Alpha subunit is detectable in significant quantities throughout pregnancy, whereas CG and free βCG levels are low in the third trimester. It appears that α-subunit production during pregnancy is more than five-fold that of holoCG, suggesting that β-subunit synthesis limits CG formation. The free subunits found in the circulation are secreted from trophoblast cells and are not derived from dissociation of holoCG.

FIGURE 124–12. Mean levels ± SEM of CG, free α- and free β-subunits in maternal serum between 5 and 22 weeks after the last menstrual period (LMP) in normal pregnancies. (From Ozturk M et al: Physiological studies of human chorionic gonadotropin, (hCG), αhCG and βhCG as measured by specific monoclonal immunoradiometric assays. Endocrinology 120:549–558, copyright © 1987 by the Endocrine Society.)

When α-subunits are not combined intracellularly with CGβ subunits, they undergo a post-translational modification.[85] Thus the free α subunit is distinguished from the α subunit bound to the CGβ subunit because it is more sialylated than α of holoCG and has a different pattern of N-glycosylation. The Asn-linked oligosaccharides of free α are more branched (triantennary or larger).[86, 87] The pattern of glycosylation of the free α-subunit changes with increased incorporation of more highly branched fucosylated oligosaccharides as gestation progresses.[87, 88] The biological significance of these changes remains to be determined.

Free βCG subunits usually are present in very low levels after the first eight weeks of pregnancy.[82–84] From eight weeks of pregnancy to term free βCG subunit is 1 per cent or less of total βCG immunoreactivity in serum. Early in gestation, however, free βCG is present as a greater fraction of immunoreactive CG (see Fig. 124–12). In patients undergoing in vitro fertilization and embryo transfer who have been monitored serially, free βCG subunit may account for as much as 50 per cent of total immunoreactive CG 8 to 10 days after embryo transfer, with 4 to 10 per cent of total immunoreactive CG being free βCG subunit between four and six weeks of pregnancy.

Regulation of CG Synthesis

The factors that control CG production, and in particular the unique pattern of secretion during pregnancy, remain to be elucidated. Several models have been suggested to account for this pattern, including differentiation-modulated gene expression and the sequential action of stimulating and inhibiting factors (see Fig. 124–9). Boime[89] has suggested that differentiation of the trophoblast cells may be responsible for this pattern, with the formation of syncytia being tied to CG production. Observations consistent with this notion include the findings that in vitro, isolated cytotrophoblast cells increase CG secretion as they spontaneously form syncytial structures.[43] This relation could be explained by a rise in cellular cAMP levels as cytotrophoblast fuse.[11] However, the trophectoderm, consisting of mononucleate cells, produces CG before implantation.[41] Therefore, the formation of a syncytium is not an absolute prerequisite for CG expression.

Alternatively, CG secretion may be under the control of tropic and inhibitory factors. Because trophoblast cells do not store CG in typical secretory granules, the action of these factors is probably at the level of synthesis of the CG subunits, through control of the contents of the respective mRNAs. The substances that are known to increase CG production by trophoblast cells include GnRH,[89a] EGF,[30] CSF-1[33] agents that stimulate adenylate cyclase,[11, 89b] and the cytokines interleukin (IL)-1[89c] and IL-6.[89d]

Cyclic AMP acts by increasing transcription of the CG subunit genes. The α-subunit gene contains tandem CRE's in its 5' flanking region as well as other elements that confer cAMP regulation.[11, 48, 89e] The βCG genes are also transcriptionally regulated by cAMP but respond more slowly.[89g] The cAMP response elements in the βCG gene promoters are different from those of the α subunit gene. However, the activation of cAMP-dependent protein kinase appears to be essential for the stimulation of both α and β subunit genes' cAMP-responsive enhancer elements. The transfactor, CREB, that binds to the CRE's is certainly one of the substrates phosphorylated in response to cAMP-dependent protein kinase activation.

The observations that the placenta expresses the GnRH gene,[89h] possesses GnRH receptors, and responds to GnRH in vitro, probably by way of calcium or phospholipid-derived second messengers with increased CG secretion, suggest the possibility that villous cytotrophoblast cells govern syncytiotrophoblast CG secretion through a paracrine mechanism mediated by GnRH.[89a] The correspondence of the peak of placental CG secretion with the greatest abundance of villous cytotrophoblast relative to syncytiotrophoblast, and the greater responsiveness of first-trimester placental tissue to GnRH than term placenta, are consistent with this idea. However, the administration of GnRH to a pregnant woman does not increase serum CG levels,[89i] perhaps because the placental GnRH receptors are low affinity compared with pituitary GnRH receptors and would not be activated at the concentrations of GnRH administered, or because the trophoblast GnRH response systems are saturated by endogenous hormone.

One possible stimulator of trophoblast adenylyl cyclase that would lead to increased cAMP formation, and hence increased transcription of the α and β subunit genes, is CG itself. CG is known to activate placental cyclase,[89j] and trophoblastic cells have been reported to express LH-CG receptors.[89k] Thus a positive feedback might exist whereby CG augments its own production. Glucocorticoids can modify the response to cAMP, increasing the response in normal trophoblast cells.[90] Alternatively, as noted above, trophoblast cAMP levels may be increased by the cell fusion event that occurs as the syncytial form. This could account for the observation of CG synthesis by syncytiotrophoblast but not cytotrophoblast in first-trimester villi.[11]

Petraglia et al.[91, 92] have proposed that inhibin and activin, also produced by the placenta, may contribute to the biphasic pattern of CG secretion. In vitro studies carried out by these investigators indicate that inhibin blocks GnRH stimulation of CG secretion, whereas activin stimulates it.

Progesterone has been found to reduce CG secretion by placental explants, and it has been suggested that the decline in CG secretion is coupled to increasing placental progestin biosynthesis.[93, 94] A 7- to 10-kDa protein of decidual origin has also been reported to inhibit CG secretion.[95] This could be a known growth factor–cytokine or a novel factor.

The apparent mimicry of the neuroendocrine system with respect to placental CG regulation is appealing. Based on the existing literature, it is possible to construct a model in which stimulators working in a paracrine mode, including EGF, GnRH, activin, and CG, functioning as an autocrine regulator, increase CG synthesis, whereas inhibin and progesterone suppress it (see Fig. 124–9). This concept is based almost exclusively on in vitro studies and does not yet account for the differential patterns of α and βCG gene expression during pregnancy.

Metabolism and Clearance of CG and Its Subunits

The clearance of holoCG from the circulation has two components: a fast half-life of about 7 hours and a slow component of 39 hours.[96] The half-life of CG is considerably longer than that of the pituitary glycoprotein hormones primarily because of the glycosylated carboxy-terminal peptide of the β subunit. The metabolic clearance rate of CG, or volume of plasma cleared of CG per unit of time, is about 4.4 L/d. Renal clearance, a major pathway of removal of CG from maternal circulation, is unchanged during pregnancy. Because rates of clearance of CG do not change significantly during pregnancy, steady-state CG levels in maternal blood are directly related to CG synthesis and secretion.

The half-lives of the free α subunits and βCG subunits are short compared with that of holoCG.[96] The fast and slow components for α subunits and βCG subunits have been estimated to be 13 and 94 minutes and 43 and 239 minutes, respectively. Thus the metabolic clearance rate for α subunit is about three-fold greater than for βCG, but the free subunits are eliminated at a rate that is 10- to 30-fold faster than holoCG. Although the metabolic clearance rates of the subunits are much greater than holoCG, the renal clearances of the free subunits are much lower (less than 1 per cent of free subunits are excreted in urine) so that rapid renal excretion does not account for their shorter half-lives.

The βCG subunit is subject to proteolytic processing. Nicking of the βCG subunit by protease between residues 44 and 45 or 47 and 48 markedly reduces biological activity.[97] A unique form of the β subunit, consisting of βCG residues 6 to 40 with a disulfide bond link to residues 55 to 92, called the β–core fragment, is the predominant immunoreactive βCG in urine during pregnancy, accounting for as much as 90 per cent of the urinary immunoreactive βCG.[98, 99] The β–core fragment is apparently a catabolite of CG that is generated largely in the kidneys after uptake of CG from the plasma. There is a possibility that some of this material is secreted from the placenta.[99a] However, serum levels of β–core fragment during pregnancy are very low.

CG Actions

The primary action of CG in the maternal organism is to serve as a signal to the ovary to maintain the corpus luteum, which would regress if it were not rescued by CG. In keeping with this notion, administration of antiserum against CG causes pregnancy termination in primate models.[100] As noted above, CG may also have an autocrine-paracrine role in the placenta, since LH-CG receptors are expressed on trophoblastic cells, and in vitro studies suggest that CG can stimulate trophoblast adenylyl cyclase and progestin secretion.[89j, 89k, 101]

Other functions for CG in the maternal organism have been proposed, including effects on the endometrium, which possibly are related to implantation. The endometrium has been shown to express LH-CG receptors.[102] CG has been suggested to be a stimulant of maternal thyroid function.[103] The hormone binds to thyroid-stimulating hormone (TSH) receptors and stimulates thyroid adenylyl cyclase.[104] Hence one of the factors that contribute to increased maternal thyroxine secretion during pregnancy may be CG.

In the fetus, CG derived from the trophoblast or, possibly, produced by fetal kidneys or other fetal tissues[80] may have a role in regulating fetal testicular testosterone secretion, which is needed to drive differentiation of the inter-

nal and external genitalia. CG may also stimulate dehydroepiandrosterone production by the fetal adrenal gland.[105]

Although it is held that the free CG subunits do not possess biological activity, reports have linked the α-subunit to the growth of nontrophoblastic tumors.[106, 107] This is of particular interest given the not uncommon expression of the α-subunit gene by malignant cells. Neutralization of α-subunits by antisera or inhibition of α-subunit synthesis by antisense methods reduces the growth of lung tumor cells. However, the mechanisms by which free α-subunit affects tumor cell growth have not been elucidated, and it is not known if similar actions of free α-subunit could influence proliferation of normal or malignant trophoblast cells.

Free α-subunit has been shown to be a potent stimulator of decidual prolactin secretion in vitro.[108] Given the proximity of the trophoblast to the decidua and the substantial levels of free α-subunit produced, it is reasonable to propose that free α-subunit could play a key role in controlling decidual prolactin release in vivo.

Clinical Utility of CG Assays

Standardization of Assays

Chorionic gonadotropin levels in biological fluids usually are reported in international units (IU) per liter or in mass units (e.g., nanograms per milliliter). Two standards have been used for CG assays reported in international units: the 1st International Reference Preparation (IRP) of hCG for Immunoassay (1974) and the 2nd International Standard of hCG for Bioassay (1964).[109, 110] These materials are not equivalent, having been characterized for immunoassays and bioassays, respectively. One microgram of the 2nd International Standard corresponds to 5.7 IU of the IRP, whereas 1 μg of the IRP equals 12 IU. Thus immunoassays standardized to the 2nd International Standard give values in international units that are about 50 per cent of those standardized to the IRP. The CG levels given in this chapter are based on the IRP.

Pregnancy Tests

The detection of CG in serum or urine serves as the basis of contemporary pregnancy tests, reflecting the significant contribution of Aschheim and Zondek in 1927, who developed the first bioassay for this pregnancy-associated factor.[111, 112] Current serum CG assays have a sensitivity of about 25 IU/L and can detect pregnancy within 8 to 12 days after ovulation, whereas urinary CG assays detect CG 14 to 18 days after ovulation in a fertile cycle.

Monitoring Pregnancy

Quantitative CG assays can provide an estimate of gestational age, and sequential monitoring of maternal serum CG provides a biochemical index of growth of the conceptus. In normal pregnancies CG titers in maternal serum double every 1.3 to 2.3 days. This pattern of CG increase in maternal serum is abnormal in pregnancies that subsequently fail or when implantation of the embryo occurs at an ectopic site.[68–70, 113, 114]

By determining maternal CG levels and assessing the uterus and adnexa by ultrasonography, it is possible to rule in or rule out intra-uterine versus ectopic pregnancies once CG titers have reached certain threshhold values.[114, 115] Table 124–2 provides a summary of early events in pregnancy observed by ultrasonography and corresponding CG levels.

The presence of CG in the blood of a woman who has been pregnant reflects either the presence of viable trophoblast tissue and/or the kinetics of CG clearance. The time for clearance depends in part on the level of CG. For example, CG can be found in maternal serum or urine for up to 24 days after normal delivery. Because of the very high levels of CG in the circulation during the first 13 weeks of pregnancy, CG may be detected in maternal blood or urine for as many as 60 days after pregnancy termination in the first trimester.[111]

Prenatal Genetic Screening

Measurements of serum CG in conjunction with α-feto-protein and plasma unconjugated estriol have been used in the prenatal diagnosis of chromosomal abnormalities in so-called "triple screening."[116] In pregnancies in which the fetus is aneuploid, CG levels and free αCG values frequently are elevated at or after 18 weeks of pregnancy. This may be a consequence of altered growth of the extra-embryonic tissues when chromosomal abnormalities are present.

Gestational Trophoblastic Disease and Nontrophoblastic Tumors

Chorionic gonadotropin measurements are used to diagnose and monitor therapy of gestational trophoblastic disease as well as numerous CG-secreting nontrophoblastic neoplasms (Table 124–3).[117] Molar pregnancies are associated with extremely high levels of CG that may reach into the millions of IU per liter. These concentrations typically are much greater than those found in women with chorio-carcinomas. Serial monitoring of CG can provide an index of the success of extirpation and chemotherapy.

Testicular tumors (about 5 per cent of seminomas and 66 per cent of nonseminoma germ cell tumors) produce immunoreactive CG.[118] In addition, 10 to 16 per cent of other nontrophoblastic cancers are associated with immunoreactive CG in blood, including a high percentage of islet cell tumors, epithelial ovarian tumors, carcinoids, breast and gastrointestinal cancers, and nonovarian gynecological cancers.[116, 118] The levels of CG found in these instances usually are modest (10 to 340 IU/L).

CG in Normal Nonpregnant Subjects

Immunoreactive CG has been found in low concentrations in normal men and women.[119–121] This immunoreactive CG is probably produced by the pituitary gland and may be under GnRH regulation. Normal men have been reported to have immunoreactive CG levels of 0.02 to 0.8 IU/L in serum, and normal premenopausal women have levels between 0.02 and 0.2 IU/L. Postmenopausal women have higher levels, ranging from less than 0.02 to 2.8 IU/L. Therefore, the presence of low levels of immunoreactive CG in a nonpregnant subject does not necessarily indicate the presence of an occult tumor.

Aberrant CG Assay Results

False-positive pregnancy tests or discordant quantitative CG levels can occur as a result of assay interference by anti-CG antibodies present in people who have been treated with CG or heterophilic antibodies that react with animal antibodies used in immunoassays.[111, 112] Other factors, such as hyperlipidemia and elevated immunoglobulin levels, can interfere with some CG assays. Discordant results often can be identified by performing assays on serial dilutions of the specimen.[122, 123] If values do not decline in relation to the dilutions, assay interference can be inferred.

TABLE 124–2. EVENTS EARLY IN PREGNANCY OBSERVED BY ULTRASOUND AND THE CORRESPONDING MEAN CG LEVELS

AUTHOR	EVENT	DAYS	CG (IU/L)
Cacciatore et al (1990) Br J Obstet Gynaecol 97:678–681	Gestational sac 1–3 mm	31	730 (467–935)
	Yolk sac apparent	36	4103 (1120–7280)
	Heart action seen	41	12,050 (5280–22,950)
Goldstein et al (1988) Obstet Gynecol 71:747–750	Gestational sac 1 cm		>6000
Bernaschek et al (1988) Am J Obstet Gynecol 158:608–612	Gestational sac seen		>600
Nyberg et al (1988) Radiology 167:619–622	Gestational sac seen:		
	20% of cases		<1000
	80% of cases		1000–2000
	100% of cases		>1000
Fossum et al (1988) Fertil Steril 49:788–791	Gestational sac seen	34.8 ± 2.2	1398 ± 155
	Fetal pole seen	40.3 ± 3.4	5113 ± 298
	Fetal heart seen	46.9 ± 6	17,208 ± 3772
Daya et al (1991) J Clin Ultrasound 19:139–142	Yolk sac first seen	36	1900
	Yolk sac always seen	40	5800
	Heart action first seen	41	9200
	Heart action always seen	46	24,000

Modified from Chard T: Pregnancy tests: A review. Hum Reprod 7:701–710, 1992.

TABLE 124–3. IMMUNOREACTIVE CG IN SERA OF PATIENTS WITH CANCER

TUMOR OR SITE	N		PERCENTAGE POSITIVE	
Islet cell	104		39.4	
Gynecologic	2010		28.9	
Ovary		633		28.6
Endometrium		348		16.7
Cervix		976		33.8
Vulva/vagina		37		27.0
Carcinoid	41		26.8	
Gastrointestinal	2165		18.0	
Oropharynx		298		14.8
Esophagus		124		17.7
Gastric		232		20.7
Small intestine		24		16.7
Colon/rectum		693		9.8
Hepatic		281		22.1
Biliary		26		30.7
Pancreatic		200		20.0
Lung	1365		17.4	
Breast	3031		16.8	
Melanoma	244		13.9	
Genitourinary	658		11.8	
Renal		119		6.7
Bladder		176		23.3
Prostate		363		8.0
Sarcoma	136		11.8	
Hematopoietic	544		6.1	
Lymphoma	339		5.3	
Miscellaneous	576		10.4	
Total	11,213		18.0	

Reproduced with permission from Braunstein GD: Placental proteins as tumor markers. *In* Heberman RB, Mercer DW (eds): Immunodiagnosis of Cancer. New York, Marcel Dekker, 1991, pp 673–701.

CHORIONIC SOMATOMAMMOTROPIN (CS) AND VARIANT GROWTH HORMONE (GH-V)

CS/GH Gene Cluster

The CS-GH gene family is represented by five linked genes that are located on human chromosome 17q22-24 (Fig. 124–13).[124–126] These genes share a similar structure consisting of five exons and four introns and probably arose from a common ancestral precursor by gene duplication.[124, 127] The CS-A and CS-B genes (also referred to as hCS-1 or hPL4 and hCS-2 or hPL3, respectively) encode CS, also called human placental lactogen (hPL). These genes are 98 per cent identical, and their products differ in only one amino acid that resides in the signal peptide. The GH-N (N for normal) gene encodes pituitary GH. The GH-V (V for variant) gene is located between the CS-A and CS-B genes.[128] It encodes a protein whose amino acid sequence differs from the GH-N product in 13 residues (nonconservative substitutions) dispersed throughout the protein. It is expressed in the placenta and appears in maternal serum from the second trimester through term. The fifth gene, called CS-L, gives rise to an mRNA that could encode a CS-like protein of unknown function.[129]

CS Structure and Sites of Synthesis

Chorionic somatomammotropin is a 191–amino acid protein that is 96 per cent homologous, including conser-

vative substitutions, to pituitary GH.[130, 131] It is synthesized with a 26–amino acid signal sequence that is cleaved co-translationally. The syncytiotrophoblast and extravillous intermediate trophoblasts, or X cells, are the sites of CS synthesis.[42, 132, 133] CS can be detected by immunofluorescence in the syncytiotrophoblast by the second week after conception. The hormone is measurable in maternal serum by the third week after conception, and concentrations of CS rise progressively until 34 weeks, reaching levels of 5 to 15 mg/L by term (Fig. 124–14).[134–136] The maternal serum levels of CS parallel changes in placental mass.

CS is one of the major secretory products of the trophoblast. At term the placenta secretes from 1 to 3 g of CS per day, which represents about 10 per cent of placental protein production.[137–139] It has a half-life in maternal serum of 10 to 30 minutes.[139, 140] CS accumulates in amniotic fluid by routes that have not yet been clarified but could include passive diffusion.[141] The levels of CS in amniotic fluid are nearly similar to those in maternal serum early in pregnancy and gradually increase until term, but the increase is less than that observed in serum. The concentrations of CS in fetal blood are 300- to 1000-fold lower than those in maternal serum.[142, 143]

Two mRNA's from the CS-L gene have been detected in placental tissue. These appear to arise from alternative splicing.[129] The mRNA's encode *putative* proteins of 174 and 197 amino acids, respectively, after cleavage of the signal peptide, which share 91 per cent amino acid identity with CS. The smaller transcript is most abundant relative to the larger mRNA (called hCS-L'). The proteins encoded by these mRNA's have not been isolated, so it is not certain that the messages are translated.

Regulation of CS Synthesis and Secretion

The factors that regulate CS secretion include the differentiation of trophoblast cells, transcriptional activation, and, possibly, the action of secretagogues that enhance CS release.[127, 128, 144, 145] CS is usually considered to be a product of the syncytiotrophoblast of the chorionic villi. The increased capacity of the placenta to elaborate this hormone is directly related to the mass of syncytiotrophoblast in the placenta. However, CS is also found in extravillous trophoblast cells and villous cytotrophoblast cells very early in pregnancy.

The CS-A and CS-B genes are expressed differentially during pregnancy.[129] They are transcribed at nearly equal levels at eight weeks of pregnancy, but by term CS-A transcripts are about five-fold more abundant than CS-B transcripts. Between eight weeks and term CS-B mRNA increases 5- to 10-fold in villous tissue, whereas CS-A mRNA rises 30-fold. This shift in expression of the two CS genes occurs as CS production by the placenta increases. Because the two genes encode identical mature proteins, the significance of this shift in expression is unclear. It could possibly reflect the position of the genes in the CS-GH cluster.

Some of the promoter elements of the CS-B gene have been mapped.[126] Sequences between -142 and -129 bp were found to be important in regulating transcription. In addition, Harper et al.[126] identified an enhancer element in the ~2 kb 3′ to the CS-B gene that was contained in a 210-bp sequence. This sequence formed up to three spe-

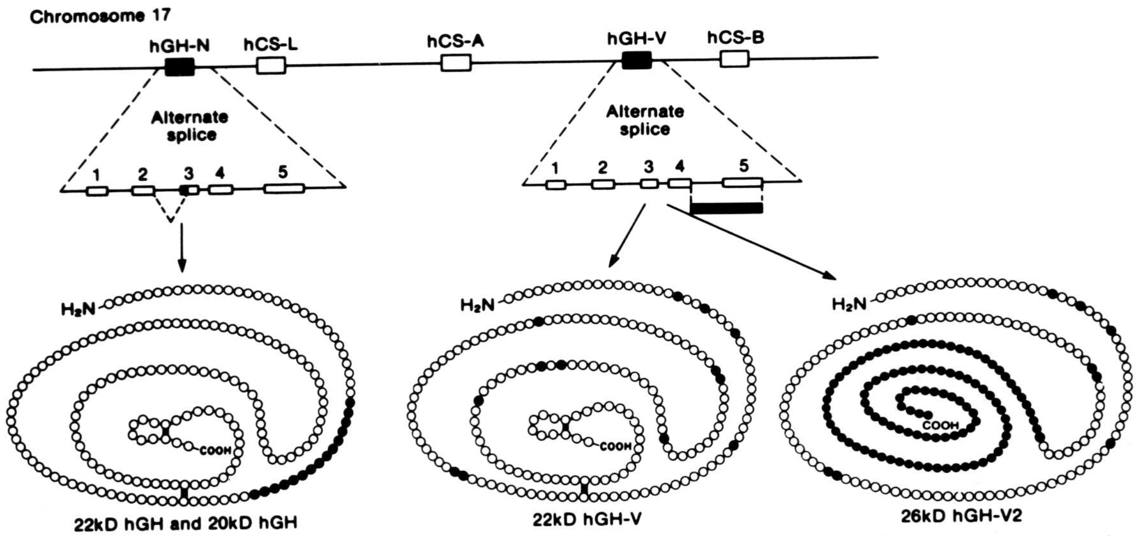

FIGURE 124–13. **Genes in the GH-CS gene cluster.** The position of each of the genes in the cluster is represented on the top line. The exon-intron structure of the GH-N and GH-V genes is shown below the respective genes. The alternatively spliced region at the 5′ end of exon 3 in GH-N and the 3′ end of exon 4 in GH-V are both shown as black rectangles connected to the gene by dotted lines. The 22- and 20-kDa GH-N proteins and the predicted 22- and 26-kDa proteins of the GH-V genes are shown below the respective genes. The 15 amino acids deleted in the GH-N 20-kDa protein by usage of the alternative splice site are shown in black in the left protein (GH-N), the amino acid differences between the 22-kDa GH-N and GH-V proteins are darkened in the middle protein (GH-V), and the region at the C-terminus of the GH-V2 protein that diverges from GH-V is shown in the right protein (GH-V2). The existence of the GH-V2 protein remains to be established. (From Cooke NE et al: Placental expression of the human growth hormone-variant gene. Troph Res 5:61–74, 1991.)

cific DNA–protein complexes with nuclear protein extracts from trophoblastic tissue, suggesting interactions of specific trans-acting factors with the enhancer element.

Evidence suggests that GRF, which is found in trophoblast cells, stimulates CS production and that somatostatin, which is also found in cytotrophoblast cells, may inhibit CS release. GRF has been shown to stimulate CS secretion by trophoblast cells in vitro.[146] Somatostatin immunostaining in human placenta is most intense early in pregnancy,[147] declining as gestation progresses. The inverse relation between somatostatin immunostaining intensity and CS secretion raises the possibility of an inhibitory action of somatostatin on CS expression. However, somatostatin does not inhibit CS secretion by term placental cells.[147a]

Neurotransmitters that regulate pituitary prolactin and GH secretion do not appear to affect placental CS production in vivo. The dopamine agonist bromocriptine, which profoundly suppresses pituitary prolactin secretion, has no effect on CS levels early in pregnancy.[148] Although some in vitro studies have suggested roles for dopamine and β-adrenergic agents in regulating CS production,[149–151] these findings contrast with the in vivo observations noted above and are in conflict with other reports on actions of β-adrenergic agents.

CS is not stored in classic secretory granules, and it appears that most of this hormone is rapidly secreted after synthesis. Data have been presented indicating that some CS is present in a storage pool and that CS secretion in vitro can be affected by various substances in a calcium-dependent manner.[144, 145] Apolipoproteins (apolipoprotein A-I) and chorion-derived factor have been reported to stimulate CS secretion by placental cells.[144] The second messengers that could mediate the actions of these substances include cAMP and the protein kinase C system. Phospholipase A_2 treatment of placental cells increases CS release, as do diacylglycerols and phorbol esters.[152, 153] Despite the extensive literature on in vitro effects of these agents, there is little evidence to support the idea that apolipoproteins or a decidual factor have a physiological role in the regulation of CS secretion in vivo.

A number of observations indicate that placental CS secretion is under metabolic regulation. Prolonged fasting in the first half of pregnancy has been reported to lead to an increase in CS in maternal blood.[154, 155] The specific mechanisms underlying the fasting-induced changes in maternal CS are unknown. Conflicting data have been published on the effects of hyperglycemia and hypoglycemia on CS levels.[145] Some authors have concluded that hyperglycemia causes a transient decline in CS, whereas insulin-induced hypoglycemia increases CS. Nonetheless, the existing data collectively suggest that glucose, insulin, amino acids, or lipids are not major short-term regulators of CS secretion. Thus Tyson et al.[154] reported that the ingestion of protein or protein- and glucose-rich meals did not have a marked effect on maternal CS levels. Moreover, in reports describing changes in CS levels in response to glucose infusions, the changes have been modest and have occurred in temporal patterns that are not entirely consistent with the alterations in glucose concentrations.[156, 157]

Activities of CS

The biological activities of CS have been explored relative to GH and prolactin. Most emphasis has been placed on CS's regulation of lipid and carbohydrate metabolism,

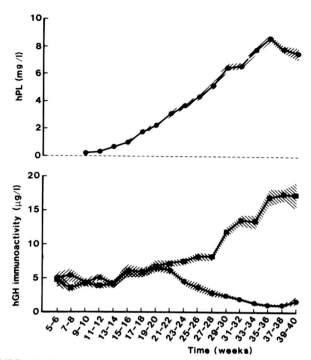

FIGURE 124–14. Levels of CS (hPL, *upper panel*), pituitary *(solid circles, lower panel)*, and placental GH-V *(solid squares, lower panel)* during pregnancy. (From Frankenne F et al: The physiology of growth hormones in pregnant women and partial characterization of a placental variant. J Clin Endocrinol Metab 66:1171, copyright © 1988 by the Endocrine Society.)

organ growth, and mammary gland function (Fig. 124–15).[127, 144, 145]

CS and Lipid Metabolism

The actions of CS on lipolysis have been examined in the most comprehensive manner. The majority of studies conducted in humans and animals have documented an increase in free fatty acids, ketones, and glycerol in blood after the administration of CS.[158, 159] These findings are all consistent with a stimulatory effect of CS on lipolysis. Moreover, in vitro studies with human and rat adipose tissue and isolated adipocytes have revealed a stimulatory effect of CS on lipolysis.[160–162] CS has been shown to increase theophylline-stimulated lipolysis, suggesting that the hormone also enhances adipocyte sensitivity to other lipolytic agents.[160]

The effects of CS on adipocytes extend to increased glucose uptake and oxidation and the incorporation of glucose carbon into fatty acids and glycerol.[163, 164] These are insulin-like actions, and subsequent studies have indicated that CS augments adipocyte sensitivity to insulin in the rat. In many of the in vitro studies on adipose tissue, very high (and in some cases nonphysiological) concentrations of CS have been used. The net effect of the lipolytic activity of CS, its actions to increase adipocyte sensitivity to other lipolytic agents, and its insulin-like effects and presumed ability to enhance insulin sensitivity is to increase adipocyte basal metabolic activity, particularly turnover of fatty acids. This is concordant with data indicating increased lipolysis and fatty acid esterification in human adipose tissue collected at the end of pregnancy. The consequences of these actions of CS are increased fatty acid mobilization in the fasting state and increased glucose uptake and fatty acid storage in the fed state when glucose and insulin levels are high.

CS and Carbohydrate Metabolism

The effects of CS on carbohydrate metabolism have been studied in human and animal models. Hypopituitary humans respond to CS administration with increases in basal insulin levels, but a number of investigators have found no effects of CS on basal insulin levels in normal subjects.[165–168] Enhancement of carbohydrate-stimulated insulin secretion by CS has been documented in normal, diabetic, and hypopituitary humans.[166, 169] The effects of CS on insulin levels could be due in part to direct effects of CS on the

FIGURE 124–15. Proposed actions for CS in the mother and fetus. (From Handwerger S: Clinical counterpoint: The physiology of placental lactogen in human pregnancy. Endocr Rev 12:329–336, copyright © 1991 by the Endocrine Society.)

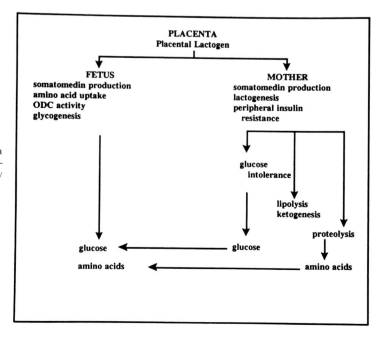

pancreas because studies have demonstrated that CS stimulates insulin secretion by rodent pancreas in vitro.[170] In addition, CS may have indirect effects through its modulation of other fuels (e.g., fatty acids and amino acids).

The disposal of plasma glucose may also be influenced by CS. CS has been reported to reduce carbohydrate tolerance in diabetics.[168, 169] In some studies similar effects have been reported in normal subjects.[140, 166] These actions have been attributed to an increase in insulin resistance.[171, 172] The specific organs involved in the insulin resistance have not been identified but probably include the liver. In contrast, adipose tissue sensitivity to insulin, as discussed above, is increased. Thus there may be tissue-specific responses to CS. The mechanisms for insulin resistance have not been defined and could include direct effects of CS or be secondary to CS effects on nonesterified fatty acid levels.

The integrated role of CS in modulating maternal intermediary metabolism is probably of a long-term nature, since acute changes in nutrients do not have a significant effect on CS levels. Thus this hormone may function to dampen swings in maternal nutrient levels or alter the sensitivity of specific maternal organs to key regulators as pregnancy progresses and maternal and fetal metabolic demands change. Maternal metabolic changes during pregnancy are the result of the actions of many hormones, including sex steroids and glucocorticoids, and any of the proposed actions of CS that have not been placed in the context of the changes in the aforementioned hormones may have to be re-evaluated.

CS as a Fetal Growth Hormone

There has been considerable interest in the potential role of CS in fetal growth. The effects of CS in the maternal compartment could have important consequences for fetal growth. Whether the hormone has a direct role in the fetus in this regard is less certain. Evidence that is compatible with a role for CS as a growth hormone includes its anabolic effects in vivo and its in vitro effects in GH bioassays. The administration of CS to humans at concentrations found during pregnancy has been reported to promote a slight increase in nitrogen retention in children and adults in some studies.[166, 169, 174] CS has also been shown to have growth-promoting effects in certain bioassays in rodents, but its activity in this regard is about 1 per cent of that of GH.[175–178] Moreover, CS has been shown to increase DNA synthesis in fetal fibroblasts and myoblasts, IGF production by fetal cells, and neutral amino acid uptake and DNA synthesis in fetal hepatocytes.[158, 167, 179–181] Because levels of CS in the fetus are quite low, fetal tissues would have to be very sensitive to CS for this hormone to have an effect on fetal growth.

CS and Mammary Gland Function

The role of CS in controlling mammary gland function remains to be clarified. In vitro, CS acts on human breast epithelium to stimulate growth, and it stimulates DNA synthesis in epithelial cells in breast explants in nude mice.[182, 183] Its role in lactation is less clear. Whereas animal studies suggest some lactogenic activity, CS failed to maintain established lactation in an in vitro system, whereas ovine prolactin did.[184] Thus CS's action on the mammary gland may be primarily to stimulate cell proliferation rather than milk secretion.[185]

Mutations in the CS-GH Gene Cluster

Several cases of normal gestation in the presence of low levels or the absence of serum and placental CS have been reported. These cases are due to partial or complete fetal CS gene deletions.[186–190] The women had normal glucose tolerance during pregnancy and normal placental function as assessed by measurements of CG, estriol, and progesterone. The women also experienced normal lactation after delivery, and their offspring were of normal size and had normal postnatal growth patterns. Although these data suggest that CS may not be required for normal pregnancy, fetal growth and development, and lactation, hormones with similar activities, including GH-V, may have subsumed CS functions. Indeed, in one well-studied case in which the CS-A, CS-B, and GH-V genes were deleted, a GH-CS hybrid protein was detected that may have compensated for the absence of CS and GH-V. Moreover, the expression of CS-L was not explored.[190, 191]

GH-V Structure

The GH-V gene gives rise to two mRNAs generated by alternative splicing of the fourth exon (see Fig. 124–13).[127–129] One gene product, GH-V, consists of 191 amino acids. It contains a consensus N-glycosylation signal, and two glycosylated forms of GH-V have been described. Through an alternative splicing mechanism, the GH-V gene yields a product with a frameshift so that the 104–amino acid carboxyl-terminus of the molecule diverges completely from GH-V. This 25-kDa protein, named GH-V2, lacks the N-glycosylation site and instead has a hydrophobic "tail" that may serve to anchor the molecule to the plasma membrane.

Regulation of GH-V Expression

The GH-V gene is expressed in the same pattern as the CS genes but at levels that are several orders of magnitude lower than CS (see Fig. 124–14).[128, 129, 192, 193] This parallel pattern suggests that similar regulatory mechanisms govern the expression of these related genes. GH-V levels in maternal blood increase as pregnancy progresses, and it becomes the predominant GH in maternal blood by the second trimester. Like GH-N, it binds to the circulating GH binding protein, which is a secreted form of the GH receptor.

GH-V appears to be secreted from the placenta in a relatively constant manner, and levels do not change episodically or in a pulsatile manner as do levels of GH-N. GRH has been detected in placental tissue. It can stimulate CS secretion, but it is not known whether GH-V production is regulated by GRH.[194]

The GH-V2 mRNA is expressed at levels of 5 to 7 per cent of GH-V mRNA in the first trimester but increases to about 15 to 20 per cent at term, suggesting a developmental pattern of alternative splicing of the GH-V gene that could reflect changes in splice site selection or mRNA stability.[128, 129]

GH-V Actions

Variant growth hormone has growth-promoting bioactivity in animal bioassays. It is equivalent to 22-kDa GH as a somatogen but 10- to 20-fold less potent than GH-N as a lactogen.[195, 196] The bioactivity of GH-V in humans has not been reported.

The placental-derived GH molecules could have an action in the maternal compartment as well as directly on the placenta. The latter possibility is supported by the discovery of GH receptor protein and mRNA in human placenta.[192, 193] Hill et al.[197] detected GH receptor by immunocytochemistry in the syncytiotrophoblast as early as eight weeks of pregnancy. Immunoreactive receptor was not found in cytotrophoblasts. Urbaneck et al.[198] have cloned cDNA's for the GH receptor from a human placental cDNA library. The placental GH receptor sequence reported by these authors was identical to that of the human liver GH receptor, with the exception that it lacked the sequences encoded by exon 3 of the receptor gene. The mRNA lacking the exon 3 sequences is exclusively expressed in chorionic villi and amnion, whereas choriocarcinoma cells contain an mRNA that includes the third exon sequences. The alternatively spliced chorionic villus receptor would have a 22–amino acid deletion in the extracellular segment that contains one N-linked glycosylation site. Although the absence of the exon 3 sequences does not appear to affect the ability of this alternative receptor form to bind GH when expressed in bacteria, it could have some impact on receptor function in situ.[199] The role of this GH receptor in mediating GH effects on the placenta remains to be elucidated.

In the one reported case in which the GH-V gene as well as CS-A and CS-B genes were deleted in the conceptus, there were no abnormalities in fetal growth or postnatal development.[186] Although this case suggests that the GH-V gene products are not crucial for pregnancy and fetal growth, a hybrid GH-CS molecule found in this pregnancy may have assumed GH-V functions.[191] The role of GH-V2

in pregnancy is not known. Its presumed location at the plasma membrane raises the possibility that it functions in cell-to-cell communication.

Clinical Utility of CS Assays

Low levels of CS have been associated with intra-uterine growth retardation and fetal distress.[200, 201] Most obstetricians, however, believe that the quantitation of CS in maternal serum does not provide clinically useful information regarding the condition of the fetus or the prognosis for outcome in high-risk pregnancies compared with biophysical profiles or other analyses that directly assess fetal function in real time (e.g., ultrasonography).[200, 201]

PLACENTAL CRH

Structure and Site of Synthesis

Corticotropin-releasing hormone and prepro-CRH mRNA have been found in human placenta.[202–205] The placental CRH is identical to hypothalamic CRH, but two larger CRH polypeptides isolated from placenta have not been detected in the hypothalamus.[202, 203] Immunoreactive CRH protein and CRH mRNA have been localized in intermediate trophoblasts, syncytiotrophoblast, amnion and the musculature of the umbilical vessels, and decidua.[204] Some investigators have suggested that villous cytotrophoblast elaborate CRH.[205a]

Immunoreactive CRH in the plasma of nonpregnant women is low, and concentrations remain in the range of 2 to 9 pmol/L in the first trimester but begin to increase in the middle of the second trimester to reach concentrations of around 55 pmol/L early in the third trimester.[206–208] There is a striking increase (20-fold) in CRH mRNA in the placenta during the last five weeks of pregnancy that parallels an increase in CRH in placental tissue and maternal blood (Fig. 124–16).[209, 210] In the last weeks of pregnancy CRH concentrations rise to 250 to 300 pmol/L (Fig. 124–17). Within 20 to 30 minutes after delivery maternal pe-

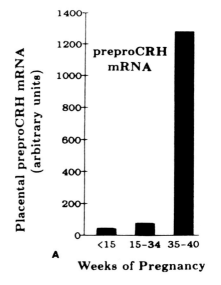
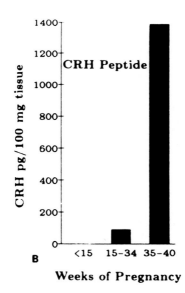

FIGURE 124–16. Relative changes in CRH mRNA (A) and CRH levels (B) in the placenta during pregnancy. (From Frim DM et al: Characterization and gestational regulation of corticotropin-releasing hormone messenger RNA in human placenta. J Clin Invest 82:290, 1988, by copyright permission of the American Society for Clinical Investigation.)

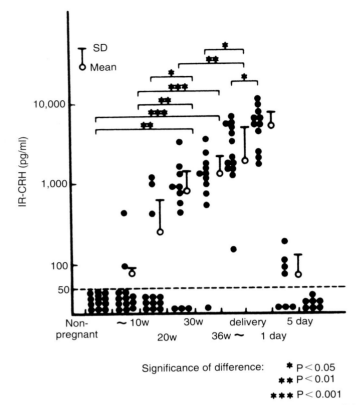

IR-CRH (pg/ml)

Significance of difference: * P < 0.05
** P < 0.01
*** P < 0.001

FIGURE 124–17. Maternal plasma levels of CRH during pregnancy. Solid points represent individual values; open circles and bars are means ± SD. (From Okamoto E et al: Immunoreactive corticotropin-releasing hormone, adrenocorticotrophin and cortisol in human plasma during pregnancy, delivery and post partum. Horm Metab Res 21:566, 1989.)

ripheral plasma and uterine venous plasma CRH levels fall to one half of predelivery concentrations, and within one to five days after parturition maternal plasma CRH concentrations decline to values seen in nonpregnant women.[206, 209–213]

In general, placental CRH content, maternal and fetal blood CRH concentrations, and amniotic fluid CRH levels are highly correlated, with the exception that amniotic fluid CRH does not increase during labor, whereas maternal plasma CRH levels rise.[214]

Maternal CRH levels increase earlier in gestation and rise to higher levels in twin pregnancies, reflecting in part the greater trophoblast mass and earlier time of delivery.[215–217] In gestations complicated by pregnancy-induced hypertension, intrauterine fetal growth retardation, fetal asphyxia, premature rupture of membranes, and premature labor, maternal plasma CRH levels are also increased.[208, 216, 217] The rise in maternal plasma CRH before delivery has raised the possibility that sequential monitoring of this hormone could predict onset of premature labor.

CRH Binding Proteins

Much of the CRH in the maternal circulation (67 to 90 per cent) is associated with a high-affinity binding protein. Maternal plasma concentrations of the binding protein are

similar to those of nonpregnant women during the first half of gestation, but they decline during the second half of pregnancy.[218] Nonetheless, the binding protein is present at a 10-fold molar excess over CRH in the third trimester (2.7 nmol/L for the binding protein compared with 270 pmol/L for CRH).[219, 220] The 37-kDa CRH binding protein is also present in amniotic fluid but at lower concentrations than in plasma.[221] CRH bound to the carrier protein is biologically inert, since the binding protein inhibits the stimulatory effects of CRH on pituitary cell ACTH release. Because of the presence of the CRH binding protein, the maternal pituitary gland is apparently not subject to stimulation by placental CRH. Thus maternal ACTH and β-endorphin levels are not correlated with circulating CRH. The gene encoding the binding protein is expressed in the placenta, liver, and brain.[222]

Regulation of Placental CRH Synthesis and Secretion

The regulation of placental CRH secretion has been studied primarily with in vitro systems, and a number of neurotransmitters and peptide hormones have been shown to increase CRH secretion by trophoblast and amnion preparations.[223] Several of these factors can be placed in a physiological or pathophysiological context with respect to regulation of CRH production by the placenta and fetal membranes.

Glucocorticoids stimulate trophoblast CRH gene expression in vitro, whereas they inhibit it in the hypothalamus.[224, 225] Jones et al.[226] also reported that glucocorticoids stimulate CRH secretion by amnion, chorion, and decidua cells, whereas progesterone inhibits it. The observations of positive rather than negative feedback by dexamethasone on placental CRH led Robinson et al.[225] to propose that the increase in CRH near the end of pregnancy may be driven by glucocorticoids. They raised the possibility of a short-loop feed-forward system in which glucocorticoids stimulate placental CRH production, which in turn stimulates fetal pituitary and placental ACTH production, which increases glucocorticoid output from fetal adrenals, which in turn drives more placenta CRH secretion. This feed-forward system could help the fetus respond to stress or be a preliminary to parturition. It remains to be established that this system functions in vivo, especially since the administration of betamethasone to women in premature labor at 28 to 32 weeks of pregnancy has no effect on maternal CRH levels, even though plasma ACTH and cortisol are suppressed.[227]

In experimental sheep models of acute fetal hypoxemia induced by compression of the uterine artery or by infusion of adrenaline into the fetal circulation, CRH concentrations rise in the fetal and maternal plasma.[228] The increase in CRH in the fetus is probably due to a reduction in uteroplacental blood flow, with the subsequent release of catecholamines triggering CRH secretion in both the fetus and the placenta.[222] A role for catecholamines is suggested by the fact that norepinephrine and epinephrine stimulate CRH release by human placental cells.[229] The stimulatory actions of these catecholamines are mimicked by α_1- and α_2-adrenergic receptor agonists (metoxamine, clonidine) and blocked by α_1- and α_2-receptor antagonists (prazosin, yohimbine). Arginine vasopressin is increased in the fetal sheep circulation in response to hypoxemia, and arginine vasopressin also stimulates CRH production by cultured human placental cells.[230, 231]

The rise in CRH in response to hypoxemia may be an adaptation to counteract reductions in uteroplacental blood flow, since CRH has significant vasodilatory actions on the mesenteric circulation.[232, 233] This hypothesis is consistent with the elevations in maternal CRH found in pregnancies complicated by preeclampsia and other conditions in which placental blood flow is reduced.

Prostaglandins (PG) E_2 and $F_{2\alpha}$ stimulate CRH secretion by cultured human placental cells.[223, 224] These prostanoids also promote ACTH secretion, but the ACTH release provoked by prostaglandins can be blocked by a CRH antagonist. CRH stimulates PGE_2 and $PGF_{2\alpha}$ release from amnion, chorion, decidual, and placental cells, presumably acting through lRH receptors on these tissues. The stimulation of prostanoid production by CRH in term placental and decidual cells is blocked by an antiserum to ACTH.[234, 235] Based on these observations, Jones and Challis[234, 235] proposed a model in which placental CRH, ACTH, and prostaglandins interact in a feed-forward regulatory loop. They suggest that the stimulation of prostanoid production by CRH may in part be controlled by ACTH. The rise in prostanoids stimulates more CRH release, leading to greater ACTH secretion and augmented prostaglandin formation. They suggest that this cycle of increasing prostanoid production may be critical to the initiation of labor.

CRH interacts with oxytocin at the level of the myometrium, and oxytocin stimulates CRH secretion from cultured human placental cells.[229] CRH also has both priming and potentiating actions on myometrial contractile activity at term. The exposure of myometrial strips, removed at the time of cesarean section, to CRH enhanced the ionotropic action of oxytocin, and pre-exposure of the strips to CRH primed the strips to the subsequent response to oxytocin.[236] The rise in oxytocin at parturition may, therefore, stimulate CRH release, which would augment the actions of oxytocin on the myometrium and collaborate with the above-noted relations between CRH and prostaglandin production to promote labor.

Cytokines, including IL-1α and -1β, stimulate the secretion of CRH by cultured human placental cells.[229, 237] These cytokines may be derived from decidual cells, trophoblast, or Hofbauer cells in the chorionic villi.[238-240] An increase in cytokine release has been associated with premature labor caused by infection and may also be a precedent to normal term labor.[241] A direct link between onset of infection and release of cytokines and increased CRH remains to be established.

CHORIONIC PROOPIOMELANOCORTIN PEPTIDES

The placenta contains the proopiomelanocortin (POMC) peptides ACTH, β-lipotropin, β-endorphin, and three forms of dynorphin.[242-245] Maternal plasma ACTH concentrations increase during pregnancy, presumably reflecting a placental contribution (Fig. 124–18).[246, 247] In vitro, CRH stimulates the secretion of ACTH by trophoblast cells.[234, 235] Moreover, the placental content of dynorphin is relatively

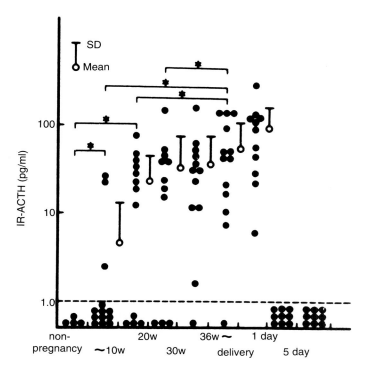

FIGURE 124–18. Maternal plasma levels of ACTH during pregnancy. Solid points represent individual values; open circles and bars are means ± SD. (From Okamoto E et al: Immunoreactive corticotrophin-releasing hormone, adrenocorticotrophin and cortisol in human plasma during pregnancy, delivery and post partum. Horm Metab Res 21:566, 1989.)

high at term, and high levels of dynorphin have been found in amniotic fluid and umbilical venous plasma.[245, 248] Dynorphin concentrations in maternal plasma in the third trimester and at delivery are higher than those found in nonpregnant women. Beta-endorphin levels in maternal plasma are relatively low during pregnancy, but they rise late in labor and rise further during delivery.[249]

The role that chorionic ACTH and other placental POMC peptides play during pregnancy has not been elucidated. It has been suggested that chorionic ACTH, β-endorphin, and other POMC-derived peptides might function in fetal responses to stress, including hypoxia and acidosis, and in the initiation of labor.[234, 235, 250] In addition, dynorphin binds to the kappa opiate receptors that are abundant in the placenta, suggesting that dynorphin could have a paracrine role in modulating placental function.[251]

PLACENTAL NEUROPEPTIDE Y

Neuropeptide Y, a 36–amino acid molecule, is found in the cytotrophoblast and intermediate trophoblast cells.[252] Levels of neuropeptide Y in maternal blood rise early in pregnancy and remain elevated at term, increasing further during labor, but not in women who deliver by cesarean section. Levels of this peptide fall precipitously after delivery (Fig. 124–19). Neuropeptide Y is also found in amniotic fluid.[253]

Neuropeptide Y receptors have been detected in the placenta, and the peptide has been reported to stimulate

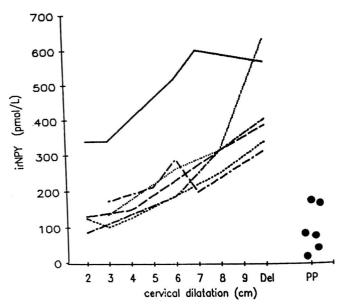

FIGURE 124–19. Plasma immunoreactive neuropeptide Y (irNPY) levels in six women during labor according to cervical dilation, at delivery (Del), or two hours postpartum (pp). (From Petraglia F et al: Plasma and amniotic fluid immunoreactive neuropeptide-Y level changes during pregnancy, labor and at parturition. J Clin Endocrinol Metab 69:324–328, copyright © 1989 by the Endocrine Society.)

release of CRH from placental cells.[252] Thus it could have a role in controlling the secretion of this hormone.

PLACENTAL INHIBINS/ACTIVINS

The inhibin/activin family consists of dimeric glycoprotein hormones composed of subunits encoded by three genes (α, βA, and βB) that are linked by disulfide bonds. These hormones are members of the transforming growth factor-β family of polypeptides. Inhibin consists of an α-subunit and a βA or βB subunit, whereas activins are homodimers or heterodimers of βA and/or βB. These hormones were first characterized by their ability to inhibit (inhibin) or stimulate (activin) pituitary FSH secretion. It is now clear that they have functions in various processes, including morphogenesis, and gonadal and placental function.

Alpha inhibin subunit mRNA can be found in placental tissue early in pregnancy.[254, 255] Beta gene expression is also detectable but at much lower levels than α-inhibin subunit. Both α-inhibin subunit and βA subunit mRNA levels increase in the placenta during gestation. Low levels of βB mRNA are found in placenta only in the third trimester. All three subunits have been localized by immunocytochemistry in the syncytiotrophoblast. Other studies indicate that βA subunit expression may be more widespread.[256] A monoclonal antibody recognizing the βA homodimer, called activin A, revealed by immunocytochemistry that this hormone is present in both cytotrophoblast and syncytiotrophoblast throughout gestation, in the Hofbauer cells in the first- and second-trimester chorionic villi, and in the amniotic epithelium and cytotrophoblast cells of the chorion.[256] The placenta's secretory pattern of

inhibin/activin has not been fully elucidated. Circulating immunoreactive inhibin α levels increase in pregnancy as a result of placental production of the hormone and decline rapidly after delivery (Fig. 124–20).[257–260]

Inhibin secreted by the placenta could play a role in modulating maternal pituitary FSH secretion during pregnancy (see Fig. 124–20), participating in the suppression of this gonadotropin and, hence, follicular development. As noted in the discussion of CG, the inhibin/activin peptides have also been postulated to have a role in governing trophoblast function.[91, 92] Neutralization of inhibin with antibodies has been shown to increase CG secretion. Conversely, exogenous activin increased GnRH and progesterone secretion by placental cells. The actions of activin were blocked by inhibin. Activins have also been postulated to play roles in stem cell differentiation and morphogenesis, so these compounds could have unappreciated roles in placental differentiation and control of decidual function.[261]

STEROID HORMONES

The placenta produces progestins and estrogens but is incapable of synthesizing androgens because the enzyme P45017α (17α-hydroxylase/17-20 desmolase) is not expressed.[262, 263] Hence placental estrogen formation depends on a supply of androgen precursors from the fetus and mother. The syncytiotrophoblast of the chorionic villi is the primary site of steroidogenesis, and the capacity of the placenta to produce steroids increases progressively during gestation as the placenta grows in size and syncytiotrophoblast accumulates. The steroidogenic activity of the placenta is sufficient to assume the full support of gestation by the eighth week of gestation.[264–267]

PROGESTINS

Biosynthesis of Progesterone

Progesterone is synthesized mainly from cholesterol circulating in maternal blood.[268–270] This steroid precursor is transported in lipoproteins that are taken up by trophoblast cells by way of lipoprotein receptors. At least five receptor systems could contribute to the uptake of maternal cholesterol carried by low-density lipoproteins (LDL), very low-density lipoproteins (VLDL), oxidized LDL, and high-density lipoproteins (HDL).[271] These include (1) the LDL receptor,[272–274] (2) the LDL receptor–related protein (LRP),[275] (3) a recently described VLDL/apoE receptor, (4) the scavenger receptor,[271] and (5) the HDL receptor,[276] respectively. Each of these receptors has been described on placental cells and membranes. The uptake of LDL, oxidized LDL, and VLDL all entail absorptive endocytosis, whereas HDL receptors seem to mediate the transport of cholesterol by way of a nonendocytotic process.[271, 277] The relative quantitative significance of each of these pathways to the supply of steroidogenic substrate to the placenta has not been determined. It is likely, however, that LDL and VLDL could be major sources, especially since VLDL lipid levels increase more than two-fold during pregnancy.[278] Because LDL receptor gene expression in placenta falls as

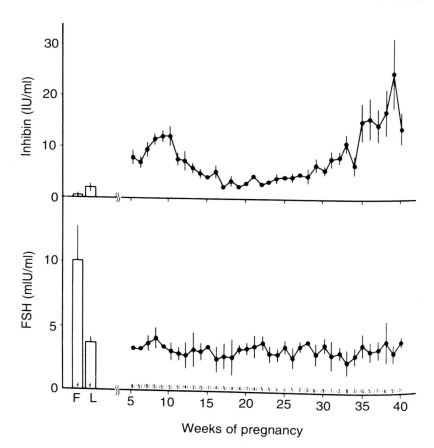

FIGURE 124–20. Mean ± SE blood inhibin *(upper panel)* and FSH *(lower panel)* concentrations in the midfollicular (F) and midluteal (L) phases of the cycle and normal pregnancy. (From Abe Y et al: High concentrations of plasma immunoreactive inhibin during normal pregnancy in women. J Clin Endocrinol Metab 71:133, copyright © 1990 by the Endocrine Society.)

gestation progresses,[279] and whereas LRP gene expression increases, VLDL may be the primary source of sterol substrate late in pregnancy.

De novo cholesterol synthesis by placental tissue is modest as assessed by ^{14}C-acetate incorporation into cholesterol. In keeping with this finding, the activity of the rate-limiting enzyme in de novo cholesterol biosynthesis, 3-hydroxy-3-methylglutaryl coenzyme A reductase, is low in placental microsomes.[280]

Women with homozygous hypobetalipoproteinemia have markedly reduced levels of progesterone during pregnancy, consistent with a role for apolipoprotein B–containing particles in the supply of cholesterol for steroidogenesis.[281] On the other hand, women with homozygous familial hypercholesterolemia are able to produce sufficient levels of progesterone to maintain pregnancy, so that mechanisms other than the LDL receptor (e.g., LRP and the VLDL/apoE receptors) must be able to supply sufficient cholesterol for steroid synthesis.

The accumulation of syncytiotrophoblast is correlated with increased placental progestin synthesizing capacity. The enzymes responsible for progestin synthesis, including P450scc and its associated electron transport chain of adrenodoxin and adrenodoxin reductase and 3β-hydroxysteroid dehydrogenase, are most abundant in syncytiotrophoblast cells.[282, 283] There are two genes that encode 3β-hydroxysteroid dehydrogenase in the human genome.[284] The type I and type II genes on human chromosome 1p11-13 code for proteins of 372 and 371 amino acids, respectively. The type I gene is expressed in the placenta, whereas the type II gene is expressed in the gonads and adrenal

gland.[285] cAMP causes mRNA's for all the placental steroidogenic enzymes noted above to increase. Hence the expression of the steroidogenic machinery in syncytiotrophoblast may be a consequence of activation of the cAMP signaling pathway during the process of cytotrophoblast cell terminal differentiation into syncytia.[286, 287]

Others have suggested on the basis of in vitro studies that placental progesterone synthesis could be modulated by endogenous steroids affecting activities of steroidogenic enzymes.[288] If these mechanisms are indeed operative, they are likely to be of lesser significance compared with control of steroidogenesis at the level of enzyme protein content.

Placental Progesterone Secretion

The pre-implantation embryo does not appear to produce significant amounts of progesterone, and progesterone secretion by the placenta is generally thought to be insufficient to maintain gestation until some 40 days of pregnancy have passed.[264–267] Before this time the corpus luteum is the primary source of progesterone, and its removal before the sixth week of pregnancy can result in abortion.[264–267] After 45 days of pregnancy the placenta is secreting sufficient progesterone to maintain gestation in the face of removal of the corpus luteum of pregnancy (Fig. 124–21). This transition to independence from ovarian function is referred to as the "luteoplacental shift." By 10 weeks of pregnancy placental secretion of progesterone surpasses that of the corpus luteum. At term the placenta produces more than 200 mg of progesterone per day in single pregnancies, and maternal progesterone concen-

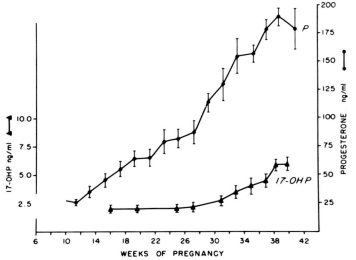

FIGURE 124–21. Progesterone and 17α-hydroxyprogesterone levels in maternal serum during pregnancy. (From Tulchinsky D et al: Plasma estrone, estradiol, progesterone and 17-hydroxyprogesterone in human pregnancy. I. Normal pregnancy. Am J Obstet Gynecol 112:1095, 1972, with permission.)

trations range from 100 to 300 μg/L.[289–292] In multiple gestations placental production of progesterone may be as much as 600 mg/d. Eighty-five per cent or more of the progesterone produced by the placenta enters the maternal compartment. Progesterone is also present in amniotic fluid, but concentrations decline as pregnancy advances.[292]

The amount of placentally (and perhaps ovarian) derived progesterone required to sustain gestation may be far less than is produced in a normal pregnancy. The data that support this notion include the fact that women with hypobetalipoproteinemia maintain pregnancies despite circulating levels of progestin that are 50 per cent of normal.[281] Ongoing pregnancies have also been reported in assisted reproductive technology programs in which women have had "anovulatory" levels of progesterone in early pregnancy. In addition, pregnancies associated with fetal congenital lipoid adrenal hyperplasia (presumed P450scc deficiency) go to term.[293] Because there is only a single P450scc gene in the human genome, these pregnancies are likely to be associated with low progesterone levels because the placenta would be deficient in the activity catalyzing the key step in hormone formation, unless alternative mechanisms for conversion of cholesterol to pregnenolone exist.

The existence of two 3β-hydroxysteroid dehydrogenase genes, one expressed in the placenta and the other in the gonads and adrenals, means that deficiency of the type II gene can occur without compromising placental progesterone production.[285] A deficiency of the placental 3β-hydroxysteroid dehydrogenase (type I gene) has not been described.

Progesterone Metabolism

Ring A and 20α-reduced metabolites of progesterone are secreted by the corpus luteum of pregnancy and the placenta and are formed from progesterone in peripheral tissues (Fig. 124–22).[294] Levels of 5α-dihydroprogesterone are 12 to 33 per cent of those of progesterone in the luteal phase and during pregnancy.[295] The ratio of progesterone to 5α-dihydroprogesterone falls as pregnancy advances, suggesting that either there are changes in the pattern of progesterone metabolism or the compound is not produced from plasma progesterone.

On the basis of recent findings, about 60 to 65 per cent of the secreted progesterone undergoes 5α-reduction, much of it at extrahepatic sites. The remainder is converted to 5β-pregnane compounds, the most prominent being pregnenediol.[294, 296] The discovery of greater 5α-reduction contrasts with the formerly held notion that most of the progesterone was metabolized into 5β-reduced compounds. The 5α-reduced steroids are sulfurylated and mostly excreted into bile.[297] Intestinal micro-organisms further degrade these compounds, with subsequent excretion of the catabolites in feces. Urinary excretion of the end products is not the major route of disposal of the 5α-reduced steroids.[298]

21-Hydroxylation of progesterone metabolites also takes place in peripheral tissues.[299, 300] The reaction probably is mediated by an enzyme other than P450c21.[301] Deoxycorticosterone, an active mineralocorticoid, is also formed in this way.

Actions of Progesterone

The primary function of progesterone is to support pregnancy. Progesterone is believed to have a number of significant roles in this regard, including preparation of the endometrium for implantation of the embryo (e.g., decidualization of endometrial stromal cells) and the maintenance of endometrial integrity during gestation. These actions of progesterone are mediated by the progesterone receptor and can be blocked by progesterone antagonists like RU 486.[302]

Progesterone has been proposed to play a role in the maternal acceptance of the fetal semiallograft by suppressing T lymphocyte–mediated tissue rejection. This idea is based on studies that demonstrate prolongation of xenografts and enhanced survival of trophoblastic tissue transplants in rodents by progesterone.[303]

A major locus of action of progesterone during pregnancy is the myometrium. Progesterone, probably in concert with other hormones, reduces myometrial contractility. This response is due in part to diminished prostaglandin formation and inhibition of gap junction formation between myometrial cells.[304] The withdrawal of progesterone's influence on the myometrium, through either local metabolism or antagonism of its action, is postulated to be a key step in the initiation of labor.

The A-ring–reduced progestin metabolites may have significant nongenomic actions (i.e., not mediated by the progesterone receptor) during pregnancy.[294] In particular, these compounds are known to modify γ-aminobutyric acid (GABA) receptor function. The progestin metabolites, depending on their structure, can act as agonists, partial agonists, or antagonists of the GABA$_A$ receptor.[294, 305–307] These steroids interact with the GABA$_A$ receptor at a site different from the GABA binding domain and either enhance or reduce the affinity of the receptor for GABA. The compounds that increase the affinity of the receptor for GABA (e.g., 3α,21-dihydroxy-5α-pregnan-20-one) have anesthetic and anxiolytic activity.[307]

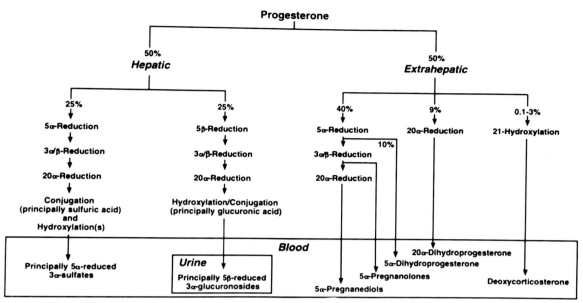

Metabolism of Plasma Progesterone

FIGURE 124–22. Pathways of progesterone catabolism. (From MacDonald PC et al: Recurrent secretion of progesterone in large amounts: An endocrine/metabolic disorder unique to young women? Endocr Rev 12:372–401, copyright © 1991 by the Endocrine Society.)

Progesterone metabolites may also have a number of other effects in the maternal organism and fetus, including regulation of heme synthesis.[294] The ring A–reduced progestins, particularly the 5β-compounds, stimulate formation of δ-aminolevulinic acid synthase.[308]

Clinical Utility of Progesterone Assays

Early in pregnancy (the first 50 days) abnormal gestations, including ectopic pregnancies and abortive gestations, frequently are associated with low serum progesterone levels (less than 15 μg/ml). When levels are less than 10 μg/ml the predictive value of the assay of serum progesterone for identifying abnormal pregnancy is greater than 90 per cent.[309] Abortion occurs in about 80 per cent of patients with progesterone concentrations less than 10 μg/ml at the time of initial evaluation.[310] The low progesterone values during this time reflect deficient stimulation of the corpus luteum, presumably caused by lower CG secretion and, to a lesser extent, diminished trophoblast progestin production.

Maternal progesterone levels are higher in pregnancies that are complicated by Rh sensitization, probably reflecting the increased placental mass associated with erythroblastosis.[311]

17α-Hydroxyprogesterone and 16α-Hydroxyprogesterone

Early in pregnancy 17α-hydroxyprogesterone is secreted by the corpus luteum.[312] The placenta does not express the cytochrome P45017α gene and is thus incapable of synthesizing this steroid de novo. The placenta, however, is capable of converting 17α-hydroxypregnenolone, usually presented as a sulfoconjugate synthesized by the fetal adrenal

cortex, into 17α-hydroxyprogesterone.[313] This process occurs in the third trimester and accounts for a progressive increase in maternal serum 17α-hydroxyprogesterone as term approaches (see Fig. 124–21).[291] A related steroid, 16α-hydroxyprogesterone, is produced by the same pathway and also increases in maternal blood near term.[291, 314]

ESTROGENS

Estrogen Synthesis

The biosynthesis of estrogens during pregnancy involves a complex interplay between the placenta and the fetal adrenal cortex (Fig. 124–23).[315] The placenta is capable of carrying out the initial and terminal steps in estrogen synthesis but is incapable of producing androgens. The immediate precursors of the estrogens are provided mainly by the fetal adrenal cortex.

The fetal adrenal cortex consists of a fetal zone, or X-zone, which at term constitutes 85 per cent of the volume of the cortex, the remainder being the neocortex.[316–318] The X-zone markedly increases in volume during the third trimester (32 to 37 weeks of pregnancy). At term the fetal adrenal glands weigh about 10 g. Relative to body weight, they are 25 times larger than the adult adrenal glands. The growth and function of the fetal zone of the adrenal cortex seems to be governed by a number of hormones. Fetal pituitary hormones, particularly ACTH, are essential. A role for the fetal pituitary is supported by the fact that the fetal zone undergoes atrophy after the 20th week of pregnancy when the fetus is anencephalic and fetal plasma ACTH levels are low or undetectable.[319] ACTH is known to stimulate steroidogenesis by the fetal zone.[320] The administration of pharmacological doses of glucocorticoids to the mother causes fetal pituitary ACTH suppression and atro-

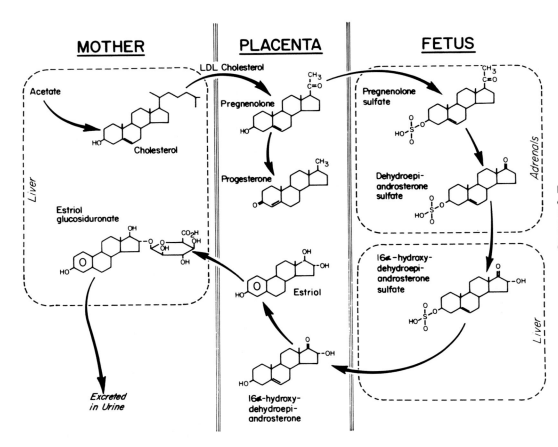

FIGURE 124–23. Schematic view of estriol biosynthesis in late pregnancy. (From Jaffe RB. *In* Yen SSC, Jaffe RB [eds]: Reproductive Endocrinology [ed 3]. Philadelphia, WB Saunders Co, 1991.)

phy of the fetal adrenals. The most rapid phase of fetal adrenal cortex growth occurs while fetal ACTH levels decline,[321] and the architecture of the fetal zone is normal in anencephalic fetuses during the first 14 weeks of pregnancy.[319] Hence roles for other hormones, including GH and prolactin, in regulating fetal adrenal growth and steroidogenesis have been suggested but not proven.[105, 322–324] Alternatively, growth of the fetal zone early in development may depend on nonpituitary hormones (e.g., CG, CS) or local growth factors. This would account for the initial normal growth and development of the fetal adrenals in anencephaly. Later the fetal zone may become dependent on fetal pituitary ACTH.

The growth-promoting effects of ACTH or other hormones on the fetal zone are likely to be mediated by growth factors produced locally in response to the tropic actions of these hormones.[325–327] Both EGF and fibroblast growth factor stimulate mitosis in fetal zone and definitive zone fetal adrenal cells. Moreover, IGF-II is expressed in the fetal adrenal gland, and the expression of this growth factor is increased by ACTH.[328]

The steroidogenic capacity of the fetal adrenal cortex is remarkable. These glands secrete 100 to 200 mg of steroid per day, which accounts for 90 per cent of the precursor of estriol formed in the placenta at term.[329] The fetal zone is deficient in 3β-hydroxysteroid dehydrogenase,[330] and therefore, Δ5-3β-hydroxysteroids are formed. These steroids are mostly sulfated, and dehydroepiandrosterone (DHEA) sulfate is the primary product of the fetal zone. It is derived from pregnenolone sulfate synthesized in the fetal adrenals from fetal LDL-carried cholesterol and, to a

lesser extent, from pregnenolone secreted by the placenta into the fetal compartment.[331] The levels of LDL cholesterol in fetal plasma decline as the fetal zone increases in size and steroidogenic activity, but LDL cholesterol levels are elevated in the anencephalic fetus, presumably reflecting the diminished metabolism of plasma cholesterol into steroids when the fetal zone is atrophic.[332–334]

DHEA sulfate can be secreted from the fetal adrenal cortex as such or as 16-hydroxy-DHEA-sulfate.[335] DHEA sulfate can also be metabolized to 16-hydroxy-DHEA-sulfate in the fetal liver.[336] Further metabolism of DHEA sulfate and 16-hydroxy-DHEA-sulfate takes places in the placenta, which rapidly removes DHEA and its sulfate from the circulation. The eight-fold increase in DHEA sulfate clearance during pregnancy parallels placental growth.[325] The first metabolic step in this process is the removal of the sulfate group by sulfatase, which is followed by aromatization. These reactions take place primarily in the syncytiotrophoblast.[336–338]

The key enzyme in placental estrogen synthesis, aromatase, is localized to the syncytiotrophoblast. Aromatase is encoded by a large (greater than 72-kb) gene, P450aro, on human chromosome 15q21. The gene contains 10 exons and has several promoters, including two that appear to be operative in placental tissue.[339] At the ultrastructural level the enzyme has been found to be associated with the endoplasmic reticulum and inner surface of the microvilli.[340] As pregnancy progresses there is a substantial increase in placental aromatase activity as syncytiotrophoblast accumulates. The increased activity directly parallels the increase in cytochrome P450aro content, which rises more than 15-fold between the first (11 to 18 weeks) and third trimesters (37 to 39 weeks). The large amount of aromatase in the placenta effectively prevents androgenic steroids from the maternal compartment from reaching the fetus. Hence aromatase activity is not rate-limiting in placental estrogen synthesis from maternal C19 steroid precursors.

An NADPH-dependent enzyme, 17β-hydroxysteroid dehydrogenase, catalyzes the interconversion of estrone and estradiol. It functions as a homodimer of 34-kDa subunits, and is localized primarily in the villous syncytiotrophoblast but is also found in cytotrophoblast cells at some stages of pregnancy.[341] This enzyme is encoded by tandem genes on human chromosome 17q.[342] The expression of aromatase and 17β-hydroxysteroid dehydrogenase is regulated by cAMP, and the abundance of these enzymes in villous syncytiotrophoblast could reflect the action of this cyclic nucleotide on expression of the respective genes during the terminal steps of trophoblast differentiation.[343–345]

The factors that determine rates of estrogen synthesis include the size of the fetal adrenal cortex, the extent of stimulation of the fetal zone by tropic hormones, the availability of cholesterol substrate (e.g., fetal LDL), and the mass and function of the syncytiotrophoblast.

Because of the critical role of the fetal adrenal cortex, estrogen synthesis depends on fetal viability.[346] Moreover, factors that affect growth of the fetal adrenal cortex, including the absence of tropic support in the case of anencephaly or generalized fetal growth retardation, are associated with low estrogen formation.[346–348] Fetal pituitary ACTH stimulation of the adrenal cortex is also significant because the administration of glucocorticoids to pregnant women results in a marked reduction in estrogen production, reflecting suppression of fetal as well as maternal ACTH secretion.[348, 349]

Estrogen Levels During Pregnancy

Early in pregnancy estradiol is the major estrogen produced, and it is derived from the ovaries (Fig. 124–24).[290] After the sixth week of pregnancy the placenta begins to produce increasing amounts of estradiol from maternal and fetal DHEA sulfate. By term about equal amounts of maternal and fetal DHEA sulfate serve as substrate for placental estradiol formation.[338, 350] After the first trimester the placenta is the major site of estradiol synthesis. Estradiol levels in the maternal circulation rise from values of 0.5 μg/L in the first weeks of pregnancy to values in the range of 15 μg/L by term.[351–353]

Estrone production parallels that of estradiol, with the placenta becoming the primary site of formation of this hormone after the sixth to seventh week of pregnancy (see Fig. 124–24). Estrone levels rise from 0.3 μg/L early in pregnancy to concentrations in the range of 8 μg/L at term.[290, 311, 353]

Estriol is essentially produced only by the placenta.[354] This hormone is first detectable in maternal plasma by nine weeks of pregnancy, and the increase in estriol levels parallels the growth of the fetal adrenal cortex, which provides 90 per cent of the estriol precursor at term (see Fig. 124–24).[290, 346, 355] Unconjugated estriol in maternal blood increases from negligible levels to levels averaging 13 μg/L at term. Because estradiol is bound to sex hormone–binding globulin (SHBG), concentrations of this estrogen usu-

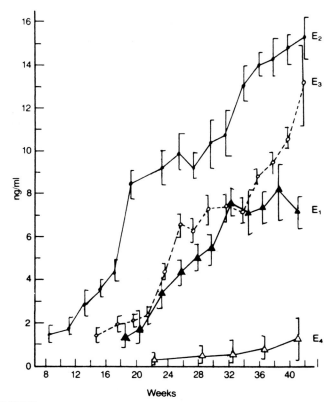

FIGURE 124–24. Mean plasma concentrations ± SEM of unconjugated estrone (E1), estradiol (E2), estriol (E3) and estetrol (E4) during pregnancy. (From Levitz M, Young BK: Estrogens in pregnancy. Vitam Horm 35:109, 1977.)

ally are higher than those of estrone and estriol, which are not effectively bound to SHBG.[356] However, the production of estriol far exceeds that of estradiol and its levels in the circulation are lower than estradiol because of its more rapid clearance. Estriol also accumulates in high quantities in amniotic fluid.[357]

Estetrol

Hydroxylation of estriol at the 15 position yields a compound called estetrol. The 15α-hydroxylation occurs exclusively in the fetal compartment.[358] Maternal estetrol levels rise from 22 weeks to term (see Fig. 124–24).

Estriol Metabolism

More than 90 per cent of the estrogen formed by the placenta is secreted into the maternal compartment. The metabolic clearance of estriol is rapid, with a plasma half-life of about 5 to 8 minutes.[359] Estriol is converted first to a sulfoconjugate and subsequently to a glucosiduronate or mixed conjugate.[360] It is excreted into the urine mostly as a glucosiduronate. At term 35 to 45 mg of estriol per day is excreted in the urine.

Defects in Estrogen Synthesis During Pregnancy

SULFATASE DEFICIENCY. Abnormally low amounts of estrogen are produced in pregnancy when placental sulfatase is deficient. The sulfatase enzyme is encoded by a gene that resides on Xp22.3.[361] Sulfatase deficiency is not uncommon (1 in 2000 to 6000 live-born males), and it frequently is the result of deletion of the entire gene, although other mutations occur.[361–363] In pregnancies associated with a male fetus bearing an abnormal sulfatase gene, the placenta is unable to cleave DHEA sulfate or 16-hydroxy-DHEA-sulfate and thus cannot aromatize these steroids, resulting in minimal estrogen production.[363–365] Urinary excretion of estriol is about 5 per cent of that found in normal pregnancies, and the excretion of estrone and estradiol is in the range of 15 per cent of normal. Moreover, the intravenous administration of DHEA sulfate to the mother is not accompanied by an increase in estrogen excretion, whereas estrogen excretion increases markedly after the administration of DHEA.[366, 366a] This in vivo test establishes the defect in sulfatase in the presence of active aromatase. In vitro assay of the various enzymes has confirmed the selective deficiency of sulfatase in several of these cases.

The major consequence of the low estrogen production in placental sulfatase deficiency is a failure of cervical ripening and onset of spontaneous labor. These observations suggest that the high estrogen levels during late pregnancy are most important for the preparation of the reproductive tract for labor and not for fetal growth or development, as was once assumed.

AROMATASE DEFICIENCY. Rare instances of fetoplacental aromatase deficiency have been described.[367] These pregnancies were associated with low urinary estrogen excretion and deficient placental aromatase activity. Maternal and fetal virilization have been reported in these situations. Biochemical analysis of placental tissue from one such case revealed that microsomes had 0.3 per cent of normal aromatase activity.[368, 368a] The mRNA encoding the mutant aromatase was found to have an insertion of 87 bp at the splice point between exon 6 and intron 6 such that splicing did not occur at the correct position. This resulted in translation of a mutant protein with 29 extra amino acids. The expression of a cDNA corresponding to the mutant mRNA yielded an aromatase with only trace enzymatic activity.

Estrogen Action in Pregnancy

Estrogens have been postulated to have a number of important functions in maintaining pregnancy and preparing the reproductive tract for parturition. Estrogens alter uterine blood flow in nonpregnant and pregnant animals.[369] Estradiol is most active in this regard, but estrone and estriol also have similar actions. Because the uterine vessels would be exposed to relatively high concentrations of estriol synthesized in the placenta, it has been argued that augmentation of uterine blood flow is a principal function of estriol in pregnancy. The effects of estrogens on the vascular system are thought to be mediated by prostanoids.

There is strong evidence that estrogens have a key role in the preparation of the cervix for labor and in the initiation of myometrial contractions.[304, 363, 364] Among the most convincing evidence supporting this notion is the observed failure of cervical ripening and spontaneous labor in women bearing a fetus with sulfatase deficiency. Estrogens may also be critical for inducing sensitivity to oxytocin and the peripartal increase in myometrial gap junctions required for coordinated muscle contraction.[370]

Clinical Utility of Estrogen Assays

For nearly two decades measurements of urinary total estriol or plasma unconjugated estriol were used as biochemical indices of pregnancy well-being.[351–353, 358] The wide range of normal values, day-to-day variations of as much as 40 per cent, and the influence of other factors, including maternal disease and drug therapy, on estrogen metabolism restricted the usefulness of these assays. With the advent of biophysical profiles and improved ultrasound technology, estrogen assays have been abandoned as a tool to assess high-risk pregnancy. The exception is the recent use of plasma unconjugated estriol assays in prenatal genetic screening in conjunction with CG and α-fetoprotein assays. In pregnancies complicated by chromosomal abnormalities (e.g., Down's syndrome) there is a low plasma unconjugated estriol level in the second trimester, which can be used to increase the sensitivity of the α-fetoprotein analysis.[371, 372]

ENDOCRINE ACTIVITY OF THE CHORION LAEVE AND AMNION

The cytotrophoblast cells of the chorion laeve produce protein and steroidal hormones and prostaglandins.[373–376] The endocrine repertoire of these cells includes synthesis of GnRH, CRH, relaxin, prorenin, progesterone, and PGE. In combination with the amnion, the chorion laeve is believed to play a key role in the initiation of labor, with its secretory products acting on the myometrium. The production of some of these hormones can be stimulated by angiotensin, in the case of GnRH, or agents that increase cAMP levels, in the case of progesterone.

The amnion expresses several vasoactive peptides, including endothelin-1 and parathyroid hormone–related protein.[377, 378] The expression of the genes encoding these proteins is increased by TGFβ. It has been suggested that the amnion may influence fetoplacental blood flow through elaboration of these factors.

OTHER PLACENTAL PROTEINS

A large number of proteins have been identified in human placental extracts by immunochemical methods. Some of these have been purified and their cDNAs cloned.[379–381] Several of the proteins have subsequently been found to be of decidual origin (e.g., placental protein [PP] PP12 and PP14) or to be produced by uterine tissues as well as the trophoblast. Certain proteins that originate from the placenta have been detected in maternal plasma, including pregnancy-associated plasma protein A (PAPP-A) and pregnancy-specific β₁-glycoprotein (PSG), also known as Schwangerschaff's proteins-1 (SP1) and PP5 and PP10. The characteristics of some of the proteins that are believed to be produced by the placenta and are found in the maternal circulation are summarized in Table 124–4.

TABLE 124–4. CHARACTERISTICS OF SOME SECRETED PLACENTAL PROTEINS

NAME/SYNONYM		ELECTROPHORETIC MOBILITY	MOLECULAR WEIGHT (DALTONS)	CARBOHYDRATE (%)	MAJOR SITES OF SYNTHESIS
PAPP-A	Pregnancy-associated plasma protein A	α_2	750,000	19.2	Syncytiotrophoblasts
PAPP-B	Pregnancy-associated plasma protein B	β_1	1,000,000	?	Syncytiotrophoblasts and amnion
PP5	Placental protein 5	β_1	36,600	19.8	Syncytiotrophoblasts
PP10	Placental protein 10	α_1	48,000	6.6	Villous and decidual histiocytes
MBP	Eosinophil granule major basic protein		14,000	0	Extravillous trophoblasts

Modified from Wasmoen TL: Placental Proteins. Vol 1. Philadelphia, WB Saunders Co, 1992, pp 87–95.

Pregnancy-Associated Plasma Protein A

Pregnancy-associated plasma protein A is a 750,000-Da glycoprotein (~19.27 carbohydrate) that is structurally related to α_2-macroglobulin, which binds and inactivates serine proteases.[382–385] The molecule is isolated in a dimer of homologous subunits. PAPP-A is produced primarily by the syncytiotrophoblast but is also apparently synthesized by ovarian granulosa cells as well as other tissues of the reproductive tract. Some PAPP-A is present in the serum of nonpregnant women, and levels rise progressively through pregnancy, with an accelerated increase after 30 weeks until term. PAPP-A is rapidly lost from maternal blood after parturition, declining with an estimated half-life of 55 to 73 hours.

The function of PAPP-A in pregnancy is not known, but it has been suggested that it may function to modulate coagulation because of its ability to bind heparin and to block thrombin-induced coagulation of fibrin.[386, 387] Hence PAPP-A could participate in the maintenance of blood flow in the intervillous space. PAPP-A has also been proposed to be immunosuppressive in pregnancy because of its ability to inhibit lymphocyte transformation.[388] Contaminating heparin in the preparations of PAPP-A used in these studies may have been responsible for these actions.[383] PAPP-A is reportedly deficient in pregnancies in which the fetus is affected with Cornelia de Lange's syndrome (includes severe fetal growth retardation, oligodactyly or phocomelia of upper extremities, and mental retardation), but the pregnancies are normal.[389]

Pregnancy-Specific β_1-Glycoproteins

The PSG's are members of a family of related proteins encoded by a cluster of closely linked genes on chromosome 19q13.2-13.3.[390–392] There may be as many as 20 distinct PSG genes that have marked sequence similarities (greater than 90 per cent homology) with the exception of variability in the carboxy termini. The PSG's are related to carcinoembryonic antigens, which are in turn similar to immunoglobulins. They are primarily produced by the syncytiotrophoblast, but other placental cell types are capable of producing isoforms of this glycoprotein.

PSG, which consists of 28 to 32 per cent carbohydrate, is detectable in maternal serum by one to two weeks after conception, and concentrations increase as pregnancy progresses, reaching levels of 200 to 400 mg/L by term.[393, 394] This pattern is similar to that of CS. The role of PSG in pregnancy is not known. The fact that abortion occurs in 80 per cent of monkeys treated with antibodies to PSG

suggests that it has some important function.[395] Proposed roles for PSG include a carrier protein for hormones and iron, regulation of carbohydrate metabolism, prevention of rejection of the fetus, and as a matrix molecule because of the presence of the tripeptide Arg-Gly-Asp in the amino termini of some PSG forms.[381, 392, 395–398]

Although some of these proteins, particularly PSG's, are more or less pregnancy-specific, qualitative or quantitative assays of these proteins have not proved to be superior to the assay of CG as a biochemical test of pregnancy. Assay of PSG has, however, been applied in monitoring therapeutic response in choriocarcinoma and other cancers.[399]

Placental Enzymes

At least two enzymes are released from syncytiotrophoblast into the maternal circulation: placental-type alkaline phosphatase and leucine aminopeptidase, also known as oxytocinase.[400, 401] Alkaline phosphatase is a glycoprotein expressed by syncytiotrophoblast. The enzyme protein and its mRNA are detectable in placenta by seven weeks of pregnancy, and levels continue to rise throughout gestation.[402] Alkaline phosphatase is localized to the plasma membrane of syncytiotrophoblast, bound by a phosphatidylinositol glycan anchor. It is shed into the maternal circulation in a pattern that parallels growth of the placenta. The function of the enzyme remains to be elucidated, although it has been suggested that it plays a role in placental nutrient transport.

Leucine aminopeptidase also accumulates in the maternal circulation as pregnancy progresses. This enzyme may participate in oxytocin, vasopressin, and angiotensin degradation.[401]

REFERENCES

1. Moore KL: The Developing Human: Clinically Oriented Embryology. Philadelphia, WB Saunders Co, 1982.
2. Aplin JD: Implantation, trophoblast differentiation and hemochorial placentation: Mechanistic evidence in vivo and in vitro. J Cell Sci 99:681–692, 1991.
3. Boyd JD, Hamilton WJ: The Human Placenta. Cambridge, England, Heffer & Sons, 1970.
4. Knoth M, Larsen JF: Ultrastructure of a human implantation site. Acta Obstet Gynecol Scand 51:385–393, 1972.
5. Kaufmann P, Scheffen I: Placental development. In Polin RA, Fox WW (eds): Fetal and Neonatal Physiology. Vol 1. Philadelphia, WB Saunders Co, 1992, pp 47–56.
6. Leiser R, Kosanke G, Kaufmann P: Human placental vascularization. Structural and quantitative aspects. In Soma H (ed): Placenta Basic Research for Clinical Application. Basel, Karger, 1991, pp 32–45.

7. Rhodin JAG, Terzakis J: The ultrastructure of the human full-term placenta. J Ultrastruct Res 6:88–106, 1962.

8. Terzakis J: The ultrastructure of the normal human first trimester placenta. J Ultrastruct Res 9:268–284, 1963.

9. Coutifaris C, Kao L-C, Sehdev HM, et al: E-cadherin expression during the differentiation of human trophoblasts. Development 113:767–777, 1991.

10. Benirschke K, Kaufmann P: Pathology of the Human Placenta (ed 3). New York, Springer, 1990.

11. Strauss JF III, Kido S, Sayegh R, et al: The cAMP signalling system and human trophoblast function. Placenta 13:389–403, 1992.

12. Damsky CH, Fitzgerald ML, Fisher SJ: Distribution patterns of extracellular matrix components and adhesion receptors are intricately modulated during first trimester cytotrophoblast differentiation along the invasive pathway, in vivo. J Clin Invest 89:210–222, 1992.

13. Castellucci M, Classen-Linke I, Muhlhauser J, et al: The human placenta: A model for tenascin expression. Histochemistry 95:449–458, 1991.

14. Kurman RJ, Main CS, Chen H-C: Intermediate trophoblasts: A distinctive form of trophoblast with specific morphological, biochemical and functional features. Placenta 5:349–370, 1984.

15. Kaufmann P: Basic morphology of the fetal and maternal circuits in the human placenta. In vitro perfusion of human placental tissue. Contrib Gynecol Obstet 13:77–86, 1985.

16. Pijnenborg R, Dixon G, Robertson WB, Brosens I: Trophoblastic invasion of the human decidua from 8 to 18 weeks of pregnancy. Placenta 1:3–9, 1991.

17. Pijnenborg R, Bland JM, Robertson WB, Brosens I: Uteroplacental arterial changes related to interstitial trophoblast migration in early human pregnancy. Placenta 4:397–414, 1991.

18. Brosens I: The utero-placental vessels at term: The distribution and extent of physiological changes. Trophoblast Res 3:61–68, 1988.

19. Bourne GL: The Human Amnion and Chorion. London, Lloyd-Luke, 1962.

20. Simpson RA, Mayhew TM, Barnes PR: From 13 weeks to term, the trophoblast of human placenta grows by continuous recruitment of new proliferative units: A study of nuclear number using the disector. Placenta 13:501–512, 1992.

21. Pfeifer-Ohlsson S, Goustin AS, Rydnert J, et al: Spatial and temporal pattern of cellular *myc* oncogene expression in developing human placenta: Implications for embryonic cell proliferation. Cell 38:585–596, 1984.

22. Maruo T, Mochizuki M: Immunohistochemical localization of epidermal growth factor receptor and *myc* oncogene product in human placenta: Implication for trophoblast proliferation and differentiation. Am J Obstet Gynecol 156:721–727, 1987.

23. Ohlsson R: Growth factors, protooncogenes and human placental development. Cell Diff Dev 28:1–16, 1989.

23a. Prager D, Weber MM, Herman-Bonert V: Placental growth factors and releasing/inhibiting peptides. Semin Reprod Endocrinol 10:83–94, 1992.

24. Ohlsson R, Holmgren L, Glaser A, et al: Insulin-like growth factor 2 and short-range stimulatory loops in control of human placental growth. EMBO J 8:1993–1999, 1989.

25. Glaser A, Luthman H, Stern I, Ohlsson R: Spatial distribution of active genes implicated in the regulation of insulin-like growth factor stimulatory loops in human decidua and placental tissue of first-trimester pregnancy. Mol Reprod Dev 33:7–15, 1992.

26. Fazleabas AT, Bell SC, Verhage HG: Insulin-like growth factor binding proteins: A paradigm for conceptus-maternal interactions in the primate. In Strauss JF III, Lyttle CR (eds): Uterine and Embryonic Factors in Early Pregnancy. New York, Plenum Press, 1991, pp 157–166.

27. Ohlsson R, Franklin G, Donovan M, et al: The molecular and cellular biology of growth stimulatory pathways during human placental development. In Strauss JF III, Lyttle CR (eds): Uterine and Embryonic Factors in Early Pregnancy. New York, Plenum Press, 1991, pp 219–233.

27a. Graham CH, Lysiak JJ, McCrae KR, Lala PK: Localization of transforming growth factor β at the human fetal-maternal interface: Role in trophoblast growth and differentiation. Biol Reprod 46:561–572, 1992.

28. Hofmann GE, Drews MR, Scott RT Jr, et al: Epidermal growth factor and its receptor in human implantation trophoblast: Immunohistochemical evidence for autocrine/paracrine function. J Clin Endocrinol Metab 74:981–988, 1992.

29. Ladines-Llave CA, Maruo T, Manalo A, Mochizuki M: Cytologic local-

ization of epidermal growth factor and its receptor in developing human placenta varies over the course of pregnancy. Am J Obstet Gynecol 165:1377–1382, 1991.

30. Morrish DW, Bhardwaj D, Dabbagh LK, et al: Epidermal growth factor induces differentiation and secretion of human chorionic gonadotropin and placental lactogen in human placenta. J Clin Endocrinol Metab 65:1282–1290, 1987.

31. Daiter E, Pampfer S, Yeung YG, et al: Expression of colony-stimulating factor-1 in the human uterus and placenta. J Clin Endocrinol Metab 74:850–858, 1942.

32. Pampfer S, Daiter E, Barad D, Pollard JW: Expression of the colony stimulating factor-1 receptor (c-fms proto-oncogene product) in the human uterus and placenta. Biol Reprod 46:48–57, 1992.

33. Saito S, Saito M, Motoyoshi K, Ichijo M: Enhancing effects of human macrophage colony-stimulating factor on secretion of human chorionic gonadotropin by human chorionic villous cells and tPA30-1 cells. Biochem Biophys Res Commun 178:1099–1104, 1991.

34. Castellucci M, Kaufmann P, Bischof P: Extracellular matrix influences hormone and protein production by human chorionic villi. Cell Tissue Res 262:135–142, 1990.

35. Emonard H, Christiane Y, Smet M, et al: Type IV and interstital collagenolytic activities in normal and malignant trophoblast cells are specifically regulated by extracellular matrix. Invest Metast 10:170–177, 1990.

36. Fox H: Effects of hypoxia on trophoblast in organ culture. Am J Obstet Gynecol 107:1058–1064, 1970.

37. Kaufmann P: Untersuchungen uber die langhanszellen in der menschlichen placenta. Z Zellforsch 128:283–302, 1972.

38. Ringler GE, Strauss JF III: In vitro systems for the study of human placental endocrine function. Endocrine Rev 11:105–123, 1990.

39. Sasagawa M, Yamazaki T, Endo M, et al: Immunohistochemical localization of HLA antigens and placental proteins αhCG, βhCG, CTP, hPL, and SP1 in villous and extravillous trophoblast in normal human pregnancy: A distinctive pathway of differentiation of extravillous trophoblast. Placenta 8:515–528, 1987.

40. Fishel SB, Edwards RG, Evans CHJ: Human chorionic gonadotropin secreted by pre-implantation embryos cultured in vitro. Science 223:816–818, 1984.

41. Ohlsson R, Larsson E, Nilsson O, et al: Blastocyst implantation precedes induction of insulin-like growth factor II gene expression in human trophoblasts. Development 106:555–559, 1989.

42. Hoshina M, Boothby M, Boime I: Cytological localization of chorionic gonadotropin and placental lactogen mRNA during development of the human placenta. J Cell Biol 93:190–198, 1982.

43. Kliman HJ, Nestler JE, Sermasi E, et al: Purification, characterization and in vitro differentiation of cytotrophoblasts from human term placentae. Endocrinology 118:1567–1582, 1986.

44. Kao L-C, Caltabiano S, Wu S, et al: The human villous cytotrophoblast: Interactions with extracellular matrix proteins, endocrine function and cytoplasmic differentiation in the absence of syncytium formation. Dev Biol 130:693–702, 1988.

45. Petraglia F, Volpe A, Genazzani AR, et al: Neuroendocrinology of the human placenta. Front Neuroendocrinol 11:6–13, 1990.

46. Jaffe RB: Protein hormones of the placenta, decidua, and fetal membranes. In Yen SSC, Jaffe RB (eds): Reproductive Endocrinology (ed 3). Philadelphia, WB Saunders, 1991, pp 920–935.

46a. Morrish DW, Marusyk H, Siy O: Demonstration of specific secretory granules for human chorionic gonadotropin in placenta. J Histochem Cytochem 36:193–197, 1988.

46b. Schlafke S, Lantz KC, King BR, Enders AC: Ultrastructural localization of pregnancy-specific β₁-glycoprotein (SP1) and cathepsin B in villi of early placenta of the macaque. Placenta 13:417–428, 1992.

46c. Belisle S, Tulchinsky D: Amniotic fluid hormones. In Tulchinsky D, Ryan KJ (eds): Maternal-Fetal Endocrinology. Philadelphia, WB Saunders Co, 1980, pp 169–195.

47. Knoll BJ: Gene expression in the human placental trophoblast: A model for developmental gene regulation. Placenta 13:311–327, 1992.

47a. Salem HT, Menabawey M, Seppala M, et al: Human seminal plasma contains a wide range of trophoblast "specific" proteins. Placenta 5:413–418, 1984.

48. Nilson JH, Bokar JA, Clay CM, et al: Different combinations of regulatory elements may explain why placenta-specific expression of the glycoprotein hormone α-subunit gene occurs only in primates and horses. Biol Reprod 44:231–237, 1991.

49. Nachtigal MW, Nickel BE, Cattini PA: Pituitary-specific repression of placental members of the human growth hormone gene family. A

possible mechanism for locus regulation. J Biol Chem 268:8473–8479, 1993.

50. Hay DL, Lopata A: Chorionic gonadotropin secretion by human embryos in vitro. J Clin Endocrinol Metab 67:1322–1324, 1988.
51. Fiddes JC, Goodman HM: The gene encoding the common alpha subunit of the four human glycoprotein hormones. J Mol Appl Genet 1:3–18, 1981.
52. Naylor SL, Chin WW, Goodman HM, et al: Chromosome assignment of genes encoding the alpha and beta subunits of glycoprotein hormones in man and mouse. Somat Cell Mol Genet 9:757–770, 1983.
53. Policastro PF, Daniels-McQueen S, Caple G, Boime I: A map of the hCGβ-LHβ gene cluster. J Biol Chem 261:5907–5916, 1986.
54. Graham MY, Otani T, Boime I, et al: Cosmid mapping of the human chorionic gonadotropin β subunit genes by field-inversion gel electrophoresis. Nucleic Acids Res 15:4432–4448, 1987.
55. Hulsebos T, Brunner H, Wireinga B, et al: Regional assignment of C3, GP1, APOC2, and beta-HCG and their linkage relationships with DM and 91 cen. Cytogenet Cell Genet 40:658, 1985.
56. Brook JD, Shaw DJ, Meredith AL, et al: A somatic cell hybrid panel for chromosome 19: Localization of known genes and RFLP's and orientation of the linkage groups. Cytogenet Cell Genet 40:590–591, 1985.
57. Jameson JL, Lindell CM: Isolation and characterization of the human chorionic β subunit (CGβ) gene cluster: Regulation of a transcriptionally active CGβ gene by cyclic AMP. Mol Cell Biol 8:5100–5107, 1988.
58. Otani T, Otani F, Bo M, et al: Promoter sequences in the chorionic gonadotropin β subunit gene. In Mochizuki M, Hussa R (ed): Placental protein hormones. Amsterdam, Elsevier, 1988, pp 87–100.
59. Talmadge K, Vamvakopoulos NC, Fiddes JC: Evolution of the genes for the β subunits of human chorionic gonadotropin and luteinizing hormone. Nature 307:37–40, 1984.
60. Fares FA, Suganuma N, Nishimori K, et al: Design of a long-acting follitropin agonist by fusing the c-terminal sequence of the chorionic gonadotropin β subunit to the follitropin β subunit. Proc Natl Acad Sci USA 89:4304–4308, 1992.
61. Matzuk MM, Biome I: The role of the asparagine-linked oligosaccharides of the α subunit in the secretion and assembly of human chorionic gonadotropin. J Cell Biol 106:1049–1059, 1988.
62. Matzuk MM, Boime I: Site-specific mutagenesis defines the intracellular role of the asparagine-linked oligosaccharides of chorionic gonadotropin β subunit. J Biol Chem 263:17106–17111, 1988.
63. Matzuk MM, Keene JL, Boime I: Site-specificity of the chorionic gonadotropin N-linked oligosaccharides in signal transduction. J Biol Chem 264:2409–2414, 1989.
64. Braunstein GD, Rasor J, Adler D, et al: Serum human chorionic gonadotropin levels throughout normal pregnancy. Am J Obstet Gynecol 126:678–681, 1976.
65. Lenton EA, Neal LM, Sulaiman R: Plasma concentrations of human chorionic gonadotropin from the time of implantation until the second week of pregnancy. Fertil Steril 37:773–778, 1982.
66. Gosseye S, Fox H: An immunocytochemical comparison of the secretory capacity of villous and extravillous trophoblast in the human placenta. Placenta 5:329–348, 1984.
67. Beck T, Schweikhart G, Stolz E: Immunohistochemical localization of HPL, SP1 and βHCG in normal placentas of varying gestational age. Arch Gynecol 239:63–74, 1986.
68. Kadar N, Romero R: Observations on the log human chorionic gonadotropin–time relationship in early pregnancy and its practical implications. Am J Obstet Gynecol 157:73–78, 1987.
69. Pittaway DE, Reish RL, Wentz AC: Doubling times of human chorionic gonadotropin increase in early viable intrauterine pregnancies. Am J Obstet Gynecol 152:299–302, 1985.
70. Lenton EA, Woodward AJ: The endocrinology of conception cycles and implantation in women. J Reprod Fertil (Suppl) 36:1–15, 1988.
71. Rizkallah T, Gurpide E, Vande Wiele RL: Metabolism of HCG in man. J Clin Endocrinol Metab 29:92–100, 1969.
72. Jovanovic L, Landesman R, Saxena BB: Screening for twin pregnancies. Science 198:738, 1977.
73. Hussa RO: Clinical utility of human chorionic gonadotropin and α-subunit measurements. Obstet Gynecol 60:1–12, 1982.
74. Bogart MH, Pandian MR, Jones OW: Abnormal maternal serum chorionic gonadotropin level in pregnancies with fetal chromosome abnormalities. Prenat Diagn 7:623–630, 1987.
75. Bogart MH, Golbus MS, Sorg DS, Jones OW: Human chorionic gonadotropin levels in pregnancies with aneuploid fetuses. Prenat Diagn 9:379–384, 1989.

76. Obiekwe BC, Chard T: Placental proteins in late pregnancy: Relation to fetal sex. Br J Obstet Gynaecol 3:163–164, 1983.
77. Nakajima ST, McAuliffe T, Gibson M: The 24-hour pattern of the levels of serum progesterone and immunoreactive human chorionic gonadotropin in normal early pregnancy. J Clin Endocrinol Metab 71:345–353, 1990.
78. Houghton DJ, Newnham JP, Lo K, et al: Circadian variation of circulating levels of placental proteins. Br J Obstet Gynaecol 89:831–835, 1982.
79. Wathen NC, Cass PL, Kitau MJ, Chard T: Human chorionic gonadotropin and alpha-fetoprotein levels in matched samples of amniotic fluid, extraembryonic coelomic fluid and maternal serum in the first trimester of pregnancy. Prenat Diagn 11:145–151, 1991.
80. McGregor WG, Kuhn RW, Jaffe RB: Biologically active chorionic gonadotropin: Synthesis by the human fetus. Science 220:306–309, 1983.
81. Rothman PA, Chao VA, Taylor MR, et al: Extraplacental human fetal tissues express mRNA transcripts encoding the human chorionic gonadotropin-β subunit protein. Mol Reprod Dev 33:1–6, 1992.
82. Cole LA, Kroll TG, Ruddon RW, Hussa RO: Differential occurrence of free beta and free alpha subunits of human chorionic gonadotropin (hCG) in pregnancy sera. J Clin Endocrinol Metab 58:1200–1202, 1980.
83. Hay DL: Discordant and variable production of human chorionic gonadotropin and its free α- and β-subunits in early pregnancy. J Clin Endocrinol Metab 61:1195–1200, 1985.
84. Ozturk M, Bellet D, Manil L, et al: Physiological studies of human chorionic gonadotropin (hCG), αhCG and βhCG as measured by specific monoclonal immunoradiometric assays. Endocrinology 120:549–558, 1987.
85. Blithe DL: N-linked oligosaccharides on free α interfere with its ability to combine with the human chorionic-β subunit. J Biol Chem 265:21951–21956, 1990.
86. Blithe DL, Nisula BL: Variations in the oligosaccharides on free and combined α subunits of human chorionic gonadotropin in pregnancy. Endocrinology 117:2218–2228, 1985.
87. Blithe DL: Carbohydrate composition of the α subunit of human chorionic gonadotropin (cCG-α) and the free α molecule produced in pregnancy: Most free α and some hCG α molecules are fucosylated. Endocrinology 126:2788–2799, 1990.
88. Skarulis MC, Wehmann RE, Nisula BC, Blithe DL: Glycosylation changes in human chorionic gonadotropin and free alpha subunit as gestation progresses. J Clin Endocrinol Metab 75:91–96, 1992.
89. Boime I: Human placental hormone production is linked to the stage of trophoblast differentiation. Troph Res 5:57–60, 1991.
89a. Siler-Khodr TM, Kang IA, Khodr GS: Effects of chorionic GNRH on intrauterine tissues and pregnancy. Placenta 12:91–103, 1991.
89b. Nulsen JE, Woolkalis MJ, Kopf GS, Strauss JF III: Adenylate cyclase in human cytotrophoblasts: Characterization and its role in modulating chorionic gonadotropin secretion. J Clin Endocrinol Metab 66:258–265, 1988.
89c. Masuhiro K, Matsuzaki N, Nishino E, et al: Trophoblast-derived interleukin-1 (IL-1) stimulates the release of human chorionic gonadotropin by activating the IL-6 and IL-6 receptor system in first trimester human trophoblasts. J Clin Endocrinol Metab 72:594–601, 1991.
89d. Nishino E, Matsuzaki N, Masuhiro K, et al: Trophoblast-derived interleukin-6 (IL-6) regulates human chorionic gonadotropin release through IL-6 receptor on human trophoblasts. J Clin Endocrinol Metab 71:436–441, 1990.
89e. Delegeane AM, Ferland LH, Mellon PL: Tissue-specific enhancer of the human glycoprotein hormone α-subunit gene: Dependence on cyclic AMP-inducible elements. Mol Cell Biol 7:3994–4002, 1987.
89f. Deutsch PJ, Jameson JL, Habener JF: Cyclic AMP responsiveness of human gonadotropin-α gene transcription is dissected by a repeated 18-base pair enhancer. J Biol Chem 262:12669–12174, 1987.
89g. Jameson JL, Hollenberg AN: Regulation of chorionic gonadotropin gene expression. Endocr Rev 14:203–221, 1993.
89h. Kelly AC, Rodgers A, Dong Xe-Wan, et al: Gonadotropin-releasing hormone and chorionic gonadotropin gene expression in human placental development. DNA Cell Biol 10:411–421, 1991.
89i. Tamada T, Akabori A, Konuma S, Araki S: Lack of release of human chorionic gonadotropin by gonadotropin-releasing hormone. Endocrinol Jpn 23:531–533, 1976.
89j. Menon KMJ, Jaffe RB: Chorionic gonadotropin-sensitive adenylate cyclase in human term placenta. J Clin Endocrinol Metab 36:1104–1109, 1973.
89k. Lei ZM, Rao ChV, Ackerman DM, Day TG: The expression of hu-

man chorionic gonadotropin/human luteinizing hormone receptors in human gestational trophoblastic neoplasms. J Clin Endocrinol Metab 74:1236–1241, 1992.

90. Ringler GE, Kallen CB, Strauss JF III: Regulation of human trophoblast function by glucocorticoids: Dexamethasone promotes increased secretion of chorionic gonadotropin. Endocrinology 124:1625–1631, 1989.

91. Petraglia F, Vaughan J, Vale W: Inhibin and activin modulate the release of GnRH, hCG and progesterone from cultured human placental cells. Proc Natl Acad Sci USA 86:5114–5117, 1989.

92. Petraglia F, Sawchenko PA, Lim ATW, et al: Localization, secretion and action of inhibin in human placenta. Science 237:187–189, 1987.

93. Wilson EA, Jawad MJ, Powell DE: Effect of estradiol and progesterone on human chorionic gonadotropin secretion in vitro. Am J Obstet Gynecol 149:143–148, 1984.

94. Maruo T, Matsuo H, Ohtani T, et al: Differential modulation of chorionic gonadotropin (CG) subunit messenger ribonucleic acid levels and CG secretion by progesterone in normal placenta and choriocarcinoma cultured in vitro. Endocrinology 119:855–864, 1986.

95. Ren SG, Braunstein GD: Decidua produces a protein that inhibits choriogonadotrophin release from human trophoblasts. J Clin Invest 87:326–330, 1991.

96. Nisula BL, Wehmann RE: Distribution, metabolism and excretion of human chorionic gonadotropin and its subunits in man. In Segal SJ (ed): Chorionic Gonadotropin. New York, Plenum Press, 1980, pp 199–212.

97. Zirken S, Gawinowicz MA, Kardana A, Cole LA: The heterogeneity of human chorionic gonadotropin (hCG). II. Characteristics and origin of nicks in hCG reference standards. Endocrinology 29:1551–1558, 1991.

98. Kato Y, Braunstein GD: β-Core fragment is a major form of immunoreactive urinary chorionic gonadotropin in human pregnancy. J Clin Endocrinol Metab 66:1197–1201, 1988.

99. Wehmann RE, Blithe DL, Akar AH, Nisula BC: Disparity between β-core levels in pregnancy urine and serum: Implications for the origin of urinary β-core. J Clin Endocrinol Metab 70:371–378, 1990.

99a. de Medeiros SF, Amato F, Bacich D, et al: Distribution of the β-core human chorionic gonadotrophin fragment in human body fluids. J Endocrinol 135:175–188, 1992.

100. Stevens VC: Potential control of fertility in women by immunization with hCG. Res Reprod 7:1–9, 1985.

101. Bhattacharyya S, Chaudhary J, Das C: Antibodies to hCG inhibit progesterone production from human syncytiotrophoblast cells. Placenta 13:135–139, 1992.

102. Reshef E, Lei ZM, Rao CV, et al: The presence of gonadotropin receptors in nonpregnant human uterus, human placenta, fetal membranes and decidua. J Clin Endocrinol Metab 70:421–430, 1990.

103. Kennedy RL, Darne J: The role of hCG in regulation of the thyroid gland in normal and abnormal pregnancy. Obstet Gynecol 78:298–307, 1991.

104. Tomer Y, Huber GK, Davies TF: Human chorionic gonadotropin (hCG) interacts directly with recombinant human TSH receptors. J Clin Endocrinol Metab 74:1477–1479, 1992.

105. Seron-Ferre M, Lawrence CC, Jaffe RB: Role of hCG in the regulation of the fetal zone of the human fetal adrenal gland. J Clin Endocrinol Metab 46:834–837, 1978.

106. Rivera RT, Pasion SG, Wong DT, et al: Loss of tumorigenic potential by human lung tumor cells in the presence of antisense RNA specific to the ectopically synthesized alpha subunit of human chorionic gonadotropin. J Cell Biol 108:2423–2434, 1984.

107. Kumar S, Talwar GP, Biswas DK: Necrosis and inhibition of growth of human lung tumor by anti-α-human chorionic gonadotropin antibody. J Natl Cancer Inst 84:42–47, 1992.

108. Blithe DL, Richards RG, Skarulis MC: Free alpha molecules from pregnancy stimulate secretion of prolactin from human decidual cells: A novel function for free alpha in pregnancy. Endocrinology 129:2257–2259, 1991.

109. Bangham DR, Grab B: The second international standard for chorionic gonadotropin. Bull WHO 31:111–125, 1964.

110. Storring PC, Gaines D, Das RE, Bangham DR: International reference preparation of human chorionic gonadotropin for immunoassay: Potency estimates in various bioassay and protein binding assay systems and international reference preparation of the α and β subunits of human chorionic gonadotropin for immunoassay. J Endocrinol 84:295–310, 1980.

111. Ren GS, Braunstein GD: Human chorionic gonadotropin. Sem Reprod Endocrinol 10:95–105, 1992.

112. Chard T: Pregnancy tests: A review. Hum Reprod 7:701–710, 1992.

113. Batzer FR, Schlaff S, Goldfarb AF, Corson SL: Serial beta-subunit human chorionic gonadotropin doubling time as a prognosticator of pregnancy outcome in an infertile population. Fertil Steril 35:307–312, 1981.

114. Holman J, Tyrey ER, Hammond C: A contemporary approach to suspected ectopic pregnancy with use of quantitative and qualitative assays for the beta subunit of human chorionic gonadotropin and sonography. Am J Obstet Gynecol 130:151–157, 1984.

115. Daya S, Woods S, Ward S, et al: Transvaginal ultrasound scanning in early pregnancy and correlation with human chorionic gonadotropin levels. J Clin Ultrasound 19:139–142, 1991.

116. White I, Papiha SS, Magnay D: Improved methods of screening for Down's syndrome. N Engl J Med 320:401–402, 1989.

117. Braunstein GD: hCG expression in trophoblastic and nontrophoblastic tumors. In Fishman WH (ed): Oncodevelopmental Markers. Biologic Diagnostic and Monitoring Aspects. New York, Academic Press, 1983, p 351.

118. Braunstein GD, Thompson R, Prinder SL, McIntire KR: Trophoblastic proteins as tumor-markers in nonseminomatous germ cell tumors. Cancer 57:1842–1845, 1986.

119. Borkowski A, Puttaert V, Gyling M, et al: Human chorionic gonadotropin-like substances in plasma of normal nonpregnant subjects and women with breast cancer. J Clin Endocrinol Metab 58:1171–1178, 1984.

120. Odell WD, Griffin J: Pulsatile secretion of chorionic gonadotropin during the normal menstrual cycle. J Clin Endocrinol Metab 69:528–532, 1989.

121. Odell WD, Griffin J, Bashey HM, Snyder PJ: Secretion of chorionic gonadotropin by cultured human pituitary cells. J Clin Endocrinol Metab 71:1318–1321, 1990.

122. Filstein MR, Cullinan JA, Strauss JF III: Aberrant results of serum β-human chorionic gonadotropin assays: An infrequent but vexing problem. Fertil Steril 39:714–716, 1983.

123. Hussa RO, Rinke ML, Schweitzer P: Discordant hCG results: Causes and solutions. Obstet Gynecol 65:211–219, 1985.

124. Barsch GS, Seeburg PH, Gelinus RE: The human growth hormone gene family: Structure and evolution of the chromosomal locus. Nucleic Acids Res 11:3939–3958, 1983.

125. George DL, Phillips J, Francke U, Seeburg PH: The genes for growth hormone and chorionic somatomammotropin are on the long arm of human chromosome 17 in the region q21 to pter. Hum Genet 57:138–141, 1981.

126. Harper ME, Barrera-Saldana HA, Saunders GF: Chromosomal localization of the human placental lactogen-growth hormone gene cluster to 17q22-24. Am J Hum Genet 34:227–234, 1982.

127. Walker WH, Fitzpatrick AL, Barrera-Saldana HA, et al: The human placental lactogen genes: Structure, function, evolution and transcriptional regulation. Endocrinol Rev 12:316–328, 1991.

128. Cooke NE, Emery JG, Ray J, et al: Placental expression of the human growth hormone-variant gene. Troph Res 5:61–74, 1991.

129. MacLeod JN, Lee AK, Liebhaber A, Cooke NE: Developmental control and alternative splicing of the placentally expressed transcripts from the human growth hormone gene cluster. J Biol Chem 267:14219–14226, 1992.

130. Li CH, Dixon JS, Chung D: Amino acid sequence of human chorionic somatomammotropin. Arch Biochem Biophys 155:95–110, 1973.

131. Bewley TA, Dixon JS, Li CH: Sequence comparison of human pituitary growth hormone, human chorionic somatomammotropin, and nine pituitary growth and lactogenic hormones. Int J Pept Protein Res 4:281–287, 1972.

132. Beck JA: Time of appearance of human placental lactogen in the embryo. N Engl J Med 283:189–190, 1970.

133. Sciarra JJ, Kaplan SL, Grumbach MM: Localization of anti-human growth hormone serum within the human placenta: Evidence for a human chorionic growth hormone prolactin. Nature 199:1005–1006, 1963.

134. Braunstein GD, Rasor JL, Engvall E, Wade ME: Interrelationships of human chorionic gonadotropin, human placental lactogen, and pregnancy-specific β₁-glycoprotein throughout normal human gestation. Am J Obstet Gynecol 138:1205–1213, 1980.

135. Sciarra JJ, Sherwood LM, Varma AA, Lunberg WB: Human placental lactogen (HPL) and placental weight. Am J Obstet Gynecol. 101:413–416, 1968.

136. Spellacy WN, Carlson KL, Birk SA: Dynamics of human placental lactogen. Am J Obstet Gynecol 96:1164–1173, 1966.

137. Seeburg PH, Shine J, Martial JA, et al: Nucleotide sequence of part of the gene for human chorionic somatomammotropin: Purification of DNA complementary to predominant mRNA species. Cell 12:157–165, 1977.

138. Barrera-Saldana HA, Robberson DL, Saunders GL: Transcriptional products of the human placental lactogen gene. J Biol Chem 257:12399–12404, 1982.

139. Kaplan SL, Gurpide E, Sciarra JJ, Grumbach MM: Metabolic clearance rate and production rate of chorionic growth hormone-prolactin in late pregnancy. J Clin Endocrinol Metab 28:1450–1460, 1968.

140. Beck P, Daughaday WH: Human placental lactogen: Studies on its acute metabolic effects and disposition in normal men. J Clin Invest 46:103–110, 1967.

141. Beck P: Pattern of the human chorionic somatomammotropin (HCS) concentration ratio in maternal serum and amniotic fluid during normal pregnancy. Acta Endocrinol (Copenh) 76:364–368, 1974.

142. Kaplan SL, Grumbach MM: Serum chorionic "growth hormone prolactin" and serum pituitary growth hormone in mother and fetus at term. J Clin Endocrinol Metab 25:1370–1374, 1965.

143. Houghton DJ, Shackleton P, Obiekwe BC, Chard T: Relationship of maternal and fetal levels of human placental lactogen to the weight and sex of the fetus. Placenta 5:455–458, 1984.

144. Handwerger S: The physiology of placental lactogen in human pregnancy. Endocrinol Rev 12:329–336, 1991.

145. Talamantes F, Ogren L: The placenta as an endocrine organ: Polypeptides. In Knobil E, Neill JD (eds): The Physiology of Reproduction. New York, Raven Press, 1988, pp 2093–2144.

146. Hochberg Z, Bick T, Perlman R: Two pathways of placental lactogen secretion by cultured human trophoblast. Biochem Med Metab Biol 39:111–116, 1988.

147. Watkins WB, Yen SSC: Somatostatin in cytotrophoblast of the immature human placenta: Localization by immunoperoxidase cytochemistry. J Clin Endocrinol Metab 50:969–971, 1980.

147a. Macaron C, Kynel M, Rutsky L: Failure of somatostatin to affect human chorionic somatomammotropin and human chorionic gonadotropin secretion in vitro. J Clin Endocrinol Metab 47:1141–1143, 1978.

148. Ylikorkala O, Kivinen S, Ronnberg L: Bromocryptine treatment during early human pregnancy: Effects on the levels of prolactin, sex steroids and placental lactogen. Acta Endocrinol (Copenh) 95:412–415, 1980.

149. Macaron C, Famuyiwa O, Singh SP: In vitro effects of dopamine and pimozide on human chorionic somatomammotropin (hCS) secretion. J Clin Endocrinol Metab 47:168–170, 1978.

150. Belleville F, Lasbennes A, Nabet P, Paysant P: HCS-HCG regulation in cultured placenta. Acta Endocrinol (Copenh) 88:169–181, 1978.

151. Shu-ronj Z, Bremme K, Eneroth P, Nordberg A: The regulation in vitro of placental release of human chorionic gonadotropin, placental lactogen and prolactin. Effects of an adrenergic beta-receptor agonist and antagonist. Am J Obstet Gynecol 143:444–450, 1982.

152. Zeitler P, Markoff E, Handwerger S: Characterization of the synthesis and release of human placental lactogen and human chorionic gonadotropin by an enriched population of dispersed placental cells. J Clin Endocrinol Metab 57:812–818, 1983.

153. Harman I, Zeitler P, Ganong B, et al: Sn 1,2 diacylglycerols and phorbol esters stimulate the synthesis and release of human placental lactogen from placental cells: A role for protein kinase C. Endocrinology, 119:1239–1244, 1986.

154. Tyson JE, Austin KL, Farinholt JW: Prolonged nutritional deprivation in pregnancy: Changes in chorionic somatomammotropin and growth hormone secretion. Am J Obstet Gynecol 109:1080–1082, 1971.

155. Kim YJ, Felig P: Plasma chorionic somatomammotropin levels during starvation in midpregnancy. J Clin Endocrinol Metab 32:864–867, 1971.

156. Burt RL, Leake NH, Rhyne AL: Human placental lactogen and insulin-blood glucose homeostasis. Obstet Gynecol 36:233–237, 1970.

157. Gaspard U, Sandront H, Luyckz A: Glucose-insulin interaction and the modulation of human placental lactogen (HPL) secretion during pregnancy. J Obstet Gynaecol Br Commonw 81:201–209, 1974.

158. Grumbach MM, Kaplan SL, Abrams CL, et al: Plasma free fatty acid response to the administration of chorionic "growth hormone-prolactin." J Clin Endocrinol Metab 26:478–482, 1966.

159. Beck P: Comparative studies on the metabolic effects of some param-

eters of carbohydrate and lipid metabolism after intravenous administration of human placental lactogen, human prolactin and growth hormone. Acta Endocrinol [Suppl] (Copenh) 173:104, 1973.

160. Williams C, Coltart TM: Adipose tissue metabolism in pregnancy: The lipolytic effect of human placental lactogen. Br J Obstet Gynaecol 85:43–46, 1978.

161. Turtle JR, Kipnis DM: The lipolytic action of human placental lactogen on isolated fat cells. Biochim Biophys Acta 144:583–593, 1967.

162. Genazzani AR, Benuzzi-Badoni M, Felber JP: Human chorionic somatomammotropin (HCSM): Lipolytic action of a pure preparation of isolated fat cells. Metabolism 18:593–598, 1969.

163. Genazzani AR, Zaragoza N, Neri P, Felber JP: Human chorionic somatomammotropin (HCS): Effects on glucose metabolism in rat epididymal adipose tissue. Ital J Biochem 19:230–240, 1970.

164. Felber JP, Zaragoza N, Benuzzi-Badoni M, Genazzani AR: The double effect of human chorionic somatomammotropin (HCS) and pregnancy in lipogenesis and on lipolysis in the isolated rat epididymal fat pad and fat pad cells. Horm Metab Res 4:293–296, 1972.

165. Kalkhoff RK, Kissebah AH, Kim HJ: Carbohydrate and lipid metabolism during normal pregnancy: Relationship to gestational hormone action. Semin Perinatol 2:291–307, 1978.

166. Grumbach MM, Kaplan SL, Sciarra JJ, Burr IM: Chorionic growth hormone–prolactin (CGP): Secretion, disposition, biological activity in man and postulated function as the "growth hormone" of the second half of pregnancy. Ann NY Acad Sci 148:501–531, 1968.

167. Josimovich JB, Mintz DH: Biological and immunochemical studies on human placental lactogen. Ann NY Acad Sci 148:488–500, 1968.

168. Kalkhoff RK, Richardson BL, Beck P: Relative effects of pregnancy, human placental lactogen and prednisolone on carbohydrate tolerance in normal and subclinical diabetic subjects. Diabetes 18:153–163, 1969.

169. Samaan N, Yen SCC, Gonzalez D, Pearson OH: Metabolic effects of placental lactogen (HPL) in man. J Clin Endocrinol Metab 28:485–491, 1968.

170. Nielsen JH: Effects of growth hormone, prolactin and placental lactogen on insulin content and release and deoxyribonucleic acid synthesis in cultured pancreatic islets. Endocrinology 110:600–606, 1982.

171. Beck P: Reversal of progesterone enhanced insulin production by human chorionic somatomammotropin. Endocrinology 87:311–315, 1970.

172. Sladek CD: The effects of human chorionic somatomammotropin and estradiol on gluconeogenesis and hepatic glycogen formation in the rat. Horm Metab Res 7:50–54, 1975.

173. Leake NH, Burt RL: Effects of HPL and pregnancy on glucose uptake in rat adipose tissue. Am J Obstet Gynecol 103:39–43, 1969.

174. Shultz RB, Blizzard RM: A comparison of human placental lactogen (HPL) and human growth hormone (HGH) in hypopituitary patients. J Clin Endocrinol Metab 26:921–924, 1966.

175. Friesen H: Purification of a placental factor with immunological and chemical similarity to human growth hormone. Endocrinology 76:369–381, 1965.

176. Florini JR, Tonelli G, Breuer CB, et al: Characterization and biological effects of purified placental protein (human). Endocrinology 79:692–708, 1966.

177. Kaplan SL, Grumbach MM: Studies of a human and simian placental hormone with growth hormone-like and prolactin-like activities. J Clin Endocrinol Metab 24:80–100, 1964.

178. Murakawa S, Raben MS: Effect of growth hormone and placental lactogen on DNA synthesis in rat costal cartilage and adipose tissue. Endocrinology 83:645–650, 1968.

179. Hill DJ, Crace CJ, Milner RDG: Incorporation of [³H]-thymidine by isolated human fetal myoblasts and fibroblasts in response to human placental lactogen (HPL): Possible mediation of HPL action by release of immunoreactive SM-C. J Cell Physiol 125:337–344, 1985.

180. Hill DJ, Crace CJ, Strain AJ, Milner RDG: Regulation of amino acid uptake and deoxyribonucleic acid synthesis in isolated human fetal fibroblasts and myoblasts: Effects of human placental lactogen, somatomedin-C, multiplication-stimulating activity, and insulin. J Clin Endocrinol Metab 62:753–761, 1986.

181. Strain AJ, Hill DJ, Swenne I, Milner RDG: Regulation of DNA synthesis in human fetal hepatocytes by placental lactogen, growth hormone, and insulin-like growth factor I/somatomedin-C. J Cell Physiol 132:33–40, 1987.

182. Welsch CW, McManus MJ: Stimulation of DNA synthesis by human placental lactogen or insulin in organ cultures of benign human breast tumors. Cancer Res 37:2257–2261, 1977.

183. McManus MJ, Dembroske SE, Pienkowski MM, et al: Successful transplantation of human benign breast tumors into the athymic nude mouse and demonstration of enhanced DNA synthesis by human placental lactogen. Cancer Res 38:2343–2349, 1978.

184. Beck P: Lactogenic activity of human chorionic somatomammotropin in rhesus monkeys. Proc Soc Exp Biol Med 140:183–187, 1972.

185. Thordarson G, Talamantes F: Role of the placenta in mammary gland development and function. In Neville MC, Daniel C (eds): The Mammary Gland: Development, Regulation, and Function. New York, Plenum Press, 1986, pp 459–498.

186. Parks JS, Nielsen PV, Sexton LA, Jorgensen EH: An effect of gene dosage on production of human chorionic somatomammotropin. J Clin Endocrinol Metab 60:994–997, 1985.

187. Hubert C, Descombey D, Mondon F, Daffos F: Plasma human chorionic somatomammotropin deficiency in a normal pregnancy is the consequence of low concentration of messenger RNA coding for human chorionic somatomammotropin. Am J Obstet Gynecol 147:676–678, 1983.

188. Simon P, Decoster C, Brocas H, et al: Absence of human chorionic somatomammotropin during pregnancy associated with two types of gene deletion. Hum Genet 74:235–238, 1986.

189. Nielsen PV, Pedersen H, Kampmann EM: Absence of human placental lactogen in an otherwise uneventful pregnancy. Am J Obstet Gynecol 135:322–326, 1976.

190. Wurzel JM, Parks JS, Herd JE, Nielsen PV: A gene deletion is responsible for absence of human chorionic somatomammotropin. DNA 1:251–257, 1982.

191. Frankenne F, Hennen G, Parks JS, Nielsen PV: A gene deletion in the hCH/hCS gene cluster could be responsible for the placental expression of hCH and/or hCS like molecules absent in normal subjects. Endocrinology 118(Suppl):128, 1986.

192. Frankenne F, Rentier-Delrue F, Scippo ML, et al: Expression of the growth hormone variant gene in human placenta. J Clin Endocrinol Metab 64:633–637, 1987.

193. Frankenne F, Closset J, Gomez F, et al: The physiology of growth hormones in pregnant women and partial characterization of a placental variant. J Clin Endocrinol Metab 66:1171–1175, 1986.

194. Berry SA, Srivastava CH, Rubin LR, et al: Growth hormone-releasing hormone-like messenger ribonucleic acid and immunoreactive peptide are present in human testes and placenta. J Clin Endocrinol Metab 75:281–284, 1992.

195. Ray J, Okamura H, Kelly PA, et al: Human growth hormone-variant demonstrates a receptor binding profile distinct from that of normal pituitary growth hormone. J Biol Chem 265:7939–7944, 1990.

196. MacLeod JN, Worsley I, Ray J, et al: Human growth hormone-variant is a biologically active somatogen and lactogen. Endocrinology 128:1298–1302, 1991.

197. Hill DJ, Riley SC, Bassett NS, Waters MJ: Localization of the growth hormone receptor, identified by immunocytochemistry in second trimester human fetal tissues and in placenta throughout gestation. J Clin Endocrinol Metab 75:646–650, 1992.

198. Urbaneck M, MacLeod JN, Cooke NE, Liebhaber SA: Expression of a human growth hormone (hGH) receptor isoform is predicted by tissue-specific alternative splicing of exon 3 of the hCG receptor gene transcript. Mol Endocrinol 6:279–287, 1992.

199. Bass SH, Mulkerrin MG, Wells JA: A systematic mutational analysis of hormone-binding determinants in the human growth hormone receptor. Proc Natl Acad Sci USA 88:4498–4502, 1991.

200. Spellacy WN, Buhi WC, Birk SA: The effectiveness of human placental lactogen measurements as an adjunct in decreasing perinatal deaths. Am J Obstet Gynecol 121:835–844, 1975.

201. Polin JI, Frangipane WL: Current concepts in management of obstetric problems for pediatricians. I. Monitoring the high risk fetus. Pediatr Clin North Am 33:621–647, 1986.

202. Sasaki A, Tempst P, Liotta AS, et al: Isolation and characterization of a corticotropin-releasing hormone-like peptide from human placenta. J Clin Endocrinol Metab 67:768–773, 1988.

203. Robinson BG, D'Angio LA Jr, Pasieka KB, Majzoub JA: Preprocorticotropin releasing hormone: cDNA sequence and in vitro processing. Mol Cell Endocrinol 61:175–180, 1989.

203a. Chan E-C, Thomson M, Madsen G, et al: Differential processing of corticotropin-releasing hormone by the human placenta and hypothalamus. Biochem Biophy Res Commun 153:1229–1235, 1988.

204. Riley SC, Walton JC, Herlick JM, Challis JRG: The localization and distribution of corticotropin-releasing hormone in the human placenta and fetal membranes throughout gestation. J Clin Endocrinol Metab 72:1001–1007, 1991.

205. Okamoto E, Takagi T, Azuma C, et al: Expression of the corticotropin-releasing hormone (CRH) gene in human placenta and amniotic membrane. Horm Metab Res 22:394–397, 1990.

205a. Petraglia F, Sawchenko PE, Rivier J, Vale W: Evidence for local stimulation of ACTH secretion by corticotropin-releasing factor in human placenta. Nature 328:717–719, 1987.

206. Goland RS, Wardlaw SL, Stark RI, et al: High levels of corticotropin-releasing hormone immunoreactivity in maternal and fetal plasma during pregnancy. J Clin Endocrinol Metab 63:1199–1203, 1986.

207. Sasaki A, Shinkawa O, Margioris AN, et al: Immunoreactive corticotropin-releasing hormone in human plasma during pregnancy, labor, and delivery. J Clin Endocrinol Metab 64:224–229, 1987.

208. Campbell EA, Linton EA, Wolfe CD, et al: Plasma corticotropin-releasing hormone concentrations during pregnancy and parturition. J Clin Endocrinol Metab 64:1054–1059, 1987.

209. Frim DM, Emanuel RL, Robinson BG, et al: Characterization and gestational regulation of corticotropin-releasing hormone messenger RNA in human placenta. J Clin Invest 82:287–292, 1988.

210. Schulte HM, Healy DL: Corticotrophin releasing hormone and adreno-corticotrophin-like immunoreactivity in human placenta, peripheral and uterine vein plasma. Horm Metab Res [Suppl]16:44–46, 1987.

211. Economides D, Linton E, Nicolaides K, et al: Relationship between maternal and fetal corticotropin-releasing hormone-41 and ACTH levels in human mid-trimester pregnancy. J Endocrinol 114:497–501, 1987.

212. Maser-Gluth C, Lorenz U, Vecsei P: In pregnancy, corticotropin-releasing factor in maternal blood and amniotic fluid correlates with the gestational age. Horm Metab Res [Suppl] 16:42–44, 1987.

213. Laatikainen T, Virtanen T, Raisanen I, Salminen K: Immunoreactive corticotrophin releasing factor and corticotrophin in plasma during pregnancy, labor and puerperium. Neuropeptides 10:343–353, 1987.

214. Petraglia F, Giardino L, Coukos G, et al: Corticotropin-releasing factor and parturition: Plasma and amniotic fluid levels and placental binding sites. Obstet Gynecol 75:784–789, 1990.

215. Wolfe CDA, Patel SP, Campbell EA, et al: Plasma corticotrophin-releasing factor (CRF) in normal pregnancy. Br J Obstet Gynaecol 95:997–1002, 1988.

216. Wolfe CDA, Patel SP, Linton EA, et al: Plasma corticotrophin-releasing factor (CRF) in abnormal pregnancy Br J Obstet Gynaecol 95:1003–1006, 1988.

217. Okamoto E, Takagi T, Sath H, et al: Immunoreactive corticotrophin-releasing hormone, adrenocorticotrophin and cortisol in human plasma during pregnancy, delivery and post partum. Horm Metab Res 21:566–572, 1989.

218. Suda T, Iwashita M, Tozawa F, et al: Characterization of corticotrophin releasing hormone binding protein in human plasma by chemical cross-linking and its binding during pregnancy. J Clin Endocrinol Metab 67:1278–1283, 1988.

219. Orth DN, Mount CD: Specific high-affinity binding protein for human corticotropin-releasing hormone in normal human plasma. Biochem Biophys Res Commun 143:411–417, 1987.

220. Linton EA, Wolfe CDA, Behan DP, Lowry PJ: A specific carrier substance for human corticotrophin releasing factor in late gestational maternal plasma which could mask the ACTH-releasing activity. Clin Endocrinol (Oxf) 28:315–324, 1988.

221. Behan DP, Linton EA, Lowry PJ: Isolation of the human plasma corticotrophin-releasing factor-binding protein. J Endocrinol 122:23–31, 1989.

222. Potter E, Behan DP, Fischer WH, et al: Cloning and characterization of the cDNAs for human and rat corticotropin releasing factor-binding proteins. Nature 349:423–426, 1991.

223. Riley SC, Challis JRG: Corticotrophin-releasing hormone production by the placenta and fetal membranes. Placenta 12:105–119, 1991.

224. Jones SA, Challis JRG: Steroid, corticotropin-releasing hormone, ACTH and prostaglandin interactions in the amnion and placenta of early pregnancy in man. J Endocrinol 125:153–159, 1970.

225. Robinson BG, Emanuel RL, Frim DM, Majzoub JA: Glucocorticoids stimulate expression of corticotrophin-releasing hormone gene in human placenta. Proc Natl Acad Sci U.S.A. 85:5244–5248, 1988.

226. Jones SA, Brooks AW, Challis JRG: Steroids modulate corticotrophin-releasing factor production in human fetal membranes and placenta. J Clin Endocrinol Metab 68:825–830, 1989.

227. Troper PJ, Goland RS, Wardlaw SL, et al: Effects of betamethasone on maternal plasma corticotropin releasing factor, ACTH and cortisol during pregnancy. J Perinatol Med 15:221–225, 1987.

228. Jones CT, Gu W, Parer JT: Production of corticotrophin releasing

hormone by the sheep placenta in vivo. J Develop Physiol 11:97–101, 1989.
229. Petraglia F, Sutton S, Vale W: Neurotransmitters and peptides modulate the release of immunoreactive CRH from cultured human placental cells. Am J Obstet Gynecol 160:247–251, 1989.
230. Stark RI, Wardlaw SL, Daniel SS, et al: Vasopressin secretion induced by hypoxia in sheep: Developmental changes and relationship to β-endorphin. Am J Obstet Gynecol 143:204–215, 1982.
231. Oosterbaan HP, Swaab DF: Amniotic oxytocin and vasopressin in relation to human fetal development and labour. Early Hum Dev 19:253–262, 1989.
232. MacCannell KL, Lederis K, Hamilton PL, Rivier J: Amunine (ovine CRF) urotensin I and sauvagine, three structurally related peptides, produce selective dilation of the mesenteric circulation. Pharmacology 25:116–120, 1982.
233. Fisher LA, Jessen G, Brown MR: Corticotrophin-releasing factor (CRF): Mechanism to elevate mean arterial pressure and heart rate. Regul Pept 5:153–161, 1983.
234. Jones, SA, Challis JRG: Local stimulation of prostaglandin production by corticotrophin-releasing hormone in human fetal membranes and placenta. Biochem Biophys Res Commun 159:192–199, 1989.
235. Jones SA, Challis JRG: Effects of corticotrophin-releasing hormone and adrenocorticotrophin on prostaglandin output by human placenta and fetal membranes. Gynecol Obstet Invest 29:165–168, 1990.
236. Quartero HWP, Fry CH: Placental corticotrophin-releasing factor may modulate human parturition. Placenta 10:439–440, 1989.
237. Petraglia F, Garuti GC, De Ramundo B, et al: Mechanism of action of interleukin-1β in increasing corticotrophin-releasing factor and adrenocorticotrophin hormone release from cultured human placental cells. Am J Obstet Gynecol 163:1307–1312, 1990.
238. Romero R, Wu YK, Brody DT, et al: Human decidua: A source of interleukin-1. Obstet Gynecol 73:31–34, 1989.
239. Main EK, Strizki J, Schochet P: Placental production of immunoregulatory factors: Trophoblast is a source of interleukin-1. Troph Res 2:149–152, 1987.
240. Flynn A, Finke J, Hilfinker ML: Placental mononuclear phagocytes as a source of interleukin-1. Science 218:475–476, 1982.
241. Romero R, Brody DT, Oyarzun E, et al: Interleukin-1: A signal for the onset of parturition. Am J Obstet Gynecol 160:1117–1123, 1989.
242. Liotta A, Osanthanondh R, Ryan KJ, Krieger DT: Presence of corticotrophin in human placenta: Demonstration of in vitro synthesis. Endocrinology 101:1552–1558, 1977.
243. Liotta AS, Houghten R, Krieger DT: Identification of a β-endorphin-like peptide in cultured human placental cells. Nature 195:593–595, 1982.
244. Odagiri ED, Sherrell BJ, Mount CD, et al: Human placental immunoreactive corticotropin, lipotropin and β-endorphin: Evidence for a common precursor. Proc Natl Acad Sci USA 76:2027–2031, 1977.
245. Lemaire S, Valette A, Chouinard L, et al: Purification and identification of multiple forms of dynorphin in human placenta. Neuropeptides 3:181–191, 1983.
246. Carr BR, Parker CR, Madden JD, et al: Maternal plasma adrenocorticotrophin and cortisol relationships through human pregnancy. Am J Obstet Gynecol 139:416–422, 1981.
247. Okamoto E, Takagi T, Sata H, et al: Immunoreactive corticotrophin-releasing hormone, adrenocorticotrophin and cortisol in human plasma during pregnancy and delivery and postpartum. Horm Metab Res 21:566–572, 1989.
248. Valette A, Desprat R, Cros J, et al: Immunoreactive dynorphine in maternal blood, umbilical vein and amniotic fluid. Neuropeptides 7:145–151, 1986.
249. Goland RS, Wardlaw SL, Stark RI, Frantz AG: Human plasma β-endorphin during pregnancy, labor and delivery. J Clin Endocrinol Metab 52:74–78, 1981.
250. Wardlaw SL, Stark RI, Baxi L, Frantz AG: Plasma β-endorphin and β-lipotropin in the human fetus at delivery. Correlation with arterial pH and pO₂. J Clin Endocrinol Metab 49:888–891, 1979.
251. Belisle S, Petit A, Gallo-Payet N, et al: Functional opioid receptor sites in human placentas. J Clin Endocrinol Metab 66:283–289, 1988.
252. Petraglia F, Calza L, Giardino L, et al: Identification of immunoreactive neuropeptide Y in human placenta: Localization, secretion and binding sites. Endocrinology 124:2016–2022, 1989.
253. Petraglia F, Coukos G, Battaglia C, et al: Plasma and amniotic fluid immunoreactive neuropeptide-Y level changes during pregnancy, labor and at parturition. J Clin Endocrinol Metab 69:324–328, 1989.
254. Petraglia F, Garuti GC, Calza L, et al: Inhibin subunits in human placenta: Localization and messenger ribonucleic acid levels during pregnancy. Am J Obstet Gynecol 165:750–758, 1991.
255. Mayo KE, Cerelli GM, Speiss J, et al: Inhibin A-subunit cDNAs from porcine ovary and human placenta. Proc Natl Acad Sci USA 83:5849–5852, 1986.
256. Rabinovici J, Goldsmith PC, Librach CL, Jaffe RB: Localization and regulation of the activin-A dimer in human placental cells. J Clin Endocrinol Metab 75:571–576, 1992.
257. McLachlan RI, Healy DL, Lutjen PJ, et al: The maternal ovary is not the source of circulating inhibin levels during human pregnancy. Clin Endocrinol (Oxf) 27:663–668, 1987.
258. McLachlan RI, Healy DL, Robertson DM, et al: Circulating immunoreactive inhibin in the luteal phase, early gestation of women undergoing ovulation induction. Fertil Steril 48:1001–1005, 1987.
259. Abe Y, Hasegawa Y, Miyamoto K, et al: High concentration of plasma immunoreactive inhibin during normal pregnancy in women. J Clin Endocrinol Metab 71:133–137, 1990.
260. Abe Y, Hasegawa Y, Miyamoto K, et al: Activin-A in urine and amniotic fluid of pregnancy women. 71st Annual Meeting of the Endocrine Society, 1989, Abstr 1590.
261. Petraglia F, Calza L, Garuti GC, et al: Presence and synthesis of inhibin subunits in human decidua. J Clin Endocrinol Metab 71:487–492, 1990.
262. Diczfalusy E: Endocrine functions of the human fetoplacental unit. Fed Proc 23:791–798, 1964.
263. Albrecht ED, Pepe GJ: Placental steroid hormone biosynthesis in primate pregnancy. Endocrinol Rev 11:124–150, 1990.
264. Csapo A, Knobil E, Van der Molen HJ, Wiest WG: Peripheral plasma progesterone levels during human pregnancy and labor. Am J Obstet Gynecol 110:630–632, 1971.
265. Csapo AI, Pulkkinen MO, Ruttner B, et al: The significance of the human corpus luteum in pregnancy maintenance. I. Preliminary studies. Am J Obstet Gynecol 112:1061–1067, 1972.
266. Csapo AI, Pulkkinen MO, Wiest WG: Effects of luteectomy and progesterone replacement therapy in early pregnant patients. Am J Obstet Gynecol 115:759–765, 1973.
267. Csapo AI, Pulkkinen M: Indispensability of the human corpus luteum in the maintenance of early pregnancy: Luteectomy evidence. Obstet Gynecol Surv 83:69–81, 1978.
268. Cassmer O: Hormone production of the isolated human placenta. Studies on the role of the foetus in the endocrine functions of the placenta. Acta Endocrinol 32(Suppl 45):9–12, 1959.
269. Bloch K: Biological conversion of cholesterol to pregnanediol. J Biol Chem 157:661–666, 1945.
270. Hellig H, Gattereau D, Lefebvre Y, et al: Steroid metabolism from plasma cholesterol. I. Conversion of plasma cholesterol to placental progesterone in humans. J Clin Endocrinol Metab 30:624–631, 1970.
271. Alsat E, Malassiné A, Cédard L: Low density lipoprotein receptor function. A review. Troph Res 2:17–27, 1991.
272. Simpson R, Billheimer DR, MacDonald PC, et al: Uptake and degradation of plasma lipoproteins by human choriocarcinoma cells in culture. Endocrinology 104:8–16, 1979.
273. Winkel CA, Gilmore J, MacDonald PC, Simpson ER: Uptake and degradation of lipoproteins by human trophoblastic cells in primary culture. Endocrinology 107:1892–1898, 1980.
274. Henson MC, Pepe GJ, Albrecht ED: Developmental increase in placental low density lipoprotein uptake during baboon pregnancy. Endocrinology 130:1698–1706, 1992.
275. Gafvels ME, Coukos G, Sayegh R, et al: Regulated expression of the trophoblast α₂-macroglobulin receptor/low density lipoprotein receptor-related protein. Differentiation and cAMP modulate protein and mRNA levels. J Biol Chem 267:21230–21234, 1992.
276. Cummings SW, Hatley W, Simpson ER, Ohashi M: The binding of high and low density lipoproteins to human placental membrane fractions. J Clin Endocrinol Metab 54:903–908, 1982.
277. Nestler JE, Takagi K, Strauss JF III: Lipoprotein and cholesterol metabolism in cells that synthesize steroid hormones. In Estahani M, Swaney JB (eds). Advances in Cholesterol Research. Caldwell, NJ, Telford Press, 1991, pp 135–167.
278. Warth MR, Arky RA, Knopp RH: Lipid metabolism in pregnancy. III. Altered lipid composition in intermediate, very low, low and high density lipoprotein fractions. J Clin Endocrinol Metab 41:649–655, 1975.
279. Furuhashi M, Seo H, Mizutani S, et al: Expression of low density lipoprotein receptor gene in human placenta. Mol Endocrinol 3:1252–1256, 1989.

280. Van Leusden H, Villee CA: The de novo synthesis of sterols and steroids from acetate by preparations of human term placenta. Steroids 6:31–45, 1965.

281. Parker CR Jr, Illingworth DR, Bissonnette J, et al: Endocrine changes during pregnancy in a patient with homozygous familial hypobetalipoproteinemia. N Engl J Med 314:557–560, 1986.

282. Nulsen JC, Silavin SL, Kao LC, et al: Control of the steroidogenic machinery of the human trophoblast by cyclic AMP. J Reprod Fertil [Suppl]37:147–153, 1989.

283. Riley SC, Dupont E, Walton JC, et al: Immunohistochemical localization of 3β-hydroxy-5-ene-steroid dehydrogenase/Δ⁵-Δ⁴ isomerase in human placenta and fetal membranes throughout gestation. J Clin Endocrinol Metab 75:956–961, 1992.

284. Luu-The V, Lachance Y, Labrie C, et al: Full length cDNA structure and deduced amino acid sequence of human 3β-hydroxy-5-ene steroid dehydrogenase. Mol Endocrinol 3:1310–1312, 1989.

285. Rhaume E, Lachance Y, Zhao HF, et al: Structure and expression of a new complementary DNA encoding the almost exclusive 3β-hydroxysteroid dehydrogenase/Δ⁵-Δ⁴-isomerase in human adrenals and gonads. Mol Endocrinol 5:1147–1157, 1991.

286. Ringler GE, Kao L-C, Miller WL, Strauss JF III: Effects of 8-bromo-cAMP on expression of endocrine functions by cultured human trophoblast cells. Regulation of specific mRNAs. Mol Cell Endocrinol 6:13–22, 1989.

287. Picado-Leonard J, Voutilainen R, Kao LC, et al: Human adrenodoxin: Cloning of three cDNAs and cycloheximide enhancement in JEG-3 cells. J Biol Chem 263:3240–344, 1988.

288. Rabe T, Kiesel L, Runnebaum B: Regulation of human placental progesterone synthesis in vitro by naturally occurring steroids. J Steroid Biochem 22:657–664, 1985.

289. Lin TJ, Lin SL, Erlenmyer F, et al: Progesterone production rates during the third trimester of pregnancy in normal women, diabetic women and women with abnormal glucose tolerance. J Clin Endocrinol Metab 34:287, 1972.

290. Tulchinsky D, Hobel CJ: Plasma human chorionic gonadotropin, estrone, estradiol, estriol progesterone and 17α-hydroxyprogesterone in human pregnancy. III. Early normal pregnancy. Am J Obstet Gynecol 117:884–893, 1973.

291. Buster JE, Change RJ, Preston DL, et al: Interrelationships of circulating maternal steroid concentrations in third trimester pregnancies. I. C21 Steroids:Progesterone, 16α-hydroxyprogesterone, 17α-hydroxyprogesterone, 20α-dihydroprogesterone, Δ⁵-pregnenolone, Δ⁵-pregnenolone sulfate, and 17-hydroxy-Δ⁵-pregnenolone. J Clin Endocrinol Metab 48:133–138, 1979.

292. Johansson ED, Johansson LE: Progesterone levels in amniotic fluid and plasma from women. I. Levels during normal pregnancy. Acta Obstet Gynecol Scand 50:339–343, 1971.

293. Lin D, Gitelman SE, Saenger P, Miller WL: Normal genes for the cholesterol side chain cleavage enzyme, P450scc, in congenital lipoid hyperplasia. J Clin Invest 88:1955–1962, 1991.

294. MacDonald PC, Dombroski RA, Casey ML: Recurrent secretion of progesterone in large amounts: An endocrine/metabolic disorder unique to young women? Endocrinol Rev 12:372–401, 1991.

295. Milewich L, Gomez-Sanchez C, Madden JD, MacDonald PC: Isolation and characterization of 5α-pregnane-3,20-dione and progesterone in peripheral blood of pregnant women. Measurement throughout pregnancy. Gynecol Invest 6:291–306, 1975.

296. Anderson RA, Baellie TA, Axelson M, et al: Stable isotope studies on steroid metabolism and kinetics: Sulfates of 3α-hydroxy-5α-pregnane derivatives in human pregnancy. Steroids 55:443–457, 1990.

297. Laatikainen T, Karjalainen O: Excretion of conjugates of neutral steroids in human bile during late pregnancy. Acta Endocrinol (Kbh) 69:775–788, 1972.

298. Bradlow HL, Fukushima DK, Zumoff B, et al: Studies on 3α-hydroxy-5α-pregnan-20-one 4-14C. Steroids 10:389–396, 1967.

299. Parker CR Jr, Winkel CA, Rush AJ Jr, et al: Plasma concentrations of 11-deoxycorticosterone in women during the menstrual cycle. Obstet Gynecol 58:26–30, 1981.

300. Winkel CA, Milewich L, Parker CR Jr, et al: Conversion of plasma progesterone to deoxycorticosterone in men, nonpregnant and pregnant women, and adrenalectomized subjects: Evidence for steroid 21-hydroxylase activity in non-adrenal tissues. J Clin Invest 66:803–812, 1980.

301. Mellon SH, Miller WL: Extraadrenal steroid 21-hydroxylation is not mediated by P45021. J Clin Invest 84:1497–1502, 1989.

302. Baulieu EE: The steroid hormone antagonist RU486. Mechanism at the cellular level and clinical applications. Endocrinol Metab Clin North Am 20:873–891, 1991.

303. Siiteri PK, Febres F, Clemens S, et al: Progesterone and maintenance of pregnancy: Is progesterone nature's immunosuppressant? Ann NY Acad Sci 286:384–396, 1977.

304. Huszar G: The Physiology and Biochemistry of the Uterus in Pregnancy and Labor. Boca Raton, CRC Press, 1986.

305. Holzbauer M: Physiological aspects of steroids with anaesthetic properties. Med Biol 54:227–242, 1976.

306. Paul SM, Purdy RH: Neuroactive steroids. FASEB J 6:2311–2322, 1992.

307. Harrison NL, Majewska MD, Harrington JW, Barker JL: Structure-activity relationships for steroid interaction with the γ-aminobutyric acid A receptor complex. J Pharmacol Exp Ther 241:346–353, 1987.

308. Kappas A, Sassa S, Galbraith RA, Nordmann Y: The porphyrias. In Scriver CR, Beaudet AC, Sly WS, Vale D (eds): The Metabolic Basis of Inherited Disease. Vol 1. New York, McGraw-Hill, 1989, p 1305.

309. Cowan BD, Vandermolen DT, Long CA, Whitworth NJ: Receiver-operator characteristic, efficiency analysis, and predictive value of serum progesterone concentration as a test of abnormal gestations. Am J Obstet Gynecol 166:1729–1737, 1992.

310. Nygren KG, Johansson EDB, Wide L: Evaluation of the prognosis of threatened abortion from the peripheral plasma levels of progesterone, estradiol, and human chorionic gonatotropin. Am J Obstet Gynecol 116:916–922, 1973.

311. Tulchinsky D, Hobel CJ, Yeager E, Marshall JR: Plasma estradiol, estriol and progesterone in human pregnancy. Am J Obstet Gynecol 113:766–778, 1972.

312. Yoshimi T, Strott CA, Marshall JR, Lipsett MB: Corpus luteum function in early pregnancy. J Clin Endocrinol Metab 29:225–230, 1969.

313. Tulchinsky D, Simmer HH: Sources of plasma 17α-hydroxyprogesterone in human pregnancy. J Clin Endocrinol Metab 35:799–808, 1972.

314. Abraham GE, Samojlik E: Correlation between plasma unconjugated estriol and 16α-hydroxyprogesterone during human pregnancy. Obstet Gynecol 44:767–768, 1974.

315. Ryan KJ: Placental synthesis of steroid hormones. In Tulchinsky D, Ryan KJ (eds): Maternal-Fetal Endocrinology. Philadelphia, WB Saunders Co, 1980, pp 3–16.

316. Jost A: The fetal adrenal cortex. In Greep RO, Astwood WB (eds): Handbook of Physiology. Vol 6. Endocrinology. Washington, DC, American Physiological Society 1975, pp 107–115.

317. Spector WS (ed): Handbook of Biological Data. Philadelphia, WB Saunders Co, 1956.

318. Bethune JE (ed): The Adrenal Cortex: A Scope Monograph. Kalamazoo, UpJohn Co, 1974.

319. Benirschke K: Adrenals in anencephaly and hydrocephaly. Obstet Gynecol 8:412–425, 1956.

320. Seron-Ferre M, Lawrence CC, Siiteri PK, Jaffe RB: Steroid production by the definitive and fetal zones of the human fetal adrenal. J Clin Endocrinol Metab 47:603–609, 1978.

321. Winters AJ, Oliver C, Colston C, et al: Plasma ACTH levels in the human fetus and neonate as related to age and parturition. J Clin Endocrinol Metab 39:269–273, 1974.

322. Seron-Ferre M, Lawrence CC, Jaffe RB: Role of hCG in regulation of the fetal zone of the human fetal adrenal gland. J Clin Endocrinol Metab 46:834–837, 1978.

323. Davies IJ: The fetal adrenal. In Tulchinsky D, Ryan KJ (eds): Maternal-Fetal Endocrinology. Philadelphia, WB Saunders Co, 1980, pp 242–251.

324. Winters AJ, Colston C, MacDonald PC, Porter JC: Fetal plasma prolactin levels. J Clin Endocrinol Metab 4:626–629, 1975.

325. Jaffe RB, Seron-Ferre M, Crickard K, et al: Regulation and function of the primate fetal adrenal gland and gonad. Recent Prog Horm Res 37:41, 1981.

326. Simonian MH, Gill GN: Regulation of the fetal human adrenal cortex: Effects of adrenocorticotropin on growth and function of monolayer cultures of fetal and definitive zone cells. Endocrinology 108:1769–1779, 1981.

327. Crickard K, Ill CR, Jaffe RB: Control of proliferation of human fetal adrenal cells in vitro. J Clin Endocrinol Metab 53:790–800, 1981.

328. Voutilainen R, Miller WL: Coordinate tropic hormone regulation of mRNAs for insulin-like growth factor II and cholesterol side-chain cleavage enzyme, P450scc, in human steroidogenic tissues. Proc Natl Acad Sci USA 84:1590–1594, 1987.

329. Siiteri RK, MacDonald PC: Placental estrogen biosynthesis during human pregnancy. J Clin Endocrinol Metab 26:751–761, 1966.

330. Doody KM, Carr BR, Rainey WE, et al: 3-β-Hydroxysteroid dehydrogenase/isomerase in fetal zone and neocortex of the human fetal adrenal gland. Endocrinology 126:3487–3492, 1990.

331. Carr BR, Simpson ER: Lipoprotein utilization and cholesterol synthesis by the human fetal adrenal gland. Endocrinol Rev 2:306–326, 1981.

332. Parker CR Jr, Carr BR, Winkel CA, et al: Decline in the concentration of low-density lipoprotein-cholesterol in human fetal plasma near term. Metabolism 32:919–923, 1983.

333. Parker CR Jr, Carr BR, Winkel CA, et al: Hypercholesterolemia due to elevated low-density lipoprotein-cholesterol in newborns with anencephaly and adrenal atrophy. J Clin Endocrinol Metab 57:37–43, 1983.

334. Parker CR Jr, Simpson ER, Billheimer DW, et al: Inverse relation between low density lipoprotein-cholesterol and dehydroisoandrosterone sulfate in human fetal plasma. Science 208:512–514, 1980.

335. Gant NF, Hutchinson HT, Siiteri PK, MacDonald PC: Study of the metabolic clearance rate of dehydroisoepiandrosterone sulfate in pregnancy. Am J Obstet Gynecol 111:555–563, 1971.

336. Diczfalusy E: Steroid metabolism in the foeto-placental unit. In Pecile A, Finzi C (eds): The Foeto-Placental Unit. Amsterdam, Excerpta Medica, 1969, pp 65–109.

337. Inkster SE, Brodie AM: Immunocytochemical studies of aromatase in early and full-term human placental tissue: Comparison with biochemical assays. Biol Reprod 41:889–898, 1989.

338. Siiteri PK, MacDonald PC: Placental estrogen biosynthesis during human pregnancy. J Clin Endocrinol Metab 26:751–761, 1966.

339. Simpson ER, Mahendroo MS, Means GD, et al: Tissue-specific promoters regulate aromatose cytochrome P450 expression. J Steroid Biochem 44:321–330, 1993.

340. Kitawaki J, Inoue S, Tamura T, et al: Increasing aromatase cytochrome P-450 level in human placenta during pregnancy: Studied by immunohistochemistry and enzyme-linked immunosorbent assay. Endocrinology 130:2751–2757, 1992.

341. Dupont E, Labrie F, Luu-The V, Pelletier G: Localization of 17β-hydroxysteroid dehydrogenase throughout gestation in human placenta. J Histochem Cytochem 9:1403–1407, 1991.

342. Luu-The V, Labrie C, Simard J, et al: Structure of two in tandem human 17β-hydroxysteroid dehydrogenase genes. Mol Endocrinol 4:268–275, 1990.

343. Lobo JO, Bellino FL: Oestrogen synthetase (aromatase) and hormone secretion in primary cultures of human placental trophoblast cells. Effects of cyclic AMP addition at the start of culture in attached and unattached cell populations. Placenta 10:377–385, 1989.

344. Tremblay Y, Ringler GE, Morel Y, et al: Regulation of the gene for estrogenic 17-ketosteroid reductase lying on chromosome 17 cen-q25. J Biol Chem 264:20458–20462, 1989.

345. Ritvos O, Voutilainen R: Regulation of aromatase P-450 and 17β-hydroxysteroid dehydrogenase messenger ribonucleic acid levels in choriocarcinoma cells. Endocrinology 130:61–67, 1992.

346. Tulchinsky D, Hobel CJ, Korenman SG: A radioligand assay for plasma unconjugated estriol in normal and abnormal pregnancies. Am J Obstet Gynecol 111:311–318, 1971.

347. Loriaux DL, Ruder HJ, Knab DR, Lipsett MB: Estrone sulfate, estrone, estradiol and estriol plasma levels in human pregnancy. J Clin Endocrinol Metab 35:887–891, 1972.

348. Arai K, Kuwabara Y, Okinaga S: The effect of adrenocorticotropic hormone and dexamethasone, administered to the fetus in utero, upon maternal and fetal estrogens. Am J Obstet Gynecol 113:316–322, 1972.

349. Simmer HH, Frankland M, Greipel M: On the regulation of fetal and maternal 16α-hydroxydehydroepiandrosterone and its sulfate by cortisol and ACTH in human pregnancy at term. Am J Obstet Gynecol 121:646–652, 1975.

350. MacDonald PC, Siiteri PK: Origin of estrogen in woman pregnant with an anencephalic fetus. J Clin Invest 44:465–474, 1965.

351. Tulchinsky D, Korenman SG: The plasma estradiol is an index of fetoplacental function. J Clin Invest 50:1490–1497, 1971.

352. Abraham GE, Odell WD, Swerdloff RS, Hopper K: Simultaneous radioimmunoassay of plasma FSH, LH, progesterone, 17-hydroxyprogesterone, and estradiol-17β during the menstrual cycle. J Clin Endocrinol Metab 34:312–318, 1972.

353. Lindberg BS, Johansson EDB, Nilsson BA: Plasma levels of nonconjugated oestrone, oestradiol-17β and oestriol during uncomplicated pregnancy. Acta Obstet Gynecol Scand [Suppl] 32:21–36, 1974.

354. Klopper A, Masson G, Campbell D, Wilson G: Estriol in plasma: A compartmental study. Am J Obstet Gynecol 117:21–26, 1973.

355. Johannisson E: The foetal adrenal cortex in the human. Acta Endocrinol [Suppl] (Kbh) 130:1–107, 1968.

356. Goebelsmann U, Chen LC, Saga M, et al: Plasma concentration and protein binding of oestriol and its conjugates in pregnancy. Acta Endocrinol (Kbh) 74:592–604, 1973.

357. Schindler AE, Siiteri PK: Isolation and quantitation of steroids from normal human amniotic fluid. J Clin Endocrinol Metab 28:1189–1198, 1968.

358. Tulchinsky D, Frigoletto FD, Ryan KJ, Fishman J: Plasma estetrol as an index of fetal well-being. J Clin Endocrinol Metab 40:560–567, 1975.

359. Klopper A, Buchan P, Wilson G: The plasma half-life of placental hormones. Br J Obstet Gynaecol 85:738–747, 1978.

360. Diczfalusy E, Levitz M: Formation, metabolism, and transport of estrogen conjugates. In Bernstein S, Solomon S (eds): Chemical and Biological Aspects of Steroid Conjugates. New York, Springer-Verlag, 1970, pp 291–320.

361. Yen PH, Allen E, Marsh B, et al: Cloning and expression of steroid sulfatase cDNA and the frequent occurrence of deletions in STS deficiency: Implications for X-Y interchange. Cell 49:443–454, 1987.

362. Basler E, Grompe M, Parenti G, et al: Identification of point mutations in the steroid sulfatase gene of three patients with X-linked ichthyosis. Am J Hum Genet 150:483–491, 1992.

363. France JT, Liggins GC: Placental sulfatase deficiency. J Clin Endocrinol Metab 29:138–141, 1969.

364. France JT, Seddon RJ, Liggins GC: A study of pregnancy with low estrogen production due to placental sulfatase deficiency. J Clin Endocrinol Metab 36:1–9, 1973.

365. Bedin M, Alsat E, Tanguy G, Cédard L: Placental sulfatase deficiency: Clinical and biochemical study of 16 cases. Eur J Obstet Gynaecol Reprod Biol 10:21–34, 1980.

366. Lauritzen C: Conversion of DHA-sulfate to estrogens as a test of placental function. Horm Metab Res 1:96, 1969.

366a. Madden JD, Siiteri PK, MacDonald PC, et al: The pattern and rates of metabolism of maternal plasma dehydroisoandrosterone sulfate in human pregnancy. Am J Obstet Gynecol 125:915–920, 1976.

367. Shozu M, Akasofu K, Harada T, Kubota Y: A new cause of female pseudohermaphroditism: Placental aromatase deficiency. J Clin Endocrinol Metab 72:560–566, 1991.

368. Harada N, Ogawa H, Shozu M, et al: Biochemical and molecular genetic analyses in placental aromatase (P-450arom) deficiency. J Biol Chem 4781–4785, 1992.

368a. Harada N: Genetic analysis of human placental aromatose deficiency. J Steroid Biochem 44:331–340, 1993.

369. Resnik R, Killam AP, Battaglia FC, et al: The stimulation of uterine blood flow by various estrogens. Endocrinology 94:1192–1196, 1974.

370. Garfield RE, Kannan MS, Daniel EE: Gap junction formation in myometrium. Control by estrogens, progesterone, and prostaglandins. Am J Physiol 238:81–89, 1980.

371. Canick JA: Screening for Down syndrome using maternal serum alpha-feta-protein, unconjugated estriol and hCG. J Clin Immunoassay 13:30–33, 1990.

372. Wald NJ, Cuckle HS, Densem JW, et al: Maternal serum unconjugated oestriol as an antenatal screening test for Down's syndrome. Br J Obstet Gynaecol 95:334–341, 1988.

373. Sakbun V, Ali SM, Greenwood FC, Bryant Greenwood GD: Human relaxin in amnion, chorion, decidua parietalis, basal plate and placental trophoblast by immunohistochemistry and northern analysis. J Clin Endocrinol Metab 70:508–514, 1990.

374. Medina-Gomez P, Espinosa de-los Monteros A, Belmont J, Martinez E: Hormone release by primary amniotic fluid cell cultures. J Perinat Med 16:477–484, 1988.

375. Mitchell BF, Challis JRCT, Lukash L: Progesterone synthesis by human amnion, chorion and decidua at term. Am J Obstet Gynecol 157:349–353, 1987.

376. Poisner A: Storage, processing and release of chorionic renin and LHRH activity. In Mochizuki M, Hussa R (eds): Placental Protein Hormones. Amsterdam, Excerpta Medica, 1988, pp 161–170.

377. Sunnergren K, Sambrook JF, MacDonald PC, Casey ML: Expression and regulation of endothelin precursor mRNA in avascular human amnion. Mol Cell Endocrinol 68:R7–R14, 1990.

378. Germain AM, Aharoglu H, MacDonald PC, Casey ML: Parathyroid hormone-related protein mRNA in avascular human amnion. Endocrinology 75:1173–1175, 1992.

379. Bohn H: Biochemistry of placental proteins. In Bischof P, Klopper A (eds): Proteins of the Placenta. 5th Int Congress on Placental Proteins. Basel, S. Karger, 1984, pp 1–25.

380. Bischof P: Placental proteins. Contrib Gynecol Obstet 12:1–96, 1984.

381. Lin TM, Halbert SP, Kiefer D, et al: Characterization of four human pregnancy-associated plasma proteins. Am J Obstet Gynecol 118:223–236, 1974.

382. Bischof P: Purification and characterization of pregnancy associated plasma protein A (PAPP-A). Arch Gynecol 227:315–326, 1979.

383. Bischof P: Pregnancy-associated plasma protein-A. Semin Reprod Endocrinol 10:127–135, 1992.

384. Klopper A: Observations on the function of pregnancy associated plasma protein A. Placenta 4(Suppl):83, 1982.

385. Bischof P, DuBerg S, Schindler AM, et al: Endometrial and plasma concentrations of pregnancy-associated plasma protein-A (PAPP-A). Br J Obstet Gynaecol 89:701–703, 1982.

386. Westergaard JG, Hau J, Teisner B, Grudzinskas JG: Specific and reversible interaction between pregnancy-associated plasma protein A and heparin. Placenta 4:13–18, 1983.

387. Bischof P, Meisser A, Haenggeli L, et al: Pregnancy-associated plasma protein-A (PAPP-A) inhibits thrombin-induced coagulation of plasma. Thromb Res 32:45–55, 1983.

388. Bischof P, Lauber K, de Wurstemberger B, Girard JP: Inhibition of lymphocyte transformation by pregnancy-associated plasma protein A. J Clin Lab Immunol 7:61–65, 1982.

389. Westergaard JG, Chemnitz J, Teisner B: Pregnancy-associated plasma protein A: A possible marker in the classification and prenatal diagnosis of Cornelia de Lange syndrome. Prenat Diagn 3:225–232, 1983.

390. Thompson J, Koomari R, Wagner K, et al: The human pregnancy-specific glycoprotein genes are tightly linked on the long arm of chromosome 19 and are coordinately expressed. Biochem Biophys Res Commun 167:848–859, 1990.

391. Zheng Q-X, Tease LA, Shupert WL, Chan W-Y: Characterization of cDNAs of the human pregnancy-specific β_1 glycoprotein family: A new subfamily of the immunoglobulin gene superfamily. Biochemistry 29:2845–2852, 1990.

392. Chou JY, Plouzek CA: Pregnancy-specific β_1 glycoprotein. Semin Reprod Endocrinol 10:116–124, 1992.

393. Lin TM, Halbert SP, Spellacy WN: Measurement of pregnancy-associated plasma proteins during human gestation. J Clin Invest 54:576–582, 1974.

394. Lee JN, Grudzinskas JG, Chard T: Circulating levels of pregnancy proteins in early and late pregnancy in relation to placental tissue concentration. Br J Obstet Gynaecol 86:888–890, 1979.

395. Bohn H, Weinmann E: Immunologische unterbrechung der schwangerschaft bei affen mit antikorpern gegen das menschliche schwangershafts-spezifische β_1-glykoprotein (SP1). Arch Gynaek 217:209–218, 1974.

396. Bohn H: Untersuchungen uber das schwangerschaffs-spezifische β_1-glykoprotein (SP1). Arch Gynaek 216:347–358, 1974.

397. Gordon YB, Chard T: The specific proteins of the human placenta: Some new hypotheses. *In* Klopper A, Chard T (eds): Placental Proteins. New York, Springer-Verlag, 1979, pp 1–27.

398. Cerni C, Tatra G, Bohn H: Immunosuppression by human placental lactogen (hPL) and the pregnancy-specific β_1-glycoprotein (SP1). Inhibition of mitogen-induced lymphocyte transformation. Arch Gynaek 223:1–7, 1977.

399. Sakuragi N, Ohkubo H, Yamamoto R, et al: The serum pregnancy-specific β_1-glycoprotein to beta-human chorionic gonadotropin ratio as an index of prognosis in patients with choriocarcinoma. Br J Obstet Gynaecol 95:614–618, 1988.

400. Narisawa S, Millan JL: Placental alkaline phosphatase. Semin Reprod Endocrinol 10:136–145, 1992.

401. Mizutani S, Tomoda Y: Oxytocinase: Placental cystine aminopeptidase or placental leucine aminopeptidase (P-LAP). Semin Reprod Endocrinol 10:146–153, 1992.

402. Okamoto T, Seo H, Mano H, et al: Expression of human placenta alkaline phosphatase in placenta during pregnancy. Placenta 11:319–327, 1990.

125

Endocrinology of Parturition

GRAHAM C. LIGGINS

When the child has grown large, the mother cannot supply him with enough nourishment, he looks for more and he becomes agitated. Moving around and waving his arms and legs, the infant ruptures one of the internal membranes—Hippocrates, translated by Littre, 1851.

For more than 2000 years the determinants of the time of birth have excited the curiosity of physicians and philosophers. Hippocrates unequivocally designated an active role to the fetus, a view that held sway until Fabricius ab Aquapendente (1533–1619) accurately described the mechanics of labor and attributed its onset to the limits of uterine distensibility being reached as a result of fetal growth. William Harvey's (1578–1657) view that the fetus had no active part in the timing of labor was exemplified by a poem written of him by Martin Llewellyn (1653):

That both the Hen and the Housewife are so matcht
That her Son born is only her Son hatcht.

The theories abounding until recently invariably attributed the cause of labor to some aspect of maternal physiology, and they received powerful support with the advent of endocrinology. The discovery of estrogen, progesterone, and oxytocin, together with experiments showing that removal of the corpus luteum in animals caused abortion, appeared to confirm that control of the pregnant uterus resided in the maternal pituitary and ovary. By 1960, however, circumstantial evidence coming from two directions pointed to a fetal role as well. First, interbreeding of breeds with differing gestation lengths resulted in durations of intermediate length. The classic examples are the crosses between horses and donkeys (Table 125–1). Other less dramatic examples of crossbreeding have been described, ranging down to eastern and western Australian gray kangaroos, in which an intermediate gestation length is discernible despite the length of pregnancy being little more than the nonpregnant luteal phase.[1] Clearly, the fetal genotype influences gestation length. Second, experiments of nature in which greatly extended lengths of pregnancy were associated with defective development of the fetal pituitary gland gave a clue as to how the fetal genotype might be expressed. In sheep, ingestion of a teratogen contained in a weed, *Veratrum californicum*, on day 14 causes

cyclopean malformation, pituitary hypoplasia, and retention of the fetus for many weeks post term.[2] Likewise, an inherited defect of fetal pituitary development in cattle is characterized by enormously prolonged pregnancies.[3] Surgical hypophysectomy in fetal sheep[4] demonstrated directly both the obligatory contribution of the fetus to the initiation of parturition and the key role of the fetal pituitary. In twin pregnancies the presence of an intact fetus ensures delivery of both fetuses at normal term. Subsequent experiments, in which bilateral fetal adrenalectomy caused prolonged pregnancy[5] and infusion of ACTH or glucocorticoids caused premature delivery,[6] demonstrated that the adrenal secretion of cortisol mediates the action of the pituitary (Fig. 125–1). Section of the pituitary stalk[7] or destruction of the paraventricular nuclei[8] reproduces the effects of hypophysectomy, but the factors responsible for hypothalamic activation at term are uncertain.

Hopes that the understanding of the role of the fetal hypothalamic-pituitary-adrenal system in sheep would lead to rapid progress toward a similar understanding of the mechanism of parturition in humans proved to be groundless. Evidence was already available to indicate that humans and sheep differed fundamentally. A human fetus lacking a pituitary[9] or adrenals[10] may deliver spontaneously at term. Furthermore, treatment of pregnant women with corticosteroids in doses sufficient to inhibit fetal adrenal production of dehydroepiandrosterone (DHEA) and to accelerate maturation of fetal organs[11] does not shorten pregnancy. The mechanism that initiates parturition in human pregnancy remains enigmatic, although there is general agreement that it lies inside rather than outside the uterus.

TABLE 125–1. LENGTH OF PREGNANCY IN HORSE-DONKEY CROSSBREEDING

MATING	DURATION OF PREGNANCY (DAYS)
Stallion × mare	340
Stallion × jenny	350
Jack × mare	355
Jack × jenny	365

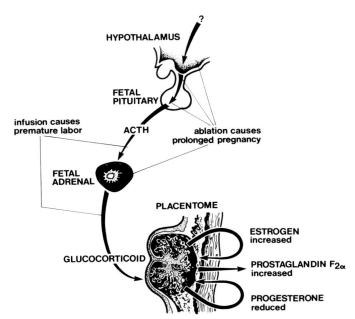

FIGURE 125–1. Diagram of the mechanism that initiates parturition in sheep. Interventions that increase glucocorticoid levels in the fetal circulation cause premature delivery, whereas those that prevent adrenal activation cause prolonged pregnancy.

COMPARATIVE ENDOCRINOLOGY

The species can be classified according to whether or not progesterone secreted by the corpus luteum is essential for the maintenance of pregnancy to term. Accordingly, the species can be sharply divided into corpus luteum–dependent and placenta-dependent; in the latter the placenta takes over as the major source of progesterone, usually before midpregnancy, and luteectomy is not followed by abortion. In human pregnancy the transition from luteal dependence to independence occurs at seven weeks.[12] The placenta-dependent species can be further subdivided in a way that is fundamental to understanding not only the nature of the fetoplacental unit but also the differing mechanisms of parturition: the placenta may or may not contain a functional steroid 17α-hydroxylase (cytochrome P-450 17α-hydroxylase). Examples of the classification are listed in Table 125–2. When the placental trophoblast contains an active 17α-hydroxylase, side-chain cleavage of progesterone by 17,20-desmolase can be achieved and the synthesis of androgens and estrogens from cholesterol can occur entirely within the placenta. In the absence of 17α-hydroxylase the synthesis of estrogen by the placenta requires an extraplacental source of an androgen precursor. In primates the precursor is DHEA secreted by the fetal zone of the fetal adrenal, which is sulfoconjugated in the fetal liver (see Ch. 127). In some species, such as horses and seals, the adrenal lacks a fetal zone, the source of androgen being the gonads, which are large, active, and visually indistinguishable between the sexes.

In relation to the initiation of parturition, the important property of 17α-hydroxylase is inducibility of activity by cortisol.[13] Thus activation of the fetal hypothalamic-pituitary-adrenal system at term (as in sheep) stimulates the conversion of progesterone to estrogen, resulting in a fall in placental secretion of progesterone and a rise in the production of estrogen.

These changes lead in turn to the release of prostaglandins and parturition. In contrast, a placenta that lacks 17α-hydroxylase activity (as in human pregnancy) is unable to respond to rising concentrations of cortisol by a fall in the ratio of progesterone-estrogen production. Indeed, the response to administered corticosteroid is the reverse of that in sheep; fetal adrenal secretion of DHEA is inhibited, leading to a fall in placental production of estrogen, whereas the production of progesterone is unchanged. Thus corticosteroid in human pregnancy increases, rather than reduces, the ratio of progesterone to estrogen.

In corpus luteum–dependent species, parturition is invariably preceded by luteolysis and a profound fall in progesterone production. The luteolytic signal is poorly understood but probably involves both withdrawal of a luteotrophic complex and release of a luteolysin, probably prostaglandin $F_{2\alpha}$ ($PGF_{2\alpha}$). The relative importance of the two components appears to vary between species, and the manner in which the conceptus contributes is uncertain. An interesting transitional species is the goat, which, although closely related to the sheep, is corpus luteum–dependent, but the placenta produces some steroids and has an active 17α-hydroxylase.[14] Rising concentrations of fetal cortisol induce the enzyme, stimulate estrogen production, release $PGF_{2\alpha}$, and cause luteolysis.

HUMAN PARTURITION

The time of onset of labor in women usually is defined by the beginning of regular, painful contractions at intervals of less than 10 minutes. This arbitrary definition has clinical utility but obscures the fact that less obvious events that are necessary for the normal progress of labor begin hours, days, or even weeks earlier. These changes involve the two cell types (smooth muscle cells and fibroblasts) responsible for expulsion of the conceptus from the uterus. Although labor often is considered solely in terms of smooth muscle contractions, the contribution of fibroblasts to connective tissue changes that convert the cervix from a firm, indistensible structure to a soft, compliant ring capable of stretching sufficiently to allow the passage of the fetus is of equal importance. Even the most forceful contractions are incapable of overcoming the resistance of the "unripe" cervix, and uterine rupture is a possible outcome.

TABLE 125–2. CLASSIFICATION OF SPECIES ACCORDING TO SOURCE OF PROGESTERONE IN LATE PREGNANCY AND PRESENCE OR ABSENCE OF PLACENTAL 17α-HYDROXYLASE

SOURCE OF PROGESTERONE	PLACENTAL 17α-HYDROXYLASE	EXAMPLES
Placenta	Present	Sheep
		Cattle
Placenta	Absent	Humans
		Primates
		Guinea pigs
Corpus luteum		Rabbits
		Rats
		Dogs

Connective Tissue Changes

Cervical Ripening

The time course of ripening varies from a few hours in some multigravid women to weeks in some primigravid women. The connective tissue changes involve the whole reproductive tract, including the vagina, but are most evident in the cervix because at least 80 per cent of its bulk is collagenous tissue, compared with about 5 per cent in the uterine body. The altered physical properties of the cervix result from well-defined biochemical events that differ only quantitatively from those that occur in connective tissues elsewhere in response to injury, inflammation, or remodeling.[15]

The morphological appearances during the ripening process have been studied by electron microscopy in animals.[16] The most prominent feature is dissolution, splitting up and dissociation of collagen fibers, and expansion of the interfibrillar space because of edema (Fig. 125–2). The fibroblasts are highly active with cytoplasmic components typical of secretory cells. Infiltration with polymorphonuclear granulocytes, macrophages, and mast cells is extensive. Biochemically, the morphological appearances are explained by a five-fold increase in collagenolytic activity and a 50 per cent reduction in the concentration of both collagen and sulfated glycosaminoglycans.[17] The latter, highly charged components of the proteoglycan matrix, bind collagen bundles tightly; a reduction in their concentration allows loosening of the bundles and more ready access of proteases secreted by the fibroblasts. The remaining collagen is mainly extractable, indicating recently synthesized protein with weak cross-links.

The physiological stimulus of cervical ripening is uncertain. In some animals, such as the sow, parturition is preceded by a marked rise in circulating relaxin,[18] but plasma concentrations are falling at term in women.[19] The source of circulating relaxin is the corpus luteum, but its removal during pregnancy has no ill effects on the dilatation of the cervix at term, despite unmeasurably low concentrations in plasma.[20] Nevertheless, local application of porcine relaxin to the cervix in women at term causes rapid ripening of the cervix.[21] Relaxin is also synthesized in the decidua only

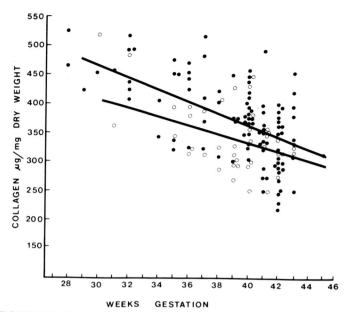

FIGURE 125–3. Concentration of collagen in amnion according to gestational age and whether the membranes ruptured prematurely (○) or not (●). (From Skinner SJM et al: Collagen content of human amniotic membranes: Effect of gestation length and premature rupture. Obstet Gynecol 57:487–489, 1981. Reprinted with permission from the American College of Obstetricians and Gynecologists.)

in small amounts, but it may be sufficient to diffuse to the cervix.[22] Prostaglandins (both PGE_2 and $PGF_{2\alpha}$) applied to the cervix are equally effective in promoting ripening[23] and are the likeliest candidates for the physiological stimulus by analogy with their well-established role in inflammatory conditions.

Rupture of the Membranes

The amnion is a remarkably robust membrane that will withstand pressures of up to 100 mm Hg until near term.[24] The membrane weakens as part of the preparations for the onset of labor to the extent that normal labor contractions of 15 to 20 mm Hg are sufficient to burst the amnion and the relatively weak chorion. Weakening of the amnion results from collagenolysis similar to that in the cervix, and the time courses of collagenolysis in the two tissues are similar; in primigravid women cervical ripening and effacement may be progressive over the last four to six weeks of pregnancy, and there is a 20 per cent loss of collagen in the amnion during this time.[25] The concentration of sulfated glycosaminoglycans falls in parallel with collagen (Fig. 125–3).

Uterine Contractility

The sympathetic nerve supply of the human uterus degenerates progressively through pregnancy, and there is no intrinsic neural network.[26] Thus propagation of spike potentials depends on the formation of points of low electrical resistance between smooth muscle cells. Until near term, gap junctions are sparse and uterine contractions are incoordinate. Gap junctions appear in term and preterm labor[27] when uterine contractions become coordinate (Ta-

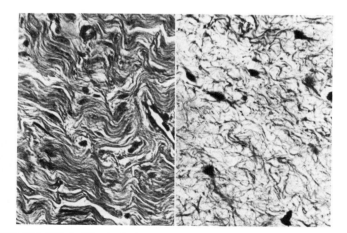

FIGURE 125–2. Histological appearance of the nonpregnant *(left)* and postpartum *(right)* cervix. ×835. (From Danforth DN et al: Connective tissue changes incident to cervical effacement. Am J Obstet Gynecol 80:939–945, 1960.)

ble 125–3). The stimulus to the formation of gap junctions is uncertain. In laboratory animals formation is promoted by estrogen or prostaglandins and inhibited by progesterone.[28] In the absence of prepartum changes in the concentrations of estrogen and progesterone (see below), prostaglandins are the likeliest stimulus to gap junction synthesis. At least in laboratory animals nonsteroidal antiinflammatory agents inhibit development of gap junctions.[29] As a consequence of gap junction formation, the myometrium functions as a syncytium, and spike potentials generated at a pacemaker site spread rapidly over the uterus.

Activation of the Uterus

Throughout pregnancy the uterus is relatively quiescent and is refractory to oxytocics such as oxytocin. Irregular, painless contractions, referred to as Braxton-Hicks contractions, are felt by the mother as "tightenings" in the latter half of pregnancy. Their duration may be as long as three to four minutes, possibly reflecting poor propagation, and they have no known function. Uterine quiescence is favored by the absence of gap junctions and by degeneration of the nerve supply, but, in addition, certain endocrine factors markedly reduce the excitability of the smooth muscle. Removal of these inhibitory factors is likely to make an important contribution to activation of the uterus at term.

Nonprostanoid Agonists of Uterine Functions

PROGESTERONE. Maintenance of pregnancy depends on progesterone in most—if not all—species, as is readily demonstrable by removal of the corpus luteum before placental production becomes an alternative source. Until recently the importance of progesterone throughout human pregnancy has been unclear, but with the advent of pharmacological inhibitors of progesterone synthesis and of receptor antagonists, a clearer picture is emerging. Epostane, an inhibitor of 3β-hydroxysteroid dehydrogenase, has been studied in the first and second trimesters[30] and was found to be ineffective in inducing abortion, although plasma concentrations of progesterone were maintained for several days at less than 20 per cent of pretreatment values. The synthesis of estrogen, as well as of progesterone, is inhibited by epostane, and the ratio of the two hormones is unaltered, perhaps explaining the failure to induce abortion. Alternatively, relatively low concentrations of proges-

TABLE 125–4. ACTIONS OF PROGESTERONE ON THE PREGNANT UTERUS

Promotes smooth muscle hypertrophy
Promotes formation of decidua
Promotes degeneration of uterine nerves
Promotes β-adrenergic response (relaxation)
Inhibits phospholipase A_2 activity and prostanoid synthesis
Increases capacity for prostanoid synthesis
Inhibits formation of gap junctions
Inhibits collagenolysis
Down-regulates oxytocin receptors
Down-regulates estrogen receptors
Down-regulates prostanoid receptors?
Inhibits immunological responses

terone may be sufficient to maintain pregnancy, a possibility that is supported by a report of a normal pregnancy despite very low levels of progesterone throughout pregnancy in a woman with abetalipoproteinemia.[31] The potent progesterone receptor antagonist mifepristone (RU486) is considerably more effective than epostane in inducing abortion in early pregnancy[32] but is increasingly less so after eight weeks unless followed by the administration of a prostaglandin analogue.[33, 34] These observations suggest that maintenance of human pregnancy, at least late pregnancy, is less dependent on progesterone compared with other species and that a fall in progesterone concentration is not in itself a stimulus of prostanoid synthesis.

The plasma concentration of progesterone rises linearly in the second half of pregnancy to reach values of 500 to 1000 mmol/L at term. Numerous investigators have sought evidence of a fall in concentration near term without success.[35, 36] The concentration of progesterone in fetal plasma obtained in utero by cordocentesis is in a similar range to that of the mother and likewise shows no fall at term.[37] Endometrial and myometrial nuclear receptors are saturated at term, and the concentrations of neither progesterone nor its receptors fall prepartum.[38–40] Challis and Mitchell[40] propose that progesterone is synthesized and metabolized near the site of action and that significant local changes in concentration may not be reflected in the plasma. In support of the hypothesis, they demonstrated that explant cultures of amnion, chorion, or decidua convert pregnenolone to progesterone and that activity is less in preparations taken after the onset of labor.

Progesterone has multiple actions that relate to the maintenance of pregnancy (Table 125–4). In vitro experiments with strips of human myometrium demonstrate that progesterone inhibits both spontaneous and oxytocin-induced contractions.[41] The inhibitory effect was attributed by some electrophysiologists to hyperpolarization of the cell membrane,[42] but this was not confirmed subsequently,[43, 44] and the question remains unresolved. There is agreement that progesterone attenuates action potentials and impairs the coupling of action potentials and mechanical activity. Other actions of progesterone have been demonstrated in laboratory animals and can only be assumed to apply to the human uterus. Inhibition of gap junction formation has been referred to above.[29] Inhibitory effects on the formation of oxytocin receptors and estrogen receptors and on prostaglandin synthesis are considered below. The key role of Ca^{2+} as a second messenger in mediating the contractile response to agonists suggests several post-

TABLE 125–3. GAP JUNCTIONS IN HUMAN MYOMETRIUM BEFORE AND DURING LABOR

SOURCE OF TISSUE	NO.	NO. WITH GJ's
Term labor	39	17
Spontaneous	22	12
Oxytocin-induced	17	5
Term prelabor	30	2
Preterm prelabor	6	0

GJ's, gap junctions.
Adapted with permission from Garfield RE, Hagashi RH: Appearance of gap junctions in the myometrium of women during labor. Am J Obstet Gynecol 140:257, 1981.

receptor sites at which progesterone might act. Preliminary work indicates an action of progesterone on G proteins.[45] In addition, progesterone inhibits adenosine triphosphate (ATP)–dependent calcium binding in a microsomal preparation of pregnant human myometrium.[46] Clearly, a better understanding of the regulation of smooth muscle contraction by progesterone at a molecular level awaits further investigations, but this may do little to explain how the actions of progesterone appear to be reversed at term with no apparent fall in the concentrations of progesterone or its receptors.

ESTROGEN. Human pregnancy is characterized by massive production of estrogen, much of it in the form of the weak estrogen estriol. Total estrogen concentrations in plasma rise from less than 10 ng/ml in early pregnancy to 100 to 200 ng/ml at term, the ratio of estriol–estradiol-17β–estrone being about 10:1:5. The pattern of placental estrogen production is dominated by the nature of the precursor and by the presence in the fetal liver of a very active 16α-hydroxylase; as a result, the major substrate for aromatization is 16-hydroxy DHEA and the product is estriol. Labor in women is not preceded by a rise in estrogen levels,[35, 36, 47, 48] in contrast to the sharp rise observed in species with an active 17α-hydroxylase. The concentration of the estradiol-17β in myometrium is low throughout pregnancy,[49] probably because of down-regulation of receptors by progesterone, and estradiol receptors increase in laboring women.[50] The concentrations of the catechol estrogens 2-hydroxyestradiol and 2-hydroxyestrone in amniotic fluid double with the onset of labor.[51] The source is unknown but could be a fetal urinary constituent, since levels in cord blood are high after spontaneous delivery.[52]

The actions of estrogen on the uterus are controversial because of contrasting responses in vitro and in vivo. The contractility of strips of human[53] or animal[54] myometrium is inhibited by estrogen with a potency greater than that of progesterone, yet in many species estrogen stimulates uterine activity in vivo. The paradox probably is resolved by the ability of estrogen to stimulate prostaglandin synthesis in the endometrium,[55] which is absent from muscle strips.

Estrogen production is readily manipulated in pregnant women by either suppressing fetal adrenal production of DHEA with corticosteroid or by administering DHEA to the mother. Prednisone in dosages of 20 mg/d or equivalent dosages of other glucocorticoids depress circulating estrogen levels to less than 10 per cent of normal values but do not prolong pregnancy. Conversely, intravenous infusions of DHEAS markedly increase plasma estradiol-17β and estriol levels but do not stimulate uterine activity. Placental sulfatase deficiency, a recessive X-linked chromosomal disorder that limits the conversion of DHEAS to DHEA and is associated with very low production of estrogen, is compatible with term delivery.[56] These observations do not encourage the view that placental estrogens have an active role in parturition. A paracrine mechanism whereby the abundant estrogen sulfates present in amniotic fluid are converted locally in the membranes to free estrogens has recently been postulated. A steroid sulfatase capable of hydrolyzing estrone sulfate is present in chorion and decidua and is more active in tissues obtained in labor.[57] These tissues also contain 17β-hydroxysteroid dehydrogenase, which converts estrone to estradiol-17β.

Although estrogen is unlikely to be active in promoting labor, a permissive role is possible. Animal experiments have shown that estrogen has several actions that enhance myometrial responsiveness. These include formation of gap junctions,[27] increasing oxytocin receptors,[58, 59] and release of $PGF_{2\alpha}$.[60] Caution must be exercised in extrapolating from animals to humans because of species variability. For example, in the guinea pig, a species in which the endocrinology of pregnancy shares many features with human pregnancy, estrogen inhibits both the onset of labor induced by the progesterone antagonists mifepristone and epostane and the release of $PGF_{2\alpha}$.[61] Estrogen stimulates prostaglandin production from nonpregnant human endometrium,[56, 62] but pregnant tissues have not been investigated. Indeed, no clear evidence exists of estrogen actions on the intact pregnant human uterus other than growth of muscle and connective tissues.

OXYTOCIN. The discovery of the potent oxytocic action of extracts of the posterior pituitary and the ability of infusions of Pituitrin to augment or induce labor in women led to the belief that the release of oxytocin from the maternal pituitary constituted the physiological stimulus that initiated labor. With the advent of sensitive immunoassays, attempts to show an increase in the concentration of oxytocin in jugular venous blood early in labor were unsucccessful.[63, 64] The measurement of oxytocin in plasma is difficult because the concentration usually is below the limits of sensitivity of the assay, release is pulsatile, and plasma contains an active L-cystine aminopeptidase that rapidly degrades oxytocin unless inactivated during the collection of samples. A recent study[65] using a highly specific antibody, frequent sampling (every minute for 30 minutes), and inactivation of oxytocinase found measurable pulses of one to three minutes' duration in women both before and during labor. The frequency of pulses increased from about one pulse every 30 minutes in women at term but not in labor to four pulses every 30 minutes in the first stage of labor. The amplitude of pulses (about 1 U/ml) did not differ in women before labor or during labor. These observations lend little support to the idea that the release of oxytocin initiates labor, although the increase in pulse frequency during labor may augment uterine contractility. The stimulus to increased pulse frequency is unknown, since there is no evidence of the existence in human pregnancy of the Ferguson reflex, a neural reflex that arises from cervical stretching that releases oxytocin in some laboratory animals.

The apparent absence of significantly increased oxytocin release at the onset of labor does not rule out a role for it, since greater sensitivity could have the same effect as greater concentration. A progressive increase in the response to oxytocin as pregnancy advances, reaching a peak near term, is well known to obstetricians who attempt to induce labor.[66] Theobald, who first observed the phenomenon, postulated that labor begins when the uterus becomes sufficiently sensitive to circulating oxytocin.[67] The molecular basis of increasing sensitivity is explained at least in part by rising concentrations of uterine oxytocin receptors. Myometrial oxytocin receptor concentration is 150 times greater in labor than in the nonpregnant uterus, which corresponds to a 100-fold increase in sensitivity.[68] The concentration of receptors during labor is twice that in myometrial samples taken before the onset of labor (Fig. 125–4). The up-regulation of oxytocin receptors probably is explained by the effects of rising concentrations of estrogen throughout pregnancy, but it is difficult to attribute

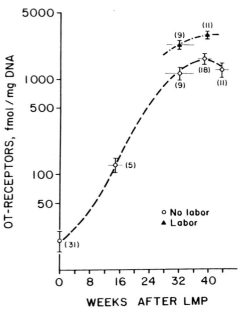

FIGURE 125–4. Concentration of oxytocin-binding sites in human myometrium throughout pregnancy and parturition. Note logarithmic scale. ○, before labor; ●, during labor. (From Fuchs A-R et al: Oxytocin receptors in human uterus during pregnancy and parturition. Am J Obstet Gynecol 150:734–741, 1984.)

the further rise during labor to estrogen, which remains unchanged at that time. The possibility that postreceptor events also mediate increased myometrial sensitivity has not been explored but may account for enhanced sensitivity to oxytocin observed during the administration of prostaglandins[69] or in muscle strips exposed to PGE_2.[70]

Despite its potency as an oxytocic and its ability to stimulate uterine activity throughout pregnancy, oxytocin is incapable of inducing labor except close to term. However, prior treatment with locally applied PGE_2 to ripen the cervix not only sensitizes the uterus but also facilitates induction of labor with oxytocin infusions earlier in pregnancy. Likewise, oxytocin is capable of inducing labor when preceded by amniotomy, a procedure that is known to cause the release of prostaglandins.[71] These observations emphasize the fact that the action of oxytocin on the uterus (decidua excepted) is limited to the smooth muscle and that labor cannot progress in the absence of changes in the connective tissue.

Receptor sites are present in the decidua as well as the myometrium, and their concentrations are highest during labor.[68, 72] The significance of this finding was greatly enhanced when it was demonstrated that oxytocin stimulates the release of $PGF_{2\alpha}$ and PGE_2 from explants of term decidua in culture[68] and of arachidonic acid and $PGF_{2\alpha}$ from superfused dispersed decidual cells[73] (Fig. 125–5). Assuming that prostaglandins generated by the decidua can diffuse into the myometrium, the uterine responsiveness to oxytocin could be amplified by a postreceptor action of decidual prostaglandin.

The second messenger mediating the interaction of oxytocin and its receptor is uncertain, but the action of oxytocin on both the contractile apparatus of the smooth muscle cells and the synthesis of prostaglandins almost certainly involves an increase in the intracellular concentration of

free calcium. Calcium-channel blockers of the dihydropyridine group inhibit both spontaneous and oxytocin-stimulated uterine contractions.[74] The nature of the coupling between oxytocin receptors and calcium channels is unknown. A G protein linked to the oxytocin receptor has yet to be demonstrated, but there is evidence for activation of phospholipase C and increased phosphatidylinositol turnover. The Ca^{2+}-mediated stimulation of phosphatidylinositol turnover depends only in part on the entry of extracellular Ca^{2+}.[75] In addition, Ca^{2+} is released from sarcoplasmic reticulum by inositol triphosphate and probably, therefore, by oxytocin.[76]

A further mechanism of oxytocin action has been demonstrated in rats and rabbits, but the applicability to the human uterus is uncertain.[77] Oxytocin inhibits (Ca^{2+})ATPase in the myometrial plasma membrane fraction. Presumably the lower rate of extrusion of Ca^{2+} by a calcium pump results in higher concentrations of intracellular Ca^{2+}.

The oxytocin story has been further complicated by the recent demonstration that human chorion contains oxytocin mRNA, the concentration of which is three to four times higher in tissue obtained during labor than in tissue obtained before labor.[78] The possibility that oxytocin released by the chorion has a paracrine action on the contiguous decidua remains speculative.

A competitive inhibitor of oxytocin, CAP 440 (1-deamino-2-D-Tyr(OEt)-4-Thr-8-Orn-oxytocin), is being used to investigate whether oxytocin has an obligatory role in the initiation of labor. Studies of human muscle strips in vitro show that CAP 440 abolishes oxytocin-stimulated contractions.[79] Uncontrolled trials in women in preterm labor indicate that it may be effective in stopping labor,[80] but the results of controlled trials are awaited before the question can be confidently addressed. Clinical reports of normal labor at term in hypophysectomized women do not necessarily exclude a permissive role for oxytocin, since hypothalamic release may provide sufficient amounts to activate a highly sensitive uterus.

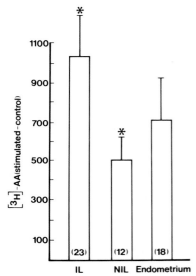

FIGURE 125–5. Effect of pulses of oxytocin on the release of labeled arachidonic acid from perfused decidual cells obtained either before (NIL) and after (IL) the onset of labor and from non-pregnant endometrium. (From Wilson T et al: Oxytocin stimulates the release of arachidonic acid and prostaglandin $F_{2\alpha}$ from human decidual cells. Prostaglandins 35:771–780, 1988.)

RELAXIN. The structure of the gene encoding human relaxin, a protein of about 6 kDa molecular weight, has been determined,[81] and recombinant material is available. Relaxin is a member of a family of structurally related peptides that includes insulin and insulin-like growth factors. The source of circulating relaxin in human pregnancy is the ovary, as in several animal species, and it disappears from the circulation after removal of the corpus luteum.[20] In some corpus luteum–dependent species, such as the pig and rat, parturition is preceded by a marked rise in the plasma concentration of relaxin preceding luteolysis,[18] which is thought to have profound effects on the pelvic and uterine connective tissues and on myometrial contractility. In human pregnancy, concentrations are lowest in the third trimester and unchanged at term,[82] which does not encourage the idea that systemic relaxin is relevant to parturition. Furthermore, labor begins normally at term and progresses without cervical dystocia in women who have been subjected to removal of the corpus luteum in midpregnancy. Recombinant human relaxin is not yet available in sufficient quantities to allow investigations of biological activities in vivo, but porcine relaxin applied to the cervix causes softening and effacement.[21] Although it is active in inhibiting contractility in rat myometrium in vitro, synthetic relaxin has little activity on human myometrium, suggesting that the latter lacks receptors. The pattern of circulating relaxin levels coupled with the absence of effects on the myometrium are in keeping with the proposal that the action of relaxin in human pregnancy is paracrine and mainly, if not exclusively, on the connective tissue of the cervix and membranes.[19] The decidua and, to a lesser extent, the chorion and amnion contain relaxin and express mRNA for both the H1 and H2 relaxin genes.[83] All these tissues contain high-affinity binding sites for porcine relaxin, and the membranes respond in vitro to relaxin with increased release of both plasminogen activator and collagenase.[84] Nothing is known of the factors that regulate relaxin production by the decidua, and a paracrine role for relaxin in the collagenolytic activity in the fetal membranes and cervix—although appealing—has yet to be firmly established.

CORTICOTROPIN-RELEASING HORMONE. The placenta and fetal membranes secrete large quantities of corticotropin-releasing hormone (CRH) predominantly into the maternal circulation but also into the amniotic fluid and fetal blood.[85, 86] The concentration in maternal plasma increases exponentially from less than 10 pg/ml in the first trimester to 2000 to 5000 pg/ml at delivery,[87] equaling that in pituitary portal blood of nonpregnant subjects (Fig. 125–6). Cord blood concentrations are 100- to 1000-fold lower than maternal values. A high-affinity binding protein of 37 kDA that has been sequenced[88] binds most of the CRH until near term, when the capacity of the binding protein falls and the levels of free CRH are greatly increased. In vitro the placental secretion of CRH is stimulated by oxytocin, prostaglandins, cytokines, catecholamines, and glucocorticoids[89] and inhibited by progesterone.[90]

The possible relevance to the initiation of parturition comes from two unusual actions of CRH. The release of PGE$_2$ by amnion in vitro is stimulated by CRH, and it has been proposed that CRH in amniotic fluid has a similar action in vivo.[90] Furthermore, CRH potentiates the contractile response of human myometrial strips to oxytocin, although it has no effect alone on contractility.[91] It is unlikely

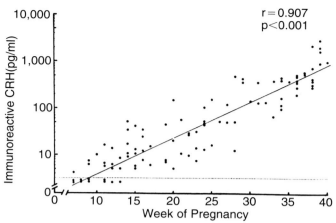

FIGURE 125–6. Concentration of immunoreactive corticotropin-releasing hormone throughout pregnancy. Note logarithmic scale. (From Sasaki A et al: Immunoreactive corticotropin-releasing hormone in human plasma during pregnancy, labor and delivery. J Clin Endocrinol Metab 64:224–229, 1987. © The Endocrine Society.)

that placental CRH in the fetal circulation has a major action on the pituitary-adrenal system, since anomalous fetuses that lack a hypothalamus have hypoplasia of the pituitary and adrenals. In addition, treatment of the fetus with corticosteroids causes marked inhibition of adrenal activity as judged by estriol production.

CYTOKINES. The part that cytokines play in the etiology of preterm labor is described in the section on preterm labor. At this point consideration is given only to those cytokines that may be part of the mechanism of normal labor at term.

Interleukin-8 (IL-8) is produced in large amounts by cultured decidual cells obtained from fetal membranes at elective cesarean section or spontaneous delivery.[92] Release is inhibited by progesterone and stimulated by the progesterone receptor antagonist mifepristone.

IL-8 is primarily a neutrophil chemotactic agent, but it also activates neutrophils. The products of neutrophil activation include collagenases and platelet-activating factor (PAF), which can stimulate prostaglandin synthesis. The hypothesis linking IL-8 to the onset of parturition comes from the observation that cervical biopsies taken during labor show infiltration with neutrophils,[93] suggesting a sequence of events beginning with the release of IL-8 and proceeding through neutrophil infiltration and activation, the release of collagenases and PAF, the release of prostaglandins, cervical ripening, and uterine contractions. The weakness of the hypothesis is that evidence does not support increased production of decidual IL-8 at the onset of labor, since the rates of release from tissue obtained before and during labor do not differ.[92]

Parathyroid hormone–related protein (PTHrP) has been identified in a number of human and animal reproductive tissues, including sheep placenta,[94] pregnant rat myometrium,[95] and human breast cancer.[96] The human myometrium has yet to be studied. The concentration of PTHrP in rat myometrium rises sharply from day 19 of pregnancy and is accompanied by a similar increase in levels of PTHrP mRNA.[95] Levels of the message are modulated by treatment with estradiol-17β but not by glucocorticoids. The contractility of rat myometrial strips in vitro is inhibited by PTHrP,[97] suggesting that the peptide may have functions similar to those of relaxin in maintaining uterine quiescence until overridden by oxytocin and $PGF_{2\alpha}$ at the start of labor.

ENDOTHELIN-1. This potent vasoactive peptide is present in amniotic fluid and probably arises from the amnion in which mRNA for the precursor is expressed in response to IL-1.[98] Amnion is an avascular tissue that lacks smooth muscle, and the target for endothelin may be the uterine smooth muscle. A direct action is possible, since it has been shown to increase cytoplasmic Ca^{2+} and myosin phosphorylation in human myometrium[99] and to stimulate contractions of the rat uterus.[100] An indirect action mediated by prostaglandin synthesis is an alternative possibility, since endothelin activates phospholipases A and C in vascular tissue.[101] Endothelin-1 has no effect on prostaglandin synthesis in cultures of decidua or amnion.[102] Endothelin-1 stimulates prostaglandin synthesis in nonpregnant proliferative endometrium but not in secretory endometrium,[113] which is consistent with the lack of response in pregnant tissues being attributable to inhibition by progesterone.

Endocrine Functions of the Decidua

The decidua occupies a crucial anatomical position, lying in apposition to the outer layer of the conceptus (the chorionic membrane and placenta) on the one hand and to the contractile tissue of the uterus on the other. Given that current hypotheses for the mechanism that initiates parturition in human pregnancy are invariably based on a paracrine relation of the conceptus and the maternal tissues, it is inevitable that the decidua is seen as the tissue that receives and relays signals emanating from the conceptus. Whereas little is known of the nature of the fetal signals, the decidua has a surprisingly wide range of potential transduction mechanisms. This specialized epithelium is analogous to the endothelium of blood vessels, which generates messengers, such as prostacyclin and endothelin, that mediate the effect of chemical and physical stimuli in the blood on the surrounding smooth muscle. Unlike the vascular endothelium, the decidua has a prominent stroma that contains large, lipid-filled cells, many of which may be derived from macrophages[104] and are the source of many of the decidual products.

Hormones and molecules with possible endocrine functions identified in decidua include prolactin, relaxin, human placental lactogen, prostanoids, somatostatin-like peptide, platelet-activating factor (PAF), and β-endorphin[22] (Table 125–5). Some of the products, such as prolactin, may be concerned primarily with regulation of the movement of fluid and electrolytes across the amniotic membrane. Others, particularly the prostanoids and relaxin, are directed toward the smooth muscle and connective tissue of the uterus. The remainder await designation of functions.

Prostanoids

Almost without exception, current hypotheses place prostanoids in a central position in the mechanism that initiates human parturition. The evidence supporting an obligatory role for prostanoids comes partly from clinical observations, partly from laboratory studies of human tissues in vitro, and partly from extrapolation of studies in laboratory animals, which include such diverse species as primates, ungulates, rodents, carnivores, lagomorphs, and marsupials. Evidence of a clinical nature includes the following:

1. Prostanoids are the only physiological agonists that induce abortion or labor at any stage of pregnancy from implantation to term. Administration of $PGF_{2\alpha}$, PGE_2, or one of their analogues by the parenteral, intravaginal, or intrauterine route is effective with a latent period of 8 to 24 hours.[23]

2. The clinical features of prostaglandin-induced labor mimic those of spontaneous labor in regard to both cervical and myometrial function.

3. Prostaglandin antagonists, such as indomethacin and fenamic acid derivatives, inhibit established labor. Withdrawal of the antagonist is followed by resumption of labor.[105]

4. Continuous administration of aspirin or salicylates is associated with prolonged pregnancy.[106]

5. The concentrations of $PGF_{2\alpha}$ and PGE_2 in amniotic fluid rise steeply during labor.[107, 108]

6. Attempted induction of labor with oxytocin at term is associated with a sustained increase in circulating PGFM only when induction is successful.[58]

7. Intra-amniotic injection of arachidonic acid causes abortion.[109]

8. Amniotomy and other mechanical methods of inducing labor are preceded by increased concentrations of $PGF_{2\alpha}$ in amniotic fluid[71] or PGFM in the circulation.[110]

Synthesis of Prostanoids

Prostaglandins are ubiquitous molecules synthesized in every tissue in the body by pathways that are common to all, although the end products vary in different tissues. The major precursor of the prostanoids is arachidonic acid, which is available in relatively large amounts from the glycerophospholipids of cell membranes, from triglycerides, and, probably, from circulating low-density lipoproteins (LDL) by way of the LDL receptor.[111] The phospholipids of fetal membranes are highly enriched in arachidonic acid,[112] which accounts for one seventh of the total content of fatty acids. In labor the fraction of arachidonic acid falls and is replaced by palmitic acid.[113] At least part of the arachidonic acid appears to enter the amniotic fluid during labor, the concentration rising up to 10-fold.[109] Intracellular concentrations of free arachidonic are maintained

TABLE 125–5. HORMONES, PEPTIDES, AND OTHER AGENTS PRODUCED BY OR ACTING ON THE DECIDUA

PRODUCT	AGONIST
Prostaglandins	Progesterone
Prolactin	Estrogen
Placental lactogen	Oxytocin
Protein 12	Gravidin
Protein 14	Bradykinin
Ca 125 antigen	Histamine
Cytokines	Interleukins
Oncofetal protein	Tumor necrosis factor
Platelet-activating factor	Prolactin

at very low levels by rapid re-incorporation into stores or by metabolism. Because prostanoids are not stored in cells, the rate of their release mainly depends on the rate of release of arachidonic acid from the various lipid stores. In some tissues the rate of synthesis of prostanoids may be controlled by the rate of reacylation,[114] but there is no evidence that this acyltransferase pathway is important in uterine tissues.

LIBERATION OF FREE ARACHIDONIC ACID. The rate of release of arachidonic acid from phospholipids, in which it occupies the *sn*-2 position, is catalyzed either by phospholipase A$_2$ (PLA$_2$) acting on the various phospholipids or by phospholipase C (PLC) acting specifically on phosphatidylinositol (Fig. 125–7). The relative proportions of arachidonic acid that arise from these two sources are uncertain and may vary according to whether release is basal or stimulated and to the nature of the stimulus. Both PLA$_2$ and PLC are Ca^{2+}-dependent.

Phospholipase C is activated by means of a G protein by the binding of certain agonists to their receptors. The products of hydrolysis of phosphatidylinositol-4,5-biphosphate by PLC are diacylglycerol (DAG) and inositol phosphates. Sequential hydrolysis of DAG by DAG-lipase and of monoacylglycerol (MAG) by MAG-lipase liberates arachidonic acid.[115] Activation of PLC leads to the release of arachidonic acid by two additional indirect mechanisms. Increased concentration of cytosolic Ca^{2+} in response to 1,4,5-inositol triphosphate liberated by phosphatidylinositol may stimulate PLA$_2$, which in turn releases arachidonic acid from phosphatidylcholine and phosphatidylethanolamine. In addition, DAG activates protein kinase C (PKC), which may be directly involved in phosphorylation of contractile proteins.[116] Phorbol esters that mimic the action of PKC stimulate prostaglandin synthesis in dispersed human endometrial cells.[55]

The activity of PLA$_2$ in fetal membranes and decidua increases through gestation, but there is no further increase with labor.[117] The enzyme is membrane-bound and inactive in vivo, activation occurring instantaneously without a requirement for synthesis of new protein. Thus assays in vitro determine enzyme content rather than activity in vivo. For the same reason, assays of the concentration of prostaglandins in tissues are indicative only of capacity for synthesis, since the trauma of tissue handling leads to activation of PLA$_2$ and the rapid synthesis of arachidonic acid metabolites.

At least near term the rate-limiting step in prostanoid synthesis is almost certainly the rate at which arachidonic acid is released by one or the other or both phospholipases rather than the rate of metabolism of arachidonic acid by cyclooxygenase or lipoxygenase. The rapidity with which substantial quantities of prostaglandins are released into the amniotic fluid by amniotomy,[71] which probably activates PLA$_2$, is consistent with the unimpeded further metabolism of arachidonic acid.

If it is accepted that phospholipases control the rate of synthesis of prostaglandins, it follows that factors that inhibit or stimulate phospholipase activity are crucial in the mechanism that initiates parturition. Apart from the many mechanical, chemical, and bacteriological factors that stimulate PLA$_2$ under pathological conditions, several agonists have physiological significance. Of these, oxytocin may be the most important. Oxytocin receptors in human term decidua mediate stimulation of PLC, as evidenced by an increase in the turnover of phosphatidylinositol with liberation of inositol phosphates and by inhibition of this response by the oxytocin antagonist CAP 440.[118] Explants of decidua release PGE and PGF$_{2\alpha}$ in response to oxytocin, but production is no greater from decidua obtained after labor than from that obtained before.[68] Dispersed decidual cells release both arachidonic acid and PGF$_{2\alpha}$, and the response is greater when the cells are harvested from fetal membranes after spontaneous delivery.[73] The relative contribution of arachidonic acid from hydrolysis of DAG or

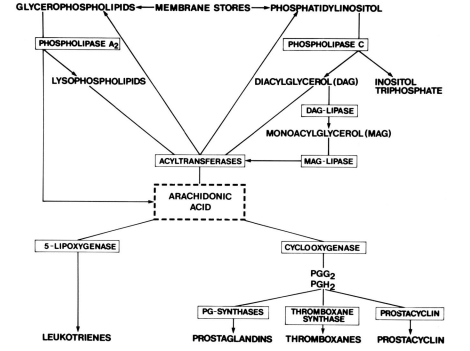

FIGURE 125–7. **Arachidonic acid cascade.** Arachidonic acid released from glycerophospholipids is either metabolized or immediately reincorporated.

from activation of PLA_2 by products of phosphatidylinositol turnover is unknown. Clearly, however, the observed increase in the concentration of oxytocin receptors in labor has the potential for playing an important part in stimulating production of prostaglandins at term, but it leaves unanswered the nature of the stimulus to receptor synthesis. A possible alternative is that prostaglandins enhance the sensitivity of the decidua to oxytocin, as they do in myometrium, thus creating a positive feedback loop in which increased production of prostaglandin is the primary event.

PAF is found in most samples of amniotic fluid from women in labor but is absent before labor.[120] The source of PAF is uncertain, since it is not released by amnion in culture, but the fluid secreted by the fetal lungs contains PAF associated with the lamellar body fraction. This bioactive lipid is known to increase cytosolic Ca^{2+}, which in turn can activate phospholipases, and it can also directly stimulate smooth muscle contraction. It has been speculated that the lung signals its maturity at term with increased PAF secretion into amniotic fluid, which then stimulates prostaglandin production and parturition. However, labor occurs normally at term in fetuses with anomalies such as pulmonary aplasia and tracheal atresia that prevent entry of lung fluid into the amniotic fluid. Constituents of fetal urine, including epidermal growth factor and an uncharacterized protein,[121] stimulate production of PGE_2 by amnion in vitro, but clinical evidence does not support the idea of the fetal kidneys sending a signal for parturition, since pregnancies are not prolonged in Potter's syndrome, in which the kidneys are absent. Estrogen stimulates a modest increase in prostaglandin production by amnion and decidual cells in culture, but the mode of action is unknown. The relevance of the observation that steroid sulfates, but not free steroids, stimulate PLA_2 activity[122] remains obscure.

A number of substances that inhibit release of arachidonic acid have been identified. At least part of the inhibitory action of progesterone may depend on the inhibition of PLA_2.[123] Lipocortins are abundant in human placenta,[124] suggesting that their inhibitory effects on PLA_2 could be relevant to intrauterine prostaglandin production, but available evidence is not supportive. Parturition is not delayed in women receiving corticosteroid treatment, and uterine tissues respond to rising plasma corticosteroid levels in labor with an increase, rather than a decrease, in the release of prostaglandin.[125] Renin, a chorionic product, inhibits amnion PGE_2 production in vitro by a mechanism that is not mediated by angiotensin II.[126] Prolactin, which is produced in abundance by decidua, inhibits production of PGE_2 by amnion but only in concentrations that greatly exceed those in amniotic fluid.[127] Gravidin, an 80-kDa protein that is a potent inhibitor of PLA_2, has been isolated from amniotic fluid and identified as the secretory component of immunoglobulin A.[128] Of the intrauterine tissues, gravidin is produced in vitro in greatest quantity by chorion (Fig. 125–8). The feature of gravidin that gives it particular relevance to parturition is the finding that the protein secreted by chorion, obtained after the onset of labor, no longer inhibits PLA_2.[129] Although the mechanism by which gravidin is inactivated is unknown, it possibly involves phosphorylation.

METABOLISM OF ARACHIDONIC ACID. The metabolism of free arachidonic acid can proceed through either the 5-

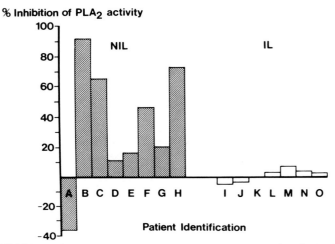

FIGURE 125–8. Effect on phospholipase A_2 activity of gravidin obtained from incubated chorion recovered from individual patients before (NIL) or after (IL) the onset of labor. (From Wilson T et al: Purification and characterization of a uterine phospholipase inhibitor that loses activity after labor onset in women. Am J Obstet Gynecol 160:602–606, 1989.)

lipoxygenase pathway to leukotrienes or the cyclooxygenase pathway to prostanoids. Although leukotrienes have been identified in uterine tissues,[119] there is little evidence of their involvement in the initiation of parturition. Arachidonic acid is converted by cyclooxygenase through PGG_2 to PGH_2, the common precursor of the prostaglandins. Specific prostacyclin synthetase and thromboxane synthetase form prostacyclin (PGI_2) and thromboxane, respectively (see Fig. 125–7). A specific isomerase and reductase form PGE_2 and $PGF_{2\alpha}$, respectively. Cyclooxygenase, a microsomal enzyme, usually is not regarded as rate-limiting for prostaglandin production, but there is evidence in some animal species that it may limit the rate of metabolism of arachidonic acid in intrauterine tissues.[130] The concentration of cyclooxygenase in human placental and myometrial microsomes increases three-fold through pregnancy, suggesting that the enzyme may be rate-limiting early in pregnancy.[131] The rate at which the enzyme in human chorioamnion is regenerated after irreversible inactivation by aspirin is five-fold greater in tissues obtained after spontaneous labor.[132]

Cyclooxygenase activity is self-regulating to the extent that one of the products (oxygen-derived free radicals) stimulates activity[133] and, possibly, contributes subsequently to rapid destruction of the enzyme. The activity may also be subject to regulation by PKC. Phorbol esters and synthetic DAG stimulate cyclooxygenase in dispersed amnion, and this action as well as that of dexamethasone and EGF is blocked by staurosporine, an inhibitor of PKC.[134] Increased activity by these means depends on protein synthesis, suggesting that activity is promoted by de novo synthesis of enzyme. Synthesis of the enzyme is probably stimulated also by estrogen, which may account for the increased release of prostaglandin in laboratory animals treated with estrogen.

The enzyme is best known as the site of the inhibitory action of aspirin on prostaglandin synthesis, but no endogenous inhibitors have been fully characterized. Endogenous inhibitor of prostaglandin synthase (EIPS), a protein-like material of about 30 kDa, is present in maternal and fetal plasma and in amniotic fluid.[135] The source of EIPS is unknown, but it might correspond to an as yet uncharacterized cyclooxygenase inhibitor generated by amnion.[136]

METABOLISM OF PROSTANOIDS. Prostanoids are metabolized to inactive products in or near their site of synthesis. Any residual active material that enters the circulation is cleared completely in a single passage through the lungs. This generalization holds also for the intrauterine tissues. Chorion is relatively low in synthetic capacity but is very active in metabolizing prostaglandins,[137] thereby limiting the diffusion of prostaglandins outward from the amnion or inward from the decidua, but there is no evidence that metabolism regulates the levels of biologically active prostaglandin. The relatively stable inactive metabolites that enter the circulation and are useful for immunoassay reflecting the rates of synthesis are 13,14-dihydro-15-keto-$PGF_{2\alpha}$ (PGFM), 13,14-dihydro-15-keto-PGE (PGEM), 11-deoxy-13, 14-dihydro-15-keto-11,16-cyclo-prostaglandin E_2 (PGEM-II), 6-keto-PGI_2, and thromboxane B_2. Plasma $PGF_{2\alpha}$ and PGE_2 are unstable and decompose during extraction, but PGE_2 can be stabilized by methoximation before extraction.

Sites of Prostanoid Synthesis

The fetal membranes, decidua, and myometrium all synthesize all the prostanoids as well as various lipoxygenase products, but the spectrum of products is characteristic of each tissue, reflecting varying activities of specific synthases. The predominant in vitro product of myometrium is PGI_2 and of decidua, $PGF_{2\alpha}$, whereas the amnion produces mainly PGE_2.[138] The cervix also releases prostaglandins in substantial amounts.[139] Overall, the amnion and cervix have the greatest capacity for synthesis of prostaglandins, at least in vitro, suggesting that the amnion is the source of prostaglandins that initiate labor. Although the amnion is the likely source of prostaglandins in amniotic fluid where PGE_2 predominates, several observations argue in favor of decidua rather than amnion as being the more important source.

1. Labor is associated with a marked increase in the plasma concentration of PGFM, whereas PGE_2 metabolite levels do not rise.[140, 141]

2. After delivery of the placenta and membranes, the plasma concentration of PGEM falls rapidly, whereas PGFM levels persist for several hours, pointing to a decidual source of PGFM.[142]

3. The conversion of PGE_2 formed in the amnion to $PGF_{2\alpha}$ in the decidua is unlikely because PGE_2 is metabolized by chorion during passage,[127] and the decidua has relatively low 9-keto-reductase activity, which converts PGE_2 to $PGF_{2\alpha}$.[143]

4. Amnion obtained during labor releases more PGE_2 in culture than amnion obtained before labor,[136, 144] perhaps reflecting collagenolysis during weakening of the membranes. The function of the active synthesis of PGE_2 by the amnion remains obscure.

Both components of decidua, the epithelium and the stromal cells, produce $PGF_{2\alpha}$ and serve as the major source of prostaglandin in labor. It has been proposed that the stromal cells are macrophage-like[104] and are derived in part from bone marrow cells.[145] Common features of macrophages and stromal cells include 1-hydroxylation of 25-OH-

vitamin D_3, production of β-endorphin, and release of prostaglandins and cytokines in response to bacterial endotoxin. The decidua is ideally situated as a source of prostaglandins that can diffuse outward into the myometrium, inward to the membranes and amniotic fluid, and even downward to the cervix. Furthermore, the endometrium is the source of the $PGF_{2\alpha}$ that causes luteolysis in many domestic and laboratory animals. In sheep and cattle the luteolytic signal is inhibited early in pregnancy by interferons released by the conceptus.[146] Menstrual cramps undoubtedly have their origin in the decidual production of prostaglandins and possibly leukotrienes.[147] The decidua is well placed also to receive signals from chorionic membrane or placenta with which it is in intimate contact. The rate of uterine synthesis of $PGF_{2\alpha}$ has been calculated from values for the plasma concentration of PGFM and its rate of clearance.[104] The rate obtained in this way is similar to the rate at which $PGF_{2\alpha}$ must be infused intravenously to induce labor when allowance is made for the large proportion of infused $PGF_{2\alpha}$ that is cleared by the lungs.

Prostacyclin produced by the myometrium derives in part from the vasculature and in part from the nonvascular smooth muscle.[131] As judged by little[148] or no[149] rise in the concentration of PGI_2 in amniotic fluid during labor, myometrial production of prostaglandins does not increase markedly with contractile activity.

All the intrauterine tissues release lipoxygenase products during culture with labeled arachidonic acid. The major products are 12-hydroxyeicosatetraenoic acid (12-HETE) and 15-HETE.[150] Amniotic fluid at term contains 12-HETE in a concentration similar to that of $PGF_{2\alpha}$ with lesser amounts of 15-HETE and leukotriene B_4. The concentrations in samples obtained during labor are increased at least two-fold.[151]

Actions of Prostanoids

The therapeutic use of prostaglandins in medical practice is restricted almost entirely to stimulating the pregnant uterus either early in pregnancy (abortion) or late in pregnancy (induction of labor). To a large extent, this restricted use is a consequence of unpleasant and potentially dangerous adverse effects associated with parenteral administration of prostaglandins or their analogues that act on many organs in addition to the target organ. In the case of the pregnant uterus, however, local application intravaginally, intracervically, or intra-amniotically elicits a therapeutic response without sufficient uptake of prostaglandin into the circulation to cause other than minor adverse effects. The clinical utility of local prostaglandin treatment is a major advance in relaxing the cervix before surgical abortion, in conjunction with mifepristone as a medical abortifacient and in the induction or augmentation of labor. Prostaglandins can also be injected directly into the myometrium to arrest uncontrollable postpartum hemorrhage caused by uterine atony.

PROSTANOID RECEPTORS. The study of prostaglandin receptors has proved difficult, and reports of work in the pregnant human uterus are sparse. Receptors for both PGE_2 and $PGF_{2\alpha}$ are present in cell membrane fractions, and the concentration shows little change through pregnancy and labor.[152] PGE_1 and PGE_2 appear to bind to the same receptors, but $PGF_{2\alpha}$ has a separate receptor with an affinity 10 to 20 times less than that of PGE$_2$ and its receptor.[152] Three separate receptors for PGE$_1$, termed EP1, EP2, and EP3, have been proposed to explain the opposing effects of PGE$_2$ in different tissues.[153] The EP1 receptors are thought to work through the inositol triphosphate pathway, whereas EP2 and EP3 may be linked through G proteins to the adenylate cyclase system to either increase or decrease cAMP concentrations. This finding may help to explain the paradox that PGE$_2$ inhibits the spontaneous contractility of human nonpregnant myometrial strips, whereas contractility of pregnant myometrium is stimulated both in vitro and in vivo.[154] Binding sites of the same affinity as those in cell membranes have been identified in fractions of sarcoplasmic reticulum.[155]

ACTIONS ON CONNECTIVE TISSUE. The application of PGE$_2$ and PGF$_{2\alpha}$ to the cervix undoubtedly causes it to ripen, and it usually is assumed that this reflects collagenolysis resulting from increased collagenase activity, as occurs in the spontaneously ripening cervix (Table 125–6). The most recent study of this question[156] failed to find either increased collagenase activity or increased collagen breakdown products. An alternative mode of action of PGE$_2$ is on the glycosaminoglycan (GAG) component of the cervical matrix. If the highly charged sulfated GAG's are replaced by less sulfated GAG or hyaluronic acid, the collagen fibrils are less tightly bound and can disperse and destabilize with a resulting increase in compliance. Support for this mechanism comes from the finding that PGE$_2$-induced cervical ripening is accompanied by a rise in the circulating levels of sulfated GAG's.[157]

ACTIONS ON SMOOTH MUSCLE. The actions of cyclooxygenase and lipoxygenase metabolites on the uterine tissue at a cellular level are complex and poorly understood. Although receptors have been identified, it is uncertain whether or not all the actions of prostanoids are mediated by receptors. Compared with oxytocin, prostaglandins are relatively weak stimuli of uterine contractions; their major effect on contractility probably lies in potentiation of the response to oxytocin. Both oxytocin and prostaglandins increase the intracellular concentrations of Ca^{2+}, but they appear to do this by different mechanisms. Whereas oxytocin increases concentration of Ca^{2+} in cells in a calcium-free medium, this effect of prostaglandin is apparent in human myometrial cells only at very high concentrations.[75] Thus stimulation of Ca^{2+} uptake into the myometrial cell is the major avenue by which prostaglandin raises intracellular concentrations of Ca^{2+}; the ability of prostaglandin to inhibit ATP-dependent microsomal uptake of Ca^{2+}[158] and to release microsomal Ca^{2+}[159] plays a minor part. The mechanism by which prostaglandin increases entry of Ca^{2+} is uncertain, but it is likely that it is at least partly attributable to passage through voltage-gated Ca^{2+} channels.[75] In addition, PGF$_{2\alpha}$ may enhance Ca^{2+} entry by virtue of its ionophoretic properties.[160] Interaction of oxytocin and prostaglandins probably occurs at the level of Ca^{2+}, but additional mechanisms, such as prostaglandin-induced gap junction formation, which enhances the response to oxytocin, may contribute.

SUMMARY

The mechanism that initiates labor in human pregnancy appears to be a complex paracrine-autocrine system within the uterus to which hormones such as estrogen, progesterone, and oxytocin in the maternal circulation contribute in no more than a permissive way. Four tissues (amnion, chorion, decidua, and myometrium) that lie in intimate contact with one another interact by means of messengers that are poorly understood. Current hypotheses identify prostanoids (particularly PGF$_{2\alpha}$) and oxytocin receptors as the main players. Labor may begin with increasing release of PGF$_{2\alpha}$, which increases responsiveness to oxytocin, directly stimulates smooth muscle, induces gap junction formation, and increases the compliance of the collagenous connective tissue of the cervix. The main sources of prostanoids are amnion, which mainly releases PGE$_2$, and decidua, which mainly releases PGF$_{2\alpha}$. Further understanding depends on elucidating the factors that control prostaglandin release and stimulate formation of oxytocin receptors. Various potential inhibitory and stimulatory factors have been identified, but their physiological roles remain uncertain. Whatever the signals, the source is almost certainly the conceptus, but whether it arises from a trophoblastic genetic clock or reflects maturation of the fetus as a whole is an unanswered question.

PRETERM LABOR

Preterm labor constitutes the major complication of modern obstetrics, accounting for about 75 per cent of neonatal morbidity and mortality in Western societies.[161] Preterm infants who survive are at risk for cerebral palsy, hydrocephalus, blindness, and deafness.[162] Despite intense clinical and laboratory research, the incidence of preterm labor in the United States has persisted at 6 to 10 per cent for the past 35 years. Progress in neonatal intensive care has been dramatic to the extent that an infant born after 30 weeks is almost certain to survive unless malformed, but mortality is maintained by unsuccessful attempts at salvage of infants born as early as 24 weeks. Prevention of preterm labor has the potential to make a profound impact on human health in the early years.

Etiology

Parturition before term may mimic term parturition, except for inappropriate timing, or the smooth muscle and connective tissue components of parturition may be dissociated.

Premature Connective Tissue Changes

The collagenous structure of either the cervix or the membranes may undergo changes before term that nor-

TABLE 125–6. ACTIONS OF PROSTAGLANDINS ON UTERINE TISSUES

Potentiates response to oxytocin
Stimulates contractions
Increases flux of Ca^{2+} into cells
Stimulates collagenolysis
Modifies glycosaminoglycans
Induces gap junction formation
Induces oxytocin receptor formation

mally are seen only at term, but there is no increase in the frequency of contractions.

FETAL MEMBRANES. For reasons that are not understood, the fetal membranes may rupture prematurely without warning and in the absence of contractions. Labor ensues within a few days in most of the women, but in the remainder, pregnancy may continue for many weeks, even to term. Studies of the composition of prematurely ruptured amnion shows that it undergoes the same changes in connective tissue composition normally seen at term: the concentrations of both collagen and sulfated GAG's are reduced.[25, 163]

CERVIX. Recurrent midtrimester abortion of normally formed live fetuses is likely to be caused by a disorder known as incompetent cervix. The onset of abortion is heralded by increasing vaginal discharge but no discomfort. On examination the cervix is soft, effaced, and dilated and the exposed membranes bulge into the vagina. Unless treated, the fetus is extruded with little or no sign of uterine contractions until the second stage of labor. Biomechanical measurements both in vivo[164] and in vitro[17] confirm the low strength and high distensibility of the cervix. Biochemical studies of biopsies of incompetent cervices show no loss of total collagen, but mature collagen is replaced by new collagen with fewer crosslinks, and collagenolytic activity is increased.[17] Cervical incompetence has a strong association with a past history of trauma resulting from complicated delivery or therapeutic abortion, suggesting that scar tissue may serve as a nidus that liberates substances, such as PGE$_2$, that act on adjacent normal connective tissue. The condition is treated by closing the canal with a tape tied around the cervix at its junction with the lower segment. Success rates are high, provided that the surgical procedure is performed before the membranes are widely exposed.

Premature Myometrial Activation

Many obstetrical complications (e.g., uterine malformations, placental bleeding, trauma, severe maternal infections, specific fetal infections, such as listeriosis, and multiple pregnancy) can cause preterm labor. In general, it usually is a plausible hypothesis to attribute premature myometrial contractility to release of prostaglandins in response to damage or stress in the decidua and/or the fetal membranes.

IDIOPATHIC PRETERM LABOR. In the absence of a recognizable cause, preterm labor is said to be idiopathic, although it is recognized that sometimes an underlying complication may be present. In particular, the extent to which low-grade infection causes preterm labor is controversial (see below). The major risk factor predicting preterm labor is a previous history of preterm labor; otherwise, associations such as low socioeconomic status are too weak to be useful in predicting preterm labor with the reliability needed to undertake intervention.[165] The cause of recurrent idiopathic preterm labor usually is assumed to be a disorder of the timing mechanism; until the timing mechanism in term parturition is elucidated, it is likely that the disorder in preterm labor will remain obscure.

INFECTIVE PRETERM LABOR. Chorioamnionitis diagnosed histologically is present in 20 to 33 per cent of women with preterm deliveries, compared with 5 to 10 per cent of those

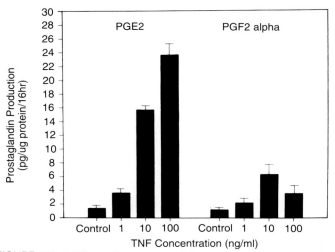

FIGURE 125–9. Effects of tumor necrosis factor on prostaglandin production by cells from decidua. (From Mitchell MD et al: Prostaglandin biosynthesis by human decidual cells: Effects of inflammatory mediators. Prostaglandins Leukotrienes Essent Fatty Acids 41:35–38, 1990.)

delivered at term.[166, 167] Most such women have no clinical signs of infection, and bacteria have been recovered from the membranes in some studies[168, 169] but not others.[170, 171] The most commonly isolated organisms are *Ureaplasma urealyticum*, *Mycoplasma hominis*, and *Gardnerella vaginalis*.[169] Although there is no doubt that certain specific organisms, such as *Listeria monocytogenes*, can be the primary agent causing preterm labor, whether low-grade chorioamnionitis is the cause or the consequence of preterm labor remains unresolved. Nevertheless, it appears likely that the development of chorioamnionitis creates an irreversible situation that rapidly progresses to delivery.[172] Controlled clinical trials of antibiotics in arresting progress of early preterm labor have so far proved inconclusive.[173]

The mechanism by which chorioamnionitis could stimulate preterm labor has been extensively investigated. Not surprisingly, various products of inflamed fetal membranes have been identified that stimulate prostaglandin production and could cause the increased concentrations of PGFM and PGEM-II found in amniotic fluid.[174] Lipopolysaccharide bacterial endotoxin is present in amniotic fluid in women in preterm labor with chorioamnionitis but not in normal amniotic fluid,[175] and it stimulates the production of PGF$_{2\alpha}$ and cytokines by decidual cells and explants[176] and the production of PGE$_2$ by amnion cells.[177] The cytokines generated by decidua include IL-1[178] and tumor necrosis factor-β (TNF-β).[176] IL-1α, IL-1β, IL-6, and TNF-β are potent stimuli of PGF$_{2\alpha}$ by decidual cells[176, 179, 180] (Fig. 125–9) and of PGE$_2$ by amnion cells[126] and have been identified in amniotic fluid in preterm labor associated with chorioamnionitis.[176, 181] Although these observations clearly establish a mechanism by which low-grade infection can cause preterm labor, their full significance awaits resolution of the question of how frequently the association of chorioamnionitis and preterm labor is causal.

REFERENCES

1. Poole WE: Reproduction in the two species of grey kangaroo, *Macropus giganteus* Shaw, and *M. fuliginosus* (Desmarest). II. Gestation, parturition and pouch life. Aust J Zool 23:333–353, 1975.

2. Binns W, Shupe JL, Keeler RF, James LF: Chronologic evaluation of teratogenicity in sheep fed *Veratrum californicum.* J Am Vet Assn 147:839–842, 1965.

3. Kennedy PC, Kendrick JW, Stormont C: Adenohypophyseal aplasia, an inherited defect associated with abnormal gestation in Guernsey cattle. Cornell Vet 47:160–165, 1957.

4. Liggins GC, Kennedy PC, Holm LW: Failure of initiation of parturition after electrocoagulation of the pituitary of the fetal lamb. Am J Obstet Gynecol 98:1080–1086, 1966.

5. Drost M, Holm LW: Prolonged gestation in ewes after foetal adrenalectomy. J Endocrinol 40:293–298, 1968.

6. Liggins GC: Premature parturition following infusion of corticotrophin or cortisol into foetal lambs. J Endocrinol 42:323–329, 1968.

7. Antolovich GC, Clark IJ, McMillen IC, et al: Hypothalmo-pituitary disconnection in the fetal sheep. Neuroendocrinology 51:1–9, 1990.

8. McDonald TJ, Nathanielsz PW: Bilateral destruction of the fetal paraventricular nuclei prolongs gestation in sheep. Am J Obstet Gynecol 165:764–770, 1991.

9. Milic AB, Adamsons K: The relationship between prolonged pregnancy and anencephaly. J Obstet Gynaecol Br Commonw 76:102–108, 1969.

10. O'Donohoe NW, Holland PDJ: Familial congenital adrenal hypoplasia. Arch Dis Child 43:717–722, 1968.

11. Liggins GC: Adrenocortical-linked maturational events in the fetus. Am J Obstet Gynecol 126:931–939, 1976.

12. Csapo AI, Pulkkinen MO, Weist WG: Effects of lutectomy and progesterone replacement therapy in early pregnant patients. Am J Obstet Gynecol 115:759–765, 1973.

13. Flint APF, Anderson ABM, Steele PA, Turnbull AC: The mechanism by which foetal cortisol controls the onset of parturition in the sheep. Biochem Soc Trans 3:1189–1194, 1975.

14. Flint APF, Kingston EJ, Robinson JS, Thorburn GD: The initiation of parturition in the goat: Evidence for control by fetal glucocorticoid through activation of placental C21-steroid 17α-hydroxylase. J Endocrinol 78:367–378, 1978.

15. Liggins GC: Cervical ripening as an inflammatory reaction. In Ellwood DA, Anderson ABM (eds): The Cervix in Pregnancy and Labor. Edinburgh, Churchill Livingston, 1981, pp 1–9.

16. Chwalisz K, Hegale-Hartung Ch, Schulz R, et al: Progesterone control of cervical ripening—experimental studies with the progesterone antagonists onapristone, liloprostone and mifepristone. In Leppert PC, Woessner J (eds): The Extracellular Matrix of the Uterus, Cervix and Fetal Membranes. Ithaca, Perinatology Press, 1991, pp 119–131.

17. Rechberger T, Uldbjerg N, Oxlund H: Connective tissue changes in the cervix during normal pregnancy and pregnancy complicated by cervical incompetence. Obstet Gynecol 71:563–567, 1988.

18. Sherwood OD, Chang CC, Bevier GW, Dziuk PJ: Radioimmunoassay of plasma relaxin levels throughout pregnancy and at parturition in the pig. Endocrinology 97:834–839, 1975.

19. Bryant-Greenwood GD: The human relaxin: Concensus and dissent. Mol Cell Endocrinol 79:C125–C132, 1991.

20. Weiss G, O'Byrne EM, Steinetz BG: Relaxin: A product of the human corpus luteum of pregnancy. Science 194:948–949, 1976.

21. MacLennan AH, Green RC, Bryant-Greenwood GD, et al: Ripening of the human cervix and induction of labour with purified porcine relaxin. Lancet 1:220–223, 1980.

22. Bryant-Greenwood GD, Greenwood FC: The human fetal membranes and decidua as a model for paracrine interactions. In McNellis D, Challis J, MacDonald P, et al (eds): The Onset of Labor: Cellular and Integrative Mechanisms. Ithaca, Perinatology Press, 1988, pp 253–273.

23. Liggins GC: Controlled trial of induction of labor by vaginal suppositories containing prostaglandin E₂. Prostaglandins 18:167–172, 1979.

24. Al-Zaid NS, Bou-Resli MN, Goldspink R: Bursting pressure and collagen content of fetal membranes and their relation to premature rupture of the membranes. Br J Obstet Gynaecol 87:227–229, 1980.

25. Skinner SJM, Campos GA, Liggins GC: Collagen content of human amniotic membranes: Effect of gestation length and premature rupture. Obstet Gynecol 57:487–489, 1981.

26. Morizaki N, Morizaki J, Hayashi RH, Garfield RE: A functional and structural study of the innervation of the human uterus. Am J Obstet Gynecol 160:218–228, 1989.

27. Garfield RE, Blennerhassett MG, Miller SM: Control of myometrial contractility: Role and regulation of gap junctions. Oxford Rev 10:436–490, 1988.

28. Garfield RE, Rabideau S, Challis JR, Daniel EE: Ultrastructural basis

29. Garfield RE, Kannan MS, Daniel EE: Gap junction formation in myometrium: Control by estrogens, progesterone and prostaglandins. Am J Physiol 238:C81–C89, 1980.

30. Pattison NS, Webster MA, Phipps SL, et al: Inhibition of 3β-hydroxysteroid dehydrogenase (HSD) activity in first- and second-trimester human pregnancy and the luteal phase using epostane. Fertil Steril 42:875–881, 1984.

31. Parker CR, Illingworth DR, Bissonnette J, Carr BR: Endocrine changes during pregnancy in a patient with homozygous familial hypobetalipoproteinemia. N Engl J Med 314:557–560, 1986.

32. Kovacs L, Sas M, Resch BA, et al: Termination of very early pregnancy by RU486—an antiprogestational compound. Contraception 29:339–410, 1984.

33. Roger MW, Baird DT: Induction of therapeutic abortion in early pregnancy with mifepristone in combination with prostaglandin pessary. Lancet 2:1415–1418, 1987.

34. Baulieu EE, Ulman A, Philibert D: Contragestion by antiprogestin RU 486: A review. Arch Gynaecol Obstet 241:73–85, 1987.

35. Block BSB, Liggins GC, Creasy RK: Preterm delivery is not predicted by serial plasma estradiol or progesterone concentration measurements. Am J Obstet Gynecol 150:716–721, 1984.

36. Hartikainen-Sorri AL, Kauppila A, Tuimala R, et al: The lack of significant change in plasma progesterone and estradiol-17β before the onset of human labor. Acta Obstet Gynecol Scand 60:497–499, 1981.

37. Donaldson A, Nicolini U, Symes EK, et al: Changes in the concentrations of cortisol, dehydroepiandrostenedione sulphate and progesterone in fetal and maternal serum during pregnancy. Clin Endocrinol 35:447–451, 1991.

38. Kreitmann B, Bayard F: Oestrogen and progesterone receptor concentration in human endometrium during gestation. Acta Endocrinol 92:547–552, 1979.

39. Batra S, Bengtsson LP: 17β-Estradiol and progesterone concentrations in myometrium and their relationships to concentrations in peripheral plasma. J Clin Endocrinol Metab 46:622–626, 1978.

40. Challis JRG, Mitchell BF: Steroid production by the fetal membranes in relation to the onset of parturition. In McNellis D, Challis J, MacDonald P, et al (eds): The Onset of Labor: Cellular and Integrative Mechanisms. Ithaca, Perinatology Press, 1988, pp 233–246.

41. Kumar D, Sullivan WJ, Wagatsuma T: The mechanism of action of progesterone on human myometrium. Am J Obstet Gynecol 98:1055–1060, 1967.

42. Daniel EE, Singh H: Electrical properties of the smooth muscle cell membrane. Can J Physiol Pharmacol 36:959–966, 1958.

43. Kao CY, Nishiyama A: Ovarian hormones and resting potential of rabbit smooth muscle. Am J Physiol 207:793–798, 1964.

44. Jung H: Electrophysiology of the uterus and electrohysterography. J Obstet Gynaecol 69:1040–1044, 1962.

45. Roberts JM, Reimer RK, Bottari SP, et al: Myometrial postreceptor responses: Targets for steroidal regulation. In McNellis D, Challis J, MacDonald P, et al (eds): The Onset of Labor: Cellular and Integrative Mechanisms. Ithaca, Perinatology Press, 1988, pp 37–50.

46. Carsten ME: Calcium accumulation by human uterine microsomal preparations: Effects of progesterone and oxytocin. Am J Obstet Gynecol 133:598–601, 1979.

47. Chew PCT, Ratnam J: Serial levels of plasma oestradiol-17β at the approach of labour. J Endocrinol 71:267–268, 1976.

48. Boroditzky RS, Reyes FI, Winter JSD, Faiman C: Maternal serum estrogens and progesterone concentrations preceding normal labor. Obstet Gynecol 51:686–691, 1978.

49. Haukkamea M, Lahteenmaki P: Steroids in human myometrium and maternal and umbilical cord plasma before and during labor. Obstet Gynecol 53:617–622, 1979.

50. Hilary HK, Cohen SL: The changing estrogen content of the nuclear fraction of human myometrium during labor. Steroids 38:175–184, 1981.

51. Biswas A, Chaudhury A, Chattoraj SC, Dale SL: Do catechol estrogens participate in the initiation of labor? Am J Obstet Gynecol 165:984–987, 1991.

52. Gross GL, Chattoraj SE, Schinfield JS, et al: Catechol estrogen concentration in maternal and umbilical circulation at different modes of delivery. Am J Obstet Gynecol 158:1196–1200, 1988.

53. Barnafi L, Larraguibel R: The in vitro effect of progesterone and oestrogens on the spontaneous and oxytocin-induced activity of the human myometrium. Acta Endocrinol 76:172–177, 1974.

54. Hempel R, Newmann F: Hemming der Uteruswirkung von Oxytocin durch wasserlosliche Steroid. Acta Endocrinol 48:656–663, 1965.

55. Skinner SJM, Liggins GC, Wilson T, Neale G: Synthesis of prostaglandin F by cultured human endometrial cells. Prostaglandins 27:821–828, 1984.
56. France JT, Liggins GC: Placental sulphatase deficiency. J Clin Endocrinol Metab 29:138–141, 1969.
57. Romano W, Lukash L, Challis JRG, Mitchell BF: Substrate utilization for estrogen synthesis by human fetal membranes and decidua. Am J Obstet Gynecol 155:1170–1175, 1986.
58. Fuchs A-R, Goeschen K, Husslein P, et al: Oxytocin and the initiation of human parturition. III. Plasma concentrations of oxytocin and 13,14-dihydro-15-keto-prostaglandin F$_2$ alpha in spontaneous and oxytocin induced labor at term. Am J Obstet Gynecol 147:497–502, 1983.
59. Soloff MS, Fernstrom MA, Periyasamy S, et al: Regulation of oxytocin receptor concentration in rat uterine explants by estrogen and progesterone. Can J Biochem Cell Biol 61:625–630, 1983.
60. Liggins GC, Fairclough RJ, Grieves SA, et al: The mechanism of initiation of parturition in the ewe. Recent Prog Horm Res 29:111–150, 1973.
61. Elger W, Churalisz K, Fahnrich M, et al: Studies on labor-conditioning and labor-inducing effects of antiprogesterones in animal models. In Garfield RE (ed): Uterine Contractility. Norwell, Serono Symposia, 1990, pp 153–175.
62. Schatz F, Markiewic L, Gurpide E: Differential effects of estradiol, arachidonic acid and A23187 on prostaglandin F$_{2\alpha}$ output by epithelial and stromal cells of human endometrium. Endocrinology 120:1465–1471, 1987.
63. Dawood MY, Ylikorkala O, Trivedi D, Fuchs F: Oxytocin in maternal circulation and amniotic fluid during pregnancy. J Clin Endocrinol Metab 49:429–434 1979.
64. Sellars SM, Hodgson HT, Mountford LA, et al: Is oxytocin involved in parturition? Br J Obstet Gynaecol 88:725–729, 1981.
65. Fuchs A-R, Romero R, Keefe D, et al: Oxytocin secretion and human parturition: Pulse frequency and duration increase during spontaneous labor in women. Am J Obstet Gynecol 165:1515–1523, 1991.
66. Caldeyro-Barcia R, Sereno J: The response of the human uterus to oxytocin throughout pregnancy. In Caldeyro-Barcia R, Sereno J (eds): Oxytocin. Oxford, Pergamon Press, 1961, pp 177–202.
67. Theobald GW: The choice between death from postmaturity, of prolapsed cord and life from induction of labour. Lancet 1:59–65, 1959.
68. Fuchs A-R, Fuchs F, Husslein P, et al: Oxytocin receptors and human parturition: A dual role for oxytocin in the initiation of labor. Science 215:1396–1398, 1982.
69. Gillespie A: Prostaglandin–oxytocin enhancement and potentiation and their clinical application. Br Med J 1:150–152, 1972.
70. Brummer HC: Interaction of E prostaglandins and Syntocinon on the pregnant human myometrium. J Obstet Gynaecol Br Common 78:305–309, 1971.
71. Mitchell MD, Keirse MJNC, Anderson ABM, Turnbull AC: Evidence for a local control of prostaglandins within the pregnant human uterus. Br J Obstet Gynaecol 84:35–38, 1977.
72. Fuchs A-R, Fuchs F, Husslein P, Soloff MS: Oxytocin receptors in human uterus during pregnancy and parturition. Am J Obstet Gynecol 150:734–741, 1984.
73. Wilson T, Liggins GC, Whittaker DJ: Oxytocin stimulates release of arachidonic acid and prostaglandin F$_{2\alpha}$ from human decidual cells. Prostaglandins 35:771–781, 1988.
74. Forman A, Gantrup P, Andersen KE, Ulmsten U: Effects of nifedipine on oxytocin- and prostaglandin F$_{2\alpha}$-induced activity in the postpartum uterus. Am J Obstet Gynecol 144:665–670, 1982.
75. Molnar M, Hertelendy F: Regulation of intracellular free calcium in human myometrial cells by prostaglandin F$_{2\alpha}$: Comparison with oxytocin. J Clin Endocrinol Metab 71:1243–1250, 1990.
76. Carsten ME, Miller JD: Ca^{2+} release by inositol triphosphate from Ca^{2+}-transporting microsomes derived from uterine sarcoplasmic reticulum. Biochem Biophys Res Commun 130:1027–1031, 1985.
77. Enyedi A, Minami J, Caride AJ, Penniston JT: Characteristics of the Ca^{2+} pump and Ca^{2+} "ATPase" in the plasma membrane of rat myometrium. Biochem J 252:215–220, 1988.
78. Chibbar R, Miller FD, Mitchell BF: Oxytocin is synthesized in human fetal membranes. Proceedings of the 38th Annual Meeting of the Society for Gynecologic Investigation, San Antonio, Society for Gynecologic Investigation, March 20–23, 1991, p 102, Abstr 7.
79. Melin P, Trojnar J, Johansson B, et al: Synthetic antagonists of the myometrial response to vasopressin and oxytocin. J Endocrinol 111:125–131, 1986.
80. Akerlund M, Stromberg P, Hanksson A, et al: Inhibition of uterine contractions of premature labour with an oxytocin analogue. Results from a pilot study. Br J Obstet Gynaecol 94:1040–1044, 1987.

81. Hudson P, Haley J, John M, et al: Structure of a genomic clone encoding biologically active human relaxin. Nature 301:628–631, 1983.
82. Bell RJ, Eddie LW, Lester AR, et al: Relaxin in human pregnancy serum measured with an homologous RIA. Obstet Gynecol 69:585–589, 1987.
83. Hansell DJ, Bryant-Greenwood GD, Greenwood FC: Expression of the human relaxin HI gene in the decidua, trophoblast, and prostate. J Clin Endocrinol Metab 72:899–904, 1991.
84. Koay ESC, Bryant-Greenwood GD, Yamamoto SY, Greenwood FC: The human fetal membranes: A target tissue for relaxin. J Clin Endocrinol Metab 62:513–521, 1986.
85. Sasaki A, Tempst P, Liotta AS, et al: Isolation and characterization of a corticotropin-releasing hormone-like peptide from human placenta. J Clin Endocrinol Metab 67:768–773, 1988.
86. Riley SC, Challis JRG: Corticotrophin-releasing hormone production by the placenta and fetal membranes. Placenta 12:105–119, 1991.
87. Wolfe CDA, Patel SP, Linton EA, et al: Plasma corticotrophin-releasing factor (CRF) in normal pregnancy. Br J Obstet Gynaecol 95:997–1002, 1988.
88. Potter E, Behan DP, Fischer WH, et al: Cloning and characterization of the cDNAs for human and rat corticotropin releasing factor-binding proteins. Nature 349:423–426, 1991.
89. Petraglia F, Giardino L, Coukos G, et al: Corticotropin-releasing factor and parturition: Plasma and amniotic fluid levels and placental binding sites. Obstet Gynecol 75:784–789, 1990.
90. Jones SA, Challis JRG: Effects of corticotropin-releasing hormone and adrenocorticotropin on prostaglandin output by human placenta and fetal membranes. Gynecol Obstet Invest 29:165–168, 1990.
91. Quartero HWP, Fry CH: Placental corticotrophin releasing factor may modulate human parturition. Placenta 10:439–443, 1989.
92. Kelly RW, Leask R, Calder AA: Choriodecidual production of interleukin-8 and mechanism of parturition. Lancet 339:776–777, 1992.
93. Junquiera LCU, Zugaib M, Montes GS, et al: Morphological and histochemical evidence for the occurrence of collagenolysis and for the role of neutrophilic polymorphonuclear leukocytes during cervical dilation. Am J Obstet Gynecol 138:273–281, 1980.
94. Rodda CP, Kubota M, Heath JA, et al: Evidence for a novel parathyroid hormone–related protein in fetal parathyroid glands and sheep placenta. J Endocrinol 117:261–271, 1988.
95. Theide MA, Daifotis AG, Weir EC, et al: Intrauterine occupancy controls expression of the parathyroid hormone–related gene in preterm rat myometrium. Proc Natl Acad Sci USA 87:6969–6973, 1990.
96. Southby J, Kissin MW, Danks JA, et al: Immunohistochemical localization of parathyroid hormone–related protein in human breast cancer. Cancer Res 50:7710–7716, 1990.
97. Shew RL, Robinson MF, Olansky L, Yee JA: Inhibitory effect of [Tyr 34] b PTH-(7-34)-amide on b PTH-(1-34) ability to reduce uterine contraction. Peptides 11:583–589, 1989.
98. Sunnergren KP, Word RA, Sambrook JF, et al: Expression and regulation of endothelin precursor mRNA in avascular human amnion. Mol Cell Endocrinol 68:R7–R14, 1990.
99. Word RA, Kamm KE, Stull JT, Casey ML: Endothelin increases cytoplasmic calcium and myosin phosphorylation in human myometrium. Am J Obstet Gynecol 162:1103–1108, 1990.
100. Kozuka M, Ito T, Hirose S, et al: Endothelin induces two types of contractions of rat uterus. Biochem Biophys Res Commun 159:317–323, 1989.
101. Resink TJ, Scott-Burden T, Buhler FR: Activation of phospholipase A$_2$ by endothelin in cultured vascular smooth muscle cells. Biochem Biophys Res Commun 158:279–282, 1989.
102. Mitchell MD, Romero RJ, Lepera R, et al: Actions of endothelin-1 on prostaglandin production by gestational tissues. Prostaglandins 40:627–635, 1990.
103. Cameron IT, Davenport AP, Brown MJ, Smith SK: Endothelin-1 stimulates prostaglandin F$_{2\alpha}$ release from human endometrium. Prostaglandins Leukotrienes Essent Fatty Acids 42:155–157, 1991.
104. Casey ML, MacDonald PC: Decidual activation: The role of prostaglandins in labor. In McNellis D, Challis J, MacDonald P, et al (eds): The Onset of Labor: Cellular and Integrative Mechanisms. Ithaca, Perinatology Press, 1988, pp 141–156.
105. Amy JJ, Volckaert M, Foulon W, et al: The use of prostaglandin inhibitors in obstetrics. In Bottari JP, Thomas JP, Vokaer A, Vokaer R (eds): Uterine Contractility. New York, Masson, 1984, pp 146–160.
106. Collins E, Turner G: Maternal effects of regular salicylate ingestion in pregnancy. Lancet 2:335–337, 1975.
107. Salmon JA, Amy JJ: Levels of prostaglandin F$_{2\alpha}$ in amniotic fluid during pregnancy and labor. Prostaglandins 4:523–533, 1973.

108. Keirse MJNC, Turnbull AC: E prostaglandins in amniotic fluid during late pregnancy and labour. J Obstet Gynaecol Br Commonw 80:970–973, 1973.

109. MacDonald PC, Schultz FM, Duenhoelter JH, et al: Initiation of human parturition. I. Mechanism of action of arachidonic acid. Obstet Gynecol 44:629–636, 1978.

110. Davidson BJ, Murray RD, Challis JRG: Estrogen, progesterone, prolactin prostaglandin E_2, prostaglandin $F_{2\alpha}$ and 6-keto-prostaglandin $F_{1\alpha}$ gradients across the uterus in women in labor and not in labor. Am J Obstet Gynecol 157:54–58, 1987.

111. Habenicht AJR, Salbach P, Gaerig M: The LDL receptor pathway delivers arachidonic acid for eicosanoid formation in cells stimulated by platelet-derived growth factor. Nature 345:634–636, 1990.

112. Schwartz BE, Schultz FM, MacDonald PC, Johnston JM: Initiation of human parturition. III. Fetal membrane content of prostaglandin E_2 and $F_{2\alpha}$ precursor. Obstet Gynecol 46:564–568, 1975.

113. Okita JR, MacDonald PC, Johnston JM: Mobilization of arachidonic acid from specific glycerophospholipids of human fetal membranes during early labor. J Biol Chem 257:14029–14034, 1982.

114. Irvine RF: How is the level of free arachidonic acid controlled in mammalian cells? Biochem J 204:3–16, 1982.

115. Okazaki T, Sagawa N, Okita JR, et al: Diacylglycerol metabolism and arachidonic acid release in human fetal membranes and decidua vera. J Biol Chem 256:7316–7321, 1981.

116. Carsten ME, Miller JD: Calcium control mechanisms in the myometrial cell and the role of the phosphoinositide cycle. In Carsten ME, Miller JD (eds): Uterine Function: Molecular and Cellular Aspects. New York, Plenum, 1990, pp 121–168.

117. Okazaki T, Sagawa N, Bleasdale JE, et al: Initiation of human parturition. XIII. Phospholipase C, phospholipase A_2 and diacylglycerol lipase activities in fetal membranes and decidua vera from early and late gestation. Biol Reprod 25:103–109, 1981.

118. Schrey MP, Read AM, Steer PJ: Oxytocin and vasopressin stimulate inositol phosphate production in human gestational myometrium and decidua cells. Biosci Rep 6:613–619, 1986.

119. Lopez-Bernal A, Canete-Soler R, Turnbull AC: Are leukotrienes involved in human uterine contractility? Br J Obstet Gynaecol 96:568–573, 1989.

120. Billah MM, Johnston JM: Identification of phospholipid platelet-activating factor (1-0-alkyl-2-acetyl-sn-glycero-3-phospholcholine) in human amniotic fluid and urine. Biochim Biophys Res Commun 113:51–58, 1983.

121. Casey ML, MacDonald PC, Mitchell MD: Stimulation of prostaglandin E_2 production in amnion cells in culture by a substance(s) in human fetal and adult urine. Biochem Biophys Res Commun 114:1056–1063, 1983.

122. Saitoh H, Hirato K, Tahara R, Ogawa K: Enhancement of human amniotic phospholipase A_2 activity by steroid-sulphate derived from the foeto-placental unit. Acta Endocrinol 107:420–426, 1984.

123. Wilson T, Liggins GC, Aimer GP, Watkins EJ: The effect of progesterone on the release of arachidonic acid from human endometrial cells stimulated by histamine. Prostaglandins 31:343–360, 1986.

124. Wallner BP, Mattaliano RJ, Hesslon C, et al: Cloning and expression of human lipocortin, a phospholipase A_2 inhibitor with potential anti-inflammatory activity. Nature 320:77–81, 1986.

125. Casey ML, MacDonald PC, Mitchell MD: Despite a massive increase in cortisol secretion in women during parturition, there is an equally massive increase in prostaglandin synthesis: A paradox? J Clin Invest 75:1852–1857, 1985.

126. Lundin-Schiller S, Mitchell MD: Renin increases human amnion cell prostaglandin E_2 biosynthesis. J Clin Endocrinol Metab 73:436–440, 1991.

127. Tyson JE, Dubin NH, McCoshen JA: Inhibition of fetal membrane prostaglandin production by prolactin: Relative importance in the initiation of labor. Am J Obstet Gynecol 151:1032–1038, 1985.

128. Wilson T, Christie DL: Gravidin, an endogenous inhibitor of phospholipase A_2 activity, is a secretory component of IgA. Biochem Biophys Res Commun 176:447–452, 1991.

129. Wilson T, Liggins GC, Joe L: Purification from incubated chorion of a phospholipase A_2 inhibitor active before but not after the onset of labor. Am J Obstet Gynecol 160:602–606, 1989.

130. Rice GE, Wong MH, Hollingsworth S, Thorburn GD: Prostaglandin G/H synthase activity in ovine cotyledons: A gestational profile. Eicosanoids 3:231–236, 1990.

131. Keirse MJNC, Moonen P, Klok G: Prostaglandin synthesis in pregnant human myometrium is not confined to the uteroplacental vasculature. IRCS Med Sci 12:824–825, 1984.

132. Gaffney RC, Rice GE, Brennecke SP: Is human labour triggered by an increase in the rate of synthesis of prostaglandin G/H synthase? Reprod Fertil Dev 2:603–606, 1990.

133. Hemmler ME, Cook MW, Lands WEM: Prostaglandin biosynthesis can be triggered by lipid peroxides. Arch Biochem Biophys 193:340–347, 1979.

134. Zaker T, Olson DM: Dexamethasone stimulates arachidonic acid conversion to prostaglandin E_2 in human amnion cells. J Dev Physiol 12:269–272, 1989.

135. Saeed SA, Strickland DM, Young DC, et al: Inhibition of prostaglandin synthesis by human amniotic fluid: Acute reduction in inhibitory activity of amniotic fluid obtained during labor. J Clin Endocrinol Metab 55:801–803, 1982.

136. Manzai M, Liggins GC: Inhibitory effects of dispersed human amnion cells on production rates of PGE and F by endometrial cells. Prostaglandins 28:297–307, 1984.

137. Keirse MJNC, Turnbull AC: Metabolism of prostaglandins within the pregnant uterus. Br J Obstet Gynaecol 82:887–893, 1975.

138. Mitchell MD: Sources of eicosanoids within the uterus during pregnancy. In McNellis D, Challis J, MacDonald P, et al (eds): The Onset of Labor: Cellular and Integrative Mechanisms. Ithaca, Perinatology Press, 1988, pp 165–181.

139. Ellwood DA, Mitchell MD, Anderson ABM, Turnbull AC: In vitro production of prostanoids by the human cervix during pregnancy: Preliminary observations. Br J Obstet Gynaecol 87:210–214, 1980.

140. Husslein P: Concentration of 13,14-dihydro-15-keto-prostaglandin E_2 in the maternal peripheral plasma during labour of spontaneous onset. Br J Obstet Gynaecol 91:228–231, 1984.

141. Brennecke SP, Castle BM, Demers LM, Turnbull AC: Maternal plasma prostaglandin E_2 metabolite levels during human pregnancy and parturition. Br J Obstet Gynaecol 92:345–349, 1985.

142. Fuchs A-R, Husslein P, Sumulong L, Fuchs F: The origin of 13,14-dihydro-15-keto-$PGF_{2\alpha}$ during delivery. Prostaglandins 24:715–722, 1982.

143. Niesert S, Christopherson W, Korte K, et al: Prostaglandin E_2 9-ketoreductase activity in human decidua vera tissue. Am J Obstet Gynecol 155:1348–1352, 1986.

144. Skinner KA, Challis JRG: Changes in the synthesis and metabolism of prostaglandins by human fetal membranes and decidua at labor. Am J Obstet Gynecol 151:519–523, 1985.

145. Bulmer J, Sutherland CA: Bone marrow origins of endometrial granulocytes in the early human placental bed. J Reprod Immunol 5:383–387, 1983.

146. Imakawa K, Anthony RV, Kazemi M, et al: Interferon-like sequence of ovine trophoblast protein secreted by embryonic trophectoderm. Nature 330:377–379, 1987.

147. Rees MCP, Di Marzo V, Tippins JR, et al: Leukotriene release by endometrium and myometrium throughout the menstrual cycle in dysmenorrhea and menorrhagia. J Clin Endocrinol Metab 113:291–295, 1987.

148. Makarainen L, Ylikorkala O: Amniotic fluid 6-keto-prostaglandin $F_{1\alpha}$ and thromboxane B_2 during labor. Am J Obstet Gynecol 150:765–768, 1984.

149. Mitchell MD, Keirse MJNC, Anderson AGM, Turnbull AC: Concentrations of the prostacyclin metabolite, 6-keto-prostaglandin $F_{1\alpha}$ in amniotic fluid during late pregnancy and labour. Br J Obstet Gynaecol 86:350–353, 1979.

150. Mitchell MD, Grzyboski CF: Arachidonic acid metabolism by lipoxygenase pathways in intrauterine tissues of women at term of pregnancy. Prostaglandins Leukotrienes Med 28:303–312, 1987.

151. Romero R, Emamian M, Wan M, et al: Increased concentrations of arachidonic acid lipoxygenase metabolites in amniotic fluid during parturition. Obstet Gynecol 70:849–853, 1987.

152. Giannopoulos G, Jackson K, Kredentser J, Tulchinsky D: Prostaglandin E and $F_{2\alpha}$ receptors in human myometrium during the menstrual cycle and in pregnancy and labor. Am J Obstet Gynecol 153:904–910, 1985.

153. Coleman RA, Humphrey PPA, Kennedy I: Prostanoid receptors in smooth muscle: Further evidence for a proposed classification. In Kalsner S, Taylor W, Francis J (eds): Trends in Autonomic Pharmacology. Vol 3. London, Taylor & Francis, 1985, pp 35–49.

154. Wikland M, Lindblom B, Wilhelmsson L, Wiqvist N: Oxytocin, prostaglandins, and contractility of the human uterus at term pregnancy. Acta Obstet Gynecol Scand 61:467–472, 1982.

155. Carsten ME, Miller JD: Prostaglandin E_2 receptor in the myometrium: Distribution in subcellular fractions. Arch Biochem Biophys 212:700–716, 1981.

156. Rath W, Adelmann-Grill BC, Pieper U, Kuhn W: The role of collagenases and proteases in prostaglandin induced cervical ripening. Prostaglandins 34:119–127, 1987.

157. Calder AA, Greer IA: Prostaglandins and the biological control of cervical function. Reprod Fertil Dev 2:459–465, 1990.
158. Carsten ME, Miller JD: Effects of prostaglandins and oxytocin on calcium release from a uterine microsomal fraction. J Biol Chem 252:1576–1581, 1977.
159. Carsten ME: Prostaglandins and oxytocin: Their effects on uterine smooth muscle. Prostaglandins 5:33–40, 1974.
160. Deleers M, Grognet P, Brasseur R: Structural considerations for calcium ionophoresis by prostaglandins. Biochem Pharmacol 34:3831–3836, 1985.
161. Rush RW, Keirse MJNC, Howat P, et al: Contribution of preterm delivery to perinatal mortality. Br Med J 2:965–968, 1976.
162. McCormick MC: The contribution of low birthweight to infant mortality and childhood morbidity. N Engl J Med 312:82–90, 1985.
163. Artal R, Sokol RJ, Neuman M, et al: The mechanical properties of prematurely and non-prematurely ruptured membranes. Am J Obstet Gynecol 125:655–659, 1976.
164. Neuman MR, Merkatz IR, Selim MA, et al: Continuous monitoring of cervical dilatation during labor and measurement of cervical compliance in the human. In Naftolin F, Stubblefield PG (eds): Dilatation of the Uterine Cervix. New York, Raven Press, 1980, pp 233–264.
165. Creasy RK, Gummer BA, Liggins GC: System for predicting spontaneous preterm birth. Obstet Gynecol 55:692–698, 1980.
166. Russell P: Inflammatory lesions of the human placenta. I. Clinical significance of acute chorioamnionitis. Am J Diagn Gynecol Obstet 1:127–137, 1979.
167. Guzick DS, Winn K: The association of chorioamnionitis with preterm delivery. Obstet Gynecol 65:11–16, 1985.
168. Pankuch GA, Appelbaum PC, Lorenz RD, et al: Placental microbiology and histology and the pathogenesis of chorioamnionitis. Obstet Gynecol 64:802–806, 1984.
169. Hillier SL, Martius J, Krohn M, et al: A case-control study of chorioamniotic infection and histologic chorioamnionitis in prematurity. N Engl J Med 319:972–987, 1988.
170. Svenson L, Ingemarsson I, Mardh P-A: Chorioamnionitis and the isolation of microorganisms from the placenta. Obstet Gynecol 67:403–409, 1986.
171. Dong Y, St. Clair PJ, Ramzy I, et al: A microbiologic and clinical study of placental inflammation at term. Obstet Gynecol 70:175–182, 1987.
172. Gravett MG, Hummel D, Eschenbach DA, Holmes KK: Preterm labor associated with subclinical amniotic fluid infection and with bacterial vaginosis. Obstet Gynecol 67:229–237, 1986.
173. Newton ER, Dinsmoor MJ, Gibbs RS: A randomized, blinded, placebo-controlled trial of antibiotics in idiopathic preterm labor. Obstet Gynecol 74:562–566, 1989.
174. Romero R, Wu YK, Sirtori M, et al: Amniotic fluid concentrations of prostaglandin $F_{2\alpha}$, 13,14-dihydro-15-keto-prostaglandin $F_{2\alpha}$ (PGFM) and 11-deoxy-13,14-dihydro-15-keto-11,16-cyclo-prostaglandin E_2 (PGEM-LL) in preterm labor. Prostaglandins 37:149–156, 1989.
175. Cox SM, MacDonald PC, Casey ML: Assay of bacterial endotoxin (lipopolysaccaride) in human amniotic fluid: Potential usefulness in diagnosis and management of preterm labor. Am J Obstet Gynecol 159:99–106, 1988.
176. Casey ML, Cox SM, Beutler B, et al: Cachectin/tumor necrosis factor formation in human decidua. J Clin Invest 83:430–436, 1989.
177. Romero R, Hobbins JC, Mitchell MD: Endotoxin stimulates prostaglandin E_2 production by human amnion. Obstet Gynecol 71:227–232, 1988.
178. Romero R, Wu YK, Brody DT, et al: Human decidua: A source of interleukin-1. Obstet Gynecol 73:31–34, 1989.
179. Mitchell MD, Edwin S, Romero RJ: Prostaglandin biosynthesis by human decidual cells: Effects of inflammatory mediators. Prostaglandins Leukotrienes Essent Fatty Acids 41:35–38, 1990.
180. Romero R, Avila C, Santhanam U, Sehgal PB: Amniotic fluid interleukin 6 in preterm labor: Association with infection. J Clin Invest 85:1392–1396, 1990.
181. Romero R, Brody DT, Oyarzun E, et al: Interleukin-1: A signal for the onset of parturition. Am J Obstet Gynecol 160:1117–1123, 1989.

126

Endocrinology of Lactation and Nursing: Disorders of Lactation

VALERIANO LEITE
ELIZABETH ANNE COWDEN
AND HENRY G. FRIESEN

Lactation is the final phase of the complete reproductive cycle of mammals. In almost all species the newborn are dependent on maternal milk during the neonatal period; in most, the young are dependent for a considerable time. Adequate lactation is therefore essential for reproduction and the survival of the species; biologically, failure to lactate can be just as much a cause of failure to reproduce as is failure to mate or to ovulate. Milk provides both a source of nutrients and protection against infections because of the immunoglobulins and other antibacterial elements present. Other significant constituents in milk are being recognized, including many hormones and trace elements. The importance of these to the growth and well-being of the suckling infant in many cases is not fully appreciated.

The process of lactation may be divided into at least three stages: mammogenesis, that is, mammary growth and development; lactogenesis, or milk formation and secretion; and milk ejection, or removal. The hormonal mechanisms that regulate each of these three processes are considered. Lactation demands appropriate adaptive changes in the mother. The metabolic cost of producing more than 1 liter of milk daily may require substantial dietary modification to balance the maternal loss of protein, calories, fluids, and minerals while maintaining ideal body weight. In addition to metabolic adaptations there are alterations in ovarian function secondary to breastfeeding. In the initial postpartum period lactational amenorrhea is present, and its duration is directly related to the extent and frequency of breastfeeding. Thus lactation is nature's contraceptive.

Lactation can be suppressed either by terminating breastfeeding alone or with the use of pharmacological agents that inhibit prolactin secretion or the action of prolactin. Inappropriate lactation, or galactorrhea, and its diagnosis and treatment is considered at the end of the chapter.

MORPHOLOGICAL AND FUNCTIONAL DEVELOPMENT OF THE BREAST

Morphological Development of the Breast (Mammogenesis)

The mammary gland, which is derived from ectoderm, first is evident in the 4-mm embryo as a mammary bud from which the mammary crest, or milk line, develops. After several modifications the epithelial nodule is recognizable buried in mesenchyme. At this early stage of development there is an interesting interaction between epithelial and surrounding mesenchymal cells. Fetal hormones, testosterone for example, act on the mesenchymal cells, which by a paracrine mechanism affect the differentiation of the neighboring mammary epithelial elements.[1] In the 120- to 150-mm embryo secondary epithelial buds develop, forming cellular cords that lengthen and bifurcate, and give rise, by reabsorption of the internal cells, to the excretory and lactiferous ducts of the mammary gland.

The human mammary gland is a compound tubuloalveolar gland consisting of 15 to 25 irregular lobes radiating from the mammary papilla or nipple. The lobes are separated by a layer of dense connective tissue and are embedded in an abundance of adipose tissue. Each lobe is subdivided into a series of lobules from which emerge lactiferous ducts lined by stratified squamous epithelium. Loose intralobular connective tissue surrounds the system of ducts, permitting greater distensibility as the epithelial portion of the gland develops during pregnancy and lactation.

At birth the mammary structures are still rudimentary, but in some newborns, particularly prematures, a slight degree of secretory function is observed (witch's milk) within a few days after birth. When this occurs the mammary gland appears enlarged and the epithelial ducts expand into milk sinuses. Secretory activity results from high prolactin levels in the newborn. Subsequently the breast enters a quiescent state (Fig. 126–1A). With the onset of puberty in the female the areola enlarges and becomes more pigmented, and further growth occurs (Fig. 126–1B). The growth of the breast at puberty is essentially due to rapid growth of the mammary stroma. The ductal system, however, also proliferates. These changes are related to the onset of estrogen and progesterone secretion by the ovary.

There is in fact considerable variation in the development of mammary gland function among different species, acinar development being more pronounced in species with a long progestational phase. In species with short estrous cycles (e.g., mouse and rat) in which the follicular phase of the cycle is predominant and the luteal phase almost nonexistent, only the duct system develops, and in these species, complete development of the mammary gland occurs only in pregnancy. In species with a long luteal phase, such as primates, mammary development during each menstrual cycle is considerable and, in a limited sense, similar to the changes during pregnancy.

Breast Changes During the Menstrual Cycle

During each menstrual cycle, cyclic proliferative changes and active growth of duct tissues occur; these changes progress during the follicular and periovulatory phases, reach a maximum in the late luteal phase, and then regress. Clinically, evidence of these changes is supported by a history of increased tenderness and even painful enlargement of the breasts during the luteal phase of the cycle. Histological examination of the normal breast reveals that after puberty, mammary development consists of a slow, progressive increase in glandular tissue brought about by

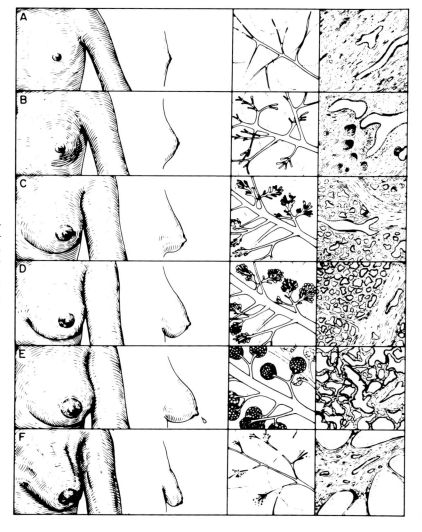

FIGURE 126–1. **Phases of mammary gland development.** Anterior and lateral views of the breast on the left side and microscopic appearance of ducts and lobules on the right side. **A**, Prepuberty (childhood). **B**, Puberty. **C**, Maturity (reproductive). **D**, Pregnancy. **E**, Lactation. **F**, Postmenopausal (senescent) state. (Adapted from Copeland EM, Bland KI: The breast. *In* Sabiston DC [ed]: Essentials of Surgery. Philadelphia, WB Saunders, 1987, p 294.)

epithelial outgrowths that lengthen, hollow out, and form further subdivisions of the ducts (Fig. 126–1C). The complex groupings of ductules, surrounded by loose and delicate stroma, thus form rudimentary lobules. Normal growth goes no further in nonpregnant subjects, and it is generally agreed that true alveoli usually are not present until the third month of pregnancy. Thus between puberty and adult life limited development of the mammary gland occurs, accompanied by cyclic changes, but complete development of mammary function occurs only in pregnancy.

Breast Changes During Pregnancy and Lactation

The development of the human mammary gland during pregnancy has been reviewed elsewhere.[2, 3] At the beginning of pregnancy there is rapid growth and branching from terminal portions of the gland at least in part at the expense of interstitial adipose tissue. Increased vascularity accompanies the infiltration of interstitial tissue by lymphocytes, eosinophils, and plasma cells. True glandular acini, the basic components of a functional mammary gland, appear at the beginning of the third month. The hollow alveolus is lined by a single layer of myoepithelial cells. The highly branched myoepithelial cells enclose the glandular alveolus in a loosely meshed network surrounded by capillaries, with the lumen of the alveolus connected by an intralobular duct. In the second trimester of pregnancy alveolar secretion begins and then increases further during the third trimester (Fig. 126–1D). In the last month of pregnancy the enlargement of the breasts results largely from hypertrophy of parenchymal cells and distention of the alveoli with a hyaline, eosinophilic secretion termed colostrum. During lactation the glandular tissue increases further with milk accumulating in the alveoli (Fig. 126–1E). After cessation of breastfeeding the mammary gland rapidly regresses but the alveoli persist. The result of this is that the histological pattern of the breast is no longer identical to the pattern found in the breast of the nulligravida.[4] With menopause there is regression of the epithelium and fibrosis of the stroma (Fig. 126–1F).

Hormonal Effects on Mammary Growth

There is a vast literature dealing with the hormonal control of mammary growth and function. In these studies attempts have been made to establish the simplest hormonal combinations required for duct and lobuloalveolar growth, principally using hypophysectomized, adrenalectomized, and oophorectomized rats. Using this experimental model Lyons et al,[5] in their classic experiments, demonstrated that a number of hormones were involved, including six pituitary hormones: prolactin, adrenocorticotropin (ACTH), growth hormone (GH), thyrotropin (TSH), follicle-stimulating hormone (FSH), and luteinizing hormone (LH). In addition, the placenta secretes a prolactin-like hormone, placental lactogen (PL), and, in humans, a placental growth hormone–variant (hGH-V). Moreover, steroid hormones from the ovary, adrenal, and placenta, plus thyroid hormones and insulin, are involved in mammary growth and function. In several cases (TSH, FSH, and LH)

the hormones listed do not act directly on the gland; their effects result from the secretion of hormones from target glands they stimulate. Despite the fact that these classic studies were performed on rats, the conclusions derived frequently have been applied to many species, including humans.

The role of ovarian hormones in mammogenesis in women is clearly established on clinical grounds because gonadal failure in the prepubertal period results in absence of mammary gland development. Once mammary development is complete, oophorectomy has a much less obvious effect. Among the ovarian hormones, estrogens appear to be associated with the proliferation of the ductal system, as pointed out in the studies of Folley[6] and Meites[7] in the rat and mouse and by others[3] in humans, whereas progesterone appears to be necessary for complete mammogenesis by stimulating alveolar proliferation. During pregnancy, progesterone, estradiol, estrone, and estriol blood concentrations increase markedly, indicating higher production of these steroids by the fetal-placental unit. Furthermore, high levels of human chorionic gonadotropin (hCG), prolactin, hPL, and hGH-V are found. It is likely that all these hormonal factors work in concert to provide the mature alveolar system in human mammary glands.

Despite its direct effect on the development of the mammary gland, prolactin also induces the liver to release additional factors known to enhance the action of prolactin on the breast.[8, 9] This is analogous to insulin-like growth factor (IGF-I) induction by GH.

The growth factors that may play a role in mammogenesis include IGF-I, epidermal growth factor (EGF), and transforming growth factor α (TGF-α). The first is a potent mitogen of mammary tissue from a variety of species.[10–12] Like IGF-I, EGF is able to stimulate lobuloalveolar development and epithelial cell proliferation.[13] TGF-α may play a role in the morphogenesis of the mouse mammary ductal system.[14] TGF-α expression has also been identified in human mammary epithelial cells.[15, 16] The actions of these growth factors in the stimulation of the normal mammary tissue probably encompass endocrine as well as paracrine mechanisms, since they have been reported to be synthesized in the mammary gland.[15–18] The stimulatory action of these factors may be balanced by other factors, such as TGF-β, which inhibit mammary development.[19]

In summary, three classes of hormones are important for mammary development and growth: (1) steroids, estradiol, progesterone, and glucocorticoids; (2) the pituitary and placental protein hormone family of prolactin, GH, and PL (other protein hormones include insulin, IGF-I, EGF, and TGF-α); and (3) thyroid hormones, which are important to mammary gland growth.

CELLULAR AND HORMONAL MECHANISMS OF LACTATION

Cellular Mechanisms

By means of morphological and biochemical approaches, it has been possible to gain an understanding of the major pathways involved in milk secretion. As shown in Figure 126–2, four transcellular pathways are used to pro-

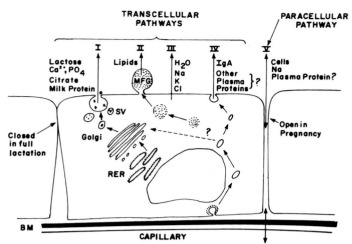

FIGURE 126–2. **Pathways for milk synthesis and secretion in the mammary alveolus.** Pathway I: Exocytosis of milk protein and lactose in Golgi-derived secretory vesicles. Pathway II: Milk fat secretion by way of the milk fat globule. Pathway III: Secretion of ions and water across the apical membrane. Pathway IV: Pinocytosis-exocytosis of immunoglobulins. Pathway V: The paracellular pathway for plasma components and leukocytes. SV, secretory vesicle; RER, rough endoplasmic reticulum; BM, basement membrane; MFG, milk fat globule. (Adapted from Neville MC et al: The mechanisms of milk secretion. *In* Neville MC, Neifert MR [eds]: Lactation: Physiology, Nutrition, and Breast-Feeding. New York, Plenum Press, 1983, p 50.)

mote secretion of the major constituents of milk.[3] The first pathway involves an exocytotic mechanism. Proteins, lactose, calcium, phosphate, and citrate are packaged into secretory vesicles in the Golgi system. Calcium and phosphate combine with caseins to form micelles. The combined action of galactosyltranferase and α-lactalbumin on appropriate substrates leads to the formation of lactose. The Golgi vesicle is impermeable to lactose, an osmotically active sugar, so that water is drawn into the vesicle. Indeed, the volume of milk is directly related to its lactose content. As the secretory vesicle matures it moves toward the apical surface of the alveolar cell, where its contents are discharged into the lumen. Pathway II involves milk lipids, which are synthesized in the cytoplasm and on the smooth endoplasmic reticulum. The lipids initially aggregate into droplets that coalesce to form fat globules that ultimately are discharged into the alveolar lumen. Pathway III promotes the secretion of monovalent ions and water. Water moves across the cell drawn by the osmotic gradient generated by lactose, while ions follow water moving down electrochemical gradients. Pathway IV is used for transport of immunoglobulins. Immunoglobulin A (IgA) enters the cell by a specific receptor-mediated process. The receptor immunoglobulin complex becomes internalized in endocytotic vesicles and is transported either to the Golgi vesicle or to the apical membrane of the cell for secretion into milk.

Pathway V, unlike the first four transcellular mechanisms, is a paracellular route. Substances normally have limited passage between alveolar cells because of the presence of tight junctions, but during active milk secretion the junctions become leaky, allowing plasma constituents to pass directly into milk. During pregnancy and lactation the breast is infiltrated by leukocytes and especially gut-derived immunoblasts that secrete IgA. The entry of these immunological cells into the mammary tissue is a hormone-dependent event. Prolactin, estrogen, and progesterone all combine to produce a chemotactic signal that favors migration of these cellular elements into the breast.

Hormones and Lactation

We have considered the hormones that are involved in the development and growth of the mammary gland. We propose now to consider the hormones that are necessary for lactation and to review the cellular and molecular mechanisms by which they exert their effects. Much of our knowledge is derived from studies in species other than the human, and hence we are forced to extrapolate from this knowledge to the human. The reader should appreciate that this extension may not always be warranted. Folley,[6] along with Lyons et al,[5] was among the first to stress that lactation results from the interaction of many hormones acting on the breast. The list includes many, if not all, of the hormones listed in the section on hormones and mammogenesis.

Prolactin

Of all the hormones necessary for lactation, none is more important than prolactin. Human prolactin was identified as a separate pituitary hormone in the early 1970s[20, 21]; since that time a large body of information has accumulated about the physiological and pharmacological factors that control its secretion. The gene coding for prolactin is 10 Kb in length and is located on chromosome 6.[22]

During pregnancy there is a gradual and progressive increase in serum prolactin concentrations from a mean before pregnancy of 7 to 10 ng/ml to values above 200 ng/ml in maternal serum at term. Despite the fact that the decidua is capable of producing prolactin, the pituitary is the source of the increased levels of prolactin found in maternal serum during pregnancy. In fact, during pregnancy there is hyperplasia of lactotrophs[23] that is accompanied by a decrease in the number of somatotrophs[23, 24] and, possibly, a decrease in the secretion of hGH by the pituitary.[25] The latter is still a matter of controversy.[26] Whether these hyperplastic prolactin-producing cells arise from pre-existing lactotrophs, from stem cells, or from somatotrophs is also unclear.

In the case of decidual prolactin, it is known that this hormone is released into the amniotic fluid. It has been shown that the transcription initiation site for decidual prolactin is 5 Kb upstream from that used in the pituitary; hence many of the 5′ regulatory sites used in the pituitary are in the extra 5′ untranslated region of the decidual prolactin gene.[27] This may explain why some modulators of the synthesis of prolactin by the pituitary are ineffective in the decidua. In the postpartum period in women who are not breastfeeding, prolactin concentrations gradually decrease to nonpregnant levels by three to six weeks. In contrast, in women who are breastfeeding, prolactin levels remain elevated for several months postpartum.[28–32] Even in these women there is a progressive decline in serum prolactin despite continued breastfeeding. This decline apparently is due to a decrease in the amount of prolactin released in each secretory episode (Fig. 126–3) and not to

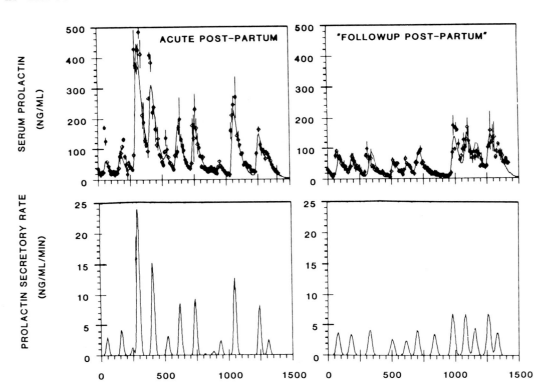

FIGURE 126–3. Deconvolution analysis of episodic prolactin secretion in one lactating woman studied at three weeks (*left panels*, **acute**) **and three months** (*right panels*, **follow-up**) **postpartum.** The upper panels depict the serial serum prolactin concentrations measured by RIA of blood collected at 10-minute intervals for 24 hours. The curve through the observed prolactin values is the computer-predicted fit of the data. The lower panels show the calculated prolactin secretory rates. (Adapted from Nunley WC et al: Dynamics of pulsatile prolactin release during the postpartum lactational period. J Clin Endocrinol Metab 72:291, 1991. ©The Endocrine Society.)

a decrease in the number or duration of the prolactin bursts. The concentrations of serum prolactin determined by radioimmunoassay (RIA) are, in most circumstances, identical with those estimated by bioassay using an Nb2-lymphoma cell bioassay.[33] In some patients with macroprolactinemia, where large molecular weight variants of prolactin predominate in the circulation, the estimates of prolactin by RIA and Nb2 bioassay are poorly correlated, although a significant correlation exists between the measurements of prolactin by Nb2 bioassay and by an immunoradiometric method.[34]

With the use of the dopamine agonist bromocriptine, which specifically inhibits prolactin secretion, it has been possible to clarify the role of this hormone in human lactation. When bromocriptine is administered in the immediate postpartum period, the elevated prolactin concentrations decline within hours to nonpregnant values, and breast engorgement and lactation are abolished.[35] This clinical experiment demonstrates that prolactin is essential for the initiation of lactation. In women with Sheehan's syndrome, lactation presumably does not occur because prolactin disappears from the circulation after pituitary infarction in the immediate postpartum period. On the other hand, if estrogens are used to suppress lactation and breast engorgement in the postpartum period, serum prolactin values actually are raised slightly above those seen in nursing subjects but no milk is formed. These observations

demonstrate that the action of prolactin in the breast is inhibited by high concentrations of estrogens. It is likely that the same mechanism is responsible for preventing milk formation during pregnancy. Similar interaction may account for the initiation of lactation. With the rapid decline in estrogens and progesterone in the immediate postpartum period, the inhibitory effects of steroids are removed, allowing prolactin to act unimpeded on the fully developed and primed mammary gland.

Quite possibly the surge of prolactin secretion that follows each episode of suckling serves to stimulate maximal milk formation and readies the breast for the next feeding. Similarly in monkeys a single large increase in serum prolactin produces histologically recognizable lactational changes in the mammary gland within hours. It is clear from anecdotal accounts that breast engorgement and milk formation can occur with surprising rapidity after a variety of events, including surgical procedures, or more gradually after repeated nipple stimulation, as occurs in wet nurses, some of whom have been in the postmenopausal age group. It is assumed that these events are accompanied by increases in serum prolactin, but thus far no systematic studies have been conducted.

In most species prolactin is essential for the onset of lactation, but there are considerable species differences. In the cow, for example, prolactin is crucial for the initiation of lactation, whereas subsequently, when serum prolactin concentrations are reduced with bromocriptine, milk yield declines only 10 to 20 per cent.[2] Thus far there have been few studies in which attempts have been made to determine whether milk yield and the concentration of prolactin values can be correlated. In one study[36] no correlation of basal prolactin values with milk yield was found, but there appeared to be a positive correlation between the magnitude of the increase in prolactin after breastfeeding and milk yield. Others have attempted to increase milk production with the use of agents that increase serum prolactin, such as thyrotropin-releasing hormone (TRH). Although milk yield was not increased, fat and protein content were raised. Similar studies with TRH in cows failed to produce any effect on milk yield and composition. Moreover, earlier studies with exogenous administration of prolactin to cows also failed to demonstrate any striking effects on milk production. It appears, therefore, that prolactin plays an important—indeed crucial—role in the initiation of lactation in many species, including humans, but its role in maintaining lactation is more variable. In women the secretion of prolactin in the postpartum period gradually declines. Nevertheless, the low levels in serum late in the postpartum period remain crucial for the maintenance of lactation.

It is generally accepted that in mammals, one of the principal target tissues for prolactin is the mammary gland. The direct effects and mechanism of action of prolactin on mammary gland differentiation, growth, and function have been examined extensively in animal models. Like other polypeptide hormones, prolactin exerts its effects on mammary cells through receptor-mediated mechanisms. The nature and role of prolactin receptors have been clarified to a degree.[37–43] Structural analysis of prolactin receptors indicates that they belong to a superfamily of receptors that includes cytokines, GH, and prolactin receptors.[41, 42] All these forms have a single transmembrane domain, a large extracellular ligand-binding domain, and a cytoplasmic domain of variable length. After interaction of the hormone with its receptor, the receptor hormone complex is rapidly internalized into an endocytotic vesicle. The complex may then directly follow a pathway to the lysosomes or the Golgi complex, where hormone and receptor dissociate, with the latter being recycled. By using hormone labelled with iodine-125, it is evident that the internalized prolactin is degraded. Evidence that the internalized fragments of prolactin do not appear to be mediators of the action of the hormone is provided by experiments using antibodies to prolactin receptors. With antibodies to prolactin receptors one can block the action of prolactin on the mammary gland, indicating the obligatory role of the receptor in mediating the action of prolactin. Moreover, other antibodies have been generated that can mimic the action of prolactin, demonstrating that appropriate receptor activation is a sufficient signal to reproduce the action of prolactin itself.[37, 44, 45] The entirely different chemical structure of prolactin and antibodies would suggest that a component of internalized, degraded prolactin was not an essential mediator of the action of prolactin. The discovery that certain fragments of prolactin (16K prolactin) can bind to specific receptors[46] not shared by the intact hormone may question that possibility. It is presumed that the cleavage of prolactin by target tissues represents a normal mechanism to create diversity in the actions of the hormone. In the case of 16K prolactin the specific receptors may mediate at least one specific action of 16K prolactin: the inhibition of the proliferation of capillary endothelial cells.[47] Depending on the concentration and timing, prolactin can induce, or up-regulate, the number of prolactin receptors, whereas under other experimental conditions prolactin may down-regulate, or cause a decrease in, its own receptor number. In addition, other hormones, estrogens, and GH can increase the number of prolactin receptors, whereas androgens decrease the prolactin receptor number. Nutritional states and age-dependent factors also may modulate receptor number.

Implicit in all these considerations is the view that hormonal effects are a function of hormone concentration and tissue responsiveness and that the latter is determined by receptor number and postreceptor mechanisms. In the case of prolactin the postreceptor mechanisms are still not well understood, although several intracellular mediators (cAMP, cGMP, calcium ions, phospholipids, polyamines) have been implicated in the actions of prolactin. In addition to its role in promoting mammary growth, prolactin stimulates the synthesis of casein,[48, 49] α-lactalbumin,[50, 51] lactose,[52] and milk fat.[53] The synthesis of casein has been studied extensively.[54] The gene structure for casein has been elucidated. With the availability of cDNA probes for casein it has been possible to examine the hormonal control of gene expression. Prolactin stimulates casein gene transcription several-fold, but a much greater effect of prolactin is to stabilize mRNA for casein, enhancing its half-life some eight-fold. These effects of prolactin can be inhibited by progesterone in rat mammary gland explants.

Human Growth Hormone, Human Growth Hormone–Variant, and Human Placental Lactogen

Human growth hormone and hPL have been termed lactogenic because of their activity in various bioassay systems. For example, they induce lactational changes in the rabbit mammary gland, cause luteotropic effects in rats, stimulate proliferation of pigeon crop-sac epithelium, and stimulate the growth of Nb2-node rat lymphoma cells in tissue culture—the latter being a sensitive and specific bioassay for lactogenic hormones.[55] Moreover, there is considerable chemical homology among prolactin, hGH, and hPL, suggesting a common ancestral precursor for these molecules.

It is possible that hGH may play a permissive role in augmenting milk production, since Lyons et al.,[5] for example, demonstrated that hGH administration enhanced milk yield, as judged by an accelerated weight gain in infants whose mothers were treated with hGH. hGH-V is a recently characterized placental hormone[25] that appears to be unique to humans. The levels of hGH-V in maternal circulation progressively rise during the second half of pregnancy, when it becomes the predominant form of hGH in serum.[56] The somatogenic activity of these two hormones is similar. The lactogenic activity of hGH-V, however, measured by its capacity to stimulate division of Nb2 lymphoma cells, is about 20-fold lower than that of the normal pituitary hGH.[57]

Concentrations of hPL gradually increase throughout the first two trimesters of pregnancy, reaching average concentrations of 5 to 8 μg/ml; these values, unlike those of hGH, are maintained throughout the last trimester until they disappear completely within 24 hours of delivery. Available data would suggest that hPL primarily facilitates mammary growth and development rather than lactation per se. The report of rare people who lack the hPL gene yet have an uneventful pregnancy and appear to have normal lactation suggests that the role of hPL may be of relatively little importance.[58] In rat models it has been demonstrated that major reduction in PL secretion during pregnancy results in impaired mammary development and subsequent poor lactation, and it has been suggested that the effects of PL on mammary development may themselves be indirect—perhaps by stimulation of formation of estrogen receptors in breast tissue, thus sensitizing it to the growth-promoting effects of estrogen itself.

Thyroid Hormones

Thyroid hormones are important for adequate milk secretion in many species.[2] In rats the degree of lactation is directly related to thyroid secretion, whereas supraphysiological concentrations of T_4 and T_3 depress milk yield in both rats and rabbits.

Insulin, Serum, and Tissue Growth Factors

There are large numbers of specific insulin-binding sites in human mammary tissue, but the precise role insulin plays in stimulating human mammary function has not been defined. It is likely that insulin's stimulation of glucose entry into the cell accelerates lipogenesis and protein synthesis.

It is also clear that in tissue culture of mouse and rat mammary epithelial cells, insulin at high concentrations acts as a mitogen.[1] It is possible that some of the mitogenic effects of insulin are mediated by IGF receptors. The latter have been demonstrated on human breast cancer cells in which IGF-I has been shown to have a direct mitogenic effect.[59, 60]

EGF, a single-chain polypeptide isolated from male mouse submaxillary gland, has been reported in serum of pregnant women and in human milk. In fact, EGF is present in human milk at concentrations well above those found in plasma.[61] Whether EGF and platelet-derived growth factor, which also has been identified in human milk, stimulate milk formation is not clear. Additional locally generated tissue growth factors may act by a paracrine or autocrine effect, including TGF-α and -β, fibroblast growth factor, and IGF-binding proteins.

Estrogen and Progesterone

Although oophorectomy has no detrimental effects on established lactation, estrogen is thought to have a major impact on lactation both by its direct action on mammary tissue (causing suppression of lactation when present in high concentration) and by its indirect action in stimulating prolactin secretion. In turn prolactin is known to modulate estrogen receptors in the rat, both in vitro and in vivo, adding a further level of complexity to the interaction of these hormones at target tissue level. In cultured mammary glands from subhuman primates estradiol has been

shown to inhibit the action of prolactin on stimulating casein synthesis.

In addition to its role in mammogenesis, progesterone can inhibit the onset of lactation[62] while not affecting established lactation.

Adrenal Steroids

Once again, although the presence of adrenal steroids is a prerequisite for the induction and maintenance of milk secretion in many species (rat, mouse, goat), their role in human lactation remains to be documented.

Parathyroid Hormone, Parathyroid Hormone–Like Peptide, and Vitamin D

Despite the large amounts of calcium secreted in human milk, parathyroid gland activity in cows appears depressed at the height of lactation, but removal of these glands causes depression of lactation—in other animals as well as in cows. The relation between parathyroid activity and lactation in the human is unclear. Parathyroid hormone–like peptide (PTH-LP) is a calcium-mobilizing hormone that has been detected in human milk at concentrations about 10,000 times higher than in serum.[63] PTH-LP mRNA is expressed in mammary tissue of the rat in response to suckling, and this effect may be mediated by prolactin. In fact, serum levels of prolactin are correlated with the expression of PTH-LP mRNA in mammary tissue, and injections of prolactin induce PTH-LP mRNA in puerperal glands of the rat.[64] This suggests that prolactin may have a regulatory role in the transport of calcium into milk by stimulating the synthesis of PTH-LP by the mammary gland. During pregnancy the serum concentrations of vitamin D levels are increased. There are indications that prolactin may be one of the mediators of the increased blood levels of vitamin D.[65, 66]

LACTATION

Initiation

There is considerable variation among different species in the time when milk can first be detected in mammary alveoli during pregnancy. In ruminants considerable quantities of milk may be produced before parturition, and indeed, milk production continues uninterrupted during the early stages of pregnancy. In the rat and rhesus monkey copious milk secretion does not occur until two days after parturition. Similarly in humans the alveoli become distended with colostrum in the last third of pregnancy, but mammary secretion does not appear until three to four days after childbirth. There are numerous theories concerning the possible involvement of endocrine mechanisms in the initiation of lactation. It has been suggested that the secretory activity of the alveolar epithelium during pregnancy is inhibited by steroids from the fetal-placental unit that exert an inhibitory effect directly on mammary epithelial cells, rendering them less responsive to lactogenic hormones. The observations that serum prolactin levels reach their peak shortly before delivery, when no lactation occurs, and that estrogen treatment inhibits puer-

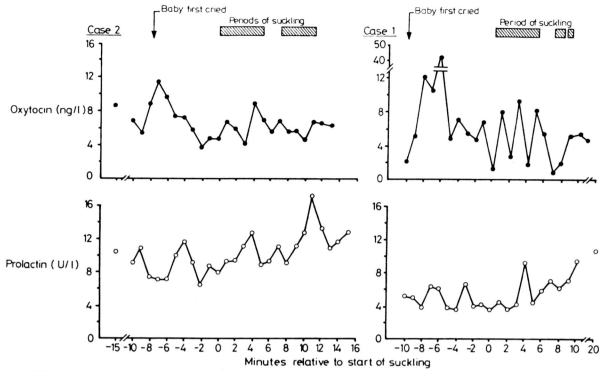

FIGURE 126–4. **Changes in plasma oxytocin (●) and prolactin (○) concentrations before and during suckling in two women on day four postpartum.** Note the release of oxytocin before the baby is attached to the breast and the increase in prolactin concentrations with suckling. (Adapted from McNeilly AS et al: Release of oxytocin and prolactin in response to suckling. Br Med J 286:258, 1983.)

peral lactation in the presence of elevated serum prolactin levels support this hypothesis. At parturition a fall in the concentration of steroids in blood permits the mammary gland to respond to the "lactogenic complex."

Effect of Breastfeeding on Prolactin and Oxytocin

The mechanisms involved in the maintenance of milk production have been defined in part. One of the most potent factors that favor the establishment of lactation is suckling. There are many anecdotal reports in which non-pregnant women have been able to produce an adequate supply of milk within a few days of taking a baby to the breast. When the newborn suckles, a complex chain of events is initiated. A neural stimulus is transmitted to the brain, where it results in the secretion of prolactin and oxytocin. The exact anatomical pathways that mediate the release of prolactin and oxytocin have not been defined in humans, but some experimental data are available in animals. With the availability of specific and sensitive RIA's increases in serum prolactin with suckling have been observed in cows, goats, sheep, and humans. When nursing women were allowed to hold their infants but not to breastfeed, prolactin did not increase despite the occurrence of the milk let-down reflex. The application of a breast pump at regular periods of breastfeeding caused prolactin elevations similar in timing and magnitude to those that occur during suckling. Hence it is concluded that neither psychological factors associated with expectation of nursing nor

the presumed release of oxytocin, as evidenced by milk let-down, is effective in stimulating the release of prolactin.[29]

The milk ejection caused by posterior pituitary extracts was first observed in 1910 in lactating goats. Both posterior pituitary hormones, oxytocin and vasopressin, cause milk ejection, but oxytocin is five times more active than vasopressin. Oxytocin exerts a direct effect on the myoepithelial elements surrounding the alveoli of the breast, causing them to contract and force milk into the mammary ducts, where it is more readily available to the suckling infant.

Although suckling is the primary stimulus in the milk ejection reflex, it may be conditioned by factors such as the sight of the baby, scheduled time of feeding, and breast preparation. Pain, distraction, embarrassment, and anesthetics inhibit the reflex. As shown in Figure 126–4, oxytocin release takes place in most women before the baby is attached to the nipple.

Caldeyro Barcia[67] has carried out extensive studies on the milk let-down reflex in humans. He catheterized human mammary ducts and measured intraductal pressure under various physiological circumstances. Injection of oxytocin and suckling of the nipple on the opposite breast or dilation of the cervix produced a marked increase in ductal pressure. The rhythmic contraction induced by suckling was closely mimicked by successive intravenous injections of oxytocin given at frequent intervals in an appropriate dose, whereas a continuous intravenous infusion or a single intravenous or intramuscular injection of a high dose of oxytocin evoked nonphysiological responses, suggesting that oxytocin release occurs in repeated spurts in women.

Serum oxytocin concentrations have been determined during periods of breastfeeding in both animals and humans where rapid intermittent spurts of oxytocin are detected. These spurt discharges of oxytocin also occur during the resting phase but with reduced frequency.

Breastfeeding and Lactational Amenorrhea

Breastfeeding is associated with a period during which ovarian function is inhibited. The duration of the period of lactational amenorrhea is related to the frequency and intensity of the suckling stimulus. The endocrine mechanisms leading to the inhibition of normal ovulatory cycles have been the subject of a number of studies.[68–70] Breastfeeding in some cultures is widely recognized to be nature's contraceptive, and epidemiological studies have documented a wide variation in birth intervals, depending on the type of breastfeeding that is practiced. In primitive tribes, such as the Kung hunter-gatherers in Africa, babies frequently are nursed for as long as three to four years. Birth intervals are spaced at four years, with a mean live birth number of five during the reproductive cycle of the women. In another cultural group, the Hutterite farmers of North America, supplemental feeding is offered a few months after birth. In this group the birth interval is reduced to two years, allowing a mean of 11 births in the reproductive period of women. In women who do not breastfeed, the duration of postpartum amenorrhea is reduced to two to three months on average. Clearly breastfeeding has a profound effect on inhibition of ovulatory cycles and the duration of birth intervals.

On closer examination of the patterns of breastfeeding used in these groups, important variations in the practice of breastfeeding are seen. For example, in more primitive cultures the frequency of suckling is much greater than commonly accepted schedules in North America. Robyn and Meuris[68] have reported that in one African tribe, the average number of feedings per day during the first year is around 13. In Bangladesh the number reported is 15 to 18 times per day.[69] In Europe and North America the number of breastfeedings seldom exceeds six per day and commonly decreases to three or four. There is a fairly close correlation among the milk volume, the frequency of suckling, and persistent elevation of prolactin levels in the postpartum period.[68] It has been suggested that six feedings per day is the minimum required for maintenance of hyperprolactinemia and suppression of ovulation.

The endocrine changes that contribute to postpartum amenorrhea have been examined both in cross-sectional and in longitudinal studies.[70] In women who choose to bottlefeed, ovulatory cycles usually resume by 70 to 100 days post partum. The initial cycles often are associated with inadequate corpus luteum functions. In contrast, women who breastfeed exhibit suppression of follicular development. Although plasma FSH levels return to normal by 30 days post partum, pulsatile LH secretion in the majority does not.[70] Suckling appears to suppress the pulsatile secretion of gonadotropin hormone–releasing hormone (GnRH) from the hypothalamus with resultant cessation of follicle growth. Although this inhibition of GnRH secretion may be mediated by the increased levels of prolactin associated with suckling, no correlation has been found between suckling-induced prolactin pulses and LH release.[32] Several other factors may play a role in the

suppression of gonadotropic function during lactation. These include opioids[71] and pituitary unresponsiveness caused by a deprivation of endogenous GnRH during pregancy.[72]

Despite all the studies done so far, the mechanism responsible for this lactational amenorrhea remains elusive.

CLINICAL ASPECTS OF LACTATION

Composition of Colostrum and Milk

Colostrum

In the last weeks of pregnancy and in the first few days after delivery, a small amount of fluid usually can be expressed from the mammary gland. This opalescent fluid, which is small in volume, yellowish, and contains fat globules, is called colostrum. Microscopic examination of this fluid reveals multinucleated cells loaded with particles of fat. These "foam cells" are derived from alveolar and ductal cells that have been shed into the lumen. Colostrum contains about 8 per cent protein, including lactalbumin, immunoglobulins (lactoglobulin), and lactoferrin, but it contains fat and lactose but little or no casein.

Milk

Usually two to four days after delivery colostrum is replaced by milk. Physiochemically, milk is an emulsion of fat in water, and the relative proportion of each component varies throughout a period of breastfeeding. This fact was appreciated as early as 1473, when wet nurses were advised to first milk the breast to drain the watery fluid before allowing the infant to nurse. Together with water and fat droplets in suspension (3 to 4 per cent), milk contains 1 per cent proteins (casein, lactalbumin, and lactoglobulin) and 7 per cent lactose, as well as electrolytes in solution, minerals, and vitamins. Human milk contains more than 100 known constituents, and additional components constantly are being identified. Of considerable interest are the varieties of hormones and neuropeptides that are found in milk,[73, 74] some at concentrations exceeding those found in serum. These include hypothalamic hormones (GnRH, TRH, growth hormone–releasing factor), pituitary hormones (hGH, prolactin, TSH), calcium-regulating hormones (PTH, PTH-LP, calcitonin), and growth factors (IGF, EGF). If these hormones are absorbed by the gastrointestinal tract of the neonate, they may exert biological effects in the infant. For instance, milk EGF was shown to have a role in the neonatal development of the gastrointestinal tract in rats.[75]

Evidence is accumulating of the great importance of a balanced diet for optimal nutrition of the infant. Although there is little difference between the caloric energy provided by human and cow's milk (about 70 kcal/100 ml), there must be an overall balance of nutrients as well as of individual constituents in the infant's diet. One example that illustrates this point is the fact that infantile tetany is reported to occur almost exclusively in formula-fed babies.[76, 77] This results from the very different calcium and phosphorus content in human milk compared with those in various widely used formulas. Furthermore, formula-fed infants seem more susceptible to infection in infancy, including gastroenteritis, recurrent respiratory infection, and various viral diseases. This problem is especially acute in underdeveloped countries where hygienic measures are not widely used, but it is also recognized in certain disadvantaged groups in industrialized countries.[78]

Specific properties of human milk that increase resistance to infection have in fact been reported.[3, 79] One of these is a nitrogen-containing polysaccharide that favors the growth of *Lactobacillus bifidus*. The presence of this organism confers a protective effect against invasive enteropathogenic organisms such as *Escherichia coli*. Furthermore, antibodies (IgA), lysozyme (300 times more than in cow's milk), and interferon produced by the lymphocytes of the milk itself may also have a protective effect. Human milk also contains chemotactic factors for blood monocytes that may aid in attracting macrophages to the mucosa of the infant's gastrointestinal tract. Tumor necrosis factor-α may be one of these factors.[80]

Milk, by itself, combined with fetal stores and sunlight, usually is adequate to sustain growth and nutrition in the infant. At the end of the first week postpartum 550 ml/d of milk are produced. By two to three weeks this increases to 800 ml/d, with maximal rates as great as 1.5 to 2 L/d.

With the advances in neonatal intensive care more and more premature infants, even when born at earlier gestational periods, are surviving. Early nutritional support is particularly important to premature infants because they are born without the nutritional reserves of the term infant, and growth is at an accelerated pace. It has been established that the milk of mothers who give birth prematurely differs in composition from the milk of women who give birth at term.[81] Preterm milk contains higher concentrations of protein, fat, elemental sodium, and chloride but lower levels of lactose. These differences begin to disappear by four weeks postpartum. Possible explanations for the differences in composition may involve reduced mammary gland blood flow and hence milk volume, incomplete differentiation of mammary epithelial cells, and absence of tight junctions between epithelial cells.

Maternal Dietary Requirements for Milk Production and Composition

To avoid major depletion of maternal tissue reserves, the diet of the lactating woman must be adequate. Within reason she may eat her usual diet, but the ingestion of meat, fish, and eggs is important, and fresh fruit, green vegetables, and salads are recommended. Fluid intake should be liberal. Supplemental iron often is prescribed, and during lactation there should be adequate dietary intake of calcium. Recommended daily caloric intake as well as useful information with regard to the composition of human and cow's milk may be found elsewhere.[82] Many attempts have been made to assess the effects of maternal food restriction on lactation. It is generally agreed that lactation persists despite severe malnutrition; however, with extreme maternal deprivation the protein and fat contents of human milk are lower. Severe dehydration also decreases milk yield.

The fat content in milk over a 24-hour period is relatively constant, but a diurnal variation has been reported, with minimal values occurring in the first morning feeding and highest at midmorning. These changes are not influenced by the mother maintaining a uniform distribution of calories and fat intake over a 24-hour period. Dietary fat composition does influence the types of fatty acids that are found in milk.

There is a considerable difference in the fat content of the initial and final phases of milk produced with each breastfeeding, with higher concentrations in the latter. It has been suggested[82] that this change in biochemical composition is a cue for the baby to stop feeding. No such cue would be received by a bottlefed baby because neither taste nor flavors change during the feeding.

In the last weeks of gestation pregnant women may express colostrum from the nipples twice a day, and it may be helpful if the woman learns how to empty the breast manually antepartum before the breasts become engorged and painful.

A final cautionary note must be added about drug ingestion and breastfeeding. It has become apparent that a number of drugs should not be given to the mother while she is nursing.[83] These include bromocriptine, cocaine, cyclophosphamide, doxorubicin, methotrexate, cyclosporine, ergotamine, lithium, phencyclidine, and phenidione. In practical terms, all drugs should be avoided whenever possible during pregnancy and breastfeeding. It was shown[84] that even small amounts of ethanol in the milk can alter the behavior of the breastfed infant. Lactating women should be aware of this and avoid alcohol or at least limit their intake during breastfeeding.

It is useful to consider the general problem of contraception in the postpartum period. In the past, breastfeeding was the principal means by which child spacing was attempted; it is evident that the protection against a new pregnancy is quite inadequate when breastfeeding as practiced in the industrialized world is used. More reliable contraception can be provided by mechanical methods, intrauterine devices (IUD's), or oral agents. The IUD has the advantage of not interfering with lactation. It must be pointed out, however, that the rate of expulsion of the IUD may be rather high. (Contraception is discussed in detail in Ch. 123.) Previously when contraceptives containing large amounts of estrogens and progestagens were used, breastfeeding was inhibited. With the lower steroid content of oral contraceptives currently in use, including the progestagen-only preparations, lactation is not impaired (especially when the oral agents are started after lactation is well established.) The use of GnRH long-acting agonists also proved to be an acceptable method of contraception during breastfeeding.[85] Effective contraception can also be achieved by breastfeeding alone, provided women remain amenorrheic and do not feed their babies with supplements until six months after delivery. This method of family planning is called lactational amenorrheic method.[86, 87]

Benefits Associated with Breastfeeding

Apart from the economic benefits associated with breastfeeding and its usefulness as a contraceptive method, breastfeeding may also be the best way of satisfying the nutritional needs of an infant for the first months of life. In fact, morbidity and mortality rates are lower in breastfed than in artificially fed infants. At least in part, this is due to higher prevalence of infections among non-breastfed babies.[88] It was even suggested that breast milk may favorably affect the development of the nervous system. In this study children fed with mother's milk had significantly higher IQ's at 7½ to 8 years of age than those fed by commercial formulas alone.[89]

Breastfeeding is also believed to foster bonding between mother and infant and, as a consequence, to be beneficial for the development and growth of children. Some of the hormones found in milk may play a role in the development of the bonding process. That might be the case with the opioid peptides that may be responsible for the infant's becoming addicted to their own mother's milk, as suggested by others.[73]

The positive impact of breastfeeding in the development, growth, and survival of children was recognized in 1990 in the World Summit for Children, which took place at the United Nations. Among the goals for children adopted in this summit and to be reached by the year 2000 was a recommendation for all women to breastfeed their children exclusively for four to six months and to continue breastfeeding with complementary food well into the second year.

Another potential benefit of breastfeeding is the negative association reported between lactation and the subsequent risk of breast cancer.[90–93] Some studies, however, have found little evidence in favor of such protective effect,[94, 95] and more work needs to be done before advising women to breastfeed specifically to decrease their risk of developing cancer of the breast.

DISTURBANCES OF LACTATION

Engorgement

A common complication, engorgement usually affects both breasts and typically occurs between days two and four postpartum. The condition results from milk retention and vascular and lymphatic stasis accompanied by tissue edema. During this period the breasts become firm, tense, and swollen and the areolae become edematous, resulting in less nipple protrusion, which makes it difficult for the infant to suckle. Although there may be considerable local discomfort, systemic symptoms, including slight temperature elevation, are uncommon. A much less pronounced degree of engorgement may occur after weaning.

Failing Lactation

The absence of lactation (agalactia) is the hallmark of patients who suffer from Sheehan's syndrome (postpartum pituitary necrosis) and results from prolactin deficiency. Because of improved obstetrical care, this situation is now rare in developed countries. Agalactia should be differentiated from conditions in which failure of the milk ejection reflex, rather than of milk production, constitutes the basis for unsuccessful breastfeeding. These include anxiety, breast engorgement, sore or inverted nipples, and inadequate suckling by the baby because of cleft palate or prematurity.

Attempts to increase milk yield with hormonal therapy date back to 1896, when it was reported that thyroid extracts increased milk yield in both women and cows. More recently hGH preparations have been used to increase milk yield, but neither treatment has general application. Pharmacological agents, including sulpiride, metoclopramide, phenothiazines, and TRH, have been shown to increase serum prolactin concentrations, and attempts have been made to enhance milk production in both animals and humans.[96–98] Intranasal oxytocin spray also has been reported to increase milk yield in women.[99]

In some conditions it may be inadvisable for the mother to breastfeed. These include the presence of serious infectious diseases, such as tuberculosis, hepatitis, and acquired immunodeficiency syndrome,[100] and the ingestion of certain drugs that are excreted in the milk.[83] In addition, various conditions that affect the baby, such as prematurity, cleft palate, esophageal defects, and mental deficiency, may limit the infant's ability to suckle. Because of the importance of breastfeeding in the bonding between mother and infant, a decision not to breastfeed when mothers suffer from debilitating or life-threatening diseases should be made only after careful evaluation of the potential risks or benefits associated with breastfeeding.

SUPPRESSION OF LACTATION

Before the introduction of estrogens to suppress lactation, a variety of empirical measures were tried, including the application of breast binders along with restriction of fluid intake, as well as the use of laxatives and diuretics. At times the treatment was worse than the problem, because, despite the application of all these measures, the breasts became engorged and painful. Suppression of lactation with estrogens began in the late 1930's, and subsequently a variety of estrogen preparations were used. A common practice was to give ethinyl estradiol (0.25 mg) three times daily for five days, or longer if necessary. With any of the regimens used a failure rate of 10 to 20 per cent was seen.

The inhibitory action of estrogen on lactation appears to be exerted at the mammary gland by blocking the action of prolactin. For some patients the administration of estrogen enhances the risk of thromboembolic complications in the puerperium. In addition, estrogen may potentially interfere with proper uterine involution. The potential risks of estrogen use have led to a search for effective, safe alternatives. With the demonstration that bromocriptine inhibits prolactin secretion with few adverse effects, this agent is now the treatment of choice for suppression of lactation. Bromocriptine therapy (2.5 mg two or three times a day) initiated immediately postpartum should be continued for a 10- to 14-day period to prevent rebound engorgement. It may also be used in women who experience engorgement after spontaneous or therapeutic abortion. In addition to bromocriptine, other dopamine agonists (cabergoline, CV 205-502) have been successfully used in the suppression of puerperal lactation.[101, 102] A long-acting injectable form of bromocriptine is also effective in preventing postpartum lactation and can be used as an alternative to the oral preparation.[103]

ABNORMAL LACTATION (GALACTORRHEA)

Definition

Galactorrhea is the secretion of milk from the breast under nonphysiological circumstances. It may be unilateral or bilateral, and the amount of milk secreted may vary from as little as a drop, which can be expressed manually, to continuous, copious, and spontaneous milk leakage. It is important to remember that small amounts of serous fluid may be expressed from the breasts of the vast majority of women who have previously been pregnant and that this discharge does not constitute galactorrhea.

It is a common clinical occurrence for women who have noted a slight discharge from the breast, in their concern and fear that this may be abnormal, to considerably aggravate the situation by repeatedly squeezing and examining the breast. This is akin to the effect of constant suckling in the maintenance of normal lactation, and unless the patient is reassured and discouraged from this practice, it simply ensures the persistence and increase of discharge from the breast.

Classification

Perhaps the most clinically useful classification of galactorrhea is the one that incorporates only two entities: galactorrhea in the presence and galactorrhea in the absence of hyperprolactinemia.

Hyperprolactinemic galactorrhea constitutes the minority of those cases with abnormal milk secretion (30 per cent).[104] Nevertheless, it is by far the one that has received the greatest attention in recent years. Patients whose galac-

torrhea is but one manifestation of hyperprolactinemia usually provide some other clue in the history or physical examination to suggest the presence of an elevated prolactin level. For example, on questioning, the patient may also complain of oligomenorrhea or amenorrhea, of infertility, or of sexual dysfunction.[105] Abnormalities in prolactin secretion are dealt with in considerable detail in another chapter, but it is important to reiterate that irrespective of the cause of hyperprolactinemia (and there are many causes), the clinical manifestations of this biochemical disorder are remarkably consistent. Galactorrhea is but one of these manifestations, but it may be the one that causes the patient to seek medical advice.

The vast majority of patients who have galactorrhea have normal circulating prolactin levels, and it is suggested that these women may be excessively sensitive to normal circulating prolactin concentrations. They are characteristically healthy with no history of menstrual irregularity or of infertility, and on physical examination no abnormality is detected other than the presence of abnormal milk discharge. It is also common in these patients to identify some specific event from which the symptom dates—most commonly after the birth of a child or weaning or after commencement or cessation of oral contraceptive therapy.

Approach to the Patient with Galactorrhea

A scheme that may be useful in the assessment of patients with galactorrhea is outlined in Figure 126–5. Of prime importance is the distinction of those patients who are hyperprolactinemic from those who are not, and to this end a simple serum prolactin estimation should suffice. Because stress-induced hyperprolactinemia is so common,[106] it is prudent to confirm its presence before attrib-

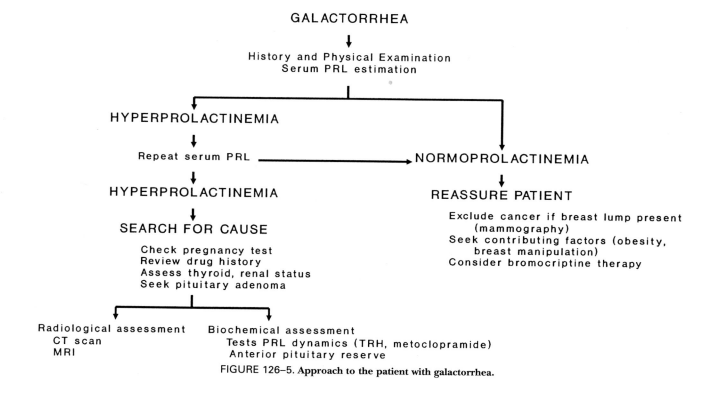

FIGURE 126–5. Approach to the patient with galactorrhea.

uting any clinical findings such as galactorrhea to it. If hyperprolactinemia is indeed present, then a careful search for its cause is mandatory, remembering that when secondary causes (e.g., pregnancy, drugs, hypothyroidism, and renal disease) have been excluded, the most likely cause is a prolactin-secreting pituitary tumor.

When prolactin levels are normal, simply reassuring the patient that no major endocrine dysfunction exists usually is sufficient. Many of these women fear that their breast discharge is a sign of breast cancer, and specific reassurance on this point is warranted after mammography if any breast lumps are present. In those very rare patients in whom galactorrhea is severe and intractable despite attention to all these factors, consideration should be given to therapy with bromocriptine. There is no question that this treatment is effective even in patients with normal prolactin levels.[107]

ACKNOWLEDGMENT: Valeriano Leite is a recipient of a fellowship (BD/845/90-ID) from Junta Nacional de Investigação Científica e Tecnológica, Portugal.

REFERENCES

1. Topper YJ, Freeman CS: Multiple hormone interactions in the developmental biology of the mammary gland. Physiol Rev 60:1049–1106, 1980.
2. Cowie AT, Forsyth IA, Hart IC: The Hormonal Control of Lactation. Berlin, Springer-Verlag, 1980, pp 1–274.
3. Neville MC, Neifert MR: Lactation: Physiology, Nutrition and Breast Feeding. New York, Plenum Press, 1983.
4. Glasier A, McNeilly AS: Physiology of lactation. Baillière's Clin Endocrinol Metab 4:379–395, 1990.
5. Lyons WR, Li CH, Johnson RE: The hormonal control of mammary growth and lactation. Recent Prog Horm Res 14:219–254, 1958.
6. Folley SJ: Endocrine control of the mammary gland. II. Lactation. Br Med Bull 5:135–142, 1948.
7. Meites J: Maintenance of the mammary lobulo-alveolar system in rats after adreno-orchidectomy by prolactin and growth hormone. Endocrinology 76:1220–1223, 1965.
8. Anderson TR, Rodriguez J, Nicoll CS: The synlactin hypothesis: Prolactin's mitogenic action may involve synergism with a somatomedin-like molecule. In Spencer EM (ed): Insulin-Like Growth Factors/Somatomedins. Berlin, Walter deGruyter, 1983, pp 71–78.
9. Anderson TR, Pitts DS, Nicoll CS: Prolactin's mitogenic action on the pigeon crop sac mucosal epithelium involves direct and indirect mechanisms. Gen Comp Endocrinol 54:236–246, 1984.
10. Imagawa W, Spencer EM, Larson L, Nandi S: Somatomedin-C substitutes for insulin for the growth of mammary epithelial cells from normal virgin mice in serum-free collagen gel cell culture. Endocrinology 119:2695–2699, 1986.
11. Deeks S, Richards J, Nandi S: Maintenance of normal rat mammary epithelial cells by insulin and insulin-like growth factor 1. Exp Cell Res 174:448–460, 1988.
12. Shamay A, Cohen N, Niwa M, Gertler A: Effect of insulin-like growth factor I on deoxyribonucleic acid synthesis and galactopoiesis in bovine undifferentiated and lactating mammary tissue in vitro. Endocrinology 123:804–809, 1988.
13. Tonelli QJ, Sorof S: Epidermal growth factor requirement for development of cultured mammary gland. Nature 285:250–252, 1980.
14. Snedeker SM, Brown CF, DiAugustine RP: Expression and functional properties of transforming growth factor α and epidermal growth factor during mouse mammary gland ductal morphogenesis. Proc Natl Acad Sci USA 88:276–280, 1991.
15. Zajchowski D, Band V, Pauzie N, Tager A, et al: Expression of growth factors and oncogenes in normal and tumor-derived human mammary epithelial cells. Cancer Res 48:7041–7047, 1988.
16. Valverius EM, Bates SE, Stampfer MR, et al: Transforming growth factor α production and epidermal growth factor receptor expression in normal and oncogene transformed human mammary epithelial cells. Mol Endocrinol 3:203–214, 1989.
17. Brown CF, Teng CT, Pentecost BT, DiAugustine RP: Epidermal growth factor precursor in mouse lactating mammary gland alveolar cells. Mol Endocrinol 3:1077–1083, 1989.
18. Campbell PG, Skaar TC, Vega JR, Baumrucker CR: Secretion of insulin-like growth factor I (IGF-I) and IGF-binding proteins from bovine mammary tissue in vitro. J Endocrinol 128:219–228, 1991.
19. Daniel CW, Silberstein GB, VanHorn K, et al: TGF-β1–induced inhibition of mouse mammary ductal growth: Developmental specificity and characterization. Dev Biol 135:20–30, 1989.
20. Hwang P, Guyda H, Friesen HG: Purification of human prolactin. J Biol Chem 247:1955–1958, 1972.
21. Lewis UJ, Singh RNP, Seavey BK: Problems in the purification of human prolactin. In Boyns AR, Griffiths K (eds): Prolactin and Carcinogenesis. Cardiff, Wales, Alpha Omega Alpha, 1972, p 4.
22. Truong AT, Duez C, Belayeu A, et al: Isolation and characterization of the human prolactin gene. EMBO J 3:429–437, 1984.
23. Scheithauer BW, Sano T, Kovacs KT, et al: The pituitary gland in pregnancy: A clinicopathologic and immunohistochemical study of 69 cases. Mayo Clin Proc 65:461–474, 1990.
24. Goluboff LG, Ezrin L: Effect of pregnancy on the somatotroph and the prolactin cell of the human adenohypophysis. J Clin Endocrinol 29:1533–1538, 1969.
25. Frankenne F, Rentier-Delrue F, Scippo ML, et al: Expression of the growth hormone variant in human placenta. J Clin Endocrinol Metab 64:635–637, 1987.
26. Luthman M, Bremme K, Jonsdottir I, et al: Serum levels and molecular sizes of growth hormone during pregnancy in relation to levels of lactogens, insulin-like growth factor I and insulin-like growth factor binding protein-1. Gynecol Obstet Invest 31:67–73, 1991.
27. DiMattia GE, Gellersen B, Duckworth ML, Friesen HG: Human prolactin gene expression. The use of an alternative noncoding exon in decidua and the IM-9-P3 lymphoblast. J Biol Chem 265:16412–16421, 1990.
28. Tyson JE, Hwang P, Guyda H, et al: Studies of prolactin secretion in human pregnancy. Am J Obstet Gynecol 113:14–20, 1972.
29. Noel GL, Suh HK, Frantz AG: Prolactin release during nursing and breast stimulation in postpartum and non-postpartum subjects. J Clin Endocrinol Metab 38:413–423, 1974.
30. Battin DA, Marrs RP, Fleiss PM, Mishell DR: Effect of suckling on serum prolactin, luteinizing hormone, follicle-stimulating hormone, and estradiol during prolonged lactation. Obstet Gynecol 65:785–788, 1985.
31. Nunley WC, Urban RJ, Kitchin JD, et al: Dynamics of pulsatile prolactin release during the postpartum lactational period. J Clin Endocrinol Metab 72:287–293, 1991.
32. Kremer JAM, Borin G, Schellekens LA, et al: Pulsatile secretion of luteinizing hormone and prolactin in lactating and nonlactating women and the response to naltrexone. J Clin Endocrinol Metab 72:294–300, 1991.
33. Rowe RC, Cowden EA, Faiman C, Friesen HG: Correlation of Nb2 bioassay and radioimmunoassay values for human serum prolactin. J Clin Endocrinol Metab 57:942–946, 1983.
34. Leite V, Cosby H, Sobrinho LG, et al: Characterization of big-big prolactin in patients with hyperprolactinaemia. Clin Endocrinol 37:365–372, 1992.
35. Brun Del Re R, Del Pozo E, De Grandi P, et al: Prolactin inhibition and suppression of puerperal lactation by Br-ergocryptine (CB-154): A comparison with estrogen. Obstet Gynecol 41:884–890, 1973.
36. Aono T, Shioji T, Shoda T, Kurachi K: The initiation of human lactation and prolactin response to suckling. J Clin Endocrinol Metab 44:1101–1106, 1977.
37. Posner B, Khan MN, Bergeron JJM: Endocytosis of peptide hormones and other ligands. Endocr Rev 3:280–298, 1982.
38. Hughes JP, Elsholtz HP, Friesen HG: Growth hormone and prolactin receptors. In Posner B (ed): Polypeptide Hormone Receptors. New York, Marcel Dekker, 1985, pp 157–199.
39. Boutin JM, Edery M, Shirota M: Identification of a cDNA encoding a long form of prolactin receptor in human hepatoma and breast cancer cells. Mol Endocrinol 3:1455–1461, 1989.
40. Shirota M, Banville D, Ali S: Expression of two forms of prolactin receptor in rat ovary and liver. Mol Endocrinol 4:1136–1143, 1990.
41. Cosman D, Lyman SD, Idzerda RL, et al: A new cytokine receptor superfamily. Trends Biochem Sci 15:265–270, 1990.
42. Thoreau E, Petridou B, Kelly PA, et al: Structural symmetry of the extracellular domain of the cytokine growth hormone/prolactin receptor family and interferon receptors revealed by hydrophobic cluster analysis. FEBS Lett 282:26–31, 1991.

43. Kelly PA, Djiane J, Postel-Vinay M-C, Edery M: The prolactin growth hormone receptor family. Endocr Rev 12:235–251, 1991.
44. Djiane J, Houdebine LM, Kelly PA: Prolactin-like activity of anti-prolactin receptor antibodies in casein and DNA synthesis in the mammary gland. Proc Natl Acad Sci USA 78:7445–7448, 1981.
45. Djiane J, Dusanter-Fourt I, Katoh M, Kelly PA: Biological activities of binding site specific monoclonal antibodies to prolactin receptors of rabbit mammary gland. J Biol Chem 260:11430–11435, 1985.
46. Clapp C, Sears PS, Nicol CS: Binding studies with intact rat prolactin and a 16K fragment of the hormone. Endocrinology 125:1054–1059, 1989.
47. Ferrara N, Clapp C, Weiner R: The 16K fragment of prolactin specifically inhibits basal or fibroblast growth factor stimulated growth of capillary endothelial cells. Endocrinology 129:896–900, 1991.
48. Matusik RJ, Rosen JM: Prolactin induction of casein mRNA in organ culture. J Biol Chem 253:2343–2347, 1978.
49. Matusik RJ, Rosen JM: Prolactin regulation of casein gene expression: Possible mediators. Endocrinology 106:252–259, 1980.
50. Kleinberg DL, Todd J, Niemann W: Prolactin stimulation of α-lactalbumin in normal primate mammary gland. J Clin Endocrinol Metab 47:435–441, 1978.
51. Goodman GT, Akers RM, Friderici KH, Tucker HA: Hormonal regulation of α-lactalbumin secretion from bovine mammary tissue cultured in vitro. Endocrinology 112:1324–1330, 1983.
52. Delonis C, Denamur R: Induction of lactose synthesis by prolactin in rabbit mammary gland explants. J Endocrinol 52:311–319, 1972.
53. Forsyth IA, Strong CR, Dils R: Interaction of insulin, corticosterone and prolactin in promoting milk-fat synthesis by mammary explants from pregnant rabbits. Biochem J 129:929–935, 1972.
54. Rosen JM, Jones WK, Rodgers JR, et al: Regulatory sequences involved in the hormonal control of casein gene expression. Ann NY Acad Sci 464:87–99, 1986.
55. Tanaka T, Shiu RPC, Gout PN, et al: A new sensitive and specific bioassay for lactogenic hormones: Measurement of prolactin and growth hormone in human serum. J Clin Endocrinol 51:1058–1063, 1980.
56. Frankenne F, Closset J, Gomez F, et al: The physiology of growth hormones (GHs) in pregnant women and partial characterization of the placental GH variant. J Clin Endocrinol Metab 66:1171–1180, 1988.
57. MacLeod JN, Worsley I, Ray J, et al: Human growth hormone-variant is a biologically active somatogen and lactogen. Endocrinology 128:1298–1302, 1991.
58. Wurzel JM, Parks JS, Herd JE, Nielsen PV: Gene deletion is responsible for absence of immunoassayable human chorionic somatomammotropin. DNA 1:251–257, 1982.
59. Furlanetto RW, DiCarlo JN: Somatomedin C receptors and growth effects in human breast cells maintained in long term tissue culture. Cancer Res 44:2122–2128, 1984.
60. Myal Y, Shiu RPC, Bhaumick B, Bala M: Receptor binding and growth promoting activity of insulin-like growth factors in human breast cancer cells (T47D) in culture. Cancer Res 44:5486–5490, 1984.
61. Starkey RH, Orth DN: Radioimmunoassay of human epidermal growth factor (urogastrone). J Clin Endocrinol Metab 45:1144–1153, 1977.
62. Davis JW, Wikman-Coffelt J, Eddington CL: The effect of progesterone on biosynthetic pathways in mammary tissue. Endocrinology 91:1011–1019, 1972.
63. Budayr AA, Halloran BP, King JC, et al: High levels of parathyroid hormone-like protein in milk. Proc Natl Acad Sci USA 86:7183–7185, 1989.
64. Thiede MA: The mRNA encoding a parathyroid hormone-like peptide is produced in mammary tissue in response to elevations in serum prolactin. Mol Endocrinol 3:1443–1447, 1989.
65. Robinson CJ, Spanos E, James MF, et al: Role of prolactin in vitamin D metabolism and calcium absorption during lactation in the rat. J Endocrinol 94:443–453, 1982.
66. Brommage R, Jarmagin K, DeLuca HF: 1,25-Dihydroxyvitamin D$_3$ normalizes maternal food consumption and pup growth in rats. Am J Physiol 246E:227–231, 1984.
67. Caldeyro Barcia R: Milk ejection in women. In Reynolds M, Folley S (eds): Lactogenesis. Philadelphia, Oxford Press, 1969, pp 229–243.
68. Robyn C, Meuris S: Pituitary, prolactin, lactational performance and puerperal infertility. Semin Perinatol 6:254–264, 1982.
69. Short RV: Breast feeding. Sci Am 250:35–41, 1984.
70. McNeilly AS: Endocrine control of lactational infertility in women. In Labrie F, Proulx L (eds): Endocrinology. 1984 ICS Series. New York, Elsevier Science Publishers, 1984, pp 803.
71. Ishizuka B, Quigley ME, Yen SSC: Postpartum hypogonadotrophinism: Evidence for increased opioid inhibition. Clin Endocrinol 20:573–578, 1984.
72. Sheehan KL, Yen SSC: Activation of pituitary gonadotropic function by an agonist of luteinizing hormone–releasing factor in the puerperium. Am J Obstet Gynecol 135:755–758, 1979.
73. Hazum E: Neuroendocrine peptides in milk. Trends Endocrinol Metab 2:25–28, 1991.
74. Koldovsky O, Thornburg W: Hormones in milk. J Pediatr Gastroenterol Nutr 6:172–196, 1987.
75. Berseth CL: Enhancement of intestinal growth in neonatal rats by epidermal growth factor in milk. Am J Physiol 253:G662–G665, 1987.
76. Oppe TE, Redstone D: Calcium and phosphorus levels in healthy newborn infants given various types of milk. Lancet 1:1045–1048, 1968.
77. Baum D, Cooper L, Davies PA: Hypocalcaemic fits in neonates. Lancet 1:598, 1968.
78. Ellestad-Sayed J, Coodin FJ, Dilling LA, Haworth JC: Breast-feeding protects against infection in Indian infants. Can Med Assoc J 120:295–298, 1979.
79. Jelliffe DB: Unique properties of human milk (remarks on some recent developments). J Reprod Med 14:133–137, 1975.
80. Mushtaha AA, Schmalstieg FC, Hughes TK, et al: Chemokinetic agents for monocytes in human milk: Possible role of tumor necrosis factor-α. Pediatr Res 25:629–633, 1989.
81. Anderson GH: The effect of prematurity on milk composition and its physiological basis. Fed Proc 43:2438–2442, 1984.
82. Hall B: Changing composition of human milk and early development of an appetite control. Lancet 1:779–781, 1975.
83. American Academy of Pediatrics, Committee on Drugs: Transfer of drugs and other chemicals into human milk. Pediatrics 84:924–936, 1989.
84. Mennella JA, Beauchamp GK: The transfer of alcohol to human milk. Effects on flavor and the infant's behavior. N Engl J Med 325:981–985, 1991.
85. Fraser HM, Dewart PJ, Smith SK, et al: Luteinizing hormone releasing hormone agonist for contraception in breast feeding women. J Clin Endocrinol Metab 69:996–1002, 1989.
86. Kennedy KI, Visness CM: Contraceptive efficacy of lactational amenorrhoea. Lancet 339:227–230, 1992.
87. Perez A, Labbok M, Queenan JT: Clinical study of the lactational amenorrhoea method for family planning. Lancet 339:968–970, 1992.
88. Victora CG, Smith PG, Vaughan JP, et al: Evidence for protection by breast-feeding against infant deaths from infectious diseases in Brazil. Lancet 2:319–322, 1987.
89. Lucas A, Morley R, Cole TJ, et al: Breast milk and subsequent intelligence quotient in children born preterm. Lancet 339:261–264, 1992.
90. McTiernan A, Thomas DB: Evidence for a protective effect of lactation on risk of breast cancer in young women. Am J Epidemiol 124:353–358, 1986.
91. Byers T, Graham S, Rzepka T, Marshall J: Lactation and breast cancer, evidence for a negative association in premenopausal women. Am J Epidemiol 121:664–674, 1985.
92. Yuan J-M, Yu MC, Ross RK, et al: Risk factors for breast cancer in Chinese women in Shanghai. Cancer Res 48:1949–1953, 1988.
93. MacMahon B, Lin TM, Lowe CR, et al: Lactation and cancer of the breast: A summary of an international study. Bull WHO 42:185–194, 1970.
94. Kvale G, Hench I: Lactation and cancer risk: Is there a relation specific to breast cancer? J Epidemiol Community Health 42:30–37, 1987.
95. London SJ, Colditz, GA, Stampfer MJ, et al: Lactation and risk of breast cancer in a cohort of US women. Am J Epidemiol 132:17–26, 1990.
96. Aono T, Shioji T, Aki K, et al: Augmentation of puerperal lactation by oral administration of sulpirides. J Clin Endocrinol Metab 48:478–482, 1979.
97. Guzman V, Toscano G, Canales ES, Zarate A: Improvement of defective lactation by using oral metoclopramide. Acta Obstet Gynecol Scand 58:53–55, 1979.
98. Peters F, Schulze-Tollert J, Schuth W: Thyrotrophin-releasing hormone—a lactation promoting agent? Br J Obstet Gynaecol 98:880–885, 1991.
99. Luhman L: The effect of intranasal oxytocin on lactation. Obstet Gynecol 21:713–717, 1963.
100. Van-de-Perre P, Simonon A, Msellati P, et al: Postnatal transmission

of human immnodeficiency virus type I from mother to infant: A prospective cohort study in Kigali, Rwanda. N Engl J Med 325:593–598, 1991.

101. European Multicentre Study Group for Cabergoline in Lactation Inhibition: Single dose cabergoline versus bromocriptine in inhibition of puerperal lactation: Randomised, double blind multicentre study. Br Med J 302:1367–1371, 1991.
102. Van-Der Heijden PFM, Kremer JAM, Brownell J, Rolland R: Lactation inhibition by the dopamine agonist CV 205–502. Br J Obstet Gynaecol 98:270–276, 1991.
103. Kremer JAM, Rolland R, Van-Der Heijden PFM, et al: Lactation inhibition by a single injection of a new depot—bromocriptine. Br J Obstet Gynaecol 97:527–532, 1990.
104. Frantz A, Kleinberg DL, Noel G: Studies on prolactin in man. Recent Prog Horm Res 28:527–590, 1972.
105. Sobrinho LG, Sá-Melo P, Nunes MCP, et al: Sexual dysfunction in hyperprolactinaemic women. Effect of bromocriptine. J Psychosom Obstet Gynaecol 6:43–48, 1987.
106. Cowden EA, Ratcliffe WA, Beastall GH, Ratcliffe JG: Laboratory assessment of prolactin status. Ann Clin Biochem 16:113–121, 1979.
107. Friesen HG, Tolis G: The use of bromocriptine in the galactorrhea amenorrhea syndromes: The Canadian Cooperative Study. Clin Endocrinol 6(Suppl):91–99, 1977.

Fetal and Neonatal Endocrinology

DANIEL H. POLK
DELBERT A. FISHER

The intrauterine environment and fetal growth and development are conditioned and maintained by the interaction of a complex array of maternal, placental, and fetal hormones and endocrine systems. The placental hormones play a unique role in fetal metabolism or have been uniquely adapted to fetal metabolic needs. In addition, a variety of hormones and their metabolites are particularly prominent in the fetus. Some represent ontogeny recapitulating phylogeny, whereas others reflect pathways of hormone inactivation unique to or characteristic of the fetal environment. Finally, growth and development in the fetus are not mediated by hormones as in childhood. Rather, a complex interaction of growth factors, acting predominantly by autocrine and paracrine routes, appears to be largely responsible for the extraordinary rates of growth and differentiation characteristic of the mammalian fetus.

At parturition, the neonate is faced with the abrupt termination of placental support and rapid transition to the extrauterine environment, in which air breathing, circulatory adjustments, endogenous thermogenesis, free water conservation, and mobilization of energy substrates are required for survival. The adrenal cortex and the autonomic nervous system play key roles in neonatal transitional physiology, but other endocrine systems are required for optimal homeostasis. Understanding the fetal endocrine milieu and neonatal adaptations has contributed importantly to our improved management of premature infants, infants of diabetic mothers, infants with abnormal sexual differentiation, and infants with pituitary, thyroid, or parathyroid gland dysfunction. In addition, this understanding allows more effective diagnostic and therapeutic approaches to the fetus and its intrauterine milieu.

THE PLACENTAL ROLE IN ENDOCRINE HOMEOSTASIS

Fetal homeostasis is inextricably dependent on placental development and function. By the first week after conception in the human, the blastocyst consists of an inner cell mass destined to form the embryo and an outer trophoblast that implants into the maternal myometrium. In the ensuing several days, the trophoblast differentiates into two distinct layers. These consist of an inner cytotrophoblast layer and an outer, thicker layer of continuous cytoplasm, the syncytiotrophoblast, which serves as the early fetal-maternal interface. Interspecies differences in placental development allow for varied placental structure. Thus, while human placentation is hemomonochorial, with three tissue layers between maternal and fetal circulations (syncytiotrophoblast, fetal basement membrane, and fetal vascular endothelium), placentation in the rat is hemotrichorial, with four tissue layers separating maternal from fetal circulations (chorionic epithelium, syncytiotrophoblast, cytotrophoblast, and fetal vascular endothelium). Ovine placentation is characterized as epitheliochorional, with six tissue layers separating the circulations (maternal endothelium, connective tissue, endometrial syncytium, cytotrophoblast, fetal basement membrane, and vascular epithelium). These differences to some extent likely result in interspecies variation in placental permeability, which should be considered when extrapolating experimental results to human pregnancy. In the human, the syncytiotrophoblast is the major site of diffusion between the maternal venous lacunae and fetal capillaries. The syncytiotrophoblast also synthesizes large amounts of steroids and many diverse peptide hormones and, by the end of the first trimester, is the most active fetal (or maternal) endocrine organ.

Placental Transfer of Hormones

Transplacental transfer of molecules may occur via either extracellular or transcellular routes. The rate of extracellular transfer is proportional to the size and charge of intercellular channels, as well as the size (roughly correlated with molecular weight) and lipid solubility of the transferred molecule.[1, 2] Generally, the placenta is more permeable to lipid-soluble molecules, and this permeability is inversely correlated with molecular weight. Table 127–1 summarizes data regarding the transfer of a variety of hormones. These data are derived from a variety of human and animal models and, while interspecies differences are likely, are probably applicable in most cases to the human. As indicated, placental transfer decreases with increasing molecular mass, with an upper threshold in the range of 700 to 1200 Da. Larger hormones have no significant access to the fetal compartment.

Steroid Hormones

The placenta is permeable to adrenal corticosteroids. While no direct human measurements are available, studies in developing sheep and monkeys demonstrate a maternal-fetal transfer rate for cortisol of roughly 0.5 mg/d and a fetal-maternal cortisol transfer rate of nearly 1.5 mg/d.[3, 4] However, the placenta expresses an active 11β-hydroxysteroid dehydrogenase that facilitates conversion of most of the maternally derived cortisol to cortisone, resulting in a cortisol:cortisone ratio of less than 1 in near-term human placental tissue.[5] In the baboon, oxidation of cortisol by the utero-placental-decidual unit is seven-fold that of the reverse reaction. Aldosterone, progesterone, and androgenic or estrogenic steroids also cross the placenta.[6, 7] However, the quantity of transferred estrogen or progesterone is small in comparison with the amount of these hormones derived from placental synthesis.

Polypeptide Hormones

The relative size of most of the polypeptide hormones precludes much placental transfer. Extensive data indicate that the placenta is impermeable to hormones secreted from the anterior pituitary, including growth hormone, adrenocorticotropic hormone, gonadotropins, and thyrotropin.[8–12] Available evidence suggests that there is no transfer of the posterior pituitary hormones vasopressin and oxytocin.[13, 14] While the tripeptide thyrotropin-releasing hormone (TRH) does cross the human placenta, the other hypothalamic releasing factors do not.[15] The placenta is also impermeable to insulin, glucagon, parathyroid hormone, and calcitonin.[16–19] The absence of demonstrable plasma renin activity in the anephric fetus suggests little placental transfer.[20] Finally, placental cell membranes express a variety of receptors for the polypeptide hormones and growth factors, including the insulin-like growth factors (IGF-I and IGF-II) and epidermal growth factor (EGF). These receptors bind and, in some cases, degrade their respective ligands but do not facilitate placental transfer.[21]

Thyroid Hormones

Extensive data document that the placenta is relatively impermeable to thyroid hormones in the euthyroid state.[12, 22] While there is a gradient in maternal-fetal serum T_4 and free T_4 concentration which favors maternal to fetal transfer, this gradient is abolished by about 35 weeks' gestation. Fetal serum T_3 and free T_3 levels are lower than maternal values throughout gestation. Some placental transfer of radiolabeled T_4 occurs early in gestation; moreover, administration of large quantities of T_4 (1600 to 1800 μg) or T_3 (300 μg) to pregnant women near term demonstrates significant maternal to fetal transfer.[23, 24] This is likely due, in part, to placental expression of an inner ring monodeiodinase, which converts T_4 to the inactive metabolite $3,3',5'$-triiodothyronine (rT_3) and T_3 to inactive diiodothyronine.[25] In addition, the levels of T_4 in cord serum of athyrotic infants or in infants with a total inability to organify iodide are about half the maternal level, indicating a significant contribution of maternal thyroid hormone to circulating T_4 levels in the fetal hypothyroid state.[26] Maternal to fetal T_4 transfer also has been described in the pregnant rat, and this maternal transfer is associated with normalized brain T_3 levels when the fetal thyroid is chemically ablated.[27] Such data suggest that fetal brain development may rely in part on a maternal contribution of thyroid hormone, especially in the hypothyroid fetus.

Catecholamines

Epinephrine and norepinephrine do cross the placenta.[28] Maternal administration of norepinephrine results in a significant transient reflex fetal bradycardia, while maternal epinephrine infusion results in fetal tachycardia and hyperglycemia.[29, 30] Only about 50 per cent of the hormone crosses the placenta intact; the balance is degraded by placental catechol O-methyltransferase and monoamine oxi-

TABLE 127–1. PLACENTAL TRANSFER OF HORMONES

HORMONE	APPROXIMATE MOLECULAR SIZE (Da)	TRANSFER
Catecholamines	180	Yes
Melatonin	230	Yes
Steroid hormones	350	Yes
Vitamin D	350	Yes
Thyrotropin-releasing hormone	360	Yes
Thyroid hormones	800	Limited
Oxytocin	1000	No
Vasopressin	1100	No
Luteinizing hormone–releasing hormone	1200	Yes
Calcitonin	3400	No
Glucagon	3600	No
Corticotropin	4500	No
Corticotropin-releasing hormone	4800	No
Insulin	6000	No
Parathyroid hormone	9000	No
Growth hormone	22,000	No
Thyrotropin	27,000	No
Luteinizing hormone	30,000	No
Renin	40,000	No

dase.[31] The catecholamine metabolites normetanephrine, metanephrine, dihydroxymandelic acid, and vanillylmandelic acid are demonstrable in placental homogenates.[28]

Placental Production of Hormones

The human placenta subserves an important endocrine role during fetal development. It is the major source of estrogens and progesterone during pregnancy, synthesizes several polypeptide hormones which are either similar or identical to those secreted from the anterior pituitary, and is also a source of many of the hypothalamic neuropeptides. These diverse hormones are secreted into both the maternal and the fetal circulations. We are just beginning to understand the roles which these substances play during development, but their contribution to the unique endocrine environment is substantial.

Steroid Hormones

PLACENTAL ESTROGEN PRODUCTION. Estrogen production in nonpregnant women is less than 1 mg/d. The human placenta near term, however, secretes large amounts of estrogens, including estrone, estradiol, and estriol. Daily secretion of these steroids approximates 2, 1, and 30 to 40 mg, respectively.[32] Placental estrogen production relies on precursors derived from the fetal adrenal gland, a process characterized as the human fetoplacental unit.[33] The process of placental estrogen synthesis is summarized in Figure 127–1. The major substrates for placental estrogen synthesis are dihydroepiandrosterone (DHEA) and androstenedione. These biologically inactive adrenal steroids are derived from both fetal and maternal adrenal sources. The fetal zone of the adrenal cortex is deficient in 3β-hydroxysteroid dehydrogenase (3β-HSD) and $\Delta^{4,5}$-isomerase activities, but it has high steroid sulfokinase activity.[32–34] Thus the conversion of pregnenolone to progesterone is limited in this tissue, and the major secretory product of fetal adrenal steroidogenesis is DHEA sulfate (DHEAS), which is transported to the liver for 16-hydroxylation. The placenta is deficient in 17-hydroxylase activity but sufficient in 3β-HSD and sulfatase activities and also expresses an aromatase that converts androstenedione and testosterone to estrone and estradiol, respectively.[32, 34] DHEAS and 16-OH-DHEAS are hydrolyzed in the placenta by steroid sulfatase; DHEA serves as a substrate for placental estrone and estradiol biosynthesis, while 16-OH-DHEA is the major substrate for placental estriol synthesis. Placental estrogen biosynthesis is a function of placental mass and the provision of steroid precursors by the fetal adrenal gland.

Most of the placentally derived estrogen is secreted into the maternal circulation, but fetal concentrations and levels in amniotic fluid are also quite high. The physiological significance of the large amounts of placental estrogen produced during pregnancy remains somewhat obscure for both the mother and the fetus. Estrogens stimulate uterine and mammary growth and have other metabolic effects in the mother. Estriol is a relatively weak estrogen in many biological systems and may have a unique role in the maintenance of uteroplacental blood flow. However, estrogen production and circulating estrogen levels (especially estriol) are markedly reduced in pregnancies in which the fetus (including the placenta) has an X-linked steroid sulfatase deficiency. In these infants, the placenta is unable to convert DHEAS to free DHEA for estrogen biosynthesis. Only about 10 per cent of normal estrogen biosynthesis continues in such pregnancies, relying on maternal DHEA and androstenedione as substrates. Although parturition may be somewhat delayed, the pregnancy proceeds normally and the fetus seems to be otherwise normal.[35]

PLACENTAL PROGESTERONE PRODUCTION. During normal pregnancy, there is a marked and progressive increase in progesterone production.[32, 34, 36] The maternal corpus luteum is the major source of plasma progesterone during the first 5 to 6 weeks of gestation; after 12 weeks, the placenta is the major source. The principal substrate for placental progesterone synthesis is circulating maternal low-density lipoprotein (LDL) cholesterol; de novo placental synthesis of cholesterol from acetate is limited.[32, 34] Placental progesterone production occurs largely independent of the maternal pituitary or adrenal glands, and fetal death in utero has little acute effect on maternal progesterone levels. Placental progesterone production is regulated by the number of LDL receptors and thus placental mass.[32, 34] There is evidence that estrogens may stimulate placental progesterone production via effects on placental LDL receptors and the conversion of cholesterol to pregnenolone. Estrogens also have a negative-feedback effect on adrenal DHEA production. Human chorionic gonadotropin (hCG) and the insulin-like growth factors also may have a role in autoregulation of progesterone synthesis.[32, 34]

The production of progesterone approximates 200 mg/d during the third trimester, a value some 10-fold higher than that during the midluteal phase of the normal menstrual cycle; 90 per cent of this amount is secreted into the maternal circulation. Progesterone acts on the uterine musculature to maintain a state of quiescence and may inhibit maternal cell-mediated immune responses to foreign (fetal) antigens.[37] Despite the predominant secretion of progesterone into the maternal circulation, fetal blood progesterone levels are two- to three-fold higher than maternal values because of a lower metabolic clearance of progesterone in the fetus.[32, 34] The significance of this progesterone to fetal homeostasis is not clear.

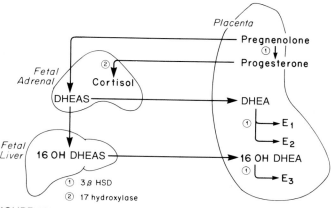

FIGURE 127–1. Estrogen production by the fetal-placental unit (see text for details). (DHAS, dihydroepiandrosterone; E_1, estrone; E_2, estradiol; E_3, estriol.)

Polypeptide Hormones

The placenta produces several pituitary-like hormones. The most abundant are hCG and human placental lactogen (hPL, also called *human chorionic somatomammotropin*, hCS).[38] Placental hCG is a glycoprotein of 36 to 40 kDa with structural, biological, and immunological similarities to the pituitary gonadotropins and thyrotropin (TSH). Placental hPL is a 191-amino acid protein with 96 per cent amino acid homology to human pituitary growth hormone (GH). It has 3 per cent or less of the growth-promoting bioactivity of GH and equivalent prolactin (PRL)–like effects. Placental hCG is secreted predominantly during the first half of gestation and hPL during the second half. The control of placental synthesis and secretion of these peptide hormones is not well understood. Hormone secretion is related to placental mass and continues for some time in the event of a fetal demise. Chorionic luteinizing hormone–releasing hormone (LHRH), also called *gonadotropin-releasing hormone* (GnRH), may have a paracrine role in modulating hCG production.[39, 40] In addition, glucocorticoids and cAMP increase hCG production by placental cells in vitro; progesterone decreased hCG production in some studies.[41, 42]

The probable roles of hCG are the maintenance of the corpus luteum during the early part of pregnancy, stimulation of the fetal testes to produce androgens, and stimulation of placental progesterone production.[43] Placental hCG has TSH-like activity, but this activity is weak (less than 0.5 μU of TSH per unit of hCG), and hCG produces minimal changes in maternal thyroid function during normal pregnancy. Placental lactogen has weak GH-like and PRL-like bioactivities and has been proposed to exert an anti-insulin effect on maternal carbohydrate and lipid metabolism. This effect would tend to increase maternal glucose and amino acid levels, thus augmenting maternal to fetal substrate flow.[36] In addition, hPL appears to be an important stimulus of fetal growth.

The placenta also may produce a separate chorionic TSH. Pregnant women demonstrate significant levels of a circulating substance which immunoreacts with antibodies raised to bovine TSH.[44] Complete characterization and the physiological significance of this TSH, however, remain unclear; most of the thyrotropic activity in placental tissue and that in maternal plasma during pregnancy are attributable to the inherent TSH bioactivity of hCG.[45]

The human placenta synthesizes a proopiomelanocortin (POMC) and a material similar to corticotropin (ACTH) referred to as *human chorionic corticotropin* (hCC).[46, 47] Cleavage products of placental POMC, including β-endorphin, α-melanocyte-stimulating hormone (α-MSH), and α- and β-lipotropin, have been isolated from placental tissue extracts.[48] These peptides have been localized to the syncytiotrophoblast.[49] The control of hCC production is not understood, but corticotropin-releasing hormone (CRH) is also produced by the placenta, and CRH has been observed to stimulate hCC production from perfused human placental fragments, supporting a possible paracrine role for placental CRH in modulating placental hCC production.[48] Glucocorticoids and oxytocin stimulate placental POMC release while having an opposite or no effect on the pituitary release of ACTH.[48, 50] β-Endorphin and α-MSH are released from placental tissue in larger amounts than ACTH, suggesting that control of placental POMC production and

processing differs from that in the anterior pituitary. The significant increases in plasma levels of POMC-derived peptides in pregnant women and the resistance of maternal plasma ACTH to glucocorticoid suppression in pregnancy suggest that the placenta may be involved in regulation of the maternal pituitary-adrenal axis during pregnancy.[49–51]

Renin activity is present in homogenates and in cultured explants of placenta and has been localized to chorionic tissue by immunohistochemistry.[52] The amino acid composition and NH_2-terminal sequence of chorionic renin are identical to those of kidney renin. Renin mRNA has been demonstrated in the chorion throughout pregnancy with no mRNA detectable in decidua, amnion, or myometrium.[52, 53] Placental renin mRNA concentrations at term are about 10 per cent of kidney levels, and the total placental renin mRNA level approximates 20 per cent of kidney content. Angiotensinogen mRNA has not been detected in placenta.[53]

Placental renin probably influences the production of fetal angiotensin II and may have a role in fetal skin and carcass growth. Functional angiotensin II receptors are present in skeletal muscle and connective tissue of the late-gestation rat embryo.[54] In fetal skin fibroblasts these receptors are coupled with membrane phospholipid turnover and mediate increases in cellular inositol phosphate and cytosolic calcium concentrations. Moreover, injection of angiotensin II into 18-day-old rat fetuses increases amino acid incorporation into skin protein.

The sheep placenta produces a parathyroid hormone (PTH)–like protein that is similar in composition and bioactivity to the PTH-related peptide produced by tumors associated with hypercalcemia.[55] Bioactivity of the partially purified sheep placental PTH-like protein is inhibited by antisera against synthetic human PTH-related peptide (PTHrP). However, antisera that neutralize bovine PTH bioactivity have no effect on the ovine PTH-like bioactivity. The ovine placental PTH-like bioactivity is highest during midgestation. Similar material is present in fetal and maternal ovine parathyroid glands. Calcitonin (CT) mRNA is also present in the rat placenta, in association with a CT-like immunoreactivity.[56] The significance of these proteins is discussed later in the section describing the fetal PTH-CT system.

Neuropeptides

The human placenta contains and produces LHRH, thyrotropin-releasing hormone (TRH), somatostatin (SRIF, somatotropin release inhibitory factor), CRH, growth hormone-releasing hormone (GHRH), and oxytocin (OT). Chorionic LHRH has not been purified, but by high-performance liquid chromatography (HPLC) analysis, chorionic LHRH is similar to or identical with synthetic hypothalamic LHRH; LHRH mRNA is present in placental tissue.[57] The structure of chorionic LHRH predicted from human placental cloned cDNA is identical with that of the hypothalamic peptide.[58] LHRH is produced in the cytotrophoblast and can bind to receptors in the syncytiotrophoblast. The placental LHRH receptor has lower affinity and less selectivity for LHRH analogues than the pituitary receptor. Because synthetic LHRH increases in vitro production of hCG, and perhaps progesterone, estrone, estradiol, and estriol from placental explants, endogenous chorionic LHRH may have a paracrine role in the regulation of placental hCG and steroid hormone production.

Placental TRH immunoreactivity has not been completely characterized, nor has its site of production been identified. In most studies its immunoreactivity and chromatographic characteristics are similar to those of synthetic TRH, and bioactivity has been demonstrated.[59] Sheep placental TRH has immunological identity with synthetic TRH and coelutes with synthetic TRH by HPLC.[60] A single 1.6-kilobase TRH mRNA is expressed in both ovine placental and hypothalamic tissue. Placental TRH peptide levels vary with the thyroid status of the fetus, increasing with hypothyroidism and decreasing after administration of T_3 to the fetus.[60] These data suggest that regulation of placental TRH gene transcription, at least in the ovine species, resembles that for hypothalamic TRH.

Immunoreactive chorionic somatostatin, like LHRH, is localized in the cytotrophoblast.[61] The observations that the somatostatin-containing cells in the placenta disappear as pregnancy progresses and that hPL production increases progressively during the second half of gestation led to the speculation that chorionic somatostatin may exert negative paracrine control on production of hPL by the syncytiotrophoblast. No data for or against this hypothesis are available.

Immunoreactive CRH and CRH mRNA have been identified in human placental extracts.[62, 63] CRH immunoreactivity is also detectable in third-trimester human pregnancy plasma but not in plasma of pregnant women during the first or second trimesters; immunoreactivity disappears postpartum.[63, 64] The lack of correlation of maternal plasma ACTH or cortisol and CRH levels has suggested that placental CRH is not primarily involved in maternal pituitary ACTH regulation. However, maternal CRH levels are strongly correlated with gestational age, which suggests a relationship to placental function. Moreover, studies with the baboon (which resembles the human with regard to CRH metabolism during pregnancy) have shown a blunted maternal pituitary ACTH response to CRH after CRH infusion.[65] These studies were interpreted to support a role of placental CRH in modulating maternal pituitary and adrenal function during pregnancy. In contrast to the negative-feedback effect of glucocorticoid on hypothalamic CRH production, glucocorticoid stimulates placental CRH mRNA and CRH production.[50] This observation and the parallel increases in placental CRH and CRH mRNA concentrations during the last 5 weeks of pregnancy suggest that the increase in fetal glucocorticoid production near term may stimulate placental CRH and POMC production, thus further augmenting prenatal fetal cortisol production. A role for placental CRH has been implicated in the pathogenesis of preterm labor.

Immunoreactive GHRH and biologically active GHRH are present in rat placenta.[66] Two forms of GHRH activity were identified by HPLC: one eluting identically with synthetic GHRH and one similar to the methionine sulfoxide analogue. By analogy with other placental releasing factors, chorionic GHRH may be involved in paracrine control of hPL or placental GH production. Plasma GHRH levels, like CRH concentrations, are elevated during the third trimester of human gestation, correlate with gestational age and hPL concentrations, and become undetectable 3 days postpartum.[67]

Finally, immunoreactive oxytocin (OT) has been identi-

fied in human, primate, and rodent placenta.[68-70] An OT mRNA of 0.66 kilobase has been isolated from rat placenta. While this transcript is smaller than that expressed in rat hypothalamus, the difference is due to dissimilar polyadenylated tail lengths.[70] HPLC analysis of rat placental extracts demonstrates two immunoreactive peaks which coincide with synthetic OT and an OT-neurophysin complex similar to that previously described for the bovine ovary. The physiological role for placental OT, like most of the other placental neuropeptides, remains uncertain. Placental OT effects on prostacyclin synthesis, as well as a paracrine effect on placental POMC synthesis, have been postulated.

FETAL ENDOCRINE SYSTEMS

General

Hormone systems can be classified into two major groups, as shown in Table 127-2. The neuroendocrine hormone systems transduce or convert neural into endocrine information. Three such mechanisms have been identified: (1) the hypothalamic–anterior pituitary system, (2) the hypothalamic–posterior pituitary system, and (3) the autonomic nervous system. The insulin-glucagon and parathyroid hormone–calcitonin systems function as autonomous endocrine systems. In these systems, hormone secretion is largely regulated by local feedback mechanisms. During fetal life, neither the neuroendocrine transducer systems nor the autonomous endocrine systems seem to be of vital importance to survival or growth. Certain aspects of fetal metabolism may be influenced, however, by fetal or placental hormones, and fetal pituitary–target organ function (particularly the adrenal glands and gonads) may be pituitary trophic hormone–dependent.

The events of parturition abruptly terminate this period of dependent development and precipitate a series of profound metabolic stresses. As indicated earlier, extrauterine survival requires autonomous thermogenesis and alimentation, as well as autonomous respiratory and excretory activities, and these activities are largely dependent on the functional state of the endocrine systems. The neuroendocrine transducer systems appear to be well developed at birth and function smoothly to defend against the stresses of extrauterine exposure. The autonomous endocrine systems regulating blood sugar and calcium levels, however, are relatively less mature and/or are suppressed in utero. Thus abnormalities related to homeostasis of blood sugar and serum calcium concentrations are relatively frequent in the early neonatal period.

TABLE 127-2. TYPES OF FETAL ENDOCRINE SYSTEMS

Neuroendocrine hormone systems
    Hypothalamus–anterior pituitary–target organs
    Hypothalamus–posterior pituitary
    Sympathetic nervous system
Autonomous endocrine systems
    Endocrine pancreas (insulin-glucagon)
    Parathyroid gland–thyroid C cells (parathyroid hormone-calcitonin)

TABLE 127–3. HUMAN FETAL PITUITARY HORMONE CONTENT

GESTATIONAL AGE (WEEKS)	MEAN PITUITARY WEIGHT (mg)	GH (ng)	PRL (ng)	LG (ng)		FSH (ng)		TSH (mU)	ACTH (mU)	AVP (mU)	OXYTOCIN (mU)
				M	F	M	F				
10–14	3.4	0.44	4.1	21	88	1.8	7.4	0.21	—	0.07	—
15–19	6.7	9.2	14.8	165	797	13	316	0.69	496	0.25	12
20–24	16.0	59.4	405	490	3940	51	3726	3.3	—	1.0	33
25–29	36.4	256	542	1222	4983	149	5789	—	—	1.5	110
30–34	49.7	578	872	—	2353	—	2010	1.1	—	—	—
35–40	99.1	675	2039	1590	—	361	—	—	—	4.65	250

Numbers reported as mean values.
M, male; F, female.

Neuroendocrine Transducer Systems

Anterior Pituitary Systems

DEVELOPMENT. The human fetal forebrain begins to differentiate by 3 weeks of gestation.[71, 72] The hypothalamus is identifiable by 7 weeks above the bony floor of the sella turcica. Rathke's pouch, the buccal component of the anterior pituitary gland, has developed by 5 weeks and migrates cephalad as the pituitary stalk grows caudally from the hypothalamus. By 11 to 12 weeks of gestation, Rathke's pouch is obliterated by the developing sphenoid bone, and the pituitary gland becomes partially encapsulated within the sella turcica. Intact pituitary-portal blood vessels are present by 12 to 17 weeks. Maturation and function of the pituitary-portal system continue through 30 to 35 weeks of gestation. There is a parallel development of the hypothalamic nuclei, and the median eminence and supraoptic tract are identifiable by 20 to 21 weeks. Thus by midgestation the fetal hypothalamic–anterior pituitary complex is well differentiated anatomically.[71, 72]

By 8 to 10 weeks of gestation, the fetal hypothalamus contains significant concentrations of releasing hormones.[22, 73–79] Secretory granules have been identified within anterior pituitary cells by 10 to 12 weeks. In addition, GH, follicle-stimulating hormone (FSH), luteinizing hormone (LH), TSH, ACTH, PRL, OT, vasotocin (AVT), and vasopressin (VP) can be identified in significant concentrations in pituitary tissue at this time. Table 127–3 summarizes changes in hormone content in the pituitary gland throughout gestation. Changes in pituitary serum hormone concentrations during gestation are summarized in Table 127–4. Hormone concentrations within the pituitary increase progressively, whereas concentrations in fetal serum tend to peak near midgestation and decrease progressively toward term.

It has been postulated that anterior pituitary hormone synthesis and secretion are low in the first-trimester fetus. During the second trimester, maturation of the hypothalamus and pituitary–portal vascular system occurs, and an unrestrained release of hypothalamic hormones has been postulated to account for the high fetal circulating levels of anterior pituitary hormones.[22, 73, 74] However, placental and/or fetal extrahypothalamic production of releasing hormones also may influence release of anterior pituitary hormones during development.

During the third trimester, anterior pituitary hormone secretion is progressively modulated. In part this is due to maturation of negative-feedback control systems. In addition, there seems to be a progressive maturation of inhibitory electrical activity in the neocortex during the latter half of gestation.[73, 74] The low levels of serum GH and TSH in the anencephalic infant support the view that anterior pituitary hormone secretion is dependent on an intact hypothalamus. The late increase in fetal serum PRL concentrations (see Table 127–4) does not seem to be dependent on hypothalamic function, since serum PRL concentrations in cord blood of normal and anencephalic infants are similar.[4] Rather, the increase in fetal serum PRL has been postulated to be due to the progressive increase in maternal and/or fetal estrogen levels. However, incomplete integration of hypothalamic mechanisms may contribute.[74] There is considerable indirect evidence that negative-feedback control of TSH, ACTH, FSH, and LH secretion develops during the last half of gestation.[22, 73, 74] The control systems for TSH and ACTH secretion seem to be mature or largely so at birth. However, the neuroendocrine control systems for GH, FSH, and LH continue to mature during the early weeks, months, and years of extrauterine life.

PITUITARY-ADRENAL AXIS. During the third week of gestation, the bilateral adrenal primordia are discernible cephalad to the developing mesonephros. By the eighth week of gestation, adrenal differentiation has proceeded to a stage in which two distinct zones of developing adrenal cortex are distinguishable: an inner fetal zone which comprises most of the glandular cortex and a subcapsular rim of immature cells known as the outer or definitive zone. Adrenal growth is rapid; adrenal cortical mass at term averages 8 g, and the fetal zone accounts for nearly 80 per cent.[32, 34, 80] The regulation of fetal adrenal growth is complex and dependent on a variety of fetal pituitary and placental factors. In addition, growth factors acting via paracrine and autocrine routes are probably also involved. The major stimulus to fetal adrenal function is fetal pituitary ACTH. While placental hCG may support early growth, the involution of the adrenal which occurs after 15 weeks in the anencephalic fetus suggests the crucial role of pituitary-derived factors.[81] Moreover, other pituitary peptides, including β-endorphin, β-lipotropin, α-MSH, and corticotropin-like intermediate peptide, have little adrenocorticotropic effect.[82] In the midgestation fetus, plasma ACTH levels average 55 pmol/L, and while concentrations decline toward birth, fetal ACTH levels exceed those later in life.

The control of fetal ACTH secretion, in turn, is complex. Circulating CRH levels are elevated in the fetus and likely result from both hypothalamic and ectopic (placental) sources.[63, 64, 83] Arginine vasopressin (AVP) and catecholamines are also significant stimuli for fetal ACTH secretion.[84, 85] Finally, epidermal growth factor (EGF) has been shown to stimulate ACTH release in vivo in the late gestation ovine fetus.[86] The relative physiological importance of these various ACTH secretogogous is unknown. Maternal levels of CRH are also elevated in the latter half of gestation and continue to rise until term. This observation may account for the relative lack of suppression of ACTH secretion (by cortisol) in the pregnant female near term. Feedback control of fetal ACTH release is not well characterized in the human. While exogenous dexamethasone administered in pharmacological doses to term infants is associated with short-term pituitary-adrenal suppression, a similar phenomenon is not noted in the fetus.[87, 88] This may be due, in part, to altered pituitary glucocorticosteroid receptor binding characteristics of the fetus.[89]

The fetal adrenal expresses the same five steroidogenic apoenzymes as the adult gland: two mitochondrial cytochrome P450 enzymes for cholesterol side-chain cleavage (P450$_{SCC}$) and C11/C18 hydroxylation of the parent steroid structure (P450$_{C11/C18}$) and two microsomal enzymes with 17-hydroxylase and 17,20-desmolase (P450$_{C17}$) and 21-hydroxylase (P450$_{C21}$) activities. A fifth enzyme, expressed by the smooth endoplasmic reticulum, exhibits both 3β-HSD and Δ^{4,5}-isomerase activities. However, there are quantitative differences in the relative activities of these enzymes between cells derived from the fetal versus definitive zones of the adrenal cortex: little 3β-HSD is expressed in the fetal zone.[32, 80] The fetal zone also expresses relatively high steroid sulfotransferase activities. Thus the major steroid products of the fetal adrenal are DHEA, DHEAS, pregnenolone sulfate, and several Δ^5-3β-hydroxysteroids. Limited amounts of the Δ^5-3-ketosteroids (such as cortisol or aldosterone) are produced by the fetal zone of the adrenal cortex.[32, 90] Cholesterol, the major substrate for fetal adrenal steroidogenesis, is derived from circulating LDL cholesterol, primarily of hepatic origin. Some de novo adrenal synthesis also occurs.[91, 92]

As discussed earlier (see section on placental hormone production and Fig. 127–1), the major fetal adrenal secretory product is DHEA, which is converted to 16-OH-DHEAS by the fetal adrenal and liver and serves largely as a precursor for placental estrogen production. About two thirds of the circulating cortisol in the fetus is derived autonomously from fetal adrenal gland synthesis; the remainder results from transplacental transfer. Fetal cortisol is rapidly metabolized to inactive cortisone via an 11β-hydroxysteroid dehydrogenase expressed in a variety of fe-

tal tissues, resulting in circulating fetal cortisone levels that are four- to five-fold higher than cortisol concentrations. As term approaches, selected fetal tissues express increased levels of 11-ketosteroid reductase activity and are thus able to convert cortisone to cortisol locally. Glucocorticoid receptors are present in responsive tissues at birth; significant glucocorticoid receptor activities are present at midgestation in a variety of fetal tissues including placenta, brain, liver, lung, and gut.[93, 94] Cortisol serves as an important maturational stimulus to facilitate the fetal transition to extrauterine homeostasis. Increases in circulating and local cortisol concentrations over the final 10 weeks of gestation lead to maturation of a variety of key effector systems, including the thyroid gland, sympathoadrenal activity, cardiovascular and pulmonary adaptation, hepatic glycogenolysis and gluconeogenesis, and alterations in renal blood flow and renal tubular function.[95, 96] Finally, the preparturient rise in cortisol has been implicated as a critical event in the onset of labor in a variety of mammalian species.[34] The link between prenatal increases in cortisol and birth in the human is less distinct.

The human fetal adrenal gland is capable of aldosterone secretion near term; cord plasma levels of aldosterone exceed maternal levels three- to five-fold.[80] This increased secretion of aldosterone continues throughout the first year of life.[97] Fetal aldosterone secretion is low in midgestation and is relatively unresponsive to changes in plasma renin or angiotensin.[98] In the developing ovine fetus, furosemide stimulates plasma renin without much effect on aldosterone secretion. Aldosterone influences renal sodium excretion during the perinatal period.[80, 98] Relatively reduced glomerular filtration rates in the newborn limit sodium loss, but by 1 week of age, salt loss due to aldosterone deficiency produces clinically significant hyponatremia, hyperkalemia, and intravascular volume depletion.

PITUITARY-GONADAL AXIS. Male differentiation of the primitive gonads begins at 7 weeks of gestation when interstitium and germ cell–containing testicular cords are identifiable.[99, 100] Leydig cells are visible during the eighth week and are capable of androgen biosynthesis at that time. By 14 weeks, the fetal testicular mass approximates 20 mg, increasing to 800 mg at term. Female differentiation also begins during the seventh week with appearance of interstitium and medullary cords containing the oogonia. Primitive granulosa cells are visible by 12 weeks.[99, 100] With further maturation many oogonia degenerate, whereas those surviving undergo the first meiotic division to become primary oocytes. Primordial follicles can be identified at 5 months, and primary follicles, with their

TABLE 127–4. HORMONE CONCENTRATIONS IN HUMAN FETAL SERUM

GESTATIONAL AGE (WEEKS)	GH (μg/ml)	PRL (μg/ml)	LH (μg/ml) M	LH (μg/ml) F	FSH (μg/L) M	FSH (μg/L) F	TSH (mU/L)	ACTH (pmol/L)
10–14	65	25	—	—	10	15	—	—
15–19	115	17	—	12	—	—	2.4	54.8
20–24	132	—	7	—	17	24	—	—
25–29	54	18	—	—	—	—	9.6	—
30–34	43	208	—	—	—	—	—	—
35–40	35	268	ND*	ND*	1.8	1.8	8.9	31.4

Numbers reported as mean values.
*ND, not detected.

thecal cell investment, are present by 7 months. The combined ovarian tissue mass approximates 30 mg at 14 weeks and 600 to 700 mg at birth.

In the male fetus there is an increase in testicular testosterone production between 10 and 20 weeks, stimulated by the high levels of circulating placental hCG.[99, 100] Fetal pituitary LH may contribute to the fetal Leydig cell stimulation, but the predominant gonadotropic effect at this time is hCG. Fetal testosterone stimulates male sexual differentiation of the primitive mesonephric ducts (to form the ductus deferens, epididymis, seminal vesicles, and ejaculatory ducts) and masculinizes the urogenital sinus and external genitalia (to form the prostate gland, phallus, and penile urethra). Enzymatic conversion of testosterone to dihydrotestosterone is necessary for male differentiation of the urogenital sinus and external genitalia.[99, 100]

The fetal testes, in addition to testosterone, synthesize a müllerian-inhibiting substance (MIS), which dedifferentiates the primitive müllerian duct system.[101–103] MIS, a glycoprotein approximately 72 kDa in size, is produced by Sertoli cells; the hormone reaches the müllerian duct cells via local diffusion. Production continues throughout gestation, is maximal at the time of müllerian duct regression, and then decreases after birth. MIS also may facilitate testicular descent into the scrotum.[101, 102] In the female fetus, müllerian duct differentiation proceeds in the absence of MIS, and the primitive mesonephric duct system dedifferentiates in the absence of testosterone. In the absence of dihydrotestosterone, the urogenital sinus and external genitalia differentiate to the female phenotype.

Thus placental hCG and, to a lesser extent, fetal pituitary LH evoke male sexual differentiation in the XY genetic male via stimulation of the differentiating testes to produce testosterone. MIS also plays a role, but the factors stimulating its production are not clear. There is evidence that MIS production may be modulated by FSH and testosterone.[102] Sexual differentiation in the XX genetic female occurs normally in the absence of testicular hormones. Gonadal hormones in the fetus also determine sexual differentiation of the developing brain and hypothalamus.[104–106] The female hypothalamus is programmed for the pulsatile release of gonadotropin-stimulating hormone and for feedback modulation of the gonadotropic hormone secretion profiles that allow for cyclic ovarian function postpubertally. Testosterone administration during this crucial programming period inhibits this cyclic response.[104] However, the mechanisms for sexual hypothalamic dimorphic differentiation of the fetus remain unclear.[105]

PITUITARY-THYROID AXIS. Development of fetal pituitary-thyroid function is discussed in detail in Chapter 47. A brief overview of this process is presented here. The fetal thyroid gland develops from contributions of two anlagen: a midline thickening of the pharyngeal floor (median anlage) and paired caudal extensions derived from the fourth branchial pouch. These structures, discernible by day 17 of human gestation, fuse and migrate caudally over the next month of development, such that by day 50 of gestation the thyroid gland has lost its connection to the posterior pharynx and has assumed its definitive position in the anterior neck. By 10 weeks of gestation, colloid formation is demonstrable, and by 12 weeks the gland weighs about 80 mg. At term gestation, the gland weighs about 2 g.[107] Pituitary and plasma TSH concentrations increase during the second trimester in the human fetus, coincident with the

development of the pituitary portal circulation. Plasma total T_4 concentrations increase progressively from low levels at 16 weeks of gestation to plateau by 36 to 38 weeks of gestation at about 130 nmol/L. While plasma levels of thyroxine-binding globulin also increase concurrently with the increases in T_4 secretion, circulating free T_4 levels also increase progressively due to maturation of thyroidal hormone production.[25] These increases in circulating T_4 and TSH levels represent a progressive maturation of feed-forward hypothalamic control of TSH secretion, as well as feedback inhibitory effects of thyroid hormones on TSH release. The TSH response to TRH is clearly present early in the third trimester, while T_4 feedback inhibition develops progressively during this period.

In contrast to T_4, fetal serum T_3 levels remain low until the final weeks of gestation. Plasma T_3 levels are less than 0.2 nmol/L before 30 weeks of gestation and then increase slowly to levels averaging 0.7 nmol/L at term. The disparity between circulating T_4 and T_3 levels is largely due to low peripheral conversion of T_4 to T_3.[25, 107] Several different monodeiodinases catalyze the deiodination of T_4 to the triiodothyronines.[25] T_4 can be monodeiodinated to either 3′,3,5-triiodothyronine (T_3) or 3,3′,5′-triiodothyronine (reverse T_3, rT_3). Only T_3 demonstrates biological activity due to the stereospecificity of the T_3 receptor. Deiodination of the outer (phenolic) ring of T_4 is catalyzed by either of two 5′-monodeiodinases, which differ in several important respects. Type I outer ring monodeiodinase (MDI) is principally expressed in the adult by hepatic and renal tissues, while type II outer ring MDI is expressed in brain, pituitary, and brown adipose tissues. The type I MDI has a high capacity for T_4, is inhibited by propylthiouracil (PTU), and its expression is stimulated by T_4; type II MDI has a low capacity for T_4 conversion, is relatively insensitive to PTU, and its expression is inhibited by T_4. A third enzyme (type III MDI) catalyzes the deiodination of the inner (tyrosyl) ring of T_4 to produce inactive rT_3. In the adult, most of the circulating T_4 is deiodinated by the type I MDI to provide circulating T_3. Type II MDI functions principally to provide local T_3 in brain and brown adipose tissues.[25, 107]

Fetal thyroid hormone metabolism is characterized by low levels of type I MDI activity and high levels of type III MDI activity, principally expressed in placental as well as a variety of other fetal tissues. Thus, in the fetus, there is little conversion of T_4 to active T_3; instead, rT_3 levels are elevated, ranging from 2 to 4 nmol/L. In the developing ovine fetus, the daily T_4 production rate averages 50 nmol/kg of body weight, while the daily T_3 production rate is only about 7 nmol/kg. In this species, the T_3 production rate parallels circulating T_3 levels, and both increase in the final weeks of gestation, principally due to maturation of hepatic type I MDI activity; rT_3 levels fall during this time. Significant levels of type II MDI activity are expressed in fetal brain and brown adipose tissues at midgestation (prior to the increases in plasma T_3 levels), and it is likely that expression of type II MDI activity provides for a local source of T_3 during this period. While fetal thyroid development occurs largely independent of maternal influences, maternal sources of thyroid hormone may play a role in certain pathophysiological circumstances. Infants born with a complete inability to organify iodide due to an inborn error of metabolism demonstrate cord blood levels of T_4 which range from 30 to 70 nmol/L. This T_4, presumably of maternal origin, may serve as an important substrate for local T_3 production by type II MDI expressing tissues (e.g., brain).[26, 27]

Physiological effects of thyroid hormone are dependent on expression of functional thyroid hormone receptors. Levels of T_3 nuclear receptors are developmentally regulated in all mammalian species studied to date. There is a paucity of data regarding the maturation of thyroid hormone receptors in developing humans. Nuclear T_3 receptor binding has been described in fetal lung, brain, heart, and liver by the twentieth week of gestation, but little ontogenic data are available.[107] Relatively high levels of nuclear T_3 receptors are present in the cerebral cortex of the fetal sheep at midgestation and during the final third of gestation. Hepatic nuclear T_3 receptors are expressed at adult levels only near term in the ovine fetus.[108] Similar differential tissue expression of T_3 nuclear receptors has been described in developing rats.[107] The size, weight, appearance, behavior, biochemical parameters, extrauterine adaptation, and early neonatal course are usually normal in the congenitally hypothyroid infant. This lack of signs and symptoms in the athyroid human neonate may relate to differential tissue expression of T_3 receptors, to low levels of circulating T_3, or to developmental regulation of T_3-mediated transcriptional events. Maternal T_4 acquired transplacentally also might ameliorate some of the fetal manifestations of congenital hypothyroidism. However, during the first months of postnatal life, growth, brain development, and metabolism become importantly dependent on thyroid hormones.

Posterior Pituitary System

Arginine vasopressin (AVP) is detectable after 10 to 12 weeks of gestation in the human fetal neurohypophysis. By 40 weeks, the level approximates 20 per cent of that of adults (see Table 127–3). Fetal pituitary oxytocin (OT) levels, detectable by 11 to 15 weeks, exceed AVP concentrations by 19 weeks. The AVP:OT ratio falls progressively thereafter (see Table 127–3). At 11 to 19 weeks of gestation, immunoreactive arginine vasotocin (AVT) is found in the human fetal pituitary in approximately two thirds the concentration of AVP and is secreted by cultured human fetal pineal cells during the second trimester.[109–111] In addition, AVT is found in mammalian cerebrospinal fluid, fetal pituitary, and adult pineal but not in the adult pituitary.[111, 112] The role of AVT in mammals is not known, but the hormone is known to bind to and activate AVP receptors.[111, 112] There is little information regarding AVP secretion in the human fetus, but considerable data are available in the sheep model. During the final third of gestation, the sheep fetus responds to hemorrhage, hypertonic saline, angiotensin II, and hypoxia with increased AVP secretion.[110, 113] The responses to hypertonicity and dehydration in the newborn lamb are quantitatively comparable with the adult responses, while the response to hypoxia greatly exceeds that of the adult. The ability of the newborn infant to respond to isotonic dextran or hypertonic saline with appropriate alterations in kidney free-water clearance indicate that human volume and osmolar control systems for AVP secretion also are mature at birth.[114]

Fetal serum AVP and OT also increase in response to parturition in the human neonate.[115–117] Newborn serum AVP levels are not increased after cesarean section delivery, whereas OT levels are. Serum levels of AVP in vaginally delivered infants are variable and seem to relate to the degree of fetal stress, probably including hypoxia and head compression.[115, 116] The mechanism for the OT release at birth is not known, but elevated levels after cesarean section delivery indicate that the stimuli for release of AVP and OT differ at the time of parturition.

As noted, the most potent stimulus for AVP release in the fetus is hypoxia, suggesting that AVP in the fetus functions as a stress hormone. Plasma levels of AVP in the human neonate are elevated in response to intrauterine bradycardia and meconium passage.[116] Moreover, AVP appears to be important to fetal circulatory homeostasis during hemorrhage or hypoxia.[118, 119] Hypoxia also stimulates catecholamine release in the fetus, and hypoxia and AVP have been known to stimulate pituitary ACTH release.[120–122] AVP is known to function as a corticotropin-releasing factor (CRF) in adults, and the third-trimester ovine fetal pituitary has been shown to respond to CRF and AVP separately and synergistically with regard to ACTH release.[120–122]

Both AVP and AVT evoke antidiuretic effects and inhibit lung fluid production in fetal sheep during the last third of gestation.[123, 124] These actions serve to conserve water for the fetus by inhibiting water loss into amniotic fluid. These effects are summarized in Figure 127–2. Maximal renal concentrating ability is limited in the fetus and newborn due to inherent immaturity of the renal tubules.[114] However, hypertonic saline administration evokes maximal antidiuresis in the human neonate, while isotonic dextran (volume expansion) evokes a maximal water diuresis.[114] Thus volume and osmolar control of AVP release are mature at birth.

Autonomic Nervous System

Functional development of the sympathoadrenal system is critical to both fetal and neonatal adaptation to stress. By 6 weeks of gestation, the primordia of the sympathetic ganglia are discernible. These are composed of primitive sympathetic neurons and chromaffin cells which coalesce into paired cell masses along the descending aorta. The paired adrenal medullary masses are well developed by 12 weeks of gestation; however, most of the chromaffin tissue in the fetus is present in scattered extramedullary para-aortic paraganglia, the largest of which are termed the

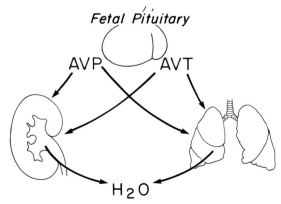

FIGURE 127–2. The effects of arginine vasopressin (AVP) and vasotocin (AVT) on water balance in the developing fetus (see text for details).

organs of Zuckerkandl. After birth, these paraganglia gradually atrophy, disappearing by 2 to 3 years of age.[125]

Catecholamines (epinephrine and norepinephrine) are demonstrable in chromaffin tissue by 15 weeks of gestation, with concentrations increasing to term. Para-aortic tissue contains predominantly norepinephrine, due to diminished activity of phenylethanolamine *N*-methyl transferase (PNMT), which converts norepinephrine to epinephrine.[126] In contrast, epinephrine is the predominant catecholamine secreted by the adrenal medulla. Developmental induction of adrenal medullary PNMT activity occurs in response to locally elevated glucocorticoid levels derived from surrounding adrenal cortical tissues.[127] Prior to complete splanchnic innervation, which occurs near term, the immature fetus cannot activate catecholamine release via the usual cholinergic mechanisms. However, the immature fetus does release catecholamines in response to hypoxia. This non-neurally mediated response occurs principally in paraganglionic tissues, resulting in relatively increased levels of circulating norepinephrine; as maturation continues, the response includes adrenal medullary secretion of epinephrine as well.[128] The physiological consequences of increased catecholamine secretion differ in the fetus and in adults. The fetus responds with metabolic effects (increased circulating glucose and free fatty acids) and fewer cardiovascular actions, while hemodynamic responses predominate in the adult.[129] In the fetus, circulating catecholamines rise acutely in response to maternal hypoglycemia and are accompanied by increases in fetal circulating free fatty acids and glucose.[130] These changes occur in the absence of any demonstrable change in fetal plasma insulin or glucagon levels, suggesting that the fetus may uniquely alter its metabolic environment via activation of the sympathetic-adrenal nervous system.

There is a significant increase in fetal circulating catecholamines during the final hours of labor; a logarithmic increase in plasma epinephrine and norepinephrine occurs at the time of parturition coincident with severing the placental circulation.[131] These changes are noted in Figure 127–3. It is likely that this postnatal surge in circulating catecholamines is an integrated response to a variety of stimuli, including head compression, mild asphyxia, tactile stimulation, hypothermia, and afferent baroreceptor activity. The physiological significance of the increases in circulating catechols at birth is complex and referenced in more

detail in the section dealing with newborn adaptations. However, when the surge is obtunded via surgical extirpation of fetal adrenal medullary tissues, profound cardiovascular and metabolic derangements ensue, and the transition from the intrauterine to the extrauterine environment is markedly altered.[131] Preterm infants respond to birth with augmented (in comparison with term infants) levels of circulating catecholamines[132] (see Fig. 127–3). The significance of this observation is uncertain, but it may represent an adaptive response by the preterm newborn in the face of immaturity of catecholamine-stimulated effector systems.

Autonomous Endocrine Systems

The Fetal Pancreas

The fetal pancreas is identifiable by the fourth week of gestation, with pancreatic islets, including alpha and beta cells, present by the ninth week.[133] Early in gestation, alpha cells predominate, while beta cells proliferate during the latter half of gestation; roughly equal numbers of alpha and beta cells are present at term. The beta cell is functional by 14 weeks of gestation, and fetal pancreatic insulin content exceeds that of the adult throughout most of gestation; circulating insulin levels are comparable with those seen in the postprandial adult. However, fetal glucose metabolism is largely independent of the glucoregulatory hormones insulin and glucagon.[134, 135] In studies involving euglycemic clamped fetal sheep, insulin infusion increases glucose utilization only about two-fold, in contrast to the almost five-fold increase observed in similarly euglycemic-hyperinsulinemic clamped adult sheep, suggesting that insulin is less important as a regulator of fetal glucose metabolism.[134] In physiological doses, glucagon does not increase hepatic glucose production, probably due to a paucity of hepatic glucagon receptors in the fetus.[135, 136] Insulin receptors are present in a variety of fetal tissues, at levels generally exceeding those of the adult.[135] In addition, downregulation of insulin receptor binding characteristics does not occur during fetal hyperinsulinemia, again in contrast with observations in adult animals. Acute hypoglycemia or hyperglycemia are not associated with significant alterations in either insulin or glucagon levels. However, chronic fetal hyperglycemia does evoke hyperinsulinemia and glucagon suppression, and chronic hypoglycemia may inhibit fetal insulin and promote fetal glucagon release.[137] The relative tachyphylaxis of fetal pancreatic insulin secretion appears to involve beta cell metabolic immaturity. Augmentation of the cAMP-generating systems in the fetus is associated with a more robust response of plasma insulin in response to hyperglycemia.

In studies involving pregnant sheep, net fetal umbilical glucose uptake from the placenta matches the fetal glucose utilization; it is difficult to document fetal hepatic gluconeogenesis under most physiological conditions.[135, 136] This may be explained by the finding of low levels of phosphoenolpyruvate carboxykinase (PEPCK) activity in the fetal liver; PEPCK is the rate-limiting enzyme for gluconeogenesis. Interestingly, inhibition of the transcription of the PEPCK gene may occur in response to the sustained fetal insulin levels.[138] Taken together, the consistent fetal insulin levels, which are relatively insensitive to changes in fetal plasma glucose concentration but present in association

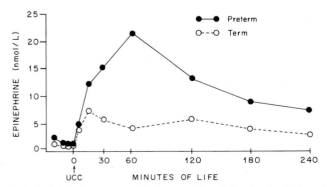

FIGURE 127–3. The pattern of plasma epinephrine levels during the perinatal period in term and preterm sheep. UCC denotes the time of umbilical cord cutting. (Data from Padbury JF, Martinez AM: Sympathoadrenal system activity at birth: Integration of postnatal adaptation. Semin Perinatol 12:163–172, 1988.)

with increased insulin receptors in many fetal tissues, probably serve to facilitate anabolic deposition of glucose, protein, and fat in fetal tissues. Low levels of circulating glucagon and decreased fetal glucagon receptor binding characteristics limit glycogenolysis and catabolism in fetal tissues.

During the newborn period, placental sources of glucose are abolished and plasma glucagon levels rise in association with a rapid increase in functionally coupled glucagon receptors, thus tending to promote glucose homeostasis. Increases in plasma catecholamines coincident with parturition may be responsible for some of these changes; catecholamines both stimulate glucagon release and inhibit insulin release.[135, 136] PEPCK activity also rises during this period. Thus gluconeogenesis is readily demonstrable in the newborn and in neonates; nearly 10 per cent of glucose utilization is accounted for by gluconeogenesis from alanine.[139] Plasma free fatty acid concentrations also rise postnatally, due to effects of catecholamines and chemical thermogenesis. Oxidation of fatty acids probably provides cofactors (acetyl-CoA and NAHD) required for gluconeogenesis, as well as sparing glucose for utilization by crucially dependent tissues such as brain.[135, 136]

Parathyroid Hormone–Calcitonin–Vitamin D System

The parathyroid glands are derived from the paired third and fourth pharyngeal pouches. These pouches are identifiable on the lateral wall of the pharyngeal gut by 4 to 5 weeks of gestation. The third pouches are destined to form the thymus and inferior parathyroid glands, and the fourth pouches form the superior parathyroid gland. The fifth pharyngeal pouches form the paired ultimobranchial bodies, which are incorporated into the thyroid gland during embryogenesis as the perifollicular calcitonin-secreting (C) cells. The parathyroid glands develop between 5 and 14 weeks of gestation and increase from a diameter of less than 0.1 mm at 14 weeks to 1 to 2 mm at birth. Adult glands measure 2 to 5 mm in width and 3 to 8 mm in length. Near term, fetal parathyroid cells are composed largely of inactive chief cells; there are few intermediate chief cells containing occasional secretory granules. C cells are particularly prominent in the neonatal thyroid gland, and the calcitonin content is as high as 540 to 2100 mU/g of tissue, values as much as 10 times those observed in the normal adult gland.[140, 141]

Information regarding function of the human fetal parathyroid glands or thyroid C cells is limited. Human fetal parathyroid glands from 12- to 13-week fetuses in heterologous explant systems cause resorption of the fetal bone, suggesting that such glands contain bioactive PTH-like activity.[142] The third-trimester human fetus at term is characterized by low circulating concentrations of PTH and relatively high levels of calcitonin;[140, 143, 144] the PTH response to hypocalcemia is somewhat obtunded. Presumably this is due to the prevailing high levels of total and ionized calcium maintained in fetal blood by active placental transport from maternal blood.[140, 145] Placental transport of calcium occurs across the syncytiotrophoblast, which contains a calcium-binding protein in association with an ATP-dependent calcium pump.[55] Vitamin D levels and metabolites in the fetus are derived, in significant part, from the mater-

nal circulation.[140, 145] However, the levels of free or unbound vitamin D metabolites are higher than maternal concentrations, implying active placental transport and/or fetal synthesis.[145] It has been postulated that the high levels of total and ionized calcium in the fetal circulation, maintained by placental transport, tend to suppress fetal PTH secretion and stimulate fetal calcitonin production.[140]

Studies in the fetal sheep model have contributed important observations to our understanding of fetal calcium metabolism. The fetal sheep has low circulating levels of PTH but can increase serum PTH concentrations in response to a fall in serum calcium concentrations induced by EDTA.[146] The third-trimester sheep fetus also can respond promptly to infused calcium with increased serum calcitonin levels.[147] In this model, fetal parathyroidectomy decreases placental calcium transport and lowers fetal serum calcium.[55] While PTH has no effect on placental calcium transport, PTH-related peptide (PTHrP) is present in fetal parathyroid tissue and stimulates calcium transport in isolated, perfused placental tissue derived from thyroparathyroidectomized fetuses.[85] Moreover, placental PTH receptors, which bind both PTH and PTHrP, are present on the brush borders and apical plasma membranes of human placental cells.[148] These data suggest that PTHrP from the fetal thyroid gland modulates placental calcium transport to maintain the high levels of fetal serum calcium. In addition, the placenta also produces PTHrP, which also may play a role.[55]

Nephrectomy in the fetal sheep reduces fetal serum calcium concentrations, and this hypocalcemia can be prevented by prior administration of 1,25(OH)$_2$ vitamin D.[55] The fetal kidney can produce 1,25(OH)$_2$ vitamin D, and the placenta contains 1,25,(OH)$_2$ vitamin D receptors as well as a vitamin D–dependent calcium-binding protein.[55, 145] Dihydroxy vitamin D production in the fetal sheep is sixfold greater than in the maternal ewe.[149] Although not entirely clear, it seems likely that fetal PTH and presumably PTHrP act on the fetal kidney to stimulate 1-hydroxylation of 25(OH) vitamin D and that the 1,25(OH)$_2$ vitamin D participates in modulating placental calcium transport. Thus the parathyroid glands in the fetus appear to augment maternal to fetal calcium transport across the placenta, providing for the high rate of bone mineral acceleration in the latter half of pregnancy. The high serum calcium, in turn, chronically stimulates fetal calcitonin secretion. Since calcitonin inhibits bone resorption, high blood levels would help to promote bone calcium accretion. Placental calcitonin production also has been demonstrated and also may contribute.[56] These effects are summarized in Figure 127–4.

NEUTRALIZATION OF HORMONE ACTIONS IN THE FETUS

Another of the unique aspects of the fetal endocrine milieu is the observation that the biological actions of a variety of otherwise potent hormones are neutralized in utero. During the latter half of gestation, cortisol is neutralized in most fetal tissues by conversion to inactive cortisone via 11β-hydroxysteroid dehydrogenase. This enzyme activity in placental tissue is relatively low until midgestation and increases progressively to term, resulting in a pro-

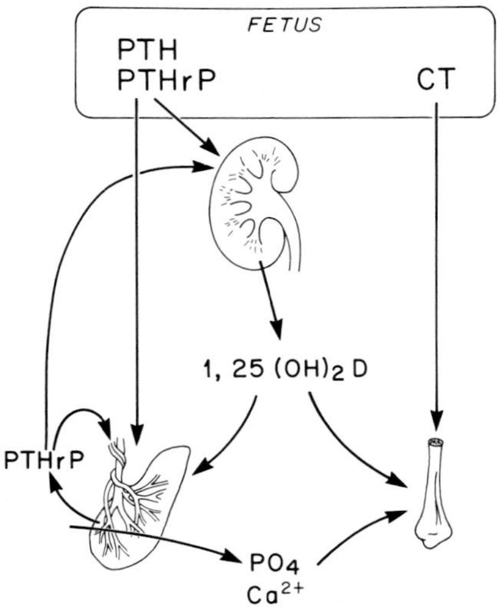

FIGURE 127–4. Hormonal modulation of fetal calcium homeostasis. Parathyroid hormone (PTH) and PTH-related peptide (PTHrP) are derived from both fetal parathyroid and placental tissues and act to promote the actions of dihydroxy vitamin D [1,25(OH)$_2$ vitamin D]. Fetal thyroidal calcitonin (CT) facilitates bone mineralization (see text for details).

gressive decrease in maternal to fetal transfer of active cortisol.[32, 150] Many adult tissues are capable of converting cortisone to cortisol via expression of an 11-ketosteroid reductase. Fetal tissues, in contrast, express low levels of this enzyme activity. As a result, the ratio of cortisone to cortisol in fetal blood are in the range of 3 to 4:1.[32, 150] Near term the ratio of cortisol to cortisone increases due to increased fetal adrenal secretion of cortisol and decreased 11-ketosteroid reductase activities in fetal tissues.[32, 151]

As indicated earlier (Ch. 47), the actions of the thyroid hormones are largely neutralized in the fetus. Placental tissue contains an active iodothyronine inner ring monodeiodinase (MDI), which converts thyroxine to inactive reverse triiodothyronine (rT$_3$). In addition, fetal tissue levels of outer ring iodothyronine MDI activities are low so that conversion of thyroxine to active triiodothyronine (T$_3$) is limited.[152] As a consequence, the ratio of rT$_3$:T$_3$ is high (15 to 20:1) in fetal plasma. Fetal plasma levels of thyroxine sulfate and T$_3$ sulfate also are relatively high, and these metabolites also are biologically inactive.[153] Fetal brain and brown adipose tissue, in contrast with other fetal tissues, do manifest significant levels of outer ring iodothyronine MDI activity, and this activity is augmented in the hypothyroid fetus.[152] This type II MDI activity contributes to local T$_3$ production and may be important to protect fetal brain development, particularly in hypothyroxinemic fetuses. During the perinatal period, fetal T$_3$ conversion from T$_4$ increases, and there is a marked stimulation of thyroidal T$_3$ secretion at birth. Both pathways increase fetal and neonatal blood T$_3$ levels.

A second mechanism for neutralizing the biological activity of potent hormones in the fetus is the delayed appearance of tissue receptors or postreceptor responsiveness. Studies in fetal sheep have shown a relative unresponsiveness of fetal liver and kidney Na$^+$,K$^+$-ATPase and mitochondrial α-glycerophosphate activities to T$_3$ during the latter third of gestation.[152] The appearance of other enzyme, receptor, and growth factor responses to thyroid hormones also is delayed until the neonatal period.[152]

These delayed responses appear to be due to the late appearance of T$_3$ nuclear receptors in selected tissues, as well as an apparent delay in maturation of post-nuclear receptor responsiveness. Growth hormone also is inactive in the fetus due to the delayed appearance of plasma membrane receptors, and a relative deficiency of prolactin receptors may contribute to limited prolactin bioactivity in the fetus.[154]

There are limited data regarding fetal hormone responsiveness in other systems. Beta-adrenergic receptor binding in heart and lungs of fetal sheep is relatively reduced during the latter third of gestation, increasing in the perinatal period.[155] The appearance of estrogen receptors in the neonatal rat uterus, cervix, oviduct, and vagina is delayed until 10 days after birth.[156] The newborn human infant may demonstrate evidence of an estrogen effect on vaginal and breast tissues at birth, but in general, the effects of the high estrogen levels in fetal and neonatal blood are limited.

FETAL GROWTH

The factors modulating fetal growth are only partially understood. It is clear that the hormones most important for postnatal growth, including thyroxine, growth hormone, and gonadal steroids, have a very limited role in fetal growth.[157] Genetic factors appear to play a role, but the mechanism(s) remain obscure. During the past decade, evidence has accumulated suggesting that the insulin-like growth factors (IGF-I and IGF-II) play a major role in modulating fetal growth.[157–159] Both IGF-I and IGF-II are expressed in placental tissue and in a variety of fetal tissues early in gestation.[2–4, 160] Protein and mRNA levels are most abundant in fetal tissues of mesenchymal origin but are also identified in tissues of ectodermal and endodermal origin.[158, 161, 162] In addition, the type I IGF receptor, which mediates most of the biological actions of the IGF's, is present early in gestation in a wide variety of fetal tissues. Type II IGF receptors and insulin receptors also are present in fetal tissues but probably have a limited role in fetal growth.[158, 159]

An endocrine role for the IGF's in the fetus is possible. Circulating IGF binding proteins are present early in gestation, and total plasma concentrations of the IGF's are high compared with tissue concentrations. However, the levels of both IGF's in fetal and cord blood are relatively low compared with childhood or adult values.[158, 163] The predominant IGF in fetal blood is IGF-II, in keeping with its prominent role in fetal growth. It seems likely, however, that the major routes of IGF actions in the fetus are autocrine or paracrine. The co-localization of IGF and IGF receptors in growing fetal tissues and the widespread tissue distributions of the IGF and IGF-I receptor mRNA species would favor this view. In the midgestation fetus, both IGF-I and IGF-II are abundant in gut, liver, kidney, skeletal and cardiac muscle, skin, hematopoietic tissues, lung, and adrenal tissues.[158, 159] The predominant localization of both IGF-I and IGF-II mRNA levels to mesenchymal connective tissues around and within these organs suggests their largely paracrine roles on adjacent target cells.[158, 162]

The control of IGF production in the fetus is not entirely clear. Growth hormone, which stimulates IGF-I production after birth, has little or no role in fetal IGF production.[157–159] Human placental lactogen (hPL), via unique fetal receptors, stimulates IGF-I production and DNA synthesis in human fetal muscle cells and fetal fibroblasts.[164, 165] There also is evidence that insulin may play a role in modulating IGF synthesis in the fetus.[166] Finally, nutrition has been shown to modulate IGF levels in developing and postnatal mammals. Plasma IGF concentrations are reduced in fetuses of protein-deficient pregnant rats, and IGF-I levels are reduced in suckling rats deprived of milk.[158, 167] Moreover, the effect in starved pregnant rats can be reversed by hPL.[167] There is evidence to suggest that glucocorticoids limit fetal growth by inhibiting IGF actions at the tissue level.[168]

Insulin, too, has been suggested to stimulate fetal growth, particularly late in gestation.[166] The hyperinsulinemia commonly observed in the fetus of the diabetic mother is associated with increased body weight and increased body fat deposition.[166] The fetus with pancreatic agenesis and hypoinsulinemia is small and relatively devoid of body fat. Insulin infusion to fetal monkeys near term increases body weight, with prominent anabolic effects on heart, liver, and spleen.[169] Insulin may act directly and/or by stimulating IGF production and may act via insulin receptors or type I IGF receptors.[166]

Other growth factors probably also play a role in modulating fetal growth and differentiation. The epidermal growth factor (EGF)–transforming growth factor alpha (TGFα) family of growth factors, acting through EGF receptors, is known to stimulate precocious eyelid opening and tooth eruption in neonatal rodents and to stimulate palatal development, gastrointestinal maturation, and lung maturation. EGF/TGFα also appears to play an important role in kidney, liver, and thyroid and adrenal gland growth.[170–172] Maternal salivary gland and plasma EGF concentrations increase four- to five-fold in the mouse during pregnancy, and removal of the maternal salivary glands reduces litter size and fetal weight; the administration of exogenous EGF reverses these effects.[173] The mechanism(s) of these EGF effects remain unclear, but an effect on maternal or placental metabolism is likely. The placenta is a rich source of EGF receptors. EGF receptors are present in many fetal tissues early in gestation, but EGF and EGF precursor mRNA have not been identified in most fetal tissues or in fetal blood of rodents.[171, 174–176] Low levels of pro-EGF mRNA have been characterized in tooth, dermis, spleen, and lung tissues of embryonic mice.[177] However, the predominant fetal species of this family of growth factors in the developing fetus appears to be TGFα.[171, 178, 179] The control of TGFα production in the fetus is not understood. Thyroid and steroid hormones and growth hormone play a role in the control of EGF production in the neonatal period but not in the fetus; there is little information regarding regulation of TGFα production in the fetus.[171]

Other growth factors are involved in fetal growth and maturation, but data and our understanding of their role are limited. Hematopoietic growth factors play a role in the fetus.[180, 181] Erythropoietin (EP) is produced by the liver during fetal development, and there is a switch to renal EP production shortly after birth in sheep and other mammals.[181, 182] Postnatal renal EP production is modulated by oxygen tension in blood and by thyroid hormones and testosterone; oxygen tension also regulates hepatic EP production in the fetus.[181, 182] The thyroid hormone and testosterone regulatory roles become manifest in the neonatal period.

Fibroblast growth factors (FGF) probably play a role in fetal development. Infusion of FGF into renal arteries of rats containing a renal subcapsular transplant of a 10-day rat embryo has been shown to stimulate growth of the embryo.[183] The major effects were on tissues of endodermal and mesodermal origin; moreover, FGF antiserum inhibited growth of endodermal tissues in the transplanted embryos, as well as in some of the mesodermal-derived tissues.[183]

Nerve growth factor (NGF) is known to stimulate growth and differentiation of the autonomic nervous system in developing rodents. NGF injection in neonatal mice increases the size of the superior cervical ganglia. Selected enzyme activities also increase in response to NGF infusion, including RNA polymerase, ornithine carboxylase, and tyrosine hydroxylase; NGF antiserum injection, in contrast, results in permanent sympathectomy.[184, 185] Studies involving induction of autoantibodies of NGF in rats and rabbits have shown that mothers with high titers to NGF antibody deliver fetuses with significantly impaired autonomic nervous system development.[186, 187] This includes small dorsal root ganglia and decreased autonomic innervation of peripheral organs. NGF-like activity is produced by neonatal mouse brain astroglial cells maintained in tissue culture, suggesting that an NGF-like molecule may be involved in fetal brain maturation.[188]

Other growth factors almost surely will be shown to have a role in fetal mammalian organ maturation and overall fetal growth and differentiation. For example, the production and action of a variety of factors have been demonstrated in the developing kidney.[189] These include the IGF and EGF families, TGFβ, platelet-derived growth factor (PDGF), FGF, and NGF. The list of possible factors is increasing rapidly. It is of interest that a growing number of these factors have been shown to be produced by the placenta. Thus, as is the case for the insulin-like growth factors, both endocrine and autocrine-paracrine routes of production and action of a variety of growth factors may prove to be important in individual fetal organ development and in overall fetal growth and differentiation.

ADAPTATION TO EXTRAUTERINE LIFE

Successful transition to extrauterine life requires that the fetus, previously poikilothermic with the placenta subserving most of its metabolic needs, becomes homeothermic and self-sustaining. Crucial integration of a variety of neural and endocrine events is a prerequisite for this transition. Appropriate adrenal cortical and medullary functions are crucial to the immediate processes of thermoregulation, transition to air breathing, and cardiovascular adaptation. Longer term transition requires adaptation to intermittent substrate supply (with concomitant transient substrate deficiency), as well as calcium homeostasis.

The Catecholamine Surge

As indicated, parturition is associated with enormous increases in circulating catecholamine levels (see Fig. 127–

3). That the newborn is physiologically dependent on appropriate sympathoadrenal activity is supported by the following observations. In the fetal sheep, adrenalectomy (with subsequent cortisol replacement) is associated with profound alterations in cardiovascular and metabolic responses during the immediate postnatal period. Adrenalectomized newborns have an obtunded surge in plasma epinephrine levels and fail to demonstrate the expected increases in a variety of cardiovascular responses. These newborns are hypotensive, with low cardiac outputs due to poor myocardial contractility. They fail to mobilize endogenous energy substrates, resulting in postnatal hypoglycemia as well as blunted metabolism of free fatty acids. Thermogenesis also is affected, as is pulmonary adaptation, including poor mobilization of pulmonary fluid and altered surfactant synthesis and secretion.[129, 131, 190] Effects of catecholamines on a variety of physiological processes are summarized in Figure 127–5.

The Cortisol Surge

A modest increase in circulating cortisol levels occurs prenatally in a variety of primate and other mammalian species.[32, 34] This occurs primarily as a result of increased fetal adrenal cortisol production and decreased metabolism of cortisol to cortisone. Plasma ACTH levels tend to remain stable, although the pulsatility of ACTH secretion also may increase during this period. These prenatal increases in circulating cortisol concentrations are associated with a variety of physiological responses and are summarized in Figure 127–5. These include (1) induction and maturation of a variety of gut enzymes for nutrient absorption, as well as promoting maturation of gut transport processes, motility, and structure, (2) increased conversion of T_4 to T_3 by hepatic outer ring iodothyronine deiodinase

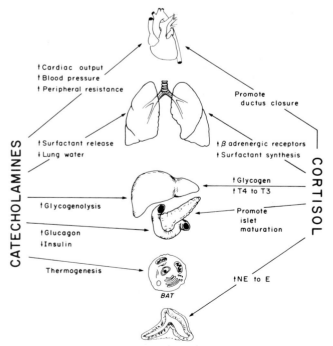

FIGURE 127–5. The roles of catecholamines and cortisol during the transition to extrauterine life (see text for details).

leading to increased circulating T_3 levels, (3) increased epinephrine secretion by sympathetic chromaffin tissue (including adrenal medulla) due to augmented phenylethanolamine transferase activity (which converts norepinephrine to epinephrine), (4) stimulation or maturation of a variety of hepatic enzyme activities, (5) augmented surfactant synthesis, secretion, and maturation of surfactant composition, and (6) increased beta-adrenergic receptor density in a variety of tissues, including lung, heart, and brown adipose tissue.[25, 32, 34, 96, 129, 191, 192] These myriad and beneficial effects of the prenatal cortisol surge have led to the current therapy of prenatal corticosteroid therapy in pregnancies threatened by the risk of preterm delivery. Generally, preterm infants prenatally exposed to augmental glucocorticoid levels have lower overall morbidity and mortality than untreated infants.[193] Finally, activation of the hypothalamic-pituitary-adrenal axis has been proposed as a principal mechanism for the induction of the processes leading to parturition.[191] While this is certainly true for the ovine species, the role of augmented adrenal cortical activity in human parturition is less clear.[32, 34, 194]

Brown Adipose Tissue Thermogenesis

Brown adipose tissue is the major site for newborn thermogenesis. The mass of brown adipose tissue peaks at birth and involutes in most species after the first weeks of life. Extirpation of brown adipose tissue during fetal life is associated with profound neonatal hypothermia. Regulation of brown adipose tissue function is coordinated through several endocrine systems. Catecholamines, via β-adrenergic receptors, stimulate fatty acid oxidation and thermogenesis; this response is also thyroid hormone–dependent.[195] Mitochondria in brown adipose tissue express a unique protein (thermogenin or uncoupling protein, UCP) which uncouples oxidation from subsequent ADP phosphorylation, thus promoting the release of heat. Thermogenin is T_3-dependent; brown adipose tissue expresses an iodothyronine monodeiodinase which provides for local T_3 synthesis from T_4.[196] In the ovine fetus, fetal thyroidectomy leads to hypothermia and low plasma free fatty acid concentrations despite increased circulating levels of catecholamines.[197] In vitro, brown adipocyte basal O_2 consumption, as well as catechol and dibutyryl cAMP-stimulated O_2 consumption, is markedly diminished after fetal thyroidectomy.[197] Thus thyroid hormones and catecholamines are essential for optimal brown adipose tissue function and euthermia in the transition to extrauterine life. Placental factors, including adenosine and PGE_2, may serve to inhibit brown adipose tissue thermogenesis in the fetus while allowing for normal development of the tissue in preparation for the transition to extrauterine life.[198]

Glucose Homeostasis

The abrupt withdrawal of placental glucose transport leads to a prompt fall in plasma glucose immediately after birth. This relative hypoglycemia, along with augmented catecholamine levels, stimulates pancreatic glucagon secretion. These early glucagon and catecholamine surges rapidly deplete available hepatic glucagon stores so that maintenance of blood glucose levels in the 12 to 24 hours following birth requires increased hepatic gluconeogenesis.[134, 137] Infants born prior to term have a more severe and prolonged neonatal hypoglycemia because of reduced hepatic glycogen stores and relatively impaired hepatic gluconeogenesis. While the healthy term infant achieves adultlike regulation of glucose homeostasis within days of birth, the preterm infant may require several weeks to autonomously regulate endogenous glucose levels.

Other Hormonal Adaptations

Delivery of the infant and severing of the placental circulation result in abruptly decreased levels of estrogens, progesterone, hCG, and hPL in the newborn. The decrease in estrogens removes a major stimulus to newborn prolactin release, and prolactin levels remain low over the next several weeks of life. GH levels also are low in the postnatal period due to delayed hypothalamic-pituitary feedback and control.[199, 200] These probably involve changes in the GH sensitivity to both GHRH and somatostatin. Newborn IGF levels fall to low values, presumably due to removal of placental hPL stimulation and placental somatomedin production. The dramatic increases in neonatal TSH secretion are due to influences of cooling and augmented circulating catechols. The increases in TSH and catecholamine activity, in turn, increase thyroidal T_4 and T_3 secretion and enhance peripheral T_4 to T_3 conversion. Re-equilibrium of neonatal serum TSH levels requires altered feedback inhibition by prevailing circulating T_4 levels. Reverse T_3 production slowly ceases in most neonatal tissues by 3 to 4 weeks of age, at which time rT_3 values approximate those in the adult.[22, 25, 107]

SUMMARY

We have reviewed our current level of understanding of the perinatal endocrine milieu. Recent progress has remarkably improved our ability to manage infants born with a variety of endocrine disorders, including infants of diabetic mothers, infants with ambiguous or disordered sexual differentiation, and infants born with congenital thyroid, parathyroid, pituitary, and adrenal disorders. Moreover, we have learned to recognize important maturational differences leading to altered endocrine function in preterm infants. Obstetrical and neonatal management of these infants continues to provide clinical challenges for the practitioner.

We are entering a new era in which direct fetal access and manipulation of the intrauterine environment are not only feasible but commonplace. Manipulation of maternal fertility, artificial insemination, and in vitro fertilization are now routine. Expanded ultrasound-guided techniques to obtain fetal tissue, fluid, or blood as early as the first trimester of pregnancy are now possible, leading to initial diagnosis and resultant intrauterine therapies of fetal disorders, including abnormalities in adrenal and thyroid function. Precocious maturation of the preterm fetus at risk for premature delivery via exogenous maternal corticosteroid administration has had a significant impact on neonatal morbidity and mortality. Indwelling catheterization and chronic pump implantation are used routinely for therapy in a variety of fetal animals, and these techniques may be co-opted for human use. It has been suggested that intrauterine fetal growth retardation might respond to exogenous administration of growth factors, including the IGF's or EGF. Techniques of molecular biology will allow for precise antenatal diagnosis of a variety of endocrine defects; direct fetal access and recombinant technology may allow for fetal cure prior to irreversible developmental defects arising as a consequence of inborn errors of metabolism.

Finally, transplantation of a variety of fetal neuroendocrine tissues may be key in the therapies of several adult diseases, including diabetes mellitus, diabetes insipidus, and Parkinson's disease. While the ethical considerations must be addressed, continuing progress in this area serves as an important adjunct to present medical management. Thus the next decades will witness continued expansion of our understanding of perinatal endocrinology, leading to increased effectiveness in the diagnosis and management of abnormal pregnancies, as well as preterm and term infants.

REFERENCES

1. Sibley CP, Boyd RDH: Mechanism of transfer across the human placenta. In Polin RA, Fox WW (eds): Fetal and Neonatal Physiology. Philadelphia, WB Saunders Co, 1992, pp 62–74.
2. Robinson WR, Atkinson DE, Jones CIP, Sibley CP: Permeability of the near-term rat placenta to hydrophilic solutes. Placenta 9:361–372, 1988.
3. Beitins IZ, Kowarski A, Shermeta DW, et al: Fetal and maternal secretion rate of cortisol in sheep, diffusion resistance of the placenta. Pediatr Res 4:129–134, 1970.
4. Mitchell BF, Seron-Ferre M, Hess DL, Jaffe RB: Cortisol production and metabolism in the late gestation Rhesus monkey fetus. Endocrinology 108:916–924, 1981.
5. Murphy BEP: Cortisol and cortisone in human fetal development. J Steroid Biochem 11:509–513, 1979.
6. Bayard F, Ances IG, Tapper AJ, et al: Transplacental passage and fetal secretion of aldosterone. J Clin Invest 49:1389–1392, 1970.
7. Lauritzen C, Klopper A: Estrogens and androgens. In Fuchs F, Klopper A (eds): Endocrinology of Pregnancy. Hagerstown, MD, Harper & Row, 1983, pp 73–91.
8. Sopelak VM, Hodgen GD: Infusion of gonadotropin releasing hormone agonist during pregnancy: Maternal and fetal responses in primates. Am J Obstet Gynecol 156:755–760, 1987.
9. Miyakawa I, Ikeda I, Maegama M: Transport of ACTH across human placenta. J Clin Endocrinol Metab 39:440–442, 1974.
10. King KC, Adam PAJ, Schwartz R, Teramo K: Human placental transfer of human growth hormone-I[125]. Pediatrics 48:534–539, 1971.
11. Foster DL, Karsch FJ, Nalbandov AV: Regulation of luteinizing hormone (LH) in the fetal and neonatal lamb: II. Study of placental LH transfer in the sheep. Endocrinology 90:589–592, 1972.
12. Roti E, Gnudi A, Braverman LE: The placental transport, synthesis and metabolism of hormones and drugs which affect thyroid function. Endocr Rev 4:131–149, 1983.
13. Glatz TH, Weitzman RE, Nathanielz PW, Fisher DA: Metabolic clearance rate and transplacental passage of oxytocin in the pregnant ewe and fetus. Endocrinology 106:1006–1011, 1980.
14. Stegner H, Leake RD, Palmer SM, et al: Permeability of the sheep placenta to ^{125}I arginine vasopressin. Dev Pharmacol Ther 7:140–144, 1984.
15. Ballard RA, Ballard PL, Creasy R, et al: Respiratory disease in very low birth weight infants after prenatal thyrotropin-releasing hormone and glucocorticoid. Lancet 339:510–515, 1992.
16. Wolf H, Salsata V, Frerichs H, Stubbe P: Evidence for the impermeability of human placenta for insulin. Horm Metab Res 1:274–275, 1969.
17. Sperling MA, Erenberg, Fiser RH, et al: Placental transfer of glucagon in sheep. Endocrinology 93:1435–1438, 1973.

18. Balabanova S, Lang T, Wolf AS, et al: Placental transfer of parathyroid hormone. J Perinat Med 14:243–250, 1986.
19. Garel JM, Milhaud G, Sizonenko PC: Inactivation de la calcitonin porcine par differents organes foetaux et maternals du rat. C R Acad Sci Paris 270:2469–2471, 1970.
20. Symonds EM, Furler I: Plasma renin levels in the normal and anephric fetus at birth. Biol Neonate 23:133–138, 1973.
21. Blay J, Hollenberg MD: The nature and function of the polypeptide growth factor receptors in the human placenta. J Dev Physiol 12:237–248, 1989.
22. Fisher DA, Dussault JH, Sack J, Chopra IJ: Ontogenesis of hypothalamic-pituitary-thyroid function and metabolism in man, sheep and rat. Recent Prog Horm Res 33:59–116, 1977.
23. Fisher DA, Lehman H, Lackey C: Placental transfer of thyroxine. J Clin Endocrinol Metab 24:393–400, 1964.
24. Raiti S, Holzman CB, Scott RL, Blizzard RM: Evidence for the placental transfer of triiodothyronine in human beings. N Engl J Med 277:456–459, 1967.
25. Wu SY, Fisher DA, Polk DH, Chopra IJ: Maturation of thyroid hormone metabolism. In Wu SY (ed): Thyroid Hormone Metabolism: Regulation and Clinical Implications. Boston, Blackwell Scientific, 1991, pp 293–320.
26. Vulsma T, Gons MH, DeViljder JJM: Maternal-fetal transfer of thyroxine in congenital hypothyroidism due to a total organification defect or thyroid agenesis. N Engl J Med 321:13–16, 1989.
27. Ruiz de Ona C, Obregon MJ, Escobar del Rey F, Morreale de Escobar G: Developmental changes in rat brain 5′-monodeiodinase and thyroid hormones during the fetal period: The effects of fetal hypothyroidism and maternal thyroid hormones. Pediatr Res 24:588–594, 1988.
28. Sodha RJ, Proegler M, Schneider H: Transfer and metabolism of norepinephrine studied from maternal-to-fetal and fetal-to-maternal sides in the in vitro perfused human placental lobe. Am J Obstet Gynecol 148:474–481, 1984.
29. Beard RW: Response of the human foetal heart and maternal circulation to adrenaline and noradrenaline. BMJ 1:443–446, 1962.
30. Zuspan FP, Whaley WH, Nelson GH, Ahlquist RP: Placental transfer of epinephrine: I. Maternal-fetal metabolic alterations of glucose and non-esterified fatty acids. Am J Obstet Gynecol 95:284–289, 1966.
31. Luschinsky HL, Singher HO: Identification and assay of monoamine oxidase in the human placenta. Arch Biochem 19:95–107, 1948.
32. Albrecht ED, Pepe GJ: Placental steroid hormone biosynthesis in primate pregnancy. Endocr Rev 11:124–150, 1990.
33. Diczfalusy E: Endocrine functions of the human fetoplacental unit. Fed Proc 23:791–798, 1964.
34. Challis JRG, Brook AN: Maturation and activation of hypothalamic-pituitary-adrenal function in fetal sheep. Endocr Rev 10:182–204, 1989.
35. Ryan KJ: Placental synthesis of steroid hormones. In Tulchinsky D, Ryan KJ (eds): Maternal-Fetal Endocrinology. Philadelphia, WB Saunders Co, 1980, pp 3–16.
36. Buster JE, Simon JA: Placental hormones, hormonal preparation for and control of parturition and hormonal diagnosis of pregnancy. In DeGroot LJ, Besser GM, Cahill GF Jr (eds): Endocrinology (ed 2). Philadelphia, WB Saunders Co, 1989, pp 2043–2073.
37. Siiteri PK, Febres F, Clemens LE, et al: Progesterone and the maintenance of pregnancy: Is progesterone nature's immunosuppressant? Ann NY Acad Sci 286:384–387, 1977.
38. Siler-Khoder T: Endocrine and paracrine function in the human placenta. In Polin RA, Fox WW (eds): Fetal and Neonatal Physiology. Philadelphia, WB Saunders Co, 1992, pp 74–85.
39. Siler-Khoder T: Hypothalamic-like releasing hormones of the placenta. Clin Perinatol 10:553–566, 1983.
40. Radovick S, Wornisford FE, Nakayama Y, et al: Isolation and characterization of the human gonadotropin releasing hormone gene in the hypothalamus and placenta. Mol Endocrinol 4:476–480, 1990.
41. Ringler GE, Kallen CB, Strauss JF III: Regulation of human trophoblast function by glucocorticoids: Dexamethasone promotes increased secretion of chorionic gonadotropin. Endocrinology 124:1625–1631, 1989.
42. Maruo T, Matsuo H, Ohtani T, et al: Differential modulation of chorionic gonadotropin (CG) subunit ribonucleic acid levels and CG secretion by progesterone in normal placenta and choriocarcinoma cultured in vitro. Endocrinology 119:855–864, 1986.
43. Abu-Hakima M, Branchaud CL, Goodyear CG, et al: The effects of human chorionic gonadotropin on growth and steroidogenesis of the human fetal adrenal gland in vitro. Am J Obstet Gynecol 156:681–687, 1987.
44. Harada A, Hershman JM, Reed AW, et al: Comparison of thyroid stimulators and thyroid hormone concentrations in the serum of pregnant women. J Clin Endocrinol Metab 48:793–797, 1979.
45. Pekonen F, Alfthan H, Stenman UH, Ylikorkala O: Human chorionic gonadotropin (hCG) and thyroid function early in pregnancy: Circadian variation and evidence for intrinsic thyrotropic activity of hCG. J Clin Endocinol Metab 66:853–856, 1988.
46. Chen CLC, Chang CC, Krieger DT, Bardin CW: Expression and regulation of proopiomelanocortin-like gene in the ovary and placenta: Comparison with the testis. Endocrinology 118:2382–2389, 1986.
47. Petraglia F, Sawchenko PE, Rivier J, Vale WW: Evidence for local stimulation of ACTH secretion by corticotropin-releasing factor in human placenta. Nature 9:373–375, 1987.
48. Margioris AN, Grino M, Protos P, et al: Corticotropin-releasing hormone and oxytocin stimulate the release of placental proopiomelanocortin peptides. J Clin Endocrinol Metab 66:922–926, 1988.
49. Laatikainen T, Saijonmaa O, Salminen K, Wahlstrom T: Localization and concentrations of β-endorphin and β-lipotropin in human placenta. Placenta 8:381–387, 1987.
50. Robinson BG, Emanuel RL, Frim DM, Majzoub JA: Glucocorticoid stimulates expression of corticotropin-releasing hormone gene in human placenta. Proc Natl Acad Sci USA 85:5244–5248, 1988.
51. Abboud TK: Maternal and fetal β-endorphin: Effects of pregnancy and labor. Arch Dis Child 63:707–709, 1988.
52. Egan DA, Grzegorczyk V, Tricarico KA, et al: Placental chorionic renin: Production, purification and characterization. Biochim Biophys Acta 965:68–75, 1988.
53. Ihara Y, Taii S, Mori T: Expression of renin and angiotensinogen genes in human placental tissues. Endocrinol Jpn 34:887–896, 1987.
54. Millan MA, Carvallo P, Izumi SI, et al: Novel sites of expression of functional angiotensin II receptors in the late gestation fetus. Science 244:1340–1342, 1989.
55. Care AD: Development of endocrine pathways in the regulation of calcium homeostasis. Baillieres Clin Endocinol Metab 3:671–688, 1989.
56. Jousset V, Legendre B, Besnard P, et al: Calcitonin-like immunoreactivity and calcitonin gene expression in the placenta and in the mammary gland of the rat. Acta Endocrinol 119:443–451, 1988.
57. Lee J, Seppala M, Chard T: Characterization of placental luteinizing hormone releasing factor-like material. Acta Endocrinol 96:394–397, 1981.
58. Seeburg PH, Adelman J: Characterization of cDNA for precursor of human luteinizing hormone releasing hormone. Nature 311:666–668, 1984.
59. Schambaugh GD, Kubek M, Wilber JF: Thyrotropin releasing hormone activity in the human placenta. J Clin Endocrinol Metab 48:483–486, 1979.
60. Polk DH, Rev-iczky A, Lam RW, Fisher DA: Thyrotropin releasing hormone in ovine fetus: Ontogeny and effect of thyroid hormone. Am J Physiol 260(Endocrinol Metab 23):E53–E58, 1991.
61. Wattkins WB, Yen SSC: Somatostatin in cytotrophoblast of the immature human placenta: Localization by immunoperoxidase cytochemistry. J Clin Endocrinol Metab 50:969–971, 1980.
62. Frim DM, Emanuel RL, Robinson BG, et al: Characterization and gestational regulation of corticotropin-releasing hormone messenger RNA in human placenta. J Clin Invest 82:287–292, 1988.
63. Sasaki A, Shinkawa O, Margioris A, et al: Immunoreactive corticotropin-releasing hormone in human plasma during pregnancy, labor and delivery. J Clin Endocrinol Metab 64:224–229, 1987.
64. Goland RS, Wardlow SL, Stark RI, et al: High levels of corticotropin releasing hormone immunoreactivity in maternal and fetal plasma during pregnancy. J Clin Endocrinol Metab 63:1199–1203, 1986.
65. Goland RS, Stark RI, Wardlaw SL: Response to corticotropin-releasing hormone during pregnancy in the baboon. J Clin Endocrinol Metab 70:925–929, 1990.
66. Baird A, Wehrenberg WB, Bohlen P, Ling N: Immunoreactive and biologically active growth hormone releasing factor in rat placenta. Endocrinology 117:1598–1601, 1985.
67. Jeske W, Soszynski P, Rogozinski W, et al: Plasma GHRH, CRH, ACTH, β-endorphin, human placental lactogen, GH and cortisol concentrations at the third trimester of pregnancy. Acta Endocrinol 120:785–789, 1989.
68. Fields PA, Eldridge RK, Fuchs AR, et al: Human placental and bovine corpora luteal oxytocin. Endocrinology 112:1544–1546, 1983.
69. Amico JA: Oxytocin and oxytocin-like peptides in primate tissues and body fluids. In Yoshida S, Share L (eds): Recent Progress in Posterior Pituitary Hormones. New York, Elsevier, 1988, pp 207–213.

70. Lefebvre DA, Giaid A, Zingg HH: Expression of the oxytocin gene in rat placenta. Endocrinology 130:1185–1192, 1992.

71. Falin LI: The development of human hypophysis and differentiation of cells of the anterior lobe during embryonic life. Acta Anat (Basel) 44:188–205, 1961.

72. Conklin JL: The development of the human fetal adenohypophysis. Anat Rec 110:79–91, 1968.

73. Kaplan SL, Grumbach MM, Aubert ML: The ontogenesis of pituitary hormones and hypothalamic factors in the human fetus: Maturation of central nervous system regulation of anterior pituitary function. Recent Prog Horm Res 32:111–243, 1976.

74. Gluckman PD, Grumbach MM, Kaplan SL: The neuroendocrine regulation and function of growth hormone and prolactin in the mammalian fetus. Endocr Rev 4:363–395, 1981.

75. Levina SE: Endocrine features in development of human hypothalamus, hypophysis and placenta. Gen Comp Endocrinol 11:151–159, 1968.

76. Fukuchi M, Inoe T, Abe H, Kumahara Y: Thyrotropin in human fetal pituitaries. J Clin Endocrinol Metab 31:565–569, 1970.

77. Pavlova EB, Pronina TS, Skebelskaya YB: Histostructure of adenohypophysis of human fetuses and contents of somatotropic and adrenocorticotropic hormones. Gen Comp Endocrinol 10:269–276, 1968.

78. Allen JP, Cook DM, Kendall JM, McGilvra R: Maternal-fetal ACTH relationship in man. J Clin Endocrinol Metab 37:230–234, 1973.

79. Winters AJ, Oliver C, Colston C, et al: Plasma ACTH levels in the human fetus and neonate as related to age and parturition. J Clin Endocrinol Metab 39:269–273, 1974.

80. Winter JSD: Fetal and neonatal adrenocortical physiology. In Polin RA, Fox WW (eds): Fetal and Neonatal Physiology. Philadelphia, WB Saunders Co, 1992, pp 1829–1841.

81. Gray ES, Abramovitch DR: Morphologic features of the anencephalic adrenal gland in early pregnancy. Am J Obstet Gynecol 137:491–495, 1980.

82. Walsh SW, Norman RL, Novy MJ: In utero regulation of rhesus monkey fetal adrenals: Effect of dexamethasone, adrenocorticotropin, thyrotropin-releasing hormone, prolactin, human chorionic gonadotropin, and α-melanocyte-stimulating hormone on fetal and maternal plasma steroids. Endocrinology 104:1805–1813, 1979.

83. Thomson M, Smith R: The action of hypothalamic and placental corticotropin releasing factor on the corticotrope. Mol Cell Endocrinol 62:1–12, 1989.

84. Rivier C, Vale W: Neuroendocrine interaction between corticotropin releasing factor and vasopressin on adrenocorticotropic hormone secretion in the rat. In Schrier RW (ed): Vasopressin. New York, Raven Press, 1985, pp 181–188.

85. Al-Damluji S: Adrenergic mechanisms in the control of corticotropin secretion. J Endocrinol 119:5–14, 1988.

86. Polk DH, Ervin MG, Padbury JF, et al: Epidermal growth factor acts as a corticotropin-releasing factor in chronically catheterized fetal lamb. J Clin Invest 79:984–988, 1987.

87. Dorr HG, Versmold HT, Sippell WG, et al: Antenatal betamethasone therapy: Effects on maternal, fetal and neonatal mineralocorticoid, glucocorticoids and progestins. J Pediatr 108:990–993, 1986.

88. Wilson D, Baldwin R, Ariagno R: A randomized, placebo-controlled trial of dexamethasone on the hypothalamic pituitary adrenal axis in preterm infants. J Pediatr 113:764–768, 1988.

89. Yang K, Jones SA, Challis JRG: Changes in glucocorticoid receptor number in the hypothalamus of the sheep fetus with gestational age and after adrenocorticotropin treatment. Endocrinology 123:1307–1313, 1990.

90. Nelson HP, Kuhn RW, Deyman ME, Jaffe RB: Human fetal adrenal definitive and fetal zone metabolism of pregnenolone and corticosterone: Alternative biosynthetic pathways and absence of detectable aldosterone synthesis. J Clin Endocrinol Metab 70:693–698, 1990.

91. Carr BR, Simpson ER: De novo synthesis of cholesterol by human fetal adrenal gland. Endocrinology 108:2154–2162, 1981.

92. Carr BR, Ohashi M, Simpson ER: Low-density lipoprotein binding and de novo synthesis of cholesterol in the neocortex and fetal zones of the human fetal adrenal gland. Endocrinology 110:1994–1998, 1982.

93. Ballard PL: Glucocorticoids and differentiation. In Baxter JD, Rousseau GG (eds): Monographs on Endocrinology, Vol 12: Glucocorticoid Action. Berlin, Springer-Verlag, 1979, pp 493–575.

94. Pavlik A, Buresova M: The neonatal cerebellum: The highest level of glucocorticoid receptors in the brain. Dev Brain Res 12:13–20, 1984.

95. Liggins GC: Adrenocortical-related maturational events in the fetus. Am J Obstet Gynecol 126:931–941, 1976.

96. Fisher DA: The unique endocrine milieu of the fetus. J Clin Invest 78:603–611, 1986.

97. Beitens IZ, Graham GG, Kowarski J, Migeon CJ: Adrenal function in normal infants and in marasmus and kwashiorkor: Plasma aldosterone concentration and aldosterone secretion rate. J Pediatr 84:444–451, 1974.

98. Siegel SR, Fisher DA: Ontogeny of the renin-angiotensin-aldosterone system in the fetal and newborn lamb. Pediatr Res 14:99–102, 1980.

99. Wilson JD: Sexual differentiation. Annu Rev Physiol 40:279–306, 1978.

100. Pelliniemi LJ, Dym M: The fetal gonad and sexual differentiation. In Tulchinsky D, Ryan KJ (eds): Maternal-Fetal Endocrinology. Philadelphia, WB Saunders Co, 1980, pp 252–280.

101. Josso N: Antimüllerian hormone and intersex states. Trends Endocrinol 2:227–233, 1991.

102. Kuroda T, Lee MM, Ragin RC, et al: Müllerian inhibiting substance production and cleavage is modulated by gonadotropins and steroids. Endocrinology 129:2985–2992, 1991.

103. Behringer RR, Cote RL, Frochik GJ, et al: Abnormal sexual development in transgenic mice chronically expressing müllerian inhibiting substance. Nature 345:167–170, 1990.

104. Barraclough CA, Gorski RA: Evidence that the hypothalamus is responsible for androgen-induced sterility in the female rat. Endocrinology 68:68–79, 1961.

105. Naftolin F, Brawer JB: The effect of estrogens on hypothalamic structure and function. Am J Obstet Gynecol 132:758–765, 1978.

106. Sholl SA, Gay RW, Kin KL: 5α-Reductase, aromatase and androgen receptor levels in the monkey brain during fetal development. Endocrinology 124:627–634, 1989.

107. Polk DH, Fisher DA: Fetal and neonatal thyroid physiology. In Polin RA, Fox WW (eds): Fetal and Neonatal Physiology. Philadelphia, WB Saunders Co, 1992, pp 1842–1850.

108. Polk D, Cheromcha D, Reviczky A, Fisher DA: Nuclear thyroid hormone receptors: Ontogeny and thyroid hormone effects in sheep. Am J Physiol 256:E543–E549, 1989.

109. Artman HG, Leake RD, Weitzman RE, et al: Radioimmunoassay of vasotocin, vasopressin and oxytocin in human neonatal cerebrospinal and amniotic fluid. Dev Pharmacol Ther 7:39–49, 1984.

110. Fisher DA: Maternal fetal neurohypophyseal system. Clin Perinatol 10:695–708, 1983.

111. Ervin MG, Leake RD, Ross MG, et al: Arginine vasotocin in ovine maternal and fetal blood, fetal urine, and amniotic fluid. J Clin Invest 75:1696–1701, 1985.

112. Perks AM: Developmental and evolutionary aspects of the neurohypophysis. Am Zool 17:833–849, 1977.

113. Stegner H, Leake RD, Palmer SM, et al: The effect of hypoxia on neurohypophyseal hormone release in fetal and maternal sheep. Pediatr Res 18:188–191, 1984.

114. Fisher DA, Pyle HR Jr, Porter JC, Panos TC: Control of water balance in the newborn. Am J Dis Child 106:137–146, 1963.

115. Hadeed AJ, Leake RD, Weitzman RE, Fisher DA: Possible mechanism of high blood levels of vasopressin during the neonatal period. J Pediatr 94:805–808, 1979.

116. DeVane GW, Porter JC: An apparent stress-induced release of arginine vasopressin in human neonates. J Clin Endocrinol Metab 51:1412–1416, 1980.

117. Leake RD, Weitzman RE, Fisher DA: Oxytocin concentrations during the neonatal period. Biol Neonate 39:127–131, 1981.

118. Kelly RT, Rose JC, Meis PJ, et al: Vasopressin is important for restoring cardiovascular homeostasis in fetal lambs subjected to hemorrhage. Am J Obstet Gynecol 146:807–812, 1983.

119. Jones CT, Ritchie JW: The effects of adrenergic blockade on fetal response to hypoxia. J Dev Physiol 5:211–222, 1983.

120. Norman LJ, Challis JRG: Dose-dependent effects of arginine vasopressin on endocrine and blood gas responses on fetal sheep during the last third of pregnancy. Can J Physiol Pharmacol 65:2291–2296, 1987.

121. Brooks AN, White A: Activation of pituitary adrenal function in fetal sheep by corticotropin-releasing factor and arginine vasopressin. J Endocrinol 124:27–35, 1990.

122. Norman LJ, Challis JRG: Synergism between systemic corticotropin-releasing factor and arginine vasopressin on adrenocorticotropin release in vivo varies as a function of gestational age in the ovine fetus. Endocrinology 120:1052–1058, 1987.

123. Ervin MG, Ross MG, Leake RD, Fisher DA: Changes in steady state plasma arginine vasotocin levels affect ovine fetal renal and cardiovascular function. Endocrinology 118:759–765, 1986.

124. Ross MG, Ervin MG, Leake RD, et al: Fetal lung fluid regulation by neuropeptides. Am J Obstet Gynecol 150:421–425, 1984.

125. Coupland RE, Kent C, Kent SE: Normal function of extra-adrenal

chromaffin tissues in the young rabbit and guinea pig. J Endocrinol 92:433–442, 1982.

126. Padbury JF, Diakomanoles ES, Lam RW, Fisher DA: Ontogenesis of tissue catecholamines in fetal and neonatal rabbits. J Dev Physiol 3:297–303, 1981.
127. Bohn MC, Goldstein M, Black IB: Role of glucocorticoids in expression of the adrenergic phenotype in rat embryonic adrenal gland. Dev Biol 82:1–10, 1981.
128. Slotkin TA, Seidler FJ: Adrenomedullary catecholamine release in the fetus and newborn: Secretory mechanisms and their role in stress and survival. J Dev Physiol 10:1–6, 1988.
129. Padbury JF: Functional maturation of the adrenal medulla and peripheral sympathetic nervous system. Baillieres Clin Endocrinol Metab 33:689–705, 1989.
130. Harwell C, Padbury JF, Anand RS, et al: Fetal catecholamine responses to maternal hypoglycemia. Am J Physiol 259:1126–1130, 1990.
131. Padbury JF, Martinez AM: Sympathoadrenal system activity at birth: Integration of postnatal adaptation. Semin Perinatol 12:163–172, 1988.
132. Newnham JP, Marshall CJ, Padbury FJ, et al: Fetal catecholamine release with preterm delivery. Am J Obstet Gynecol 149:888–893, 1984.
133. Liu HM, Potter EL: Development of the human pancreas. Arch Pathol 74:439–452, 1962.
134. Hay WW Jr, Meznarich HK: The effect of hyperinsulinemia on glucose utilization and oxidation and oxygen consumption in the fetal lamb. Q J Exp Physiol 71:689–698, 1986.
135. Menon RK, Sperling MA: Carbohydrate metabolism. Semin Perinatol 12:157–162, 1988.
136. Girard J: Control of fetal and neonatal glucose metabolism by pancreatic hormones. Ballieres Clin Endocrinol Metab 3:817–836, 1989.
137. Hay WW Jr, Sparks JW, Wilkening RB, et al: Fetal glucose uptake and utilization as functions of maternal glucose concentrations. Am J Physiol 246:E237–242, 1984.
138. Granner D, Andreone T, Sasaki K, Beale E: Inhibition of transcription of the phosphenol pyruvate carboxykinase gene by insulin. Nature 305:549–551, 1983.
139. Frazer TE, Karl IE, Hillman LS, Bier D: Direct measurement of gluconeogenesis from $(2,3-^{13}C_2)$-alanine in the human neonate. Am J Physiol 240:E615–E621, 1981.
140. Schedewie HK, Fisher DA: Perinatal mineral homeostasis. In Tulchinsky D, Ryan KJ (eds): Maternal Fetal Endocrinology. Philadelphia, WB Saunders Co, 1980, pp 355–386.
141. Wolfe HJ, DeLellis RA, Voelkel EF, Tashjian AH Jr: Distribution of calcitonin containing cells in the normal neonatal human thyroid gland: A correlation of morphology and peptide content. J Clin Endocrinol Metab 41:1076–1081, 1975.
142. Scotthorne RJ: Functional capacity of the fetal parathyroid glands with reference to their clinical use as homografts. Ann NY Acad Sci 120:669–676, 1964.
143. David L, Anast CS: Calcium metabolism in newborn infants. J Clin Invest 54:287–296, 1974.
144. Samaan NA, Anderson GD, Adam-Mayne ME: Immunoreactive calcitonin in the mother, neonate, child, and adult. Am J Obstet Gynecol 121:622–625, 1975.
145. Bouillon R, Van Assche FA: Perinatal vitamin D metabolism. Dev Pharmacol Ther 4(Suppl 1):38–44, 1982.
146. Smith GH Jr, Alexander DP, Buckle RM, et al: Parathyroid hormone in fetal and adult sheep: The effect of hypocalcemia. J Endocrinol 53:339–348, 1972.
147. Littledike ET, Arnaud CD, Whipp SC: Calcitonin secretion in ovine, porcine and bovine fetuses. Proc Exp Biol Med 139:428–433, 1972.
148. Lafond J, Auger D, Fortier J, Brunette MG: Parathyroid hormone receptor in human placental syncytiotrophoblast brush border and basal plasma membranes. Endocrinology 123:2834–2840, 1988.
149. Ross R, Halbert K, Tsang RC: Determination of the production and metabolic clearance rates of 1,25-dihydroxy vitamin D_3 in the pregnant sheep and its chronically catheterized fetus by primed infusion technique. Pediatr Res 26:633–638, 1989.
150. Baggia S, Albrecht ED, Babischkin S, Pepe GJ: Interconversion of cortisol and cortisone in baboon trophoblast and decidua cells in culture. Endocrinology 127:1735–1741, 1990.
151. Murphy BEP: Cortisol and cortisone in human fetal development. J Steroid Biochem 11:509–513, 1979.
152. Fisher DA, Polk DH: Development of the thyroid. Baillieres Clin Endocrinol Metab 3:627–657, 1989.
153. Wu SY, Polk D, Wong S, et al: Thyroxine sulfate (T_4S) is a major

thyroid hormone metabolite and a potential intermediate in the monodeiodination pathways on fetal sheep. Endocrinology 131:1751–1756, 1992.
154. Hill DJ, Freemark M, Strain AH, et al: Placental lactogen and growth hormone receptors in human fetal tissues: Relationship to fetal plasma hPL concentrations and fetal growth. J Clin Endocrinol Metab 66:1283–1290, 1988.
155. Padbury JF, Klein AH, Polk DH, et al: The effect of thyroid status on lung and heart beta adrenergic receptors in fetal and newborn sheep. Dev Pharmacol Ther 9:44–53, 1986.
156. Yamashita S, Newbold RR, McLachlan JA, Korach K: Developmental pattern of estrogen receptor expression in female mouse genital tracts. Endocrinology 125:2888–2896, 1989.
157. Fisher DA: Endocrinology of fetal development. In Wilson J, Foster D (eds): Textbook of Endocrinology. Philadelphia, WB Saunders Co, 1991, pp 1049–1077.
158. D'Ercole AJ: The insulin-like growth factors and fetal growth. In Spencer EM (ed): Modern Concepts of Insulin-Like Growth Factors. New York, Elsevier, 1991, pp 9–24.
159. Wang HS, Chard T: The role of insulin-like growth factor I and insulin-like growth factor binding protein I in the control of fetal growth. J Endocrinol 132:11–19, 1992.
160. Spaventi R, Antica M, Pavelic K: Insulin and insulin-like growth factors I (IGF-I) in early mouse embryogenesis. Development 108:491–495, 1990.
161. D'Ercole AJ, Applewhite GT, Underwood LE: Evidence that somatomedins are synthesized by multiple tissues in the fetus. Dev Biol 75:315–318, 1980.
162. Han VKM, D'Ercole AJ, Lung PK: Identification of somatomedin (insulin-like growth factor) messenger RNA in the human fetus. Pediatr Res 22:245–249, 1987.
163. Bennett A, Wilson D, Liu F, Nagashima R, et al: Levels of insulin-like growth factors I and II in human cord blood. J Clin Endocrinol Metab 57:609–612, 1983.
164. Freemark M, Comer M: Purification of a distinct placental lactogen receptor, a new member of the growth hormone/prolactin receptor family. J Clin Invest 83:883–889, 1989.
165. Hill DJ, Crace CJ, Strain AJ, Milner RDG: Regulation of amino acid uptake and deoxyribonucleic acid synthesis in isolated human fetal fibroblasts and myoblasts: Effects of human placental lactogen, somatomedin-C, multiplication stimulating activity, and insulin. J Clin Endocrinol Metab 62:753–760, 1986.
166. Hill DJ, Milner RDG: Insulin as a growth factor. Pediatr Res 19:879–886, 1985.
167. Pilistine SJ, Moses AC, Munro HN: Placental lactogen administration reverses the effect of low protein diet on maternal and fetal somatomedin levels in the pregnant rat. Proc Natl Acad Sci USA 81:5853–5857, 1984.
168. Johnson JW, Mitzner W, Beck JC, et al: Long-term effects of betamethasone in fetal development. Am J Obstet Gynecol 141:1053–1064, 1981.
169. Susa JB, McCormick KL, Widness JA, et al: Chronic hyperinsulinemia in the fetal rhesus monkey: Effects on fetal growth and composition. Diabetes 28:1058–1063, 1979.
170. Carpenter G, Cohen S: Epidermal growth factor. Annu Rev Biochem 48:193–216, 1979.
171. Fisher DA, Lakshmanan J: Metabolism and effects of EGF and related growth factors in mammals. Endocr Rev 11:418–442, 1990.
172. Thorburn GD, Waterns MJ, Young IR: Epidermal growth factor: A critical factor in fetal maturation? CIBA Found Symp 86:172–198, 1981.
173. Tsutumi O, Oka T: Epidermal growth factor deficiency during pregnancy causes abortion in mice. Am J Obstet Gynecol 156:241–244, 1987.
174. Adamson ED, Meek J: Epidermal growth factor receptors during mouse development. Dev Biol 103:62–70, 1984.
175. Adamson ED, Deller MJ, Warshaw JB: Functional EGF receptors are present in mouse embryonal tissues. Nature 291:656–659, 1981.
176. Gubits RM, Shaw PA, Gresik EW, et al: Epidermal growth factor gene expression is regulated differently in mouse kidney and submandibular gland. Endocrinology 119:1382–1387, 1986.
177. Snead ML, Luo W, Oliver P, et al: Localization of epidermal growth factor precursor in tooth and lung during embryonic mouse development. Dev Biol 134:420–429, 1989.
178. Brown PI, Lam R, Lakshmanan J, Fisher DA: Transforming growth factor alpha in the developing rat. Am J Physiol 259:E256–E260, 1990.
179. Freemark M, Comer M: Epidermal growth factor-like transforming

growth factor (TGF) activity and EGF receptors in ovine fetal tissues: Possible role for TGF in ovine fetal development. Pediatr Res 22:609–615, 1987.

180. Sieff CA: Hematopoietic growth factors. J Clin Invest 79:1549–1557, 1987.

181. Zanjani ED, Ascensau JL, McGlave PG: Studies on the liver to kidney switch of erythropoietin production. J Clin Invest 67:1183–1188, 1981.

182. Eckardt KU, Ratcliffe PJ, Tan CC, et al: Age dependent expression of the erythropoietin gene in rat liver and kidneys. J Clin Invest 89:753–760, 1992.

183. Liu L, Nicoll CS: Evidence for a role of basic fibroblast growth factor in rat embryonic growth and differentiation. Endocrinology 123:2027–2031, 1988.

184. Gospodarowicz D: Epidermal and nerve growth factors in mammalian development. Annu Rev Physiol 43:251–263, 1981.

185. Levi-Montalcini R, Angeletti PU: Nerve growth factor. Annu Rev Physiol 48:534–569, 1968.

186. Gorin PD, Johnson EM: Effects of exposure to nerve growth factor antibodies on the developing nervous system of the rat—an experimental autoimmune approach. Dev Biol 80:313–323, 1980.

187. Padbury JF, Lam RW, Polk DH, et al: Autoimmune sympathectomy in fetal rabbits. J Dev Physiol 8:369–376, 1986.

188. Tarris RH, Weichsel ME Jr, Fisher DA: Synthesis and secretion of a nerve growth stimulating factor by neonatal mouse astrocyte cells in vitro. Pediatr Res 20:367–372, 1986.

189. Hammerman MR, Rogers SA, Ryan G: Growth factors and metanephrogenesis. Am J Physiol 262:523–532, 1991.

190. Padbury JF, Agata Y, Ludlow J, et al: Effect of fetal adrenalectomy on catecholamine release and physiologic adaptation at birth in sheep. J Clin Invest 80:1096–1103, 1987.

191. Ballard P: Hormonal control of lung maturation. Ballieres Clin Endocrinol Metab 3:723–753, 1989.

192. Birk E, Iwamoto HS, Heymann M: Hormonal effects on circulating changes during the perinatal period. Ballieres Clin Endocrinol Metab 3:795–815, 1989.

193. Ballard RA: Antenatal glucocorticoid therapy: Clinical effects. Monogr Endocrinol 28:137–172, 1986.

194. Challis JRG, Hooper S: Birth: Outcome of a positive cascade. Ballieres Clin Endocrinol Metab 3:781–793, 1989.

195. Polk DH: Thyroid hormone effects on neonatal thermogenesis. Semin Perinatal 12:151–156, 1988.

196. Wu SY, Polk DH, Fisher DA: Biochemical and ontogenic characterization of thyroxine 5′-monodeiodinase in brown adipose tissue from fetal and newborn lambs. Endocrinology 118:1334–1339, 1986.

197. Polk DH, Callegari CC, Newnham J, et al: Effect of fetal thyroidectomy on newborn thermogenesis in lambs. Pediatr Res 21:453–457, 1987.

198. Gunn TR, Gluckman PD: The endocrine control of the onset of thermogenesis at birth. Ballieres Clin Endocrinol Metab 3:869–886, 1989.

199. Gluckman PD, Grumbach MM, Kaplan SL: The neuroendocrine regulation and function of growth hormone and prolactin in the mammalian fetus. Endocr Rev 2:363–395, 1981.

200. deZegher F, Daaboul J, Grumbach MM, Kaplan SL: Hormone ontogeny in the ovine fetus and neonate: XXII. The effect of somatostatin on the growth hormone response to growth hormone releasing factor. Endocrinology 124:1114–1117, 1989.

128

Metabolic Aspects of Fuel Homeostasis in the Fetus and the Neonate

DOMINIQUE DARMAUN
MOREY W. HAYMOND
DENNIS M. BIER

During the transition from intrauterine to extrauterine life, a variety of metabolic changes and adaptations occur in fuel homeostasis. These adaptations allow the fetus to convert from a state of total dependence on maternal fuel sources delivered intravenously to a state in which it must rely on alimentation and endogenous substrate supplies to maintain normal cellular function and growth.

This chapter will deal with (1) placental substrate transport and fetal fuel storage, (2) the development of certain key enzymatic and hormonal systems that modulate substrate mobilization, interconversion, and utilization, and (3) how defects in normal development of these systems may result in pathology. We recognize that a variety of inborn errors in metabolism (synthetic and catabolic disorders of amino acids, glycoproteins, and lipids) may affect fuel homeostasis, but it is beyond the scope of this chapter to consider this material in detail. Since the most common consequence of abnormalities in fuel regulation in the neonatal period is hypoglycemia, primary attention will be given to factors affecting glucose homeostasis. Several reviews of these topics have been published recently, and we would recommend them to the interested reader.[1–8]

PLACENTAL TRANSPORT OF METABOLIC FUELS AND NUTRIENTS

The placenta is no longer considered solely as an organ of transfer. Besides its endocrine functions (reviewed in Ch. 124), it is involved in both the transport and metabolism of nutrients.

The structure and functions of the placenta have many similarities with those of the small intestine: the trophoblast comprises a polarized epithelium, with a microvillous apical membrane on the maternal side and a basolateral membrane on the fetal side. In addition, the placenta is active in the metabolism of carbohydrate, fat, and amino acids. Its oxygen consumption is as high as that of liver or brain.[7]

Normal fetal growth and development are wholly dependent on the placenta for respiration, nutrition, and excretion. Unless the transplacental lifeline to the fetus can be established early and effectively maintained, pregnancy will terminate with absorption or expulsion of the embryo. Numerous substances are transferred from the maternal to the fetal circulation, and with regard to all aspects of energy metabolism, the fetus is solely dependent on maternal sources. Physiological or pathological abnormalities inherent within the mother, fetus, or placenta may act to limit the availability of various substances for normal fetal development, which, in turn, results in fetal wastage or neonatal defects. Since placental transport is intimately involved with normal fetal metabolism and development, selected aspects of this process will be considered briefly. For additional aspects of placental transport, the interested reader is referred to papers addressing the mechanisms of transport,[7] transport of gases,[13-16] water, and electrolytes[17-20] and to the excellent reviews by Longo,[9] Hay,[7] and Smith et al.[10]

Amino Acids, Polypeptides, and Proteins

It is well established that the free alpha amino nitrogen concentration is higher in fetal than in maternal extra- and intracellular fluids in pregnant women, rhesus monkeys, sheep, rodents, and dogs, and it has been shown that each individual amino acid contributes differently to the high fetal/maternal ratio. The normal fetal/maternal alpha amino nitrogen ratio varies from about 1.2 to 5.0, with a mean of 1.8 in humans.[21] Amino acid transport across the placenta has all the characteristics of active transport, including (1) competition among certain amino acids such as histidine and glycine, (2) saturation at high concentrations of amino acids, (3) inhibition of transport by metabolic inhibitors, and (4) finally, amino acid uptake from the maternal plasma against a concentration gradient into the intracellular matrix of the trophoblast. From the trophoblast to fetal plasma, amino acid transfer then occurs following a decreasing concentration gradient. The transport draws its energy from Na^+, K^+-ATPase for Na^+- and H^+-dependent transport.[7] This subject has been reviewed recently.[10, 21] Several amino acid transport systems have been identified in the placenta.[7-10] These systems seem to be regulated through changes in the synthesis rates of the transporters to maintain optimal amino acid transfer; thus it was found in rats that even when prolonged hypoaminoacidemia is maintained in the mother, fetal amino acid concentrations are preserved.[22] In the ovine placental unit, there is net transfer of basic and neutral amino acids to the fetus but a net flux of the acidic amino acid glutamate from the fetus to the placenta.[23, 24] In fetal sheep, placental-fetal interorgan cycling has been documented for glutamine, asparagine, and glycine. These three amino acids are taken up by the fetal liver, while glutamate, aspartate, and serine (i.e., their respective metabolic products) are released by fetal liver and taken up by the placenta.[25] Recent tracer studies performed in fetal sheep showed that both the placenta and the fetus deaminate leucine to its ketoacid ketoisocaproate (KIC), yet the fetus was the main site of ultimate decarboxylation of KIC, since 20 per cent of the infused leucine load was converted to CO_2 within the fetus.[26] Maternal fasting results in a sig-

nificant reduction in the fetal uptake of essential amino acids.[27]

Placental transfer of the polypeptide hormones is considered in detail in Chapter 124. Polypeptides cross the placenta poorly, if at all, and for all practical purposes, the fetus is dependent on its own production and secretion of these compounds. The majority of evidence is consistent with a placental barrier to the transport of the two polypeptides of major interest in this chapter—insulin[28] and glucagon.[29] Transplacental passage of antibody-bound insulin has been observed, however, in fetuses of insulin-dependent diabetic mothers with high titers of anti-insulin antibodies.[30] Although albumin, 7S gamma globulin, 19S macroglobulin, fibrinogen, transferrin, and acid glycoproteins have been demonstrated to cross the placenta by pinocytosis, the fetus probably synthesizes the vast majority of its structural and enzymatic proteins from amino acids derived from the maternal circulation.[9]

Lipid Transport

Placental transport of lipids (Fig. 128–1) has been reviewed by Robertson and Sprecher[31] and discussed in detail by others.[1, 32-38] Fetal fat is the product of synthesis from carbohydrate and acetate and from free fatty acids (FFA's) transferred across the placenta. Fatty acids transferred from maternal blood contribute approximately 50 per cent of the total fetal fatty acid requirements.[38] Free fatty acids exchange rapidly across the placenta by simple diffusion.[34, 35]

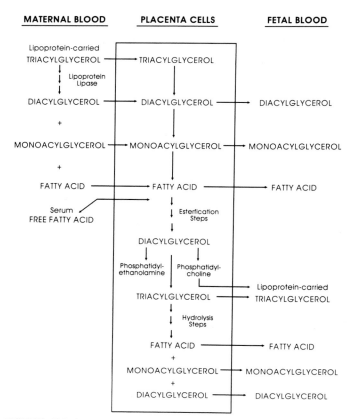

FIGURE 128–1. Possible routes of lipid transport across the placenta. (Adapted from Coleman RA: Placental metabolism and transport of lipid. Fed Proc 45:2519, 1986.)

Their rate of transfer depends on the transplacental fatty acid concentration gradient; accordingly, increases in the circulating levels of fatty acids in maternal blood result in enhanced fat incorporation into fetal rodents.[38] Since non-esterified fatty acids are carried by albumin, fetal albumin concentration may be a limiting factor for the rate of transplacental fatty acid transfer.[38] In a study of 26 healthy women and infants at parturition, it was found that the fetal uptake of several essential fatty acids, as calculated from whole-blood fatty acid concentrations, largely exceeds the uptake based on measurement of concentrations in plasma alone, suggesting that red blood cells may participate in the transport of essential FFA into the fetus.[36] There appears to be no difference in the total amount of fatty acid transferred regardless of degree of saturation, carbon chain length, or whether the fatty acid is given singly or in combination with other fatty acids in studies utilizing the perfused guinea pig placenta.[34] In the human placenta, however, short- and medium-chain fatty acids are transferred faster than long-chain fatty acids.[38] Complex lipids such as triacylglycerol do not cross the placenta. The placenta has, however, a high lipoprotein lipase activity so that fatty acids carried by maternal lipoprotein can be transferred to the fetus. This could explain the observation that the fatty acids from a complex mixture of triglycerides (Intralipid) could be detected in the fetal circulation or in cord venous blood when Intralipid is infused into pregnant rabbits or humans. The transit times for free (albumin-bound) ^{14}C-labeled palmitate and for ^{14}C-palmitate incorporated in a triacylglycerol were compared in pregnant guinea pigs; although both tracers appeared in the fetal circulation, the lag time was longer for the labeled triglyceride.[32] Other studies suggest that transport of triglyceride fatty acids into fetal blood involves hydrolysis, re-esterification followed by subsequent hydrolysis, and finally, release of FFA into fetal blood.[32]

Unlike FFA, very little or no direct transport of complex lipids (e.g., cholesterol, phospholipids, or triglycerides) occurs across the guinea pig placenta,[34] while maternal cholesterol accounts for only 10 to 20 per cent of the total fetal cholesterol pool in the fetal rat.[39] The placental transfer of cholesterol is thought to contribute around 40 to 50 per cent of fetal cholesterol in primates,[40] and uptake and degradation of low- and high-density lipoprotein has indeed been documented in cultured human trophoblast.[41] Fetal plasma cholesterol concentrations are lower than those of the mothers. This is considered to be related to the low β-lipoprotein content of fetal plasma. In contrast, α-lipoprotein content is the same in both maternal and fetal blood.[42] The cause of the low fetal β-lipoprotein could be a result of placental impermeability or of catabolism of the β-lipoprotein–cholesterol complex. Although ketone bodies are not considered significant fuels for the fetus, the placenta appears more permeable to β-hydroxybutyrate in the baboon and in humans than in the sheep, since the maternal/fetal ratio of β-hydroxybutyrate is approximately 2 in the former versus more than 4 to 5 in the latter.[43] Acute hyperketonemia, whether induced by maternal starvation or by infusion of β-hydroxybutyrate in fed pregnant rats, decreases the rate of glucose utilization in most tissues of fetal rats, implying that ketone bodies affect glucose metabolism in the fetus.[44]

As considered in Chapters 124 and 127, estrogens, progesterone, and cortisol readily cross the placenta. Besides transport of steroid hormones, the placenta enzymatically alters steroid structure as well, and such alteration may play a major role in the transport process. The placenta also converts inactive steroid precursors (i.e., cholesterol, pregnenolone, and dehydroepiandrosterone) to progesterone and estrogen.

Carbohydrate Transport

Glucose is the principal fetal fuel, although not the sole fuel source of the fetus, as previously thought. Fetal glucose uptake is a function of the maternal plasma glucose concentration.[45] In a variety of species, the maternal-to-fetal transfer approximates 4 to 7 mg glucose/min/kg of fetal weight.[5–8, 46] In a 3-kg human fetus at term, this would amount to about 25 g glucose daily and would yield only 33 kcal/kg of body weight per day if completely oxidized. Thus glucose could account for only approximately 60 per cent of the minimal or basal energy requirements of a nongrowing term fetus in a thermoneutral environment but only about one-quarter to one-third the necessary energy for growth and development.[47] While adult kidney and intestine may concentrate glucose against a concentration gradient and possess an active sodium-glucose co-transporter, the placenta lacks this ability. Recent publications[48–51] support previous articles[52–55] which strongly suggest that the mechanism by which the placental transport of glucose occurs is facilitated diffusion, which is now known to be mediated by glucose transporters.

Besides the *active* sodium-glucose transporters described in kidney and intestine, five *facilitative* glucose transporters (GLUT-1 through GLUT-5) have been described in adult human tissues. GLUT-1 is especially abundant in red cells and is not insulin-responsive; in contrast, GLUT-4 predominates in fat and muscle, two insulin-sensitive tissues. The majority of fetal tissues express mostly GLUT-1 and are less sensitive to insulin than the corresponding adult tissues; expression of GLUT-4 only increases after birth to reach adult levels after weaning.[48]

Placental glucose transporters are present on both the maternal-facing microvillous membrane and the basolateral fetal-facing side of the trophoblast. Although insulin receptors have been found on the maternal side, the uptake of glucose is found to be insensitive to insulin (0 to 1200 μU/ml) in the human placenta perfused in vitro.[49] It has been demonstrated recently that the insulin-independent GLUT-1 and GLUT-3 systems are the predominant glucose transporters in placenta.[48]

In contrast, when *fetal* insulin deficiency was produced in vivo by streptozotocin injection into near-term fetal sheep, a marked rise (approximately 50 per cent) in fetal blood glucose and a 66 per cent reduction in umbilical glucose uptake were observed; this suggests that the normal fetal insulin concentration *indirectly* determines net umbilical glucose uptake by regulating fetal glucose concentration[51] and thus maternal-fetal glucose transfer.

Maternal and fetal glucose concentrations are similar in early gestation.[28, 45] At term, a concentration gradient across the placenta from maternal artery to umbilical vein of about 10 to 30 per cent has been observed repeatedly. The variability in this gradient is most likely related to the stress of delivery and may reflect the net result of increased glucose utilization by the fetus and the release of glucose from fetal hepatic glycogen stores.

The placenta synthesizes large amounts of glycogen from maternal glucose. The role, if any, of this glycogen in transport and metabolism of glucose is unknown. Placental glycogen concentration changes during pregnancy and is highest at 8 weeks. This gradually declines until 18 to 20 weeks and is maintained at a level of 15 to 20 mg/100 mg dry weight until term. There is a continuous exchange between maternal glucose, placental glycogen, and fetal glucose.[56] At the present time, there is no clear explanation for either the role or the necessity of placental glycogen in the face of normal concentrations of maternal blood glucose. However, in situations of substrate limitation to the fetus, such as those secondary to hypoxia, fetal hepatic glycogen may be an important energy reserve, since the fetal liver is capable of augmented glycogenolysis under these circumstances.[16]

In human fetal blood, a small amount of fructose (5 mg/100 ml) is present. Fetal fructose is produced by the placenta from glucose.[57] In sheep, although maternal levels of fructose are low, the fetal and newborn lamb have high plasma levels which disappear slowly after birth. Since the placenta of ungulates contains only small amounts of glycogen, it has been suggested that this may be an important reserve nutrient for these species,[56] although fructose is oxidized at 20 per cent the rate of glucose in fetal sheep.[8]

Contribution of Transported Substrates to Fetal Energy Metabolism

It has become increasingly clear that glucose is not the sole fetal fuel source, as had been believed previously. In carefully studied, unstressed fetal lambs, the respiratory quotient of the fetal lamb is significantly less than 1.0,[3, 58, 59] and glucose oxidation could account for only about half of total fetal oxygen consumption. Furthermore, in this species, the contribution of glucose to total oxygen consumption declines with gestational age[58] and maternal starvation.[60] In humans, obviously, data are less firm. However, the human umbilical glucose/oxygen quotient is about 0.8,[61] an observation in general agreement with the ovine data, which suggests that the human fetus, too, is not solely dependent on glucose for its energy requirements.

Further, Battaglia and co-workers[45, 62] and Char and Creasy[63] have shown that lactate is quantitatively second to glucose as a fetal fuel source and that lactate oxidation accounts for 20 to 25 per cent of total fetal oxygen consumption. Fisher, Heymann, and Rudolph[64] have confirmed that lactate is a major fuel source of the fetal lamb myocardium, but soon after birth, it becomes a minor fuel source.[65] The human placenta perfused in vitro also releases lactate from glucose metabolism.[7] Likewise, the ovine fetal liver, which is responsible for as much as 20 to 25 per cent of fetal oxygen consumption, takes up only a trivial amount of glucose.[15] Hepatic lactate uptake, on the other hand, accounts for most of the fetal-umbilical lactate uptake and suggests that lactate is a major hepatic fuel as well.

Amino acids provide the remaining 20 to 25 per cent of the fetal fuel,[66] while fructose, fatty acids, and glycerol account for negligible amounts of oxygen consumed by the ovine fetus. Intravenous infusion of [1-^{14}C]-leucine into fetal sheep revealed that under normal conditions, approximately half the leucine delivered to the fetus via the placenta is oxidized and half is utilized for protein synthesis.[67] Of the total substrate transported, 40 and 60 per cent of the carbon and nitrogen, respectively, are retained for growth. Of this, amino acids represent about 80 per cent of the total nitrogen and 55 per cent of the total carbon content of the fetus.[68] Although active fetal swallowing of amniotic fluid occurs and the intestinal transport systems for amino acids and glucose are present, the contribution of nutrients absorbed from the fetal gastrointestinal tract to fetal metabolism is considered negligible.[7] These data collectively underscore the importance of normal placental function, since alterations in the transport of a diverse group of substrates by a variety of mechanisms may have adverse effects on fetal growth and development.

DEVELOPMENT OF FETAL AND NEONATAL INSULIN AND GLUCAGON SECRETION

Growth and development of the fetus require a complex system of regulatory controls, and the fetal endocrine system becomes active in early fetal life (see Ch. 127). The role of some of these organs and their secretions in normal development is clear, while in other cases the hormones are known to be present in both fetal tissues and blood but there is only a limited knowledge of their function.[69] Further, it is not necessary to assume a priori that the presence of a hormone in utero dictates the same function or degree of activity observed for that hormone in the child or adult. For example, even though fetal and adult beta-adrenergic receptors appear identical, isoproterenol is a potent vasoconstrictor in the early avian embryo but is an inotropic agent with vasodilator activity in chicks or adult birds. Similarly, Jost and Jacquot[70] have demonstrated that animals deprived of growth hormone and thyroid-stimulating hormone by fetal decapitation grow normally in utero, and infants with hypothalamic or pituitary hypoplasia generally are of normal weight and length at birth.[71] Shortly after birth, however, deficiencies of pituitary function become obvious when the infant fails to grow and develop normally. Furthermore, it is not clear whether insulin and/or glucagon are absolutely necessary for maintenance of fetal glucose homeostasis or whether secretagogues controlling their release in utero are the same as in the adult. However, it is quite clear from observations in the infant of the diabetic mother and in the infant born with transient diabetes that postnatal control of insulin release must develop rapidly.

Fetal Pancreatic Insulin and Glucagon

Two successive generations of islets have been described in the developing human pancreas.[72, 73] The first generation, observed at the eighth week, grows out from solid cords of cells that will form the primitive pancreatic tubules; the second generation begins to develop at the third month of gestation and is formed from acinar cells or from cells of the pancreatic ductules. The first generation progressively involutes after the third month.

At 8 to 9 weeks' gestation beta cells and alpha$_1$ or alpha$_2$ cells, the latter containing glucagon, can be seen with the electron microscope and quantitated by immunofluorescence.[74] In fetal life, alpha cells are more numerous than beta cells, but the former reach their relative peak at midgestation.[74–76] Thereafter, the insulin/glucagon cell ratio increases three- to four-fold. Cells containing immunoreactive somatostatin and pancreatic polypeptide also can be identified as early as 8 to 10 weeks' gestation but constitute a minor fraction of islet cell mass. However, from midgestation until term, somatostatin cells are the second most abundant cell type after the beta cell. Total pancreatic insulin content increases during pregnancy from 6 ± 1 U/g between 20 and 32 weeks to 13 ± 3 U/g between 34 and 40 weeks as compared with 2.1 ± 0.3 U/g in the adult pancreas.[77]

Control of Fetal and Neonatal Insulin and Glucagon Secretion

Numerous studies of fetal plasma insulin responses to a glucose load have yielded conflicting results in the same as well as in different species. A combination of factors most likely accounts for the discrepant results: species differences, the type of infusion (i.e., acute or chronic), the route of administration (i.e., fetal versus maternal infusion), and the age of the fetus. These data have been reviewed in detail by others.[2, 78–80]

In vitro studies with cultured explants of rat fetal pancreas[81] and 12-week-old human pancreas[82] have demonstrated that glucose and tolbutamide are poor stimulators of insulin release. However, in the presence of caffeine, insulin secretion is markedly potentiated by both agents. Milner et al.,[83] utilizing incubated pancreatic pieces from human fetuses of 12 to 24 weeks' gestation, demonstrated that both glucose and tolbutamide were ineffective as insulin secretagogues, while agents considered to increase intracellular levels of 3',5',-cyclic adenosine monophosphate (i.e., glucagon, theophylline, and dibutyl–cyclic adenosine monophosphate) stimulated insulin release in the presence or absence of glucose. The amino acids leucine and arginine differed from glucose in that each stimulated insulin release alone; however, the pattern of release differed between the two: arginine consistently stimulated insulin release from the pancreas of larger fetuses (e.g., >200 g), whereas leucine was more effective in the pancreas of a fetus weighing less than 200 g. These data make it possible to speculate on the times in fetal life when different stimuli of insulin release become effective. At 12 to 14 weeks of gestation, the beta cell is capable of releasing insulin to substances that work via generation of cAMP either by stimulating plasma membrane adenyl cyclase (e.g., glucagon) or by increasing intracellular concentrations of this nucleotide through inhibition of phosphodiesterase (e.g., caffeine and theophylline). At this early stage in development, leucine also stimulates insulin release. At 18 to 20 weeks, arginine becomes an effective stimulus, but glucose does not result in significant insulin secretion until approximately the 24th week of fetal life.

Further insight into the decreased sensitivity of fetal beta cells to glucose was gained from recent studies. Postnatal (and adult) rat and human islets respond to glucose with a biphasic pattern: an initial insulin peak, thought to arise from closure of membrane K^+ channels, followed by a slow, sustained second phase, believed to be the result of the opening of the cell membrane Ca^{2+} channels, since the latter response is inhibited by verapamil, a Ca^{2+} channel blocker. In contrast, in 3-day prenatal rat islets and 17- to 20-week human fetal pancreas, glucose only elicits a monophasic response. This pattern is not specific for glucose (it is also observed for α-ketoisocaproate, another insulin secretagogue) nor due to defective metabolism of glucose. Incubation with quinine, a blocker of the K^+ channels, both potentiates insulin secretion and confers sensitivity to verapamil.[84, 85] Thus the lack of a biphasic response is not due to a lack of K^+ or Ca^{2+} channels in fetal islets but rather to a lack of coupling between glucose metabolism and closing of the K^+ channels.[86]

In agreement with the preceding in vitro studies are the observations obtained in the primate fetus near term which show that induction of fetal hyperglycemia is ineffective in elevating plasma insulin levels,[87] while glucagon injected directly into the fetus is associated with an increase.[88] Furthermore, theophylline, in concentrations that are ineffective alone in mediating insulin secretion, potentiates fetal insulin responses to glucagon and results in insulin secretion to glucose stimulation. Insulin secretion is also stimulated by the dibutyryl derivative of cAMP and tolbutamide. Following birth, the fetal pancreatic beta-cell responses rapidly change, and glucose becomes the primary secretagogue.[87, 88]

In premature newborns, both theophylline and glucagon[89] are potent insulinogenic secretagogues, whereas glucose alone has little or no effect.[90, 91] In contrast to glucose, administration of arginine[90] or a mixture of naturally occurring amino acids[91] results in insulin secretion. Both arginine and a mixture of amino acids in low concentrations, which individually have little or no effect on insulin release, act synergistically when administered in combination with glucose.

In the normal full-term human, several studies have shown that the fetal and newborn pancreas reacts only sluggishly, if at all, to hyperglycemia.[92–94] However, in a recent in vivo study, human newborns were challenged with glucose infusion rates of 8 or 16 mg/kg/min via the intravenous or the enteral route, respectively.[94] The responses of plasma insulin and the insulin/glucose ratio were higher when glucose was administered enterally than parenterally, although both groups achieved similar plasma glucose concentrations. This suggests that insulin secretion may be stimulated more effectively by enteral glucose, implying that the enteroinsular axis is functional in full-term newborn infants.[94] Intravenous glucose given to the mother during the second stage of labor results in maternal hyperglycemia, a rapid and appropriate rise in maternal plasma insulin (Fig. 128–2), and a fall in FFA concentration.[92] The maternal hyperglycemia is reflected in the fetal serum glucose concentration (see Fig. 128–2), but this change has no effect on fetal serum insulin for the first 30 minutes and only later causes a small increase in plasma insulin.

At birth, the maternal supply of glucose to the fetus ceases abruptly, and the neonatal blood glucose concentration, which is normal by adult standards, declines to a mean level of 50 mg/dl (2.8 mM) by 2 hours of age. Sub-

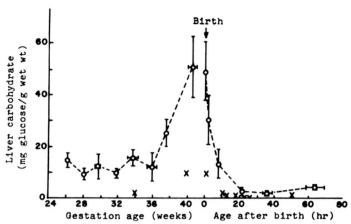

FIGURE 128–2. Liver carbohydrate (CHO) concentrations in human fetuses during the last trimester and in babies after birth. The data were derived from autopsies performed on 15 fresh stillbirths, 32 babies 4 hours old, and 40 babies up to 70 hours old of >37 weeks' gestation. Dashed line indicates accumulation of liver CHO before birth and disappearance after birth; open circles represent values in babies of normal birth weight for gestation; crossed lines represent values of individual babies of low birth weight for gestation. (From Shelley JH, Neligan GA: Neonatal hypoglycemia. Br Med Bull 22:34, 1966, by permission of the Medical Department, the British Council.)

sequently, this level rises and is stabilized at approximately 70 mg/dl (3.9 mM) by the third day of life.[2, 95] Unstimulated, postabsorptive plasma insulin concentrations from birth through 7 days of age are relatively stable.[2, 96, 97] During this time interval there is a decreased rate of glucose disappearance following intravenous glucose administration, which is correlated with a reduced and delayed rate of insulin secretion. But by the third to seventh day of life, the plasma glucose removal rate following IV administration increases toward that observed in older children and adults. When portal vein blood is sampled by umbilical vein catheter, both first and second phases of insulin release to intravenous glucose challenge have been observed; the total amount of insulin released during the first phase increases from day 1 to day 7. Oral glucose challenge also results in a delayed release of insulin.[98, 99]

As discussed in Chapters 78 and 79, the concept that glucagon plays an important role in adult glucose homeostasis is well accepted. Glucagon plays a role in maintaining basal hepatic glucose output, is suppressed by hyperglycemia, and is stimulated by hypoglycemia and gluconeogenic amino acids, resulting in potent stimulation of glycogenolysis and gluconeogenesis. The predominance of fetal pancreatic glucagon in early gestation suggests that it might play a role in embryonic differentiation via a cAMP-dependent mechanism.[100] Whether this hormone is of major importance to fuel homeostasis late in gestation remains under active investigation.

In vitro studies[101] utilizing the splenic lobe of newborn rat pancreas have demonstrated that glucagon release is not modified by changes in glucose concentrations. Similar to the beta cell, the fetal alpha-cell secretion of glucagon to amino acid stimulation is potentiated by factors that elevate intracellular cAMP. Investigations utilizing the chronically catheterized sheep fetus also have demonstrated that plasma glucagon concentrations are independent of acute changes in circulating blood glucose and are

unresponsive to alanine stimulation.[102] Subsequent studies in this model have shown that theophylline administered along with alanine produces marked augmentation of glucagon secretion.[103] When fetal hyperglycemia or hypoglycemia is produced by infusing the pregnant rat with glucose or insulin, appropriate fetal insulin responses are observed without changes in circulating fetal glucagon. In contrast to these acute manipulations, marked elevations of fetal glucagon occur in response to chronic fetal hypoglycemia induced by fasting pregnant rats for 96 hours, by inducing intrauterine growth retardation, or by maternal treatment with phloridzin, a potent inhibitor of renal glucose reabsorption.[104, 105]

Furthermore, membrane glucagon receptors in several fetal animal species are diminished compared with the adult, and progressive postnatal maturation of receptors and receptor-mediated cAMP production occur.[105–107] Functionally, this receptor deficit is reflected by the impaired ability of the fetus to increase glucose production when exposed to plasma glucagon levels in the high physiological range.[108]

Less information is available relevant to glucagon release in the human fetus. Human pancreatic slices release glucagon when incubated in the presence of alanine or arginine,[109, 110] and basal plasma glucagon concentrations in three second-trimester fetuses were in the adult range.[109] Intraperitoneal injection of arginine in the 25-week fetus had no effect on glucagon release, and similarly, no change in concentration occurred from basal levels over a 4-hour period of observation in a 26-week fetus. However, maternal alanine infusion during labor significantly increased the glucagon level in the umbilical cord,[111] and arginine stimulated glucagon secretion in the term infant immediately after birth.[112]

Immediately after birth in mammalian species, including humans,[113] a significant increase in plasma glucagon occurs which is closely correlated with the characteristic fall in plasma glucose during the first 2 hours of life. Despite the persistence of relative hypoglycemia, plasma glucagon concentrations remain stable and do not significantly change between 2 and 24 hours of life. A further significant elevation in plasma glucagon occurs from day 1 to day 3 of life, associated with the return of glucose to what is considered in the older child to be euglycemic levels. This change occurs simultaneously with the establishment of a routine feeding pattern.

Whereas a 30-minute infusion of the gluconeogenic amino acid alanine into normal 1-hour-old infants increases plasma glucagon threefold, it is ineffective in increasing plasma glucose.[112] However, 6-hour-old human infants have detectable incorporation of alanine carbon into circulating blood glucose.[113, 114] These observations suggest that gluconeogenesis is not fully established in utero or at the time of birth in humans but becomes operative soon thereafter.[115]

In summary,

1. Carbohydrate metabolism in utero is less dependent on fetal insulin and glucagon than on the maternal supply of glucose, and perhaps lactate.

2. There is no a priori reason to believe that fetal insulin secretagogues nor the metabolic consequences of released fetal insulin are the same as those in the adult. Since the fetus is growing rapidly, amino acid stimulation of insulin

release with consequent augmented cellular amino acid uptake and protein synthesis would be a more appropriate role for fetal insulin than the control of glucose homeostasis. Conversely, release of the catabolic hormone glucagon would be counterproductive for growth, yet it could be important for maintaining blood glucose during periods of placental insufficiency.[104]

3. The adenylate cyclase–cAMP system is of primary importance in both insulin and glucagon release, and the transition from fetal to mature hormone secretory responses parallels maturation of this system.

4. Although there is some evidence for anti-insulin effects of growth hormone on fat and glucose metabolism in fetal sheep similar to those observed in adult life,[116, 117] the role of insulin-like growth factors (IGF's) in the regulation of fetal energy metabolism is not known with certainty.

HEPATIC ENZYME SYSTEMS AND SUBSTRATE REGULATION

Throughout gestation the fetus is dependent solely on maternal supply and placental transfer of nutrients to meet the cellular metabolic demands for differentiation and growth. At the time of delivery, the fetal organism loses its constant source of intravenous substrates and must be metabolically prepared to enter its first fast. To maintain normal cellular metabolism and anabolic growth, the newborn, like the older child and adult, must meet at least three requirements: (1) have adequate stores of hepatic glycogen, muscle protein, and fat from which substrates can be mobilized, (2) have or rapidly acquire the enzymatic capacity to release, interconvert, and utilize these substrates, and (3) release regulatory hormones in an appropriate manner to modulate enzyme activities, substrate mobilization, and peripheral utilization of metabolic fuels. Since the liver plays a central role in regulation of substrate interconversions, primary attention will be given to its role in fetal and neonatal glucose homeostasis.

The net result of these various interacting processes is an initial fall in plasma glucose following delivery with subsequent recovery of normoglycemia. This fall in plasma glucose is associated with increased concentrations of cortisol, glucagon, and presumably epinephrine and a subsequent rise in plasma FFA and ketone bodies.[97, 118, 119] A failure in substrate delivery, interconversion, or utilization could lead to hypoglycemia and subsequent cellular dysfunction, including central nervous system (CNS) symptoms, which, if sustained or profound, could result in permanent CNS damage or death.

One of the primary differences between the fetus and the older child or adult is the absence or very low activities of a number of key hepatic enzymes (particularly gluconeogenic enzymes) necessary for fuel homeostasis in the fasting state.[120] Teleologically, there should be no need for hepatic gluconeogenesis in a fetus receiving constant "hyperalimentation," and in fact, in vivo tracer studies in the ovine fetus demonstrate that gluconeogenesis is minimal or virtually absent.[17, 39, 45] The appropriate temporal induction or activation of these enzymes may involve one or more mechanisms: transcription and/or translation from DNA or RNA, respectively, to form the nascent enzyme peptides or allosteric activation of pre-existing enzymes by

changes in co-factors or intracellular substrate concentrations. The induction of these enzymes may involve genetically predetermined factors, the maturity of the organism, differentiation of cellular sensitivity to circulating hormones or substrates, or some combination of these factors. It is not the purpose of this chapter to evaluate in depth these various possibilities.

The majority of data on substrates and enzymatic systems have been derived from the rat and a variety of other mammalian species, and much less is available from subhuman primates and humans. Patterns of enzyme activities and substrate availability are similar in many species, despite the marked variability in relative maturity of these organisms at the time of delivery. For this reason, although caution should be applied, analogies from the rat or other mammalian species to humans may provide a framework upon which to examine human physiology.

Fetal and Neonatal Carbohydrate Metabolism

The enzymatic and substrate regulatory control of glycogen synthesis, glycogenolysis, and gluconeogenesis is beyond the scope of this chapter but is well reviewed elsewhere.[121–131]

Fetal Glycogen Metabolism

It is well documented that hepatic stores of glycogen are assimilated rapidly during the last third of gestation in all mammalian species examined including humans[131, 132] (Figs. 128–2 and 128–3). In the human fetus, hepatic glycogen is detectable as early as 8 to 10 weeks of gestation,[54, 132] which of necessity implies the presence of hepatic glycogen synthetic enzymes. This early presence of hepatic glycogen differs from lower mammalian species

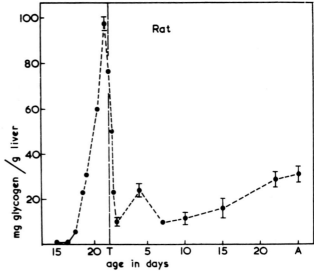

FIGURE 128–3. Neonatal rat liver glycogen content (*T*, term; *A*, adult). Limits of ± SEM are shown where they are large enough to be drawn. (From Ballard FJ, Oliver IT: Glycogen metabolism in embryonic chick and neonatal rat liver. Biochem Biophys Acta 71:578, 1963.)

(rat, rabbit, dog, and guinea pig), in which the fetal liver is devoid of glycogen until just prior to term.[131]

Phosphorylase is present in the preimplantation morula stage of the embryo,[133] but whether this cellular phosphorylase activity is maintained in the differentiating liver remains unknown. Following differentiation of the liver, phosphorylase activity in the rat is detectable prior to accumulation of hepatic glycogen.[131] However, even following the appearance of hepatic glycogen, phosphorylase would appear to have little role in maintenance of fetal plasma glucose, since glucose-6-phosphatase, a key enzyme necessary for glucose production from either glycogenolysis or gluconeogenesis, does not appear until the 19th to 20th day of gestation.[134]

Although the rate-limiting enzyme systems necessary for both hepatic glycogen synthesis and glycogen degradation are present prior to the accumulation of glycogen,[135] the mechanism by which glycogen accumulation occurs, as well as the source of substrate, remains somewhat vague. During the period of rapid glycogen accumulation, increases in hepatic glycogen synthetic enzymes occur.[131] Utilizing labeled incubation studies, the source of substrate for glycogen is most likely glucose, not pyruvate, in the rat. However, in the guinea pig, incorporation of ^{14}C-labeled glucose, pyruvate, and fructose was found to be low even near term, at a time when hepatic glycogen stores were rapidly increasing.[135] In the adult, recent studies suggest that under physiological conditions in vivo, hepatic glycogen is formed both from direct uptake of glucose (direct pathway) and via three carbon precursors (indirect pathway),[136] both routes contributing approximately 50 per cent.[137] The contributions of the direct and indirect pathways are not established in the fetus. Isotopic studies performed in fetal lambs suggest that glycogen synthesis occurs at least in part via the indirect pathway and that lactate is a major precursor of glycogen in that species.[138] In neonatal rats, glucose incorporation into glycogen seems to occur mainly through the indirect pathway, while galactose may be used preferentially for neonatal glycogen synthesis.[139]

A variety of factors have been shown to alter fetal hepatic glycogen content. Jost and Jacquot[70] provided the first evidence that fetal endocrine function was necessary for normal enzymic differentiation of the liver. In utero decapitation of fetal rabbits prevented the accumulation of glycogen and the increase in enzymes necessary for glycogen formation.[70, 140] Treatment of the fetus with glucocorticoids corrected this abnormality.[140] In rats, both fetal decapitation and maternal adrenalectomy are necessary to create similar findings.[141] Treatment of the normal rat fetus with glucocorticoids results in glycogen accumulation at an earlier time in gestation.[120] Thus it would appear that glucocorticoids are involved in fetal glycogen metabolism. Catecholamines are known to affect glycogen metabolism in older children and adults by altering both hepatic glycogen synthetase and phosphorylase activities. Accumulation of epinephrine in the fetal adrenal gland is apparently controlled by the pituitary, since decapitation depletes adrenal epinephrine. ACTH or cortisone treatment of the fetus restores these concentrations by increasing the activity of phenylethanol amino N-methyl transferase, the enzyme necessary for conversion of norepinephrine to epinephrine.[142, 143]

Hepatic phosphorylase and glucose-6-phosphatase are necessary for hydrolysis of glycogen and release of glucose into the systemic circulation (Fig. 128–4). The activity of rat hepatic glucose-6-phosphatase is very low until the 19th to 20th day of gestation, at which time its activity increases rapidly,[134] whereas phosphorylase activity, as already discussed, is detectable as early as the 17th day of gestation.[131] Adrenalectomy in adult rats is known to inhibit phosphorylase activity and glycogenolysis to cyclic AMP stimulation and in newborn rats results in a 30 per cent decrease in phosphorylase activity.[144] How much of the increase in phosphorylase activity is activation of existing enzyme or de novo synthesis is not clear. In contrast, the mechanism of normal induction of fetal glucose-6-phosphatase is dependent on de novo protein synthesis. Intrauterine injection of glucagon or thyroxine results in a prompt (3 hours) increase in the activity of glucose-6-phosphatase, whereas similar injections of these hormones along with the protein synthetic inhibitor actinomycin D results in no increase.[120] In utero fetal decapitation also prevents the normal increase in glucose-6-phosphatase.[140]

In contrast to the in vitro enzymatic data, in vivo stimulation with glucagon or dibutyryl–cAMP has little effect on mobilization of hepatic glycogen and elevation of plasma glucose until several hours following parturition.[144] Two explanations for this refractory period have been suggested, including incomplete postnatal induction of glycogenolytic enzymes and end-organ resistance to hormonal stimulation. Recent investigations in the rat have demonstrated low adenylate cyclase responsiveness of fetal hepatic

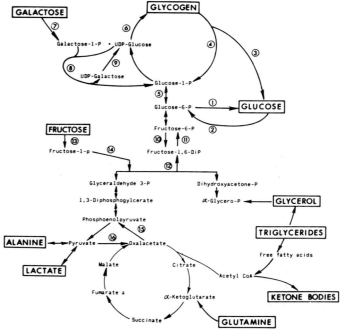

FIGURE 128–4. Metabolic pathways involved in glycogen synthesis and degradation and gluconeogenesis. Key enzymes are designated by number: (1) glucose-6-phosphate, (2) glucokinase, (3) amylo-1,6-glucosidase, (4) phosphorylase, (5) phosphoglucomutase, (6) glycogen synthetase, (7) galactokinase, (8) galactose-1-phosphate uridyl transferase, (9) uridine diphosphogalactose-4-epimerase, (10) phosphofructokinase, (11) fructose-1,6-diphosphatase, (12) fructose-1,6-diphosphate aldolase, (13) fructokinase, (14) fructose-1-phosphate aldolase, (15) phosphoenolypyruvate carboxykinase, and (16) pyruvate carboxylase. (Adapted from Dekaban A, Baird R: The outcome of pregnancy in diabetic women: I. Fetal wastage, mortality and morbidity in the offspring of diabetic and normal control mothers. J Pediatr 55:563, 1959.)

membranes to glucagon stimulation. Adenylate cyclase activity increases to adult levels only following 30 days of extrauterine life. Similarly, hormone-binding studies with fetal hepatic membranes showed decreased binding of both insulin and glucagon when compared with hepatic membranes of adult controls. Insulin binding reached mature values by 20 days of fetal life, whereas glucagon binding did not attain adult levels until the 30th postnatal day. The demonstration of significant insulin binding, which is relatively unopposed by glucagon binding, may have physiological importance for rapid fetal growth and protection from in utero fetal catabolism.

If one can equate the relative amounts of hepatic membrane–bound hormone to biological activity, glycogen accumulation would be favored and gluconeogenesis inhibited despite significant concentrations of plasma insulin and glucagon in the fetus. Similarly, this could explain the refractory response of glycogen and plasma glucose to pharmacological doses of glucagon in the early postnatal period,[144] as well as the apparent dichotomy of rising glucagon concentrations in the presence of a falling plasma glucose level following delivery in the neonate.[113]

Fetal and Neonatal Gluconeogenesis

Throughout gestation, glucose is transported rapidly across the placenta so that fetal glucose concentration approximates the maternal concentration. As a result, the fetus is protected from catabolic processes, such as gluconeogenesis, during the period of most rapid growth. There is considerable evidence in the literature from a variety of species that the enzymes necessary for gluconeogenesis have very low or absent activities in early and midgestation.[120] During the latter portion of gestation, there is some increase in one or more of the key rate-limiting gluconeogenic enzyme(s) prior to parturition (see Fig. 128–4). However, in every species examined, at least one enzyme maintains low activity in utero until the immediate postnatal period.[120, 145] This functional block in gluconeogenesis is further supported by in vitro liver-slice studies in which there is minimal conversion of labeled lactate, pyruvate, or alanine to glucose.[131, 145, 146] Consistent with the data obtained in vitro, in vivo tracer kinetic studies in the normal ovine fetus demonstrate little active gluconeogenesis[39, 42, 147]; significant production of glucose by the fetal lamb has been observed, however, when pregnant sheep were made chronically hypoglycemic (22 mg/dl [1.2 mM]) by insulin infusion.[148, 149] Although limited, studies in human infants using stable isotopic tracer are consistent with the virtual absence of gluconeogenesis at birth, and presumably during fetal life, in the human as well.[150]

A number of factors have profound effects on enzyme activities in the fetal and neonatal liver. Glucose-6-phosphatase activity is known to be extremely low during gestation in the rat and increases somewhat during the last 2 to 3 days prior to parturition, with a marked increase following delivery.[120, 134] Early induction of this enzyme can be accomplished by premature delivery or intrauterine treatment of the fetus with glucagon, thyroxine or epinephrine, and cAMP.[120] Decreased activity has been observed with postmaturity, intrauterine fetal decapitation, and intrauterine administration of glucose or actinomycin D.[110] Although

the aforementioned situations may be artificial and pharmacological, several conclusions are warranted: (1) increased activity of glucose-6-phosphatase requires a translational or transcriptional step; (2) at least one stimulus for increased enzyme activity and/or synthesis is cAMP, since hormones that stimulate this nucleotide, as well as cAMP itself, increase enzyme activity; and (3) glucose appears to be a potent inhibitor of the induction of this enzyme, presumably by inhibiting protein synthesis. Whether this effect is mediated by glucose directly, via insulin, or via other mechanisms remains unknown. The mechanisms through which thyroxine or fetal pituitary hormones affect the induction of glucose-6-phosphatase are unknown, but these hormones may play a permissive role.

In most animal species, fructose-1,6-diphosphatase and pyruvate carboxylase (see Fig. 128–4) have low fetal activities which rapidly increase prior to delivery. Since the activities of these two enzymes are increasing prior to parturition, they would not appear to be rate-limiting.

In contrast, in most species, phosphoenolpyruvate carboxykinase (PEPCK) would appear to be the last rate-limiting gluconeogenic enzyme induced in fetal or neonatal liver. This is demonstrated most clearly in the crossover studies of Ballard,[151] in which there was a marked increase in substrate concentrations just proximal to PEPCK (Fig. 128–5). In the rat, induction of PEPCK has many parallels to that of glucose-6-phosphatase, but the mechanisms have been more precisely defined. The activity of this enzyme is not only inhibited by actinomycin D but by puromycin and amino acid analogues.[152] Therefore, de novo protein syn-

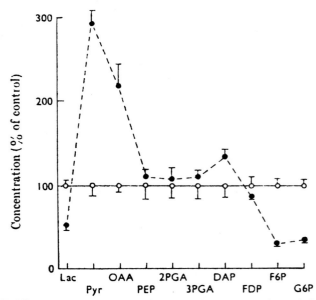

FIGURE 128–5. Crossover plot comparing the concentrations of gluconeogenic intermediates in livers of 1-hour-old rats (●), with the respective compounds in livers of fetal rats (○). Values shown are the means ± SEM for 8 to 10 determinations. Abbreviations used and the concentrations of each intermediate in fetal liver are: lactate (*Lac*), 5.74 pmol/g; pyruvate (*Pyr*), 0.074 μmol/g; oxaloacetate (*OAA*), 0.0075 μmol/g; phosphoenolpyruvate (*PEP*), 0.033 μmol/g; 2-phosphoglycerate (*2PGA*), 0.012 pmol/g; 3-phosphoglycerate (*3PGA*), 0.82 μmol/g; dihydroxyacetone phosphate (*DAP*), 0.12 μmol/g; fructose 1,6-diphosphate (*FDP*), 0.0059 μmol/g; fructose 6-phosphate (*F6P*), 0.113 μmol/g; glucose-6-phosphate (*G6P*), 0.406 μmol/g. (Used, with permission, from Ballard FJ: The development of gluconeogenesis in rat liver: Controlling factors in the newborn. Biochem J 124:265, 1971.)

thesis is necessary for induction. cAMP, dibutyl–cAMP, epinephrine, and glucagon stimulate the activity of this enzyme in vivo in rats[152, 153] and in vitro in rats[154] and human fetal liver.[155] Protection of the animal from hypoglycemia by glucose injection at the time of delivery as well as the administration of a variety of substrates (i.e., lactate, pyruvate, glycerol, galactose, fructose, mannose, and ribose) inhibited its induction.[152]

Both epinephrine and norepinephrine stimulate PEPCK activity in the neonatal rat.[152] This implies that the autonomic nervous system may have a role in the induction of this enzyme. It has been established that vagal stimulation in adult rats results in an increase in hepatic output of glucose and a remarkable increase in glucose-6-phosphatase activity.[156] It would be difficult to conceive that the "trauma" of delivery and readjustment of a variety of physiological parameters to extrauterine life would not be associated with a marked increase in epinephrine secretion and autonomic nervous system activity. The precise role of the autonomic nervous system in hepatic enzyme induction must await further studies.

The normal neonatal increase in PEPCK activity is preceded by an accumulation of PEPCK in messenger RNA in the liver, which is presumably the result of an increase in PEPCK gene transcription. Transcription of the PEPCK gene is believed to be triggered immediately after birth by (1) the fall in blood glucose concentration, (2) the rise in the glucagon/insulin ratio, (3) the rise in hepatic cAMP concentration, and (4) the change in the redox state of liver.[157] The gene for cystosolic PEPCK has been isolated, and a short sequence of its promoter-regulatory region carries all the information for the response of the gene to hormones; the major factor stimulating transcription appears to be cAMP, while insulin is able to suppress transcription even in the presence of cAMP.[158–161] If activity of PEPCK is required for the incorporation of 3-carbon precursors into glycogen, and if the latter enzyme is not present until birth, this implies that fetal glycogen must be synthesized via the direct pathway.

The increased activity of PEPCK in humans is even more complex than in the rat model, since two gene loci are most likely involved, one for mitochondrial and the other for cytosolic enzyme. If the induction of PEPCK in humans is similar to that in the pig, the primary increase in activity in the neonatal liver would be in the mitochondrial fraction.[162]

An additional rate-limiting factor which must be considered in the establishment of neonatal gluconeogenesis is tissue oxygenation. Hypoxemia even in the face of maximal glucagon-stimulated PEPCK activity is associated with suppressed gluconeogenesis.[163] Since gluconeogenesis is an energy-requiring process, concentrations of high-energy phosphates become rate-limiting. Birth is associated with some degree of hypoxemia in all mammals, whether due to delivery of the intact fetal-placental unit as in the rat, compromised blood flow to the infant with cord compression during passage through the birth canal, or in conditions in which decreased fetal oxygenation is due to maternal or placental pathology (e.g., toxemia, maternal hypertension, long-standing maternal diabetes).

Normal fetal liver has a highly reduced redox potential and relatively low concentrations of ATP, a condition resembling hypoxemia in older animals and not favorable for gluconeogenesis.[151] Since hypoxemia in the adult and fetus is a potent stimulus for glycogenolysis and glycolysis, the observation of increased hepatic glycogen stores in the fetus at term would appear paradoxical. In the rat, immediately following delivery, there is increased activity of tricyclic acid (TCA) cycle enzymes,[120] a fall in ADP and AMP, and increasing ATP concentrations,[151] conditions favorable for gluconeogenesis.

In summary, following delivery and with Pa_{O_2} values significantly higher than in the fetus, every mammalian species experiences a fall in plasma glucose during the early hours of life. The plasma glucose concentration subsequently increases even in the absence of oral alimentation and is associated with a decrease in hepatic glycogen and an increase in gluconeogenic enzyme activity. This period of "physiological" hypoglycemia is associated with the secretion of a variety of hormones (glucagon, cortisol, growth hormone, and presumably epinephrine and norepinephrine), but whether their secretion is the result of the hypoglycemia or secondary to the stresses of delivery and of extrauterine life remains to be determined.

The activity and regulation of gluconeogenesis in the newborn are more complex than those for mature animals. The process involves not only the relative rates and controls of glycolysis and gluconeogenesis known to exist in adults but also the induction of one or more key rate-limiting enzymes in gluconeogenesis (PEPCK and glucose-6-phosphatase), as well as improvement in systemic oxygenation.

Nevertheless, these activities are integrated almost immediately after birth in the human infant. Thus, whereas infused alanine elicits no glycemic response in the 1-hour-old infant,[112] recycling of gluconeogenic carbon occurs by 2 hours of age,[164] isotopic alanine carbon can be found in circulating glucose by 6 hours of age,[114] and gluconeogenesis from glycerol is established before the end of the first postnatal day.[165–167]

Fatty Acid and Ketone Body Metabolism

The majority of fat stores in the fetus are accumulated during the last 5 weeks of gestation[168] (Fig. 128–6). Following delivery, the respiratory quotient of the newborn falls from above 0.8 to near 0.7 in the first days of life,[169] indicating conversion from a primarily glucose-based fuel economy to one of fatty acid metabolism. The human neonate has two types of fat stores: a unilocular white adipose tissue composed of cells with single fat vacuoles and a multilocular brown adipose tissue containing multivacuolated cells. Both are sensitive to circulating norepinephrine and other lipolytic hormones (i.e., growth hormone, cortisol, and glucagon) and are innervated by sympathetic fibers. The primary difference in the two tissues is their response to stimulation. In white fat, hydrolysis of stored triglycerides results in the release of FFA and glycerol, whereas in brown fat, fatty acids are oxidized within the adipocyte, the primary result being the generation of heat. The brown color is due to high mitochondrial content and capillaries. Since the neonate does not respond to hypothermia with shivering, as in the older child and adult, the brown fat plays an important role in thermal homeostasis.[170]

In the fetus and the normal neonate immediately following delivery, circulating concentrations of FFA are low and

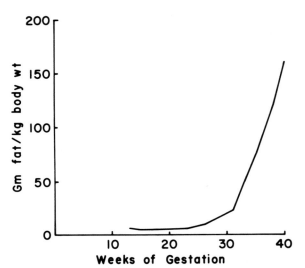

FIGURE 128–6. Human fetal fat content (g/kg of body weight) throughout gestation. (From Shaffer AJ, Avery ME: Diseases of the Newborn (ed 3). Philadelphia, WB Saunders Co, 1971, p 21.)

rise progressively over the early hours of extrauterine life.[171] This is accomplished by an accelerated lipolytic rate which is several-fold that of the adult and comparable with that found only after prolonged fasting in mature individuals.[165–167] These events occur in the absence of a demonstrable fall in plasma insulin but in the presence of increased glucagon, growth hormone, cortisol, presumably epinephrine secretion, and increased sympathetic tone. Cold or relative cold exposure is associated with a marked reduction in adipose tissue stores and increased oxygen consumption in neonatal rabbits.[170] Recent in vitro studies performed on isolated adipocytes obtained from neonates show that thyroid-stimulating hormone (TSH) has a much more powerful lipolytic effect than catecholamines; this suggests that the peak elevation of circulating TSH observed at birth may be essential to stimulate lipolysis.[172] In humans, cold exposure results in a two- to three-fold increase in circulating FFA within 30 minutes.[173]

FFA's can be utilized directly by heart, kidney, and muscle,[174] thus decreasing glucose utilization. A portion of FFA undergoes ketogenesis within the liver with the generation of ketone bodies, β-hydroxybutyrate, and acetoacetate. As pointed out earlier, this not only supplies the energy for hepatic gluconeogenesis but also provides acetyl-CoA to activate pyruvate carboxylase and shares with gluconeogenesis the mutual production and utilization of oxidized pyridine nucleotide. There is no enzymatic limitation to hepatic ketogenesis, since addition of fatty acids to fetal hepatocytes or hepatic homogenates from both human and rat sources results in acetoacetate formation.[175]

At the time of delivery, cord blood β-hydroxybutyrate concentrations are often moderately elevated, reflecting transplacental transfer of maternal ketoacids.[97] Within the first 2 hours of life, plasma ketone body concentrations decrease, most likely secondary to neonatal utilization, since the immature human brain has the functional capacity to use ketones as a fuel.[176–179] Thereafter, ketone body levels increase to the 1 to 2 mM range,[152, 180–184] a range found in adults only after 1 to 2 days of starvation. This increase in plasma ketone body concentration is presumed to be the result of high rates of ketone body production.[183]

Obviously, early infant feeding and/or intravenous glucose infusion will stimulate insulin secretion and inhibit lipolysis, resulting in lower ketone concentrations. Ketones may play an important alternate fuel role in the neonate,[183] since ketones might supply the energy equivalent of about 10 kcal/kg per day to human neonates if ketone body oxidation in the newborn is similar to that of the adult.

METABOLIC DERANGEMENTS OF FUEL HOMEOSTASIS IN THE NEONATE

General Considerations

In utero, the entire fuel needs of the fetus are supplied from maternal sources delivered intravenously. During transition from intra- to extrauterine existence, however, a number of metabolic changes occur because the infant must make immediate adjustments to the abrupt cessation of its "foreign fuel" supply. These sudden adjustments include activation of an enteral fuel axis and adaptation to a lipid fuel economy from one almost entirely carbohydrate-based.

The profound physiological burden of these adjustments can be appreciated from the following considerations. (1) On a weight basis, the energy needs of the infant are greater than those of the adult. (2) Nonetheless, the newborn infant is only 5 per cent the size of an adult and has, therefore, limited endogenous fuel reserves. (3) Oral food intake is generally inadequate to meet energy demand in the immediate postnatal period. (4) Specific metabolic pathways that are minimally functional in utero must suddenly bear a major fuel transport burden. (5) And finally, the developmental maturity of various regulatory systems may not be complete.

Derangements of fuel metabolism in the neonate are manifested, as in the growing child or adult, by disturbances in blood glucose homeostasis. In contrast to the adult, when diabetes (and hence hyperglycemia) is the most prevalent disorder, hypoglycemia is very common in the neonate and hyperglycemic syndromes are rare (Table 128–1).

Definition, Signs, and Symptoms of Hypoglycemia

The clinical symptomatology associated with a rapid and acute fall in the blood glucose in the older child and adult is usually easily interpreted and reflects excessive epinephrine secretion (i.e., sweating, weakness, tachycardia, nervousness, and hunger). In the neonate, hypoglycemic symptoms are nonspecific, are less obvious, and may be completely overlooked or absent. Hypoglycemia should be suspected in any neonate with poor feeding, jitteriness, perioral cyanosis, lethargy, or seizures. Further, hypoglycemia should be anticipated in any infant known to be at high risk, e.g., infants of diabetic mothers, small-for-gestational-age infants, and infants with neonatal asphyxia (see below).

Children and adults are usually symptomatic when the true blood glucose reaches a concentration of approximately 40 mg/dl (2.2 mM). Symptoms are frequently un-

TABLE 128–1. DISORDERS OF FUEL HOMEOSTASIS IN
THE NEONATE

Transient
SGA infant
   Hypoglycemia
   Hyperglycemia
Infant of the diabetic mother
Erythroblastosis
Beckwith-Wiedemann syndrome
Miscellaneous: sepsis, hypoxemia, hypothermia
Chronic
Sustained hyperinsulinemia
Endocrine deficiencies
   Growth hormone
   ACTH
   Cortisol
   Glucagon
Hepatic enzyme deficiencies of carbohydrate metabolism
   Glucose-6-phosphatase
   Glucose-6-phosphate translocase
   Fructose-1,6-diphosphatase
   Glycogen synthetase
   Galactose-1-phosphate uridyl transferase
   Fructose-1-phosphate aldolase
Defects in amino acid metabolism
Defects in fatty acid metabolism

recognized despite extremely low blood glucose levels in newborn infants.

The precise concentration of blood glucose that is detrimental to neonatal brain is unknown. Recent studies using cerebral nuclear magnetic resonance (NMR) imaging suggest that brain glucose concentration reaches 0 when plasma glucose is less than 40 mg/dl (2.2 mM).[185] The data on "normal" glucose levels in neonates have accumulated over the last 30 years.[184, 186–192] In view of this sum of information, and although nadir plasma glucose concentrations less than 45 mg/dl (2.5 mM) are commonly observed in healthy babies 2 to 3 hours after birth, it seems prudent to recommend that every effort should be made to maintain the plasma glucose concentrations above 40 mg/dl (2.3 mM), and the authors of a recent review[95] on this question concur with our previous recommendations.[189]

Therapy

It is the authors' current policy to monitor the blood glucose level of all high-risk infants (i.e., small-for-gestational-age infants, premature infants, infants of diabetic mothers, and so on) at 1- to 2-hour intervals with blood glucose monitoring reagents. Since variable and inconsistent results are frequently observed with these methods at low blood glucose concentrations, "low" test results should be verified frequently with plasma glucose values determined by a reliable laboratory method. If the blood glucose estimate is 45 mg/dl (2.5 mM) or less, a blood specimen is obtained for measurement of glucose by the glucose oxidase method, and the infant is started immediately on a feeding of 5 per cent glucose followed subsequently at 2- to 3-hour intervals with standard formula feedings. Throughout this time, the blood glucose concentration is monitored before each feeding. In the large majority of instances, adequate glucose concentrations are maintained by this practice. If, however, the plasma glucose value remains below 40 mg/dl (2.2 mM) by specific measurement,

an intravenous infusion of 10 to 20 per cent glucose is begun at a rate equivalent to normal neonatal hepatic glucose production (4 to 8 mg/kg per min).[164, 165, 193, 194] However, the variability in requirements between patients is large enough that the rate of administration needs to be individualized and the patient given an amount of glucose that will maintain plasma glucose above 40 to 50 mg/dl (2.2 to 2.8 mM). This approach to therapy requires frequent monitoring of the blood glucose and close observation of the volume of fluid being administered. On rare occasions, hypoglycemia persists despite this infusion, and then cortisone acetate is administered intramuscularly at 8-hour intervals (total dosage is 5 mg/kg of body weight per day). Using this regimen, the blood glucose concentration is readily stabilized in the vast majority of infants. Usually, the intravenous infusion of glucose can be tapered after 48 hours, and cortisone acetate therapy can be gradually eliminated during the subsequent 4 to 5 days. If hypoglycemia persists for more than 72 hours on this regimen or is recurrent following cessation of therapy, causes for chronic hypoglycemia should be considered.

TRANSIENT DISORDERS

The Small-for-Gestational-Age (SGA) Infant

Infants whose weights are below the 10th percentile for gestational age[195] have been found to have an increased risk of both hypoglycemia and transient neonatal hyperglycemia. These infants have been termed *intrauterine-growth-retarded* or *small-for-gestational-age* (SGA) *infants*. The cause of the growth retardation is frequently not clear but may be related to placental insufficiency; however, chromosomal defects and congenital viral syndromes have been implicated.[196]

Hypoglycemia in the SGA Infant

Lubchenco and Bard[195] showed that the risk for the development of blood sugar levels less than 30 mg/dl (1.7 mM) in the SGA infant was correlated with the degree of maturation of the infant—i.e., the incidence of hypoglycemia was 67 per cent in premature, 25 per cent in term, and 18 per cent in post-term SGA infants. Theoretically, the factors predisposing these infants to the development of hypoglycemia could be a defect in any one of the essential requirements for the maintenance of normal glucose homeostasis, including the integrity of the hepatic gluconeogenic and glycogenolytic pathways, sufficient endogenous gluconeogenic substrate, adequate alternative fuel sources, and appropriate hormonal secretion to modulate these processes.

A number of studies have demonstrated elevated plasma concentrations of growth hormone and cortisol in low-birth-weight infants.[69, 97] Therefore, it must be concluded that the pituitary gland and the pituitary-adrenal axis are responding appropriately in the early hours of life. Insulin has been implicated in a variety of specific clinical and pathological disorders in the newborn (see below), but hyperinsulinemia has not been found in SGA infants, and these neonates have an appropriate hyperglucagonemic response to alanine infusion.[197–200] These observations collectively speak against abnormal pancreatic hormone regulation as an etiological factor in the hypoglycemia of these infants.

With regard to substrate availability, several reports have indicated that FFA, glycerol, and ketone body concentrations are lower in SGA infants when compared with normal infants.[97, 201–204] Both fatty acid and ketone body turnover rates are proportional to their circulating concentrations in the normal newborn.[165, 183] Recently, Fjeld et al.[167] showed that lipolysis is very active in SGA infants with blood glucose concentrations of 2.0 to 2.4 mM, as attested by increased rates of glycerol turnover. Thus there is no clear evidence for a decreased "alternate fuel" supply in the SGA infant. Nonetheless, in the newborn rat and pig, the energy supplied by adequate FFA availability is essential to sustain high gluconeogenic rates,[206–210] and the augmented lipid supply in the small human infant increases the plasma glucose concentration.[204, 211, 212] Oral administration of medium-chain triglycerides was shown recently to enhance hepatic glucose production in premature and SGA babies as well as in term neonates.[213]

Hyperlactacidemia and hyperalaninemia are well-established findings in patients with defects in hepatic gluconeogenesis, either congenital in origin (i.e., glucose-6-phosphatase or fructose-1,6-diphosphatase deficiencies[128, 129] or acquired (i.e., lactic acidosis[214]). Similarly, hyperlactacidemia and hyperalaninemia have been found consistently in the SGA infant[97, 197] (Fig. 128–7). The persistence of hyperlactacidemia and hyperalaninemia is most compatible with a defect in gluconeogenesis compromising the ability of the infant to utilize gluconeogenic substrates entering at or below pyruvate. With decreased hepatic gluconeogenesis, a larger proportion of hepatic glucose release must be derived from stored glycogen, which results in rapid depletion of this substrate reservoir (see Fig. 128–2) and would explain the poor glycemic responses observed in these infants upon challenge with glucagon.[215]

However, Frazer et al.[114] could find no correlation between the plasma alanine concentration and the rate of [2,3-$^{13}C_2$]-alanine incorporation into plasma glucose in normoglycemic SGA infants. Whether this lack of relationship exists in the hypoglycemic SGA infant remains to be determined.

Since hypoglycemia develops in only 40 to 50 per cent of SGA infants,[97, 195] there is obviously a spectrum of clinical and biochemical findings. Nevertheless, (1) significant inverse correlations between glucose and lactate or alanine, (2) lowered fatty acid, glycerol, and ketone levels and their consequent effects on gluconeogenesis, and (3) the diminished ability of the SGA infant to utilize alanine as a gluconeogenic substrate[197, 216] strongly support the hypothesis that hypoglycemia in the SGA newborn results from a transient defect in hepatic gluconeogenesis. Unfortunately, measurement of gluconeogenic kinetic rates would not only be ethically unacceptable in the hypoglycemic SGA infant, but they would also be uninterpretable because there is no reliable means to quantify hepatic gluconeogenesis in the nonsteady state. Thus direct confirmation of the preceding hypothesis will not be forthcoming soon.

Hyperglycemia in the SGA Infant

In normal adults, hepatic glucose production is so finely regulated that when exogenous glucose is infused at a rate

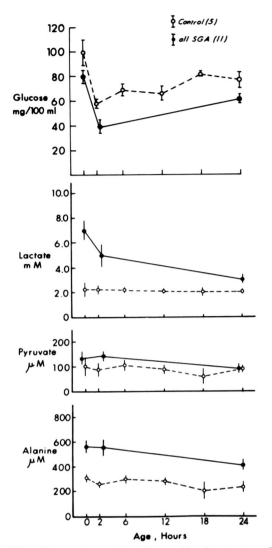

FIGURE 128–7. Plasma glucose, blood lactate, blood pyruvate, and plasma alanine concentrations of the normal and SGA infants during the first 24 hours of life (mean ± SEM). (Used, with permission, from Haymond MW, Karl IE, Pagliara AS: Increased gluconeogenesis substrates in the small-for-gestational-age infant. N Engl J Med 291:322, 1974.)

equal to basal glucose production, the endogenous production is suppressed so as to maintain plasma glucose concentrations in the normal range. In contrast, in both term and premature neonates, endogenous glucose production persists during glucose infusion[217, 218]; this may account for the common occurrence of hyperglycemia in neonates receiving parenteral glucose.

Transient hyperglycemia is indeed common in the first 24 hours of life in premature and SGA infants weighing less than 1300 g and receiving parenteral nutrition, since it was reported in 20 per cent of babies weighing less than 1300 g and in 70 per cent of those weighing less than 1000 g. In addition to exogenous glucose infusion, etiological factors associated with elevation of plasma glucose include lipid infusion, sepsis, hypoxia, and treatment with theophylline.[217, 219]

Sustained, spontaneous hyperglycemia and glycosuria occurring in the absence of intravenous glucose infusion during the first month of life are uncommon. An occasional case may represent the initial episode of true insulin-dependent diabetes mellitus or pancreatic dysplasia,[220] while others have been associated with overwhelming infection and/or CNS disease ending in death. In 1926, Ramsey[221] described the first well-documented case of a clinical entity simulating true diabetes mellitus which subsequently has been referred to as *transient diabetes in the newborn, pseudodiabetes of the newborn, infantile glucosuria,* and *temporary neonatal hyperglycemia.* Characteristically, the disorder presents within the first 6 weeks of life with hyperglycemia, glycosuria, and dehydration, but ketonuria, if present, is minimal. This disorder most commonly affects the SGA infant, and recovery appears to be complete.

The causes of this syndrome and its association with other forms of diabetes mellitus remain obscure. In approximately one third of cases there is a positive family history of diabetes mellitus.[222] In a few patients studied at autopsy, no characteristic abnormalities have been found in the pancreas.[222] A flat oral glucose tolerance test has been observed in the mothers of some of these infants. It has been suggested that the beta cells of these infants are hypoplastic due to the lack of a normal glucose stimulus in utero, which, in light of the data presented on insulin secretion in the fetus, would make this postulate highly unlikely. Further, several mothers have given birth to infants with this syndrome[223, 224] who have had normal or diabetic carbohydrate tolerance.

Few studies dealing with glucose-insulin relationships have been reported in these infants. Gentz and Cornblath[222] reported two patients, one of whom had plasma insulin concentrations of 6 and 17 μU/ml when the blood glucose was 1280 and 2300 mg/dl, respectively. Following remission of the hyperglycemia in these infants, oral and intravenous glucose tolerance tests were normal.

In an infant with this syndrome, intramuscular injection of caffeine, a potent nucleotide phosphodiesterase inhibi-

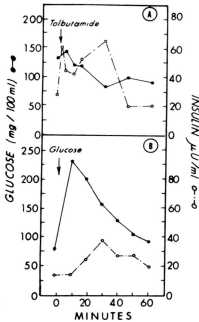

FIGURE 128–9. *A,* Response to intravenous sodium tolbutamide (20 mg/kg) at 52 days of age. *B,* Response to intravenous glucose (0.75 g/kg) at 59 days of age in an infant with transient neonatal diabetes. (Used, with permission, from Pagliara AS, Karl IE, Kipnis DM: Transient neonatal diabetes: Delayed maturation of the pancreatic beta cell. J Pediatr 81:97, 1973.)

tor, caused an increase in plasma insulin from 12 to 50 μU/ml with only a slight decrease in plasma glucose[225] (Fig. 128–8). Tolbutamide administration during the hyperglycemic phase resulted in neither a detectable increase in circulating insulin nor a decrease in plasma glucose and suggests that the pancreatic beta cells of this patient were insensitive to tolbutamide- and glucose-mediated insulin release and therefore similar to the in vitro human fetal pancreas.[81–83, 221] Following resolution of the hyperglycemia, repeat tolbutamide testing revealed a normal glucose response with an appropriate increase in plasma insulin (Fig. 128–9). In addition, the infant demonstrated a normal tolerance during an intravenous glucose challenge.

As considered in detail earlier, normal neonates also demonstrate varying degrees of decreased sensitivity of insulin release to glucose. Thus the defect seen in infants with transient neonatal diabetes may be quantitative in nature. Since caffeine, a phosphodiesterase inhibitor, is capable of releasing insulin during the transient diabetic phase, it is postulated that the defect may be related to delayed maturation of the adenyl cyclase–cyclic adenosine monophosphate system as a result of either a deficiency of beta-cell adenyl cyclase or of an increased activity of the nucleotide phosphodiesterase. This hypothesis is consistent with the transient nature of the disorder.

Infant of the Diabetic Mother

While the ability to conceive does not apparently differ between diabetic and nondiabetic women, teratogenesis, fetal wastage, neonatal mortality, and morbidity are significantly higher than in the normal population. Defects in

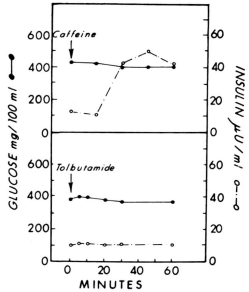

FIGURE 128–8. Responses to intramuscular caffeine benzoate (4 mg/kg) at 9 days of age and intravenous sodium tolbutamide (20 mg/kg) at 18 days of age in an infant with transient neonatal diabetes. (Used, with permission, from Pagliara AS, Karl IE, Kipnis DM: Transient neonatal diabetes: Delayed maturation of the pancreatic beta cell. J Pediatr 81:97, 1973.)

organogenesis occur prior to the seventh week of gestation.[226] While there is limited information on the benefit of strict normalization of maternal metabolic milieu on teratogenesis in the human infant of a diabetic mother, there appears to be little doubt that careful control of maternal diabetes during the period of organogenesis in the rat reduces malformation rates.[226–229]

The remaining complications, however, are directly related to maternal vascular disease and metabolic normalcy but not to the degree of insulin dependence, age of onset, or duration of diabetes. Furthermore, sustained fetal hyperinsulinemia per se can decrease fetal arterial oxygen content,[230] which, when coupled with the consequences of maternal vascular insufficiency, might augment the pathophysiological factors contributing to fetal wastage. White's classification[231] of the severity of maternal vascular compromise has subsequently been modified by Cornblath and Schwartz[95] (Table 128–2). Class A in this schema includes women with gestational diabetes and prediabetes. The *gestational diabetic* is defined as the woman who develops abnormal glucose tolerance during pregnancy and postpartum reverts to a normal tolerance; the *prediabetic* includes pregnant women with a genetic predisposition to the disease, including a strong family history of diabetes, a history of previously overweight infants (>4000 g), or unexplained stillbirth beyond 28 weeks' gestation.[95] By definition, the pregnant prediabetic has a normal glucose tolerance, and neither subclass is symptomatic or is receiving insulin therapy during pregnancy. A glycosylated hemoglobin determination in the suspected but unproven gestational diabetic mother at the time of delivery may prove to be helpful in the management of an infant with hypoglycemia.

In a retrospective study by Dekaban and Baird,[232] abortions, stillbirths, neonatal deaths, and abnormal survivors were significantly higher in overt and prediabetics as compared with control individuals. When the diabetic mothers were classified according to the criteria given in Table 128–2, fetal loss was 14.5 per cent for combined classes B and C and 29 per cent for combined classes D through F. In a recent study, however, the risk of malformation was not correlated with glycohemoglobin[233] during early gestation. Other factors that have been shown to affect the outcome of the pregnancy are toxemia and hydramnios.[95]

TABLE 128–2. MODIFIED WHITE CLASSIFICATION OF DIABETES AND PREGNANCY

Class A	High fetal survival, no insulin, minimal dietary regulation
	Gestational diabetes: Abnormal glucose tolerance test during pregnancy which reverts to normal within a few weeks after delivery
	Prediabetes: Normal glucose tolerance test, but family history of diabetes, previous large infants, or unexplained stillbirths
Class B	Onset of diabetes in adult life after age 20, duration less than 10 years, no vascular disease
Class C	Diabetes of long duration (10–19 years) with onset during adolescence (over 10 years) with minimal vascular disease
Class D	Diabetes of 20 years or more duration, onset before age 10, evidence of vascular disease (i.e., retinitis, albuminuria, hypertension)
Class E	Patients with diabetes, plus demonstrable calcification of pelvic vessels
Class F	Patients with diabetes plus nephritis

It is generally accepted that the neonates of overt insulin-dependent diabetics (classes B to F) have increased survival if the pregnancy is interrupted between 35 and 37 weeks of gestation. Delivery prior to 35 weeks is associated with excessive neonatal mortality and delivery after 37 weeks with an increased incidence of stillbirths.

The infant of the diabetic mother is generally a "large for date" infant. In a recent study of 127 infants of diabetic mothers, 43 per cent were large for gestational age, and the degree of macrosomia correlated with maternal glycohemoglobin levels measured in the last (yet not in the first and second) trimester of gestation.[234] However, despite their size, these infants are physiologically immature. Diabetic mothers with severe vascular disease may give birth to SGA infants. The excessive weight in the majority of the infants of diabetic mothers is due to increased body fat and enlargement of certain viscera, primarily liver and heart.[235, 236] They often exhibit several clinical problems associated with their prematurity, including respiratory distress due to hyaline membrane disease (the leading cause of death), nonhemolytic hyperbilirubinemia, hypocalcemic tetany, polycythemia, and rarely, renal vein thrombosis.[236] Congenital anomalies are three times more frequent among these infants than among normal controls.

In 1954, Pedersen et al.[237] suggested that prolonged and excessive exposure of the fetus in a diabetic mother to hyperglycemia resulted in stimulation of the pancreatic beta cell to synthesize and secrete excessive insulin. The high level of glucose and insulin would thus result in increased synthesis and storage of fat, glycogen, and protein in utero. The last 30 years have seen no serious challenge to this hypothesis, although it is now clear that Pedersen's scheme must be modified to include derangements in all insulin-dependent maternal fuels and their consequent effects on the fetus.[238] Furthermore, the last several years have seen experimental verification of this hypothesis with demonstration that chronic hyperinsulinemia in the primate fetus can produce the macrosomia, organomegaly, altered enzyme activities, and substrate changes characteristic of the human circumstance.[239–242] Fetal hyperinsulinemia also was found to increase rates of protein synthesis in the brain, heart, and liver of rat fetuses.[243] Recently, it was observed that significant amounts of antibody-bound insulin can be transferred from insulin-treated diabetic mothers to their fetuses; although the degree of newborn macrosomia correlated with the amount of insulin transfer, the effect of this placentally transported gamma globulin–bound insulin on fetal substrate metabolism is unknown.[30]

Soon after birth, severe symptomatic hypoglycemia occurs in 10 to 20 per cent and asymptomatic hypoglycemia in up to 50 per cent of these infants. The substrate fuel concentrations during the first day of life have been carefully recorded[244–248] and include, in addition to hypoglycemia, lowered levels of FFA and selected amino acids as well. These changes are secondary to the transient postnatal persistence of hyperinsulinemia[235, 249, 250] and, possibly, to suppression of glucagon secretion as well.[251, 252] The net effect of combined hyperinsulinemia and relative hypoglucagonemia is attenuation of hepatic glucose production[253] with consequent hypoglycemia. Rigorous antenatal control of maternal hyperglycemia normalizes neonatal hepatic glucose production[254] and circulating substrate levels,[255] presumably the result of preventing dysfunction in the secretion of fetal pancreatic hormones.

Erythroblastosis

Infants with erythroblastosis fetalis also have a high incidence of hypoglycemia which is secondary to hyperinsulinemia.[256] Beta-cell hyperplasia has been found at postmortem examination in these infants. No etiology is apparent that accounts for the beta-cell hyperplasia and subsequent hyperinsulinemia observed in these patients. However, with the advent of preventive therapy, erythroblastosis and the uncommonly associated hypoglycemia are rarely seen.

Beckwith-Wiedemann Syndrome

Beta-cell hyperplasia has been observed in the Beckwith-Wiedemann syndrome. This disorder is characterized by macroglossia, omphalocele, hyperplastic visceromegaly, and frequently, hypoglycemia. Subsequent to the original descriptions of this syndrome, a large number of additional somatic abnormalities have been described; the interested reader is referred to several reviews.[257, 258] The hypoglycemia, when it occurs in these neonates, is profound but improves spontaneously over the first few days of life. Hyperinsulinemia and elevated insulin-like activity have been documented in a number of these infants, and the Beckwith-Wiedemann gene is located on the short arm of chromosome 11, adjacent to the location of the insulin and insulin-like growth factor II genes, as reported in two children with the Beckwith-Wiedemann syndrome.[259] Recent studies suggest that at least some patients with Beckwith-Wiedemann syndrome carry two copies of the corresponding father's gene (uniparental paternal disomy), similar to the uniparental disomy observed in Prader-Willi and Angelman syndromes.[260, 261] Any newborn with macroglossia and/or omphalocele should be prospectively followed for the development of hypoglycemia so that prompt therapy can be instituted to minimize the CNS dysfunction so frequently observed with this disorder.

Sepsis, Hypoxemia, and Hypothermia

Neonatal bacterial sepsis is associated with hypoglycemia and accelerated rates of glucose disappearance to IV glucose administration.[262, 263] Whether the hypoglycemia is secondary to poor antecedent caloric intake or to the effects of circulating endotoxins on glucose homeostatic mechanisms has not been established. However, hypoglycemia has been observed in adults with gram-negative bacteremia.[264] In animal studies, gram-negative infection and exogenously administered endotoxins have been associated with hypoglycemia, hepatic glycogen depletion, and decreased rates of gluconeogenesis.[265]

Neonatal hypoxemia frequently is associated with hypoglycemia in the early hours of life.[266] In neonatal animal studies, it has been observed that tissue oxygenation is a prerequisite for the establishment of hepatic gluconeogenesis.[151] Therefore, under the stress of hypoxemia, hepatic glycogen stores would be depleted rapidly, and with a superimposed functional defect in gluconeogenesis, hypoglycemia would ensue.

Hypoglycemia also has been associated with hypothermia in the newborn infant.[267] Cause and effect are not clear, since hypothermia is a common finding in adults with hypoglycemia.

CHRONIC HYPOGLYCEMIA

Sustained Hyperinsulinemia

Absolute or relative hyperinsulinism is a relatively common cause of persistent hypoglycemia in the neonate or young infant. Hyperinsulinism seems to occur either as a familial form or as a sporadic disease. However, Thornton et al.[268] recently reviewed their series of 26 patients with hyperinsulinism, composed of 21 simplex families (when only one child is affected) and 5 multiplex families (when more than one sibling was affected). They proposed that in most or all cases—even the apparently sporadic ones—hyperinsulinism may be an inherited disease with an autosomal recessive transmission.

That the hypoglycemia is a consequence of inappropriate insulinemia is supported by observations that these infants have low circulating FFA and ketone levels,[269] retain glycogen reserves in the face of hypoglycemia,[270, 271] and require infusion of exogenous glucose at rates far higher than normal hepatic glucose output in order to maintain normoglycemia. Furthermore, hepatic glucose production in these infants is reduced as a consequence of the hyperinsulinemia,[272] as it is in the infant of the diabetic mother.[253] Somewhat surprisingly, however, Bougnères et al.[272] demonstrated that a ketone body infusion in hyperinsulinemic children restored normoglycemia not by reducing glucose utilization as a consequence of an increased supply of "alternate fuel" but rather by restoring hepatic glucose production. The mechanism of this remains to be elucidated.

Chronic, inappropriate hypersecretion of insulin can be seen with a variety of histological abnormalities of the pancreatic islets, including beta-cell adenoma, beta-cell hyperplasia, and nesidioblastosis (or neoformation of beta cells from ductal epithelial cells). In children, true islet cell tumors are relatively rare[271, 273] and are invariably adenomas rather than carcinomas. No gross pancreatic pathology is typical in the infant or young child with hypoglycemia secondary to sustained hyperinsulinemia. Beta-cell hyperplasia, focal adenomatosis and nesidioblastosis, and normal pancreatic pathology have been reported. Quantitative studies have shown that the total mass of pancreatic endocrine cells is not increased in hyperinsulinemic infants.[274] However, all these pathological findings have now been reported in the pancreata of nonhypoglycemic infants.[275-277] A subtle finding may characterize the islets of the hyperinsulinemic, hypoglycemic infants in that the nuclei of the islet cells are larger and less well defined and provide the basis for the application of the term *endocrine cell dysplasia*.[275]

Despite the presence or absence of pancreatic pathology, these children have a functional defect in insulin secretion. At the present time, it is impossible to distinguish the etiology of hyperinsulinemia in these children on the basis of plasma insulin responses to fasting or to provocative challenge with insulin secretagogues or on the basis of pathological findings. Decreased somatostatin secretion could result in hypersecretion of insulin through disturbed paracrine regulation of the beta cell (see Ch. 77). The 50 per cent decrease in pancreatic somatostatin content and decreased secretion of somatostatin in vitro from islets from infants and young children with hypoglycemia and hyperinsulinemia,[278, 279] together with their hyperglycemic response to exogenous infusion of somatostatin, would support this hypothesis.[280, 281] Further studies will be required to clarify the pathophysiological process resulting in the abnormal insulin secretion in these children.

As adenomas are generally less than 1 cm in size and are rare in children less than 1 year of age, celiac arteriography is of little use and only adds to the morbidity and cost of the evaluation.[282] The authors have not found high-resolution computed axial tomography to be of value in these patients. Transhepatic catheterization of the right portal vein with selective sampling for plasma insulin concentrations has been reported to detect focal zones of insulin secretion in 15 of 30 cases of hyperinsulinemic hypoglycemic infants.[283] However, this invasive procedure requires general anesthesia and must be considered experimental until further independent validation is provided. Preoperative and intraoperative ultrasonography is clearly of great value in locating and resecting insulin-secreting (and non-insulin-secreting) tumors, which may not be palpable.[284] Recent reports suggest that in adult patients small pancreatic adenomas could be visualized using endoscopic ultrasonography[285] or scanning with ^{123}I-labeled octreotide, a somatostatin analogue, since pancreatic adenomas possess receptors to somatostatin.[286] To the authors' knowledge, these techniques have yet to be evaluated in pediatric-age patients. Should an islet-cell adenoma be found, a search for other endocrine abnormalities (hyperparathyroidism, hypergastrinemia, and pituitary tumors) must be made in both the patient and family members to exclude multiple endocrine neoplasia syndrome type I.[271]

The ultimate aim of therapy is to prevent seizures, permanent neurological sequelae, and in extreme situations, death. Medical management of hyperinsulinemia has included the long-term use of glucocorticoids or the use of zinc-protamine glucagon, a long-acting form of glucagon,[287] and dietary manipulations. In general, the response to such treatment has been poor.

The hyperglycemic effect of diazoxide is due, at least in part, to suppression of pancreatic insulin secretion.[288] However, in a number of infants with proven hyperinsulinemia, diazoxide is ineffective in controlling hypoglycemia. Unfortunately, too, there has been surprisingly little written about the long-term follow-up and outcome of "successfully" treated patients. In the authors' experience, no proven diazoxide-controlled hyperinsulinemic infant has been able to be weaned successfully from diazoxide treatment without subsequent predilection to develop recurrent hypoglycemia. In a dosage range of 10 to 15 mg/kg of body weight daily (maximum dose of 20 mg/kg of body weight daily), the common side effects of diazoxide therapy consist of hypertrichosis, advancement of bone age, mild hyperuricemia, and depressed serum IgG. A less common but potentially more serious side effect is the retention of sodium and fluid with resulting congestive heart failure. On occasion, sudden unexplained cardiac arrest has occurred which might be a consequence of the latter mechanism. Reversible hypertrophic cardiomyopathy also has been described in patients suffering from hyperinsulinism and treated with diazoxide.[289, 290] The respective roles of elevated insulin level per se and diazoxide in the pathophysiology of this complication are unclear, since the cardiomyopathy resolved following radical treatment, which permitted weaning the patients from the diazoxide. Diazoxide has a particularly long biological half-life, on the order of 18 to 24 hours, and this rate is prolonged further in the neonate. Thus one must wait a number of days to achieve a new steady-state blood level after altering the dose. Due caution is required in the frequency of dosage increases based on apparent unresponsiveness, since toxic drug levels will likewise not be corrected for several days.

Recent preliminary studies suggest that long-term treatment with octreotide, a long-acting somatostatin analogue, given as thrice-daily subcutaneous injections at doses of 15 to 40 μg/kg per day, may control blood glucose in a sizable subset of patients with no obvious deceleration of growth.[291, 292]

There is no uniform agreement on the therapeutic effectiveness of pancreatic surgery in children with hyperinsulinism. Obviously, it can be cured with the removal of a beta-cell adenoma. The variable results reported with this procedure reflect, at least in part, the heterogeneity of the underlying pathology and the extent of the pancreatectomy.[129] Since subtotal pancreatectomy in a child performed by an experienced surgeon carries relatively little risk[129, 271, 294, 295] and the pathological basis for hyperinsulinism cannot be defined by clinical testing, the authors feel that any infant with hypoglycemia and proven hyperinsulinemia persisting beyond the age of 2 weeks that is not responding to standard medical measures is a candidate for pancreatic exploration. If an adenoma is not found after careful inspection and palpation and intraoperative ultrasonography,[284] a subtotal pancreatectomy is indicated, in which about 85 to 90 per cent of the pancreas is removed, but sparing the spleen. Following the procedure, exogenous insulin may be required for a period of time (one day to several months) to control hyperglycemia. Sufficient exocrine pancreas is preserved to avoid fat malabsorption.

Despite subtotal pancreatectomy, frequent feedings, diazoxide, and/or octreotide may be required. If the hypoglycemia cannot be controlled adequately with medical management, reoperation and near-total pancreatectomy should be considered. Obviously, long-term follow-up of these patients is required before definitive conclusions on the efficacy of surgical therapy can be made. However, current results would indicate that a significant number of children can benefit by this form of therapy.[129, 271, 282, 294, 295]

Endocrine Deficiencies

Hypoglycemia is a frequent occurrence in neonates and children with primary and secondary adrenal insufficiency, i.e., Addison's disease,[129] congenital adrenal hyperplasia,[296] and isolated ACTH deficiency.[297] A 20 per cent incidence has been noted in panhypopituitarism, monotrophic growth hormone, or various combinations of trophic hormonal deficiencies including growth hormone (GH) and ACTH.[298] The pathophysiology of hypoglycemia in these disorders is generally assumed to be the consequence of diminished substrate mobilization and gluconeogenic enzyme activity due to cortisol insufficiency and/or augmented glucose utilization secondary to GH inadequacy. Studies based on circulating substrate levels alone support this view.[299] Conflicting data have been reported on the effects of GH deficiency on glucose kinetics in humans; although GH treatment increased plasma glucose concentration, it failed to affect the glucose production rate in 10 euthyroid GH-deficient children studied by Dahms et al.[300] In contrast, Bougnères et al.[301] reported that hepatic glucose production and peripheral glucose utilization were reduced in GH-deficient children and that replacement therapy produced normoglycemia principally by restoring hepatic glucose output. Until further study, the etiology of hypoglycemia in these children remains to be determined.

The entity of isolated glucagon deficiency has not been clearly established. The absence of alpha cells in pancreatic tissue from infants and young children with intractable hypoglycemia has been reported, but measurements of plasma immunoreactive glucagon were not performed (see ref. 302). Two children with severe hypoglycemia have been reported with decreased plasma immunoreactive glucagon concentrations, significant hyperglycemic response to exogenous glucagon, and clinical improvement with the institution of long-term protamine zinc glucagon therapy.[302, 303] In both patients, insulin values were inappropriately high (at least 10 μU/ml) at the time of hypoglycemia; in addition, one patient had low concentrations of plasma FFA. These data suggest a primary abnormality in the regulation of insulin secretion. Since the metabolic response of patients with hyperinsulinemia to exogenous glucagon is similar to that reported in children with purported glucagon deficiency, further documentation of glucagon deficiency as a clearly defined entity may be necessary to separate this condition from the more common hyperinsulinemia of infants and children.

Hepatic Enzyme Deficiencies

Glucose-6-Phosphatase Deficiency (Glycogen Storage Disease Type I)

The glycogen storage diseases are inherited defects characterized by either a deficient or abnormally functioning enzyme involved in the degradation of glycogen. Glycogen storage diseases type II (deficient lysosomal α-1,4-glucosidase) and type IV (amylo-1,4$\rightarrow$1,6-transglucosidase brancher enzyme), as well as those due to specific muscle enzyme defects, are not considered in this chapter because they are not associated with hypoglycemia. In addition, deficiencies of amylo-1,6-glucosidase and phosphorylase (glycogen storage diseases type III and type VI, respectively) rarely present with neonatal hypoglycemia and usually present with asymptomatic hepatomegaly at an older age. The interested reader is referred to recent reviews of these topics.[304]

The first case of hypoglycemia associated with hepatomegaly and ketonuria was reported by Snapper and van Creveld in 1928.[305] The following year, Von Gierke[306] demonstrated increased glycogen deposition in the liver and kidney of a similar patient, and 23 years later Cori and Cori[307] reported the absence of glucose-6-phosphatase in patients with the hepatic form of glycogen storage disease.

Since hydrolysis of glucose-6-phosphatase is the final common enzymatic event in the release of glucose from either the gluconeogenic or glycogenolytic pathway, the absence of glucose-6-phosphatase typically results in severe hypoglycemia. Surprisingly, however, glucose production is on the order of 60 per cent or more of the rate found in age-matched controls.[308, 309] The reasons for this apparent discrepancy are not entirely clear, but there is some evidence to support the hypothesis that residual glucose-6-phosphatase activity could be sufficient to account for the observed rates of glucose production.[309]

Hepatomegaly, growth retardation, lacticacidemia, ketonemia, hypertriglyceridemia, and hyperuricemia are also common clinical features of this disorder. Chronic hypoglycemia provokes the increased secretion of various hormones (i.e., catecholamines, glucagon, and cortisol) and suppresses insulin secretion. The hyperlactacidemia is most likely the result of increased lactate formation from glucose and decreased lactate clearance as a result of a defective gluconeogenesis. However, since lactate can serve as an alternate CNS fuel in children with type I glycogen storage disease, lacticacidemia may play a beneficial role.[310] Ketonemia in these children is a more complex problem. In the first several hours of fasting, their circulating ketone body levels are elevated compared with normal children. However, children with type I glycogen storage disease are actually hypoketonemic if their ketone body concentrations are compared with children who are matched on the basis of blood sugar level or glucose production rate or with normal children after a prolonged fast.[309, 311, 312] To the authors' knowledge, ketone body kinetics have not been quantified in children with this disorder, but Havel et al.[308] measured hepatic ketone body balance in overnight-fasted adults with type I glycogen storage disease and found near-normal production rates when circulating FFA's were elevated, implying a relative defect in ketogenesis.

The hyperuricemia is the result of both decreased renal clearance secondary to elevated blood lactate and ketone body concentrations, which compete for a common renal tubular secretory site, and increased de novo uric acid production,[313, 314] which may result in chronic gouty arthritis. Hypercholesterolemia and hypertriglyceridemia together with increased lipid stores in the liver appear related to increased lipogenesis.[314, 315] Despite marked hepatomegaly due to excessive lipid and glycogen storage, there is generally little impairment of other hepatic functions.[314]

Glucose-6-phosphatase is also normally present in kidney and intestinal mucosa. Although the kidneys demonstrate excessive storage of glycogen, renal function is normal at the time of diagnosis, except for occasional glycosuria and aminoaciduria.[315] Several young adults have been reported with impending renal failure with focal glomerulosclerosis which cannot be attributed to uric acid nephropathy. While the etiology of the renal dysfunction remain to be determined, its prevalence seems to be high. In a recently reported series of 20 patients 13 years old or older, 14 had renal failure.[315]

Although occasional patients present with only mild clinical biochemical abnormalities (hypoglycemia after 15 to 20 hours of fasting) and subnormal but detectable glycemic responses to glucagon, fructose, and galactose administration[316] (see Fig. 128–4), glucose-6-phosphatase activity cannot be demonstrated in liver biopsy specimens. Conversely, a number of well-studied cases, presenting with all the clinical features of glucose-6-phosphatase deficiency and biopsy-proved hepatic glycogen storage disease, have been reported in which normal levels of this enzyme have been found in vitro.[309, 316] It has been established recently that individuals similar to those described in the past have a defect in the glucose-6-phosphatase translocase present in microsomal membranes and are designated as type Ib (G-6-P'tase translocase defect)[317–319] or type Ic (defective in G-6-P'tase translocase and in translocase for P_i, PP_i, and carbamyl-P).[320] In addition, children with type Ib frequently have granulocytopenia, absence of leukocyte chemotaxis, and are prone to mucocutaneous and occasionally deep-seated and life-threatening infections.

Fructose-1,6-Diphosphatase Deficiency

Hepatic fructose-1,6-diphosphatase deficiency is a gluconeogenic enzyme defect with presenting signs and symptoms similar to those of glycogen storage disease type I. However, excessive glycogen storage does not occur, since the glycogenolytic pathway is intact. Hepatomegaly is secondary to lipid storage, but liver function studies are generally normal. Lactic acidosis, ketoacidosis, hyperlipidemia, and hyperuricemia in this condition are presumed to have the same pathogenesis as in glucose-6-phosphatase deficiency.

The first report of this entity by Baker and Winegrad[321] was followed within a few months by the description of four additional cases.[322–325] The five children ranged in age from 5 months to 5.5 years at the time of diagnosis. Several of these patients presented with hypoglycemia and acidosis in the neonatal period. In three of the five families there were five affected siblings who presented with hepatomegaly and died in the neonatal or early childhood period from unexplained metabolic acidosis. Consanguinity was noted in two of the five families,[323, 324] and on the basis of available data, this disorder appears to be inherited as an autosomal recessive trait.

Since the glycogenolytic system is intact, glucagon administration produces a hyperglycemic response in the immediate postprandial period but not after a short fast.[322, 324] Glucose, galactose, maltose, and lactose are utilized carbohydrates and can be stored as glycogen and metabolized. Since fructose, glycerol, and the gluconeogenic amino acids enter the gluconeogenic pathway at or below the level of fructose-1,6-diphosphatase (see Fig. 128–4), these substances cannot be converted to glucose. Infusions of these substrates cause the accumulation of lactate and consequent lactic acidosis and produce a rapid fall in the blood glucose level. The mechanism of this hypoglycemic effect has not been clarified, but one possibility is that the accumulation of triose phosphates below the level of fructose-1,6-diphosphatase may acutely inhibit glycogenolysis in a manner similar to that resulting from the accumulation of fructose-1-phosphate in patients with hereditary fructose intolerance.

Diagnosis and Treatment of Glycogen Storage Disease Type I and Fructose-1,6-Diphosphate Deficiency

The diagnosis and management of these two disorders is described in detail elsewhere.[186] However, definitive diagnosis is made by determining specific enzyme activities and glycogen content in liver biopsy specimens. Management consists of proper dietary constituents and maintenance of a normal plasma glucose concentration via frequent meals or nasogastric infusion, as well as the use of oral uncooked cornstarch.[326–332]

Glycogen Synthetase Deficiency

Fasting hypoglycemia from birth has been reported in identical twins and their younger siblings, in whom liver biopsy studies in one twin demonstrated fatty metamorphosis, absence of glycogen, and a lack of glycogen synthetase activity.[333] Parr and associates[334] observed a 4-month-old infant with hypoglycemia in whom no glycogen was demonstrable in muscle, liver, kidney, and adrenal glands. The liver showed fatty infiltration, absent hepatic glycogen synthetase and phosphorylase, and markedly diminished glucose-6-phosphatase. Similar histological findings also were observed in two siblings who had clinical hypoglycemia. It is of interest that hepatic glycogen synthetase deficiency has been reported in a 9-year-old child who was managed successfully on four around-the-clock feedings of protein-rich meals.[336]

Galactose-1-Phosphate Uridyl Transferase Deficiency (Galactosemia) and Fructose-1-Phosphate Aldolase Deficiency (Hereditary Fructose Intolerance)

Infants with the classical form of galactosemia due to a deficiency of the gene for galactose-1-phosphate uridyl transferase, located on chromosome 9,[336] are intolerant to products containing lactose and galactose and present with hypoglycemia, diarrhea, and vomiting following meals and failure to thrive. The accumulation of galactose-1-phosphate in tissue reflects the inability to convert this substrate to glucose-1-phosphate (see Fig. 128–4) and results in hepatosplenomegaly, jaundice, lenticular cataracts, mental retardation, and renal tubular abnormalities. The occurrence of postprandial hypoglycemia in this disorder appears to be due to inhibition of phosphoglucomutase by galactose-1-phosphate, thereby resulting in acute inhibition of glycogenolysis. Diagnosis is relatively easy and should be considered in all infants with failure to thrive together with any of the preceding physical manifestations or symptoms. This topic has been reviewed extensively.[337, 338] While elimination of galactose from the diet in early life is lifesaving and essentially curative, some of these children still suffer developmental[339, 340] or endocrinological[341] sequelae.

Fructose-1-phosphate aldolase deficiency (hereditary fructose intolerance) is dominated by symptoms of hypoglycemia and vomiting following ingestion of foods containing fructose. Fructosuria is present only after meals, and these patients frequently manifest hepatomegaly, jaundice, aminoaciduria, and failure to thrive. Several comprehensive reviews have been published.[342–344] The hypoglycemia following fructose ingestion is a result of accumulation of fructose-1-phosphate which inhibits the phosphorylase system and gluconeogenesis at the level of fructose-1,6-diphosphate aldolase (see Fig. 128–4). Since most neonates are not exposed to fructose in the first weeks to months of life, this diagnosis can be entertained only in those special circumstances in which an infant is receiving sucrose-containing foods or formulas. The latter include most soy protein–based formulas.

The diagnosis of galactosemia or hereditary fructose intolerance should be considered in infants presenting with hypoglycemia, hepatomegaly, and failure to thrive; these infants also may have non–glucose-reducing substances (i.e., galactose, fructose) in the urine following meals in the immediate postprandial period. The definitive diagnosis of galactosemia is made by determining the galactose-1-phosphate uridyl transferase activity in red blood cells; a galactose infusion test is not required and is contraindicated. Hereditary fructose intolerance is classically diagnosed by the hypoglycemic and hypophosphatemic responses produced by the cautious intravenous infusion of fructose (0.25 g/kg of body weight); the intravenous route of fructose administration obviates the distressful symptoms of nausea or vomiting associated with oral ingestion.[342–344] A recent report suggests that infusion of ^{13}C-labeled fructose in tracer amounts with monitoring of ^{13}C appearance into plasma glucose can identify patients with aldolase deficiency and may be a diagnostic tool in the future.[345] Finally, the human gene for hepatic aldolase was recently found to be located on chromosome 9 and subsequently sequenced; although several mutations have been described,[346] three missense mutations account for most cases of the diseases, which may provide a new diagnostic tool in the future.

Defects in Amino Acid Metabolism

Branched-Chain Ketoacid Dehydrogenase Deficiency

Maple syrup urine disease (MSUD) is an autosomal recessive disorder resulting from deficiency of the enzyme that decarboxylates the α-ketoacids of leucine, isoleucine, and valine. Hypoglycemia and profound hypoalaninemia are observed in patients with classical MSUD at times when their branched-chain amino acids and α-ketoacids are markedly elevated.[347, 348] With dietary therapy and correction of the plasma branched-chain amino acid abnormalities, fasting plasma alanine and glucose values have been observed to increase toward normal. Glycogen metabolism and the gluconeogenic enzyme pathways seem to be intact. It appears that an enzyme(s) regulating TCA cycle homeostasis is affected, which may divert substrates away from gluconeogenesis.

Defects in Fatty Acid Metabolism

A new group of metabolic disorders resulting from abnormalities in fatty acid transport and/or oxidation has been identified and is associated with hypoglycemia and ketone deficiency. During periods of fasting or catabolic stress, FFA's are mobilized from adipose stores and are oxidized directly by body tissue (heart, muscle, intestine) or undergo β-oxidation in the liver with the subsequent release of ketone bodies. For hepatic ketogenesis to occur, long-chain FFA's are converted to their acyl-CoA esters, transported across the mitochondrial membrane via the acylcarnitine transport system, and reconverted to the acyl-CoA derivative. This process involves (1) sodium-dependent uptake of the free carnitine molecule at the level of the cell plasma membrane, (2) formation of acylcarnitine from acyl-CoA and carnitine, catalyzed by carnitine-palmitoyltransferase type 1 (CPT1) on the inner aspect of the outer mitochondrial membrane, (3) translocation of the acylcarnitine complex across the inner mitochondrial membrane, catalyzed by the carnitine-acylcarnitine translocase, and (4) release of the acyl-CoA and free carnitine on the inner aspect of the inner mitochondrial membrane, catalyzed by carnitine-palmitoyltransferase type 2 (CPT2).[349, 350] The long-chain CoA is subsequently catabolized to acetyl-CoA, acetoacetyl-CoA, and ketone bodies (Fig. 128–10).

Systemic Carnitine Deficiency

Although the entity of systemic carnitine deficiency has been recognized for a number of years,[349, 351, 352] no reports exist that demonstrate a biosynthetic defect in carnitine. An infusion of methyl ^{3}H-trimethyl lysine, a precursor of carnitine, resulted in production of ^{3}H-carnitine in patients with systemic carnitine deficiency.[352] Although carnitine is synthesized from lysine and methionine, a significant source of carnitine is from the diet.[353, 354] Young infants have lower plasma concentrations of both free and total (free + acyl carnitine) carnitine when compared with adults, so some care must be taken in the interpretation of plasma carnitine values in this age group.[355] In addition,

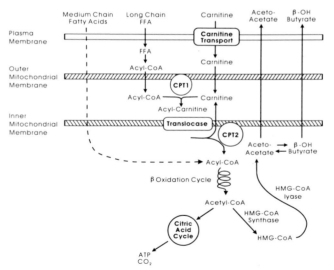

FIGURE 128–10. Pathway of mitochondrial fatty acid oxidation. In contrast to medium-chain fatty acids, long-chain free fatty acids (FFA's) cannot enter mitochondria directly. After its activation to an acylcoenzyme A (CoA) ester at the outer mitochondrial membrane, the FFA molecule is transesterified by carnitine palmitoyltransferase type 1 (CPT1) to form an acylcarnitine on the inner aspect of the outer mitochondrial membrane. Carnitine is supplied by a plasma membrane carnitine transporter. Acylcarnitine is then transported across the inner mitochondrial membrane by a translocase in exchange for free carnitine. On the inner aspect of the inner mitochondrial membrane, carnitine palmitoyltransferase type 2 (CPT2) releases free carnitine and converts the acylcarnitine to an acyl-CoA. The acyl-CoA molecule can then enter the β-oxidation cycle. The β-oxidation cycle involves four consecutive steps (catalyzed by an acyl-CoA dehydrogenase, an acyl-CoA hydratase, a 3-hydroxyacyl-CoA dehydrogenase, and a thiolase) and shortens the fatty acid chain by two carbons with the release of acetyl-CoA. Acetyl-CoA can either be oxidized in the citric acid cycle or enter the pathway for ketone body synthesis. (Adapted, with permission, from Stanley CA, Hale DE, Berry GT, et al: Brief report: A deficiency of carnitine-acylcarnitine translocation in the inner mitochondrial membrane. N Eng J Med 327:19, 1992.)

low plasma carnitine has been observed in infants subsisting totally on nonmilk base protein diets and children on long-term total parenteral nutrition. Whether this presumed ''dietary'' deficiency of carnitine is associated with any clinical symptoms is unknown.

Children with systemic carnitine deficiency present with profound hypoglycemia, hypotonia, encephalopathy, hepatomegaly with microvesicular fat, increased plasma concentrations of FFA, and NH_3 and liver and muscle enzymes (LDH and CPK)—a clinical presentation similar to Reye's syndrome. In addition, the long-term neurological sequellae are most likely due to inadequate cerebral perfusion secondary to cerebral edema. It is becoming increasingly clear that at least the majority of these patients have enzymatic defects in the catabolism of acyl-CoA compounds. Accumulation of these compounds most likely leads to increased formation and excretion of acylcarnitine.

Disorders so far identified associated with abnormalities in fatty acid metabolism include (1) primary defects of fatty acid β-oxidation, i.e., long-, medium-, and short-chain acyl-dehydrogenase deficiencies, (2) defects of the free carnitine transporter, (3) defects of the acylcarnitine transport system, i.e., carnitine-palmitoyltransferase deficiencies, and (4) secondary defects of fatty acid metabolism presumably due to carnitine depletion secondary to abnormal amino acid metabolism, such as isovaleric acidemia, proprionic acidemia, and methylmalonic aciduria.

Primary Defects of β-Oxidation (Table 128–3)

Medium-chain acyl-CoA dehydrogenase (MCAD) deficiency has been diagnosed in about 100 patients and is the most commonly recognized defect of β-oxidation.[349, 352, 356, 357] Its frequency has been estimated to be 1 in 10,000 to 1 in 25,000, and it is transmitted as an autosomal recessive disorder. Thus the frequency of heterozygotes may approach 1 in 100 in the general population. The clinical presentation is extremely variable from sudden death (especially during the second year of life) to asymptomatic disease.[357] Children with this disorder usually present before 2 years of age with profound hypoglycemia, vomiting, and lethargy, frequently reminiscent of classical Reye's syndrome. The CNS symptoms may not be attributable to hypoglycemia but rather to CNS toxicity of fatty acid inter-

mediates resulting in many cases of cerebral edema. These children frequently present with mild hepatomegaly and mild hepatic dysfunction (increased transaminases and ammonium levels).

Long-chain acyl-CoA dehydrogenase (LCAD) deficiency has only been described in eight patients. It is characterized by an earlier and more severe presentation, with skeletal muscle hypotonia and myoglobinuria and heart (cardiomyopathy) involvement, and it is also thought to be transmitted as an autosomal recessive disorder.[349, 358–360]

Short-chain acyl-CoA dehydrogenase (SCAD) deficiency is still less frequent; four patients presenting with lethargy and metabolic acidosis have been diagnosed.[349, 352, 361]

Finally, urinary excretion of long-chain dicarboxylic acids with a hydroxyl group in position 3 led to the diagnosis of 3-hydroxy acyl-CoA dehydrogenase deficiency in an infant with cardiomyopathy and hypoketotic hypoglycemia.[362]

Defects of Carnitine Transport

Cardiomyopathy, profound hypoglycemia, and coma have been reported in children with a defect in the plasma membrane transport system that takes up free carnitine.[363, 364]

Defects of the Acylcarnitine Transport System

Although children with acylcarnitine transferase deficiency can present with hypoglycemia, hypoketonemia, and lactic acidemia, in general they differ from those with carnitine deficiency in that they may have myalgias, rhabdomyolysis, and myoglobinuria and do not present with metabolic acidosis.[352]

Carnitine-palmitoyltransferase consists of two enzymes distributed in the outer (CPT1) and the inner (CPT2) mitochondrial membrane; CPT1 deficiency is thought to be responsible for the hepatic form of the disease, while CPT2 deficiency is responsible for the muscular form of the disease.[365–367] Only the hepatic form (CPT1 deficiency) was thought to be associated with hypoglycemia.[367] However, hypoketotic hypoglycemia also was reported in infants with near-total CPT2 deficiency.[368] A patient was recently described with hypoglycemia and severe cardiac arrhythmia due to carnitine-acylcarnitine translocase deficiency.[350]

Secondary Defects of Fatty Acid Metabolism

Hypoglycemia and carnitine deficiency have been observed in patients with methylmalonic aciduria, isovaleric acidemia, and proprionic acidemia during episodes of metabolic acidosis.[370–372] Detailed studies of urinary metabolites have identified methylated products of the TCA cycle (methyl citrate) that may competitively inhibit normal cycle activity and lead to profound cellular dysfunction.[371, 372] Accumulation of circulating potential gluconeogenic substrates (lactate, pyruvate, and alanine) observed during these episodes is compatible with a secondary defect in hepatic glucose production.

These patients, and perhaps children with defects in branched-chain amino acid metabolism as well, are potentially at risk for the development of acute hypoglycemia, encephalopathy, and a Reye's-like presentation during cat-

TABLE 128–3. FEATURES OF MEDIUM- (MCAD), LONG- (LCAD), AND SHORT-CHAIN (SCAD) ACYL-CoA DEHYDROGENASE DEFICIENCIES

	MCAD	LCAD	SCAD
Induced by fasting			
Vomiting	+	+	+
Coma	+	+	+
Nonketotic hypoglycemia	+	+	−
Fatty hepatomegaly	+	+	?
Dicarboxylic aciduria	+	+	+/−
Chronic abnormalities			
Carnitine deficiency	+	+	+
Cardiomyopathy	−	+	−
Muscle weakness	−	+	+
Retardation	−	−	+
Autosomal recessive inheritance	+	+	+

From Stanley CA: New genetic defects in mitochondrial fatty acid oxidation and carnitine deficiency. Adv Pediatr 34:59, 1987.

abolic illness which may be life-threatening or result in severe permanent neurologic damage.

Another secondary disorder of fatty acid metabolism is hydroxymethylglutaryl-CoA (HMG-CoA) lyase deficiency. A defect in this enzyme on the pathway of ketogenesis (see Fig. 128–10) can lead to lethal hypoglycemia.[373]

Diagnosis of Fatty Acid Metabolism Defects

The diagnosis of the preceding primary and secondary defects in fatty acid oxidation is predicated on a high index of suspicion and a thorough laboratory evaluation. Acyl-CoA dehydrogenase deficiencies and other inborn errors of fatty acid metabolism should be considered whenever hypoglycemia is not accompanied by significant ketosis (hypoketotic hypoglycemia), in the absence of increased insulin concentrations, and is accompanied by signs of mild liver dysfunction or continued encephalopathy following correction of hypoglycemia (hyperammonemia and elevated plasma transaminase activities). Measurement of urinary organic acids by gas chromatography/mass spectrometry (GCMS) should be performed in these cases as a screening test and will detect adipic (C_6), suberic (C_8), and sebacic (C_{10}) acids produced via ω-oxidation in cases of MCAD deficiency.[349, 352] Glycine conjugates (phenylpropionyl-, hexanolyl-, and suberylglycine) are also increased.[374] Carnitine assay reveals an increase in acylcarnitine with a decrease in both total and free plasma carnitine concentrations. During an acute episode, plasma carnitine may be normal, and therefore, determination should be repeated several weeks following recovery. If the suspicion of a defect in fatty acid metabolism is reinforced by any of the screening tests, more specific diagnostic procedures will help establish the diagnosis: (1) identification of urinary acylcarnitine by fast atom bombardment mass spectrometry (FAB-MS), (2) fibroblast culture with measurement of rates of $^{14}CO_2$ production from ^{14}C-labeled fatty acids or rates of ^3H_2O from 9,10-^3H-labeled fatty acids or rates of ^3H_2O from 9,10-^3H-labeled palmitate,[375] (3) oxidation of ^{14}C-labeled fatty acids by circulating leukocytes,[376] and/or (4) formal enzyme analysis on skin fibroblasts.

Asymptomatic siblings affected by the disease may be identified by measurement of acylcarnitines in the urine after an oral dose of L-carnitine.[349, 352] Finally, it should be noted that the gene coding for medium-chain acyldehydrogenase deficiency has been located on chromosome 1.[377] A single point mutation has been found in most patients. Polymerase chain reaction has been used to amplify a small genomic DNA sample, and it is now possible to identify the mutation in tissues obtained from biopsies as well as from postmortem specimens. Seven families have been identified in which the proband child died of an unknown cause and in which a living sibling was diagnosed as having MCAD deficiency. It was found that all the dead siblings had indeed undiagnosed MCAD deficiency.[378] However, the prevalence of the MCAD mutation was the same as that of controls in 397 children dying of sudden infant death syndrome (SIDS), implying that MCAD deficiency is not a common cause of SIDS.[379]

The pathophysiology of the hypoglycemia in children with fatty acid metabolism defects is not known, since no systematic study of their carbohydrate metabolism has been undertaken. Two mechanisms might be considered: First,

they may suffer decreased glucose production, since both gluconeogenesis and ketogenesis are linked by the production and utilization of phosphopyridine nucleotides. Besides, since acetyl-CoA is the obligatory activator of pyruvate carboxylase, a block in the production of acetyl-CoA would decrease the activity of pyruvate-carboxylase and thus the production of oxaloacetate, the direct precursor of PEP and a main entry point of substrates into the gluconeogenetic pathway (see Fig. 128–4). Second, the mechanism may involve accelerated rates of glucose utilization. In the presence of defective ketogenesis, ketone bodies, which normally can meet up to 50 per cent of brain metabolic needs during fasting, would not be available, and thus high rates of glucose utilization would be sustained by the brain under circumstances normally accompanied by ketogenesis and decreased glucose utilization.

Management of these disorders should be directed to the correction of both hypoglycemia and increased intracranial pressure and carried out by experienced individuals. At the time of diagnosis, parenteral glucose should be infused at rates sufficient to maintain normal plasma concentrations, stimulate endogenous insulin secretion, and suppress lipolysis (5 to 10 mg/kg per min). Once the diagnosis has been established, periods of fasting should be avoided, and frequent high-carbohydrate feedings should be given during any catabolic stress. If the child is unable to take carbohydrate orally, parenteral glucose therapy should be initiated to avoid the development of symptoms. If carnitine deficiency is identified, oral and/or IV carnitine replacement should be initiated in an effort to "trap" potentially toxic fatty acid metabolites. However, normalization of the plasma (or even tissue) carnitine should not be construed as curative, since both the underlying enzyme defect persists and the pathophysiology of the devastating encephalopathy remains to be determined. As a result, when these children are unable to take adequate carbohydrate orally during periods of catabolic stress (i.e., most commonly illness associated with nausea or vomiting), they should be electively admitted early in the course of their illness for intravenous glucose therapy.

REFERENCES

1. Adam PAJ, Felig P: Carbohydrate, fat and amino acid metabolism in the pregnant woman and fetus. In Faulkner F, Tanner JM (eds): Human Growth, Vol 1. New York, Plenum Press, 1978.
2. Aynsley-Green A: Metabolic and endocrine interrelations in the human fetus and neonate. Am J Clin Nutr 41:399–417, 1985.
3. Battaglia FC, Meschia G: Principal substrates of fetal metabolism. Physiol Rev 58:499–521, 1978.
4. Battaglia FC: Commonality and diversity in fetal development: Bridging the interspecies gap. Pediatr Res 12:736–745, 1978.
5. Girard JR: Metabolic fuels of the fetus. Isr J Med Sci 11:591, 1975.
6. Girard J, Ferré P, Pégorier JP, et al: Adaptations of glucose and fatty acid metabolism during perinatal period and suckling-weaning transition. Physiol Rev 72:507, 1992.
7. Hay WH: The placenta: Not just a conduit for maternal fuels. Diabetes 40(2):44–50, 1991.
8. Battaglia FC, Meschia G: Fetal nutrition. Annu Rev Nutr 8:43, 1988.
9. Longo LD: Disorders of placental transfer. In Assali NS (ed): Pathophysiology of Gestation, vol 2. New York, Academic Press, 1972, p 1.
10. Smith CH, Moe AJ, Ganapathy V: Nutrient transport pathways across the epithelium of the placenta. Annu Rev Nutr 12:183, 1992.
11. Dancis J, Olsen G, Folkart G: Transfer of histidine and xylose across the placenta and into the red blood cell and amniotic fluids. Am J Physiol 194:44, 1958.

12. Stephens RJ: The development and fine structure of the allantoic placental barrier in the bat *Tadarida brasiliensis cynocephala*. J Ultrastruct Res 28:371, 1969.

13. Holzman I, Philipps AF, Battaglia FC: Glucose metabolism, lactate, and ammonia production by the human placenta in vitro. Pediatr Res 13:117, 1979.

14. Hauguel S, Challier JC, Cedard L, Olive G: Metabolism of the human placenta perfused in vitro: Glucose transfer and utilization, O₂ consumption, lactate and ammonia production. Pediatr Res 17:729, 1983.

15. Holzman I, Lemons JA, Meschia G, et al: Ammonia production by the pregnant uterus. Proc Soc Exp Biol Med 156:27, 1977.

16. Bristow J, Rudolph AM, Itskovitz J, et al: Hepatic oxygen and glucose metabolism in the fetal lamb: Response to hypoxia. J Clin Invest 71:1047, 1983.

17. Vosburgh GJ, Flexner LB, Cowie DB, et al: The rate of renewal in women of the water and sodium of the amniotic fluid as determined by tracer techniques. Am J Obstet Gynecol 56:1156, 1948.

18. Comar CL: Radiocalcium studies in pregnancy. Ann NY Acad Sci 64:281, 1956.

19. Bothwell TH, Pribilla WF, Mebust W, et al: Iron metabolism in the pregnant rabbit: Iron transport across the placenta. Am J Physiol 192:615, 1958.

20. Logothetopoulos J, Scott RF: Concentration of iodine-131 across the placenta of the guinea pig and the rabbit. Nature (London) 175:775, 1955.

21. Lemons JA: Fetal placental nitrogen metabolism. Semin Perinatol 3:177, 1979.

22. Domenech M, Gruppuso PA, Nishino VT, et al: Preserved fetal plasma amino acid concentrations in the presence of maternal hypoaminoacidemia. Pediatr Res 20:1071–1076, 1986.

23. Lemons JA, Adcock EW III, Jones AD, Jr, et al: Umbilical uptake of amino acids in the unstressed fetal lamb. J Clin Invest 58:1428, 1976.

24. Holzman IR, Lemons JA, Meschia G, et al: Uterine uptake of amino acids and placental glutamine-glutamate balance in the pregnant ewe. J Dev Physiol 1:137, 1979.

25. Marconi AM, Sparks JW, Battaglia FC, Meschia G: A comparison of amino acid arteriovenous differences across the liver, hindlimb and placenta in the fetal lamb. Am J Physiol 258:E2508–E2512, 1989.

26. Loy GL, Quick AN, Hay WW, et al: Fetoplacental deamination and decarboxylation of leucine. Am J Physiol 259:E492, 1990.

27. Morriss FH, Rosenfeld CR, Crandell SS, et al: Effects of fasting on uterine blood flow and substrate uptake in sheep. J Nutr 110:2433, 1980.

28. Adam PAJ, Teramo K, Raiha N, et al: Human fetal insulin metabolism early in gestation response to acute elevation of the fetal glucose concentration and placental transfer of human insulin I-131. Diabetes 18:409, 1969.

29. Adam PAJ, King KC, Schwartz R: Human placental barrier to ¹²⁵I-glucagon early in gestation. J Clin Endocrinol Metab 34:772, 1972.

30. Menon RK, Cohen RM, Sperling MA, et al: Transplacental passage of insulin in pregnant women with insulin-dependent diabetes mellitus. N Engl J Med 323:309, 1990.

31. Robertson AF, Sprecher H: A review of human placental lipid metabolism and transport. Acta Paediatr Scand 57(suppl 183):1, 1968.

32. Kimura RE: Lipid metabolism in the fetal-placental unit. *In* Cowett RM, ed., Principles of Perinatal-Neonatal Metabolism. New York, Springer-Verlag, 1991, p 291.

33. Knopp RH, Magee MS, Bonet B, et al: Lipid metabolism in pregnancy. *In* Cowett RM (ed): Principles of Perinatal-Neonatal Metabolism. New York, Springer-Verlag, 1991, p 177.

34. Kayden HJ, Dancis J, Money WL: Transfer of lipids across the guinea pig placenta. Am J Obstet Gynecol 104:564, 1969.

35. Portman OW, Behrman RE, Soltys P: Transfer of free fatty acids across the primate placenta. Am J Physiol 216:143, 1969.

36. Ruyle M, Connor WE, Anderson GJ, et al: Placental transfer of essential fatty acids in humans: Venous-arterial difference for docosahexaenoic acid in fetal umbilical erythrocytes. Proc Nat Acad Sci USA 87:7902, 1990.

37. Coleman RA: Placental metabolism and transport of lipid. Fed Proc 45:2519, 1986.

38. Coleman RA: The role of the placenta in lipid metabolism and transport. Semin Perinatol 13:180, 1989.

39. Gelfand MM, Strean GJ, Pavilanis V, et al: Studies in placental permeability: Transmission of poliomyelitis antibodies, lipoproteins, and cholesterol in single and twin newborn infants. Am J Obstet Gynecol 79:117, 1960.

40. Pitkin RM, Connor WE, Lins DS: Cholesterol metabolism and placental transfer in the pregnant rhesus monkey. J Clin Invest 51:2584, 1972.

41. Cummings SW, Hatley W, Simpson ER, et al: The binding of high and low density lipoproteins to human placental membrane fractions. J Clin Endocrinol Metab 54:903, 1982.

42. Goldwater WH, Stetten DW Jr: Studies in fetal metabolism. J Biol Chem 169:723, 1947.

43. Paton JB, Levitsky LL, Fisher DE: Placental transfer and fetal effects of maternal sodium β-hydroxybutyrate infusion in the baboon. Pediatr Res 25:435, 1989.

44. Leturque A, Hauguel S, Revelli JP, et al: Fetal glucose utilization in response to maternal starvation and acute hyperketonemia. Am J Physiol 256:E699, 1989.

45. Hay WH Jr, Sparks JW, Wilkening RB, et al: Fetal glucose uptake and utilization as function of maternal glucose concentration. Am J Physiol 246:E237, 1984.

46. Hay WW Jr, Sparks JW, Quissell BJ, et al: Simultaneous measurements of umbilical uptake, fetal utilization rate, and fetal turnover rate of glucose. Am J Physiol 240:E662, 1981.

47. Sparks JW, Girard JR, Battaglia FC: An estimate of the caloric requirements of the human fetus. Biol Neonate 38:113, 1980.

48. Devaskar SU, Mueckler MM: The mammalian glucose transporters. Pediatr Res 31:1, 1992.

49. Challier JC, Hauguel S, Demaizieres V: Effect of insulin in glucose uptake and metabolism in the human placenta. J Clin Endocrinol Metab 672:803, 1986.

50. Kahn BB, Flier JS: Regulation of glucose transporter gene expression in vitro. Diabetes Care 13:548, 1990.

51. Hay WW, Meznarich HK: Use of streptozotocin injection to determine the role of normal levels of fetal insulin in regulating uteroplacental and umbilical glucose exchange. Pediatr Res 24:312, 1988.

52. Widdas WF: Inability of diffusion to account for placental glucose transfer in the sheep and consideration of the kinetics of a possible carrier transfer. J Physiol (Lond) 118:23, 1952.

53. Widdas WF: Transport mechanisms in the foetus. Br Med Bull 17:107, 1961.

54. Howard JM, Krantz KE: Transfer and use of glucose in the human placenta during in vitro perfusion and the associated effects of oxytocin and papaverine. Am J Obstet Gynecol 98:445, 1967.

55. Longo LD, Kleinzeller A: Transport of monosaccharides by placental cells. Fed Proc 29:802, 1970.

56. Villee CA: Regulation of blood glucose in the human fetus. J Appl Physiol 5:437, 1953.

57. Hagerman DD, Villee CA: The transport of fructose by human placenta. J Clin Invest 31:911, 1953.

58. Boyd RDH, Morriss FH, Meschia G, et al: Growth of glucose and oxygen uptakes by fetuses of fed and starved ewes. Am J Physiol 225:897, 1973.

59. James EJ, Raye JR, Gresham EL, et al: Fetal oxygen consumption, carbon dioxide production, and glucose uptake in a chronic sheep preparation. Pediatrics 50:361, 1972.

60. Tsoulos NG, Colwill JR, Battaglia FC, et al: Comparison of glucose, fructose, and O₂ uptakes by fetuses of fed and starved ewes. Am J Physiol 221:234, 1971.

61. Morris FH, Makowski EL, Meschia G, et al: The glucose/oxygen quotient of the term human fetus. Biol Neonate 25:44, 1975.

62. Sparks JW, Hay WW Jr, Bonds D, et al: Simultaneous measurements of lactate turnover rate and umbilical lactate uptake in the fetal lamb. J Clin Invest 70:179, 1982.

63. Char V, Creasy R: Lactate and pyruvate as fetal metabolic substrates. Pediatr Res 10:231, 1976.

64. Fisher DJ, Heymann MA, Rudolph AM: Myocardial consumption of oxygen and carbohydrates in newborn sheep. Pediatr Res 15:843, 1981.

65. Fisher DJ, Heymann MA, Rudolph AM: Myocardial oxygen and carbohydrate consumption in fetal lambs in utero and in adult sheep. Am J Physiol 238:H399, 1980.

66. Gresham EL, James EJ, Raye JR, et al: Production and excretion of urea by the fetal lamb. Pediatrics 50:372, 1972.

67. Van Veen LCP, Teng C, Hay WW, et al: Leucine disposal and oxidation rates in the fetal lamb. Metabolism 36:48, 1987.

68. Meier P, Teng C, Battaglia FC, et al: The rate of amino acid nitrogen and total nitrogen accumulation in the fetal lamb. Proc Soc Exp Biol Med 167:463, 1981.

69. Tulchinsky D, Ryan KJ: Maternal-Fetal Endocrinology. Philadelphia, WB Saunders Co, 1980, pp 169–293.

70. Jost A, Jacquot R: Recherches sur les facteurs endocriniens de la charge en glycogène du foie foetal chez le lapin. Ann Endocrinol (Paris) 16:849, 1955.

71. Kaplan SA: Hypopituitarism. *In* Gardner LI (ed): Endocrine and Genetic Diseases of Childhood. Philadelphia, WB Saunders Co, 1969.
72. Liu HM, Potter EL: Development of the human pancreas. Arch Pathol 74:439, 1962.
73. Emergy JL, Bary HPR: Involutionary changes in the islets of Langerhans. Biol Neonate 6:15, 1964.
74. Stefan Y, Grasso S, Perrelet A, et al: A quantitative immunofluorescent study of the endocrine cell populations in the developing human pancreas. Diabetes 32:293, 1983.
75. Goldman H, Wong I, Patel YC: A study of the structural and biochemical development of human fetal islets of Langerhans. Diabetes 31:987, 1982.
76. Wirdman PK, Milner RDG: Quantitation of β and α cell functions in human pancreas from early fetal life to puberty. Early Human Dev 5:299, 1981.
77. Steinke J, Driscoll S: The extractable insulin content of pancreas from fetuses and infants of diabetic and control mothers. Diabetes 14:573, 1965.
78. Ktorza A, Bihoreau MT, Nurjhan N, et al: Insulin and glucagon during the neonatal period: Secretion and metabolic effects on the liver. Biol Neonate 48:204, 1985.
79. Sperling MA: Integration of fuel homeostasis by insulin and glucagon in the newborn. Monogr Paediatr 16:39, 1982.
80. Sperling MA: Carbohydrate metabolism: Glucagon, insulin and somatostatin. *In* Tulchinsky D, Ryan KJ (eds): Maternal-Fetal Endocrinology. Philadelphia, WB Saunders Co, 1980.
81. Lambert AE, Juno A, Stauffacher W, et al: Organ culture of fetal rat pancreas: I. Insulin release induced by caffeine and by sugars and some derivatives. Biochim Biophys Acta 184:529, 1969.
82. Espinosa MMA, Driscoll SG, Steinke J: Insulin release from isolated human fetal pancreas. Science 168:1111, 1970.
83. Milner RDG, Ashworth MA, Barson AJ: Insulin release from human foetal pancreas in response to glucose, leucine and arginine. J Endocrinol 52:497, 1972.
84. Hole RH, Pian-Smith MCM, Sharp GWP: Development of the biphasic response to glucose in fetal and neonatal pancreas. Am J Physiol 254:E167, 1988.
85. Otontoski T: Insulin and glucagon secretory responses to arginine, glucagon, and theophylline during perifusion of human fetal islet-like cell clusters. J Clin Endocrinol Metab 67:734, 1988.
86. Rorsman P, Arkhammar P, Hellerstrom C, et al: Failure of glucose to elicit a normal secretory response in fetal pancreatic β-cell results from glucose insensitivity of the ATP-regulated K+ channels. Proc Natl Acad Sci USA 86:4505, 1989.
87. Mintz DH, Chez RA, Horger EO: Fetal insulin and growth hormone metabolism in the subhuman primate. J Clin Invest 48:176, 1969.
88. Chez RA, Mintz DH, Hutchinson DL: Effect of theophylline on glucagon and glucose mediated plasma insulin responses in subhuman primate fetus and neonate. Metabolism 20:806, 1971.
89. Grasso S, Messina A, Saporito N: Effect of theophylline, glucagon and theophylline plus glucagon on insulin secretion in the premature infant. Diabetes 19:837, 1970.
90. Reitano G, Grasso S, Distefano G, et al: The serum insulin and growth hormone response to arginine and to arginine with glucose in the premature infant. J Clin Endocrinol 33:924, 1971.
91. Grasso S, Messina A, Distefano G, et al: Insulin secretion in the premature infant, response to glucose and amino acids. Diabetes 22:349, 1973.
92. Tobin JD, Roux JF, Soeldner JS: Human fetal insulin response after acute maternal glucose administration during labor. Pediatrics 44:668, 1969.
93. Milner RDG, Hales CN: Effect of intravenous glucose on concentration of insulin in maternal and umbilical cord plasma. Br Med J 1:2849, 1965.
94. King KC, Oliven A, Kalhan SC: Functional enteroinsular axis in full-term newborn infants. Pediatr Res 25:490, 1989.
95. Cornblath M, Schwartz R: Disorders of Carbohydrate Metabolism in Infancy (ed 3). Boston, Blackwell Scientific, 1991.
96. Joassin G, Parker ML, Pildes RS, et al: Infants of diabetic mothers. Diabetes 16:306, 1967.
97. Haymond MW, Karl IE, Pagliara AS: Increased gluconeogenic substrates in the small-for-gestational infant. N Engl J Med 291:322, 1974.
98. Adam PA: Control of glucose metabolism in the human fetus and newborn infant. Adv Metab Disord 5:183, 1971.
99. Falorni A, Fracassini F, Masi-Benedetti F, et al: Glucose metabolism and insulin secretion in the newborn infant. Diabetes 23:19729, 1974.
100. Rall LB, Pictet RL, Williams RH, et al: Early differentiation of glucagon-producing cells in embryonic pancreas: A possible developmental role of glucagon. Proc Nat Acad Sci USA 70:3478, 1973.
101. Jarrousse C, Rosselin G: Interaction of amino acids and cyclic AMP on the release of insulin and glucagon by newborn rat pancreas. Endocrinology 96:168, 1975.
102. Fiser RH Jr, Erenberg A, Sperling MA, et al: Insulin-glucagon substrate interrelationships in the fetal sheep. Pediatr Res 8:951, 1974.
103. Fiser RH, Williams PR, Sperling MA, et al: Glucagon secretory maturation in the neonatal sheep: Relationship to cyclic AMP. Pediatr Res 9:350, 1975.
104. Girard JR, Kervran A, Soufflet E, et al: Factors affecting secretion of insulin and glucagon by the rat fetus. Diabetes 23:310, 1973.
105. Ganguli S, Sinha MK, Sterman B, et al: Ontogeny of hepatic insulin and glucagon receptors and adenylate cyclase in rabbit. Am J Physiol 244:E624, 1983.
106. Ganguli S, Sinha M, Sperling MA, et al: Ontogeny of insulin and glucagon receptors and the adenylate cyclase system in guinea pig liver. Pediatr Res 18:558, 1984.
107. Vinicor F, Higdon G, Clark JF, et al: Development of glucagon sensitivity in neonatal rat liver. J Clin Invest 58:571, 1976.
108. Devaskar SU, Ganguli S, Styer D, et al: Glucagon and glucose dynamics in sheep: Evidence for glucagon resistance in the fetus. Am J Physiol 246:E256, 1984.
109. Schaeffer LD, Wilder ML, Williams RH: Secretion and content of insulin and glucagon in human fetal pancreas slices in vitro. Proc Soc Exp Biol Med 143:314, 1973.
110. Assan R, Boillot J: Pancreatic glucagon and glucagon-like material in tissues and plasmas from human foetuses 6-26 weeks old. *In* Jonxis JHP, Visser HKA, Troestra JA (eds): Metabolic Processes in the Foetus and Newborn Infant. Baltimore, Williams & Wilkins, 1971, p 210.
111. Wise JK, Lyall SS, Hendler R: Evidence of stimulation of glucagon secretion by alanine in the human fetus at term. J Clin Endocrinol Metab 37:345, 1973.
112. Lowry MF, Adams PAJ: Lack of gluconeogenesis from alanine at birth. Pediatr Res 9:353, 1975.
113. Sperling MA, DeLamater PV, Phelps D, et al: Spontaneous and amino acid stimulated glucagon secretion in the immediate postnatal period. J Clin Invest 53:1159, 1974.
114. Frazer TE, Karl IE, Hillman LS, et al: Direct measurement of gluconeogenesis from [2,3-^{13}C$_2$]alanine in the human neonate. Am J Physiol 240:E615, 1981.
115. Williams PR, Fiser RH Jr, Sperling MA, et al: Effects of oral alanine feedings on blood glucose, plasma glucagon and insulin concentrations in small for gestational age infants. N Engl J Med 292:612, 1975.
116. Parkes MJ, Bassett JM: Antagonism by growth hormone of insulin action in fetal sheep. Endocrinology 105:379, 1985.
117. Stevens D, Alexander G: Lipid deposition after hypophysectomy and growth hormone treatment in the sheep fetus. J Dev Physiol 8:139, 1986.
118. Harris RJ: Plasma nonesterified fatty acids and blood glucose levels in healthy and hypoxemic newborn infants. J Pediatr 84:578, 1974.
119. Alexander G, Bell AW, Hales JRS: The effect of cold exposure on the plasma levels of glucose, lactate, free fatty acids, and glycerol on the blood gases and acid-base status in young lambs. Biol Neonate 20:9, 1972.
120. Greengard O: The developmental formation of enzymes in rat liver. *In* Litwack G (ed): Biochemical Actions of Hormones. London, Academic Press, 1970, p 53.
121. Newsholme EA, Leech AR (eds): Biochemistry for the Medical Sciences. New York, John Wiley and Sons, 1983.
122. Hems DA, Whitton PD: Control of hepatic glycogenolysis. Physiol Rev 60:1, 1980.
123. Hers HG, Van Schaftingen E: Fructose 2,6-biphosphate 2 years after its discovery. Biochem J 206:1–12, 1982.
124. Hanson RW, Mehlman MA (eds): Gluconeogenesis: Its Regulation in Mammalian Species. New York, Wiley-Interscience, 1976.
125. Larner J, Lawrence JC, Walkenbach RJ, et al: Insulin control of glycogen synthesis. Adv Cyl Nucleotide Res 9:425, 1978.
126. Rizza RA, Gerich JE: Hypoglycemia: Physiology and pathophysiologic considerations. In Service FJ (ed): Hypoglycemic Disorders: Pathogenesis, Diagnosis and Treatment. New York, GK Hall Medical Publishers, 1983, p 1.
127. Radziuk J: Sources of carbon in hepatic glycogen synthesis during absorption of an oral glucose load in humans. Fed Proc 41:110–116, 1982.
128. Pagliara AS, Karl IE, Haymond MW, et al: Hypoglycemia in infancy and childhood, part I. J Pediatr 82:365–379, 1973.

129. Pagliara AS, Karl IE, Haymond MW, et al: Hypoglycemia in infancy and childhood, part II. J Pediatr 82:558–577, 1973.

130. Exton JH, Mallette LE, Jefferson LS, et al: The hormonal control of hepatic gluconeogenesis. Recent Prog Horm Res 26:411, 1970.

131. Ballard FJ, Oliver IT: Glycogen metabolism in embryonic chick and neonatal rat liver. Biochem Biophys Acta 71:578, 1963.

132. Shelley HJ, Neligan GA: Neonatal hypoglycemia. Br Med Bull 22:34, 1966.

133. Barbehenn EK, Wales RG, Lowry OH: The explanation for the block-ade of glycolysis in early mouse embryos. Proc Natl Acad Sci USA 71:1056, 1974.

134. Burch HB, Kulman M, Skerjance J, et al: Changes in patterns of enzymes of carbohydrate metabolism in the developing rat kidney. Pediatrics 47:119, 1971.

135. Lea MA, Walker DG: Glycogenesis in the guinea pig liver during development. Dev Biol 15:51, 1967.

136. Katz J, McGarry JD: The glucose paradox: Is glucose a substrate for liver metabolism? J Clin Invest 74:1901, 1984.

137. Shulman GI, Cline G, Schumann WC, et al: Quantitative comparison of pathways of hepatic glycogen repletion in fed and fasted humans. Am J Physiol 259:E335, 1990.

138. Levitsky LL, Paton JB, Fisher DE: Precursors to glycogen in ovine fetuses. Am J Physiol 255:E743, 1988.

139. Kunst C, Kliegman R, Trindade C: The glucose paradox in neonatal murine hepatic glycogen synthesis. Am J Physiol 257:E697, 1989.

140. Jacquot R, Kretchmer N: Effect of fetal decapitation on enzymes of glycogen metabolism. J Biol Chem 239:1301, 1964.

141. Jacquot R: Recherches sur le contrôle endocrinien de l'accumulation de glycogène dans le foie chez 6 foetus de rat. J Physiol (Paris) 51:655, 1959.

142. Margolis FL, Roffi J, Jost A: Norepinephrine methylation in fetal rat adrenals. Science 154:275, 1966.

143. Parker LN, Nobel EP: Prenatal glucocorticoid administration and the development of the epinephrine-forming enzyme. Proc Soc Exp Biol Med 126:734, 1967.

144. Snell K, Walker DG: Glucose metabolism in the newborn rat: Hor-monal effects in vivo. Biochem J 134:889, 1973.

145. Mersmann HJ: Glycolytic and gluconeogenic enzyme levels in pre- and postnatal pigs. Am J Physiol 220:1297, 1971.

146. Philippidis H, Ballard FJ: The development of gluconeogenesis in rat liver: Experiments in vivo. Biochem J 113:651, 1969.

147. Palacin M, Lasucion MA, Herrera E: Lactate production and absence of gluconeogenesis from placental transferred substrates in fetuses from fed and 48-h starved rats. Pediatr Res 22:6, 1987.

148. DiGiacomo JE, Hay WW: Regulation of placental glucose transfer and consumption by fetal glucose production. Pediatr Res 25:429, 1989.

149. DiGiacomo JE, Hay WW: Fetal glucose metabolism and oxygen con-sumption during sustained hypoglycemia. Metabolism 39:193, 1990.

150. Kalhan SC, D'Angelo LJ, Savin SM, et al: Glucose production in pregnant women at term gestation. J Clin Invest 63:388, 1979.

151. Ballard FJ: The development of gluconeogenesis in rat liver: Con-trolling factors in the newborn. Biochem J 124:265, 1971.

152. Yeung D, Oliver IT: Factors affecting the premature induction of phosphopyruvate carboxylase in neonatal rat liver. Biochem J 108:325, 1968.

153. Yeung D, Oliver IT: Induction of phosphopyruvate carboxylase in neonatal rat liver by adenosine-3′,5′-cyclic monophosphate. Bio-chemistry 7:3231, 1968.

154. Wicks WD: Regulation of hepatic enzyme synthesis by cyclic AMP. Ann NY Acad Sci 185:152, 1971.

155. Kirby L, Hahn P: Enzyme induction in human fetal liver. Pediatr Res 7:75, 1973.

156. Shimazu T, Amakawa A: Regulation of glycogen metabolism in liver by the autonomic nervous system: II. Neural control of glycogenolytic enzymes. Biochim Biophys Acta 165:335, 1968.

157. Lamers WH, Hanson RW, Meisner H: CAMP stimulates transcription of the gene for cystolic PEPCK in rat liver nuclei. Proc Natl Acad Sci USA 79:5137, 1982.

158. Wynshaw-Boris A, Short JM, Loose DS, et al: Characterization of the PEPCK promoter-regulatory region. J Biol Chem 261:9414, 1986.

159. Lyonnet S, Coupe C, Girard J, et al: In vivo regulation of glycolytic and gluconeogenic enzyme gene expression in newborn rat liver. J Clin Invest 81:1682, 1988.

160. O'Brien RM, Lucas PS, Forest CD, et al: Identification of a sequence in the PEPCK gene that mediates a negative effect of insulin on transcription. Science 249:533, 1990.

161. Magnuson MA, Quinn PG, Granner DK: Multihormonal regulation of PEPCK-chloramphenicol acetyltransferase fusion genes—Insulin's effects oppose those of CAMP and dexamethasone. J Biol Chem 262:14917, 1987.

162. Helmrath TA, Bieber L: Development of gluconeogenesis in neona-tal pig liver. Am J Physiol 227:1306, 1974.

163. Philippidis H, Ballard RJ: The development of gluconeogenesis in rat liver: Effects of glucagon and ether. Biochem J 120:385, 1970.

164. Kalhan SC, Bier DM, Savin SM, et al: Estimation of glucose turnover and ^{13}C recycling in the human newborn by simultaneous [1-^{13}C]glucose and [6,6-$^2H_2$]glucose tracers. J Clin Endocrinol Metab 50:456, 1980.

165. Bougnères PF, Karl IE, Hillman LS, et al: Lipid transport in the human newborn: Palmitate and glycerol turnover and the contribu-tion of glycerol to neonatal hepatic glucose output. J Clin Invest 70:262, 1982.

166. Patel D, Kalhan S: Glycerol metabolism and triglyceride/fatty acid cycling in the human newborn: Effect of maternal diabetes and intrauterine growth retardation. Pediatr Res 31:52, 1992.

167. Fjeld CR, Cole FS, Bier DM: Energy expenditure, lipolysis, and glu-cose production in preterm infants treated with theophylline. Pediatr Res 32:693, 1992.

168. Schaffer AJ, Avery ME: Diseases of the Newborn (ed 3). Philadelphia, WB Saunders Co, 1971, p 21.

169. Windle WF: Physiology of the Fetus. Springfield, IL, Charles C Thomas, 1971, p 34.

170. Dawes GS: Foetal and Neonatal Physiology. Chicago, Year Book Med-ical Publishers, 1968, p 247.

171. Milichar V, Novak M, Zoula J, et al: Energy sources in the newborn. Biol Neonate 9:298, 1965/66.

172. Marcus C, Ehren H, Bolme P, et al: Regulation of lipolysis during the neonatal period: Importance of thyrotropin. J Clin Invest 82:1793, 1988.

173. Pribylova H, Rylander E: Free fatty acids, glycerol, glucose and α-hydroxybutyrate in plasma of infants protected from cooling and exposure to cold at various times after birth. Biol Neonate 20:425, 1972.

174. Lockwood EA, Bailey E: Some aspects of fatty acid oxidation and ketone body formation and utilization during development of the rat. Enzyme 15:239, 1973.

175. Ferre P, Satabin P, Decaux JF, et al: Development and regulation of ketogenesis in hepatocytes isolated from newborn rats. Biochem J 214:937, 1983.

176. Persson B, Settergren G, Dahlquist G: Cerebral arteriovenous differ-ence of acetoacetate and D-β-hydroxybutyrate in children. Acta Pae-diatr Scand 61:273–278, 1972.

177. Kraus H, Schlenker S, Schwedesky D: Developmental changes of cerebral ketone body utilization in human infants. Hoppe-Seylers Z Physiol Chem 355:164, 1974.

178. Adam PAJ, Raiha N, Rahiala EL, et al: Oxidation of glucose and D-β-OH-butyrate by the early human fetal brain. Acta Paediatr Scand 64:17, 1975.

179. Settergren G, Lindblad BS, Persson B: Cerebral blood flow and ex-change of oxygen, glucose, ketone bodies, lactate, pyruvate and amino acids in infants. Acta Paediatr Scand 65:343, 1976.

180. Melichar V, Drahota V, and Hahn P: Ketone bodies in the blood of full term newborns, premature and dysmature infants and infants of diabetic mothers. Biol Neonate 11:23, 1967.

181. Persson B, Gertz J: The pattern of blood lipids and ketone bodies during the neonatal period, infancy, and childhood. Acta Paediatr Scand 55:353, 1976.

182. Anday EK, Stanley CA, Baker L, et al: Plasma ketones in newborn infants: Absence of suckling ketosis. J Pediatr 98:628, 1981.

183. Bougneres PF, Lemmel C, Ferre P, et al: Ketone body transport in the human neonate and infant. J Clin Invest 77:42, 1986.

184. Hawdon JM, Ward Platt MP, Aynsley-Green A: Patterns of metabolic adaptation for preterm and term infants in the first neonatal weeks. Arch Dis Child 67:357, 1992.

185. Rothman DL, Novotny EJ, Shulman GI, et al: ^1H-[^{13}C]NMR measure-ments of [4-^{13}C] glutamate turnover in human brain. Proc Nat Acad Sci USA 89:9603, 1992.

186. Haymond MW: Hypoglycemia in infants and children. Endocrinol Metab Clin North Am 18:211, 1989.

187. Cornblath M, Odell GB, Levin EY: Symptomatic neonatal hypoglyce-mia associated with toxemia of pregnancy. J Pediatr 55:545, 1959.

188. Creery RDG, Parkinson TJ: Blood glucose changes in the newborn. Arch Dis Child 28:134, 1953.

189. Pagliara AS, Karl I, Haymond MW, et al: Hypoglycemia in infancy and childhood (Reply). J Pediatr 83:694, 1973.

190. Ward OC: Blood sugar studies on premature babies. Arch Dis Child 28:194, 1953.
191. Baens SG, Lundeen E, Cornblath M: Studies of carbohydrate metabolism in the newborn infant. Pediatrics 31:580, 1963.
192. Ditchburn RK, Wilkinson RH, Davies PA, et al: Plasma glucose levels in infants 2500 g and less fed immediately after birth with breast milk. Biol Neonate 11:29, 1967.
193. Bier DM, Leake RD, Haymond MW, et al: Measurement of "true" glucose production rates in infancy and childhood with 6,6-dideuteroglucose. Diabetes 26:1016, 1977.
194. Kalhan SC, Savin SM, Adam PAJ: Measurement of glucose turnover in the human newborn with glucose-1-^{13}C. J Clin Endocrinol Metab 43:704, 1976.
195. Lubchenco LL, Bard H: Incidence of hypoglycemia in newborn infants classified by birthweight and gestational age. Pediatrics 47:831, 1971.
196. Drillien CM: The small-for-date infant: Etiology and prognosis. Pediatr Clin North Am 17:9, 1970.
197. Williams PR, Fiser RH Jr, Sperling MA, et al: Effects of oral alanine feeding on blood glucose, plasma glucagon and insulin concentrations in small for gestational age infants. N Engl J Med 292:612, 1975.
198. DeLamater PV, Sperling MA, Fiser RH, et al: Plasma alanine: Relation to plasma glucose, glucagon, and insulin in the neonate. J Pediatr 85:702, 1974.
199. Fiser RH, Williams PR, Fisher DA, et al: The effect of oral alanine on blood glucose and glucagon in the human newborn infant. Pediatrics 56:78, 1975.
200. Salle BL, Ruiton-Ugliengo AR: Effects of oral glucose and protein load on plasma glucagon and insulin concentrations in small for gestational age infants. Pediatr Res 11:108, 1977.
201. Gertz JC, Warner R, Persson BE, et al: Intravenous glucose tolerance, plasma insulin free fatty acids and beta-hydroxybutyrate in underweight newborn infants. Acta Pediatri Scand 58:481, 1969.
202. De Leeuw R, de Vries IJ: Hypoglycemia in small-for-date newborn infants. Pediatrics 58:18, 1976.
203. Stanley CA, Anday EK, Baker L, et al: Metabolic fuel and hormone responses to fasting in newborn infants. Pediatrics 64:613, 1979.
204. Sann L, Divry P, Lasne Y, et al: Effect of oral lipid administration on glucose homeostasis in small-for-gestational age infants. Acta Paediatr Scand 71:923, 1982.
205. Ferre P, Pegorier JP, Marliss EB, et al: Influence of exogenous fat and gluconeogenic substrates on glucose homeostasis in the newborn rat. Am J Physiol E129, 1978.
206. Ferre P, Pegorier JP, Williamson DH, et al: Interactions in vivo between oxidation of nonesterified fatty acids and gluconeogenesis in the newborn rat. Biochem J 182:593, 1979.
207. Ferre P, Satabin P, El Manoubi L, et al: Relationship between ketogenesis and gluconeogenesis in isolated hepatocytes from newborn rats. Biochem J 200:429, 1981.
208. Pegorier JP, Duee PH, Assan R, et al: Changes in circulating fuels, pancreatic hormones and liver glycogen concentration in fasting or suckling newborn pigs. J Dev Physiol 3:203, 1981.
209. Pegorier JP, Duee PH, Girard J, et al: Development of gluconeogenesis in isolated hepatocytes from fasting or suckling newborn pigs. J Nutr 112:1038, 1982.
210. Pegorier JP, Duee PH, Girard J, et al: Metabolic fate of nonesterified fatty acids in isolated hepatocytes from newborn and young pigs. Biochem J 212:93, 1983.
211. Sann L, Mathieu M, Lasne Y, et al: Effect of oral administration of lipids with 67% medium chain triglycerides on glucose homeostasis in preterm neonates. Metabolism 30:712, 1981.
212. Vileisis RA, Cowett RM, Oh W: Glycemic response to lipid infusion in the premature neonate. J Pediatr 100:108, 1982.
213. Bougneres PF, Castano L, Rocchiccioli F, et al: Medium-chain fatty acids increase glucose production in normal and low birth weight newborns. Am J Physiol 256:E692, 1989.
214. Marliss EB, Aoki TT, Toews CH, et al: Amino acid metabolism in lactic acidosis. Am J Med 52:474, 1972.
215. Cornblath M, Wybregt SH, Baens GS: Studies of carbohydrate metabolism in the newborn infant: VII. Tests of carbohydrate tolerance in premature infants. Pediatrics 32:1007, 1963.
216. Mastyan J, Schultz K, Horvath M: Comparative glycemic responses to alanine in normal term and small for gestational age infants. J Pediatr 85:276, 1974.
217. Pildes RS: Neonatal hyperglycemia. J Pediatr 109:905, 1985.
218. Cowett RM, Oh W, Schwartz R: Persistent glucose production during glucose infusion in the neonate. J Clin Invest 71:467, 1983.
219. Cowett RM, Andersen GE, Maguire CA, et al: Ontogeny of glucose homeostasis in low birth weight infants. J Pediatr 112:462, 1988.
220. Howard CP, Go VLW, Infante AJ, et al: Long-term survival in a case of functional pancreatic agenesis. J Pediatr 97:786, 1980.
221. Ramsey WR: Glucosuria of the newborn treated with insulin. Trans Am Pediatr Soc 38:100, 1926.
222. Gentz JCH, Cornblath M: Transient diabetes of the newborn. Adv Pediatr 16:345, 1969.
223. Coffey JD, Wormack NC: Transient neonatal diabetes in half sisters. Am J Dis Child 45:480, 1967.
224. Hager H, Herbst R: Das transitorische diabetes mellitus syndrom des neuge borenen ein Krankbeutsbild sue generes. Z Kinderheilk 95:3324, 1966.
225. Pagliara AS, Karl IE, Kipnis DM: Transient neonatal diabetes: Delayed maturation of the pancreatic beta cell. J Pediatr 81:97, 1973.
226. Mills JL, Baker L, Goldman AS: Malformations in infants of diabetic mothers occur before the seventh gestational week. Diabetes 28:292, 1979.
227. Baker L, Egler JM, Klein SH, et al: Meticulous control of diabetes during organogenesis prevents congenital lumbosacral defects in rats. Diabetes 30:955, 1981.
228. Eriksson U, Dahlstrom E, Larsson KS, et al: Increased incidence of congenital malformations in the offspring of diabetic rats and their prevention by maternal insulin therapy. Diabetes 31:1, 1982.
229. Sadler TW, Horton WE Jr: Effects of maternal diabetes on early embryogenesis: The role of insulin and insulin therapy. Diabetes 32:1070, 1983.
230. Carson BS, Philipps AF, Simmons MA, et al: Effects of a sustained insulin infusion upon glucose uptake and oxygenation of the ovine fetus. Pediatr Res 14:147, 1980.
231. White P, Kosby P, Duckers J: The management of pregnancy complicating diabetes and of children of diabetic mothers. Med Clin North Am 37:1481, 1953.
232. Dekaban A, Baird R: The outcome of pregnancy in diabetic women: I. Fetal wastage, mortality and morbidity in the offspring of diabetic and normal control mothers. J Pediatr 55:563, 1959.
233. Mills JL, Knopp RH, Simpson JL, et al: Lack of relation of increased malformation rates in infants of diabetic mothers to glycemic control during organogenesis. N Engl J Med 318:671, 1988.
234. Berk MA, Mimouri F, Miodovnik M, et al: Macrosomia in infants of insulin-dependent diabetic mothers. Pediatrics 83:1029, 1989.
235. Pildes RS: Infants of diabetic mothers. N Engl J Med 289:902, 1973.
236. Pedersen J: The Pregnant Diabetic and Her Newborn: Problems and Management. Baltimore, Williams & Wilkins, 1967.
237. Pedersen J, Bojsen-Moller B, Poulsen H: Blood sugar in newborn infants of diabetic mothers. Acta Endocrinol (Copenh) 15:33, 1954.
238. Freinkel N: Banting lecture 1980: Of pregnancy and progeny. Diabetes 29:1023, 1980.
239. McCormick KL, Susa JB, Widness JA, et al: Chronic hyperinsulinemia in the fetal rhesus monkey: Effects on hepatic enzymes active in lipogenesis and carbohydrate metabolism. Diabetes 28:1064, 1979.
240. Susa JB, McCormick KL, Widness JA, et al: Chronic hyperinsulinemia in the fetal rhesus monkey: Effects on fetal growth and composition. Diabetes 28:1058, 1979.
241. Susa JB, Neave C, Sehgal P, et al: Chronic hyperinsulinemia in the fetal rhesus monkey: Effects of physiologic hyperinsulinemia on fetal growth and composition. Diabetes 33:656, 1984.
242. Susa JB, Gruppuso PA, Widness JA, et al: Chronic hyperinsulinemia in the fetal rhesus monkey: Effects of physiologic hyperinsulinemia on fetal substrates, hormones and hepatic enzymes. Am J Obstet Gynecol 150:415, 1984.
243. Johnson JD, Dunham T, Wogenrich FJ, et al: Fetal hyperinsulinemia and protein turnover in fetal rat tissues. Diabetes 39:541, 1990.
244. Andersen GE, Hertel J, Kuhl C, et al: Metabolic events in infants of diabetic mothers during first 24-hours after birth: II. Changes in plasma insulin. Paediatr Scand 71:27, 1982.
245. Chen CH, Adam PAJ, Laskowski DE, et al: Plasma free fatty acid composition and blood glucose of normal and diabetic pregnant women and their newborns. Pediatrics 36:843, 1965.
246. Gentz J, Kellum M, Persson B: The effect of feeding on oxygen consumption, RQ, and plasma levels of glucose, FFA, and D-β-hydroxybutyrate in newborn infants of diabetic mothers and small for gestational age infants. Acta Paediatr Scand 65:445, 1976.
247. Hertel J, Andersen GE, Brandt NJ, et al: Metabolic events in infants of diabetic mothers during first 24 hours after birth: III. Changes in plasma amino acids. Acta Paediatr Scand 71:33, 1982.
248. Kuhl C, Andersen GE, Hertel J, et al: Metabolic events in infants of diabetic mothers during first 24 hours after birth: I. Changes in plasma glucose. Paediatr Scand 71:19, 1982.

249. Heding LG, Persson B, Stangenberg M: B-cell function in newborn infants of diabetic mothers. Diabetologia 19:427, 1980.

250. Sosenko IR, Kitzmiller JL, Loo SW, et al: The infant of the diabetic mother. N Engl J Med 301:859, 1979.

251. Bloom SR, Johnston DI: Failure of glucagon release in infants of diabetic mothers. Br Med J 4:453, 1972.

252. Williams PR, Sperling MA, Racasa Z: Blunting of spontaneous and alanine-stimulated glucagon secretion in newborn infants of diabetic mothers. Am J Obstet Gynecol 133:51, 1979.

253. Kalhan SC, Savin SM, Adam PAJ: Attenuated glucose production rate in newborn infants of insulin-dependent diabetic mothers. N Engl J Med 296:375, 1977.

254. King KC, Tserng KY, Kalhan SC: Regulation of glucose production in newborn infants of diabetic mothers. Pediatr Res 16:608, 1982.

255. Persson B, Gentz J, Kellum M, et al: Metabolic observations in infants of strictly controlled diabetic mothers: Plasma levels of glucose, FFA, glycerol, and D-β-hydroxybutyrate during the first two hours after birth. Acta Paediatr Scand 62:465, 1973.

256. Barnett CT, Oliver TK Jr: Hypoglycemia and hyperinsulinisms in infants with erythroblastosis fetalis. N Engl J Med 278:1260, 1968.

257. Grunt JA, Enriquez AR: Further studies of hypoglycemia in children with exomphalos-macroglossia-gigantism syndrome. Yale J Biol Med 45:15–21, 1972.

258. Sotelo-Avila C, Gonzalex-Crussi F, Fowler JW: Complete and incomplete forms of Beckwith-Wiedemann syndrome: Their oncogenic potential. J Pediatr 96:47–50, 1980.

259. Waziri M, Patil SR, Hanson JW, et al: Abnormalities of chromosome 11 in patients with features of Beckwith-Wiedemann syndromes. J Pediatr 102:873–876, 1983.

260. Henry I, Bonaiti-Pellie C, Chehensse V, et al: Uniparental paternal disomy in a genetic cancer-predisposing syndrome. Nature 351:665, 1991.

261. Little M, VanHeyningen V, Hastie N: Dads and disomy and disease. Nature 351:609, 1991.

262. Yeung CY: Hypoglycemia in neonatal sepsis. J Pediatr 77:812, 1970.

263. Yeung CY, Lee VWY, Yeung MB: Glucose disappearance rate in neonatal infection. J Pediatr 82:486, 1973.

264. LaNone KF, Mason AD Jr, Daniels JP: The impairment of gluconeogenesis by gram-negative infection. Metabolism 17:606, 1968.

265. Shands JW Jr, Miller V, Martin H: The hypoglycemic activity of endotoxin: I. Occurrence in animals hyperreactive to endotoxin. Proc Soc Exp Biol Med 130:413, 1969.

266. Harris RJ: Plasma nonesterified fatty acid and blood glucose levels in healthy and hypoxemic newborn infants. J Pediatr 84:578, 1974.

267. Greenberg RE, Christiansen O: The critically ill child: Hypoglycemia. Pediatrics 46:915, 1970.

268. Thornton PS, Summer AE, Ruchelli ED: Familial and sporadic hyperinsulinism histopathologic findings and segregation analysis support a single autosomal disorder. J Pediatr 119:721, 1991.

269. Stanley CA, Baker L: Hyperinsulinism in infancy: Diagnosis by demonstration of abnormal response to fasting hypoglycemia. Pediatrics 57:702, 1976.

270. Finegold DN, Stanley CA, Baker L: Glycemic response to glucagon during fasting hypoglycemia: An aid in the diagnosis of hyperinsulinism. J Pediatr 96:257, 1980.

271. Simmons PS, Telander RL, Carney JA, et al: Surgical management of hyperinsulinemic hypoglycemia in children. Arch Surg 119:520, 1984.

272. Bougnères PF, Ferre P, Chaussain JL, et al: Glucose metabolism in +hyperinsulinemic infants: The effects of fasting and sodium DL-Γ-hydroxybutyrate on glucose production and utilization rates. J Clin Endocrinol Metab 57:1054, 1983.

273. Schwartz JF, Zwiren GT: Islet cell adenomatosis and adenoma in an infant. J Pediatr 79:232, 1971.

274. Rahier J, Falt K, Muntefering H, et al: The basic structural lesion of persistent neonatal hypoglycemia with hyperinsulinism: Deficiency of pancreatic D cells or hyperactivity of B cells? Diabetologia 26:282, 1984.

275. Jaffe R, Hashida Y, Yunis EJ: Pancreatic pathology in hyperinsulinemic hypoglycemia in infants. Lab Invest 42:356, 1980.

276. Rahier J, Wallon J, Henquin EJ: Cell populations in the endocrine pancreas of human neonates and infants. Diabetologia 20:540, 1981.

277. Wilte DP, Greider MH, DeSchryver-Kecskemeti K, et al: The juvenile human endocrine pancreas: Normal vs idiopathic hyperinsulinemic hypoglycemia. Semin Diagn Pathol 1:30, 1984.

278. Bishop AE, Polak JM, Garin-Chesa P, et al: Decrease of pancreatic somatostatin in neonatal nesidioblastosis. Diabetes 20:122, 1981.

279. Upp JR, Ishizuka J, Lobe T, et al: Somatostatin secretion in cultured human islet cells from patients with nesidioblastosis: A compensatory mechanism? J Pediatr Surg 22:1185, 1987.

280. Hirsch HJ, Loo S, Evans N, et al: Hypoglycemia of infancy and nesidioblastosis: Studies with somatostatin. N Engl J Med 296:1323, 1977.

281. Becker K: β-cell nesidioblastosis. Eur J Pediatr 127:75, 1978.

282. Stanley CA, Baker L: Hyperinsulinism in infants and children: Diagnosis and therapy. Adv Pediatr 23:315, 1976.

283. Brunelle F, Negre V, Barth MO, et al: Pancreatic venous sampling in infants and children with primary hyperinsulinism. Pediatr Radiol 19:100, 1989.

284. Telander RL, Charboneau JW, Haymond MW: Intraoperative ultrasonography of the pancreas in children. J Pediatr Surg 21:262, 1986.

285. Rosch T, Lightdale CJ, Botet JF, et al: Localization of pancreatic endocrine tumors by endoscopic ultrasonography. N Engl J Med 326:1721, 1992.

286. Lamberts SWJ, Bakker WH, Reubi JC, et al: Somatostatin-receptor imaging in the localization of endocrine tumors. N Engl J Med 323:1246, 1990.

287. Rose SR, Chrovsos GC, Cornblath M, et al: Management of postoperative nesidioblastosis with zinc protamine glucagon and oral starch. J Pediatr 108:97, 1986.

288. Mereu TR, Kassoff A, Goodman D: Diazoxide in the treatment of infantile hypoglycemia. N Engl J Med 275:1455, 1966.

289. Parker JJ, Allen DB: Hypertrophic cardiomyopathy after prolonged diazoxide therapy for hyperinsulinemic hypoglycemia. J Pediatr 118:906, 1991.

290. Harris JP, Ricker AT, Gray RS, et al: Reversible hypertrophic cardiomyopathy associated with nesidioblastosis. J Pediatr 120:272, 1992.

291. Delemare-van de Waal HA, Veldkamp EJM, Schrander-Stumpel CTRM: Long-term treatment of an infant with nesidioblastosis using a somatostatin analogue. N Engl J Med 317:222, 1987.

292. DeClue TJ, Malone JI, Cercu BB: Linear growth during long-term treatment with somatostatin analogue for persistent hyperinsulinemic hypoglycemia of infancy. J Pediatr 116:747, 1990.

293. Thornton PS, Alter CA, O'Neill JA, et al: Octreotide therapy in hyperinsulinism (abstract). Pediatr Res 31:189A, 1992.

294. Hamilton JP, Baker L, Kaye R, et al: Subtotal pancreatectomy in the management of severe persistent idiopathic hypoglycemia in children. Pediatrics 39:49, 1967.

295. Thomas CG, Underwood LE, Carney CN, et al: Neonatal and infantile hypoglycemia due to insulin excess: New aspects of diagnosis and surgical management. Ann Surg 185:505, 1977.

296. Gemelli M, De Luca F, Barberio G: Hypoglycaemia and congenital adrenal hyperplasia. Acta Paediatr Scand 68:285, 1979.

297. Aynsley-Green A, Moncrieff MW, Ratter S, et al: Isolated ACTH deficiency. Arch Dis Child 53:499, 1975.

298. Goodman HG, Grumbach MM, Kaplan SL: Growth and growth hormone: II. A comparison of isolated growth hormone deficiency and multiple pituitary-hormone deficiencies in 35 patients with idiopathic dwarfism. N Engl J Med 278:57, 1968.

299. Haymond MW, Karl IE, Weldon VV, et al: The role of growth hormone and cortisone on glucose and gluconeogenic substrate regulation in fasted hypopituitary children. J Clin Endocrinol 42:846, 1976.

300. Dahms WT, Owens RP, Kalhan SC, et al: Urea synthesis, nitrogen balance, and glucose turnover in growth-hormone deficient children before and after growth hormone administration. Metabolism 38:197, 1989.

301. Bougnères PF, Artavia-Loria E, Ferre P, et al: Effects of hypopituitarism and growth hormone replacement therapy on the production and utilization of glucose in childhood. J Clin Endocrinol Metab 61:1152, 1985.

302. Vidnes J, Oyasaeter S: Glucagon deficiency causing severe neonatal hypoglycemia in a patient with normal insulin secretion. Pediatr Res 11:943, 1977.

303. Kollee LA, Monnens LA, Cejka V, et al: Persistent neonatal hypoglycaemia due to glucagon deficiency. Arch Dis Child 53:422, 1978.

304. Hers HG, VanHoof F, deBarsy T: Glycogen storage diseases. In Scriver CR, Beaudet AL, Sly WS, Valle D (eds): The Metabolic Basis of Inherited Disease. New York, McGraw-Hill, 1989, p 425.

305. Snapper I, van Creveld S: Un cas de'hypoglycemic acetonie chez un enfant. Bull Soc Med Hop Paris 52:1315, 1928.

306. Von Gierke E: Hepato-nephromegalia glykogenica (glykogenspeicherkrankheitden leber nieren). Beitr Pathol Anat 82:497, 1929.

307. Cori GT, Cori CF: Glucose-6-phosphatase in the liver in glycogen storage disease. J Biol Chem 199:661, 1952.

308. Havel RJ, Balasse EO, Williams HE, et al: Splanchnic metabolism in von Gierke's disease (glycogenosis type 1). Trans Assoc Am Physicians 82:305, 1969.

309. Tsalikian E, Simmons P, Gerich JE, et al: Glucose production and utilization in children with glycogen storage disease type I. Am J Physiol 247:E513, 1984.

310. Fernandes J, Berger R, Smit GPA: Lactate as a cerebral metabolic fuel for glucose-6-phosphatase deficient children. Pediatr Res 18:335, 1984.

311. Fernandes J, Pikaar NA: Ketosis in hepatic glycogenosis. Arch Dis Child 47:41, 1972.

312. Binkiewicz A, Senior B: Decreased ketogenesis in von Gierke's disease (type 1 glycogenosis). J Pediatr 83:973, 1973.

313. Cohen JL, Vinik A, Faller J, et al: Hyperuricemia in glycogen storage disease type I. J Clin Invest 75:251, 1985.

314. Ockerman PA: In vitro studies of adipose tissue metabolism of glucose, glycerol and free fatty acids in glycogen storage disease type I. Clin Chem Acta 12:383, 1965.

315. Chen YT, Coleman RA, Scheinman, et al: Renal disease in type I glycogen storage disease. N Engl J Med 318:7, 1988.

316. Spencer-Peet J, Norman ME, Lake BD, et al: Hepatic glycogen storage disease, clinical and laboratory; findings in 23 cases. Q J Med 40:95, 1971.

317. Narisawa K, Igarashi Y, Otomo H, et al: A new varient of glycogen storage disease type I probably due to a defect in the glucose-6-phosphate transport system. Biochem Biophys Res Commun 83:1360, 1978.

318. Lange AJ, Arion WJ, Beaudet AL: Type 1b glycogen storage disease is caused by a defect in the glucose-6-phosphate translocase of the microsomal glucose-6-phosphatase system. J Biol Chem 255:8381, 1980.

319. Narisawa K, Otomo H, Igarashi Y, et al: Glycogen storage disease type 1b: Microsomal glucose-6-phosphatase system in two patients with different clinical findings. Pediatrics 17:545, 1983.

320. Nordlie RC, Sukalski KA, Munoz JM, et al: Type Ic: A novel glycogenosis. J Biol Chem 258:9739, 1983.

321. Baker L, Winegrad AI: Fasting hypoglycemia and metabolic acidosis associated with deficiency of hepatic fructose-1,6-diphosphatase activity. Lancet 2:13, 1970.

322. Pagliara AS, Karl IE, Keating J, et al: Hepatic fructose-1,6-diphosphatase deficiency: A cause of lactic acidosis and hypoglycemia in infancy. J Clin Invest 51:2115, 1972.

323. Baerlocher K, Gitzelman R, Nussli R, et al: Infantile lactic acidosis due to hereditary fructose-1,6-diphosphatase deficiency. Helv Paediatr Acta 26:489, 1971.

324. Hulsmann WC, Fernandes J: A child with lacticidemia and fructose dephosphatase deficiency in the liver. Pediatr Res 5:633, 1971.

325. Melancon SB, Khachadurian AK, Nadler HL, et al: Metabolic and biochemical studies in fructose 1,6-diphosphatase deficiency. J Pediatr 82:650, 1973.

326. Folkman J, Philippart A, Tze WJ, Crigler J: Portocaval shunt for glycogen storage disease: Value of prolonged intravenous hyperalimentation before surgery. Surgery 73:306, 1972.

327. Schwenk WF, Haymond MW: Optimal rate of enteral glucose administration in children with glycogen storage disease type I. N Engl J Med 314:682, 1986.

328. Burr IM, O'Neil JA, Karzon JA, et al: Comparison of the effects of total parenteral nutrition, continuous intragastric feeding and portocaval shunt on a patient with type I glycogen storage disease. J Pediatr 85:792, 1974.

329. Erlich RM, Robinson BH, Freedman MH, et al: Nocturnal intragastric infusion of glucose in management of defective gluconeogenesis with hypoglycemia. Am J Dis Child 132:241, 1978.

330. Fernandes J, Jansen H, Jansen TC: Nocturnal gastric drip feedings in glucose-6-phosphatase deficient children. Pediatr Res 13:225, 1979.

331. Greene HL, Slonim AE, Burr IM, et al: Type I glycogen storage disease: Five years of management with nocturnal intragastric feeding. J Pediatr 96:590, 1980.

332. Chen Y, Cornblath M, Sidbury J: Cornstarch therapy in type I glycogen storage disease. N Engl J Med 310:171, 1984.

333. Lewis GM, Spencer-Peet J, Stewart KM: Infantile hypoglycemia due to inherited deficiency of glycogen synthetase in liver. Arch Dis Child 38:40, 1963.

334. Parr J, Teree TM, Larner J: Symptomatic hypoglycemia, visceral fatty metamorphosis and aglycogenosis in an infant lacking glycogen synthetase and phosphorylase. Pediatrics 35:770, 1965.

335. Aynsley-Green A, Williamson DH, Gitzelman R: Hepatic glycogen synthetase deficiency. Arch Dis Child 52:573, 1977.

336. Mohandas T, Sparkes RS, Sparkes MC, et al: Assignment of the human gene for galactose-1-phosphate uridyl transferase to chromosome 9: Studies with Chinese hamster-human somatic cell hybrids. Proc Natl Acad Sci USA 74:5628, 1977.

337. Komrower GM: Galactosaemia—Thirty years on. The experience of a generation. J Inherited Metab Dis 5(suppl 2):96, 1982.

338. Kliegman RM, Sparks JW: Perinatal galactose metabolism. J Pediatr 107:831, 1985.

339. Fishler K, Koch R, Donnell GN, et al: Developmental aspects of galactosemia from infancy to childhood. Clin Pediatr 19:38, 1980.

340. Lo W, Packman S, Nash S, et al: Curious neurologic sequelae in galactosemia. Pediatrics 73:309, 1984.

341. Kaufman FR, Kogut MD, Donnell GN, et al: Hypergonadotropic hypogonadism in female patients with galactosemia. N Engl J Med 304:994, 1981.

342. Baerlocher K, Gitzelmann R, Steinmann B, et al: Hereditary fructose intolerance in early childhood: A major diagnostic challenge. Helv Paediatr Acta 33:465, 1978.

343. Odievre M, Gentil C, Gautier M, et al: Hereditary fructose intolerance in childhood. Am J Dis Child 132:605, 1978.

344. Steinmann B, Gitzelmann R: The diagnosis of hereditary fructose intolerance. Helv Paediatr Acta 36:297, 1981.

345. Gopher A, Vaisman N, Mandel H, et al: Determination of fructose metabolic pathways in normal and fructose-intolerant children: A ^{13}C NMR study using [U-^{13}C]fructose. Proc Natl Acad Sci USA 87:5449, 1990.

346. Cross NCP, deFranchis R, Sebastio G, et al: Molecular analysis of aldolase B genes in hereditary fructose intolerance. Lancet 335:306, 1990.

347. Donnell GN, Lieberman E, Shaw KNF, et al: Hypoglycemia in maple syrup urine disease. Am J Dis Child 113:60, 1967.

348. Haymond MW, Karl IE, Feigin RD, et al: Hypoglycemia and maple syrup urine disease: Defective gluconeogenesis. Pediatr Res 7:500, 1973.

349. Stanley CA: New genetic defects in mitochondrial fatty acid oxidation and carnitine deficiency. Adv Pediatr 34:59, 1987.

350. Stanley CA, Hale DE, Berry GT, et al: Brief report: A deficiency of carnitine-acylcarnitine translocase in the inner mitochondrial membrane. N Engl J Med 327:19, 1992.

351. Engel AG, Bankers BQ, Eiben RM: Carnitine deficiency: Clinical, morphological and biochemical observations in a fetal case. J Neurol Neurosurg Psychiatry 40:313, 1977.

352. Roe CR, Coates PM: Acyl-coA dehydrogenase deficiencies. In Scriver SR, Beaudet AL, Sly WS, Valle D (eds): The Metabolic Basis of Inherited Disease (ed 6). New York, McGraw-Hill, 1989, pp 889–914.

353. Rebouche CJ, Peter Bosh E, Chanard CA, et al: Utilization of dietary precursors for carnitine synthesis in human adults. J Nutr 119:1907, 1989.

354. Rebouche CJ: Quantitative estimation of absorption and degradation of a carnitine supplement by human adults. Metabolism 40:1305, 1991.

355. Shenai JP, Borum PR, Mohan P, et al: Carnitine status at birth of newborn infants of varying gestation. Pediatr Res 17:579, 1983.

356. Stanley CA, Hale DE, Coates PM, et al: Medium chain acyl-CoA dehydrogenase deficiency in children with non-ketotic hypoglycemia and low carnitine levels. Pediatr Res 17:877, 1983.

357. Roe CR, Millington DC, Maltby DA, et al: Recognition of medium chain acyl-CoA dehydrogenase deficiency in asymptomatic siblings of children dying of sudden infant death or Reye-like syndromes. J Pediatr 108:13, 1986.

358. Glasgow AM, Engel AG, Bier DM, et al: Hypoglycemia, hepatic dysfunction, muscle weakness, cardiomyopathy, free carnitine deficiency and long-chain acylcarnitine excess responsive to medium chain triglyceride diet. Pediatr Res 17:319, 1983.

359. Hales DE, Coates PM, Stanley CA: Long chain acyl-CoA dehydrogenase deficiency. Pediatr Res 17:290A, 1983.

360. Treem WR, Stanley CA, Hale DE, et al: Hypoglycemia, hypotonia, and cardiomyopathy: The evolving clinical picture of long-chain acyl-CoA dehydrogenase deficiency. Pediatrics 87:328, 1991.

361. Amendt BA, Greene C, Sweetman L, et al: Short-chain acyl-coenzyme A deficiency: Clinical and biochemical studies in two patients. J Clin Invest 79:1303, 1987.

362. Rocchiccioli F, Wanders RJA, Aubourg P, et al: Deficiency of long-chain 3-hydroxyacyl-CoA dehydrogenase: A cause of lethal myopathy and cardiomyopathy in early childhood. Pediatr Res 28:657, 1990.

363. Treem WR, Sanley CA, Finegold DN, et al: Primary carnitine deficiency due to a failure of carnitine transport in kidney, muscle and fibroblasts. N Engl J Med 319:1331, 1988.

364. Stanley CA, DeLeeuw S, Coates PM, et al: Chronic cardiomyopathy and weakness or acute coma in children with a defect in carnitine uptake. Ann Neurol 30:709, 1991.

365. Bougnères PF, Saudubray JM, Marsac C, et al: Decreased ketogenesis

due to deficiency of hepatic carnitine acyl transferase. N Engl J Med 302:123, 1980.

366. Bougnères PF, Saudubray JM, Marsac C, et al: Fasting hypoglycemia resulting from hepatic carnitine palmityle transferase deficiency. J Pediatr 98:742, 1981.

367. Demaugre F, Bonnefont JP, Mitchel G, et al: Hepatic and muscular presentations of carnitine palmitoyltransferase deficiency: Two distinct entities. Pediatr Res 24:308, 1988.

368. Demaugre F, Bonnefond JP, Colonna M, et al: Infantile form of carnitine palmitoyltransferase II deficiency with hepatomuscular symptoms and sudden death. J Clin Invest 87:859, 1991.

369. Hug G, Bove KE, Soukup S: Lethal neonatal multiorgan deficiency of carnitine palmitoyltransferase II. N Engl J Med 325:1862, 1991.

370. Cheema-Madli S, Lernoff CC, Haperin ML: Effect of methylcitrate on citrate metabolism: Implications for the management of patients with proprionic acidemia and methylmalonic aciduria. Pediatr Res 9:905, 1975.

371. Stanley CA, Berry GT, Yudkoff M, et al: Urine carnitine excretion in secondary carnitine deficiency. Pediatr Res 18:300A, 1984.

372. Roe CR, Millington DS, Maltby DA, et al: L-Carnitine enhances excretion of propionyl coenzyme A as propionylcarnitine in proprionic acidemia. J Clin Invest 73:1785, 1984.

373. Schutgens RBH, Heymans H, Ketel A, et al: Lethal hypoglycemia in a child with deficiency of 3-hydroxy-3-methyl glutaryl coenzyme A lyase. J Pediatr 94:89, 1979.

374. Rinaldo P, O'Shea J, Coates PM, et al: Medium-chain acyl-coA dehydrogenase deficiency: Diagnosis by stable-isotope dilution measurement of urinary n-hexanoylglycine and 3-phenylpropionylglycine. N Engl J Med 319:1308, 1988.

375. Moon A, Rhead WJ: Complementation analysis of fatty acid oxidation disorders. J Clin Invest 79:59–64, 1987.

376. Wanders RJA, Ijlst L, VanEltz E, et al: Octanoate and palmitate β-oxidation in human leukocytes: Implications for the rapid diagnosis of fatty acid β-oxidation disorders. J Inherited Metab Dis 14:317, 1991.

377. Yokota I, Indo Y, Coates P, et al: Molecular basis of MCAD deficiency. J Clin Invest 86:1000, 1990.

378. Ding JH, Roe CR, Iafolla AK, et al: Medium-chain acyl-coenzyme A dehydrogenase deficiency and sudden infant death. N Engl J Med 325:61, 1991.

379. Miller ME, Brooks JH, Forbes N, et al: Frequency of medium-chain acyl-CoA dehydrogenase deficiency G985 mutation in sudden infant death syndrome. Pediatr Res 31:305, 1992.

Pitfalls in Endocrine Tests and Testing in Pregnancy

MARK E. MOLITCH

Pregnancy alters normal physiology and endocrine testing in a number of ways as a result of a variety of factors (Table 129–1). Pregnancy results in an expansion of plasma and red blood cell volume; the former predominates, causing a mild hemodilution of substances present in the blood. The increase in plasma volume begins at about 6 to 8 weeks' gestation, and the maximum volume is about 40 per cent increased by 30 to 34 weeks.[1] The increase in plasma volume is accompanied by an increase in cardiac output of 30 to 50 per cent, initially due to an increase in stroke volume and subsequently to an increase in heart rate.[2, 3] Along with the increase in cardiac output

TABLE 129–1. CHANGES IN NORMAL PHYSIOLOGY THAT MAY AFFECT ENDOCRINE TESTS

Cardiovascular
Increased plasma and RBC volume
Increased cardiac output
  Lowered "osmostat" for vasopressin release and thirst
Renal
Increased GFR and renal plasma flow
  Increased hormone and substrate clearance
Altered renal tubular function
  Decreased T_m for glucose
Placental Hormone Production
Increased estrogen and progesterone production
  Increased hormone binding globulin production
  Stimulation of pituitary lactotrophs
Production of peptide hormones
  ACTH, CRH, GnRH, HCG, GH variant, HPL, cTSH, PRL
Placental Enzyme Production
Vasopressinase

there is an increase in renal plasma flow and glomerular filtration rate (GFR) of similar proportions. The increase in GFR is apparent by week 4 and between the 6th and 12th weeks of gestation increases to about 140 to 150 per cent of the nonpregnant state.[4–6] The GFR increases by another 10 per cent over the remainder of the second trimester, stabilizes in the third trimester, and sometimes falls in the last 4 weeks of gestation.[6, 7] These changes in GFR may result in altered clearance of various hormones, causing changes in their serum and urinary levels.

Renal tubular function is also altered. This has importance with respect to glucose, in that tubular reabsorption of glucose is decreased, resulting in a low tubular maximum for glucose transport and significant glycosuria despite normal plasma glucose levels.[8] Although the tubular handling of bicarbonate is normal, because of the mild hyperventilation and respiratory alkalosis present during gestation, serum bicarbonate levels generally are decreased, the normal levels being 18 to 22 mEq/L. Thus the patient suspected of developing alcoholic or diabetic ketoacidosis normally has a lower bicarbonate, and confirmation of the acidotic state with arterial blood gas measurements is crucial. Tubular reabsorption of sodium is increased substantially due to numerous factors, including the increased GFR, increased progesterone production by the placenta, increased concentrations of aldosterone and cortisol, and exaggerated postural effects.[6]

Hormone production by the placenta may have profound effects on other hormonal systems. Estradiol levels increase 100-fold, beginning at about 6 to 8 weeks of gestation[9] (Fig. 129–1). These elevated estrogen levels cause an increase in concentration of the hormone-bind-

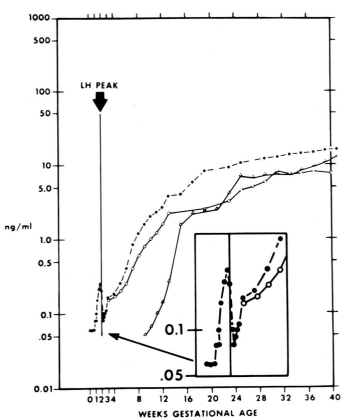

FIGURE 129-1. Maternal serum levels of unconjugated estrone (○—○), estradiol (●—●), and estriol (△—△) from last menstrual flow through a conceptual cycle to term pregnancy. The points represent mean steroid hormone levels compiled from four separate studies. (From Buster JE, Abraham GE: The applications of steroid hormone radioimmunoassays to clinical obstetrics. Obstet Gynecol 46:489–499, 1975. Reprinted with permission of the American College of Obstetricians and Gynecologists.)

ing globulins thyroid-hormone binding globulin (TBG), corticosteroid-binding globulin (CBG), and sex hormone–binding globulin (SHBG). This causes an increase in the total bound plus free measurements of these hormones, although free hormone levels are only minimally affected (see below). Estrogens also have a direct stimulatory effect on the pituitary lactotrophs, causing an increased production of prolactin (PRL). A number of peptide hormones are produced by the placenta, including chorionic gonadotropin (hCG), chorionic somatomammotropin (placental lactogen), placental growth hormone (GH) variant, chorionic thyrotropin, chorionic adrenocorticotropic hormone (ACTH), chorionic corticotropin-releasing hormone (CRH), chorionic gonadotropin-releasing hormone (GnRH), and chorionic somatostatin (see Ch. 124). Although most of these do not interfere with normal circulating blood levels of the hormones present before gestation, some do. For example, the placental growth hormone variant appears to have a negative-feedback action, suppressing pituitary GH secretion. Also, the placental CRH may influence pituitary ACTH secretion. Although hCG does not affect the pituitary, its structure is so similar to luteinizing hormone (LH) that it cross-reacts in some LH assays, and this fact may cause diagnostic problems if unanticipated. The placenta also can produce 1,25-dihydroxyvitamin D, which may have importance in calcium homeostasis during pregnancy.

Placental estrogen, progesterone, lactogen, and possibly GH variant also function as counterregulatory hormones with respect to insulin, causing insulin resistance and accelerated lipolysis. These phenomena are dealt with fully in Chapter 128.

The placenta produces enzymes which may affect normal endocrine function. Placental vasopressinase is so potent that the production rate of vasopressin in normal individuals must increase substantially. In patients with mild, subclinical diabetes insipidus, this accelerated metabolism of vasopressin may make this subclinical condition manifest.

This chapter will review the changes in normal physiology that occur during pregnancy and result in altered hormone levels that may create diagnostic difficulties when attempting to evaluate endocrine disorders in the pregnant patient. Specific aspects of pregnancy as it interacts with intermediary metabolism and diabetes mellitus are dealt with in other chapters (see also Chs. 85 and 128).

PITUITARY

Prolactin

Changes in Prolactin Physiology During Pregnancy

Estrogens produced by the placenta stimulate lactotroph DNA synthesis and mitotic activity, prolactin (PRL) mRNA levels, and PRL synthesis.[10–13] Progesterone also has been shown to stimulate PRL secretion.[14, 15] During pregnancy, there is a progressive rise in serum PRL levels[16, 17] (Fig. 129–2) that parallels an increase in the size and number of pituitary lactotroph cells.[18–21] By term, PRL levels may be increased 10-fold to levels over 200 ng/ml.[16, 17] These elevated PRL levels found at term prepare the breast for lactation. Thus the finding of amenorrhea associated with hyperprolactinemia could well be due to pregnancy and not due to pathological hyperprolactinemia.

It should be noted that PRL identical to pituitary PRL is also produced by the human decidua during pregnancy and causes high amniotic fluid PRL levels.[22] However, this decidual PRL is not present in maternal blood, and its physiological role may be limited to regulation of water

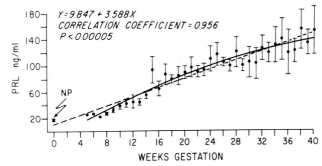

FIGURE 129-2. Mean ± SEM (n = 4) serum PRL concentrations measured serially at weekly intervals as a function of duration of gestation. Dashed line represents the linear regression, and solid line represents second-order regression (NP = nonpregnant PRL value). (From Rigg LA, Lein A, Yen SCC: Pattern of increase in circulating prolactin levels during human gestation. Am J Obstet Gynecol 129:454–456, 1977.)

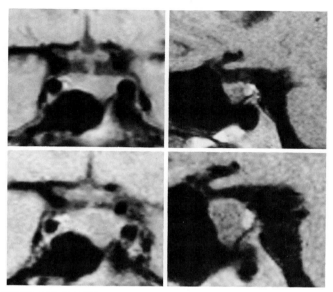

FIGURE 129–3. MRI scans with coronal (left) and sagittal (right) views demonstrating enlargement of a prolactin-secreting macroadenoma (above) before pregnancy and (below) in the third trimester of pregnancy. The patient had been complaining of increasing headaches.

and ion transport across extraembryonic membranes.[22] The placenta makes another hormone called *placental lactogen* (also known as *chorionic somatomammotropin*) which has lactogenic activity but is more structurally related to GH than PRL and also does not contribute to blood PRL levels during pregnancy.[22]

Prolactinomas

The normal pituitary enlarges during pregnancy, predominantly due to hyperplasia of the PRL-producing lactotroph cells.[18–21] A magnetic resonance imaging (MRI) scan performed during pregnancy will often reveal an enlarged pituitary due to this hyperplasia, but careful review of the scan will show no evidence of a pituitary tumor.[23]

However, the finding of an enlarged sella during pregnancy may not be due just to normal lactotroph hyperplasia but also could be due to the stimulatory effect of pregnancy on a pre-existing prolactinoma (Fig. 129–3). In two series of cases collected from the literature composed of 187[24] and 246[25] patients with prolactinomas who became pregnant, it was found that the risks of significant tumor enlargement were 1.6 per cent[25] and 4.4 per cent[24] for microadenomas, 15.5 per cent[25] and 33.9 per cent[24] for macroadenomas that had not been subjected to prior treatment by surgery or irradiation, and 4.3 per cent[25] and 7.1

per cent[24] for macroadenomas that had been subjected to prior surgery and/or irradiation (Table 129–2).

Lymphocytic Hypophysitis

Pituitary enlargement during pregnancy also may be due to lymphocytic hypophysitis. Lymphocytic hypophysitis is characterized by massive infiltration of the pituitary by lymphocytes and plasma cells with destruction of the normal parenchyma. The disorder is thought to have an autoimmune basis. Most cases occur in association with pregnancy, and women present during pregnancy or postpartum either with symptoms of varying degrees of hypopituitarism or with symptoms related to the mass lesion, such as headaches or visual field defects. Mild hyperprolactinemia and diabetes insipidus also may be found. On computed tomographic (CT) or MRI scan, a sellar mass is found which may extend in an extrasellar fashion and may cause visual field defects. The condition is usually confused with that of a pituitary tumor and, in fact, cannot be distinguished from a tumor except by biopsy. By virtue of the hypopituitarism it produces, lymphocytic hypophysitis also can be confused clinically with Sheehan's syndrome postpartum, except that there is no history of obstetrical hemorrhage.[26–29] The diagnosis of lymphocytic hypophysitis should be entertained in women with symptoms of hypopituitarism and/or mass lesions of the sella during pregnancy or postpartum, especially in the absence of a history of obstetrical hemorrhage. An evaluation of pituitary function is warranted as well as a CT or MRI scan. If PRL levels are only modestly elevated (<150 ng/ml) in the presence of a large mass, the diagnosis is unlikely to be an enlarging prolactinoma and more likely to be hypophysitis or a nonsecreting tumor.[30]

Growth Hormone

Changes in Growth Hormone Physiology During Pregnancy

In the second half of pregnancy, pituitary growth hormone (GH) secretion falls and a GH variant made by the syncytiotrophoblastic epithelium of the placenta increases in the circulation[31, 32] (Fig. 129–4). The episodic secretion of pituitary GH is replaced with a constant, nonpulsatile secretion of this variant at the rather high levels of 10 to 20 ng/ml.[32, 33] The production of the placental variant is accompanied by decreased production of normal pituitary GH, presumably because of negative-feedback effects.[34] Evidence in favor of this feedback effect of placental GH on pituitary GH secretion includes the fact that in patients

TABLE 129–2. EFFECT OF PREGNANCY ON PROLACTINOMAS

TUMOR TYPE	PRIOR THERAPY	NUMBER	SYMPTOMATIC ENLARGEMENT*	ASYMPTOMATIC ENLARGEMENT†
Microadenomas	None	246	4	11
Macroadenomas	None	45	7	4
Macroadenomas	Yes	46	2	0

*Requiring intervention: surgery or bromocriptine.
†Determined by postpartum CT scanning.
Adapted with permission, from Molitch ME: Pregnancy and the hyperprolactinemic woman. N Engl J Med 312:1364–1370, 1985.

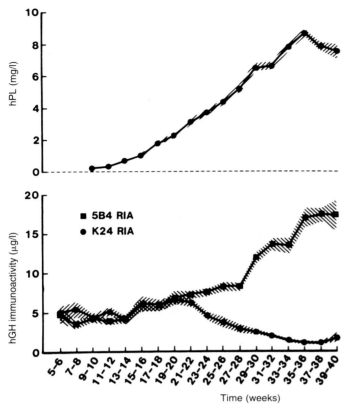

FIGURE 129–4. Mean (±SD) serum GH and placental lactogen levels in women throughout pregnancy. The 584 RIA antibody is specific for the GH placental variant, whereas the K24 RIA antibody is specific for pituitary GH. Note the rise in serum levels of the GH placental variant coinciding with the fall in serum levels of pituitary GH. (From Frankenne F, Closset J, Gomez F, et al: The physiology of growth hormones (GHs) in pregnant women and partial characterization of the placental GH variant. J Clin Endocrinol Metab 66:1171–1180, Copyright © 1978, the Endocrine Society.)

with acromegaly who have autonomous GH secretion and who become pregnant, both forms of GH persist in the blood throughout pregnancy.[35]

The GH variant differs from pituitary GH by 13 amino acids and has similar somatogenic but less lactogenic bioactivity than pituitary GH,[36] reflecting differences in binding to somatogenic versus lactogenic GH receptors.[37] On the other hand, the placental GH variant binds equipotently with pituitary GH to the high-affinity GH-binding protein which is thought to be the extracellular domain of the GH receptor,[38] and in the second half of pregnancy, overall GH bioactivity is considerably elevated, as measured by a radioreceptor assay.[39] Although one report suggested that the GH variant is considerably less able to stimulate insulin-like growth factor I (IGF-I, also known as somatomedin C), IGF-I levels in the last trimester of pregnancy being just minimally elevated,[39] most other reports have demonstrated considerably elevated IGF-I levels during pregnancy, commensurate with the elevated GH variant levels measured by radioimmunoassay and radioreceptor assay.[40–42] The GH variant also has similar activity to normal pituitary with respect to carbohydrate and lipid metabolism.[47]

At present, the physiological significance of the change in the source of circulating GH during pregnancy is not known. However, the elevated levels of the placental variant with elevated levels of IGF-I may account for the coarsening of features occasionally seen in some pregnant women, and such women may be suspected of having acromegaly. It is not clear as to whether these elevated placental GH variant levels contribute to the insulin resistance of pregnancy.

Acromegaly

Standard radioimmunoassays for GH usually cannot distinguish between normal pituitary GH and the placental GH variant and, therefore, may give misleading results with respect to the assessment of pituitary GH secretion during the latter half of pregnancy. Basal levels of the variant are considerably higher than normal, nonpregnant GH levels and therefore may erroneously indicate excessive pituitary GH secretion. Special radioimmunoassays utilizing antibodies that recognize specific epitopes on the two hormones[32] or an immunoradiometric assay (IRMA)[39] are necessary to distinguish normal from placental GH. When such specific assays are not available, it may be necessary to wait until infant delivery to assess pituitary GH secretion accurately, because levels of the placental GH variant fall to undetectable levels within 24 hours.[32] However, there are two differences between placental GH variant secretion and pituitary GH secretion in acromegaly that may allow a distinction to be made during pregnancy: (1) pituitary GH secretion in acromegaly is highly pulsatile, with 13 to 19 pulses per 24 hours,[44, 45] whereas pregnancy GH variant secretion is nonpulsatile,[33] and (2) in acromegaly, about 70 per cent of patients have a GH response to thyrotropin-releasing hormone (TRH),[46–49] whereas the placental GH variant does not respond to TRH.[35]

Actual reports of pregnancies in acromegalic patients are uncommon,[35, 50–53] perhaps because of the fact that about 40 per cent of such patients are hyperprolactinemic.[39] Indeed, correction of the hyperprolactinemia with bromocriptine may be necessary to permit ovulation and conception in these patients.[50, 53] It is possible that in a patient initially diagnosed with acromegaly during pregnancy, the finding of hyperprolactinemia may be due to the stimulated production of PRL by the normal lactotrophs and not be due to tumor production.

Vasopressin

Changes in Vasopressin Physiology During Pregnancy

The primary regulator of vasopressin secretion is the osmolality of the plasma, sensed by the osmoreceptors (see Ch. 25). The osmotic threshold for vasopressin release in nonpregnant subjects is about 280 to 285 mOsmol/kg, with a normal range of 275 to 290 mOsmol/kg. Thirst is generally stimulated at a plasma osmolality level about 5 mOsmol/kg above that for vasopressin release, a level near which maximum concentration of urine will already have been achieved.

In pregnancy there is a lowering of the "osmostat," the setpoint for serum osmolality, by about 10 mOsmol/kg. The decline in plasma osmolality begins by the time of the first missed menstrual period and gradually increases until the tenth week of gestation, after which there is little fur-

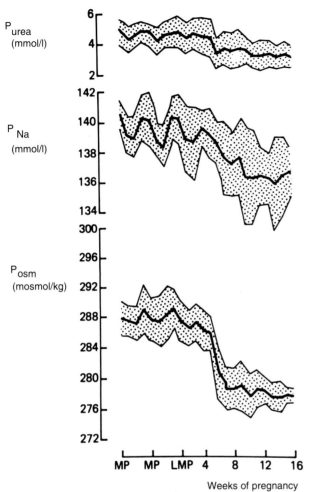

FIGURE 129–5. Mean values ($\pm$ SD) for plasma urea (P_{urea}), sodium (P_{Na}), and osmolality (P_{osmol}) measured at weekly intervals from before conception to the first trimester in nine women with successful obstetric outcome (MP = menstrual period; LMP = last menstrual period). (From Davison JM, Vallotton MB, Lindheimer MD: Plasma osmolality and urinary concentration and dilution during and after pregnancy: Evidence that lateral recumbency inhibits maximal urinary concentrating ability. Br J Obstet Gynaecol 88:472–479, 1981.)

ther change[54] (Fig. 129–5). Pregnant women experience thirst and release vasopressin at lower levels of serum osmolality than do nonpregnant individuals to maintain this lower osmolality[55] (Fig. 129–6). A water load will suppress vasopressin secretion appropriately, resulting in dilute urine and excretion of this water load, thereby maintaining this lower osmolality.[55, 56] This reset osmostat results in a lowering of the serum sodium by about 4 to 5 mEq/ml.[54, 56] The physiological basis for this reset osmostat is not clear. However, recent experiments in humans have shown that hCG injected into nonpregnant women lowers their osmostat by 5 mOsmol/kg.[57] Furthermore, a case has been described in which a woman with a hydatidiform mole had a lower osmostat which returned to normal only when hCG levels in the serum finally became undetectable 40 days after evacuation of the mole.[57] Evidence from rat studies and from human studies in which pregnant women were immersed in water to expand the central blood volume suggest that a decreased "effective" blood volume does not play a role in this resetting of the osmostat.[56]

The placenta produces vasopressinase, a cystine amino-

peptidase that rapidly inactivates vasopressin. Vasopressinase levels increase 1000-fold between the fourth and 38th weeks of gestation.[58] How much this increase in vasopressinase activity contributes to the increased clearance of endogenous vasopressin during pregnancy is not clear, however.[58] The placenta itself is also able to metabolize vasopressin.[59] Overall, the combination of increased vasopressinase levels and increased placental metabolism of vasopressin results in a two- to four-fold increased metabolic clearance rate for vasopressin.[58, 60]

Diabetes Insipidus

In a patient with pre-existing diabetes insipidus (DI) this increased metabolism of vasopressin during pregnancy results in a worsening of the DI.[61] Thus mild cases treated with either increased fluids or chlorpropamide will likely experience considerable worsening. Women being treated with pitressin tannate in oil or lysine vasopressin spray also may experience such worsening. The vasopressin analogue dDAVP (desmopressin) is not affected by vasopressinase, and a number of women have been treated quite satisfactorily with this medication.[61] Rarely, asymptomatic women will experience symptomatic DI only during pregnancy.[62, 63]

When a pregnant patient presents with polyuria and polydipsia, the finding of lower than expected serum sodium levels should not therefore exclude the diagnosis of DI.[54, 61] Testing for DI (see Ch. 25) in a pregnant woman should be performed in the sitting position because the lateral recumbent position results in an inhibition of maximal urinary concentrating ability.[54, 64] The increased metabolism of vasopressin also limits the rise in plasma vaso-

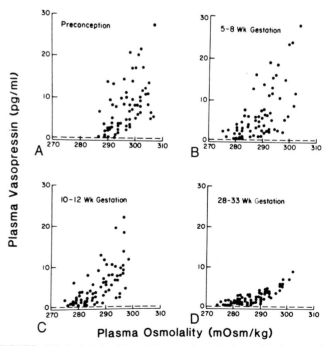

FIGURE 129–6. Relationship of P_{AVP} to P_{osmol} during a 2-h hypertonic saline infusion in eight women studied serially before and during pregnancy. Each point is an individual plasma determination. Dashed lines indicate lower limit of detection for AVP. (From Lindheimer MD, Barron WM, Davison JM: Osmoregulation of thirst and vasopressin release in pregnancy. Am J Physiol 257(Renal Fluid Electrolyte Physiol 26):F159–F169, 1989. Reproduced with permission of the Society for Clinical Investigation and the American Society of Physiology.)

pressin levels during testing, especially in the last trimester.[55, 57] Therefore, the levels of vasopressin and osmolality used in nomograms for nonpregnant patients cannot be used for pregnant patients, and an extrapolation from Figure 129–6 can be used. When obtained for vasopressin measurement during pregnancy, blood should be drawn into syringes containing orthophenanthroline (0.1 ml in a 10-ml syringe) to inactivate vasopressinase activity and then rapidly transferred to chilled heparinized tubes, centrifuged in the cold, and extracted within 3 hours.[55, 58]

THYROID

Thyroid Hormones and Thyroid Regulation

Changes in Normal Thyroid Physiology During Pregnancy

A number of changes occur in the thyroid and the measurement of thyroid hormones during pregnancy. It is widely believed that a goiter commonly develops during pregnancy. This belief stems from uncontrolled early observations and other studies such as one in Scotland in which goiters were found in 70 per cent of 184 pregnant women but only in 37 per cent of nonpregnant controls.[65] It appears, however, that most such studies were done in iodine-deficient regions. In iodine-replete regions, there is no increase in the frequency of goiters during pregnancy.[66–68] In a recent study of Belgian women with borderline iodine status, thyroid volume was found to increase about 18 per cent during pregnancy,[69] a change that would not be clinically apparent. Of 309 pregnant adolescents evaluated by Long et al.,[68] 18 were found to have goiters; 2 had Graves' disease and were hyperthyroid, 3 had Hashimoto's thyroiditis, 1 being hyperthyroid, and 4 had subacute thyroiditis, 1 being hyperthyroid. The other 9 with goiters were thought to have simple nontoxic goiters. Thus, although thyroid volume does increase slightly during pregnancy, perhaps due to relative iodine deficiency and/ or the stimulatory effect of hCG (see below), the presence of a palpable goiter in iodine-replete areas indicates significant disease in about 50 per cent of patients and should always be evaluated. In one third of patients found to have goiters, an increase in size of 17 to 55 per cent may be expected over the course of gestation.[70]

The renal clearance of iodine is increased because of the increased GFR that occurs with pregnancy. When iodine intake is marginal, this increased loss may result in iodine deficiency.[69] Even in the absence of hypothyroidism, the total-body iodine pool becomes decreased, resulting in an increased radioactive iodine uptake.[71] Radioactive iodine uptakes are, of course, contraindicated during pregnancy because the placenta is freely permeable to iodine and the fetal thyroid is 20 to 50 times more avid for iodine than the maternal thyroid.[72] However, the tracer dose used in these studies is so small that it is not sufficient to cause concern if given inadvertently during pregnancy.[72] Generally, the iodine in iodized salt and prenatal vitamins prevents iodine deficiency. Excessive iodine ingestion is to be avoided, however, because it crosses the placenta and may cause neonatal goiter.

The fetal thyroid and the fetal hypothalamic-pituitary-thyroid axis develop independently of maternal thyroid status (see Ch. 127). At 11 to 12 weeks of gestation, the fetal thyroid begins to concentrate iodine. In addition to iodine, the placenta is freely permeable to medications used to treat hyperthyroidism, such as propylthiouracil (PTU), methimazole, and propranolol; triiodothyronine (T_3) and thyroid-stimulating hormone (TSH) cross the placenta only minimally.[73] Thyroxine (T_4) crosses the placenta in somewhat larger (although still small) amounts, and late in gestation, large doses are able to ameliorate the effects of hypothyroidism in infants with congenital hypothyroidism due to enzyme defects or agenesis of the thyroid.[74]

Bioassayable thyroid-stimulating activity in serum is increased in the first trimester due to intrinsic thyroid-stimulating activity of hCG.[69, 75–78] The hCG may cause increased T_4 and T_3 levels and may cause a transient hyperthyroidism associated with hyperemesis gravidarum (see below). Markedly elevated levels of hCG seen in trophoblastic neoplasms also may cause hyperthyroidism.[79, 80] There also may be a human chorionic thyrotropin made by the placenta with little thyroid-stimulating activity, and it probably plays no physiological role.[76]

Alterations in Thyroid Function Tests During Pregnancy

The basal metabolic rate (BMR) is increased by about 15 to 20 per cent during pregnancy, about 70 to 80 per cent of the increment being attributable to the placenta and fetus and the remainder to increased maternal cardiac output.[81] This test is rarely done at present.

T_4 is about 85 per cent bound to thyroxine-binding globulin (TBG) and about 15 per cent bound to thyroxine-binding prealbumin; only 0.04 per cent is unbound or "free." The increased estrogens of the placenta result in increased TBG levels in the blood as a result of increased production by hepatocytes,[82] as well as decreased degradation owing to altered glycosylation.[83] The increased TBG levels result in increased bound T_4 measurements, beginning by 4 to 6 weeks of gestation[75, 84] (Fig. 129–7). The amount of binding of hormone to TBG may be estimated using the resin uptake test, which decreases as TBG increases.

The metabolic activity of the hormones correlates best with the free hormone levels. Free T_4 levels may be estimated indirectly using the resin uptake test to compensate for the increase in TBG and the total T_4 levels (frequently referred to as the *free T_4 index*), or they may be measured directly by equilibrium dialysis. The latter is more accurate but more difficult to perform. When there is any question, free T_4 measurements by dialysis should be performed. Free T_4 levels have been reported to be unchanged,[85] increased,[75] or decreased[69, 86] during pregnancy, although they usually remain within the normal range[77] (Fig. 129–8). These differences may relate to relative iodine deficiencies in the populations studied[69] and what stage of pregnancy is being assessed. Harada et al.[75] have postulated that the slightly elevated free T_4 levels they found may be due to the stimulating activity of the high levels of hCG, and free T4 levels have been shown to correlate well with serum hCG levels[69] (Fig. 129–9). The elevation of free T_4 levels, when reported, peaks near the end of the first trimester and then falls back toward baseline, in parallel with changes in hCG.[69]

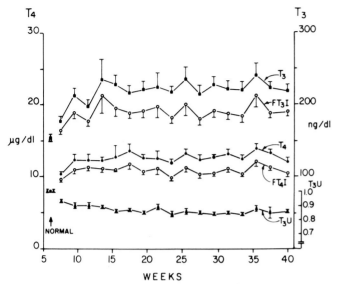

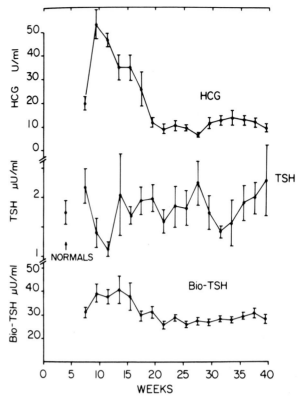

FIGURE 129-7. Serum T$_4$, serum T$_3$, T$_3$ uptake (T$_3$U), FT$_4$I, and FT$_3$I at various weeks of pregnancy (±SE). (Left) Nonpregnant control values. Serum T$_4$, T$_3$, FT$_4$I, and FT$_3$I were significantly elevated, and T$_3$U was reduced throughout pregnancy. (From Harada K, Hershman JM, Reed AW, et al: Comparison of thyroid stimulators and thyroid hormone concentrations in the sera of pregnant women. J Clin Endocrinol Metab 48:793–797, copyright © 1979 by the Endocrine Society.)

FIGURE 129-9. Serum hCG, hTSH (RIA), and bioassayable thyroid-stimulating activity (bio-TSH; ±SE) during pregnancy. Bioassayable thyroid-stimulating activity was significantly elevated from 9 to 16 weeks compared with the remainder of pregnancy. Human TSH (by RIA) was significantly lower at 9 to 12 weeks compared with the rest of pregnancy. (From Harada K, Hershman JM, Reed AW, et al: Comparison of thyroid stimulators and thyroid hormone concentrations in the sera of pregnant women. J Clin Endocrinol Metab 48:793–797, copyright © 1979 by the Endocrine Society.)

T$_4$ turnover is increased during pregnancy,[86] and in the patient receiving thyroxine replacement, TSH levels should be checked each trimester to determine if there is a need to increase the dose.[87] In one study, 75 per cent of patients needed to increase their thyroxine doses during pregnancy[87] (Fig. 129-10). T$_3$ is bound to TBG with somewhat less affinity than T$_4$, but the same increase in total T$_3$ measurements is seen as with T$_4$ during pregnancy.[75] TSH levels

are minimally decreased during the first trimester of pregnancy (see Fig. 129–9), possibly due to the increased free T$_4$ levels.[75]

Hyperthyroidism

Because of the hyperdynamic state of pregnancy, the clinical diagnosis of hyperthyroidism may prove difficult. The features of tachycardia, warm skin, systolic flow murmurs, and heat intolerance are common to both. Even the finding of a goiter may not be specific. Weight loss, a marked tachycardia, eye signs, and a bruit over the thyroid are more suggestive of hyperthyroidism.[88] Infiltrative dermopathy or ophthalmopathy is specific for Graves' disease but does not indicate the degree of hyperthyroidism.

The changes in thyroid hormones already discussed may cause further diagnostic difficulty. Because of the elevation of TBG in blood, total T$_4$ and T$_3$ levels are elevated. If the free T$_4$ index that has been calculated by the laboratory from the total T$_4$ and the resin uptake test is not elevated, despite a strong clinical suspicion, then a free T$_4$ done by dialysis should be performed. However, in normal pregnancy, free T$_4$ levels also may be mildly elevated,[76] and TSH levels may be suppressed to below the level of detectability with older assays and below normal with the newer, ultrasensitive assays due to the high levels of free T$_4$ and hCG

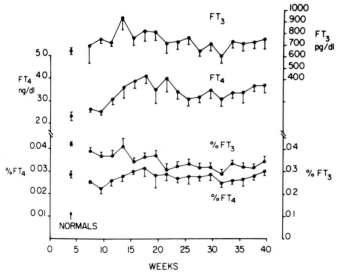

FIGURE 129-8. Serum free T$_4$ (FT$_4$) and free T$_3$ (FT$_3$), %FT$_4$, and %FT$_3$ (±SE) during pregnancy; values in nonpregnant controls are at the left. Serum %FT$_3$ was significantly lower than control throughout pregnancy, but %FT$_4$ was not reduced during pregnancy. Free T$_4$ was significantly elevated after 10 weeks of pregnancy and free T$_3$ was significantly elevated only at 13 to 20 weeks. (From Harada K, Hershman JM, Reed AW, et al: Comparison of thyroid stimulators and thyroid hormone concentrations in the sera of pregnant women. J Clin Endocrinol Metab 48:793–797, copyright © 1979 by the Endocrine Society.)

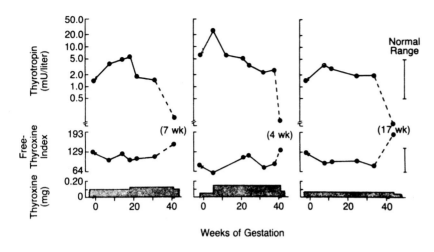

FIGURE 129-10. Representative patterns of changes in thyroid function and thyroxine dose during pregnancy in women with hypothyroidism. The left-hand and middle panels show the results for two women who required an increased dose of thyroxine during pregnancy. The right-hand panel shows the results for a woman whose thyroxine dose was not changed during pregnancy. The normal ranges for serum thyrotropin and the free thyroxine index are indicated by the vertical bars on the right side of the figure. The discontinuity marks indicate the beginning and end of pregnancy. The dashed line represents the change between the last gestational and the first postpartum values (the number of weeks postpartum is noted in parentheses). (Reproduced with permission from Mandel SJ, Larsen PR, Seely EW, Brent EA: Increased need for thyroxine during pregnancy in women with primary hypothyroidism. N Engl J Med 323:91–96, 1990.)

(see above). However, the TSH levels will not be *undetectable* with these newer assays in pregnancy,[69] as they are with typical hyperthyroidism,[89] making this the critical assessment when other levels are borderline. It is important to make the diagnosis of hyperthyroidism accurately and carefully, since untreated hyperthyroidism clearly has an adverse consequence on fetal outcome.[90]

Hyperthyroidism and Hyperemesis Gravidarum

Nausea and vomiting occasionally may be the predominant presenting symptom in patients with hyperthyroidism. When this occurs during pregnancy, it may present as hyperemesis gravidarum.[91, 92] In one series of patients with hyperemesis gravidarum, 2 of 39 patients were found to be thyrotoxic.[93] However, elevated free T$_4$ and T$_3$ levels may be found transiently in up to one third of subjects presenting with hyperemesis gravidarum.[94] These increased thyroid hormone levels are likely due to stimulation by hCG because serum hCG levels were increased by about 50 per cent in those subjects with elevated free T$_4$ levels and correlated with the free T$_4$ levels.[94] On the other hand, there

is considerable overlap of hCG levels with those of normal individuals so that some authors have postulated that in these particular cases associated with transient hyperthyroidism, the hCG may have some structural variation resulting in increased biological activity.[94] In most patients, the free T$_4$ levels fall to normal over 6 to 133 days (mean 35.1 days) while still pregnant[94] (Fig. 129–11). Therefore, patients with hyperemesis and elevated free T$_4$ and T$_3$ levels present a considerable diagnostic dilemma. In prior studies, TSH levels in those patients thought to be hyperthyroxinemic usually were not suppressed,[93] but this may have been due to cross-reactivity of very high levels of hCG in those TSH assays. Although data using the newer, highly sensitive TSH assays are lacking in these patients, it would be expected that their increased specificity as well as sensitivity[94a] would result in the finding of undetectable TSH levels in those women who become truly thyrotoxic. Because of the increased morbidity to mother and fetus of untreated hyperthyroidism, it appears to be safest to treat with antithyroid drugs any woman with symptomatic hyperthyroidism or those in whom thyroid hormone levels do not spontaneously revert to normal over 1 to 3 weeks and

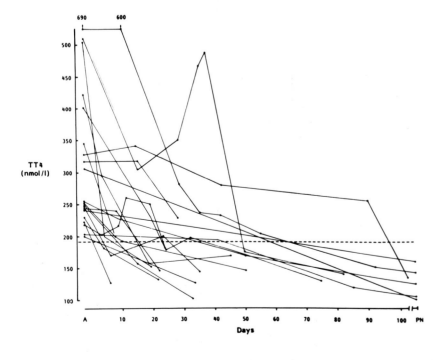

FIGURE 129–11. Changes in plasma total thyroxine concentration in 20 hyperemesis subjects on admission *(A)* and during the course of their pregnancy. The interrupted line represents the mean ± SD value seen in normal pregnancy (PN = postnatal). (From Swaminathan R, Chin RK, Lao TTH, et al: Thyroid function in hyperemesis gravidarum. Acta Endocrinol 120:155–160, 1989.)

in whom TSH levels are suppressed below detectability using a highly sensitive assay. Careful follow-up and adjustment of medications may allow stopping of antithyroid medication in those with transient hormonal abnormalities.

Hypothyroidism

The clinical picture of the patient developing spontaneous hypothyroidism during pregnancy may be confusing because of the tendency of pregnancy to cause tachycardia, fatigue, warm skin, and heat intolerance. However, other typical findings of hypothyroidism should gradually become apparent, such as muscle cramps, excessive fatigue, dry skin, etc. The elevated TBG levels may cause total T_4 levels to be normal, but free T_4 levels will be low and TSH levels will be elevated. As noted above, replacement doses of thyroxine may need to be increased[87] because of the increased clearance of thyroxine during pregnancy.

ADRENAL CORTEX

Glucocorticosteroids and Glucocorticosteroid Regulation

Changes in Adrenal Physiology During Pregnancy

Cortisol levels increase progressively over the course of gestation, resulting in a two- to three-fold increase by term[95-98] (Fig. 129–12). Most of the elevation of cortisol levels is due to the estrogen-induced increase in cortisol-binding globulin (transcortin) levels,[95, 98-100] but the biologically active "free" fraction in serum is elevated threefold as well.[95, 99-101] This is reflected in two- to three-fold elevations in urinary free cortisol levels.[102, 103] The increased CBG results in a prolonged cortisol half-life in plasma, but the cortisol production rate is also increased.[101] Urinary 17-hydroxycorticosteroid levels are decreased, however, due to a decrease in the excretion of cortisol tetrahydro metabolites.[104, 105] Cortisol can cross the placenta, and the major direction of transfer is from mother to fetus.[106]

ACTH levels have been variously reported as being normal,[107] suppressed,[97] and elevated[96, 108] early in gestation. During the pregnancy, there is a progressive rise, followed by a final surge of ACTH and cortisol levels during labor[96, 97, 107] (see Fig. 129–12). ACTH does not cross the placenta[109] but is manufactured by the placenta[107, 110] (see Ch. 124). The amounts of ACTH in serum that are due to placental versus pituitary origin at various stages of gestation are not known.

CRH is also produced by the placenta[111, 112] (see Ch. 124) and is released into maternal plasma,[113] where levels gradually increase over the course of the second and third trimesters, peaking during labor and delivery.[114, 115] This CRH is bioactive and may release ACTH both from the placenta, in a paracrine fashion,[110, 116, 117] and from the maternal pituitary,[118] although the latter is not absolutely proved. The rise in CRH over the course of gestation and delivery is highly correlated with the rise in ACTH and cortisol levels, implying cause and effect.[118, 119]

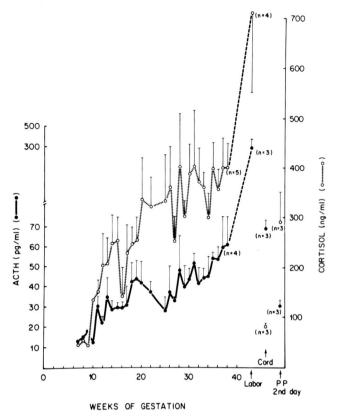

FIGURE 129–12. Plasma concentration of ACTH and cortisol during normal pregnancy. Blood samples were obtained weekly at 0800 to 0900 hours from five normal pregnant women and from three women during labor and on the second postpartum day. In addition, umbilical cord plasma was obtained from the newborn infants of three of these subjects. The mean plasma concentrations for ACTH are denoted by the solid circles, whereas plasma cortisol levels are denoted by open circles. The vertical bars correspond to the magnitude of the standard error of the mean. (From Carr BR, Parker CR Jr, Madden JD, et al: Maternal plasma adenocorticotropin and cortisol relationships throughout human pregnancy. Am J Obstet Gynecol 139:416–422, 1981.)

Neither ACTH[110] nor CRH production by the placenta[111] are suppressible in vitro with exogenous glucocorticoids. In some in vitro studies, CRH production is actually increased by exogenous glucocorticoids.[120, 121] These findings of the lack of suppressibility of placental ACTH and CRH production by glucocorticoids correlate well with the in vivo findings that ACTH and cortisol levels do not suppress normally in the third trimester, as shown in one patient with unchanging ACTH levels during treatment with 10 mg/d of prednisone at term[96] and by nonsuppressible urinary free cortisol values in six women who underwent a standard low-dose (2 mg/d for 3 days) dexamethasone test during the last trimester.[107] However, in one study, betamethasone was shown to be capable of suppressing ACTH and cortisol, but not CRH levels, very early in the third trimester (26 to 30 weeks).[121] In another study, overnight dexamethasone (1 mg) suppression tests showed normal cortisol suppression in seven normal women at unspecified portions of the second and third trimesters.[122] Thus, based on limited studies, it appears that CRH levels are nonsuppressible throughout the last trimester but that ACTH and cortisol levels become nonsuppressible only in the latter part of the third trimester. No studies in normal pregnant women have been performed with high-dose dexamethasone.

Cushing's Syndrome

The diagnosis of Cushing's syndrome should be made during pregnancy, as the untreated condition is associated with high fetal mortality and increased prematurity, as well as maternal hypertension, preeclampsia, and myopathy.[90] Although less than 70 cases of Cushing's syndrome during pregnancy have been reported,[90, 124, 125] it is apparent that the distribution of causes of Cushing's is different in pregnancy. Less than 50 per cent are due to pituitary adenomas, a like number are due to adrenal adenomas, and 10 per cent are due to adrenal carcinomas. Interestingly, in many cases Cushing's syndrome first became manifested or became exacerbated during the pregnancy, with improvement following parturition. It has been speculated that in some cases of Cushing's disease, the unregulated placental CRH was instrumental in causing this pregnancy-induced exacerbation.[124, 125]

The diagnosis of Cushing's syndrome during pregnancy may be quite difficult. Both may be associated with weight gain in a central distribution, fatigue, edema, emotional upset, glucose intolerance, and hypertension. The striae associated with the weight gain and increased abdominal girth are usually white in normal pregnancy and red or purple in Cushing's. Hirsutism and acne may point to excessive androgen production.

As can be inferred from the laboratory findings described above, the biochemical evaluation of Cushing's syndrome in pregnant women is not straightforward. The finding of a greatly elevated total serum cortisol level, increased serum and urinary free cortisol levels, and increased ACTH levels can be compatible with normal pregnancy, as well as Cushing's syndrome. Furthermore, at least in the latter part of the third trimester, these elevated levels are nonsuppressible by low-dose dexamethasone. In pregnant patients reported with Cushing's disease, plasma cortisol levels suppress minimally with 2 days of low-dose dexamethasone but suppress quite well with the high dose.[126] Pregnant patients with adrenal adenomas also do not suppress with high-dose dexamethasone,[127–130] as expected. Basal ACTH levels have been reported to be normal in two patients with Cushing's disease during pregnancy.[126, 131] However, similarly normal ACTH levels have been reported in patients with adrenal adenomas.[130, 132–134] These "normal" rather than suppressed levels of ACTH in patients with adrenal adenomas may be due to the production of ACTH by the placenta or the nonsuppressible stimulation of pituitary ACTH by placental CRH (see above). Thus the presence of "normal" levels of ACTH may be quite misleading in the differential diagnosis of Cushing's syndrome during pregnancy. Most helpful in distinguishing Cushing's syndrome from the hypercortisolism of pregnancy is the finding of a persistent diurnal variation of elevated levels of total and free serum cortisol during normal pregnancy,[98, 101, 103, 135] a finding characteristically absent in all forms of Cushing's syndrome (see Ch. 100). There has been no experience reported with more recently used techniques such as CRH stimulation testing[136] or petrosal venous sinus sampling in diagnosing Cushing's disease during pregnancy. However, CRH stimulation tests have been shown to elicit normal ACTH responses in the early second trimester but to elicit no ACTH responses in the late third trimester.[118] Thus the finding of a blunted ACTH response to CRH would be more in favor of simple pregnancy rather than Cushing's disease, in which there generally is hyperresponsiveness to CRH.[136] On the other hand, the finding of a blunted or no response to CRH also would be compatible with an adrenal adenoma or carcinoma.[136] Overall, CRH testing would appear to be of limited utility in the differential diagnosis of pregnancy versus the different causes of Cushing's syndrome. In any case, CRH testing during late gestation has the potential hazard of inducing premature labor, because CRH has been shown to potentiate the contractile response of pregnant myometrium to oxytocin and has been implicated in participating in the process of parturition.[137]

When biochemical evidence points to the presence of Cushing's syndrome and to a pituitary or adrenal origin, radiologic imaging becomes necessary. The pituitary volume is often increased during pregnancy (see above), and pituitary CT or MRI may yield a false-positive finding. However, careful review of the MRI findings may indicate a focal abnormality in a patient with a tumor compared with the diffusely enlarged, homogeneous gland seen with pregnancy (see above). Often an adrenal mass will be visible on ultrasound.[139] Usually, however, CT or MRI scanning of the pituitary or adrenal will be necessary (see Ch. 130). With the techniques and equipment available at present, CT and MRI appear to be about equal in detecting adrenal masses. Because MRI may be safer during pregnancy, it may be the technique of choice for localizing the mass. Most adrenal lesions are unilateral, so localization is important.

Adrenal Insufficiency

Adrenal insufficiency is uncommon during pregnancy[139] and usually is due to autoimmune destruction. Adrenal insufficiency caused by infiltrative diseases, such as tuberculosis, fungal diseases, and metastatic cancer, is much less common. Rarely, bilateral adrenal hemorrhage may occur in association with surgery or anticoagulant use, usually presenting as an acute adrenal crisis that is manifested by fever, abdominal or flank pain, vomiting, confusion, and hypotension.[140, 141]

Patients commonly present with fatigue, anorexia, nausea, vomiting, weight loss, depression, and nonspecific abdominal pain.[139] Obviously, it may be difficult to sort out the features of fatigue, nausea, and vomiting during the first trimester, but persistence of these symptoms should at least trigger a screening diagnostic evaluation. Patients with primary adrenal insufficiency and normal pituitaries respond by increasing ACTH and lipotropin secretion, resulting in increased pigmentation in skin creases, scars, and mucous membranes. However, a similar increased pigmentation also may be seen during normal pregnancy.[142] On examination, patients will usually display evidence of orthostatic hypotension. Mild cases may go undetected during pregnancy, only to go into adrenal crisis with the stress of labor or other illness, such as a urinary tract infection or dehydration from excessive sun exposure.[139, 143] In some cases, severe adrenal insufficiency may not develop until the postpartum period, possibly due to maintenance of maternal cortisol levels by fetal adrenal production.[144] Maternal adrenal insufficiency has been associated with intrauterine growth retardation in some cases.[143, 144]

Laboratory features of adrenal insufficiency include hyperkalemia due to aldosterone deficiency, hyponatremia due to an inability to excrete free water by the kidney, mild azotemia, eosinophilia, and a lymphocytosis. Fasting hypoglycemia also may be present. However, fasting hypoglycemia also may be present during normal pregnancy, especially in the first trimester. Basal cortisol levels may appear "normal" but really are inappropriately low when corrected for the stage of gestation. The finding of an inappropriately normal or low cortisol level with a substantially elevated ACTH level makes the diagnosis of primary and not secondary adrenal insufficiency. A stimulation test with Cortrosyn (synthetic $ACTH_{1-24}$) 25 μg should be performed immediately after obtaining the preceding baseline measurements, without waiting for the results. In primary adrenal insufficiency, the second cortisol level obtained 60 minutes later will show an inadequate increment [i.e., less than a doubling of the basal levels and/or an increase to >18 μg/dl in nonpregnant individuals (see Ch. 99); normal values have not been established for pregnant women]. In patients with suspected pituitary disease as the cause of the adrenal insufficiency, the cortisol and ACTH responses to insulin-induced hypoglycemia should be obtained, using for normal the same parameters as given above for the ACTH stimulation test. Because of the insulin resistance associated with pregnancy, a dose of 0.15 or 0.20 U/kg of insulin may be needed to induce hypoglycemia instead of the standard 0.1 U/kg. Standard metyrapone testing (750 mg every 4 hours for 6 doses) also has been performed during pregnancy, and 75 per cent of normal pregnant subjects showed diminished responses, while the other 25 per cent had normal responses.[145] Therefore, such testing does not appear to be valid during pregnancy.

Aldosterone and Renin and Aldosterone and Renin Regulation

Changes in Aldosterone and Renin Physiology During Pregnancy

During pregnancy, the blood pressure falls, reaching a nadir at about 28 weeks and then gradually returning to close to prepregnancy levels by term.[146] This fall in blood pressure is accompanied by an increase in heart rate, which

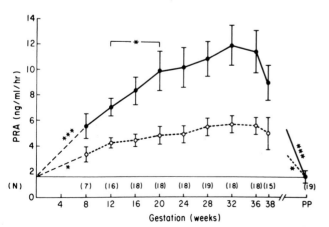

FIGURE 129–13. Sequential changes in PRA (●) and in PRA normalized to the postpartum substrate values (○) (mean ±SE) throughout pregnancy (*$p < 0.05$, ***$p < 0.001$). (From Wilson M, Morganti AA, Zervondakis I, et al: Blood pressure, the renin-aldosterone system and sex steroids throughout normal pregnancy. Am J Med 68:97–104, 1980.)

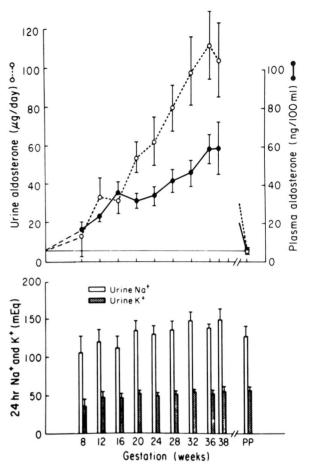

FIGURE 129–14. Sequential changes throughout pregnancy in plasma aldosterone, urine aldosterone, urinary sodium, and potassium (mean ± SE). (From Wilson M, Morganti AA, Zervondakis I, et al: Blood pressure, the renin-aldosterone system and sex steroids throughout normal pregnancy. Am J Med 68:97–104, 1980.)

increases by 20 to 25 beats/min by week 32.[146] Plasma renin activity increases four-fold by 8 weeks and then increases only minimally over the subsequent 32 weeks of gestation (Fig. 129–13), whereas plasma renin substrate (angiotensinogen) levels increase four-fold over the course of the first 20 weeks of gestation and then increase only minimally over the subsequent 20 weeks of gestation.[146, 147] Angiotensin II levels double early in pregnancy and eventually are increased three- to four-fold by term.[147] Similar increases occur in plasma aldosterone levels (Fig. 129–14), a five-fold increase occurring by 16 weeks and ultimately a seven- to ten-fold elevation occurring by term.[123, 146–150] This increase in plasma aldosterone levels is reflected in a seven-fold elevation in urinary aldosterone levels by 12 weeks and ultimately a 20- to 25-fold elevation by term.[146] There are significant correlations between plasma aldosterone and plasma renin activity; plasma progesterone, plasma estriol, and plasma estradiol levels; and urine aldosterone levels.[146] Furthermore, plasma renin substrate also correlates with estradiol levels.[146] Individual levels of urinary sodium and potassium did not correlate with aldosterone or plasma renin activity.[146] Wilson et al.[146] calculated that about 50 per cent of plasma renin activity was due to the increased renin substrate concentration, but that the remaining 50 per cent represented a real increase in renin concentration. This activation of the renin-angiotensin-aldosterone axis during pregnancy has been hypothesized to be secondary to the fall in blood pressure, which may be due to vasodilatation secondary to decreased vascular responsiveness to angiotensin II[151] and decreased vascular resistance caused by altered prostaglandins.[152] The high progesterone levels from placental production block aldosterone action, in part, preventing kaliuresis and hypokalemia.[153, 154]

Primary Hyperaldosteronism

Primary hyperaldosteronism has been reported in pregnant women rarely.[155-160] Whereas the elevated aldosterone levels found in patients with these tumors are similar to those found in pregnancy, in hyperaldosteronism there should be suppression of plasma renin activity rather than the elevated levels normally found. Both patients reported in whom simultaneous renin and aldosterone levels were determined during pregnancy had markedly elevated levels of aldosterone with low renin levels.[157, 160]

In addition to measuring simultaneous plasma aldosterone and renin levels, diagnostic testing also may involve determining whether the aldosterone levels can be suppressed with salt loading or by the administration of exogenous mineralocorticoid (see Ch. 102). During normal pregnancy, the basal elevated aldosterone levels also fall normally with such maneuvers[150, 154] so that these maneuvers can be of diagnostic utility. Both pregnant patients with aldosteronomas put through such maneuvers failed to demonstrate normal suppressibility of aldosterone levels.[157, 158] If results of baseline renin and aldosterone levels or suppression tests are equivocal and/or CT or MRI scanning does not suggest unilateral disease, it has been recommended that patients be treated medically until delivery, when more definitive isotope scanning can be done and when aldosterone and renin levels should fall.[160] Spironolactone, the aldosterone antagonist usually used for such treatment, can cross the placenta. Since spironolactone is a potent antiandrogen, it may cause abnormal development of genitalia[161] and thus is contraindicated during pregnancy.

ADRENAL MEDULLA

Pheochromocytomas

Pheochromocytomas are found uncommonly during pregnancy. The maternal mortality rate from undiagnosed pheochromocytomas is about 50 per cent; this rate falls to 11 per cent if the diagnosis is made antepartum.[162, 163] The fetal loss rate is similar, even if the diagnosis is made during pregnancy.[163] Catecholamines cross the placenta only minimally[164]; therefore, the fetus appears to be unaffected by the high maternal levels. However, there may be some element of hypoxia due to vasoconstriction of the uterine vascular bed.[165] Because of this high maternal and fetal mortality in the undiagnosed and untreated patient, it is critical to make the diagnosis antepartum.

Symptoms may be vague, or there may be classic symptoms due to episodic secretion of catecholamines, as in the nonpregnant state (see Ch. 106). Some patients may have episodes that are very infrequent, and therefore, the first suspicion of the pheochromocytoma may occur with a

blood pressure rise during the induction of anesthesia or during labor or surgery. Failure to recognize this possibility may result in death of the patient.[166] Some patients present with sudden shock appearing spontaneously or induced by anesthesia or labor and delivery.[162]

Extra-adrenal tumors, which comprise about 10 per cent of cases, may provoke paroxysmal symptoms after particular activities. A frequent site is the organ of Zuckerkandl, located at the bifurcation of the aorta, and the enlarging uterus may cause pressure on such a tumor, with hypertensive episodes occurring with changes in position, uterine contractions, fetal movement, and Valsalva maneuvers.[90, 167] Although about 10 per cent of pheochromocytomas are found to be malignant, this frequency appears to be considerably less when the diagnosis is made in a pregnant woman, since only four such cases have been reported.[168]

A key consideration in diagnosing pheochromocytomas during pregnancy is to differentiate them from preeclampsia. Onset of hypertension in the first two trimesters, of course, would not be characteristic of preeclampsia. Careful evaluation will reveal the absence of proteinuria, edema, or hyperuricemia. Urinary and plasma epinephrine and norepinephrine levels are normal in uncomplicated pregnancy,[169-173] as well as in preeclampsia.[169, 170] However, urinary and plasma catecholamines are two- to four-fold elevated for more than 24 hours following a seizure in eclampsia.[174, 175] Therefore, to make a diagnosis in a woman not having eclampsia, measurement of 24-hour urinary collections for vanillylmandelic acid and fractionated metanephrines and catecholamines can be used as for the nonpregnant patient (see Ch. 106). Stimulation tests have been associated with fetal demise, and their use has been discouraged.[162, 163]

Once the diagnosis is made biochemically, then efforts should be made to localize the tumor. Both CT and MRI are excellent in detecting the presence of tumors, but MRI has been preferred during pregnancy because of the lack of exposure of the fetus to ionizing irradiation.[176] Recently, ^{131}I-MIBG scanning has proved to be quite useful in localizing tumors (see Ch. 106). However, it should be noted that false-negative results occur with this technique. Isotopic scanning is, in general, contraindicated during pregnancy,[72] and there have been no reported cases of its use during pregnancy.

PARATHYROID GLANDS

Calcium and Calcium Regulation

Changes in Calcium Metabolism During Pregnancy

About 25 to 30 g of calcium is transferred from mother to fetus during gestation, about 300 mg/d being transferred in the third trimester.[177] In addition to the net transfer of calcium from the mother to the fetus, there is a net loss of calcium into the urine resulting in a 24-hour urinary calcium that may be over 600 mg[178-180] (Fig. 129–15). In some series, over 20 per cent of women had urinary calcium levels greater than 350 mg/24 hours.[178, 179] The hypercalciuria is in part due to the increased glomerular filtration but is primarily due to increased gastrointestinal absorption of calcium, i.e., absorptive hypercalciuria, that

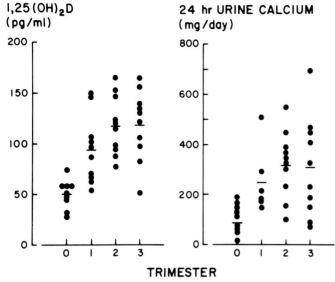

FIGURE 129–15. Circulating 1,25-dihydroxyvitamin D concentration and 24-h calcium excretion during pregnancy, by trimester. The values for both determinations were significantly increased ($p < 0.05$) during pregnancy (trimesters 1 to 3) as compared with postpartum values (trimester 0). The horizontal bars represent mean values. The upper-normal limit for plasma 1,25-dihydroxyvitamin D is 66 pg/ml. (From Gertner JM, Couston DR, Kliger AS, et al: Pregnancy as state of physiologic absorptive hypercalciuria. Am J Med 81:451–456, 1986.)

is likely due to the increase in $1,25(OH)_2D_3$ levels[180] (see below). Total serum calcium levels decrease modestly from about 2.4 to about 2.2 mmol/L, in parallel with a fall in serum albumin from about 4.7 to 3.2 g/dl.[182] Ionized calcium levels, however, remain unchanged throughout gestation[181, 182] (Fig. 129–16).

A number of changes in maternal calcium homeostasis occur during pregnancy that prevent the mother from going into markedly negative calcium balance from the increased urinary and fetal calcium losses. The primary adaptational event appears to be an increase in circulating 1,25-dihydroxyvitamin D levels.[179, 183–187] (see Fig. 129–15), while 25-hydroxyvitamin D levels remain unchanged.[184, 186] Levels of vitamin D–binding protein also increase during gestation, but it appears that both the bound and free fractions of 1,25-dihydroxyvitamin D increase by 50 to 100 per cent.[184, 187] Although this increased formation of 1,25-dihydroxyvitamin D has been thought to be due to increases in parathyroid hormone (PTH) levels of 30 to 50 per cent found in some series,[181, 182, 186] in other series PTH levels have been reported as being decreased.[179, 183, 188] These discrepancies in PTH results may be due to differences in various assays in their detection of PTH cleavage products whose clearance will increase along with the increased GFR.[179] When the biological effect of PTH is measured by measuring nephrogenous cAMP levels, this activity is normal despite lowered immunoreactive PTH levels in the serum.[179] Thus the results of measurement of PTH levels in normal pregnancy are highly variable and very much dependent on the type of assay used.

Although the kidney is the predominant site of 1-hydroxylation in the formation of 1,25-dihydroxyvitamin D, a significant amount of 1-hydroxylation of 25-OH vitamin D also occurs in the placenta.[185] 1,25-Dihydroxyvitamin D levels are increased during pregnancy in nephrectomized rats.[189] In humans with pseudohypoparathyroidism, in

whom the renal response to PTH is reduced, serum calcium and 1,25-dihydroxyvitamin D levels are normal during pregnancy as a result of placental production.[190, 191] Therefore, the source and stimulus for the elevated 1,25-dihydroxyvitamin D levels remain unknown.

Hypercalcemia

Most patients found to be hypercalcemic are asymptomatic, the condition being discovered on routine screening with a multichannel autoanalyzer. It is uncommon now for patients to present because of renal calculi, peptic ulcer disease, bone disease, or mental dysfunction. This is especially true of women in the reproductive age. Rarely, the diagnosis in the mother is made only postpartum after an evaluation is done because of hypocalcemia in the neonate.[192] The neonatal hypocalcemia is due to the placental transfer of the elevated calcium levels with suppression of the fetal parathyroid glands. At delivery, the calcium transfer stops, but the involuted parathyroid glands cannot maintain adequate calcium levels. Rarely, women may develop severe hypercalcemia (''hypercalcemic crisis''), presenting with rapidly progressive anorexia, nausea, vomiting, weakness, fatigue, dehydration, and stupor. More common clinical findings include hypertension, nausea, and vomiting. The latter two may be mistaken for hyperemesis gravidarum.[193] In general, pregnancy has an ameliorating affect on the hypercalcemia due to a shunting of calcium from mother to fetus. This may lead to a dramatic worsening and even hypercalcemic crisis postpartum when such shunting is lost.[193–195]

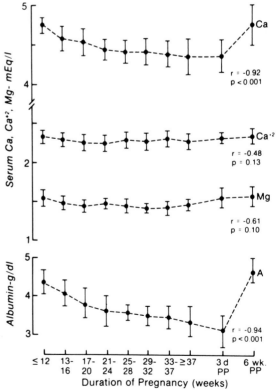

FIGURE 129–16. Mean ($\pm$SD) levels of Ca (total calcium), Ca^{2+} (ionized calcium), Mg, and albumin during pregnancy and the puerperium. (From Pitkin RM, Reynolds WA, Williams GA, et al: Calcium metabolism in normal pregnancy: A longitudinal study. Am J Obstet Gynecol 133:781–787, 1979.)

Because serum total calcium levels decrease (see above), the finding of a serum calcium level that is only slightly elevated or is even at the upper limit of normal may indicate significant hypercalcemia. Ionized calcium levels are helpful in establishing the diagnosis of hypercalcemia, since they remain normal during pregnancy. During pregnancy, immunoreactive PTH levels have been reported as being normal, low, or elevated (see above) depending on the assay used, but even when they have been reported as being elevated, the increase was only 30 to 50 per cent. Therefore, the finding of a markedly elevated PTH level in the setting of pregnant hypercalcemic woman would indicate the presence of hyperparathyroidism. Measurement of nephrogenous cAMP levels also may be helpful, since they have been reported to be normal during pregnancy (see above). The finding of low-normal PTH and cAMP levels in a pregnant hypercalcemic woman will necessitate an investigation for the other myriad causes of hypercalcemia (see Ch. 63).

REFERENCES

1. Brown MA: Sodium and plasma volume regulation in normal and hypertensive pregnancy: A review of physiology and clinical implications. Clin Exp Hypertens [B] 7:265–282, 1988.
2. Lee W, Rokey R, Cotton DB: Noninvasive maternal stroke volume and cardiac output determinations by pulsed Doppler echocardiography. Am J Obstet Gynecol 158:505–510, 1988.
3. Robson S, Hunter S, Boys RJ, et al: Serial study of factors influencing changes in cardiac output during human pregnancy. Am J Physiol 256(Heart Circ Physiol 25):H1060–H1065, 1989.
4. Dunlop W: Serial changes in renal haemodynamics during normal human pregnancy. Br J Obstet Gynaecol 88:1–9, 1981.
5. Davison JM, Noble MCB: Serial changes in 24 hour creatinine clearance during normal menstrual cycles and the first trimester of pregnancy. Br J Obstet Gynecol 88:10–17, 1981.
6. Lindheimer MD, Davison JM: Renal disorders. In Barron WM, Lindheimer MD (eds): Medical Disorders During Pregnancy. St. Louis, Mosby–Year Book, 1991, pp 42–72.
7. Davison JM, Dunlop W, Ezimokhai M: 24-hour creatinine clearances during the third trimester of normal pregnancy. Br J Obstet Gynaecol 87:106–109, 1980.
8. Davison JM, Lovedale C: The excretion of glucose during normal pregnancy and after delivery. J Obstet Gynaecol Br Commw 81:30–34, 1974.
9. Buster JE, Abraham GE: The applications of steroid hormone radioimmunoassays to clinical obstetrics. Obstet Gynecol 46:489–499, 1975.
10. Vician L, Shupnik Ma, Gorski J: Effects of estrogen on primary ovine pituitary cell cultures: Stimulation of prolactin secretion, synthesis, and preprolactin messenger ribonucleic acid activity. Endocrinology 104:736–743, 1979.
11. Shupnik MA, Baxter LA, French LR, et al: In vivo effects of estrogen on ovine pituitaries: Prolactin and growth hormone biosynthesis and messenger ribonucleic acid translation. Endocrinology 104:729–735, 1979.
12. West B, Dannies PS: Effects of estradiol on prolactin production and dihydroergocryptine-induced inhibition of prolactin production in primary cultures of rat pituitary cells. Endocrinology 106:1108–1113, 1980.
13. Maurer RA: Relationship between estradiol, ergocryptine, and thyroid hormone: Effects on prolactin synthesis and prolactin messenger ribonucleic acid levels. Endocrinology 110:1515–1520, 1982.
14. Rakoff JS, Yen SSC: Progesterone induced acute release of prolactin in estrogen primed ovariectomized women. J Clin Endocrinol Metab 47:918–921, 1978.
15. Bohnet HG, Naber NG, del Pozo E, et al: Effects of synthetic gestagens on serum prolactin and growth hormone secretion in amenorrheic patients. Arch Gynecol 226:233–240, 1978.
16. Tyson JE, Hwang P, Guyda H, et al: Studies of prolactin secretion in human pregnancy. Am J Obstet Gynecol 113:14–21, 1972.
17. Rigg LA, Lein A, Yen SSC: Pattern of increase in circulating prolactin levels during human gestation. Am J Obstet Gynecol 129:454–456, 1977.
18. Goluboff LG, Ezrin C: Effect of pregnancy on the somatotroph and the prolactin cell of the human adenohypophysis. J Clin Endocrinol Metab 29:1533–1538, 1969.
19. Pasteels JL, Gausset P, Danguy A, et al: Morphology of the lactotropes and somatotropes of man and rhesus monkeys. J Clin Endocrinol Metab 34:959–967, 1972.
20. Asa SL, Penz G, Kovacs K, et al: Prolactin cells in the human pituitary: A quantitative immunocytochemical analysis. Arch Pathol Lab Med 106:360–363, 1982.
21. Scheithauer BW, Sano T, Kovacs KT, et al: The pituitary gland in pregnancy: A clinicopathologic and immunohistochemical study of 69 Cases. Mayo Clin Proc 65:461–474, 1990.
22. Soares MJ, Faria TN, Roby KF, Deb S: Pregnancy and the prolactin family of hormones: Coordination of anterior pituitary, uterine and placental expression. Endocr Rev 12:402–423, 1991.
23. Elster AD, Sanders TG, Vines FS, Chen MYM: Size and shape of the pituitary gland during pregnancy and post partum: Measurement with MR imaging. Radiology 181:531–535, 1991.
24. Gemzell C, Wang CF: Outcome of pregnancy in women with pituitary adenoma. Fertil Steril 31:363–372, 1979.
25. Molitch ME: Pregnancy and the hyperprolactinemic woman. N Engl J Med 312:1364–1370, 1985.
26. Quencer RM: Lymphocytic adenohypophysitis: Autoimmune disorder of the pituitary gland. AJNR 1:343–345, 1980.
27. Asa SL, Bilbao JM, Kovacs K, et al: Lymphocytic hypophysitis of pregnancy resulting in hypopituitarism: A distinct clinicopathologic entity. Ann Intern Med 95:166–171, 1981.
28. Baskin DS, Townsend JJ, Wilson CB: Lymphocytic adenohypophysitis of pregnancy simulating a pituitary adenoma: A distinct pathological entity. J Neurosurg 56:148–153, 1982.
29. Cosman F, Post KD, Holub DA, et al: Lymphocytic adenohypophysitis: Report of 3 new cases and review of the literature. Medicine 68:240–256, 1989.
30. Molitch ME, Reichlin S: Neuroendocrine studies of prolactin secretion in hyperprolactinemic states. In Mena F, Valverde-Rodriguez C (eds): Prolactin Secretion: A Multidisciplinary Approach. New York, Academic Press, 1984, pp 393–421.
31. Frankenne F, Rentier-Delrue F, Scippo M-L, et al: Expression of the growth hormone variant gene in the human placenta. J Clin Endocrinol Metab 64:635–637, 1987.
32. Frankenne F, Closset J, Gomez F, et al: The physiology of growth hormones (GHs) in pregnant women and partial characterization of the placental GH variant. J Clin Endocrinol Metab 66:1171–1180, 1988.
33. Eriksson L, Frankenne F, Eden S, et al: Growth hormone 24-h serum profiles during pregnancy: Lack of pulsatility for the secretion of the placental variant. Br J Obstet Gynaecol 96:949–953, 1989.
34. Abe H, Molitch ME, Van Wyk JJ, Underwood LE: Human growth hormone and somatomedin C suppress the spontaneous release of growth hormone in unanesthetized rats. Endocrinology 113:1319–1324, 1983.
35. Beckers A, Stevenaert A, Foidart J-M, et al: Placental and pituitary growth hormone secretion during pregnancy in acromegalic women. J Clin Endocrinol Metab 71:725–731, 1990.
36. MacLeod JN, Worsley I, Ray J, et al: Human growth hormone-variant is a biologically active somatogen and lactogen. Endocrinology 128:1298–1302, 1991.
37. Ray J, Okamura H, Kelly PA, et al: Human growth hormone-variant demonstrates a receptor binding profile distinct from that of normal pituitary growth hormone. J Biol Chem 265:7939–7944, 1990.
38. Baumann G, Davila N, Shaw M, et al: Binding of human growth hormone (GH)-variant (placental GH) to GH-binding proteins in human plasma. J Clin Endocrinol Metab 73:1175–1179, 1991.
39. Daughaday WH, Trivedi B, Winn HN, Yan H: Hypersomatotropism in pregnant women, as measured by a human liver radioreceptor assay. J Clin Endocrinol Metab 70:215–221, 1990.
40. Furlanetto RW, Underwood LE, Van Wyk JJ, Handwerger S: Serum immunoreactive somatomedin-C is elevated late in pregnancy. J Clin Endocrinol Metab 47:695–698, 1978.
41. Wilson DM, Bennett A, Adamson GD, et al: Somatomedins in pregnancy: A cross-sectional study of insulin-like growth factors I and II and somatomedin peptide content in normal human pregnancies. J Clin Endocrinol Metab 55:858–869, 1982.
42. Caufriez A, Frankenne F, Enlert Y, et al: Placental growth hormone as a potential regulator of maternal IGF-I during human pregnancy. Am J Physiol 258:E1014–E1019, 1990.

43. Goodman HM, Tai L-R, Ray J, et al: Human growth hormone variant produces insulin-like and lipolytic responses in rat adipose tissue. Endocrinology 129:1779–1783, 1991.
44. Barkan AL, Stred SE, Reno K, et al: Increased growth hormone pulse frequency in acromegaly. J Clin Endocrinol Metab 69:1225–1233, 1989.
45. Hartman ML, Veldhuis JD, Vance ML, et al: Somatotropin pulse frequency and basal concentrations are increased in acromegaly and are reduced by successful therapy. J Clin Endocrinol Metab 70:1375–1384, 1990.
46. Irie M, Tsushima T: Increase of serum growth hormone concentration following thyrotropin-releasing hormone injection in patients with acromegaly or gigantism. J Clin Endocrinol Metab 35:97–100, 1972.
47. Faglia G, Beck-Pecoz P, Ferrari C, et al: Plasma growth hormone response to thyrotropin-releasing hormone in patients with active acromegaly. J Clin Endocrinol Metab 36:1259–1262, 1973.
48. Hanew K, Kokubun M, Sasaki A, et al: The spectrum of pituitary growth hormone responses to pharmacological stimuli in acromegaly. J Clin Endocrinol Metab 51:292–297, 1980.
49. Molitch ME: Growth hormone hypersecretory states. In Raiti S, Tolman RA (eds): Human Growth Hormone. New York, Plenum Press, 1986, pp 29–50.
50. Bigazzi M, Ronga R, Lancranjan I, et al: A pregnancy in an acromegalic woman during bromocriptine treatment: Effects on growth hormone and prolactin in the maternal, fetal, and amniotic compartments. J Clin Endocrinol Metab 48:9–12, 1979.
51. Abelove WA, Rupp JJ, Paschkis KE: Acromegaly and pregnancy. J Clin Endocrinol 14:32–44, 1954.
52. Finkler RS: Acromegaly and pregnancy: Case report, J Clin Endocrinol 14:1245–1246, 1954.
53. Luboshitzky R, Dickstein G, Barzilai D: Bromocriptine-induced pregnancy in an acromegalic patient. JAMA 244:584–586, 1980.
54. Davison JM, Vallotton MB, Lindheimer MD: Plasma osmolality and urinary concentration and dilution during and after pregnancy: Evidence that lateral recumbency inhibits maximal urinary concentrating ability. Br J Obstet Gynaecol 88:472–479, 1981.
55. Davison JM, Gilmore EA, Durr J, et al: Altered osmotic thresholds for vasopressin secretion and thirst in pregnancy. Am J Physiol 246(Renal Fluid Electrolyte Physiol 15):F105–F109, 1984.
56. Lindheimer MD, Barron WM, Davison JM: Osmoregulation of thirst and vasopressin release in pregnancy. Am J Physiol 257(Renal Fluid Electrolyte Physiol 26):F159–F169, 1989.
57. Davison JM, Shiells EA, Philips PR, Lindheimer MD: Serial evaluation of vasopressin release and thirst in human pregnancy: Role of chorionic gonadotropin in the osmoregulatory changes of gestation. J Clin Invest 81:798–806, 1988.
58. Davison JM, Shiells EA, Barron WM, et al: Changes in the metabolic clearance of vasopressin and of plasma vasopressinase throughout human pregnancy. J Clin Invest 83:1313–1318, 1989.
59. Landon MJ, Cspas DK, Shiells EA, Davison JM: Degradation of radiolabeled arginine vasopressin (125I-AVP) by the human placenta perfused in vitro. Br J Obstet Gynaecol 95:488–492, 1988.
60. Davison JM, Barron WA, Lindheimer MD: Metabolic clearance rates of vasopressin increase markedly in late gestation: A possible cause of polyuria in pregnant women. Trans Assoc Am Physicians 100:91–98, 1987.
61. Durr JA: Diabetes insipidus in pregnancy. Am J Kidney Dis 9:276–283, 1987.
62. Barron WM, Cohen LH, Ulland LA, et al: Transient vasopressin-resistant diabetes insipidus of pregnancy. N Engl J Med 310:442–444, 1984.
63. Iwasaki Y, Oiso Y, Kondo K, et al: Aggravation of subclinical diabetes insipidus during pregnancy. N Engl J Med 324:522–526, 1991.
64. Miller M, Dalakos T, Moses AM, et al: Recognition of partial defects in antidiuretic hormone secretion. Ann Intern Med 73:721–729, 1970.
65. Crooks J, Aboul-Khair SA, Turnbull AC, Hytten FE: The incidence of goitre during pregnancy. Lancet 2:334–336, 1964.
66. Crooks J, Tulloch MI, Turnbull AC, et al: Comparative incidence of goitre in pregnancy in Iceland and Scotland. Lancet 2:625–627, 1967.
67. Levy RP, Newman DM, Rejai LS, et al: The myth of goiter in pregnancy. Am J Obstet Gynecol 137:701–703, 1980.
68. Long TJ, Felice ME, Hollingsworth DR: Goiter in pregnant teenagers. Am J Obstet Gynecol 152:670–674, 1985.
69. Glinoer D, De Nayer P, Bourdoux P, et al: Regulation of maternal thyroid during pregnancy. J Clin Endocrinol Metab 71:276–297, 1990.
70. Glinoer D, Soto MF, Bourdoux P, et al: Pregnancy in patients with mild thyroid abnormalities: Maternal and neonatal repercussions. J Clin Endocrinol Metab 73:421–427, 1991.
71. Halnan KE: The radioiodine uptake of the human thyroid in pregnancy. Clin Sci 17:281–290, 1958.
72. Brent RL: The effect of embryonic and fetal exposure to x-ray, microwaves, ultrasound, magnetic resonance, and isotopes. In Barron WM, Lindheimer MD (eds): Medical Disorders of Pregnancy. St. Louis, Mosby–Year Book, 1991, pp 568–604.
73. Thomas R, Reid RL: Thyroid disease and reproductive dysfunction: A review. Obstet Gynecol 70:789–798, 1987.
74. Vulsma T, Gons MH, de Vijlder JJM: Maternal-fetal transfer of thyroxine in congenital hypothyroidism due to a total organification defect or thyroid agenesis. N Engl J Med 321:13–16, 1989.
75. Harada K, Hershman JM, Reed AW, et al: Comparison of thyroid stimulators and thyroid hormone concentrations in the sera of pregnant women. J Clin Endocrinol Metab 48:793–797, 1979.
76. Pekonen F, Alfthan H, Stenman UH, Ylikorkala O: Human chorionic gonadotropin (hCG) and thyroid function in early human pregnancy: Circadian variation and evidence for intrinsic thyrotropic activity of hCG. J Clin Endocrinol Metab 66:853–856, 1988.
77. Yoshikawa N, Nishikawa M, Horimoto M, et al: Thyroid-stimulating activity in sera of normal pregnant women. J Clin Endocrinol Metab 69:891–895, 1989.
78. Kimura M, Amino N, Tamaki H, et al: Physiologic thyroid activation in normal early pregnancy is induced by circulating hCG. Obstet Gynecol 75:775–778, 1992.
79. Higgins HP, Hershman JM, Kenimer JG, et al: The thyrotoxicosis of hydatidiform mole. Ann Intern Med 83:307–311, 1975.
80. Rajatanavin R, Chailurkit LO, Srisupandit S, et al: Trophoblastic hyperthyroidism: Clinical and biochemical features of five cases. Am J Med 85:237–241, 1988.
81. Burrow GN: Thyroid diseases. In Burrow GN, Ferris TF (eds): Medical Complications During Pregnancy (ed 3), Philadelphia, WB Saunders Co, 1988, pp 224–253.
82. Glinoer D, Gershengorn MC, Dubois A, Robbins J: Stimulation of thyroxine-binding globulin synthesis by isolated rhesus monkey hepatocytes after in vivo β-estradiol administration. Endocrinology 100:807–813, 1977.
83. Ain KB, Mori Y, Refetoff S: Reduced clearance rate of thyroxine-binding globulin (TBG) with increased sialylation: A mechanism for estrogen-induced elevation of serum TBG concentration. J Clin Endocrinol Metab 65:686–696, 1987.
84. Robbins J, Nelson JH: Thyroxine-binding by serum protein in pregnancy and the newborn. J Clin Invest 37:153–159, 1958.
85. Osathanondh R, Tulchinsky D, Chopra IJ: Total and free thyroxine and triiodothyronine in normal and complicated pregnancy. J Clin Endocrinol Metab 42:98–104, 1976.
86. Dowling JT, Appleton WG, Nicoloff JT: Thyroxine turnover during human pregnancy. J Clin Endocrinol 27:1749–1750, 1967.
87. Mandel SJ, Larsen PR, Seely EW, Brent GA: Increased need for thyroxine during pregnancy in women with primary hypothyroidism. N Engl J Med 323:91–96, 1990.
88. Van der Spuy ZM, Jacobs HS: Management of endocrine disorders in pregnancy: 1. Thyroid and parathyroid disease. Postgrad Med J 60:245–252, 1984.
89. Spencer CA, LoPresti JS, Patel A, et al: Applications of a new chemiluminometric thyrotropin assay to subnormal measurement. J Clin Endocrinol Metab 70:453–460, 1990.
90. Molitch ME: Pituitary, thyroid, adrenal, and parathyroid disorders. In Barron WM, Lindheimer MD (eds): Medical Disorders of Pregnancy. St. Louis, Mosby–Year Book, 1991, pp 102–147.
91. Dozeman R, Kaiser FE, Cass O, et al: Hyperthyroidism appearing as hyperemesis gravidarum. Arch Intern Med 143:2202–2203, 1983.
92. Jeffcoate WJ, Bain C: Recurrent pregnancy-induced thyrotoxicosis presenting as hyperemesis gravidarum: Case report. Br J Obstet Gynaecol 92:413–415, 1985.
93. Lao TT, Chin RKH, Chang AMZ: The outcome of hyperemetic pregnancies complicated by transient hyperthyroidism. Aust NZ J Obstet Gynaecol 27:99–101, 1987.
94. Swaminathan R, Chin RK, Lao TTH, et al: Thyroid function in hyperemesis gravidarum. Acta Endocrinol 120:155–160, 1989.
94a. Billabio M, Poshyachinda M, Ekins RP: Pregnancy-induced changes in thyroid function: Role of human chorionic gonadotropin as putative regulator of maternal thyroid. J Clin Endocrinol Metab 73:824–831, 1991.
95. Rosenthal HE, Slaunwhite WR Jr, Sandberg AA: Transcortin: A corticosteroid-binding protein of plasma: X. Cortisol and progesterone

interplay and unbound levels of these steroids in pregnancy. J Clin Endocrinol 29:352–367, 1969.

96. Genazzani AR, Fraioli F, Hurlimann J, et al: Immunoreactive ACTH and cortisol plasma levels during pregnancy: Detection and partial purification of corticotrophin-like placental hormone: the human chorionic corticotrophin. Clin Endocrinol 4:1–14, 1975.

97. Carr BR, Parker CR Jr, Madden JD, et al: Maternal plasma adrenocorticotropin and cortisol relationships throughout human pregnancy. Am J Obstet Gynecol 139:416–422, 1981.

98. Demey-Ponsart E, Foidart JM, Sulon J, Sodoyez JC: Serum CBG, free and total cortisol and circadian patterns of adrenal function in normal pregnancy. J Steroid Biochem 16:165–169, 1982.

99. DeMoor P, Steeno O, Brosens I, et al: Data on transcortin activity in human plasma as studied by gel filtration. J Clin Endocrinol 26:71–78, 1966.

100. Doe RP, Dickinson P, Zinneman HH, et al: Elevated nonproteinbound cortisol (NPC) in pregnancy, during estrogen administration and in carcinoma of the prostate. J Clin Endocrinol 29:757–766, 1969.

101. Nolten WE, Lindheimer MD, Rueckert PA, et al: Diurnal patterns and regulation of cortisol secretion in pregnancy. J Clin Endocrinol Metab 51:466–472, 1980.

102. Murphy BE: Clinical evaluation of urinary cortisol determinations by competitive protein-binding radioassay. J Clin Endocrinol 28:343–348, 1968.

103. Burke CW, Roulet F: Increased exposure of tissues to cortisol in late pregnancy. Br Med J 1:657–659, 1970.

104. Cohen M, Stiefel M, Reddy WJ, et al: The secretion and disposition of cortisol during pregnancy. J Clin Endocrinol 18:1076–1092, 1958.

105. Migeon CJ, Kenny FM, Taylor FH: Cortisol Production rate: VIII. pregnancy. J Clin Endocrinol 28:661–666, 1968.

106. Beitins IZ, Bayard F, Anges IG, et al: The metabolic clearance rate, blood production, interconversion and transplacental passage of cortisol and cortisone in pregnancy near term. Pediatr Res 7:509–519, 1973.

107. Rees LH, Burke CW, Chard T, et al: Possible placental origin of ACTH in normal human pregnancy. Nature 254:620–622, 1975.

108. Genazzani AR, Felber JP, Fioretti P: Immunoreactive ACTH, immunoreactive human chorionic somatomammotrophin (HCS) and 11-OH steroids plasma levels in normal and pathological pregnancies. Acta Endocrinol 83:800–810, 1977.

109. Allen JP, Cook DM, Kendall JW, et al: Maternal-fetal ACTH relationship in man. J Clin Endocrinol Metab 37:230–234, 1973.

110. Petraglia F, Sutton S, Vale W: Neurotransmitters and peptides modulate the release of immunoreactive corticotropin-releasing factor from cultured human placental cells. Am J Obstet Gynecol 160:247–251, 1989.

111. Shibisaki T, Odagiri E, Shizume K, Ling N: Corticotropin-releasing factor-like activity in human placental extracts. J Clin Endocrinol Metab 55:384–386, 1982.

112. Frim DM, Emanuel RL, Robinson BG, et al: Characterization and gestational regulation of corticotropin-releasing hormone messenger RNA in human placenta. J Clin Invest 82:287–292, 1988.

113. Sasaki A, Liotta AS, Luckey MM, et al: Immunoreactive corticotropin-releasing factor is present in human maternal plasma during the third trimester of pregnancy. J Clin Endocrinol Metab 59:812–814, 1984.

114. Sasaki A, Shinkawa O, Margioris AN, et al: Immunoreactive corticotropin-releasing hormone in human plasma during pregnancy, labor and delivery. J Clin Endocrinol Metab 64:224–229, 1987.

115. Campbell EA, Linton EA, Wolfe CDA, et al: Plasma corticotropin-releasing hormone concentrations during pregnancy and parturition. J Clin Endocrinol Metab 65:1054–1059, 1987.

116. Sasaki A, Tempst P, Liotta AS, et al: Isolation and characterization of a corticotropin-releasing hormone–like peptide from human placenta. J Clin Endocrinol Metab 67:768–773, 1988.

117. Margioris A, Grino M, Protos P, et al: Corticotropin-releasing hormone and oxytocin stimulate the release of placental proopiomelanocortin peptides. J Clin Endocrinol Metab 66:922–926, 1988.

118. Sasaki A, Shinkawa O, Yoshinaga K: Placental corticotropin-releasing hormone may be a stimulator of maternal pituitary adrenocorticotropic hormone secretion in humans. J Clin Invest 84:1997–2001, 1989.

119. Okamoto E, Takai T, Makino T, et al: Immunoreactive corticotropin-releasing hormone, adrenocorticotropin and cortisol in human plasma during pregnancy and delivery and postpartum. Horm Metab Res 21:566–572, 1989.

120. Robinson BG, Emanuel RL, Frim DM, Majzoub JA: Glucocorticoid stimulates expression of corticotropin-releasing hormone gene in human placenta. Proc Natl Acad Sci USA 85:5244–5248, 1988.

121. Jones SA, Brooks AN, Challis JRG: Steroids modulate corticotropin-releasing hormone production in human fetal membranes and placenta. J Clin Endocrinol Metab 68:825–830, 1989.

122. Goland RS, Wardlaw SL, Blum M, et al: Biologically active corticotropin-releasing hormone in maternal and fetal plasma during pregnancy. Am J Obstet Gynecol 159:884–890, 1988.

123. Nolten WE, Lindheimer MD, Oparil S, Ehrlich EN: Desoxycorticosterone in normal pregnancy: I. Sequential studies of the secretory patterns of desoxycorticosterone, aldosterone, and cortisol. Am J Obstet Gynecol 132:414–420, 1978.

124. Aron DC, Schnall AM, Sheeler LR: Cushing's syndrome and pregnancy. Am J Obstet Gynecol 162:244–252, 1990.

125. Buescher MA, McClamrock HD, Adashi EY: Cushing syndrome in pregnancy. Obstet Gynecol 79:130–137, 1992.

126. Casson IF, Davis JC, Jeffreys RV, et al: Successful management of Cushing's disease during pregnancy by transsphenoidal adenectomy. Clin Endocrinol 27:423–428, 1987.

127. Gormley MJJ, Hadden DR, Kennedy TL, et al: Cushing's syndrome in pregnancy: Treatment with metyrapone. Clin Endocrinol 16:283–293, 1982.

128. Connell JMC, Cordiner J, Davies DL, et al: Pregnancy complicated by Cushing's syndrome: Potential hazard of metyrapone therapy. Case report. Br J Obstet Gynaecol 92:1192–1195, 1985.

129. Koerten JM, Morales WJ, Washington SR, et al: Cushing's syndrome in pregnancy: A case report and literature review. Am J Obstet Gynecol 154:626–628, 1986.

130. Barasch E, Sztern M, Spinrad S, et al: Pregnancy and Cushing's syndrome: Example of endocrine interaction. Isr J Med Sci 24:101–104, 1988.

131. Semple CG, McEwan H, Teasdale GM, et al: Recurrence of Cushing's disease in pregnancy: Case report. Br J Obstet Gynaecol 92:295–298, 1985.

132. Bevan JS, Gough MH, Gillmer MDG, et al: Cushing's syndrome in pregnancy: The timing of definitive treatment. Clin Endocrinol 27:225–233, 1987.

133. Cook DJ, Riddell RH, Booth JD: Cushing's syndrome in pregnancy. Can Med Assoc J 141:1059–1061, 1989.

134. Pricolo VE, Monchik JM, Prinz RA, et al: Management of Cushing's syndrome secondary to adrenal adenoma during pregnancy. Surgery 108:1072–1078, 1990.

135. Cousins L, Rigg L, Hollingsworth D, et al: Qualitative and quantitative assessment of the circadian rhythm of cortisol in pregnancy. Am J Obstet Gynecol 145:411–416, 1983.

136. Nieman LK, Chrousos GP, Oldfield EH, et al: The ovine corticotropin-releasing hormone stimulation test and the dexamethasone suppression test in the differential diagnosis of Cushing's syndrome. Ann Intern Med 105:862–867, 1986.

137. Quartero HWP, Fry CH: Placental corticotrophin releasing factor may modulate human parturition. Placenta 10:439–443, 1989.

138. Abrams HL, Siegelman SS, Adams DF, et al: Computed tomography versus ultrasound of the adrenal gland: A prospective study. Radiology 143:121–128, 1982.

139. Brent F: Addison's disease and pregnancy. Am J Surg 79:645–652, 1950.

140. Portnay GI, Vagenakis AG, Braverman LE, et al: Anticoagulant therapy and acute adrenal insufficiency. Ann Intern Med 81:115, 1974.

141. Xarli VP, Steele AA, Davis PJ, et al: Adrenal hemorrhage in the adult. Medicine 57:211–221, 1978.

142. Aronson IK, Halaska B: Dermatologic diseases. In Barron WM, Lindheimer MD (eds): Medical Disorders of Pregnancy. St. Louis, Mosby-Year Book, 1991, pp 534–550.

143. O'Shaughnessy RW, Hackett KJ: Maternal Addison's disease and fetal growth retardation. J Reprod Med 29:752–756, 1984.

144. Drucker D, Shumak S, Angel A: Schmidt's syndrome presenting with intrauterine growth retardation and postpartum addisonian crisis. Am J Obstet Gynecol 149:229–230, 1984.

145. Beck P, Eaton CJ, Young IS, Kupperman HS: Metyrapone response in pregnancy. Am J Obstet Gynecol 100:327–330, 1968.

146. Wilson M, Morganti AA, Zervoudakis I, et al: Blood pressure, the renin-aldosterone system and sex steroids throughout normal pregnancy. Am J Med 68:97–104, 1980.

147. Weir RJ, Brown JJ, Fraser R, et al: Relationship between plasma renin, renin-substrate, angiotensin II, aldosterone and electrolytes in normal pregnancy. J Clin Endocrinol Metab 40:108–115, 1975.

148. Smeaton TC, Andersen GJ, Fulton IS: Study of aldosterone levels in plasma during pregnancy. J Clin Endocrinol Metab 44:1–7, 1977.

149. Bay WH, Ferris TF: Factors controlling plasma renin and aldosterone during pregnancy. Hypertension 1:410–415, 1979.

150. Brown MA, Sinosich MJ, Saunders DM, Gallery EDM: Potassium regulation and progesterone-aldosterone interrelationships in human pregnancy: A prospective study. Am J Obstet Gynecol 155:349–353, 1986.

151. Gant NF, Daley GL, Chand S, et al: A study of angiotensin II pressor response throughout primigravid pregnancy. J Clin Invest 52:2682–2689, 1973.

152. Lindheimer MD, Katz AI: The kidney and hypertension in pregnancy. In Brenner BM, Rector FC Jr (eds): The Kidney (ed 4). Philadelphia, WB Saunders Co, 1991, pp 1551–1595.

153. Landau RL, Lugibihl K: Inhibition of the sodium-retaining influence of aldosterone by progesterone. J Clin Endocrinol 18:1237–1245, 1958.

154. Ehrlich EN, Lindheimer MD: Effects of administered mineralocorticoids on ACTH in pregnant women: Attenuation of kaliuretic influence of mineralocorticoids during pregnancy. J Clin Invest 51:1301–1309, 1972.

155. Crane MG, Andes JP, Harris JJ, Slate WG: Primary aldosteronism in pregnancy. Obstet Gynecol 23:200–208, 1964.

156. Boucher BM, Mason AS: Conn's syndrome with associated pregnancy. Proc Roy Soc Med 58:575–576, 1965.

157. Gordon RD, Fishman LM, Liddle GW: Plasma renin activity and aldosterone secretion in a pregnant woman with primary aldosteronism. J Clin Endocrinol 27:385–388, 1967.

158. Biglieri EG, Slaton PE Jr: Pregnancy and primary aldosteronism. J Clin Endocrinol 27:1628–1632, 1967.

159. Merrill RH, Dombroski RA, MacKenna JM: Primary hyperaldosteronism during pregnancy. Am J Obstet Gynecol 150:786–787, 1984.

160. Lotgering FK, Derkx FMH, Wallenburg HCS: Primary aldosteronism in pregnancy. Am J Obstet Gynecol 155:986–988, 1986.

161. Tremblay RR: Treatment of hirsutism with spironolactone. J Clin Endocrinol Metab 15:363–371, 1986.

162. Schenker JG, Chowers I: Pheochromocytoma and pregnancy. Obstet Gynecol Surv 26:739–747, 1971.

163. Schenker JG, Granat M: Phaeochromocytoma and pregnancy: An updated appraisal. Aust NZ J Obstet Gynaecol 22:1–10, 1982.

164. Thiery M, Derom RMJ, van Kets HE, et al: Pheochromocytoma in pregnancy. Am J Obstet Gynecol 97:21–29, 1967.

165. Griffith MI, Felts JH, James FM, et al: Successful control of pheochromocytoma in pregnancy. JAMA 229:437–439, 1974.

166. Cross DA, Meyer JS: Postoperative deaths due to unsuspected pheochromocytoma. South Med J 70:1320–1323, 1977.

167. Levin N, McTighe A, Abdel-Aziz MIE: Extra-adrenal pheochromocytoma in pregnancy. Md State Med J 32:377–379, 1983.

168. Ellison GT, Mansberger JA, Mansberger AR Jr: Malignant recurrent pheochromocytoma during pregnancy: Case report and review of the literature. Surgery 103:484–489, 1988.

169. Burn GP: Urinary excretion of the pressor amines in relation to phaeochromocytoma. Br Med J 1:697–699, 1953.

170. Castren O: Urinary excretion of noradrenaline and adrenaline in late normal and toxemic pregnancy. Acta Pharmacol Toxicol 20(Suppl 2):1–98, 1963.

171. Jaffe RB, Harrison TS, Cerny JC: Localization of metastatic pheochromocytoma in pregnancy by caval catheterization: Including urinary catecholamine values in uncomplicated pregnancies. Am J Obstet Gynecol 104:939–944, 1969.

172. Zuspan FP: Urinary excretion of epinephrine and norepinephrine during pregnancy. J Clin Endocrinol 30:357–360, 1970.

173. Tunbridge RDG, Donnai P: Plasma noradrenaline in normal pregnancy and in hypertension of late pregnancy. Br J Obstet Gynaecol 88:105–108, 1981.

174. Zuspan FP: Adrenal gland and sympathetic nervous system response in eclampsia. Am J Obstet Gynecol 114:304–311, 1972.

175. Moodley J, McFadyen ML, Dilraj A, Rangiah S: Plasma noradrenaline and adrenaline levels in eclampsia. S Afr Med J 80:191–192, 1991.

176. Greenberg M, Moawad AH, Wieties BM, et al: Extraadrenal pheochromocytoma: Detection during pregnancy using MR imaging. Radiology 161:475–476, 1986.

177. Pitkin RM: Calcium metabolism in pregnancy and the perinatal period: A review. Am J Obstet Gynecol 151:99–109, 1985.

178. Howarth AT, Morgan DB, Payne RB: Urinary excretion of calcium in late pregnancy and its relation to creatinine clearance. Am J Obstet Gynecol 129:499–502, 1977.

179. Gertner JM, Couston DR, Kliger AS, et al: Pregnancy as state of physiologic absorptive hypercalciuria. Am J Med 81:451–456, 1986.

180. Maikranz P, Holley JL, Parks, JH, et al: Gestational hypercalciuria causes pathological urine calcium oxalate supersaturation. Kidney Int 36:108–113, 1989.

181. Pitkin RM, Reynolds WA, Williams GA, et al: Calcium metabolism in normal pregnancy: A longitudinal study. Am J Obstet Gynecol 133:781–787, 1979.

182. Rasmussen N, Rolich A, Hornnes Pj, Hegedus L: Serum ionized calcium and intact parathyroid hormone levels during pregnancy and postpartum. Br J Obstet Gynecol 97:857–862, 1990.

183. Whitehead M, Lane G, Young O, et al: Interrelations of calcium-regulating hormones during normal pregnancy. Br Med J 283:10–12, 1981.

184. Bouillon R, van Assche FA, van Baelen H, et al: Influence of the vitamin D–binding protein on the serum concentration of 1,25-dihydroxyvitamin D_3: Significance of the free 1,25-dihydroxyvitamin D_3 concentration. J Clin Invest 67:589–596, 1981.

185. Gray TK, Lowe W, Lester GE: Vitamin D and pregnancy: The maternal-fetal metabolism of vitamin D. Endocr Rev 2:264–274, 1981.

186. Reddy GS, Norman AW, Willis DM, et al: Regulation of vitamin D metabolism in normal human pregnancy. J Clin Endocrinol Metab 56:363–370, 1983.

187. Wilson SG, Retallack RW, Kent JC, et al: Serum free 1,25-dihydroxyvitamin D and the free 1,25-dihydroxyvitamin D index during a longitudinal study of human pregnancy and lactation. Clin Endocrinol 32:613–622, 1990.

188. Davis OK, Hawkins DS, Rubin LP, et al: Serum parathyroid hormone (PTH) in pregnant women determined by an immunoradiometric assay for intact PTH. J Clin Endocrinol Metab 67:850–852, 1988.

189. Weissman Y, Vargas A, Duckett G, et al: Synthesis of 1,25-dihydroxyvitamin D in the nephrectomized pregnant rat. Endocrinology 103:1992–1996, 1978.

190. Breslau NA, Zerwekh JE: Relationship of estrogen and pregnancy to calcium homeostasis in pseudohypoparathyroidism. J Clin Endocrinol Metab 62:45–51, 1986.

191. Zerwekh JE, Breslau NA: Human placental production of 1,25-dihydroxyvitamin D_3: Biochemical characterization of production in normal subjects and patients with pseudohypoparathyroidism. J Clin Endocrinol Metab 62:192–196, 1986.

192. Salem R, Taylor S: Hyperparathyroidism in pregnancy. Br J Surg 66:648–650, 1979.

193. Shangold MM, Dor N, Welt SI, et al: Hyperparathyroidism and pregnancy: A review. Obstet Gynecol Surv 37:217–228, 1982.

194. Croom RD, Thomas CG: Primary hyperparathyroidism during pregnancy. Surgery 96:1109–1117, 1984.

195. Matthias GSH, Helliwell TR, Williams A: Postpartum hyperparathyroid crisis: Case report. Br J Obstet Gynaecol 94:807–810, 1987.

PART X

MALE REPRODUCTION

Basic Endocrinology of the Testis

DAVID M. De KRETSER
GAIL P. RISBRIDGER
JEFFREY B. KERR

FUNCTIONAL MORPHOLOGY

Macroscopic Organization

The testis lies within the scrotum and is covered on its anterolateral and medial surface by apposed serous membranes that form a closed cavity termed the *tunica vaginalis,* an isolated outpocketing of the peritoneum reflecting the retroperitoneal origin of the testis. The posterior border of the testis is associated with the epididymis and with the spermatic cord, the latter incorporating the ductus deferens, together with neurovascular structures running to and from the middle and upper ends of the posterior border of the testis.[1] Nerves and vessels of the spermatic cord exit and enter the testis through a thick, fibrous connective tissue capsule deep to the tunica vaginalis, termed the *tunica albuginea,* semitransparent in many species but opaque in the human testis. Upon entering the testis posteriorly, the testicular artery descends toward the inferior pole just deep to the tunica albuginea, giving rise to the region termed the *tunica vasculosa.* In the human testis the main stem of the artery ascends beneath the anterior surface before smaller branches penetrate the parenchyma. Incisions of the tunica albuginea of the human testis which are least likely to encounter a major arterial branch are the medial and lateral aspects of the upper pole.[2] Posteriorly the tunica albuginea is thickened and projects into the parenchyma of the testis to form the mediastinum, a honeycomb-like structure providing a passageway linking the seminiferous tubules with the efferent ductules and the epididymis. Numerous imperfect thin connective tissue septa extend inwardly from the tunica albuginea toward the mediastinum, thereby establishing incomplete pyramidal lobules of loose connective tissue which support the seminiferous tubules, the terminal ends of which empty into the mediastinum by straight tubular extensions termed *tubuli recti.* Depending on the species, individual seminiferous tubules may be highly convoluted (human), or they may form numerous relatively linear segments linked by cranial and caudal hairpin turns, as seen in rodent testes.[3]

Spermatozoa and fluid produced by the seminiferous tubules enter the rete testis, a maze of anastomosing corridors within the mediastinum which provide a route toward the epididymis. The morphology of the rete is species-specific,[4, 5] although three principal zones (Fig. 130–1) have been described: the *septal* rete, consisting of the straight tubules which empty into the *mediastinal* rete, a network of anastomosing passages and channels that in turn drain into the *extratesticular* rete, characterized by still wider spaces in continuity with the 6 to 12 fine efferent ductules leading to the head of the epididymis.

Seminiferous Tubules

Peritubular Tissue

The seminiferous tubules owe their cylindrical shape to multiple layers of cellular and extracellular elements collectively known as the lamina propria, tunica propria, or peritubular tissue (Figs. 130–2 and 130–3). Of variable thickness, up to six or more concentric cellular layers are seen in the human testis,[6] whereas only two to three layers are noted in the majority of mammals.[7–10] The innermost layer commences with the thin basement membrane apposed to the basal surfaces of the cells of the seminiferous epithelium. Collagen fibers lie external to this, followed by one or more layers of very attenuated myofibroblastic cells, which, by virtue of their microfibrillar and elastic fiber components, are responsible for the contractile activity of the tubules.[11–14] A thin outermost layer of endothelium or fibroblast cytoplasm marks the boundary between the peri-

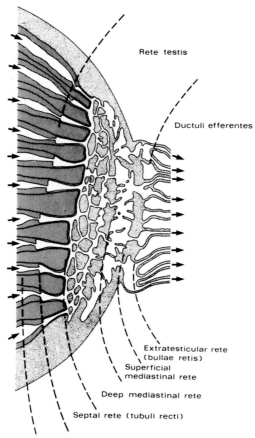

FIGURE 130–1. Relationship between the seminiferous tubules and the rete testis within the mediastinum. Zones of the rete testis are indicated. (From de Kretser DM, et al: Anatomical and functional aspects of the male reproductive organs. *In* Bandhauer K, Frick J (eds): Handbook of Urology, vol XVI, Disturbances in Male Fertility. Berlin, Springer-Verlag, 1982, pp 1–131.)

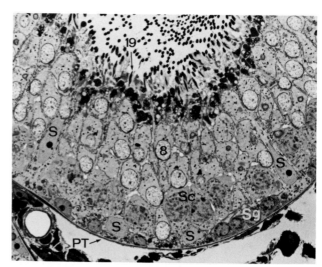

FIGURE 130–2. Seminiferous epithelium of the rat testis, illustrating Sertoli cell nuclei (S), spermatogonia (Sg), primary spermatocytes (Sc), step eight spermatids (8), and step 19 spermatids (19). Peritubular tissue (PT) is shown.

tubular tissue and the connective tissues of the intertubular region. The passage of macromolecules from the intertubular tissue into the seminiferous tubules is partly restricted by the peritubular tissues in some rodents.[7–9] Extracellular tracers introduced into the monkey and human testis[15–17] via the vascular system or into fresh tissue biopsies diffuse freely through the peritubular tissue, suggesting that it does not restrict entry of macromolecules into the basal aspect of the seminiferous tubules.

Spermatogenesis

Within the seminiferous tubules the germ cells and the Sertoli cells make up the seminiferous epithelium, a complex stratified arrangement of germ cells supported by the tall columnar Sertoli cells, which rest upon the basement membrane and extend apically toward the tubule lumen (Figs. 130–2 and 130–3). The germ cells are highly synchronized in their proliferation and development and form distinct cellular associations, establishing a precisely coordinated "cycle of the seminiferous epithelium" believed to be regulated in part by the Sertoli cells (see below).

Spermatogenesis commences with the replication of stem cells or spermatogonia which, by a complex series of cell divisions and maturation, ultimately give rise to sper-

matozoa (Fig. 130–4). The duration of the entire process of spermatogenesis varies between species, for example, 35 days in the mouse and hamster, approximately 50 days in the rat, and 70 days in the human.[28] Three main phases of spermatogenesis are identified: (a) proliferation and differentiation of spermatogonia; (b) meiotic maturation of spermatocytes; (c) transformation of spermatids into spermatozoa.

SPERMATOGONIAL STEM CELLS. Spermatogonia are basally positioned within the seminiferous epithelium and are in contact with the basement membrane of the tubule. Two main classes of spermatogonia are recognized in all mammals: type A exhibiting fine pale-staining nuclear chromatin and type B with coarse granules or more heavily stained chromatin associated with the nuclear membrane and nucleolus.[23] Type A can be further divided into several subtypes, which are thought to represent steps in proliferation to ensure the preservation of stem cells together with

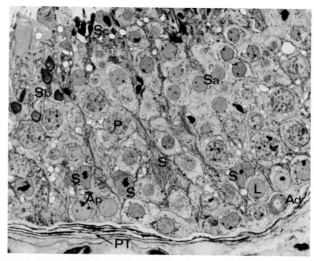

FIGURE 130–3. Seminiferous epithelium of the human testis, illustrating Sertoli cell nuclei (S): spermatogonial types (Ap, Ad); primary spermatocytes, leptotene (L), pachytene (P); spermatids at various stages (Sb, Sc, Sd). Note multiple layers of the peritubular tissue (PT).

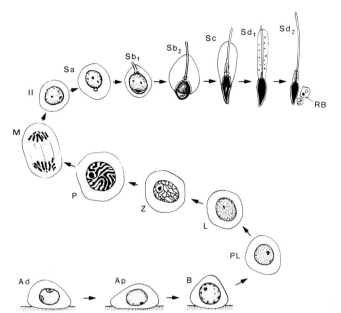

FIGURE 130–4. Sequence of germ cell types in the spermatogenic process in man. Spermatogenesis commences with a spermatogonium and progresses through an orderly sequence of cell proliferations and maturation, terminating with a mature spermatozoon. Explanation of symbols: spermatogonial cells, dark type A and pale type A (Ad, Ap), type B (B); primary spermatocytes, preleptotene (PL), leptotene (L), zygotene (Z), pachytene (P), meiotic division (M); secondary spermatocyte (II); spermatids (Sa, Sb, Sc, Sd); excess spermatid cytoplasm or residual body (RB).

DNA synthesis and with condensation of their chromatin into thin filaments, the leptotene stage is identified. Thickening and pairing of homologous chromosomes are recognized in the zygotene stage, progressing to the pachytene primary spermatocytes in which the nucleus is enlarged and the paired chromosomes are visible as thick threads within the nucleus. Each chromosome pair consists of four chromatids, referred to as bivalents. At this time exchange of genetic material between homologous chromosomes (maternal and paternal) is achieved by crossing over, marked by the appearance of chiasmata. Partial separation of homologous pairs still joined at their chiasmata occurs at the diplotene stage; the chromosomes then shorten, lose contact with the nuclear membrane, and the bivalents, recognizable as pairs, mark the diakinetic stage. Subsequently the nuclear membrane disappears, a spindle forms to which each bivalent gains attachment, thereby forming an equatorial plate at metaphase. Movement of each member of the bivalent to the opposite pole of the spindle occurs in anaphase. Following the reappearance of a nuclear membrane around the chromosomes at telophase, the intervening cytoplasm constricts but maintains a cytoplasmic bridge between the resulting secondary spermatocytes, now containing a haploid number of chromosomes (each composed of a pair of chromatids) but a diploid DNA content. In the second meiotic division the conjoined secondary spermatocytes divide to form spermatids, which have both a haploid chromosomal and DNA content.

SPERMIOGENESIS. In this terminal phase of spermatogenesis, the young round spermatids are transformed, without further cell replication, into spermatozoa that require condensation and remodeling of the nucleus into a shape unique to each species, together with the development of a flagellum and divestment of most of the cytoplasm. The major morphological features of spermiogenesis are common to all species, and in the context of this chapter a description of spermiogenesis in the human is considered to be a suitable model applicable to the same process in mammals. Reviews on spermiogenesis in mammals and man are numerous,[29–34] and in the human the sequence of changes proposed by Clermont[21] is designated in six steps illustrated in Figure 130–5. These steps may be conveniently followed in four main phases, that is, the Golgi, cap, acrosome, and maturation phases.

Early in the Golgi phase, the spermatids show a prominent Golgi complex in proximity to the nuclear membrane, to which it contributes a large vacuole containing dense material. The vacuole is designated the acrosomal vesicle, and the association with the nucleus establishes the cranial pole of the spermatid, which becomes covered by the flattening and conformation of the acrosomal vesicle. Centrioles within the cytoplasm provide a focal point for the development of a primitive axial filament or axoneme consisting of a 9 + 2 arrangement of peripheral doublets and a central pair of microtubules. Moving to the nuclear membrane opposite to the acrosomal vesicle, the centrioles with their protruding axoneme (the future flagellum) then articulate with the nucleus to establish the caudal pole of the spermatid.

Accumulation of dense glycoprotein material within the acrosome occurs in the cap phase; that is, the acrosome now covers the cranial half to two thirds of the elongating spermatid nucleus. During fertilization the acrosome re-

a process of differentiation toward the development of type B spermatogonia, which subsequently differentiate into spermatocytes.[29] In the human testis, type A spermatogonia occur in two main categories, referred to as the dark type A cell containing dense chromatin with a small central nuclear pale area and a pale type A spermatogonium showing pale-staining chromatin and one or two nucleoli along the nuclear membrane. Long type A spermatogonia (elongated nuclei) and cloudy type A spermatogonia (mixture of dark and pale chromatin) have also been described, although their functional significance is uncertain.[28] Because of incomplete cytokinesis during mitosis, the spermatogonia are joined by intercellular bridges, which persist between all their progeny through subsequent steps of spermatogenesis. These intercellular connections are severed just prior to the release of individual spermatozoa into the lumen of the tubule. This "clonal-type" development contributes to the observed synchrony of germ cell maturation, and growing evidence indicates that biochemical interactions between the germ cells and the Sertoli cells are essential for maintenance of normal spermatogenesis (see below).

MEIOTIC MATURATION OF SPERMATOCYTES. Division of type B spermatogonia and their detachment from the basement membrane provide the preleptotene primary spermatocytes which represent the first step in the long process of meiotic maturation characterized by reduction of the chromosomal number from diploid to haploid, involving two cell divisions: primary spermatocytes dividing into secondary spermatocytes and the latter into spermatids. Identification of spermatocytes is based upon their size and the characteristic and changing appearance of their chromatin.[29] During prophase of the first meiotic division, preleptotene primary spermatocytes engage in

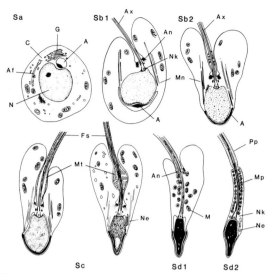

FIGURE 130–5. The process of spermiogenesis in the human testis, as observed by electron microscopy. A, Acrosome or acrosomic vesicle; Af, developing axial filament; An annulus; Ax, axoneme; C, centrioles; Fs, fibrous sheath; G, Golgi complex; M mitochondria; Mn, manchette; Mp, middle piece; Mt; microtubules in spindle-shaped body; N, nucleus; Ne, redundant nuclear envelope; Nk, neck; Pp, principal piece. (From Kerr JB: Functional cytology of the human testis. *In* de Kretser DM (ed): Bailliere's Clin Endocrinol Metab 6:235–250, 1992.)

leases enzymes in the zona pellucida of the egg, assisting sperm penetration. With the whole cell now beginning to change to an elliptical shape the nucleus rotates to face the basement membrane of the tubule and the flagellum and caudal cytoplasm point adluminally.

The acrosome phase is marked by nuclear condensation and cell elongation. With the considerable shrinkage and remodeling of nuclear volume, excess nuclear membrane is discarded, the DNA becomes cross-linked, most nonhistone nuclear proteins are lost, and gene transcription is ultimately suppressed. In the cytoplasm long parallel arrays of microtubules form a cylindrical sheath around the flagellum, termed the manchette, which is possibly involved in the redistribution of organelles and inclusions toward the caudal regions of the elongated cytoplasm. The pair of centrioles bridging the nucleus and the developing flagellum become embedded in a connecting piece or neck shaped like a truncated cone. Details of the formation of the neck have been discussed elsewhere.[29–31] An outer set of nine coarse fibers extend caudally from the neck and stiffens the flagellum. Their assembly is related to significant protein synthetic activity in midspermiogenesis.[35] Distal displacement of the spermatid cytoplasm is associated with the helical orientation of mitochondria that surround the tail, thereby forming the midpiece. Beyond this, the principal piece consists of the axoneme, two of the coarse fibers, and an outer fibrous sheath of rib-like fibers that branch perpendicular to the axoneme.

Commencement of the maturation phase is identified by the separation of the caudal cytoplasm from the head and tail of the mature spermatid. This so-called excess residual cytoplasm is formed in response to penetration by slender invaginations of Sertoli cell cytoplasm into the spermatids, which cleave off their cytoplasm in lobes to be surrounded and eventually phagocytosed by the adluminal cytoplasm of the Sertoli cells. At this time the lobes of residual cyto-

plasm round up to form the residual bodies containing many of the organelles and inclusions previously found in the caudal spermatid cytoplasm. Release of the spermatids from the tips of the Sertoli cell is referred to as *spermiation* and is achieved via at least three mechanisms: adluminal displacement of the spermatids toward the lumen, detachment from surface specializations between the spermatid acrosome and the Sertoli cells, and disengagement of slender tubular invaginations into the Sertoli cell cytoplasm arising from the thin mantle of cytoplasm covering the head of the spermatid. The spermatids are released as spermatozoa, whereas the retained residual bodies undergo autolysis and lysosomal degradation within the Sertoli cells.

COORDINATION OF SPERMATOGENESIS. The germ cells are aggregated into morphologically distinct associations or groups of cells classified into histological stages unique to each species. The precise and repeatable occurrence of certain types of germ cells has been recognized since the nineteenth century, most notably by von Ebner[18] and Benda,[19] who contributed to the idea of the spermatogenic cycle, that is, recognizable cell associations succeeding one another along the length of the seminiferous tubule. Extensive histological and radioautographic studies by Clermont,[21, 23] Leblond and Clermont,[20] and Heller and Clermont[22] defined the cycle of the seminiferous epithelium as "the series of changes in a given area of the seminiferous epithelium between two appearances of the same developmental stage." The orderly sequence of complete sets of stages along the seminiferous tubules was initially referred to as a "spermatogenic wave,"[18] which lead Regaud[27] to propose that "the wave is in space what the cycle is in time." For a given species, the number of stages of the cycle is usually determined by the PAS histochemical reaction to stain the acrosomes of the spermatids. Fourteen stages are described in the rat, 13 in the hamster and guinea pig, 12 in the mouse and monkey, 8 in the ram and bull, and 6 in the human.[23] In most mammals, coordination of spermatogenesis is found about a radial axis with the entire tubule cross-section showing the same stage of the seminiferous cycle (Fig. 130–6). However, in the testes of two species of monkey[24, 25] and the human,[22] the position of the stages noted in a cross-sectioned tubule gives the impression of a rather irregular pattern of germ cell development in which several stages occur adjacent to each other (Figs. 130–7 and 130–8). Recently Schulze and Reh-

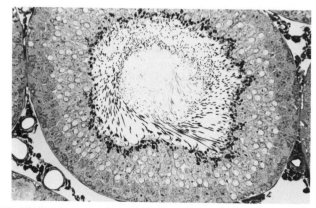

FIGURE 130–6. Cross-sectioned seminiferous tubule of the rat testis. Note that the development of particular types of germ cells is synchronized around a radial axis from the center to the periphery of the tubule.

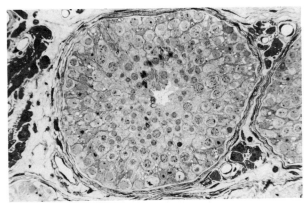

FIGURE 130-7. Cross-sectioned seminiferous tubule of the human testis. The development of germ cells appears irregular owing to some areas containing densely staining Sc spermatids *(upper region)*, whereas the lower region contains round Sa spermatids.

Helical organization pattern of the human seminiferous epithelium

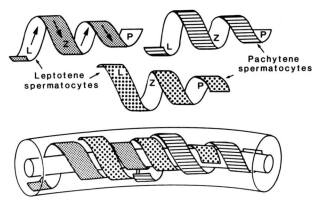

FIGURE 130-9. Helical arrangement of the development of primary spermatocytes of the human testis [leptotene (L), zygotene (Z), pachytene (P)] drawn as strips that overlap and gyrate toward the lumen of the seminiferous tubule.

der[26] reinvestigated the topographic arrangement of stages along the human seminiferous tubule and showed that the stages were not positioned randomly but formed an orderly sequence oriented in an oblique plane in relation to the longitudinal axis of the tubule. Analysis of serial sections and computer-assisted three-dimensional reconstructions of primary spermatocytes in the human testis have shown that germ cell development follows a helical pattern (Fig. 130–9). The diameter of the helix decreases toward the lumen, with a successive helix overlapping the external surface of the previous spiral, allowing multiple spirals to gyrate in a concentric pattern, similar to an archimedian spiral. When this mathematical model is viewed in two dimensions, the germ cells of the human seminiferous epithelium are seen to be precisely ordered and coordinated in their development (Fig. 130–10). A similar helical continuity of germ cell stages also has been confirmed in the nonhuman primate species already referred to.

The Sertoli Cell

The relationship between the structure and function of the Sertoli cell has been considered extensively in the literature, and several reviews are available[29, 36–40] which provide detailed information beyond the scope of this chapter. The aim of this discussion is to focus attention on those aspects of Sertoli cell morphology believed to be involved in the development of germ cells which provide a basis for reviewing cell-cell interactions considered later in the chapter.

SHAPE AND DISTRIBUTION. Sertoli cells resemble the shape of a tree, being tall columnar cells, resting upon

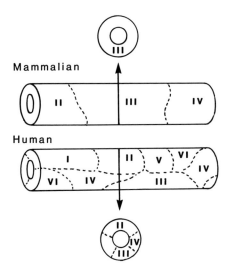

FIGURE 130-8. Comparison of the organization of the stages of spermatogenesis in mammals (including numerous primates) and in man. In mammals the stages occupy longitudinal segments along the seminiferous tubules, whereas in the human they occur as discrete patches. When transverse sections of tubules are examined, two or more stages are noted in the human seminiferous epithelium.

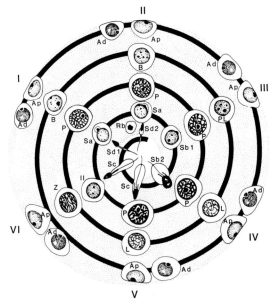

FIGURE 130-10. Representation of the six stages of the spermatogenic cycle of the human testis with their complement of germ cells arranged to show how their sequence of development corresponds to the geometry of spirals gyrating conically toward the lumen. In actual tubules some of the stages would be positioned at more superficial or deeper levels along the seminiferous tubule. Symbols are as defined in Figure 130–4. (From Kerr JB: Functional cytology of the human testis. *In* de Kretser DM (ed): Bailliere's Clin Endocronol Metab 6:235–250, 1992.)

the basement membrane, and extending lateral and apical cytoplasmic branches from the body or trunk of the cell, which overarch the spermatogonia and interdigitate and surround all other germ cells (Fig. 130–11). Depending upon the species, they occupy 14 to 43 per cent of the volume of the seminiferous epithelium.[41] By providing physical support to the germ cells, the Sertoli cell must maintain a degree of rigidity while retaining the capacity to change shape in synchrony with the division, enlargement, and metamorphic alterations of the germ cells. The attainment of quantitatively normal spermatogenesis in the adult depends upon an adequate number of Sertoli cells[42, 43] which is achieved by their proliferative activity during the growth of the fetal and postnatal testis and depends upon FSH stimulation.[44, 45] Quantitative histological studies of the human testis have reported that Sertoli cell numbers may increase up to 15 years of age.[46] At its base each Sertoli cell is in contact with five or six adjacent Sertoli cells, and each cell supports up to 50 germ cells throughout the depth of the seminiferous epithelium.[41, 47]

BLOOD-TESTIS BARRIER. Where the plasma membranes of adjacent Sertoli cells are apposed in the basolateral regions of the cell, they form special occluding tight junctions (Fig. 130–11), which in freeze-fracture preparations resemble multiple parallel rows of spot fusions, forming a band or zone of adhesion around the circumference of the cell.[7, 36, 48] The junctions form the blood-testis barrier and are stabilized by subsurface actin filaments and smooth membranous cisternae.[47] Their unusual position at the base of the seminiferous epithelium is known to subdivide the epithelium into basal and adluminal regions, which partition young and more mature germ cells into two distinct anatomical and functional compartments. Spermato-

gonia and early spermatocytes (up to leptotene) reside within the basal compartment and may be exposed to the biochemical environment maintained by the intertubular tissue. The strategic position of the tight junctions between adjacent Sertoli cells and above these germ cells prevents intercellular transport between Sertoli cells and thus creates an adluminal compartment thought to provide a unique physiological environment for all other germ cells. Completion of meiotic maturation and spermiogenesis therefore occurs within a special epithelial domain created and regulated by the Sertoli cells. Upward displacement of germ cells from the basal to the adluminal compartment is achieved by a synchronized dissolution and reassembly of tight junctions above and below the migrating germ cells. The blood-testis barrier exists in all animals[29] and is formed during the initiation of spermatogenesis[49] in response to gonadotrophic stimulation[50] and the appearance of zygotene-pachytene primary spermatocytes.[51]

PLASTICITY AND LINKS WITH GERM CELLS. Sertoli cells exhibit an elaborate and dynamic cytoskeleton that serves to maintain the columnar shape of the cell, to determine the intracellular distribution of organelles, and to provide intercellular adhesion with germ cells. The supranuclear regions of the Sertoli cell cytoplasm are supplied with microtubules (chiefly α-tubulin and dynein), which are especially abundant in the crypts surrounding elongating spermatids.[52] Together with intermediate filaments,[53] these cytoskeletal elements are believed to influence the shape and position of the germ cells in concert with the spermatogenic cycle. A further component of the cytoskeleton of the Sertoli cells is evident at the interface between the plasma membranes of Sertoli cells and germ cells and is identified as an ectoplasmic specialization. This appears to be identical to one half of the inter-Sertoli tight junction and consists of a dense mat of actin filaments sandwiched between the plasma membrane and a cistern of smooth endoplasmic reticulum.[47, 54] Only rarely associated with zygotene primary spermatocytes, they are more frequently observed facing pachytene primary spermatocytes and always occur in association with round and elongating spermatids, forming a mantle around the heads of the latter germ cells.[29] The presence of vinculin with these ectoplasmic specializations[55] suggests that the Sertoli cells adhere to the plasma membrane of germ cells and thus play a role in determining the shape of the elongating sperm head and in adjusting the orientation of the germ cells within the seminiferous epithelium. Atypical desmosome-gap junctions exist between Sertoli cells and all round germ cells, between spermatogonia of the same type, and rarely between primary spermatocytes.[56–58] Their functional significance is not yet clear.

PHAGOCYTOSIS, ENDOCYTOSIS, AND SECRETION. It is the duty of the Sertoli cells to dispose of the excess residual cytoplasm of spermatids shed at spermiation and to eliminate degenerating germ cells, which is a naturally occurring phenomenon during spermatogenesis. With the exception of mature spermatids, initial disintegration of residual bodies and germ cells occurs via autolysis and is soon supplemented by the lysosomal system within the cytoplasm of the Sertoli cells.[29] Lysosomal numbers and enzymatic activities vary throughout the spermatogenic cycle[59–62] and serve to dispose of degenerative germ cell products. The endocytosis of tracers such as ferritin has suggested that the lysosomal system also participates in

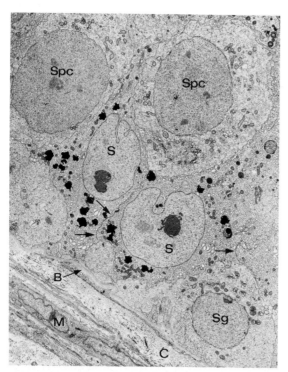

FIGURE 130–11. Ultrastructure of human seminiferous epithelium showing Sertoli cell nuclei (S), a spermatogonium (Sg), and primary spermatocytes (Spc). Electron-dense lines represent inter–Sertoli cell tight junctions (*arrows*). In the peritubular tissue, the basal lamina (B), collagen fibers (C), and a myoid cell (M) are indicated.

reduction of excess plasma membrane and the absorption of luminal fluid through the apical cytoplasm.[59] Sertoli cells show receptor-mediated endocytosis of macromolecules via their apex and base,[63, 64] and recent studies both in vivo and in vitro have demonstrated that this is the mechanism by which the Sertoli cells deliver iron to the germ cells from the serum.[65, 66] Although the Sertoli cells are known to secrete many proteins and are capable of limited synthesis and secretion of steroids,[67] little is currently known about their physiological significance. Sertoli cells do not exhibit a well-defined secretory apparatus, and thus links between specific secretory products and cytoplasmic organelles or inclusions have not been established.[29, 36–40] It is known that the Sertoli cells show significant alterations of cell volume, number, and type of cytoplasmic components at each stage of the spermatogenic cycle.[29, 41, 59–62] These variations provide the morphological counterparts for the alterations in responsiveness to hormonal stimulation and interactions with specific germ cells at given stages of the spermatogenic cycle (see below).

Intertubular Tissue

Organization

The region between the seminiferous tubules, termed the *intertubular* or *interstitial tissue*, consists of loose connective tissue, the cellular and extracellular components of which are qualitatively similar in the mammalian testis, although its quantitative composition is species-specific. Detailed discussions of the structure-function relationships of the intertubular tissue are available in several reviews.[10, 29, 68, 69] The most remarkable histological variation of the intertubular tissue is the relative proportion of Leydig cells[10] known for many years to synthesize and secrete androgens, chiefly testosterone, which is essential for the maintenance of spermatogenesis. As a general rule, testes in which the Leydig cells occupy only 10 to 20 per cent of the intertubular tissue (rat, guinea pig, ram, human) can show extensive intertubular lymphatic spaces or edematous connective tissue (Fig. 130–12), in contrast to other species such as the boar, zebra, and numerous marsupial species, in which this ratio is reversed.[10, 29] The relative paucity of Leydig cells in some species, compared with others in which the Leydig cells are extraordinarily abundant, has implications for the interpretation of Leydig cell size, position, and interactions with other intertubular cells, the peritubular tissue, and the cells of the seminiferous epithelium, where the overwhelming focus of attention is confined to the rat testis. Blood vessels occur randomly throughout the intertubular tissue, and capillaries are non-fenestrated. Lymphatic vessels and large lymphatic sinusoids are seen in several rodent species (mouse, rat, guinea pig) in contrast to the human testis, in which these vessels exist only in the main connective tissue septa extending inward from the tunica albuginea.[69] Fibroblasts and macrophages are also found in the intertubular tissue, whereas lymphocytes, plasma cells, and mast cells are generally confined to the region of the tunica vasculosa.

Leydig Cells

The morphology of Leydig cells in the mammalian testis presents a consistent architecture devoted to the synthesis

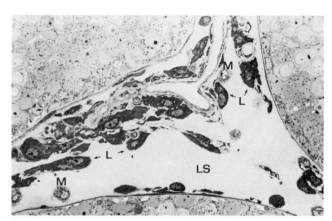

FIGURE 130–12. Intertubular tissue of the rat testis illustrating basophilic Leydig cells (L), macrophages (M), and an extensive lymphatic sinusoid (LS).

and secretion of steroids, notably testosterone.[68, 71] Fetal, immature, and adult-type Leydig cells are epithelioid in shape (Fig. 130–13), and their basophilic staining property is attributed to the dominant organelle within their cytoplasm, the smooth endoplasmic reticulum, whose surface provides binding sites for numerous enzymes catalyzing a variety of steroidogenic conversions. The pathway leading to the secretion of testosterone commences with exogenous acetate or cholesterol, taken into the cytoplasm where, depending on the species and/or the extent of cell maturation, it may be stored within lipid droplets containing esterified cholesterol and triglycerides. The subsequent steps in the steroidogenic pathway and its control are discussed below. Leydig cells contain Golgi membranes, microtubules, individual smooth vesicles, mitochondria with tubular cristae (unique in steroidogenic cells), and small quantities of rough endoplasmic reticulum. The mechanism by which testosterone leaves the Leydig cell remains unclear, and it is assumed that this occurs via diffusion, because typical secretory vacuoles or granules have not been observed. Leydig cells are capable of endocytotic activity via fluid-phase or adsorptive endocytosis, the ingested materials entering the lysosomal pathway.[29]

Peroxisomes have been identified in Leydig cells, and their content of a sterol carrier protein suggests their involvement with the intracellular transport of cholesterol to

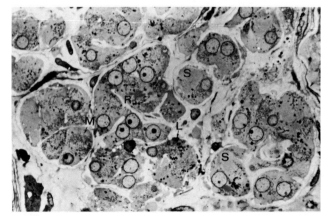

FIGURE 130–13. High magnification of a cluster of human Leydig cells containing mitochondria (M), areas of smooth endoplasmic reticulum (S), crystals of Reinke (R), and lipofuscin granules (L).

the mitochondria for subsequent side-chain cleavage to pregnenolone.[72] Undigested materials appear as lipofuscin pigment granules, which are prevalent in human Leydig cells. Crystals of Reinke composed of globular protein subunits are frequently noted in human Leydig cells, and although similar crystalline inclusions increase in abundance in the Leydig cells of a seasonally breeding wild rat, their functional significance is unknown.[29]

Interstitial Cells

The ability of the intertubular tissue to retain exogenously administered dyes is attributable to the presence of macrophages, which have been characterized for several species using histochemical, immunological, and ultrastructural techniques.[68, 71, 73–76] In most species the ratio of macrophages to Leydig cells is in the range of 1:10 or even 1:50, whereas in the rat testis they are especially abundant, with one macrophage for every four Leydig cells. This relatively large proportion has prompted further investigation of their functional activities, particularly in relation to the finding that tissue allografts or xenografts are rejected by the ram testis but survive for long periods in the rat testis,[76] suggesting that the latter represents an immunologically privileged tissue. The possibility that macrophages contribute to immune privilege in the testis and their interactions with Leydig cells and other interstitial cells is discussed below.

The populations of mesenchymal or fibroblast-type cells in the intertubular tissue serve not only as loose connective tissue cells but are also the source of new Leydig cells. These precursor or stem cells are found in peritubular and perivascular locations. They are capable of producing testosterone via LH stimulation and ultimately differentiate into Leydig cells.[77–79] Studies of the endocrine and paracrine factors that influence the development of Leydig cells are discussed later in this chapter.

CONTROL OF TESTICULAR FUNCTION

The major factors that control the production of testosterone by the Leydig cells and spermatozoa by the seminiferous tubules are the gonadotrophic hormones FSH and LH. These two hormones are secreted by the anterior pituitary gland under the control of the episodic secretion of gonadotrophin-releasing hormone (GnRH) into the pituitary portal vessels. In addition to GnRH, the secretion of FSH and LH is controlled by the level of negative feedback from the testis via its secretion of testosterone and inhibin (see below).

Although it is useful to consider the control of the compartments of the testis as separate entities, increasing evidence indicates that their functions are intimately related through known and unknown factors operating through paracrine mechanisms.[80–83] Furthermore, a substantial body of evidence now indicates that the stimulatory action of FSH and LH, the latter through testosterone, on seminiferous tubule function is modulated by local factors. The actions of the gonadotrophic hormones are considered first, and the interaction between the Leydig cells, Sertoli cells, and germ cells in modulating the actions of FSH and LH is considered later in this chapter.

Leydig Cell Function and Control

The intimate location of the Leydig cells in the intertubular tissue adjacent to the seminiferous tubules places them in an excellent position to influence spermatogenesis by paracrine mechanisms. The close association of these cells with the vasculature of the testis enables them to perform one of their major functions, namely the secretion of androgens to influence the secondary sex characteristics of the male. In addition to androgen secretion, the Leydig cells are the source of a range of hormones that may have significance in the local control of testicular function. These hormones are considered in the section concerning the interrelationships between the compartments of the testis. Although a number of naturally occurring steroids have the capacity to exhibit androgen action, testosterone is the major product of the Leydig cells with the most potent androgenic action.[84, 85] The adult human testis produces approximately 7 mg of testosterone daily. In addition, the testis produces smaller amounts of weaker androgens, such as androstenedione and dehydroepiandrosterone (DHEA). As discussed later, testosterone exerts its action by binding to specific intracellular androgen receptors, and the weaker androgens, androstenedione and DHEA, have a lower binding affinity for the androgen receptor. The testis also produces small amounts of dihydrotestosterone, which has a very strong affinity for the androgen receptor. In addition to androgens, the testis produces approximately 25 per cent of the total daily production of 17β-estradiol,[86] with the remainder (both estradiol and estrone) being derived by conversion of both testicular and adrenal androgens, such as androstenedione and DHEA, by the enzyme aromatase in peripheral tissues.

Biosynthetic Pathway

The major substrate for steroid production by the Leydig cell is cholesterol. Cholesterol can be derived from two sources, the first consisting of an uptake mechanism by which circulating low-density lipoprotein can bind to specific receptors on Leydig cells, and by internalization can thereby provide a ready source of cholesterol. In the rat, Leydig cell receptors for high-density lipoprotein have also been found.[87] The other source of cholesterol represents de novo synthesis from acetate by the Leydig cell. It is likely that the proportion of cholesterol obtained by these two pathways may vary, depending on the species and the state of stimulation of the Leydig cells. Some estimates have suggested that more than half of the cholesterol required by the Leydig cells comes from the low-density lipoprotein.[88] The conversion of cholesterol to testosterone involves a number of steps that are catalysed by hemoprotein mixed function oxidases, which predominantly belong to the cytochrome P450 family. The steps in the steroidogenic pathway are illustrated in Figure 130–14.

The first step in this pathway is the mobilization of cholesterol from pools of cholesterol esters by a testicular cholesterol ester hydrolase[84, 85] and the conversion of cholesterol to pregnenolone. The free cholesterol is transported to mitochondria, where it passes from the outer to the inner mitochondrial membrane with the aid of a 30-amino acid steroidogenic activator peptide.[89] The enzyme, cholesterol side-chain cleavage, which converts cholesterol to

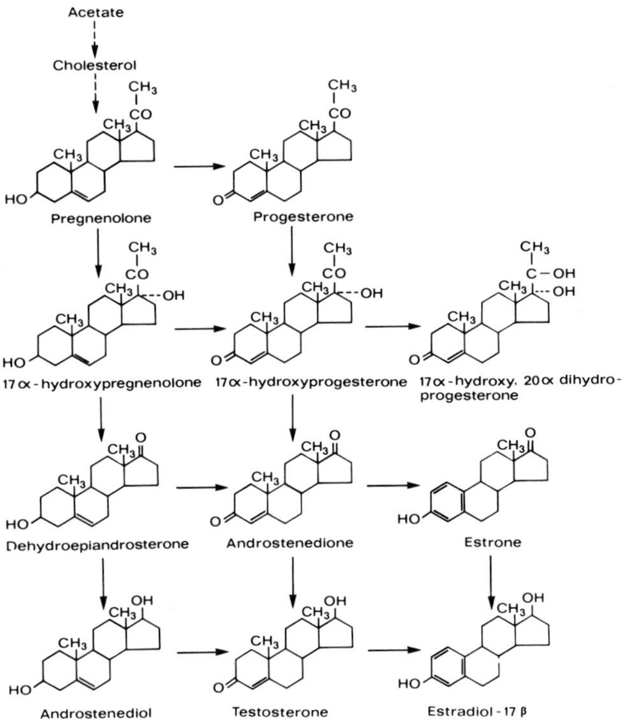

FIGURE 130–14. The steroid biosyntheic pathways leading to testosterone and estradiol production.

pregnenolone, is located on the inner mitochondrial membrane and catalyses three separate reactions. Two hydroxylations occur at the C20 and C22 positions and a cleavage of the cholesterol side-chain at the C20-22 carbon bond to form pregnenolone with the release of the six-carbon compound, isocaproic acid. The enzyme catalyzing this reaction is termed cytochrome $P450_{SCC}$. It is likely that stimulation of this reaction is crucial in the regulation of steroidogenesis, with cholesterol substrate being a rate-limiting step. The cytochrome $P450_{SCC}$ is encoded for by a single gene that transcribes a single species of mRNA, and it is likely that the testicular and adrenal enzymes are identical.[90]

The pregnenolone formed may be converted to progesterone through the enzyme 3β-hydroxysteroid hydrogenase (3βHSD) or can be hydroxylated at the 17α position by 17α-hydroxylase. The pathways taken by pregnenolone either through progesterone (the Δ_4 pathway) or through 17α-hydroxypregnenolone (the Δ_5 pathway) may vary between species and the physiological state of the mammal. In the human, the Δ_5 pathway appears to predominate in both the adult and fetal testis.[91, 92]

In following the Δ_5 pathway, pregnenolone is hydroxylated to 17α-hydroxy pregnenolone, which subsequently undergoes cleavage to form the C_{19} steroid, dehydroepiandrosterone, by the enzyme 17,20 lyase. Both steps appear to be catalyzed by a single microsomal enzyme, cytochrome P450c17. A single copy gene on chromosome 10 encodes for this enzyme in both the adrenal and testis.[93, 94] A further conversion of dehydroepiandrosterone to androstenediol is mediated by the enzyme 17β-hydroxysteroid dehydrogenase, which is a microsomal enzyme that does not belong to the cytochrome P450 series.[95] There appears to be a single gene for 17β-hydroxysteroid dehydrogenase on chromosome 17.[96]

The conversion of substrates in the Δ_5 pathway to the Δ_4 pathway (Fig. 130–14) involves the enzyme 3βHSD. It is possible that more than one copy of the human 3βHSD gene may be found on chromosome 1.[97] In addition to the conversion of pregnenolone to progesterone, 3βHSD has the capacity to convert other precursors in the Δ_5 pathway to the Δ_4 pathway, namely the conversion 17α-hydroxy pregnenolone to 17-hydroxy progesterone, the conversion of dehydroepiandrosterone to androstenedione and the conversion of androstenediol to testosterone.

As indicated earlier, the testis has the capacity to produce 17β-estradiol, and this reaction is catalyzed by the enzyme cytochrome P450 aromatase. This conversion involves a series of reactions resulting in hydroxylation at C_3, and loss of the methyl side chain at C_{10}. Two cytochrome P450 aromatase genes have been found on chromosome 15.[98]

The testis has the capacity to secrete small amounts of dihydrotestosterone, and the enzyme catalyzing the conversion of testosterone to dihydrotestosterone is 5α reductase. The testicular level of this enzyme is much lower than that found in genital skin or prostatic tissue. The enzyme, encoding human 5α-reductase, has been cloned and catalyzes a reduction of the unsaturated C4-5 double bond of testosterone to form 5α-dihydrotestosterone.[99]

The cellular localization of these enzymes has been determined with the conversion of cholesterol to pregnenolone occurring within the mitochondria through the localization of cytochrome $P450_{SCC}$ on the inner mitochondrial membrane.[100] Pregnenolone is transported from the mitochondrion to the smooth endoplasmic reticulum, where the remaining enzymes necessary for the conversion of pregnenolone to testosterone are located. Numerous studies have demonstrated that the smooth endoplasmic reticulum gives rise to the microsomal fraction that contains the necessary enzymes.

Regulation of Testicular Steroidogenesis

The control of testosterone production is by the gonadotrophin LH, through the presence of specific receptors on the surface of Leydig cells.[102] The LH receptor has been recently isolated, sequenced, and cloned and its structure characterized.[101]

Considerable evidence indicates that interaction of LH with its receptor activates the cAMP pathway through a GTP-binding protein.[84, 103] Some concern about signal transduction through the protein kinase A pathway existed, because LH could stimulate submaximal testosterone production without any significant changes in cAMP concentrations.[104] More recent data have suggested the possibility that changes in intracellular calcium concentrations may be involved in the action of LH by activating phospholipases in the lipoxygenase pathway.[105] This would provide an alternative pathway for the control of steroidogenesis in Leydig cells. In addition, the changes in calcium may regulate adenylate cyclase via the protein kinase C pathway.[84, 103, 105]

The action of LH leads to a number of events that result in the provision of cholesterol substrate and in the stimulation of the side-chain cleavage enzyme to convert cholesterol to pregnenolone. This involves mobilization of cholesterol from cholesterol stores and stimulation of cholesterol ester hydrolase.[84] The resultant production of pregnenolone is rapidly translated into a release of testosterone within the 30 to 60 minutes of LH stimulation. This acute response varies in magnitude between species, being very clear in the rat and the ram, but less so in the human.[106, 107] A much longer response can be seen with repeated stimuli using LH or by a single injection of hCG, the latter having a considerably longer half-time.[106, 107] In experiments utilizing hCG, the initial rise in testosterone peaks within 12 hours, and the levels subsequently decline to an elevated plateau at 24 hours, rising again to a peak some 48 to 72 hours after the initial injection. This biphasic response of testosterone secretion to hCG stimulation of Leydig cells does not occur with LH and probably results from a number of factors. Following acute stimulation of Leydig cells with high doses of LH or hCG, receptors are lost from the surface of Leydig cells.[108] This is also accompanied by a refractoriness of the Leydig cells to further LH/hCG stimulation for approximately 48 to 72 hours,[109] probably as a result of the conversion of testosterone to estradiol and a feedback inhibition of the C17-20 lyase enzyme.[110] The second phase of testosterone secretion at 72 hours after an hCG injection is likely to be due to a recovery from this inhibition of steroid biosynthesis, and the long half-life of hCG ensures that following high doses, adequate levels of hCG are still present in the circulation to result in the reactivation of steroid secretion. However, other factors are also likely to play a role, because LH and hCG are trophic hormones and their action results in stimulation of a range of enzyme synthesis, cellular hypertrophy, and hyperplasia.[111, 112] Thus in states of chronic Leydig cell stimulation, LH enhances transcription of genes encoding the range of enzymes in the steroidogenic pathway.[113] In the normal physiological state, it is unlikely that the phenomenon of down-regulation of receptors and refractoriness to further LH stimulation occurs. This results predominantly from the fact that LH stimulation of the testis is episodic and pulsatile in nature, resulting from the pulsatility of GnRH stimulation of the pituitary gland. Nevertheless, increases in pulse frequency can result in the augmentation of the testosterone secretory responses, although the size of the LH pulses decreases.[114]

Control of Seminiferous Tubule Function

The intimate association of the germ cells and Sertoli cells described earlier in this chapter emphasizes the need to consider the hormonal control of spermatogenesis in conjunction with the factors modulating Sertoli cell function. There is general agreement that the seminiferous tubule is controlled by FSH and LH, the latter acting via the local secretion of testosterone. However, the specific cell types and processes influenced by these hormones are still debated, particularly the role of FSH in the maintenance of spermatogenesis. Furthermore, increasing evidence suggests that local factors may modulate the actions of FSH and testosterone; these are considered later in this chapter.

Localization of Receptors

Receptors for FSH on the seminiferous tubules were demonstrated by Means and Vaitukaitis,[115] and a more detailed cellular localization was established by autoradiographic studies showing receptors on Sertoli cells and spermatogonia.[116, 117] No germ cells other than spermatogonia have been shown to contain FSH receptors.

LH receptors have not been demonstrated on seminiferous tubule cells, and consequently the hormonal requirement of LH for tubule function has been presumed to result from LH stimulation of Leydig cell testosterone production. Several studies have failed to identify receptors for testosterone on germ cells.[118, 119] However functional androgen receptors have been localized to Sertoli cells, Leydig cells, and peritubular cells.[118–121]

The localization of FSH and androgen receptors to Sertoli cells and the absence of these hormonal receptors on germ cells other than spermatogonia emphasize the key role of the Sertoli cell as an intermediary of FSH and androgen action on spermatogenesis. As discussed below, although aspects of Sertoli cell function are clearly controlled by FSH and testosterone, the molecules or mechanisms by which these hormones exert an influence on spermatogenesis remain unknown. Even the recently described process by which androgen action on peritubular cells influences seminiferous tubule function involves the Sertoli cells; a protein P-Mod-S produced by peritubular cells under androgen stimulation acts by stimulating Sertoli cell inhibin and transferrin production.[122, 123] Whether this recently purified protein[123] acts directly on germ cells requires further study.

In view of the importance of the Sertoli cell as a key intermediary in hormonal action on spermatogenesis, the mechanisms and effects of FSH and androgen action on this cell are considered prior to discussion of their role in spermatogenesis.

Hormonal Control of Sertoli Cell Function

MECHANISM OF FSH ACTION. Following the demonstration of FSH receptors on Sertoli cells,[115–117] several studies demonstrated that FSH exerts its action via the adenylate cyclase–protein kinase system.[124, 125] FSH stimulation results in an increase in cAMP, which in turn results in phosphorylation of a number of Sertoli cell proteins.[125–127] Evidence indicates that FSH modulates intracellular free calcium levels.[128, 129] These actions lead to modification of cellular processes, which in turn change a number of functions of Sertoli cells. This view is consistent with numerous studies demonstrating that FSH stimulates mRNA and protein synthesis by Sertoli cells.[125, 130]

Stimulation by FSH, like a number of trophic hormones, results in a desensitization of its target tissue, the Sertoli cell, making it less sensitive to further stimulation. This process involves a loss of receptors,[131] a reduced response by adenylate cyclase,[132] and increased phosphodiesterase production.[133, 134]

Stimulation of immature Sertoli cell cultures by FSH results in an increase in a number of proteins secreted by these cells, such as androgen binding protein (ABP) secretion,[135] transferrin,[136] inhibin,[137, 138] aromatase,[139] and plasminogen activators.[140] However, this effect of FSH is specific, as some Sertoli cell proteins do not respond to FSH stimulation.[141]

Other Sertoli cell functions are also influenced by FSH stimulation. It is recognized that glucose transport is influenced by FSH,[142] as is the conversion of glucose to lactate.[143] The dependence of germ cells on Sertoli cell–lactate production is one mechanism by which FSH can indirectly influence germ cell development.[144] FSH, cAMP, and calcium have also been shown to stimulate the phosphorylation of cytoskeletal proteins such as vimentin in Sertoli cells, and these actions are likely to be responsible for the changes in their morphology in culture in the presence of FSH.[145, 146]

FSH also stimulates immature Sertoli cells to divide mitotically.[44, 45] Because the major proliferation of Sertoli cells takes place in late gestation and the early postnatal period in the rat, the adequacy of FSH stimulation during this time significantly influences the total Sertoli cell complement of the adult testis.[42] Little is known about the kinetics of Sertoli cell division in other species, but a recent study in humans demonstrated an increase in Sertoli cell number from 260 million in the late fetal testis to 1500 million by 10 years.[46] In the adult, the Sertoli cells represent a stable cell population, and some studies have emphasized the temporal dependence of certain aspects of their function. Some investigators have claimed that the mature Sertoli cell is resistant to FSH stimulation based on the failure of FSH to stimulate Sertoli cell function in whole adult testis preparations.[125] However, the studies of Parvinen[147] have shown that FSH action is stage dependent, with the highest levels of FSH receptors being found at stage 1 and FSH-dependent cAMP production being greatest at stages 1 to 3. The failure of some investigators to demonstrate effects of FSH in the whole testis may have been due to the mixture of responsive and nonresponsive stages of the seminiferous cycle. More recent studies have shown that parameters such as inhibin production by adult seminiferous tubules in culture[148] and by adult Sertoli cells in culture[149] can be stimulated by FSH.

MECHANISM OF ANDROGEN ACTION. Although the effects of FSH on a range of Sertoli cell functions have been well established, those modulated by androgen are not well defined. In vivo, seminiferous tubule fluid production is disrupted if androgens are removed and is stimulated in hypophysectomized rats treated with testosterone.[150, 151] In vitro, testosterone stimulates RNA polymerase II with both a rapid and prolonged phase (3 to 6 hours).[152] Despite this stimulation very few of the well-known Sertoli cell proteins are stimulated by androgens. ABP secretion is one such protein, but androgens either have no effect[132, 136] or inhibit factors such as plasminogen activator[153] or β nerve growth factor mRNA levels.[154] Roberts and Griswold,[155] using two-dimensional gel electrophoresis, noted two proteins that were induced by testosterone. Among the proteins stimulated by testosterone are the testins.[156] Recently Sharpe et al.[157] have shown that depletion of testosterone resulting from Leydig cell destruction by ethane dimethane sulphonate (EDS) caused a 60 per cent reduction in protein synthesis in seminiferous tubules at stage VII of the cycle. Further studies are necessary to identify the nature of these proteins and their role.

Despite the failure of testosterone to stimulate inhibin and transferrin secretion in cultures of immature Sertoli cells, the addition to these cells of P-Mod-S, the androgen-induced protein secreted by peritubular myoid cells, caused a significant stimulation of both transferrin and inhibin production.[123, 158] Thus androgens may exert a dual action on Sertoli cells both directly and indirectly via P-Mod-S. Isolation and characterization of P-Mod-S have shown that it consists of two forms with molecular weights of 56 kDa and 59 kDa.[122]

Although no evidence indicates that the androgen receptor in the testis differs from that found in other tissues,[159] intratesticular testosterone concentrations are 50 times greater than in peripheral blood, and the levels of testosterone required to maintain spermatogenesis in hypophysectomized rats caused hypertrophy of the prostate and seminal vesicles.[160] The androgen receptor within the testis must be continually saturated and although the 5α-reductase levels in the testis are low relative to those in the prostate, dihydrotestosterone levels are also sufficiently high to saturate the androgen receptor. What mechanisms are involved in the modulation of androgen action in the presence of saturated receptor sites are unknown, but it is recognized that androgen treatment of immature Sertoli cell cultures stimulates androgen receptor levels.[161]

Hormonal Control of Spermatogenesis

Despite the absence of FSH and testosterone receptors on germ cells, successful completion of spermatogenesis is under the control of these substances. The relative importance of these two hormones is still unclear, particularly in the adult, in which the requirement for FSH has been questioned. The latter issue arose from the observation that in hypophysectomized rats, testosterone alone could maintain spermatogenesis if commenced immediately after hypophysectomy.

INITIATION OF SPERMATOGENESIS. There is general agreement that successful commencement of spermatogenesis requires both FSH and LH secretion by the pituitary gland. The failure of these hormones to show their pubertal rise is associated with the maintenance of the prepubertal state. The progressive rise of FSH and LH during sexual maturation has been documented in humans[162] and in other species.[163, 164] In disorders such as hypogonadotrophic hypogonadism (Kallmann's syndrome), in which the absence of GnRH stimulation is associated with the failure of FSH and LH secretion, treatment with FSH and LH[165] or pulsatile GnRH initiates spermatogenic development.[166]

Experimental evidence to support the need for a fully functional hypothalamohypophyseal unit emerges from the regression of testes in animals immunized against GnRH.[167] Furthermore the temporal decrease and increase in FSH and LH that precede seasonal cessation and onset of fertility add further support for this view.[168]

The view that the role of LH in the control of spermatogenesis is mediated via the stimulation of Leydig cell testosterone production is supported by the observation that Leydig cell adenomas in prepubertal boys are associated with a stimulation of spermatogenesis in the vicinity of the tumor but not at a distance.[170]

MAINTENANCE OF SPERMATOGENESIS. In the human and primate testis a strong case can be made that both FSH and testosterone are required for the maintenance of full spermatogenesis. Immunization of monkeys against FSH either actively[170] or passively[171] was associated with disruption of fertility and a decline in sperm concentrations, albeit not to zero. Furthermore, patients in whom pituitary tumors interrupted gonadotrophic secretion required both FSH and LH to cause a return of fertility.[172]

More recently, several studies by Bremner et al.[173] and Matsumoto and colleagues[174, 175] have supported the need for FSH but also posed several interesting and unanswered questions. They administered testosterone to normal men, causing a suppression of LH and FSH and resulting in a progressive decrease in sperm concentrations to azoospermic or severely oligospermic levels. In this model they noted that the additional stimulus of LH caused sperm counts to rise, presumably by stimulating intratesticular testosterone concentrations, but the sperm concentrations achieved did not reach normal. Thus stimulation of testosterone could, in the absence of detectable FSH, partially restore spermatogenesis. However, in the same model, if instead of hCG treatment FSH was administered, a similar increase in sperm count occurred.[173] This partial restoration of spermatogenesis occurred presumably in association with markedly suppressed endogenous intratesticular testosterone concentrations. As a result of these studies, it is reasonable to conclude that both FSH and LH (testosterone) are required to quantitatively stimulate spermatogenesis in man.

Studies of spermatogenesis in rats have questioned the requirement of FSH in view of the capacity of testosterone to maintain sperm production in hypophysectomized rats.[176] If the seminiferous epithelium was allowed to regress after hypophysectomy, however, testosterone was unable to restore spermatogenesis.[177] More recently these results have been challenged by studies which indicate that high-dose testosterone could restore spermatogenesis after posthypophysectomy regression in rats and monkeys.[178-180] All these studies suggested that the high local intratesticular concentrations of testosterone were sufficient to maintain spermatogenesis. This view was supported by observations in normal rats which showed that at low doses of testosterone administered by Silastic implants, spermatogenesis was disrupted but that as the testosterone dose was increased, spermatogenesis was maintained despite suppressed LH levels.[181, 182] However, Cunningham and Huckins[183] confirmed the results of the earlier study by Clermont and Harvey,[176] by the use of quantitative techniques which demonstrated that testosterone could maintain spermatogenesis at about 80 per cent of normal in hypophysectomized rats. It is significant, however, that this study demonstrated that intratesticular testosterone levels in these rats were only 10 to 20 per cent of normal, raising doubts about the specific requirement of high intratesticular concentrations of testosterone for the maintenance of spermatogenesis. A number of recent studies, using both intact and hypophysectomized rats, have reached similar conclusions concerning the concentrations of testosterone within the testis at which spermatogenesis was maintained.[179, 185, 186] A detailed dose-response study by Sun et al.[160] showed that the doses of testosterone required to take spermatogenesis from the suppressed state to the well-maintained range was relatively small (Fig. 130–15). The serum testosterone levels in these animals were equivalent to twice normal and resulted in intratesticular testosterone levels that were 10 to 20 per cent of normal. Although these doses of testosterone were required to maintain spermatogenesis, another androgen-dependent organ, the prostate gland, was grossly hypertrophied by the same levels of testosterone.[160] The differing responses in the prostate and seminiferous epi-

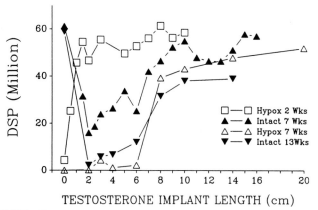

FIGURE 130–15. The relationship between daily sperm production (DSP) in intact and hypophysectomized adult rats maintained with differing doses of testosterone. The latter were achieved by the use of Silastic implants of different sizes. (From de Kretser DM (ed): Control of spermatogenesis by follicle stimulating hormone and testosterone. Bailliere's Clin Endocrinol Metab 6:335–354, 1992.)

thelium to these doses of testosterone raise questions as to the nature of the androgen receptors at each site and make it likely that other factors interact with testosterone or its receptors to maintain normal function at one site and yet cause hypertrophy at another.

The majority of the studies defining the role of testosterone in the maintenance of spermatogenesis have been relatively short term. In longer-term studies extending over 7 to 13 weeks, Sun et al.[160] showed that while testosterone could maintain spermatogenesis in hypophysectomized or intact rats at serum testosterone levels that were approximately twice normal, prolongation of the experiment led to failure of these doses to maintain daily sperm production in the normal range. Similar results demonstrating a subnormal maintenance of spermatogenesis in hypophysectomized rats were also noted in a study by Santulli et al.[186] These observations suggested that a pituitary factor, which was most likely to be FSH, was likely to be involved in the long-term maintenance of spermatogenesis. This possibility is supported by the increasing evidence that high doses of testosterone, rather than suppressing FSH further, cause the stimulation of FSH secretion.[160, 187, 188]

The site at which testosterone exerts its action on spermatogenesis still remains somewhat controversial. It was claimed that testosterone influenced a range of germ cell types, but these earlier studies did not use precise quantitative techniques.[177, 189-192] Other factors contributing to the varying results were the range of doses of testosterone used and the differing experimental designs. A recent study, utilizing morphometric techniques to define the stages of germ cell development that were influenced by testosterone and FSH, compared the responses of normal and hypophysectomized male rats to different doses of testosterone.[193] The results demonstrated that the transformation of round spermatids to spermatozoa, namely spermiogenesis, was highly dependent on testosterone, with lower doses of testosterone supporting the survival of round spermatids but higher doses being required to enable these cells to proceed to spermatozoa (Fig. 130–16). The studies demonstrated that the conversion of spermatogonia to spermatocytes and the latter to round spermatids were also testosterone dependent. However, the results of these studies, by comparing the responses of hypophysectomized to intact rats, strongly suggested that FSH was also likely to be required for the conversion of spermatogonia to spermatocytes, but particularly for the conversion of spermatocytes to round spermatids.

Several other studies have used models in which intact or hypophysectomized rats were treated with differing doses of testosterone and estradiol implants or were actively immunized against LH or GnRH.[194, 195] In their studies of hypophysectomized rats, they showed only limited recovery of spermatogenesis when high doses of testosterone were used, supporting the concept that a pituitary factor, probably FSH, was required for spermatogenic restoration. However, these results contrast with their studies using active immunization against GnRH in which they demonstrated that high doses of testosterone alone could fully restore, in a quantitative sense, spermatogenesis in these animals. These results contrast with the study by Sun et al.[193] and conclusions reached by Matsumoto.[196] Further studies are clearly required to clarify these issues.

In summary, it is clear that testosterone is an important factor in the maintenance of spermatogenesis, despite the absence of receptors on germ cells for this substance. Although still a matter of controversy, it is likely that FSH is required for the maintenance of spermatogenesis, but the relative amounts of FSH or testosterone may vary in different pathological states. The requirement for FSH is more evident in studies using primates and humans.

Feedback Control of FSH and LH by the Testis

The demonstration that FSH and LH secretion by the pituitary gland rises rapidly after castration establishes the existence of a negative feedback control by the testis on the production of the gonadotrophins. As the secretion of FSH and LH depend on the stimulation of the gonadotrophins by GnRH, these feedback effects may be exerted at the hypothalamus, resulting in a change in GnRH secretion, or may result from a direct action at the pituitary. The demonstration that FSH and LH are co-secreted by the majority of gonadotrophs raises intriguing questions about the manner in which stimulatory (GnRH) and inhibitory substances regulate their differential secretion.

Control of LH Secretion

Numerous studies have shown that testosterone, estradiol, and dihydrotestosterone exert a negative modulation of LH secretion.[197, 198] Controversy existed about whether testosterone could directly exert this action or had to be metabolized to estradiol or dihydrotestosterone.[199] The demonstration that nonaromatizable androgens could inhibit LH secretion resolved this issue.[200] This careful study by Santen[200] showed that estradiol probably acted at the pituitary by decreasing LH pulse amplitude without changing pulse frequency, whereas testosterone probably acted at the hypothalamus by decreasing pulse frequency without a change in pulse amplitude. In a recent study, experimental proof of this concept was provided by demonstrating that the pulse frequency of GnRH secretion in portal blood was decreased by the treatment of castrated animals with

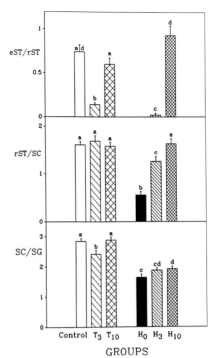

FIGURE 130–16. The conversion ratios for spermatogonia (SG) to primary spermatocytes (SC), primary spermatocytes to round spermatids (rST), and round spermatids to elongated spermatids (eST) are shown in intact (control) and hypophysectomized (H_o) rats treated for 13 weeks with testosterone-containing Silastic implants of 3 or 10 cm. (From Sun YT, Wreford NG, Robertson DM, de Kretser DM: Quantitative cytological studies of spermatogenesis in intact and hypophysectomized rats: Identification of androgen-dependent stages. Endocrinology 127:1215–1223, 1990, © 1990 by the Endocrine Society.)

testosterone.[201] These studies also showed no change in portal blood GnRH secretory patterns during treatment with estradiol, which lowered LH levels by decreasing LH pulse amplitude.[201]

Control of FSH Secretion

The factors involved in the control of FSH have been a matter of some controversy for many years. This debate has centered on the concept that the steroid hormones testosterone and estradiol could account for the entire negative feedback exerted by the testis[202] on FSH secretion and that there was no need to postulate the presence of a specific FSH feedback substance, namely inhibin.[203] The existence of inhibin[204] has been established as discussed earlier in this book (see Ch. 114), and this section explores the roles of testosterone and inhibin in the control of FSH secretion.

ROLE OF TESTOSTERONE. Several studies have shown that testosterone could suppress FSH secretion in a number of species when administered at amounts equivalent to or greater than its production rate.[197, 198] When administered to castrated rats,[202] increasing doses of testosterone suppressed both FSH and LH secretion. However, in their study and those of others,[205] the highest doses of testosterone decreased LH to the undetectable range, but the FSH levels plateaued in the normal range and could not be suppressed further. More recently, several investigators have shown that at very high doses of testosterone, FSH levels increased,[160, 187] indicating a complex relationship between testosterone and FSH secretion. Perhaps the most convincing data supporting a physiological role for testosterone in the control of FSH emerged from the experiments in rats in which the Leydig cells were destroyed by the cytotoxin ethane dimethane sulphonate (EDS). EDS treatment resulted in a rapid decline in testosterone levels and a rapid increase in FSH concentrations.[77, 206] It is important to note that the FSH levels in these experiments reached only 50 per cent of castrate levels, and it is likely that the continuing feedback control was achieved by inhibin, which was maintained after EDS treatment.[207] In fact, when EDS was given to rats in which the induction of cryptorchidism had resulted in increased FSH levels associated with decreased inhibin concentrations,[208] the removal of testosterone feedback increased FSH levels to the castrate range.[209] It is clear from this brief summary of a number of papers that testosterone can exert an inhibitory control on FSH secretion, but its precise role relative to inhibin may vary according to the physiological circumstances and the species concerned. In the rat, about 50 per cent of the feedback may result from testosterone and 50 per cent from inhibin.

ROLE OF INHIBIN. The isolation of inhibin A[204] and inhibin B[210] from follicular fluid was associated with the demonstration that these two forms of inhibin are equally potent in suppressing FSH. Both inhibin A and inhibin B are disulfide-linked dimers consisting of a common α-subunit with specific β-subunits termed β_A and β_B. Further details of the structure of these subunits and their secretion as larger precursor proteins secreted under the control of separate genes are discussed earlier, in Chapter 114.[211, 212] In the male, inhibin has been isolated to homogeneity from ram rete testis fluid and has been shown to have a structure identical to that of ovine inhibin isolated from ovarian follicular fluid.[213, 214]

Following the isolation of inhibin, dimers of the β-subunit, termed activin, were also isolated from porcine follicular fluid on the basis of their ability to stimulate FSH, in contrast to the effect of inhibin, which suppresses this hormone.[215, 216] Two forms of activin were identified, namely activin A ($\beta_A \beta_A$) and activin AB ($\beta_A \beta_B$). Activin B has been produced by recombinant DNA technology and has also been shown to have the capacity of stimulating FSH.[217] Subsequent studies demonstrated the existence of a further suppressor of FSH, namely follistatin or FSH-suppressing protein.[218, 219] This protein is unrelated to inhibin and was isolated in three molecular weight forms—39, 35, and 31 kDa—all of which shared a common N-terminal sequence. These forms may arise by alternative splicing from the multiple exons contributing to this protein which bears no structural homology to inhibin.[220] The three forms of follistatin that are identified in these studies had 10 to 30 per cent of the biopotency of inhibin in the rat pituitary cell bioassay.[219] However, more recently, the production of follistatin by recombinant DNA technology has demonstrated a 288-amino acid form that has a similar biopotency to inhibin.[221] It is still unclear whether follistatin acts directly on the pituitary gonadotroph or through another property, namely that of its capacity to bind activin.[222] In regard to the latter, several studies have demonstrated that follistatin binding can neutralize the biopotency of activin, and because both of these substances are produced within the pituitary gland, these results question whether follistatin has a direct action at that level.[223]

In the male, several earlier studies using bioassay measurements demonstrated that inhibin was produced by immature Sertoli cells in culture.[137, 224] These results were subsequently confirmed by the demonstration that immature Sertoli cell cultures secrete immunoassayable inhibin.[138] Further confirmation of this secretory capacity of the Sertoli cells came from the demonstration that mRNA for the α, β_A, and β_B subunits was found in the Sertoli cell.[225] These studies suggested that the predominant form of inhibin in the adult rat testis may be inhibin B, as the predominant β-subunit message in the adult testis was β_B.[226] Several studies in intact and hypophysectomized rats have suggested that FSH stimulates α-subunit production without altering β-subunit message.[226, 227] It is important to note that excessive FSH stimulation leads to the production of an α-subunit, pro-α_C, which is immunoactive but not bioactive.[228, 229]

In addition to a Sertoli cell source of inhibin, Leydig cells have now been shown to secrete both immunoactive and bioactive inhibin.[230] LH stimulation leads to an increase in immunoactive inhibin but not bioactive inhibin, raising the possibility that α-subunit products may be the result of LH stimulation. The relative contribution of the Leydig cells to inhibin secretion is still unclear, although some investigators have suggested that this may be a minor component.[231]

The failure of bioactive levels to rise following LH stimulation may result from the production of activins, because Lee et al.[232] have suggested that Leydig cell lines and Leydig cells in culture have the capacity to secrete a substance with the capability of increasing FSH, namely activin. Further studies are necessary to confirm the site of activin production within the testis. This may be of some importance in view of the demonstrated capacity of activin to stimulate spermatogonial mitosis[233] and the presence of activin receptors on primary spermatocytes, round spermatids, and Sertoli cells.[235] Similarly, the source of testicular follistatin needs to be clarified. mRNA for follistatin has been detected in the testis,[235] but its cellular site has not been specifically identified.

It is clear that the production by the testis of substances that are capable of suppressing or stimulating FSH further complicates our understanding of the mechanisms of feedback control of this gonadotrophic hormone. The description of the changes in FSH secretion in rats following EDS treatment provides convincing evidence for a role of inhibin in the control of FSH secretion. Further support for this concept has emerged from the studies of Dubey et al.[236] in primates. They showed that in arcuate nucleus–lesioned monkeys maintained on a constant GnRH pulse regimen, testosterone could prevent the postcastration rise in LH but not FSH. In subsequent experiments they demonstrated that partially purified inhibin from porcine follicular fluid could prevent this postcastration rise in FSH secretion.[237]

Further support for a role of inhibin in the control of FSH emerged from passive immunization experiments in male monkeys wherein administration of an antiserum to inhibin raised by immunization against an α-subunit peptide resulted in a monotropic increase in FSH secretion.[238] Some evidence for a species difference emerged from the observation that the same antiserum, when given to rats, could cause an increase only in immature rats but not in adults[239] unless they were rendered testosterone deficient by prior treatment with EDS.[240]

The capacity of recombinant human inhibin (rh-inhibin) to suppress FSH has been shown in 30-day-old rats,[241] with the nadir occurring 6 to 8 hours after injection (Fig. 130–17).[242] Similar actions of rh-inhibin have been shown in castrate rams,[243] and synergism in the control of FSH was found when the animals were pretreated with testosterone. No effect of inhibin on LH secretion was demonstrable in these studies.

Because the purification of inhibin utilized a rat anterior pituitary cell bioassay, it is evident that this glycoprotein acts at the pituitary cell through a receptor yet to be identified. At the pituitary it decreases FSH β-subunit mRNA.[244, 245] To date no convincing evidence has emerged to support a hypothalamic action of inhibin.

The isolation of dimers of the β-subunit of inhibin, termed activins,[215, 216] which raise FSH have complicated the control of FSH further, especially in view of the presence of α- and β-subunit mRNA in the pituitary gland, particularly in gonadotrophs.[246] That this mRNA functions emerged from the data of Corrigan et al.,[247] who showed that a monoclonal antibody to activin B, when added to

pituitary cells in culture, causes a suppression of FSH secretion. However in these experiments they noted that inhibin, when added to these cultures, produced a suppression of FSH despite the presence of the activin antiserum demonstrating an action of inhibin independent of activin.

The data supporting a role for inhibin in the control of FSH are consistent with the decrease in inhibin secretion by Sertoli cells and the rise in FSH in a number of models of spermatogenic damage such as cryptorchidism[208] and intratesticular glycerol treatment.[248] However, in infertile men, a surprising finding was the normal levels of serum inhibin in men with severe damage to the seminiferous epithelium.[249] In patients with Klinefelter's syndrome, the elevated FSH levels were associated with low, normal, or high inhibin levels; the latter observation was surprising in view of the severe degree of seminiferous tubule damage in which germ cells and, frequently, Sertoli cells were absent.

Two possibilities may account for these unexpected observations: (1) Leydig cells recently have been shown to produce inhibin,[230] and the source of inhibin in Klinefelter's syndrome patients may be the Leydig cells, but this would still not explain the elevated FSH levels. (2) Several studies have shown that products of the α subunit alone (pro-α_C) may be found at sources where mRNA's for the inhibin subunits are localized.[250, 251] Pro-α_C cross-reacts (288 per cent) with the antiserum used to measure inhibin but has no capacity to suppress FSH, and consequently the inhibin produced by the testis in Klinefelter's syndrome may represent pro-α_C.

INTERACTIONS BETWEEN CELL TYPES WITHIN THE TESTIS

Interactions Within the Tubules

The anatomical description of the seminiferous epithelium which precedes this section has discussed the structural organization of the cellular components of the epithelium. That section of this chapter described the intimate association of the Sertoli cells with the germ cells and the presence of the blood-testis barrier, which effectively creates a specialized intratubular environment. In addition, the basal aspect of the epithelium is in continuous contact with the basal lamina, being directly in contact with the basement membrane and interstitial fluids. Hence at least four different types of interactions can occur in the epithelium; these are between (1) Sertoli cells, (2) germ cells, (3) Sertoli and germ cells, or (4) Sertoli cells and peritubular cells.

Sertoli–Sertoli Cell Interactions

Ultrastructural details of the junctional specializations between adjacent Sertoli cells have been discussed previously, and the junctional complexes are thought to be composed of occluding, gap, and close junctions. The occluding junctions result, in part, in the formation of the blood-testis barrier in the mammalian testis. In addition, processes from one Sertoli cell can invaginate the cytoplasm of an adjacent Sertoli cell to give rise to a structure

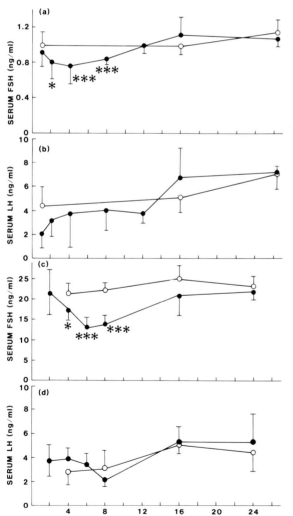

FIGURE 130–17. The responses of serum FSH and LH (●) in 35-day-old three-day castrate rats treated with bovine follicular fluid (100 μl/100 g body wt; *a* and *b*) or human recombinant inhibin (10 μg/100 g body wt; *c* and *d*) are shown relative to the number of hours after administration. Saline-injected controls are also shown (○). (From Robertson DM, Prisk M, McMaster J, et al: Serum FSH suppressing activity of human recombinant inhibin A in male and female rats. J Reprod Fertil 91:321–328, 1991.)

termed the *tubulobular complex,* which provides another form of physical interaction between Sertoli cells in vivo.

The junctional particles involved in these physical interactions between cells have been suggested to consist of protein or lipid.[252-255] The strongest evidence that proteins are involved in the occluding junction complexes has come from the observation that inhibitors of protein synthesis increase their permeability of the occluding junctions.[256, 257] More recently it has been shown that a polypeptide ZO-1 (zona occludens 1) is present in the immature mouse testis on Sertoli cell plasma membrane prior to the formation of the blood-testis barrier. Following formation of a competent barrier, ZO-1 is found only at the site of the junctional specializations associated with tight junctions[258] and is thought to have a role in linking the submembrane cytoskeleton and membrane components of the occluding junction.

Other molecules that may be associated with cell junctions between these epithelial Sertoli cells include cingulin and the cadherin class of cell-adhesion molecules. The formation of intercellular junctions requires cell adhesion, and the cadherins L-CAM and N-CAM have been detected in the testis, but at present no other adhesion molecules commonly localized to adhering junctions in other epithelia have been identified in the testis. The means by which the Sertoli cell regulates the expression of ZO-1 and other junctional molecules remains to be determined, especially during the dismantling and reformation of the occluding junctions.

Sertoli Cell–Germ Cell Interactions

There are a number of consequences of the structural communications between Sertoli cells; the barrier so formed is selectively permeable to the entry and exit of some substances so that a unique microenvironment for the developing germ cell populations is provided as well as presenting an immunological barrier in the testis. Therefore, the Sertoli cells must communicate with the germ cells. Specialized cell junctions (tight junctions, gap junctions, and adhering junctions) between Sertoli cell membrane segments that face adjoining germ cell membranes provide structural sites of communication between these cell types, as do the tubulobular complexes. It is believed that through these sites the germ cells can directly or indirectly influence the function of the Sertoli cells and vice versa.

All germ cells, particularly those in the luminal compartment, are dependent on the Sertoli cells for survival; therefore they must influence Sertoli cell function so that adequate provision is made for their development. This influence on Sertoli cell function ensures that serum proteins, nutrients, hormones, and metabolic activities required for germ cell survival, development, and function are procured at the correct time by the appropriate cell types.

The data providing evidence that these interactions occurred in vivo were initially derived from microscopic examinations showing that Sertoli cell structure changed in a cyclic manner with the stages of the seminiferous epithelium. These studies noted changes in the volume of Sertoli cells,[259] the organization of the cytoplasmic components

of the cell,[62, 63, 260] and the shape and position of the nuclei.[261, 262]

Unequivocal evidence that the Sertoli cells modulate their secretory functions according to the developmental stage of the germ cells has been provided by the identification of a number of Sertoli cell secretory products, together with the demonstration that their production occurs in a cyclical fashion. The acquisition of much of this knowledge was made possible with the pioneering technique of transillumination-assisted dissection of each individual stage of the seminiferous tubule as developed and modified by Parvinen.[147] More sophisticated techniques of cell isolation and culture have also been employed to study specific interactions between germ cells and Sertoli cells in vitro.[263, 264] Using these techniques the Sertoli cell products have been identified as binding protein or transport molecules that are involved in the delivery of essential chemicals or hormones to the germ cells, or as hormones or cytokines thought to have an integral role in the local regulation of seminiferous tubule function.[265, 266] Many of these protein products and numerous mRNA species have been shown to be produced in a cyclical manner.

The general *metabolic* requirements of the Sertoli cells can vitally influence germ cell survival, and it was demonstrated that Sertoli cells could produce glucose metabolites such as inositol[267] and pyruvate and lactate.[144, 268] Both pyruvate and lactate are efficient energy sources for the germ cells, and it was postulated that the Sertoli cells could provide these metabolites to the germ cells; furthermore, the transport and metabolism of glucose by the Sertoli cells was stimulated by FSH.[142, 143] The means by which the metabolites are then delivered to the germ cells across the physical barriers between the germ cells and Sertoli cells remain to be determined.

Other nutritional requirements of the germ cells such as essential *ions* and *vitamins* are transported from outside the blood-testis barrier to the germ cells via the action of binding or transport proteins. Testicular transferrin is an iron-binding protein that delivers iron to the cell through a receptor-mediated endocytotic process.[269, 270] Transferrin is a secretory product of the Sertoli cell regulated by FSH, and although all cells have transferrin receptors, particularly high concentrations of transferrin receptors have been localized to pachytene spermatocytes.[271, 272] Ceruloplasmin is a binding and transport protein for copper that is thought to act in a manner similar, but not identical, to that of transferrin in the delivery of copper to the germ cells.[273] All cells require iron to maintain respiration and cytochrome function, and copper is required as a coenzyme for proteins and feroxidase. More recently Cheng[274] isolated a protein (SPARC) from primary Sertoli cell culture which is believed to be involved in the binding and transport of calcium. The role of vitamins in the maintenance of testis function has led to numerous studies of vitamin A retinoids. Sertoli cells respond to vitamin A by increased synthesis of secretory products such as transferrin, and retinoid-binding proteins are localized in Sertoli cells themselves. But vitamin A is essential for germ cells, and deprivation results in a disruption of spermatogenesis,[275] suggesting a direct effect on the germ cells themselves. The means by which retinoid transport to germ cells is facilitated remains to be determined.

The transport of *lipids* has not been examined thoroughly in the testis, although it has been demonstrated that lipid inclusions in the Sertoli cell cytoplasm show significant stage-dependent variation.[261] Sulfated glycoprotein 1 (SGP-1) is a specific lipid-binding protein that is secreted by Sertoli cells.[276] It has been identified as a form of sphingolipid-binding protein,[277] but the lipid specificity of SGP-1 is still unclear. Lipid-binding proteins are also thought to be required in the metabolism and degradation of residual bodies by Sertoli cells during spermatogenesis.

Numerous serum-derived hormones and locally produced factors present in interstitial fluid are required by the germ cell populations in the adluminal compartment but are accessible via the Sertoli cell. Thus many *receptors* or *binding proteins* for these substances are also present on Sertoli cells. Androgens essential for the maintenance of the seminiferous epithelium can enter the Sertoli cells by binding to the androgen receptor or androgen-binding protein (ABP), both of which are located on the Sertoli cell. ABP was initially thought to transport androgens to the germ cells, but it is now considered to be involved in transporting androgens to the luminal surface of the epithelium and thence to the male reproductive tract, which contains androgen-dependent tissues.[278] Nevertheless, based on observations using transillumination-assisted microdisections of rat seminiferous tubules, ABP production has been shown to be stage specific; this suggests that ABP may have a role in the epithelium that is regulated by the germ cell populations contained within.[279] Production of the androgen receptor is also stage dependent (based on mRNA levels or binding studies) and, as may be expected, the highest levels of receptor binding are detected at stages seven and eight, which are the most sensitive to the effects of androgen withdrawal. FSH is another serum-derived hormone that is required for spermatogenesis, and the FSH receptor has been localized to Sertoli cells. Both the level of FSH binding and mRNA receptor levels have been shown to be stage-dependently regulated.[280] Accordingly, a number of Sertoli cells products known to be regulated by FSH have been shown to be stage-specifically produced or localized, for example, inhibin, testibumin clusterin, and α_2 macroglobulin.[281, 282] α_2 Macroglobulin is a protease inhibitor and may be involved in the epithelial cell remodeling as well as playing a major role in inhibiting the release of sperm through its action on proteases. It also binds growth factors or cytokines such as TGF-β and interleukin-1α and hence could affect the production and local action of these cytokines in vivo. The stage-specific distribution of other substances such as SGP-2, decarboxylase, and cyclic protein-2 would indicate that there is a specific requirement for these products at particular stages of germ cell development.[283, 284] Because the precise function of some of these substances remains to be determined, it can only be postulated at the present time that the germ cells regulate these Sertoli cells products for this purpose.

Although some *hormones* or *cytokines* required by the germ cells may be serum derived, a number of substances thought to be involved in Sertoli–germ cell interactions are synthesized by Sertoli cells themselves. Although these substances may be secreted through the basal surface of the epithelium and into the interstitium and peripheral circulation, or secreted apically, they may also act directly on the germ cells in the epithelium itself.

GONOCYTE/SPERMATOGONIAL CELL–SERTOLI CELL INTERACTIONS. In the developing testis, Orth and her co-workers[285, 286] have investigated the functional coupling of neonatal Sertoli cells and gonocytes in co-cultures and have produced data to suggest that gap junction–mediated communication between these cells may be involved in stimulating and regulating changes in the gonocyte population during postnatal development of the testis. In the adult testis, the existence of a positive promotor of spermatogonial cell proliferation was first suggested by Dym and Clermont.[287] Seminiferous growth factor (SGF) was one of the first factors to be identified with mitogenic properties that could potentially act on spermatogenic cells.[288] However mitogenicity was demonstrated on somatic but not spermatogenic cells, and further studies are required to determine if SGF can indeed promote germ cell proliferation. Since then, a number of cytokines have been identified with inhibitory or stimulatory actions on germ cell proliferation. An interleukin-1–like factor (tIL-1) originates from the seminiferous tubules, most probably from the Sertoli cells,[289, 290] and it has been postulated that tIL-1 is a spermatogonial growth factor. Along the wave of the seminiferous epithelium, tIL-1 secretion and content were found to correlate with spermatogonial DNA synthesis.[291] More specifically, Parvinen et al.[292] have shown that tIL-1 stimulates spermatogonial DNA synthesis in both meiotic and mitotic phases; although these effects are mainly stimulatory, inhibitory effects can be demonstrated under specific conditions, indicating a further degree of complexity in the regulation of these events. Most recently Woodruff et al.[293] have identified stage-specific binding of inhibin and activin to subpopulations of rat germ cells. FITC-labeled inhibin-A, activin-A, and activin-B were used to localize binding to germ cells in co-culture. Inhibin-A binding was to spermatogonia, spermatocytes, and early spermatids, whereas activin binding was greater to spermatogonia. These data are consistent with a previous observation[233] that activin stimulates spermatogonial cell proliferation in vitro; the demonstration that receptors are present on the spermatogonia indicates that this is a direct action of activin.

SPERMATOCYTE–SERTOLI CELL INTERACTIONS. In contrast to Sertoli cell–derived products, nerve growth factor (NGF) is the only putative germ cell product that has been postulated to mediate the interaction between germ cells and Sertoli cells through binding to Sertoli cells. β-NGF gene expression and NGF immunoreactivity have been localized to spermatocytes and early spermatids[294, 295]; NGF receptor gene expression has been identified in Sertoli cells and is under androgen regulation.[154] Together this suggests that germ cells produce NGF, which may bind to NGF receptors on the Sertoli cell to mediate an effect, but the production of the NGF peptide itself and the demonstration of an action on Sertoli cells remain to be elucidated.

Co-cultures of germ cells and Sertoli cells have been used to demonstrate direct actions of germ cells on Sertoli cell functions, although in many cases the means by which these interactions occur is not known. Galdieri et al.[296] reported that pachytene primary spermatocytes that were directly in contact with Sertoli cells stimulated the production of ABP. Numerous reports since then have shown that different types of germ cells, spermatocytes, and spermatids can influence immature Sertoli cell function by direct or indirect contact, using a variety of in vitro culture conditions. Rat pachytene primary spermatocytes stimulate Sertoli cell protein synthesis, specifically transferrin, proteins S1 and S2, and ABP, but inhibit estradiol production.[297, 298] These general effects are observed in co-cultures or with the addition of spent media to conventional Sertoli cell cultures or polarized layers of Sertoli cells cultured in bicameral chambers on extracellular matrix,[299] although variations in the responses were reported with Sertoli cells prepared from different ages of animals.[300] Contact between these cells may involve binding interactions and Le Magueresse and Jégou[298] showed that primary spermatocytes adhered to Sertoli cells through a specific binding process that was time and temperature dependent and required the viability of the cells to be retained; this binding could be regulated hormonally by, for example, FSH. A further analysis of the binding kinetics by Enders and Millette[301] demonstrated that binding of pachytene spermatocytes to Sertoli cells was different from that between spermatids and Sertoli cells.

SPERMATID–SERTOLI CELL INTERACTIONS. The involvement of step one to eight spermatids in the production of substances which influence Sertoli cell ABP, transferrin, inhibin, γ-glutamyl transpeptidases, ceruloplasmin, SGP1 and 2, or aromatase activity has been clearly demonstrated.[302] Whether or not late spermatids are also able to secrete factors that regulate Sertoli cell function is unknown. Nevertheless, Jégou has speculated that this may be possible; in discussing potential ways in which this interaction could occur, he has proposed that residual bodies may be involved. Specifically, he suggests that residual bodies may contain mRNA species which control Sertoli cell gene expression or that the act of phagocytosis of residual bodies by the Sertoli cell may be analogous to the monocyte/macrophage system and trigger the release of potent cytokines such as interleukins.[302, 303] Additionally, alterations in the type of adhesive contact between late spermatids and Sertoli cells or an effect of late spermatids on the cytoskeletal organization of the Sertoli cell could provide other means of influencing Sertoli cell gene expression.

Conversely, the role of Sertoli cell products in the regulation of spermatid function has been discussed and reviewed. The direction of this interaction is achieved through the secretion of a number of putative Sertoli cell factors which may also involve the structural points of contact between these cells.[82, 303] However, this control may be via the action of systemic hormones such as FSH and testosterone. In this context Cameron and Muffly[304] have recently shown that spermatid binding to Sertoli cells is stimulated by a combination of FSH and testosterone. FSH is required to obtain peripheral distribution of junction-related actin around the Sertoli-spermatid junctional complex. This reorganization of the cytoskeleton then optimizes and stabilizes the actual cell-cell binding event between the Sertoli cells and spermatids.

An alternative approach to investigate the role of germ cells in the regulation of Sertoli cell function is to observe the effects of germ cell depletion by damage to the seminiferous epithelium. A variety of means to achieve this effect are available, including heat treatment of the testis, which results in the loss of the most heat-sensitive stages, the primary spermatocytes and round spermatids.[305] The consequent changes in Sertoli cell function correspond with the temporal loss and recovery of the spermatid population.[306, 307] Similarly, the temporary disruption of the seminiferous epithelium by the withdrawal of testosterone, following the administration of EDS (see review by

Sharpe[308]) has yielded further evidence that specific interactions occur between the germ cells and Sertoli cells and that these are hormonally regulated in vivo. The development of more sophisticated culture techniques should allow revelation of the exact means by which these interactions occur. Given the complexity and organization of the epithelium, a combination of endocrine and paracrine factors is probably involved in maintaining the interaction.

Sertoli–Peritubular Cell Interactions

The stromal cells that surround the basal surface of the Sertoli cells in the seminiferous tubule are peritubular myoid cells.[9] These cells contact the basal surface of the Sertoli cells and provide another means of cellular interaction with the tubule. It is believed that these cells provide the structural integrity for the tubule and are involved in the contractile motions of the tubules, as well contributing to the blood-testis barrier.

The structural integrity of the tubules is vitally important to the maintenance of testis function and is mediated by extracellular matrix. The extracellular matrix is co-operatively produced by both the Sertoli cells and the peritubular cells. Sertoli cells produce laminin, collagen types I and IV, and proteoglycans; peritubular cells produce collagen type I, proteoglycans, and fibronectin.[309] Therefore from the individual components of the two cell types a fully functional basement membrane can be synthesized. The importance of the deposition of extracellular matrix has been convincingly demonstrated by the culture of Sertoli cells, either on matrix-coated surfaces or with peritubular cells, and the subsequent determination of their structure and function in vitro.[310, 311] Sertoli cells cultured on ECM, as opposed to plastic, form tight junctions, and a polarized layer of cells develop and exhibit many of the features of Sertoli cells in the epithelium in vivo.[311] Bidirectional, that is, basal or apical, secretion of Sertoli cell secretory products such as inhibin, transferrin, and ABP has been demonstrated in association with these structural features.[312–314]

A number of other products of the peritubular cells could influence Sertoli cell function because co-culture with peritubular cells themselves or with peritubular cell–conditioned media increases the production of a number of Sertoli cell proteins such as ABP and transferrin.[315–319] Proteins termed P-Mod-S have been purified from peritubular cell culture media and shown to stimulate most functions of Sertoli cells such as ABP, transferrin, and inhibin production[122, 123, 320] but to inhibit others such as aromatase activity.[321] It has also been postulated that P-Mod-S may be involved in the action of androgens on Sertoli cells because androgens enhance the productions of P-Mod-S, which, in turn, can regulate Sertoli cell functions as discussed above. This provides an alternative means of androgen action on the Sertoli cells, and peritubular cells are known to possess receptors for androgens.[120] The specificity of the androgen-dependent interaction between the peritubular stromal cells and the epithelial Sertoli cells was raised by the interesting report from Swinnen et al.[322] Stromal cells from another androgen-dependent tissue, the prostate, could alter Sertoli cell functions in a manner similar to that of peritubular stromal cells, but footsole fibroblasts, which are unresponsive to androgens, could not. Proteins such as P-Mod-S may be important in the induction and differentiation of Sertoli cells but may also represent a more general class of proteins involved in mediating stromal-epithelial cell interactions in other tissues under androgenic regulation. The purification of these proteins is required in order to test these hypotheses and to determine their actions in vivo.

Peritubular cells also produce a number of growth factors that may represent paracrine agents of communication between the Sertoli cells and peritubular cells; these include the EGF, TGF-α, TGF-β, and IGF-I. TGF-α is synthesised by both Sertoli cells and peritubular cells, but functional receptors have been located only on the peritubular cells.[323] TGF-α/EGF stimulates peritubular cell growth and can alter some Sertoli cell functions,[323–325] but its exact role remains to be elucidated. TGF-β is produced by both Sertoli cells and peritubular cells and inhibits the growth-promoting action of TGF-α.[326] TGF-β itself has significant effects on peritubular cell migration and colony formation in vitro and may be involved in the structural organization of the tubules; Sertoli cell functions do not appear to respond to TGF-β. Even less information is available on the site of production and action of IGI 1 and its role in the interaction between Sertoli cells and peritubular cells. Such a role can only be postulated in view of the reports that IGI-I and its binding proteins and receptors are present in the testis and IGF can influence some Sertoli cell functions.[327–329]

As previously discussed, the Sertoli cell produces plasminogen activator, and peak levels of this protein coincide with the translocation of germ cells from the basal to the apical region of the epithelium. This requires the dismantling and reformation of the tight junctions between the Sertoli cells, and it has been suggested that plasminogen activator may influence the modulation of Sertoli cell tight junctions.[330–332] A protease inhibitor is produced by peritubular cells which inhibits plasminogen activator activity,[333] so the peritubular cells may play a role in the regulation of protease activity in the seminiferous tubule, as well as controlling the level of degradation of the extracellular matrix.[331]

Interactions Within the Interstitium

The space separating individual seminiferous tubules contains numerous cell types, lymphatic and vascular vessels, and fluids including Leydig cells, macrophages, vascular, and lymphatic endothelial cells. Local interactions in the interstitium have focused mainly on the Leydig cells and have been associated with either the regulation of steroidogenesis, the mediation of inflammatory response, or the development of Leydig cells. In the rat the notion of a functional interaction between Leydig cells and macrophages was suggested by the previous observation that these cells can be observed in intimate association in vivo via specialized points of contact.[334] The local regulation of Leydig cell steroidogenesis was suggested[335] by the demonstration that isolated media from macrophage cultures could stimulate Leydig cell testosterone production in vitro. The stimulatory action of testicular macrophage products on steroidgenesis was specific and not exhibited using peritoneal macrophage products; it was also stimulated by FSH, which can be endocytosed by testicular macro-

phages.[335] A number of other substances secreted by macrophages have the potential to regulate steroidogenesis by Leydig cells, including interleukins. In vitro these are potent regulators of testosterone, but there are discrepant reports in the literature concerning their effects. Hence IL-1α has been reported as an inhibitor[336] or stimulator of testosterone synthesis.[337–339]

IL-1, as well as TNF-α and IFN-γ, are mediators of inflammation, and although macrophage products may be involved in inflammation-like responses in the testis, this response can be induced by hyperstimulation of the Leydig cells with hCG.[340] Because hCG binds principally to the Leydig cells, it has been suggested that the Leydig cell had a role in the mediation of the inflammatory response involving mast cell secretion, infiltration of PMN cells and increased blood flow, capillary permeability, and interstitial fluid accumulation.[341–343] This was confirmed by the demonstration that the selective removal of Leydig cells using the cytotoxic drug ethane dimethane sulfonate prevented the inflammation-like changes induced by hCG administration.[340] These findings suggest that hyperstimulation of Leydig cells, which provokes an inflammatory response, can involve an interaction between the Leydig cells and macrophages. The testis is considered to be an immunologically privileged site and a further consequence of Leydig cell–macrophage interactions is thought to include a role in immunoprotection; macrophages in other tissues have been shown to secrete immunosuppressive factors as well as activate T-cells. Therefore Leydig cells may regulate the macrophages by inhibiting antigen-presenting functions as well as inducing immunosuppressive functions.[344]

The origin of Leydig cells, either during fetal life or at puberty, is currently believed to be from mesenchymal stem cells located in the peritubular or perivascular regions of the testis.[29, 345] In vivo studies have suggested that local interactions are involved in this process based on several interesting observations. First, FSH administration has been reported to induce the differentiation of Leydig cells in the immature rat testis.[346] Because the Sertoli cells are target tissues for FSH in the testis, it was proposed that FSH stimulation of seminiferous tubule factors may induce the differentiation of Leydig cells. This view was contested by Molenaar et al.,[347] who were able to induce the differentiation of Leydig cells (after the destruction of the existent population of Leydig cells with EDS treatment) with the administration of LH/hCG. Although these data appear to be contradictory, an explanation may lie in the proposal that the development of fetal or adult Leydig cells is a multistep process. The recruitment of mesenchymal cells from the perivascular or peritubular regions of the testis is first stimulated by unknown factors into the pathway leading to the development of intermediate Leydig cell precursors; this involves proliferation of these cell types as has been observed in vivo.[348] The proliferation of these cells can be advanced by the induction of seminiferous tubule damage, indicating that local factors can regulate mitosis of these cells.[347, 349] The next phase involves differentiation of Leydig cell precursors to fetal or adult Leydig cells and is considered to be controlled by LH. This latter process has been investigated more thoroughly in vitro; the Leydig cell precursors have been isolated and a role for LH together with the androgen DHT has been established.[350, 351] Finally a detailed stereological study of rat Leydig cell development at puberty has shown that the

Leydig cells present in the 28-day-old rat testis must divide mitotically in order to achieve the full number of Leydig cells in the adult testis[352] at 56 days of age. Although the administration of LH can stimulate Leydig cell mitosis in the adult rat testis,[112] Kahn et al.[353] have recently demonstrated that locally produced factors such as TGF-β and IGF-I can stimulate DNA synthesis by immature Leydig cells. Thus local interactions may determine the proliferative state of Leydig cells during development. Further progress requires the unique characteristics of the Leydig cell precursors to be identified and used as markers in order to explore the process of Leydig cell development and its regulation by peripheral and local hormones or factors.

Interactions Between the Tubules and Interstitium

The major cellular components of these compartments are the Sertoli cells and the Leydig cells, respectively. These cells are not in physical contact with one another, but through the action of secreted proteins each can profoundly influence the functional activity and morphology of the other.

A number of recent reviews have discussed in detail the considerable body of evidence that interactions occur between the Sertoli cells and Leydig cells.[354, 355] This interaction is viewed as being bidirectional, so that not only do Leydig cell products influence Sertoli cell (and more generally seminiferous tubule) function, but Sertoli cell products influence Leydig cell functions.

The endocrine control of Leydig cell testosterone secretion by LH, and the subsequent paracrine action of testosterone on the process of spermatogenesis, is unequivocal. The paracrine action of other Leydig cell–derived products is not as well investigated or understood. It is believed that the Leydig cells can secrete a number of peptides and proteins; some of these that could potentially have a regulatory action on Sertoli cells include renin[356] and angiotensin,[357] oxytocin,[358] and prodynorphin,[359] but the functional and physical roles of these substances are not understood at the present time. More is known about the action of POMC and related peptides such as α-MSH, β-endorphin, and ACTH.[360, 361] Minor stimulatory actions of α-MSH and ACTH on Sertoli cells have been recorded in vitro which may suggest roles in vivo.[362] On the other hand, β-endorphin synthesis and secretion have been detected in fetal Leydig cell preparations,[361] receptors for opiates have been localized to Sertoli cells,[363] and β-endorphin has been shown to influence Sertoli cell division in the postnatal testis[285, 364] and inhibin production in the immature testis.[362] These data suggest that the paracrine actions of β-endorphin on Sertoli cells are important during fetal and postnatal development of the testis.

The hypothesis that Sertoli cell products could exert a paracrine influence on Leydig cell activity and particularly testosterone production was not seriously investigated until the 1970's. This concept was advanced by Aoki and Fawcett[365] to explain their observations that damage to the seminiferous tubule and a disruption of spermatogenesis resulted in morphological changes to the Leydig cells. This concept was novel, as it was generally believed that LH was the only regulator of Leydig cell function; since then a

number of studies have provided both morphological and functional evidence of support. Several methods of experimentally induced disruption of spermatogenesis have been used, including vitamin A deficiency, X-irradiation in utero, cryptorchidism, efferent duct ligation, and heat treatment, all of which have resulted in abnormal Leydig cell function and cytological features.[275, 366–369] Histological examination of abnormal and normal interstitial tissues has also implied that such a regulatory interaction exists and that it is stage dependent.[370, 371] These studies were extended in vitro by using cultures of Sertoli cells or seminiferous tubules to examine the action on Leydig cell steroidogenesis, and both inhibitory and stimulatory actions on Leydig cells were reported.[38, 372]

As evidence for the hypothesis continued to accumulate, many laboratories turned their efforts to the task of identifying the agents of communication between the Sertoli cells and Leydig cells. Two main approaches were used; either the action of substances known to be produced locally in the tubule was shown to regulate Leydig cell steroidogenesis, or gonadal fluids such as interstitial fluid or media from Sertoli cell or seminiferous tubule cultures were fractionated in order to identify novel factors.

According to the original observations that Leydig cell hypertrophy and hyper-responsiveness occurred following seminiferous tubule damage, it was postulated that either inhibitory or stimulatory factors could regulate the Leydig cells. If an inhibitor was produced, it was necessary to postulate that less of the inhibitor was present in the damaged testis, allowing the cells to be released from the inhibition that controlled them in the normal testis. Alternatively, if stimulatory activity regulated the Leydig cells in the normal testis, it was necessary to postulate that production of that factor declined under conditions of seminiferous tubule damage. The capacity to produce steroids is commonly used as an index of Leydig cell function, and many locally synthesized hormones or factors have been tested for their ability to inhibit or stimulate steroidogenesis.

The inhibitory action of testicular estrogens was one of the first effects thought to be involved in the local regulation of testosterone, but debate arose about whether this was a paracrine or autocrine effect, as the main source of estrogens in the adult (as opposed to the immature testis) was the Leydig cells themselves.[373, 374] These studies were followed by the report that an GnRH-like factor had been isolated from the testis which could inhibit testosterone synthesis.[375] The absolute levels of GnRH material in the testis was finally determined to be approximately 1 pg,[376] and the role of these low levels of peptide remains to be established. These studies stimulated great interest and led to the subsequent identification of local synthesis or production of many other different hormones and peptides not classically thought to be of testicular origin. Most of these are growth factors that have an inhibitory effect on steroid biosynthesis and include TGF-α/EGF,[377] TGF-β,[378, 379] IL-1α, IL-β, and IL-2,[336, 380, 381] FGF,[382, 383] CRF,[384] TNF-α,[385] and activin.[386, 387] The mechanism of action of some of these factors has been examined, particularly IL-1α, which causes a reduction in the level of LH binding to the Leydig cells, an inhibition of gonadotrophin-stimulated cAMP formation, and an inhibition of cholesterol cytochrome P450 expression.[336, 388] The inhibiting action of IL-1β is apparently more complex and appears to involve the down-regulation of mRNA levels of IGF-1, which can enhance androgen production.[389]

It must be remembered that most of these studies have been conducted in vitro, and a wide range of Leydig cell preparations and bioassays have been developed and used in this context. A number of variable parameters are important in the preparation and performance of Leydig cell bioassays, the end-point of which is an alteration in the steroid production.[390] Therefore as the list of actions of putative paracrine agents with inhibitory effects continues to grow, discrepant reports in the literature have appeared. Accordingly, it has also been reported that some growth factors such as IL-1[337–339] and EGF[391] can stimulate Leydig cell steroidogenesis. These apparent discrepancies are probably due to the diverse nature of the Leydig cell bioassays that have been used to detect the effects on steroidogenesis.

The observations that Sertoli cell–conditioned media or seminiferous tubule culture media could inhibit Leydig cell testosterone production was initially received with caution, but these reports have been confirmed.[392, 393] Previous studies had clearly shown stimulatory action by the same type of preparations owing to the presence of undetermined factors.[394–397] More recently, further purification of Sertoli cell media has been undertaken by Papadopoulus[398] and Zwain et al.[399] Interestingly, one report is of inhibitory and the other of stimulatory activity. Using purified media from a rat Sertoli cell clonal cell line (TM4), Zwain et al.[399] have partially purified a novel inhibitory factor that inhibits cAMP and testosterone levels in vitro by 80 per cent or more, although 400 μg/ml of this protein is required to observe this effect. Purification of conditioned media from human Sertoli cells has led to the identification of an 80-kDa active principle hSCSP-80, which stimulates Leydig cell steroidogenesis 25-fold at picomolar concentrations.[398] Both of these substances represent potent sources of Sertoli cell–derived regulatory activities that may be involved in the local control of Leydig cell steroidogenesis.

As well as these two factors, a large number of reports documented the presence of novel regulatory proteins in other biological fluids, including interstitial fluid (IF), albumin, and human follicular fluid (hFF). Initial findings that the stimulatory action of IF was due to novel factor(s)[400, 401] were vigorously pursued by Melsert et al.,[402] who proposed that albumin was the major component of IF that could stimulate steroidogenesis in vitro. Subsequent studies have indicated that although the overall effect of IF is stimulatory, this is due to the combined action of several inhibitory and stimulatory factors, including lipoproteins.[403] Human and bovine follicular fluids have been used as alternative sources of starting material for the purification of paracrine factors,[404–406] based on the assumption that the same factors are common to both the testis and ovary. However, comparison of steroid-stimulating activities in rat interstitial fluid with bovine and human ovarian follicular fluids has clearly shown that the principal steroidogenesis-regulating factors are biochemically and/or functionally distinct from one another.[407]

Despite more than a decade of research to resolve the identity of putative paracrine agents responsible for the communication between the Sertoli cells and Leydig cells, the results are equivocal and the substances responsible remain elusive. In part this is due to the multiplicity of peptides that could fulfil a paracrine role in the testis in vivo but may also lie in the variation in bioassays and procedures used to detect these activities. More recently, procedures used for the isolation and culture of highly purified preparations of Leydig cells have been developed and reported[408, 409]; the ability to maintain these Leydig cells in vitro and to demonstrate that steroid production is similar to that observed in vivo has led to the hypothesis that inhibitors rather than stimulators provide the more relevant means of regulating steroidogenesis.[355] It has always been known that intratesticular levels of testosterone exceed those required to maintain spermatogenesis and that spermatogenesis can be qualitatively maintained with 15 per cent of normal intratesticular testosterone levels. Although it has been suggested that the fine regulation of Leydig cell testosterone levels is not in fact required,[410] it can be argued that other Leydig cell products (about which very little is known) could be equally necessary for the maintenance of normal testicular function and that paracrine control of these products is important in vivo.

REFERENCES

1. de Kretser DM, Temple-Smith PD, Kerr JB: Anatomical and functional aspects of the male reproductive organs. In Bandhauer K, Frick J (eds): Handbook of Urology, vol XVI, Disturbances in Male Fertility. Berlin, Springer-Verlag, 1982, pp 1–131.
2. Jarow JP: Intratesticular arterial anatomy. J Androl 11:255–259, 1990.
3. Clermont Y, Huckins C: Microscopic anatomy of the sex cords and seminiferous tubules in growing and adult male albino rats. Am J Anat 108:79–97, 1961.
4. Dym M: The mammalian rete testis—a morphological examination. Anat Rec 186:493–524, 1976.
5. Roosen-Runge EC, Holstein AF: The human rete testis. Cell Tissue Res 189:409–433, 1978.
6. Bustos-Obregon E, Holstein AF: On structural patterns of the lamina propria of human seminiferous tubules. Z Zellforsch 131:413–425, 1973.
7. Dym M, Fawcett DW: The blood-testis barrier in the rat and the physiological compartmentation of the seminiferous epithelium. Biol Reprod 3:308–326, 1970.
8. Fawcett DW, Heidger PM, Leak LV: Lymph vascular system of the interstitial tissue of the testis as revealed by electron microscopy. J Reprod Fertil 19:109–119, 1969.
9. Fawcett DW, Leak LV, Heidger PM: Electron microscopic observations on the structural components of the blood-testis barrier. J Reprod Fertil 10(Suppl): 105–122, 1970.
10. Fawcett DW, Neaves WB, Flores MN: Comparative observations on intertubular lymphatics and the organization of the interstitial tissue of the mammalian testis. Biol Reprod 9:500–532, 1973.
11. Virtanen I, Kallojoki M, Narvanen O: Peritubular myoid cells of human and rat testis are smooth muscle cells that contain desmin-type intermediate filaments. Anat Rec 215:10–20, 1986.
12. Clermont Y: Contractile elements in the limiting membrane of the seminiferous tubules of the rat. Exp Cell Res 15:438–440, 1958.
13. Hovatta O: Contractility and structure of adult rat seminiferous tubule in organ culture. Z Zellforsch 130:171–179, 1972.
14. Ross MH, Long IR: Contractile cells in human seminiferous tubules. Science 153:1271–1273, 1966.
15. Dym M, Cavicchia JC: Further observations on the blood-testis barrier in monkeys. Biol Reprod 17:390–403, 1977.
16. Landon GV, Pryor JP: The blood-testis barrier in men of diverse fertility status: An ultrastructural study. Virchows Arch [A] 392:355–364, 1981.
17. Bergmann M, Nashan D, Nieschlag E: Pattern of compartmentation in human seminiferous tubules showing dislocation of spermatogonia. Cell Tissue Res 256:183–190, 1989.
18. von Ebner V: Untersuchungen uber den Bau der Samenkanalchen und die Entwicklung der Spermatozoiden bei den Saugentieren und beim Menschen. In Rollet's Untersuchungen aus dem Institut fur Physiologie und Histologie in Graz. Leipzig, 1871, pp 200–236.
19. Benda C: Untersuchungen uber den Bau des funktionierenden Sa-

menkanalchens einiger Saugetiere und Folgerungen fur die Spermatogenese dieser Wirbeltierklasse. Arch Mikrobiol Anat 30:49–76, 1887.

20. Leblond CP, Clermont Y: Definition of the stages of the cycle of the seminiferous epithelium in the rat. Ann NY Acad Sci 55:548–573, 1952.

21. Clermont Y: The cycle of the seminiferous epithelium man. Am J Anat 112:35–51, 1963.

22. Heller CG, Clermont Y: Kinetics of the germinal epithelium in man. Recent Prog Horm Res 20:545–575, 1964.

23. Clermont Y: Kinetics of spermatogenesis in mammals: Seminiferous epithelium cycle and spermatogonial renewal. Physiol Rev 52:198–236, 1972.

24. Chowdhury AK, Marshall G: Irregular pattern of spermatogenesis in the baboon (Papio anubis) and its possible mechanism. In Steinberger A, Steinberger E (eds): Testicular Development, Structure and Function. New York, Raven Press, 1980, pp 129–137.

25. Dietrich T, Schulze W, Riemer M: Untersuchung zur Gliederung des Keimepithiels beim Javaneraffen (Macaca cynomolgus) mittels digitaler Bildverarbeifung. Urologe [A] 25:179–186, 1986.

26. Schulze W, Rehder U: Organization and morphogenesis of the human seminiferous epithelium. Cell Tissue Res 237:395–407, 1984.

27. Regaud C: Etudes sur la structure des tubes seminiferes et sur la spermatogenese chez les mammiferes. Arch Anat Microsc 4:101–156, 1901.

28. Kerr JB: Functional cytology of the human testis. In Burger H (ed): Bailliere's Clinical Endocrinology and Metabolism, vol 6, no 2. London, Bailliere Tindall, 1992, pp 235–250.

29. de Kretser DM, Kerr JB: The cytology of the testis. In Knobil E, Neill J (eds): The Physiology of Reproduction. New York, Raven Press, 1988, pp 837–932.

30. Holstein AF, Roosen Runge EC: Atlas of Human Spermatogenesis. Berlin, Grosse Verlag, 1981.

31. de Kretser DM: Ultrastructural features of human spermiogenesis. Z Zellforsch 98:477–505, 1969.

32. Holstein AF: Ultrastructural observations on the differentiation of spermatids in man. Andrologia 8:157–165, 1976.

33. Fawcett DW: The mammalian spermatozoon. Dev Biol 44:394–436, 1975.

34. Clermont Y, Leblond CP: Spermiogenesis of man, monkey, ram and other mammals as shown by the periodic acid–Schiff technique. Am J Anat 96:229–253, 1955.

35. Irons MJ, Clermont Y: Formation of the outer dense fibers during spermiogenesis in the rat. Anat Rec 202:463–471, 1982.

36. Fawcett DW: Ultrastructure and function of the Sertoli cell. In Hamilton DW, Greep RO (eds): Handbook of Physiology, Section 7, Endocrinology, vol 5, Male Reproductive System. Baltimore, Williams & Wilkins, 1975, pp 21–55.

37. Bardin CW, Cheng CY, Musto NA: The Sertoli cell. In Knobil E, Neill J (eds): The Physiology of Reproduction. New York, Raven Press, 1988, pp 933–974.

38. Skinner MK: Cell-cell interactions in the testis. Endocr Rev 12:45–77, 1991.

39. Tindall D, Rowley D, Murthy L, et al: Structure and biochemistry of the Sertoli cell. Int Rev Cytol 94:127–149, 1985.

40. Griswold MD, Morales C, Sylvester SR: Molecular biology of the Sertoli cell. Oxford Rev Reprod Biol 10:124–161, 1988.

41. Russell LD, Ren HP, Sinha Hikim I, et al: A comparative study in twelve mammalian species of volume densities, volumes, and numerical densities of selected testis components, emphasizing those related to the Sertoli cell. Am J Anat 188:21–30, 1990.

42. Orth JM, Gunsalus GL, Lamperti AA: Evidence from Sertoli cell–depleted rats indicates that spermatid number in adults depends on numbers of Sertoli cells produced during perinatal development. Endocrinology 122:787–794, 1988.

43. Johnson L, Zane RS, Petty CS, Neaves WB: Quantification of the human Sertoli cell population: Its distribution, relation to germ cell numbers, and age-related decline. Biol Reprod 31:785–795, 1984.

44. Orth JM: Proliferation of Sertoli cells in fetal and postnatal rats: A quantitative autoradiographic study. Anat Rec 203:485–492, 1982.

45. Orth JM: The role of follicle-stimulating hormone in controlling Sertoli cell proliferation in testes of fetal rats. Endocrinology 115:1248–1255, 1984.

46. Cortes D, Muller J, Skakkebaek NE: Proliferation of Sertoli cells during development of the human testis assessed by stereological methods. Int J Androl 10:589–596, 1987.

47. Vogl AW, Soucy LJ: Arrangement and possible functions of actin filament bundles in ectoplasmic specializations of ground squirrel Sertoli cells. J Cell Biol 100:814–825, 1985.

48. McGinley D, Posalaky Z, Porvaknik M: Intercellular junctional complexes of the rat seminiferous tubules: A freeze-fracture study. Anat Rec 189:211–232, 1977.

49. Setchell BP, Zupp JP, Pollanen P: Blood-testis barrier at puberty. In Parvinen M, Huhtaniemi I, Pelliniemi LJ (eds): Development and Function of the Reproductive Organs. Rome, Serono Symp Rev No 14, 1988, pp 77–84.

50. de Kretser DM, Burger HG: Ultrastructural studies of the human Sertoli cell in normal men and males with hypogonadotrophic hypogonadism before and after gonadotrophic treatment. In Saxena BB, Beling CG, Gandy HM (eds): Gonadotrophins. New York, Wiley-Interscience, 1972, pp 640–656.

51. Cavicchia JC, Sacerdote FL: Correlation between blood-testis barrier development and onset of the first spermatogenic wave in normal and in busulfan-treated rats: A lanthanum and freeze-fracture study. Anat Rec 230:361–368, 1991.

52. Vogl AW: Changes in the distribution of microtubules in rat Sertoli cells during spermatogenesis. Anat Rec 222:34–41, 1988.

53. Paranko J, Kallajoki M, Pelliniemi LJ, et al: Transient coexpression of cytokeratin and vimentin in differentiating rat Sertoli cells. Dev Biol 117:35–44, 1986.

54. Oko R, Hermo L, Hecht NB: Distribution of actin isoforms within cells of the seminiferous epithelium of the rat testis: Evidence for a muscle form of actin in spermatids. Anat Rec 231:63–81, 1991.

55. Pfeiffer DC, Vogl AW: Evidence that vinculin is codistributed with actin bundles in ectoplasmic ("junctional") specializations of mammalian Sertoli cells. Anat Rec 231:89–100, 1991.

56. Altorfer J, Fukuda T, Hedinger C: Desmosomes in human seminiferous epithelium. Virchows Arch [B] 16:181–194, 1974.

57. McGinley DM, Posalaky Z, Porvaznik M, Russell LD: Gap junctions between Sertoli cells and germ cells of rat seminiferous tubules. Tissue Cell 11:741–754, 1979.

58. Russell LD, Tallon-Doran M, Weber JE, et al: Three-dimensional reconstruction of a rat stage V Sertoli cell, III: A study of specific cellular relationships. Am J Anat 167:181–192, 1983.

59. Morales C, Clermont Y, Nadler NJ: Cyclic endocytic activity and kinetics of lysosomes in Sertoli cells of the rat: A morphometric analysis. Biol Reprod 34:207–218, 1986.

60. Chemes H: The phagocytic function of Sertoli cells: A morphological, biochemical and endocrinological study of lysosomes and acid phosphatase localization in the rat testis. Endocrinology 119:1673–1681, 1986.

61. Ueno H, Mori H: Morphometrical analysis of Sertoli cell ultrastructure during the seminiferous epithelial cycle in rats. Biol Reprod 43:769–776, 1990.

62. Kerr JB: An ultrastructural and morphometric analysis of the Sertoli cell during the spermatogenic cycle in the rat. Anat Embryol 179:191–203, 1988.

63. Morales C, Clermont Y, Hermo L: Nature and function of endocytosis in Sertoli cells of the rat. Am J Anat 173:203–217, 1985.

64. Rong-Xi D, Djakiew D, Dym M: Endocytic activity of Sertoli cells grown in bicameral culture chambers. Anat Rec 218:306–312, 1987.

65. Petrie RG, Morales CR: Receptor-mediated endocytosis of testicular transferrin by germinal cells of the rat testis. Cell Tissue Res 267:45–55, 1992.

66. Segretain D, Egloff M, Gerard N, et al: Receptor-mediated and adsorptive endocytosis by a male germ cells of different mammalian species. Cell Tissue Res 268:471–478, 1992.

67. Fawcett DW: The ultrastructure and functions of the Sertoli cell. In Greep RO, Koblinsky MA (eds): Frontiers in Reproduction and Fertility Control. Cambridge, MA, MIT Press, 1977, pp 302–320.

68. Christensen AK: Leydig cells. In Hamilton DW, Greep RO (eds): Handbook of Physiology, Section 7, Endocrinology, vol 5, Male Reproductive System. Baltimore, Williams & Wilkins, 1975, pp 57–94.

69. Schulze C: Sertoli cells and Leydig cells in man. Adv Anat Embryol Cell Biol 88:1–104, 1984.

70. Holstein AF, Orlandini GE, Moller R: Distribution and fine structure of the lymphatic system in the human testis. Cell Tissue Res 200:15–27, 1979.

71. Christensen AK, Gillim SW: The correlation of the fine structure and function in steroid-secreting cells, with emphasis on those of the gonads. In McKerns KW (ed): The Gonads. New York, Appleton-Century-Crofts, 1969, pp 415–488.

72. Mendis-Handagama SMLC, Zirkin BR, Scallen TJ, Ewing LL: Studies on peroxisomes of the adult rat Leydig cell. J Androl 11:270–278, 1990.

73. Miller SC: Localization of plutonium-241 in the testis: An interspecies comparison using light and electron microscope autoradiography. Int J Radiat Biol 41:633–643, 1982.

74. Miller SC, Bowman BM, Rowland HG: Structure, cytochemistry, endocytic activity and immunoglobulin (Fc) receptors of rat testicular interstitial tissue macrophages. Am J Anat 168:1–13, 1983.

75. Hutson JC: Development of cytoplasmic digitations between Leydig cells and testicular macrophages of the rat. Cell Tissue Res 267:385–389, 1992.

76. Pollanen P, Maddocks S: Macrophages, lymphocytes and MHC II antigen in the rat and ram testis. J Reprod Fertil 82:437–445, 1988.

77. Jackson AE, O'Leary PC, Ayers MM, de Kretser DM: The effects of ethylene dimethanesulphate (EDS) on rat Leydig cells: Evidence to support a connective tissue origin of Leydig cells. Biol Reprod 35:425–437, 1986.

78. Kerr JB, Bartlett JMS, Donachie K, Sharpe RM: Origin of regenerating Leydig cells in the testis of the adult rat. Cell Tissue Res 249:367–377, 1987.

79. Chemes H, Cigorraga S, Bergada C, et al: Isolation of human Leydig cell mesenchymal precursors from patients with the androgen insensitivity syndrome: Testosterone production and response to human chorionic gonadotropin stimulation in culture. Biol Reprod 46:793–801, 1992.

80. Sharpe RM: Intratesticular factors controlling testicular function. Biol Reprod 30:29–49, 1984.

81. de Kretser DM: Local regulation of testicular function. Int Rev Cytol 10:89–112, 1987.

82. de Kretser DM: Germ cell–Sertoli cell interactions. Reprod Fertil Dev 2:225–235, 1990.

83. Parvinen M, Vihko KK, Topari J: Cell interactions during the seminiferous epithelial cycle. Int Rev Cytol 104:115–151, 1987.

84. Hall PF: Testicular steroid synthesis: Organisation and regulation. *In* Knobil E, Neill J (eds): The Physiology of Reproduction. New York, Raven Press, 1988, pp 975–998.

85. Rommerts FFG, van der Molen HJ: Testicular steroidogenesis. In Burger HG, de Kretser DM (eds): The Testis. New York, Raven Press, 1989, pp 303–328.

86. Baird DT, Galbraith A, Fraser IS, Newsam JE: The concentration of oestrone and oestradiol-17β in spermatic venous blood in man. J Endocrinol 57:285–288, 1973.

87. Chen YI, Kraemer FB, Reaven GM: Identification of specific HDL-binding sites in rat testis. J Biol Chem 255:9162–9169, 1980.

88. Freeman DA, Ascoli M: The LDL pathway of cultured Leydig tumour cells. Biochem Biophys Acta 754:72–79, 1983.

89. Mertz LM, Pedersen RC: The kinetics of steroidogenesis activator polypeptide in the rat adrenal cortex. J Biol Chem 264:15274–15279, 1989.

90. Chung B, Matteson KJ, Voutilainen R, et al: Human cholesterol side-chain cleavage enzyme P450 scc: cDNA cloning, assignment of the gene to chromosome 15 and expression in the placenta. Proc Natl Acad Sci USA 83:8962–8966, 1986.

91. Weinsten JJAM, Sunals AGM, Hofman JA, et al: Early time sequence in pregnenolone metabolism to testosterone in homogenates of human and rat testis. Endocrinology 120:1909–1913, 1987.

92. Huhtaniemi I: Studies on steroidogenesis and its regulation in human fetal adrenal and testis. J Steroid Biochem 8:491–497, 1977.

93. Matteson KJ, Picardo-Leonard J, Chung B, et al: Assignment of the gene for adrenal P450c17 (steroid 17α hydroxylase/17,20 lyase) to human chromosome 10. J Clin Endocrinol Metab 63:789–791, 1986.

94. Chung B, Picardo-Leonard J, Haniu M, et al: Cytochrome P450c17 (steroid 17α hydroxylase/17, 20 lyase): Cloning of human adrenal and testis cDNA indicates the same gene is expressed in both tissues. Proc Natl Acad Sci USA 84:407–411, 1987.

95. Inano H, Ishii-Ohba H, Sugimoto Y, et al: Purification and properties of enzymes related to steroid hormone synthesis. Ann NY Acad Sci 595:17–25, 1990.

96. Luu-The V, Labrie C, Simard J, et al: Structure of two in tandem 17β human hydroxysteroid dehydrogenase genes. Mol Endocrinol 4:268–275, 1990.

97. Lorence MC, Corbin CG, Kamimura N, et al: Structural analysis of the gene encoding human 3β hydroxysteroid dehydrogenase/delta 5-4 isomerase. Mol Endocrinol 4:1850–1855, 1990.

98. Chen S, Besman MJ, Sparks RS, et al: Human aromatases: cDNA cloning, Southern analysis and assignment of the gene to chromosome 15. DNA 7:27–38, 1988.

99. Andersson S, Russel DW: Structural and biochemical properties of cloned and expressed human and rat steroid 5 alpha reductases. Proc Natl Acad Sci USA 87:3640–3644, 1990.

100. Christensen AK: Leydig Cells. *In* Greep RO, Astwood EB (eds): Handbook of Physiology, Section 7, vol 5. Baltimore, Williams & Wilkins, 1975, pp 57–94.

101. Loosefelt H, Misrahi M, Atger M, et al: Cloning and sequencing of porcine LH-hCG receptor cDNA: Variants lacking transmembrane domain. Science 245:525–528, 1989.

102. de Kretser DM, Catt KJ, Paulsen CA: Studies on the *in vitro* testicular binding of iodinated luteinizing hormone in rats. Endocrinology 88:332–337, 1971.

103. Dufau ML: Endocrine regulation and communicating functions of the Leydig cell. Ann Rev Physiol 50:483–508, 1988.

104. Dufau ML, Tsuruhara T, Horner KA, et al: Intermediate role of adenosine 3'5'-cyclic monophosphate and protein kinase during gonadotrophin induced steroidogenesis in testicular interstitial cells. Proc Natl Acad Sci USA 74:3419–3423, 1977.

105. Cooke BA: Is cyclic AMP an obligatory second messenger for luteinizing hormone? Mol Cell Endocrinol 69:C11–C115, 1990.

106. Hodgson YM, de Kretser DM: Serum testosterone response to single injection of hCG ovine-LH and LHRH in male rats. Int J Androl 5:81–91, 1982.

107. Padron RS, Wischusen J, Hudson B, et al: Prolonged biphasic response of plasma testosterone to single intramuscular injections of human chorionic gonadotrophin. J Clin Endocrinol Metab 50:1100–1104, 1980.

108. Sharpe RM: hCG-induced decrease in availability of rat testis receptors. Nature 264:644–646, 1976.

109. Haour F, Saez JM: hCG-dependent regulation of gonadotrophin receptor sites: Negative control in testicular Leydig cells. Mol Cell Endocrinol 7:17–24, 1977.

110. Cigorraga SB, Sorell S, Bator J, et al: Estrogen dependence of a gonadotrophin-induced steroidogenic lesion in rat testicular Leydig cells. J Clin Invest 65:699–705, 1980.

111. Hodgson YM, de Kretser DM: Acute responses of Leydig cells to hCG: Evidence for early hypertrophy of Leydig cells. Mol Cell Endocrinol 35:75–82, 1984.

112. Christensen AK, Peacock KL: Increase in Leydig cell number in testes of adult rats treated chronically with an excess of human chorionic gonadotropin. Biol Reprod 22:383–391, 1980.

113. Waterman MR, Simpson ER: Regulation of steroid hydroxylase gene expression is multifactorial in nature. Recent Prog Horm Res 45:533–566, 1989.

114. Wu FCW, Irby DC, Clarke IJ, et al: Effects of gonadotropin-releasing hormone pulse-frequency modulation on luteinizing hormone, follicle stimulating hormone and testosterone secretion in hypothalamo/pituitary-disconnected rams. Biol Reprod 37:501–510, 1987.

115. Means AR, Vaitukaitis J: Peptide hormone receptors: Specific binding of ^{131}I-FSH to testis. Endocrinology 90:39–46, 1972.

116. Orth J, Christensen AK: Localization of ^{125}I-labelled FSH in the testes of hypophysectomized rats by autoradiography at the light and electron microscopic levels. Endocrinology 101:262–278, 1977.

117. Orth J, Christensen AK: Autoradiographic localization of specifically bound ^{125}I-labelled follicle stimulating hormone on spermatogonia of the rat testis. Endocrinology 103:1944–1951, 1978.

118. Mulder E, Peters MJ, de Vries J, van der Molen HJ: Characterization of a nuclear receptor for testosterone in seminiferous tubules of mature rat testes. Mol Cell Endocrinol 2:171–182, 1975.

119. Sanborn BM, Steinberger A, Tcholakian RK, Steinberger E: Direct measurement of androgen receptors in cultured Sertoli cells. Steroids 29:493–502, 1977.

120. Verhoeven G: Androgen receptor in cultured interstitial cells derived from immature rat testis. J Steroid Biochem 13:469–473, 1980.

121. Namiki M, Yokokawa K, Okuyama A, et al: Evidence for the presence of androgen receptors in human Leydig cells. J Steroid Biochem Mol Biol 38:79–82, 1991.

122. Skinner MK, Fetterolf PM, Anthony CT: Purification of a paracrine factor, P-Mod-S, produced by testicular peritubular cells that modulates Sertoli cell function. J Biol Chem 25:2884–2890, 1988.

123. Skinner MK, McLachlan RI, Bremner WJ: Stimulation of Sertoli cell inhibin secretion by the testicular paracrine factor P-Mod-S. Mol Cell Endocrinol 66:239–249, 1989.

124. Heindel JJ, Rothenberg R, Robinson GA, Steinberger A: LH and FSH stimulation of cyclic AMP in specific cell types isolated from the testes. J Cyclic Nucleotide Res 1:69–79, 1975.

125. Means AR: Biochemical effects of FSH on the testis. *In* Greep RO, Hamilton DW (eds): Handbook of Physiology, Section 7, vol 5. Baltimore, Williams & Wilkins, 1975, pp 203–218.

126. Conti M, Toscano MV, Geremia R, Stefanini M: Follicle stimulating hormone regulates *in vivo* phosphodiesterase. Mol Cell Endocrinol 29:79–90, 1983.

127. Ireland ME, Rosenblum BB, Welsh MJ: Two dimensional gel analysis of Sertoli cell protein phosphorylation: Effects of short-term expo-

sure to follicle stimulating hormone. Endocrinology 118:526–532, 1986.

128. Grasso P, Joseph MP, Reichert LE: A new role for follicle stimulating hormone in the regulation of calcium flux in Sertoli cells: Inhibition of Na$^+$/Ca^{++} exchange. Endocrinology 128:158–164, 1991.

129. Gorczynska E, Handelsman DJ: The role of calcium in follicle-stimulating hormone (FSH) signal transduction in Sertoli cells. J Biol Chem 266:23739–23744, 1991.

130. Dorrington JH, Roller NF, Fritz IB: Effects of follicle stimulating hormone on cultures of Sertoli cell preparations. Mol Cell Endocrinol 3:57–70, 1975.

131. Attramadal H, Le Gac F, Jahnsen T, Hansson V: β adrenegic regulation of Sertoli cell adenylate cyclase: Desensitization by homologous hormone. Mol Cell Endocrinol 34:1–6, 1984.

132. Le Gac F, Attramadal H, Jahsen T, Hansson V: Studies on the mechanism of follicle stimulating hormone–induced desensitization of Sertoli cell adenyl cyclase in vitro. Biol Reprod 32:916–924, 1985.

133. Conti M, Toscano MV, Petrelli L, et al: Involvement of phosphodiesterase in the refractoriness of the Sertoli cell. Endocrinology 113:1845–1853, 1983.

134. Conti M, Monaco L, Geremia R, Stefanini M: Effect of phosphodiesterase inhibitors on Sertoli cell refractoriness: Reversal of impaired androgen aromatization. Endocrinology 118:901–908, 1986.

135. Hansson V, Reusch E, Trygstad O, et al: FSH stimulation of testicular androgen binding protein. Nature (New Biol) 246:56–58, 1973.

136. Skinner MK, Griswold MD: Secretion of testicular transferrin by cultured Sertoli cells is regulated by hormones and retinoids. Biol Reprod 27:211–221, 1982.

137. Le Gac F, de Kretser DM: Inhibin production by Sertoli cells. Mol Cell Endocrinol 28:487–498, 1982.

138. Bicsak T, Vale W, Vaughan J, et al: Hormonal regulation of inhibin production by cultured Sertoli cells. Mol Cell Endocrinol 49:211–217, 1987.

139. Dorrington JH, Armstrong DT: Follicle stimulating hormone stimulates estradiol-17β synthesis in cultured Sertoli cells. Proc Natl Accad Sci USA 72:2677–2681, 1975.

140. Lacroix M, Smith FE, Frtiz IB: Secretion of plasminogen activator by Sertoli cell enriched culture. Mol Cell Endocrinol 9:227–236, 1977.

141. Cheng CY, Mather JP, Byer AL, Bardin CW: Identification of hormonally responsive proteins in primary Sertoli cell culture medium by high performance liquid chromatography. Endocrinology 118:480–488, 1986.

142. Hall PF, Mita M: Influence of FSH on glucose transport by cultured Sertoli cells. Biol Reprod 31:863–869, 1984.

143. Mita M, Price JM, Hall PF: Stimulation by FSH of synthesis of lactate by Sertoli cells from rat testis. Endocrinology 110:1535–1541, 1982.

144. Jutte NHPM, Hansen R, Grottegoed JA, et al: FSH stimulation of the production of pyruvate and lactate by rat Sertoli cells may be involved in hormonal regulation of spermatogenesis. J Reprod Fertil 68:219–226, 1983.

145. Spruill WA, Steiner AL, Tres LL, Kierszenbaum AL: Follicle stimulating hormone dependent phosphorylation of vimentin in cultures of rat Sertoli cells. Proc Natl Acad Sci USA 80:993–997, 1983.

146. Spruill WA, Zysk JR, Tres LL, Kierszenbaum AL: Calcium/calmodulin dependent phosphorylation of vimentin in rat Sertoli cells. Proc Natl Acad Sci USA 80:760–764, 1983.

147. Parvinen M: Regulation of the seminiferous epithelium. Endocr Rev 3:404–417, 1982.

148. Gonzales GF, Risbridger GP, de Kretser DM: In vitro synthesis and release of inhibin in response to FSH stimulation by isolated segments of seminiferous tubules from normal adult male rats. Mol Cell Endocrinol 59:179–185, 1988.

149. Simpson BJ, Hedger MP, de Kretser DM: Characterization of adult Sertoli cell cultures from cryptorchid rats: Inhibin secretion in response to FSH stimulation. Mol Cell Endocrinol 87:167–177, 1993.

150. Jégou B, Le Gac F, Irby D, de Kretser DM: Studies on seminiferous tubule fluid production in the adult rat: Effect of hypophysectomy and treatment with FSH, LH and testosterone. Int J Androl 6:249–260, 1983.

151. Au CL, Irby DC, Robertson DM, de Kretser DM: Effects of testosterone on testicular inhibin and fluid production in intact and hypophysectomized adult rats. J Reprod Fertil 76:257–266, 1986.

152. Lamb DJ, Wagle JR, Tsai YH, et al: Specificity and nature of the rapid steroid stimulated increase in Sertoli cell nuclear RNA polymerase activity. J Steroid Biochem 116:653–660, 1982.

153. Ailenberg M, McCabe D, Fritz IB: Androgens inhibit plasminogen activator activity secreted by Sertoli cells in culture in a two-chambered assembly. Endocrinology 126:1561–1568, 1990.

154. Persson H, Ayer-Le Lievre C, Soder O, et al: Expression of beta-nerve growth factor receptor mRNA in Sertoli cells is down regulated by testosterone. Science 247:704–707, 1990.

155. Roberts K, Griswold MD: Testosterone induction of cellular proteins in cultured Sertoli cells from hypophysectomized rats and rats of different ages. Endocrinology 125:1174–1179, 1989.

156. Cheng CY, Grima J, Stahler MS, et al: Testins are structurally related Sertoli cell proteins whose secretion is tightly coupled to the presence of germ cells. J Biol Chem 264:21386–21393, 1989.

157. Sharpe RM, Maddocks S, Millar M, et al: Testosterone and spermatogenesis: Identification of stage-specific, androgen regulated proteins secreted by adult rat seminiferous tubules. J Androl 13:172–184, 1992.

158. Skinner MK, Fritz IB: Testicular peritubular cells secrete a protein under androgen control that modulates Sertoli cell function. Cell Biol 82:114–118, 1985.

159. Tan J, Joseph DR, Quarmby VE, et al: The rat androgen receptor primary structure, autoregulation of its messenger ribonucleic acid and immunocytochemical localization of the receptor protein. Mol Endocrinol 2:1276–1285, 1988.

160. Sun YT, Irby DC, Robertson DM, de Kretser DM: The effects of exogenously administered testosterone on spermatogenesis in intact and hypophysectomized rats. Endocrinology 125:1000–1010, 1989.

161. Verhoeven G, Cailleau J: Follicle stimulating hormone and androgens increase the concentration of the androgen receptor in Sertoli cells. Endocrinology 122:1541–1550, 1988.

162. Boyar RJ, Finkelstein H, Roffwarg S, et al: Synchronization of augmented luteinizing hormone secretion with sleep during puberty. N Engl J Med 287:582–586, 1972.

163. Lee VWK, de Kretser DM, Hudson BH, Wang C: Variations in serum FSH, LH and testosterone levels in male rats from birth to sexual maturity. J Reprod Fertil 42:121–126, 1975.

164. Lee VWK, Cumming IA, de Kretser DM, et al: Regulation of gonadotrophin secretion in rams from birth to sexual maturity: I. Plasma LH, FSH and testosterone levels. J Reprod Fertil 46:1–6, 1976.

165. Paulsen CA, Espeland DH, Michals EL: Effects of hCG, HMG, HLH and HGH administration on testicular function. In Rosenberg E, Paulsen CA (eds): The Human Testis. New York, Plenum Press, 1970, pp 547–562.

166. Finkel DM, Phillips JL, Synder PJ: Stimulation of spermatogenesis by gonadotropins in men with hypogonadotropic hypogonadism. N Engl J Med 313:651–655, 1985.

167. Fraser HM, Gunn A, Jeffcoate SL, Holland DT: Effect of active immunization to luteinizing hormone releasing hormone on serum and pituitary gonadotropins, testes and accessory sex organs in the male rat. J Endocrinol 63:399–401, 1974.

168. Lincoln GA, Short RV: Seasonal breeding: Nature's contraceptive. Recent Prog Horm Res 36:1–43, 1980.

169. Steinberger E, Root A, Ficher M, Smith KD: The role of androgens in the initiation of spermatogenesis in man. J Clin Endocrinol Metab 37:746–751, 1973.

170. Srinath BR, Wickings EJ, Witting C, Nieschlag E: Active immunization with follicle stimulating hormone for fertility control: A 4 1/2 year study in male rhesus monkeys. Fertil Steril 40:110–117, 1983.

171. Murty GSRC, Sheela Rani CS, Moudgal NR, Prasad MRN: Effect of passive immunization with specific antiserum to FSH on the spermatogenic process and fertility of adult male bonnet monkeys (Macaca radiata). J Reprod Fertil 26:147–163, 1979.

172. MacLeod J, Pazianos A, Ray B: The restoration of human spermatogenesis and of the reproductive tract with urinary gonadotropins following hypophysectomy. Fertil Steril 17:7–23, 1986.

173. Bremner WJ, Matsumoto AM, Sussman AM, Paulsen CA: Follicle stimulating hormone and spermatogenesis. J Clin Invest 68:1044–1052, 1981.

174. Matsumoto AM, Karpas AE, Paulsen CA, Bremner WJ: Reinitiation of sperm production in gonadotropin-suppressed normal men by administration of follicle stimulating hormone. J Clin Invest 72:1005–1015, 1983.

175. Matsumoto AM, Paulsen CA, Bremner WJ: Stimulation of sperm production by human luteinizing hormone in gonadotropin-suppressed normal men. J Clin Endocrinol Metab 59:882–887, 1984.

176. Clermont Y, Harvey SG: Duration of the cycle of the seminiferous epithelium of normal hypophysectomized and hypophysectomized-hormone treated albino rats. Endocrinology 76:80–89, 1965.

177. Steinberger E: Hormonal control of mammalian spermatogenesis. Physiol Rev 51:1–22, 1971.

178. Boccabella AV: Reinitiation and restoration of spermatogenesis with testosterone propionate and other hormones after a long-term post-

hypophysectomy regression period. Endocrinology 72:787–791, 1963.

179. Huang HFS, Nieschlag E: Suppression of the intratesticular testosterone is associated with quantitative changes in spermatogonial populations in intact adult rats. Endocrinology 118:619–627, 1986.
180. Marshall GR, Wickings EJ, Ludecke DK, Nieschlag E: Stimulation of spermatogenesis in stalk-sectioned rhesus monkeys by testosterone alone. J Clin Endocrinol Metab 57:152–159, 1983.
181. Walsh PC, Swerdloff RS: Biphasic effect of testosterone on spermatogenesis in the rat. Invest Urol 11:190–193, 1973.
182. Berndtson WE, Desjardins C, Ewing LL: Inhibition and maintenance of spermatogenesis in rats implanted with polydimethylsiloxane capsules containing various androgens. J Endocrinol 62:125–135, 1974.
183. Cunningham GR, Huckins C: Persistence of complete spermatogenesis in the presence of low intra-testicular concentration of testosterone. Endocrinology 105:177–186, 1979.
184. Sharpe RM: Testosterone and spermatogenesis. J Endocrinol 113:1–2, 1987.
185. Zirkin BR, Santulli R, Awoniyi CA, Ewing LL: Maintenance of advanced spermatogenic cells in the adult rat testis: Quantitative relationships to testosterone concentration within the testis. Endocrinology 124:3043–3049, 1989.
186. Santulli R, Sprando RL, Awoniyi CA, et al: To what extent can spermatogenesis be maintained in the hypophysectomized adult rat testis with exogenously administered testosterone? Endocrinology 126:95–101, 1990.
187. Rea MA, Marshall GR, Weinbauer GF, Nieschlag E: Testosterone maintains pituitary and serum FSH and spermatogenesis in gonadotropin-releasing hormone antagonist suppressed rats. J Endocrinol 108:101–103, 1986.
188. Bhasin S, Fielder TJ, Swerdloff RS: Testosterone selectively increases serum follicle stimulating hormone (FSH) but not luteinizing hormone (LH) in gonadotropin-releasing hormone antagonist–treated male rats: Evidence for differential regulation of LH and FSH secretion. Biol Reprod 37:55–59, 1987.
189. Elkington JSH, Blackshaw AW: Studies on testicular function: 1. Quantitative effects of FSH, LH, testosterone and dihydrotestosterone on restoration and maintenance of spermatogenesis in the hypophysectomized rat. Aust J Biol Sci 27:47–57, 1974.
190. Vernon RG, Go VLW, Fritz IB: Hormonal requirements of the different cycles on the seminiferous epithelium during reinitiation of spermatogenesis in long-term hypophysectomized rats. J Reprod Fertil 42:77–94, 1975.
191. Chowdhury AK: Dependence of testicular germ cells on hormones: A quantitative study in hypophysectomized testosterone treated rats. J Endocrinol 82:331–340, 1979.
192. Bartlett JMS, Weinbauer GF, Nieschlag E: Differential effects of FSH and testosterone on the maintenance of spermatogenesis in the adult hypophysectomized rat. J Endocrinol 121:49–58, 1989.
193. Sun YT, Wreford NG, Robertson DM, de Kretser DM: Quantitative cytological studies of spermatogenesis in intact and hypophysectomized rats: Identification of androgen-dependent stages. Endocrinology 127:1215–1223, 1990.
194. Awoniyi CA, Santulli R, Chandrashekar V, et al: Quantitative restoration of advanced spermatogenic cells in adult male rats made azoospermic by active immunization against luteinizing hormone or gonadotropin-releasing hormone. Endocrinology 125:1303–1309, 1990.
195. Awoniyi CA, Sprando RL, Santulli R, et al: Restoration of spermatogenesis by exogenously administered testosterone in rats made azoospermic by hypophysectomy or withdrawal of luteinizing hormone alone. Endocrinology 127:177–184, 1990.
196. Matsumoto AM: Hormonal control of human spermatogenesis. In Burger HG, de Kretser DM (eds): The Testis (ed 2). New York, Raven Press, 1989, pp 181–196.
197. Lee PA, Jaffe RB, Midgeley, et al: Regulation of human gonadotropins VIII: Suppression of serum LH and FSH in adult males following exogenous testosterone administration. J Clin Endocrinol Metab 35:636–641, 1972.
198. Sherins RJ, Loriaux DL: Studies on the role of sex steroids in the feedback control of FSH concentrations in men. J Clin Endocrinol Metab 36:886–893, 1973.
199. Naftolin F, Ryan KJ, Petro Z: Aromatization of androstenedione by the diencephalon. J Clin Endocrinol Metab 33:368–370, 1971.
200. Santen RJ: Is aromatization of testosterone to estradiol required for inhibition of luteinizing hormone secretion in man? J Clin Invest 56:1555–1563, 1975.
201. Tilbrook AJ, de Kretser DM, Cummins JT, Clarke IJ: The negative

feedback effects of the testicular steroids are predominantly at the hypothalamus in rams. Endocrinology 129:3080–3092, 1991.
202. Decker MH, Loriaux DL, Cutler GB: A seminiferous tubular factor is not obligatory for regulation of plasma follicle-stimulating hormone in the rat. Endocrinology 108:1035–1039, 1981.
203. McCullagh DR: Dual endocrine activity of the testes. Science 76:19–20, 1932.
204. Robertson DM, Foulds LM, Leversha L, et al: Isolation of inhibin from bovine follicular fluid. Biochem Biophys Res Commun 126:220–226, 1985.
205. de Kretser DM, Au CL, Robertson DM: The physiology of inhibin in the male. In Burger HG, de Kretser DM, Findlay JK, Igarashi M (eds): Inhibin—Non Steroidal Regulation of Follicle Stimulating Hormone Secretion, Serono Symposia. New York, Raven Press, 1987, pp 149–161.
206. Jackson CM, Morris ID: Gonadotrophin levels in male rats following impairment of Leydig cell function by ethylene dimethanesulphonate. Andrologia 9:29–32, 1977.
207. de Kretser DM, O'Leary PO, Irby DC, Risbridger GP: Inhibin secretion is influenced by Leydig cells: Evidence from studies using the cytotoxin ethane dimethane sulphonate (EDS). Int J Androl 12:273–280, 1988.
208. Gonzales GF, Risbridger GP, de Kretser DM: In vivo and in vitro production of inhibin by cryptorchid testes from adult rats. Endocrinology 124:1661–1668, 1989.
209. O'Leary P, Jackson AE, Averill S, de Kretser DM: The effects of ethane dimethane sulphonate (EDS) on bilaterally cryptorchid rat testes. Mol Cell Endocrinol 45:183–190, 1986.
210. Ling N, Ying SY, Ueno N, et al: Isolation and partial characterization of a MW 32,000 protein with inhibin activity from porcine follicular fluid. Proc Natl Acad Sci USA 82:7217–7221, 1985.
211. Mason AJ, Hayflick JS, Esch F, et al: Complementary DNA sequences of ovarian follicular fluid inhibin show precursor structure and homology with transforming growth factor β. Nature 318:659–663, 1985.
212. Forage RG, Ring JM, Brown RW, et al: Cloning and sequence analysis of cDNA species coding for the two subunits of inhibin from bovine follicular fluid. Proc Natl Acad Sci USA 83:3091–3095, 1986.
213. Bardin CW, Morris PL, Chen CL, et al: Testicular inhibin: Structure and regulation by FSH, androgens and EGF. In Burger HG, de Kretser DM, Findlay JK, Igarashi M (eds): Inhibin—Non-Steroidal Regulation of Follicle Stimulating Hormone Secretion, Serono Symposia. New York, Raven Press, 1987, pp 179–190.
214. Leversha LJ, Robertson DM, de Vos FL, et al: Isolation of inhibin from ovine follicular fluid. J Endocrinol 112:213–221, 1987.
215. Vale W, Rivier J, Vaughan J, et al: Purification and characterization of an FSH releasing protein from porcine follicular fluid. Nature 321:776–779, 1986.
216. Ling N, Ying SY, Ueno N, et al: Pituitary FSH is released by a heterodimer of the β subunits of the two forms of inhibin. Nature 321:782–779, 1986.
217. Mason AJ, Berkanmeier L, Schmelzer C, Schwall R: Activin B: Precursor sequences, genomic structure and in vitro activities. Mol Endocrinol 3:1352–1358, 1989.
218. Ueno N, Ling N, Ying SY, et al: Isolation and partial characterization of follistatin: A single-chain Mr 35000 monomeric protein that inhibits the release of follicle stimulating hormone. Proc Natl Acad Sci USA 84:8282–8286, 1987.
219. Robertson DM, Klein R, de Vos FL, et al. The isolation of polypeptides with FSH suppressing activity from bovine follicular fluid which are structurally different from inhibin. Biochem Biophys Res Commun 149:744–749, 1987.
220. Shimasaki S, Koga M, Esch F, et al: Porcine follistatin gene structure supports two forms of mature follistatin produced by alternative splicing. Biophys Biochem Res Commun 152:717–723, 1988.
221. Inouye S, Guo Y, de Paolo L, et al: Recombinant expression of human follistatin with 315 and 288 amino acids: Chemical and biological comparison with native porcine follistatin. Endocrinology 129:815–822, 1991.
222. Nakamura T, Takio K, Eto Y, et al: Activin binding protein from rat ovary is follistatin. Science 247:836–838, 1990.
223. Gospodarowicz D, Lau K: Pituitary follicular cells secrete both vascular endothelial growth factor and follistatin. Biochem Biophys Res Commun 165:292–298, 1989.
224. Steinberger A, Steinberger E: Secretion of a FSH-inhibiting factor by cultured Sertoli cells. Endocrinology 99:918–921, 1976.
225. Toebosch AMW, Robertson DM, Trapman J, et al: Effects of FSH and IGF₁ on immature Sertoli cells: Inhibin α and β subunits mRNA levels and inhibin secretion. Mol Cell Endocrinol 55:101–105, 1988.

226. Klaij I, Timmerman MA, Blok LJ, et al: Regulation of inhibin β_B subunit mRNA expression in rat Sertoli cells: Consequences for the production of bioactive and immunoactive inhibin. Mol Cell Endocrol 85:237–246, 1992.

227. Krummen LA, Toppari J, Kim WH, et al: Regulation of testicular inhibin subunit messenger ribonucleic acid levels in vivo: Effects of hypophysectomy and selective follicle-stimulating hormone replacement. Endocrinology 125:1630–1637, 1989.

228. Grootenhuis AJ, van Beurden WMO, Timmerman MA, de Jong FH: Follicle stimulating hormone stimulation secretion of an immunoreactive 29 kDa inhibin alpha-subunit complex, but not of 32 kDa bioactive inhibin from cultured immature rat Sertoli cells. Mol Cell Endocrinol 74:125–132, 1990.

229. Hancock AD, Robertson DM, de Kretser DM: Inhibin and inhibin α chain precursors are produced by immature Sertoli cells in culture. Biol Reprod 46:155–161, 1992.

230. Risbridger GP, Clements J, Robertson DM, et al: Immuno bioactive inhibin and inhibin α subunit expression in rat Leydig cell cultures. Mol Cell Endocrinol 66:119–122, 1989.

231. Maddocks S, Sharpe RM: Assessment of the contribution of Leydig cells to the secretion of inhibin by the rat testis. Mol Cell Endocrinol 67:113–118, 1989.

232. Lee W, Mason AJ, Schwall R, et al: Secretion of activin by interstitial cells in the testis. Science 243:396–398, 1989.

233. Mather JP, Attie KM, Woodruff TK, et al: Activin stimulates spermatogonial proliferation in germ cell–Sertoli cell cocultures from immature rat testis. Endocrinology 127:3206–3214, 1990.

234. de Winter JP, Themmen APN, Hoogerbrugge JW, et al: Activin receptor mRNA expression in rat testicular cell types. Mol Cell Endocrinol 83:R1–R8, 1992.

235. Michel U, Albiston A, Findlay JK: Rat follistatin: Gonadal and extragonadal expression and evidence for alternative splicing. Biochem Biophys Res Commun 173:401–407, 1990.

236. Dubey AK, Zeleznik AJ, Plant TM: In the Rhesus monkey (Macaca mulatta), the negative feedback regulation of follicle stimulating hormone secretion by an action of testicular hormone directly at the level of the anterior pituitary gland cannot be accounted for by either testosterone or estradiol. Endocrinology 121:2229–2237, 1987.

237. Abeyawardene SA, Plant TM: Institution of combined treatment with testosterone and charcoal-extracted follicular fluid immediately after orchidectomy prevents the post castration hypersecretion of follicle stimulating hormone in the hypothalamus-lesioned rhesus monkey (Macaca mulatta) receiving an invariant intravenous gonadotropin releasing hormone infusion. Endocrinology 124:1310–1318, 1989.

238. Medhamurty R, Abeywardene SA, Culler MD, et al: Immunoneutralization of circulating inhibin in the hypophysiotropically clamped male Rhesus monkey (Macaca mulatta) results in a selective hypersecretion of follicle-stimulating hormone. Endocrinology 126:2116–2124, 1990.

239. Culler MD, Negro-Vilar A: Passive immunoneutralization of endogenous inhibin: Sex-related differences in the role of inhibin during development. Mol Cell Endocrinol 58:263–273, 1988.

240. Culler MD, Negro-Vilar A: Destruction of testicular Leydig cells reveals a role of endogenous inhibin in regulating FSH secretion in the male rat. Mol Cell Endocrinol 70:89–98, 1990.

241. Tierney ML, Goss NH, Tomkins SM, et al: Physiochemical and biological characterization of recombinant human inhibin A. Endocrinology 126:3268–3270, 1990.

242. Robertson DM, Prisk M, McMaster J, et al: Serum FSH suppressing activity of human recombinant inhibin A in male and female rats. J Reprod Fertil 91:321–328, 1991.

243. Tilbrook AJ, de Kretser DM, Clarke IJ: Plasma concentrations of FSH are suppressed by the direct pituitary actions of human recombinant inhibin A and testosterone in castrated rams. J Endocrinol, in press.

244. Carroll RS, Corrigan AZ, Gharib SD, et al: Inhibin, activin and follistatin: Regulation of follicle stimulating hormone messenger ribonucleic acid levels. Mol Endocrinol 3:1969–1976, 1989.

245. Mercer JE, Clements JA, Funder JW, Clarke IJ: Rapid and specific lowering of FSH β mRNA levels by inhibin. Mol Cell Endocrinol 53:251–254, 1987.

246. Roberts V, Meunier H, Vaughan J, et al: Production and regulation of inhibin subunits in pituitary gonadotropes. Endocrinology 124:552–554, 1989.

247. Corrigan AZ, Bilezikjian LM, Carroll RS, et al: Evidence for an autocrine role of activin B within the rat anterior pituitary cultures. Endocrinology 128:1682–1685, 1991.

248. Weinbauer GF, Behre HM, Fingscheidt U, Nieschlag E: Human follicle stimulating hormone exerts a stimulatory effect on spermato-

249. de Kretser DM, McLachlan RI, Robertson DM, Burger HG: Serum inhibin in normal men and men with testicular disorders. J Endocrinol 120:517–523, 1989.

250. Robertson DM, Giacometti M, Foulds LM, et al: Isolation of inhibin α-subunit precursor proteins from bovine follicular fluid. Endocrinology 125:2141–2149, 1989.

251. Sugino K, Nakamura T, Takio J, et al: Inhibin alpha subunit monomer is present in bovine follicular fluid. Biochem Biophys Res Commun 159:1323–1329, 1989.

252. Staehelin LA: Further observations on the fine structure of freeze-cleaved tight junctions. J Cell Sci 13:763–786, 1973.

253. van Deurs B, Koehler JK: Tight junctions in the choroid plexus epithelium: A freeze-fracture study including complementary replicas. J Cell Biol 80:662–673, 1979.

254. Pinto da Silva P, Kachar B: On tight junction structure. Cell 28:441–450, 1982.

255. Kacher B, Reese TS: Evidence for the lipidic nature of tight junction strands. Nature 296:464–466, 1982.

256. Cereijido M, Robbins ES, Dolan WJ, et al: Polarized monolayers formed by epithelia cells on a permeable and translucent support. J Cell Biol 77:853–880, 1978.

257. Meza I, Sabenero M, Stefoni E, Cereijido M: Occluding junctions and cytoskeletal components in a cultured transporting epithelium. J Cell Biol 87:746–754, 1982.

258. Byers SW, Graham R, Dai HN, Hoxter B: Development of Sertoli cell junctional specializations and distribution of the tight-junction-associated protein ZO-1 in the mouse testis. Am J Anat 191:35–47, 1991.

259. Kerr JB: A light microscope and morphometric analysis of the Sertoli cell during the spermatogenic cycle of the rat. Anat Embryol (Berl) 177:341–348, 1988.

260. Ueno H, Nishimune Y, Mori H: Cyclic localization change of Gogli apparatus in Sertoli cells induced by mature spermatids in rats. J Biol Reprod 44:656–662, 1991.

261. Kerr JB, de Kretser DM: Cyclic variations in Sertoli cell lipid content throughout the spermatogenic cycle of the rat. J Reprod Fertil 43:1–8, 1975.

262. Ulvik NM, Dahl E: Stage-dependent variation in volume density and size of Sertoli cell vesicles in the rat testis. Cell Tissue Res 221:311–320, 1981.

263. Hadley MA, Djakiew D, Byers SW, Dym M: Polarized secretion of androgen binding protein and transferrin by Sertoli cells grown in bicameral culture system. Endocrinology 120:1097–1103, 1987.

264. Janecki A, Jakubowiak A, Steinberger A: Study of the dynamics of Sertoli cell secretions in a new superfusion, two compartment culture system. In Vitro 23:492–500, 1987.

265. Griswold MD: Protein secretions of Sertoli cells. Int Rev Cytol 110:133–156, 1988.

266. Jégou B: The Sertoli cell. Baillieres Clin Endocrinol Metab 6:273–311, 1992.

267. Robinson R, Fritz B: Myoinositol biosynthesis by Sertoli cells and levels of myoinositol biosynthesis enzymes in testis and epididymis. Can J Biochar 57:962–974, 1979.

268. Jutte NHPM, Jansen R, Grootegoed AJ, et al: Regulation of survival of rat pachytene spermatocytes by lactate supply from Sertoli cells. J Reprod Fertil 65:431–438, 1982.

269. Djakiew D, Hadley MA, Byers SW, Dym M: Transferrin-mediated transcellular transport of 59_{Fe} across confluent epithelial sheets of Sertoli cells grown in bicameral cell culture chambers. J Androl 7:355–366, 1986.

270. Djakiew D, Griswold MD, Lewis DM, Dym M: Micropuncture studies of receptor-mediated endocytosis of transferrin in the rat epididymis. Biol Reprod 34:691–700, 1986.

271. Holmes D, Bucci LR, Lipshultz LI, Smith RG: Transferrin binds specifically to pachytene spermatocytes. Endocrinology 113:1916–1918, 1983.

272. Morales C, Sylvester SR, Griswold MD: Transport of iron and transferrin synthesis by the seminiferous epithelium of the rat in vitro. Biol Reprod 37:995–1005, 1987.

273. Skinner MK, Griswold MD: Sertoli cells synthesize and secrete a ceruloplasmin-like protein. Biol Reprod 28:1225–1229, 1983.

274. Cheng CY: Purification of calcium binding protein (rat SPARC) from primary Sertoli cell enriched medium. Biochem Biophys Res Commun 167:1393–1399, 1990.

275. Rich K, de Kretser DM: Effect of differing degrees of distinction of the rat seminiferous epithelium on levels of serum follicle stimulat-

ing hormone and androgen binding protein. Endocrinology 101: 959, 1977.

276. Sylvester SR, Skinner MK, Griswold MD: A sulfated glycoprotein synthesized by Sertoli cells and by epididymal cells is a component of the sperm membrane. Biol Reprod 31:1087, 1984.

277. O'Brien JS, Kretz KA, Dewji N, et al: Coding of two sphingolipid activator proteins (SAP-1 and SAP-2) by same genetic locus. Science 241:1098, 1988.

278. Hagenas L, Ritzen EM, Ploen L, et al: Sertoli cell origin of testicular androgen-binding protein (ABP). Mol Cell Endocrinol 2:339, 1975.

279. Linder CC, Heckert LL, Roberts KP, et al: Expression of receptors during the cycle of the seminifarous epithelium. Ann Acad Sci 637:313–321, 1991.

280. Kangasneimi M, Kaipia A, Toppari J, et al: Cellular regulation of follicle-stimulating hormone (FSH) binding in rat seminiferous tubules. J Androl 11:336–343, 1990.

281. Kaipia A, Blaüer M, Parvinen M, et al: Expression of inhibin α and β$_A$ peptides in staged rat seminiferous tubules. 11th North American Testis Workshop, Montreal, Canada, A24, 1991.

282. Kangasneimi M, Cheng CY, Toppari J, et al: Cyclic secretion and hormonal stimulation of testibumin, clusterin and² α₂-macroglobulin by staged rat seminiferous tubules. 11th North American Testis Workshop, Montreal, Canada, A27, 1991.

283. Erickson-Lawrence M, Zabludoff SD, Wright WW: Cyclic protein-2, a secretory product of rat Sertoli cells, is the proenzyme form of cathepsin-L. J Cell Biol 111:107A, 1990.

284. Wright WW, Parvinen M, Musto NA, et al: Identification of stage-specific proteins synthesized by rat seminiferous tubules. Biol Reprod 29:257–270, 1983.

285. Orth J, Boehm R: Functional coupling of neonatal rat Sertoli cells and gonocytes in co-culture. Endocrinology 127:2812–2820, 1990.

286. Orth J, McGuiness MP: Neonatal gonocytes co-cultured with Sertoli cells on a laminin containing matrix resume mitosos and elongate. Endocrinology 129:1119–1121, 1991.

287. Dym M, Clermont Y: Role of spermatogonia in the repair of the seminiferous epithelium following X-irradiation of the rat testis. Am J Anat 128:265–282, 1970.

288. Feig LA, Bellve AR, Horbach-Erickson N, Klagsbrun M: Sertoli cells contain a mitogenic polypeptide. Proc Natl Acad Sci USA 77:4774–4778, 1980.

289. Khan S, Soder O, Gustafsson K, et al: The rat testis produces large amounts of interleukin-1–like factor. Int J Androl 10:494–503, 1987.

290. Soder O, Syed V, Pollanen P, et al: Testicular interleukin-1–like factor. In Cooke BA, Sharpe RM (eds): The Molecular and Cellular Endocrinology of the Testis, Serono Symposia, vol 50. New York, Raven Press, 1988, pp 325–332.

291. Soder O, Syed V, Callard GV, et al: Production and secretion of an interleukin-1–like factor is stage-dependent and correlates with spermatogonial DNA synthesis in the rat seminiferous epithelium. Int J Androl 14:223–231, 1991.

292. Parvinen M, Soder O, Mali P, et al: In vitro stimulation of stage-specific deoxyribonucleic acid synthesis in rat seminiferous tubule segments by interleukin-1-α. Endocrinology 129:1614–1620, 1991.

293. Woodruff TK, Borree J, Attie KM, et al: Stage-specific binding of inhibin and activin to subpopulations of rat germ cells. Endocrinology 130:871–881, 1992.

294. Ayer-LeLievre C, Olsen L, Ebendal T, et al: Nerve growth factor mRNA and protein in the testis and epididymis of mouse and rat. Proc Natl Acad Sci USA 85:2628, 1988.

295. Olsen L, Ayer-LeLievre C, Ebendal T, Seiger A: Nerve growth factor-like immunoreactivities in rodent salivary glands and testis. Cell Tissue Res 248:275, 1987.

296. Galdieri M, Monaco L, Stefanini M: Secretion of androgen binding protein by Sertoli cells is influenced by contact with germ cells. J Androl 5:409, 1984.

297. Djakiew D, Dym M: Pachytene spermatocyte proteins influence Sertoli cell function. Biol Reprod 39:1193, 1988.

298. Le Magueresse B, Jégou B: Paracrine control of immature Sertoli cells by adult germ cells, in the rat (an in vitro study): Cell-cell interactions within the testis. Mol Cell Endocrinol 58:65, 1988.

299. Janecki A, Jakubowiak A, Steinberger A: Effect of germ cells on vectorial secretion of androgen binding protein and transferrin by immature rat Sertoli cells in vitro. J Androl 9:126, 1988.

300. Le Magueresse B, Jégou B: In vitro effects of germ cells on the secretory activity of Sertoli cells recovered from rats of different ages. Endocrinology 122:1672, 1988.

301. Enders GC, Millette CF: Pachytene spermatocyte and round spermatid binding to Sertoli cells in vitro. J Cell Sci 90:105–114, 1988.

302. Jégou B, Syed V, Sourdaine P, et al: The dialogue between late spermatids and Sertoli cells in vertebrates: A century of research. In Neischalg E, Habenicht V (eds): Schering Foundation Workshop, vol 4, Spermatogenesis-Fertilization-Contraception. Berlin, Springer-Verlag, 1992.

303. Jégou B: Spermatids are regulators of Sertoli cell function. In Robaire B (ed): The male germ cell spermatozonium to fertilization. Ann NY Acad Sci 637:340–353, 1991.

304. Cameron D, Muffly K: Hormonal regulation of spermati binding. J Cell Sci 100:623–633, 1991.

305. Chowdhury AK, Steinberger E: A quantitative study of the effects of heat on the germinal epithelium of rat testes. Am J Anat 115:509–524, 1964.

306. Jégou B, Laws A, de Kretser DM: Changes in testicular function induced by short-term exposure to the rat testis to heat: Further evidence for interaction of germ cells, Sertoli cells and Leydig cells. Int J Androl 7:244–257, 1984.

307. Au CL, Robertson DM, de Kretser DM: Changes in testicular inhibin after a single episode of heating of rat testes. Endocrinology 120:973–977, 1987.

308. Sharpe RM: Intratesticular control of steroidogenesis. Clin Endocrinol 33:787–807, 1990.

309. Skinner MK, Tung PS, Fritz IB: Cooperativity between Sertoli cells and testicular peritubular cells in the production and deposition of extracellular matrix components. J Cell Biol 100:941, 1985.

310. Tung PS, Fritz IB: Extracellular matrix promotes rat Sertoli cell histotype expression in vitro. Biol Reprod 30:213, 1984.

311. Hadley MA, Byers SW, Suarez-Quian CA, et al: Extracellular matrix regulates Sertoli cell differentiation, testicular cord formation and germ cell development in vitro. J Cell Biol 101:1511, 1985.

312. Handelsman DJ, Spaliviero JA, Kidston E, Robertson DM: Highly polarized secretion of inhibin by Sertoli cells in vitro. Endocrinology 125:721–729, 1989.

313. Hadley MA, Djakiew D, Byers SW, Dym M: Polarized secretion of androgen-binding protein and transferrin by Sertoli cells grown in a bicameral culture system. Endocrinology 120:1097, 1987.

314. Anthony CT, Skinner MK: Action of extracellular matrix on Sertoli cell morphology and function. Biol Reprod 40:691–702, 1989.

315. Tung PS, Fritz IB: Interactions of Sertoli cells with myoid cells in vitro. Biol Reprod 23:207, 1980.

316. Hutson JC, Stocco DM: Peritubular cell influence on the efficiency of androgen-binding protein secretion by Sertoli cells in culture. Endocrinology 108:1362, 1981.

317. Holmes SD, Lipshultz LI, Smith RG: Regulation of transferrin secretion by human Sertoli cells cultured in the presence or absence of human peritubular cells. J Clin Endocrinol Metab 59:1058, 1984.

318. Hutson JC, Yee JA: Peritubular cells influence Sertoli cells at the level of translation. Mol Cell Endocrinol 52:11, 1987.

319. Ailenberg M, Tung PS, Pelletier M, Fritz IB: Modulation of Sertoli cell functions in the two-chamber assembly by peritubular cells and by extracellular matrix. Endocrinology 122:2064, 1988.

320. Skinner MK, Fritz IB: Identification of a non-mitogenic paracrine factor involved in mesenchymal-epithelial cell interactions between testicular peritubular cells and Sertoli cells. Mol Cell Endocrinol 44:85, 1986.

321. Verhoeven G, Cailleau J: Testicular peritubular cells secrete a protein under androgen control that inhibits induction of aromatase activity in Sertoli cells. Endocrinology 123:2100–2110, 1988.

322. Swinnen K, Cailleau J, Heyns W, Verhoeven G: Stromal cells from the rat prostrate secrete androgen-regulated factors which modulate Sertoli cell function. Mol Cell Endocrinol 62:147–152, 1989.

323. Skinner MK, Takacs K, Coffey RJ: Cellular localization of transforming growth factor-alpha gene expression and action in the seminiferous tubule: Peritubular cell–Sertoli cell interactions. Endocrinology 124:845, 1989.

324. Morris PH, Vale WW, Cappel S, Bardin CW: Inhibin production by primary Sertoli cell–enriched cultures: Regulation by follicle-stimulating hormone, androgens, and epidermal growth factor. Endocrinology 122:717, 1988.

325. Mallea LE, Machado AJ, Navaroli F, Rommerts FFG: Epidermal growth factor stimulates lactate production and inhibits aromatisation in cultured Sertoli cells from immature rats. Int J Androl 9:201–208, 1986.

326. Skinner MK, Moses HL: Transforming growth factor-beta gene expression and action in the seminiferous tubule: Peritubular cell–Sertoli cell interactions. Mol Endocrinol 3:625, 1989.

327. Cailleau J, Vermaire S, Verhoeven G: Independent control of the production of insulin-like growth factor 1 and its binding protein by cultured testicular cells. Mol Cell Endocrinol 69:79–89, 1990.

328. Oonk RB, Grootegoed JA: Insulin-like growth factor 1 (IGF-1) receptors on Sertoli cells from immature rats and age-dependent testicular binding of IGF-I and insulin. Mol Cell Endocrinol 55:33, 1988.

329. Hall K, Ritzen EM, Johnsonbaugh RE, Parvinen M: Secretion of somatomedin-like compound from Sertoli cells *in vitro*. *In* Spencer EM (ed): Insulin-like Growth Factors/Somatomedins. New York, DeGruyter, 1983, pp 611–644.

330. Fritz IB, Tung PS: Role of interactions between peritubular cells and Sertoli cells in mammalian testicular functions. *In* Gall JG (ed): 44th Symposium of the Society for Developmental Biology: Gametogenesis and the Early Embryo. New York, Alan R. Liss, 1986, pp 151–173.

331. Ailenberg M, Fritz IB: Influences of follicle-stimulating hormone, proteases and antiproteases on permeability of the barrier generation by Sertoli cells in a two-chambered assembly. Endocrinology 124:1399–1407, 1989.

332. Pelletier RM, Byers SW: The blood-testis barrier and Sertoli cell junctions: Structural considerations. Mic Res Tech 20:3–33, 1992.

333. Hettle JA, Waller EK, Fritz IB: Hormonal stimulation alters the type of plasminogen activator produced by Sertoli cells. Biol Reprod 34:895–909, 1986.

334. Miller SC, Bowman BM, Roberts LK: Identification and characterization of mononuclear phagocytes isolated from rat testicular interstitial tissues. J Leukoc Biol 36:679–687, 1984.

335. Yee JB, Hutson JC: Effects of testicular macrophage-conditioned medium on Leydig cells in culture. Endocrinology 116:268–274, 1985.

336. Calkins JH, Sigel MM, Nankin HR, Lin T: Interleukin-1 inhibits Leydig cell steroidogenesis in primary culture. Endocrinology 123:1605–1610, 1988.

337. Verhoeven G, Kayo J, van Damme J, Billiau A: Interleukin-1 stimulates steroidogenesis in cultured rat Leydig cells. Mol Cell Endocrinol 57:51–60, 1988.

338. Moore C, Moger WH: Interleukin-1 α induced changes in androgen and cyclic adenosine 3′,5′-monophosphate release in adult rat Leydig cells in culture. J Endocrinol 129:381–390, 1991.

339. Warren DW, Pasupupeti V, Lu Y, et al: Tumour necrosis factor and interleukin-1 stimulate testosterone secretion in adult rat Leydig cells *in vitro*. J Androl 11:353–360, 1990.

340. Setchell BP, Rommerts FFG: The importance of the Leydig cells in the vascular response to hCG in the testis. Int J Androl 8:436–440, 1985.

341. Sharpe RM, Doogan DG, Cooper I: Direct effects of a luteinizing hormone–releasing hormone agonist on intratesticular levels of testosterone and interstitial formation in intact male rats. Endocrinology 113:1306–1313, 1983.

342. Sowerbutts SF, Jarvis LG, Setchell BP: The increase in testicular permeability induced by human chorionic gonadotrophin involves 5-hydroxy tryptamine and possibly estrogens, but not testosterone, prostaglandins, histamine or bradykinin. Aust J Exp Biol Med Sci 64:137–147, 1986.

343. Bergh A, Rooth P, Widmark A, Damber J: Treatment of rats with hCG induced inflammation by changes in the testicular circulation. J Reprod Fertil 79:135–143, 1987.

344. Hedger MP, Qin J, Robertson DM, de Kretser DM: Intragonadal regulation of immune system function. Reprod Fertil Dev 2:263–280, 1990.

345. Wartenberg H: Differentiation and development of the testis. *In* Burger HG, de Kretser DM (eds): The Testis. New York, Raven Press, 1989, pp 67–118.

346. Kerr JB, Sharpe R: Follicle stimulating hormone induction of Leydig cell maturation. Endocrinology 116:2592–2604, 1985.

347. Molenaar R, de Rooij DG, Rommerts FFG, van der Molen HJ: Repopulation of Leydig cells in mature rats after selective destruction of the existent Leydig cell population with ethylene dimethane sulphonate (EDS) is dependent on LH but not FSH. Endocrinology 118:2546–2554, 1986.

348. Teerds KJ, de Rooij DG, Rommerts FFG, Wensing GJG: The regulation of proliferation and differentiation of rat Leydig cell precursor cells after EDS administration or daily hCG treatment. J Androl 9:343–351, 1989.

349. Risbridger GP, Kerr JB, de Kretser DM: Influence of the seminiferous epithelium on the regeneration of Leydig cells after the administration of ethane dimethane sulphonate. J Endocrinol 112:197–204, 1987.

350. Hardy MP, Kelce WR, Klinefelter G, Ewing LL: Differentiation of Leydig cell precursors *in vitro*: Role for androgen. Endocrinology 127:488–490, 1990.

351. Murono EP, Washburn AL: Evidence that Leydig cell precursors localise in immature band two cells isolated on Percoll gradients. J Steroid Biochem Mol Biol 37:675–680, 1990.

352. Hardy MP, Zirkin B, Ewing LL: Kinetic studies on the development of the adult population of Leydig cells in testes of the pubertal rat. Endocrinology 124:762–770, 1989.

353. Kahn S, Teerds K, Dorrington J: Growth factor requirements for DNA synthesis by Leydig cells from the immature rat. Biol Reprod 146:335–341, 1992.

354. Risbridger GP, de Kretser DM: Paracrine regulation of the testis. *In* Burger HG, de Kretser DM (eds): The Testis. New York, Raven Press, 1989, pp 255–268.

355. Risbridger GP: Local regulation of Leydig cell function by inhibitors of steroidogenic activity. Cell Biol Int Rep 16:399–406, 1992.

356. Parmentier M, Inagani T, Pochat R, Dasclin JC: Pituitary-dependent renin immunolike immunoreactivity in the rat testis. Endocrinology 112:1318–1323, 1983.

357. Pandey KN, Inagami T: Regulation of renin angiotesin by gonadotrophic hormones in culture cell tumor cells. J Biol Char 261:3934–3938, 1986.

358. Nicholson HD, Hardy MP: Luteinizing hormone differentially regulates the secretion of testicular oxytocin and testosterone by purified adult rat Leydig cells *in vitro*. Endocrinology 130:671–677, 1992.

359. Douglass J, Cox B, Quinn B, et al: Expression of the prodynorphin gene in male and female mammalian tissues. Endocrinology 120:707–713, 1987.

360. Bardin C, Shara C, Mathar J, et al: Identification and possible function of pro-opiomelanocortin–derived peptides in the testis. *In* Catt KI, Dufau ML (eds): Hormone Action and Testicular Function. New York, NY Academy of Science, 1984, pp 346–364.

361. Fabbri A, Knox G, Buczko E, de Foe ML: Beta-endorphin production by the foetal Leydig cell: Regulation and implications for paracrine control of Sertoli cell function. Endocrinology 122:749–755, 1988.

362. Morris PL, Vale WW, Bardin CW: Beta-endorphin regulation of FSH stimulated inhibin production is a component of short-loop system in the testis. Biochem Biophys Res Commun 148:1513–1519, 1987.

363. Fabbri A, Tsai-Morris CH, Luna S, et al: Opiate receptors are present in the rat testis, identification and localization in Sertoli cells. Endocrinology 117:2544–2546, 1985.

364. Orth JN: FSH-induced Sertoli cell proliferation in the developing rat is modified by β-endorphin. Endocrinology 119:1876–1878, 1986.

365. Aoki A, Fawcett D: Is there a local feedback from the seminiferous tubules effecting activity of the Leydig cells? Biol Reprod 19:144–158, 1978.

366. Rich KA, Kerr JB, de Kretser DM: Evidence for Leydig cell dysfunction in rats with seminiferous damage. Mol Cell Endocrinol 13:123, 1979.

367. Risbridger GP, Kerr JB, de Kretser DM: Evaluation of Leydig cell function and gonadotrophin binding in unilateral and bilateral cryptorchidism: Evidence for local control of Leydig cell function by seminiferous tubules. Bio Reprod 24:534, 1981.

368. Risbridger GP, Kerr JB, Peake RA, de Kretser DM: An assessment of Leydig cell function after bilateral or unilateral effect duct ligation—further evidence for local control of Leydig cell function. Endocrinology 109:1234, 1981.

369. Jégou B, Laws AO, de Kretser DM: Changes in testicular function induced by short-term exposure of rat to heat: Further evidence for interaction of germ cells, Sertoli cells and Leydig cells. Int J Androl 7:244–257, 1984.

370. Bergh A: Local differences in Leydig cell morphology in the adult rat testes: Evidence for a local control of Leydig cells by adjacent seminiferous tubules. Int J Androl 5:325, 1982.

371. Bergh A: Development of stage-specific paracine regulation of Leydig cells by the seminiferous tubules. Int J Androl 8:80, 1985.

372. Risbridger GP, de Kretser DM: Paracrine regulation of the testes. *In* Burger HG, de Kretser DM (eds): The Testis (ed 2). New York, Raven Press, 1989, pp 255–268.

373. Valadares LE, Payne AH: Induction of testicular aromatization by luteinizing hormone in mature rats. Endocrinology 105:431–436, 1979.

374. Mogret WH: Temporal changes in testicular estradiol and testosterone concentrations, cytoplasmic estradiol binding and desensitization after human chorionic gonadotrophin administration to the immature rat. Endocrinology 106:496–503, 1980.

375. Sharpe RM, Fraser HM, Cooper I, Rommerts FF: Sertoli-Leydig cell communication via an LHRH like factor. Nature 290:785, 1981.

376. Hedger MP, Robertson DM, Browne CA, et al: The isolation and measurement of luteinizing hormone releasing hormone (LHRH) from the rat testis. Mol Cell Endocrinol 42:163–174, 1985.

377. Hsueh HJW, Welsh TH, Jones PBC: Inhibition of ovarian and testicular steroidogenesis by epidermal growth factor. Endocrinology 108:2002–2004, 1981.

378. Avallet O, Vigier M, Perrard-Sapori M, Saez JM: Transforming growth factor β inhibits Leydig cell functions. Biochem Biophys Res Commun 146:575–581, 1987.
379. Lin T, Blaisdell J, Haskell JF: Transforming growth factor β inhibits Leydig cell steroidogenesis. Biochem Biophys Res Commun 146:387–394, 1987.
380. Fauser CJM, Galway AB, Hsueh AJW: Inhibitory actions of interleukin-1β on steroidogenesis on primary cultures of neonatal testicular cells. Acta Endocrinol 120:401–408, 1989.
381. Guo H, Calkins J, Seegal LT: Interleukin-2 is a potent inhibitor of Leydig cell steroidogenesis. Endocrinology 127:1234–1239, 1990.
382. Murono EP, Washburn AL: Fibroblast growth factor inhibits 5α-reductase activity in cultured immature Leydig cells. Mol Cell Endocrinol 68:R19–R23, 1990.
383. Fauser BCJM: Fibroblast growth factor inhibits luteinizing hormone–stimulated androgen production by cultured rat testicular cells. Endocrinology 123:2935–2941, 1988.
384. Ulisse S, Fabbri A, Dutan ML: Corticotrophin releasing factor receptors and action in rat Leydig cells. J Biol Chem 264:2156–2163, 1989.
385. Maudit C, Hartmann DJ, Chauvin MA, et al: Tumour necrosis factor α inhibits gonadotrophin action in cultured porcine Leydig cells: Sites of action. Endocrinology 129:2930–2940, 1991.
386. Hsueh AJ, Dahl KD, Vaughan J, et al: Heterodimers and homodimers of inhibin subunits have different paracrine action in the modulation of luteinizing hormone–stimulated androgen biosynthesis. Natl Acad Sci USA 84:5082–5086, 1987.
387. Lin T, Calkins JH, Morris PL, et al: Regulation of Leydig cell function in primary culture and activin. Endocrinology 125:2134–2140, 1989.
388. Lin T, Wang D, Nagpal NL, et al: Interleukin-1 inhibits cholesterol side-chain cleavage cytochrome P450 expression on primary cultures of Leydig cells. Endocrinology 129:1305–1311, 1991.
389. Lin T, Wang D, Nagpal ML, et al: Down regulation of Leydig cell insulin-like growth factor 1 gene expression by interleukin-1. Endocrinology 130:1217–1224, 1992.
390. Abeyasekara DRE, Kurlak LO, Band AM, et al: Effect of cell purity, cell concentration, and incubation conditions on rat testis Leydig cell steroidogenesis in vitro. Dev Biol 27:253–259, 1991.
391. Verhoeven G, Caillieau J: Stimulatory effects of epidermal growth factor on steroidogenesis in Leydig cells. Mol Cell Endocrinol 47:99–106, 1986.
392. Syed V, Kahn SA, Ritzen EM: Stage specific inhibition of interstitial cell testosterone secretion by rat seminiferous tubules in vitro. Mol Cell Endocrinol 40:257–264, 1985.
393. Vihko KK, Huhtaniemi I: A rat seminiferous epithelial factor inhibits Leydig cell cyclic AMP and testosterone production: Mechanism of action stage-specific secretion and partial characterization. Mol Cell Endocrinol 65:119–127, 1989.
394. Papadopoulus V, Camtchouing P, Drosdowski MA, et al: Adult rat Sertoli cells secrete a factor or factors which modulate Leydig cell function. J Endocrinol 114:459–467, 1987.
395. Verhoeven G, Cailleau J: A Leydig cell stimulatory factor produced by human testicular tubules. Mol Cell Endocrinol 48:137–142, 1987.
396. Janecki A, Jakubowiak A, Lukaszyk A: Stimulatory effect of Sertoli cell secretory products on testosterone secretion by purified Leydig cells in primary culture. Mol Cell Endocrinol 42:235–243, 1985.
397. Parvinen M, Nikula H, Huhtaniemi I: Influence of rat seminiferous tubules on Leydig cells in primary culture. Mol Cell Endocrinol 37:331–336, 1984.
398. Papadopoulus V: Identification and purification of a human Sertoli cell—secreted protein (hSCSP-80) stimulating Leydig cell steroid biosynthesis. J Clin Endocrinol Metab 72:1332–1339, 1991.
399. Zwain IH, Morris PL, Cheng CY: Identification of an inhibitory factor from a Sertoli clonal cell line (TM4) that modulates Leydig cell steroidogenesis. Mol Cell Endocrinol 80:115–126, 1991.
400. Risbridger GP, Jenkin GJ, de Kretser DM: The interaction of hCG, hydroxysteroids and interstitial fluid on Leydig cell steroidogenesis in vitro. J Reprod Fertil 77:239–245, 1986.
401. Sharpe RM, Cooper I: Intratesticular secretion of a factor(s) with major stimulatory effects on Leydig cell testosterone secretion in vitro. Mol Cell Endocrinol 37:159–168, 1984.
402. Melsert R, Huggerbrugge JW, Rommerts FFG: The albumin fraction of rat testicular fluid stimulates steroid production by isolated Leydig cells. Mol Cell Endocrinol 59:221–231, 1988.
403. Hedger MP, Risbridger GP: Effect of serum and serum lipoproteins on testosterone production by adult rat leydig cells in vitro. J St Biochem Molec Biol 43:581–589 1992.
404. Risbridger GP, Averill S, de Kretser DM: Leydig cells are stimulated by follicular fluid. In Spera G, de Kretser DM (eds): Morphological Basis of Human Reproduction. New York, Plenum Press, 1987, pp 63–64.
405. Kahn SA, Hallin P, Bartlett TTJ, et al: Characterization of a factor from human ovarian follicular fluid which stimulates Leydig cell testosterone production. Acta Endocrinol 118:283, 1988.
406. Kahn SA, Keck C, Gudermann T, Nieschlag E: Isolation of a protein from human ovarian follicular fluid which exerts major stimulatory effects on in vitro steroid production of testicular, ovarian and adrenal cells. Endocrinology 126:3043–3052, 1990.
407. Hedger MP, Leung A, Robertson DM, et al: Steroidogenesis-stimulating activity in the gonads: Comparison of rat testicular interstitial fluid with bovine and human ovarian follicular fluid. Biol Reprod 44:937–944, 1991.
408. Klinefelter GR, Ewing LL: Maintenance of testosterone production by purified adult rat Leydig cells for 3 days in vitro. Cell Devel Biol 25:282–288, 1989.
409. Risbridger GP, Hedger MP: Adult rat Leydig cell cultures: Minimum requirements for the maintenance of LH-responsiveness and testosterone production. Mol Cell Endocrinol 83:125–132, 1992.
410. Rommerts FFG: How much androgen is required for maintenance of spermatogenesis? J Endocrinol 116:7–9, 1988.

131

Androgen Physiology

ANDROGEN RECEPTORS AND ACTION

RICHARD A. HIIPAKKA
SHUTSUNG LIAO

Amino-Terminal Domain
DNA-Binding Domain
Steroid-Binding Domain
ANDROGEN RECEPTOR MUTATIONS
MECHANISM OF ANDROGEN ACTION
5α-Reductase and Androgen Action
   Mutations in the Gene for
   5α-Reductase
   Inhibitors of 5α-Reductase
Antiandrogens
Activation of Androgen Receptors
Androgen Response Elements
Post-transcriptional Role for Androgen
   Receptors
GENES REGULATED BY ANDROGENS
**DETECTION AND MEASUREMENT OF
ANDROGEN RECEPTORS**

**ANDROGEN RECEPTOR GENE AND
mRNA**
**ANDROGEN RECEPTOR STRUCTURE AND
FUNCTION**

Androgens are steroids that are responsible for the development and maintenance of the male phenotype. Androgens affect the development, growth, and function of a wide variety of cell types and tissues, and these effects are due in large part to the interaction of androgens with an intracellular component, the androgen receptor.[1, 2] The androgen receptor is a member of a growing family of transcription factors that share common structural motifs and are regulated by specific ligands. Other members of this class of ligand-activated transcription factors include receptors for estrogens, progestins, glucocorticoids, mineralocorticoids, vitamin D, thyroid hormones, retinoic acids, and so-called orphan receptors whose natural ligands remain unknown.[3–5] Androgen receptor complexes bind to specific sequences of DNA in those genes regulated by androgens and modulate the rate of specific gene transcription, perhaps through interactions with other components of the transcriptional apparatus. Androgens also have post-transcriptional effects on gene expression, such as increasing the stability of specific mRNA. These changes in gene expression ultimately produce the characteristic effects of androgens on an organism.

ANDROGEN RECEPTOR GENE AND mRNA

Androgen receptors are minor components of even those cells in which they are relatively abundant, comprising less than 0.01 per cent of the total protein, or about 50,000 molecules per cell. The low level of androgen receptors in target tissues long prevented their isolation and structural characterization. However, when the sequence

of receptors for other steroids (estrogens, progestins, glucocorticoids, and mineralocorticoids) became available through DNA cloning, a common structural design of these receptors was observed. In particular, the amino acid sequence of a region of these receptors required for DNA binding was highly conserved in this family of proteins. Several laboratories constructed DNA probes based on the amino acid sequence of this region and used these probes to clone the mRNA for androgen receptors.[6–12]

Androgen receptor mRNA is transcribed from a single copy gene present on the q11–12 region of the X chromosome and covers more than 90 kilobases (Kb) of DNA.[13, 14] The androgen receptor gene contains eight exons, with each exon contributing to the protein-coding sequence.[14–16] The 5′ and 3′-noncoding regions of androgen receptor mRNA are derived from single exons.[17, 18] The exon/intron boundaries of the androgen receptor gene are similar to those found in the genes for other steroid receptors, indicating that the genes for steroid hormone receptors diverged from a common ancestral gene. A single promoter is used to transcribe androgen receptor mRNA in a variety of cell types producing a 10.6-Kb mRNA, but only 2.8 Kb of this mRNA contains the open-reading frame for the receptor.[19, 20, 20a] The mRNA contains 5′ and 3′-noncoding regions of about 1 and 7 Kb, respectively. Low levels of androgen receptor mRNA smaller than 10.6 Kb have been observed and in one case an 8.5-Kb mRNA was the result of alternative splicing within the 3′-noncoding sequence.[18] Androgen receptor mRNA isoforms have also been observed in the rat central nervous system and the larynx of male *Xenopus laevis*.[20b, 20c] These smaller AR mRNA's appear to lack portions of the 5′-noncoding region of the mRNA.

Other smaller uncharacterized forms of androgen receptor mRNA may be due to alternative splicing within coding exons or the result of different transcriptional initiation sites. These mRNA's could encode for androgen receptors with different amino acid sequences and perhaps different functions than the full-length receptor.

ANDROGEN RECEPTOR STRUCTURE AND FUNCTION

The human androgen receptor contains some 918 amino acids, although the exact number may vary from individual to individual owing to variations in the length of polyglycine and polyglutamine stretches found in the amino-terminal region of the receptor.[6–12] The molecular weight of the receptor based on its amino acid sequence is about 98,000; however, estimates of its molecular weight by techniques such as denaturing polyacrylamide gel electrophoresis yield values near 110,000.[22, 23] This difference may reflect post-translational modifications or an unusual mobility of androgen receptors on gel electrophoresis. The only post-translational modification known for this receptor is phosphorylation; its role in receptor function is unknown, but it may regulate steroid-binding activity of the receptor.[24–26] Phosphorylation of the androgen receptor occurs predominantly in the amino-terminal domain.[26a]

Androgen receptors, like other steroid receptors, are composed of three functional domains—an amino-terminal domain that is important for transcriptional activation, a central DNA-binding domain, and a carboxyl-terminal ligand-binding domain. The roles of these various domains in the mechanism of androgen action have been investigated by determining the effect of deletion mutations on the function of androgen receptors.[27–30] Most of these studies involve the co-transfection of cells that do not express androgen receptors with expression vectors encoding normal or mutant receptors, as well as with a plasmid that contains an easily monitored reporter gene, such as the gene encoding the enzyme chloramphenicol acetyltransferase (CAT), linked to a promoter known to be regulated by the androgen receptor.[31] A well-studied promoter is the mouse mammary tumor virus (MMTV) long terminal repeat, which contains a promoter that is active in many cells and is responsive to androgen, as well as glucocorticoid, mineralocorticoid, and progestin receptors. The MMTV promoter contains specific DNA sequences called hormone response elements (HRE), which androgen and other steroid receptors bind and through which these receptors enhance the transcription of genes.[32] Transcriptional activation of the MMTV CAT reporter gene by androgen and other steroid receptors requires that the receptor be bound to its respective ligand in order to activate gene transcription.

Amino-Terminal Domain

The amino-terminal domain of the androgen receptor makes up more than half of the receptor, and a single exon encodes most of this domain.[17] The amino-terminal domain is poorly conserved among all members of the steroid receptor family in both sequence and length (Fig.

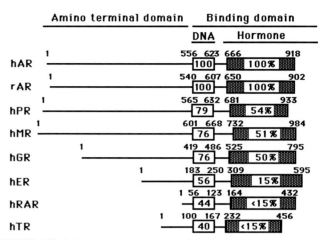

FIGURE 131–1. Schematic comparison of the domain structures of various receptors. Numbers above refer to amino acid positions of the receptors. Numbers within rectangles are the per cent identity of the amino acid sequence of the particular receptor domain with regard to the same domain in the human androgen receptor. The amino-terminus of the receptors is on the left. h, human; r, rat; AR, PR, MR, GR, ER, RAR, TR: androgen, progestin, mineralocorticoid, glucocorticoid, estrogen, retinoic acid, and thyroid hormone receptors, respectively.

131–1). Only 116 of the 555 amino acids comprising this region are conserved between androgen receptors from humans and rats.[7] A striking feature of this domain in the human androgen receptor is the presence of two homopolymeric stretches of glycine and glutamine (Fig. 131–2). The length of these stretches has been found to vary in normal individuals from 17 to 23 residues for glutamine and 16 to 27 for glycine in the human androgen receptor.[6–12, 21] Androgen receptors from mice and rats have much shorter glutamine and glycine repeats (Fig. 131–2). Not all steroid receptors contain these homopolymeric repeats, and their role in androgen receptor function remains unknown. However, similar homopolymeric repeats have been found in other classes of proteins regulating gene expression, and so these repeats may be important for transcriptional regulation. The amino-terminal domain also contains short runs (three to eight residues long) of other amino acids including alanine, leucine, proline, and serine (Fig. 131–2). Androgen receptors with deletions of up to 140 amino acids from the amino terminus (which

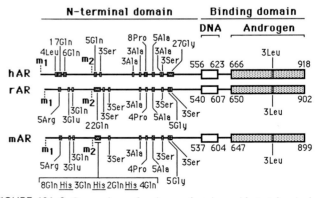

FIGURE 131–2. Comparison of various polyamino acid stretches in human, rat, and mouse androgen receptor domains. Numbers flanking the DNA and androgen-binding domains refer to amino acid positions of the androgen receptor. m_1 and m_2 indicate positions of possible initiator methionines.

includes the polyglutamine repeat) activate reporter gene transcription at levels similar to the full-length receptor.[30] More extensive deletions from the amino-terminus (210 to 337 amino acids) produce androgen receptors that bind androgens, interact with cellular DNA, but activate reporter gene transcription at levels less than 5 per cent of the full-length receptor.[30]

The amino-terminus of the androgen receptor has not been determined by direct sequencing of the isolated receptor. A putative translation initiation point that conforms to consensus sequences for translation initiation has been adopted from the cDNA sequence. However, it is not known if this initiation site is correct, if alternative initiation codons are used, or if processing of the androgen receptor amino-terminus occurs after synthesis of the primary translation product. The size of the androgen receptor in various tissues, however, is consistent with translation initiation from the first methionine codon (Fig. 131–2).

DNA-Binding Domain

The androgen receptor DNA-binding domain consists of about 70 amino acids (Fig. 131–3) and is located between the amino-terminal domain and the carboxyl-terminal androgen-binding domain. Steroid receptors as a group have the greatest amino acid sequence similarity in the DNA-binding domain; the identity in this region between androgen receptors and receptors for estrogens, glucocorticoids, mineralocorticoids, and progestins is 56, 76, 76, and 79 per cent, respectively.[7] Androgen receptors from humans,[6, 10–12] mice,[33] and rats[6, 9] have identical amino acid sequences in this region. A variety of studies, including x-ray crystallography[34] and two-dimensional ^{1}H NMR of glucocorticoid[35] and estrogen receptors,[36] have shown that the sulfurs of eight cysteines in this domain coordinate two Zn^{+2} ions in a tetrahedral configuration, forming motifs that are called *zinc fingers*. The two zinc finger motifs fold to form a single

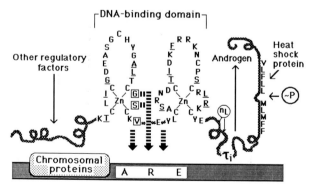

FIGURE 131–3. Sequence of the DNA-binding domain of androgen receptors and location of the two "zinc fingers." The sulfurs from four cysteines in each finger coordinate a single Zn^{2+} ion. Amino acids that are not conserved in human androgen, glucocorticoid, mineralocorticoid, and progesterone receptors are underlined. Amino acids conserved in human androgen and three other steroid receptors are underlined bold letters. The boxed amino acids are residues important for HRE-binding specificity. n_L, nuclear localization signal; τ_i: transcriptional inactivation domain; V, L, F, and M, amino acid residue involved in possible "leucine zipper"–like structures between different transcription factors. The androgen receptor is a phosphoprotein but the phosphorylation (P) site(s) on the androgen receptor is unknown. The HSP 90 binding site is not well-defined but involves amino acids in the amino-terminal half of the ligand-binding domain.

structural domain, which consists in part of two overlapping perpendicular helices. Part of the amino terminal zinc finger defines one helix whose amino acids interact with bases of the HRE in the major groove of the DNA. Three amino acids in this helical region, which are conserved among androgen, glucocorticoid, mineralocorticoid, and progestin receptors, define the HRE-binding specificity of a steroid receptor[37–39]; therefore, it is not surprising that androgen, glucocorticoid, mineralocorticoid, and progestin receptors recognize similar HRE's.[32] The carboxyl-terminal zinc finger includes the other helical segment that folds back over the helix in the first finger, and hydrophobic contacts between the helices help to stabilize the overall structure of this domain. This second zinc finger also includes amino acids that interact during head-to-head receptor dimerization on DNA.[34, 40] Deletion of the DNA-binding domain from the androgen receptor yields a receptor that does not bind to DNA, does not activate transcription but does bind androgens.[29, 30] Two exons encode the DNA-binding domain of the androgen receptor, one for each zinc finger.

A nuclear localization signal that functions independently of the DNA-binding domain is present in the androgen receptor and is located adjacent (carboxyl-terminal) to the DNA-binding domain.[29, 30, 30a] A related amino acid sequence is found in other steroid receptors and some other nuclear proteins. This signal sequence may help to localize receptor in the nucleus in the absence of ligand.

Steroid-Binding Domain

The carboxyl-terminal androgen-binding domain represents some 30 per cent of the receptor. The amino acid sequence of this domain is the second most highly conserved region among the steroid receptors, with overall identity between androgen and other steroid receptors ranging from 15 to 54 per cent and certain subregions being highly conserved.[6] The amino acid sequences of the ligand-binding domain of androgen receptors from humans, mice, and rats are identical. Little is known about the secondary and tertiary structure of this domain for any steroid receptor. Deletion of as little as 20 or as much as 120 amino acids from the carboxyl-terminus of the androgen receptor destroys the receptors' ability to bind steroid and activate transcription.[27–30] A region near the carboxyl-terminus that is conserved in the steroid receptor family has been defined as having a role in transcriptional activation of steroid receptors, perhaps through interactions with other transcriptional activators or components of the transcriptional machinery.[41] Deletion of 200 to 270 amino acids from the carboxyl-terminus produces androgen receptors that do not bind steroid, but these truncated receptors constitutively activate transcription at levels of 40 to 100 per cent of the full-length receptor. Therefore, a region in the steroid-binding domain inhibits the transcriptional activating properties of androgen receptors, but this inhibition can be relieved by steroid binding to the full-length receptor or by deletion of this part of the receptor. Part of this region is conserved among members of the steroid receptor family and is important for interaction of androgen and other steroid receptors with heat shock protein 90 (HSP 90), and this region also has been implicated in dimerization of some members of this class of transcription factors.[42–44] The role of HSP 90 in receptor function is unclear, but it may maintain proper steroid receptor structure until ligand binds or may have a regulatory role in the mechanism of action of androgen and other steroid receptors.[45, 46] The ligand-binding domain of the androgen receptor contains several heptad repeats of leucine and other small hydrophobic amino acids. These heptad repeats have been implicated in protein-protein interactions through structures called *leucine zippers* and may be important for interaction of receptors with other transcription factors.[47] The hormone-binding domain of the androgen and other steroid receptors are rich in methionine, and 5 of the 13 methionines in this domain of the androgen receptor are conserved in other steroid receptors. These methionines may play a role in structures, such as leucine zippers, important in receptor function.

ANDROGEN RECEPTOR MUTATIONS

More than 50 different naturally occurring mutations in the androgen receptor gene have been described in individuals with complete or partial insensitivity to androgens. These mutations are summarized in Table 131–1. Individuals with these androgen receptor mutations have a 46 X, Y genotype, testes, and normal to high circulating testosterone levels, but vary from phenotypic females to undervirilized or infertile men. Clinical observations, biochemical analysis of androgen receptors in genital skin fibroblasts, and sequencing of the androgen receptor gene in these individuals have provided additional information with regard to structure and function of androgen receptors.

Only a few mutations causing abnormal androgenic responses have been described for the amino-terminal domain of the androgen receptor. The rarity of described mutations in this domain compared with the other domains may reflect the insensitivity of androgen receptor function to mutations in this region. Expansion of the polyglutamine stretch in this domain, which in normal individuals varies from 17 to 23 residues to 40 to 50 residues, has been linked to the rare X chromosome–linked disease, spinal and bulbar muscular atrophy (SBMA, Kennedy disease).[50, 51] Affected males have progressive muscular weakness secondary to neural degeneration, reduced fertility, and gynecomastia. The role of the polyglutamine stretch in receptor function is unknown; however, androgen receptors containing polyglutamine stretches of 46 to 50 residues transactivate less efficiently an MMTV growth hormone reporter gene in transfected COS-1 cells.[84] The polyglutamine stretch is not required for transcriptional activation of a reporter gene because androgen receptors with deletions encompassing the polyglutamine stretch activate transcription from an MMTV CAT reporter gene in COS-1 cells as well as the normal full-length receptor.[30] Expansion of the polyglutamine stretch of the androgen receptor may produce a gain-in-function mutation in which the mutant receptor acquires a new property resulting in the observed phenotype. Individuals with complete deletions of the androgen receptor gene have complete androgen insensitivity as expected but are otherwise healthy individuals and in particular do not exhibit symptoms of SBMA. An individual with partial androgen insensitivity

who responded to high-dose androgen therapy had an androgen receptor with a relatively short (12 residues) polyglutamine stretch in the amino-terminus, as well as a point mutation in exon 5, encoding part of the steroid-binding domain.[52] Both of these mutations contribute to defective androgen receptor function based on transfection studies with androgen receptors containing these mutations, individually or in combination.

Three naturally occurring point mutations in the amino-terminal domain of the androgen receptor in individuals with androgen insensitivity have been described. These mutations introduce premature translation termination signals and a change in reading frame of the receptor mRNA, which result in truncated proteins that do not bind steroids or DNA.[53–57] The testicular feminized (Tfm) mouse, which has been used extensively in laboratory experiments as a model system of androgen insensitivity, has a deletion mutation (a single C residue) in the DNA encoding the amino-terminal domain of the androgen receptor.[54–56] This deletion changes the reading frame of the receptor mRNA, introducing 41 missense amino acids before a premature termination codon. Kidney tissue from Tfm mice has approximately 10 per cent of the androgen-binding activity of normal littermates. This residual androgen-binding activity may be due to translation initiation downstream of the normal point of translational initiation, producing amino-terminal–truncated receptors with steroid-binding activity.

Four individuals with partial or complete insensitivity to androgens have been found to have point mutations in the DNA-binding domain of the androgen receptor. One of these mutations is in the receptor dimerization interface,[58] two are mutations in residues making phosphate contacts in the DNA HRE backbone,[60, 61] and the last mutation introduces a premature translation termination codon, which results in the deletion of the second zinc finger and the steroid-binding domain.[16] Two siblings with complete androgen insensitivity due to deletion of exon 3 of the androgen receptor gene have been described.[59] This mutation produces an androgen receptor in which the second zinc finger of the DNA-binding domain is missing. Individuals with this mutation have supranormal levels of androgen-binding activity in genital skin fibroblasts, and surprisingly, their androgen receptors are localized in nuclei by immunocytochemistry. A putative nuclear localization signal adjacent to the DNA-binding domain may be responsible for this nuclear localization.[29, 30]

Numerous (more than 30) point mutations in the four exons encoding the androgen receptor steroid-binding domain have been described in individuals with androgen insensitivity. Many of these mutations destroy or diminish steroid-binding activity of the androgen receptor. The Tfm rat, another experimental model system of androgen insensitivity similar to the Tfm mouse, has a point mutation in the DNA encoding the ligand-binding domain that changes an arginine residue, which is conserved in several members of this family of transcription factors, to a glutamine.[69] The same mutation has been described in humans.[70] CV-1 cells expressing this mutant androgen receptor have a much lower androgen-binding capacity than cells expressing wild-type receptor; however, the mutant receptor has a normal affinity for androgens. This mutation alters a putative phosphorylation recognition signal, and phosphorylation of this site may be required for ste-

TABLE 131–1. NATURALLY OCCURRING MUTATIONS IN THE ANDROGEN RECEPTOR

LESION*	MUTATION†	DOMAIN‡	PHENOTYPE§	COMMENTS (REFERENCE)
Total gene deletion	—	N, D, L	C	(48)
Partial gene deletion	—	L	C	(49)
Insertion at Q58-73	+ (CAG)25	N	P	Linked to spinal and bulbar muscular atrophy (50, 51)
Deletion at Q58-73	− (CAG)12	N	P	Additional mutation present: Y762C (52)
Q114Stop	C to T	N, D, L	C	Low level of initiation downstream (53)
P372Nonsense	−C	N	C	Tfm mouse; low level of initiation downstream (54–56)
Y533Stop	A to G	N	C	(57)
K589Stop	A to T	D	C	(16)
A595T	*G to A	D	P/R	Mutation in receptor dimerization interface (58)
Deletion of exon 3	—	D	C	Second zinc finger deleted (59)
K608R	A to G	D	P	Phosphate contact in ARE (60)
K614P	G to C	D	C	Phosphate contact in ARE (61)
Deletion of amino acids 674–714	G to T	L −	C	Splice donor mutation; use of cryptic splice site (62)
D689H	G to C	L ±	C	(63)
D689N	G to A	L ±	C	(64)
D694H	G to C	L −	C	Amino acid conserved in SR (64)
D694N	*G to A	L −	C	Amino acid conserved in SR (64)
N704S	A to G	L −	C	Amino acid conserved in SR (65)
W717Stop	G to A	L −	C	(66)
L727S	T to C	L ±	P	(67)
V729M	*G to A	L	?	Human prostate tumor (68)
W740R	T to C	L −	C	(67)
A747D	C to A	L ±	P/R	Amino acid conserved in SR (67)
M748S	A to G	L	C	(65)
R751Q	*G to A	L −	C	Tfm rat; amino acids conserved in SR (69, 70)
S758F	C to T	L −	C	Amino acid conserved in MR (65)
Y762C	A to G	L ±	P	Additional mutation (insertion) at Q58 (52)
F763L	C to A,G	L −	C	Amino acid conserved in SR (67)
A764V	C to T	L −	C	Amino acid conserved in SR (71)
P765S	C to T	L ±	C	(67)
E771A	A to C	L +	P	Amino acid conserved in SR (71)
E771G	A to G	L	P	Amino acid conserved in SR (72)
R773C	*C to T	L −	C	Amino acid semiconserved in SR (Lys or Arg) (73–75)
R773H	*G to A	L ±	C	Amino acid semiconserved in SR (Lys or Arg) (73)
M786V	A to G	L −	C	Amino acid conserved in SR (76)
W795Stop	*G to A	L −	C	(77)
S813N	G to A	L ±	P	(78)
R830Q	*G to A	L −	C	Amino acid conserved in SR (67)
R830Stop	*C to T	L −	C	Amino acid conserved in SR (65)
Y833C	A to G	L −	C	(67)
R839C	*C to T	L ±	P/R	Amino acid semiconserved in SR (Lys or Arg) (67)
R839H	*G to A	L ±	P/R/C	Variable phenotype; amino acid semiconserved in SR
R853K	G to A	L ±	P	(67)
R854H	*G to A	L +	P/R/C	Variable phenotype (67)
R854C	*C to T	L −	C	Amino acid conserved in SR (65)
D863G	A to G	L −	C	Amino acid conserved in SR (65)
V865L	G to T	L +	P	Leu or Met in other SR (79)
V865M	G to A	L ±	P/C	Leu or Met in other SR (15, 79)
V865E	T to A	L −	C	(67)
I868M	T to G	L −	P	(80)
T876A	A to G	L +		LNCaP; altered hormone-binding specificity (81, 82)
K882Stop	A to T	L −	C	(83)
P903H	C to A	L −	C	(67)
V901M	G to A	L ±	P/R	(67)

*Single letter amino acid code is used for wild-type and mutants; numbers indicate amino acid position as published by Chang et al.[16]

†Base change to produce given mutation; *denotes mutations at CpG dinucleotides which are hot spots for mutations due to the prevalence of methylation of C residues at this dinucleotide.

‡Domain affected by mutation: N, amino-terminal; D, DNA binding; L, androgen-binding; +, quantitatively normal androgen-binding activity; ±, qualitatively or quantitatively abnormal androgen-binding activity compared with wild-type androgen receptor; −, very little or no androgen-binding activity.

§Androgen insensitivity phenotype: C, complete, P, partial, R, Reifenstein syndrome. SR, steroid receptor; MR, mineralocorticoid receptor; ARE, androgen response element.

roid-binding activity of the receptor.[69] Androgen receptors with this mutation have a reduced ability to activate gene transcription from reporter genes linked to an MMTV promoter. Mutations in the androgen receptor steroid-binding domain have also been found in DNA from human prostate tumors.[68, 81, 82] In the human prostate cancer cell line, LNCaP (lymph node cancer of the prostate), a mutation in the steroid-binding domain alters the steroid-binding specificity of the androgen receptor (Table 131–2) such that estrogens, progestins, and certain antiandrogens have agonist activity.[81, 82] Mutations like the one found in LNCaP cells may have medical significance because some treatments for androgen-dependent prostatic cancer, such as antiandrogen therapy, could actually promote cancer growth. Also, the progression of prostatic cancer from an androgen-dependent to an androgen-independent form could conceivably be related in some cases to mutations in the androgen receptor.

TABLE 131–2. COMPARISON OF THE RELATIVE BINDING AFFINITIES OF VARIOUS STEROIDS AND ANTIANDROGENS FOR NORMAL AND LNCaP ANDROGEN RECEPTORS

STEROID/ANTIANDROGEN	NORMAL ANDROGEN RECEPTOR	LNCaP ANDROGEN RECEPTOR
Dihydrotestosterone	1.18	0.49
Testosterone	0.52	0.32
Dimethylnortestosterone	1.00	0.41
Methyltrienolone	1.06	0.56
Progesterone	0.12	0.56
Estradiol	0.13	0.18
Dexamethasone	0.07	0.07
Cyproterone acetate	0.25	0.26
Hydroxyflutamide	0.10	0.23

Androgen receptors were produced by in vitro translation in a rabbit reticulocyte lysate. A relative competition index was determined by analyzing the effect of various unlabeled steroids on binding of labeled dimethylnortestosterone to the androgen receptor. All values are normalized relative to dimethylnortestosterone, which is given a value of 1.0.

MECHANISM OF ANDROGEN ACTION

The two principal androgens active in target cells are testosterone and 5α-dihydrotestosterone (Fig. 131–4). These two steroids have the highest affinity for the androgen receptor among various steroids present in the blood of men (Table 131–3). Testosterone is the most abundant androgen circulating in the blood of men and is principally derived from testicular secretions. The adrenals provide a small amount of the circulating testosterone, either directly or from the peripheral conversion of secreted androstenedione and dehydroepiandrosterone. 5α-Dihydrotestosterone is also produced by the testis, but most of the circulating 5α-dihydrotestosterone results from the peripheral metabolism of testosterone in various tissues. Both testosterone and 5α-dihydrotestosterone are present in blood at concentrations far exceeding their dissociation constants for the androgen receptor; however, the availability of these two androgens to target tissues or sites of metabolic degradation is limited by the binding of these steroids to blood proteins, such as the specific high-affinity carrier, sex hormone–binding globulin (SHBG).[85] Only 1 to 2 per cent of the total blood testosterone and 5α-dihydrotestosterone is available for uptake into cells. Although there is some evidence for receptor-mediated uptake of SHBG, free and loosely bound (such as to albumin) steroids are thought to be the active hormone fraction in blood.[86] Although little is known about the transport of free steroids into the cell, given their hydrophobic nature, steroids probably diffuse freely through the plasma membrane.[87]

A complex interplay of enzymatic activation and inactivation inside the cell also may limit the availability of androgens in certain cell types.[88] Some steroids, such as androstenedione and dehydroepiandrosterone, secreted by the testis or adrenals, are not active androgens but can be converted to testosterone in certain cells. Therefore, these steroids can promote androgenic effects, especially when the synthesis of these steroids is elevated (as in congenital adrenal hyperplasia). Testosterone and dihydrotestosterone are metabolized in various cells to less active androgens, such as androstanediols and androsterone, which may be conjugated to glucuronic acid and ultimately excreted.[89]

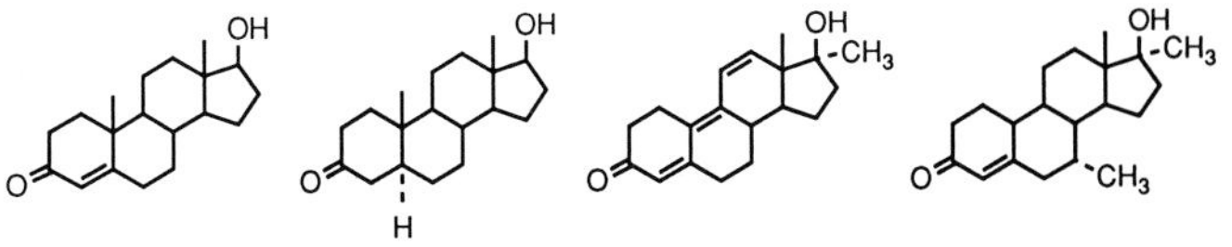

FIGURE 131–4. Structure of natural and synthetic ligands for androgen receptors. Testosterone and 5α-dihydrotestosterone are potent naturally occurring ligands for the androgen receptor. R1881 (methyltrienolone) and DMNT (dimethylnortestosterone; Mibolerone) are synthetic androgens resistant to metabolic inactivation and are often used in radioactive forms as labeling agents for androgen-receptor studies.

5α-Reductase and Androgen Action

Once inside a cell, testosterone may be metabolized to a variety of steroids, but in most androgen-sensitive cells testosterone is converted to the more potent androgen, 5α-dihydrotestosterone, by the NADPH-dependent enzyme 5α-reductase, which is located in the endoplasmic reticulum and nuclear membrane.[90] 5α-Dihydrotestosterone is the predominant steroid present in extracts of nuclei of androgen-sensitive tissues exposed to labeled testosterone.[91, 92] Two different genes for 5α-reductase have been characterized in rats and humans.[93–96] The human 5α-reductase type 1 gene is located on band p15 of chromosome 5.[97] A processed pseudogene related to this type 1 reductase is also present on q24-qter of the X chromosome, but no evidence for its expression has been found. Transcription and processing of the five exons of the type 1 gene produce a 2.5-Kb mRNA in various rat tissues, which codes for a hydrophobic 29,400-dalton protein. The human 5α-reductase type 2 gene is located on band p23 of chromosome 2 and has five exons with similar exon/intron boundaries as the type 1 gene.[98] Transcription of the type 2 gene produces a 3.6-Kb mRNA, which codes for a hydrophobic 28,300-dalton protein. The type 1 and 2 5α-reductases share 50 per cent identity in their amino acid sequences and differ in several biochemical parameters. The rat and human type 1 enzymes have broad neutral to basic pH optima compared with the sharp acidic pH optima of the type 2 enzymes, and the type 1 5α-reductases have higher Michaelis constants for testosterone and lower affinities for the 4-azasteroid 5α-reductase inhibitor finasteride (Fig.

TABLE 131–3. APPROXIMATE BLOOD STEROID CONCENTRATIONS AND RELATIVE BINDING AFFINITIES OF VARIOUS STEROIDS FOR THE ANDROGEN RECEPTOR

STEROID	RELATIVE BINDING AFFINITY*	BLOOD CONCENTRATION (nM)
5α-Dihydrotestosterone	1.0	2
Testosterone	0.2	20
Progesterone	0.02	1
Estradiol	0.015	0.15
Cortisol	<0.0001	300
Aldosterone	<0.0001	4

*The dissociation constants for testosterone and 5α-dihydrotestosterone binding to the androgen receptor are in the range of 0.2 to 0.4 nM and 0.5 to 1.0 nM, respectively. Relative binding affinity is the concentration of steroid required to block 50 per cent of the binding of a labeled androgen, such as ³H-R1881, to the androgen receptor, and are normalized relative to 5α-dihydrotestosterone, which is given a value of 1.0.

131–5) compared with the type 2 5α-reductases. The tissue distribution of the mRNA (and presumably the protein) for these two enzymes in various rat tissues is also different. The mRNA for the type 1 enzyme, which is postulated to have a catabolic role in metabolism of testosterone, predominates in rat tissues such as liver, kidney, intestine, brain, adrenal, and lung, whereas the mRNA for the type 2 enzyme, which is postulated to have an anabolic role, is relatively more abundant in rat epididymis, testis, and vas deferens. The rat prostate and seminal vesicle have mRNA for both enzymes and the type 1 mRNA is present in three- to five-fold excess over the type 2 mRNA in these tissues. The tissue-specific and developmental expressions (mRNA and protein) of the different 5α-reductase enzymes have also been studied in humans.[98a] The type 1 enzyme is immunologically detected in skin and liver and the mRNA for the type 1 enzyme is found in brain (pons, cerebellum, medulla oblongata, and hypothalamus), liver, and skin. The mRNA for the type 2 enzyme is present in epididymis, seminal vesicle, prostate, and liver. Expression of both types of reductase in liver does not begin until birth. Both enzymes are found in the skin of the chest and scalp of the neonate, but only the type 1 enzyme is expressed in skin after puberty. The type 1 enzyme is also expressed in balding scalp. The type 2 but not the type 1 enzyme is present in hyperplastic and neoplastic prostatic tissue. The kinetic parameters for 5α-reductase from human prostatic stromal and epithelial cells are different, perhaps indicative of different cellular locations for these two enzymes in this tissue.[99] The subcellular location of these enzymes may also differ because rat liver 5α-reductase (type 1 enzyme) is found predominantly in microsomes derived from the endoplasmic reticulum, whereas human and rat prostatic 5α-reductases are found associated with nuclei as well as microsomes.[100, 101] 5α-Reductase is associated with nuclei in many androgen-sensitive tissues, a location that may facilitate subsequent interaction of 5α-dihydrotestosterone with the androgen receptor because androgen receptors may reside in nuclei even in the absence of ligand.

Certain tissues, such as mouse kidney or muscle of most animals, contain little or no 5α-reductase but respond to androgens. In these tissues testosterone may be the active androgen and may bind directly to the androgen receptor to elicit a response.

Mutations in the Gene for 5α-Reductase

The importance of 5α-reductase to a cell's response to circulating testosterone has become evident from studies of the effects of a deficiency in the activity of this enzyme on the development of the male phenotype.[102] A 5α-reductase deficiency causes a form of male pseudohermaphroditism, in which testosterone levels are adequate for development of the epididymis, vas deferens, and seminal vesicle from the wolffian ducts but are inadequate for complete virilization of the urogenital sinus and genital tubercle, swellings and folds from which the prostate and external genitalia develop. At puberty, some growth of the urogenital tract and external genitalia occurs, and a male pattern of musculoskeletal development takes place; however, other aspects of sexual maturation, including growth of beard and body hair, development of acne, and temporal hairline recession are missing or minimal. The ability of testosterone to support the development of reproductive tract tissues from the wolffian duct, but not from the urogenital sinus, may reflect a high local intracellular concentration of testosterone in the wolffian duct but not in the urogenital sinus or external genital anlagen, perhaps as the result of proximity to the developing testis. During the early stages of normal wolffian duct differentiation, 5α-reductase activity is very low or absent; testosterone may therefore be the active androgen in this tissue at this time.[103]

Twenty different mutations in the 5α-reductase type 2 gene have been described in individuals with a diagnosis of 5α-reductase deficiency and male pseudohermaphroditism from 25 families of various ethnic backgrounds.[98, 104] Six of these mutations were recurrent in 19 different ethnic backgrounds, indicative of mutational hot spots. No mutations in the type 1 gene have been linked to this disorder. These mutations occur in each of the five exons of the 5α-reductase gene and include total and partial gene deletions, nonsense and missense mutations, and a mutation in a splice junction. Some of the individuals with these mutations were simple (four families) and compound (six families) heterozygotes. One of these mutations is present in a well-characterized kindred composed of 29 families with 47 affected individuals from the Dominican Republic, in which arginine 246 is replaced by tryptophan as the result of a C to T mutation.[104] Affected individuals have ambiguous external genitalia at birth but exhibit partial virilization at puberty. The mutant enzyme expressed in cultured cells had a V_{max} that was 5 to 10 per cent of the normal gene product, perhaps the result of a higher Michaelis constant (600 μM for mutant versus 10 μM for wild-type) for the substrate NADPH. Three individuals from different ethnic backgrounds had a mutation which changed glycine 34 to arginine. The mutant enzyme expressed in cultured cells has a 10-fold higher Michaelis constant for testosterone than the wild-type enzyme. Individuals with this mutation have a female phenotype with only minor virilization at puberty. In contrast to the severe effects of this mutation, an individual with a mutation that changed glycine 196 to serine had a predominantly male phenotype and variable expression of 5α-reductase deficiency. The mutant enzyme, expressed in cultured cells, has a 10-fold higher Michaelis constant for NADPH than the wild-type enzyme.

Inhibitors of 5α-Reductase

The importance of 5α-reductase in a tissue's response to testosterone has led to the development of natural and synthetic inhibitors (Fig. 131–5) of this enzyme, which may be useful for the selective treatment of conditions such as benign prostatic hyperplasia, hirsutism, alopecia, and acne that may depend on 5α-dihydrotestosterone for their development. Of the various inhibitors under development, 4-azasteroids, such as finasteride (N-[2-methyl-2-propyl]-3-oxo-4-aza-5α-andorst-1-ene-17β-carboxamide, Proscar), are orally active inhibitors of 5α-reductase and have shown some clinical efficacy in treatment of benign prostatic hyperplasia.[105] The 4-azasteroid 17β-N,N diethylcarbamoyl-4-aza-5α-androstan-3-one (4-MA) is also an inhibitor of 5α-reductase (K_i, 5 nM), and ^{3}H-4-MA is useful for quantitation of 5α-reductase in a simple binding assay.[106] The 4-azasteroid 21-diazo-4-methyl-4-aza-5α-pregnane-3, 20-dione (diazo

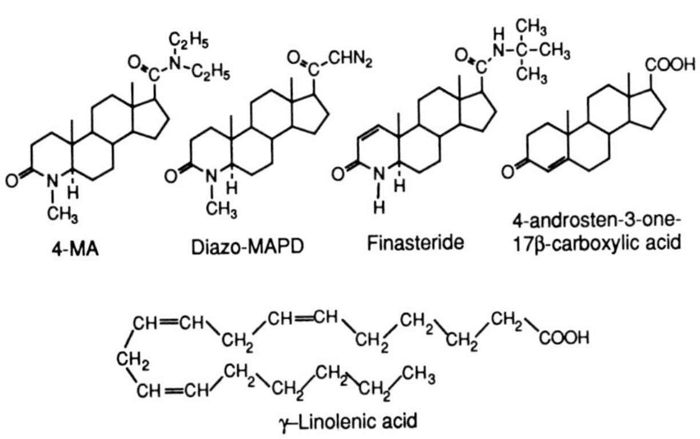

FIGURE 131–5. Natural and synthetic inhibitors of the enzyme 5α-reductase.

MAPD) binds to 5α-reductase (K_i, 8 nM) and contains a photoreactive group, which allows covalent labeling and inactivation of 5α-reductase.[107] Other irreversible inhibitors of 5α-reductase include 17-acetoxy-6-methylene-4-pregnene-3, 20-dione (K_i, 1 μM),[108] 5α-4-diazo-21-hydroxy-20-methylpregnan-3-one (K_i, 35 nM),[109] and the allenic seco-steroid 5, 10-seco-19-norpregna-4,5-diene-3,10,20-trione (K_i, 1 μM).[110] A well-studied competitive inhibitor of 5α-reductase is androst-4-ene-3-one-17β-carboxylic acid (K_i, 1 μM).[111] Specific aliphatic unsaturated fatty acids, such as γ-linolenic acid, also inhibit 5α-reductase (50 per cent inhibition at 10 μM).[112] It remains to be established if unsaturated fatty acids have a physiological role in modulating androgen action; however, unsaturated fatty acids may find use in the pharmacological control of certain androgenic responses.

Antiandrogens

Some synthetic compounds compete for binding to androgen receptors, but do not elicit androgenic effects. These antagonists are called *antiandrogens* and are clinically useful in some circumstances, such as for treatment of acne, alopecia, seborrhea, hirsutism, and androgen-dependent prostatic cancer, where they are used to block possible agonist effects of adrenal androgens after castration or in conjunction with a GnRH superagonist, which pharmacologically blocks testicular secretion of androgens.[113] Clinical use of antiandrogens in women of reproductive age carries the risk of feminization of male fetuses, and use in men has limitations due to effects on sexual function. Both steroidal and nonsteroidal antiandrogens are in clinical use (Fig. 131–6). Flutamide is a pure androgen antagonist (that is, it produces no androgenic or other steroidal effects) and is metabolized to hydroxyflutamide, which has a higher affinity for the androgen receptor and may be the active form of this antiandrogen.[114] The antiandrogen anandron is structurally related to flutamide and binds to the androgen receptor with an affinity similar to that of hydroxyflutamide.[115] Both flutamide and anandron are used clinically for treatment of disseminated androgen-dependent prostatic cancer. Use of pure antiandrogens in noncastrated men produces a surge in androgen secretion by the testis because these antiandrogens block the negative feedback effect of androgens on the hypothalamus and pituitary. Cyproterone acetate has both antagonist and ag-

onist (progestational, adrenocortical) activities that enhance and limit its clinical usefulness.[116] Spironolactone, an aldosterone antagonist, also has antiandrogenic properties. It is widely used in some countries in the management of hirsutism, although it does have some side effects.[117] Certain H_2 receptor antagonists, such as cimetidine, have weak antiandrogenic effects and occasionally produce gynecomastia in individuals taking this drug.[118] The compound RU 3882 is a potential topical antiandrogen that has little or no systemic activity and may find use in treating androgen-dependent skin disorders without affecting other tissues sensitive to androgens.[119, 120] Dihydrophenanthrene is also an antiandrogen, and unlike most active androgens is devoid of keto- and hydroxy- functional groups.[121] It is unclear at present how antiandrogens and other antisteroids function because they bind to receptors but do not activate gene transcription. It is uncertain if there is a common mechanism of action for all steroid antagonists; however, in some cases steroid antagonists are unable to elicit a conformational change in the receptor that may be required for transcriptional activation of genes.[122]

Activation of Androgen Receptors

The point of interaction of androgen receptors with their ligands inside the cell is not entirely clear, but early models of androgen action pictured androgen receptors, free of ligand, as components of the cell cytoplasm that translocated into nuclei after binding steroid. These models were based on cell fractionation studies which showed that androgen receptors were in the cytosol fraction of disrupted cells, if cells were not exposed to steroid but were found in nuclei after exposure of cells to steroids. These results have been reinterpreted in light of recent immuno-localization and other studies which indicate that unliganded steroid receptors are present in nuclei.[123] In recent models of steroid hormone action, steroid receptors are loosely associated with nuclei in the absence of hormone and upon disruption of the cell leak out of nuclei into the cytosol fraction, whereas in the presence of ligand, receptors are tightly bound to nuclear components and fractionate with nuclei after cell disruption. In some circumstances, androgen and other steroid receptors have been found in

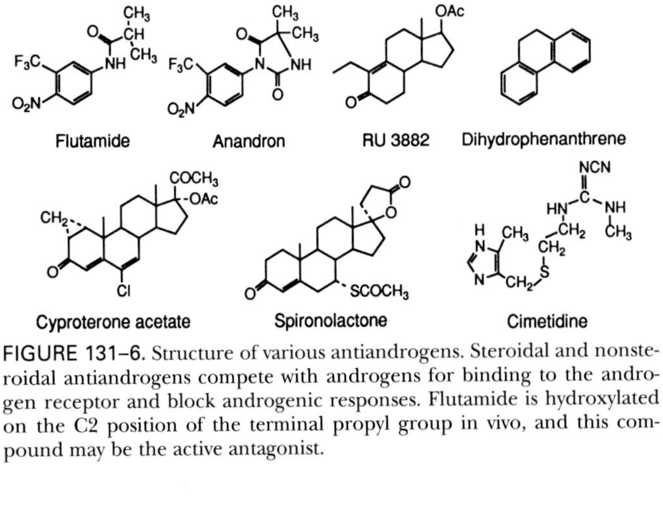

FIGURE 131–6. Structure of various antiandrogens. Steroidal and nonsteroidal antiandrogens compete with androgens for binding to the androgen receptor and block androgenic responses. Flutamide is hydroxylated on the C2 position of the terminal propyl group in vivo, and this compound may be the active antagonist.

the cytoplasm of cells, observations which ensure that the subcellular location of steroid receptors remains a controversial subject. Given the post-transcriptional effects of steroid hormones, for example on mRNA stability, a cytoplasmic role for steroid receptors is not out of the question.

It is not known at this time what changes occur in vivo to cause the increased affinity of receptors for nuclei after binding steroid; however, most models of steroid hormone action include a receptor transformation or activation step to signify this change in affinity for nuclei or DNA. Transformation of steroid receptors can be observed in vitro and can be induced by high salt concentrations and increases in temperature. Transformation is accompanied by a decrease in size of the steroid receptor as measured by sedimentation rate in a sucrose gradient. Steroid receptors in cytoplasmic extracts of cells are usually present as a complex with a variety of proteins and other factors, such as RNA. Some of the proteins associated with untransformed steroid receptors are HSP 70, HSP 90, and a peptidyl-prolyl cis-trans isomerase.[46] Transformation of steroid receptors to the DNA-binding state is accompanied by the loss of HSP 90 from the complex. The physiological significance of the association of steroid receptors in cell extracts with other components has been questioned. However, in a yeast model system, HSP 90 (or the yeast homologue HSP 82) is required for efficient hormone-dependent activation of gene transcription,[124] and steroid receptors can be cross-linked to some of these proteins in intact cells.[125] It has been proposed that HSP 70, HSP 90, and peptidyl-prolyl cis-trans isomerase function in protein folding and transport in the cell.[45] Association of steroid receptors with these proteins may be necessary for maintaining a conformation of the receptor that facilitates steroid binding or some other receptor function. Because steroid receptors free of these accessory proteins can bind to DNA in the absence of ligand, the role of ligand in the mechanism of action of steroid receptors involves steps prior to or after DNA binding.[126] Steroid binding to the receptor may facilitate removal of factors (HSP 90) that inhibit DNA binding or may provide a receptor conformation important for transcriptional activation, perhaps by enhancing receptor interaction with other transcriptional factors.

Androgen Response Elements

Several genes regulated by androgens have been characterized in sufficient depth to show that these genes contain DNA elements that confer androgen-regulated expression of linked reporter genes (Table 131–4). These DNA sequence elements are called androgen response elements (ARE) and have been shown to interact directly with the androgen receptor by DNase I footprinting or gel-shift assays. Progestin, glucocorticoid, and mineralocorticoid receptors regulate gene expression through an HRE that has the consensus sequence 5'-AGTACANNNTGTTCT-3', which is very similar to the sequence of various naturally occurring ARE's (Table 131–4).[32] A consensus DNA-binding site for the androgen receptor, determined by in vitro binding of random oligonucleotides, has a sequence similar to the above consensus HRE.[134] Estrogen receptors activate gene transcription by binding to the similar yet distinct sequence 5'-AGGTCANNNTGACCT-3'.[32] Given the

TABLE 131–4. FUNCTIONAL ANDROGEN RESPONSE ELEMENTS OF VARIOUS ANDROGEN-REGULATED GENES AND PROMOTERS

GENE	RESPONSE ELEMENT
Rat dorsal prostate probasin (proximal)[127]	ATACAAataGGTTCT
Rat dorsal prostate probasin (distal)[127]	ATAGCAtctTGTTCT
Rat ventral prostate C3[128, 129]	AGTACGtgaTGTTCT
Rat liver tyrosine aminotransferase[130]	TGTACAggaTGTTCT
Human prostate-specific antigen[131]	AGCACTtgcTGTTCT
Mouse liver sex-limited protein[132]	AGAACAggcTGTTTC
MMTV (distal)[133]	GTTACAaacTGTTCT
MMTV (proximal no. 1)[133]	GGTATCaaaTGTTCT
MMTV (proximal no. 2)[133]	AGCTCTtagTGTTCT
MMTV (proximal no. 3)[133]	ATTTTCctaTGTTCT
Consensus ARE/GRE/PRE[32]	AGTACAnnnTGTTCT
Consensus ERE[32]	AGGTCAnnnTGACCT

Lower-case letters in the response element sequence signify the three nucleotide spacer found in all HRE's. Proximal and distal indicate a specific HRE in promoters containing multiple HRE's.

similarity of natural ARE's to the consensus GRE, it is not surprising that androgen receptors can activate gene transcription through glucocorticoid response elements in the MMTV promoter and in the tyrosine aminotransferase gene (Table 131–4).[130, 133] The nearly palindromic nature of an HRE is consistent with the observation that steroid receptors bind to DNA as homodimers. However, HRE's that are perfect palindromes are not the best steroid response elements, and some strong HRE's are very imperfect palindromes. Receptor dimers may be flexible enough to accommodate these nonpalindromic binding sites provided one member can bind tightly to the HRE.[34] Androgen and other steroid response elements are often found in the 5'-flanking region of a gene, but are also effective when present in introns and 3'-flanking DNA. Multiple HRE's have a synergistic effect on the activation of gene transcription by steroid receptors and the spacing of individual HRE's and their topology often affect the degree of transcriptional activation.[135]

The ability of androgen, progestin, glucocorticoid, and mineralocorticoid receptors to activate transcription through very similar HRE's is inconsistent with the specificity of the effects of steroid hormones in vivo. It is conceivable that minor sequence differences may alter the receptor specificity of an HRE, but no evidence for this has been found from comparisons of various natural and synthetic HRE's. Naturally occurring HRE's are usually part of complex transcriptional regulatory elements that contain binding sites for other regulatory factors that could cooperate with steroid receptors in controlling the specificity of gene transcription.[32] Cell-specific factors may also bind to steroid receptors directly and modulate their activity. Evidence for both of these possibilities has been presented. For example, each of the four HRE's of the MMTV LTR contribute to the activation of transcription by androgens, progestins, and glucocorticoids. However, various mutations in the MMTV LTR outside the receptor binding sites differentially affect the hormone inducibility of a linked reporter gene.[136, 137] In particular, mutations in the binding site for the transcription factor NF-1 reduce the level of activation of transcription by androgens and glucocorticoids but not progestins. Mutations in the binding sites for the transcriptional factor OTF-1 in the MMTV LTR significantly reduce transactivation by progestin receptors. The mouse sex-limited protein (Slp) gene, a duplicated complement C4 gene, is expressed in male but not female mice and contains a proviral insert with an HRE, similar to the GRE consensus, in its 5′-LTR. Androgens, progestins, and glucocorticoids stimulate transcription from reporter gene constructs containing only the Slp HRE, although androgens are much less effective than the other two steroids. However, androgens but not glucocorticoid and progestins activate transcription from constructs containing a 120-base pair segment of the LTR containing the HRE, indicating that the exclusive transcriptional response to androgens in vivo is probably due to interactions of the androgen receptor with factors outside the HRE.[132] Testosterone may also produce its effects on Slp expression indirectly through hormonal control of growth hormone secretion.[132a] Transcriptional activation by androgen and other steroid hormones appears to be modulated by the proto-oncogenes c-*fos* and c-*jun*.[138] These proteins combine to form the transcription factor AP-1, which in some cases competes for overlapping binding sites with steroid receptors or binds to adjacent sites to affect gene transcription. c-*Jun* may form complexes with steroid receptors, perhaps through leucine zipper motifs found in both proteins, and affect transcription in this manner. The relative levels of c-*fos* and c-*jun* appear to determine whether they inhibit or enhance transcription activation by steroid hormones.

The mechanism by which androgen and other steroid receptors modulate gene transcription after binding to their respective HRE's is not totally clear. Many genes that are regulated by steroid hormones show DNase I hypersensitivity upon exposure of target cells to steroid. This change may indicate an opening-up of the chromatin structure in the vicinity of the hormone-regulated gene. Steroid treatment of cells harboring minichromosomes containing the MMTV LTR leads to the displacement of nucleosomes on the MMTV LTR and increased accessibility of the basal transcription factor NF-1 for its binding site. Increased accessibility of basal and specific transcription factors to steroid-regulated genes could enhance the formation of a stable transcription initiation complex promoting the synthesis of mRNA.

Post-transcriptional Role for Androgen Receptors

Although androgens and other steroid hormones have well-documented effects on gene transcription, steroids can also have post-transcriptional effects on gene expression. For example, androgens stimulate the transcription of the gene for a secretory protein in the rat ventral prostate 5- to 10-fold but increase the mRNA level for this protein more than 50-fold.[139] Androgens therefore must increase the stability of this mRNA 5- to 10-fold. Androgens increase the level of several mRNA's and proteins in mouse kidney, and this effect is also largely post-transcriptional.[140] Androgen and other steroid receptors can bind to RNA and ribonucleoproteins[141, 142]; therefore, steroid receptors may be directly involved in post-transcriptional effects on mRNA stability. The fate of androgen receptors after activating gene transcription is unknown, but they may be involved in a recycling mechanism involving the process-

ing, transport, and utilization of mRNA.[143] The association of androgen receptors with the nuclear matrix of target cells,[144] a possible site of RNA transcription and processing, may be related to the post-transcriptional effects of androgens.

GENES REGULATED BY ANDROGENS

Given the phenotypic differences of males and females of most species, it is not surprising that androgens affect many different cell types both during development and in the adult. Androgenic effects have been documented in a wide variety of tissues, including the prostate, seminal vesicle, vas deferens, epididymis, scrotum, penis, testis, muscle, brain, spinal chord, liver, kidney, hematopoietic system, skin and appendages, salivary gland, mammary gland, and bone. Androgen receptors have been detected in cells in most of these tissues, and so many of the effects of androgens appear to be mediated through the androgen receptor. In some cases, androgens exert their effects indirectly. For example, male sexual behavior depends on the conversion of testosterone to estradiol in the brain and subsequent interactions with the estrogen receptor.[145] Cells lacking androgen receptors also respond indirectly by interacting with trophic factors that are synthesized and secreted by other cells that respond directly to androgens. Although the gross effects of androgens on various tissues is well-documented, most of the underlying changes in gene expression that bring about the tissue's response to androgen are currently unknown. However, this lack of knowledge is changing rapidly as more and more gene products regulated by androgens are discovered and studied at the molecular level.

Some of the best-documented effects of androgens on gene expression involve the effects of androgens on male accessory sex glands, although examples of androgenic effects on gene expression also have been reported for the testis, kidney, liver, and salivary glands. The mammalian prostate has been used extensively as a model system for examining androgen-regulated gene expression and so we present selected results only for this experimental system. Androgens are important both for the growth and differentiation of the prostate and for regulating the secretory activity of the mature gland. Androgen receptors are present in both the stromal and epithelial cells of the prostate of mature animals. During development, however, androgen receptors first appear in stromal cells. Prostatic stromal cells, under the influence of androgens, control epithelial cell differentiation and proliferation.[146] This effect may be mediated by a paracrine factor, such as keratinocyte growth factor (KGF), whose synthesis in prostatic stromal cells is regulated by androgens.[147] KGF, secreted by the stroma, may bind to receptors on prostatic epithelial cells and control cell differentiation and proliferation. Androgens also regulate another paracrine factor produced by peritubular cells of the testis that affects the function of neighboring Sertoli cells.[148] Androgens also have direct effects on prostatic epithelial cell function, stimulating the synthesis of several proteins that ultimately become part of the prostatic secretion, a component of semen upon ejaculation. Human, rat, and dog prostatic epithelia secrete a kallikrein-like protease thought to be involved in semen clot dissolution.[149] This protease is the major secretory product of the dog prostate[150] and the blood levels of the human enzyme, also known as prostate-specific antigen (PSA), are routinely monitored to follow the effectiveness of hormonal therapy for metastatic prostatic cancer.[151] Androgens stimulate the synthesis of mRNA for this protein, although additional post-transcriptional effects, for example on mRNA stability, may account for increased levels of this mRNA.[152] The promoter for the PSA gene contains a functional androgen response element, although additional upstream sequences are needed for optimal androgen-inducibility of linked reporter genes in transfected cells.[130]

Perhaps the most thoroughly studied androgen-regulated gene is a major secretory product of the rat ventral prostate. This protein, which represents about 50 per cent of the protein secreted by the rat ventral prostate, was identified in several laboratories and has been called α-protein,[153] prostate binding protein,[154] and prostatein.[155] The function of this protein is unknown, but it binds many steroids in vitro and appears to be complexed with cholesterol in vivo.[153] The protein may have a role in sperm capacitation.[156] α-Protein is a tetramer composed of three distinct subunits termed C1, C2, and C3. The mRNA levels for all three proteins are regulated by androgens. Normal rats contain approximately 100,000 copies of the C3 mRNA per cell, but this level falls to about 100 copies within seven days after castration. The steady-state levels of C3 mRNA are regulated at both the transcriptional and post-transcriptional levels. Putative ARE's have been found in the genes for all three proteins and an ARE in the first intron of the C3 gene can confer androgen-regulated expression of reporter genes in transfected cells.[129] The androgen-responsive unit of the C3 gene also contains binding sites for octamer transcription factor 1, nuclear factor 1, and an unidentified prostate-specific factor that may interact synergistically with androgen receptor to provide tissue-specific androgen-dependent gene expression.[156a]

A heterogeneous group of small (38 amino acids) proline-rich polypeptides, whose levels are regulated by androgens, form a 1:1 stoichiometric complex with α-protein. These heterogeneous peptides are derived from a single large precursor protein of 637 kDa encoded by a single mRNA of greater than 12.5 Kb. Proteolytic processing of repetitive units of the protein produces the proline-rich peptides. The gene for this protein contains several putative ARE's in the 5'-flanking region that may be involved in androgen-regulated expression of this unusual gene product.[157]

Another unusual androgen-regulated gene product in the rat ventral prostate is a 35-kDa secretory protein, called spermine-binding protein, which binds various polyamines, perhaps as a result of the numerous aspartic and glutamic acids in the carboxyl terminus of the protein. The mRNA level for this protein is regulated by androgens, decreasing to less than 20 per cent of control levels within two days after castration. Administration of androgens, such as 5α-dihydrotestosterone, prevents or reverses this decline in spermine-binding protein mRNA.[158]

In contrast to these positive effects of androgens on prostatic secretory protein mRNA levels, androgens appear to negatively regulate the levels of certain messages in the rat ventral prostate. After castration, the level of the mRNA for the Y_{b1} subunit of glutathione S-transferase increases in rat ventral prostate and rapidly decreases upon androgen treatment of castrated rats.[159] A similar effect is seen on the levels of the mRNA for a protein called sulfated glycoprotein-2.[160] This latter protein is found in many cells undergoing apoptosis, including those of the rat ventral prostate. The mechanism by which androgens negatively regulate the levels of these mRNA's is unknown. Gonadotropin gene expression in the pituitary also is repressed by androgens. This repression may involve direct binding of the androgen receptor to the promoter of the α subunit gene.[160a]

Androgens also control the level of mRNA for two proteins intimately connected with the androgenic response in the rat ventral prostate, the androgen receptor and 5α-reductase. Castration of rats leads to an increase in the level of mRNA for the androgen receptor in several tissues, including the rat ventral prostate, brain, kidney, epididymis, and coagulating gland.[161] Treatment of castrated rats with androgens reduces the level of androgen receptor mRNA in these various tissues. The effect of castration and androgen treatment on androgen receptor mRNA was not seen in the kidney of Tfm rats, who lack functional androgen receptors. Therefore, this effect on androgen receptor mRNA levels appears to be an androgen receptor-regulated process. Androgen withdrawal also increases the level of androgen receptor mRNA in human prostate and mammary and hepatoma cancer cells in culture.[161–163] The mechanism of down-regulation of androgen receptor mRNA by androgens in unknown, but down-regulation of other steroid receptors by their ligands has been attributed to both transcriptional and post-transcriptional effects. The activity of the enzyme 5α-reductase and the steady-state level of its mRNA, in contrast to that for androgen receptors, decreases in the rat ventral prostate after castration, although this decrease may reflect the declining population of epithelial cells and not a specific response to low androgen levels.[164, 165] Treatment of castrated rats with androgen causes a large increase in 5α-reductase mRNA levels and enzymatic activity above the levels seen in the ventral prostate of intact animals. Because androgens have no effect on prostatic 5α-reductase mRNA levels in normal animals, the androgen-induced increase in 5α-reductase mRNA or protein levels requires prostatic growth. 5α-Dihydrotestosterone appears to be more effective than testosterone for induction of 5α-reductase, an effect termed autocatalytic or feed-forward control of prostatic growth.[164] Androgen induction of 5α-reductase may be mediated by insulin-like growth factor I in some cell types.[165a]

DETECTION AND MEASUREMENT OF ANDROGEN RECEPTORS

Androgen receptors can be detected in cells or tissues by their ability to bind specifically to tritiated androgens of high specific activity, such as ³H-5α-dihydrotestosterone,[166] ³H-R1881 (methyltrienolone; 17β-hydroxy-17α-methyl-estra-4,9,11-trien-3-one)[167] and ³H-DMNT (mibolerone; 7α, 17α-dimethyl-19-nortestosterone)[168] (see Fig. 131–4). The latter two steroids have affinities for the androgen receptor equal to or greater than testosterone or 5α-dihydrotestosterone, are resistant to metabolic inactivation, and have been useful in many laboratory studies on androgen receptors. Androgen receptors can be quantitated in whole cells or tissue extracts using either a single-point saturation assay or a multiconcentration Scatchard analysis. Tritiated androgens also have been used in the cellular and subcellular localization of androgen receptors in various tissue by autoradiography,[169] but this technique is being supplanted by immunohistochemical methods of androgen receptor localization.

Several different antibodies have been produced against the androgen receptor, and in all cases, production of these antibodies has relied upon information and material garnered from the cloning of the cDNA for the androgen receptor for production of a suitable immunogen because purification of androgen receptors from target tissues has been unsuccessful. Both monoclonal and polyclonal antibodies have been produced against the androgen receptor using bacterially expressed segments of the androgen receptor or synthetic peptides as immunogens.[9, 170–172] These antibodies have been used in a variety of studies to determine the cellular and subcellular location of androgen receptors by immunohistochemical staining. In reproductive tissues (prostate, seminal vesicles, epididymis, vas deferens, penis, testis) from humans, monkeys, rats, and mice, androgen receptors have been localized by immunohistochemical staining predominantly to nuclei of secretory epithelia and in some tissues to nuclei of various stromal cells.[9, 171, 173–174] Cytoplasmic staining is minimal or lacking in most of these tissues. Castration does not appear to alter the nuclear location of androgen receptors in rat prostatic epithelia.[171] Nuclei of epithelial cells from hyperplastic and cancerous human prostatic tissue are immunohistochemically stained with antibody against androgen receptor, and this staining is more heterogeneous than the staining observed in normal tissue.[178] Most prostatic tumors are initially responsive to androgen withdrawal therapies but eventually progress to an androgen-independent form. The time to tumor progression may be affected by androgen receptor levels in tumors before therapy; however, the percentage of androgen receptor–positive cells determined by immunohistochemical staining of prostatic tumors does not correlate with response to hormonal therapy.[179] Androgen receptors also have been detected immunohistochemically in the nuclei of certain cells in various nonreproductive tissues including skin, liver, brain, and cardiac muscle.[177, 180]

REFERENCES

1. Liao S: Molecular actions of androgens. In Litwack G (ed): Biochemical Actions of Hormones, vol IV. New York, Academic Press, 1977, pp 351–406.
2. Mooradian AD, Morley JE, Korenman SG: Biological actions of androgens. Endocr Rev 8:1–28, 1987.
3. Evans RM: The steroid and thyroid hormone receptor superfamily. Science 240:889–895, 1988.
4. O'Malley B: The steroid receptor superfamily: More excitement predicted for the future. Mol Endocrinol 4:363–369, 1990.
5. Wahli W, Martinez E: Superfamily of steroid nuclear receptors: Positive and negative regulators of gene expression. FASEB J 5:2243–2249, 1991.
6. Chang C, Kokontis K, Liao S: Structural analysis of complementary DNA and amino acid sequences of human and rat androgen receptors. Proc Natl Acad Sci USA 85:7211–7215, 1988.
7. Chang C, Kokontis K, Liao S: Molecular cloning of human and rat complementary DNA encoding androgen receptors. Science 240:324–326, 1988.
8. Lubahn DB, Joseph DR, Sullivan PM, et al: Cloning of human androgen receptor complementary DNA and localization to the X chromosome. Science 240:327–330, 1988.
9. Tan J, Joseph DR, Quarmby VE, et al: The rat androgen receptor: Primary structure, autoregulation of its messenger ribonucleic acid, and immunocytochemical localization of the receptor protein. Mol Endocrinol 2:1276–1285, 1988.
10. Lubahn DB, Joseph DR, Sar M, et al: The human androgen receptor: Complementary deoxyribonucleic acid cloning, sequence analysis and gene expression in prostate. Mol Endocrinol 2:1265–1275, 1988.
11. Trapman J, Klaassen P, Kuiper GGJM, et al: Cloning, structure and expression of a cDNA encoding the human androgen receptor. Biochem Biophys Res Commun 153:241–248, 1988.
12. Tilley WD, Marcelli M, Wilson JD, McPhaul MJ: Characterization and expression of a cDNA encoding the human androgen receptor. Proc Natl Acad Sci USA 86:327–331, 1989.
13. Brown CJ, Goss SJ, Lubahn DB, et al: Androgen receptor locus on the human X chromosome: Regional localization to Xq11-12 and description of a DNA polymorphism. Am J Hum Genet 44:264–269, 1989.
14. Kuiper GGJM, Faber PW, van Rooij HCJ, et al: Structural organization of the human androgen receptor gene. J Mol Endocrinol 2:R1–R4, 1989.
15. Lubahn DB, Brown TR, Simental JA, et al: Sequence of the intron/exon junctions of the coding region of the human androgen receptor gene and identification of a point mutation in a family with complete androgen insensitivity. Proc Natl Acad Sci USA 86:9534–9538, 1989.
16. Marcelli M, Tilley WD, Wilson CM, et al: Definition of the human androgen receptor gene structure permits the identification of mutations that cause androgen resistance: Premature termination of the receptor protein at amino acid residue 588 causes complete androgen resistance. Mol Endocrinol 4:1105–1116, 1990.
17. Faber PW, Kuiper GGJM, van Rooij HCJ, et al: The N-terminal domain of the human androgen receptor is encoded by one large exon. Mol Cell Endocrinol 61:257–262, 1989.
18. Faber PW, van Rooij HCJ, van der Korput AGM, et al: Characterization of the human androgen receptor transcription unit. J Biol Chem 266:10743–10749, 1991.
19. Baarends WM, Themmen APN, Blok LJ, et al: The rat androgen receptor promoter. Mol Cell Endocrinol 74:75–84, 1990.
20. Tilley WD, Marcelli M, McPhaul MJ: Expression of the human androgen receptor gene utilizes a common promoter in diverse human tissues and cell lines. J Biol Chem 265:13776–13781, 1990.
20a. Faber PW, van Rooij HCJ, Schipper HJ, et al: Two different, overlapping pathways of transcription initiation are active on the TATA-less human androgen receptor promoter. J Biol Chem 268:9296–9301, 1993.
20b. McLachlan RI, Tempel BL, Miller MA, et al: Androgen receptor gene expression in the rat central nervous system: Evidence for two mRNA transcripts. Molec Cell Neurosci 2:17–22, 1991.
20c. Fischer L, Catz D, Kelley D: An androgen receptor mRNA isoform associated with hormone-induced cell proliferation. Proc Natl Acad Sci USA 90:8254–8258, 1993.
21. Sleddens HFBM, Oostra BA, Brinkmann AO, Trapman J: Trinucleotide repeat polymorphism in the androgen receptor gene. Nucleic Acids Res 20:1427, 1991.
22. Johnson MP, Young CYF, Rowley DR, Tindall DJ: A common molecular weight of the androgen receptor monomer in different target tissues. Biochemistry 26:3174–3182, 1987.
23. van Laar JH, Bolt-de Vries J, Voorhorst-Ogink MM, Brinkmann AO: The human androgen receptor is a 110 kDa protein. Mol Cell Endocrinol 63:39–44, 1989.
24. Kemppainen JA, Lane MV, Sar M, Wilson EM: Androgen receptor phosphorylation, turnover, nuclear transport, transcriptional activation. J Biol Chem 267:968–974, 1992.
25. van Laar JH, Berrevoets CA, Trapman J, et al: Hormone-dependent androgen receptor phosphorylation is accompanied by receptor transformation in human lymph node carcinoma of the prostate cells. J Biol Chem 266:3734–3738, 1991.
26. Rossini GP, Liao S: Intracellular inactivation, reactivation and dynamic status of prostate androgen receptors. Biochem J 208:383–392, 1982.
26a. Kuiper GGJM, De Ruiter PE, Trapman J, et al: Localization and hormonal stimulation of phosphorylation sites in the LNCaP-cell androgen receptor. Biochem J 291:95–101, 1993.
27. Rundlett SE, Wu XP, Miesfield RL: Functional characterizations of the androgen receptor confirm that the molecular basis of androgen action is transcriptional regulation. Mol Endocrinol 4:708–714, 1990.

28. Govidan MV: Specific region in hormone binding domain is essential for hormone binding and trans-activation by human androgen receptor. Mol Endocrinol 4:417–427, 1990.

29. Jenster G, van der Korput HAGM, van Vroonhoven C, et al: Domains of the human androgen receptor involved in steroid binding, transcriptional activation, and subcellular localization. Mol Endocrinol 5:1396–1404, 1991.

30. Simental JA, Sar M, Lane MV, et al: Transcriptional activation and nuclear targeting signals of the human androgen receptor. J Biol Chem 266:510–518, 1991.

30a. Jenster G, Trapman J, Brinkmann AO: Nuclear import of the human androgen receptor. Biochem J 293:761–768, 1993.

31. Alam J, Cook JL: Reporter genes: Application to the study of mammalian gene transcription. Anal Biochem 188:245–254, 1990.

32. Lucas PC, Granner DK: Hormone response domains in gene transcription. Annu Rev Biochem 61:1131–1173, 1992.

33. Faber PW, King A, van Rooij HCJ, et al: The mouse androgen receptor: Functional analysis of the protein and characterization of the gene. Biochem J 278:269–278, 1991.

34. Luisi BF, Xu WX, Otwinowski Z, et al: Crystallographic analysis of the interaction of the glucocorticoid receptor with DNA. Nature 352:497–505, 1991.

35. Härd T, Kellenbach E, Boelens R, et al: Solution structure of the glucocorticoid receptor DNA-binding domain. Science 249:157–160, 1990.

36. Schwabe JWR, Neuhaus D, Rhodes D: Solution structure of the DNA-binding domain of the oestrogen receptor. Nature 348:458–461, 1990.

37. Danielson M, Hinck L, Ringold GM: Two amino acids within the knuckle of the first zinc finger specify DNA response element activation by the glucocorticoid receptor. Cell 57:1131–1138, 1989.

38. Umesono K, Evans RM: Determinants of target gene specificity for steroid/thyroid hormone receptors. Cell 57:1139–1146, 1989.

39. Mader S, Kumar V, de Verneuil H, Chambon P: Three amino acids of the oestrogen receptor are essential to its ability to distinguish an oestrogen from a glucocorticoid-responsive element. Nature 338:271–274, 1989.

40. Dahlman-Wright K, Wright A, Gustafsson JA, Carlstedt-Duke J: Interaction of the glucocorticoid receptor DNA-binding domain with DNA as a dimer is mediated by a short segment of five amino acids. J Biol Chem 266:3107–3112, 1991.

41. Danielian PS, White R, Lees JA, Parker MG: Identification of a conserved region required for hormone dependent transcriptional activation by steroid hormone receptors. EMBO J 11:1025–1033, 1992.

42. Marivoet S, Van Dijck P, Verhoeven G, Heyns W: Interaction of the 90 kDa heat shock protein with native and in vitro translated androgen receptor and receptor fragments. Mol Cell Endocrinol 88:165–174, 1992.

43. Fawell SE, Lees JA, White R, Parker MG: Characterization and colocalization of steroid binding and dimerization activities in the mouse estrogen receptor. Cell 60:953–962, 1990.

44. Lee JW, Gulick T, Moore DD: Thyroid hormone receptor dimerization function maps to a conserved subregion of the ligand binding domain. Mol Endocrinol 6:1867–1873, 1992.

45. Gething MJ, Sambrook J: Protein folding in the cell. Nature 355:33–45, 1992.

46. Smith DF, Toft DO: Steroid receptors and their associated proteins. Mol Endocrinol 7:4–11, 1993.

47. Forman BM, Samuels HH: Interactions among a subfamily of nuclear hormone receptors: The regulatory zipper model. Mol Endocrinol 4:1293–1301, 1990.

48. Quigley CA, Friedman KJ, Johnson A, et al: Complete deletion of the androgen receptor gene: Definition of the null phenotype of the androgen insensitivity syndrome and determination of carrier status. J Clin Endocrinol Metab 74:927–933, 1992.

49. Brown TR, Lubahn DB, Wilson EM, et al: Deletion of the steroid-binding domain of the human androgen receptor gene in one family with complete androgen insensitivity syndrome: Evidence for further genetic heterogeneity in this syndrome. Proc Natl Acad Sci USA 85:8151–8155, 1988.

50. La Spada AR, Wilson EM, Lubahn DB, et al: Androgen receptor gene mutations in X-linked spinal and bulbar muscular atrophy. Nature 352:77–79, 1991.

51. Caskey CT, Pizzuti A, Fu YH, et al: Triplet repeat mutations in human disease. Science 256:784–789, 1992.

52. McPhaul MJ, Marcelli M, Tilley WD, et al: Molecular basis of androgen resistance in a family with a qualitative abnormality of the androgen receptor and responsive to high-dose androgen therapy. J Clin Invest 87:1413–1421, 1991.

53. Zoppi S, Wilson CM, Harbison MD, et al: Complete testicular feminization caused by an amino-terminal truncation of the androgen receptor with downstream initiation. J Clin Invest 91:1105–1112, 1993.

54. Charest NJ, Zhou Z, Lubahn DB, et al: A frameshift mutation destabilizes androgen receptor messenger RNA in the Tfm mouse. Mol Endocrinol 5:573–581, 1991.

55. He WW, Kumar MV, Tindall DJ: A frame-shift mutation in the androgen receptor gene causes complete androgen insensitivity in the testicular-feminized mouse. Nucleic Acids Res 19:2373–2378, 1991.

56. Gaspar ML, Meo T, Bourgarel P, et al: A single base deletion in the Tfm androgen receptor gene creates a short-lived messenger RNA that directs internal translation initiation. Proc Natl Acad Sci USA 88:8606–8610, 1991.

57. McPhaul MJ, Marcelli M, Tilley WD, et al: Androgen resistance caused by mutations in the androgen receptor gene. FASEB J 5:2910–2915, 1991.

58. Klocher H, Kaspar F, Eberle J, et al: Point mutation in the DNA binding domain of the androgen receptor in two families with Reifenstein syndrome. Am J Hum Genet 50:1318–1327, 1992.

59. Quigley CA, Evans BAJ, Simental JA, et al: Complete androgen insensitivity due to deletion of exon C of the androgen receptor gene highlights the functional importance of the second zinc finger of the androgen receptor in vivo. Mol Endocrinol 6:1103–1112, 1992.

60. Saunders PTK, Padayachi T, Tincello DG, et al: Point mutations detected in the androgen receptor gene of three men with partial androgen insensitivity syndrome. Clin Endocrinol 37:214–220, 1992.

61. Marcelli M, Zoppi S, Grino PB, et al: A mutation in the DNA-binding domain of the androgen receptor gene causes complete testicular feminization in a patient with receptor-positive androgen resistance. J Clin Invest 87:1123–1126, 1991.

62. Ris-Stalpers C, Kuiper GGJM, Faber PW, et al: Aberrant splicing of androgen receptor mRNA results in synthesis of a nonfunctional receptor protein in a patient with androgen sensitivity. Proc Natl Acad Sci USA 87:7866–7870, 1990.

63. Ris-Stalpers C, Trifiro MA, Kuiper GGJM, et al: Substitution of aspartic acid-686 by histidine or asparagine in the human androgen receptor leads to a functionally inactive protein with altered hormone-binding characteristics. Mol Endocrinol 5:1562–1569, 1991.

64. Kaufman M, Beitel LK, Trifiro M, et al: Androgen resistance: Genotype-phenotype prediction and structure-function analysis on alternative missense substitutions at four codons in the androgen-binding domain of the androgen receptor. Am J Hum Genet 51:A170, 1992.

65. DeBellis A, Quigley CA, Cariello NF, et al: Single base mutations in the human androgen receptor gene causing complete androgen insensitivity: Rapid detection by a modified denaturing gradient gel electrophoresis technique. Mol Endocrinol 6:1909–1920, 1992.

66. Sai T, Seino S, Chang C, et al: An exonic point mutation of the human androgen receptor gene in a family with complete androgen insensitivity. Am J Hum Genet 46:1095–1100, 1990.

67. McPhaul MJ, Marcelli M, Zoppi S, et al: Mutations in the ligand-binding domain of the androgen receptor gene cluster in two regions of the gene. J Clin Invest 90:2097–2101, 1992.

68. Newmark JR, Hardy DO, Tonb DC, et al: Androgen receptor gene mutations in human prostate cancer. Proc Natl Acad Sci USA 89:6319–6323, 1992.

69. Yarbrough WG, Quarmby VE, Simental JA, et al: A single base mutation in the androgen receptor gene causes androgen insensitivity in the testicular feminized rat. J Biol Chem 265:8893–8900, 1990.

70. Evans BAJ: Detection of a point mutation within the androgen receptor gene in a family with complete androgen insensitivity syndrome and subsequent prenatal diagnosis [abstract P26]. J Endocrinol (Suppl) 135:1992.

71. Trifiro MA, Vasiliou M, Kaufman M, et al: The human androgen receptor gene: Differential consequences of germinal missense mutations at 4 of 14 codons in an ultraconserved region of the androgen-binding domain. Am J Hum Genet 51:A178, 1992.

72. Tincello DG, Wu FCW, Hargreave TB, Saunders PTK: Temperature gradient gel electrophoresis can detect point mutations in the androgen receptor gene in patients with androgen insensitivity [abstract P27]. J Endocrinol (Suppl) 135:1992.

73. Prior L, Bordet S, Trifiro MA, et al: Replacement of arginine 773 by cysteine or histidine in the human androgen receptor causes complete androgen insensitivity with different receptor phenotypes. Am J Hum Genet 51:143–155, 1992.

74. Brown TR, Lubahn DB, Wilson EM, et al: Functional characterization of naturally occurring mutant androgen receptors from subjects with complete androgen insensitivity. Mol Endocrinol 4:1759–1772, 1990.

75. Marcelli M, Tilley WD, Zoppi S, et al: Androgen resistance associated with a mutation of the androgen receptor at amino acid 772 (Arg → Cys) results from a combination of decreased messenger ribonucleic acid levels and impairment of receptor function. J Clin Endocrinol Metab 73:318–325, 1991.
76. Nakao R, Haji M, Yanase T, et al: A single amino acid substitution (Met⁷⁸⁶ → Val) in the steroid-binding domain of human androgen receptor leads to complete androgen insensitivity syndrome. J Clin Endocrinol Metab 74:1152–1157, 1992.
77. Marcelli M, Tilley WD, Wilson CM, et al: A single nucleotide substitution introduces a premature termination codon into the androgen receptor gene of a patient with receptor-negative androgen resistance. J Clin Invest 85:1522–1528, 1990.
78. Mhatre A, Kazemi-Esfarjani P, Trifiro M, et al: Host cell restricted expression of a ligand-selective mutant androgen receptor phenotype. Am J Hum Genet 51:A321, 1992.
79. Kaufman M, Beitel LK, Trifiro M, et al: Androgen resistance: Genotype-phenotype prediction and structure-function analysis on alternative missense substitutions at four codons in the androgen-binding domain of the androgen receptor. Am J Hum Genet 51:A170, 1992.
80. Batch JA, Williams DM, Davies HR, et al: Androgen receptor gene mutations identified by SSCP in fourteen subjects with androgen insensitivity syndrome. Hum Molec Genet 1:497–503, 1992.
81. Veldschkolte J, Ris-Stalper C, Kuiper GGJM, et al: A mutation in the ligand binding domain of the androgen receptor of human LNCaP cells affects steroid binding characteristics and response to anti-androgens. Biochem Biophys Res Commun 173:534–540, 1990.
82. Kokontis J, Ito K, Hiipakka RA, Liao S: Expression and function of normal and LNCaP androgen receptors in androgen-insensitive human prostatic cancer cells. Receptor 1:271–279, 1991.
83. Trifiro M, Prior RL, Sabbaghian N, et al: Amber mutation creates a diagnostic Mae I site in the androgen receptor gene of a family with complete androgen insensitivity. Am J Hum Genet 40:493–499, 1991.
84. Pinsky L, Mhatre AN, Kazemi-Esfarjani P, et al: Spinal and bulbar muscular atrophy (SBMA): Characterization of mutant androgen receptors having an amplified polyglutamine tract. Am J Hum Genet 51:A41, 1992.
85. Petra PH: The plasma sex steroid binding protein (SBP or SHBG): A critical review of recent developments on the structure, molecular biology and function. J Steroid Biochem Mol Biol 40:735–753, 1991.
86. Mendel CM: The free hormone hypothesis: A physiologically based mathematical model. Endoc Rev 10:232–274, 1989.
87. Giorgi EP, Stein WD: The transport of steroids into animal cells in culture. Endocrinology 108:688–697, 1981.
88. Orlowski J, Clark AF: Epithelial-stromal interactions in the regulation of rat ventral prostate function: Identification and characterization of pathways for androgen metabolism in isolated cell types. Endocrinology 128:872–884, 1991.
89. Rittmaster RS: Androgen conjugates: Physiology and clinical significance. Endocr Rev 14:121–132, 1993.
90. Gloyna RE, Wilson JD: A comparative study of the conversion of testosterone to 17β-hydroxy-5α-androstan-3-one (dihydrotestosterone) by prostate and epididymis. J Clin Endocrinol Metab 29:970–977, 1969.
91. Anderson KM, Liao S: Selective retention of dihydrotestosterone by prostatic nuclei. Nature 219:277–279, 1968.
92. Bruchovsky N, Wilson JD: The conversion of testosterone to 5α-androstan-17β-ol-3-one by rat prostate in vivo and in vitro. J Biol Chem 243:2012–2021, 1968.
93. Andersson S, Bishop RW, Russell DW: Expression cloning and regulation of steroid 5α-reductase, an enzyme essential for male sexual differentiation. J Biol Chem 264:16249–16255, 1989.
94. Andersson S, Russell DW: Structural and biochemical properties of cloned and expressed human and rat steroid 5α-reductases. Proc Natl Acad Sci USA 87:3640–3644, 1990.
95. Andersson S, Berman DM, Jenkins EP, Russell DW: Deletion of steroid 5α-reductase 2 gene in male pseudohermaphroditism. Nature 354:159–161, 1991.
96. Normington K, Russell DW: Tissue distribution and kinetic characteristics of rat steroid 5α-reductase isozymes: Evidence for distinct physiological functions. J Biol Chem 267:19548–19554, 1992.
97. Jenkins EP, Hsieh CL, Milatovich A, et al: Characterization and chromosomal mapping of a human steroid 5α-reductase gene and pseudogene and mapping of the mouse homologue. Genomics 11:1102–1112, 1991.
98. Thigpen AE, Davis DL, Milatovich A, et al: Molecular genetics of steroid 5α-reductase deficiency. J Clin Invest 90:799–809, 1992.
98a. Thigpen AE, Silver RI, Guileyardo JM, et al: Tissue distribution and ontogeny of steroid 5α-reductase isozyme expression. J Clin Invest 92:903–910, 1993.
99. Bruchovsky N, Rennie PS, Batzold FH, et al: Kinetic parameters of 5α-reductase activity in stroma and epithelium of normal, hyperplastic, and carcinomatous human prostates. Endocrinology 67:806–816, 1988.
100. Moore RJ, Wilson JD: Localization of the reduced nicotinamide adenine dinucleotide phosphate: Δ⁴-3-ketosteroid 5α-oxidoreductase in the nuclear membrane of the rat ventral prostate. J Biol Chem 247:958–967, 1972.
101. Houston B, Chisholm GD, Habib FK: Evidence that human prostatic 5α-reductase is located exclusively in the nucleus. FEBS Lett 185:231–235, 1985.
102. Imperato-McGinley J, Gautier T: Inherited 5α-reductase deficiency in man. Trends Genet 2:130–133, 1986.
103. Wilson JD, Lasnitzki I: Dihydrotestosterone formation in fetal tissues of the rabbit and rat. Endocrinology 89:659–668, 1971.
104. Thigpen AE, Davis DL, Gautier T, et al: The molecular basis of steroid 5α-reductase deficiency in a large Dominican kindred. N Engl J Med 327:1216–1219, 1992.
105. Stoner E, The Finasteride Study Group: The clinical effects of a 5α-reductase inhibitor, finasteride, on benign prostatic hyperplasia. J Urology 147:1298–1302, 1992.
106. Liang T, Heiss CE, Ostrove S, et al: Binding of a 4-methyl-azasteroid to 5α-reductase of rat liver and prostate microsomes. Endocrinology 112:1460–1468, 1983.
107. Liang T, Cheung AH, Reynolds GF, Rasmusson GH: Photoaffinity labeling of steroid 5α-reductase of rat liver and prostate microsomes. J Biol Chem 260:4890–4895, 1985.
108. Petrow V, Wang Y, Lack L: Prostatic cancer: I. 6-methylene-4-pregnen-3-ones as irreversible inhibitors of rat prostatic Δ⁴-3 ketosteroid 5α-reductase. Steroids 38:121–140, 1981.
109. Blohm TR, Metcalf BW, Laughlin ME, et al: Inhibition of testosterone 5α-reductase by a proposed enzyme-activated, active site directed inhibitor. Biochem Biophys Res Commun 95:273–280, 1980.
110. Robaire B, Covey DF, Robinson CH, Ewing LL: Selective inhibition of rat epididymal steroid Δ⁴-5α-reductase by conjugated allenic 3-oxo-5,10-secosteroids. J Steroid Biochem 8:307–310, 1977.
111. Voigt W, Hsia SL: The antiandrogenic action of 4-androsten-3-one-17β-carboxylic acid and its methyl ester on hamster flank organ. Endocrinology 92:1216–1222, 1973.
112. Liang T, Liao S: Inhibition of steroid 5α-reductase by specific aliphatic unsaturated fatty acids. Biochem J 285:557–562, 1992.
113. Namer M: Clinical applications of antiandrogens. J Steroid Biochem 31:719–729, 1988.
114. Neri R, Peets E, Watnick A: Anti-androgenicity of flutamide and its metabolite Sch 16423. Biochem Soc Trans 7:565–569, 1979.
115. Moguilewsky M, Bouton MM: How the study of the biological activities of antiandrogens can be oriented towards the clinic. J Steroid Biochem 31:699–710, 1988.
116. Neumann F, Topert M: Pharmacology of antiandrogens. J Steroid Biochem 25:885–895, 1986.
117. Tremblay RR: Treatment of hirsutism with spironolactone. Clin Endocrinol Metab 15:363–372, 1980.
118. Sivelle PC, Underwood AH, Jelly JA: The effects of histamine H₂ receptor antagonists on androgen action in vivo and dihydrotestosterone binding to the rat prostate androgen receptor in vitro. Biochem Pharmacol 31:677–684, 1982.
119. Bouton MM, Lecaque D, Secchi J, Tournemine C: Effect of a new topically active antiandrogen (RU 38882) on the rat sebaceous gland: Comparison with cyproterone acetate. J Invest Dermatol 86:163–167, 1986.
120. Namer M: Clinical applications of antiandrogens. J Steroid Biochem 31:719–729, 1988.
121. Chang C, Liao S: Topographic recognition of cyclic hydrocarbons and related compounds by receptors for androgens, estrogens, and glucocorticoids. J Steroid Biochem 27:123–131, 1987.
122. Allan GF, Leng X, Tsai SY, et al: Hormone and antihormone induce distinct conformational changes which are central to steroid receptor activation. J Biol Chem 267:19513–19520, 1992.
123. Murdoch FE, Gorski J: The role of ligand in estrogen receptor regulation of gene expression. Mol Cell Endocrinol 78:C103–C108, 1991.
124. Picard D, Khursheed B, Garabedian MJ, et al: Reduced levels of HSP 90 compromise steroid receptor action in vivo. Nature 348:166–168, 1990.
125. Wrenn CK, Katzenellenbogen BS: Cross-linking of estrogen receptor to chromatin in intact MCF-7 human breast cancer cells: Optimization and effect of ligand. Mol Endocrinol 4:1647–1654, 1990.

126. Willmann T, Beato M: Steroid-free glucocorticoid receptor binds specifically to mouse mammary tumor virus DNA. Nature 324:688–691, 1986.

127. Rennie PS, Bruchovsky N, Leco KJ, et al: Characterization of two *cis*-acting DNA elements involved in the androgen regulation of the probasin gene. Mol Endocrinol 7:23–36, 1993.

128. Tan J, Marschke KB, Ho KC, et al: Response elements of the androgen-regulated C3 gene. J Biol Chem 267:4456–4466, 1992.

129. Claessens F, Celis L, Peeters B, et al: Functional characterization of an androgen response element in the first intron of the C3(1) gene of prostatic binding protein. Biochem Biophys Res Commun 164:833–840, 1989.

130. Denison SH, Sands A, Tindall DJ: A tyrosine aminotransferase glucocorticoid response element also mediates androgen enhancement of gene expression. Endocrinology 124:1091–1093, 1989.

131. Riegman PHJ, Vlietstra RJ, van der Korput JAGM, et al: The promoter of the prostate specific antigen gene contains a functional androgen responsive element. Mol Endocrinol 5:1921–1930, 1991.

132. Adler AJ, Danielsen M, Robins DM: Androgen-specific gene activation via a consensus glucocorticoid response element is determined by interaction with nonreceptor factors. Proc Natl Acad Sci USA 89:11660–11663, 1992.

132a. Georgatsou E, Bourgarel P, Meo T: Male-specific expression of mouse sex-limited protein requires growth hormone, not testosterone. Proc Natl Acad Sci USA 90:3626–3630, 1993.

133. Ham J, Thomson A, Needham M, et al: Characterization of response elements for androgens, glucocorticoids and progestins in mouse mammary tumour virus. Nucleic Acids Res 16:5263–5276, 1988.

134. Roche PJ, Hoare SA, Parker MG: A consensus DNA-binding site for the androgen receptor. Mol Endocrinol 6:2229–2235, 1992.

135. Beato M: Transcriptional control by nuclear receptors. FASEB J 5:2044–2051, 1991.

136. Gowland PL, Buetti E: Mutations in the hormone regulatory element of mouse mammary tumor virus differentially affect the response to progestins, androgens, and glucocorticoids. Mol Cell Biol 9:3999–4008, 1989.

137. Cato ACB, Skroch P, Weinmann J, et al: DNA sequences outside the receptor-binding sites differentially modulate the responsiveness of the mouse mammary tumour virus promoter to various steroid hormones. EMBO J 7:1403–1410, 1988.

138. Shemshedini L, Knakuthe R, Sassone-Corsi P, et al: Cell-specific inhibitory and stimulatory effects of Fos and Jun on transcription activation by nuclear receptors. EMBO J 10:3839–3849, 1991.

139. Page MJ, Parker MG: Effect of androgen on the transcription of rat prostatic binding proteins. Mol Cell Endocrinol 27:343–355, 1982.

140. Berger FG, Loose D, Meisner H, Watson G: Androgen induction of messenger RNA concentrations in mouse kidney is posttranscriptional. Biochemistry 25:1170–1175, 1986.

141. Liao S, Smythe S, Tymoczko JL, et al: RNA-dependent release of androgen and other steroid-receptor complexes from DNA. J Biol Chem 255:5545–5551, 1980.

142. Liao S, Liang T, Tymoczko JL: Ribonucleoprotein binding of steroid-receptor complexes. Nature New Biol 241:211–213, 1973.

143. Hiipakka RA, Liao S: Steroid receptor recycling and interaction of receptor with RNA. Am J Clin Oncol 11:S18–S22, 1988.

144. Getzenberg RH, Pienta KJ, Coffey DS: The tissue matrix: Cell dynamics and hormone action. Endocr Rev 11:399–417, 1990.

145. Arnold AP, Gorski RA: Gonadal steroid induction of structural sex differences in the central nervous system. Annu Rev Neurosci 7:413–442, 1984.

146. Cunha GR, Donjacour AA, Cooke PS, et al: The endocrinology and developmental biology of the prostate. Endocr Rev 8:338–362, 1987.

147. Yan G, Fukabori Y, Nikolaropoulos S, et al: Heparin-binding keratinocyte growth factor is a candidate stromal to epithelial cell andromedin. Mol Endocrinol 6:2123–2128, 1992.

148. Norton JN, Skinner MK: Regulation of Sertoli cell differentiation by the testicular paracrine factor PModS: Potential role of immediate-early genes. Mol Endocrinol 6:2018–2026, 1992.

149. Aumuller G, Seitz J: Protein secretion and secretory processes in male accessory sex glands. Int Rev Cytol 121:127–231, 1990.

150. Isaacs WB, Coffey DS: The predominant protein of canine seminal plasma is an enzyme. J Biol Chem 259:11520–11526, 1984.

151. Carter HB, Morrell CH, Pearson JD, et al: Estimation of prostatic growth using serial prostate-specific antigen measurements in men with and without prostate disease. Cancer Res 52:3323–3328, 1992.

152. Riegman PHJ, Vlietstra RJ, van der Korput HAGM, et al: Identification and androgen-regulated expression of two major human glandular kallikrein-1 (hGK-1) mRNA species. Mol Cell Endocrinol 76:181–190, 1991.

153. Chen C, Schilling K, Hiipakka RA, et al: Prostate α-protein: Isolation and characterization of the polypeptide components and cholesterol binding. J Biol Chem 257:116–121, 1982.

154. Heyns W, DeMoor P: Prostatic binding protein: A steroid-binding protein secreted by rat prostate. Eur J Biochem 78:221–230, 1977.

155. Lea OA, Petrusz P, French FS: Prostatein: A major secretory protein of the rat ventral prostate. J Biol Chem 254:6196–6202, 1979.

156. Davis BK: Timing of fertilization in mammals: Sperm cholesterol/phospholipid ratio as a determinant of the capacitation interval. Proc Natl Acad Sci USA 78:7560–7564, 1981.

156a. Celis L, Claessens F, Peeters B, et al: Proteins interacting with an androgen-responsive unit in the C3(1) gene intron. Molec Cell Endocrinol 94:165–172, 1993.

157. De Clercq N, Hemschjoote K, Devos A, et al: The 4.4 kilodalton proline-rich polypeptides of the rat ventral prostate are the proteolytic products of a 637-kilodalton protein displaying highly repetitive sequences and encoded in a single exon. J Biol Chem 267:9884–9894, 1992.

158. Chang C, Saltzman AG, Hiipakka RA, et al: Prostatic spermine-binding protein: Cloning and nucleotide sequence of cDNA, amino acid sequence and androgenic control of mRNA level. J Biol Chem 262:2826–2831, 1987.

159. Chang C, Saltzman AG, Sorensen NS, et al: Identification of glutathione S-transferase Yb$_1$ mRNA as the androgen-repressed mRNA by cDNA cloning and sequence analysis. J Biol Chem 262:11901–11903, 1987.

160. Bettuzzi S, Hiipakka RA, Gilna P, Liao S: Identification of an androgen-repressed mRNA in rat ventral prostate as coding for sulphated glycoprotein 2 by cDNA cloning and sequence analysis. Biochem J 257:293–296, 1989.

160a. Clay CM, Keri RA, Finicle AB, et al: Transcriptional repression of the glycoprotein hormone α subunit gene by androgen may involve direct binding of androgen receptor to the proximal promoter. J Biol Chem 268:13556–13564, 1993.

161. Quarmby VE, Yarbrough WG, Lubahn DB, et al: Autologous down-regulation of androgen receptor messenger ribonucleic acid. Mol Endocrinol 4:22–28, 1990.

162. Shan LX, Rodriguez MC, Janne OA: Regulation of androgen receptor protein and mRNA concentrations by androgens in rat ventral prostate and seminal vesicles and in human hepatoma cells. Mol Endocrinol 4:1636–1646, 1990.

163. Hackenberg R, Hawighorst T, Filmer A, et al: Regulation of androgen receptor mRNA and protein level by steroid hormones in human mammary cancer cells. J Steroid Biochem Mol Biol 43:599–607, 1992.

164. George FW, Russell DW, Wilson JD: Feed-forward control of prostate growth: Dihydrotestosterone induces expression of its own biosynthetic enzyme, steroid 5α-reductase. Proc Natl Acad Sci USA 88:8044–8047, 1991.

165. Moore RJ, Wilson JD: The effect of androgenic hormones on the reduced nicotinamide adenine dinucleotide phosphate: Δ^4-3-Ketosteroid 5α-oxidoreductase of rat ventral prostate. Endocrinology 93:581–592, 1973.

165a. Horton R, Pasupuletti V, Antonipillai I: Androgen induction of steroid 5α-reductase may be mediated via insulin-like growth factor-I. Endocrinology 133:447–451, 1993.

166. Liao S, Liang T, Fang S, et al: Steroid structure and androgenic activity: Specificities involved in the receptor binding and nuclear retention of various androgens. J Biol Chem 248:6154–6162, 1973.

167. Bonne C, Raynaud JP: Assay of androgen binding sites by exchange with methyltrienolone (R1881). Steroids 27:497–507, 1976.

168. Schilling K, Liao S: The use of radioactive 7α, 17α-dimethyl-19-nortestosterone (mibolerone) in the assay of androgen receptor. Prostate 5:581–588, 1984.

169. Peters CA, Barrack ER: A new method for labeling and autoradiographic localization of androgen receptors. J Histochem Cytochem 35:755–762, 1987.

170. Chang C, Whelan CT, Popovich TC, et al: Fusion proteins containing androgen receptors sequences and their use in the production of poly- and monoclonal anti-androgen receptor antibodies. Endocrinology 125:1097–1099, 1989.

171. Husmann DA, Wilson CM, McPhaul MJ, et al: Antipeptide antibodies to two distinct regions of the androgen receptor localize the receptor protein to the nuclei of target cells in the rat and human prostate. Endocrinology 126:2359–2368, 1990.

172. Zegers ND, Claessen E, Neelen C, et al: Epitope prediction and confirmation for the human androgen receptor: Generation of monoclonal antibodies for multi-assay performance following the synthetic peptide strategy. Biochim Biophys Acta 1073:23–32, 1991.

173. Takeda H, Chodak G, Mutchik S, et al: Immunohistochemical localization of androgen receptors with mono- and polyclonal antibodies to androgen receptor. J Endocrinol 126:17–25, 1990.
174. West NB, Chang C, Liao S, Brenner RM: Localization and regulation of estrogen, progestin and androgen receptors in the seminal vesicle of the Rhesus monkey. J Steroid Biochem Mol Biol 37:11–21, 1990.
175. Prins GS, Birch L, Greene GL: Androgen receptor localization in different cell types of the adult rat prostate. Endocrinology 129:3187–3199, 1991.
176. Takane KK, Husmann DA, McPhaul MJ, Wilson JD: Androgen receptor levels in the rat penis are controlled differently in distinctive cell types. Endocrinology 128:2234–2238, 1991.

177. Ruizeveld de Winter JA, Trapman J, Vermey M, et al: Androgen receptor expression in human tissues: An immunohistochemical study. J Histochem Cytochem 39:927–936, 1991.
178. Chodak G, Kranc DM, Puy LA, et al: Nuclear localization of androgen receptor in heterogeneous samples of normal, hyperplastic and neoplastic human prostate. J Urol 147:798–803, 1992.
179. Sadi MV, Walsh PC, Barrack ER: Immunohistochemical study of androgen receptors in metastatic prostate cancer. Cancer 12:3057–3064, 1991.
180. Liang T, Hoyer S, Yu R, et al: Immunocytochemical localization of androgen receptors in human skin using monoclonal antibodies against the androgen receptor. J Invest Dermatol 100:663–666, 1993.

TESTOSTERONE AND OTHER ANDROGENS: PHYSIOLOGY, PHARMACOLOGY, AND THERAPEUTIC USE

DAVID J. HANDELSMAN

Testosterone is the principal androgen in the circulation of mature male mammals. An androgen, or male sex hormone, is defined as a substance capable of developing and maintaining masculine sexual characteristics (including the genital tract, secondary sexual characteristics, and fertility) and the anabolic status of somatic tissues. Testosterone and synthetic androgens based on its structure are used clinically for androgen replacement therapy and pharmacological androgen effects. The principal goal of androgen replacement therapy is to replicate physiological levels of testosterone. Thus, an understanding of the normal physiology of testosterone is required as a basis for androgen pharmacology.[1]

TESTOSTERONE: PHYSIOLOGY

Biosynthesis

Testosterone is synthesized by an enzymatic sequence of steps from cholesterol[2] (Fig. 131–7) within the 500 million Leydig cells located in the interstitial (intertubular) compartment which constitutes about 5 per cent of mature testis volume.[3] The cholesterol is predominantly formed by de novo synthesis from acetate, although preformed cholesterol either from intracellular cholesterol ester stores or extracellular supply from circulating low-density lipoproteins also contributes.[2] Testosterone biosynthesis involves two multifunctional cytochrome P450 complexes involving hydroxylations and side-chain scissions (cholesterol side-chain cleavage [C20 and C22 hydroxylation and C20,22 lyase] and 17-hydroxylase/17,20 lyase) together with 3 and 17β-hydroxysteroid dehydrogenases and $\Delta^{4,5}$ isomerase. Regulation of the 17,20 lyase activity (active in gonads but inactive in adrenals) independently of 17-hydroxylase activity (active in all steroidogenic tissues) is thus highly selective, yet both activities reside in a single, multifunctional protein. This selectivity has yet to be fully explained. Testicular testosterone secretion is governed principally by luteinizing hormone (LH) through its regulation of the rate-limiting step, the conversion of cholesterol to pregnenolone within Leydig cell mitochondria by the cytochrome–P450 cholesterol side-chain cleavage enzyme complex located on the inner mitochondrial membrane. Cytoplasmic proteins including sterol carrier protein 2 facilitate transfer of cholesterol into mitochondria. All subsequent enzymatic steps are located in the Leydig cell endoplasmic reticulum. The high testicular production rate of testosterone creates both high local concentrations (up to 1 μg/g tissue) and

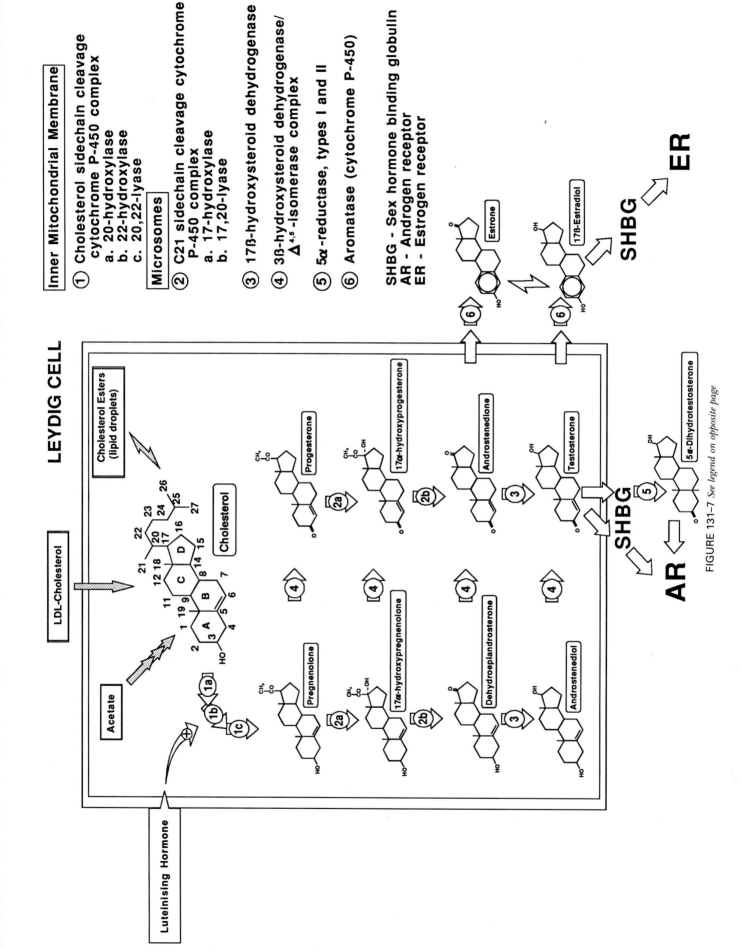

FIGURE 131–7 *See legend on opposite page*

rapid turnover (200 times per day) of intratesticular testosterone.

Secretion

Testosterone is secreted at adult levels during three epochs of male life—transiently during the first trimester of intrauterine life coinciding with genital tract differentiation, later during neonatal life for unknown physiological reasons, and continually after puberty. After middle age circulating total and free testosterone levels decline gradually as gonadotropin and sex-hormone binding globulin (SHBG) levels increase,[4, 5] with these trends being exaggerated by the coexistence of chronic illness.[5–7] These changes are attributable to both impaired hypothalamic regulation of testicular function[8–10] and to Leydig cell attrition.[3]

Testosterone and other lipophilic steroids leave the testis by diffusing down a concentration gradient across cell membranes into the bloodstream, with smaller amounts secreted into lymphatics and tubular fluid. After puberty greater than 95 per cent of circulating testosterone is derived from testicular secretion, with the remainder arising from metabolic conversion of precursors, predominantly secreted by the adrenal cortex, of low intrinsic androgenic potency such as dehydroepiandrosterone (DHA), its sulfate (DHAS), and androstenedione. These weak androgens constitute a large reservoir of precursors for extragonadal conversion to bioactive sex steroids in extragonadal tissues, including liver, kidney, muscle, and adipose tissue. Adrenal androgens contribute negligibly to direct virilization of men while making a proportionately larger contribution to lower total circulating testosterone levels in children and women in whom blood testosterone is derived about equally directly from gonadal secretion and indirectly from peripheral interconversion of adrenal androgen precursors.

Hormone production rates can be calculated either by estimating metabolic clearance rate (from bolus injection or steady-state isotope infusion) and mean circulating testosterone levels[11] or by estimating testicular arteriovenous differences and testicular blood-flow rate.[12] These methods give consistent estimates for testosterone production rate of 3 to 10 mg/d and interconversion rates of 4 per cent to dihydrotestosterone (DHT) and 0.2 per cent to estradiol under the assumption of steady-state conditions (hours to days). This assumption neglects diurnal rhythm or the fluctuation over shorter periods (minutes to hours) of circulating testosterone levels due to postural variation in hepatic blood flow and testosterone metabolic clearance rate[13] and to intermittent testosterone secretion entrained by pulsatile LH secretion.[14]

Transport

Testosterone circulates in blood at concentrations above its aqueous solubility by binding to circulating plasma proteins. Testosterone binds most avidly to SHBG, a heterodimeric glycoprotein of 95 kDa with a single high-affinity androgen-binding site. Circulating SHBG is secreted by the liver and is structurally identical to the testicular androgen binding protein.[15] Circulating SHBG (and thereby total testosterone) levels are up-regulated by estrogens, thyroxine, chronic liver disease (cirrhosis, hepatitis), and androgen deficiency and down-regulated by obesity, glucocorticoid or androgen excess, protein-losing states, and genetic SHBG deficiency.[16] Under physiological conditions, 60 to 70 per cent of circulating testosterone is SHBG-bound, with the remainder bound to lower-affinity, high-capacity binding sites (albumin, α_1-acid glycoprotein, transcortin) and 2 per cent remaining non-protein bound. The free fraction is the most biologically active, with the loosely protein-bound testosterone constituting a large and accessible buffer for the readily diffusible free fraction.[17] Free testosterone levels are calculated from total testosterone levels using tracer equilibrium dialysis or ultrafiltration methods to estimate the proportion of unbound testosterone.[18]

Circulating testosterone levels demonstrate distinct circhoral and diurnal rhythms. Circhoral LH pulsatility entrains some pulsatility in blood testosterone levels,[14] although delays in testosterone secretion and buffering effects of the circulating steroid-binding proteins cause marked dampening. Diurnal patterns of morning peak testosterone levels and nadir levels in afternoon are evident in younger men, although this pattern is lost in aging men,[19] possibly due to increased circulating SHBG levels and reduced testosterone secretion.[4]

Metabolism

A small proportion of circulating testosterone is metabolized to biologically active metabolites in certain target tissues to modulate biological effects, whereas most is converted to inactive metabolites for urinary or biliary excretion. About 4 per cent of circulating testosterone is converted to DHT, a more active androgen receptor agonist, by 5α-reductase. This occurs efficiently within the prostate stroma and to a lesser extent in other tissues (skin, liver), so that DHT circulates at 10 per cent of testosterone levels. A smaller proportion (0.2 per cent) of testosterone is converted to estradiol by aromatase in various tissues, thereby permitting action via the estrogen receptor. Aromatization of testosterone to estradiol within the brain is an important mediator of cerebral androgen effects, including regulation of gonadotropin secretion and sexual function. The significance of aromatization in mediating testosterone effects on other tissues is less clear.

Testosterone is converted mainly to inactive metabolites in the liver, kidney, muscle, and adipose tissue. Inactivation is predominantly by hepatic mixed function oxidases, lead-

FIGURE 131–7. **Pathways of testosterone biosynthesis and action.** In men, testosterone biosynthesis occurs almost exclusively in mature Leydig cells by the enzymatic sequences illustrated. Cholesterol originates predominantly by de novo synthesis pathway from acetyl-CoA with luteinizing hormone regulating the rate-limiting step, the conversion of cholesterol to pregnenolone within mitochondria, while remaining enzymatic steps occur in smooth endoplasmic reticulum. The Δ^5 and Δ^4 steroidal pathways are on the left and right, respectively. Testosterone and its androgenic metabolite, dihydrotestosterone, exert biological effects directly through binding to the androgen receptor and indirectly through aromatization of testosterone to estradiol, which allows action via binding to the estrogen receptor.

ing to oxidative degradation at most oxygen moieties of the molecule and ultimately hepatic conjugation to glucuronides, which are sufficiently hydrophilic for renal excretion. Metabolic clearance rate of testosterone is reduced by increases in circulating SHBG levels[20] or decreases in hepatic blood flow (e.g., posture)[13] or function, although theoretically drugs that influence hepatic mixed function oxidase activity could alter metabolic inactivation of testosterone. The rapid hepatic metabolic inactivation of testosterone leads to both a low oral bioavailability[21–24] and a short duration of action when injected parenterally.[25, 26] These limitations dictate the need for parenteral depot testosterone formulations (such as testosterone esters, implants, or transdermal patches) to achieve sustained androgenic effects or orally active synthetic androgens.[25–27]

Regulation

Testicular testosterone output is regulated primarily by pituitary LH secretion, which stimulates Leydig cell steroidogenesis via increasing steroid substrate availability and activity of rate-limiting steroidogenic enzymes as well as testicular blood flow. LH is a dimeric glycoprotein consisting of an α subunit common to hCG, FSH, and TSH and a β subunit providing distinctive biological specificity for each dimeric glycoprotein hormone by virtue of its specific binding to the LH/hCG, FSH, or TSH receptors.[28] These cell-surface receptors are themselves highly homologous members of the heptahelical, G-protein–linked family of membrane receptors. Functionally hCG is a natural, long-acting analogue of LH, as their β subunits are nearly identical except that hCG has a C-terminal peptide extension of 21 amino acids containing four O-linked, terminally sialic acid capped carbohydrate side chains conferring greater resistance to degradation, which prolongs circulating residence time and biological activity compared with LH. LH receptors are located exclusively on Leydig cell surface membranes and utilize signal transduction mechanisms involving both cAMP[29] and calcium[30] as second messengers to cause protein kinase–dependent phosphorylation of specific proteins that maintain testosterone secretion.

Driven by brief bursts of hypothalamic secretion of GnRH into the pituitary portal bloodstream, pituitary gonadotropes secrete LH episodically in pulses of high amplitude at about hourly intervals with little intervening interpulse basal LH secretion, so that circulating LH levels are distinctly pulsatile.[31] This pattern maintains Leydig cell sensitivity to LH as more continuous exposure causes desensitization.[2] Additional factors regulating testosterone secretion include paracrine factors originating within the testis to influence Leydig cell function, usually via indirect effects on Sertoli cells and blood vessels, respectively.[32] These include inhibin, activin, GnRH, FSH, prolactin, prostaglandins E_2 and $F_{2\alpha}$, growth hormone, insulin-like and other growth factors, and partially uncharacterized factors secreted by Sertoli cells. LH also influences testicular testosterone output by stimulation of Leydig cell secretion of vasoactive factors that promote testicular blood flow.

Testosterone participates in a negative testicular feedback cycle through its inhibition of hypothalamic GnRH and, consequently, pituitary gonadotropin secretion. Such negative feedback involves both testosterone effects on an-

drogen receptors and aromatization to estradiol within the hypothalamus. The small proportion (20 per cent) of circulating estradiol directly secreted from the testes makes it unlikely that estradiol derived from the bloodstream participates significantly in the negative feedback regulation of gonadotropin secretion in men. Extragonadal formation of bioactive steroids is not subject to known physiological regulation.

Action

Effects of testosterone, DHT, and other androgens are mediated by binding to the androgen receptor. The androgen receptor is specified by a single gene located at q11-12 on the X chromosome[33] and expressed as a protein of 919 amino acids[34] which resides in the nucleus. Androgen binding to the C-terminal hormone-binding region causes an allosteric conformational change in the androgen receptor protein which facilitates DNA binding to initiate the androgen-receptor complex's activity as a ligand-activated transcriptional factor. Mutations in the androgen receptor lead to a wide phenotypic spectrum of androgen insensitivity syndromes which parallel the variable degree of blockade of androgen action (see "Androgen Receptors and Action").

Testosterone is converted to the more active androgen DHT by the specific enzyme 5α-reductase, which originates from two genes expressed in androgen-sensitive tissues including the testis, prostate, liver, kidney, and skin. Congenital 5α-reductase deficiency due to mutation of the enzyme protein[35] leads to a distinctive form of genital ambiguity resulting in failure of masculinization in prepubertal boys who may be raised as females but in whom puberty leads to marked virilization, including phallic growth and gender reorientation.[36] This remarkable natural history reflects the predominant expression of 5α-reductase in urogenital sinus tissues largely restricting DHT effects to those structures. This physiology is exploited by the development of azasteroid 5α-reductase inhibitors[37] which capitalize on the restricted expression of 5α reduction to block testosterone action on urogenital sinus tissues such as the prostate without blocking all androgenic effects.

PHARMACOLOGY

Indications for Androgen Therapy

Androgen Replacement Therapy

The main specific clinical indication for testosterone is as androgen replacement therapy for hypogonadal men. The prevalence of male hypogonadism requiring androgen therapy in the general community can be estimated from the known prevalence of Klinefelter's syndrome (1.5 to 2.5 per 1000 male births[38]), as Klinefelter's syndrome accounts for 35 to 50 per cent of men requiring androgen replacement therapy.[39] The estimated prevalence of 5 per 1000 men in the general community makes androgen deficiency the most common hormonal deficiency disorder among men. Untreated androgen deficiency, rather than being life shortening, is compatible with a long but suboptimal quality of life. Owing to its variable and often subtle clinical features, male hypogonadism remains underdiagnosed and suboptimally managed, denying many androgen-deficient men simple and effective medical treatment, often with striking benefits.

Hypogonadism of any cause may require androgen replacement therapy depending only on whether the deficit in endogenous testosterone production is sufficient to cause clinical and/or biochemical manifestations of androgen deficiency. The clinical features of androgen deficiency vary according to the severity, chronicity, and epoch of life at presentation. These include ambiguous genitalia, microphallus, delayed puberty, sexual dysfunction, infertility, osteoporosis, anemia, flushing, excessive fatigability, or incidental biochemical diagnosis.[40] As the underlying disorders are mostly irreversible, life-long androgen replacement therapy after the age of puberty is usually required. Androgen replacement therapy can rectify most clinical features of androgen deficiency apart from inducing spermatogenesis. When fertility is required in gonadotropin-deficient men, spermatogenesis can be initiated by treatment with pulsatile GnRH[41] or gonadotropins[42] to substitute for pituitary gonadotropin secretion with LH or hCG, respectively, stimulating endogenous testosterone production. Once fertility is no longer required, androgen replacement therapy usually reverts to the simpler and cheaper use of testosterone while preserving the ability subsequently to reinitiate spermatogenesis by gonadotropin replacement.[43]

The potential role for androgen replacement therapy in men manifesting subclinical androgen deficiency as evident in biochemical features of Leydig cell dysfunction (persistently elevated LH/T ratio) seen in aging[44] or following testicular damage[45] remains uncertain. As tissue androgen levels fall with age,[5] controlled clinical trials are required to determine if androgen supplementation ameliorates the age-related changes in bone, muscle, and other androgen-dependent tissues[46] and how such benefits balance potential long-term risks of cardiovascular or prostatic disease.[47] The scope of androgen treatment may also be widened by development of hormonal male contraception because all currently envisaged regimens, aiming to suppress spermatogenesis by inhibiting gonadotropin secretion (see Ch. 137), would require testosterone either alone[48] or together with a progestin[49] or a GnRH antagonist[50, 51] in order to replace endogenous testosterone secretion.

Nonspecific or Pharmacological Androgen Therapy

Nonspecific or pharmacological uses of androgens include treatment of anemia due to marrow[52] or renal[53] failure, osteoporosis,[54] estrogen receptor–positive breast cancer[55, 56] hereditary angioedema (C1-esterase inhibitor deficiency),[57, 58] and muscular diseases.[59, 60] These applications represent second-line, empirical therapies that are eventually rendered obsolete by more specific treatments for the underlying conditions. For example, recombinant erythropoietin[61] largely supplants androgen therapy for anemias and acts primarily by stimulating endogenous erythropoietin secretion.[52, 62] The pharmacological applications have frequently involved synthetic, orally-active 17α-

alkylated androgens despite their inherent risk of hepatotoxicity.[63] In treating angioedema, oral 17α-alkylated androgens increase circulating C1-esterase inhibitor levels, which reverses the secondary depletion of serum complement factors (C4 and C2) and prevents attacks.[57, 58] These benefits may derive from hepatic effects of the 17α-alkyl androgens rather than androgen action per se.[27] Otherwise, the safer parenteral testosterone formulations are favored, although this preference must be balanced against potential benefits and life expectancy in situations in which a proven clinical role for pharmacological androgen therapy exists. In eugonadal men, androgens transiently increase positive nitrogen balance and body weight, presumably owing to increased appetite and lean mass[60, 64–66]; however, androgen therapy has no proven role in sustaining improved nitrogen balance during catabolic states (such as burns, postoperative and post-traumatic states, malignant cachexia, malnutrition, and glucocorticoid excess) or in preventing muscular atrophy during limb immobilization.[66, 67]

Androgen Misuse and Abuse

Misuse of androgens involves both the medical prescription without a legitimate clinical indication and nonmedical androgen abuse by athletes (see also Ch. 132). Among non–androgen-deficient men, androgens have no clinical role or may be deleterious in treating male sexual dysfunction or infertility. The dramatic escalation of financial rewards in competitive sports over recent decades has evolved an underground folklore among gullible athletes and trainers, particularly in power sports and body building, that androgens ("anabolic steroids") enhance sports performance. Based largely on rumor and wishful thinking promulgated in the pseudoscientific fantasies of underground publications, this credulous folklore fosters the use of prodigious doses of androgen cocktails in bizarre ("stacking") regimens. Controlled clinical studies have repeatedly failed to demonstrate significant improvement of sports performance once placebo effects including motivation, training, and diet are properly controlled.[68–70] Nevertheless, athletic abuse of androgens is epidemic among elite power sportsmen and recreational body builders,[71] who use androgens, including veterinary, inert, or counterfeit preparations, obtained mostly through illicit sales by underground networks with a small proportion obtained from compliant doctors. Although highly sensitive urinary drug screening methods for synthetic androgens have been adopted by international sporting bodies and legislation has been introduced by some governments to tightly regulate clinical use of androgens, the epidemic of androgen abuse is likely to continue, being driven by user demand until the limited efficacy of androgens is understood and the "win-at-all-costs" mentality dissipates.

Practical Goals of Androgen Replacement Therapy

The goal of androgen replacement therapy is to replicate the physiological actions of endogenous testosterone, usually for the remainder of life. This requires rectifying the deficit and maintaining androgenic/anabolic effects on bone, muscle, blood-forming marrow, and other androgen-responsive tissues[46] as well as sexual function.[72] The ideal preparation for long-term androgen replacement therapy should be safe, effective, convenient, and inexpensive, with long-acting depot properties due to reproducible, zero-order release kinetics. Androgen replacement therapy usually employs testosterone rather than synthetic androgens for reasons of safety and ease of monitoring and aims to maintain physiological testosterone levels.[40, 73] The practical goal of androgen replacement therapy is therefore to maintain stable, physiological testosterone levels for prolonged periods using convenient depot testosterone formulations, which facilitate compliance and avoid either supranormal or excessive fluctuation of androgen levels.

Pharmacological Features of Androgens

Androgens are defined pharmacologically by their binding and activation of the androgen receptor. Testosterone is the model androgen featuring a 19-carbon, 4-ring steroid structure with two oxygens (3-keto, 17β-hydroxy), including a Δ^4 nonaromatic A ring. Testosterone derivatives (Fig. 131–8) have been developed to enhance intrinsic androgenic potency, prolong duration of action, and/or improve oral bioavailability of synthetic androgens. Major structural modifications of testosterone include 17β-esterification, 19-normethyl, 17α-alkyl, 1-methyl, 7α methyl, and D-homo-androgens.[74] The identification of a single gene and protein for the androgen receptor[34] explains the physiological observation that, at equivalent doses, all androgens have essentially identical effects.[27] Consequently, the term "anabolic steroid," referring to an idealized androgen lacking virilizing features but maintaining myotrophic properties, is functionally synonymous with the term "androgen," and the false distinction perpetuates an obsolete terminology.

Formulation, Route, and Dosage

Unmodified testosterone is used in a variety of formulations. Fused implants of crystalline testosterone provide stable, physiological testosterone levels for up to six months following a single implantation procedure.[75] Despite nearly ideal depot properties, this old form of testosterone administration[76] is not widely adopted because of the cumbersome, minor surgical implantation procedure with its skill-dependent complications (extrusion 5 per cent, bleeding or infection 1 per cent).[77] Testosterone-impregnated adhesive patches can maintain physiological testosterone levels but require daily application and disproportionately increase blood DHT levels due to 5α reduction of testosterone by hair follicles and genital fibroblasts during its transdermal passage.[78] Transdermal patches applied to the highly vascular, thin scrotal skin still

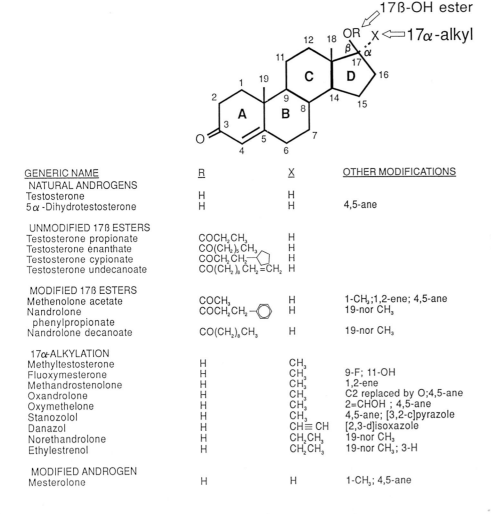

GENERIC NAME	R	X	OTHER MODIFICATIONS
NATURAL ANDROGENS			
Testosterone	H	H	
5α-Dihydrotestosterone	H	H	4,5-ane
UNMODIFIED 17β ESTERS			
Testosterone propionate	COCH₂CH₃	H	
Testosterone enanthate	CO(CH₂)₅CH₃	H	
Testosterone cypionate	COCH₂CH₂⬠	H	
Testosterone undecanoate	CO(CH₂)₉CH₂=CH₂	H	
MODIFIED 17β ESTERS			
Methenolone acetate	COCH₃	H	1-CH₃;1,2-ene; 4,5-ane
Nandrolone phenylpropionate	COCH₂CH₂—⬡	H	19-nor CH₃
Nandrolone decanoate	CO(CH₂)₈CH₃	H	19-nor CH₃
17α-ALKYLATION			
Methyltestosterone	H	CH₃	
Fluoxymesterone	H	CH₃	9-F; 11-OH
Methandrostenolone	H	CH₃	1,2-ene
Oxandrolone	H	CH₃	C2 replaced by O;4,5-ane
Oxymethelone	H	CH₃	2=CHOH ; 4,5-ane
Stanozolol	H	CH₃	4,5-ane; [3,2-c]pyrazole
Danazol	H	CH≡CH	[2,3-d]isoxazole
Norethandrolone	H	CH₂CH₃	19-nor CH₃
Ethylestrenol	H	CH₂CH₃	19-nor CH₃; 3-H
MODIFIED ANDROGEN			
Mesterolone	H	H	1-CH₃; 4,5-ane

FIGURE 131–8. Testosterone and its derivatives. Listed are the androgens in most common clinical use and their chemical relationship to testosterone.

need to be large to permit sufficient testosterone absorption,[78] whereas smaller patches used on nonscrotal skin require potentially irritating absorption enhancers.[79] Dermal gels containing either testosterone[80] or DHT[81] rubbed daily on the trunk are used in Europe and provide effective androgen replacement but may transfer androgen to the female partner by skin contact.[82] Suspensions of biodegradable microspheres, consisting of poly-glycolide-lactide matrix similar to absorbable suture material and laden with testosterone, can deliver stable, physiological levels of testosterone for two to three months following intramuscular injection.[83] The application of microsphere technology to testosterone delivery may be restricted by costs and technical limitations, including limited loading capacity, large injection volumes, and difficulty ensuring batchwise consistency as well as susceptibility to mechanical shear forces during injection. Micronized testosterone has low oral bioavailability requiring high daily doses (200 to 400 mg) to maintain physiological testosterone levels,[21] and this heavy androgen load causes prominent hepatic enzyme induction, although it is not hepatotoxic.[84] Although effective in small studies, micronized testosterone has been little used. A sublingual cyclodextrin formulation of testosterone requires multiple daily dosing to maintain physiological testosterone levels, making it unlikely to be useful for long-term androgen replacement.[85]

The most widely used testosterone formulation is intramuscular injection of testosterone esters, formed from fatty acids of various aliphatic and/or aromatic chain lengths and composition, injected in an oil vehicle. This depot formulation relies on retarded release of the testosterone ester from the oil vehicle injection depot as, following release, esters undergo rapid hydrolysis by ubiquitous esterases to liberate free testosterone into the circulation. The pharmacokinetics of testosterone esters is therefore determined primarily by ester side-chain length and hydrophobicity, which dictates rate-limiting ester release rate, which in turn is governed by the physicochemical partitioning of the testosterone ester between the hydrophobic oil vehicle and the aqueous extracellular fluid. Testosterone propionate with a short aliphatic side-chain ester has a brief duration of action requiring injections of 25 to 50 mg at one- to two-day intervals for androgen replacement. In contrast, testosterone enanthate has a longer duration of action so that it is routinely administered at doses of 200 to 250 mg every 10 to 14 days for androgen replacement therapy in hypogonadal men.[86–89] Other testosterone esters (cypionate, cyclohexanecarboxylate) have virtually identical pharmacokinetics, making them pharmacologically equivalent to the enanthate,[89] which is the most widely used testosterone ester. Mixtures of short- and longer-acting testosterone esters are available but lack a convincing rationale, as they only exaggerate the shortfall from desirable zero-order kinetics release profiles. An important recent advance is the development by public sector agencies of testosterone buciclate (trans-4-n-butyl cyclohexane carboxylate, 20 AET-1), a novel insoluble testosterone ester in an aqueous suspension. Release of testosterone from the buciclate ester is rate-limited by steric hindrance to ester side-chain hydrolysis, providing steady testosterone release for up to four months following parenteral administration in nonhuman primates[90] and hypogonadal men.[91]

Oral testosterone undecanoate, an oleic acid suspension of the ester in 40 mg capsules, is administered as 160 to 240 mg in three to four doses per day. The hydrophobic, long aliphatic chain ester in an oil vehicle favors preferential absorption into chylomicrons entering the gastrointestinal lymphatics and largely bypassing hepatic first-pass metabolism during portal absorption. Testosterone undecanoate has low and erratic oral bioavailability, short duration of action, and causes gastrointestinal intolerance, making it a second choice testosterone formulation[87, 88] unless parenteral therapy is to be avoided (for example, bleeding disorders or anticoagulation, children).[92] Most other oral androgens are 17α-alkylated (methyltestosterone, fluoxymesterone, oxymetholone, oxandrolone, ethylestranol, stanozolol, methandrostenolone, norethandrolone, danazol), making them undesirable for routine long-term androgen replacement therapy. The 1-methyl androgen, mesterolone, functionally an oral DHT analogue, is a synthetic oral androgen free of hepatotoxicity but rarely used for androgen replacement owing to the need for multiple daily dosing, its poorly described pharmacology, and limited androgenic potency.[93]

The choice of testosterone formulation for androgen replacement therapy depends primarily on physician experience and patient preference involving factors such as convenience, availability, familiarity, cost, and tolerance for frequent injections. Preparations of testosterone or its esters are increasingly favored over synthetic androgens for all androgen applications by virtue of assured safety and efficacy, ease of dose titration, and assay monitoring. The hepatotoxicity of synthetic 17α-alkylated androgens[63] makes them unsuitable for long-term androgen administration, and this is reflected in the progressive withdrawal of 17α-alkylated androgens from clinical use in most countries. Cross-over studies indicate that most experienced patients prefer formulations with stable testosterone levels and smoother clinical effects (such as implants[87, 88] or transdermal patches[78]) to the wide fluctuations in testosterone levels and effects with intramuscular injections of testosterone esters in an oil vehicle.[86, 88, 89] There are few well-established formulation or route-dependent differences between various testosterone formulations once adequate doses are administered. As with estrogen replacement, testosterone effects on SHBG may be viewed as manifestations of hepatic overdosage[16] so that oral 17α-alkylated androgens and testosterone undecanoate cause prominent lowering of SHBG levels owing to marked first-pass hepatic effects, whereas intramuscular testosterone ester injections cause transient falls that mirror testosterone levels and long-acting depot testosterone formulations (such as testosterone buciclate, implants, and microspheres) have minimal effects.[83, 88, 91, 94] Long-acting depot testosterone preparations with zero-order release patterns[75, 83, 91] that are also convenient and affordable are likely to supplant the present injectable testosterone esters as the mainstays of androgen replacement therapy.

Side Effects of Androgen Therapy

Serious adverse effects from androgens are uncommon and are mostly due to either inappropriate treatment or the hepatotoxicity of the 17α-alkylated androgens.

Steroidal Effects

Androgens can stimulate physical and mental activity (to enhance assertiveness, libido, and mood) to reverse their slowing during androgen deficiency.[95, 96] In normal, eugonadal men, however, additional androgens have negligible effect on mood or behavior.[48, 97] This contrasts with athlete abusers of androgens, among whom high levels of background psychological disturbance[98] and drug habituation[99] may predispose to behavioral disturbances reported during androgen abuse.[95, 96, 96a] Excessive or undesirable androgenic effects may be experienced during androgen therapy due to intrinsic androgenic effects in inappropriate settings (such as in women and children). In untreated older hypogonadal men, initiation of androgen treatment with standard doses occasionally produces an intolerable increase in libido and erection frequency. More gradual acclimatization to full androgen doses with counseling of men and their wives may be useful in such situations. Seborrhea and acne, with a predominantly truncal distribution after adolescence in contrast to the facial acne of adolescents, is common during androgen therapy and is related to high blood testosterone levels and so is most evident during treatment with intramuscular testosterone esters. It is usually adequately managed with topical measures or broad-spectrum antibiotics despite continuing testosterone treatment. Weight gain reflecting anabolic effects on muscle mass and/or fluid retention is also common. Increased body hair and temporal hair loss or balding may be seen. Gynecomastia may occur, especially during use of aromatizable androgens such as testosterone which increase circulating estradiol levels. As with gynecomastia in other circumstances, the exact pathophysiological mechanisms are unclear, although an excessive estrogen to androgen milieu is presumably involved. Androgenic side effects are rapidly reversible on cessation of treatment apart from changes in voice and terminal body hair, which are irreversible.

Testosterone and its esters lower total and LDL cholesterol whereas HDL levels are minimally altered,[47, 100–102] reversing the hyperlipidemic effects of chronic androgen deficiency.[103] In contrast, oral 17α-alkylated androgens markedly lower HDL cholesterol levels owing to prominent reduction in hepatic lipoprotein levels.[104] The potential long-term consequences for cardiovascular disease of such pharmacological changes are unknown, although low testosterone levels may represent another of the constellation of interrelated epidemiological risk factors for atherosclerotic cardiovascular disease.[105–107]

Hepatotoxicity

Hepatotoxicity is a well-recognized but uncommon side effect of 17α-alkylated but not with other androgens.[63] Biochemical hepatotoxicity, involving either a cholestatic or hepatic pattern, usually abates with cessation of steroid ingestion. Hepatic tumors related to androgen use include peliosis hepatis (blood-filled cysts), adenoma, and carcinoma. Prolonged use of 17α-alkylated androgens requires regular clinical examination and biochemical monitoring of hepatic function. If biochemical abnormalities are detected, treatment with 17α-alkylated androgens should cease, and safer androgens may be substituted without concern. Where structural lesions are suspected, radionuclide scan, ultrasonography, or abdominal CT scan should precede hepatic biopsy, during which severe bleeding may be provoked in peliosis hepatis. As equally effective and safer alternatives exist, the hepatotoxic 17α-alkylated androgens should be replaced in routine clinical practice, especially for long-term androgen replacement in androgen-deficient men.

Formulation Related

Complications related to testosterone formulations are related to mode of administration or idiosyncratic reactions to constituents. Intramuscular injections of oil vehicle may cause local pain (7.4 per cent), bleeding or bruising (15.2 per cent), and coughing fits or fainting, possibly due to oil microembolization (1.5 per cent).[39] Inadvertent subcutaneous administration of the oil vehicle is highly irritating and may cause pain, inflammation, or even dermal necrosis. Allergy to oil vehicle of testosterone ester injections (sesame, castor, arachis) is very rare, and even patients allergic to peanuts may tolerate arachis (peanut) oil without incident. Oral testosterone undecanoate frequently causes gastrointestinal intolerance due to the oleic acid suspension vehicle. Testosterone implants may be associated with extrusion of implants or with bleeding, infection, or scarring at implant sites.[77] Intramuscular injection of biodegradable microspheres involves a large injection volume, which may cause discomfort.[83]

Monitoring of Androgen Replacement Therapy

Monitoring of androgen replacement therapy involves clinical and biochemical observations both to optimize androgen effects and to recognize side effects, although testosterone and its esters are sufficiently safe not to require routine toxicological monitoring. Clinical monitoring depends upon judicious observation of serial improvement in the key presenting features of androgen deficiency. Androgen-deficient patients may report subjective improvements in energy, well-being, psychosocial drive, initiative, and assertiveness as well as in sexual activity (especially libido and ejaculation frequency), increased sexual hair and muscular strength and endurance. Objective measures of androgen action would be highly desirable, but suitable valid biochemical indices are not yet available for most androgen-responsive tissues.[46] The main biochemical measures available for monitoring of androgenic effects include hemoglobin (which rises by about 10 to 20 g/L when androgen dosage is adequate[108]) and circulating testosterone and gonadotropin levels (in men with hypergonadotropic hypogonadism) at appropriate times relative to testosterone doses, usually best at trough levels prior to the next dose. In the presence of normal testosterone-negative feedback on hypothalamic GnRH and pituitary LH secretion, plasma LH levels are elevated in rough proportion to the degree of androgen deficiency, with severe androgen deficiency achieving virtually castrate levels of LH hypersecretion. Thus among men with hypergonadotropic hypogonadism (with intact hypothalamopituitary function), circulating LH levels provide a sensitive and specific index of tissue testosterone effects. Suppression of LH into the eugonadal range indicates adequate androgen replacement therapy, whereas persistent nonsuppression after the first few months of treatment is an indication of inadequate dosage or pattern of testosterone levels. In hypogonadotropic hypogonadism, however, impaired hypothalamopituitary function diminishes circulating LH levels, which then do not reflect tissue androgenic effects. Plasma testosterone measurements have a limited role in routine monitoring of androgen replacement therapy, particularly during initiation of treatment or when adequacy of replacement needs clarification. During depot testosterone treatment in which quasi–steady-state plasma testosterone levels are achieved, trough plasma testosterone levels may detect patients whose treatment is suboptimal and whose dose and/or treatment interval needs modification. In some patients measurement of free testosterone and/or SHBG levels may also help clarify androgen status. Plasma testosterone levels are not helpful for routine monitoring of androgen therapy using any synthetic androgens or oral testosterone undecanoate.

Although chronic androgen deficiency is a protective factor for prostatic disease, hypogonadal men receiving androgen replacement require surveillance for prostatic disease similar to that of eugonadal men of comparable age. Evaluation of symptoms, digital rectal examination of the prostate (or preferably transrectal prostatic ultrasonography), and prostate-specific antigen measurements should be evaluated at diminishing intervals after the age of 50 years and annually among men over 60 years. Monitoring of lipids and blood pressure should be appropriate to the cardiovascular risks of individual patients. Serial evaluation of bone density (especially vertebral trabecular bone) by quantitative CT or photon absorptiometry at annual or longer intervals may be useful to verify the adequacy of tissue androgen effects.

Contraindications and Precautions of Androgen Therapy

Prostate or breast cancer in men is a contraindication to androgen therapy, as the tumors may be androgen responsive. Pregnancy is a contraindication to androgen therapy, as transplacental passage of sex steroids may disturb fetal sexual differentiation. Precautions and/or careful monitoring of androgen use is required in (1) older men starting androgen treatment, who may experience intolerable changes in sexual function or increased prostatic obstruction, (2) competitive athletes, who may be subject to disqualification, (3) women of reproductive age, especially those who use their voice professionally, who may become irreversibly virilized, (4) patients with bleeding disorders or undergoing anticoagulation, when parenteral administration may cause severe bruising or bleeding, (5) sex steroid–sensitive epilepsy or migraine, (6) those with cardiac or renal failure or severe hypertension susceptible to fluid overload from sodium and fluid retention, and (7) men with obstructive sleep apnea that may be exacerbated by exogenous androgens.[109] Excessive androgen doses prior to completion of puberty may risk premature epiphyseal closure, leading to foreshortened final adult stature and/or precocious sexual development.

REFERENCES

1. Nieschlag E, Behre HM (eds): Testosterone: Action, Deficiency, Substitution. Berlin, Springer-Verlag, 1990.
2. Hall PF: Testicular steroid synthesis: Organization and regulation. In Knobil E, Neill J (eds): The Physiology of Reproduction. New York, Raven Press, 1988, pp 975–998.
3. Neaves WB, Johnson L, Porter JC, et al: Leydig cell numbers, daily sperm production, and serum gonadotropin levels in aging men. J Clin Endocrinol Metab 55:756–763, 1984.
4. Handelsman DJ: The hypothalamo-pituitary-gonadal axis in aging. In Imura H, Shizume K, Yoshida S (eds): Progress in Endocrinology. Amsterdam, Excerpta Medica International Congress Series, 1988, pp 267–272.
5. Vermeulen A: Androgens and male senescence. In Nieschlag E, Behre HM (eds): Testosterone: Action, Deficiency, Substitution. Berlin, Springer-Verlag, 1990, pp 261–276.
6. Nieschlag E, Lammers U, Freischem CW, et al: Reproductive function in young fathers and grandfathers. J Clin Endocrinol Metab 55:676–681, 1982.
7. Handelsman DJ, Staraj S: Testicular size: The effects of aging, malnutrition and illness. J Androl 6:144–151, 1985.
8. Deslypere JP, Kaufman JM, Vermeulen T, et al: Influence of age on pulsatile luteinizing hormone release and responsiveness of the gonadotrophs to sex hormone feedback in men. J Clin Endocrinol Metab 64:68–73, 1987.
9. Vermeulen A, Desylpere JP, Kaufman JM: Influence of antiopioids on luteinizing hormone pulsatility in aging men. J Clin Endocrinol Metab 68:68–72, 1989.
10. Veldhuis JD, Urban RJ, Lizarralde G, et al: Attenuation of luteinizing hormone secretory burst amplitude as a proximate basis for the hypoandrogenism of healthy aging men. J Clin Endocrinol Metab 75:707–713, 1992.
11. Gurpide E: Tracer Methods in Hormone Research. New York, Springer, 1975.
12. Setchell BP: The Mammalian Testis. London, Paul Elek, 1978.
13. Southren AL, Gordon GG, Tochimoto S: Further studies of factors affecting metabolic clearance rate of testosterone in man. J Clin Endocrinol Metab 28:1105–1112, 1968.
14. Veldhuis JD, King JC, Urban RJ, et al: Operating characteristics of the male hypothalamo-pituitary-gonadal axis: Pulsatile release of testosterone and follicle-stimulating hormone and their temporal coupling with luteinizing hormone. J Clin Endocrinol Metab 65:929–941, 1987.
15. Petra PH: The plasma sex steroid binding protein (SBP or SHBG): A critical review of recent developments on the structure, molecular biology and function. J Steroid Biochem Molec Biol 40:735–753, 1991.
16. Schoultz BV, Carlstrom K: On the regulation of sex-hormone-binding globulin: A challenge of an old dogma and outlines of an alternative mechanism. J Steroid Biochem 32:327–334, 1989.
17. Mendel CM: The free hormone hypothesis: A physiologically based mathematical model. Endocr Rev 10:232–274, 1989.
18. Ekins R: Measurement of free hormones in blood. Endocr Rev 11:5–46, 1990.
19. Bremner WJ, Vitiello MV, Prinz PN: Loss of circadian rhythmicity in blood testosterone levels with aging in normal men. J Clin Endocrinol Metab 56:1278–1281, 1983.
20. Petra P, Stanczyk FZ, Namkung PC, et al: Direct effect of sex-steroid binding protein (SBP) of plasma on the metabolic clearance rate of testosterone in the rhesus macaque. J Steroid Biochem 22:739–746, 1985.
21. Johnsen SG, Bennet EP, Jensen VG: Therapeutic effectiveness of oral testosterone. Lancet 2:1473–1475, 1974.
22. Nieschlag E, Mauss J, Coert A, Kicovic P: Plasma androgen levels in men after oral administration of testosterone or testosterone undecanoate. Acta Endocrinol 79:1975.
23. Nieschlag E, Cuppers HJ, Wickings EJ: Influence of sex, testicular development and liver function on the bioavailability of oral testosterone. Eur J Clin Invest 7:145–147, 1977.
24. Frey H, Aakvag A, Saanum D, Falch J: Bioavailability of testosterone in males. Eur J Clin Pharmacol 16:345–349, 1979.
25. Foss GL: Clinical administration of androgens. Lancet 1:502–504, 1939.
26. Parkes AS: Effective absorption of hormones. BMJ 371–373, 1938.
27. Wilson JD: The use and misuse of androgens. Metabolism 29:1278–1295, 1980.

28. Chin WW, Boime I (eds): Glycoprotein Hormones: Structure, Synthesis and Biologic Function. Norwell, MA, Serono Symposia, 1990.
29. Dufau ML, Catt KJ: Gonadotropin receptors and regulation of steroidogenesis in the testis and ovary. Vitam Horm 36:461–592, 1978.
30. Cooke BA: Is cyclic AMP an obligatory second messenger for luteinizing hormone? Mol Cell Endocrinol 69:C11–C15, 1990.
31. Veldhuis JD, Carlson ML, Johnson ML: The pituitary gland secretes in bursts: Appraising the nature of glandular secretory impulses by simultaneous multiple-parameter deconvolution of plasma hormone concentrations. Proc Natl Acad Sci USA 84:7686–7690, 1988.
32. Skinner MK: Cell-cell interactions in the testis. Endocr Rev 12:45–77, 1991.
33. Brown CJ, Goss SJ, Lubahn DB, et al: Androgen receptor locus on the human X chromosome: Regional localization to Xq11–12 and description of a DNA polymorphism. Am J Hum Genet 44:264–269, 1989.
34. Lubahn D, Joseph DR, Sullivan PM, et al: Cloning of the human androgen receptor complementary DNA and localisation to the X-chromosome. Science 240:327–330, 1988.
35. Thigpen AE, Davis DL, Milatovich A, et al: Molecular genetics of steroid 5α-reductase 2 deficiency. J Clin Invest 90:799–809, 1992.
36. Imperato-McGinley J, Peterson RE, Gautier T, Sturla E: Androgens and the evolution of male gender identity among male pseudohermaphrodites with 5-α reductase deficiency. N Engl J Med 300:1233–1237, 1979.
37. Rasmusson GH: Biochemistry and pharmacology of 5-α reductase inhibitors. In Furr BJA, Wakeling AE (eds): Pharmacology and Clinical Uses of Inhibitors of Hormone Secretion and Action. London, Balliere Tindall, 1987, pp 308–325.
38. Sorensen K: Klinefelter's syndrome in childhood, adolescence and youth: A genetic, clinical, developmental, psychiatric and psychological study. Chippenham, Parthenon Publishing, 1987.
39. Handelsman DJ: unpublished.
40. Nieschlag E, Behre HM: Pharmacology and clinical use of testosterone. In Nieschlag E, Behre HM (eds): Testosterone: Action, Deficiency, Substitution. Berlin, Springer-Verlag, 1990, pp 92–114.
41. Spratt DI, Finkelstein JS, O'Dea LSL, et al: Long-term administration of gonadotropin-releasing hormone in men with idiopathic hypogonadotropic hypogonadism: A model for studies of the hormone's physiological effects. Ann Intern Med 105:848–855, 1986.
42. Finkel DM, Phillips JL, Snyder PJ: Stimulation of spermatogenesis by gonadotropins in men with hypogonadotropic hypogonadism. N Engl J Med 313:651–655, 1985.
43. Burger HG, de Kretser DM, Hudson B, Wilson JD: Effects of preceding androgen therapy on testicular response to human pituitary gonadotropin in hypogonadotropic hypogonadism. Fertil Steril 35:64–68, 1981.
44. Davidson JM, Chen JJ, Crapo L, et al: Hormonal changes and sexual function in aging men. J Clin Endocrinol Metab 57:71–77, 1983.
45. Booth JD, Merriam GR, Clark RV, et al: Evidence for Leydig cell dysfunction in infertile men with a selective increase in plasma follicle-stimulating hormone. J Clin Endocrinol Metab 64:1194–1198, 1987.
46. Mooradian AD, Morley JE, Korenman SG: Biological actions of androgens. Endocr Rev 8:1–28, 1987.
47. Tenover JS: Effects of testosterone supplementation in the aging male. J Clin Endocrinol Metab 75:1092–1098, 1992.
48. World Health Organisation Task Force on Methods for the Regulation of Male Fertility: Contraceptive efficacy of testosterone-induced azoospermia in normal men. Lancet 336:955–959, 1990.
49. Schearer SB, Alvarez-Sanchez F, Anselmo J, et al: Hormonal contraception for men. Int J Androl (Suppl 2):680–712, 1978.
50. Tom L, Bhasin S, Salameh W, et al: Induction of azoospermia in normal men with combined Nal-Glu GnRH antagonist and testosterone enanthate. J Clin Endocrinol Metab 75:476–483, 1992.
51. Pavlou SN, Brewer K, Farley MG, et al: Combined administration of a gonadotropin-releasing hormone antagonist and testosterone in men induces reversible azoospermia without loss of libido. J Clin Endocrinol Metab 73:1360–1369, 1991.
52. Najean Y: Long-term follow-up in patients with aplastic anemia: A study of 137 androgen-treated patients surviving more than two years. Am J Med 71:543–551, 1981.
53. Neff MS, Goldberg J, Slifkin RF, et al: Anemia in chronic renal failure. Acta Endocrinol Suppl 271:80–86, 1985.
54. Dequeker J, Geusens P: Anabolic steroids and osteoporosis. Acta Endocrinol Suppl 271:45–52, 1985.
55. Cooperative Breast Cancer Group: Testosterone propionate therapy in breast cancer. JAMA 188:1069–1074, 1964.
56. Ingle JN: Additive hormonal therapy in women with advanced breast cancer. Cancer 53:766–777, 1984.
57. Gelfand JA, Sherins RJ, Alling DW, Frank MM: Treatment of hereditary angioedema with danazol: Reversal of clinical and biochemical abnormalities. N Engl J Med 295:1444–1448, 1976.
58. Agostini A, Cicardi M: Hereditary and acquired C1-inhibitor deficiency: Biological and clinical characteristics in 235 patients. Medicine (Baltimore) 71:206–215, 1992.
59. Griggs RC, Pandya S, Florence JM, et al: Randomized controlled trial of testosterone in myotonic dystrophy. Neurology 39:219–222, 1989.
60. Welle S, Lozefowicz R, Forbes G, Griggs RC: Effect of testosterone on metabolic rate and body composition in normal men and men with muscular dystrophy. J Clin Endocrinol Metab 74:332–335, 1992.
61. Erslev AJ: Erythropoietin. N Engl J Med 324:1339–1344, 1991.
62. Gardner FH, Besa EC: Physiologic mechanisms and the hematopoietic effects of the androstanes and their derivatives. Curr Top Hematol 4:123–195, 1983.
63. Ishak KG, Zimmerman HJ: Hepatotoxic effects of the anabolic-androgenic steroids. Semin Liver Dis 7:230–236, 1987.
64. Watson RN, Bradley MH, Callahan R, et al: A six-month evaluation of an anabolic drug, norethandrolone, in underweight persons. Am J Med 26:238–248, 1959.
65. Kalliomaki JL, Pirila AM, Ruikka I: A therapeutic trial with ethylestrenol in geriatric patients. Acta Endocrinol 63(Suppl):124–131, 1962.
66. Tweedle D, Walton C, Johnston IDA: The effect of an anabolic steroid on postoperative nitrogen balance. Br J Clin Pract 27:130–132, 1973.
67. Landau RL: The metabolic effects of anabolic steroids in man. In Kochakian CD (ed): Anabolic-Androgenic Steroids. Berlin, Springer-Verlag, 1976.
68. Haupt HA, Rovere GD: Anabolic steroids: A review of the literature. Am J Sports Med 12:469–484, 1984.
69. Wilson JD: Androgen abuse by athletes. Endocr Rev 9:181–199, 1988.
70. Elashoff JD, Jacknow AD, Shain SG, Braunstein GD: Effects of anabolic-androgenic steroids on muscular strength. Ann Intern Med 115:387–393, 1991.
71. Buckley WE, Yesalis CE, Freidl KE, et al: Estimated prevalence of anabolic steroid use among male high school students. JAMA 260:3441–3445, 1988.
72. Davidson JM, Camargo CA, Smith ER: Effects of androgens on sexual behaviour in hypogonadal men. J Clin Endocrinol Metab 48:955–958, 1979.
73. Nieschlag E, Wang C, Handelsman DJ, et al (eds): Guidelines for the Use of Androgens in Men. Geneva, Special Programme of Research, Development and Research Training in Human Reproduction of the World Health Organisation, 1992.
74. Avery MA, Tanabe M, Crowe DF, et al: Synthesis and testing of 17αβ-hydroxy-7α methyl-D-homoestra-4,16-dien-3-one: A highly potent orally active androgen. Steroids 55:59–64, 1990.
75. Handelsman DJ, Conway AJ, Boylan LM: Pharmacokinetics and pharmacodynamics of testosterone pellets in man. J Clin Endocrinol Metab 71:216–222, 1990.
76. Deansley R, Parkes AS: Further experiments on the administration of hormones by the subcutaneous implantation of tablets. Lancet 2:606–608, 1938.
77. Handelsman DJ: Pharmacology of testosterone pellet implants. In Nieschlag E, Behre HM (eds): Testosterone: Action, Deficiency, Substitution. Berlin, Springer-Verlag, 1990, pp 136–154.
78. Place VA, Atkinson L, Prather DA, et al: Transdermal testosterone replacement through genital skin. In Nieschlag E, Behre HM (eds): Testosterone: Action, Deficiency, Substitution. Berlin, Springer-Verlag, 1990, pp 165–181.
79. Meikle AW, Mazer NA, Moellmer JF, et al: Enhanced transdermal delivery of testosterone across nonscrotal skin produces physiological concentrations of testosterone and its metabolites in hypogonadal men. J Clin Endocrinol Metab 74:623–628, 1992.
80. Guerin JF, Rollet J: Inhibition of spermatogenesis in men using various combinations of oral progestogens and percutaneous or oral androgens. Int J Androl 11:187–199, 1988.
81. Chemana D, Morville R, Fiet J, et al: Percutaneous absorption of 5α-dihydrotestosterone in man: II. Percutaneous administration of 5α-dihydrotestosterone in hypogonadal men with idiopathic haemochromatosis; clinical, metabolic and hormonal effectiveness. Int J Androl 5:595–606, 1982.
82. Delanoe D, Fougeyrollas B, Meyer L, Thonneau P: Androgenisation of female partners of men on medroxyprogesterone acetate/percutaneous testosterone contraception. Lancet 1:276, 1984.

83. Bhasin S, Swerdloff RS, Steiner B, et al: A biodegradable testosterone microcapsule formulation provides uniform eugonadal levels of testosterone for 10–11 weeks in hypogonadal men. J Clin Endocrinol Metab 74:75–83, 1992.

84. Johnsen SG, Kampmann JP, Bennet EP, Jorgensen F: Enzyme induction by oral testosterone. Clin Pharmacol Ther 20:233–237, 1976.

85. Stuenkel CA, Dudley RE, Yen SSC: Sublingual administration of testosterone-hydroxypropyl-β-cyclodextrin inclusion complex simulates episodic androgen release in hypogonadal men. J Clin Endocrinol Metab 72:1054–1059, 1991.

86. Snyder PJ, Lawrence DA: Treatment of male hypogonadism with testosterone enanthate. J Clin Endocrinol Metab 51:1335–1339, 1980.

87. Cantrill JA, Dewis P, Large DM, et al: Which testosterone replacement therapy? Clin Endocrinol 24:97–107, 1984.

88. Conway AJ, Boylan LM, Howe C, et al: A randomised clinical trial of testosterone replacement therapy in hypogonadal men. Int J Androl 11:247–264, 1988.

89. Behre HM, Oberpenning F, Nieschlag E: Comparative pharmacokinetics of androgen preparations: Application of computer analysis and simulation. In Nieschlag E, Behre HM (eds): Testosterone: Action, Deficiency, Substitution. Berlin, Springer-Verlag, 1990, pp 115–135.

90. Weinbauer GF, Marshall GR, Nieschlag E: New injectable testosterone ester maintains serum testosterone of castrated monkeys in the normal range for four months. Acta Endocrinol 113:128–132, 1986.

91. Behre HM, Nieschlag E: Testosterone buciclate (20 Aet-1) in hypogonadal men: Pharmacokinetics and pharmacodynamics of the new long-acting androgen ester. J Clin Endocrinol Metab 75:1204–1210, 1992.

92. Butler GE, Sellar RE, Walker RF, et al: Oral testosterone undecanoate in the management of delayed puberty in boys: Pharmacokinetics and effects on sexual maturation and growth. J Clin Endocrinol Metab 75:37–44, 1992.

93. Luisi M, Franchi E: Double-blind group comparative study of testosterone undecanoate and mesterolone in hypogonadal male patients. J Endocrinol Invest 3:305–308, 1980.

94. Small M, Beastall GH, Semple CG, et al: Alterations of hormone levels in normal males given the anabolic steroid stanozolol. Clin Endocrinol 21:49–55, 1984.

95. Hubert W: Psychotropic effects of testosterone. In Nieschlag E, Behre HM (eds): Testosterone: Action, Deficiency, Substitution. Berlin, Springer-Verlag, 1990, pp 51–71.

96. Archer J: The influence of testosterone on human aggression. Br J Psychol 82:1–28, 1991.

96a. Bahrke MS, Yesalis CE, Wright JE: Psychological and behavioral effects of endogenous testosterone levels and anabolic-androgenic steroids among males. A review. Sports Medicine 10:303–337, 1990.

97. Anderson RA, Bancroft J, Wu FCW: The effects of exogenous testosterone on sexuality and mood of normal men. J Clin Endocrinol Metab 75:1503–1507, 1992.

98. Pope HG, Katz DL: Affective and psychotic symptoms associated with anabolic steroid use. Am J Psychiatry 145:487–490, 1988.

99. Kashkin KB, Kleber HD: Hooked on hormones? An anabolic steroid addiction hypothesis. JAMA 262:3166–3170, 1989.

100. Friedl KE, Hannan CJ, Jones RE, Plymate SR: High-density lipoprotein cholesterol is not decreased if an aromatisable androgen is administered. Metabolism 39:69–74, 1990.

101. Friedl KE, Dettori JR, Hannan CJ, et al: Comparison of the effects of high dose testosterone and 19-nortestosterone to a replacement dose of testosterone on strength and body composition in normal men. J Steroid Biochem Molec Biol 40:607–612, 1991.

102. Handelsman DJ, Conway AJ, Boylan LM: Suppression of human spermatogenesis by testosterone implants in man. J Clin Endocrinol Metab 75:1326–1332, 1992.

103. Oppenheim DS, George SL, Zervas NT, et al: Elevated serum lipids in hypogonadal men with and without hyperprolactinemia. Ann Intern Med 111:288–292, 1989.

104. Thompson PD, Cullinane EM, Sady SP, et al: Contrasting effects of testosterone and stanozolol on serum lipoprotein levels. JAMA 261:1165–1168, 1989.

105. Hauner H, Stangl K, Burger K, et al: Sex hormone concentrations in men with angiographically assessed coronary artery disease—relationship to obesity and body fat distribution. Klin Wochenschr 69:664–668, 1991.

106. Barrett-Connor E: Lower endogenous androgen levels and dyslipidemia in men with non–insulin-dependent diabetes mellitus. Ann Intern Med 117:807–811, 1992.

107. Plymate SR, Swerdloff RS: Androgens, lipids and cardiovascular risk. Ann Intern Med 117:871–872, 1992.

108. Palacios A, Campfield LA, McClure RD, et al: Effect of testosterone enanthate on hematopoiesis in normal men. Fertil Steril 40:100–104, 1983.

109. Matsumoto A, Sandblom RE, Schoene RB, et al: Testosterone replacement in hypogonadal men: Effects on obstructive sleep apnea, respiratory drives and sleep. Clin Endocrinol 22:713–721, 1985.

132

Anabolic Steroids

DON H. CATLIN

PHARMACOLOGY

Definition

Anabolic androgenic steroids are a class of chemically related steroid hormones that promote both protein anabolism and masculinization. Chemically they are analogues of testosterone. Pharmacologically their dominant effect is net synthesis of protein in virtually all tissues that are capable of growth, including male reproductive tissue. Even effects that are commonly referred to as androgenic, such as regulation of male accessory sex organs, can be considered to be anabolic; in fact, an androgenic effect has been described as an anabolic effect on sex organs.[1]

Testosterone, other endogenous steroids, and hundreds of synthetic steroids fulfill this definition. However, the terms *androgen* and *anabolic* are overly simplistic and inadequate because some effects are not easily classified as anabolic or androgenic and some are clearly neither (such as decrease in sex hormone–binding globulin). In fact, a remarkable feature of the anabolic androgenic steroids is their diversity and multiplicity of effects. Virtually all tissues are affected in some manner, and often it is difficult to distinguish between primary and secondary effects.

Despite intense research efforts, no steroid has been described that is purely anabolic or androgenic. Furthermore, in healthy man there is no direct evidence for more than one receptor. Thus, the ability to both promote growth and masculinize is inherent in the same molecule;

therefore, the most appropriate designation is anabolic androgenic steroid (AAS). Nevertheless, the term is commonly shortened to "anabolic steroid" or "androgenic steroid," depending on the context. "Androgenic" is used for discussions that emphasize sexual differentiation, pubertal changes, virilization, and effects on primary and secondary organs of reproduction. This chapter focuses on anabolic effects and the use of synthetic AAS's for conditions other than hypogonadism and related endocrine disease.

The Androgen Receptor

The notion of one receptor mediating androgenic effects in male reproductive tissue and another mediating anabolic effects in muscle tissue arose from the observation in experimental animals that some compounds exert anabolic activity and relatively little androgenic activity.[2] The hope of discovering an AAS devoid of androgenic activity fueled a concerted effort to synthesize and test new agents.[1] Because nitrogen balance studies were cumbersome, a simple bioassay was developed that compared, in the same animal, the AAS-induced increases in weight of the prostate and of the levator ani muscle.[3, 4] The anabolic:androgenic ratio was interpreted to be an index of relative dissociation of anabolic from androgenic activity. Although this assay did correlate reasonably well with nitrogen retention studies, later the validity of the assay was questioned.[5–7] In addition, research on specific intracellular enzymes, differences in the affinity of compounds for receptor-binding proteins, and differences in levels of receptors in various tissues showed that the diversity of responses could be explained by other mechanisms. Moreover, recent studies provide substantial evidence for only one receptor.

The androgen receptor (AR) has been isolated and characterized,[8] and a cDNA that encodes the AR has been cloned and expressed.[9–11] Only one type has been discovered by either molecular biological techniques or receptor-binding studies. The binding characteristics of receptors isolated from reproductive tissue and from skeletal muscle are identical.[5] Antiandrogens also bind to the AR and compete with testosterone and dihydrotestosterone (DHT) for the binding sites. Perhaps the most convincing evidence for the one-receptor theory are studies describing clinical consequences of androgen receptor disorders and associated molecular biology of the androgen-receptor gene.[12] For example, patients with complete testicular feminization have high levels of testosterone, and high doses of AAS do not result in anabolic or androgenic responses.[13]

Most of the effects of AAS's are presumed to be mediated like those of testosterone in tissues that contain AR, which include reproductive organs, brain, kidney, liver, skin, skeletal muscle, cardiac muscle, bone, larynx, thymus, and hematopoietic and lipid tissue. At the subcellular level the effects are determined by the affinity-binding constant with the AR and molecular details of receptor DNA interaction, transcription, and translation. Within the target cell the effects of AAS are presumed to be influenced by the same mechanisms that control the fate and effects of testosterone. These include enzymes that activate and deactivate testosterone, enzymes that control the activity of receptor androgen interactions, and differences in receptor content.[14–16]

Absorption, Distribution, and Metabolism

None of the synthetic nonendogenous AAS's has been studied as intensively as testosterone, although the available data indicate that the basic pharmacology of anabolic steroids is analogous to that of testosterone. The synthetic agents are absorbed from the gastrointestinal tract, mucous membranes, skin, and intramuscular depots. In the circulation most testosterone is loosely bound to albumin, a smaller fraction is tightly bound to sex hormone–binding globulin (SHBG), and some is free. The synthetic agents also bind to SHBG.[5, 17] The concentration of AAS and metabolites can be measured in serum and urine, and some data are available on concentration in serum relative to therapeutic effects; however, plasma levels are not commonly used to monitor dosing.

Free testosterone diffuses into cells, where it may bind directly to the androgen receptor (AR), undergo reduction of the C4-C5 double bond to 5α-DHT by 5α-reductase, or be metabolized further. Both testosterone and DHT bind to the same AR,[18] although DHT is more tightly bound, leading to the conclusion that DHT is the most active and potent intracellular androgen.[19] Binding to the AR activates the complex, enabling it to interact specifically with DNA and to activate specific genes.[8] Some testosterone is

metabolized by aromatase to estradiol, which binds to the estrogen receptor (ER). These important features of testosterone metabolism emphasize that administration of testosterone results in a mixture of effects mediated by testosterone + AR and/or DHT + AR and estradiol + ER. In some cases the effects at one receptor may be neutralized or enhanced by effects at the other.

The extent to which the effects of AAS's are mediated at both ER and AR is less certain, in part because the metabolism of AAS's has not been studied as extensively as that of testosterone. Any synthetic AAS with a δ-4, 3-keto function is subject to metabolism by aromatase to the corresponding estrogen. A few estrogen metabolites of AAS's have been described in man, and in vitro studies indicate that many more are likely.[20] Examples of AAS's that are not substrates for aromatase are DHT, fluoxymesterone, mesterolone, and oxandrolone.

Receptor-binding studies confirm that AR's derived from muscle tissue or prostate tissue are the same, and that synthetic agents, testosterone, and DHT bind to the same AR.[5] All synthetic AAS's undergo extensive metabolism primarily to hydroxylated and 5α- and 5β-reduced metabolites. Most of these are excreted in urine as sulfates or glucuronides. Various metabolites of synthetic AAS's have been found in subcellular fractions of target tissues, and their binding to AR has been characterized.[21, 22] Unlike testosterone, however, 5α-reduced metabolites of 17α-methyl AAS's are not more active than the parent compound.

Route of Administration and Molecular Structure

A fundamental determinant of the magnitude and spectrum of effects produced by AAS's is their molecular structure, which in turn determines their metabolism, kinetics, optimal routes of administration, and efficacy.

Oral Administration

The male testis produces approximately 7 mg of testosterone per day. However, following oral administration of up to 25 mg of testosterone, plasma levels do not increase because testosterone is rapidly metabolized during its first pass through the gastrointestinal tract and liver. This led to the design and synthesis of analogues of testosterone that were resistant to metabolism. Of the hundreds of compounds developed and tested, the most resistant to first-pass metabolism are those with a methyl or other alkyl group at C17 (Fig. 132–1). Of these, methyltestosterone, methandrostenolone, oxandrolone, oxymetholone, and stanozolol are the orally active AAS's used most today. Although some of these are also active via the buccal route of administration, there is little advantage to this route and absorption is highly variable.[20]

Compared with 17α-methylated AAS, methylation at the C1 position (for example, methenolone and mesterolone) reduces oral potency; nevertheless, these agents are sufficiently resistant to metabolism to be useful by the oral route. Various additions to the ring structure (such as fluoxymesterone), substitutions in the A ring (such as oxandrolone), or even the addition of a pyrazole ring to the

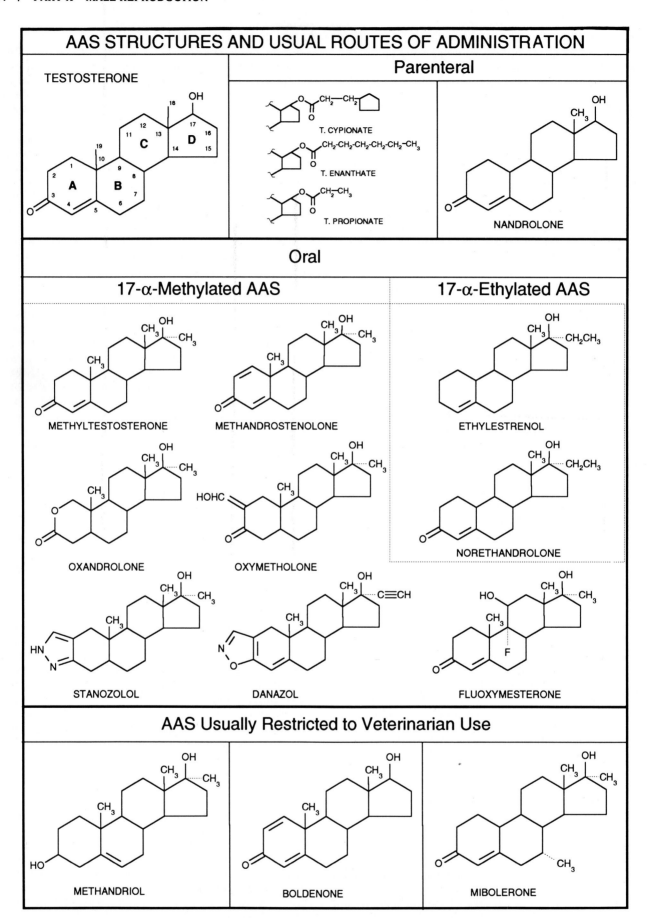

FIGURE 132–1. *See legend on opposite page*

A ring (stanozolol) result in orally active substances with preservation of anabolic and androgenic activity. However, danazol, which has both a 2,3-isoxazole group and a C17 ethinyl group, is unique in that it is a good inhibitor of gonadotropin secretion and has relatively little androgenic and anabolic activity. Accordingly danazol is useful in clinical circumstances in which androgenicity is unwanted and inhibition of gonadotropin secretion is desired.

Parenteral Administration

Parenteral administration of unmodified AAS is neither practical nor efficacious, even though first-pass metabolism is bypassed. Parenterally administered labeled testosterone has a half-life of approximately one hour. The formation of an ester in the 17β position, by increasing lipophilicity, markedly influences the duration of action and plasma levels of testosterone and other parenteral AAS. The length of the ester group correlates positively with lipid solubility, plasma half-life, and duration of action. The esterified AAS is commonly prepared in a lipid vehicle (sesame oil) and injected intramuscularly. The ester is slowly released from the site, and both the ester and the de-esterified drug may be detected in plasma. The rate-limiting step is release from the site rather than cleavage of the ester.[23] One of the most commonly prescribed AAS's is nandrolone (19 nortestosterone) esterified as decanoate (ND) or phenpropionate (NP). The plasma half-life of nandrolone after ND and NP administration is approximately 8 and 21 days, respectively.[24]

Choice of Agents and Dose

Relative to other classes of drugs, little systematic information is available on comparative dosage, potency, and efficacy of the synthetic AAS's. Unfortunately, the effects of AAS on experimental animals are not good predictors of effects in man.[1] In fact, data from receptor-binding studies with human tissue correlate better with clinical activity than do data from intact experimental animals. For most variables it is difficult to find clinical studies that provide dose-response curves that directly compare one AAS with another. This lack is related to a combination of methodological difficulties, a limited number of clinical indications, and less stringent regulatory requirements in the past. As a result, dosing regimens are generally based on clinical observation and experience.[1, 25] Despite numerous claims of differences between the various 17-alkylated AAS's, no systematic clinical data show a clear difference in the relative position of dose-response curves for any of the effects.

The dose of testosterone esters for replacement in hypogonadals is approximately 100 mg/wk (1.4 mg/kg/wk = 0.2 mg/kg/d). Because the synthetic agents are rarely used for hypogonadal syndromes, good comparative data are not available. Higher doses of testosterone, approximately 0.4 to 0.5 mg/kg/d administered weekly, are used in contraception trials in which the objective is to suppress FSH, LH, and sperm production. In order to achieve an effect equivalent to testosterone esters, it is necessary to administer a larger daily dose of an oral AAS. The dosing range is extremely broad. Doses as low as 0.05 mg/kg are effective in short stature, and the lowest effective dose has not been established. Typical doses in postmenopausal osteoporosis are 0.1 mg/kg, and in aplastic anemia trials they are 2 to 3 mg/kg. Athletes have used doses of 5 to 7 mg/kg. Of the oral agents, stanozolol may be somewhat more potent and oxymetholone less than the others. Danazol is far less potent. Maximal therapeutic doses recommended by the pharmaceutical manufacturers range from 8 to 30 mg (Fig. 132–1), yet doses of 50 to 400 mg/d are used for aplastic anemia.

Testosterone esters, particularly the enanthate, are currently the drug of choice for hypogonadal syndromes. This recommendation is based on a wealth of clinical experience, numerous successful clinical trials with various formulations of testosterone, advantages of providing the natural hormone, and of avoiding hepatotoxicity associated with 17-alkylated AAS's. For most other disorders that are treated with oral AAS's, the supporting clinical data are not sufficient to clearly distinguish one agent from another. The choice of an agent seems to depend on custom and clinical experience, with the result that oxandrolone is widely used for short stature, nandrolone and oxymetholone for anemia, and stanozolol, methandienone, or ND for osteoporosis.

EFFICACY IN VARIOUS DISORDERS

Osteoporosis

Sex steroids exert major influence on bone metabolism and homeostasis.[26-28] Postmenopausal osteoporosis is due to estrogen deficiency and is retarded by estrogen replacement therapy (see Ch. 73). Serum testosterone levels gradually decline with aging,[29] and elderly males experience a progressive decline in bone mass. Some develop osteoporosis late in life. The osteoporosis associated with hypogonadism responds to testosterone administration.[30, 31] The use of antiandrogens such as flutamide in the management of prostate carcinoma results in osteoporosis.[32] These and other observations stimulated investigations of the effects of anabolic steroids on bone and their role in the management of osteoporosis.[28, 33]

Pharmacology–Cell Culture

Until recently any effects of androgens on bone were considered indirect. Now AR's have been identified in cul-

FIGURE 132–1. Anabolic androgenic steroid structures and usual routes of administration. The solid heavy lines separate the AAS into two categories according to the usual but not exclusive route of administration (upper and middle panels) and a veterinarian group (bottom panel). For testosterone (upper left) the conventional numbering and lettering system is shown: carbon atoms are numbered and rings are designated with letters. The structure of the ester group for the three most commonly prescribed parenteral esters of testosterone (T) is shown (upper right) together with nandrolone (19-nortestosterone). The most commonly prescribed esters of nandrolone (esters not shown) are the phenpropionate and decanoate. The orally active AAS (middle panel) are subdivided (dotted lines) into a 17α-methyl group each with a methyl group on C19, and a 17α-ethyl group without a C19 methyl group. The veterinarian group (bottom panel) are formulated for parenteral administration.

tured human osteoblast-like cells,[34] and there is increasing evidence of a functional role for these AR's. Under the influence of DHT these cells proliferate and produce alkaline phosphatase.[35, 36] Moreover, testosterone stimulates growth and bone energy metabolism in vitro as measured by increased creatine kinase activity and enhanced [³H] thymidine incorporation into DNA.[37] Stanozolol also stimulates incorporation of [³H] thymidine and proliferation of cultured human bone cells.[38]

Efficacy in Postmenopausal Osteoporosis

Anabolic steroids could improve osteoporosis by a direct effect mediated by bone AR's. They might stimulate osteoblasts to increase bone formation or inhibit osteoclasts and reduce bone resorption. AAS also could improve bone indirectly by increasing renal absorption of calcium, increasing calcium uptake from the gut, or enhancing vitamin D activity. The data favor a direct effect on inhibition of bone resorption, with some support for a decrease in calcium excretion and no evidence for an influence on vitamin D.

About 10 studies of the efficacy of AAS in women with postmenopausal osteoporosis have been published since 1977. The number of treated subjects varied between 20 and 46, the length of treatment ranged from 6 to 24 months, and ND (N=6) and stanozolol (N=2) were the most commonly used drugs. Several studies were not double blind and placebo controlled. None reported a significant decrease in the incidence of new fractures, but one found no new spinal compression fractures over 29 months in the treated group.[39]

EFFECT ON BONE MINERAL CONTENT. In one double-blind study ND increased bone mineral content (BMC) in the proximal but not the distal part of the forearm and not in the spine.[40, 41] There was no change in indirect measures of bone formation: plasma bone Gla protein, serum alkaline phosphatase, and whole body retention of ^{99m}Tc-diphosphonates. During 6 to 18 months of follow-up, BMC returned to baseline. Another placebo-controlled study showed a small increase in lumbar spine BMC and trabecular bone volume and no effect on intestinal calcium absorption.[42] Of those studies reporting an increase in BMC, most concluded that it was due to inhibition of bone resorption.[33, 43–47]

INDIRECT EFFECTS. A decline in calcium excretion is generally interpreted as a decrease in the release of calcium from bone. AAS's modestly decreased urinary calcium in postmenopausal osteoporosis patients,[26, 39, 45] and it fell 20 per cent in one study,[48] although the calcium-retaining properties of estrogens are much greater.[27, 28] Plasma levels of alkaline phosphatase, calcium, phosphorus, and urinary hydroxyproline are generally unaffected by AAS.[40, 42, 45, 48] Similarly, there is little or no effect on parathyroid hormone and vitamin D.[39, 45, 49]

BONE BIOPSIES. The results of biopsies taken after a course of AAS are inconsistent. Increased turnover of trabecular bone,[48] increased endocortical apposition of bone,[48] and either no change[42] or increased bone volume[48] has been noted. Bone-resorbing surfaces of iliac crest biopsies taken from osteoporotic women were greatly increased by estrogens, whereas androgens had minimal effects.[31, 43]

Taken together, these clinical and in vitro studies provide convincing evidence that testosterone and DHT play a

role in maintaining healthy bone and correcting osteoporosis associated with hypogonadism. AAS's can increase bone mass in postmenopausal osteoporosis, but their efficacy is modest and the magnitude of the effects is mitigated by virilization and other adverse effects. On average only 10 per cent of European patients are treated with AAS's,[50] and the US Food and Drug Administration has withdrawn support. Moreover, there is convincing evidence of efficacy for alternatives such as estrogens, calcitonin, and calcitriol.[51, 52, 53] Elderly males with bona fide hypogonadism and accompanying osteoporosis are treated with testosterone esters and/or agents specific for the primary cause of the osteoporosis.[54] ND has not been shown to be efficacious for men or women with osteoporosis secondary to rheumatoid arthritis.[55, 56]

Hematopoietic Disorders

AAS's have been used for many years in the management of patients with aplastic anemia, Fanconi anemia, and the anemia associated with end-stage renal disease (ESRD). With the availability of recombinant human erythropoietin (EPO), androgens are no longer indicated for the anemia of ESRD. They are used in aplastic anemia and related disorders.

Pharmacology

The use of AAS's in the management of various types of bone marrow failure and anemia arose from observations linking androgens to erythropoiesis. The hemoglobin concentration in boys and girls is the same until puberty.[57, 58] Hypogonadism is associated with reduced red cell mass, which is corrected by replacement therapy, and castration results in a 10 per cent decline in red cell mass.[59, 60] The administration of AAS to eugonadal men and women results in a small but definite increase in hemoglobin and hematocrit.[61, 62]

Testosterone and AAS's stimulate EPO production,[60] presumably via AR's in kidney. In turn, EPO regulates RBC production by stimulating erythroid progenitor cells. In addition, experimental evidence indicates that testosterone and various 5β-reduced analogues of testosterone directly stimulate hemoglobin production by a mechanism that is independent of EPO.[63, 64] The stereochemistry of this mechanism is unusual because it is the only instance in which anabolics with the 5β configuration mediate an important effect. DHT, the most active metabolite of testosterone, is 5α-DHT. Steroids with the 5β configuration also stimulate hemoglobin synthesis in vitro.[65] More recently, extracts of cultured human erythroblasts have been found to contain binding sites that share many physicochemical characteristics of typical AR, except that the extracts bind 5β-DHT with higher affinity than 5α-DHT.[66] Taken together, it appears that AAS's enhance hemoglobin production by two mechanisms: 5α AAS's acting indirectly via EPO and possibly by a direct effect of testosterone and/or 5β-steroids on erythropoietic stem cells.

Anemia of End-Stage Renal Disease

This anemia is mainly but not entirely due to a deficiency of EPO. Prior to the availability of recombinant human EPO, androgens were used with modest success. Between 30 and 50 per cent of patients respond with an increase in hematocrit of 3 to 5 percentage points.[25, 67] The response rate is greater if AAS's are given by the parenteral route and for at least one year. Patients who have had nephrectomies or who require transfusions generally respond poorly. In some patients, hemoglobin levels may remain stable even after discontinuation of the AAS's.[25] Parenterally administered esters of testosterone and nandrolone are the most efficacious AAS's, although several oral agents have produced satisfactory results.[25] Dose-response data are not available for the individual agents.

The use of AAS in ESRD has been pre-empted by EPO, which is highly effective in virtually all patients with ESRD. The possibility of combining EPO and nandrolone (approximately 100 mg/wk) is under investigation to determine if efficacy equivalent to that of EPO alone can be achieved with smaller and less costly doses of EPO (approximately 2000 units, 3 times/wk). One study showed positive results,[68] but a controlled trial showed no potentiation.[69]

Aplastic Anemia

Nearly 40 years of investigation have established that about half the patients improve on AAS.[60, 70] Patients with severe disease have a poor prognosis even with AAS's. The anemia may not improve for three to six months even though the marrow displays changes earlier. The response often includes improvement in the neutrophil and platelet counts. Because some patients dramatically improve while on AAS's, they are often tried even though improvement may be coincidental. An occasional patient demonstrates marked androgen dependence characterized by blood counts that fluctuate in parallel with drug administration.[71] Ethical considerations preclude a comparison of AAS with placebo; thus, research designs compare AAS with other modes of therapy or are uncontrolled. It is difficult to draw conclusions regarding the relative efficacy of various AAS's. Positive and negative results are reported with virtually all parenteral and oral agents. In the United States oxymetholone (2 to 4 mg/kg) and ND (1 to 1.5 mg/kg/wk) are used most often. In a large prospective series of trials, 1 mg/kg of fluoxymesterone and norethandrolone provided much greater efficacy than doses of 0.2 mg/kg; and at doses of 1 mg/kg fluoxymesterone was superior to norethandrolone and stanozolol.[72] A prospective comparison of AAS with bone marrow transplantation (BMT) showed no benefit with oxymetholone or ND and good results with BMT.[73] If BMT is not a possibility, antilymphocyte globulin (ALG) plus AAS's is recommended.[74] A retrospective comparison found superior results with ALG plus norethandrolone compared with ALG alone,[75] and a prospective study of oxymetholone (2 mg/kg) initiated after five days of ALG and one month of methylprednisolone showed an improved response rate in the patients receiving oxymetholone.[75a]

Other Anemias

Anemias associated with myelofibrosis, myeloid metaplasia, and myelodysplastic syndromes generally respond favorably to AAS's.[76, 77] In contrast, results in myelodysplastic syndromes have been poor[70, 78] with one exception.[79] Preliminary data indicate that AAS's increase hemoglobin in patients with paroxysmal nocturnal hemoglobinuria,[70] and danazol may decrease the number of crises in sickle-cell disease.[80] Danazol has proved useful in managing autoimmune hemolytic anemia,[81] autoimmune thrombocytopenia,[82] and idiopathic thrombocytopenic purpura.[83, 84] In the latter condition danazol did not alter levels of antiplatelet antibodies, but it may have been responsible for a decrease in the number of Fc (IgG) receptors on monocytes.[84]

Hereditary Angioneurotic Edema (HANE)

This rare genetic disorder is characterized by attacks of mucosal swelling, abdominal pain, and life-threatening obstruction of the upper airways due to indiscriminant activation of the complement system. Type I HANE is due to a deficiency in an inhibitor of C1, a plasma protein that controls the activation of C1. C1 and the remainder of the complement system are not affected. In type II a C1 inhibitor is present in normal or even increased amounts but it is dysfunctional. The efficacy of 17-alkylated AAS in this disorder is dramatic and unequivocal.[85, 86] The levels of C1 inhibitor return to normal in type I and become functional in type II. AAS's that have been shown to be effective include stanozolol, methyltestosterone, oxymetholone, and danazol. Many patients respond to doses of danazol (200 mg/d) that are well tolerated and produce minimal adverse effects.

Coagulation, Fibrinolysis, and Hemophilia

Ever since a 1962 report of increased blood fibrinolytic activity in patients treated with testosterone and nandrolone esters,[87] reports periodically appear on the effects of oral AAS's on the clotting system and on efficacy in conditions in which enhanced fibrinolytic activity may be beneficial. These investigations find that AAS's increase fibrinolytic activity, decrease fibrinogen, and increase plasminogen.[88–92] However, these effects may be temporary, and the agents have not been widely used for their fibrinolytic activity. Recent reports of success with danazol in the management of EPO-induced shunt thrombosis may stimulate further studies of the role of AAS's in thrombotic disorders.[93] Danazol increased levels of Factors VIII and IX in patients with hemophilia A and B in one account,[94] although others report minimal efficacy and/or insignificant clinical improvement.[95–97]

Disorders of Growth

Constitutional Delay of Growth and Puberty (CDGP)

CDGP is the most common cause of short stature in boys during puberty. In view of the substantial psychological distress associated with CDGP[98] and despite considerable controversy,[99] both oral AAS's and testosterone esters have been used to initiate the adolescent growth spurt. Proponents of AAS's in CDGP consider that efficacy is established if height velocity is increased, ultimate height is not less than predicted height, puberty is not delayed, and no unwanted side effects occur.

These objectives have been achieved with low doses of testosterone esters, fluoxymesterone[99a] and oxandrolone administered for three months,[100, 101] six months,[102, 103] and 12 months or more.[104, 105] Although many reports are retrospective reviews, efficacy is found in prospective randomized studies with control groups[100, 101] and placebo.[100]

Minimum doses and durations have not been unequivocally established. Oxandrolone accelerated growth in doses as small as 1.25 mg/d for three months[106] or six months[102] and 2.5 mg/d (mean = 0.072 mg/kg/d[100]) for three months.[100, 101a] However, negative results have been found with similar doses.[107] Testosterone enanthate was considered efficacious in doses of 50 mg/month for three to six months[103] and 0.8 to 1.7 years.[104]

The most feared complication is that skeletal maturation will be enhanced more than linear growth and that final height will be less than predicted. This has occurred with high doses of oral AAS's[108–110] administered for one year or more.[108] Another concern is that AAS's may delay progression of puberty owing to suppression of gonadotropin required for testosterone secretion and testicular maturation. However, assessment of the effects of AAS's on pubertal stage generally finds either no effect[104, 111] or slight temporary acceleration,[102, 103, 105] although reduced testicular volume is reported.[107]

If AAS's are used to treat CDGP, it is essential to emphasize to patients and family that the effect is on short-term growth and not on final height. With the availability of synthetic growth hormone (GH), AAS's are no longer used to treat GH deficiency, and they have no effect on GH levels in this condition. Testosterone esters and oxandrolone increase insulin-like growth factor-1 and mean GH concentrations in prepubertal boys who are not deficient in GH.[100, 112]

Turner's Syndrome

Virtually 100 per cent of females with this syndrome have short stature together with sexual infantilism, webbing of the neck, and deformity of the elbows. The short stature has been treated with a variety of AAS's, testosterone esters, and estrogens with variable results.[113] The authors of a large multicenter trial recently concluded that human GH alone or in combination with oxandrolone (0.0625 mg/kg/d) results in a sustained increase in growth rate and a significant increase in adult height for most prepubertal girls with Turner's syndrome.[114]

Alcoholic Hepatitis

Various AAS's including testosterone have been used to treat patients with alcoholic hepatitis since the early 1960's under the rationale that positive nitrogen balance and perhaps appetite and well-being will be enhanced. In 1984 a comprehensive multicenter study found that oxandrolone (80 mg/d for 30 days) had no effect on short-term survival but was associated with a beneficial effect on long-term survival.[115] Most recently oxandrolone (20 mg/d for 21 days) was associated with short-term benefits as measured by laboratory parameters, but the overall results appeared to be similar to those provided by parenteral nutrition alone or with oxandrolone.[116, 117] Another study with oxan-

drolone did find improved survival in a subset of patients with moderate malnutrition.[117a]

MISUSE OF ANDROGENS

Epidemiology

Weightlifters, throwers, and body builders discovered AAS's in the early 1960's; by the mid-1970's misuse spread to elite athletes in aerobic and endurance sports; in the 1980's misuse spread to university sports, and even teenagers experimented with AAS's.[118–121] The illegal and secretive nature of the misuse defies efforts to discover its true scope and magnitude. Various testimonials suggest that in the past virtually all elite athletes in some sports used AAS's,[119–122] and at least one government imposed doping on athletes.[123] Surveys estimate that by age 17, 5 to 11 per cent of United States males and 0.5 to 2.5 per cent of females have used AAS's.[124, 125–125c] Two surveys[125, 125b] reveal that more than 25 per cent of the adolescent users consumed AAS's to enhance physical appearance, not performance, and in two[125a, 125b] an association between steroid use and use of other illicit drugs was shown.

Despite the lack of accurate usage data, it became increasingly obvious that the AAS's were having a substantial impact on sport. New records became commonplace, anecdotal reports appeared regularly, morbidity reports increased, some females appeared quite masculinized, and well-known athletes were found with positive tests. Sports authorities world wide took notice and initiated testing programs and extensive educational campaigns. Urine testing for AAS's formally began with the 1976 Olympics and has increased in sophistication and number ever since.[126] AAS's do not enhance performance in the short term. They are taken months before the event, and, if testing is anticipated, discontinued three to four weeks before the scheduled test. Recently sport authorities have imposed random-selection, year-round, short-notice (up to 48 hours) testing schedules. These programs are extremely effective deterrents yet they are complex and difficult to administer.

Drugs and Dosing Regimens

Although there is an infinite variety of regimens, typically the first-time user begins with an oral agent and graduates to parenteral formulations and multiple drugs (stacking). Doses of 25 to 100 or even 500 mg/d are consumed for several weeks or months.[118, 120, 127–130] The most sophisticated regimens include human chorionic gonadotropin to prevent testicular atrophy and antiestrogens to inhibit gynecomastia. Methandienone, stanozolol, oxandrolone, oxymetholone, and methyltestosterone are the most popular oral AAS's. Even veterinary products such as boldenone and mibolerone are used. Before drug testing was instituted, ND was widely used. However, its metabolites are detectable for several months after discontinuation, so its use has declined sharply. Parenteral formulations of methenolone, methandienone, and stanozolol clear more rapidly. Use of testosterone esters is rapidly increasing, in part because their use is more difficult to detect.[131] Another disturbing trend is the misuse of other endogenous steroids and hormones such as DHT,[130, 132] EPO, and GH.[118]

Pharmacological Basis for Use by Athletes

The most widely considered hypothesis is that AAS's act via AR's to increase muscle mass, which in turn provides greater strength and speed. Other possibilities include an anticatabolic effect mediated by glucocorticoid receptors, increased blood volume, and behavioral or motivational effects mediated by the CNS.

Muscle Androgen Receptors

AR's are found in most human skeletal muscles,[133] and like other AR's, human muscle receptors bind both testosterone and DHT. However, skeletal muscle tissue differs from other androgen-responsive tissue in that 5α-reductase activity is low,[134] and testosterone is present in greater amounts than DHT.[135] Thus testosterone is the dominant intracellular agonist in muscle. In the experimental animal the concentration of AR's varies markedly from one muscle group to another, and those with high concentrations respond the most to androgen. This parallels the observation in man that muscles of the upper arm, chest, and back are more responsive to AAS's than others.

Muscle Hypertrophy

Morphometric analysis of human skeletal muscle biopsies performed after a course of AAS's reveals an increase in muscle fiber diameter.[136–138] More detailed studies in animals show that AAS's increase and castration decreases cross-sectional area and width of muscle fibers.[139] In the normal animal testosterone produces marked hypertrophy in selected muscles.[2, 139, 140] At the subcellular level, the increased width of muscle fibers is due to an increased number of myofilaments and myofibrils,[141] and at the molecular level testosterone induces changes in the structure of myosin heavy chain isoforms.[140] These results suggest that testosterone acts directly on contractile protein gene expression.[140]

Lean Body Mass in Man

The earliest clinical investigations unequivocally established that hypogonadal men given replacement doses of testosterone undergo positive nitrogen balance accompanied by proportional retention of potassium, phosphates, and sulfates.[142–144] Total body weight and lean body mass (LBM) increase, body fat decreases, and there is growth of muscles, particularly in the upper back and shoulder regions. If the enhanced muscle mass hypothesis is correct, then AAS's also must increase muscle mass in normal men and women. Nitrogen retention is found in normal subjects treated with testosterone or methyltestosterone[142, 144, 145]; however, muscle mass is difficult to assess directly. The best estimates are derived from creatinine excretion[138, 146, 147] or from estimates of LBM based on total body [40]K counting.[147]

It has become increasingly clear that pharmacological doses of AAS's produce supranormal anabolic effects in normal men and women. Using the [40]K method for estimating LBM, increases are observed in nonathletic men,[138, 146–149] sedentary women with osteoporosis,[41, 47] and body builders and strength athletes.[148, 159] The increase in LBM appears to depend on the cumulative total dose[147, 148] and is observed with a variety of AAS's, including testosterone and nandrolone esters, methandienone, and stanozolol. Negative studies may not have administered sufficient doses. In addition to [40]K estimates of LBM, other measurements of muscle mass also increase following AAS's: creatinine excretion,[138] the rate of muscle protein synthesis measured by [^{13}C] leucine incorporation into muscle,[138] and muscle cross-sectional areas obtained from radiographs.[150]

The most comprehensive studies of body composition reveal that in addition to an increase in LBM, AAS's also decrease body fat.[41, 146–148] The pattern of increased LBM and decreased fat is not found in any other condition except GH administration, and distinguishes the effects of AAS from that of simple caloric excess, which produces both an increase in fat and LBM.[147, 151]

Increased Blood Volume

Many clinical studies report that AAS's increase body weight, but many do not describe which compartment is affected. In fact, a fraction of the increase in LBM is likely due to fluid retention and/or expanded blood volume[138, 150, 152]; however, muscle hypertrophy accounts for the most substantial portion of the increase. AAS's increase red cell mass,[62] and this could contribute to enhanced performance in aerobic sports that depend on delivery of oxygen to muscles,[118] but it is unlikely to affect performance that relies on static strength.

Taken together, studies of muscle morphology, AR's, and body composition provide strong evidence that pharmacological doses of AAS increase body weight and LBM and that the increase is due to muscle hypertrophy. However, it has been pointed out[152] that under normal physiological conditions AR's are fully saturated and therefore seemingly unable to mediate major anabolic effects.

Glucocorticoid Receptors

One alternative hypothesis that does not require AR's is that AAS's promote positive nitrogen balance and muscle growth by acting as an antagonist at glucocorticoid receptors, thereby inhibiting catabolic actions of glucocorticoids.[152] AAS's effectively compete for glucocorticoid-binding sites.[153] Moreover, in the only study that estimated the rate of muscle protein synthesis, a high rate was observed and this rate should have produced a much larger increase in muscle mass than was found; this suggested that the rate of catabolism also increased.[138] These findings are consistent with an anticatabolic effect of AAS's mediated at glucocorticoid receptors, or a dual action at both androgen and glucocorticoid receptors.

Central Nervous System

The role of the CNS has not been established. AR's are present in brain, but their function in adults is unclear. AAS's do promote aggressiveness and some athletes feel that enhanced performance is related to aggressiveness and other motivational factors. In addition neuromuscular factors such as neuronal activity are known to influence muscle strength.[154]

Efficacy

Assuming that AAS's do increase muscle mass, the question is whether this muscle is sufficient to enhance athletic performance. Although it is reasonable to speculate that larger muscles are stronger muscles, the relationship between cross-sectional area and strength is complex.[154, 155] Likewise, the relationship between muscle diameter and speed of contraction is complex. Experienced users are completely convinced that AAS's enhance performance in both strength and aerobic sports.[118, 152]

Nearly 30 studies of the effects of AAS on athletic performance of males have been conducted and reviewed, yet the results do not provide a consensus.[118, 128, 152, 156] Some show an increase in performance[150] and others do not.[157] Nevertheless various authors,[118, 128, 158] athletes who use AAS's,[120, 121] and sports medicine societies[156] conclude that AAS's probably do enhance performance. Because the effect of AAS's on LBM is related to the total dose and is not apparent if a cumulative total dose of less than 2000 g is administered, one likely explanation for the failure of some studies to demonstrate efficacy is insufficient total dose. Other explanations include design considerations, difficulty of blinding subjects, small numbers of subjects, and lack of statistical power.

TOXIC AND UNDESIRED EFFECTS

One consequence of the extensive number of effects of AAS's is difficulty distinguishing between primary and secondary effects and between specific AR-mediated and nonspecific effects. Often a specific AR action is inferred if the action is associated with a particular organ and AR's are present in the tissue. For some effects, supporting data are available from experimental animals treated with AR inhibitors alone and with AAS's. Essentially no systematic data from chronic administration studies convincingly demonstrate any difference between various oral AAS's with respect to the relative position of dose-response curves for any of the adverse effects. The agents do differ in potency based on dose, although in equipotent doses the adverse effects are similar. It is not clear if danazol is truly an exception to this.

In the case of endocrine effects involving reproductive organs and secondary sexual characteristics, adverse effects of pharmacological doses are clearly extensions of underlying normal physiological actions mediated by endogenous AAS's at AR's. At the other extreme, the mechanism of AAS-induced cholestatic hepatitis in unknown. Many effects are common to all AAS's, although others are observed only with 17-alkylated AAS's. In the latter case one hypothesis is that the alkyl group is the essential element; an alternative is that testosterone and nandrolone esters form more potent estrogenic metabolites than alkylated AAS's and that the estrogens neutralize the effect.

Endocrine Effects and Virilization

Except for the management of hypogonadism and male contraception, oral AAS's are most often used in pharmacological doses in circumstances in which the desired effects are anabolic enhancements of bone, muscle, hematopoiesis, or specific proteins. In this context most endocrine effects are undesired and adverse. In the female and young male, virilization is unavoidable and often limits treatment. The voice lowers owing to enlargement of the larynx and stiffening of the vocal cords. Muscles increase in size and strength. Hair growth is stimulated, particularly on the face, arms, and legs. Females chronically treated with high doses experience clitoral enlargement, breast atrophy, and male pattern baldness. In addition, suppression of gonadotropins leads to inhibition of ovulation and amenorrhea. In the only clinical description of adverse effects in female weight-trained athletes who self-administered AAS's, most or all experienced a low voice, menstrual irregularities, enhanced strength, clitoral enlargement, and increased facial hair.[129]

In the male, high doses of AAS's exert control over the hypothalamic-pituitary-testicular axis by inhibiting the release of LH, FSH, and probably GnRH, which progressively leads to oligospermia and aspermia. Testosterone production declines and serum levels of testosterone FSH and LH fall. The mechanism of gynecomastia is poorly understood but is presumed to be related to estrogen metabolites and an imbalance between androgens and estrogens.[159, 160] Prior to puberty AAS's both promote longitudinal bone growth and hasten the closure of the epiphyses. Accordingly administration of AAS's requires scrupulous attention to dose and growth rates because continual dosing leads to short stature.

Both males and females experience an increase in number, size, and secretions of sebaceous glands. The skin is oily, and acne results from obstructed sebaceous glands. Skin atrophy and striae have been noted.[161]

Serum Proteins and Thyroid Function

Both natural and synthetic AAS's consistently lower plasma concentrations of three binding proteins of hepatic origin—SHBG, TBG, and vitamin D–binding protein (DBG).[162–166, 166a] It is not known if these effects are primary or secondary, or if they are due to diminished synthesis, enhanced clearance, or even both enhanced synthesis and clearance.[167] Levels of corticosteroid binding protein (CBG) are not consistently altered by AAS's.[162, 166] In addition, 17-alkylated AAS's elevate plasma levels of haptoglobin, orosomucoid, protein-bound sialic acid, plasminogen, and β-glucuronidase.[88, 162]

In addition to the decrease in TBG, oral AAS's also decrease plasma levels of thyroxine (T_4) and triiodothyronine (T_3).[163–165, 168] Free T_4 and TSH levels are either unchanged[163, 164, 166] or slightly decreased.[165] The administration of AAS's may induce mild thyroidal impairment,[166a] but it is not associated with overt hyperthyroidism or hypothyroidism.

Metabolic Effects

AAS's increase the basal metabolic rate, although if the rate is calculated per gram of LBM there is no change.[146]

Insulin resistance and diminished glucose tolerance are reported with two 17-alkylated AAS's,[169, 170] but not with esters of testosterone or nandrolone.[171] Adipose tissue contains AR's, and biopsies following a course of AAS's reveal a marked decrease in lipoprotein lipase activity (LPL).[172, 173] Excessive doses result in modest increases in blood pressure due to salt and water retention.

Decrease in HDL Cholesterol

The most predictable and universal adverse effect of oral AAS's, and one that has stimulated considerable research, is a decrease in the HDL fraction of cholesterol.[174–179] The HDL-C2 fraction and accompanying A1 are most affected. The fall in HDL-C is shortly preceded by increased activity of hepatic triglyceride lipase activity (HTLA), leading to the hypothesis that the decline is due to induction of HTLA.[175, 179] In contrast to the oral AAS's, the esters of testosterone and nandrolone are not clearly associated with a decline in HDL-C.[176] In addition, AAS's often increase the LDL-C fraction, so that the combined effect is an increased LDL-C/HDL-C ratio. Because a low HDL-C and elevated ratio are risk factors for cardiovascular disease,[177, 178, 180] the possibility that athletes and medical patients have an increased risk for cardiovascular disease has been considered.[174, 177] Although several cases of stroke and myocardial infarction are associated with administration of AAS's,[177, 181] they are not common and a causal relationship has not been established.

Hepatic Effects Associated with C17-Alkylated AAS's

Virtually all AAS's alkylated on C17 are associated with modest elevations of alanine (ALT) and aspartate (AST) aminotransferases.[182–185] Such elevations are extremely common, probably dose dependent, rarely exceed twice the baseline level, and usually regress even if the AAS's are continued.[182, 183] Although the effects on ALT and AST are considered hepatic in origin and toxic, other tissues could contribute, and many other serum markers of hepatotoxicity are not affected by AAS's.[183]

Infrequently AAS's cause cholestatic jaundice characterized by elevated bilirubin, stasis of small bile ducts, and reversal after cessation of AAS's.[177, 185–187] BSP retention is more common than jaundice.[188] Cholestatic jaundice is associated with all oral AAS's and has not been convincingly linked to esters of testosterone or nandrolone. In most reviews the incidence is a few per cent, although in one series 17 per cent developed jaundice.[177, 189]

Neoplasia

Hepatocellular Adenoma and Carcinoma

AAS administration is associated with a variety of histological types of hepatic neoplasia ranging from benign adenoma to histologically malignant adenocarcinoma.[177, 184, 186, 190] A review of cancer registries and literature surveys discovered 91 androgen-associated tumors, of which 48

were discounted either because of a lack of convincing histology or because they occurred in patients with Fanconi's anemia, which itself is associated with neoplasia.[177] Despite the histological characteristics of hepatic carcinomas, their clinical behavior is benign: They do not metastasize; they are not associated with elevated α-fetoprotein; and they usually but not always regress with discontinuation of the AAS.[177, 184, 190–192] The median time of androgen exposure before diagnosis is five years, and latency is 2 to 30 years.[177] Four cases of hepatic angiosarcoma have been associated with AAS's.[193] AAS's are not mutagenic in the Ames test,[194] and in the mouse nandrolone decanoate acted like a promotor rather than an initiator of hepatocarcinogenesis.[195]

Peliosis Hepatis

This unusual lesion is characterized by microscopic and macroscopic blood-filled hepatic or splenic cysts.[186] Because of deaths and serious morbidity due to spontaneous bleeding, peliosis hepatis is the most serious complication of AAS's.[177, 196] The lesion regresses with discontinuation of the AAS.[197, 198] At least 70 cases are reported, many of whom were being treated with oxymetholone or methyltestosterone for anemia or hypogonadism.[177] Peliosis hepatis has been reported with all commonly used oral AAS's, and to a lesser extent with testosterone and nandrolone esters.[199, 200] Autopsy series report a high incidence of unrecognized peliosis in patients treated with oral AAS's.[201]

Psychiatric Effects

Most medical patients do not experience remarkable psychiatric effects while receiving AAS's, although some report a general sense of well-being and invigoration. AAS's have been used to treat depression with variable results[202–204] and less efficacy than tricyclic antidepressants. In contrast, reports of serious behavioral and psychiatric sequelae including homicide associated with misuse of AAS's are increasing.[205] Moreover, a carefully controlled study of 20 normal volunteers showed that high-dose methyltestosterone (240 mg/d) induced positive mood symptoms (euphoria, energy, and sexual arousal), negative mood symptoms (irritability, mood swings, violent feelings, hostility), and cognitive impairment (forgetfulness, confusion); one subject developed acute mania.[205a] A structured psychiatric interview of high-dose users found a high incidence of aggressive behavior, affective syndromes, and psychotic symptoms.[206] Although a correlation exists between plasma levels of testosterone and aggressive behavior in animals, a causal link has not been established in man.[204, 207] The possibility that high-dose users develop an addiction with physical dependence and a withdrawal syndrome is gaining support.[208, 209]

Drug Interactions and Contraindications

Both AAS's and isoretinoin lower HDL-C. The combination has resulted in a profound reduction in HDL-C.[210] Concurrent administration of oral anticoagulants and oral AAS's leads to prolonged prothrombin times and life-threatening bleeding.[211] The mechanism of AAS-induced potentiation of anticoagulants does not involve altered pharmacokinetics of the anticoagulant.[212] The combination of methyltestosterone and imipramine in depressed men led to an acute paranoid state in four of five patients.[213] AAS's are contraindicated in prostate cancer, mammary carcinoma in men, pregnancy, and individuals who could not tolerate a change in the quality of their voice.

Toxicity Peculiar to Athletes and Body Builders

Individuals who had taken enormous doses of AAS's have experienced an acute abdomen owing to tremendous iliopsoas hypertrophy,[214] ruptured tendons,[215] and bleeding esophageal varices secondary to liver disease.[216] HIV infection and other complications of sharing needles are reported in AAS abusers.

Reversibility

The reversibility of adverse effects is highly variable. At one extreme, diminished height resulting from premature closure of the epiphyses is completely irreversible, whereas elevated levels of ALT and AST rapidly reverse. Cholestatic jaundice and peliosis hepatis are reversible, and to some extent hepatic adenoma regresses with discontinuation of AAS's. Most of the virilizing effects in females are considered irreversible.[152] Voice changes are particularly slow to change.[217] Changes in body composition take many months to fully recover. After a 12-week course of testosterone enanthate, body fat and LBM did not return to baseline for approximately six months,[149] and after one to two years of ND the forearm fat content remained low for at least another six months.[41]

Hypogonadism induced by AAS's is reversible, but the rate of recovery may be quite slow and depends in part on the particular drug and duration of treatment. For example, following a two-week course of methandienone (30 mg/d), FSH and LH returned to baseline in seven days but testosterone levels were still low after two weeks,[166] whereas after 12 weeks of fluoxymesterone (10 to 30 mg/d) plasma levels of testosterone were back to normal in one to two weeks.[218] In contraception studies with testosterone esters lasting several months, the sperm count may not return to normal for 20 to 30 weeks after drug discontinuation.[219] Athletes taking high doses of nandrolone esters frequently experience azoospermia that may last over 20 weeks after drug discontinuation, and plasma levels of FSH, LH, and testosterone also take many weeks to recover.[220, 221] Taken together, these studies are consistent with the view that the time to full recovery of reversible effects is positively correlated with some combination of the total dose, duration of treatment, and serum half-life of the agent.

REFERENCES

1. Kopera H: The history of anabolic steroids and a review of clinical experience with anabolic steroids. Acta Endocrinol 110 (Suppl 271):11–18, 1985.
2. Kochakian CD: The effect of dose and nutritive state on the renotrophic and androgenic activities of various steroids. Am J Physiol 145:549–556, 1946.
3. Overbeek GA: Anabolic Steroids. Berlin, Springer-Verlag, 1966.
4. Hershberger LG, Shipley EG, Meyer RK: Myotrophic activity of 19-nortestosterone and other steroids determined by modified levator ani muscle method. Proc Soc Exp Biol Med 83:175–180, 1953.
5. Saartok T, Dahlberg E, Gustafsson JA: Relative binding affinity of anabolic-androgenic steroids: Comparison of the binding to the androgen receptors in skeletal muscle and in prostate, as well as to sex hormone–binding globulin. Endocrinology 114:2100–2106, 1984.
6. Kochakian CD: Definition of androgens and protein anabolic steroids. Pharmacol Ther B 1:149–177, 1975.
7. Potts GO, Arnold A, Beyler AL: Dissociation of the androgenic and other hormonal activities from the protein anabolic effects of steroids. In Kochakian CD (ed): Anabolic-Androgenic Steroids. New York, Springer-Verlag, 1976, pp 361–403.
8. Carson-Jurica MA, Schrader WT, O'Malley BW: Steroid receptor family: Structure and functions. Endocr Rev 11:201–220, 1990.
9. Chang C, Kokontis J, Liao S: Molecular cloning of human and rat complementary DNA encoding androgen receptors. Science 240: 324–326, 1988.
10. Lubahn DB, Joseph DR, Sullivan PM, et al: Cloning of human androgen receptor complementary DNA and localization to the X chromosome. Science 240:327–330, 1988.
11. Tilley WD, Marcelli M, Wilson JD, McPhaul MJ: Characterization and expression of a cDNA encoding the human androgen receptor. Proc Natl Acad Sci USA 86:327–331, 1989.
12. Griffin JE: Androgen resistance—the clinical and molecular spectrum. Sem Med Beth Israel Hospital, Boston 326:611–618, 1992.
13. Strickland AL, French FS: Absence of response to dihydrotestosterone in the syndrome of testicular feminization. J Clin Endocrinol Metab 29:1284–1286, 1969.
14. Roy AK: Regulation of steroid hormone action in target cells by specific hormone-inactivating enzymes. Proc Soc Exp Biol Med 199:265–272, 1992.
15. Evans RM: The steroid and thyroid hormone receptor suprafamily. Science 240:889–895, 1988.
16. Bardin CW, Catterall JF: Testosterone: A major determinant of extragenital sexual dimorphism. Science 211:1285–1294, 1981.
17. Pugeat MM, Dunn JF, Nisula BC: Transport of steroid hormones: Interaction of 70 drugs with testosterone-binding globulin and corticosteroid-binding globulin in human plasma. J Clin Endocrinol Metab 53:69–75, 1981.
18. Grino PB, Griffin JE, Wilson JD: Testosterone at high concentrations interacts with the human androgen receptor similarly to dihydrotestosterone. Endocrinology 126:1165–1172, 1990.
19. Wilbert DM, Griffin JE, Wilson JD: Characterization of the cytosol androgen receptor of the human prostate. J Clin Endocrinol Metab 56:113–120, 1983.
20. Krüskemper HL: Anabolic Steroids. New York, Academic Press, 1968.
21. Tóth M, Zakár T: Classification of anabolic steroids using the methods of competitive metabolism. Exp Clin Endocrinol 87:125–132, 1986.
22. Bergink EW, Geelen JA, Tutpijn EW: Metabolism and receptor binding of nandrolone and testosterone under in vitro and in vivo conditions. Acta Endocrinol 110(Suppl 271):31–37, 1985.
23. Wijnand HP, Bosch AMG, Donker CW: Pharmacokinetic parameters of nandrolone (19-nortestosterone) after intramuscular administration of nandrolone decanoate (Deca-Durabolin [R]) to healthy volunteers. Acta Endocrinol 110(Suppl 271):19–30, 1985.
24. Belkien L, Schürmeyer T, Hano R, et al: Pharmacokinetics of 19-nortestosterone esters in normal men. J Steroid Biochem 22:623–629, 1985.
25. Neff MS, Goldberg G, Slifkin RF, et al: A comparison of androgens for anemia in patients on hemodialysis. N Engl J Med 304:871–875, 1987.
26. Lafferty FW, Spencer GE, Pearson OH: Effects of androgens, estrogens and high calcium intakes on bone formation and resorption in osteoporosis. Am J Med 36:514–528, 1964.
27. Reifenstein EC Jr, Albright F: The metabolic effects of steroid hormones in osteoporosis. J Clin Invest 26:24–25, 1947.
28. Schot LPC, Schuurs AHWM: Sex steroids and osteoporosis: Effects of deficiencies and substitutive treatments. J Steroid Biochem Molec Biol 37:167–182, 1990.
29. Gray A, Feldman HA, McKinlay JB, Longcope C: Age, disease, and changing sex hormone levels in middle-aged men: Results of the Massachusetts male aging study. J Clin Endocrinol Metab 73:1016–1025, 1991.

30. Baran DT, Bergfeld MA, Teitelbaum SL, Avioli LV: Effect of testosterone therapy on bone formation in an osteoporotic hypogonadal male. Calcif Tissue Res 26:103–106, 1978.
31. Riggs BL, Jowsey J, Kelly PJ, et al: Effect of sex hormones on bone in primary osteoporosis. J Clin Invest 48:1065–1072, 1969.
32. Peters CA, Walsh PC: The effect of nafarelinacetate, a luteinizing-hormone–releasing hormone agonist, on benign prostatic hyperplasia. N Engl J Med 317:599–604, 1987.
33. Dequeker J, Geusens P: Anabolic steroids and osteoporosis. Acta Endocrinol 110(Suppl 271):45–52, 1985.
34. Colvard DS, Eriksen EF, Keeting PE, et al: Identification of androgen receptors in normal human osteoblast-like cells. Proc Natl Acad Sci USA 86:854–857, 1989.
35. Kasperk CH, Wergedal JE, Farley JR, et al: Androgens directly stimulate proliferation of bone cells in vitro. Endocrinology 124:1576–1578, 1989.
36. Fukayama S, Tashjian AH: Direct modulation by androgens of the response of human bone cells (SaOS-2) to human parathyroid hormone (PTH). Endocrinology 125:1789–1794, 1989.
37. Sömjen D, Weisman Y, Harell A, et al: Direct and sex specific stimulation by sex steroids of creatine kinase activity and DNA synthesis in rat bone. Proc Natl Acad Sci USA 86:3361–3365, 1989.
38. Vaishnav JN, Beresford JN, Gallagher JA, Russell RGG: Effects of the anabolic steroid stanozolol on cells derived from human bone. Clin Sci 74:455–460, 1988.
39. Chestnut CH III, Ivey JL, Gruber HE, et al: Stanozolol in postmenopausal osteoporosis: Therapeutic efficacy and possible mechanisms of action. Metabolism 32:571–580, 1983.
40. Johansen JS, Hassager C, Podenphant J, et al: Treatment of postmenopausal osteoporosis: Is the anabolic steroid nandrolone decanoate a candidate? Bone Miner Metab 6:77–86, 1989.
41. Hassager C, Riis BJ, Podenphant J, Christiansen C: Nandrolone decanoate treatment of post-menopausal osteoporosis for 2 years and effects of withdrawal. Maturitas 11:305–317, 1989.
42. Gennari C, AgnusDei D, Gonnelli S, Nardi P: Effects of nandrolone decanoate therapy on bone mass and calcium metabolism in women with established post-menopausal osteoporosis: A double-blind placebo controlled trial. Maturitas 11:187–197, 1989.
43. Riggs BL, Jowsey J, Goldsmith RS, et al: Short and long term effects of estrogen and synthetic anabolic hormones in postmenopausal osteoporosis. J Clin Invest 52:1659–1663, 1972.
44. Chestnut CH III, Nelp WB, Baylink DJ, Denney JD: Effect of methandrostenolone on postmenopausal bone wasting as assessed by changes in total bone mineral mass. Metabolism 26:267–277, 1977.
45. Need AG, Morris HA, Hartley TF, et al: Effects of nandrolone decanoate on forearm mineral density and calcium metabolism in osteoporotic postmenopausal women. Calcif Tissue Int 41:7–10, 1987.
46. Need AG, Horowitz M, Walker CJ, et al: Cross-over study of fat-corrected forearm mineral content during nandrolone decanoate therapy for osteoporosis. Bone 10:3–6, 1989.
47. Aloia JF, Kapoor A, Vaswani A, Cohn SH: Changes in body composition following therapy with methandrostenolone. Metab Clin Exp 30:1076–1079, 1981.
48. Beneton MNC, Yates AJP, Rogers S, et al: Stanozolol stimulates remodelling of trabecular bone and net formation of bone at the endocortical surface. Clin Sci 81:543–549, 1991.
49. Hartwell D, Hassager C, Overgaard K, et al: Vitamin D metabolism in osteoporotic women during treatment with estrogen, an anabolic steroid, or calcitonin. Acta Endocrinol 122:715–721, 1990.
50. Dequeker J, Geusens P: Treatment of established osteoporosis and rehabilitation: Current practice and possibilities. Maturitas 12:1–36, 1990.
51. Chestnut CH III: Osterporosis and its treatment. N Engl J Med 326:406–407, 1992.
52. Tilyard MW, Spears GFS, Thomson J, Dovey S: Treatment of postmenopausal osteoporosis with calcitriol or calcium. N Engl J Med 326:357–362, 1992.
53. Consensus Development Report: Prophylaxis and treatment of osteoporosis. Am J Med 90:107–110, 1991.
54. Jackson JA, Kleerekoper M: Osteoporosis in men: Diagnosis, pathophysiology, and prevention. Medicine 69:137–152, 1990.
55. Bijlsma JWJ, Duursma SA, Bosch R, Huber O: Lack of influence of the anabolic steroid nandrolone decanoate on bone metabolism. Acta Endocrinol 101:140–143, 1982.
56. Bird HA, Burkinshaw L, Pearson D, et al: A controlled trial of nandrolone decanoate in the treatment of rheumatoid arthritis in postmenopausal women. Ann Rheum Dis 46:237–243, 1987.
57. Krabbe S, Christensen T, Worm J, et al: Relationship between hae-

moglobin and serum testosterone in normal children and adolescents and in boys with delayed puberty. Acta Paediatr Scand 67:655–658, 1978.
58. Valquist B: The cause of the sexual differences in erythrocyte, hemoglobin and serum iron levels in human adults. Blood 5:874–875, 1950.
59. Hamilton JB: The role of testicular secretions as indicated by the effects of castration in man and by studies of pathological conditions and the short lifespan associated with maleness. Recent Prog Horm Res 3:257–322, 1948.
60. Shahidi NT: Androgens and erythropoiesis. N Engl J Med 289:72–80, 1973.
61. Alèn M: Androgenic steroid effects on liver and red cells. Br J Sports Med 19:15–20, 1985.
62. Gardner FH, Nathan DG, Piomelli S, Cummins JF: The erythrocythemic effects of androgens. Br J Haematol 14:611–615, 1968.
63. Gordon AS, Zanjani ED, Levere RD, Kappas A: Stimulation of mammalian erythropoiesis by 5β-H steroid metabolites. Proc Natl Acad Sci USA 65:919–924, 1970.
64. Congote IF, Solomon S: Testosterone stimulation of a rapidly labeled, low-molecular-weight RNA fraction in human hepatic erythroid cells in culture. Proc Natl Acad Sci USA 72:523–527, 1975.
65. Beckman B, Maddux B, Segaloff A, Fisher JW: Effects of testosterone and 5β androstanes on in vitro erythroid colony formation in mouse bone marrow. Proc Soc Exp Biol Med 167:51–58, 1981.
66. Claustres M, Sultan C: Androgen and erythropoiesis: Evidence for an androgen receptor in erythroblasts from human bone marrow cultures. Horm Res 29:17–22, 1988.
67. Richardson JR Jr, Weinstein MB: Erythropoietic response of dialyzed patients to testosterone administration. Ann Intern Med 73:403–407, 1970.
68. Ballal SH, Domoto DT, Polack DC, et al: Androgens potentiate the effects of erythropoietin in the treatment of anemia of end stage renal disease. Am J Kidney Dis 17:29–33, 1991.
69. Berns JS, Rudnick MR, Cohen RM: A controlled trial of recombinant erythropoietin and nandrolone decanoate in the treatment of anemia in patients on chronic hemodialysis. Clin Nephrol 37:264–267, 1992.
70. Ammus SS: The role of androgens in the treatment of hematologic disorders. Adv Intern Med 34:191–208, 1989.
71. Azen EA, Shahidi NT: Androgen dependency in acquired aplastic anemia. Am J Med 63:320–324, 1977.
72. French Cooperative Group for the Study of Aplastic and Refractory Anemia: Androgen therapy in aplastic anemia: A comparative study of high and low dose and four different androgens. Scand J Haematol 36:346–352, 1986.
73. Camitta BM, Thomas ED, Nathan DG, et al: A prospective study of androgens and bone marrow transplantation for treatment of severe aplastic anemia. Blood 53:504–514, 1979.
74. Nissen C, Gratwohl A, Speck B: Management of aplastic anemia. Eur J Haematol 46:193–197, 1991.
75. Facon T, Walter MP, Fenaux P, et al: Treatment of severe aplastic anemia with antilymphocyte globulin and androgens: A report on 33 patients. Ann Hematol 63:89–93, 1991.
75a. Bacigalupo A, Chaple M, Hows J, et al: Treatment of aplastic anaemia (AA) with antilymphocyte globulin (ALG) and methylprednisolone (MPred) with or without androgens: A randomized trial from the EBMT SAA working party. Br J Haematol 83:145–151, 1993.
76. Gardner FH, Nathan DG: Androgen and erythropoiesis: III. Further evaluation of testosterone treatment of myelofibrosis. N Engl J Med 274:420–426, 1966.
77. Besa EC, Nowel PC, Greller NL, Gardner FH: Analysis of the androgen response of 23 patients with agnogenic myeloid metaplasia: The value of chromosomal studies in predicting response and survival. Cancer 49:308–313, 1982.
78. Najean Y, Pecking A: Refractory anemia with excess of myeloblasts in the bone marrow: A clinical trial of androgens in 90 patients. Br J Haematol 37:25–31, 1979.
79. Cines DB, Cassileth PA, Kiss JE: Danazol therapy in myelodysplasia. Ann Intern Med 103:58–60, 1985.
80. Temple JD, Harrington WJ, Ahn YS, Rosenfeld E: Treatment of sickle cell disease with danazol. J Fla Med Assoc 73:847–848, 1986.
81. Ahn YS, Harrington WJ, Mylvaganam R, et al: Danazol therapy for autoimmune hemolytic anemia. Ann Intern Med 102:298–301, 1985.
82. West G, Johnson SC: Danazol for the treatment of refractory autoimmune thrombocytopenia in systemic lupus erythematosus. Ann Intern Med 108:703–706, 1988.
83. Ahn YS, Harrington WJ, Simon SR, et al: Danazol for the treatment

of idiopathic thrombocytopenic purpura. N Engl J Med 308:1396–1399, 1983.

84. Schreiber AD, Chien P, Tonaski A, Cines DB: Effect of danazol in immune thrombocytopenic purpura. N Engl J Med 316:503–508, 1987.

85. Cicardi M, Bergamaschini L, Cugna M, et al: Long-term treatment of hereditary angioedema with attenuated androgens: A survey of a 13-year experience. J Allergy Clin Immunol 87:768–773, 1991.

86. Sim TC, Grant A: Hereditary angioedema: Its diagnostic and management perspectives. Am J Med 88:656–664, 1990.

87. Fearnley GR, Chakrabarti R: Increase of blood fibrinolytic activity by testosterone. Lancet 2:128–132, 1962.

88. Barbosa J, Seal US, Doe RP: Effects of anabolic steroids on haptoglobin, orosomucoid, plasminogen, fibrinogen, transferrin, ceruloplasmin, α¹-antitrypsin, β-glucuronidase and total serum proteins. J Clin Endocrinol 33:388–398, 1971.

89. Cade JF, Stubbs KP, Stubbs AE, Clegg EA: Thrombosis, fibrinolysis and ethylestrenol. Acta Endocrinol 110(Suppl 271):53–58, 1985.

90. Mannucci PM, Kluft C, Traas DW, et al: Congenital plasminogen deficiency associated with venous thromboembolism: Therapeutic trial with stanozolol. Br J Haematol 63:753–759, 1986.

91. Walker ID, Davidson JF, Richards A, et al: The effect of the synthetic steroid ORG OD14 on fibrinolysis and blood lipids in postmenopausal women. Thromb Haemost 53:303–305, 1985.

92. Davidson JF, Lochhead M, McDonald GA, NcNicol GP: Fibrinolytic enhancement by stanozolol: A double blind trial. Br J Haematol 22:543–558, 1972.

93. Al-Momen AK, Huraib SO, Gader AMA, Sulaimani F: Low dose danazol is effective in management of erythropoietin induced thrombosis. Thromb Res 64:577–532, 1991.

94. Gralnick RH, Rick ME: Danazol increased factor VIII and factor IX in classic hemophilia and Christmas disease. N Engl J Med 308:1393–1395, 1983.

95. Greer IA, Greeves M, Madhok R, et al: Effect of stanolozol on factor VIII and IX and serum aminotransferases in hemophilia. Thromb Haemost 53:386–389, 1985.

96. Kasper CK, Boylen AL: Poor response to danazol in hemophilia. Blood 65:211–213, 1985.

97. Saidi P, Lega BZ, Kim HC, Raska K: Effect of danazol on clotting factor levels, bleeding incidence, factor infusion requirements and immune parameters in hemophilia. Blood 68:673–679, 1986.

98. Gordon M, Crouthamel C, Post EM, Richman RA: Psychosocial aspects of constitutional short stature: Social competence, behavior problems, self-esteem, and family functioning. J Pediatr 101:477–480, 1982.

99. Dannenhoffer R, Crawford JD: Testosterone need questioned [letter]. Pediatrics 71:666–667, 1983.

99a. Strickland AL: Long-term results of treatment with low-dose fluoxymesterone in constitutional delay of growth and puberty and in genetic short stature. Pediatrics 91:716–20, 1993.

100. Stanhope R, Buchanan CR, Fenn GC, Preece MA: Double blind placebo controlled trial of low dose oxandrolone in the treatment of boys with constitutional delay of growth and puberty. Arch Dis Child 63:501–505, 1988.

101. Rosenfeld RG, Northcraft GB, Hintz RL: A prospective, randomized study of testosterone treatment of constitutional delay of growth and development in male adolescents. Pediatrics 69:681–687, 1982.

101a. Malhotra A, Poon E, Tse WY, et al: The effects of oxandrolone on the growth hormone and gonadal axes in boys with constitutional delay of growth and puberty. Clin Endocrinol 38:393–398, 1993.

102. Tse WY, Buyukgebiz A, Hindmarsh PC, et al: Long-term outcome of oxandrolone treatment in boys with constitutional delay of growth and puberty. J Pediatr 117:588–591, 1990.

103. Uruena M, Pantsiotou S, Preece MA, Stanhope R: Is testosterone therapy for boys with constitutional delay of growth and puberty associated with impaired final height and suppression of the hypothalamo-pituitary-gonadal axis? Eur J Pediatr 151:15–18, 1992.

103a. Bassi F, Neri AS, Gheri RG, et al: Oxandrolone in constitutional delay of growth: Analysis of the growth patterns up to final stature. J Endocrinol Invest 16:133–137, 1993.

104. Richman RA, Kirsch LR: Testosterone treatment in adolescent boys with constitutional delay in growth and development. N Engl J Med 319:1563–1567, 1988.

105. Joss EE, Schmidt HA, Zuppinger KA: Oxandrolone in constitutionally delayed growth: A longitudinal study up to final height. J Endocrinol Metab 69:1109–1115, 1989.

106. Stanhope R, Noone C, Brook CGD: Oxandrolone in the treatment of constitutional delay of growth and puberty in boys. Arch Dis Child 60:784–785, 1985.

107. Marti-Henneberg C, Niirianen AK, Rappaport R: Oxandrolone treatment of constitutional short stature in boys during adolescence: Effect on linear growth, bone age, pubic hair, and testicular development. Adolesc Med 86:783–788, 1975.

108. Jackson ST, Rallison ML, Buntin WH, et al: Use of oxandrolone for growth stimulation in children. Am J Dis Child 126:481–484, 1973.

109. Sobel EH, Raymond CS, Quinn KV, Talbot NB: The use of methyltestosterone to stimulate growth: Relative influence on skeletal maturation and linear growth. J Clin Endocrinol 16:241–248, 1956.

110. Foss GL: The influence of androgen treatment on ultimate height in males. Arch Dis Child 40:66–70, 1965.

111. Buyukgebiz A, Hindmarsh PC, Brook CG: Treatment of constitutional delay of growth and puberty with oxandrolone compared with growth hormone. Arch Dis Child 65:448–449, 1990.

112. Ulloa-Aguirre A, Blizzard RM, Garcia-Rubi E, et al: Testosterone and oxandrolone, a nonaromatizable androgen, specifically amplify the mass and rate of growth hormone (GH) secreted per burst without altering GH secretory burst duration or frequency or the GH half-life. J Endocrinol Metab 71:846–854, 1990.

113. Lippe B: Turner syndrome. Endocrinol Metab Clin North Am 20:121–152, 1991.

114. Rosenfeld RG, Frane J, Attie KM, et al: Six-year results of a randomized, prospective trial of human growth hormone and oxandrolone in Turner syndrome. J Pediatr 121:49–55, 1992.

115. Mendenhall CL, Anderson S, Garcia-Pont P, et al: Short-term and long-term survival in patients with alcoholic hepatitis treated with oxandrolone and prednisolone. N Engl J Med 311:1464–1470, 1984.

116. Bonkovsky HL, Fiellin DA, Smith GS, et al: A randomized, controlled trial of treatment of alcoholic hepatitis with parenteral nutrition and oxandrolone: I. Short-term effects on liver function. Am J Gastroenterol 86:1200–1208, 1991.

117. Bonkovsky HL, Singh RH, Jafri IH, et al: A randomized, controlled trial of treatment of alcoholic hepatitis with parenteral nutrition and oxandrolone: II. Short-term effects on nitrogen metabolism, metabolic balance, and nutrition. Am J Gastroenterol 86:1209–1218, 1991.

117a. Mendenhall CL, Moritz TE, Roselle GA, et al: A study of oral nutritional support with oxandrolone in malnourished patients with alcoholic hepatitis: results of a Department of Veterans Affairs cooperative study. Hepatology 17:564–576, 1993.

118. Catlin DH, Hatton CK: Use and abuse of anabolic and other drugs for athletic enhancement. Adv Intern Med 36:381–405, 1990.

119. Dubin C: Commission of Inquiry into the Use of Drugs and Banned Practices Intended to Increase Athletic Performance. Ottawa, Canada, Canadian Government Publishing Center, 1990.

120. United States Senate, Committee on the Judiciary: Proper and Improper Use of Drugs by Athletes (Hearings before the Subcommittee to Investigate Juvenile Delinquency, June 18 and July 12 and 13, 1973). Washington, DC, US Government Printing Office, 1973, pp 1–843.

121. United States Senate, Committee on the Judiciary: Steroids in Amateur and Professional Sports—The Medical and Social Costs of Steroid Abuse (Hearings before the Committee on the Judiciary, April 3 and May 9, 1989). Washington, DC, US Government Printing Office, 1990, pp 1–253.

122. Parliament of the Commonwealth of Australia, Senate Committee on Environment, Recreation and the Arts: Drugs in Sport. Canberra, Aust, Australian Government Publishing Service, 1989.

123. Dickman S: East Germany: Science in the disservice of the state. Science 254:26–27, 1991.

124. Kusserow RP: Adolescent Steroid Use. Washington, DC, US Department Health and Human Services, 1990.

125. Buckley WE, Yesalis CE, Friedl KE, et al: Estimated prevalence of anabolic steroid use among male high school seniors. JAMA 260:3441–3445, 1988.

125a. DuRant RH, Rickert VI, Ashworth CS, et al: Use of multiple drugs among adolescents who use anabolic steroids. N Engl J Med 328:922–926, 1993.

125b. Whitehead R, Chillag S, Elliott D: Anabolic steroid use among adolescents in a rural state. J Fam Pract 35:401–405, 1992.

125c. Radakovich J, Broderick P, Pickell G: Rate of anabolic-androgenic steroid use among students in junior high school. J Am Board Fam Pract 6:341–345, 1993.

126. Catlin DH, Kammerer RC, Hatton CK, et al: Analytical chemistry at the games of the XXIIIrd Olympiad in Los Angeles, 1984. Clin Chem 33:319–327, 1987.

127. Duchaine D: Underground Steroid Handbook II. Venice, CA, HLR Technical Books, 1989.

128. Haupt HA, Rovere GD: Anabolic steroids: A review of the literature. Am J Sports Med 12:469–484, 1984.

129. Strauss RH, Liggett MT, Lanese RR: Anabolic steroid use and perceived effects in ten weight-trained women athletes. JAMA 253:2871–2875, 1985.

130. Yesalis CE, Herrick RT, Buckley WE, et al: Self-reported use of anabolic-androgenic steroids by elite power lifters. Phys Sportsmed 16:91–100, 1988.

131. Catlin DH, Cowan DA: Detecting testosterone administration [editorial]. Clin Chem 38:1685–1686, 1992.

132. Southan GJ, Brooks RV, Cowan DA, et al: Possible indices for the detection of the administration of dihydrotestosterone to athletes. J Steroid Biochem Molec Biol 42:87–94, 1992.

133. Snochowski M, Saartok T, Dahlberg E, et al: Androgen and glucocorticoid receptors in human skeletal muscle cytosol. J Steroid Biochem 14:765–771, 1981.

134. Krieg M, Smith K, Elvers B: Androgen receptor translocation from cytosol of rat heart muscle, bulbo-cavernosus levator ani muscle and prostate into heart muscle nuclei. J Steroid Biochem 13:577–587, 1980.

135. Deslypere JP, Vermeulen A: Influence of age on steroid concentrations in skin and striated muscle in women and in cardiac muscle and lung tissue in men. J Clin Endocrinol Metab 61:648–653, 1985.

136. Alén M, Hakkinen K, Komi PV: Changes in neuromuscular performance and muscle fiber characteristics of elite power athletes self-administering androgenic and anabolic steroids. Acta Physiol Scand 122:535–544, 1984.

137. Hosegood JL, Franks AJ: Response of human skeletal muscle to the anabolic steroid stanozolol. BMJ 297:1028–1029, 1988.

138. Griggs RC, Kingston W, Jozefowicz RF, et al: Effect of testosterone on muscle mass and muscle protein synthesis. J Appl Physiol 66:498–503, 1989.

139. Wainman P, Shipounoff GC: The effects of castration and testosterone propionate on the striated perineal musculature in the rat. Endocrinology 29:975–978, 1941.

140. Lyons GE, Kelly AM, Rubinstein NA: Testosterone-induced changes in contractile protein isoforms in the sexually dimorphic temporalis muscle of the guinea pig. J Biol Chem 261:13278–13284, 1986.

141. Venable JH: Morphology of the cells of normal, testosterone-deprived and testosterone-stimulated levator ani muscles. Am J Anat 119:271–301, 1966.

142. Kenyon AT, Knowlton K, Sandiford I, et al: A comparative study of the metabolic effects of testosterone propionate in normal men and women and in eunuchoidism. Endocrinology 26:26–45, 1940.

143. Kenyon AT, Knowlton K, Sandiford I: The anabolic effects of the androgens and somatic growth in man. Ann Intern Med 20:632–654, 1944.

144. Landau RL: The metabolic effects of anabolic steroids in man. In Kochakian CD (ed): Anabolic-Androgenic Steroids. New York, Springer-Verlag, 1976, pp 45–71.

145. Kenyon AT, Knowlton K, Lotwin G, Sandiford I: Metabolic response of aged men to testosterone propionate. J Clin Endocrinol 2:690–695, 1942.

146. Welle S, Jozefowicz R, Forbes G, Griggs RC: Effect of testosterone on metabolic rate and body composition in normal men and men with muscular dystrophy. J Clin Endocrinol Metab 74:332–335, 1992.

147. Forbes GB: Human Body Composition: Growth, Aging, Nutrition, and Activity. New York, Springer-Verlag, 1987.

148. Forbes GB: The effect of anabolic steroids on lean body mass: The dose response curve. Metabolism 34:571–573, 1985.

149. Forbes GB, Porta CR, Herr BE, Griggs RC: Sequence of body changes in body composition induced by testosterone and reversal of changes after drug is stopped. JAMA 267:397–399, 1992.

150. Hervey GR, Knibbs AV, Burkinshaw L, et al: Effects of methandienone on the performance and body composition of men undergoing athletic training. Clin Sci 60:457–461, 1981.

151. Forbes GB: Body composition as affected by physical activity and nutrition. Fed Proc 44:343–347, 1985.

152. Wilson JD: Androgen abuse by athletes. Endocr Rev 9:181–199, 1988.

153. Mayer M, Rosen F: Interaction of anabolic steroids with glucocorticoid receptor sites in rat muscle cytosol. Am J Physiol 229:1381–1386, 1975.

154. Moritani T, DeVries H: Neural factors versus hypertrophy in the time course of muscle strength gain. Am J Appl Physiol 58:115–130, 1979.

155. MacDougall J, Sale D, Elder G, Sutton J: Muscle ultrastructural characteristics of elite powerlifters and bodybuilders. Eur J Appl Physiol 48:117–126, 1982.

156. American College of Sports Medicine: Position statement on the use of anabolic-androgenic steroids in sports. Med Sci Sports Exerc 19:534–539, 1987.

157. Hervey GR, Hutchinson I, Knibbs AV, et al: Anabolic effects of methandienone in men undergoing athletic training. Lancet 2:699–702, 1976.

158. Elashoff JD, Jacknow AD, Shain SG, Braunstein GD: Effects of anabolic-androgenic steroids on muscular strength. Ann Intern Med 115:387–393, 1991.

159. Friedl KE, Yesalis CE: Self-treatment of gynecomastia in bodybuilders who use anabolic steroids. Phys Sportsmed 17:67–79, 1989.

160. Wilson JD, Aiman J, MacDonald PC: The pathogenesis of gynecomastia. Adv Intern Med 25:1–25, 1980.

161. Scott MJ Jr, Scott MJ III: Dermatologists and anabolic-androgenic drug abuse. Cutis 44:30–35, 1989.

162. Barbosa J, Seal US, Doe RP: Effects of anabolic steroids on hormone-binding proteins, serum cortisol and serum nonprotein-bound cortisol. J Clin Endocrinol 32:232–240, 1971.

163. Small M, Beastall GH, Semple CG, et al: Alteration of hormone levels in normal males given the anabolic steroid stanozolol. Clin Endocrinol 21:49–55, 1984.

164. Malarkey WB, Strauss RH, Leizman DJ, et al: Endocrine effects of female weight lifters who self-administer testosterone and anabolic steroids. Am J Obstet Gynecol 165:1385–1390, 1991.

165. Alén M, Rahkila P, Reinilä M, Vihko R: Androgenic-anabolic steroid effects on serum thyroid, pituitary and steroid hormones in athletes. Am J Sports Med 15:357–362, 1987.

166. Clerico A, Ferdeghini M, Palombo C, et al: Effect of anabolic treatment on serum levels of gonadotropins, testosterone, prolactin, thyroid hormones and myoglobin of male athletes under physical training. J Nucl Med Allied Sci 25:79–88, 1981.

166a. Deyssig R, Weissel M: Ingestion of androgenic-anabolic steroids induces mild thyroidal impairment in male body builders. J Clin Endocrinol Metabol 76:1069–1071, 1993.

167. Lee IR, Dawson SA, Wetherall JD, Hahnel R: Sex hormone–binding globulin secretion by human hepatocarcinoma cells is increased by both estrogens and androgens. J Clin Endocrinol Metab 64:825–831, 1987.

168. Federman DD, Robbins J, Rall JE: Effects of methyltestosterone on thyroid function, thyroxine metabolism, and thyroxine-binding protein. J Clin Invest 37:1024–1030, 1958.

169. Godsland IF, Shennan NM, Wynn V: Insulin action and dynamics modelled in patients taking the anabolic steroid methandienone (Dianabol). Clin Sci 71:665–673, 1986.

170. Woodard TL, Burghen GA, Kitabchi AE, Wilimas JA: Glucose intolerance and insulin resistance in aplastic anemia treated with oxymetholone. J Clin Endocrinol Metab 53:905–908, 1981.

171. Friedl KE, Jones RE, Hannan CJ Jr, Plymate SR: The administration of pharmacological doses of testosterone or 19-nortestosterone to normal men is not associated with increased insulin secretion or impaired glucose tolerance. J Clin Endocrinol Metab 68:971–975, 1989.

172. Rebuffé-Scrive M, Mårin P, Björntorp P: Effect of testosterone on abdominal adipose tissue in men. Int J Obes 15:791–795, 1991.

173. Xu X, de Pergola G, Björntorp P: The effects of androgens on the regulation of lipolysis in adipose tissue. Endocrinology 126:1229–1234, 1990.

174. Hurley BF, Seals DR, Hagberg JM, et al: High-density-lipoprotein cholesterol in bodybuilders v. powerlifters: Negative effects of androgen use. JAMA 252:507–513, 1984.

175. Applebaum DM, Haffner S, Hazzard WR: The dyslipoproteinemia of anabolic steroid therapy: Increase in hepatic triglyceride lipase precedes the decrease in high density lipoprotein-2 cholesterol. Metabolism 36:949–952, 1987.

176. Friedl KE, Hannan CJ Jr, Jones RE, Plymate SR: High-density lipoprotein cholesterol is not decreased if an aromatizable androgen is administered. Metabolism 39:69–74, 1990.

177. Friedl KE: Reappraisal of the health risks associated with the use of high doses of oral and injectable androgenic steroids. In Lin GC, Erinoff L (eds): Anabolic Steroid Abuse (Research Monograph 102). Rockville, MD, National Institute on Drug Abuse, 1990, pp 142–176.

178. Haffner SM, Kushwaha RS, Foster DM, et al: Studies on the metabolic mechanism of reduced high density lipoproteins during anabolic steroid therapy. Metabolism 32:413–420, 1983.

179. Kantor MA, Bianchini A, Bernier D, et al: Androgens reduce HDL_2-cholesterol and increase hepatic triglyceride lipase activity. Med Sci Sports Exerc 17:462–465, 1985.

180. Gordon T, Castelli WP, Hjortland MC, et al: High density lipoproteins as a protective factor against coronary heart disease: The Framingham Study. Am J Med 62:707–714, 1977.

181. McNutt RA, Ferenchick GS, Kirlin PC, Hamlin NJ: Acute myocardial infarction in a 22-year-old world class weight lifter using anabolic steroids. Am J Cardiol 62:164, 1988.

182. Petera V, Bobek K, Lahn V: Serum transaminase (GOT, GPT) and lactic dehydrogenase activity during treatment with methyltestosterone. Clin Chim Acta 7:604–606, 1962.

183. Wynn V, Landon J, Kawerau E: Studies on hepatic function during methandienone therapy. Lancet 1:69–75, 1961.

184. Zimmerman HJ: Hormonal derivatives and other drugs used to treat endocrine diseases. In Zimmerman HJ (ed): Hepatotoxicity: The Adverse Effects of Drugs and Other Chemicals on the Liver. New York, Appelton-Century-Crofts, 1978, pp 436–467.

185. Ishak KG, Zimmerman HJ: Hepatotoxic effects of the anabolic/androgenic steroids. Semin Liver Dis 7:230–252, 1987.

186. Ishak KG: Hepatic neoplasms associated with contraceptive and anabolic steroids. In Lingeman CH (ed): Carcinogenic Hormones. Berlin, Springer-Verlag, 1979, pp 73–128.

187. Foss GL, Simpson SL: Oral methyltestosterone and jaundice. BMJ 1:259–263, 1959.

188. Kory RC, Bradley MH, Watson RN: A six-month evaluation of an anabolic drug, norethandrolone, in underweight persons: II. Busulphalein (BSP) retention and liver function. Am J Med 26:243–248, 1959.

189. Pecking A, Lejolly JM, Najean Y: Hepatic toxicity of androgen therapy in aplastic anemia. Nouv Rev Fr Hematol 22:257–265, 1980.

190. Anthony PP: Hepatoma associated with androgenic steroids [letter]. Lancet 1:685–686, 1975.

191. Overly WL, Dankoff JA, Wang BK, Singh UD: Androgens and hepatocellular carcinoma in an athlete. Ann Intern Med 100:158–159, 1984.

192. Zevin D, Turani H, Cohen A, Levi J: Androgen-associated hepatoma in a hemodialysis patient. Nephron 29:274–276, 1981.

193. Falk H, Popper H, Thomas LB, Ishak KG: Hepatic angiosarcoma associated with androgenic-anabolic steroids. Lancet 2:1120–1123, 1979.

194. Ingerowski GH, Scheutwinkel-Reich M, Stan HJ: Mutagenicity studies on veterinary anabolic drugs with the salmonella/microsome test. Mutat Res 91:93–98, 1981.

195. Lesna M, Taylor W: Liver lesions in BALB/C mice induced by an anabolic androgen (DecaDurabolin), with and without pretreatment with diethylnitrosamine. J Steroid Biochem 24:449–453, 1986.

196. Taxy JB: Peliosis: A morphologic curiosity becomes an iatrogenic problem. Hum Pathol 9:331–340, 1978.

197. Lowdell CP, Murray-Lyon IM: Reversal of liver damage due to long term methyltestosterone and safety of non-17α-alkylated androgens. BMJ 291:637, 1985.

198. Nadell J, Kosek J: Peliosis hepatis: Twelve cases associated with oral androgen therapy. Arch Pathol Lab Med 101:405–410, 1977.

199. Turani H, Levi J, Zevin D, Kessler E: Hepatic lesions in patients on anabolic androgenic therapy. Isr J Med Sci 19:332–337, 1983.

200. Bagheri SA, Boyer JL: Peliosis hepatis associated with androgenic-anabolic steroid therapy—a severe form of hepatic injury. Ann Intern Med 81:610–618, 1974.

201. Wakabayashi T, Onda H, Tada T, et al: High incidence of peliosis hepatis in autopsy cases of aplastic anemia with special reference to anabolic steroid therapy. Acta Pathol Jpn 34:1079–1086, 1984.

202. Uzych L: Anabolic-androgenic steroids and psychiatric-related effects: A review. Can J Psychiatry 37:23–28, 1992.

203. Altschule MD, Tillotson KJ: The use of testosterone in the treatment of depression. N Engl J Med 239:1036–1038, 1948.

204. Bahrke MS, Yesalis CE, Wright JE: Psychological and behavioral effects of endogenous testosterone levels and anabolic-androgenic steroids among males. Sports Med 10:303–337, 1990.

205. Pope HG Jr, Katz DL: Homicide and near-homicide by anabolic steroid users. J Clin Psychiatry 51:28–31, 1990.

205a. Su TP, Pagliaro M, Schmidt PJ, et al: Neuropsychiatric effects of anabolic steroids in male normal volunteers. JAMA 269:2760–2764, 1993.

206. Pope HG, Jr, Katz DL: Affective and psychotic symptoms associated with anabolic steroid use. Am J Psychiatry 145:487–490, 1988.

207. Archer J: The influence of testosterone on human aggression. Br J Psychol 82:1–28, 1991.

208. Brower KJ, Blow FC, Young JP, Hill EM: Symptoms and correlates of anabolic-androgenic steroid dependence. Br J Addict 86:759–768, 1991.

209. Kashkin KB, Kleber HD: Hooked on hormones? An anabolic steroid addiction hypothesis. JAMA 262:3166–3170, 1989.

210. Hoag GN, Connolly VPL, Domke HL: Marked fall in high-density lipoprotein following isotretinoin therapy: Report of a case in a weight lifter on anabolic steroids. J Am Acad Dermatol 16:1264–1265, 1987.

211. McLaughlin GE, McCarty DJ, Segal BL: Hemarthrosis complication anticoagulant therapy. JAMA 196:202–203, 1966.

212. Schrogie JJ, Solomon HM: The anticoagulant response to bishydroxycoumarin: II. The effect of D-thyroxine, clofibrate, and norethandrolone. Clin Pharmacol Ther 8:70–77, 1967.

213. Wilson IC, Prange AJ, Lara PP: Methyltestosterone and imipramine in men: Conversion of depression to paranoid reaction. Am J Psychiatry 131:21–24, 1974.

214. Zeiss J, Smith RR, Taha AM: Iliopsoas hypertrophy mimicking acute abdomen in a bodybuilder. Gastrointest Radiol 12:340–342, 1987.

215. Laseter JT, Russell JA: Anabolic steroid–induced tendon pathology: A review of the literature. Med Sci Sports Exerc 23:1–3, 1991.

216. Winwood PJ, Robertson DAF, Wright R: Bleeding oesophageal varices associated with anabolic steroid use in an athlete. Postgrad Med J 66:864–865, 1990.

217. Damste PH: Voice change in adult women caused by virilizing agents. J Speech Hear Disord 32:126–132, 1967.

218. Jones TM, Fang VS, Landau RL, Rosenfield RL: The effect of fluoxymesterone administration on testicular function. J Clin Endocrinol Metab 44:121–129, 1977.

219. Mauss J, Borsch G, Bormacher K, et al: Effect of long-term testosterone oenanthate administration on male reproductive function: Clinical evaluation, serum FSH, LH, testosterone, and seminal fluid analyses in normal men. Acta Endocrinol 78:373–384, 1975.

220. Schürmeyer T, Belkien L, Knuth UA, Nieschlag E: Reversible azoospermia induced by the anabolic steroid 19-nortestosterone. Lancet 1:417–420, 1984.

221. Alèn M, Suominen J: Effect of androgenic and anabolic steroids on spermatogenesis in power athletes. Int J Sports Med 5(Suppl):189–192, 1984.

Clinical Disorders of the Testis

STEPHEN J. WINTERS

The Leydig cells of the testis are the site of testosterone synthesis, and the seminiferous tubules are the source of spermatozoa. The ability to isolate and culture testis cells has confirmed the preconceived notion that the functions of the two testicular compartments are intimately related. Thus, it is not surprising that when the testis dysfunctions, patients often develop both androgen deficiency and infertility. For conceptualization, disorders of the testis have been divided into disorders in which the gonadotropin drive to the testis is impaired (hypogonadotropic hypogonadism) and those that damage the testes directly (primary testicular failure). An increasing number of systemic illnesses have been found to have both effects, however.

HYPOGONADOTROPIC HYPOGONADISM

Hypogonadotropic hypogonadism is the term for disorders in which testicular function is impaired because gonadotropin stimulation is inadequate. Gonadotropin deficiency may occur selectively, or may coexist with a deficiency of other pituitary hormones. It may be congenital or acquired and may result from pathology intrinsic to the pituitary gland or from an impairment in the hypothalamic control of pituitary gonadotropin secretion.

Congenital Isolated Hypogonadotropic Hypogonadism

Isolated hypogonadotropic hypogonadism (IHH) is a heterogeneous disorder with a prevalence of about 1 in 10,000. Most cases are sporadic, although many affected kindreds have been described.[1] More than 90 per cent of affected individuals are males, who generally present as teenagers with deficient sexual maturation; 10 per cent are female. Affected males have a male phenotype because maternal human chorionic gonadotropin (hCG) stimulated the fetal testis to produce testosterone, thereby masculinizing the genitalia. Unilateral or bilateral cryptorchidism occurs in 10 to 25 per cent of patients, and microphallus occurs occasionally. Linear growth during childhood is normal, but the growth rate falls off in the teenage years because no adolescent growth spurt occurs.[2] In untreated young adults, the bone age is delayed compared with the chronological age. Severe osteopenia develops[3] because the sex hormone–mediated increase in bone density of adolescence fails to occur. The long bones grow in length because epiphyseal closure is delayed with resultant "eunuchoidal body proportions"; that is, the arm span exceeds the height and the upper to lower segment ratio is less than 0.9 (Fig. 133–1). Patients also tend to be tall.[4] Testis volume is variable, ranging from prepubertal values of less than 4 ml to nearly normal adult values. Gynecomastia is common. There is often some pubic hair growth which has been related to the production of dehydroepiandrosterone sulfate (DHAS).[5] Psychological problems may occur because of delayed sexual development.

The testes have a prepubertal histological appearance. Seminiferous tubules are small and contain immature Sertoli cells, which are round and may be pseudostratified. A few large spermatogonia with clear cytoplasm and a central

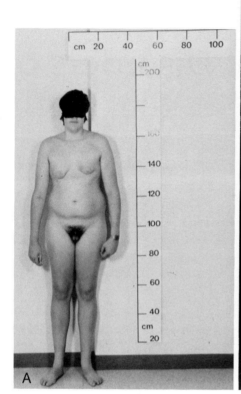
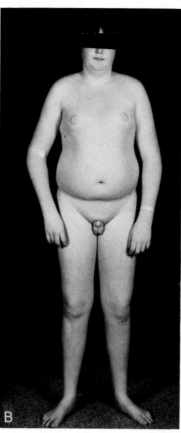
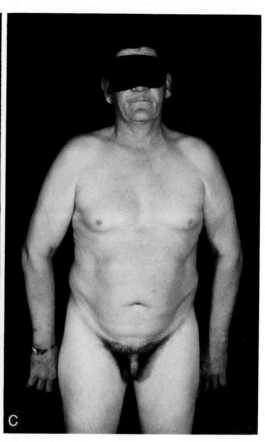

FIGURE 133–1. *A*, An 18-year-old male with isolated hypogonadotropic hypogonadism. Note the normal height, long arms and legs, poor muscular development, and prominent gynecomastia. Although his testes and phallus are small, pubic hair is present. It is very unusual for normal boys to have pubic hair growth before the genitalia have begun to develop. *B*, A 13½-year-old boy with underdeveloped genitals, absent pubic hair, and gynecomastia. The normal relationship between genital development and pubic hair growth is preserved, and over the ensuing year spontaneous testis growth began, indicating constitutional delay of puberty. *C*, A 51-year-old man with incomplete gonadotropin deficiency who presented with osteoporosis. He had life-long hypogonadism, including two infertile marriages. His serum testosterone level was 125 ng/dl, and serum LH and FSH levels were in the low normal range. His testes were 10 ml in volume.

nucleolus are present in the center of the seminiferous tubule. The interstitium is composed of loose connective tissue. Mature Leydig cells are absent, but fibroblast-like precursor cells are found (Fig. 133–2*B*).

Serum testosterone levels in most patients with IHH are at the low levels characteristic of prepubertal boys, and serum luteinizing hormone (LH) levels are barely detectable even with new, highly sensitive two-site immunoassays[6] (Table 133–1). Twenty-four–hour concentration profiles reveal that the nocturnal rise in serum LH levels characteristic of normal prepubertal boys is absent in IHH[7] (Fig. 133–3). Some patients have low-amplitude fluctuations in serum LH levels which may reflect episodes of gonadotropin-releasing hormone (GnRH) secretion. Moreover, in most patients LH and α-subunit are present in the pituitary and can be released into the circulation following GnRH stimulation, although the magnitude of the response is much less than that of normal adult men. Prolonged pulsatile administration of GnRH induces full pubertal development, indicating that IHH is due to a lack of normal stimulation of the pituitary by endogenous GnRH.[8] The secretion of other pituitary hormones is normal.[9] GH and prolactin (PRL) secretion are at or below the levels of prepubertal children because of the impact of sex steroid

deficiency, and increase to adult values during treatment with testosterone or hCG.[10, 11] Serum DHA and DHAS levels in adult men with IHH are only slightly less than those of normal men, indicating that the production of adrenal androgenic precursor steroids is independent of GnRH secretion.[5]

Other patients present with less pronounced clinical signs of congenital eunuchoidism and variable testis enlargement, and sometimes presentation is delayed until adulthood[12] (see Fig. 133–1*C*). Although the prevalence of subtle gonadotropin deficiency in the population at large is unknown, men with some evidence of testis growth comprise about 25 per cent of hypogonadotropic patients seeking specialty care in the United States, although the proportion in the Middle East may be higher.[13] Basal LH, follicle-stimulating hormone (FSH), and testosterone levels and the gonadotropin response to GnRH stimulation are greater in these men than in those with complete gonadotropin deficiency.[12, 14] Spontaneous LH pulses of reduced amplitude and/or frequency can often be detected in the circulation, providing insight into the pathophysiology of their disorder.[14, 15] Testicular biopsies reveal incomplete spermatogenesis and sparse Leydig cells (see Fig. 133–2*C*). Because there is evidence for testis growth and spermato-

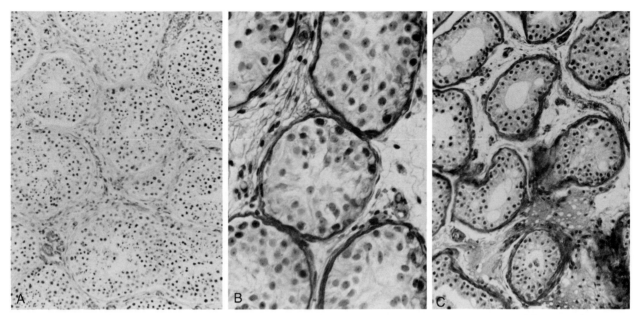

FIGURE 133–2. *A*, Parenchyma of the normal adult testis. Seminiferous tubules have a cross-sectional diameter of 150 to 300 μ and are surrounded by a basement membrane and several layers of peritubular myoid cells. Sertoli cells, which extend from the basement membrane to the tubular lumen, have polygonal nuclei located at the basal portion of the cell which contain a prominent nucleolus. There is an organized arrangement of germ cells with various cell types predominating in different portions of the tubule. Spermatozoa predominate in some portions and spermatids in others. Between the seminiferous tubules is loose connective tissue containing single cells and clusters of Leydig cells (H&E, × 50). *B*, Testicular biopsy from a patient with isolated hypogonadotropic hypogonadism. Seminiferous tubules are small (mean tubular diameter 50 μ) and are lined by immature Sertoli cells and spermatogonia. A few primary spermatocytes are also present. The tunica propria is delicate. Interstitial cells are immature and resemble undifferentiated mesenchymal cells (H&E, × 125). *C*, Testicular biopsy from a patient with partial GnRH deficiency. Seminiferous tubules are reduced in diameter (50 to 80 μ) and have incomplete spermatogenesis. Leydig cells are reduced in number (H&E, × 50).

genesis but incomplete androgenization, the term *fertile eunuch* has been applied to these men, but the term *partial GnRH deficiency* is preferred.

Kallmann's Syndrome

Male hypogonadism with anosmia was first described by Maestre de San Juan in 1856. The designation *olfactogenital dysplasia* was introduced to emphasize the association between agenesis of the olfactory bulbs and hypogonadism, and the first familial cases were reported by Kallmann and co-workers[16] in 1944. Among affected kindreds, the high male:female ratio is consistent with an X-linked trait, although kindreds with apparent autosomal dominant or recessive modes of inheritance with variable penetrance have also been described, implying that familial IHH is also a heterogeneous disorder.[17] Peripheral leukocyte karyotypes are generally normal.

Anosmia or hyposmia is present in 33 to 50 per cent of men with complete IHH and less frequently with partial IHH. Magnetic resonance imaging reveals that the anosmia results from hypoplasia of the olfactory nerves and tracts.[18] Genital, somatic, and neurological abnormalities may also be present (Table 133–2).[19] Cryptorchidism and microphallus may be explained by androgen deficiency in utero. The somatic and neurological abnormalities may be expressed in patients with apparently normal reproductive function, but their frequent coexistence with GnRH deficiency suggests that these traits are somehow related.

Immunocytochemical studies in the fetal mouse showed that GnRH neurons migrate from the olfactory placode to the hypothalamus together with the central processes of olfactory nerves.[20] These findings and the awareness that olfactory bulb development depends upon contact be-

TABLE 133–1. SERUM LEVELS OF LH, FSH, AND TESTOSTERONE IN PREPUBERTAL BOYS AND GIRLS AND PATIENTS WITH KALLMANN'S SYNDROME

	MEAN AGE (YEARS)	TESTOSTERONE/ ESTRADIOL	LH(U/L)	FSH (U/L)
Boys	6.6 ± 0.3	≤0.3 nmol/L	0.10 ± 0.03	0.46 ± 0.07
Girls	6.2 ± 0.4	≤30 pmol/L	0.19 ± 0.80	1.95 ± 0.88
Kallmann's	23.1 ± 3.8	≤0.3 nmol/L	0.14 ± 0.06	0.29 ± 0.06

Results are from Wu FCW, Butler GE, Kelnar CJH, et al: Patterns of pulsatile luteinizing hormone and follicle-stimulating hormone secretion in prepubertal (midchildhood) boys and girls and patients with idiopathic hypogonadotropic hypogonadism (Kallmann's syndrome): A study using an ultrasensitive time-resolved immunofluorometric assay. J Clin Endocrinol Metab 72:1229–1237, 1991. Plasma LH and FSH levels were measured by DELFIA immunofluorometric assays.

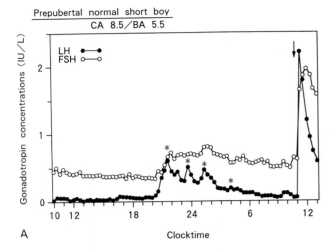

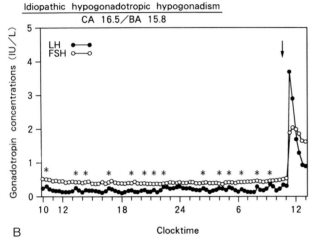

FIGURE 133–3. LH and FSH levels in blood samples drawn every 20 minutes for 25 hours beginning at 10:00 AM in a prepubertal normal boy (A) and an untreated 16½-year-old with hypogonadotropic hypogonadism (B). The arrows indicate the intravenous administration of GnRH at a dose of 25 ng/kg. Plasma LH and FSH levels were measured by DELFIA time-resolved immunofluorometric assays. Asterisks indicate pulses scored by the cluster algorithm. (From Goji K, Tanikaze S: Comparison between spontaneous gonadotropin concentration profiles and gonadotropin response to low-dose gonadotropin-releasing hormone in prepubertal and early pubertal boys and patients with hypogonadotropic hypogonadism: Assessment by using ultrasensitive, time-resolved immunofluorometric assay. Pediatr Res 31:535–539, 1992.)

tween central projections of olfactory neurons and forebrain anlage led to the hypothesis that Kallmann's syndrome results from a neuron migration defect. Studies of a 19-week stillborn male fetus from a kindred with apparent Kallmann's syndrome associated with a deletion of the short arm of the X chromosome advanced this hypothesis further.[21] Whereas GnRH-containing cells were present in the median eminence and preoptic area of age-matched fetuses, no GnRH cells were found in this fetal brain. Instead, dense clusters of GnRH cells were found in his nose, GnRH containing fibers terminated abruptly on the cribriform plate, and the olfactory bulbs and tracts were absent. There is evidence that a neural-cell adhesion protein, coded for by genes on the short arm of the X chromosome, guides the growth of axons and is abnormal in some patients with Kallmann's syndrome. This defect could prevent the entry of GnRH neurons into the brain, producing ap-

TABLE 133–2. CONGENITAL DEFECTS ASSOCIATED WITH HYPOGONADOTROPIC HYPOGONADISM

NEUROLOGICAL DEFECTS	GENITAL DEFECTS	SOMATIC DEFECTS
Anosmia	Cryptorchidism	Cleft lip
Nystagmus	Microphallus	Cleft palate
Sensorineural hearing loss		Renal agenesis
Cerebellar ataxia		Horseshoe kidney
Spastic paraplegia		Pes cavus
Learning disability		
Color blindness		
Synkinesia		
Seizures		

parent GnRH deficiency.[22] The GnRH gene, by contrast, appears to be normal in IHH.[23]

Hypogonadism with Other Central Nervous System Disorders

A variety of other syndromes occur in which neurological abnormalities are associated with hypogonadism (Table 133–3). In some conditions in which the patients may not reach adulthood, delayed puberty rather than hypogonadism may be present. In those disorders with documented gonadotropin deficiency, the pathogenesis of the syndrome remains undefined.

The Prader-Willi syndrome (PWS) is characterized by neonatal hypotonia, obesity, short stature, small hands and feet, mental retardation, and hypogonadism.[24] Most patients are diagnosed in childhood. The prevalence of PWS has been estimated to be 1 in 25,000. Males and females are affected equally, and most cases are sporadic. Deletions of chromosome 15 of paternal origin are generally present. The extent of spontaneous sexual maturation is variable. Most males have cryptorchidism and a small penis. Total testosterone levels are very low but exceed those of prepubertal boys. Basal LH and FSH concentrations are reduced, and the acute response to GnRH is attenuated.[25] Treatment with clomiphene may stimulate gonadotropin secretion (Fig. 133–4), as may long-term treatment with GnRH.[26] These data are consistent with a suppression of GnRH secretion in PWS through an obesity-associated increase in circulating estrogen concentrations, but this proposed mechanism would not explain the findings of cryptorchidism and microphallus in PWS which imply an intrauterine disturbance. Cryptorchidism may further damage the testes, explaining the subnormal testosterone response to long-term treatment with hCG. Treatment is therefore usually with topical or parenteral androgens. In-

TABLE 133–3. CLINICAL SYNDROMES OF HYPOGONADISM AND NEUROLOGICAL DYSFUNCTION

Kallmann's syndrome
Prader-Willi syndrome
Laurence-Moon-Biedl syndrome
Moebius syndrome
Lowe syndrome
Multiple lentigenes (LEOPARD) syndrome
Carpenter's syndrome
Rud syndrome

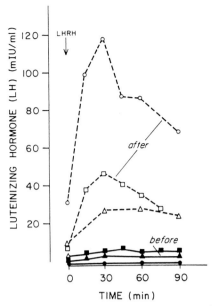

FIGURE 133–4. Effects of clomiphene treatment for 28 to 70 days on the LH response to 100 μg intravenous GnRH in three subjects older than 16 years with the Prader-Willi syndrome. Basal LH levels increased in all three patients. In the one male, clomiphene increased serum testosterone levels from 46 to 247 ng/dl. After termination of therapy, values returned to pretreatment controls. (From Bray GA, Dahms WT, Swerdloff RS, et al: The Prader-Willi syndrome: A study of 40 patients and a review of the literature. Medicine 62:59–80, 1983.)

sulin secretion increases in proportion to obesity, and many patients with PWS have diabetes mellitus.

The Laurence-Moon-Biedl syndrome is characterized by pigmented retinal dystrophy, obesity, mental retardation, polydactyly, renal structural abnormalities, spastic paraparesis, and hypogonadism. The designation Bardet-Biedl syndrome is often used in the absence of spastic paraparesis.[27] Microphallus and small testes are found in most men, and almost all men are sterile. Delayed pubertal development is common. Hypospermatogenesis, including tubular hyalinization, has been found in testicular biopsy specimens. Total testosterone levels are generally normal, and FSH and LH levels are increased or normal.[28] The disorder is often inherited as an autosomal recessive trait, but its cause is unknown.

Congenital oculofacial paralysis (Moebius syndrome) is characterized by cranial nerve paralyses and includes eye-movement disorders, seizures, mental retardation, gait disturbance, limb anomalies (Poland syndrome), and hypogonadism.[29] Several patients have documented gonadotropin deficiency.[30] In a few cases, a deletion of band 12.2 on chromosome 13 has been identified. Brain stem ischemia has also been suggested.

Lowe's oculocerebral-renal syndrome is an X-linked disorder that has been ascribed alternatively to an Xp25 or Xq24–26 locus. These patients have lenticular opacities, hypotonia, mental retardation, renal tubular acidosis, and hypogonadism.

The multiple lentigines (LEOPARD) syndrome is characterized by lentigines (L), electrocardiographic conduction defects (E), ocular hypertelorism (O), pulmonic stenosis (P), abnormal genitalia (A), retarded growth (R), and deafness (D).

In Carpenter's syndrome, hypogonadism is associated with obesity, acrocephaly, craniosynostosis, and agenesis of the hands and feet. Rud's syndrome describes the association of hypogonadism with ichthyosis and epilepsy.

Hypogonadotropic hypogonadism also occurs with X-linked congenital adrenal hypoplasia.[31] Combined glucocorticoid and mineralocorticoid deficiency leads to severe salt loss in infancy and unresponsiveness to ACTH. In some cases glycerol kinase deficiency and Duchenne muscular dystrophy have also been present, disorders that have been linked to X-short arm genes. Pituitary hypoplasia and the failure of GnRH to stimulate LH secretion suggest that HH in these patients may be due to a developmental defect in the pituitary rather than to GnRH deficiency, however.[32]

Idiopathic Panhypopituitarism

Hypogonadotropic hypogonadism may occur together with other pituitary hormone deficiencies, of which growth hormone (GH) deficiency is the most common. Although birth trauma has been suggested to cause this syndrome, the finding of micropenis in some patients suggests a disturbance in utero. The sella turcica is often small, and MR scans reveal a small pituitary gland, a poorly developed pituitary stalk, and superior dislocation of the neurohypophysis.[33] Little is known about the endocrine disturbance in these patients in adulthood. Patients with isolated GH deficiency enter puberty spontaneously, but at a delayed chronological age.[34]

Acquired Hypogonadotropic Hypogonadism

Mass Lesions of the Sella and Suprasellar Region

Gonadotropin deficiency may result from space-occupying lesions of the sella which compress and destroy the normal pituitary gland, or from suprasellar lesions that interrupt the nerve fibers bringing GnRH to the hypophyseal portal circulation. In addition to hypogonadism, these patients present with headaches and visual disturbances, characteristic symptoms of a cranial base mass lesion, and with variable manifestations of panhypopituitarism. External beam radiation therapy to the hypothalamus-pituitary may damage further the endocrine function of the pituitary.[35] ACTH or prolactin-secreting pituitary tumors produce hypogonadism by specific hormonal mechanisms, as described below.

Cushing's Syndrome

Decreased libido, impotence, and infertility are common complaints among men with Cushing's syndrome due to ACTH-producing pituitary adenomas as well as adrenal tumors or tumors outside the pituitary which produce ACTH. Serum testosterone levels are usually low, and basal and GnRH-stimulated LH concentrations are frequently suppressed.[36] Reduced SHBG levels further lower total testosterone concentrations. Increased cortisol production appears to be responsible for the gonadotropin deficiency inasmuch as adrenalectomy or treatment with mitotane or

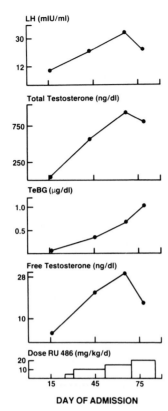

FIGURE 133–5. Restoration of LH secretion and Leydig cell function in a 25-year-old man with a metastatic ACTH-secreting carcinoid tumor of the lung treated with mifepristone (RU 486) for 10 weeks. (From Nieman LK, Chrousos GP, Kellner C: Successful treatment of Cushing's syndrome with the glucocorticoid antagonist RU 486. J Clin Endocrinol Metab 61:536–540, 1985. © 1985 by the Endocrine Society.)

the glucocorticoid antagonist mifepristone (RU 486) restores LH secretion and gonadal function (Fig. 133–5).[37] The action of glucocorticoids to induce aromatase activity in fibroblasts[38] may also contribute to the hypogonadism and gynecomastia. Prolonged glucocorticoid treatment of men with otherwise normal testicular function also produces gonadotropin deficiency.[39]

Prolactin-producing Pituitary Adenomas

Men with prolactinomas have classically presented late in the course of their disease with headaches and disturbed vision secondary to enlargement of the adenoma and with panhypopituitarism.[40, 41] But there is often a protracted history of reduced libido and potency, clinical hypogonadism, and gynecomastia. Prolactinomas in teenagers delay pubertal development.[42] The frequent finding of eunuchoidal body proportions in adult men with prolactinomas dates the onset of the tumor to adolescence. In spite of very high levels of prolactin in serum, only about 10 to 20 per cent of men with prolactinomas have galactorrhea, presumably because circulating estrogens are too low to stimulate sufficiently mammary gland growth and development. Increased awareness among physicians of the association between male hypogonadism and prolactin hypersecretion, as well as the greater willingness of patients to seek medical attention for these symptoms, has led to earlier diagnosis.

Serum testosterone levels are generally low in men with prolactinomas. Twenty-four-hour blood sampling studies indicate a pronounced diurnal change in testosterone concentrations with highest levels in the early morning hours as in normal pubertal boys (Fig. 133–6).[43] Thus, the level of testosterone in a morning blood sample may significantly overestimate the daily production rate of testosterone in these men. The LH concentration profile parallels that of testosterone, indicating that a decline in LH secretion is responsible for the reduced testosterone production, and the pulsatile pattern of LH secretion is attenuated.[44] The nature of the defect appears to be in GnRH secretion because pulsatile treatment with GnRH can restore testicular function to normal.[45] Studies in rats with experimental hyperprolactinemia using in situ hybridization techniques have demonstrated a reduction in GnRH mRNA levels per cell[46] and a resulting decline in GnRH receptor concentration. But there is at present no explanation for the reversion to a pubertal pattern of LH secretion.

The semen analysis is characterized by a reduction in sperm production, abnormal sperm morphology, and reduced sperm motility.[47] Semen volume may be reduced.

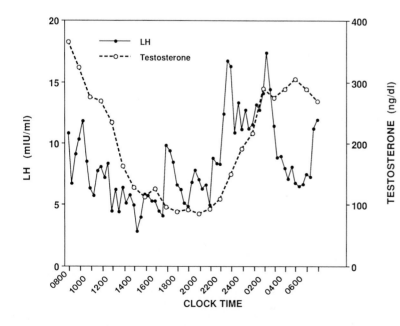

FIGURE 133–6. Serum LH levels in blood samples drawn every 20 minutes for 24 hours and testosterone concentrations in hourly serum pools in a 34-year-old man with a prolactinoma. The serum prolactin level was 195 ng/ml. (From Winters SJ: Diurnal rhythm of testosterone and luteinizing hormone in hypogonadal men. J Androl 12:185–190, 1991.)

Hyperprolactinemia is a rare finding among infertile men with normal sexual function, however.

Small prolactinomas can be cured by transsphenoidal adenomectomy with restoration of testicular function and sexual potency.[48] There may be a lag of several months before maximum testosterone levels are achieved. In many patients, however, serum prolactin levels fail to normalize in spite of apparently successful pituitary surgery. In these men, medical therapy with dopamine agonists generally results in a prompt decline in serum PRL levels with a subsequent rise in LH and testosterone concentrations (Fig. 133–7).[44] In men with large pituitary tumors and hypopituitarism, medical therapy may not increase LH and testosterone production because few normal gonadotrophs remain. In these patients, residual sexual dysfunction may not improve with testosterone replacement alone, whereas co-administration of dopamine agonists and testosterone may increase libido and potency.[40] These data suggest a direct inhibitory action of PRL on a CNS center controlling sexual arousal. If sperm production remains abnormal when prolactinomas are incompletely cured, spermatogenesis can be stimulated with gonadotropins.

Miscellaneous Causes of Gonadotropin Deficiency

Although reproductive function is commonly abnormal in women with congenital adrenal hyperplasia (CAH), testicular function is more variable. In one survey of 11 men with 21-hydroxylase deficiency, sperm density was less than 20 million/ml in only one subject, three men who were receiving no glucocorticoid treatment had normal semen analyses, and two of them had each fathered three children.[49] On the other hand, patients have been described with small testes, oligospermia or azoospermia, and decreased gonadotropin secretion in whom optimized therapy for CAH increased testosterone secretion and sperm production.[50] Clinically palpable testicular tumors occur occasionally in CAH.[51] This finding has been attributed to the presence of adrenocortical cells in the testis which are stimulated by ACTH. Glucocorticoid treatment may sup-press these tumors and restore spermatogenesis, but in other patients irreversible, unexplained damage to the seminiferous tubules and elevated serum FSH levels are found.

The massive production of hCG by choriocarcinomas may increase circulating levels of estrone and estradiol sufficiently to produce gynecomastia and suppress pituitary gonadotropin secretion.[52] Because hCG also stimulates Leydig cell testosterone production, but the testis may be replaced by tumor or damaged by X-irradiation or chemotherapy, serum testosterone levels are variable. The production of hCG can be recognized hormonally by the characteristic pattern of high LH and undetectable FSH levels when polyclonal antisera and double-antibody radioimmunoassays (RIA's) are used. With newer two-site immunoradiometric assays, however, increased specificity limits the cross-reactivity of hCG in the LH assay so that serum LH as well as FSH levels are low.[53] Gonadotropin deficiency may also occur in men with Leydig cell tumors of the testis[54] or with benign or malignant tumors of the adrenal cortex.[55] These tumors produce estradiol, or estradiol and estrone, respectively, and testosterone levels may be reduced.[56] Gynecomastia may be the presenting complaint in these men. Leydig cell function may be altered directly by high levels of circulating estrogens. Measurement of hCG in serum, CT scans of the adrenal glands, and testicular sonography[54] can be used to distinguish among these disorders.

Selective Abnormalities of LH or FSH

Because LH and FSH are products of the same pituitary cell, and the synthesis and secretion of both hormones are stimulated by GnRH, a selective deficiency of either gonadotropin would be predicted to be uncommon. Mutations in the LHβ or FSHβ gene leading to premature termination of subunit synthesis or to structural alterations precluding β-subunit to α-subunit combination could produce selective LH or FSH deficiency. Mutations in the 5' regulatory regions could markedly reduce subunit synthesis. In

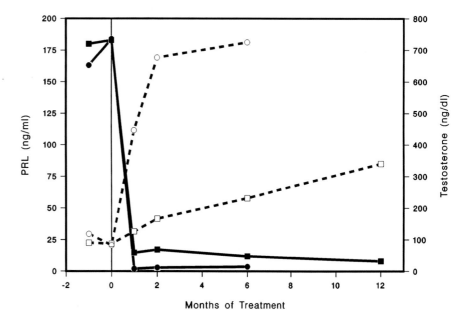

FIGURE 133–7. Changes in serum testosterone levels during bromocriptine treatment in two men with prolactin (PRL)-producing microadenomas. Solid symbols indicate PRL and open symbols are the testosterone levels. The data emphasize the variable response to PRL lowering in these men.

such patients, fetal sexual differentiation would be expected to be relatively normal because of the action of maternal hCG to stimulate fetal testicular function, whereas pubertal development and/or spermatogenesis would be impaired. Normally virilized but infertile men are occasionally found to have consistently low serum FSH levels, and a few such patients have been treated with FSH with improvement in sperm output.[57] But because FSH levels may be barely detectable in normal men, these results remain preliminary, and the nature of the defect in FSH secretion has not been established. A patient with cryptorchidism and hypospadias, normal serum LH and testosterone concentrations, and undetectable levels of FSH which normalized after three daily injections of GnRH has also been described.[58]

A series of case reports have described a man with sexual infantilism and a low serum testosterone and elevated serum LH level.[59] But unlike patients with testicular failure, the serum testosterone level increased dramatically following stimulation with hCG and was sufficient to produce sexual maturation and even some spermatogenesis. No measurable LH bioactivity was found in the patient's serum using the dispersed Leydig cell bioassay. Study of polymerase chain reaction products of genomic DNA revealed that this biologically inactive LH molecule was the consequence of a missense mutation in the coding sequence of exon 3, leading to the replacement of glutamine by arginine at amino acid 54. This region of the normal LHβ chain is believed to be important in receptor binding and activation of the signal transduction mechanism. This patient was homozygous for the mutant LHβ, having inherited abnormal alleles from consanguineous parents. Additional studies are required to demonstrate the prevalence of this abnormality in the general population and to clarify the abnormalities that result from the heterozygous state. Preliminary data suggesting a similar syndrome in a second kindred have been reported.[60]

LH and FSH are glycoproteins that exist in the pituitary and in the circulation as a series of charge isoforms that vary in carbohydrate structure. Both hormone clearance from the circulation and biological activity in vivo and in vitro are influenced by the oligosaccharide moieties of the molecule. Regulatory hormones such as GnRH and gonadal steroids have been reported to alter gonadotropin function by modifying the nature of the charge isomers secreted. Gonadotropin deficiency or hypersecretion, aging, and impotence are among the clinical conditions in men in which differences from normal in the ratios of LH or FSH measured by in vitro bioassays and immunoassays have been proposed to contribute to an endocrine disturbance. It is now evident that the purity of the standards used for the various immunoassays and bioassays, technical problems in the bioassay of the low concentrations of gonadotropins in serum, and especially the overstimulation of immunoreactive potency by double-antibody immunoassays necessitate a re-evaluation of the conclusions from many of these investigative studies.[61, 62]

A selective disorder of LH or FSH action on the testis might produce male pseudohermaphroditism or hypospermatogenesis, respectively. A deficiency of testicular LH receptors has been found in patients with sexual ambiguity due to Leydig cell hypoplasia, but the cause of these abnormalities has not been defined.[63] With the recent cloning of the FSH receptor, molecular biology strategies can be used to examine this protein in human male infertility.

Treatment of Gonadotropin-Deficient Men

Androgen deficiency in men with HH is generally treated with parenteral testosterone. In teenagers with congenital HH, androgen treatment stimulates body and beard hair growth, phallus enlargement, muscle development, voice deepening, libido and potency, morning erections, and nocturnal emissions and increases the hematocrit. Androgen treatment stimulates GH production by increasing the amplitude of spontaneous secretory episodes[11] and contributes to the adolescent growth spurt. In addition to the psychological impact of these physical changes, important dose-dependent side effects include acne and gynecomastia. Accordingly, treatment with testosterone cypionate or enanthate at a reduced initial dose of 75 mg monthly is recommended, with gradual increase to a full replacement dose of 200 mg every two weeks over two to three years. Orally administered testosterone derivatives can also be used initially but are less useful when higher doses are needed because they are more costly, less effective, and more prone to side effects. Historically, androgen treatment was often postponed until age 18 years to exclude the possibility of constitutional delay of puberty. Given the pronounced impact of androgen deficiency on bone mass and the social ridicule to which androgen-deficient teenagers are exposed, it seems more appropriate to begin androgen treatment by age 14 to 15 years to produce clinical changes and to withdraw therapy sometime thereafter to re-evaluate endogenous androgen production.

hCG, purified from pregnancy urine, can also be used to stimulate testicular testosterone production with effective virilization. In contrast to treatment with testosterone, hCG stimulates testis growth. Generally, doses of 1500 to 2000 U intramuscularly twice weekly are used because this dose sustains adult serum testosterone levels for four to seven days. Because of cost factors and the need for frequent injections, hCG treatment is usually initiated when fertility is desired. Treatment with testosterone for many years does not preclude a favorable response to hCG.[64] Antibodies to hCG may develop, but resistance to therapy is rare.[65] Induction of testicular aromatase during hCG treatment may produce high serum estradiol levels and gynecomastia; improvement may follow dose reduction.

Although LH and FSH are both required for complete spermatogenesis to occur, selected patients with IHH may produce spermatozoa and successfully impregnate their partners when treated with hCG alone (Fig. 133–8). Responders can be identified by pretreatment testis size which is beyond the 3-ml volume characteristic of prepubertal boys, indicating some endogenous gonadotropin secretion and therefore partial gonadotropin deficiency.[66] Treatment efficacy can be assessed by clinical observation and laboratory studies. Careful measurement of testis size and sequential determination of serum testosterone and inhibin levels can be used to predict which men will produce sperm.[67] In responders, testes grow to a volume of 12 to 15 ml and spermatozoa usually appear in the ejaculate within 12 months of starting treatment. hCG is generally successful in restoring spermatogenesis in men with pitui-

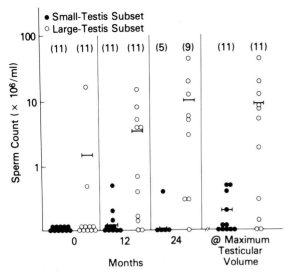

FIGURE 133–8. Mean sperm concentration during hCG therapy in 22 men with isolated hypogonadotropic hypogonadism. Men in the small testis subset (n-11) had a mean testis volume of 3 ml or less at the start of the study, consistent with complete IHH. (From Burris AS, Robard HW, Winters SJ, Sherins RJ: Gonadotropin therapy in men with isolated hypogonadotropic hypogonadism: The response to human chorionic gonadotropin is predicted by initial testicular size. J Clin Endocrinol Metab 66:1144–1151, 1988. © 1988 by the Endocrine Society.)

tary or suprasellar tumors which develop postpubertally (Fig. 133–9).[68] hCG may also sustain sperm production in men with IHH who require both hCG and FSH to initiate spermatogenesis.[69]

The majority of patients with IHH require treatment with FSH as well as hCG to induce spermatogenesis. This group includes patients with complete HH whose pretreatment testis volume is less than 4 ml and those men whose testes fail to grow to volumes of 12 to 15 ml after 12 months of hCG treatment and remain azoospermic.[66] FSH is currently prepared from the urine of postmenopausal women (human menopausal gonadotropin, hMG), although recombinant hFSH is currently being developed. The usual

dose of FSH is 75 IU three times weekly. With this approach a pregnancy rate exceeding 90 per cent has been reported.[70] The sperm concentration at the time of conception may be as low as 1 million/ml, however. Patients with IHH and cryptorchidism respond poorly to therapy (Fig. 133–9). Because Kallmann's syndrome is a genetic disorder, the offspring may be affected, but neither the rate of spontaneous abortion nor the prevalence of somatic abnormalities appears to be increased.

GnRH can also be used to stimulate spermatogenesis in men with GnRH deficiency.[71] Programmable portable infusion pumps are used to provide pulses of GnRH. The intravenous route of administration produces LH pulses of physiological contour, but this approach is dangerous and impractical for long-term use. Instead, the drug is delivered into the subcutaneous tissues of the abdomen. The frequency of administration has been every two hours because most studies in normal men indicate that LH pulses occur at this frequency. A starting dose of 4 μg per pulse is often used, with increments of 2 μg every four weeks if LH and FSH secretions do not rise. Doses as high as 16 μg per pulse have been required in selected patients. Serum testosterone levels are usually in the normal adult range by six to eight weeks. Pulsatile GnRH increases testis size, sometimes dramatically, within three to six months of beginning treatment. As with hCG/FSH treatment, final testicular volume is greater in those patients with partial GnRH deficiency. The testes rarely grow to truly normal adult size, however. Although changes in GnRH dose, frequency, or route of administration may alter this outcome, poor patient compliance is a major limitation of pulsatile GnRH therapy. Impaired Sertoli cell maturation related to an absent or attenuated postnatal surge in gonadotropin secretion or to the effect of prolonged gonadotropin deficiency may also limit the testicular response to GnRH therapy in adulthood. Allergic reactions[72] and GnRH-binding antibodies[73] may develop with long-term GnRH treatment.

Sperm appear in the ejaculate in approximately two thirds of men treated with pulsatile GnRH. In one study,[71] the interval between initiating treatment and the appear-

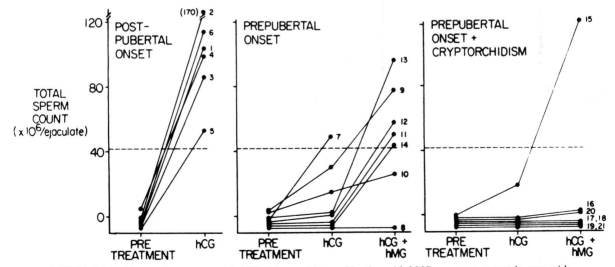

FIGURE 133–9. Effects of treatment with hCG alone and in combination with hMG on sperm output in men with gonadotropin deficiency (GD). Men with GD of postpubertal onset had pituitary adenomas (2), craniopharyngioma (3), or unknown cause (1). Cryptorchidism (unilateral in six of seven) had been treated in childhood in men with GD of prepubertal onset. (Reprinted with permission from Finkel DM, Phillips JL, Snyder PJ: Stimulation of spermatogenesis by gonadotropins in men with hypogonadotropic hypogonadism. N Engl J Med 313:651–655, 1985.)

ance of sperm in the ejaculate ranged from 18 to 139 weeks. The sperm density is most often in the range of 1 to 10 million/ml in men with complete IHH, but sperm counts may reach 60 to 100 million/ml in men with partial gonadotropin deficiency. The pregnancy rate among the partners in the latter subgroup has been reported to exceed 80 per cent,[13] whereas limited information is available for men with complete IHH. One relatively large prospective but nonrandomized study compared treatment with hCG/FSH to that with pulsatile GnRH.[74] Testis size was increased more by GnRH than by hCG/FSH in men with complete IHH, and the time until spermatozoa first appeared in the ejaculate was less for GnRH than for hCG/FSH, 12 versus 20 months. There was no difference in sperm count between the two treatment groups, however (Fig. 133–10), and very few subjects were attempting to conceive. Given the cost, complexity, and inconvenience of pulsatile GnRH therapy, hCG/FSH continues to be recommended. GnRH can be tried with treatment failures. As further data accumulate and treatment approaches are refined, pulsatile GnRH may become the treatment of first choice.

PRIMARY TESTICULAR FAILURE

In men with disorders that affect the testes directly, gonadotropin production increases because of a decline in negative feedback inhibition by testicular steroids and peptides. Thus, elevated LH and FSH levels are markers for primary testicular failure. The testes are usually reduced in size, men are infertile, and symptomatic androgen deficiency is common. When testicular failure develops rapidly, as with orchitis, vasomotor symptoms comparable to those of the female climacteric may occur.[75] In some patients, FSH levels are increased selectively. Although basal serum LH and testosterone levels are normal in these men, a disturbance in LH feedback control is suggested by the exaggerated LH response to stimulation with GnRH.[76]

Moment-to-moment changes in circulating LH levels indicate that the frequency and amplitude of LH secretory episodes are increased in men with testicular failure (Fig. 133–11).[77] Direct sampling of GnRH in hypothalamic-por-

tal blood in orchidectomized rams has confirmed that GnRH pulse frequency increases with testosterone deficiency, but GnRH pulse amplitude remains unchanged. Experiments in rats reveal that castration increases GnRH receptor number and the responsiveness of pituitary cells to GnRH, providing an explanation for the increase in gonadotropin pulse amplitude in men with testicular failure.

Increased FSH concentrations in testicular failure are partly due to increased GnRH secretion inasmuch as GnRH increases FSHβ mRNA, and immunoneutralization of circulating GnRH blocks the castration-induced rise in FSHβ mRNA and FSH secretion. But experiments in male monkeys reveal that testicular inhibin plays an important role in the regulation of FSH in male primates as well.[78] With currently available inhibin assays, however, the expected inverse correlation between serum inhibin and FSH levels in testicular failure patients has not been demonstrated.[79] Low circulating inhibin levels and the lack of specificity of current assays appear to explain these findings. There is evidence for a high molecular weight form of inhibin in serum when FSH levels are increased, and inhibin may bind to serum proteins under certain conditions. Thus, the presence in serum of a mixture of immunologically active moieties with variable biological activity may explain the normal inhibin levels in testicular failure patients and the unanticipated finding of a positive correlation between inhibin and FSH in the serum of men with germinal aplasia. Pituitary activin increases FSH in the rat, but the applicability of this finding to humans is unknown.

Klinefelter's Syndrome and its Variants

The association between small atrophic testes, gynecomastia, variable manifestations of eunuchoidism, and increased urinary gonadotropin excretion was recognized by Klinefelter et al in 1942, and the 47,XXY karyotype was established in 1959.[80] Klinefelter's syndrome occurs in 1 per 500 to 2000 male births, with a similar prevalence among abortuses. Nondysjunction during the meiotic division of gametogenesis leads to the formation of spermatozoa containing both X and Y chromosomal material, or to

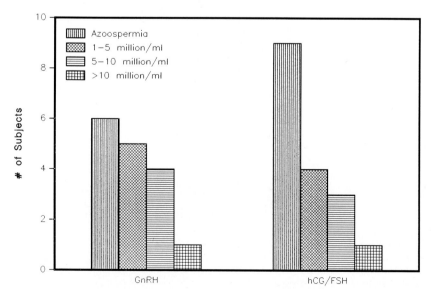

FIGURE 133–10. Histogram showing the results of treatment of men with congenital GnRH deficiency with pulsatile GnRH subcutaneously or hCG/hMG intramuscularly for 4 to 27 months. (Data from Schopohl J, Mehltretter G, von Zumbusch R, et al: Comparison of gonadotropin-releasing hormone and gonadotropin therapy in male patients with idiopathic hypothalamic hypogonadism. Fertil Steril 56:1143–1150, 1991.)

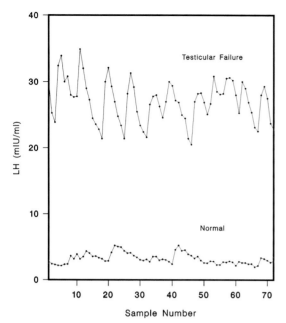

FIGURE 133–11. LH levels in serum samples drawn every 10 minutes for 12 hours beginning at 8:00 AM in a normal adult man aged 21 years and a 35-year-old man with bilateral cryptorchidism.

TABLE 133–4. CLINICAL FEATURES IN PATIENTS WITH KLINEFELTER'S SYNDROME INCLUDING 47,XXY AND VARIANT KARYOTYPES

	BIRTH	CHILD-HOOD	PUBERTY	ADULT-HOOD
Cryptorchidism	x			
Microphallus	x			
Hypospadias	x			
Somatic anomalies	x			
Learning disabilities		x	x	x
Behavioral disorders		x	x	x
Mental retardation		x	x	x
Tall stature			x	x
Eunuchoid habitus			x	x
Delayed puberty			x	
Small testes			x	x
Delayed sex characteristics			x	x
Gynecomastia			x	x
Infertility				x
Impaired libido				x
Thyroid dysfunction				x

24,XX ova. Southern blotting using DNA probes to detect restriction site polymorphisms of the X chromosome in men with Klinefelter's syndrome indicates that the additional X is about as likely to be of maternal as of paternal origin.[81] These gametes may fuse with a normal ovum or spermatozoon, respectively, producing a 47,XXY or variant karyotype. There is a marked association between advanced maternal age and maternally derived Klinefelter's syndrome.

The clinical features of 47,XXY males[82] are summarized in Table 133–4. Small testes and phallus and a tall, thin body habitus are clues to the diagnosis of Klinefelter's syndrome in childhood, although these findings overlap with normal.[83] Behavioral problems may also occur. The diagnosis of Klinefelter's syndrome is generally made, however, in teenage boys who present with gynecomastia, incomplete pubertal development, or small testes (Fig. 133–12). Some patients present in adulthood with similar complaints or with impotence or infertility. Virtually all patients with Klinefelter's syndrome are azoospermic.[85] A testicular biopsy from a man with Klinefelter's syndrome is shown in Figure 133–13. There is tubular sclerosis and apparent Leydig hyperplasia. A few tubules may contain Sertoli cells and sparse germ cells. Large clumps of Leydig cells are present between the sclerotic tubules.[84] A subtle reduction in mean seminiferous tubule diameter and in the number of germ cells has been demonstrated in young boys with Klinefelter's syndrome. By adolescence, loss of germ cells, Sertoli cell atrophy, and thickening of the tunica propria occur. Estimates of the prevalence of gynecomastia range from 25 to 88 per cent, depending upon the method of examination. Immune disorders such as thyroiditis, systemic lupus, and progressive systemic sclerosis appear to be more common in Klinefelter's syndrome than in normal men, and an association with leg ulcers and CNS germinomas has been reported. Gonadotroph hyperplasia and hypertrophy producing pituitary enlargement and simulating a pituitary

adenoma have been reported in untreated patients.[86] Somatic growth may be abnormal even before adolescence, including increased stature and long limbs.[80] In adults, not only are the limbs long, but the arm span often exceeds the height, presumably because of delayed epiphyseal fusion. Profound hypogonadism in men is associated with osteopenia and increased fracture rate. Bone density may be reduced in men with Klinefelter's syndrome,[87] but it is uncertain whether this difference results in symptomatic bone disease. The pathophysiology of the osteopenia is unknown, and it is uncertain whether testosterone influences bone matrix and mineral directly. Although testosterone treatment increased total and free plasma 1,25-dihydroxyvitamin D levels as well as calcium absorption,

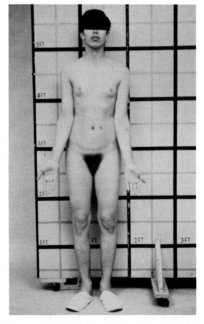

FIGURE 133–12. A 19-year-old patient with Klinefelter's syndrome (47,XXY). The testes were small (1.8 cm in length) and firm, the phallus was small (4 cm stretched), and gynecomastia was present. The arm span exceeded the height, and crown to pubis length was less than that of the lower body segment (0.9).

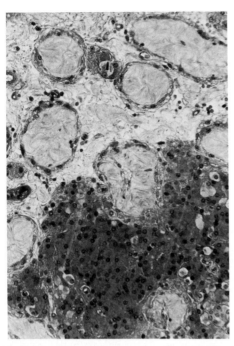

FIGURE 133–13. Testicular biopsy from a patient with Klinefelter's syndrome. Seminiferous tubules are reduced in diameter and are hyalinized. In many biopsies, a few tubules containing Sertoli cells can be identified, however. The Leydig cells form large clumps between the sclerosed tubules. (Courtesy of C. A. Paulsen.)

these parameters do not appear to be abnormal in untreated patients.[88]

The data in Table 133–5 reveal that serum LH and FSH levels are uniformly increased in men with Klinefelter's syndrome, indicating Leydig cell as well as seminiferous tubular dysfunction.[89] But it remains to be determined whether Leydig cell dysfunction results from the paracrine effects of germ cell or Sertoli cell damage, or some other mechanism. Mean serum testosterone levels are reduced, but in as many as one third of patients, total testosterone levels are in the low-normal range. Both the testosterone production rate and the free testosterone concentration are uniformly low, however. Increased SHBG production is the best explanation for these findings, although not all studies have found SHBG to be increased in Klinefelter's syndrome.[90] Inadequate Leydig cell function is confirmed by the attenuated testosterone response to hCG stimulation. The secretion of 17-hydroxyprogesterone following hCG stimulation is not diminished, however, suggesting an impairment in C17–20 lyase activity.[91] Serum estradiol levels are generally within the range of normal, although the conversion rate of radiolabeled testosterone to estradiol is greater than normal, perhaps because of the effects of high LH levels on testicular aromatase activity.[89] The rise in estradiol relative to testosterone secretion may explain the exaggerated PRL response to thyrotropin-releasing hormone (TRH) administration.[92] Leydig cell function declines further with aging, as in normal men.

Although men with Klinefelter's syndrome are permanently sterile, androgen deficiency can be treated successfully with testosterone. No controlled studies provide guidance as to when to initiate treatment, however, and this decision relies heavily on clinical judgment. Follow-up of testosterone-treated patients suggests that treatment is as-

sociated with better mood, better school performance, increased work capacity, and less irritability, as well as increased strength, libido, and potency.[93] Testosterone treatment may worsen gynecomastia, however, because of the aromatization of injected testosterone to estradiol.[94] Clinical responses and circulating steroid concentrations, but not gonadotropin levels, should be used to monitor therapy because testosterone suppresses gonadotropin secretion less effectively in men with Klinefelter's syndrome than in normal men.[94, 95]

46,XY/47,XXY mosaicism is the most common cytogenetic variant of Klinefelter's syndrome, accounting for approximately 20 per cent of X-chromatin–positive patients.[85] The karyotype of cultured skin fibroblasts or of testicular cells may reveal a mosaic pattern not identified in peripheral leukocytes. Clinical abnormalities are generally less pronounced and seminiferous tubular damage is less severe in these men.[96] Fertility has been reported. Males with other sex chromosomal abnormalities, including 48,XXYY, 48,XXXY, and 49,XXXXY, have been reported.[97, 98] Like patients with 47,XXY, they have primary testicular failure, but they are more likely to be short and mentally retarded and to have unusual facies.

Approximately 1 per 20,000 men has a female (46,XX) sex chromosome constitution.[99] The phenotype of these men is similar to that of men with Klinefelter's syndrome, but short stature and hypospadias are more common. The paradox of the 46,XX male has been explained for most patients by the observation that DNA sequences normally found on the short arm of the Y chromosome are present instead on the short arm of the X, although routine chromosomal banding methods are unable to detect the abnormality. This interchange results from the frequent X-Y recombinations that occur during normal male meiosis.[100] Some subjects appear to lack Y sequences, however.[100a]

The 47,XYY karyotype occurs in 1 to 2 per 1000 men. They are phenotypically normal males but are often tall and thin. Testicular function is usually normal, although patients with impaired spermatogenesis have been reported.[101] Most 47,XYY men are fertile and produce chromosomally normal 46,XX daughters and 46,XY sons. Preliminary data indicate that the prevalence of chromosomal abnormalities in sperm from 47,XYY men is similar to that of normal men, suggesting that the extra Y chromosome is eliminated in germ cells.[102] Psychological problems are increased, because the prevalence of this abnormality in mental and mental-penal institutions is 10-fold greater than in the general population. It has been estimated, however, that these men have only a 1 per cent incidence of criminal behavior, compared with a 0.1 per cent risk for normal men.

TABLE 133–5. RANGE OF HORMONE VALUES IN MEN WITH KLINEFELTER'S SYNDROME COMPARED WITH HEALTHY MEN

	KLINEFELTER'S SYNDROME	HEALTHY MEN
Serum LH (mIU/ml)	4.25–12.7 (7.8)	0.62–2.81 (1.8)
Serum FSH (mIU/ml)	12.1–61.2 (29.4)	0.51–5.2 (2.7)
Plasma testosterone (ng/dl)	81–849 (316)	346–1075 (990)
Plasma estradiol (pg/ml)	3–65 (34)	UD–34 (16)

From Wang C, Baker HWG, Burger HG, et al: Hormonal studies in Klinefelter's syndrome. Clin Endocrinol 4:399–411, 1975. Values in parentheses are the population means.

Cryptorchidism

Cryptorchidism is a common congenital anomaly with a prevalence of 2.7 per cent at birth.[103] But because testicular descent may occur in the newborn, this figure declines to about 1 per cent at age three months, where it remains into adulthood. Although it is clear that men with cryptorchidism are often infertile, neither the pathogenesis of cryptorchidism nor the impact of surgery or medical therapy on the natural history of this disorder is known with certainty. It is also unclear to what extent the hypospermatogenesis, abnormal androgen secretion, and predilection for testicular cancer to develop is due to an underlying disorder of the testis or is the consequence of its cryptorchid location. Biopsies of the contralateral scrotal testis in adulthood, which are normal only 25 per cent of the time, indicate that most cases of unilateral cryptorchidism are not simply an anatomical failure of testicular descent.[104, 105]

Cryptorchidism is generally classified anatomically, although various nomenclatures are used. Approximately 10 per cent of cryptorchid testes are intra-abdominal, 20 per cent are within the inguinal canal, 66 per cent have passed through the external inguinal ring but remain high in the scrotum, and 3 per cent are absent at surgical exploration.[106] Cryptorchidism is bilateral in 10 to 15 per cent of cases. Hypertrophy of a solitary scrotal testis is occasionally found and has been suggested to predict monorchism,[107] but the scrotal testis is sometimes enlarged in cryptorchidism as well.[108] Studies in prepubertal experimental animals undergoing unilateral orchidectomy suggest that decreased inhibin production leading to increased FSH secretion could be responsible for this finding under conditions in which the contralateral testis is otherwise normal.

Most high scrotal testes are retractile; that is, they ascend when the patient is examined but are found in the scrotum when the patient is completely relaxed, such as in the bathtub. The retraction is thought to be due to an active cremasteric reflex that attenuates at puberty. High scrotal testes may also be ectopic, a situation in which the gubernaculum is attached outside the normal pathway of testicular descent, such as on the inner surface of the thigh or in the perineum, or they may be associated with a hernia or hydrocele. Finally, the testicular pathway may be obstructed by fascia. The high scrotal testis is sometimes associated with ipsilateral scrotal hypoplasia. It is generally written that most patients with retractile testes are fertile and need no treatment, although some data are conflicting.[109] Difficulty distinguishing the retractile from the cryptorchid testis has been a major impediment to understanding the natural history of cryptorchidism and to analyzing the results of treatment.

Hormonal mechanisms are thought to be important in the normal descent of the testis into the scrotum and in the pathogenesis of some forms of cryptorchidism.[110] A role for testosterone is supported by the finding that antiandrogen treatment of pregnant dams blocks testicular descent in rat pups.[111] Moreover, cryptorchidism occurs in patients with congenital HH, defects in testosterone biosynthesis, and androgen resistance syndromes. But cryptorchidism is unusual among boys with HH, and in the latter two conditions, abnormal scrotal development could also limit testicular descent. The finding of low postnatal testosterone and LH levels has led to the proposal that gonadotropin secretion in cryptorchid boys is defective in late fetal and neonatal life through a mechanism that permits normal activation of gonadotropin secretion at puberty,[112] but this mechanism has not been established. Moreover, the results of newer, more sensitive immunoradiometric assays suggest that LH and FSH levels are often increased rather than decreased in prepubertal boys with cryptorchidism. Müllerian inhibitory factor (MIF) is a differentiation factor produced by the fetal and prepubertal testis which is structurally related to transforming growth factor-β. MIF leads to regression of müllerian ducts during the embryonic development of the male reproductive tract and could play a role in testicular descent. Among cryptorchid boys, MIF levels are less than normal, but the differences are small and inconsistent.[113] In the prune belly syndrome, the abdominal muscles are incomplete and cryptorchidism is common, suggesting that increased intra-abdominal pressure is required for testicular descent to occur. The frequent occurrence of cryptorchidism in patients with spina bifida suggests that spinal nerves are important in transmitting the signal for testicular descent. Although 95 per cent of patients with cryptorchidism have a 46,XY karyotype, cryptorchidism is common in boys with major autosomal abnormalities and other congenital malformations. The incidence of cryptorchidism is also increased several-fold by premature birth of whatever cause.

Because testicular function is frequently abnormal in adult men with cryptorchidism, orchidopexy is almost always performed in childhood. Testicular biopsies of boys undergoing orchidopexy provide evidence for damage to the seminiferous tubules by age one year.[114] Accordingly, surgery is currently recommended between ages 12 and 18 months, to allow for those testes that descend spontaneously in the first year of life. Although an anatomical success, surgical correction of cryptorchidism has not been convincingly shown to alter testicular function.[115] The size of the previously undescended testis is almost always reduced in adulthood, and serum FSH levels and the FSH response to GnRH stimulation are increased.[116] In patients with a history of unilateral cryptorchidism, Leydig cell function is relatively normal with normal total and free testosterone and basal LH levels, but the LH response to GnRH may be exaggerated. High LH and low testosterone levels are common in men with surgically corrected bilateral cryptorchidism.[116]

The most clinically important aspect of cryptorchidism is its impact on fertility. Most patients with bilateral cryptorchidism are infertile, with sperm counts of less than 20 million spermatozoa/ml, and orchidopexy appears to have little influence on these results (Table 133–6).[115, 116] The outlook is much better for men with unilateral cryptorchidism, in whom fertility rates approximating 60 per cent are reported, although the impact of orchidopexy is again unproven.[115, 117] In many studies, a sperm density of 20 million/ml has been used to define fertility, with no attention to sperm motility or morphology, and no direct information on pregnancy rate is provided.

Experience in treating cryptorchidism with hCG is extensive.[118] The success rate is variable, however, and ranges from 14 to 50 per cent. Differences in dose and duration of treatment, definitions of success, and the percentage of patients with retractile and not cryptorchid testes probably account for this variability. Because long-term hCG treatment produces unacceptable masculinization in prepuber-

TABLE 133–6. SPERM COUNTS IN PATIENTS WITH A HISTORY OF CRYPTORCHIDISM*

TREATMENT POLICY	AZOOSPERMIC TOTAL (%)	OLIGOSPERMIC TOTAL (%)	AZOOSPERMIC + OLIGOSPERMIC TOTAL† (%)
Bilateral			
None	16/20 (75)	4/20 (25)	20/20 (100)
Orchidopexy	65/156 (42)	49/156 (31)	114/154 (74)
hCG ± opxy	28/50 (56)	9/50 (18)	72/99 (73)
Opxy ± hCG	12/42 (29)	18/42 (43)	63/78 (81)
All treatments	105/248 (42)	76/248 (31)	249/331 (75)
Unilateral			
None	1/14 (7)	9/14 (64)	27/61 (44)
Orchidopexy	66/379 (17)	98/308 (32)	157/384 (41)
hCG ± opxy	2/43 (5)	15/43 (35)	56/115 (49)
Opxy ± hCG	4/97 (4)	11/55 (20)	44/101 (44)
All treatments	72/519 (14)	124/406 (31)	257/600 (43)

*Excludes studies of cases presenting at infertility clinics or for vasectomy. Oligospermic is defined as a sperm density > zero and < 20×10^6/ml.
†Some authors do not distinguish between azoospermic and oligospermic patients; hence the numbers in the final column may be larger than the sum of the azoospermic and oligospermic columns.
From Chilvers C, Dudley NE, Gough MH, et al: Undescended testis: The effect of treatment on subsequent risk of subfertility and malignancy. J Pediatr Surg 8:691–696, 1986.

tal boys, cumulative doses of 6000 to 13,500 U over six weeks have been recommended. Treatment with intranasal GnRH has also been advocated, with success rates ranging from 20 to 78 per cent. With this therapy, there is generally little evidence of sexual maturation, and intramuscular injections are avoided. Studies with favorable results have been criticized, however, because of the inclusion of patients with retractile testes, and because they lack an appropriate control group. In a double-blind placebo-controlled study, success with intranasal GnRH was only slightly greater than success with placebo and was less than the 21 per cent response rate for hCG.[119] The results of several other studies are in agreement. According to one interpretation, successful hormonal treatment distinguishes retractile from cryptorchid testes and obviates the need for surgery in the former. Thus, when the undescended testis is extra-abdominal and is in a path of normal descent into the scrotum, a trial of hCG treatment prior to surgery is recommended.

The incidence of testicular cancer is increased in patients with cryptorchidism. Among men with testis cancer, about 10 per cent have a history of cryptorchidism, compared with the expected figure of 1 per cent. Cancer risk is highest in those men with abdominal testes, and the entire spectrum of malignant germ cell tumors is observed. Sometimes testicular cancer occurs in the contralateral scrotal testis. Orchidopexy does not prevent the development of testis cancer, and no data indicate that orchidopexy at any age reduces the risk of cancer.[115] But the follow-up of boys who have undergone early orchidopexy is too short to allow for a final conclusion at present. Testicular cancer occurs most often between ages 20 and 44 years and is much less common in the elderly.[120] Thus, young adults with abdominal testes are usually referred for orchiectomy because of the risk for occult malignant degeneration, whereas surgery is generally not performed in older men. An adult with an inguinal testis can probably be followed with yearly evaluations.

Noonan's Syndrome

Patients with Noonan's syndrome have multiple congenital anomalies, including a characteristic facies, valvular heart disease, short stature, and hypogonadism (Table 133–7). In one series, 77 per cent of affected males had cryptorchidism.[121] Because of the resemblance of these phenotypic features to those of girls with Turner's syndrome, the term *male Turner's syndrome* has been used. However, the karyotype of males with Noonan's syndrome is 46,XY. Most cases are sporadic, but affected families have been described in which the disorder is inherited as an autosomal dominant trait.[122] The karyotype of affected females is also normal. The most characteristic cardiac lesion is pulmonary valvular stenosis with dysplastic valve leaflets, which often requires valvuloplasty. The aortic coarctation and renal abnormalities found in Turner's syndrome do not occur in Noonan's syndrome. Short stature and delayed puberty are common. Cryptorchidism is generally associated with the endocrine findings of primary testicular

TABLE 133–7. CLINICAL FINDINGS IN PATIENTS WITH NOONAN'S SYNDROME

Facial abnormalities
  Hypertelorism, down-slanting palpebral fissures
  High arched eyebrows, ptosis
  Low-set prominent ears, thickened helix
  Depressed nasal bridge
  High arched palate
  Dental malocclusion
  Broad, short, webbed neck
  Low posterior hairline
Cardiac defects
  Pulmonary valvular stenosis
  Hypertrophic cardiomyopathy
  Atrial septal defect
  Ventricular septal defect
  Conduction defects
  Coronary artery anomalies
Short stature
Delayed puberty
Cryptorchidism
Pectus excavatum
Bleeding diathesis
Lymphedema
Hypotonia
Hyperextensible joints
Neurofibromas
Hepatosplenomegaly

failure, including hypospermatogenesis and androgen deficiency,[123] although a patient with idiopathic hypopituitarism and Noonan's syndrome has been reported.[124] Rarely are adult men fertile, but father-to-son transmission of the trait can occur.

Congenital Anorchia

Congenital anorchia (vanishing testis syndrome) is the term used for the absence of testicular tissue in 46,XY phenotypic males. The condition is unilateral in 97 per cent of cases. Müllerian structures are absent and wolffian structures are normal, but the vas deferens is often rudimentary and the epididymis is absent. Instead, the vas deferens ends in a fibrovascular bundle that may be calcified and contain iron pigment.[125] There are also phenotypic males with bilateral anorchia. Anorchia is a sporadic disorder, and bilateral anorchia has been reported in an identical twin whose brother was normal. Testicular function must be normal in the first trimester in these men, and one hypothesis is that descent into the scrotum is accompanied by testicular torsion. The sequence of the SRY gene, which codes for the testis determining factor, appears to be normal.[125a] At birth the penis and scrotum are small. Boys with congenital anorchia are distinguished from those with bilateral abdominal cryptorchidism by MR scanning, laparoscopy, surgical exploration, or the failure of serum testosterone levels to increase after stimulation with hCG.[126] Puberty fails to occur, and serum LH and FSH levels are in the castrate range. Rarely, there is evidence for limited Leydig cell function, although no testes are found at surgery.[127] Therefore, the finding of a spermatic-peripheral gradient in testosterone levels, suggesting functional Leydig cells, does not guarantee that a testis is present. Testosterone treatment is begun in the early teenage years and is lifelong.

Germinal Cell Aplasia

Del Castillo et al.[128] described five sexually mature young adult men with small testes and azoospermia in whom testis biopsies revealed seminiferous tubules with no spermatogenic cells, but only Sertoli cells, and Leydig cells had a normal morphological appearance (Fig. 133–14). These men have a normal 46,XY karyotype and increased serum FSH levels, but LH and testosterone concentrations are normal. The LH response to GnRH stimulation is exaggerated, however, suggesting that Leydig cell function is somewhat impaired.[75] The cause of the ''Sertoli-cell–only'' syndrome remains unknown. Focal germinal cell aplasia is also observed in the testes of patients with cryptorchidism, chronic renal failure, Klinefelter's syndrome, 47,XYY karyotype, hypogonadotropic hypogonadism, and following estrogen treatment.[129] The largest patient population with germinal cell aplasia, however, is men who have received cancer chemotherapy.

Orchitis

The incidence of mumps in the United States has declined dramatically since the introduction of the live atten-

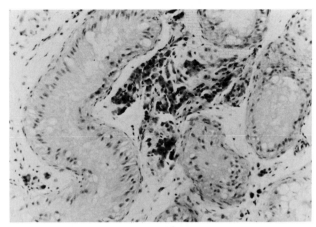

FIGURE 133–14. Testicular biopsy revealing germinal cell aplasia. Seminiferous tubules are reduced slightly in diameter and contain only Sertoli cells. Ultrastructural studies have revealed immature Sertoli cells in certain patients. (H&E, × 40).

uated mumps vaccine. Nevertheless, mumps can be a severe illness in adults. Orchitis typically develops within one week of, but may precede, parotitis. Although clinical orchitis is rare in prepubertal boys, orchitis occurs in 15 to 35 per cent of adolescents and adult men infected with the mumps virus, and in 25 per cent of them orchitis is bilateral. Most often, focal testicular lesions occur which appear to be without long-term clinical sequelae. In severe cases distention of the seminiferous tubules with leukocytes is followed by necrosis and atrophy. In one survey, testicular atrophy and/or azoospermia developed in 22 per cent of men with mumps orchitis.[130] Clinical hypogonadism and gynecomastia occur because circulating testosterone declines to very low levels, but estradiol and estrone, which are primarily produced in peripheral tissues, are normal. Serum LH and FSH increase markedly.[131] Testicular failure involving both the seminiferous tubules and Leydig cells also occurs occasionally in men with leprosy, syphilis, tuberculosis, brucellosis, nocardiosis, salmonellosis, schistosomiasis, and filariasis. Epididymo-orchitis is also a complication of gonorrhea.

Testes from men infected with the human immunodeficiency virus (HIV) frequently have absent or reduced spermatogenesis, tubular basement membrane thickening, and mild inflammation.[132] There are case reports of HIV-associated orchitis from toxoplasmosis, cryptococcus, tuberculosis, or cytomegalovirus. Men affected with HIV may complain of decreased libido, loss of body hair, muscle wasting, and gynecomastia. Serum sex hormone concentrations are normal in apparently healthy HIV seropositive patients, whereas low testosterone together with elevated LH and FSH levels occur quite often in men with more advanced AIDS.[133–135] The role of viral infection or cytokines released from lymphocytes and microphages in the development of testicular failure is unknown. With further disease progression to lymphocyte depletion and weight loss, gonadotropin deficiency occurs.

Immune disorders may affect the testis. Hypogonadism occurs in 7 per cent of patients with polyendocrine deficiency types I and II.[136] As in other autoimmune disorders, males are less frequently affected than are females. Primary testicular failure is generally observed, but gonadotropin deficiency has also been reported.[137] Men with testicular failure together with primary systemic sclerosis[138] or idiopathic retroperitoneal fibrosis[139] have also been described. PSS may be associated with Klinefelter's syndrome.[140] Most patients with polyarteritis have lesions of the internal spermatic artery and histological evidence of testicular infarcts and hemorrhage with focal degeneration of the seminiferous tubules, but clinical orchitis and hypogonadism are unusual.[141] There is limited information on testicular function in men with systemic lupus erythematosus, although evidence for increased circulating levels of estrone and estradiol has been presented.[142] Drugs used to treat these illnesses may also impair testicular function.

Miscellaneous Causes of Testicular Failure

Myotonic muscular dystrophy is an autosomal dominant, multisystem disorder in which myotonia is accompanied by weakness. Systemic abnormalities include frontal balding, cataracts, cardiac conduction defects, insulin resistance, and testicular insufficiency. The symptom complex ranges from asymptomatic adults to newborns with hypotonia and mental retardation, and the severity of myotonic dystrophy increases over generations. Mean serum LH and FSH levels are increased and testosterone is reduced, but many patients have normal values and are fertile. In one study, testicular atrophy was found in two thirds of patients.[143] Serum testosterone levels do not correlate with diminished muscle mass.

Testicular trauma and the vascular insufficiency that accompanies testicular torsion in pubertal boys may produce hypogonadism.[144] In keeping with the greater sensitivity of the seminiferous tubules than the Leydig cells to sustain damage, these conditions may produce oligospermia or azoospermia and elevated FSH levels but normal LH and testosterone concentrations. The occurrence of infertility and abnormal semen analyses in adult men who had undergone successful early unilateral detorsion suggests that torsion may occur in patients with an underlying disorder of the testes.

Patients with spinal cord injuries and paraplegia or quadriplegia are commonly unable to sustain an erection or to ejaculate. Small testes and elevated FSH and LH levels are common in these men.[145] Serum testosterone levels are generally normal. Spermatogenesis is almost always abnormal, and some men are azoospermic. The condition appears to worsen as the time elapsed after spinal cord injury increases.

Exposure of the testes to external radiation damages spermatogenesis.[146] Transiently reduced sperm counts are observed with exposures as low as 15 rads, and permanent sterility may occur with exposure to 1000 rads.

SYSTEMIC DISORDERS THAT AFFECT TESTICULAR FUNCTION

Aging

The normal aging process in men is associated with a gradual decline in testicular function, which contrasts with the abrupt cessation of ovarian function that defines the female climacteric.[147] The dominant process leading to these changes is primary testicular failure.[148] Gonadotropin secretion is also altered by aging, however, leading to a "double defect."[149] Early reports of hormone changes with aging in men provided misleading results because hospitalized or nursing home subjects rather than healthy older men were studied, so that the effects of illness as well as aging were examined. Nevertheless, it is now evident that serum total, free, and bioavailable (not bound to SHBG) testosterone levels fall with aging, although there is a wide range of variation.[150–153] The decline is most pronounced when morning plasma samples are examined because testosterone levels are highest in the morning in young adult men, whereas there is less circadian variation in the elderly.[151] Leydig cell reserve is reduced inasmuch as the testosterone response to hCG stimulation is blunted. Most, but not all, studies report that the mean LH level increases with age, but the rise is moderate, and most values in elderly men overlap with the normal range for young men.[147–153] The rise of serum FSH is more constant and correlates with an impairment in germ cell maturation[154] which may relate to atherosclerotic changes in testicular arterioles. A decline in LH and FSH metabolic clearance may also contribute to the elevated serum gonadotropin levels. Circulating inhibin levels are reduced, indicating that Sertoli cell function also decreases in elderly men.[155, 156]

The absence of a pronounced increase in LH secretion when free and bioavailable testosterone levels are low suggests that gonadotropin secretion is impaired with aging.[157] A defect in GnRH signal transduction is suggested by the delayed release of LH into the circulation following GnRH stimulation,[149, 153] although a reduction in the clearance of LH with aging may also contribute to this finding. LH pulse frequency does not appear to change appreciably with aging.[149] The number of large LH pulses per 12 hours appears to decline, however, and the magnitude of the LH response to submaximal doses of GnRH appears to be unchanged in elderly men.[158, 159] Together, these data suggest that the mass of GnRH secreted per burst may decrease with aging. The blunted diurnal rhythm in testosterone secretion observed in aging men appears to have a primary testicular basis because young men with testicular insufficiency demonstrate a similar change.[43]

One explanation for a reduction in GnRH secretion in aged men is enhanced feedback inhibition by testosterone. Indeed, infusion of the nonaromatizable androgen, dihydrotestosterone, in amounts equivalent to the physiological production rate of testosterone suppressed LH secretion more in elderly than in young men.[160] Serum levels of DHT were similar in both groups, as was the suppression of SHBG concentrations. The feedback effects of estradiol on LH secretion, by contrast, were comparable in both groups, as was production of LH when estrogen feedback was blocked by clomiphene.[148, 160]

The decrease in sexual performance which occurs in elderly men is an important health concern.[152] Multiple factors including medications taken, chronic illness, vascular disease, neurological degeneration and depression, and decreased testosterone production could contribute to the development of erectile dysfunction. At present little evidence indicates that testosterone treatment benefits the otherwise healthy elderly impotent man.[161]

TABLE 133–8. Testicular Function in Healthy Distance Runners

	WEIGHT (kg)	BMI (kg/m²)	SPERM COUNT (10⁶/ml)	TESTOSTERONE (ng/ml)
Normospermic runners (n = 18)	65.6	24.9	134	4.45
Patient				
A	51	17.8	6.0	1.0
B	62.7	21.7	5.0	1.2

From Ayers JWT, Komesu Y, Romani T, Ansbacher R: Anthropomorphic, hormonal, and psychologic correlates of semen quality in endurance trained male athletes. Fertil Steril 43:917–921, 1985. Patients A and B are 2 of 20 runners examined who were found to have severe oligospermia.

Stress, Exercise, and Illness

Short-term, intensive exercise in men is associated with a 10 to 25 per cent rise in serum testosterone levels.[162] Contributing factors are hemoconcentration and an exercise-related decline in testosterone metabolic clearance because of decreased hepatic blood flow. After several hours of heavy exercise serum testosterone levels are significantly reduced,[163] and during prolonged, intensive physical exercise with weight loss and sleep deprivation, testosterone concentrations may fall into the profoundly hypogonadal range.[164] Under these conditions LH deficiency can be clearly documented. Treatment with a GnRH agonist prevented the decline in serum testosterone which followed four hours of bicycling, suggesting that short-term exercise suppresses GnRH secretion.[163]

Mean LH, FSH, and testosterone levels in long-term regularly exercising marathon runners, by contrast, are generally similar to or only slightly less than those of normal men, although some data are conflicting.[165-169] The intensity of training, variable weight loss, and the delay between the completion of exercise and blood sampling may contribute to the varying results. In one study, fewer LH pulses and a reduction in LH pulse amplitude were found in runners, but the physiological significance of these findings is uncertain because mean LH and testosterone levels were normal.[167] In a second study, normal pulsatile LH secretion was found in men who were running at least 50 miles per week and who were 90 to 95 per cent of ideal body weight.[166] In a third study of 20 marathon runners, 18 had a normal semen analysis. In two men whose body mass index was less than 20 kg/m², however, oligospermia and low serum testosterone levels were observed (Table 133–8).[169] Thus, sustained high-level training producing thinness may cause hypogonadism in men, but in most men, participation in competitive athletics does not significantly impair testicular function.

HH occurs following surgery, burn trauma, head injury, and myocardial infarction, with changes evident within 24 hours (Fig. 133–15).[170-174] Among intensive care unit patients, very low testosterone levels are a predictor of mortality.[173] Psychological stress may also reduce serum testosterone levels.[175] Illness-related gonadotropin deficiency makes it difficult to evaluate clinically the pituitary-testicular function of patients who also have acute or chronic illness.

Stresses are often associated with a reduction in food intake, so that nutritional factors may contribute to the disturbance in testicular function. LH, FSH, and testosterone levels decline during brief periods of fasting in normal

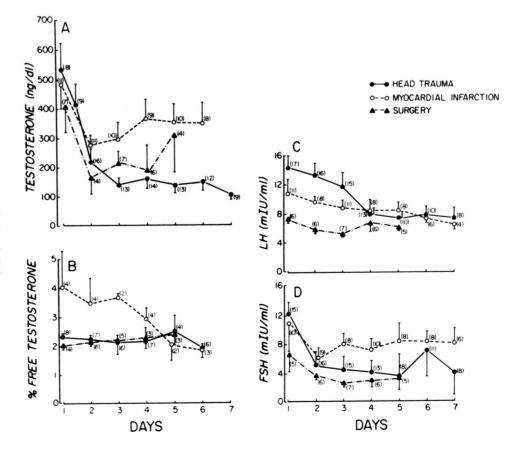

FIGURE 133–15. Daily plasma total and per cent ultrafilterable testosterone, LH, and FSH levels in 17 men with traumatic brain injury, 11 men with myocardial infarction, and 7 men undergoing elective surgery. (From Wolff PD, Hamill RW, McDonald JV, et al: Transient hypogonadotropic hypogonadism caused by critical illness. J Clin Endocrinol Metab 60:444–450, 1985. © by the Endocrine Society.)

adult men. It has been alternatively claimed that fasting decreases LH pulse frequency[176] or amplitude.[176a] Decreased GnRH secretion is suggested because short-term fasting increases the LH and FSH response to GnRH stimulation.[177]

Anorexia nervosa develops in teenage boys about one tenth as often as in girls. Testicular growth may occur, but testosterone and LH concentrations are very low and are often in the prepubertal range. Many of the symptoms of anorexia nervosa are reminiscent of hypopituitarism. Dry skin covered with lanugo-type hair, bradycardia, and a distorted attitude toward food and body image are clues to the diagnosis. In otherwise normal men with severe chronic malnutrition, by contrast, serum testosterone levels are often reduced, but LH levels are normal or increased with equal frequency.[178]

Among the factors with antigonadotropic activity which may be responsible for the suppression of testicular function during stress are ACTH, cortisol, CRF, PRL, opiate peptides, and interleukin-1 (IL-1).[179] Basal ACTH and cortisol levels are higher in trained athletes than in untrained controls, and acute exercise further stimulates ACTH and cortisol release.[180, 181] Plasma cortisol levels are increased in patients with anorexia nervosa, whereas ACTH levels are normal and the ACTH response to CRF stimulation is attenuated.[182] Increased CRF secretion has been suggested to explain these findings. Injections of CRF into the ventricles of the CNS in rodents and primates suppressed GnRH secretion, and CRF antagonists prevent the stress-induced suppression of LH secretion. PRL levels also increase during acute exercise, but serum PRL levels are normal or reduced in endurance-trained athletes or patients with anorexia nervosa.[181] Opiates reduce gonadotropin secretion, and opiate antagonists appear to increase GnRH secretion. Thus it is generally accepted that endogenous opioid peptides exert a tonic inhibitory tone on GnRH secretion which is increased during stress. Acute exercise stimulates the production by lymphocytes of several cytokines, including IL-1. The injection of pharmacological amounts of IL-1 into the cerebral ventricles (icv) of rats decreases LH secretion, and IL-1 antisera or receptor antagonists partially block the suppression of LH secretion which results from icv injection of *Escherichia coli* lipopolysaccharide. In monkeys there is evidence that CRF mediates the antigonadotropic effect of IL-1. Insulin-like growth factor I (IGF I) levels decline during starvation in experimental animals and humans, and IGF I has been reported to augment LH secretion by cultured pituitary cells, but no evidence at present indicates that gonadotropin deficiency is related to decreased IGF I production.[183, 184]

Obesity

Hypogonadism is often suspected clinically in obese men, and circulating testosterone levels are often reduced.[185] Total testosterone levels decrease as body mass index increases, partly because SHBG concentrations decline. Hyperinsulinism due to peripheral insulin resistance is believed to suppress hepatic SHBG production.[186] Free and non–SHBG-bound testosterone levels may also decline with massive obesity, however (Fig. 133–16).[187] Interestingly, sperm output in obese men is usually normal.[188]

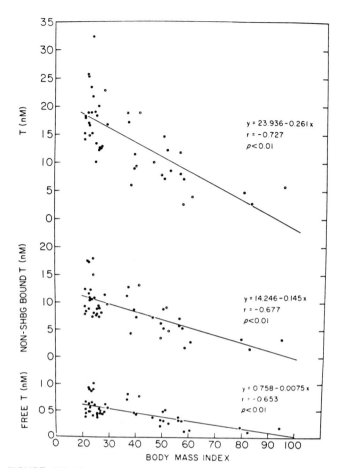

FIGURE 133–16. Relationship between body mass index (kg/m²) and total, non–SHBG-bound and free testosterone levels in 48 healthy male volunteers aged 33.2 ± 12.0 (SD) years. (From Zumoff B, Strain GW, Miller LK, et al: Plasma free and non–sex-hormone-binding-globulin–bound testosterone are decreased in obese men in proportion to their degree of obesity. J Clin Endocrinol Metab 71:929–931, 1990. © by the Endocrine Society.)

Mean serum estrone and estradiol levels are often increased several-fold.[189] One proposal is that increased estrogen production due to aromatase in adipose tissue inhibits gonadotropin pulse amplitude.[189a] With weight loss, circulating estrone falls and testosterone levels increase.[190] Low gonadotropins together with low testosterone levels may be interpreted to reflect a mass lesion of the pituitary or hypothalamus. Because these findings are anticipated with obesity, caution is advised before beginning an extensive evaluation of pituitary function in obese men.

Thyroid Disease

Hyperthyroid men may complain of gynecomastia, impotence, and infertility, and several hormonal abnormalities have been identified which may explain these symptoms. Total testosterone and estradiol levels are higher than normal, in part because of the effect of thyroxine to increase SHBG production.[191] Free testosterone levels are maintained within the range of normal, but free estradiol levels are elevated because the peripheral bioconversion of testosterone to estradiol is increased.[192] Basal and GnRH-stimulated LH and FSH levels are elevated, which may be an adaptation to the increased binding of circulating testosterone to SHBG. A second explanation is that higher-than-normal circulating serum free estradiol concentrations impair testicular function. In support of this hypothesis, sperm motility and density may be reduced, and the hormonal and seminal abnormalities are corrected by curing the hyperthyroxinemia.[193]

Men with primary hypothyroidism may experience a decrease in libido, but there is at present no adequate explanation for this symptom. Although total testosterone levels may be reduced and correct to normal with thyroxine treatment, this change is primarily in response to changes in SHBG concentrations with seemingly unchanged testosterone production.[194] Testicular failure has been associated with primary hypothyroidism but the patients reported were elderly, and L-thyroxine treatment did not correct the gonadal dysfunction.[195] Serum testosterone and T_4 levels are also reduced in chronic illness and in men with lesions of the hypothalamic-pituitary unit.

Renal Failure

Decreased libido, impotence, and gynecomastia are common complaints among men with chronic renal failure, and nearly all men are infertile in spite of effective dialysis. Sperm output and motility are markedly reduced in those few men who can provide an ejaculate. Testicular biopsies reveal arrested sperm maturation and sometimes germinal aplasia.[196] The hypogonadism in these men is complex, and its pathophysiology is incompletely understood.[197] Primary testicular failure is suggested by low serum testosterone and high serum LH levels and an attenuated testosterone response to hCG stimulation. But unlike the case in primary testicular failure, FSH levels are only slightly increased and may be normal.[198] The LH and FSH responses to clomiphene stimulation are usually normal, and the rise in LH and FSH after GnRH administration is normal or exaggerated and is prolonged. The LH pulse profile reveals low-amplitude secretory episodes.[199] The difference between the LH response to endogenous and exogenous GnRH suggests reduced GnRH secretion. Chronic illness, poor nutrition, and increased production of cortisol, estrogen, or prolactin may each suppress the GnRH signal.

Decreased renal function may directly contribute to the endocrine disturbance in these men. Glomerular filtration makes a more important contribution to the metabolism of LH than of FSH such that prolonged LH clearance could explain the elevated LH levels, the delayed LH response to GnRH, and the attenuated LH pulse amplitude. Glycoprotein α-subunit levels are also markedly increased in CRF,[200] perhaps because the excretion of this 23-kDa peptide is impaired. Cross-reactivity of α-subunit in solid-phase polyclonal antibody RIA's also contributes to the disproportionate rise in LH concentrations. Following successful renal transplantation, serum testosterone levels and sperm production often increase and LH levels decline. FSH levels may increase, then decrease.[201] In some patients, however, FSH levels remain elevated and hypospermatogenesis persists, particularly in those men who have had many years of dialysis. Both before and after transplantation, medications, including antihypertensives, glucocorticoids, and alkylating agents, may contribute to gonadal dysfunction.

Diabetes Mellitus

Erectile and ejaculatory function are often abnormal in men with diabetes mellitus. Although a complex disturbance involving neural, vascular, metabolic, and medication-related abnormalities occurs in diabetes, primary testicular failure may also be present, characterized by reduced testis size, semen volume, sperm output and motility, and increased serum LH and FSH levels, although some data are conflicting.[202–204] Testosterone therapy has been reported to improve erectile dysfunction in selected patients.[204] The low testosterone levels sometimes observed in men with insulin-dependent diabetes at the time of initial diagnosis no doubt reflect the suppressive effect of acute illness on GnRH secretion.[205]

Sickle Cell Disease

Delayed puberty and adult hypogonadism are common sequelae of sickle cell anemia. Most adult men have suppressed spermatogenesis. In one series, 25 per cent of men had hormonal evidence of primary testicular failure, but gonadotropin deficiency has also been reported.[206] Both lesions may result from vaso-occlusion of small blood vessels. Stress, pain, and use of narcotic analgesics may also contribute to gonadotropin deficiency. A functional suppression of gonadotropin secretion is suggested by the report of normalized serum gonadotropin and testosterone levels during treatment with clomiphene.[207]

Alcoholic Liver Disease

Hypogonadism is common among men with chronic liver disease. Most studies have been in alcoholic men, among whom gynecomastia, small testes, decreased body hair, and reduced libido and potency are common clinical findings.[208] When testicular biopsies were performed, incomplete spermatogenesis was often found. The hypogonadism in these men is multifactoral.[209] Free and total testosterone levels are usually reduced, and LH and FSH levels are generally increased, suggesting primary testicular failure. Experimental evidence in animals and in cultured Leydig cells indicates that alcohol damages the testes. In men with severe clinical hypogonadism, however, LH and FSH levels may be normal in spite of very low testosterone concentrations, and the LH pulse pattern is suppressed.[210] Moreover, the LH and FSH response to clomiphene stimulation is impaired, whereas the increases in LH and FSH after GnRH administration overlap with normal responses.[209, 211] These data suggest suppressed GnRH secretion. Increased estrogens, PRL, cortisol, CRF, and IL-1 have been reported in alcoholic cirrhosis, and these hormonal abnormalities as well as poor nutrition could inhibit GnRH.[212–215] Moreover, gonadotropin insufficiency may result partly from the ingestion of alcohol,[216] and hypogonadism may occur with normal liver histology. Cessation of alcohol consumption has been reported to increase sperm output and motility.[217]

The prominent feminization often observed in men with alcoholic cirrhosis is explained by reduced testosterone together with increased estrogen production.[218] The source of the estrogen appears to be the adrenal gland. Estrone levels are increased more uniformly than is estradiol, and the suppressive and stimulatory effects of dexamethasone and ACTH, respectively, on serum estrone levels are greater than the effects of fluoxymesterone and hCG.[219] The bioconversion of androstenedione to estrone is enhanced, perhaps because the clearance of androstenedione by the liver is decreased, but other factors may be operative.[220]

SHBG is markedly increased in alcoholic liver disease, and because SHBG binds testosterone more avidly than it does estradiol or estrone, the availability of estrogens relative to testosterone to the target tissues is increased. Increased SHBG may increase the total testosterone level into the normal range when bioavailable testosterone is low. Thus, bioavailable testosterone provides a better estimate than does total testosterone levels of testosterone production in men with liver disease. Alcohol may contribute to the high SHBG by increasing hepatic estrogen receptors.[221] Moreover, the SHBG produced by the liver of alcoholic cirrhotics may be abnormally glycosylated, further influencing sex steroid transport and target tissue delivery.[222]

Oral testosterone has been used to treat men with alcoholic liver disease. Hemoglobin levels increased but testosterone was without effect on the hepatic biochemical abnormalities, complications, or death from cirrhosis.[223]

Hemochromatosis

Hemochromatosis is an autosomal recessive disorder in which excessive iron is absorbed from the intestine and deposited in parenchymal cells. The classic signs of hemochromatosis are skin pigmentation, hepatomegaly, and diabetes mellitus.[224] Although unexplained, selective HH is a common early finding. In some adult men, serum testosterone levels are so low as to approach the values of castrated men. The LH and FSH responses to GnRH stimulation are blunted or absent,[225] and the anterior pituitary gland, especially the gonadotroph, contains stainable iron. Unlike the case in alcoholic liver disease, serum androstenedione, estrone, and SHBG levels are normal, and gynecomastia is uncommon (Table 133–9).[226] Although iron is deposited in most endocrine glands, adrenal insufficiency, primary gonadal failure, hypothyroidism, and hypoparathyroidism

rarely occur. The diabetes mellitus and hepatic cirrhosis that occur in hemochromatosis may also contribute to the endocrine disturbance and sexual dysfunction in these patients.[227] Intensive phlebotomy may reverse the hypogonadism, but results are conflicting.[228, 229] Chronic iron overload from transfusional hemosiderosis also produces HH.[230]

X-Linked Spinal and Bulbar Muscular Atrophy

Men with spinal and bulbar muscular atrophy (Kennedy disease) present with weakness, muscle atrophy, and fasciculations at age 20 to 40 years.[231] The weakness progresses and swallowing becomes difficult, and patients may die of aspiration. Many cases are sporadic, but familial clustering suggests an X-linked recessive disorder. Although initially fertile, affected men later in life develop gynecomastia, clinical signs of androgen deficiency, and small testes with hypospermatogenesis which may precede the onset of the neurological syndrome. Serum LH levels are usually increased, suggesting testicular failure, but total testosterone levels are normal or increased.[232] The knowledge that androgen receptors (AR) are present in spinal and bulbar motor neurons led to the proposal of an AR defect.[232] Through the use of PCR to amplify each of the eight exons of the AR gene, enlargement of a CAG repeat that codes for a polyglutamine tract has been found in exon 1.[233, 234] This portion of the gene codes for a region of the AR that is not involved in steroid or DNA binding but may be important for the function of transcription factors.

Miscellaneous Causes

Adrenoleukodystrophy is a sex-linked recessive disorder in the oxidation of very long chain fatty acids by peroxisomes. In affected children, the accumulation of fatty acids leads to demyelination of the cerebral hemispheres and to Addison's disease. Adrenomyeloneuropathy appears to be a milder and more slowly progressive form of this disorder, with clinical symptoms beginning in adolescence or young adulthood. Primary testicular insufficiency may occur.[235] Evidence also indicates that peroxisomes in Leydig cells

TABLE 133–9. A COMPARISON OF THE ENDOCRINE PROFILES IN MEN WITH CIRRHOSIS OF THE LIVER DUE TO ALCOHOLISM OR HEMOCHROMATOSIS

	ALCOHOLISM (n = 6)	HEMOCHROMATOSIS (n = 6)	NORMAL MEN (n = 6)
Testosterone (ng/ml)	2.78 ± 0.63*	2.79 ± 0.79*	5.90 ± 1.20
Androstenedione (ng/ml)	1.67 ± 0.28*,†	0.90 ± 0.23*	1.23 ± 0.10
Estradiol (pg/ml)	38.0 ± 5.3*,†	16.2 ± 4.6	20.3 ± 3.7
Estrone (pg/ml)	68.5 ± 17.2*,†	32.2 ± 4.6	26.8 ± 3.1
Cortisol (μg/dl)	12.5 ± 3.8	13.3 ± 2.5	11.1 ± 4.2
LH (mIU/ml)	10.5 ± 3.5*,†	5.5 ± 2.0*	21.0 ± 6.5
SHBG (nM/l)	80 ± 30*	35 ± 10	25 ± 10
PRL (ng/ml)	9 ± 4.5	3.0 ± 1.5*	6 ± 2

Data are mean ± SD.
*$P < 0.05$ vs normal men.
†$P < 0.05$, hemochromatosis vs alcoholism.
Data are from Kley HK, Niederau C, Stremmel W, et al: Conversion of androgens to estrogens in idiopathic hemochromatosis: Comparison with alcoholic liver cirrhosis. J Clin Endocrinol Metab 61:1–6, 1985.

are under LH control and play a role in testosterone biosynthesis.

Histiocytic granulomas may involve the basal hypothalamus, producing diabetes insipidus and hypopituitarism, as well as the bones, skin, and lung. Hypogonadotropic hypogonadism has been reported.[236] Magnetic resonance scans may demonstrate thickening of the pituitary stalk with contrast enhancement.

Sarcoidosis of the hypothalamus-pituitary region is uncommon but may cause diabetes insipidus, hyperprolactinemia, and anterior pituitary hormone deficiency. Affected patients usually have widespread disease, but endocrine symptoms may predominate. The finding of low testosterone and low LH levels which increased significantly after GnRH stimulation suggested a hypothalamic disturbance.[237]

DRUGS THAT ADVERSELY AFFECT TESTICULAR FUNCTION

Cytotoxic Chemotherapy

Patients with cancer or immunological disorders who are treated with chemotherapeutic drugs, particularly alkylating agents, frequently develop testicular dysfunction.[238] Treatment in adolescence or adulthood is more damaging than is treatment in childhood.[239] Chemotherapy-induced testicular damage is characterized by an increase in serum FSH levels and by oligospermia or azoospermia. Among men with Hodgkin's disease receiving repeated cycles of mechlorethamine hydrochloride (nitrogen mustard), vinblastine, procarbazine, and prednisone, the prevalence of azoospermia or severe oligospermia approaches 100 per cent.[240] Testicular toxicity is directly proportional to the accumulated dose of drug received. Recovery of spermatogenesis is rare. Testosterone production may decline, LH concentrations may rise, and gynecomastia may develop, particularly when total body irradiation is used together with chemotherapy.[241] Efforts to protect the testis from damage by suppressing testicular function with gonadal steroids or with GnRH analogues have so far produced disappointing results.[242] Gonadotropin deficiency from acute and chronic illness may explain the testosterone deficiency and oligospermia that sometimes occur in men with Hodgkin's disease before chemotherapy is begun.[243]

Amiodarone

Sexual dysfunction has been reported in elderly men treated with the antiarrhythmic drug amiodarone. LH and FSH levels were increased substantially compared with levels in an age-matched control group who also had cardiac disease.[244] Testicular damage is probably due to the accumulation of this lipophilic drug in testis tissue.

Antiandrogens

Antiandrogens block the action of androgens by binding to androgen receptors and may limit androgen metabolism in target cells. Thus, effects on androgen-dependent tissues throughout the body might be anticipated. Antiandrogens may be steroidal or nonsteroidal compounds. Steroidal antiandrogens may also interact with progesterone and glucocorticoid receptors and may be weak agonists in the absence of testosterone, whereas nonsteroidal antiandrogens tend to be more receptor selective and to lack agonist activity.[245]

Spironolactone is a steroid analogue that binds to mineralocorticoid receptors and is used as a diuretic and antihypertensive. Spironolactone also binds to androgen receptors and reduces the concentration of the cytochrome P450 17α-hydroxylase/C17-20 lyase enzyme complex in testicular microsomes.[246] The result is not only a partial blockade of androgen action but also a decline in testosterone biosynthesis and an increase in circulating progesterone levels. The fall in circulating testosterone levels leads to increased LH and FSH secretion, which returns serum testosterone to normal values, however. Aromatization of testosterone to estradiol is also enhanced, producing gynecomastia.[247]

Cimetidine is a histamine H_2 receptor antagonist that reduces gastric acid production and is used to treat patients with duodenal and gastric ulcer, esophagitis due to gastroesophageal reflux, and many other conditions. Gynecomastia and breast tenderness occur commonly in patients with the Zollinger-Ellison syndrome who are treated with large doses of cimetidine, but in only approximately 1 per cent of patients with duodenal ulcers who are treated with substantially smaller doses of the drug.[248] Impotence has also been reported with cimetidine therapy. No significant changes occur in serum testosterone, estradiol, LH, FSH, or prolactin levels during cimetidine treatment.[249] Instead, impotence and gynecomastia appear to be due to the action of this nonsteroid to occupy androgen receptors and block the action of testosterone on its target tissues, which include the breast.[250] The claim that cimetidine reduces sperm output was not substantiated in subsequent controlled studies.

Flutamide is a nonsteroidal antiandrogen approved recently in the United States for use in combination therapy with GnRH analogues for the treatment of metastatic prostatic carcinoma.[251] It has also been used to treat benign prostatic hyperplasia and together with oral contraceptives to treat hyperandrogenism in women. Flutamide lacks agonist activity, competes only weakly for androgen receptor binding in vitro, and is believed to be hydroxylated in vivo for full biological activity.[252] In the absence of concurrent treatment with GnRH analogues, flutamide increases LH and FSH secretion and thereby increases testosterone and estradiol production by blocking testosterone-negative feedback inhibition.[253] Tender gynecomastia may occur. Flutamide is hepatotoxic, and it occasionally produces a syndrome of clinical hepatitis.

Ketoconazole

Ketoconazole is a synthetic imidazole introduced as an oral antifungal agent. It inhibits cytochrome P450 enzyme systems not only in fungi, but also in mammalian testis, ovary, adrenal, kidney and liver.[254] Its effect on C17-20 lyase activity in the biosynthetic pathway to testosterone leads to a dose-dependent reduction in circulating testosterone levels and to an increase in serum 17α-hydroxyprogesterone concentrations in men.[255] Serum LH and FSH levels also rise. Because of ketoconazole's short serum half-life, serum testosterone levels may be normal when the drug is administered once daily. High-dose ketoconazole treatment causes gynecomastia. Although there are no reports of infertility among ketoconazole-treated men, very high doses impair sperm motility in experimental animals. Because it suppresses testosterone biosynthesis, ketoconazole has been used to treat males with gonadotropin-independent precocious puberty or prostatic cancer, and hyperandrogenic women. Ketoconazole also inhibits cortisol synthesis and has been used to treat patients with Cushing's syndrome. Recognized adverse effects of ketoconazole include nausea and hepatocellular injury.

Finasteride

Finasteride is a 4-azasteroid inhibitor of 5α-reductase activity which was recently introduced as a treatment for prostatic hyperplasia because drug treatment is associated with a reduction in prostate size and an improvement in clinical symptoms. In approved doses, finasteride decreases prostatic and serum dihydrotestosterone levels by approximately 85 per cent and 70 per cent, respectively.[256] At the same time, prostatic testosterone levels increased 7-fold but serum testosterone levels rose marginally. Basal and GnRH-stimulated LH and FSH levels are unaffected by finasteride treatment.[257] Inhibition of 5α-reductase activity does not appear to adversely influence spermatogenesis.

Sulfasalazine

Sulfasalazine is an anti-inflammatory agent used to treat patients with ulcerative colitis or Crohn's disease. Sulfasalazine is cleaved by intestinal flora into 5-aminosalicylic acid, which remains in the colon, and sulfapyridine, which may be absorbed into the circulation. Oligospermia, poor sperm motility, abnormal sperm morphology, and fertility disturbance are common during sulfasalazine treatment but appear to be reversible when treatment is discontinued.[258] The endocrine function of the testis appears to be unchanged.

Cannabinoids

Gynecomastia has been described in heavy marijuana users. Whether cannabinoids adversely affect testicular function is uncertain, however, because both suppressed and unchanged serum testosterone levels have been reported.[259] Early claims that cannabinoids interact with estrogen receptors were not substantiated, although marijuana extracts may have contaminants with estrogenic activity.[260] Marijuana and its constituents have also been reported to interact with androgen receptors.[261] Administration of cannabinoids to pregnant female mice alters testicular function in their male offspring, but these findings are of unknown clinical significance.

REFERENCES

1. Santen RJ, Paulsen CA: Hypogonadotropic eunuchoidism: I. Clinical study of the mode of inheritance. J Clin Endocrinol Metab 36:47–54, 1973.
2. van Dop C, Burstein S, Conte FA, Grumbach MM: Isolated gonadotropin deficiency in boys: Clinical characteristics and growth. J Pediatr 111:684–692, 1987.
3. Finkelstein JS, Klibanski A, Neer RM, et al: Osteoporosis in men with idiopathic hypogonadotropic hypogonadism. Ann Intern Med 106:354–361, 1987.
4. Uriarte MM, Baron J, Garcia HB, et al: The effect of pubertal delay on adult height in men with isolated hypogonadotropic hypogonadism. J Clin Endocrinol Metab 74:436–440, 1992.
5. Counts DR, Pescovitz OH, Barnes KM, et al: Dissociation of adrenarche and gonadarche in precocious puberty and in isolated hypogonadotropic hypogonadism. J Clin Endocrinol Metab 64:1174–1178, 1987.
6. Wu FCW, Butler GE, Kelnar CJH, et al: Patterns of pulsatile luteinizing hormone and follicle-stimulating hormone secretion in prepubertal (midchildhood) boys and girls and patients with idiopathic hypogonadotropic hypogonadism (Kallmann's syndrome): A study using an ultrasensitive time-resolved immunofluorometric assay. J Clin Endocrinol Metab 72:1229–1237, 1991.
7. Goji K, Tanikaze S: Comparison between spontaneous gonadotropin concentration profiles and gonadotropin response to low-dose gonadotropin-releasing hormone in prepubertal and early pubertal boys and patients with hypogonadotropic hypogonadism: Assessment by using ultrasensitive, time-resolved immunofluorometric assay. Pediatr Res 31:535–539, 1992.
8. Hoffman AR, Crowley WF Jr: Induction of puberty in men by long-term pulsatile administration of low-dose gonadotropin-releasing hormone. N Engl J Med 307:1237–1241, 1982.
9. Lieblich JM, Rogol AD, White BJ, Rosen SW: Syndrome of anosmia with hypogonadotropic hypogonadism (Kallmann syndrome). Am J Med 73:506–519, 1982.
10. Winters SJ, Johnsonbaugh RE, Sherins RJ: The response of prolactin to chlorpromazine stimulation in men with hypogonadotropic hypogonadism and early pubertal boys: Relationship to sex steroid exposure. Clin Endocrinol 16:321–330, 1982.
11. Liu L, Merriam GR, Sherins RJ: Chronic sex steroid exposure increases mean plasma growth hormone concentration and pulse amplitude in men with isolated hypogonadotropic hypogonadism. J Clin Endocrinol Metab 64:651–656, 1987.
12. Smals AGH, Kloppenborg PWC, van Haelst UJG, et al: Fertile eunuch syndrome versus classic hypogonadotropic hypogonadism. Acta Endocrinol 87:389–399, 1978.
13. Shargil AA: Treatment of idiopathic hypogonadotropic hypogonadism in men with luteinizing hormone–releasing hormone: A comparison of treatment with daily injections and with the pulsatile infusion pump. Fertil Steril 47:492–501, 1987.
14. Boyar RM, Wu RHK, Kapen S, et al: Clinical and laboratory heterogeneity in idiopathic hypogonadotropic hypogonadism. J Clin Endocrinol Metab 43:1268–1275, 1976.
15. Spratt DI, Carr DB, Merriam GR, et al: The spectrum of abnormal patterns of gonadotropin-releasing hormone secretion in men with idiopathic hypogonadotropic hypogonadism: Clinical and laboratory correlations. J Clin Endocrinol Metab 64:283–291, 1987.
16. Kallmann FJ, Schoenfeld WA, Barrera SE: Genetic aspects of primary eunuchoidism. Am J Ment Deficiency 48:203–236, 1944.
17. White BJ, Rogol AD, Brown KS, et al: The syndrome of anosmia with hypogonadotropic hypogonadism: A genetic study of 18 new families and a review. Am J Med Genet 15:417–435, 1983.
18. Klingmuller D, Dewes W, Krahe T, et al: Magnetic resonance imaging of the brain in patients with anosmia and hypothalamic hypogonadism (Kallmann's syndrome). J Clin Endocrinol Metab 65:581–584, 1987.
19. Schwankhaus JD, Currie J, Jaffe MJ, et al: Neurologic findings in men with isolated hypogonadotropic hypogonadism. Neurology 39:223–226, 1989.
20. Schwanzel-Fukuda M, Pfaff DW: Origin of luteinizing hormone–releasing hormone neurons. Nature 338:161–164, 1989.
21. Schwanzel-Fukuda M, Bick D, Pfaff DW: Luteinizing hormone–releasing (LHRH)–expressing cells do not migrate normally in an inherited hypogonadal (Kallmann) syndrome. Mol Brain Res 6:311–326, 1989.

22. Bick D, Franco B, Sherins RJ, et al: Brief Report: Intragenic deletion of the Kalig-1 gene in Kallmann's syndrome. N Engl J Med 326:1752–1755, 1992.
23. Weiss J, Adams E, Whitcomb RW, et al: Normal sequence of the gonadotropin-releasing hormone gene in patients with idiopathic hypogonadotropic hypogonadism. Biol Reprod 45:743–747, 1991.
24. Butler MG: Prader-Willi syndrome: Current understanding of cause and diagnosis. Am J Med Genet 35:319–332, 1990.
25. Jeffcoate WJ, Laurance BM, Edwards CRW, Besser GM: Endocrine function in Prader-Willi syndrome. Clin Endocrinol 12:81–89, 1980.
26. Bray GA, Dahms WT, Swerdloff RS, et al: The Prader-Willi syndrome: A study of 40 patients and a review of the literature. Medicine 62:59–80, 1983.
27. Green JS, Parfrey PS, Harnett JD, et al: The cardinal manifestations of the Bardet-Biedl syndrome, a form of Laurence-Moon-Biedl syndrome. N Engl J Med 321:1002–1009, 1989.
28. Toledo SPA, Medeiros-Neto GA, Knobel M, Mattar E: Evaluation of the hypothalamic-pituitary-gonadal function in the Bardet-Biedl syndrome. Metabolism 26:1277–1291, 1977.
29. Olson WH, Bardin CW, Walsh GO, Engel WK: Moebius syndrome. Lower motor neuron involvement and hypogonadotropic hypogonadism. Neurology 20:1002–1008, 1970.
30. Brackett LE, Demers LM, Mamourian AC, et al: Moebius syndrome in association with hypogonadotropic hypogonadism. J Endocrinol Invest 14:599–607, 1991.
31. Zachmann M, Illig R, Prader A: Gonadotropin deficiency and cryptorchidism in three prepubertal brothers with congenital adrenal hypoplasia. J Pediatr 97:255–257, 1980.
32. Kikuchi K, Kaji M, Mamoi T, et al: Failure to induce puberty in a man with X-linked congenital adrenal hypoplasia and hypogonadotropic hypogonadism by pulsatile administration of low dose gonadotropin-releasing hormone. Acta Endocrinol 114:153–160, 1987.
33. Maghnie M, Triulzi F, Larizza D, et al: Hypothalamic-pituitary dysfunction in growth hormone–deficient patients with pituitary abnormalities. J Clin Endocrinol Metab 73:79–83, 1991.
34. Tanner JM, Whitehouse RH: A note on the bone age at which patients with true isolated growth hormone deficiency enter puberty. J Clin Endocrinol Metab 41:788–790, 1975.
35. Littley MD, Shalet SM, Beardwell CG, et al: Hypopituitarism following external radiotherapy for pituitary tumors in adults. QJ Med 70:145–160, 1989.
36. Luton JP, Thieblot P, Valcke J-C, et al: Reversible gonadotropin deficiency in male Cushing's disease. J Clin Endocrinol Metab 45:488–495, 1977.
37. Nieman LK, Chrousos GP, Kellner C: Successful treatment of Cushing's syndrome with the glucocorticoid antagonist RU 486. J Clin Endocrinol Metab 61:536–540, 1985.
38. Nawata H, Ono K, Ohashi M, et al: RU 486 inhibits induction of aromatase by dexamethasone via glucocorticoid receptor in cultured human skin fibroblasts. J Steroid Biochem 29:63–68, 1986.
39. MacAdams MR, White RH, Chipps BE: Reduction of serum testosterone levels during chronic glucocorticoid therapy. Ann Intern Med 104:648–651, 1986.
40. Carter JN, Tyson JE, Tolis G, et al: Prolactin-secreting tumors and hypogonadism in 22 men. N Engl J Med 299:847–852, 1978.
41. Franks S, Jacobs HS, Martin N, Nabarro JD: Hyperprolactinemia and impotence. Clin Endocrinol 8:277–287, 1978.
42. Patton ML, Woolf PD: Hyperprolactinemia and delayed puberty: A report of three cases and their response to therapy. Pediatrics 71:572–575, 1983.
43. Winters SJ: Diurnal rhythm of testosterone and luteinizing hormone in hypogonadal men. J Androl 12:185–190, 1991.
44. Winters SJ, Troen P: Altered pulsatile secretion of luteinizing hormone in hypogonadal men with hyperprolactinemia. Clin Endocrinol 21:257–263, 1984.
45. Bouchard P, Lagoguey M, Brailly S, Schaison G: Gonadotropin-releasing hormone pulsatile administration restores luteinizing hormone pulsatility and normal testosterone levels in males with hyperprolactinemia. J Clin Endocrinol Metab 60:258–262, 1985.
46. Selmanoff M, Shu C, Petersen SL, et al: Single cell levels of hypothalamic messenger ribonucleic acid encoding luteinizing hormone-releasing hormone in intact, castrated, and hyperprolactinemic male rats. Endocrinology 128:459–466, 1991.
47. Murray FT, Cameron DF, Ketchum C: Return of gonadal function in men with prolactin-secreting pituitary tumors. J Clin Endocrinol Metab 59:79–85, 1984.
48. Pont A, Shelton R, Odell WD, Wilson CB: Prolactin-secreting tumors in men: Surgical cure. Ann Intern Med 91:211–213, 1979.

49. Urban MD, Lee PA, Migeon CJ: Adult height and fertility in men with congenital virilizing adrenal hyperplasia. N Engl J Med 299:1392–1396, 1978.
50. Wischusen J, Baker HWG, Hudson B: Reversible male infertility due to congenital adrenal hyperplasia. Clin Endocrinol 14:571–577, 1981.
51. Cutfield RG, Bateman JM, Odell WD: Infertility caused by bilateral testicular masses secondary to congenital adrenal hyperplasia (21-hydroxylase deficiency). Fertil Steril 40:809–813, 1983.
52. Stepanas AV, Samaan NA, Schultz PN, Holoye PY: Endocrine studies in testicular tumor patients with and without gynecomastia: A report of 45 cases. Cancer 41:369–376, 1978.
53. Saller B, Clara R, Spottl G, et al: Testicular cancer secretes human choriogonadotropin (hCG) and its free β-subunit: Evidence that hCG (+hCG-β) assays are the most reliable in diagnosis and followup. Clin Chem 36:234–239, 1990.
54. Kuhn JM, Mahoudeau JA, Billaud L, et al: Evaluation of diagnostic criteria for Leydig cell tumors in adult men revealed by gynaecomastia. Clin Endocrinol 26:407–416, 1987.
55. Gabrilove JL, Sharma DC, Wotiz HH, Dorfman RI: Feminizing adrenocortical tumors in the male: A review of 52 cases. Medicine 44:37–79, 1965.
56. Veldhuis JD, Sowers JR, Rogol AD, et al: Pathophysiology of male hypogonadism associated with endogenous hyperestrogenism: Evidence for dual defects in the gonadal axis. N Engl J Med 312:1371–1375, 1985.
57. Al-Ansari AA, Khalil TH, Kelani Y, Mortimer CH: Isolated follicle-stimulating hormone deficiency in men: Successful long-term gonadotropin therapy. Fertil Steril 42:618–626, 1984.
58. Mozaffarian GA, Higley M, Paulsen CA: Clinical studies in an adult male patient with "isolated follicle stimulating hormone (FSH) deficiency." J Androl 4:393–398, 1983.
59. Weiss J, Axelrod L, Whitcomb RW, et al: Hypogonadism caused by a single amino acid substitution in the β subunit of luteinizing hormone. N Engl J Med 326:179–183, 1991.
60. Gattuccio F, Lo Bartolo G, Orlando G, Janni A: Hypogonadism in a male with immunologically active, biologically inactive luteinizing hormone. Acta Eur Fertil 11:259–268, 1980.
61. Jeffcoate SL: What are we measuring in gonadotropin assays? Acta Endocrinol (Suppl) 288:28–30, 1988.
62. Chappel S: Biological to immunological ratios: Reevaluation of a concept [editorial]. J Clin Endocrinol Metab 70:1494–1495, 1990.
63. David R, Yoon DJ, Landin L, et al: A syndrome of gonadotropin resistance possibly due to a luteinizing hormone receptor defect. J Clin Endocrinol Metab 59:156–160, 1984.
64. Burger HG, deKretser DM, Hudson B, Wilson JD: Effects of preceding androgen therapy on testicular response to human pituitary gonadotropin in hypogonadotropic hypogonadism: A study of three patients. Fertil Steril 35:64–68, 1981.
65. Claustrat B, David L, Faure A, Francois R: Development of anti-human chorionic gonadotropin antibodies in patients with hypogonadotropic hypogonadism: A study of four patients. J Clin Endocrinol Metab 57:1041–1047, 1983.
66. Burris AS, Rodbard HW, Winters SJ, Sherins RJ: Gonadotropin therapy in men with isolated hypogonadotropic hypogonadism: The response to human chorionic gonadotropin is predicted by initial testicular size. J Clin Endocrinol Metab 66:1144–1151, 1988.
67. McLachlan RI, Finkel DM, Bremner WJ, Snyder PJ: Serum inhibin concentrations before and during gonadotropin treatment in men with hypogonadotropic hypogonadism: Physiological and clinical implications. J Clin Endocrinol Metab 70:1414–1419, 1990.
68. Finkel DM, Phillips JL, Snyder PJ: Stimulation of spermatogenesis by gonadotropins in men with hypogonadotropic hypogonadism. N Engl J Med 313:651–655, 1985.
69. Johnsen SG: Maintenance of spermatogenesis induced by HMG treatment by means of continuous HCG treatment in hypogonadotropic men. Acta Endocrinol 89:763–769, 1978.
70. Burris AS, Clark RV, Vantman DJ, Sherins RJ: A low sperm concentration does not preclude fertility in men with isolated hypogonadotropic hypogonadism after gonadotropin therapy. Fertil Steril 50:343–347, 1988.
71. Whitcomb RW, Crowley WF Jr: Diagnosis and treatment of isolated gonadotropin-releasing hormone deficiency in men. J Clin Endocrinol Metab 70:3–7, 1990.
72. Popovic V, Milosevic Z, Djukanovic R, et al: Hypersensitivity reaction with intravenous GnRH after pulsatile subcutaneous GnRH treatment in male hypogonadotropic hypogonadism. Postgrad Med J 64:245–246, 1988.

73. Blumenfeld Z, Frisch L, Conn PM: Gonadotropin-releasing hormone (GnRH) antibodies formation in hypogonadotropic azoospermic men treated with pulsatile GnRH—diagnosis and possible alternative treatment. Fertil Steril 50:622–629, 1988.

74. Schopohl J, Mehltretter G, von Zumbusch R, et al: Comparison of gonadotropin-releasing hormone and gonadotropin therapy in male patients with idiopathic hypothalamic hypogonadism. Fertil Steril 56:1143–1150, 1991.

75. Feldman JM, Postlethwaite RW, Glenn JF: Hot flashes and sweats in men with testicular insufficiency. Arch Intern Med 136:606–608, 1976.

76. Mecklenberg RS, Sherins RJ: Gonadotropin response to luteinizing hormone–releasing hormone in men with germinal aplasia. J Clin Endocrinol Metab 38:1005–1008, 1974.

77. Winters SJ, Troen P: A reexamination of pulsatile luteinizing hormone secretion in primary testicular failure. J Clin Endocrinol Metab 57:432–435, 1983.

78. Medhamurthy R, Culler MD, Gay VL, et al: Evidence that inhibin plays a major role in the regulation of follicle-stimulating hormone in the fully adult male rhesus monkey (Macaca mulatta). Endocrinology 129:389–395, 1991.

79. de Kretser DM, McLachlan RI, Robertson DM, Burger HG: Serum inhibin levels in normal men and men with testicular disorders. J Endocrinol 120:517–523, 1989.

80. Jacobs PA, Strong JA: A case of human intersexuality having a possible XXY sex-determining mechanism. Nature 83:302–303, 1959.

81. Jacobs PA, Hassold TJ, Whittington E, et al: Klinefelter's syndrome: An analysis of the origin of the additional sex chromosome using molecular probes. Ann Hum Genet 52:93–109, 1988.

82. Bandmann HJ, Breit R (eds): Klinefelter's Syndrome. Berlin, Springer-Verlag, 1984.

83. Caldwell PD, Smith DW: The XXY (Klinefelter's) syndrome in childhood: Detection and treatment. J Pediatr 80:250–258, 1972.

84. Wong TW, Horvath KA: Pathological changes of the testis in infertility. In Gondos B, Riddick DH (eds): Pathology of Infertility: Clinical Correlations in the Male and Female. New York, Thieme Medical Publishers, 1987, p 265.

85. Paulsen CA, Gordon DL, Carpenter RW, et al: Klinefelter's syndrome and its variants: A hormonal and chromosomal study. Recent Prog Horm Res 24:321–363, 1968.

86. Samaan NA, Stepanas AV, Danziger J, Trujillo J: Reactive pituitary abnormalities in patients with Klinefelter's and Turner's syndrome. Arch Intern Med 139:198–201, 1979.

87. Foresta C, Ruzza G, Mioni R, et al: Testosterone and bone loss in Klinefelter syndrome. Horm Metab Res 15:56–57, 1983.

88. Francis RM, Peacock M, Aaron JE, et al: Osteoporosis in hypogonadal men: Role of decreased plasma 1,25 dihydroxyvitamin D, calcium malabsorption, and low bone formation. Bone 7:261–268, 1986.

89. Wang C, Baker HWG, Burger HG, et al: Hormonal studies in Klinefelter's syndrome. Clin Endocrinol 4:399–411, 1975.

90. Plymate SR, Leonard JM, Paulsen CA, et al: Sex hormone–binding globulin changes with androgen replacement. J Clin Endocrinol Metab 57:645–648, 1983.

91. Smals AGH, Kloppenborg PWC, Pieters GFFM, et al: Basal and human chorionic gonadotropin–stimulated 17α-hydroxyprogesterone and testosterone levels in Klinefelter's syndrome. J Clin Endocrinol Metab 47:1144–1147, 1978.

92. Spitz IM, Zylber E, Cohen H, et al: Impaired prolactin response to thyrotropin-releasing hormone in isolated gonadotropin deficiency and exaggerated response in primary testicular failure. J Clin Endocrinol Metab 48:941–945, 1979.

93. Nielsen J, Pelsen B, Sorensen K: Follow-up of 30 Klinefelter males treated with testosterone. Clin Genet 33:262–269, 1988.

94. Caminos-Torres R, Ma L, Snyder PJ: Testosterone-induced inhibition of the LH and FSH responses to gonadotropin-releasing hormone occurs slowly. J Clin Endocrinol Metab 44:1142–1153, 1977.

95. Capell PT, Paulsen CA, Derleth D, et al: The effect of short-term testosterone administration on serum FSH, LH and testosterone levels: Evidence for selective abnormality in LH control in patients with Klinefelter's syndrome. J Clin Endocrinol Metab 37:752–759, 1973.

96. Gordon DL, Krmpotic E, Thomas W, et al: Pathologic testicular findings in Klinefelter's syndrome: 47,XXY vs 46,XY/47,XXY. Arch Intern Med 130:726–729, 1972.

97. Hook EB: Extra sex chromosomes and human behavior: The nature of the evidence regarding XYY, XXY, XXYY, and XXX genotypes. In Valet HL, Porter IH (eds): Genetic Mechanisms of Sexual Development. New York, Academic Press, 1979, p 437.

98. Bloomgarden ZT, Delozier CD, Cohen MP, et al: Genetic and endocrine findings in a 48,XXYY male. J Clin Endocrinol Metab 50:740–743, 1980.

99. de la Chapelle A: The etiology of maleness in XX men. Hum Genet 58:105–116, 1981.

100. Page DC, Brown LG, de la Chapelle A: Exchange of terminal portions of X- and Y-chromosomal short arms in human XX males. Nature 328:437–440, 1987.

100a. Fechner PY, Marcantonio SM, Jaswaney V, et al: The role of sex-determining region Y genes in the etiology of 46,XX maleness. J Clin Endocrinol Metab 76:690–695, 1993.

101. Ishida H, Isurugi K, Fukutani K, et al: Studies on pituitary-gonadal endocrine function in XYY men. J Urol 121:190–193, 1979.

102. Benet J, Martin RH: Sperm chromosome complements in a 47,XYY man. Hum Genet 78:313–315, 1988.

103. John Radcliffe Hospital Cryptorchidism Study Group: Cryptorchidism: An apparent substantial increase since 1960. BMJ 293:1401–1404, 1986.

104. Scott LS: Unilateral cryptorchidism: Subsequent effects on fertility. J Reprod Fertil 2:54–60, 1962.

105. Nistal M, Paniagua R: Testicular and Epididymal Pathology. New York, Thieme Stratton, 1984, p 120.

106. Moul JW, Belman AB: A review of surgical treatment of undescended testes with emphasis on anatomical position. J Urol 140:125–128, 1988.

107. Koff SA: Does compensatory testicular enlargement predict monorchism? J Urol 146:632–633, 1991.

108. Tato L, Corgnati A, Boner A, et al: Unilateral cryptorchidism with compensatory hypertrophy of descended testicle in prepubertal boys. Horm Res 9:185–193, 1978.

109. Nistal M, Paniagua R: Infertility in adult males with retractile testes. Fertil Steril 41:395–403, 1984.

110. Hutson JM, Donahoe PK: The hormonal control of testicular descent. Endocr Rev 7:270–283, 1986.

111. Husmann DA, McPhaul MJ: Time-specific androgen blockade with flutamide inhibits testicular descent in the rat. Endocrinology 129:1409–1416, 1991.

112. Gendrel D, Roger M, Job J-C: Plasma gonadotropin and testosterone values in infants with cryptorchidism. J Pediatr 97:217–220, 1980.

113. Yamanaka J, Baker M, Metcalfe S, Hutson JM: Serum levels of müllerian inhibiting substance in boys with cryptorchidism. J Pediatr Surg 26:621–623, 1991.

114. Cendron M, Keating MA, Huff DS, et al: Cryptorchidism, orchiopexy and infertility: A critical long-term retrospective analysis. J Urol 142:559–562, 1989.

115. Chilvers C, Dudley NE, Gough MH, et al: Undescended testis: The effect of treatment on subsequent risk of subfertility and malignancy. J Pediatr Surg 21:691–696, 1986.

116. Bramble FJ, Eccles S, Houghton AL, et al: Reproductive and endocrine function after surgical treatment of bilateral cryptorchidism. Lancet 2:311–314, 1974.

117. Lipshultz LI, Caminos-Torres R, Greenspan CS, Snyder PJ: Testicular function after orchiopexy for unilaterally undescended testis. N Engl J Med 295:15–18, 1976.

118. Rajfer J, Handelsman DJ, Swerdloff RS: Hormonal therapy of cryptorchidism: A randomized, double-blind study comparing human chorionic gonadotropin and gonadotropin-releasing hormone. N Engl J Med 314:466–470, 1986.

119. Christiansen P, Muller J, Buhl S, et al: Treatment of cryptorchidism with human chorionic gonadotropin (hCG) or gonadotropin-releasing hormone (GnRH). Horm Res 30:187–192, 1988.

120. Gilbert JB, Hamilton JB: Studies on malignant testis tumors: III. Incidence and nature of tumors in ectopic testes. Surg Gynecol Obstet 71:731–743, 1940.

121. Sharland M, Burch M, McKenna WM, Paton MA: A clinical study of Noonan syndrome. Arch Dis Child 67:178–183, 1992.

122. Mendez HMM, Opitz JM: Noonan syndrome: A review. Am J Med Genet 21:493–506, 1985.

123. Theintz G, Savage MO: Growth and pubertal development in five boys with Noonan's syndrome. Arch Dis Child 57:13–17, 1982.

124. Ross JL, Shenkman L: Noonan's syndrome and hypopituitarism. Am J Med Sci 279:47–52, 1980.

125. Smith NM, Byard RW, Bourne AJ: Testicular regression syndrome—a pathological study of 77 cases. Histopathology 19:269–272, 1991.

125a. Lobaccaro J-M, Medlej R, Borta P, et al: PCR analysis and sequencing of the SRY sex determining gene in four patients with bilateral congenital anorchia. Clin Endocrinol (Oxf) 38:197–201, 1993.

126. Aynsley-Green A, Zachmann M, Illig R, et al: Congenital bilateral anorchia in childhood: A clinical, endocrine and therapeutic evaluation of twenty-one cases. Clin Endocrinol 5:381–391, 1976.

127. Kirschner MA, Jacobs JB, Fraley EE: Bilateral anorchia with persistent testosterone production. N Engl J Med 282:240–244, 1970.

128. del Castillo EB, Trabucco A, de la Balze FA: Syndrome produced by absence of the germinal epithelium without impairment of the Sertoli or Leydig cells. J Clin Endocrinol Metab 7:493–502, 1947.

129. Nistal M, Jimenez F, Paniagua R: Sertoli cell type in the Sertoli-cell-only syndrome: Relationship between Sertoli cell morphology and aetiology. Histopathology 16:173–180, 1990.

130. Petersdorf RG, Bennett IL Jr: Treatment of mumps orchitis with adrenal hormones. Arch Intern Med 99:222–233, 1957.

131. Aiman J, Brenner PF, MacDonald PC: Androgen and estrogen production in elderly men with gynecomastia and testicular atrophy after mumps orchitis. J Clin Endocrinol Metab 50:380–386, 1980.

132. Dalton AD, Harcourt-Webster JN: The histopathology of the testis and epididymis in AIDS—a post-mortem study. J Pathol 163:47–52, 1991.

133. Brown LS Jr, Singer F, Killian P: Endocrine complications of AIDS and drug addiction. Endocrinol Metab Clin North Am 20:655–673, 1991.

134. Croxson TS, Chapman WE, Miller LK, et al: Changes in the hypothalamic-pituitary-gonadal axis in human immunodeficiency virus–infected homosexual men. J Clin Endocrinol Metab 68:317–321, 1989.

135. Dobs AS, Dempsey MA, Ladenson PW, Polk BF: Endocrine disorders in men infected with human immunodeficiency virus. Am J Med 84:611–615, 1988.

136. Neufeld M, Maclaren NK, Blizzard RM: Two types of autoimmune Addison's disease associated with different polyglandular autoimmune (PGA) syndromes. Medicine 60:355–362, 1981.

137. Barkan AL, Kelch RP, Marshall JC: Isolated gonadotrope failure in the polyglandular autoimmune syndrome. N Engl J Med 312:1535–1540, 1985.

138. Howlin NS, Zwillich SH, Brick JE, Carlson HE: Male hypogonadism and scleroderma. J Rheumatol 12:605–606, 1985.

139. Grossman A, Gibson J, Stansfed AG, Besser GM: Pituitary and testicular fibrosis in association with retroperitoneal fibrosis. Clin Endocrinol 12:371–374, 1980.

140. O'Donoghue DJ: Klinefelter's syndrome associated with systemic sclerosis. Postgrad Med J 58:575–576, 1982.

141. Dahl EV, Baggenstoss AH, DeWeerd JH: Testicular lesions of periarteritis nodosa, with special reference to diagnosis. Am J Med 28:222–228, 1960.

142. Inman RD, Janovic L, Dawood MY, Longcope C: Systemic lupus erythematosus in the male: A genetic and endocrine study [abstract]. Arthritis Rheum 22:624, 1979.

143. Vazquez JA, Pinies JA, Martul P, et al: Hypothalamic-pituitary-testicular function in 70 patients with myotonic dystrophy. J Endocrinol Invest 13:375–379, 1990.

144. Bartsch G, Frank ST, Marberger H, Mikuz G: Testicular torsion: Late results with special regard to fertility and endocrine function. J Urol 124:375–378, 1980.

145. Morley JE, Distiller LA, Lissoos I, et al: Testicular function in patients with spinal cord damage. Horm Metab Res 11:679–682, 1979.

146. Lushbaugh CC, Casarett GW: The effects of gonadal irradiation in clinical radiation therapy: A review. Cancer 37:1111–1120, 1976.

147. Deslypere JP, Vermeulen A: Leydig cell function in normal men: Effect of age, lifestyle, residence, diet and activity. J Clin Endocrinol Metab 59:955–962, 1984.

148. Tenover JS, Matsumoto AM, Plymate SR, Bremner WJ: The effects of aging in normal men on bioavailable testosterone and luteinizing hormone secretion: Response to clomiphene citrate. J Clin Endocrinol Metab 65:1118–1126, 1987.

149. Winters SJ, Troen P: Episodic luteinizing hormone (LH) secretion and the response of LH and follicle-stimulating hormone to LH-releasing hormone in aged men: Evidence for coexistent primary testicular insufficiency and an impairment in gonadotropin secretion. J Clin Endocrinol Metab 55:560–565, 1982.

150. Zumoff B, Strain GW, Kream J, et al: Age variation of the 24-hour mean plasma concentrations of androgens, estrogens, and gonadotropins in normal adult men. J Clin Endocrinol Metab 54:534–538, 1982.

151. Tenover JS, Matsumoto AM, Clifton DK, Bremner WJ: Age-related alterations in the circadian rhythms of pulsatile luteinizing hormone and testosterone secretion in healthy men. J Gerontol 43:M163–M169, 1988.

152. Davidson JM, Chen JJ, Crapo L, et al: Hormonal changes and sexual function in aging men. J Clin Endocrinol Metab 57:71–77, 1983.

153. Harman SM, Tsitouras PD, Costa PT, Blackman MR: Reproductive hormones in aging men: II. Basal pituitary gonadotropins and gonadotropin response to luteinizing hormone–releasing hormone. J Clin Endocrinol Metab 56:547–552, 1982.

154. Neaves WB, Johnson L, Porter JC, et al: Leydig cell numbers, daily sperm production, and serum gonadotropin levels in aging men. J Clin Endocrinol Metab 59:756–763, 1984.

155. Tenover JS, McLachlan RI, Dahl KD, et al: Decreased serum inhibin levels in elderly men: Evidence for a decline in Sertoli cell function with aging. J Clin Endocrinol Metab 67:455–459, 1988.

156. MacNaughton JA, Bangah ML, McCloud PI, Burger HG: Inhibin and age in men. Clin Endocrinol 35:341–346, 1991.

157. Korenman SG, Morley JE, Mooradian AD, et al: Secondary hypogonadism in older men: Its relation to impotence. J Clin Endocrinol Metab 71:963–969, 1990.

158. Deslypere JP, Kaufman JM, Vermeulen T, et al: Influence of age on pulsatile luteinizing hormone release and responsiveness of the gonadotrophs to sex hormone feedback in men. J Clin Endocrinol Metab 64:68–73, 1987.

159. Kaufman JM, Giri M, Deslypere JM, et al: Influence of age on the responsiveness of the gonadotrophs to luteinizing hormone–releasing hormone in males. J Clin Endocrinol Metab 72:1255–1260, 1991.

160. Winters SJ, Sherins RJ, Troen P: The gonadotropin-suppressive activity of androgen is increased in elderly men. Metabolism 33:1052–1059, 1984.

161. Tenover JS: Effects of testosterone (T) and 5α-reductase inhibitor (5-AR) administration on the responses to a sexual function questionnaire in older men [abstract]. J Androl 13:50, 1992.

162. Wilkerson JE, Horath SM, Gutin B: Plasma testosterone during treadmill exercise. J Appl Physiol 49:249–253, 1980.

163. Kujala UM, Alen M, Huhtaniemi IT: Gonadotropin-releasing hormone and human chorionic gonadotropin tests reveal that both hypothalamic and testicular endocrine functions are suppressed during acute prolonged physical exercise. Clin Endocrinol 33:219–225, 1990.

164. Opstad PK: Androgenic hormones during prolonged physical stress, sleep and energy deficiency. J Clin Endocrinol Metab 74:1176–1183, 1992.

165. Wheeler GD, Wall SR, Belcastro AN, Cumming DC: Reduced serum testosterone and prolactin levels in male distance runners. JAMA 252:514–516, 1984.

166. Rogol AD, Veldhuis JD, Williams FA, Johnson ML: Pulsatile secretion of gonadotropins and prolactin in male marathon runners. J Androl 5:21–27, 1984.

167. MacConnie SE, Barkan A, Lampman RM, et al: Decreased hypothalamic gonadotropin-releasing hormone secretion in male marathon runners. N Engl J Med 315:411–417, 1986.

168. Wheeler GD, Singh M, Pierce WD, et al: Endurance training decreases serum testosterone levels in men without change in luteinizing hormone pulsatile release. J Clin Endocrinol Metab 72:422–425, 1991.

169. Ayers JWT, Komesu Y, Romani T, Ansbacher R: Anthropomorphic, hormonal, and psychologic correlates of semen quality in endurance-trained male athletes. Fertil Steril 43:917–921, 1985.

170. Nakashima A, Koshiyama K, Uozumi T, et al: Effects of general anesthesia and severity of surgical stress on serum LH and testosterone in males. Acta Endocrinol 78:258–269, 1975.

171. Semple CG, Robertson WR, Mitchell R, et al: Mechanisms leading to hypogonadism in men with burn injuries. BMJ 295:403–407, 1987.

172. Woolf PD, Hamill RW, McDonald JV, et al: Transient hypogonadotropic hypogonadism caused by critical illness. J Clin Endocrinol Metab 60:444–450, 1985.

173. Luppa P, Munker R, Nagel D, et al: Serum androgens in intensive-care patients: Correlations with clinical findings. Clin Endocrinol 34:305–310, 1991.

174. Dong Q, Hawker F, McWilliam D, et al: Circulating immunoreactive inhibin and testosterone in men with critical illness. Clin Endocrinol 36:399–404, 1992.

175. Kreuz LE, Rose RM, Jennings JR: Suppression of plasma testosterone levels and psychological stress. Arch Gen Psychiatry 26:479–482, 1972.

176. Cameron JL, Weltzin TE, McConaha C, et al: Slowing of pulsatile luteinizing hormone secretion in men after forty-eight hours of fasting. J Clin Endocrinol Metab 73:35–41, 1991.

176a. Veldhuis JD, Icanmanesh A, Evans WS, et al: Amplitude suppression of the pulsatile mode of immunoradiometric luteinizing hormone release in fasting-induced hypoandrogenemia in normal men. J Clin Endocrinol Metab 76:587–593, 1993.

177. Rojdmark S: Increased gonadotropin responsiveness to gonadotropin-releasing hormone during fasting in normal subjects. Metabolism 36:21–26, 1987.

178. Smith SR, Chhetri MK, Johanson AJ, et al: The pituitary-gonadal axis in men with protein-calorie malnutrition. J Clin Endocrinol Metab 41:60–69, 1975.
179. Rivier C, Rivest S: Effect of stress on the activity of the hypothalamic-pituitary-gonadal axis: Peripheral and central mechanisms. Biol Reprod 45:523–532, 1991.
180. Luger A, Deuster PA, Kyle SB, et al: Acute hypothalamic-pituitary-adrenal responses to the stress of treadmill exercise: Physiologic adaptations to physical training. N Engl J Med 316:1309–1315, 1987.
181. Smoak B, Deuster P, Rabin D, Chrousos G: Corticotropin-releasing hormone is not the sole factor mediating exercise-induced adrenocorticotropin release in humans. J Clin Endocrinol Metab 73:302–306, 1991.
182. Gold PW, Gwirtsman H, Avgerinos PC, et al: Abnormal hypothalamic-pituitary-adrenal function in anorexia nervosa: Pathophysiologic mechanisms in underweight and weight-corrected patients. N Engl J Med 314:1335–1342, 1986.
183. Kanematsu T, Irahara M, Miyake T, et al: Effect of insulin-like growth factor I on gonadotropin release from the hypothalamus-pituitary axis in vitro. Acta Endocrinol 125:227–233, 1991.
184. Ziegler TR, Barbieri RL, Young LS, et al: Effects of growth hormone administration on dehydroepiandrosterone sulphate, androstenedione, testosterone and cortisol metabolism during nutritional repletion. Clin Endocrinol 34:281–287, 1991.
185. Glass AR, Swerdloff RS, Bray GA, et al: Low serum testosterone and sex hormone binding–globulin in massively obese men. J Clin Endocrinol Metab 45:1211–1219, 1977.
186. Plymate SR, Matej LA, Jones RE, Friedl KE: Inhibition of sex hormone–binding globulin production in the human hepatoma (Hep G2) cell line by insulin and prolactin. J Clin Endocrinol Metab 67:460–464, 1988.
187. Zumoff B, Strain GW, Miller LK, et al: Plasma free and non–sex-hormone-binding-globulin–bound testosterone are decreased in obese men in proportion to their degree of obesity. J Clin Endocrinol Metab 71:929–931, 1990.
188. Strain GW, Zumoff B, Kream J, et al: Mild hypogonadotropic hypogonadism in obese men. Metabolism 31:871–875, 1982.
189. Schneider G, Kirschner MA, Berkowitz R, Ertel NH: Increased estrogen production in obese men. J Clin Endocrinol Metab 48:633–638, 1979.
189a. Vermeulen A, Kaufman JM, Deslypere JP, Thomas G: Attenuated luteinizing hormone (LH) pulse amplitude but normal LH pulse frequency, and its relation to plasma androgens in hypogonadism of obese men. J Clin Endocrinol Metab 70:1140–1146, 1993.
190. Stanik SS, Dornfeld LP, Maxwell MH, et al: The effect of weight loss on reproductive hormones in obese men. J Clin Endocrinol Metab 53:828–832, 1981.
191. Kidd GS, Glass AR, Vigersky RA: The hypothalamic-pituitary-testicular axis in thyrotoxicosis. J Clin Endocrinol Metab 48:798–802, 1979.
192. Southren AL, Olivo J, Gordon GG, et al: The conversion of androgens to estrogens in hyperthyroidism. J Clin Endocrinol Metab 38:207–214, 1974.
193. Hudson RW, Edwards AL: Testicular function in hyperthyroidism. J Androl 13:117–124, 1992.
194. Cavaliere H, Abelin N, Medeiros-Neto G: Serum levels of total testosterone and sex hormone binding globulin in hypothyroid patients and normal subjects treated with incremental doses of L-T4 or L-T3. J Androl 9:215–219, 1988.
195. Wortsman J, Rosner W, Dufau ML: Abnormal testicular function in men with primary hypothyroidism. Am J Med 82:207–212, 1987.
196. Holdsworth S, Atkins RC, de Kretser DM: The pituitary testicular axis in men with chronic renal failure. N Engl J Med 296:1245–1249, 1977.
197. Handelsman DJ: Hypothalamic-pituitary gonadal dysfunction in renal failure, dialysis and renal transplantation. Endocr Rev 6:151–182, 1985.
198. Mastrogiacomo I, Feghali V, De Besi L, et al: Prolactin, gonadotropins, testosterone, and estrogens in uremic men undergoing periodic hemodialysis. Arch Androl 9:279–282, 1982.
199. Rodger RSC, Morrison L, Dewar JH, et al: Loss of pulsatile luteinizing hormone secretion in men with chronic renal failure. BMJ 291:1598–1600, 1985.
200. Blackman MR, Weintraub BD, Kourides IA, et al: Discordant elevation of the common α-subunit of the glycoprotein hormones compared to β-subunits in serum of uremic patients. J Clin Endocrinol Metab 50:846, 1980.
201. Lim VS, Kathpalia SC, Frohman LA: Hyperprolactinemia and impaired pituitary response to suppression and stimulation in chronic

renal failure: Reversal after transplantation. J Clin Endocrinol Metab 48:101–107, 1979.
202. Distiller LA, Sagel J, Morley JE, et al: Pituitary responsiveness to luteinizing hormone–releasing hormone in insulin-dependent diabetes mellitus. Diabetes 24:378–380, 1975.
203. Handelsman DJ, Conway AJ, Boylan LM, et al: Testicular function and glycemic control in diabetic men: A controlled study. Andrologia 17:488–496, 1985.
204. Murray FT, Wyss HU, Thomas RG, et al: Gonadal dysfunction in diabetic men with organic impotence. J Clin Endocrinol Metab 65:127–135, 1987.
205. Gluud C, Madsbad S, Krarup T, Bennett P: Plasma testosterone and androstenedione in insulin dependent patients at time of diagnosis and during the first year of insulin treatment. Acta Endocrinol 100:406–409, 1982.
206. Osegbe DN, Akinyanju OO: Testicular dysfunction in men with sickle cell disease. Postgrad Med J 63:95–98, 1987.
207. Landfeld CS, Schambelan M, Kaplan SL, Embury SH: Clomiphene-responsive hypogonadism in sickle cell anemia. Ann Intern Med 99:480–483, 1983.
208. Lloyd CW, Williams RH: Endocrine changes associated with Laennec's cirrhosis of the liver. Am J Med 4:315–330, 1948.
209. Van Thiel DH, Lester R, Sherins RJ: Hypogonadism in alcoholic liver disease: Evidence for a double defect. Gastroenterology 67:1188–1199, 1974.
210. Bannister P, Handley T, Chapman C, Losowsky MS: Hypogonadism in chronic liver disease: Impaired release of luteinizing hormone. BMJ 293:1191–1193, 1986.
211. Van Thiel DH, Lester R, Vaitukaitis J: Evidence for a defect in pituitary secretion of luteinizing hormone in chronic alcoholic men. J Clin Endocrinol Metab 47:499–507, 1978.
212. Bertello P, Agrimonti F, Gurioli L, et al: Circadian patterns of plasma cortisol and testosterone in chronic male alcoholics. Alcoholism (NY) 6:475–481, 1982.
213. Kirkman S, Nelson DH: Alcohol-induced pseudo–Cushing's disease: A study of prevalence with review of the literature. Metabolism 37:390–394, 1988.
214. Van Thiel DH, McClain CJ, Elson MK, et al: Evidence for autonomous secretion of prolactin in some alcoholic men with cirrhosis and gynecomastia. Metabolism 27:1778–1784, 1978.
215. Gluud C: Testosterone and alcoholic cirrhosis. Epidemiologic, pathophysiologic and therapeutic studies in men. Dan Med Bull 35:564–574, 1988.
216. Gordon GG, Altman K, Southren AL, et al: Effect of alcohol (ethanol) administration on sex-hormone metabolism in normal men. N Engl J Med 295:793–797, 1976.
217. Brzek A: Alcohol and male fertility (preliminary report). Andrologia 19:32–36, 1987.
218. Baker HWG, Burger HG, de Kretser DM, et al: A study of the endocrine manifestations of hepatic cirrhosis. QJ Med 45:145–178, 1976.
219. Van Thiel DH, Loriaux DL: Evidence for an adrenal origin of plasma estrogens in alcoholic men. Metabolism 28:536–541, 1979.
220. Gordon GG, Olivo J, Rafii F, Southren L: Conversion of androgens to estrogens in cirrhosis of the liver. J Clin Endocrinol Metab 40:1018–1026, 1975.
221. Cronholm T, Eriksson H: Effects of prolonged ethanol administration on the hepatic estrogen receptor in the rat. FEBS Lett 133:272–274, 1981.
222. Terasaki T, Nowlin DM, Pardridge WM: Differential binding of testosterone and estradiol to isoforms of sex hormone-binding globulin: Selective alteration of estradiol binding in cirrhosis. J Clin Endocrinol Metab 67:639–643, 1988.
223. The Copenhagen Study Group for Liver Diseases: Testosterone treatment of men with alcoholic cirrhosis: A double-blind study. Hepatology 6:807–813, 1986.
224. Milder MS, Cook JD, Stray S, Finch CA: Idiopathic hemochromatosis, an interim report. Medicine 59:34–49, 1980.
225. Bezwoda WR, Bothwell TH, Van der Walt LA, et al: An investigation into gonadal dysfunction in patients with idiopathic haemochromatosis. Clin Endocrinol 6:377–385, 1977.
226. Kley HK, Niederau C, Stremmel W, et al: Conversion of androgens to estrogens in idiopathic hemochromatosis: Comparison with alcoholic liver cirrhosis. J Clin Endocrinol Metab 61:1–6, 1985.
227. Cundy T, Bomford A, Butler J, et al: Hypogonadism and sexual dysfunction in hemochromatosis: The effects of cirrhosis and diabetes. J Clin Endocrinol Metab 69:110–116, 1989.
228. Kelly TM, Edwards CQ, Meikle AW, Kushner JP: Hypogonadism in hemochromatosis: Reversal with iron depletion. Ann Intern Med 101:629–632, 1984.

229. Lufkin EG, Baldus WP, Bergstralh EJ, Kao PC: Influence of phlebotomy treatment on abnormal hypothalamic-pituitary function in genetic hemochromatosis. Mayo Clin Proc 62:473–479, 1987.
230. Wang C, Tso SC, Todd D: Hypogonadotropic hypogonadism in severe β-thalassemia: Effect of chelation and pulsatile gonadotropin-releasing hormone therapy. J Clin Endocrinol Metab 68:511–516, 1989.
231. Kennedy WR, Alter M, Sung JH: Progressive proximal spinal and bulbar muscular atrophy of late onset. Neurology 18:671–680, 1968.
232. Arbizu T, Santamaria J, Gomez JM, et al: A family with adult spinal and bulbar muscular atrophy, X-linked inheritance and associated testicular failure. J Neurol Sci 59:371–382, 1983.
233. Fischbeck KH, Souders D, La Spada A: A candidate gene for X-linked spinal muscular atrophy. Adv Neurol 56:209–213, 1989.
234. La Spada AR, Wilson EM, Lubahn DB, et al: Androgen receptor gene mutations in X-linked spinal and bulbar muscular atrophy. Nature 352:7–79, 1991.
235. Libber SM, Migeon CJ, Brown FR III, Moser HW: Adrenal and testicular function in 14 patients with adrenoleukodystrophy or adrenomyeloneuropathy. Horm Res 24:1–8, 1986.
236. Braunstein GD, Kohler PO: Endocrine manifestations of histiocytosis. Am J Pediatr Hematol Oncol 3:67–75, 1981.
237. Stuart CA, Neelon FA, Lebovitz HE: Hypothalamic insufficiency: The cause of hypopituitarism in sarcoidosis. Ann Intern Med 88:589–594, 1978.
238. Schilsky RL, Lewis BJ, Sherins RJ, Young RC: Gonadal dysfunction in patients receiving chemotherapy for cancer. Ann Intern Med 93:109–114, 1980.
239. Sherins RJ, Olweny CLM, Ziegler JL: Gynecomastia and gonadal dysfunction in adolescent boys treated with combination chemotherapy for Hodgkin's disease. N Engl J Med 299:12–16, 1978.
240. Chapman RM, Sutcliffe SB, Malpas JS: Male gonadal dysfunction in Hodgkin's disease: A prospective study. JAMA 245:1323–1328, 1981.
241. Friedman NM, Plymate SR: Leydig cell dysfunction and gynaecomastia in adult males treated with alkylating agents. Clin Endocrinol 12:553–556, 1980.
242. Morris ID, Shalet SM: Endocrine-mediated protection from cytotoxic-induced testicular damage. J Endocrinol 120:7–9, 1989.
243. Vigersky RA, Chapman RM, Berenbery J, Glass AR: Testicular dysfunction in untreated Hodgkin's Disease. Am J Med 73:482–486, 1982.
244. Dobs AS, Sarma PS, Guarnieri T, Griffith L: Testicular dysfunction with amiodarone use. J Am Coll Cardiol 18:1328–1332, 1991.
245. Raynaud J-P, Ojasoo T: The design and use of sex-steroid antagonists. J Steroid Biochem 25:811–833, 1986.
246. Loriaux DL, Menard R, Taylor A, et al: Spironolactone and endocrine dysfunction. Ann Intern Med 85:630–636, 1976.
247. Rose LI, Underwood RH, Newmark SR, et al: Pathophysiology of spironolactone-induced gynecomastia. Ann Intern Med 87:398–403, 1977.
248. Jensen RT, Collen MJ, Pandol SJ, et al: Cimetidine-induced impotence and breast changes in patients with gastric hypersecretory states. N Engl J Med 308:883–887, 1983.
249. Carlson HE, Ippoliti AF, Swerdloff RS: Endocrine effects of acute and chronic cimetidine administration. Dig Dis Sci 26:428–431, 1981.
250. Winters SJ, Banks JL, Loriaux DL: Cimetidine is an antiandrogen in the rat. Gastroenterology 76:504–508, 1979.
251. Crawford ED, Eisenberger MA, McLeod DG, et al: A controlled trial of leuprolide with and without flutamide in prostatic carcinoma. N Engl J Med 321:419–424, 1989.
252. Kemppainen JA, Lane MV, Sar M, Wilson EM: Androgen receptor phosphorylation, turnover, nuclear transport, and transcriptional activation: Specificity for steroids and antihormones. J Biol Chem 267:968–974, 1992.
253. Veldhuis JD, Urban RJ, Dufau ML: Evidence that androgen negative feedback regulates hypothalamic gonadotropin-releasing hormone impulse strength and the burst-like secretion of biologically active luteinizing hormone in men. J Clin Endocrinol Metab 74:1227–1235, 1992.
254. Sonino N: The use of ketoconazole as an inhibitor of steroid production. N Engl J Med 317:812–818, 1987.
255. Pont A, Williams PL, Azhar S, et al: Ketoconazole blocks testosterone biosynthesis. Arch Intern Med 142:2137–2140, 1982.
256. McConnell JD, Wilson JD, George FW, et al: Finasteride, an inhibitor of 5α-reductase, suppresses prostatic dihydrotestosterone in men with benign prostatic hyperplasia. J Clin Endocrinol Metab 74:505–508, 1992.
257. Rittmaster RS, Lemay A, Zwicker H, et al: Effect of finasteride, a 5 alpha-reductase inhibitor, on serum gonadotropins in normal men. J Clin Endocrinol Metab 75:484–488, 1992.
258. Toovey S, Hudson E, Hendry WF, Levi AJ: Sulphasalazine and male infertility: Reversibility and possible mechanism. Gut 22:445–451, 1981.
259. Schaefer CF, Gunn CG, Dubowski KM: Normal plasma testosterone concentrations after marijuana smoking. N Engl J Med 292:867–868, 1975.
260. Sauer MA, Rifka SM, Hawks RL, et al: Marijuana: Interaction with the estrogen receptor. J Pharmacol Exp Ther 224:404–407, 1983.
261. Purohit V, Ahluwahlia BS, Vigersky RA: Marijuana inhibits dihydrotestosterone binding to the androgen receptor. Endocrinology 107:848–850, 1980.

134

Male Infertility

H. W. GORDON BAKER

Historical Aspects

There have been major advances in the management of infertility over the past 20 years, particularly with the introduction and widespread use of assisted reproductive technology (ART)—artificial insemination with husband's semen (AIH), donor insemination, in vitro fertilization (IVF), and gamete intrafallopian transfer (GIFT)—such that now most couples can be assured of having a child if they are prepared to undertake one or more of these treatments. Despite these advances the causes of most types of male infertility remain mysterious, and the results of treatment of specific conditions are still relatively poor. For example, there are still many failures after epididymal surgery and medical treatment for sperm autoimmunity. Also, although claiming to adhere to universal declarations of human rights recognizing the right of couples to found a family, many governments and health insurance companies fail to accept treatments of infertility as legitimate rebatable items. Furthermore, some governments have introduced restrictive legislation to regulate the clinical practice and research aspects of ART. In addition to this discrimination, infertile men often are afforded little compassion by their friends and relatives.

Many of the syndromes and specific diseases that cause male infertility have been recognized for some time; for example, various forms of gonadotropin deficiency were described early this century, and successful treatment with gonadotropins was reported from the mid-1960's.[1, 2] Klinefelter's syndrome was described in 1942,[3] and the relationship between undescended testes and infertility has been recognized from antiquity. Varicocele surgery for infertility is discussed in a book published in 1877, although it is only since the mid-1950's that the procedure has become popular.[4–6] The first surgery for epididymal obstructions was performed in 1905.[7] John Hunter is supposed to have been the first to have performed AIH in 1785 and William Pancoast, donor insemination in 1884.

There has been concern that male fertility may be declining because evidence exists in the literature reported over the 20th century of reduced average sperm concentrations. It is suggested that this reduction is related to environmental pollution.[8, 9, 9a] However, there does not appear to be any evidence of declining human fertility.[10]

Male infertility management as a specialty has evolved differently in various countries; for example, dermatologists and venereologists particularly in Europe and urologists and endocrinologists in many countries have mainly been involved. Plastic surgeons have recently taken an active role in epididymal and vasal surgery. The development of ART predominantly has involved gynecologists, and this group has become increasingly interested in male infertility. In the future it is likely that the clinical management of male infertility will be taken over by infertility subspecialists trained to deal with both sexes. There are now societies of andrology in many countries, and the scientific meetings usually encompass male infertility, coital disorders, and the endocrine management of prostatic disease.

NATURE AND CAUSES OF MALE INFERTILITY

Definitions

Although the terms infertility, sterility, and subfertility are used interchangeably to indicate difficulty conceiving, in this chapter they are used more specifically as follows. Infertility is a state in which there is a failure to produce a pregnancy within a reasonable period of trying, usually 12 months. Sterility is the inability to produce a pregnancy, and this may be reversible or irreversible. Subfertility is a state of infertility but not clearly sterility because of the absence of an absolute barrier to reproduction, such as azoospermia.

The time trying, 12 months, used to define infertility in couples who are not suspected of having a major cause of infertility, is reasonable. The average pregnancy rates in most human communities range from 15 to 25 per cent per month, such that about 50 per cent have conceived by 5 months and 85 per cent by 12 months.[10] Couples trying for a subsequent pregnancy have higher rates: 33 per cent in the first month and 50 per cent within two months.[11, 12] Demographic studies of Western communities indicate that about 5 per cent of married women have not produced children after five years of marriage, and it is assumed that infertility is the cause in at least one half of these cases. The remainder are actively avoiding conception by contraceptive practices.[10, 13–15]

Pregnancy rate data often were not analyzed effectively in the past. Floating numerator pregnancy rates, in which a percentage of patients pregnant is given without regard for time of exposure, have been recorded in the infertility literature despite the use of real rates for other fertility measurements, for example, the Pearl index for contraceptive failures. There has recently been much greater use of statistical methods for regression analysis with censored data—survival analysis and graphs derived in the same way as life tables.[12, 16–18] Although these were developed to examine death or other event rates particularly for cancer therapy trials, they do appear to be valid and applicable to pregnancy rates. Survival analysis methods are especially useful for assessing the impact of groups of variables on pregnancy rates, for analysis of prognostic factors, and for testing results of therapeutic trials.

The World Health Organization (WHO)[19] has provided a manual with specific nomenclature for semen defects such as aspermia, no ejaculate, and azoospermia, no sperm present in the semen or in a centrifuged deposit of the semen. Others include oligozoospermia, sperm concentration less than 20 million/ml; asthenozoospermia, sperm motility less than 50 per cent total and less than 25 per cent with rapid progressive motility; and teratozoospermia, fewer than 30 per cent of sperm with normal morphology. Compound terms are possible, such as oligoasthenoteratozoospermia, but in common parlance most leave out the "zoo" for the sake of euphony. Because of the variability of semen analysis results from day to day within one man and the lack of clinical importance, these terms do not need to be overemphasized. Abnormal semen samples do not necessarily equate with infertility or sterility because many fertile men have semen variables outside the "normal" cutoff values.

Definitions of clinical terms also require some attention. *Hypogonadism* is a relatively nonspecific term for decreased testicular or ovarian function that could include a disorder of gamete production or function and/or a disorder of sex hormone production or action. Some investigators reserve the term in men for testicular failure associated with androgen deficiency resulting in reduced virilization. Primary hypogonadism results from disorders that affect the gonads directly, and secondary hypogonadism results from defective pituitary gonadotropin secretion (see Ch. 133).

Incidence and Distribution

In most Western countries about one in seven couples, or 15 per cent, do not conceive within one year of trying for a pregnancy. In the United Kingdom about 24 per cent (95 per cent CL 22 to 27 per cent) of women experience infertility at some stage in their lives.[12] Types of infertility include female factors (ovulatory disorder, tubal obstruction, or other pelvic pathology; see Chs. 118 and 119) in about 50 per cent and, depending on the definition of abnormality, a semen disorder in 50 per cent. Analysis of detected abnormalities in the female partners of men being investigated for infertility showed that the frequency increased in parallel with semen quality; 25 per cent of women with azoospermic partners had abnormalities, whereas more than 50 per cent of women with normospermic partners had abnormalities.[20] Thus with the milder disorders there frequently are abnormalities in both partners.[20–22] The WHO Special Program of Research, Development, and Research Training in Human Reproduction has made major contributions to the standardization of the investigation of infertility. A large clinical study of more than 8500 infertile couples in 25 countries has been published, and this also showed abnormalities in both partners in 26.5 per cent.[22]

Variation in Infertility in Different Regions

Marked differences in the frequency of some causes of infertility exist in different regions of the world. For example, in Africa tubal disease in women and postinflammatory epididymal obstructions are frequent, whereas the latter are rare in Western countries, where venereal diseases are treated promptly and effectively.[23] Chromosomal disorders, such as Klinefelter's syndrome, are probably equally frequent the world over. Genetic diseases—for example, Kallmann's syndrome and congenital absence of the vasa associated with cystic fibrosis mutations—are expected to show some racial variation.[24, 25, 25a] It is curious that epididymal obstruction associated with chronic sinopulmonary disease (Young's syndrome) is diagnosed frequently in Australia and the United Kingdom yet is rare or unrecognized in the United States.[26–28]

Relation with Female Disorders

Although the interaction between male and female factors in the ease of conception is intuitive, its extent is not clear and the operating mechanisms are not understood.

As already mentioned, the finding in both partners of minor pathology that might contribute to infertility is common, for example, mild endometriosis, variably poor semen results, and a small varicocele. The frequency of these abnormalities in the fertile populations is not well known but could be considerable.[22] That the female partners of subfertile men are, as a group, subfertile is shown by the lower pregnancy rates achieved by donor sperm in comparison with those obtained in women whose husbands are sterile.[29] On the other hand, pregnancies that occur with men with poor semen quality might be explained by a greater fertility in the women, for example, pregnancies that occur during gonadotropin treatment of men with Kallmann's syndrome or during testosterone suppression for male contraception (see Ch. 137).[30–32] These aspects of fertility do not appear to be evaluated by current tests and might involve superior gamete transport in the female genital tract. The complexity of the relation between tests and outcomes is exemplified by this anecdote. The man had isolated gonadotropin deficiency. Treatment with gonadotropins resulted in spermatogenesis, but the sperm concentration was 5 million/ml, motility 20 per cent, and abnormal morphology 90 per cent at the time both children were conceived. His wife had a unicornuate uterus and oligomenorrhea probably caused by mild polycystic ovary disease. After ovulation induction with clomiphene, conception occurred within three months of the appearance of sperm in the semen on both occasions. Further understanding of this area might have great relevance to the management of infertility. Also, it is crucial that both partners of the infertile couple are investigated and managed together as a unit (see Ch. 119).

Etiology and Classification of Male Infertility

Various causes of male infertility are known, from genetic to psychological, but in most men who are investigated for infertility the precise cause and mechanisms involved in the case cannot be determined.[20] Even when a condition exists that probably caused testicular damage, such as past undescended testes or orchitis, it is not known why some men with the same history have better semen quality and are not infertile. Some of the conditions associated with infertility are more like risk factors than causative factors. Although it usually is presumed that oligospermia must result from a defect of development or subsequent damage, it is possible that some men with oligospermia could represent the lower end of the normal range, in a similar way that short stature is not always the result of a disease process.

The classification of causes of male infertility based on the effectiveness of treatment is shown in Table 134–1. Other classifications of causative mechanisms are possible.[20] WHO has developed a practical, polyglot classification to go with their standard investigation of the infertile couple,[33] and computer software has been developed (MIDACO, Amsatec Corp., Belgium). Classification on the basis of prognosis may be particularly useful in the subfertile group, and this may have several layers, including duration of infertility, female factors, and severity of semen abnormality. The results of research on ART should

TABLE 134–1. CLASSIFICATION OF MALE INFERTILITY BY POTENTIAL FOR TREATMENT

TYPE OF INFERTILITY	FREQUENCY (%)
Untreatable Sterility	12.8
Primary seminiferous tubule failure	12.1
Total teratospermia or immotile sperm	0.7
Treatable Conditions	12.1
Gonadotrophin deficiency	0.6
Obstructive azoospermia	5.0
Sperm autoimmunity	6.0
Disorders of sexual function	0.5
Reversible toxic effects	0.02
Untreatable Subfertility	75
Oligospermia	38
Asthenospermia, teratospermia	37

broaden understanding of the mechanisms by which sperm defects interfere with fertility. This may provide new modes of classifying sperm disorders, for example, defects of zona binding, zona penetration, oolemma fusion, and pronucleus formation (see below).

CLINICAL EVALUATION

The WHO task force on infertility developed a standardized procedure for the clinical assessment of infertile couples.[33] In a modification of this, basic historical data are elicited by questionnaire that the patients complete before being seen.[20] This makes it easier to find and enter information into a computer data base.

A practical approach can be recommended to separate irreversible sterility from potentially treatable conditions and those conditions that cause subfertility, for which there is no treatment of proven value (see Table 134–1). It cannot be overemphasized that both members of the couple need to be involved in the assessment and discussion of the results. An awareness of the emotional reaction of the couple to the diagnosis of infertility is crucial. An understanding of the evolution of this emotional reaction is also important because this may interfere with investigations and clinical evaluation. From the earliest stages a couple needs to be given clear information about the prognosis and the alternatives of accepting childlessness and considering donor insemination or adoption. Historical details may need to be elicited on several occasions because such intimate information may not be disclosed while the couple is embarrassed, hostile, or confused. Previous venereal disease or pregnancy may be concealed from the partner.

History

Duration and Nature of Infertility

Details of previous pregnancies in the current or other relationships, including the time taken to conceive each pregnancy, should be recorded because this is important for the prognosis. Also, if the infertility is of short duration, the couple may be concerned about a known infertility-related problem, such as past undescended testes or orchitis, or they may be unaware of the normal human fertility

rates. The speed with which further investigations are undertaken depends heavily on the possibility of finding remediable abnormalities and on the age of the female partner.

Family History

For most of the common types or associations of male infertility, such as idiopathic oligospermia, varicocele, and past undescended testes, there may be some familial aggregation, but this does not appear to be important. Young's syndrome has been described in twin brothers.[34] Men with sperm autoimmunity have increased frequencies of family histories of organ-specific autoimmune diseases and increased frequencies of autoantibodies to thyroid and gastric parietal cells in their serum, compared with control infertile men without sperm autoimmunity.[35, 36] More than 50 per cent of men with congenital absence of the vasa have one of the common cystic fibrosis gene mutations. Because some have been shown to be compound heterozygotes, it has been suggested that this condition is a genital form of cystic fibrosis.[25, 25a] Some boys with cystic fibrosis, however, have normal vasa; thus it is possible that the reason for the failure of development of the wolffian duct structures in the common cystic fibrosis phenotype and congenital absence of the vasa without clinical features of cystic fibrosis is more complicated.[37] There is also the possibility that other epididymal disorders, such as necrospermia, idiopathic obstruction, and Young's syndrome, are due to cystic fibrosis gene mutations. Kallmann's syndrome and dystrophia myotonica are rare but well characterized genetic diseases (see Ch. 133).[38, 39]

Coital Adequacy and Timing

Intravaginal deposition of semen near the time of ovulation is crucial for fertility. Infrequent coitus is quite common in couples seen for infertility. This may be a result of the emotional reaction to infertility. Rarely, couples are seen who are using some popular media advice on predetermining the sex of the child by timing intercourse before or after ovulation. Itinerant and shiftworkers may have problems in timing coitus with time of ovulation. Low libido may result from androgen deficiency, general illness, or a psychological reaction to the infertility or other stresses. Information on impotence and ejaculatory disturbances is important to elicit early in the interview (see Ch. 135).

Childhood and Pubertal Development

In utero exposure to diethylstilbestrol may have caused epididymal malformations, undescended testes, and reduced sperm production in adult life in some male offspring.[40] Treatment in childhood for penile or scrotal disorders (e.g., hypospadias, epispadias, urethral valves, undescended testes, inguinal hernia, or hydroceles) could be relevant (see Ch. 109). The timing of sexual maturation and its completeness are important for men with primary or secondary hypogonadism. There may have been associated growth problems that required treatment (see Ch. 111). Early puberty and growth resulting in short stature suggest congenital adrenal hyperplasia (see Ch. 104).[41]

General Health

Any illness, acute or chronic, could impair sperm production in a nonspecific manner.[42] Acute fevers are reputed to produce transient declines of a few months' duration.[43] Diabetes mellitus may be associated with impotence in early uncontrolled stages, with ejaculatory disorders resulting from autonomic neuropathy, and with sperm autoimmunity. Men with renal disease may have infertility of multifactorial origin, including testicular failure from chronic illness, cytotoxic drug exposure, zinc deficiency, and damage to the vasa or penile blood supply during kidney transplantation. However, as with cirrhosis, provided that metabolic decompensation is not severe, semen quality often is adequate for fertility.[42] Most men with chronic spinal cord damage cannot ejaculate, and sperm obtained by electroejaculation often have poor motility. The cause of this is unknown but does not appear to be related to defective spermatogenesis.

Respiratory Disease

Pneumonia in childhood, bronchiectasis or surgery for bronchiectasis, chronic productive cough, frequent attacks of bronchitis or pneumonia, and chronic sinusitis or surgery for sinusitis are characteristic of men with Young's syndrome.[26-28] Physical examination usually shows some evidence of the chronic lung disease with rhonchi or rales at the lung bases or in the lingula. Evidence of nasal obstruction is common, but clubbing of the fingers is rare. Bronchiectasis, sinusitis, and occasionally situs inversus are also common in men with immotile sperm from cilial defects.[44, 45] Rarely, men with cystic fibrosis present with infertility.[37]

Undescended Testes

Previously undescended testes are common in men being investigated for infertility (see Ch. 133).[20, 46, 47] In the Melbourne survey 7.7 per cent of men seen for infertility had a history of undescended testes: 11 per cent of those with average sperm concentrations of 0 or less than 1 million/ml and 3 per cent of those with more than 20 million/ml. Because less than 1 per cent of boys do not have both testes in the scrotum by age 1 year, the undescended testis is an important risk factor for infertility.[47] It is rare in Western countries that this condition has not been treated in childhood. The main concerns are cosmetic and that early detection of a testicular tumor is difficult if the testes remain undescended.[48]

Bilateral undescended testes, particularly if transplantation of testes was necessary, carry a worse outlook for fertility than unilateral undescended testes, but otherwise, the position of testes does not appear to have any prognostic significance.[49, 50] Rarely, the testes atrophy after surgery. Undescended testes may be associated with disorders of testicular hormone production or action during fetal development, such as Kallmann's syndrome, defects of androgen receptors or metabolism, and diethylstilbestrol exposure in utero.[51] Whether those children who had hormone treatment for undescended testes have any subsequent infertility problems is uncertain because there is a general feeling that those testes that descended with hormonal treatment were probably only retractile.[52] With unilateral

undescended testes the possibility of a difference in the degree of impairment of spermatogenesis on the two sides should be borne in mind. For example, a man with an atrophic right testis after orchidopexy and a left varicocele might benefit from varicocele surgery. Alternatively, a man with an atrophic right testis after bilateral orchidopexy might have an epididymal obstruction on the left side as a result of the surgery. It is still undetermined whether early surgery for undescended testes reduces the severity of the subsequent spermatogenic disorder. It is possible that the dystrophic testis fails to descend and also fails to produce sperm well into adult life despite early surgery. It is difficult to explain otherwise how men with unilateral undescended testes are so overrepresented in the infertile population.

Testicular Pain and Swelling

Episodes of severe testicular pain and swelling may result from torsion, infarction, orchitis, epididymitis, or epididymo-orchitis and may be followed by loss or atrophy of the testis. Postinflammatory atrophy is particularly frequent with mumps orchitis and rare with other illnesses such as glandular fever and brucellosis. Epididymitis or epididymo-orchitis of bacterial origin more commonly is associated with episodes of dysuria, urethritis, or urinary tract infections and may follow straining with heavy lifting. Episodes of urethritis associated with sexually transmitted diseases are important to evaluate, particularly whether or not there was associated epididymal pain or swelling and the duration of the symptoms. Some patients have postgonococcal obstructions in the tails of the epididymides without clear or admitted histories of epididymal pain or swelling.

Other Testicular Problems

Failure of development and a decrease in size of one or both testes are important symptoms of spermatogenic defects. Torsion of the testes or surgery for torsion and its outcome are important because on occasion the testes atrophy despite surgery. Fixation of the testes may also cause epididymal obstruction. Surgery in the pelvic or scrotal region may cause genital tract obstruction or infarction of the testes; for example, vas damage may occur with hernia repairs and kidney transplantation. Testicular biopsy may inadvertently damage the epididymis. Similarly, surgery for hydroceles or epididymal cysts may result in the obstruction of the epididymis. Hematomas in the scrotum and infarction of the testes may follow interference with the vascular supply of the testes. Rarely, autoimmune orchitis results from testicular injury or inflammation. Testicular tumors, including carcinoma in situ, may occur with increased frequency in men with infertility even without previous undescended testes (see Ch. 136).[53-55]

Iatrogenic Infertility

Vasectomy and Sertoli cell–only syndrome caused by successful chemotherapy and radiation therapy for malignant tumors of the testes, leukemia, or lymphoma are the most common forms of medically induced infertility.[56-60] Cytotoxic drugs are also occasionally given for serious autoimmune diseases.[58] Although some treatment regimens allow recovery of fertility, those that involve alkylating agents usually do not, especially when given in childhood.[56–60] Alkylating agents, such as cyclophosphamide and busulfan, destroy spermatogonia.[58, 60] Antimetabolites may be used to treat psoriasis, and this could have a transient adverse effect on spermatogenesis.[61] Treatment with sulfasalazine for inflammatory bowel disease or arthritis causes a reversible impairment of semen quality.[62–64] Cessation of salazopyrin often results in a marked improvement in semen quality over several months. Many other drugs have real or potential adverse effects on spermatogenesis or sexual performance, including androgens, anabolic agents, estrogens, glucocorticoids, cimetidine, spironolactone, antibacterials (especially nitrofurantoin), antihypertensive drugs, and psychotropic agents (see Chs. 15, 24, 132, 133). However, these are not common causes of infertility in practice. It is also important to recognize that any severe illness might be associated with a reduction in semen quality and that improvement in general health may improve semen quality. These changes take place slowly over several months because the spermatogenic cycle takes an average of 74 days from the division of a stem spermatogonium until the development of its progeny into mature spermatids.[42]

Antispermatogenic Factors

Exposure to heat from frequent sauna or spa baths or microwave radiation or in those in certain occupations, such as vehicle drivers, furnace operators, and perhaps outdoor workers in the summer in hot regions, may cause a decline in spermatogenesis.[65–67] This may be more obvious in subjects with other defects that could impair testicular heat exchange, such as obesity and varicoceles. Exposure to chemicals in the workplace or elsewhere, particularly nematocides, organophosphates, estrogens, benzine, zinc, lead, cadmium, and mercury fumes, may have antispermatogenic effects, but in general these exposures are well known and closely monitored, and few workers are now at risk of occupational infertility in most Western societies.[65] Transport drivers and farmers may still have some occupationally related interference with fertility from either temperature effects in the former or agricultural chemical exposure in the latter. Various social drugs, including tobacco, alcohol, marijuana, and narcotics, are potentially antispermatogenic, but these usually require heavy usage for an adverse effect.[68, 69] Some addicts have other organ damage, such as cirrhosis, which may further impair testicular function.[42]

Physical Examination

As well as palpation of the scrotum and inspection of the development of androgen-dependent structures, full physical examination is advisable with particular emphasis on the respiratory system for those men suspected of having genital tract obstructions, on the prostate for ejaculatory duct obstruction, defects of androgen production or action, or prostatitis and on the endocrine system with testicular failure. Other systems occasionally are relevant, such as the nervous system with autonomic neuropathy or dystrophia myotonica, optic field defects with pituitary tumors, and hyposmia with Kallmann's syndrome (see Chs. 90, 109, and 133).

Virilization

Hair distribution varies markedly between men and may be hard to assess. The loss of facial, pubic, axillary, and body hair is an important feature of androgen deficiency but often is unrecognized by patients. They may, however, note a reduced frequency of the need to shave. The stages of genital and pubic hair development can be recorded according to the method of Tanner (see Ch. 111). Some atrophy with depigmentation and loss of rugae in the skin of the scrotum may occur with the development of androgen deficiency in the adult. Eunuchoidal proportions (arm span greater than 5 cm longer than height or pubis-to-floor measurement greater than 5 cm longer than one half the height) result from delayed fusion of the epiphyses in Caucasians or Asians and are a good sign of delayed or incomplete puberty.

Gynecomastia

Gynecomastia of mild degree is common in men with testicular failure of any cause.[42] Marked gynecomastia may be associated with Klinefelter's syndrome, cirrhosis, androgen receptor defects, or estrogen-producing tumors (see Ch. 139). Galactorrhea is rare in men and not always associated with hyperprolactinemia.[70]

Penis

Examination of the penis for the position of the meatus, phimosis, urethral strictures, and Peyronie's disease is important because these may influence the adequacy or completeness of ejaculation. Inadequate penile size appears to be an exceptionally rare cause of infertility.[71]

Scrotal Contents

Examination of the scrotal contents is critical in the evaluation of male infertility.

EXAMINATION TECHNIQUE. A general approach to the examination is outlined in Figure 134–1. Sometimes it is difficult to examine the scrotum thoroughly because of ticklishness or because the scrotum is very tight. Testes not present in the scrotum may be palpable in the subcutaneous tissue in the groin or, occasionally, in the inguinal canal. If remnants of the vas and epididymis can be palpated in the scrotum, it is probable that the testis atrophied completely early in life possibly as the result of torsion—the vanishing testis.[72] It usually is possible to hold the spermatic cord above the testes with the forefinger and thumb of one hand while palpating the body of the testes and the head, body, and tail of the epididymis and then, by changing hands, follow the vas up to the neck of the scrotum. This is performed on both sides. Pain on palpation or excessive tenderness suggests inflammation. Loss of normal testicular sensation may occur with chronic inflammations, neuropathy, or neoplasia.

ORCHIDOMETRY. The volume of the testes is determined by comparison with an orchidometer—a set of ellipsoids of labeled volume.[73] Other measurements with calipers or rings are less accurate. In most Western countries testicular volume averages 20 to 25 ml and ranges from 15 to 30 ml. In the absence of varicoceles the right and left testes are

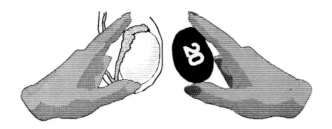

Orchidometry

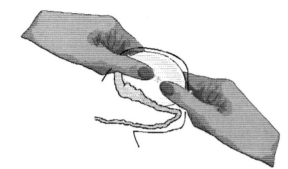

Palpation of testis

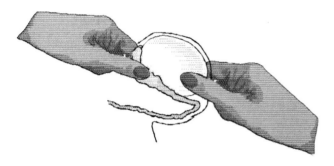

Palpation of epididymis

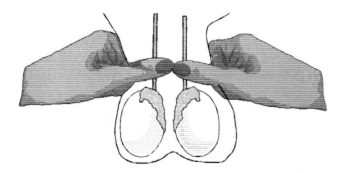

Checking for varicocele

FIGURE 134–1. Clinical examination of the scrotum.

about equal in size. With large numbers of subjects it can be shown that testicular volume is related to body size and to number of sperm per ejaculate.[22] Thus 15-ml testes may be small in a large man and 12-ml testes may be normal in a small man. Because seminiferous tubules constitute more than 90 per cent of the volume of the testes, severe impairment of spermatogenesis usually is associated with testicular atrophy.

DETECTION OF VARICOCELE. With the man standing up, the scrotum can be inspected for swelling of the pampiniform plexus and a cough or Valsalva impulse seen or palpated by holding the spermatic cords between the thumb and index finger of each hand and elevating the testes toward the external inguinal ring. This maneuver reduces the risk of confusing contractions of the cremaster muscles with venous impulses. Varicocele size can be graded into those that have only cough impulses without palpable enlargement of the spermatic cord (grade 1), palpable enlargement (grade 2), and visible enlargement (grade 3). Although predominantly a left-sided condition, varicoceles occasionally do occur on the right side, and an association between a moderate to large left-sided varicocele and a small right-sided varicocele is reasonably common. Contact thermography may be undertaken to demonstrate increased temperature of the skin over a varicocele, but this appears to be a less sensitive method of varicocele detection than palpation.[74] Many cough impulse–only (grade 1) varicoceles are not thermography positive.

TESTICULAR ABNORMALITIES. During palpation of each testis, shape, consistency, and the possibility of other abnormalities, such as tumors and scars, should be noted. Reduced consistency or softness of the testes is a feature of reduced spermatogenesis, but this is a variable sign.

EPIDIDYMAL ABNORMALITIES. While palpating the epididymis the following possibilities should be contemplated: congenital absence of the vas or other failures of development; enlargements of the heads of the epididymis in acquired epididymal obstruction; nodules in the tail of the epididymis in postinflammatory blocks; and cysts in the epididymis, particularly those that might be spermatoceles. Solid masses in the epididymis usually are adenomatoid tumors; cancer of the epididymis is extremely rare. In men with very small testes—less than 5 ml—small epididymides suggest severe androgen deficiency, as would occur with gonadotropin deficiency, whereas more normal-sized epididymides are seen with postpubertal testicular atrophy or a severe seminiferous epithelial disorder, such as Klinefelter's syndrome.

VASAL ABNORMALITIES. Abnormalities of the vas, such as nodules or the lengths of the vas segments in men with vasectomy, should be recorded. Hard thickening and beading of the vas and epididymis may indicate severe postinflammatory scarring and raise the possibility of tuberculosis.

MISCELLANEOUS ABNORMALITIES. Many often incidental scrotal abnormalities may be discovered during examination for infertility. The discovery of scars may remind the patient of forgotten surgery. Scrotal dermatitis and fat pads around the genitals in extreme obesity may disturb temperature regulation. Retroversion of the testes is common: The vas and the body and tail of the epididymis are anterior rather than posterior to the testes. Variants with the testes hanging upside down or horizontally are much less common. Testes may retract into the superficial inguinal region, especially if small. Hydroceles of mild degree are common. A tense hydrocele may hide a testicular tumor. Unilateral absence of the vas commonly is associated with absence of the kidney and ureter on the same side. Cysts include hydatids of the appendix testis (Morgagni) or epididymis. These typically are anterior to the head of the epididymis. Spermatoceles and cysts of the paradidymis (an unconnected developmental remnant tubule) may be found in the head or body of the epididymis. Inguinal hernias and nonspecific thickening, lipoma, or encysted hydroceles of the cord usually are palpated above and behind the epididymis. Many of these anomalies have little relation with infertility.

The accuracy and reproducibility of clinical examination even for structures as accessible as those in the scrotum may not be high. With practice, orchidometry can be repeated to within one to two orchidometer sizes. Varicoceles may vary in size from day to day. Even absence of the vasa may be overlooked.

LABORATORY EVALUATION

Semen Analysis

The most important laboratory investigation in male infertility is semen analysis. The variables assessed, the methods of assessment, and the acceptable ranges are contained in the WHO Laboratory Manual for the Examination of Human Semen and Semen–Cervical Mucus Interaction.[19] It is crucial that the laboratory is experienced in the performance of careful semen analyses and should have facilities nearby with adequate privacy for the collection of semen by masturbation.

The collection of semen by masturbation occasionally is impossible because of religious strictures or other reasons. In such instances semen may be obtained by coitus interruptus or by using a special nontoxic condom made of Teflon or other material.[75] Ordinary latex contraceptive condoms are unsatisfactory because the rubber usually immobilizes the sperm.[76] If these methods of collection are not possible, then postcoital examination of midcycle cervical mucus may give some information about the likelihood of adequate semen quality if many motile sperm are found.[19] In contrast, a negative postcoital test on its own is of little diagnostic value.[77] Postcoital tests may be of assistance in evaluating some rare conditions, for example, polyspermia (sperm concentration greater than 500 million/ml) and nonliquefying or extremely viscous semen; the presence of abundant motile sperm in the mucus is reassuring that these conditions are not serious.

The analysis is performed after thoroughly mixing liquefied semen—an artificial and unnatural situation. During ejaculation in most men the bulk of the sperm are contained in small volumes of liquid on the surface of each of the first two to three squirts of initially prostatic and later seminal vesicle fluid. There is in fact little mixing of the various components of the ejaculate.[78] This has been used in split ejaculate collection techniques for ART in which the semen is fractionated into two or more portions.[79] The

sperm concentration and motility often are higher in the first one third or one half of the ejaculate than in the remainder. Also, there usually is more prostatic fluid in the first part and more seminal vesicle contribution to the second.

Specimens collected by masturbation or in a nontoxic condom are preferred for semen analysis and ART. The man should be provided with a wide-mouth collection jar of a type known to be sterile and not toxic to sperm. In addition, instructions about collection and delivery to the laboratory should be provided on a written form. It is usual to request a period of abstinence from ejaculation from two to five days and to collect the sample by masturbation in a special room near the laboratory or to deliver the sperm to the laboratory within one hour of collection and without exposure to extremes of temperature.[80] In special circumstances—for example, sperm autoimmunity or necrospermia—a decreased duration of abstinence may be requested to determine if an improvement in motility is possible.[81] Other special aspects of collection include the use of lubricants. In general small amounts of K-Y jelly or other water-soluble jelly do not appear to affect sperm; on the other hand many petroleum-based jellies are toxic. To check for retrograde ejaculation, a urine collection should be provided immediately after ejaculation. Sometimes nocturnal emissions may be collected in nontoxic condoms for examination or ART in men with ejaculatory problems.

It is usual to request a semen analysis as a routine for male infertility; however, it may not be necessary in someone with severe hypogonadism, such as Klinefelter's syndrome, or hypogonadotropic hypogonadism, in which case it may be impossible for the man to ejaculate.

Because of the variability of results,[19, 82, 83] it is necessary to collect several semen samples in a man with an abnormality in the first semen test (Fig. 134–2). Three or more analyses with at least two-week intervals between commonly are required. The variability in the results is partly due to counting error—coefficient of variation: 7 per cent if 200 sperm are counted. Other technical errors and differences in the ejaculate from day to day cause within-subject coefficients of variation for repeated semen analysis results for infertile men to be large: 18 per cent for percentage normal morphology, 80 per cent for sperm concentration, and 32 per cent for percentage motile.[80] Although seasonal fluctuations in semen quality have been described, they are not important clinically if the semen is collected near the laboratory.[82] In evaluating the results of semen analysis, particularly with the first sample, it is important to question the man about the adequacy of the ejaculation and whether there were any problems with collection.

Semen constituents more or less specific to the accessory glands are available: zinc and acid phosphatase from the prostate, fructose from the seminal vesicles, and α-glucosidase and carnitine from the epididymis.[19] Prostatic fluid is acid (pH about 6.0), and in the ejaculate this is neutralized by seminal vesicle fluid. Semen biochemistry is of limited usefulness in clinical practice. Some examples are given in Table 134–2.

Tests for Sperm Antibodies

Tests for sperm antibodies should be done routinely on all men being evaluated for infertility because no semen

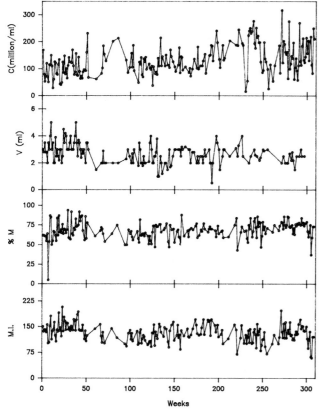

FIGURE 134–2. Variability of semen analysis results in a fertile sperm donor. C, sperm concentration; V, semen volume; M, total motility; MI, motility index—product of grade and percentage of sperm with progressive motility graded 0 to 3. (Mallidis C et al: Variation of semen quality in normal men. Int J Androl 14:99–107, 1991. Used by permission Blackwell Scientific Publications.)

pattern is characteristic of sperm autoimmunity. Semen analysis in men with sperm autoimmunity can range from azoospermic to normal. Sperm agglutination is not always present. The immunobead test (IBT) is a robust test for sperm antibodies and can be used either directly on sperm or indirectly to assess sperm antibodies in blood or seminal plasma.[19, 84, 85] Immunobeads are polyacrylamide microspheres with rabbit antihuman immunoglobulin antibodies covalently bound to the surface. Anti-IgA and anti-IgG beads are both mixed with suspensions of test sperm that have been washed to remove any free immunoglobulin in the semen that could inhibit the reaction. The beads bind to sperm coated with antibodies, and it is easy to count motile sperm with beads attached. IBT binding to more than 50 per cent of motile sperm is regarded as positive, but there usually is more than 70 to 80 per cent IgA binding with clinically significant sperm autoimmunity. Tail-tip only IBT binding is not significant.[19, 85] Azoospermic men with previous orchitis or possible obstruction must be tested for sperm antibodies. This can be performed with the indirect IBT: normal donor sperm are first exposed to test serum or seminal plasma to allow antibodies to bind to the sperm surfaces and then washed and exposed to the immunobeads.[85] An alternative screening method for men with sperm in the semen would be to perform a sperm mucus penetration test and to test for antibodies in those patients with an abnormality of sperm mucus penetration.[19] Some men, however, may have sperm autoimmunity that

fluctuates in severity, and they might be missed by relying on mucus penetration tests.

The mixed antiglobulin reaction with red blood cells or latex particles is an alternative direct test for sperm antibodies but may be less specific.[19, 86, 87] The older sperm agglutination and immobilization tests are losing favor except in research laboratories.[88] Immunofluorescence and enzyme-linked immunoassay techniques do not agree well with these tests and should not be used for screening.[89]

Sperm-mucus penetration tests can be performed by postcoital examination of sperm in cervical mucus collected at midcycle or after estrogen treatment (ethinyl estradiol, 50 μg twice daily for four days) to produce mucus of equivalent quality.[19] An alternative is the sperm mucus contact test, in which semen and mucus are mixed together and the movement of the sperm assessed by microscopy.[19] The capillary tube penetration meter (Kremer test) is probably the best method for assessing mucus penetration. Mucus penetration tests are particularly important for evaluating the significance of sperm autoantibodies; failure of sperm to penetrate more than 2 cm in one hour indicates severe sperm autoimmunity with a poor prognosis if untreated.[35]

Tests of Sperm Function

A number of tests of sperm function have been developed over the past few years. Although none is established as routine for clinical evaluation, some may become so in the near future. These include computer-assisted sperm motility analysis, assessments of the acrosomes with fluorescent dyes or antibodies, and sperm-oocyte binding and penetration tests.[19] These are summarized below, in the section on IVF for male infertility.

Interpretation of Semen Analysis Results

Table 134–2 shows a number of the patterns of abnormality of semen quality and their common causes. It is always important to ask the question, is the result spurious? Repeated tests are necessary to establish an average and to determine the variability within an individual man (Fig. 134–2).

Variations in Semen Volume and Appearance

Low semen volumes may suggest incomplete collection or short duration of abstinence from ejaculation before the test. Absence or obstruction of the seminal vesicles is a rare cause of low semen volume in an otherwise fertile man. High semen volumes (more than 8 ml) occasionally are seen, sometimes in association with oligospermia, but they are of little practical significance. Hemospermia usually is not caused by serious underlying conditions, such as tumors in the genital tract, and mostly is the result of minor bleeding from the prostatic or penile urethra. Other discoloration of the semen may indicate inflammation of accessory sex organs. Defects of liquefaction and viscosity are relatively common and presumably result from malfunction of the accessory sex organs.[22] Although these may cause problems with semen analysis and preparation of sperm for ART, they are probably of little relevance to fertility, except when associated with other abnormalities.

TABLE 134–2. COMMON OR CHARACTERISTIC PATTERNS OF SEMEN ABNORMALITY

VOL (ml) 1–6*	COUNT (10⁶/ml) 20–250*	MOTILITY (%) 50–90*	NORMAL MORPHOLOGY (%) 30–70*	COMMENT	CAUSE
0.4	0	–	–	Fructose 1 nmol/L (low); pH 6.5 (low)	Congenital absence of vasa Ejaculatory duct obstruction Partial retrograde ejaculation Testicular failure with androgen deficiency Spill
4.0	0	–	–	Fructose 15 nmol/L	Obstruction Primary seminiferous tubule failure Secondary seminiferous tubule failure with androgen treatment
3.0	100	0	35	Live 70%	(Contamination or condom collection) Immotile cilia
3.0	100	5	35	Live 20%	(Contamination or delayed examination) Necrospermia Sperm autoimmunity
3.0	100	65	0	Small round head	Total teratospermia; absent acrosomes
3.0	100	25 Progressive 10	20	Liquefaction incomplete; sperm aggregation 2+; live sperm 40%; polymorphs 1 × 10⁶/ml	Idiopathic asthenospermia Sperm autoimmunity Prostatitis (Delayed examination)
3.0	4	30 Progressive 15	10	Mixed abnormal morphology	Oligospermia of specific or nonspecific cause
3.0	<1	–	–	Some motile sperm present	Severe oligospermia of specific or nonspecific cause Primary seminiferous tubule failure Partial obstruction

*Normal range.

Sperm agglutination is common with sperm autoimmunity but can also occur for other reasons.

Oligospermia

Sperm concentrations of less than 20 million/ml are classified as oligospermic.[19] This figure probably derives mainly from the work of MacLeod, who found that only 5 per cent of fertile men had sperm concentrations less than 20 million/ml.[90] Other investigators have suggested that lower figures should be used, such as 10 million/ml. It is also important to recognize that higher sperm concentrations, up to 40 million/ml, have been suggested as the lower limit in the past, and there is a correlation between sperm concentration and other aspects of semen quality, such as percentage of motility and normal morphology. Both motility and morphology usually are poor with oligospermia. Also, many men with low sperm motility and high abnormal morphology with sperm concentrations above 20 million/ml have sperm concentrations lower than the geometric average for fertile men (80 million/ml).[80]

Asthenospermia

Asthenospermia is defined as a sperm motility of less than 50 per cent total or less than 25 per cent with rapid progressive motility.[19] Spurious asthenospermia because of exposure of sperm to rubber (particularly condoms), sper-micides, extremes of temperature, or long delays between collection and examination should be excluded before accepting that sperm motility is poor. Poor sperm motility is a frequent accompaniment of oligospermia, and there usually is a mixed picture of ultrastructural defects. It presumably arises because of defective spermatogenesis.

Severe asthenospermia usually requires evaluation with electron microscopy of the sperm.[44, 45] Specific ultrastructural defects of the axoneme typically are associated with zero sperm motility or extreme asthenospermia (less than 5 per cent motile sperm) and sterility. Those with absent dynein arms and other, less common axonemal defects may have general cilial disorders and associated bronchiectasis, situs inversus, and color blindness. Other patients have no axonemal defects but may have mitochondrial disorders or sperm with normal ultrastructure.[45] Standard semen analyses of these patients usually show normal sperm concentrations and normal sperm morphology, although some have tail abnormalities at the light microscopic level—short, straight, or thick tails or mid-piece defects. Viability tests, such as with eosin Y, usually are normal. This helps to distinguish this group of patients from those with necrospermia.[81] Patients with structural defects in the sperm that cause complete immotility are untreatable. Although it has been shown that sperm with absent dynein arms can fuse and undergo head decondensation in hamster eggs, to date no one has achieved pregnancies with microinjection of these sperm.[91]

Necrospermia is important to distinguish from other types of asthenospermia because some patients with this produce pregnancies despite low sperm motility.[81] There usually are some motile sperm (less than 20 per cent) but very poor progressive motility (less than 5 per cent) and the eosin Y test is low (less than 30 per cent), indicating a high proportion of dead sperm. The condition may fluctuate in severity, particularly with changes in coital frequency. Necrospermia may be caused by defective storage of sperm in the tails of the epididymides. There are ultrastructural features of degeneration in the ejaculated sperm but normal structure of late spermatids in testicular biopsies.[81] Characteristic of necrospermia is an improvement of sperm motility with increased frequency of ejaculation. It is also possible that the condition fluctuates in severity for other reasons. Treatment with antibiotics may have a beneficial effect, but this is not proved. The couple should have intercourse once or twice every day for three to four days up to the time of ovulation. Also, if sperm are to be prepared for ART, a period of frequent ejaculation should be practiced before the semen collection.

Asthenospermia may also be associated with sperm autoimmunity. Some rare forms of defective sperm motility have been described in which the motility looks normal under the microscope but there is defective mucus penetration (sliding sperm defect).[92] The causes of other motility defects of moderate degree are unidentified. Some suggested abnormalities of protein carboxylmethylase, lactic dehydrogenase C4, and energy generation are unconfirmed and contentious.[93, 94]

Teratospermia

If there are less than 30 per cent of sperm with normal morphology, the classification of teratospermia is used.[19] The assessment of sperm morphology is highly subjective, however, and difficult to standardize between laboratories. Various approaches to assessing morphology are used. The simplest is to assign defects with a priority, in order head, mid-piece, and tail, and to record as normal only those that conform to ideal shape with no defects in any region. It is important to distinguish mixed abnormalities of sperm morphology from those in which all or the majority of sperm show a single uniform defect, such as spherical heads with absence of the acrosomes and pin head sperm, which are produced by defective spermiogenesis.[45] Pin head sperm result when the centrioles from which the sperm tails develop are not correctly aligned opposite the developing acrosome so that the sperm heads are lost and absorbed during epididymal transit. Both these conditions are extremely rare. Mixed defects of sperm morphology have become important with the use of IVF for male infertility. The percentage of normal sperm morphology is one of the most important prognostic factors for fertilization in vitro (see below). In our clinic sperm morphology is assessed critically with the internal structure of the head as well as the silhouette taken into consideration, and the average normal morphology in the patients undergoing IVF is only 30 per cent.[95] Some fertile men are seen with a percentage of normal morphology less than 20 per cent.

Other methods for assessing morphology are used. Differential counts give the proportions of abnormal sperm with large, small, tapered, pyriform, or amorphous heads;

normal heads but mid-piece defects; or normal heads and mid-pieces but abnormal tails.[19] It has been suggested, however, that indices based on the average number of defects per spermatozoon may give more useful information (the teratospermia index).[96] Computer image analysis is being developed for objective quantification of sperm morphology.

Leukocytospermia and Semen Microbiology

To have more than 1 million polymorphs per milliliter in semen is considered abnormal.[19] Although the standard method for counting leukocytes involves staining peroxidase-positive cells, the use of monoclonal antibodies to panleukocyte or specific subset antigens is becoming popular.[19, 97] It is possible that leukocytes in the semen could interfere with sperm function.[98, 99] However, there is a poor relation between leukocytospermia and other features of supposed genital tract inflammation, such as variations in semen volume, viscosity, pH, and sperm agglutination, and the results of culture of semen.[100] Male accessory sex organ inflammation and infertility may be more important in some countries than in others, but it does not appear to be a significant problem in most parts of the United States.[22] Routine cultures of semen are probably unwarranted except for sperm donors. Patients with clinical evidence of recurrent bacterial prostatitis require full urological assessment.[101]

Hormone Assessment

It is not necessary to perform hormone measurements routinely. Measurement of follicle-stimulating hormone (FSH) is worthwhile in patients with azoospermia, normal testicular volume, and virilization to distinguish obstruction from seminiferous tubule failure or to support the presumption of normal spermatogenesis with clinical diagnoses of epididymal obstruction or congenital absence of the vasa. Measurement of FSH, luteinizing hormone (LH), and testosterone is useful in men with azoospermia and reduced testicular volume with signs of androgen deficiency to distinguish primary from secondary hypogonadism (see Ch. 133). Normal serum FSH in patients with severe oligospermia may indicate partial obstruction, seminiferous tubule failure, or different patterns in the two testes, for example, testicular failure on one side and obstruction on the other. Isolated FSH deficiency, if it exists, must be extremely uncommon.[102, 103] Rarely, high FSH levels are seen with normal spermatogenesis.[104, 105]

Measurement of prolactin should be performed in men with galactorrhea or androgen deficiency and loss of libido (see Ch. 24).[70, 106] Other hormone investigations occasionally are required, for example, thyroid function tests with hyperprolactinemia, 17-hydroxyprogesterone measurements with congenital adrenal hyperplasia, estradiol with liver disease or tumors, human chorionic gonadotropin (hCG) with tumors and estrogen excess, and pituitary function tests for panhypopituitarism (see Ch. 31).[41, 42, 107, 108] Inhibin measurement in infertile men appears to be of little clinical value.[109]

Genetic Studies

Karyotypes are performed in men with clinical evidence of primary testicular failure and small testes to confirm a clinical diagnosis of Klinefelter's syndrome, in which the karyotype usually is 47,XXY, but there may be higher numbers of X chromosomes or a sex-reversal 46,XX karyotype. Other chromosomal abnormalities have been related to defective spermatogenesis—for example, 47,XYY—but the clinical picture is much less uniform than it is for Klinefelter's syndrome.[110, 111] Cystic fibrosis gene studies are important for evaluation of patients with congenital absence of the vas.[23]

Testicular Biopsy

Testicular biopsies have been performed much less frequently over the past 20 years because of the availability of serum FSH measurements.[112] Biopsy is still necessary to assess spermatogenesis in men with potential obstruction and may be performed at the time of attempting bypass surgery. A significant proportion of men with a clinical picture of obstruction—azoospermia, normal testicular size, and normal FSH—have severe spermatogenic disorders, such as severe hypospermatogenesis and germ cell arrest.[20] Open biopsies may be performed under local or general anesthesia. It is most important that the tissue be removed from the testes with minimal damage and placed in a suitable fixative, such as Bouin's or Steive's solution; the latter is preferred if immunocytochemistry is to be performed.

Needle biopsy procedures have become popular, and although many obtain only isolated cells, these cells may be sufficient for diagnosis on the basis of cytology or for flow cytometry assessment. A technique for obtaining small amounts of tissue by needle aspiration biopsy under local anesthesia has been developed (Fig. 134–3) that usually provides sufficient material for a histological diagnosis of the state of the seminiferous epithelium and could be used for research purposes.[111a] The aspiration biopsy techniques do produce some deformation artefacts in the tissue.

Assessment of testicular histology usually is not quantitative because of the laboriousness and lack of obvious clinical benefit over a qualitative approach. The system promoted by de Kretser[112] is of clinical utility (Fig. 134–4). Spermatogenesis is divided into normal, slight, moderate, or severe hypospermatogenesis in which the cellular elements of spermatogenesis are all present but in progressively lower numbers. Germ cell arrest has the initial cellular elements of spermatogenesis present in quantitatively normal numbers, but at a certain stage the process stops. This typically is at the primary spermatocyte stage, suggesting that there is a defect of meiosis. The Sertoli cell–only syndrome is the presence of tubules that contain Sertoli cells but no germ cells; this is also called germ cell aplasia. Hyalinization is an appearance of seminiferous tubules in which all the cellular elements have disappeared and only thickened walls represent the seminiferous tubules. This pattern commonly is seen with Klinefelter's syndrome. Finally, there is the immature testis in which gonadotropin

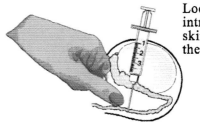

Local anaesthetic introduced into the skin and around the vas.

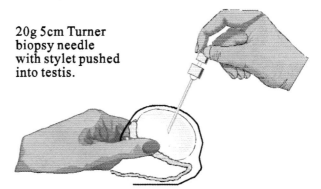

20g 5cm Turner biopsy needle with stylet pushed into testis.

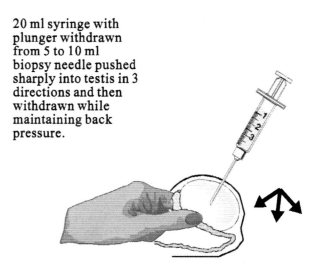

20 ml syringe with plunger withdrawn from 5 to 10 ml biopsy needle pushed sharply into testis in 3 directions and then withdrawn while maintaining back pressure.

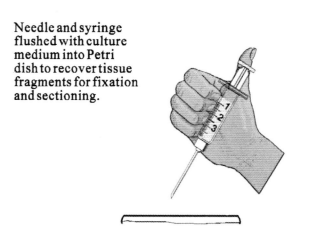

Needle and syringe flushed with culture medium into Petri dish to recover tissue fragments for fixation and sectioning.

FIGURE 134–3. Fine-needle tissue aspiration biopsy of the testis. (From Mallidis C, Baker HWG: Fine needle tissue aspiration biopsy of the testis. Fertil Steril, in press.)

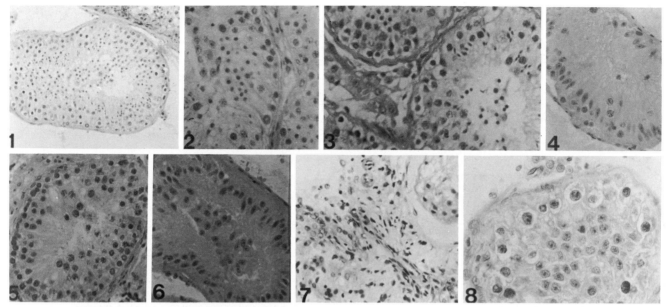

FIGURE 134–4. Testicular histology from fine-needle aspiration samples. 1. Normal (×200). 2. Mild hypospermatogenesis (×500). 3. Moderate hypospermatogenesis. 4. Severe hypospermatogenesis. 5. Germ cell arrest at the primary spermatocyte stage. 6. Sertoli cell–only syndrome. 7. Leydig cell tumor in an undescended testis with hyalinized Sertoli cell–only tubules. 8. Carcinoma in situ, only transformed spermatogonia and Sertoli cells present.

stimulation is absent, and the appearance is that of a testis from a normal prepubertal boy. As knowledge of the molecular biology of defects of spermatogenesis is gained, the use of testicular biopsy in the diagnosis of the cause of male infertility may become popular again.

Other Investigations

Ultrasonography is useful for measuring testicular size, particularly when the testes are difficult to palpate because of a tense hydrocele, for example.[113] It is also helpful for confirming the presence of cysts or other abnormalities in the scrotum and especially for checking for tumors in the testes. The procedure may demonstrate a varicocele or other abnormalities that are easily detectable clinically. In the future ultrasonic blood flow measurements of the testes may be of some value in assessing varicoceles.[114] Other tests of a varicocele, including thermography, Doppler flow studies, technetium scans, and venography, may be performed.[74] Clinical suspicion of the presence of a pituitary tumor should be followed up by appropriate radiology (see Ch. 30). Abdominal scanning is necessary to check the position of an impalpable testis.

MANAGEMENT OF SPECIFIC CONDITIONS

In this section the management of sperm autoimmunity, male genital tract obstructions, coital disorders, genital tract inflammation, and varicocele are discussed. Treatment of gonadotropin deficiency and testicular suppression are covered in Chapters 15, 109, and 133 and androgen replacement therapy, in Ch. 131.

Sperm Autoimmunity

Clinical Characteristics

Sperm autoimmunity is present in 6 to 10 per cent of men seen for treatment of infertility.[35, 115] About 5 per cent of men seen for infertility have spontaneously occurring sperm autoimmunity, and the remainder have the autoimmunity associated with genital tract obstruction either continuing or treated, particularly failed, vasovasostomy. The obstruction occasionally is one-sided.[115] Very rarely men are seen with a condition that appears to be autoimmune orchitis. This may follow an episode of epididymo-orchitis or occur spontaneously. Characteristically, there are inflammatory cell infiltrates in the testis.[116] Men with spontaneously occurring autoimmunity have a higher frequency of family histories of other autoimmune diseases, particularly of the organ-specific type (see Ch. 160).[35] They also have a greater frequency of the presence of thyroid and gastric autoantibodies in their serum.[36] This may indicate a familial predisposition to develop sperm autoantibodies.

The types of genital tract obstruction associated with sperm autoimmunity appear to be those that have occurred after puberty, such as postgonococcal epididymitis, vasectomy, or traumatic obstructions. Patients with sperm autoimmunity associated with genital tract obstruction most commonly are those with persisting infertility after vasectomy reversal procedures. About 70 per cent of men develop sperm antibodies in their serum within 12 months of vasectomy.[117] The presence of these antibodies is an adverse factor in the success of vasovasostomy. Sperm autoimmunity is uncommon with congenital epididymal obstructions, Young's syndrome, and congenital absence of the vasa. In the latter the appearance of sperm antibodies may be related to the length of epididymis present—the longer the epididymis the more likely antibodies develop.

Differential Diagnosis

The main concerns are to distinguish those men with severe sperm autoimmunity from those with low-level sperm autoantibodies that are not relevant to the infertility. These usually have IBT results with less than 70 per cent IgA binding to the sperm heads and mucus penetration tests that are normal or only marginally impaired.[34] Treatment of this situation is not warranted, and the investigation should be continued for other causes of the couple's infertility. Many patients with low-level sperm antibodies have the immunobead binding only to the tail tips.[118] In situations where there are few or no sperm present in the semen, the main problem is to determine whether the sperm antibodies are the only cause of the problem or whether there is some element of obstruction or spermatogenic disorder. In these cases it may be necessary to resort to a therapeutic trial of glucocorticoids. A final problem is the combination of sperm autoimmunity with another defect, such as teratospermia. At this stage the prognostic significance of other factors is not clearly understood, but it seems likely that the additional abnormalities, such as obstruction or spermatogenic disorders, further reduce the success of treatment of the sperm autoimmunity. This requires consideration before treatment is commenced.

Pathophysiology of Sperm Autoantibodies

Despite extensive study, it is still not clear what the epitopes are for the autoantibodies.[119] It is not clear whether the antibodies are directed against peptide or carbohydrate or even lipid constituents. It is even unknown whether the different patterns of immunobead binding to the sperm surface result from different types of antibodies binding to different binding sites, or whether these merely reflect differences in density of sperm antibody binding to the surface membrane of the sperm.[85] Also contentious is the site of entry of the autoantibodies into the genital tract. It may be that the blood-testis barrier or other mechanisms that make the testis an immunologically privileged organ are defective or that the antibodies may be produced on site, for example, by lymphocytes resident in the epithelium of the epididymis. On the other hand, it is clear that the sperm antibodies interfere with fertility at a multitude of levels—interference with spermatogenesis, sperm agglutination in the male genital tract; interference with sperm mucus penetration, blocking sperm binding to the zona pellucida; and interference with sperm motility. Although sperm antibodies of different immunoglobulin classes can be found in serum and seminal plasma, the IgG and IgA antibody classes appear to be most important, and in particular it may be secretory IgA, locally produced in the male genital tract, that causes the greatest interference with sperm function.[85, 118]

Natural History of Sperm Autoimmunity

Patients with spontaneous sperm autoimmunity may have fluctuations of the severity of the disease, and those rare patients who produce pregnancies without glucocorticoid treatment appear to have improvements in the sperm autoimmunity with a fall in IBT binding or a change to tail-tip–only binding and increased sperm mucus penetration.

The pregnancy rate for patients with untreated spontaneously occurring sperm antibodies and no sperm-mucus penetration is less than 0.5 per cent per month.[35, 120] Patients with obstructions may have an improvement in the sperm antibody problem after relief of the obstruction—for example, after vasovasostomy—but this may take many months or years to occur.[115] In most patients the severity of the sperm autoimmunity appears to be constant, and after successful glucocorticoid treatment the sperm antibody levels rise and the mucus penetration falls within a few months.

Treatment Groups

For the standard couple with sperm autoimmunity as the only obvious cause for their infertility—healthy man and normal wife—glucocorticoid treatment in the hope of achieving a natural pregnancy seems reasonable. On the other hand, if the wife has abnormalities prejudicial to fertility or the man has other illnesses—particularly peptic ulcer disease, hypertension, obesity, or diabetes mellitus—then the risks of serious adverse effects may contraindicate long-term glucocorticoid treatment. Short-term treatment with IVF may be worth considering, or alternatively, the couple may be better off accepting the infertility or pursuing donor insemination.

Treatment

Various regimens of prednisolone or other glucocorticoid therapy have been used: intermittent high dose, intermittent escalating medium dose, continuous low or medium dose, and short-term medium dose for a therapeutic trial or pre-IVF treatment.[115] Because a number of cases of aseptic necrosis of the femoral head have been associated with the high-dose methylprednisolone, this regimen has lost popularity.[121]

PREDNISOLONE THERAPY. Both continuous and intermittent prednisolone therapy regimens have been shown to be effective in placebo controlled trials[122] (Baker HWG, unpublished observations, 1992), although some small trials have produced negative results.[123] Continuous therapy is 0.75 mg/kg or 50 mg/d given as a single dose each morning with breakfast until a pregnancy occurs or for four to six months, depending on the semen quality and adverse effects. The intermittent regimen is to give 20 to 25 mg of prednisolone each day from day 1 through 10 or day 4 through 14 of the wife's cycle. If the semen quality and mucus penetration have not improved by three months, then the dosage can be doubled to 50 mg. If there is still no improvement by six months, then the dosage should be increased to 75 mg/d. Whether this intermittent regimen is better than the continuous treatment is under investigation. For a therapeutic trial, for example, in men with severe oligospermia or azoospermia after a vasovasostomy or before IVF, prednisolone 50 mg/d is given for four to eight weeks.

MONITORING. Patients are carefully monitored for improvement in semen quality and for adverse effects. Semen tests are performed monthly about the time of the wife's menses. If semen quality improves significantly, sperm are cryopreserved during the nonfertile phase of the wife's cycle. Semen analysis is performed together with IBT and sperm mucus penetration tests with the Kremer procedure to assess progress. Promising signs are increased sperm concentration, motility, and mucus penetration and decreased IBT binding, particularly IgA levels falling to less than 70 per cent binding to the heads of the motile sperm.[35]

ADVERSE EFFECTS. Adverse effects of prednisolone treatment are common (see Ch. 100). Insomnia and dyspepsia are frequent early problems. After two to three months of treatment, cushingoid appearance, muscle weakness, and joint aches are common. Occasional adverse effects resulting from depressed immunity are herpes zoster, severe folliculitis, and bronchitis. Although other serious adverse effects are possible, such as depression, cataracts, addisonian crisis after cessation of treatment, and aggravation of peptic ulcer disease, these seem to be rare. The main serious adverse effect is aseptic necrosis of the femoral head.[35, 115, 121, 122] This effect has been described in a number of men being treated for sperm autoimmunity and may be predisposed to by heavy alcohol drinking. (Patients need to be advised carefully of this adverse effect because it has led to a number of litigation actions.) It is also important to remember that other common illnesses, such as asthma and psoriasis, although improved during glucocorticoid treatment, may flare up after withdrawal. Rarely, semen quality deteriorates during glucocorticoid treatment. Whether this is fortuitous is unknown. It has been reported that normal men given glucocorticoids and men with Cushing's syndrome have poor sperm production (see Ch. 100).

GENERAL MANAGEMENT. The couple are advised to have intercourse frequently at midcycle, daily or, at a minimum, every 48 hours. Semen is cryopreserved if the quality improves. Also, if semen quality improves but there is no pregnancy after a four- to six-month course, then IVF could be attempted using fresh semen in the last month of treatment. IVF could also be performed with frozen semen.

OTHER TREATMENTS. There have been attempts to use other treatments for sperm autoimmunity—testosterone suppression of spermatogenesis, AIH, treatment of the sperm by washing to remove sperm antibodies, antibiotic therapy, and IVF without prior prednisolone therapy—but none appears to be effective.[35, 115, 124] Sperm microinjection in IVF may be an alternative, but this requires further investigation. Other immunomodulating agents, including cyclosporine and levamisole, have been used, but their value is unclear.[125, 126] Surgery to relieve obstructions, such as repeat vasovasostomy and vasoepididymostomy, or removal of an orchitic testis could also be considered.[115] Because of the uncertain results of these procedures, they could be deferred until a therapeutic trial of prednisolone was unsuccessful.

RESULTS. About 50 per cent of men treated with glucocorticoids for sperm autoimmunity have a reduction in sperm antibody levels and an increase in sperm concentration, motility, and mucus penetration.[35, 122] Sperm morphology is not changed (Baker, unpublished observations). Pregnancies occur in 25 per cent of couples during a four- to six-month course of prednisolone or after a longer period of intermittent prednisolone therapy (122, Baker unpublished observations). IVF with semen stored or fresh during prednisolone therapy may provide a few additional pregnancies.[124] Sometimes artificial insemination is successful with stored semen from a previous course of prednisolone therapy. Infertility problems in the wife—for example, ovulatory disorders, endometriosis, or non-obstructing tubal abnormalities—are negative prognostic factors, and in these couples it may be preferable to perform IVF with a shorter course of prednisolone therapy. The success rates of short-term prednisolone therapy and IVF are unknown.

Genital Tract Obstruction

Clinical Characteristics

Most men with genital tract obstruction have azoospermia, normal testicular size, normal virilization, and normal serum FSH levels. Some have combined obstruction and spermatogenic disorders or partial obstructions and severe oligospermia. There may be a history of an event that caused the obstruction, such as epididymitis after gonorrhea, or of an associated condition, such as bronchiectasis or chronic sinopulmonary symptoms associated with Young's syndrome.[20, 26–28] Although the serum FSH level usually is normal, a few men with normal spermatogenesis have elevated FSH levels, and therefore a strong clinical presumption of an obstruction should be further investigated.[104, 105] Sperm antibodies may be present, and they should be tested in all men with possible obstruction because they are probably an adverse prognostic factor.[115] Rare patients have different problems on the two sides, for example, a spermatogenic disorder on one side and an obstruction on the other side. In these patients sperm may be present in the semen. This clinical situation is very rare. In men with congenital absence of the vas or ejaculatory duct obstruction, the semen volume and the pH and fructose levels are low. The semen also does not have its characteristic smell and does not form a gel after ejaculation because it contains only prostatic and urethral fluid. Although a number of chemical markers of Sertoli and epididymal cells are present in semen, none of these has any clear clinical utility for determining the level of obstruction in the epididymis.[127, 128] Testicular biopsy usually is normal, although there may be some reduction in spermatogenesis either as a coincidence or as a result of the obstruction. The latter is particularly true in men who have had vasectomies performed.[129]

Pathophysiology

The association of congenital absence of the vas with cystic fibrosis and of the increased frequency of cystic fibrosis gene mutations in men with congenital absence of the vas without clinical cystic fibrosis has already been mentioned.[25] Other epididymal disorders, particularly Young's syndrome, may also be associated with some abnormalities of the chloride channel gene related to cystic fibrosis. With Young's syndrome the men may have developed the block after puberty because some have had children in the past.[27] The pathology shows inspissated material in the head of the epididymis, and there are lipid inclusions in the epithelial cells.[26] Postinflammatory obstructions after gonorrhea typically occur in the tail of the epididymis for unknown reasons, whereas nonspecific bacterial inflammation produces more widespread destruction, and tuberculosis, although rare in Western communities, usually causes multiple obstructions in the epididymides and vasa. Back pressure blowout obstructions are not infrequent after vasectomy and may occur at any level in the epididymis.[130]

Differential Diagnosis

Men with persistent azoospermia, normal testicular size, normal virilization, and normal FSH levels can be assumed to have obstruction until proved otherwise. The clinical diagnosis is further strengthened by a history of chronic sinopulmonary disease or an event that might have produced the obstruction. Up to one third of men with this clinical picture are found to have a serious spermatogenic disorder on testicular biopsy despite the normal serum FSH level.[20] There are rare instances of normal men who show azoospermia on single occasions or over a short period.[22, 131] The reason for this is not understood, but it is important that several sperm tests are performed before accepting that there is complete and persistent azoospermia. There are also some azoospermic men who have had recent epididymitis or prostatitis who recover with time or after antibiotic treatment. This "spurious azoospermia" must be excluded before surgery is contemplated. Once there is a confirmed or likely diagnosis of obstruction, it is then necessary to separate those patients with potentially treatable conditions from those with untreatable conditions. A proportion of men have intratesticular blocks associated with congenital absence of the vas or Young's syndrome. Those patients with high obstructions, particularly with Young's syndrome, have a poor prognosis for vasoepididymostomy, whereas those men with vasal or cauda-epididymal obstructions have a relatively good prognosis with surgery.[130, 132, 133] Although distal obstructions are very rare, they are important to diagnose because they often are easily reversed; for example, a cyst of the prostatic utricle may be treated by simple incision at panendoscopy.[134] The characteristics of ejaculatory duct obstruction are azoospermia or severe oligospermia with low semen volume, pH, and fructose in the presence of normal scrotal contents. Other ejaculatory duct obstructions not related to prostatic cysts may not be treatable. In those men in whom reconstructive surgery is not possible, the consideration is then whether sperm could be aspirated from the genital tract for ART.[130, 135] If a natural spermatocele is present, it may be possible to obtain sperm by direct puncture through the scrotal skin. Otherwise, it usually is necessary to open the scrotum under general anesthesia and collect sperm from individual epididymal tubules or from the vas.

General Management

Genetic abnormalities associated with the cystic fibrosis gene need to be considered if a pregnancy is to be attempted using the husband's sperm. The wife should be screened for cystic fibrosis gene abnormalities and the couple counseled accordingly. The wife should be investigated in detail to ensure her potential fertility before extensive epididymal surgery is contemplated in the husband. The prognosis of the procedure and the availability of other forms of treatment, including donor insemination, should be discussed realistically with the couple. It may be possible to combine vasoepididymostomy with sperm aspiration and IVF. The coexistence of other problems, such as sperm autoimmunity and defects of spermatogenesis, should be considered.

Epididymal and Vasal Surgery

These procedures are best undertaken by surgeons who specialize in male infertility surgery.[130, 132–134] The testis usually is exposed and the most proximal (to the testis) level obstruction determined. A testicular biopsy is obtained and the patency of the vas distally determined by syringing with saline or by vasography. The vas or epididymal tubule is opened proximal to the obstruction, and if possible, the presence of motile sperm is demonstrated. Then microsurgical anastomosis between the ends of the vas or between the vas and the epididymal tubule is undertaken. For epididymal sperm aspiration for IVF, single tubules are opened, the testis and epididymis are squeezed gently, and the epididymal fluid is sucked into a fine plastic tube known to be nontoxic to sperm. Later the tubules are closed to permit repeated aspiration procedures. At this stage, cryopreservation of sperm collected from the epididymis is under development. Artificial spermatoceles have been implanted into the epididymis or vas for uncorrectable obstructions and sperm obtained by needling the reservoir.[136, 137]

RESULTS. Vasovasostomy and vasoepididymostomy for caudal blocks produce relatively good results—50 to 80 per cent of patients having sperm present in the semen; however, less than one half of these produce a pregnancy within the first year.[130, 132, 133] The poor results may be related to continuing obstruction, sperm autoimmunity, or coexisting spermatogenic disorders. There may also be adverse female factors, especially with the vasovasostomy patients; for example, many wives are older than the wives of other patients. The results of vasoepididymostomy for proximal blocks are poor.[130, 133] Although sperm appear in the semen of about 30 per cent of men after vasoepididymostomy for caput epididymal blocks associated with Young's syndrome, pregnancies are extremely uncommon (fewer than 10 per cent in one year).[130]

The results of microepididymal sperm aspiration and IVF are also variable. Some groups claim good results with congenital absence of the vasa, but most find poor results, particularly with aspiration of sperm from high in the head of the epididymis.[130, 135] Using the sperm from natural or artificial spermatoceles for AIH has produced few pregnancies.[136–138] IVF may be more successful. Intracytoplasmic sperm injection (ICSI) produces good results with epididymal and testicular sperm obtained from men with caput epididymal and intratesticular obstruction[138a] (Baker, unpublished observation, 1993).

Coital Disorders

Male coital disorders important for infertility include impotence, failure of ejaculation, and retrograde ejaculation (see Ch. 135).

Impotence

Impotence may be associated with low libido from androgen deficiency as part of primary or secondary hypogonadism. Treatment of the underlying condition or replacement of androgens is highly effective. Impotence related to organic neurological or vascular abnormalities is uncommon in the age group of men presenting with infertility. Most patients in this group have diabetes with autonomic neuropathy, spinal cord injury, or pelvic trauma causing nerve damage.[20] Impotence of unknown cause or related to psychological disturbance is a common cause of infertility in some societies.[22] Many men have some problems with sexual performance for a variable period after first learning about the infertility, but this usually ameliorates with time. Occasional men with more deep-seated psychological problems and ambivalence about having children may have specific defects of intercourse at the time of ovulation, although semen can be collected by masturbation or from nocturnal emissions.

Failure of Ejaculation

Failure of ejaculation is a common problem after spinal cord injuries, but otherwise, it is an infrequent cause of infertility in most societies. Healthy men who cannot ejaculate with intercourse may be able to produce an ejaculate by masturbation with a vibrator or other stimulation, but most cannot.[139] This group of men appear to have a relatively intractable problem; few appear to respond to psychotherapy or drug therapy. However, many have nocturnal emissions that may be collected in a nontoxic condom for storage or artificial insemination. Antihypertensive and psychotropic drugs used in the past that interfered with ejaculation, causing anejaculation or retrograde ejaculation, seldom are used now.

Retrograde Ejaculation

Retrograde ejaculation occurs when the bladder neck fails to contract at the time of ejaculation so that the semen passes into the bladder. Retrograde ejaculation is diagnosed by examination of postejaculatory urine. It occasionally is partial, there being some antegrade ejaculate as well as the retrograde passage of the bulk of the ejaculate. This condition is mainly caused by neurological disorders, particularly diabetic neuropathy and pelvic nerve damage. The ejaculate produced by electroejaculation in men with spinal cord injuries is also often retrograde.[140]

Differential Diagnosis

Recognition of a coital disorder is crucial; thus all infertile patients must discuss their sexual history in detail. Once recognized, the contribution of organic and psychological factors needs to be evaluated.

General Treatment

Overall, a reasonably optimistic prognosis can be given, provided that sperm of adequate quality can be obtained. The couple needs to be advised about the various techniques that might be used for collecting the sperm for AIH or other ART. The wife's potential fertility must be evaluated.

Specific Treatment

If a drug may be contributing to the sexual disorder, such as an antihypertensive or a tranquilizer, then the possibility of stopping the drug temporarily can be considered. Various treatments for impotence could be considered, from sex behavior therapy through techniques involving rubber bands and vacuum pumps to initiate and maintain erections, intrapenile injections of vasodilators, and penile implants, but these seldom are needed in patients with infertility. Some men with failure of ejaculation or retrograde ejaculation may be able to ejaculate during intercourse with a full bladder or after the administration of cholinergic antihistamines such as brompheniramine or ephedrine.[141]

COLLECTION OF SEMEN. Some men with coital disorders may be able to collect semen by masturbation, but others may require more powerful stimulation with vibrators or even electroejaculation under general anesthesia. If these are unsuccessful, it may be possible to collect sperm from the vas or tail of the epididymis by direct puncture or surgery. Some men with failure of ejaculation or impotence may still have nocturnal emissions at relatively regular intervals, and therefore it is not necessary for them to wear condoms every night. The nocturnal emissions may occur more frequently after erotic stimulation.

Use of Collected Semen. If possible, the couple can be taught to inseminate samples at midcycle, the timing of ovulation being determined by calendar and either mucus symptoms or urinary LH surge, detected with an LH dipstick kit. Although this depends on the lucky coincidence of the collection of semen and ovulation, pregnancies often can be achieved by the couples themselves. Cryopreservation of samples for AIH in the clinic is also worth contemplating.

ELECTROEJACULATION. In early attempts to obtain semen by electroejaculation in men with spinal cord injuries, veterinary equipment was used and the results often were poor. More recently improved button and bar electrode probes have been developed that produce better results.[140] Semen obtained by electroejaculation frequently has low volume, high sperm concentration, and poor motility. The pattern may be similar to that of necrospermia, and increasing the frequency of electroejaculation might improve sperm motility. Semen quality is too poor for cryopreservation, and few pregnancies are achieved by AIH. A number of groups are claiming better results by performing IVF with electroejaculated semen, either antegrade or recovered from the bladder by catheterization.[142] The risks of electroejaculation include perforation of the rectum with the probes and thermal damage to the rectum. Modern electroejaculation equipment includes a thermal sensor in the probe, and it is standard technique to examine the rectal mucosa by proctoscopy before and after the procedure. Autonomic hyperreflexia is also a recognized complication of electroejaculation with chronic spinal cord injuries above thoracic vertebra number 6. The resulting uncontrolled hypertension may cause cerebral hemorrhage. Careful monitoring of blood pressure and prophylactic nifedipine treatment usually prevent serious problems. Men without complete sensory deprivation require general anesthesia for electroejaculation.

RETRIEVAL OF SPERM WITH RETROGRADE EJACULATION. A method for obtaining sperm from men with retrograde ejaculation is as follows.[143] The timing of ovulation is determined as described above for AIH. Three days before ovulation the man drinks extra water (2.0 to 2.5 L) with 80 g of sodium bicarbonate each day to dilute and alkalinize the urine. On the day of ovulation the osmolality of the urine is adjusted to between 200 and 400 mOsm/kg by drinking or not drinking extra water. Then the man ejaculates and passes urine or is electroejaculated as soon as possible. Urine is centrifuged as soon as possible, the supernatant poured off, and the pellet resuspended in either human tubal fluid or Hams F10 culture medium supplemented with 7.5 per cent heat-inactivated wife's serum previously checked for sperm antibodies. The resuspended sperm are washed once with at least 5 ml of culture medium, centrifuged, and the final pellet resuspended in about 0.5 ml of culture medium for insemination. It occasionally is possible to cryopreserve the sample obtained, although post-thaw motilities often are poor. Sometimes it is not possible to get the urine osmolality between 200 and 400 mOsm/kg within two hours, and in these cases it may be possible to obtain a reasonable sperm preparation despite the extreme osmolality by preparing the sample as quickly as possible. If this method fails, the bladder can be catheterized and washed out with culture medium supplemented with serum, leaving some in the bladder. The mixed semen and culture medium is obtained after ejaculation by micturition or repeat catheterization. This method should be used only as a last resort, particularly in men with diabetes, because of the risk of introducing bacteria into the bladder.

ARTIFICIAL INSEMINATION WITH HUSBAND'S SPERM. Timing of inseminations can be undertaken by calculating the likely time of ovulation from previous cycle lengths and then determining the likely day of ovulation by symptoms and inspection of the cervical opening and mucus volume and quality. This may be excessively time-consuming or wasteful of semen because an insemination should be performed each day when cervical mucus appears optimal.[144–146] Monitoring of ovulation may be performed by measurement of LH either in urine or blood each morning near midcycle. Inseminations are timed to coincide with the LH peak, and if there is any uncertainty, a second insemination is performed on the next day. Alternatively, ultrasound examination of the ovaries can be performed in the late follicular phase between days 8 and 12 of the cycle. Once a follicle obtains a diameter of 17 mm or greater, LH measurements can be performed each day and the insemination performed on the day after commencement of the rise of LH. Ultrasonography is also useful to avoid inseminating a woman with unilateral tubal obstruction who is about to ovulate from the ovary contralateral to the patent fallopian tube and who might run an increased risk of ectopic pregnancy. Another refinement is to give an ovulating dose of hCG (5000 units) once the follicle is expected to have a diameter greater than 18 mm. Insemination follows about 42 hours after the hCG injection. Women with irregular cycles or uncertain symptoms and features of ovulation may have ovulation induced. Clomiphene may be administered from day 1 through day 5 and hCG given to stimulate ovulation around day 12 of the cycle once follicles of adequate size are demonstrated by ultrasonography.[145] These procedures should reduce the number of visits and conserve semen. The same pregnancy rates can be achieved with single inseminations after hCG-induced ovulations as are achieved with inseminations

based on symptoms or LH surge monitoring. Insemination is performed by injecting the sperm suspension or semen through a Teflon cannula into the cervical canal. Small volumes of washed sperm suspension can also be injected into the uterine cavity by way of an embryo transfer catheter.[144]

Genital Tract Inflammation

Specific inflammations of the testes—for example, mumps orchitis—may produce severe disturbance of spermatogenesis. Milder inflammations in the accessory sex organs, including the prostate gland and seminal vesicles, are of dubious importance. The WHO classification does include a category of nonspecific genital tract inflammation: male accessory gland infection.[22] The frequency of signs of this type of mild inflammation is increased in men with infertility compared with that in sperm donors or normal volunteers.[100] Some infertile men complain of chronic low back pain, intermittent dysuria, discharges from the penis on straining or defecation, and discomfort in the pelvic region or testes after prolonged sexual abstinence or ejaculation. These symptoms may be consistent with chronic prostatitis. The semen may show variations of volume, either low or high. The consistency may be abnormal with increased viscosity and defects of liquefaction. There may be some discoloration and increased numbers of white blood cells in the semen. Agglutination of sperm may occur. Bacteria commonly are seen in the semen. These frequently are not pathogens but the normal commensal organisms of the urethra. However, they may be present in large numbers. There often is little relation between symptoms and features of inflammation or infection in the semen. Although some reports suggest that the presence of bacteria could impair sperm motility, whether nonspecific genital tract inflammation contributes to male infertility remains contentious.[22, 100]

General Management

Because the organisms implicated in genital tract inflammation are quite varied from *Chlamydia* and *Mycoplasma* to bacteria, antimicrobial therapy, if it is to be given, should be broad spectrum. Many of the standard antibacterial agents and antibiotics do not enter accessory sex organ fluid, especially when the accessory sex organ is inflamed. Trimethoprim, erythromycin, doxycycline, and norfloxacin commonly are used and are at least potentially effective.[149] Advice about increased frequency of ejaculation to facilitate drainage of the accessory glands and discussion about the stresses of infertility may help. Nonsteroidal anti-inflammatory drugs have been used but are probably of no value.

Varicocele

Varicoceles are found in about 25 per cent of men being examined for infertility. An additional 15 per cent of men may have a faint cough impulse in the left spermatic cord that would equate with a subclinical varicocele.[20, 22, 138, 150] Varicoceles are also found in fertile men, possibly with equal frequency.[68] Varicoceles are more common in tall men and appear to be more common in men with larger testicular volumes.[22] They appear to be less frequent in men with severe testicular atrophy, for example, with Kallmann's syndrome or Klinefelter's syndrome. The left testis frequently is smaller than the right testis when there is a moderate to large left varicocele.

Pathophysiology

Together with the smaller testis underneath a varicocele, there is evidence to suggest that men with varicoceles have poorer semen quality than those without varicoceles.[68, 150] Thus it is reasonable to assume that the varicocele has an adverse effect on testicular function. Various theories have been advanced for the effect, including vascular stasis, back pressure, interference with oxygenation, reflux of renal or adrenal products into the pampiniform plexus, and interference with the heat exchange function of the pampiniform plexus.[150] Most of these theories do not stand up to investigation, and the precise mechanisms involved are not clear. The varicoceles usually first become noticed around the time of puberty and thereafter may increase in size but remain relatively stable in size throughout the man's lifetime. Symptoms, including swelling and a dragging sensation in the scrotum, are infrequent, and many men with large varicoceles are unaware of their presence. The sudden appearance of a varicocele in an adult should be taken seriously because it may be a feature of a renal carcinoma with extension into the left renal vein. This well-known clinical association is uncommon.

Differential Diagnosis

The semen quality in men with varicoceles varies from azoospermic to normal. In the WHO data bank there is an association between varicocele, nonspecific genital tract infection, and sperm autoimmunity.[22] This association may be more related to differences between the units providing the data in their assessment of these abnormalities rather than a true association of these conditions. Thus the varicocele might be more of an association rather than an absolute cause of a couple's infertility; therefore, full evaluation of other aspects of male infertility and of the female partner are necessary. It previously was thought that a specific semen abnormality was associated with varicocele. In this abnormality, called the stress pattern, there is low sperm motility and increased proportions of sperm with tapered heads and immature forms in the semen. Although opinion is now mainly against this association, well-controlled clinical investigations have produced contradictory results, some showing that there is no association of the semen pattern with varicocele and others showing that there is.[151, 152] In practical terms, the stress pattern is not diagnostic of a varicocele. Testicular histology is quite variable, the only common feature being that the defect in spermatogenesis is more severe on the left side than on the right side.

Treatment

Treatment is a controversial area. One view is that treating varicoceles may not improve fertility; therefore, the varicoceles should only be treated for other reasons, such as symptoms.[18, 150] The other extreme is the belief that varicocele is the most important treatable cause of male infertility; therefore, all varicoceles should be treated even though small. In the middle ground are those (I am in this group) who would advise varicocelectomy in selected cases; for example, when there is an absent, obstructed, or atrophic right testis and it is presumed that all sperm are coming from the left testis, then treatment of the varicocele may produce a reasonable result.[152a] The more radical in the middle ground group would probably treat all medium or large varicoceles in men in whom there was no other obvious cause for the infertility and in whom the semen abnormality was not too severe.

The most popular method of treatment is ligation of the spermatic veins in the retroperitoneal area above the inguinal ligament.[6, 18, 138, 150] The recurrence or failure of cure rate is at least 15 per cent, and hydroceles form in 7 to 33 per cent from interference with lymphatic damage.[138] Inguinal and scrotal approaches are also used. Although with these approaches, recurrences are less common, hydroceles appear in 4 to 15 per cent, and sacrificing the testicular artery may have more serious consequences than it does in retroperitoneal operations.[138] A relatively frequent complication is pain in the wound from cutting of branches of the sensory nerves of the lower abdominal wall. Other surgical complications are rare. Goldstein recently introduced a new operation for varicocele that involves delivery of the testis through an inguinal incision and microsurgical ligation of all veins from the testis except those that accompany the vas. The testicular artery and lymphatics and the abdominal wall sensory nerves are spared.[138] The recurrence and hydrocele rates are very low (less than 0.6 per cent). Laparoscopic surgery for varicoceles is also being developed.[153]

Alternative treatments involve the placement, under venographic control, of sclerosant, glue, or steel coils in the testicular vein to obstruct it. The radiographic techniques may carry a lower morbidity than surgery under general anesthesia, but the procedure is not possible in up to 25 per cent of patients, the failure or recurrence rate ranges from 3 to 15 per cent, and coils may move, resulting in renal vein obstruction or pulmonary embolism.[138, 150, 154]

Follow-up

If semen quality is to improve after treatment, it should do so within 6 to 12 months. Semen tests could be performed at one- to two-month intervals, and cryopreservation should be considered if there was a substantial improvement in semen quality, in case the improvement is transient. Factors believed to be important for response to varicocelectomy include effectiveness of the prevention of reflux, the degree of reduction in varicocele size, pretreatment serum FSH levels, and seminiferous tubule function.[150] It is rare for azoospermic men to respond, particularly those with elevated serum FSH levels. It remains possible that improvements in semen quality after varicocele treatment result from random fluctuations and regression toward the mean.[18, 155] WHO has attempted to set up a multicenter controlled trial of varicocelectomy, and a preliminary report from one group suggests a beneficial effect.[156] Whether or not treatment of varicoceles improves fertility will continue to be argued, but from a practical clinical perspective, it is now clear that normal fertility is not achieved in any substantial number of patients; reported floating numerator pregnancy rates average 35 per cent (range 20 to 60 per cent).[138, 150]

GENERAL MANAGEMENT

This section covers aspects of the management of couples with male infertility not amenable to specific treatment. Most patients with male infertility have conditions for which there is no clearly defined and certainly effective treatment.[20, 22] In these couples it is important to discuss the prognosis for a natural pregnancy occurring, the ineffectiveness of other treatments, and the availability of IVF, donor insemination, and adoption. The investigation of the female partner should be reviewed and abnormalities treated when possible. The timing of intercourse to coincide with ovulation should be vigorously encouraged, including emphasis on ways to recognize the fertile period.[157] Measures to ensure the couples' general health should be considered. Cessation of smoking is important because it reduces fertility in women.[158] The psychological upheaval experienced by the couple should be discussed and additional help offered if necessary.

Prognosis

Various studies indicate that a number of factors in addition to semen quality are relevant for natural pregnancies in couples with untreatable sperm defects.[15–18, 96, 158–161] Some are obvious, such as female infertility disorders and coital dysfunction, but in addition female age is significant, there being a fall in fertility after age 35. Duration of infertility is a major factor in most studies. The longer the infertility, the worse the outlook for fertility. Some investigators have attempted to divide pregnancies that occur in these follow-up studies into treatment-related and non–treatment-related, but this is difficult with male infertility when it is doubtful if any of the empirical treatments used are effective.[15] There is also the problem that paternity has to be assumed in most studies. The prognostic factors found in the study to determine the effect of varicocele surgery can be summarized as follows.[18] The main factors were duration of infertility (negative), mean sperm concentration (positive), untreated sperm autoimmunity (negative), ovulatory disorders (negative), occupational group (farmers doing better than other workers), female age (negative), and previous fertility in the couple (positive). Interestingly, varicocele presence and size were positive prognostic factors even though varicocele surgery was not significant. The pregnancy rate curves for different sperm concentration groups are shown in Figure 134–5. These factors can be used to advise patients about their chances of producing a natural pregnancy in a certain time. The accuracy of such predictions is poor because the statistically significant factors only explain a minority of the variance (in the study above, about 17 per cent). Further studies of larger data sets will be necessary to determine other prognostic factors. It is likely that many factors that are unmeasurable, such as gamete transport, have an important bear-

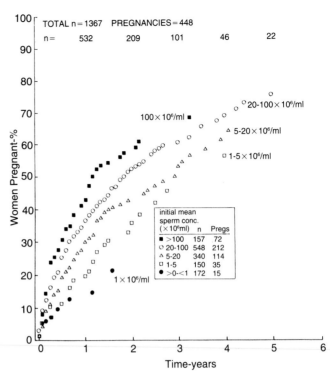

FIGURE 134–5. Pregnancy rate curves grouped according to average pretreatment sperm concentration. The number of patients followed to the beginning of each year is shown above (n). The numbers of men and pregnancies in each sperm concentration group are shown in the inset table.

ing on the ease of conception and may explain the occurrence of pregnancies in some couples despite severe oligospermia.

Psychological Aspects

Infertility causes major trauma to the ego of most patients.[161a, 162] Many undergo a grief reaction with initial denial of the problem followed by a tendency to blame others and a period of depression before final acceptance of the infertility. The reaction may take years to resolve, and it can threaten the stability of the partnership, interfere with rational investigation and management of infertility, and lead to futile involvement in expensive "cures" offered by the unscrupulous. Participation in unsuccessful treatments during this phase often is particularly difficult emotionally for the patients. Evidence suggests that anxious couples have lower fertilization rates in IVF programs.[163] An empathetic approach and involvement of independent counselors or self-help infertility groups may assist some couples. In most, the unpleasantness of the psychological reaction subsides with time.

Timing of Coitus

The timing of coitus has been poorly studied. Some recommend abstinence before ovulation in the hope of increasing the sperm number per ejaculate. This recommendation is common in the lay literature. The effect of abstinence is not great in oligospermic men.[80] Also, it is a frequent experience that many couples mistake the time of ovulation. A more practical approach is to advise intercourse each day when ovulation might occur. Ovulation can be predicted to occur about 14 days before a period is due. Alternatively, some women experience mittleschmertz or can detect mucus symptoms despite frequent intercourse.[157] Other investigators recommend the use of temperature charts; again, these may be counterproductive in couples who do not understand that the temperature rises after rather than before ovulation. Ovulation timing by measurement of urine or serum LH levels or ovarian ultrasonography is expensive and probably not warranted outside artificial insemination programs.

General Health Aspects

Although life-style factors are probably of little relevance to fertility in most Western societies, healthy living has positive long-term benefits and will not affect the semen adversely. The following are advised: weight reduction for the obese; alcohol intake reduction for the moderate to heavy drinker; avoidance of social drugs, including tobacco; reduction of stress in the workplace, marriage, and that engendered by the infertility; and avoidance of heat from frequent sauna and spa baths.

Empirical Treatments

Many treatments have been attempted for defects of sperm production. Androgens have been given to suppress spermatogenesis in the hope that there would be "rebound" improvement after the treatment is stopped. Low-dose testosterone or weak androgens, such as mesterolone, have been given in the hope of improving epididymal maturation of sperm. hCG has been given for similar reasons. Antiestrogens have been used to increase gonadotropin secretion or gonadotropins—FSH and hCG—given to "stimulate" spermatogenesis. Antibiotics and anti-inflammatory drugs have been given for subtle infections or inflammations in the accessory sex organs. Amino acids, vitamins, herbs, and minerals such as zinc pass in and out of fashion. Cold baths and testicular coolers are also being promoted enthusiastically. All these treatments either have not been submitted to adequately controlled clinical trials, or when they have, the trials have not shown any benefit.[131, 149, 164, 165] Marked improvements in semen quality can occur spontaneously (Fig. 134–6). Thus, although there is a strong urge for the medical attendant to do something and a desire of the patients for almost any form of medication, it is probably better to advise the couple of the likely ineffectiveness of these treatments. It is worth remembering that those patients treated in the past with gondotropins of pituitary origin are now at risk of developing Creutzfeldt-Jakob disease.[166] Other, apparently innocuous treatments may turn out to have long-term adverse effects.

AIH for oligospermia or other abnormalities is also widely practiced in different countries with dubious evidence of efficacy.[144–147] Many controlled trials show no benefit from AIH, and when trials have been positive it is intriguing that most of the pregnancies have occurred in the first few treatment cycles.[144, 147] This suggests that per-

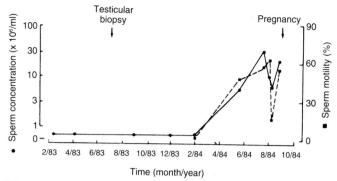

FIGURE 134–6. Sperm concentration and motility in a man with severe oligospermia and severe hypospermatogenesis included in a therapeutic trial of clomiphene. Semen quality improved and his wife conceived. He was given the placebo! (Baker HWG: Requirements for controlled therapeutic trials in male infertility. Clin Reprod Fertil 4:13–25, 1986.)

haps the couples were not having intercourse frequently. Ovulation induction with either artificial insemination, particularly intrauterine, or natural intercourse probably does increase the pregnancy rates by increasing the number of oocytes exposed to the sperm.[145] This poses a risk of multiple pregnancy, and although this may be acceptable in countries where IVF is expensive, IVF would be preferable because the number of pre-embryos placed in the uterus can be controlled and high multiple pregnancy avoided.

IVF FOR MALE INFERTILITY

Indications

In vitro fertilization has become a mainstay of management for male infertility of mild to moderate degree. Provided that more than about 2 million motile sperm can be harvested from an ejaculate, IVF can be attempted with an expectation of success close to that of IVF for other indications.[167–170] The outcome depends particularly on the sperm morphology and the ability of the sperm to bind to the zona pellucida (see below). Some groups have found that the human sperm hamster zona free oocyte penetration test is a useful predictor for success in IVF.[171] As discussed below, the clinical value of these tests is arguable, and unexpected results are common. Trial-run sperm preparations may be useful, particularly in men with severe oligospermia or asthenospermia. Patients with many inflammatory cells in the semen should be treated with antibiotics. Those with low motility or sperm autoimmunity may have better results with shorter durations of abstinence and worse results with longer periods of abstinence. Patients with fluctuating semen abnormalities may benefit from cryopreservation of semen to be used as backup if the semen is particularly poor on the day or to supplement the semen produced on the day. Those patients who produce an unexpectedly poor sample on the day of IVF might be advised to provide a second sample later to supplement the first sample. Trial-run sperm preparations also identify those patients who have difficulty collecting semen. These patients may be advised to practice collections before attending for the IVF procedure. Sperm with persistently zero motility or 100 per cent showing the same defective structure—for example, absent acrosomes—will not fertilize in vitro. In addition, men with less than 1 to 2 million motile sperm per ejaculate, less than 5 per cent of sperm with normal morphology, less than 5 per cent of sperm with progressive motility because of mixed structural defects or sperm autoimmunity with more than 80 per cent of IgA IBT binding to the heads, and zero sperm mucus penetration have poor fertilization rates.[95, 124] In these cases micromanipulation procedures could be considered or the couples could look to other alternatives, such as donor insemination.

Approaches

The standard approach is to perform IVF with transfer into the uterine cavity of two- to eight-cell pre-embryos and cryopreservation of the remaining pre-embryos. Various alternatives are also practiced. For example, GIFT has been reported to produce reasonable results for male factor infertility by some groups, but others find that the pregnancy rates are low and the information about whether or not the oocytes fertilize is lost.[172, 173] Because there is a belief that transfer of the zygote or early pre-embryo into the fallopian tube may be more physiological and result in higher pregnancy rates, procedures called pronuclear ovum stage transfer (PROST), zygote intrafallopian transfer (ZIFT), or tubal embryo stage transfer (TEST) are used by some groups. The zygotes or pre-embryos are placed in the fallopian tubes either by laparoscopy or by retrograde catheterization of the fallopian tube from the cervix and uterine cavity.[173, 174] Proof that these procedures result in higher implantation rates is still awaited.[172]

Sperm Preparation

Various procedures have been developed for sperm preparation for IVF. They are used more as they have come into vogue rather than on the basis of controlled clinical trials. Most popular are the "swim-up" procedure and centrifugation on gradients of polyvinylpyrrolidone (Percoll).[175] Other techniques involving centrifugation and resuspension in culture medium several times to remove seminal plasma have been used with success. Patients with sperm antibodies may benefit from ejaculating the semen directly into culture medium, from which the sperm are recovered. Cryopreserved samples require especially gentle handling, particularly with dilution of the semen cryoprotectant medium with culture medium. Various motility stimulants have been added to sperm, and although normal pregnancies have occurred, these treatments have not been confirmed to be beneficial by controlled clinical trials.[176, 176a]

Prediction of Results

IVF has permitted many conventional and new tests of sperm function to be examined for their ability to indicate the fertilizing potential of sperm.[95] The possible clinical value of sperm tests for predicting the results of IVF has been assessed using a statistical method named logistic regression analysis to test which groups of sperm variables are independently significantly related to the proportion of oocytes that fertilize in vitro.

Morphology

The percentage of sperm with normal morphology assessed after washing the sperm and adjusting the concentration to 80 million/ml provides one of the most useful predictors of IVF rates. There is a progressive reduction in fertilization rates from 60 per cent to 20 per cent as abnormal morphology increases from less than 70 per cent to more than 95 per cent. A few individuals fertilize all or most oocytes despite more than 95 per cent abnormal morphology. Examination of sperm bound to the zona pellucida (ZP) of oocytes that failed to fertilize indicates a selectivity of the ZP for sperm with normal morphology. A few abnormal sperm bind to the ZP but at lower rates than normal sperm, and they usually have normal acrosomal areas. It is useful to advise patients with high proportions of sperm with abnormal morphology that there may be no fertilization with standard IVF.

Motility

Measurement of various aspects of sperm motility using the Hamilton-Thorn computer-assisted sperm motility analyzer indicates that average straight line velocity and average linearity of motion are significant predictors of IVF rates.

Acrosome

Acrosome status has been examined using fluorescein-labeled antibodies or lectins, such as pisum sativum agglutinin. The higher the proportion of sperm with intact acrosomes in the insemination medium, the higher the IVF rates, particularly in men with poor sperm morphology.

Other Tests

The results of other sperm tests (hypo-osmotic swelling, amplitude of lateral head displacement, and nuclear decondensation in detergents and reducing agents) were not significantly related to IVF results when morphology, acrosomes, and motility were taken into account.

Sperm-Oocyte Interaction Tests

In a number of countries human sperm–zona free hamster oocyte penetration tests are performed to assess the ability of sperm to capacitate, acrosome react, fuse with the oolemma, and undergo nuclear decondensation in the ooplasm. This test does not evaluate sperm interaction with the ZP. Because hamsters are not permitted in Australia, I have had no practical experience with this test.

HUMAN SPERM–ZP BINDING RATIO TEST. Because the number of sperm bound to the ZP is strongly related to the IVF rate, human sperm–ZP interaction tests have been developed using oocytes that failed to fertilize. These oocytes can be used either fresh or after storage in concentrated salt solutions. Because the ZP binding capacity is variable, control (fertile donor) and test sperm are labeled with different fluorochromes (fluorescein and rhodamine). After incubation with equal numbers of control and test sperm, results are expressed as a ratio of binding to the ZP of test and control sperm for four to six oocytes. An alternative method is to cut the zonae in half and expose each to test and control sperm (Hemizona assay).[177] To date the sperm–ZP binding ratio is the most powerful predictor of IVF rates.

HUMAN SPERM–OOLEMMA BINDING RATIO TEST. Sperm–oolemma binding has been studied in the same way, but this test seems less valuable clinically than the sperm–ZP binding test. Both tests are useful for research. For example, induction of the acrosome reaction with a calcium ionophore (A23187) reduced sperm binding to the ZP but increased sperm binding to the oolemma, suggesting that human sperm bind to the ZP with the acrosome intact and that the physiological acrosome reaction occurs on the ZP.[95]

Mechanisms of Failure of Fertilization

The studies of the relationship of the results of sperm tests and IVF have increased understanding of the mechanisms by which defects of sperm contribute to failure of fertilization in vitro. Defects in the number of motile sperm or linearity of motility result in few sperm contacting the oocyte. Abnormalities of sperm head shape, particularly in the acrosomal region reduce binding to the ZP because of the mechanical disadvantage or an associated deficiency in binding sites on the overlying plasma membrane. Premature occurrence of the acrosome reaction while the sperm is swimming in the culture medium would also prevent sperm binding to the ZP. All these abnormalities will affect the number of sperm bound to the ZP. These problems seem to explain about 75 per cent of the cases of low (less than 20 per cent) or zero fertilization in IVF programs with many male-factor patients. The percentage of sperm with normal morphology and an intact acrosome can be used to advise patients about the chances of fertilization in vitro. No single test is highly accurate in the prediction of results for IVF, and there is considerable variability of semen quality from day to day in men with sperm defects. Trials are being performed to determine if enhancing the recovery of sperm with normal morphology, an intact acrosome, high linearity of motion, and ZP binding ability will increase fertilization rates in those patients predicted to have failure of fertilization because of poor semen. In general, attempts to improve semen quality by treatment of the man are unsuccessful. However, controlled trials of hormone treatment (e.g., high-dose FSH) may show that sperm function can be improved in some men.[178]

The predictive value of failed fertilization for subsequent fertility has not been clearly defined, but in general, failed fertilization is a confirmation that a sperm defect is severe. On the other hand, unexpected failures of fertilization may be procedural in origin, and further IVF attempts are worthwhile. Some natural pregnancies have occurred despite repeated failure of fertilization in vitro.

Results

In most IVF programs about 60 per cent of oocytes fertilize and cleave normally over the first 48 hours with normal semen. With abnormal semen the fertilization and normal cleavage rates are lower, particularly when the percentage of sperm with abnormal morphology is greater than 80 per cent; on average only 35 per cent of oocytes fertilize and cleave normally. If in addition to the abnormal morphology there is low sperm concentration and low sperm motility, then the fertilization and normal cleavage rates fall to 30 per cent.[95] These overall figures conceal the fact that a substantial proportion (30 to 50 per cent) of patients with poor sperm morphology have no oocytes fertilized, many have low numbers fertilized, and only a few have good fertilization rates.

Although fetal heart–embryo rates up to 24 per cent have been claimed,[179] live birth pregnancy rates for each fresh or cryopreserved pre-embryo transferred to the uterine cavity range from 5 to 10 per cent in most IVF programs.[180, 181] If two oocytes are transferred at a time, then the chance of a successful pregnancy is about 14 per cent after one transfer, 25 per cent after two transfers, 33 per cent after three transfers, and 50 per cent after five transfers. About 15 per cent of the pregnancies resulting from transfer of two pre-embryos produce twins. Because the fertilization rate is lower with abnormal sperm morphology, the cumulative chance of having a child from each attempt at IVF is reduced. In general, once fertilization occurs with abnormal semen, the outcome for the pre-embryos appears to be no different than that for pre-embryos obtained from fertilization with normal semen.[180] The implantation rate, pregnancy wastage, perinatal mortality, and risk of congenital abnormalities are no greater than with patients who have IVF for other indications.

Evaluation of Failed Fertilization

When all oocytes fail to fertilize in IVF, the cause usually is defective sperm. On rare occasions the oocytes do not fertilize because of immaturity or abnormality, but this appears to be quite an unusual cause of total failure of fertilization. Careful evaluation of the semen quality before IVF should reveal those cases with defective sperm morphology and allow the couples to be warned that failure of fertilization is a possibility.[95] Unexpected failures of fertilization should be evaluated carefully, including examination of the number and position of sperm on the ZP and penetrating into the zona. With severe sperm defects failure of sperm to bind to the zona or reduced sperm binding to the zona is common. Other sperm defects are becoming apparent, such as failure to penetrate the zona despite reasonable sperm–zona binding. Failure of fertilization may also result from undiagnosed sperm autoimmunity, the presence of sperm antibodies in maternal serum, infected semen, or technical defects in the IVF laboratory.[124]

Reinsemination of unfertilized oocytes with husband's semen after 12 to 24 hours may result in fertilization and pregnancy, but overall, the results are poor and many units would not perform this procedure.[182] Reinsemination of failed fertilization oocytes with donor sperm is also possible for diagnostic or therapeutic purposes. This procedure is not permitted in some countries.

Micromanipulation in IVF

A number of techniques have been developed to facilitate fertilization when IVF with standard procedures is believed to be impossible or when IVF has been attempted and failed.[183–188] Because the ZP appears to represent a barrier to fertilization, attempts to bypass it have been as follows. The zona may be breeched by cutting, tearing, or dissolving part of it with dilute acid or enzymes.[184–186] These procedures are generically termed partial zona dissection (PZD). After PZD, oocytes are exposed to sperm in culture medium as in the standard IVF procedure. An alternative approach is to inject sperm either through the zona into the perivitelline space (subzonal insemination) or directly into the cytoplasm (ICSI).[138a, 185, 187] Mixed approaches are also possible, for example, the subzonal insemination of several sperm and in addition the oocytes are placed in insemination medium containing sperm. Although most of these procedures have been performed mechanically with micromanipulators, the possibility of using low-powered lasers to breech the zona and perhaps to manipulate sperm into the perivitelline space is also being investigated.[189, 190]

If subjects are selected for PZD or subzonal insemination because of sperm defects with previous failure of fertilization in vitro or extreme oligospermia (less than 1 million/ml), the fertilization rates are low, ranging from 10 to 25 per cent.[185–188] Because the zona is breeched, the mechanisms for blocking polyspermia are interrupted and the polyspermy rates usually are high (10 per cent; that is, 50 to 100 per cent of the monospermic fertilization rate). If patients with better-quality semen are admitted into these programs, then the fertilization rates are higher and may approach those obtained with standard IVF. The units that use micromanipulation for severe sperm defects have low pregnancy rates (about 5 per cent per attempt), but one half to two thirds of the patients do have some pre-embryos develop for transfer.[185] ICSI is producing better results, with greater than 50 per cent normal fertilization rates for most types of severe sperm deficit. Pregnancy and normal birth rates are also very good[138a] (Baker, unpublished observations, 1993).

Improvements in IVF technology may have an important impact on the treatment of male infertility. The implantation rates in most IVF programs are lower than those that occur with natural fertility in humans, and advances in this area will substantially improve the overall pregnancy rates. Greater understanding of how sperm characteristics are related to fertilization rates will point to improved patient selection for standard IVF or ICSI. Oocyte freezing would also assist in the management of sperm defects because smaller groups of oocytes could be exposed to sperm obtained at different times and prepared in different ways.

USE OF DONOR SPERM

Donor insemination has become a common method of managing male sterility in many Western countries.[29, 191–200] Sperm banks have been established and run successfully, so that now up to 1 in 200 children is born in these countries as a result of the use of donor sperm.

Indications

The main indications for donor insemination are sterility in the male or severe or chronic subfertility. For example, subfertile men with severe oligospermia, asthenospermia, or teratospermia have little chance of producing pregnancies either naturally or by IVF. The couple may choose donor insemination as the primary method of managing their infertility, or they may choose this after treatments have failed. Rarely, donor insemination is used because of genetic abnormalities in the male. Donor sperm may also be used in IVF when there is a combination of female infertility and male sterility. Because of the higher pregnancy rates, IVF with donor sperm may be used if donor insemination fails. Donor sperm may also be used in IVF procedures as a backup, for example, when epididymal sperm aspiration is to be attempted and there is some doubt whether sperm will be obtained from the epididymis.

Cryopreservation of Semen

Donor insemination can be performed in the setting of a specialist infertility clinic with patient counseling, ovulation monitoring, and insemination procedures available as well as the sperm bank.[29, 191] Alternatively, the sperm bank may be separate from the clinics or physicians performing the artificial insemination and only supply semen for the patient. Because of the risk of transmission of infectious diseases, particularly human immunodeficiency virus (HIV) and hepatitis B, and for convenience, most donor insemination services now use only cryopreserved semen.[29, 191, 192] Cryopreservation with glycerol–egg yolk cryoprotectant and either vapor freezing or controlled-rate freezing in plastic straws or vials produce pregnancy rates equal to those with fresh semen. Importantly, cryopreservation allows the semen to be quarantined for three to six months for donors to be recalled and retested for HIV antibodies before any is used.

Selection of Donors

Prospective donors have their medical and family history evaluated and a physical examination to exclude the possibility of transmitting serious genetic diseases and infections. In some countries donors sign a life-style declaration to indicate that they are not involved in any practices that might expose them to serious infections, such as HIV. There usually is an upper age limit in the region of 40 to 45 years because of the increasing frequency of genetic abnormalities in sperm with age. Semen quality is selected to be in the upper part of the normal range, particularly for concentration and motility.[193] The semen is cultured intermittently for bacteria and blood tested for hepatitis and HIV antibodies.

As with the transfer of infection, consideration should be given to the possibility of producing problems by the transfer of genetic determinants for thalassemia or rhesus immunization. Similarly, if stimulation of ovulation is to be used, then the risk of multiple pregnancy must be discussed with the couple. The frozen semen does not appear to cause any increase in the frequency of congenital abnormalities.[29, 194–196]

It is usual to match the physical characteristics of the recipient's husband and the donor in several broad categories, including race, complexion, build, height, hair color, and eye color. In addition, blood groups may be matched. In some programs the recipient couple may be given access to other information about the donor, such as occupation and education, and they may be allowed some say in the choice of a donor.

Known donors may also be used; these may be friends or relatives of the infertile couple. In this situation special counseling of the donors and recipients is necessary. Also, there should be a full workup of the known donor as for an anonymous donor, including cryopreservation and quarantining of the semen.

Donor factors relevant to the success of donor insemination are mainly to do with the quality of the semen. Post-thaw motility has the strongest predictive value for high fertilization rates, but sperm morphology, motility, and concentration are also significant.[193, 195] Despite selection of high-quality semen, there remains considerable variability in the pregnancy rates achieved with different donors. Thus some policy to discard semen from a donor who produces no pregnancy after a certain number (e.g., 20 to 40) of inseminations is necessary.[193]

Donor Insemination Procedure

The prospective recipients are screened for HIV, hepatitis B, rubella immunity, and blood group. Tests of tubal patency are performed if the history suggests pelvic pathology. The procedures of insemination are the same as described above for AIH.

Results

The pregnancy rates with donor insemination are about 10 to 15 per cent per month for the first five to six months and then 5 to 10 per cent thereafter, so that about 50 per cent of women are pregnant by six months.[29, 191, 194–196] One of the factors that affect the pregnancy rates is female age. Women over 35 have lower pregnancy rates than those under 35; for example, 65 per cent pregnant by one year under 35 and 50 per cent pregnant by one year over 35.[29, 191, 195] Women with subfertile male partners have on average lower pregnancy rates than those with sterile male partners, which may be taken to indicate that some female factors are involved in the infertility when the male partner is subfertile.[29, 197] Interestingly, cumulative pregnancy rates for women who have had more than one pregnancy by donor insemination indicate higher conception rates over the first few months for the second pregnancy, about 33 per cent pregnant in the first cycle and 55 per cent by the second cycle.[198] Whether this results from less stress in the repeat treatment cycle or from other factors is not known.

Ovulation induction may improve pregnancy rates but exposes the women to the risk of multiple pregnancy. There is a trend now toward using IVF if no pregnancy has occurred after a reasonable number of inseminations, for example, 6 to 12.[199] Pregnancy rates with IVF in such patients are excellent (25 to 33 per cent pregnant per attempt). By using donor sperm in IVF if artificial insemination fails to produce a pregnancy quickly, couples can now

be advised that they have an 80 per cent chance of having a child within two years.

Counseling

The special nature of the use of donor sperm needs to be discussed in detail with the couple so that they are fully aware of the implications of having a child by donor. Donor insemination is forbidden in some religions. There may be local legislation or regulations to control the use of donated gametes. In some countries special laws have been enacted that may either allow or prevent the child from obtaining identifying information about the donor. The legal position of the child may also be specified in various ways. The couple need to decide how they will handle the information about the pregnancy vis-à-vis the child, particularly whether or not and when to disclose the child's donor sperm origin. What and how much they should tell their friends and relatives about their infertility treatment should also be discussed, as should their reaction to acquaintances questioning the paternity of the child. The possibility that in the future half-siblings may unwittingly find each other and attempt to have children is a considerable worry to many prospective parents and donors. This needs to be discussed carefully and the risks explained in view of the number of pregnancies permitted per donor by the clinic. Studies of donor families indicate no problems with the children and greater stability than average.[199, 199a]

PREVENTION OF INFERTILITY

Prevention is difficult because of the lack of understanding of the causes of most types of male infertility.[200] It is important to recognize that subfertility often is a couple problem, both partners contributing. Therefore, general factors that would change a society's attitude to child-bearing could have an important impact on the frequency of infertility, for example, a trend toward having children at earlier ages. On the other hand, toxins and environmental factors known to cause defects of sperm production, such as dibromochlorobenzine, lead, benzene, ionizing radiation, and microwaves, are well controlled by environmental health measures.[8, 65]

Sexually Transmitted Diseases

Postgonococcal epididymal obstructions appear to be the most important cause of infertility from sexually transmitted diseases. A clear history of prolonged, poorly treated urethritis commonly is associated with epididymitis. In most Western countries gonorrhea is treated promptly, and postgonococcal obstructions are extremely rare complications. On the other hand, these problems appear to be a predominant cause of infertility in sub-Saharan Africa and are a relatively common cause of infertility in some Asian countries.[23]

Undescended Testes

Although undescended testes have been sought and treated aggressively in most Western countries over the past

40 years, previously undescended testes remain a common association of male infertility, affecting about 7 per cent of the men seen.[49, 50] It is, therefore, uncertain whether early surgery for undescended testes has any impact on subsequent fertility. It is possible that the failure of normal descent is a feature of testicular dystrophy and that the sperm production will be poor whether or not the testes are placed in the scrotum. Because men who have had one testis removed usually have semen quality within normal limits, men with a unilateral undescended testis would not be expected to have poor semen unless there was an additional disorder of spermatogenesis in the contralateral descended scrotal testis. Thus, although orchidopexy is important for cosmetic aspects and ease of checking the testis for malignant change, it is not certain whether early orchidopexy preserves or promotes fertility.

Varicocele

As already discussed, the effectiveness of varicocelectomy for sperm defects is controversial.[18] Varicoceles are also common abnormalities and probably appear about the time of puberty. Although some European groups believe that varicoceles should be sought actively and treated in adolescence to prevent infertility, this approach could pose a major burden on the health resources because at least 15 per cent of men have varicoceles.[201, 202] Prospective trials would be valuable in this area.

Vasectomy

Vasectomy is now a common and important method of family planning in many countries. In those with a high frequency of marriage breakdown, vasectomy reversal and continuing infertility after attempted vasectomy reversal have become common medical problems. Better counseling about the results of vasectomy reversal is needed. Cryopreservation of semen before vasectomy in men who are uncertain about their need for future fertility should be promoted. Also, cryopreservation of semen after vasectomy reversal, if the quality is adequate, is worthwhile because there is a proportion of men in whom sperm appear initially but then disappear after restenosis of the vasovasostomy sites.

Semen Cryopreservation Before Sterilizing Procedures

Semen can be cryopreserved before vasectomy; in addition, men about to have treatment for malignant conditions may have sperm cryopreserved before commencing chemotherapy or radiotherapy. However, pretreatment semen quality often is poor.[203] Semen collected during such treatment must not be used because of the likelihood of induced mutations.[60] Other illnesses that require treatment that might result in sterility include nephritis, prostatic disease, psoriasis, and inflammatory bowel diseases. Some men with Young's syndrome produce sperm and, occasionally, pregnancies when they are younger, before the epididymal obstruction develops.[27] Therefore, men with bronchiectasis discovered in childhood or adolescence might be advised to store semen frozen in case they have this condition.

REFERENCES

1. Johnsen SG: A study of human testicular function by the use of human menopausal gonadotrophin and human chorionic gonadotrophin male hypogonadotrophic eunuchordism and infertilism. Acta Endocrinol 53:315–341, 1966.
2. Martin FIR: The stimulation and prolonged maintainence of spermatogenesis by human pituitary gonadotrophin in a patient with hypogonadotrophic hypogonadism. J Endocrinol 38:431–437, 1967.
3. Klinefelter HF Jr, Reifenstein EC Jr, Albright F: Syndrome characterized by gynaecomastia, aspermatogenesis without aleydigism and increased excretion of follicle stimulating hormone. J Clin Endocrinol 2:615–627, 1942.
4. Beaney JG: The Generative System and Its Function in Health and Disease (ed 3). Melbourne, FF Bailliere, 1877.
5. Tulloch WS: Varicocele in subfertility results of treatment. Br Med J 2:356–358, 1955.
6. Dubin L, Amelar RD: Varicocelectomy. 986 cases in a twelve year study. Urology 10:446–449, 1977.
7. Jequier AM: Edward Martin (1859–1938): The founding father of modern clinical andrology. Int J Androl 14:1–10, 1991.
8. Feichtinger W: Environmental factors and fertility. Hum Reprod 6:1170–1175, 1991.
9. Bendvold E, Gottlieb C, Bygdeman M, Eneroth P: Depressed semen quality in Swedish men from barren couples: A study over three decades. Arch Androl 26:189–194, 1991.
9a. Sharpe RM, Skakkeback NE: Are oestrogens involved in falling sperm counts and disorders of the male reproductive tract? Lancet 341:1392–1395, 1993.
10. Leridon H: Human Fertility: The Basic Components. Chicago, University of Chicago Press, 1977, p 104.
11. Vessey MP, Wright NH, McPherson K, Wiggins P: Fertility after stopping different methods of contraception. Br Med J 1:265–267, 1978.
12. Greenhall E, Vessey M: The prevalence of subfertility: A review of the current confusion and a report of two new studies. Fertil Steril 54:978–983, 1990.
13. Menken J, Trussell J, Larsen U: Age and infertility. Science 233:1389–1394, 1986.
14. Spira A: Epidemiology of human reproduction. Hum Reprod 1:111–115, 1986.
15. Collins JA, Garner JB, Wilson EH, et al: A proportional hazards analysis of the clinical characteristics of infertile couples. Am J Obstet Gynecol 148:527–532, 1984.
16. Hargreave TB, Elton RA: Fecundability rates from an infertile male population. Br J Urol 58:194–197, 1986.
17. Polansky FF, Lamb EJ: Do the results of semen analysis predict future fertility? A survival analysis study. Fertil Steril 49:1059–1065, 1988.
18. Baker HWG, Burger HG, de Kretser DM, et al: Testicular vein ligation and fertility in men with varicoceles. Br Med J 291:1678–1680, 1985.
19. WHO Laboratory Manual for the Examination of Human Semen and Semen-Cervical Mucus Interaction (ed 3). Cambridge, Cambridge University Press, 1992.
20. Baker HWG, Burger HG, de Kretser DM, Hudson B: Relative incidence of etiologic disorders in male infertility. In Santen RJ, Swerdloff RS (eds): Male Reproductive Dysfunction: Diagnosis and Management of Hypogonadism, Infertility and Impotence. New York, Marcel Dekker 1986, pp 341–372.
21. Hull MG, Glazener CM, Kelly NJ, et al: Population study of causes, treatment, and outcome of infertility. Br Med J 291:1693–1697, 1985.
22. Comhaire FH, de Kretser DM, Farley TM, Row PJ: Towards more objectivity in diagnosis and management of male infertility. Int J Androl (Suppl) 7:1–53, 1987.
23. Cates W, Fairley TMM, Rowe PJ: Worldwide patterns of infertility: Is Africa different? Lancet 2:596–598, 1985.
24. Burger HG, Baker HWG: The treatment of infertility. Annu Rev Med 38:29–40, 1987.
25. Angulano A, Oates RD, Amos JA, et al: Congenital bilateral absence of the vas deferens: A primary genital form of cystic fibrosis. JAMA 267:1794–1797, 1992.

25a. Patrizio P, Asch RH, Handelin B, Silber SJ: Aetiology of congenital absence of vas deferens: Genetic study of three generations. Hum Reprod 8:215–220, 1993.

26. Hendry WF, Levison DA, Parkinson MC, et al: Testicular obstruction: Clinicopathological studies. Ann R Coll Surg Engl 72:396–407, 1990.

27. Handelsman DJ, Conway AJ, Boylan LM, Turtle JR: Young's syndrome: Obstructive azoospermia and chronic sino-pulmonary infections. N Engl J Med 310:3–9, 1984.

28. Wilton LJ, Southwick GJ, Title H: Young's syndrome (obstructive azoospsermia and chronic sino-bronchial infection): A quantitative study of axonemal ultrastructure and function. Fertil Steril 55:142–151, 1991.

29. Kovacs G, Baker G, Burger HG, et al: AID with cryopreserved semen: A decade of experience. Br J Obstet Gynaecol 95:354–360, 1988.

30. Burger HG, Baker HWG: Therapeutic considerations and results of gonadotropin treatment in male hypogonadotropic hypogonadism. Ann NY Acad Sci 438:447–453, 1984.

31. Burris AS, Clark RV, Vantman DJ, Sherins RJ: A low sperm concentration does not preclude fertility in men with isolated hypogonadotropic hypogonadism after gonadotropin therapy. Fertil Steril 50:343–347, 1988.

32. World Health Organization Task Force on Methods for the Regulation of Male Fertility: Contraceptive efficacy of testosterone-induced azoospermia in normal men. Lancet 336:955–959, 1990.

33. WHO Standardized Method for Evaluation of Infertile Couples. Cambridge, Cambridge University Press, 1988.

34. Teichtahl H, Temple-Smith PD, Johnson JL, et al: Obstructive azoospermia and chronic sinobronchial disease (Young's syndrome) in identical twins. Fertil Steril 47:879–881, 1987.

35. Baker HWG, Clarke GN, Hudson B, et al: Treatment of sperm autoimmunity in men. Clin Reprod Fertil 2:55–71, 1983.

36. Baker HWG, Clarke GN, McGowan MP, et al: Increased frequency of autoantibodies in men with sperm antibodies. Fertil Steril 43:438–441, 1985.

37. Kaplan E, Shwachman H, Perlmutter AD, et al: Reproductive failure in males with cystic fibrosis. N Engl J Med 279:65–69, 1968.

38. Radovick S, Wray S, Lee E: Migratory arrest of gonadotropin-releasing hormone neurons in transgenic mice. Proc Natl Acad Sci USA 88:3402–3406, 1991.

39. Mulley JC, Gedeon AK, White SJ, et al: Predictive diagnosis of myotonic dystrophy from flanking microsatellite markers. J Med Genet 28:448–452, 1991.

40. Gill WB, Schumacher GFB, Bibbo M: Pathological semen and anatomical abnormalities of the genital tract in human male subjects exposed to diethylstilbestrol in utero. J Urol 117:477–480, 1977.

41. Wischusen J, Baker HWG, Hudson B: Reversible male infertility due to congenital adrenal hyperplasia. Clin Endocrinol 14:571–577, 1981.

42. Baker HWG: Testicular dysfunction in systemic disease. In Becker LK (ed): Principles and Practice of Endocrinology and Metabolism. Philadelphia, JB Lippincott Co, 1990, pp 971–975.

43. MacLeod J, Hotchkiss RS: The effect of hyperpyrexia on spermatozoa counts in men. Endocrinology 28:780, 1941.

44. Eliasson R, Mossberg B, Canmer P, Afzelius B: The immotile-cilia syndrome. A congenital ciliary abnormality as an etiologic factor in chronic airway infections and male sterility. N Engl J Med 297:1–6, 1977.

45. Zamboni L: The ultrastructural pathology of the spermatozoon as a cause of infertility: The role of electron microscopy in the evaluation of semen quality. Fertil Steril 48:711–734, 1987.

46. Hargreave TB, Elton RA, Webb JA, et al: Maldescended testes and fertility: A review of 68 cases. Br J Urol 56:734–739, 1984.

47. Scorer CG: The descent of the testes. Arch Dis Child 39:605–609, 1964.

48. Palmer JM: The undescended testicle. Endocrinol Metab Clin North Am 20:231–240, 1991.

49. Hezmall HP, Lipshultz LI: Cryptorchidism and infertility. Urol Clin North Am 9:361–369, 1982.

50. Puri P, O'Donnell B: Semen analysis of patients who had orchidopexy at or after seven years of age. Lancet 2:1051–1052, 1988.

51. Rajfer J, Walsh PC: Hormonal regulation of testicular descent: Experimental and clinical observations. J Urol 188:985–990, 1977.

52. Rajfer J, Handelsman DJ, Swerdloff RS, et al: Hormonal therapy for cryptorchidism. A randomized, double-blind study comparing human chorionic gonadotrophin and gonadotrophin-releasing hormone. N Engl J Med 314:466–470, 1986.

53. Skakkebaek NA: Carcinoma in situ of the testis. Frequency and relationship to invasive germ cell tumors in infertile men. Histopathology 2:157–170, 1978.

54. Pryor JP, Cameron KM, Chilton CP, et al: Carcinoma in situ in testicular biopsies from men presenting with infertility. Br J Urol 55:780–784, 1983.

55. West AB, Butler MR, Fitzpatrick A, O'Brien A: Testicular tumors in subfertile men. Report of 4 cases with implications for management of patients presenting with infertility. J Urol 133:107–109, 1985.

56. Sanderman T: The effects of X irradiation on male fertility. Br J Radiol 39:901–907, 1966.

57. Byrne J, Mulvihill JJ, Myers MH, et al: Effects of treatment on fertility in long-term survivors of childhood or adolescent cancer. N Engl J Med 317:1315–1321, 1987.

58. Fairley KF, Barrie J, Johnson W: Sterility and testicular atrophy related to cyclophosphamide therapy. Lancet 1:568–569, 1972.

59. Berthelsen JG: Testicular cancer and fertility. Int J Androl 10:371–380, 1987.

60. Bucci LR, Meistrich ML: Effects of busulfan on murine spermatogenesis: Cytotoxicity, sterility, sperm abnormalities, and dominant lethal mutations. Mutat Res 176:259–268, 1987.

61. Sussman A, Leonard JM: Psoriasis, methotrexate and oligozoospermia. Arch Dermatol 116:215–217, 1980.

62. Wu FC, Aitken RJ, Ferguson A: Inflammatory bowel disease and male infertility: Effects of sulfasalazine and 5-aminosalicylic acid on sperm-fertilizing capacity and reactive oxygen species generation. Fertil Steril 52:842–845, 1989.

63. Schlegel PN, Chang TS, Marshall FF: Antibiotics: Potential hazards to male fertility. Fertil Steril 55:235–242, 1991.

64. Pholpramool C, Ruchirawat S, Verawatnapakul V, et al: Structural requirements of some sulphonamides that possess an antifertility activity in male rats. J Reprod Fertil 92:169–178, 1991.

65. Henderson J, Baker HWG, Hanna PJ: Occupationally related male infertility: A review. Clin Reprod Fertil 4:87–106, 1986.

66. Levine RJ, Bordson BL, Mathew RM, et al: Deterioration of semen quality during summer in New Orleans. Fertil Steril 49:900–907, 1988.

67. Brown-Woodman PDC, Post EJ, Goss GC, White IG: The effect of a single sauna exposure on spermatozoa. Arch Androl 12:9–15, 1984.

68. Handelsman DJ, Conway AJ, Boylan LM, Turtle JR: Testicular function in potential sperm donors: Normal ranges and effects of smoking and varicocele. Int J Androl 7:369–382, 1984.

69. Oldereid NB, Rui H, Clausen OP, Purvis K: Cigarette smoking and human sperm quality assessed by laser-Doppler spectroscopy and DNA flow cytometry. J Reprod Fertil 86:731–736, 1989.

70. Baker HWG, Pepperell RJ: Lack of effect of bromocriptine on semen quality in men with normal or slightly elevated prolactin levels. Aust NZ J Obstet Gynecol 20:158–161, 1980.

71. Gebhard PH, Johnson AB: The Kinsey data: Marginal tabulations of the 1938–1963 interviews conducted by the Institute for Sex Research. Philadelphia, WB Saunders Co, 1979, pp 116–120.

72. Abeyaratne MR, Aherne WA, Scott JES: The vanishing testis. Lancet 2:822–824, 1969.

73. Prader A: Testicular size: Assessment and clinical importance. Triangle 7:240–243, 1966.

74. WHO Task Force on the Diagnosis and Treatment of Infertility: Comparison among different methods for the diagnosis of varicocele. Fertil Steril 43:575–582, 1985.

75. Zavos PM: Seminal parameters of ejaculates collected from oligospermic and normospermic patients via masturbation and at intercourse with the use of Silastic seminal fluid collection device. Fertil Steril 44:517–520, 1985.

76. Jones DM, Kovacs GT, Harrison L, et al: Immobilization of sperm by condoms and their components. Clin Reprod Fertil 4:367–372, 1986.

77. Kovacs GT, Newman GB, Henson GC: Postcoital tests: What is normal? Br Med J 1:818, 1978.

78. Polak B, Daunter B: Scanning electron microscopy and histological examination of human seminal plasma coagulum. Andrologia 15:452–462, 1983.

79. Amelar RD, Hotchkiss RS: The split ejaculate; its use in the management of infertility. Fertil Steril 16:46–60, 1965.

80. Baker HWG, Burger HG, de Kretser DM, et al: Factors affecting the variability of semen analysis results in infertile men. Int J Androl 4:609–622, 1981.

81. Wilton LJ, Temple-Smith PD, Baker HWG, de Kretser DM: Human male infertility caused by degeneration and death of sperm in the epididymis. Fertil Steril 49:1050–1058, 1988.

82. Mallidis C, Howard EJ, Baker HWG: Variation of semen quality in normal men. Int J Androl 14:99–107, 1991.

83. Purvis K, Tollefsrud A, Rui H: Stability of sperm characteristics in men with disturbances in sperm quality. Int J Androl 12:171–178, 1989.

84. Bronson R, Cooper G, Rosenfeld D: Detection of sperm-specific antibodies on the spermatozoan surface by immunobead binding. Arch Androl 9:61, 1982.

85. Clarke GN: Detection of antisperm antibodies using immunobeads. In Keel BA, Webster BW (eds): Handbook of the Laboratory Diagnosis and Treatment of Infertility. Boca Raton, Fla, CRC, 1990, pp 177–192.

86. Jager J, Kremer J, van Slochteren-Draaisma T: A simple method of screening for antisperm antibodies in the human male. Detection of spermatozoal surface of IgG with mixed antiglobulin reaction carried out in untreated fresh human semen. Int J Fertil 23:12, 1978.

87. MacMillan RA, Baker HWG: Comparison of latex and polyacrylamide beads for detecting sperm antibodies. Clin Reprod Fertil 5:203–209, 1987.

88. Rose NR, Hjort T, Rumke P, et al: Techniques for detection of iso- and autoantibodies to human spermatozoa. Clin Exp Immunol 23:175–199, 1976.

89. Clarke GN: Lack of correlation between the immunobead test and the enzyme-linked immunosorbent assay for sperm antibody detection. Am J Reprod Immunol Microbiol 18:44–46, 1988.

90. MacLeod J, Gold RZ: The male factor in fertility and infertility. VI. Semen quality and certain other factors in relation to ease of conception. Fertil Steril 4:10–33, 1953.

91. Aitken RJ, Ross A, Lees MM: Analysis of sperm function in Kartagener's syndrome. Fertil Steril 40:696–698, 1983.

92. Feneux D, Serres C, Jouannet P: Sliding spermatozoa: A dyskinesia responsible for human infertility? Fertil Steril 44:508–511, 1985.

93. Cooper EJ, Baker HWG: Protein carboxyl methylase in asthenospermia. Clin Reprod Fertil 4:269–274, 1986.

94. Liu DY, Jennings MG, Baker HWG: Correlation between defective motility (asthenospermia) and ATP reactivation of demembranated human spermatozoa. J Androl 8:349–353, 1987.

95. Liu DY, Baker HWG: Tests of human sperm function and fertilization in vitro. Fertil Steril 58:465–483, 1992.

96. Jouannet P, Ducot B, Feneux D, Spira A: Male factors and the likelihood of pregnancy in infertile couples. I. Study of sperm characteristics. Int J Androl 11:379–94, 1988.

97. Wolf H, Anderson DJ: Immunohistologic characterisation and quantitation of leucocyte subpopulations in human semen. Fertil Steril 49:497–504, 1988.

98. Aitken RJ, Clarkson JS, Hargreave TB, et al: Analysis of the relationship between defective sperm function and the generation of reactive oxygen species in cases of oligozoospermia. J Androl 10:214–220, 1989.

99. Barratt CLR, Kessopoulou E, Thompson LA, et al: The functional significance of leukocytes in human reproduction. Reprod Med Rev 1:115–129, 1992.

100. McGowan MP, Burger HG, Baker HWG, et al: The incidence of non-specific infection in the semen of fertile and sub-fertile males. Int J Androl 4:657–662, 1981.

101. Meares EM, Stamey TA: Bacteriologic localisation patterns in bacterial prostatitis and urethritis. Invest Urol 5:492–518, 1968.

102. Hargreave TB, Kyle KF, Kelly AM, England P: Releasing factor tests in men with oligozoospermia. Br J Urol 51:38–42, 1979.

103. Morrow AF, Baker HWG, Burger HG: Partial gonadotrophin deficiency is infrequent in infertile men. Clin Reprod Fertil 4:319–327, 1986.

104. Baker HWG, Burger HG, de Kretser DM, et al: Changes in the pituitary-testicular system with age. Clin Endocrinol 5:349–372, 1976.

105. Karpas AE, Matsumoto AM, Paulsen CA, Bremner MJ: Elevated serum follicle-stimulating hormone levels in men with normal semen fluid analyses. Fertil Steril 39:333–336, 1983.

106. Hargreave TB, Richmond JD, Liakatas J, et al: Searching for the infertile man with hyperprolactinaemia. Fertil Steril 36:630–632, 1981.

107. Snyder PJ, Bigdali H, Gardner DF, et al: Gonadal function in fifty men with untreated pituitary adenomas. J Clin Endocrinol Metab 48:309–314, 1979.

108. Hargreave TB, Elton RA, Sweeting VM, Basralian K: Estradiol and male fertility. Fertil Steril 49:871–876, 1988.

109. Burger HG: Inhibin and its implications for clinical practice. Endocrinologist 24:240–247, 1992.

110. Chandley AC, Edmond PE, Christie S, et al: Cytogenetics and infertility in man. Results of a five year survey of men attending a subfertile clinic. Karyotype and semen analysis. Ann Hum Genet 39:231–254, 1975.

111. De Braekeleer M, Dao TN: Cytogenetic studies in male infertility: A review. Hum Reprod 6:245–250, 1991.

111a. Mallidis C, Baker HWG: Fine needle tissue aspiration biopsy of the testis. Fertil Steril, in press.

112. de Kretser DM, Burger HG, Hudson B: The relationship between germinal cells and serum FSH in men with infertility. J Clin Endocrinol Metab 37:787, 1974.

113. Middleton WD: Scrotal sonography in 1991. Ultrasound 9:61–87, 1991.

114. Nasham D, Behre HM, Grunert JH, Nieschlag E: Diagnostic value of scrotal sonography in infertile men: Report of 658 cases. Andrologia 22:387–395, 1990.

115. Hendry WF: Detection and treatment of antispermatozoal antibodies in men. Reprod Fertil Dev 1:205–220, 1989.

116. Hendry WF, Stedonska J, Hughes L, et al: Steroid treatment of male subfertility caused by antisperm antibodies. Lancet 2:498–500, 1979.

117. Hellema HWJ, Rumke P: Sperm antibodies as a consequence of vasectomy. I. Within 1 year post-operation. Clin Exp Immunol 31:18–29, 1978.

118. Wang C, Baker HWG, Jennings MG, et al: Interaction between human cervical mucus and sperm surface antibodies. Fertil Steril 44:484–488, 1985.

119. Isojima S, Kameda K, Tsuji Y, et al: Establishment and characterization of a human hybridoma secreting monoclonal antibody with high titres of sperm-immobilizing and agglutinating activities against human seminal plasma. J Reprod Immunol 10:67–78, 1987.

120. Rumke P, Van Amstel N, Messer EN, Bezemer PD: Prognosis of fertility of men with spermagglutinins in the semen. Fertil Steril 25:393–398, 1974.

121. Alert J: Nontraumatic avascular necrosis of the femoral head. Clin Orthop 277:12–21, 1992.

122. Hendry WF, Hughes L, Scammell G, et al: Comparison of prednisolone and placebo in subfertile men with antibodies to spermatozoa. Lancet 335:85–88, 1990.

123. Bals-Pratsch M, Doren M, Karbowski B, et al: Cyclic corticosteroid immunosuppression is unsuccessful in the treatment of sperm antibody-related male infertility: A controlled study. Hum Reprod 7:99–104, 1992.

124. Clarke GN, Lopata A, McBain JC, et al: Effect of sperm antibodies in males on human in vitro fertilization (IVF). Am J Reprod Immunol Microbiol 8:62–66, 1985.

125. Bouloux PMG, Wass JAH, Parslow JM, et al: Effect of cyclosporin A in male autoimmune infertility. Fertil Steril 46:81–85, 1986.

126. Luisi M, Gasperi M, Franchi F, et al: Levamisole treatment in male infertility due to spermagglutinins. Lancet 20:47, 1982.

127. Liu DY, Cooper EJ, Baker HWG: Seminal transferrin, an index of Sertoli cell function: Is it of clinical value? Clin Reprod Fert 4:191–197, 1986.

128. O'Bryan MK, Baker HWG, Saunders JR, et al: Human seminal clusterin (SP-40,40). Isolation and characterization. J Clin Invest 85:1477–1486, 1990.

129. Jarow JP, Budin RE, Dym M, et al: Quantitative pathologic changes in the human testis after vasectomy. A controlled study. N Engl J Med 313:1252–1256, 1985.

130. Southwick GJ, Temple-Smith PD: Epididymal microsurgery: Current techniques and new horizons. Microsurgery 9:266–277, 1988.

131. Baker HWG: Requirements for controlled therapeutic trials in male infertility. Clin Reprod Fertil 4:13–25, 1986.

132. Silber SJ: Results of microsurgical vasoepididymostomy: Role of epididymis in sperm maturation. Hum Reprod 4:298–303, 1989.

133. Schoysman RJ, Bedford JM: The role of the human epididymis in sperm maturation and sperm storage as reflected in the consequence of epididymovasostomy. Fertil Steril 46:293–299, 1986.

134. Pryor JP, Hendry WF: Ejaculatory duct obstruction in subfertile males: Analysis of 87 patients. Fertil Steril 56:725–730, 1991.

135. Silber SJ, Ord T, Balmaceda J, et al: Congenital absence of the vas deferens. The fertilizing capacity of human epididymal sperm. N Engl J Med 323:1788–1792, 1990.

136. Turner TT: On the development and use of alloplastic spermatoceles. Fertil Steril 49:387–395, 1988.

137. Micic S, Papic N, Mladenovic I, et al: Intrauterine insemination with spermatozoa recovered from the aspirate of artificial spermatocele. Hum Reprod 5:582–585, 1990.

138. Goldstein M: Surgery of male infertility and other scrotal conditions. In Campbell's Textbook of Urology (ed 6). Philadelphia, WB Saunders Co, 1992, pp 3114–3149.

138a. Palermo G, Joris H, Devroey P, Van Steirteghem AC: Pregnancies after intracytoplasmic injection of single spermatozoon into an oocyte. Lancet 340:17–18, 1992.

139. Wheeler JS Jr, Walter JS, Culkin DJ, Canning JR: Idiopathic anejaculation treated by vibratory stimulation. Fertil Steril 50:377–379, 1988.

140. Bennett CJ, Ayers JWT, Randolf JF, et al: Electroejaculation of paraplegic males followed by pregnancies. Fertil Steril 48:1070–1072, 1987.

141. Andaloro VA, Dube A: Treatment of retrograde ejaculation with brompheniramine. Urology 5:520–522, 1975.

142. Randolph JF Jr, Ohl DA, Bennett CJ, et al: Combined electroejaculation and in vitro fertilization in the evaluation and treatment of anejaculatory infertility. J In Vitro Fert Embryo Transfer 7:58–62, 1990.

143. Mahadevan M, Leeton JF, Trounson AO: Noninvasive method of semen collection for successful artificial insemination in a case of retrograde ejaculation. Fertil Steril 36:243–247, 1981.

144. Kerin JFP, Peak J, Warnes GM, et al: Improved conception rate after intrauterine insemination of washed spermatozoa from men with poor quality semen. Lancet 1:533–535, 1984.

145. Melis GB, Paoletti AM, Strigini F, et al: Pharmacologic induction of multiple follicular development improves the success rate of artificial insemination with husband's semen in couples with male-related or unexplained infertility. Fertil Steril 47:441–445, 1987.

146. Sunde A, Kahn JA, Molne K: Intrauterine insemination: A European collaborative report. Hum Reprod (Suppl) 2:69–73, 1988.

147. Friedman A, Haas S, Kredentser J, et al: A controlled trial of intrauterine insemination for cervical factor and male factor: A preliminary report. Int J Fertil 34:199–203, 1989.

148. Comhaire FH, Verschraegen G, Vermeulen L: Diagnosis of accessory gland infection and its possible role in male infertility. Int J Androl 3:32–45, 1980.

149. Comhaire FH, Rowe PJ, Farley TM: The effect of doxycycline in infertile couples with male accessory gland infection: A double blind prospective study. Int J Androl 9:91–98, 1986.

150. Nagler HM, Zippe CD: Varicocele: Current concepts and treatment. In Lipshultz LI, Howards SS (eds): Infertility in Men. St Louis, CV Mosby–Year Book, 1991, pp 313–336.

151. Ayodeji O, Baker HWG: Is there a specific abnormality of sperm morphology in men with varicoceles? Fertil Steril 45:839–842, 1986.

152. Naftulin BN, Samuels SJ, Hellstrom WJ, et al: Semen quality in varicocele patients is characterized by tapered sperm cells. Fertil Steril 56:149–151, 1991.

152a. Hendry WF: Effects of left varicocele ligation in subfertile males with absent or atrophic right testes. Fertil Steril 57:1342–1343, 1992.

153. Matsuda T, Horii Y, Higashi S, Oishi K, et al: Laparoscopic varicocelectomy: A simple technique for clip ligation of the spermatic vessels. J Urol 147:636–638, 1992.

154. Demas BE, Hricak H, McClure RD: Varicoceles. Radiologic diagnosis and treatment. Radiol Clin North Am 29:619–627, 1991.

155. Baker HWG, Kovacs GT: Spontaneous improvement in semen quality: Regression towards the mean. Int J Androl 8:421–426, 1985.

156. Madgar I, Lunenfeld B, Weissenberg R, Goldwasser B: Controlled trial of high spermatic vein ligation for varicocele in infertile men. Am Urol Assn. Abs 115, 1991.

157. Billings EL, Billings JJ, Brown JB, Burger HG: Symptoms and hormonal changes accompanying ovulation. Lancet 1:282–284, 1972.

158. Smith KD, Rodriguez-Rigau LJ, Steinberger E: Relation between indices of semen analysis and pregnancy rate in infertile couples. Fertil Steril 28:1314–1319, 1977.

159. Dunphy BC, Kay R, Barratt CL, Cooke ID: Female age, the length of involuntary infertility prior to investigation and fertility outcome. Hum Reprod 4:527–30, 1989.

160. Silber SJ: The relationship of abnormal semen parameters to male fertility. Hum Reprod 4:947–953, 1989.

161. Bostofte E, Bagger P, Michael A, Stakemann G: Fertility prognosis for infertile men: Results of follow-up study of semen analysis in infertile men from two different populations evaluated by the Cox regression model. Fertil Steril 54:1100–1106, 1990.

161a. Bents H. Psychology of male infertility—a literature survey. Int J Androl 8:325–336, 1985.

162. Berg BJ, Wilson JF: Psychiatric morbidity in the infertile population: A reconceptualization. Fertil Steril 53:654–661, 1990.

163. Harrison KL, Callan VJ, Hennessey JF: Stress and semen quality in an in vitro fertilization program. Fertil Steril 48:633–636, 1987.

164. World Health Organization Task Force on the Diagnosis and Treatment of Infertility: Mesterolone and idiopathic male infertility: A double-blind study. Int J Androl 12:254–264, 1989.

165. Comhaire F: Treatment of idiopathic testicular failure with high-dose testosterone undecanoate: A double-blind pilot study. Fertil Steril 54:689–693, 1990.

166. Brown P, Preece MA, Wigg RG: "Friendly fire" in medicine: Hormones, homografts and Creutzfeld-Jacob disease. Lancet 340:24–27, 1992.

167. Mahadevan MM, Trounson AO: The influences of seminal characteristics on the success rate of human in vitro fertilization. Fertil Steril 42:400–405, 1984.

168. Cohen J, Fehilly CB, Fishel SB, et al: Male infertility successfully treated by in vitro fertilisation. Lancet 1:1239–1240, 1984.

169. de Kretser DM, Yates C, Kovacs GT: The use of IVF in the management of male infertility. Clin Obstet Gynaecol 4:767, 1985.

170. Acosta AA, Chillik CF, Brugo S, et al: In vitro fertilization and the male factor. Urology 28:1–9, 1986.

171. Yanagimachi R, Yanagimachi H, Rogers BJ: The use of the zona free animal ova as a test system for the assessment of fertilising capacity of human spermatozoa. Biol Reprod 15:471–476, 1976.

172. Tanbo T, Dale PO, Abyholm T: Assisted fertilization in infertile women with patent fallopian tubes. A comparison of in-vitro fertilization, gamete intra-fallopian transfer and tubal embryo stage transfer. Hum Reprod 5:266–270, 1990.

173. Tournaye H, Camus M, Khan I, et al: In-vitro fertilization, gamete or zygote intra-fallopian transfer for the treatment of male infertility. Hum Reprod 6:263–266, 1991.

174. Jansen RP, Anderson JC: Catheterization of the fallopian tubes from the vagina. Lancet 2:309–310, 1987.

175. Ng FLH, Liu DY, Baker HWG: Comparison of Percoll, mini-Percoll and swim-up methods for sperm preparation from abnormal semen samples. Hum Reprod 7:261–266, 1992.

176. Yovich JM, Edirisinghe WR, Cummins JM, Yovich JL: Preliminary results using pentoxifylline in a pronuclear stage tubal transfer (PROST) programme for severe male factor infertility. Fertil Steril 50:179–181, 1988.

176a. Tournaye H, Janssens R, Camus M, et al: Pentoxifylline is not useful in enhancing sperm function in cases with previous in vitro fertilization failure. Fertil Steril 59:210–215, 1993.

177. Burkman LJ, Coddington CC, Franken DR, et al: The hemizona assay (HZA): Development of a diagnostic test for the binding of human spermatozoa to the human hemizona pellucida to predict fertilization potential. Fertil Steril 49:688–697, 1988.

178. Acosta AA, Oehninger S, Ertunc H, Philput C: Possible role of pure human follicle-stimulating hormone in the treatment of severe male-factor infertility by assisted reproduction: Preliminary report. Fertil Steril 55:1150–1156, 1991.

179. Cohen J, Alikani M, Trowbridge J, Rosenwaks Z: Implantation enhancement by selective assisted hatching using zona drilling of human embryos with poor prognosis. Hum Reprod 7:685–691, 1992.

180. AIHW National Perinatal Statistics Unit and Fertility Society of Australia: Assisted Conception. Australia and New Zealand 1990. Sydney, 1992.

181. Kovacs GT, Rogers P, Leeton JF, et al: In-vitro fertilization and embryo transfer. Prospects of pregnancy by life-table analysis. Med J Aust 144:682–683, 1986.

182. Ben-Rafael Z, Kopf GS, Blasco L, et al: Fertilization and cleavage after reinsemination of human oocytes in vitro. Fertil Steril 45:58–62, 1986.

183. Laws-King A, Trounson A, Sathananthan H, Kola I: Fertilization of human oocytes by microinjection of a single spermatozoon under the zona pellucida. Fertil Steril 48:637–642, 1987.

184. Gordon JW, Grunfeld L, Garrisi GJ, et al: Fertilization of human oocytes by sperm from infertile males after zona pellucida drilling. Fertil Steril 50:68–73, 1988.

185. Ng SC, Bongso A, Chang SI, et al: Transfer of human sperm into the perivitelline space of human oocytes after zona-drilling or zona-puncture. Fertil Steril 52:73–78, 1989.

186. Payne D, McLaughlin KJ, Depypere HT, et al: Experience with zona drilling and zona cutting to improve fertilization rates of human oocytes in vitro. Hum Reprod 6:423–431, 1991.

187. Cohen J, Alikani M, Malter HE, et al: Partial zona dissection or subzonal sperm insertion: Microsurgical fertilization alternatives based on evaluation of sperm and embryo morphology. Fertil Steril 56:696–706, 1991.

188. Fishel S, Timson J, Lisi F, Rinaldi L: Evaluation of 225 patients undergoing subzonal insemination for the procurement of fertilization in vitro. Fertil Steril 57:840–849, 1992.

189. Tadir Y, Wright WH, Vafa O, et al: Micromanipulation of sperm by a laser generated optical trap. Fertil Steril 52:870–873, 1989.

190. Palanker D, Ohad S, Lewis A, et al: Technique for cellular microsurgery using the 193-nm excimer laser. Lasers Surg Med 11:580–586, 1991.

191. Wood C, Leeton J, Kovacs G: Artificial Insemination by Donor. Melbourne, Brown Prior Anderson, 1980.

192. Yavetz H, Yogev L, Homonnai Z, Paz G: Prerequisites for successful

human sperm cryobanking: Sperm quality and prefreezing holding time. Fertil Steril 55:812–816, 1991.

193. McGowan MP, Baker HWG, Kovacs GT, Rennie GC: Selection of high fertility donors for artificial insemination programmes. Clin Reprod Fertil 2:269–274, 1983.

194. Peek JC, Godfrey B, Matthews CD: Estimation of fertility and fecundity in women receiving artificial insemination by donor semen and in normal fertile women. Br J Obstet Gynaecol 91:1019–1024, 1984.

195. Le Lannou D, Lansac J: Artificial procreation with frozen donor semen: Experience of the French Federation CECOS. Hum Reprod 4:757–761, 1989.

196. Amuzu B, Laxova R, Shapiro SS: Pregnancy outcome, health of children, and family adjustment after donor insemination. Obstet Gynecol 75:899–905, 1990.

197. Chauhan M, Barratt CL, Cooke SM, Cooke ID: Differences in the fertility of donor insemination recipients—a study to provide prognostic guidelines as to its success and outcome. Fertil Steril 51:815–819, 1989.

198. Kovacs GT, Baker HWG, Vaux HA: The outcome of AID in initial and subsequent courses of treatment. Clin Reprod Fertil 2:295–298, 1983.

199. Vekemans M, Englert Y, Camus M, de Maertelaer G: In-vitro fertilization with donor sperm after failure of artificial insemination. Hum Reprod 2:121–125, 1987.

199a. Kovacs GT, Mushin D, Kane H, Baker HWG: A controlled study of the psycho-social development of children conceived following insemination with donor sperm. Hum Reprod 8:788–790, 1993.

200. Soules MR: Prevention of infertility. Fertil Steril 49:582–584, 1988.

201. Sayfan J, Soffer Y, Manor H, et al: Varicocele in youth. A therapeutic dilemma. Ann Surg 207:223–227, 1988.

202. Steeno OP: Varicocele in the adolescent. Adv Exp Med Biol 286:295–321, 1991.

203. Fossa SD, Aass N, Molne K: Is routine pre-treatment cryopreservation of semen worthwhile in the management of patients with testicular cancer? Br J Urol 64:524–529, 1989.

135

Male Impotence

STANLEY G. KORENMAN

CLINICAL EPIDEMIOLOGY

The loss of erectile capacity has a debilitating psychological effect on many men that permeates their entire lives. If impotence is associated with a divorce or loss of a spouse, then the man may experience social isolation, with its attendant ills. As a result of public attention to research developments and new treatments, patients have learned to request help from their physicians. Since the most common pathophysiological bases for impotence include chronic conditions managed by internists, impotence assessment and treatment ideally should fall within the territory of internal medicine.

Definitions

From the patient's perspective, impotence may be defined as the inability to perform sexually at the expected level. From the clinical standpoint, impotence may be defined as the inability to obtain or sustain an erection satisfactory for sexual intercourse on more than 50 per cent of coital attempts or cessation of coital effort because of erectile failure. Sexual complaints not normally included in the clinical definition of impotence include a loss of erectile rigidity intravaginally and early or premature ejaculation. However, these symptoms often precede fully developed impotence and may be treated similarly. Other sexual dysfunctions, including reduced libido, ejaculatory disturbances, diminished orgasmic sensation, and infertility, may accompany impotence.

Epidemiology

Although the varied and complex definitions of impotence pose problems for epidemiologists, every carefully performed study reports a substantial prevalence of impotence in the United States. The most commonly quoted number is 10 million men, or 9 per cent of the adult male population.[1] In a recent study, 51 per cent of a community-based group of men ages 40 to 70 reported a degree of erectile dysfunction as estimated on a four-level scale, extrapolating to 30 million men so affected.[2] In young couples, the prevalence of impotence was about 7 per cent.[3, 4] More than one third of older men receiving medical treatment admitted to impotence.[5, 6]

Risk Factors

The traditional description of erectile dysfunction into predominantly organic and psychogenic varieties has given way to a risk-factor approach in which a number of etiologic contributions play roles. The relative prevalence of organic and psychogenic erectile dysfunction depends on whether the condition is primary or secondary, the average age of the patients, and in published series, the referral patterns to the authors. The changing face of medicine has brought new cases of organic impotence to therapy, including patients with heart, liver, and kidney transplants, survivors of extensive pelvic surgery and irradiation, patients rendered hypogonadal in the course of treatment, and those receiving large doses of potent cardiovascular agents. Furthermore, a significant number of men with putative psychogenic impotence on further analysis have organic risk factors.

A number of conditions have been associated with the development of impotence. Unfortunately, there have been very few studies involving age-matched control groups designed to distinguish the impact of disease versus that of age or of medications. An increased prevalence of impotence has been proposed for the conditions and drug categories found in Table 135–1, which was derived from a more detailed analysis.[7] Clinical conditions found in patients presenting with impotence in medical groups are noted in Table 135–2, which was derived from data also used in part elsewhere.[7] From these analyses one could infer that the likelihood of impotence would increase, for example, with the number of risk factors, including complications of atherosclerosis, hypertension, diabetes mellitus, depression, hypogonadism, and cardiovascular drug

TABLE 135–1. Conditions Reported to Have an Increased Prevalence of Impotence

Primarily a Vascular Pathophysiology
Diabetes mellitus
Myocardial infarction
Occlusive vascular disease, even after surgery
Hypertension
Scleroderma
Primarily a Neurologic Pathophysiology
Multiple sclerosis
Stroke
Spinal cord injury
Epilepsy, especially temporal lobe
Primarily Disruption of Local Anatomy Due to Surgery
Radical prostatectomy and cystoprostatectomy
Abdominoperineal colon resection
Transurethral prostate resection
Endocrine-Related
Hypogonadism due to pituitary or testicular disease
Graves' disease
Hypothyroidism
Hemochromatosis
Uremia on dialysis
Acromegaly and prolactinoma
Other
Obstructive and restrictive pulmonary disease
Depression
Categories of Drugs and Medications
Substances of abuse, including ethanol, nicotine, cocaine, heroin
Cardiovascular and antihypertensive drugs, including beta and alpha adrenergic blockers
Antipsychotics and antidepressants
Antiandrogens and estrogens including H_2 blockers, ketoconazole, griseofulvin

intake, but such prevalence rates have not been established.

PHYSIOLOGY AND PATHOPHYSIOLOGY

Normal Erectile Mechanism

An erection results from markedly enhanced inflow of blood to the sinusoids of the corpora cavernosa under conditions of severe penile venous outflow restriction. The corpora cavernosa expand against the unyielding tunica albuginea, resulting in increased tension and penile rigidity.

The neuroanatomy of erection, while subject to a recent

TABLE 135–2. Clinical Characteristics of Patients Presenting with Impotence

Number	301
Mean impotence duration, years	4.8
Hypertension	45.8%
Diabetes mellitus	30.0%
Atherosclerosis	33.6%
Myocardial infarction	16.3%
Stroke	9.6%
Obstructive vascular disease	7.0%
Angina	9.6%
Coronary artery bypass graft	5.3%
Transurethral prostate resection	16.9%
Arthritis	22.2%
Current smoking	39.0%
Significant alcohol intake	51.0%

in-depth review by Steers,[8] still eludes complete characterization. Nocturnal erections (nocturnal penile tumescence, NPT) take place four to eight times, usually during the rapid eye movement (REM) phase of sleep. Erotically induced erections result from external (visual, tactile, auditory, olfactory) or internal (fantasy) stimuli. The processed sensory inputs undergo integration in the medial preoptic–anterior hypothalamus. This area has projections to the spinal cord employing peptidergic and catecholaminergic neurons that control the thoracolumbar sympathetic and sacral parasympathetic erection centers to control the erectile reflex. Genital manipulation also may mediate erection through stimulating pudendal sensory neurons that activate the spinal erection center.

The autonomic nervous system regulates the erectile state of the penis through control of the vascular and sinusoidal smooth muscle.[8] Alpha-adrenergic nerves contained in the pelvic plexus maintain tonic cavernosal artery and sinusoidal vasoconstriction. Erection follows reduction of vasoconstrictor impulses and activation of the vasodilator nerves of the pelvic parasympathetic plexus. The postganglionic fibers of the cavernosal nerve are neither adrenergic nor cholinergic (NANC). They mediate smooth-muscle relaxation by generating nitric oxide (NO) as their neurotransmitter.[9–11] NO activates guanylyl cyclase, increases cyclic GMP (Fig. 135–1), and reduces Ca^{2+} access to myofibrillar proteins, mediating relaxation. Cyclic GMP-dependent protein kinase also inhibits myosin light chain kinase.

Smooth-muscle relaxation decreases arterial and sinusoidal trabecular resistance and permits blood flow through the cavernosal and helicine arteries at a greatly accelerated rate, filling the lacunar spaces with blood until sinusoidal pressure equals systemic pressure (Fig. 135–2). At that point, blood flow diminishes to very low levels. The long-standing issue of how venous return was impeded in the erect penis was finally elucidated by Lue and colleagues[13, 14] in careful anatomical and electron microscopic investigations of the flaccid and erect penis that demonstrated how sinusoidal expansion itself was responsible for venous occlusion (the corporal veno-occlusive mechanism). Each cavernosal sinusoid is drained by a venule that joins others forming a subtunical venous complex. These coalesce in emissary veins that traverse the tunica albuginea at an angle. During erection, filling of the trabecular sinusoids with

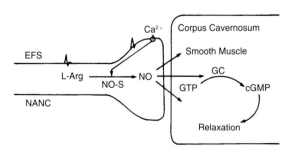

FIGURE 135–1. The role of nitric oxide (NO) as a mediator of penile erection. Electrical field stimulation (EFS) of NANC (nonadrenergic, noncholinergic) neurons triggers an influx of Ca^{2+} that activates NO synthase (NO-S) and stimulates the conversion of L-arginine (L-Arg) to NO. NO is the NANC neurotransmitter that diffuses into cavernosal vascular and sinusoidal smooth-muscle cells and activates guanylate cyclase (GC), thereby stimulating the conversion of GTP to cGMP. cGMP then causes smooth-muscle relaxation.

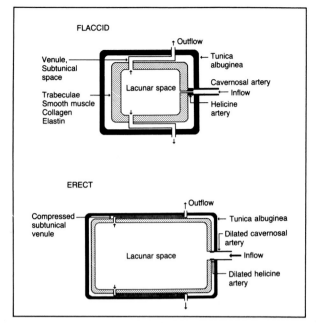

FIGURE 135–2. Mechanism of penile erection. The numerous interconnected lacunar spaces of the corpora cavernosa are represented as a single space with the trabeculae making up its wall. In the flaccid state (*upper panel*), helicine artery and cavernosal artery resistance minimize corporal blood flow, and venous drainage is prompt. In the erect state (*lower panel*), arterial and sinusoidal smooth-muscle relaxation increases arterial flow, expanding the sinusoids against the unyielding tunical wall. Compression of the subtunical venous plexus inhibits cavernosal drainage, resulting in a high intracavernosal pressure and little blood flow.

blood causes compression of the subtunical plexus and the emissary veins against the unyielding tunica, markedly reducing venous drainage.

The endocrine system plays an indirect role in erection. Androgens stimulate libido at the level of the central nervous system. They are necessary for development of the male genital structures and secretory capacity of the prostate and seminal vesicle. They also are responsible for the size and strength of the ischiocavernosus and bulbospongiosus muscles[15] in preference to other muscles. Thus the hypogonadal male usually demonstrates little interest in sex,[16] a decline in NPT, and reduced semen volume. Androgen therapy reverses these declines. However, many men castrated as adults retain erectile capacity to erotic stimuli,[16] as do hypogonadal patients withdrawn from androgens.[17] A causal relationship between impotence and hypogonadism has been impossible to establish in most cases. In fact, they appear to be independently segregating common problems of older men. Since orgasmic sensation depends on ejaculate volume, sexual pleasure depends to a degree on adequate androgen action.

Mechanisms of Erectile Dysfunction

Elucidation of the abnormalities of the erectile process associated with organic impotence depends on studies of the arterial and venous system, the nerves serving the penis, and the intrinsic structures of the corpora cavernosa. Ultrastructural examination of cavernosal tissue from impotent men demonstrated variable and focal losses of sinusoidal endothelium, degeneration of smooth muscle, an

increase of intersinusoidal collagen, and loss of neuronal bundles[18–23] in comparison with control tissue. These findings were interpreted as ischemic changes independent of the penile insult. Some reports relate the degree of smooth muscle cell damage and perisinusoidal fibrosis to the clinical severity of vascular disease as defined by the erectile response to intracavernosal vasodilator administration (see below). Subjects developing impotence from penile surgery or spinal cord injury showed corporal nerve degeneration and relatively little ischemic injury.

Arterial obstructive lesions compromising the inflow rate of blood to the corpora cavernosa have been implicated as major causes of impotence. However, neither prepenile nor severe cavernosal arterial disease are commonly seen in arteriogenic impotence, and some impotent patients have completely normal macrovascular systems.[24]

Impotent men frequently demonstrate a failure to inhibit penile venous return adequately during vasodilator-induced erections—a "venous leak." In a few instances, grossly anomalous venous flow identifies a treatable lesion whose repair results in restoration of erectile function. Most commonly, venous occlusion defects are multiple,[25] and cavernosography reveals normal venous anatomy.

However, in dogs, a small reduction of arterial inflow reduced cavernosal pressure and erectile rigidity disproportionately in the presence of a small amount of venous leakage.[26] Based on ultrastructural studies, other likely causes of veno-occlusive failure include impaired emissary vein occlusion caused by perisinusoidal fibrosis and inhibited sinusoidal filling caused by arteriolar damage. Endothelial lesions and neuronal loss may inhibit full sinusoidal and arterial vasodilatation due to reduced NO production.

The extent to which abnormal sympathetic or parasympathetic activity plays a primary role in the pathogenesis of erectile dysfunction remains unknown. One problem is that diagnostic testing for neurogenic factors fails to test the nerves stimulating or inhibiting vasodilatation in the corpora cavernosa. Alpha-adrenergic activation, however, has been implicated as an inhibitor of erection.[27]

This new understanding of the pathophysiology of impotence based on ultrastructural studies focuses attention on the structures of the penis itself and their responses to age, ischemia, and clinical conditions. It provides a rationale for the lack of effectiveness of arterial revascularization and venous ligation procedures and raises doubts as to their theoretical utility.

DIAGNOSTIC EVALUATION

The diagnostic assessment of impotence depends on a careful determination by history of the type and extent of sexual dysfunction. Cost-effective evaluation for hypogonadism should be carried out. Further assessment depends on the therapies the patient is willing to accept.

The sexual history remains the most important diagnostic tool. The physician should determine whether the problem is primary or secondary. Is the dysfunction a failure of erection? Is it persistent or intermittent, progressive or constant? Did it develop in conjunction with a medical or surgical event, with initiation of a medication, or in association with substance abuse? Has there been an associated loss of sexual interest, energy, feeling of well-being, or loss of muscle strength? To what extent has the sexual dysfunction affected the patient's relationships or been affected by them? Is he preoccupied with the problem? What therapeutic goals does the patient have, how sound are they, and what interventions is he willing to undergo to achieve them? Useful additional information includes whether there have been any changes in personal and social situation, penile sensation, ejaculate volume, and perceived health, energy, and mood. The author finds it important to assess the health, well-being, and sexual interest of the partner and the sexual repertoire of the couple. Assessing the risk factors for impotence requires a complete medical history and general medical evaluation as well as a complete history of substance intake.

The physical examination contributes to the assessment by verifying impotence risk factors and the presence of a peripheral neuropathy, documenting testicular atrophy, and determining whether depression or another psychiatric disorder accompanies the sexual dysfunction. It is also important to determine whether the fibrotic penile plaques of Peyronie's disease are present and their extent.

The general laboratory assessment should include a recent hemogram or hematocrit to identify the presence of anemia, chemistries to determine whether unexpected diabetes, renal insufficiency or liver disease is present, and a lipid profile to assess cardiovascular risk. Endocrine studies should include an ultrasensitive thyroid-stimulating hormone (TSH) test because both hypo- and hyperthyroidism have been associated with impotence.

Assessment of Hypogonadism

Depending on the definition, hypogonadism and impotence are two common conditions of the older man that may occur independently or together.[28] It is now accepted that low serum testosterone levels in aging men are rarely associated with luteinizing hormone (LH) values above the upper limit of normal[28–30] and that declines in both pituitary and testicular function commonly occur with aging. Increased testosterone binding to sex hormone–binding globulin (SHBG) commonly plays an important role in the changes in androgen availability to tissues with aging. Therefore, the author measures the non–SHBG-bound, bioavailable testosterone in all impotent patients. The author defines hypogondism as a level of bioavailable testosterone (BT) below 2.5 SD of the mean for younger men (<2.3 nM), regardless of the level of LH or follicle-stimulating hormone (FSH), reasoning that the tissues of older men cannot be expected to require less testosterone than the tissues of younger men. If the value is below normal, serum prolactin and LH determinations are obtained.

Specific diagnostic tests for impotence have evolved in the past 5 years as more knowledge has been gained as to its pathogenesis. Tests have been developed to distinguish "organic" from "psychogenic" impotence, to examine the state of the vessels supplying and draining the penis, and to characterize surgically treatable lesions.

Tests to Distinguish Functional from Organic Impotence

This group of examinations purports to distinguish organic from psychogenic impotence by assessment of nocturnal penile tumescence (NPT), which putatively is not subject to psychogenic inhibition.[31] In the stamp test and the snap gauge (Dacomed) tests, the flaccid penis has a ring placed around it at bedtime. A broken ring in the morning indicates NPT. More sophisticated and much more costly methods of measuring NPT include use of continuous monitoring of penile circumference in a sleep laboratory and use of the Rigiscan device that permits assessment of NPT at home. These procedures monitor the number of NPT episodes and the degree of penile engorgement and erectile rigidity. Recent evidence that the patient's history of nocturnal and morning erections corresponds well to NPT[32] supports the author's decision *not* to use these tests but rather to depend on the patient's history.

Tests of Vascular Integrity

Evidence of impairment of blood flow into the penis or of a venous leak strongly supports the diagnosis of vascular impotence, assists in establishing a dose for diagnostic intracavernosal vasodilator injections, and aids in therapeutic decision making. No standard algorithm for diagnostic assessment of the vascular state in impotence has been established to date.[33] Simple, relatively noninvasive tests, including the penile-brachial pressure index or duplex scanning of the penile vessels and diagnostic intracavernosal vasodilator injections, serve to make a diagnosis of vascular impotence in most cases.

THE PENILE-BRACHIAL PRESSURE INDEX (PBPI). This index is the ratio between the brachial and the penile systolic blood pressures as measured by a hand-held Doppler instrument utilizing a neonatal blood pressure cuff. With the patient supine, we measure pressures bilaterally on the lateral aspect of the flaccid penis before and after 2 minutes (if possible) of bicycling exercise, obtaining four ratios. An abnormal result is defined as any value below 0.65 or a mean fall between supine and exercise 0.15 or more. Mean values between 0.65 and 0.75 are considered indeterminate. Criticisms of this test include that it may measure pressures in the wrong arteries, that it utilizes only the flaccid penis, and that it does not correlate well with duplex scanning or other vascular study results.[34, 35] The critics never did testing after exercise, which adds 23 per cent to the abnormal values.[37] The author and colleagues have demonstrated that an abnormal PBPI relates well to future cardiovascular events,[38] that it predicts an abnormal exercise stress test,[39] that it is reproducible,[40] and that it improves with interventions that improve impotence.[40, 41]

DUPLEX ULTRASONOGRAPHY. Duplex ultrasonography examines peak systolic cavernosal arterial flow and the diameter of the cavernosal arteries with the penis both in the flaccid state and during erection induced by an intracavernosal vasodilator.[42] Veno-occlusive insufficiency also may be examined.[43] Lue et al.[42] reported their experience with duplex sonography in 687 patients. Forty-three per cent of the patients had both arterial and venous components of impotence, 32 per cent were predominantly arteriogenic, 15 per cent were predominantly venogenic, 4 per cent were neurogenic, 3 per cent were psychogenic, and 3 per cent had other causes. Corporal vasodilatation produced fully normal erections only in the neurogenic and psychogenic cases, and self-stimulation in privacy improved the quality of the induced erections. The authors recommended cavernosography and cavernosometry only for those subjects exhibiting predominantly venogenic impotence. This procedure effectively identifies vascular causes for impotence but does not assess pelvic steal.

DIAGNOSTIC INTRACAVERNOSAL VASODILATOR INJECTION. The author employs intracavernosal vasodilator injection to determine whether venogenic impotence predominates, to assess the potential of a therapeutic trial of intracavernosal therapy, and to demonstrate the procedure to assist the patient in his decision making. The author employs a mixture of prostaglandin E$_1$ (PGE$_1$) and phentolamine (500 mg PGE$_1$ and 15 mg phentolamine in 30 ml normal saline) and administers between 0.3 and 0.6 ml of solution using an insulin syringe with a no. 29 half-inch needle. The penis is massaged for 1 minute after injection to distribute the solution. The patients undertake self-stimulation 5 minutes after injection, and the degree of tumescence is recorded at 10 minutes. Subjects with an abnormal PBPI receive the full dose, and those with a normal PBPI, especially younger men, those with type I diabetes mellitus, and others with presumptive neurogenic impotence receive 0.4 ml or less. The author records the quality of erection (0 = no erection, 1 = slight tumescence, 2 = incomplete erection, 3 = complete erection with no rigidity, 4 = incomplete rigidity but usable erection, 5 = full erection) as well as the presence of any abnormal or unpleasant penile sensations. Sustained tumescence implies that the predominant lesion is not impaired corporal veno-occlusion. The degree of erectile response serves as a predictor of responsiveness to vasodilator therapy. The author's complications were two cases, about 1 per cent, of prolonged erection requiring detumescence in patients with type I diabetes receiving 1.0 ml of solution and penile burning discomfort in about 20 per cent of patients.

INVASIVE DIAGNOSTIC TESTS. Angiography, venography, and cavernosography have clinical merit if the patient is willing to undergo corrective surgery should a treatable lesion be found and if a predominantly venogenic or large-artery lesion is suspected.

TREATMENT

Therapy for impotence should not only address the restoration of erectile function but also should be directed at the risk factors leading to the impotence and toward restoration of the relationship of the couple.

Mechanical Devices

Through the ages, engineering talent has been applied toward the creation or maintenance of a usable erection. Recent attention to the problem has produced a number of effective devices to ameliorate partial or complete erectile failure. Veno-occlusive rings have been developed to sustain erections in men who obtain full but short-lived erections. They include the VED Softouch Constriction Seal, the Revive system, and the Stayerect system. In each case, application of a constricting band to the base of the penis using a rigid sleeve sustains a naturally obtained erection.

Patients with more severe impotence frequently benefit from use of a vacuum tumescence device. Two varieties are available. The most commonly employed systems, the Erecaid by Osbon; Response, Touch, and Piston, by Mentor; the Catalyst by Dacomed; and the VED by Mission, are similar in concept but differ in important details.[44, 45] In each case, the patient places a plastic cylinder over his penis tightly against the body, utilizing a water-soluble lubricant on the penis and cylinder to effect a good seal. A mechanical or electrical vacuum pump evacuates the cylinder, forcing blood into the penis. Upon achieving a full erection, the patient snaps an obstructive band which had been placed over the proximal portion of the cylinder onto the base of the penis, sustaining the erection. These devices produce a firm to rigid usable erection in about 90 per cent of cases,[41, 45] including patients with intact or explanted penile prostheses,[46, 47] and result in improved partner satisfaction.[48, 49] Vacuum tumescence devices may enhance erectile volume and occasionally cause improvement in spontaneous erections.[45] Disadvantages of the devices in a minority of patients[50] include pain or discomfort, retarded or absent ejaculation, inhibited penile circulation,[51] penile discoloration, a cool penis, and rarely, petechiae or hematoma. A second form of device, the Synergist Erection System, employs a thick, condom-like plastic sheath to which a vacuum can be applied utilizing mouth suction.[52] After lubrication, the device with the enclosed, distended penis may be inserted intravaginally. This device gives limited sexual satisfaction to the male partner and affords great protection against sexually transmitted diseases. Many patients for whom vacuum tumescence devices would successfully restore erectile function elect not to try them because they or their partners view the devices as unaesthetic or antiaphrodisiac, further supporting the view that the partner should play a decision-making role in impotence management.

Intracavernosal Injection

The therapeutic armamentarium for impotence grew dramatically with the introduction by Virag et al.[53] and Brindley[54] of intracavernosal pharmacotherapy. Although investigators employed a number of agents and mixtures, the greatest reported experience remains with papaverine alone or mixed with phentolamine or other agents. The Food and Drug Administration (FDA) has not approved any of these therapies, and patients should be so informed. Papaverine works as a combined cAMP and cGMP phosphodiesterase inhibitor, causing increases in cavernosal smooth-muscle cGMP (the effect of NO) and cAMP, prolonging beta-adrenergic relaxation. Phentolamine inhibits vasoconstrictor tone via blockade of alpha-adrenergic receptors. Self-injection with these agents produced good erections in about 70 per cent of patients with vascular impotence and in nearly 100 per cent of those with diagnoses of neurogenic or psychogenic impotence.[55] Intracavernosal papaverine caused priapism in up to 3 per cent of patients[56] but no more than 0.3 per cent of injections. Penile fibrotic nodules occur progressively more frequently with duration of therapy and frequency of use.[57] These complications led physicians to substitute prostaglandin E$_1$ (alprostadil) for papaverine when it was reported to be at least as effective[58] and to cause priapism much less frequently, but the data are not yet in. The author prescribes the same mixture for therapy as for diagnostic testing (see above) for interested patients who have not experienced significant penile pain with the diagnostic injection; 0.3 to 0.5 ml of vasodilator solution is prescribed for self-injection. Patients receive instruction to adjust the dose to produce an erection of about 1 hour in duration. In some cases, sensitization occurs and the dose may be reduced to as little as 0.1 ml.

Treatment of Hypogonadism

The author proposes a trial of testosterone enanthate or cypionate for 3 months for hypogonadal men with normal prostate-specific antigen (PSA) determinations and no significant obstructive uropathy. Oral androgens are avoided because of their hepatotoxicity. Concomitantly, a low-fat, high-fiber diet and regular aerobic exercise are recommended. At completion of the trial, changes in hematocrit, lipoprotein profile, and PSA, as well as the clinical state, are monitored. Partial restoration of erectile function may occur, but usually it is inadequate. The author's patients have not reported deterioration of urinary flow with androgen therapy. Long-term testosterone treatment is offered to those hypogonadal men demonstrating improvement in libido, well-being, or potency unless they show significant deterioration of their lipoprotein profile or PSA or an increase of their hematocrit to greater than 52 per cent. Before deciding to continue treatment, patients receive counseling as to the complications of androgen therapy, including erythremia, HDL cholesterol reduction, risk of prostatic growth, and possibly tumor promotion and as to the need for treatment directed at the impotence itself.

Penile Prostheses

Virtually every man can have erectile function restored with implantations of a penile prosthesis.[59–63] The author reserves these devices for patients who seek them or who fail with less invasive approaches to restoration of erectile function. Penile prostheses replace corpus cavernosa tissue with devices that are permanently rigid or are made rigid by the transfer of fluid from a reservoir or by manipulation of a racheting device. They require surgical implantation and are therefore quite expensive. They have undergone substantial technological improvement over the years. Unfortunately, there remain significant mechanical failure, infection, and explantation rates and the possible long-term consequences of a silicone foreign body. Penile implants should be avoided in patients with diabetes mellitus, who have an increased frequency of infection and explantation.

Arterial and Venous Surgery

Numerous ultimately disappointing attempts have been made to restore arterial flow to the penis by bypass operations or by anastomosing an artery to the dorsal vein of the penis, establishing reversal of flow. Venous insufficiency has appeared more amenable to therapy, but attempted repairs by surgical ligation or chemical ablation usually fail to restore sexual function over time. Explanations given for these failures include rapid regrowth of anomalously draining veins, failure to ablate all the offending veins, and undiagnosed arterial lesions.[25] However, our improved understanding of the pathophysiology of impotence, focusing on the intrinsic penile smooth-muscle lesion,[18–24] provides a rational basis for the expectations that surgery directed at large vessels will rarely resolve impotence.

Sex Therapy

Although other treatments have supplanted sex therapy for the majority of men experiencing erectile dysfunction, many opportunities remain to assist the dysfunctional couple in re-establishing a highly enjoyable sex life. Sex therapy focuses on sensitization of each member of the couple to the physical and emotional feelings of intimacy and of pleasuring each other.[64] It expands the sexual repertoire of the couple and redirects the focus of sexuality from simple penile-vaginal engagement. Sex therapy teaches couples about sex, and many couples, regardless of age, have much to learn about fulfilling sexuality. Therefore, couples who do not resume regular sexual activity after receiving effective treatment for erectile dysfunction should be offered sex therapy to help them re-establish intimacy.

Other Therapies

Several other agents have been proposed to help impotence. The most commonly employed is yohimbine (Yocon). This alpha$_2$-adrenergic blocking agent possesses both central and peripheral effects and was reintroduced to treat impotence and restore libido.[65] The same group subsequently found the agent no better than placebo,[66] but by then the agent was in widespread use.

Pentoxifylline (Trental) would be of theoretical benefit in that it should improve the fluidity of the blood and its ability to fill the corpora cavernosa. Two small studies revealed significant efficacy of the agent.[40, 67] Both the ability to consummate coitus and the level of the PBPI were significantly improved in half the patients in a double-blind, controlled study.[40] The drug had an expected onset of action of two to six weeks. Pentoxifylline requires further study, but it can be offered safely to those with mild to moderate vascular impotence. The author usually recommends a vacuum tumescence device at the same time, reasoning that when the man no longer needs the device, it can be stored and the patient may achieve immediate relief of his impotence. No other oral medications merit trial for the treatment of impotence despite enthusiastic endorsements.

REFERENCES

1. Krane RJ, Goldstein I, Saenz de Tejada I: Medical progress: Impotence. N Engl J Med 321:1648–1660, 1989.

2. Feldman H, Goldstein I, Krane RJ: Epidemiology of impotence in a community-based population. J Urol 147:238A, 1992.

3. Nettlebladt P, Uddenberg N: Sexual dysfunction and sexual satisfaction in 58 married Swedish men. J Psychom Res 23:141–147, 1979.

4. Frank E, Anderson C, Rubenstein D: Frequency of sexual dysfunction in normal couples. N Engl J Med 299:111–115, 1978.

5. Slag MF, Morley JE, Elson MK, et al: Impotence in medical clinic outpatients. JAMA 249:1736–1740, 1983.

6. Stanik-Davis S, Viosca SP, Guralnik M, et al: Evaluation of impotence in older men. West J Med 142:499–505, 1985.

7. Korenman SG: Sexual dysfunction. In Wilson JD, Foster DW (eds): Williams' Textbook of Endocrinology. Philadelphia, WB Saunders, 1990, pp 1033–1048.

8. Steers WD: Neural control of penile erection. Semin Urol 8:66–79, 1990.

9. Saenz de Tejada I, Goldstein I, Azadoi K, et al: Impaired neurogenic and endothelium-mediated relaxation of penile smooth muscle from diabetic men with impotence. N Engl J Med 320:1025–1030, 1989.

10. Rajfer J, Aronson WJ, Bush PA, et al: Nitric oxide as a mediator of relaxation of the corpus cavernosum in response to nonadrenergic, noncholinergic neurotransmission. N Engl J Med 326:90–94, 1992.

11. Ignarro LJ: Nitric oxide as the physiological mediator of penile erection. J NIH Res 4:59–62, 1992.

12. Burnett AL, Lowenstein CJ, Bredt DS, et al: Nitric oxide: A physiologic mediator of penile erection. Science 257:401–403, 1992.

13. Fournier GR, Juenemann KP, Lue TF, Tanagho EA: Mechanisms of venous occlusion during canine penile erection: An anatomic demonstration. J Urol 137:163–167, 1987.

14. Breza J, Aboseif SR, Orvis BR, et al: Detailed anatomy of penile neurovascular structures: Surgical significance. J Urol 141:437–443, 1989.

15. Mooradian AD, Morley JE, Korenman SG: Biological actions of androgens. Endocr Rev 8:1–28, 1987.

16. Bremer J: Asexualization: A Follow-Up Study of 244 Cases. Oslo, Norway, Oslo University Press, 1958.

17. Davidson JM, Camargo CA, Smith ER: Effects of androgen on sexual behavior in hypogonadal men. J Clin Endocrinol Metab 48:955–958, 1979.

18. Persson C, Diedrichs W, Lue TF, et al: Correlations of altered penile ultrastructure with clinical arterial evaluation. J Urol 142:1462–1468, 1989.

19. Junemann K-P, Persson-Junemann C, Alken P: Pathophysiology of erectile dysfunction. Semin Urol 8:80–93, 1990.

20. Mersdorf A, Goldsmith PC, Diedrichs W, et al: Ultrastructural changes in impotent penile tissue: A comparison of 65 patients. J Urol 145:749–758, 1991.

21. Wespes E, Goes PM, Schiffmann S, et al: Computerized analysis of smooth muscle fibers in potent and impotent patients. J Urol 146:1015–1017, 1991.

22. Jevtich MJ, Khawand NY, Vidic B: Clinical significance of ultrastructural findings in the corpora cavernosa of normal and impotent men. J Urol 143:289–293, 1991.

23. Vickers MA Jr, Seiler M, Weidner N: Corpora cavernosa ultrastructure in vascular erectile dysfunction. J Urol 143:1131–1134, 1990.

24. Bookstein JJ, Valji K: The arteriolar component in impotence: A possible paradigm shift. AJR 157:932–934, 1991.

25. Shabsigh R, Fishman IJ, Toombs BD, Skolkin M: Venous leaks: Anatomical and physiological observations. J Urol 146:1260–1265, 1991.

26. Aboseif SR, Wetterauer U, Breza J, et al: The effect of venous incompetence and arterial insufficiency on erectile function: An animal model. J Urol 144:790–793, 1990.

27. Diedrichs W, Stief CG, Benard F, et al: The sympathetic role as an antagonist of erection. Urol Res 19:123–126, 1991.

28. Korenman SG, Morley JE, Mooradian AD, et al: Secondary hypogonadism in older men: Its relation to impotence. J Clin Endocrinol Metab 71:763–769, 1990.

29. Vermeulen A, Kaaufman JM: Editorial: Role of the hypothalamo-pituitary function in the hypoandrogenism of healthy aging. J Clin Endocrinol Metab 75:704–706, 1992.

30. Tenover JS: Effects of testosterone supplementation in the aging male. J Clin Endocrinol Metab 75:1092–1098, 1992.

31. Karacan I: Diagnosis and treatment of erectile impotence. Psychiatr Clin North Am 3:97–111, 1980.

32. Ackerman MD, D'Attilio JD, Antoni MH, et al: The predictive significance of patient-reported sexual functioning in Rigiscan sleep evaluations. J Urol 146:1559–1563, 1991.

33. Seftel AD, Goldstein I: Editorial: Vascular testing for impotence. J Nucl Med 33:46, 1992.

34. Abber JC, Lue TF, Bradley R, et al: Diagnostic tests for impotence: A comparison of papaverine injection with the penile brachial pressure index and nocturnal penile tumescence. J Urol 135:923–926, 1986.

35. Aitchison M, Aitchison J, Carter R: Is the penile brachial pressure index a reproducible and useful measurement? Br J Urol 66:202–204, 1990.

36. Robinson LQ, Woodcock JP, Stephenson TP: Duplex scanning in suspected vasculogenic impotence: A worthwhile exercise? Br J Urol 63:432–436, 1989.

37. Kaiser FE, Viosca SP, Morley JE, et al: Impotence and aging: Clinical and hormonal factors. J Am Geriatr Soc 36:511–519, 1988.

38. Morley JE, Korenman SG, Kaiser FE, et al: Relationship of penile brachial pressure index to myocardial infarction and cerebrovascular accidents in older men. Am J Med 84:445–448, 1988.

39. Korenman SG, Udhoji V, Viosca SP: The relation between vascular impotence and cardiovascular ischemia. JAMA (in press).

40. Korenman SG, Viosca SP: Treatment of vasculogenic sexual dysfunction with pentoxifylline. J Am Geriatr Soc (in press).

41. Korenman SG, Viosca SP, Kaiser FE, et al: Use of a vacuum tumescence device in the management of impotence. J Am Geriatr Soc 38:217–220, 1990.

42. Lue TF, Mueller SC, Jow YR, Hwang TIS: Functional evaluation of penile arteries with duplex ultrasound in vasodilator-induced erection. Urol Clin North Am 16:799–807, 1989.

43. Bassiouny HS, Levine LA: Penile duplex sonography in the diagnosis of venogenic impotence. J Vasc Surg 13:75–83, 1991.

44. Salvatore FT, Sharman GM, Hellstrom WJ: Vacuum constriction devices and the clinical urologist: An informed selection. Urology 38:323–327, 1991.

45. Witherington R: External penile appliances for management of impotence. Semin Urol 8:124–128, 1990.

46. Korenman SG, Viosca SP: Management of impotence in men with a history of penile implant or severe pelvic disease. J Am Geriatr Soc 40:61–64, 1992.

47. Moul JW, McLeod DG: Negative pressure devices in the explanted penile prosthesis population. J Urol 142:729–731, 1989.

48. Turner LA, Althof SE, Levine SB, et al: External vacuum devices in the treatment of erectile dysfunction: A one-year study of sexual, psychosocial impact. J Sex Marital Ther 17:81–93, 1991.

49. Villeneuve R, Corcos J, Carmal M: Assisted erection follow-up with couples. J Sex Marital Ther 17:94–100, 1991.

50. Sidi AA, Becher EF, Zhang G, Lewis JH: Patient acceptance of and satisfaction with an external negative pressure device for impotence. J Urol 144:1154–1156, 1990.

51. Broderick GA, McGahan JP, Stone AR, White RD: The hemodynamics of vacuum constriction erections: Assessment by color Doppler ultrasound. J Urol 147:57–61, 1992.

52. Al-Juburi AZ, O'Donnell PD: Synergist erection system: Clinical experience. Urology 35:304–306, 1990.

53. Virag R, Frydman D, Legmann M, Floresco Bouilly P: Intracavernous injection of papaverine as a diagnostic and therapeutic method in erectile failure. Angiology 35:79–87, 1984.

54. Brindley GS: Cavernosal alpha-blockade: A new technique for investigating and treating erectile impotence. Br J Psychiatry 143:332–337, 1983.

55. Sidi AA, Chen KK: Clinical experience with vasoactive intracavernous pharmacotherapy for treatment of impotence. World J Urol 5:156–159, 1987.

56. Virag R, Shoukry K, Floresco J, et al: Intracavernous self-injection of vasoactive drugs in the treatment of impotence: 8 year experience with 615 cases. J Urol 145:287–293, 1991.

57. Levine SB, Althof SE, Turner LA, et al: Side effects of self-administration of intracavernous papaverine and phentolamine for the treatment of impotence. J Urol 141:54–57, 1990.

58. Porst H: Stellenwert von prostaglandin E₁ (PGE₁) in der diagnostik der erectilen dysfunktion (ED) im vergleich zu papaverin und papaverin/phentolamin bei 61 patienten mit ED. Urologe [A] 27:22–26, 1988.

59. Furlow WL, Motley RC: Inflatable penile prosthesis: Clinical experience with new controlled expansion cylinder. J Urol 139:945–946, 1988.

60. Stanisic TH, Dean JC, Donovan JM, Beutler LE: Clinical experience with self-contained penile implants: Flexi-Flate. J Urol 139:947–950, 1988.

61. Wilson SK, Wahman GE, Lange JL: Eleven years experience with inflatable penile prosthesis. J Urol 139:951–952, 1988.

62. Kabalin JN, Kessler R: Infectious complications of penile prosthesis surgery. J Urol 139:953–955, 1988.

63. Pendersen B, Tiefer L, Ruiz M, Melman A: Evaluation of patients and

partners 1 to 4 years after penile prosthesis surgery. J Urol 139:956–958, 1988.

64. Zilbergeld B: Alternatives to couples counseling for sex problems: Group and individual therapy. J Sex Marital Ther 6:3–18, 1980.

65. Morales A, Surridge DHC, Marshall PG, Fenemore J: Nonhormonal pharmacological treatment of organic impotence. J Urol 128:45–47, 1982.

66. Morales A, Condra MS, Owen JE, et al: Oral and transcutaneous pharmacologic agents in the treatment of impotence. Urol Clin North Am 15:87–93, 1988.

67. Korenman SG, Mooradian AD, Kaiser FE, et al: Treatment of vasculogenic sexual dysfunction with pentoxifylline. West Soc Clin Res 36:123, 1988.

136

Testicular Tumors with Endocrine Manifestations

ROBERT E. SCULLY

Over 90 per cent of testicular tumors arise from germ cells, and almost all these tumors have a potential for metastasis.[1, 2] They account for slightly over 1 per cent of all cancers in males[3] and, except for leukemia and lymphoma, are the most common malignant tumors in men between the ages of 15 and 34 years.[4] The causes of testicular cancer are unknown. Epidemiological investigations have shown that it is approximately four times more common in whites than in blacks and 10 times more frequent in cryptorchid than descended testes.[1, 2] Leydig cell tumors account for about 2 per cent of testicular neoplasms, and other tumors in the sex cord–stromal (gonadal stromal) category and lymphomas account for most of the remaining uncommon tumors.[1, 2]

Only a small proportion of germ cell tumors have endocrine manifestations, but many of them secrete hormones, mainly chorionic gonadotropin (hCG), which may serve as a marker for diagnosis and evaluation of therapy. Leydig cell tumors, as well as other tumors in the sex cord–stromal category, are often associated with clinical manifestations that result from steroid hormone secretion by the neoplastic cells; rarely, these tumors are components of a complex endocrine syndrome. Several of the tumors that may have endocrine manifestations are illustrated in Figure 136–1.

GERM CELL TUMORS

For clinical purposes, germ cell tumors are divided into two main categories: seminomas and nonseminomatous tumors. Seminomas, which account for almost 50 per cent of testicular germ cell tumors,[1, 2] are composed of primitive-appearing germ cells that fail to differentiate. Approximately 80 per cent of seminomas are "typical" or "classic," being composed of cells that resemble the primordial germ cells of the embryo. The remainder are either seminomas containing isolated syncytiotrophoblast cells or spermatocytic seminomas, which have a predominance of cells resembling spermatogonia. The nonseminomatous tumors are of four main types: teratomas, which contain a wide variety of tissues derived from one or more of the three embryonic germ layers; embryonal carcinoma, a primitive tumor composed of cells resembling those of the germ disk of the embryo and thought, on the basis of observations in animal models, to be composed of totipotential cells; choriocarcinoma, which occurs very rarely in pure form and

simulates morphologically and functionally gestational choriocarcinoma; and yolk sac tumor (endodermal sinus tumor), which recapitulates the yolk sac and its derivatives and is associated with a highly distinctive tumor marker, alpha-fetoprotein.

The seminoma reaches its peak age incidence between 35 and 40 years[1, 2] and is exceptionally rare in the first decade of life.[5] This tumor is treated optimally by radical inguinal orchidectomy followed by radiation therapy to retroperitoneal lymph nodes, with a resultant survival rate of over 95 per cent.[6] Metastatic seminoma responds to both radiation therapy and platinum-based chemotherapy.[7, 8] Most of the nonseminomatous tumors, which reach their peak age incidence between 25 and 30 years, are highly malignant and were associated with a low survival rate before the advent of combination chemotherapy, such as bleomycin, etoposide, and cisplatin; these drugs and other combinations have been curative in a high proportion of cases even in the presence of disseminated disease.[9, 10] The primary therapy of nonseminomatous germ cell tumors has generally consisted of radical inguinal orchidectomy followed by retroperitoneal lymphadenectomy. According to recent investigations,[8] however, lymphadenectomy may not be necessary in the management of stage I tumors (those confined to the testis) in this category if orchidectomy alone is followed by careful evaluation to detect early recurrence and chemotherapy is administered promptly if the findings are positive. The survival rate of patients with nonseminomatous germ cell tumors is now in the vicinity of 95 per cent.[7]

It must be emphasized that testicular germ cell tumors are often impure.[1, 2] Seminomas are combined with nonseminomatous components in approximately one third of the cases,[2] and most nonseminomatous tumors contain mixtures of two or more subtypes. The most common combination in nonseminomatous tumors is teratoma and embryonal carcinoma, sometimes referred to as *teratocarcinoma*. An additional important feature of testicular germ cell tumors is that they may be associated with metastases of other germ cell types, which are usually of a higher degree of malignancy if the patient has not received chemotherapy.[1] For example, a small seminoma may metastasize widely as embryonal carcinoma and choriocarcinoma; much less often, the reverse is true—for example, a teratocarcinoma may be complicated by a metastatic tumor composed entirely of mature teratoma. Such "maturation" of metastases has been encountered much more frequently

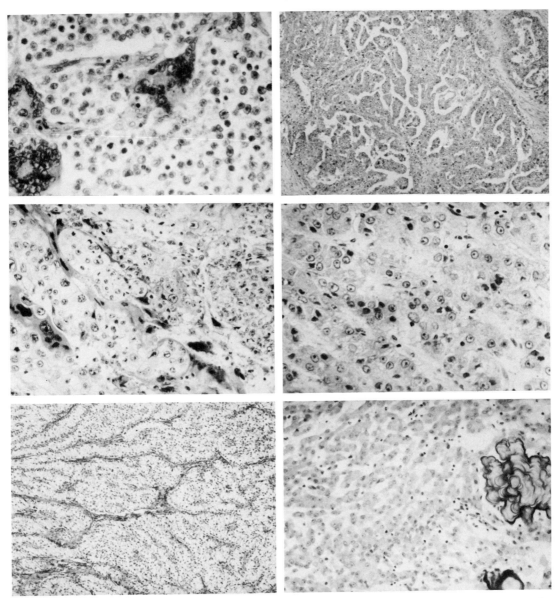

FIGURE 136–1. *(Above, left)* Seminoma with syncytiotrophoblast cells. The syncytiotrophoblast cells are large and multinucleated. *(Above, right)* Embryonal carcinoma. The tumor has a papillary glandular pattern. *(Center, left)* Chorio-carcinoma. There is a plexiform pattern of small cytotrophoblast cells and large multinucleated syncytiotrophoblast cells. *(Center, right)* Leydig cell tumor. The tumor cells have abundant cytoplasm and central nuclei with prominent nucleoli. *(Below, left)* Sertoli cell tumor. The neoplasm is composed of solid tubules containing vacuolated, lipid-rich Sertoli cells. *(Below, right)* Large-cell calcifying Sertoli cell tumor. The Sertoli cells are large and contain abundant cytoplasm. A large, laminated calcified deposit is present.

since the administration of effective chemotherapy.[14] It is uncertain whether this phenomenon indicates true maturation, is the result of destruction of the less mature elements of the tumor by chemotherapy with survival of the more mature elements, or is the effect of a combination of these mechanisms. A final important consideration is that less than 1 per cent of primary testicular tumors are clinically occult, presenting as a retroperitoneal mass or widespread hematogenous metastases.[1, 2, 15] In such cases, pathological examination of a testis may reveal a very small but grossly recognizable tumor, a microscopic focus of germ cell neoplasia, or a tumor that has undergone spontaneous regression with scar formation. High-frequency ultrasound examination can detect testicular lesions only 3 to 4 mm in diameter in this clinical setting.[16]

Gynecomastia is by far the most common endocrine manifestation of testicular germ cell tumors, occurring in 2.5 to 6 per cent of adult patients with these tumors but not occurring in affected children. The breast enlargement is usually bilateral.[17, 18] Although gynecomastia in general develops most often when the ratio of estrogens to androgens in increased,[19] investigation of patients with testicular germ cell tumors and gynecomastia has indicated the presence of a more complex endocrine background. One such study[20] has revealed high levels of prolactin, placental lactogen, hCG, estrone or estradiol, or combinations of these hormones in some patients with gynecomastia; the levels of these hormones have been normal in other patients with gynecomastia, however, and conversely, still other patients with testicular germ cell tumors without gynecomastia have had elevated values. The estrogens are thought to be secreted, at least in part, by Leydig cells in uninvolved testicular tissue that are stimulated by hCG, but in some cases the estrogen level may increase as a result of aromatization of androgens by trophoblastic cells within the tumor. Among germ cell neoplasms, gynecomastia is seen most often in association with those containing choriocarcinoma or embryonal carcinoma, the two major types of tumor that have the capacity to secrete hCG, but occasional seminomas are also associated with this manifestation.

Approximately 70 per cent of nonseminomatous germ cell tumors and 10 per cent of seminomas are accompanied by elevated levels of hCG in the serum.[21–23] In most of the cases of seminoma, the finding of high levels of hCG is attributable to initially unsampled foci of embryonal carcinoma or choriocarcinoma in the tumor specimen, the presence of scattered syncytiotrophoblast cells in the seminoma, or the existence of metastatic deposits containing embryonal carcinoma or choriocarcinoma, but in an occasional case, extensive sectioning of the primary tumor may fail to disclose an explanation for the hCG production, and metastatic tumor may not be detectable.

Several other endocrine manifestations have been attributable on rare occasions to hormone secretion by testicular germ cell tumors. One patient with an embryonal carcinoma and metastases containing teratomatous elements had elevated levels of hCG and a thyroid-stimulating hormone (TSH)–like substance in the serum, accompanied by gynecomastia and hyperthyroidism,[24] and another patient with choriocarcinomatous metastases of a testicular teratoma had hyperthyroidism with normal pituitary TSH but elevated "molar" TSH,[25] which may be identical to hCG with TSH-like activity.[26] Two patients with seminomas have had exophthalmos that resolved after orchidectomy.[27, 28] One of these tumors was a seminoma with syncytiotrophoblast cells.[27] In the other case,[28] thyroid function tests revealed a normal uptake of triiodothyronine (T_3) and normal thyroxine (T_4) and TSH levels. Carcinoid tumors develop rarely in the testis and are accompanied by teratomatous elements in approximately one fifth of cases.[1, 2] In three and possibly four cases, pure carcinoid tumors that were presumably primary in the testis were associated with manifestations of the carcinoid syndrome.[29–32]

GONADOBLASTOMA

The gonadoblastoma is a complex gonadal tumor in which germ cells, which resemble those of the testicular seminoma and the ovarian dysgerminoma, and immature sex cord elements compatible morphologically with either Sertoli or granulosa cells are arranged in discrete nests separated by stroma; in two thirds of the cases, cells resembling Leydig or lutein cells are present in the stroma.[33] This tumor is important clinically because in approximately half the cases the germ cells invade the stroma to form a germinoma (seminoma or dysgerminoma), and in less than 10 per cent of the cases, a more malignant form of germ cell tumor, such as embryonal carcinoma, choriocarcinoma, or immature teratoma, develops. Also, since gonadoblastomas contain Leydig or lutein cells, they may secrete steroid hormones.

About 80 per cent of gonadoblastomas develop in phenotypical females, who are usually virilized to some extent. The remainder arise in phenotypical males, who are mostly under 20 years of age and have cryptorchidism, which is usually bilateral, and who almost always have hypospadias and a uterus; gynecomastia is often present as well. Most males with gonadoblastomas probably have mixed gonadal dysgenesis (unilateral streak gonad and contralateral testis or unilateral or bilateral streak testes), which is most commonly associated with a 45X,46XY karyotype, or dysgenetic male pseudohermaphroditism (bilateral dysgenetic testes), which is considered by many investigators to be a variant of mixed gonadal dysgenesis. The pure gonadoblastoma is a benign tumor; its danger lies in its frequent transformation into a malignant germ cell tumor. The subject is discussed further in the Chapter 121.

LEYDIG CELL TUMORS

Leydig cell (interstitial cell) tumors account for only 1 to 3 per cent of all testicular neoplasms.[34] Eighteen per cent have been detected during the first decade, 26 per cent during the second and third decades, 30 per cent during the fourth and fifth decades, and 26 per cent in older age groups. Although the most common clinical manifestation is testicular swelling, gynecomastia is present in 30 per cent of the cases, and about a quarter of the patients with gynecomastia have an accompanying decrease in libido or potency. All prepubertal children with Leydig cell tumors have had isosexual pseudoprecocity, and a rare adult patient in whom a Leydig cell tumor has been detected gave a history of precocity. Precocity caused by Leydig cell tumors typically appears between the ages of 5 and 9 years. About 10 per cent of the precocious patients also have gynecomastia. Approximately one tenth of patients with Leydig cell tumors have no symptoms, and their tumors are discovered on physical examination performed for other reasons or at autopsy. Several cases have been reported in which an impalpable Leydig cell tumor has been detected by ultrasound examination in an adult with gynecomastia.[35]

A few reports in the literature suggest that cryptorchidism may predispose to the development of a Leydig cell tumor in view of the presence of an undescended testis or a history of it in 5 to 10 per cent of the cases.[34] Three Leydig cell tumors have occurred in patients with Klinefelter's syndrome.[34]

Testosterone is the major androgen produced by the Leydig cell tumor, but secretion of androstenedione and dehydroepiandrosterone also has been reported.[36, 37] Urinary 17-ketosteroids may be normal or high. Elevated estrogen levels have been recorded in patients with Leydig cell tumors with and without gynecomastia, and estradiol has been recovered in high concentrations from the spermatic vein blood in several cases.[38] Testosterone levels and values for gonadotropins, particularly follicle-stimulating hormone (FSH), have been low in patients with gynecomastia and elevated estradiol levels.[39, 40] In a few other cases, plasma progesterone or urinary pregnanediol values have been elevated.[41, 42] The abnormal hormonal levels may return to normal after removal of the tumor,[43] but in some cases they persist.[40]

Leydig cell tumors are unilateral in 97 per cent of the

cases. Gross pathological examination usually reveals a well-circumscribed, yellow to brown tumor, 3 to 4 cm in diameter. Microscopic examination discloses tumor cells resembling normal Leydig cells and growing diffusely or in trabeculae. Crystals of Reinke, more or less specific cytoplasmic inclusions of Leydig cells, may be found in 35 to 40 per cent of the cases[1, 34]; lipochrome pigment is often present in the cytoplasm as well. A minority of Leydig cell tumors show significant degrees of nuclear atypicality and mitotic activity as well as invasion of the adjacent tissue and blood vessels.

Approximately 10 per cent of Leydig cell tumors have a malignant clinical course, with metastases evident at the time of presentation or appearing subsequently, sometimes as long as 9 years postoperatively. Undoubtedly a higher proportion of reported tumors would have proved malignant had follow-up examination been longer at the time of publication. The average age of patients with malignant tumors is 63 years, in contrast to 40 years for Leydig cell tumors in general.[34] Only an occasional patient with a malignant tumor has presented with endocrine manifestations,[44, 45] although elevated levels of various hormones or their metabolites have been recorded in many of the cases. A malignant course in a prepubertal patient with a Leydig cell tumor is exceptional.[46]

The malignant Leydig cell tumor spreads most commonly to regional lymph nodes (72 per cent), lung (43 per cent), liver (38 per cent), and bone (28 per cent).[47] About 20 per cent of the patients have metastases at the time of diagnosis.[47] No absolute pathological criteria for malignancy of Leydig cell tumors exist, but 5 tumors that exhibited a malignant behavior in one series of 40 cases[34] had four or more of the following features: a maximal dimension of 5 cm or greater, an infiltrative margin, lymphatic or vascular invasion, necrosis, a mitotic rate of over 3 per 10 high-power fields, and moderate to marked nuclear atypicality. None of the 14 tumors in that series that had not recurred after a follow-up period of 2 or more years had more than one of these features, except for a single tumor that had three of them.

The treatment of a Leydig cell tumor is inguinal orchidectomy. If the gross or histological features indicate a likelihood of malignancy, a retroperitoneal lymphadenectomy should be considered.[34] The treatment of metastatic Leydig cell tumors has been generally unsatisfactory.[47, 48] The average length of survival of patients with a malignant Leydig cell tumor has been 4 years.[38]

TUMORS OF ADRENOCORTICAL TYPE

Testicular "tumors," which are almost always bilateral, but which may appear at different times, develop in an unknown but significant proportion of males with untreated or inadequately treated adrenogenital syndrome (TTAGs).[49–52] These "tumors," which are encountered most often in association with the salt-losing form of the syndrome (21-hydroxylase deficiency), may appear in early childhood or not until adult life. It is important to distinguish them from Leydig cell tumors because of differences in prognosis and therapy. Clinical clues to the diagnosis of TTAG include the known presence of the syndrome, a family history of it, and bilateral testicular enlargement,

which is rare in cases of Leydig cell tumor. Laboratory examination shows the features of the underlying adrenogenital syndrome, such as elevated levels of adrenocorticotropic hormone (ACTH), androstenedione, and 17-hydroxyprogesterone in the plasma and increase in 17-ketosteroids and pregnanetriol in the urine. A persistent elevation of 17-ketosteroids in the absence of detectable metastatic disease after the removal of a testicular tumor resembling a Leydig cell tumor suggests the possibility of an underlying adrenogenital syndrome. Other characteristic features of these tumors are their enlargement and enhanced hormonal secretion after the administration of ACTH and a decrease in their size and hormone output after suppression of the ACTH level by the administration of corticosteroids.

The testicular "tumor" of the adrenogenital syndrome may attain a diameter of up to 10 cm. It appears to develop in the hilar region and expand peripherally into the parenchyma and is composed of dark brown, lobulated tissue traversed by fibrous septa. Microscopic examination reveals large cells resembling Leydig cells with abundant eosinophilic cytoplasm which characteristically contains considerable lipochrome pigment but lacks crystals of Reinke. The "tumor" tissue been shown to produce cortisol and to function in the same manner as the accompanying hyperplastic adrenal glands. The nature of the "tumor" cells is controversial. Some investigators believe that they are derived from adrenocortical rests; others, that they are Leydig cells that have come under the control of ACTH; and still others, that they originate from testicular stromal cells, which are postulated to have the ability to differentiate into either Leydig or adrenocortical cells depending on the nature of the tropic stimulation.[51] Although it is arguable that these testicular masses are not true neoplasms in view of their dependence on ACTH and the absence of evidence of malignancy in the cases reported to date, they are tumors in a clinical sense and are not clearly distinguishable from Leydig cell tumors on microscopic examination alone. Since they respond to suppression of ACTH, it is not necessary to remove them except for cosmetic reasons.

A few patients with Nelson's syndrome (development of an ACTH-secreting pituitary tumor, characteristically accompanied by cutaneous hyperpigmentation, after bilateral adrenalectomy for Cushing's disease) have had testicular "tumors," paratesticular "tumors," or both resembling those of the adrenogenital syndrome.[53, 54] These "tumors" have been shown to produce corticosteroids, including cortisol, as well as androgens.

SEX CORD–STROMAL TUMORS

Although nosologically the terms *sex cord–stromal tumors*,[55] *gonadal-stromal tumors*,[1] and *androblastomas*[56] embrace neoplasms containing sex cord derivatives (Sertoli cells, granulosa cells, or both) or stromal derivatives (Leydig cells, theca cells, and stromal fibroblasts) alone or in any combination and in varying degrees of differentiation, these designations are usually applied more specifically to neoplasms that contain one or more of the preceding cell types with the exclusion of pure Leydig cell tumors, which are classified separately.[57] Sex cord–stromal tumors, of which over 100 cases have been reported in the literature, occur at all ages but are particularly common in children, in whom 38 per cent of the cases have occurred[58]; 24 per cent have been diagnosed in infants less than 1 year of age. The tumors are of clinical interest in view of their association with feminization, including gynecomastia, in about one fourth of the cases and a clinical malignancy rate of over 25 per cent in cases in which follow-up examination has been 1 year or longer.[58] Only very rare tumors diagnosed before puberty have been clinically malignant.[59, 60] If one considers only patients with sex cord–stromal tumors 10 years of age or older, almost 40 per cent of those followed for 1 year or more have had a malignant course.[58] Gynecomastia is most frequent in prepubertal patients and in those over 50 years of age and is four times more common if the tumor is clinically malignant.[58]

On gross examination, sex cord–stromal tumors range from tiny nodules to large masses that have replaced the testis. The neoplastic tissue varies from soft to firm depending on the relative quantities of neoplastic cells and collagenous stroma and gray-white to yellow depending on the amount of fat in the neoplastic cells. Microscopic examination usually discloses an admixture of sex cord and stromal elements in varying combinations and degrees of differentiation. The tumors resemble granulosa cell tumors, thecomas, and Sertoli-stromal cell tumors of the ovary but are more difficult to subclassify because differentiation is more often in the direction of both testicular and ovarian elements than it is in the ovary, where one or the other clearly predominates in the great majority of cases. Also, tubular differentiation is more frequently encountered in the testicular tumors than in their ovarian counterparts. The infantile tumors take the form of juvenile granulosa cell tumor in over three quarters of the cases[61]; indeed, this tumor is by far the most common neoplasm of the neonatal testis.

Although it is not always possible to distinguish pure Sertoli cell tumors from those containing additional cellular elements on the basis of descriptions of cases in the literature, several forms of pure Sertoli cell tumor exist as distinctive subtypes within the sex cord–stromal category. The resemblance of some of these tumors to the estrogenic Sertoli cell tumor of the canine testis led to the initial recognition of estrogenic Sertoli cell tumors of the human testis by Teilum.[56] Five cases of estrogenic Sertoli cell tumor of the testis have been reported in boys with the Peutz-Jeghers syndrome.[62, 63] This finding is not surprising in view of the frequent occurrence of sex cord tumors containing Sertoli cells in the ovaries of patients with this syndrome.[64] Some of the testicular tumors had features similar to those of the ovarian sex cord tumor with annular tubules (see Ch. 121) and the large-cell calcifying Sertoli cell tumor (discussed in the next paragraph) but were not typical of either.

A highly distinctive subtype of Sertoli cell tumor is the large-cell calcifying form,[65, 66] which is commonly multiple and bilateral, is often associated with endocrine disorders, may be familial (two brothers with cardiac myxomas and cutaneous pigmentation), and may occur in association with the Peutz-Jeghers syndrome. The accompanying endocrine abnormalities have included isosexual precocity, feminization, testicular steroid cell tumors of either Leydig or adrenocortical cell type, primary micronodular adrenocortical hyperplasia which may result in hypercortisolemia,[61] pituitary tumors accompanied by gigantism or acromegaly,[67] and the androgen insensitivity syndrome. Carney and associates[68] included the large-cell calcifying Sertoli cell tumor within "the complex of myxomas, spotty pigmentation, and endocrine overactivity" that they described.

The age range of patients with the large-cell calcifying Sertoli cell tumor has been 3 to 44 years, with all but one patient between the ages of 3 and 30 years. The 44-year-old patient was the only one described in the literature whose tumor had a malignant course, although we are aware of two additional patients in the older age category who had clinically malignant forms of the tumor. The neoplasms are typically small, with the largest recorded example 4 cm in diameter; however, multiple small nodules may enlarge the testis to a greater extent. The neoplastic tissue is characteristically hard. Because of the frequency of bilaterality, the finding of a tumor in one testis warrants careful examination of the contralateral organ by palpation and ultrasound examination to detect smaller tumors, which exhibit calcification. Microscopic examination reveals nodules of large Sertoli cells with abundant cytoplasm expanding and distorting tubules and coalescing to form large confluent masses that retain a tubular architecture to varying degrees. Rounded foci of calcification, which may become confluent, have been seen in all the tumors to date.

Sex cord–stromal tumors are generally treated by inguinal orchidectomy. If the clinical, gross, or microscopic features are suggestive of a possible malignant behavior, lymphadenectomy should be considered in view of the high frequency of lymph node spread in the clinically malignant cases.[69] Clear-cut pathological criteria of malignancy have not yet been established, however. Whether radiation therapy or chemotherapy will prove useful in the management of residual or recurrent tumor is not known at the present time.[69] The discovery of a large-cell calcifying Sertoli cell tumor should lead to a careful investigation for the presence of other endocrine abnormalities and cardiac myxomas, as well as a careful evaluation of the family history. Treatment of a unilateral tumor of this type requires orchidectomy for diagnostic purposes in most cases. If a tumor is also present in the contralateral testis, the appropriate management is not clear at the present time; it may be permissible to watch the patient carefully because of the rarity of malignant change except in older men.

PARAENDOCRINE AND RELATED DISORDERS

Disorders in this category are very rare in association with testicular tumors.[70] Two cases of seminoma have been accompanied by paraneoplastic hypercalcemia.[71, 72] One unclassifiable malignant testicular tumor resulted in Cushing's syndrome and isosexual precocity in a 3-year-old boy[73]; whether the clinical manifestations were endocrine or paraendocrine in this case, however, is unclear. Finally, one patient with a seminoma containing syncytiotrophoblast cells and producing hCG resulted in hyperandrogenism, which was attributed to hCG stimulation of Leydig cells surrounding the tumor,[74] accompanied by high plasma erythropoietin levels and mild polycythemia.

REFERENCES

1. Mostofi FK, Price EB Jr: Atlas of Tumor Pathology, series 2, fascicle 8: Tumors of the Male Genital System. Washington, Armed Forces Institute of Pathology, 1973.
2. Young RH, Scully RE: Testicular Tumors. Chicago, American Society of Clinical Pathology Press, 1990.
3. Silverberg E: Cancer statistics, 1984. CA 34:7–23, 1984.
4. Silverberg E: Cancer in young adults (ages 15 to 34). CA 32:32–42, 1982.
5. Viprakasit D, Navarro C, Guarin UK, Garnes HA: Seminoma in children. Urology 9:568–570, 1977.
6. Zagars GK: Management of stage I seminoma: Radiotherapy. In Horwich A (ed): Testicular Cancer: Investigation and Management. Baltimore, Williams & Wilkins, 1991, pp 83–107.
7. Thomas G: Management of metastatic seminoma: Role of radiotherapy. In Horwich A (ed): Testicular Cancer: Investigation and Management. Baltimore, Williams & Wilkins, 1991, pp 117–128.
8. Direx LY, Van Oosterom AT: Chemotherapy in metastatic seminoma. In Horwich A (ed): Testicular Cancer: Investigation and Management. Baltimore, Williams & Wilkins, 1991, pp 129–136.
9. Einhorn LH: Treatment strategies of testicular cancer in the United States. Int J Androl 10:399–405, 1987.
10. Nichols CR, Roth BJ: Management of metastatic non-seminoma: Development of effective chemotherapy. In Horwich A (ed): Testicular Cancer: Investigation and Management. Baltimore, Williams & Wilkins, 1991, pp 185–204.
11. Pizzocaro G: Management of stage I non-seminoma: Rationale for lymphadenectomy. In Horwich A (ed): Testicular Cancer: Investigation and Management. Baltimore, Williams & Wilkins, 1991, pp 167–174.
12. Peckham MJ, Brada M: Surveillance following orchidectomy for stage 1 testicular cancer. Int J Androl 10:247–254, 1987.
13. Cullen M: Management of stage I non-seminoma: surveillance and chemotherapy. In Horwich A (ed): Testicular Cancer: Investigation and Management. Baltimore, Williams & Wilkins, 1991, pp 149–166.
14. Ulbright TM, Roth LM: Evaluation of germ cell tumors following chemotherapy. In Talerman A, Roth LM (eds): Contemporary Issues in Surgical Pathology: Pathology of the Testis and Its Adnexa. New York, Churchill Livingstone, 1986, pp 231–241.
15. Powell S, Hendry WF, Peckham MJ: Occult germ-cell testicular tumours. Br J Urol 55:440–444, 1983.
16. Carroll B: Ultrasonography of the scrotum. In Sarti DA (ed): Diagnostic Ultrasound: Text and Cases. Chicago, Year Book Medical Publishers, 1987, pp 570–607.
17. Kurohara SS, George FW, Dykhuisen RF, Leary KL: Testicular tumors: Analysis of 196 cases treated at the US Naval Hospital in San Diego. Cancer 20:1089–1098, 1967.
18. LeFevre RE, Stewart BH, Levin HS, et al: Testis tumors: Review of 125 cases at the Cleveland Clinic. Urology 6:588–593, 1975.
19. Carlson HE: Current concepts: Gynecomastia. N Engl J Med 303:795–799, 1980.
20. Stepanas AV, Samaan NA, Schultz PN, Holoye PY: Endocrine studies in testicular tumor patients with and without gynecomastia. Cancer 41:369–376, 1978.
21. Javadpour N: Value of tumor markers in testicular cancer. In Talerman A, Roth LM (eds): Contemporary Issues in Surgical Pathology: Pathology of the Testis and its Adnexa. New York, Churchill Livingstone, 1986, pp 221–230.
22. Bosl GJ, Lange PH, Nochomovitz LE, et al: Tumor markers in advanced nonseminomatous testicular cancer. Cancer 47:572–576, 1981.
23. Mason MD: Tumour markers. In Horwich A (ed): Testicular Cancer: Investigation and Management. Baltimore, Williams & Wilkins, 1991, pp 33–50.
24. Steigbigel NH, Oppenheim JJ, Fishman LM, Carbone PP: Metastatic embryonal carcinoma of the testis associated with elevated plasma TSH-like activity and hyperthyroidism. N Engl J Med 271:345–349, 1964.
25. Karp PJ, Herschman JM, Richmond S, et al: Thyrotoxicosis from molar thyrotropin. Arch Intern Med 132:432–436, 1973.
26. Kennedy RL, Darne J: The role of hCG in regulation of the thyroid gland in normal and abnormal pregnancy. Obstet Gynecol 78:298–307, 1991.
27. Mann AS: Bilateral exophthalmos in seminoma. J Clin Endocrinol Metab 27:1500–1502, 1967.
28. Taylor JB, Solomon DH, Levine RE, Ehrlich RM: Exopthalmos in seminoma: Regression with steroids and orchiectomy. JAMA 240:860–861, 1978.
29. Wurster R, Brodner O, Rossner JA, Grube D: A carcinoid occurring in the testis. Virchows Arch [A] 370:185–192, 1976.
30. Hosking DH, Bowman DM, McMorris SL, Ramsey EW: Primary carcinoid of the testis with metastases. J Urol 125:255–256, 1981.
31. Hayes D: Primary argentaffin carcinoma of the testis. Br J Urol 54:429, 1982.
32. Leake J, Levitt G, Ramani P: Primary carcinoid of the testis in a 10-year old boy. Histopathology 19:373–375, 1991.
33. Scully RE: Gonadoblastoma: A review of 74 cases. Cancer 25:1340–1356, 1970.
34. Kim I, Young RH, Scully RE: Leydig cell tumors of the testis: A clinicopathological analysis of 40 cases and review of the literature. Am J Surg Pathol 9:177–192, 1985.
35. Haas GP, Pittabiga S, Gomella L, et al: Clinically occult Leydig cell tumor presenting with gynecomastia. J Urol 142:1325–1327, 1989.
36. Wilson BE, Netzloff ML: Primary testicular abnormalities causing precocious puberty: Leydig cell tumor, Leydig cell hyperplasia and adrenal rest tumor. Ann Clin Lab Sci 13:315–320, 1983.
37. Boulanger P, Somma M, Chevalier S, et al: Elevated secretion of androstenedione in a patient with a Leydig cell tumour. Acta Endocrinol 107:104–109, 1984.
38. Gabrilove JL, Nicolis GL, Mitty HA, Sohval AR: Feminizing interstitial cell tumor of the testis: Personal observations and review of the literature. Cancer 35:1184–1202, 1975.
39. Bercovici P, Nahoul K, Tater D, et al: Hormonal profile of Leydig cell tumors with gynecomastia. J Clin Endocrinol Metab 59:625–630, 1984.
40. Mineur P, DeCooman S, Hustin J, et al: Feminizing testicular Leydig cell tumor: Hormonal profile before and after unilateral orchidectomy. J Clin Endocrinol Metab 64:686–691, 1987.
41. Perez C, Novoa J, Alcañiz J, et al: Leydig cell tumour of the testis with gynaecomastia and elevated oestrogen, progesterone and prolactin levels: Case report. Clin Endocrinol 13:409–412, 1980.
42. Czernobilsky H, Czernobilsky B, Schneider HG, et al: Characterization of a feminizing testicular Leydig cell tumor by hormone profile, immunocytochemistry, and tissue culture. Cancer 56:1667–1676, 1985.
43. Bercovici P, Nahoul K, Ducasse M, et al: Leydig cell tumor with gynecomastia: Further studies—The recovery after unilateral orchidectomy. J Clin Endocrinol Metab 61:957–962, 1985.
44. Shapiro CM, Sankovitch A, Yoon WJ: Malignant feminizing Leydig cell tumor. J Surg Oncol 27:73–75, 1984.
45. Balsitis M, Sokal M: Ossifying malignant Leydig (interstitial) cell tumour of the testis. Histopathology 16:597–601, 1990.
46. Freeman DA: Steroid hormone-producing tumors in man. Endocr Rev 7:204–220, 1986.
47. Grem JL, Robins I, Wilson KS, et al: Metastatic Leydig cell tumor of the testis: Report of three cases and review of the literature. Cancer 58:2116–2119, 1986.
48. Bertrem KA, Bratloff B, Hodges GF, Davidson H: Treatment of malignant Leydig cell tumor. Cancer 68:2324–2329, 1991.
49. Franco-Saenz R, Antonipillai I, Tan SY, et al: Cortisol production by testicular tumors in a patient with congenital adrenal hyperplasia (21-hydroxylase deficiency). J Clin Endocrinol Metab 53:85–90, 1981.
50. Chrousos GP, Loriaux DL, Sherins RJ, Cutler GB Jr: Unilateral testicular enlargement resulting from inapparent 21-hydroxylase deficiency. J Urol 126:127–128, 1981.
51. Chakraborty J, France-Saenz R, Kropp K: Electron microscopic study of testicular tumor in congenital adrenal hyperplasia. Human Pathol 14:151–157, 1983.
52. Rutgers JL, Young RH, Scully RE: The testicular "tumor" of the adrenogenital syndrome: A report of six cases and review of the literature on testicular masses in patients with disorders of the adrenal glands. Am J Surg Pathol 12:503–513, 1988.
53. Hamwi GJ, Gwinup G, Mostow JH, Besch PK: Activation of testicular adrenal rest tissue by prolonged excessive ACTH production. J Clin Endocrinol Metab 23:861–869, 1963.
54. Johnson RE, Scheithauer B: Massive hyperplasia of testicular adrenal rests in a patient with Nelson's syndrome. Am J Clin Pathol 77:501–507, 1982.
55. Mostofi FK, Sobin LH: International Histological Classification of Tumours, No. 16. Histological Typing of Testis Tumours. Geneva, World Health Organization, 1977.
56. Teilum G: Arrhenoblastoma—androblastoma; homologous ovarian and testicular tumors; including so-called "luteomas" and "adrenal tumors" of ovary and interstitial cell tumors of testis. Acta Pathol Microbiol Scand 23:252–264, 1946.
57. Lawrence WD, Young RH, Scully RE: Sex cord-stromal tumors. In

Talerman A, Roth LM (eds): Contemporary Issues in Surgical Pathology: Pathology of the Testis and its Adnexa. New York, Churchill Livingstone, 1986, pp 67–92.

58. Gabrilove JL, Freiberg EK, Leiter E, Nicolis GL: Feminizing and non-feminizing Sertoli cell tumors. J Urol 124:757–767, 1980.

59. Rosvoll RV, Woodard JR: Malignant Sertoli cell tumor of the testis. Cancer 22:8–13, 1968.

60. Sharma S, Seam RK, Kapoor HL: Malignant Sertoli cell tumour of the testis in a child. J Surg Oncol 44:129–131, 1990.

61. Lawrence WD, Young RH, Scully RE: Juvenile granulosa cell tumor of the infantile testis: A report of 14 cases. Am J Surg Pathol 9:87–94, 1985.

62. Caccamea A, Cozzi F, Farragiana T, et al: Feminizing Sertoli cell tumor associated with Peutz-Jeghers syndrome. Tumori 71:379–385, 1985.

63. Coen P, Kulin H, Ballantine T, et al: An aromatase-producing sex-cord tumor resulting in prepubertal gynecomastia. N Engl J Med 324:317–322, 1991.

64. Young RH, Welch WR, Dickersin GR, Scully RE: Ovarian sex cord tumor with annular tubules. Cancer 50:1384–1402, 1982.

65. Proppe KH, Scully RE: Large-cell calcifying Sertoli cell tumor of the testis. Am J Clin Pathol 74:607–619, 1980.

66. Tetu B, Ro JY, Ayala AG: Large cell calcifying Sertoli cell tumor of the testis: A clinicopathologic, immunohistochemical and ultrastructural study of two cases. Am J Clin Pathol 96:717–722, 1991.

67. Rosenzweig JL, Lawrence DA, Vogel DL, et al: Adrenocorticotropin-independent hypercortisolemia and testicular tumors in a patient with a pituitary tumor and gigantism. J Clin Endocrinol Metab 55:421–427, 1982.

68. Carney JA, Gordon H, Carpenter PC, et al: The complex of myxomas, spotty pigmentation, and endocrine overactivity. Medicine 64:270–283, 1985.

69. Eble JN, Hull MT, Warfel KA, Donohue JP: Malignant sex cord-stromal tumor of testis. J Urol 131:546–550, 1984.

70. Altaffer LF: Paraneoplastic endocrinopathies associated with nonrenal genitourinary tumors. J Urol 127:411–416, 1982.

71. King WW, Cox CE, Boyce WH: Pseudohyperparathyroidism and seminoma. J Urol 107:809–811, 1972.

72. Metcalfe JB, Carey TC, Barry JM: Genitourinary malignancy and pseudohyperparathyroidism. J Urol 119:702–704, 1978.

73. Crouch RD: Adrenogenic testicular tumor. J Urol 79:527–531, 1958.

74. Reman O, Reynick Y, Casadevall N, et al: Polycythemia and steroid overproduction in a gonadotropin-secreting seminoma of the testis. Cancer 68:2224–2229, 1991.

Contraception in the Male

DAVID J. HANDELSMAN

BACKGROUND

A contraceptive for men must reduce the number of fertile sperm in the ejaculate to levels that reliably prevent fertilization. The ideal contraceptive should be safe, effective, convenient to use, affordable, widely available, and readily reversible. The risk of pregnancy can be averted by diverting or suppressing sperm output and/or inhibiting sperm-fertilizing capacity. Currently men have available traditional preindustrial methods (abstinence and withdrawal), condoms, and vasectomy, but no new methods have been introduced this century, in contrast with the highly effective, convenient, and reversible contraceptive methods developed for women over the last three decades (Tables 137–1 and 137–2). The reversible male methods have relatively high failure rates, and vasectomy has limited reversibility; yet, despite the limitations of available methods, currently male involvement in family planning remains extensive. Globally one third of contraceptors use methods requiring active male participation,[1] reflecting the traditional reliance of family planning on male involvement and the continuing willingness of men to share the burdens as well as the benefits of effective family planning. Even greater participation by men in family planning is likely if more convenient and effective methods, comparable with modern female methods, can be developed for men, allowing couples to choose the most suitable contraceptive method at various times. Although international public-sector agencies have agreed on the imperative to develop new, reversible male contraceptives, the predatory exploitation of medical product liability now poses a major disincentive to pharmaceutical research and development of new contraceptives.[2] Nevertheless, since the available male contraceptive methods are not ideal and modern chemical methods are still in early preclinical development, hormonal methods are closest to realization, with prototypes undergoing clinical testing.

NONHORMONAL METHODS

Traditional Methods

Periodic Abstinence

Celibacy and castration are the only completely reliable forms of contraception, but neither is acceptable nor practical for married couples. Apart from specific sociocultural circumstances (e.g., religious orders, lactational taboos, or social policy of delayed marriage), sexual abstinence has very limited acceptability as a form of family planning. Periodic abstinence, the limiting of sexual intercourse to days designated as "safe,"[3] has high contraceptive efficacy if the rules are followed perfectly, but the failure rates rise steeply with any rule breaking.[4] Advantages of this device-free method are its safety, reversibility, and negligible cost. The disadvantages are its limited efficacy, inflexibility, and inconvenience in disturbing the spontaneity of love making, all of which reduce its general acceptability. Nevertheless periodic abstinence is used by at least 30 million couples worldwide for family planning.[1]

Withdrawal (Coitus Interruptus)

Nearly 40 million couples rely on this traditional male method of family planning, the wide use of which is often underestimated.[1] With abortion, it was the major preindustrial method of family planning, largely responsible for the demographic transition from high to low birth rates in industrial nations. This device-free method has the advantages of being completely private, free, and without known physical side effects, but it requires skill and self-control and interferes with the pleasurability of coitus for many couples. While reasonably effective for experienced users, this method is demanding and has a correspondingly high failure rate in practice.[5]

TABLE 137–1. PREVALENCE AND TYPICAL EFFICACY OF VARIOUS CONTRACEPTIVE METHODS

CONTRACEPTIVE METHOD	COUPLES OF REPRODUCTIVE AGE* [millions, (% total couples)]			TYPICAL FAILURE RATE† (%)
	Global	Developed Countries	Developing Countries	
None	404 (46.8%)	54 (28.7%)	350 (51.9%)	85
Periodic abstinence	33 (3.8%)	17 (9.0%)	16 (2.4%)	20
Withdrawal	38 (4.4%)	26 (13.8%)	11 (1.6%)	18
Diaphragm‡	8 (0.9%)	5 (2.7%)	3 (0.4%)	18
Condom	44 (5.1%)	25 (13.3%)	18 (2.7%)	12
Intrauterine device	84 (9.7%)	11 (5.9%)	73 (10.8%)	6
Hormonal, oral	67 (7.8%)	26 (13.8%)	41 (6.1%)	3
Hormonal, injectable	8 (0.9%)	0 (0%)	8 (1.2%)	0.3
Tubal ligation	119 (13.8%)	13 (6.9%)	106 (15.7%)	0.4
Vasectomy	45 (5.2%)	7 (3.7%)	38 (5.6%)	0.15
Other§	14 (1.6%)	3 (1.6%)	11 (1.6%)	—
Total users	459 (53.2%)	134 (71.3%)	325 (48.1%)	—
TOTAL	863 (100%)	188 (100%)	675 (100%)	—

Data based on contraceptive prevalence surveys compiled by United Nations[49] based on estimates projected to 1987 and contraceptive failure rates based on typical first year of use by Trussell et al.[33, 34]
*Defined as couples, including married women aged 15 to 49 years.
†Estimates contraceptive failure rate for typical users in the first year of use based on Trussell et al.[33, 34]
‡Includes spermicide use (with a failure rate of 21 per cent used alone), but separate prevalence estimates not available.
§Includes abstinence, douching, nonvaginal intercourse, and folk methods.

Condom

About 45 million couples rely on condoms for contraception, and globally, usage is increasing for prevention of sexually transmitted disease (STD), particularly human immunodeficiency virus infection.[6] Condoms provide safe, cheap, widely available, and reversible contraception with few side effects apart from allergy to latex rubber, when nonrubber condoms can be substituted. Latex condoms are, however, perishable through tears or snagging on nails, clothing, or jewelry, as well as deterioration from exposure to light, heat, humidity, or organic oils (e.g., nonaqueous lubricants). The major limitation of condoms is their relatively high failure rates and interference with sexuality. Latex condoms are moderately effective at preventing pregnancy or STD's, although natural membrane (lamb intestine) condoms are not protective against transmission of viral STD's. The requirement for regular and correct use during sexual foreplay can intrude on the spontaneity of love making and dull erotic sensation. These aesthetic limitations contribute to the high failure rates,

which are mostly due to mis- or nonuse rather than breakage or slippage. Better design to improve tactile sensitivity and more durable polyurethane condoms could improve acceptability. Whether spermicide impregnation improves the contraceptive efficacy of condoms has not been established.

Vas Occlusion

Vasectomy is used by over 40 million couples for family planning,[7] but its popularity varies widely depending on public education and availability of convenient facilities for men.[7] Among the safest of surgical procedures for men having completed their family and fit for minor surgery, vasectomy has few relative contraindications, including bleeding disorders, scrotal pathology (hernia, hydrocele, scarring), keloid proneness, allergy to local anesthetic, and active genitourinary or groin infections. Conventional vasectomy, usually performed under local anesthesia via scrotal incisions, involves excising a segment of vas deferens and interposing a fascial barrier between the occluded cut

TABLE 137–2. CLASS OF CONTRACEPTIVE METHOD, GLOBAL USAGE, AND AVERAGE EFFICACY

CLASS OF CONTRACEPTIVE METHOD*	COUPLES OF REPRODUCTIVE AGE [millions, (% total contraceptors)]			WEIGHTED AVERAGE FAILURE RATE (%)†
	Global	Developed Countries	Developing Countries	
Sterilization	164 (35.7%)	20 (14.9%)	144 (44.3%)	0.3
Modern reversible	159 (34.6%)	37 (27.6%)	122 (37.5%)	4.4
Traditional methods	123 (26.8%)	73 (54.5%)	48 (14.8%)	16.4
Male methods	160 (34.9%)	75 (56.0%)	83 (25.5%)	11.7
Female methods	286 (62.3%)	55 (41.0%)	231 (71.1%)	3.1

Data based on contraceptive prevalence surveys compiled by United Nations[49] based on estimates projected to 1987 and contraceptive failure rates based on typical first year of use by Trussell et al.[33, 34]
*Defined as sterilization (tubal ligation, vasectomy); modern reversible (intrauterine device, hormonal methods); traditional (periodic abstinence, withdrawal, diaphragm, condom); male (periodic abstinence, withdrawal, condom, vasectomy) and female (diaphragm, intrauterine device, hormonal methods, tubal ligation).
†Average failure rate (in per cent) calculated as weighted mean failure rates for first year of use based on Trussell et al.[33, 34] and standardizing to the global pattern of contraceptive method use. These figures provide a comparative estimate of the average efficacy of classes of contraceptive methods based on type of method and category of user.

ends to minimize risk of recanalization. The "no scalpel" technique avoids skin incision and has been performed in nearly 10 million Chinese men.[7a] Novel nonsurgical vas occlusion techniques under evaluation include percutaneous injections of liquid sclerosant[7] or of polymers that harden into occluding plugs that may be later removed to restore fertility.[8]

Immediate side effects of vasectomy include bleeding and infection after 3 per cent of conventional and 0.3 per cent of "no scalpel" procedures.[7a]

Vasectomy is highly effective once sperm are cleared from the distal vas deferens; however, flushing during surgery does not accelerate clearance of sperm,[9] and additional contraception must continue until azoospermia is demonstrated or at least 10 to 20 ejaculations or 2 to 3 months have passed. Contraceptive failures are rare and are due to failure to await sperm clearance, misidentification or duplication of the vas deferens, or late spontaneous recanalization of the vas deferens (0.1 per cent). Vasectomy causes no consistent changes in circulating reproductive hormones or sexual function and does not increase the risk of cardiovascular, malignant, or other chronic diseases.[10] Sperm antibodies develop in 50 to 75 per cent of vasectomized men but have no deleterious effects on health apart from a controversial role in reducing fertility after vasectomy reversal.

The advantages of vasectomy are that it is quick, simple, highly effective, and convenient if permanent sterilization is sought. The major drawback of vasectomy is its limited reversibility. Elective prevasectomy sperm cryostorage is neither widely available nor reliable fertility insurance. Requests for reversal follow up to 1 per cent of vasectomies, mostly prompted by remarriage or the death of children. Following microsurgical vasovasostomy, between 80 and 100 per cent of men have some sperm return to the ejaculate ("patency"), but normal sperm output is less common and cumulative conception rates are only about 50 per cent. Reversibility is limited by techniques of vasectomy and of vasovasostomy, wife's age, long-term epididymal damage, and sperm antibodies.[11] Since vasectomy reversal is neither cheap, reliable, nor widely available, the intent of vasectomy must be regarded as permanent until more reversible methods supplant those presently used.

Modern Methods

Immunocontraception: Sperm Vaccines

Vaccines to interrupt male fertility by targeting sperm surface epitopes or the hormones regulating spermatogenesis have long been of interest. Sperm first appear during puberty within the immunologically protected adluminal compartment of the seminiferous tubules long after definition of immune self-tolerance, which explains their autoimmunogenicity. Sperm autoimmunity associated with subfertility is observed after vasectomy and among up to 10 per cent of spontaneously infertile men. Sperm autoantibodies have no apparent adverse effects on general health, although focal orchitis involving the rete testis may occur.[12] Experimental immunization of women with human sperm reportedly causes infertility,[13] and male and female guinea pigs immunized with a sperm surface antigen[14] exhibit effective and reversible contraception. Further steps to de-

velop a sperm vaccine include the identification of suitable surface-expressed epitopes that are sperm-specific, adequately immunogenic, and involved in fertilization.[15] Unresolved problems remain over the large antigenic burden in the male genital tract, requiring virtually complete blockade, the variability of individual immune responses, difficulties identifying an effective adjuvant safe for human use, the restricted access of antibodies into the seminiferous tubules and epididymis, and the risks of orchitis or other immune-complex disease. The smaller antigenic burden in the female reproductive tract that must be completely neutralized suggests that a sperm vaccine may be a better prospect for application in women. The improved understanding of molecular physiology of sperm function and fertilization provides new molecular targets, while improved biotechnology can supply target epitopes in unprecedented abundance, greatly improving the technical feasibility of immunological interruption of male fertility.

Chemical (Nonhormonal) Methods

The rapid proliferation of the germinal epithelium makes it highly susceptible to toxins interfering with mitosis and/or meiosis. Numerous chemical and physical cytotoxins, including alkylating drugs,[16] heat,[17] and ionizing irradiation,[18] readily abolish spermatogenesis; however, the associated mutagenic risks due to direct disruption of DNA replication make them undesirable as potentially reversible male contraceptives. Consequently, chemical methods for regulation of male fertility aim to inhibit function of postmeiotic sperm during epididymal transit, where fluid mixing permits sperm exposure to drugs.[19] A model of posttesticular chemical contraceptive is provided by alphachlorohydrin and the chlorosugars, which produced prompt and effective contraception by an irreversible effect on epididymal sperm of rodents[20] but proved too toxic for clinical development. Therapeutic drugs that impair male fertility may have potential for development as male contraceptives, although surveillance of male reproductive side effects is incomplete and unsystematic.[21] Examples include an orally active spermicidal drug concentrated in semen (e.g., ketoconazole congeners[21]) and sulphasalazine, which causes sulphonamide-related, reversible male subfertility, although the exact mechanism remains unclear.[22] Drugs that selectively prevent ejaculation without affecting sexual potency or spermatogenesis could theoretically be useful; however, a safe and effective alpha$_1$-adrenergic blocker that eliminates sperm from the ejaculate has not been developed.[23, 24]

Numerous plant products and natural medicines are reputed to inhibit male fertility and thereby have potential as chemical male contraceptives. The most widely tested is gossypol, a highly reactive polyphenolic yellow pigment identified in China as causing epidemic infertility among workers ingesting raw cottonseed oil. In over 10,000 Chinese men and smaller numbers of non-Chinese men,[25] purified gossypol reduced sperm output to below 4 million/ml in more than 98 per cent within 75 days, with suppression maintained by a lower weekly maintenance dose.[26] Although an effective male contraceptive, the systemic toxicity of gossypol (notably hypokalemia leading to muscular fatigue, paralysis, and arrhythmias) and progressively irreversible spermatogenic damage precluded further development for clinical use. Nevertheless, the contraceptive efficacy of a chemical method able to provide reliable contraception without uniformly inducing azoospermia is encouraging. *Tripterygium wilfordii* (TW) is a widely used traditional Chinese herbal medicine for rheumatoid arthritis and skin disorders, and extracts of TW inhibit fertility and impair sperm output and motility in rodents and men.[27, 28] Chemical studies are under way to determine the active components and whether they have promising posttesticular effects on sperm function.[28]

HORMONAL METHODS

Physiology: Hormonal Regulation of Spermatogenesis

The goal of hormonal male contraception is to suppress sperm production without diminishing androgen supply to the body. Spermatogenesis is pituitary-dependent, requiring secretion of follicle-stimulating hormone (FSH) to stimulate Sertoli cell support of spermatogenesis at full efficiency[29] and luteinizing hormone (LH) to stimulate Leydig cell testosterone secretion for supplying androgen to Sertoli cells in support of spermatogenesis as well as to peripheral androgen-dependent tissues. Testosterone and FSH act synergistically but indirectly to sustain spermatogenesis,[29, 30] since Sertoli cells have hormone receptors but germinal cells do not. Consequently, complete hormonal suppression of spermatogenesis needs to eliminate both FSH and testosterone action on Sertoli cells. Testicular testosterone concentrations are up to 100 times higher than in blood[31] and at least 5 to 10 times higher than the threshold required to maintain spermatogenesis,[32, 33] so eliminating androgenic support of spermatogenesis involves extensive depletion of intratesticular testosterone. Such complete inhibition of LH bioactivity makes concurrent androgen replacement necessary to avoid the systemic consequences of androgen deficiency.[34, 35] Gonadotropin action is most readily abolished by inhibiting pituitary secretion using either sex steroids or gonadotropin-releasing hormone (GnRH) analogues, while testosterone is preferred for androgen replacement. Such hormonal methods employ physiological mechanisms that recapitulate the endocrine events of puberty. Before puberty, pituitary gonadotropin secretion is absent and testes are functionally quiescent, but during puberty, spermatogenesis is initiated by increased gonadotropin and testosterone secretion. Acquired postpubertal gonadotropin deficiency abolishes spermatogenesis, which is readily restored with gonadotropin therapy regardless of the duration of gonadotropin deficiency.[36] The hormonal manipulation of spermatogenesis, therefore, affecting only Sertoli cells directly and employing physiological mechanisms activated normally during puberty (and seasonality in certain mammals[37]), is likely to be readily reversible and free of mutagenic risk.[38–41] This approach is analogous to hormonal contraception in women, in whom anovulation is the goal by analogy with pregnancy, although the degree of gonadotropin suppression required is less for women and abolition of male gamete production is more challenging, because its rate is 10^9 times greater. The recent recognition that hormonal regulation of spermatogenesis by gonadotropins is ampli-

fied by paracrine signaling between Sertoli, Leydig, and peritubular cells[42] may allow development of novel hormonal approaches to inhibit sperm production.

A key strategic issue in the development of hormonal male contraception is defining the minimum degree of suppression of sperm output required. A landmark World Health Organization (WHO) study[41] established that hormonally induced azoospermia is sufficient to provide reliable, reversible male contraception.[41] Consequently hormonal regimens achieving azoospermia uniformly in fertile men would ensure effective male contraception. No regimen yet achieves this (Fig. 137–1), although in some Asian countries (e.g., China,[41] Indonesia[43]), azoospermia rates of 90 to 100 per cent are achieved. To determine whether azoospermia is actually necessary for reliable contraception, further clinical studies are required to quantitate the contraceptive efficacy of severe oligozoospermia. Because the residual sperm of oligozoospermic men, whether spontaneously infertile[44] or during gossypol[26] or hormonal[45, 46] treatment to suppress spermatogenesis, have impaired fertilizing capacity in vivo and/or in vitro, severe oligozoospermia may be sufficient to provide reliable contraception, thereby simplifying the requirements for male contraception. Azoospermia would then be analogous to anovulation, which is sufficient but not necessary (e.g., progestin-only contraceptives[5, 47]) for effective hormonal contraception in women. If, however, severe oligozoospermia does not provide adequate contraceptive efficacy, as implied by observational studies,[48] then azoospermia will be established as a necessary prerequisite for hormonal male contraception.

Steroidal Methods

Androgen Alone

Testosterone has the unique advantage of providing simultaneously the gonadotropin suppression and androgen replacement in a single agent. This simplicity makes it an obvious first choice for a reversible hormonal male contraceptive. Reversible suppression of human spermatogenesis by androgens has long been known,[49–52] but systematic studies of androgens as a sole agent for male contraception only began in the 1970's.[53, 54] Feasibility and dose-finding studies at that time employed the most widely used androgen, testosterone enanthate (TE) in an oil vehicle, as a prototype.[39] When administered intramuscularly at doses of 100 to 200 mg weekly, TE induces azoospermia in most Caucasian men[55]; however, less frequent injections or lower weekly doses failed to sustain suppression.[56–59] Among 271 men in the WHO study having weekly injections of 200 mg TE, which moderately exceeds standard androgen replacement doses,[60] 60 per cent of non-Chinese and 91 per cent of Chinese men became azoospermic,[41] with the remainder having severe oligozoospermia. The differences within and between populations in likelihood of azoospermia are unrelated to body size but may reflect disparities in ethnopharmacology and/or kinetics of spermatogenesis.[41, 41a] As dictated by spermatogenic cycle length, azoospermia is achieved at an average of 4 months, and once attained, it is readily sustained during continuing treatment and reversed after stopping injections, with sperm reappearing at 3 months and normal output returning by 6 months. Dis-

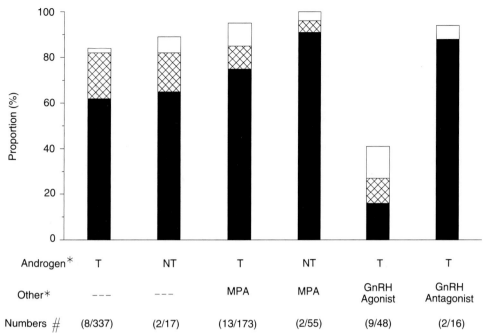

FIGURE 137–1. Percentages of men who become azoospermic *(solid fill)* or severely oligospermic (<1 million per ml *[hatched fill]* or <5 million per ml *[unfilled]*) based on nadir sperm output of healthy fertile men during various hormonal regimens to suppress spermatogenesis (T, testosterone; NT, 19-nortestosterone [nandrolone]; MPA, medroxyprogesterone acetate). Numbers are expressed in parentheses as (number of studies/number of subjects).

continuations during treatment were mainly due to intolerance of weekly injections, while discontinuations for medical side effects followed acne (4 per cent), weight gain (1 per cent), polycythemia (1 per cent), dyslipidemia (1 per cent), and behavioral effects (1 per cent) but not hepatotoxicity or overt prostatic hypertrophy. Administration of testosterone to healthy fertile men increases body weight, lean body mass, hemoglobin and prostate-specific antigen, while testis size and plasma urea decrease, with all changes being reversed after cessation of treatment.[41, 61–66] No significant change in self-reported mood or behavior (including sexuality and aggression) was observed in a placebo-controlled study.[66a]

Long-term androgen administration requires consideration of potential effects on cardiovascular and prostatic disease. No direct relationship between testosterone levels and cardiovascular disease[67, 68] or hypertension[69] has been established to explain the higher prevalence of cardiovascular mortality in men. The effects of androgen administration on plasma lipids are complex. Chronic androgen deficiency in hypogonadal men is associated with increased total and lower high-density lipoprotein (HDL) cholesterol,[70] although acute pharmacological lowering of blood testosterone increases total and HDL cholesterol in eugonadal[71, 72] and hypogonadal[73] men, with changes being normalized by physiological testosterone levels.[73] Most experimental studies of androgenic effects on lipids utilized oral 17 alpha-alkylated anabolic-androgen steroids, which have prominent hepatic toxicity, including the lowering of HDL cholesterol,[66, 74] and would be unsuitable for hormonal male contraception. In contrast, a well-controlled study demonstrated that high-dose testosterone (280 mg TE/week) administration to eugonadal men caused no change in total, HDL, and low-density lipoprotein (LDL) cholesterol, apolipoprotein A-I, triglycerides, insulin, or glucose.[62] Similarly, subdermal testosterone implants and

injectable testosterone enanthate both lowered total, HDL, and LDL cholesterol, whereas triglyceride levels were lowered during physiological testosterone levels achieved by implants but were increased by TE injections.[63] The significance of such pharmacological changes in lipids for long-term cardiovascular disease remains unclear.[75]

The long-term effects of exogenous androgens on the prostate also require monitoring, since prostatic hyperplasia and cancer are both age- and androgen-dependent. Exposure to physiological levels of testosterone in early adulthood is required for prostatic disease to develop during later decades, and prostatic disorders of aging men are androgen-sensitive.[76, 77] The precise relationship of androgens to prostatic disease, however, remains poorly understood, but there is no direct relationship between circulating testosterone levels and the occurrence of prostatic disease.[77, 78] In situ prostate cancer is common in all populations of elderly men, but rates of invasive prostate cancer differ widely between populations with similar blood testosterone levels, suggesting that early exposure to androgens may initiate prostate cancer but that later, androgen-independent environmental factors promote the outbreak of invasive prostate cancer.[76] Therefore, it is likely that maintenance of physiological androgen levels by administration of exogenous testosterone is no more hazardous than endogenous testosterone.[76] Prolonged surveillance, as undertaken for cardiovascular and breast disease in female users of hormonal contraception, would be prudent to monitor both cardiovascular and prostatic disease risk in men receiving exogenous androgens for hormonal contraception.[76a] Extensive experience with androgen use in normal men indicates no consistent changes in mood or behavior,[39, 41, 66a, 79] in contrast with observational studies of athletes and prisoners, in whom psychological preselection makes it difficult to distinguish genuine androgen effects.[79, 80]

The pharmacokinetics of testosterone esters are crucial for testosterone-induced suppression of spermatogenesis. Short-acting testosterone preparations (e.g., oral, transdermal patches, or gels) that might be satisfactory for hypogonadal men are inconvenient or unsuitable for hormonal male contraception (e.g., dermal androgen gels which risk virilizing the female partner through topical androgen transfer[81, 82]), causing dissatisfaction and higher discontinuation rates.[83] Weekly injections of TE required to provide maximal suppression of spermatogenesis[39] are inconvenient and cause supraphysiological blood testosterone levels, which risk greater androgenic side effects and may prevent adequate depletion of intratesticular testosterone required to fully suppress spermatogenesis. Since alternative oil-based testosterone esters have essentially identical kinetics to the enanthate (e.g., cypionate, cyclohexane-carboxylate) or shorter duration of action (e.g., propionate, undecanoate),[84] longer-acting, more convenient depot testosterone preparations which provide physiological testosterone levels for prolonged periods are needed. Testosterone pellets implanted subdermally by trochar provide sustained physiological testosterone levels for up to 6 months,[85, 86] and newer formulations include testosterone-loaded biodegradable microspheres[73, 87] and testosterone buciclate, an aqueous formulated testosterone ester,[88] both having up to 3 months' duration of action. Such depot androgens suppress spermatogenesis faster, at lower doses, and with fewer metabolic side effects than TE injections; however, azoospermia is still not achieved in all men.[63] The testosterone pellets require implantation by trochar under local anesthesia and occasionally extrude,[86] whereas both newer formulations require large injection volumes and microsphere synthesis has interbatch variability and is expensive. Nevertheless, such depot formulations could provide long-acting androgens for hormonal male contraception as well as improved androgen replacement for hypogonadal men.

Synthetic androgens such as methyltestosterone,[89] fluoxymesterone,[90] methandienone,[91] and danazol[92, 93] suppress spermatogenesis, but azoospermia is rarely achieved despite high doses. Numerous synthetic androgens used by athletes in idiosyncratic cocktails and dosage regimens[94, 95] also suppress spermatogenesis reversibility.[91, 95] Most synthetic androgens are 17α-alkylated androgens that are unsuitable for long-term use due to the hepatotoxicity of the 17α-alkyl substituent.[96] Synthetic androgens lacking the 17α-alkyl substituent such as mesterolone are also ineffective at suppressing spermatogenesis[97] although more potent orally active synthetic androgens lacking 17α-alkyl groups[98] might be useful if their safety and efficacy for protracted clinical use, as for male contraception, are established. The most promising synthetic androgen is 19-nortestosterone, which, lacking only the 19-methyl group of testosterone, undergoes only limited aromatization or 5α-reduction while remaining similar in safety and reversibility to testosterone. The hexoxyphenylpropionate ester, suitable for injection at 3-week intervals,[84] produces azoospermia in 88 per cent of whites[99, 100] as a sole agent and warrants further study.

Antiandrogens were proposed to inhibit selectively the epididymal and testicular effects of androgens without impeding their systemic effects.[101] Cyproterone acetate, a steroidal antiandrogen and progestin, suppresses gonadotropin secretion without achieving azoospermia and causes impotence due to androgen deficiency.[102] Pure nonsteroidal antiandrogens lacking androgenic or gestagenic effects such as flutamide, nilutamide, and casodex are ineffective at suppressing spermatogenesis.[103, 104]

Androgen Plus Progestin

Combination steroid regimens use nonandrogenic steroids to suppress gonadotropins in conjunction with testosterone for androgen replacement at lower doses than as a sole agent. In addition to reducing androgenic side effects, minimizing testosterone dosage could improve spermatogenic suppression if high blood testosterone levels counteract the maximal depletion of intratesticular testosterone.[30, 105–108] Although estradiol augments testosterone-induced suppression of primate spermatogenesis[109] and fertility,[110] estrogenic side effects, including gynecomastia and thromboembolism, are unacceptable. In contrast, progestins are potent inhibitors of pituitary gonadotropin secretion with negligible direct effect on spermatogenesis, and suitable long-acting implantation progestin formulations have been developed for female contraception. Used alone, progestins suppress spermatogenesis but cause impotence,[111, 112] so androgen replacement is necessary to avert consequences of androgen deprivation, including sexual dysfunction.[34, 35] Extensive feasibility studies concluded that progestin-androgen combination regimens had promise as hormonal male contraceptives if more potent and durable agents were developed.[39, 113] Studies using newer generations of long-acting implantation progestins such as levonorgestrel butanoate (HRP002) and nonbiodegradable implants of norgestrel (Norplant) or ketodesogestrel (Implanon) are awaited.

The most detailed information on the effects of androgen-progestin regimens is from studies with medroxyprogesterone acetate (MPA) combined with testosterone. Using either monthly injections of both agents or daily oral progestin with dermal androgen gels, azoospermia is attained by about 60 per cent of fertile men of European background, with the remainder having severe oligozoospermia and impaired sperm function.[45, 46] In contrast, virtually all Indonesian men treated with implanted MPA and androgen become azoospermic.[43, 114] Side effects related to the progestins are few, and sexual function is not impaired if the androgen replacement dosage is adequate. The major consistent metabolic effect of progestin-androgen combinations is lowering of HDL cholesterol, while total, LDL, and triglycerides remain unchanged. Following cessation of treatment, spermatogenesis recovers completely but slowly due to prolonged partial gonadotropin suppression arising from sustained low-level MPA release from secondary depots in body fat. Smaller studies of other oral progestins such as norethisterone[82, 83] and levonorgestrel,[115] in combination with testosterone, demonstrate similar efficacy, indicating that the progestin bioactivity and kinetics rather than the specific progestin determine efficacy. A nandrolone ester depot combined with depot MPA has particularly high efficacy for induction of azoospermia in 10 of 12 (84 per cent) European[116] and 44 of 45 (98 per cent) Indonesian[114] men. Overall, the theoretical benefits in safety and efficacy of progestin-androgen combinations over androgens alone await empirical confirmation, but the improved new-generation depot progestins could allow this issue to be clarified definitively.

GnRH Blockade

The pivotal role of gonadotropin-releasing hormone (GnRH) in the hormonal control of testicular function makes it an attractive target for biochemical regulation of male fertility. Inhibition of GnRH action can be achieved either by receptor blockade with synthetic GnRH analogues or by immunoneutralization of GnRH. Elimination of LH and testosterone secretion, however, requires concomitant testosterone replacement.[34, 35] Thousands of potent GnRH analogues with prolonged bioactivity due to enhanced receptor binding and resistance to proteolytic degradation have been developed. The first clinically available GnRH analogues were superactive agonists which have an established therapeutic role for inducing reversible medical castration in sex hormone–dependent diseases. The superactive GnRH agonists initially stimulate but ultimately cause a sustained, paradoxical inhibition of gonadotropin secretion and spermatogenesis due to pituitary GnRH receptor desensitization. This involves both down-regulation of GnRH receptor numbers and uncoupling of GnRH receptor–mediated signal transduction, although GnRH agonists retain partial agonist activity. When combined with testosterone, GnRH agonists partially suppress spermatogenesis but rarely achieve azoospermia,[106–108] being significantly less effective than steroidal regimens. The efficacy of GnRH agonists at spermatogenic suppression is enhanced by continuous infusion or depot implants compared with daily injections and is attenuated by concurrent testosterone administration. In contrast, GnRH antagonists create immediate and sustained competitive blockade of GnRH receptors[117] and are highly effective at suppressing spermatogenesis. Early GnRH antagonists had insufficient potency, suffered from formulation difficulties due to hydrophobicity, and caused local mast cell histamine release, making them unsuitable for clinical use. Newer generations of GnRH antagonists (e.g., Antide [Nal-Lys GnRH], Nal-Glu GnRH, Cetrorelix, detirelix, Gonirelix) with enhanced potency and causing minimal irritation produce rapid, reversible, and complete inhibition of spermatogenesis in monkeys[118–120] and men[121, 122] when combined with delayed testosterone administration. The striking superiority over GnRH agonist regimens may be due to greater inhibition of gonadotropin secretion and/or depletion of intratesticular testosterone. Because of their highly specific site of action and low effective dose, GnRH analogues have few side effects apart from those due to lowered blood testosterone levels and which are prevented by co-administration of testosterone (e.g., gynecomastia, hot flushes). Depot formulations of a GnRH antagonist and testosterone suitable for administration at up to 3-month intervals could therefore be promising as a hormonal male contraceptive regimen. Advantages for the combination in speed, degree, or uniformity of suppression to azoospermia over the simpler androgen-alone regimens are yet to be established.[122a] The drawback might be the high cost of the depot formulation and of nonnatural amino acids used to synthesize the GnRH antagonists.

Immunization against GnRH can intercept GnRH during its passage in the pituitary portal bloodstream from the hypothalamus to the anterior pituitary. Such gonadotropin-selective immunocastration abolishes pituitary gonadotropin secretion, which leads to inhibition of spermatogenesis and testosterone secretion.[123] While such a vaccine would be effective for sterilization of animals, it would require androgen replacement in humans and involves similar problems as other contraceptive vaccines. Pilot studies in men with prostate disease may clarify the safety and feasibility of this approach.[124]

FSH Blockade

Because FSH has specific receptors located only on Sertoli cell membranes, in principle, blockade of FSH bioactivity could selectively inhibit spermatogenesis without interfering with endogenous testosterone production, thereby avoiding the need for co-administration of testosterone. FSH action could be abolished by selective inhibition of pituitary secretion of FSH with inhibin or related peptides[125] or novel steroids,[126] by vaccine immunoneutralization of circulating FSH,[127] or by receptor blockade with peptide FSH antagonists.[128] Selective deficiency of FSH action in primates impairs the numbers[129] and function[127] of ejaculated sperm, so this approach might have promise. Physiologic studies, however, have cast doubt on the potential of blocking FSH action for male contraception.[130] Prolonged active or passive immunoneutralization of FSH in nonhuman primates decreases but fails to halt sperm output, suggesting that even complete FSH blockade might not produce azoospermia consistently in men.[129] This may reflect the importance of intratesticular testosterone in the dual hormonal regulation of Sertoli cell function and suggests that curtailing only FSH may not adequately reduce hormonal drive via Sertoli cells to sustain spermatogenesis. Nevertheless, since FSH-immunized primates are rendered infertile even if still oligozoospermic,[127] the fertilizing capacity of residual sperm may be diminished, and should severe oligozoospermia be adequate for effective hormonal male contraception, then selective inhibition of FSH bioactivity may still have potential as a hormonal method for male contraception. An FSH vaccine could, however, have the limitation that in addition to other drawbacks of contraceptive vaccines, including risks of autoimmune hypophysitis or orchitis,[14] pituitary FSH hypersecretion could overcome the capacity of immune blockade.

REFERENCES

1. United Nations: Levels and Trends of Contraceptive Use as Assessed in 1988. New York, Department of International Economic and Social Affairs, 1989, p 129.
2. Djerassi C: The bitter pill. Science 245:356–361, 1989.
3. Barrett JC, Marshall J: The risk of conception on different days of the menstrual cycle. Population Studies 23:455–461, 1969.
4. Trussell J, Grummer-Strawn L: Contraceptive failure of the ovulation method of periodic abstinence. Fam Planning Perspect 22:65–75, 1990.
5. Trussell J, Kost K: Contraceptive failure in the Unites States: A critical review of the literature. Stud Fam Planning 18:237–283, 1987.
6. Liskin L, Wharton C, Blackburn R, Kestelman P: Condoms—Now More Than Ever. Baltimore, Population Information Program, Center for Communication Programs, The Johns Hopkins University, 1990, p 36.
7. Liskin L, Benoit E, Blackburn R: Vasectomy: New Opportunities. Baltimore, Population Information Program, Johns Hopkins University, Baltimore, 1992, p 24.
7a. Hargreave TB: Towards reversible vasectomy. Int J Androl 15:455–459, 1992.

8. Zhao S-C: Vas deferens occlusion by percutaneous injection of polyurethane elastomer plugs: clinical experience and reversibility. Contraception 41:453–459, 1990.
9. Berthelsen JG: Preoperative irrigation of the vas deferens during vasectomy. Scand J Urol Nephrol 10:100–102, 1976.
10. Petitti DB: Epidemiologic studies of vasectomy. In Zatuchni GI, Goldsmith A, Spieler JM, Sciarra JJ (eds): Male Contraception: Advances and Future Prospects. Philadelphia, Harper & Row, 1986, pp 24–33.
11. Silber SJ: Microsurgery for vasectomy reversal and vasoepididymostomy. In Zatuchni GI, Goldsmith A, Spieler JM, Sciarra JJ (eds): Male Contraception: Advances and Future Prospects. Philadelphia, Harper & Row, 1986, pp 54–69.
12. Hendry WF, Stedronska J, Hughes L, et al: Steroid treatment of male subfertility caused by antisperm antibodies. Lancet 2:498–500, 1979.
13. Baskin MJ: Temporary sterilization by injection of human spermatozoa: A preliminary report. Am J Obstet Gynecol 24:892–897, 1932.
14. Primakoff P, Lanthrop W, Woolman L, et al: Fully effective contraception in male and female guinea pigs immunized with the sperm protein PH-20. Nature 335:543–546, 1988.
15. Aitken RJ, Peterson M, Koothan PT: Risks and benefits of immunological contraception. In Nieschlag E, Habenicht UF (eds): Spermatogenesis Fertilization Contraception: Molecular, Cellular and Endocrine Events in Male Reproduction. Berlin, Springer-Verlag, 1992, pp 461–475.
16. Meistrich ML, Finch M, da Cunha MF, et al: Damaging effects of fourteen chemotherapeutic drugs on mouse testis cells. Cancer Res 42:122–131, 1982.
17. Kandeel FR, Swerdloff RS: Role of temperature in regulation of spermatogenesis and the use of heating as a method for contraception. Fertil Steril 49:1–23, 1988.
18. Meistrich ML, Beek MEABv: Radiation sensitivity of the human testis. Adv Radiat Biol 14:227–268, 1990.
19. Cooper TG: The epididymis as a site of contraceptive attack. In Nieschlag E, Habenicht UF (eds): Spermatogenesis, Fertilization, Contraception: Molecular, Cellular and Endocrine Events in Male Reproduction. Berlin, Springer-Verlag, 1992, pp 419–460.
20. Ford WCL, Waites GMH: Cholorinated sugars: A biochemical approach to the control of male fertility. Int J Androl Suppl 2:541–564, 1978.
21. Vickery BH, Grigg MB, Goodpasture JC, et al: Towards a same-day, orally administered male contraceptive. In Zatuchni GI, Goldsmith A, Spieler JM, Sciarra JJ (eds): Male Contraception: Advances and Future Prospects. Philadelphia, Harper & Row, 1986, pp 271–292.
22. Giwercman A, Skakkebaek NE: The effect of salicylazosulphapyridine (sulphasalazine) on male fertility: A review. Int J Androl 9:38–52, 1986.
23. Hormonnai ZT, Shilon M, Paz GF: Phenoxybenzamine: An effective male contraceptive pill. Contraception 29:479–491, 1984.
24. Kjaergaard N, Kjaergaard B, Lauritsen JG: Prazosin, an adrenergic blocking agent inadequate as male contraceptive pill. Contraception 37:621–629, 1988.
25. Coutinho EM, Melo JF: Clinical experience with gossypol in non-Chinese men. Contraception 37:137–151, 1988.
26. Wu D: An overview of the clinical pharmacology and therapeutic potential of gossypol as a male contraceptive agent and in gynaecological disease. Drugs 38:333–341, 1989.
27. Qian SZ: Tripterygium wilfordii: A Chinese herb effective in male fertility regulation. Contraception 36:335–345, 1987.
28. Waites GMH: Male fertility regulation. In Diczfaluszy E, Griffin PD, Khanna J (eds): Research in Human Reproduction: WHO Biennial Report 1986–87. Geneva, World Health Organization, 1988, pp 199–227.
29. Matsumoto AM, Bremner WJ: Endocrinology of the hypothalamo-pituitary-testicular axis with particular reference to the hormonal control of spermatogenesis. In Burger HG (ed): Clinical Endocrinology and Metabolism. Paris, Balliere's, 1987, pp 71–87.
30. Marshall GR, Wickings EJ, Ludecke DK, Nieschlag E: Stimulation of spermatogenesis in stalk-sectioned rhesus monkeys by testosterone alone. J Clin Endocrinol Metab 57:152–159, 1983.
31. Morse HC, Horike N, Rowley MJ, Heller CG: Testosterone concentrations in testes of normal men: Effects of testosterone propionate administration. J Clin Endocrinol Metab 37:882–886, 1973.
32. Sharpe RM: Testosterone and spermatogenesis. J Endocrinol 113:1–2, 1987.
33. Rommerts FFG: How much androgen is required for maintenance of spermatogenesis? J Endocrinol 116:7–9, 1988.
34. Mooradian AD, Morley JE, Korenman SG: Biological actions of androgens. Endocr Rev 8:1–28, 1987.
35. Nieschlag E, Behre HM (eds): Testosterone: Action Deficiency Substitution. Berlin, Springer-Verlag, 1990, p 285.
36. Burger HG, Baker HWG: Therapeutic considerations and results of gonadotropin treatment in male hypogonadotropic hypogonadism. Ann NY Acad Sci 438:447–453, 1984.
37. Lincoln GA: Seasonal aspects of testicular function. In Burger HG, de Kretser DM (eds): The Testis, 2d ed. New York, Raven Press, 1989, pp 329–385.
38. Ketchell MM: Available clinical data concerning the effects of androgen treatment of men on outcome of subsequent pregnancies. In Patanelli DJ (ed): Hormonal Control of Male Fertility. Bethesda, MD, Department of Health Education and Welfare, 1978, pp 341–392.
39. Patanelli DJ (ed): Hormonal Control of Fertility. Washington, U.S. Department of Health Education and Welfare (NIH 78-1097), 1977, p 420.
40. Mauss J, Borsch G, Richter E, Bormacher K: Demonstration of the reversibility of spermatozoa suppression by testosterone oenanthate. Andrologia 10:149–153, 1978.
41. World Health Organization Task Force on Methods for the Regulation of Male Fertility: Contraceptive efficacy of testosterone-induced azoospermia in normal men. Lancet 336:955–959, 1990.
41a. Wallace EM, Gow SM, Wu FCW: Comparison between testosterone enanthate-induced azoospermia and oligozoospermia in a male contraceptive study I: Plasma luteinizing hormone, follicle stimulating hormone, testosterone, estradiol, and inhibin concentrations. J Clin Endocrinol Metab 77:290–293, 1993.
42. Skinner MK: Cell-cell interactions in the testis. Endocr Rev 12:45–77, 1991.
43. Pangkahila W: Reversible azoospermia induced by an androgen-progestagen combination regimen in Indonesian men. Int J Androl 44:248–256, 1991.
44. Baker HWG: Clinical evaluation and management of testicular disorders in the adult. In Burger HG, de Kretser DM (eds): The Testis, 2d ed. New York, Raven Press, 1989, pp 419–440.
45. Matsumoto AM: Is high dosage testosterone an effective male contraceptive agent? Fertil Steril 50:324–328, 1988.
46. Wu FCW, Aitken RJ: Suppression of sperm function by medroxyprogesterone acetate and testosterone enanthate in steroid male contraception. Fertil Steril 51:691–698, 1989.
47. Trussell J, Hatcher RA, Cates W, et al: Contraceptive failure in the United States: An update. Stud Fam Planning 21:51–54, 1990.
48. Barfield A, Melo J, Coutinho E, et al.: Pregnancies associated with sperm concentrations below 10 million/ml in clinical studies of a potential male contraceptive method monthly depot medroxyprogesterone acetate and testosterone esters. Contraception 20:121–127, 1979.
49. Heckel NJ: Production of oligospermia in a man by the use of testosterone propionate. Proc Soc Exp Biol Med 40:658–659, 1939.
50. McCullagh EP, McGurl FJ: The effects of testosterone propionate on epiphyseal closure, sodium and chloride balance and on sperm counts. Endocrinology 26:377–384, 1940.
51. Heller CG, Nelson WO, Hill IB, et al: Improvement in spermatogenesis following depression of the human testis with testosterone. Fertil Steril 1:415–422, 1950.
52. Heckel NJ, Rosso WA, Kestel L: Spermatogenic rebound phenomenon after administration of testosterone propionate. J Clin Endocrinol 11:235–245, 1951.
53. Reddy PRK, Rao JM: Reversible antifertility action of testosterone propionate in human males. Contraception 5:295–301, 1972.
54. Mauss J, Borsch G, Richter E, Bormacher K: Investigations on the use of testosterone oenanthate as a male contraceptive agent: A preliminary report. Contraception 10:281–289, 1974.
55. Matsumoto AM: Effects of chronic testosterone administration in normal men: Safety and efficacy of high dosage testosterone and parallel dose-dependent suppression of luteinizing hormone, follicle-stimulating hormone and sperm production. J Clin Endocrinol Metab 70:282–287, 1990.
56. Cunningham GR, Silverman VE, Thornby J, Kohler PO: The potential for an androgen male contraceptive. J Clin Endocrinol Metab 49:520–526, 1979.
57. Steinberger E, Smith KD, Rodriguez-Rigau LJ: Suppression and recovery of sperm production in men treated with testosterone enanthate for one year: A study of a possible reversible male contraceptive. Int J Androl Suppl 2:748–760, 1978.
58. Swerdloff RS, Palacios A, McClure RD, et al: Male contraception: Clinical assessment of chronic administration of testosterone enanthate. Int J Androl Suppl 2:731–747, 1978.
59. Paulsen CA: Male contraceptive development: Re-examination of tes-

tosterone enanthate as an effective single entity agent. *In* Patanelli DJ (ed): Hormonal Control of Male Fertility. DHEW Publication No (NIH) 78-1097. Washington, Department of Health Education and Welfare, 1978, pp 17–40.

60. Snyder PJ, Lawrence DA: Treatment of male hypogonadism with testosterone enanthate. J Clin Endocrinol Metab 51:1335–1339, 1980.

61. Gardner FH, Besa EC: Physiologic mechanisms and the hematopoietic effects of the androstanes and their derivatives. Curr Topic Hematol 4:123–195, 1983.

62. Friedl KE, Hannan CJ, Jones RE, Plymate SR: High-density lipoprotein cholesterol is not decreased if an aromatisable androgen is administered. Metabolism 39:69–74, 1990.

63. Handelsman DJ, Conway AJ, Boylan LM: Suppression of human spermatogenesis by testosterone implants in man. J Clin Endocrinol Metab 75:1326–1332, 1992.

64. Palacios A, McClure RD, Campfield LA, Swerdloff RS: Effect of testosterone enanthate on testis size. J Urol 126:46–48, 1981.

65. Welle S, Lozefowicz R, Forbes G, Griggs RC: Effect of testosterone on metabolic rate and body composition in normal men and men with muscular dystrophy. J Clin Endocrinol Metab 74:332–335, 1992.

66. Gooren LJ, Polderman KH: Safety aspects of androgen therapy. *In* Nieschlag E, Behre HM (eds): Testosterone: Action Deficiency Substitution. Berlin, Springer-Verlag, 1990, pp 182–203.

66a. Anderson RA, Bancroft J, Wu FCW: The effects of exogenous testosterone on sexuality and mood of normal men. J Clin Endocrinol Metab 75:1503–1507, 1992.

67. Barrett-Connor E, Khaw KT: Endogenous sex hormones and cardiovascular disease in men: A prospective population-based study. Circulation 78:539–545, 1988.

68. Donohue RP, Barrett-Connor E, Orchard TJ, Gutai JP: Endogenous insulin and sex hormones in atherosclerosis and coronary heart disease. Arteriosclerosis 8:544–548, 1988.

69. Khaw KT, Barrett-Connor E: Blood pressure and endogenous testosterone in men: An inverse relationship. J Hypertens 6:329–332, 1988.

70. Oppenheim DS, George SL, Zervas NT, et al: Elevated serum lipids in hypogonadal men with and without hyperprolactinemia. Ann Intern Med 111:288–292, 1989.

71. Moorjani S, Dupont A, Labrie F: Increase in plasma high-density lipoprotein concentration following complete androgen blockade in men with prostatic carcinoma. Metabolism 36:244–250, 1987.

72. Goldberg RB, Rabin D, Alexander AN, et al: Suppression of plasma testosterone leads to an increase in serum total and high density lipoprotein cholesterol and apolipoproteins A-I and B. J Clin Endocrinol Metab 60:203–207, 1985.

73. Bhasin S, Swerdloff RS, Steiner B, et al: A biodegradable testosterone microcapsule formulation provides uniform eugonadal levels of testosterone for 10–11 weeks in hypogonadal men. J Clin Endocrinol Metab 74:75–83, 1992.

74. Nieschlag E, Wang C, Handelsman DJ, et al (eds): Guidelines for the Use of Androgens in Men. Geneva, Special Programme of Research, Development and Research Training in Human Reproduction of the World Health Organization, 1992.

75. Godsland IF, Wynn V, Crook D, Miller NE: Sex, plasma lipoproteins, and atherosclerosis: Prevailing assumptions and outstanding questions. Am Heart J 114:1467–1503, 1987.

76. Schroeder FH: Androgens and carcinoma of the prostate. *In* Nieschlag E, Behre HM (eds): Testosterone: Action Deficiency Substitution. Berlin, Springer-Verlag, 1990, pp 245–260.

76a. Wallace EM, Pye SD, Wild SR, Wu FCW: Prostate-specific antigen and prostate gland size in men receiving exogenous testosterone for male contraception. Int J Androl 16:35–40, 1993.

77. Krieg M, Tunn S: Androgens and human benign prostatic hyperplasia. *In* Nieschlag E, Behre HM (eds): Testosterone: Action Deficiency Substitution. Berlin, Springer-Verlag, 1990, pp 219–244.

78. Nomura A, Heilbrun LK, Stemmermann GN, Judd HL: Prediagnostic serum hormones and the risk of prostate cancer. Cancer Res 48:3515–3517, 1988.

79. Hubert W: Psychotropic effects of testosterone. *In* Nieschlag E, Behre HM (eds): Testosterone: Action Deficiency Substitution. Berlin, Springer-Verlag, 1990, pp 51–71.

80. Bahrke MS, Yesalis CE, Wright JE: Psychological and behavioural effects of endogenous testosterone levels and anabolic-androgenic steroids among males: A review. Sports Med 10:303–337, 1990.

81. Delanoe D, Fougeyrollas B, Meyer L, Thonneau P: Androgenisation of female partners of men on medroxyprogesterone acetate/percutaneous testosterone contraception. Lancet 1:276, 1984.

82. Guerin JF, Rollet J: Inhibition of spermatogenesis in men using various combinations of oral progestagens and percutaneous or oral androgens. Int J Androl 11:187–199, 1988.

83. Lobel B, Olivo JF, Guille F, D Le Lanou: Contraception in men: Efficacy and immediate toxicity, a study of 18 cases. Acta Urol Belg 57:117–124, 1989.

84. Behre HM, Oberpenning F, Nieschlag E: Comparative pharmacokinetics of androgen preparations: Application of computer analysis and simulation. *In* Nieschlag E, Behre HM (eds): Testosterone: Action Deficiency Substitution. Berlin, Springer-Verlag, 1990, pp 115–135.

85. Handelsman DJ, Conway AJ, Boylan LM: Pharmacokinetics and pharmacodynamics of testosterone pellets in man. J Clin Endocrinol Metab 71:216–222, 1990.

86. Handelsman DJ: Pharmacology of testosterone pellet implants. *In* Nieschlag E, Behre HM (eds): Testosterone: Action Deficiency Substitution. Berlin, Springer-Verlag, 1990, pp 136–154.

87. Burris AS, Ewing LL, Sherins RJ: Initial trial of slow-release testosterone microspheres in hypogonadal men. Fertil Steril 50:493–497, 1988.

88. Behre HM, Nieschlag E: Testosterone buciclate (20 Aet-1) in hypogonadal men: Pharmacokinetics and pharmacodynamics of the new long-acting androgen ester. J Clin Endocrinol Metab 75:1204–1210, 1992.

89. McCullagh EP, Rossmiller HR: Methyl testosterone: I. Androgenic effects and production of gynecomastia and oligospermia. J Clin Endocrinol 1:496–502, 1941.

90. Jones TM, Fang VS, Landau RL, Rosenfield RL: The effects of fluoxymesterone administration on testicular function. J Clin Endocrinol Metab 44:121–129, 1977.

91. Holma PK: Effects of an anabolic steroid (metandienone) on spermatogenesis. Contraception 15:151–162, 1977.

92. Skoglund RD, Paulsen CA: Danazol-testosterone combination: A potentially effective means for reversible male contraception. A preliminary report. Contraception 7:357–365, 1973.

93. Sherins RJ, Gandy HM, Thorslund TW, Paulsen CA: Pituitary and testicular function studies: I. Experience with a new gonadal inhibitor, 17α-pregn-4-en-20-yno-(2,3-D) isoxazol-17-ol (Danazol). J Clin Endocrinol 32:522–531, 1971.

94. Wilson JD: Androgen abuse by athletes. Endocr Rev 9:181–199, 1988.

95. Knuth UA, Maniera H, Nieschlag E: Anabolic steroids and semen parameters in bodybuilders. Fertil Steril 52:1041–1047, 1989.

96. Ishak KG, Zimmerman HJ: Hepatotoxic effects of the anabolic-androgenic steroids. Sem Liver Dis 7:230–236, 1987.

97. Schellen TNCM, Beek JMJHA: The influence of high doses of mesterolone on the spermiogram. Fertil Steril 23:712–714, 1972.

98. Avery MA, Tanabe M, Crowe DF, et al: Synthesis and testing of 17αgb-hydroxy-7α methyl-D-homoestra-4, 16-dien-3-one: A highly potent orally active androgen. Steroids 55:59–64, 1990.

99. Knuth UA, Behre H, Belkien L, et al: Clinical trial of 19-nortestosterone hexoxyphenylpropionate (Anadur) for male fertility regulation. Fertil Steril 44:814–821, 1985.

100. Schurmeyer T, Knuth UA, Belkein L, Nieschlag E: Reversible azoospermia induced by the anabolic steroid 19-nortestosterone. Lancet 1:417–420, 1984.

101. Prasad MRN, Singh SP, Rajalakshmi M: Fertility control in male rat by continuous release of microquantities of cyproterone acetate from subcutaneous silastic capsules. Contraception 2:165–178, 1970.

102. Wang C, Yeung KK: Use of low-dosage oral cyproterone acetate as a male contraceptive. Contraception 21:245–272, 1980.

103. Chandolia RK, Weinbauer GF, Simoni M, et al: Comparative effects of chronic administration of the non-steroidal antiandrogens flutamide and casodex on the reproductive system of the male rat. Acta Endocrinol (Copenh) 125:547–555, 1991.

104. Dhar JD, Sety BS: Effect of a nonsteroidal antiandrogen, anadron, on the reproductive system and fertility in male rats. Contraception 42:121–138, 1990.

105. Frick J, Aulitzky W: Effects of potent LHRH agonist on the pituitary gonadal axis with and without testosterone substitution. Urol Res 14:261–264, 1986.

106. Bouchard P, Garcia E: Influence of testosterone substitution on sperm suppression by LHRH agonists. Horm Res 28:175–180, 1987.

107. Lunn SF, Dixson AF, Sandow J, Fraser HM: Pituitary-testicular function is suppressed by an LHRH antagonist but not by an LHRH agonist in the marmoset monkey. J Endocrinol 125:233–239, 1990.

108. Behre HM, Nashan D, Hubert W, Nieschlag E: Depot gonadotropin-releasing hormone agonist blunts the androgen-induced suppression of spermatogenesis in a clinical trial of male contraception. J Clin Endocrinol Metab 74:84–90, 1992.

109. Ewing LL, Cochran RC, Adams RJ, et al: Testis function in rhesus monkeys treated with a contraceptive steroid formulation. Contraception 27:347–362, 1983.
110. Lobl TJ, Kirton KT, Forbes AD, et al: Contraceptive efficacy of testosterone-estradiol implants in male rhesus monkeys. Contraception 27:383–389, 1983.
111. Frick J, Danner C, Joos H, et al: Spermatogenesis in men treated with subcutaneous application of levonorgestrel and estrone rods. J Androl 2:1981.
112. Heller CG, Moore DJ, Paulsen CA, et al: Effects of progesterone and synthetic progestins on the reproductive physiology of normal men. Fed Proc 18:1057–1064, 1959.
113. Schearer SB, Alvarez-Sanchez F, Anselmo J, et al: Hormonal contraception for men. Int J Androl Suppl 2:680–712, 1978.
114. World Health Organization Task Force on Methods for the Regulation of Male Fertility: Indonesian Multicenter Study: Comparison of Testosterone Enanthate plus DMPA and 19-Nortestosterone Hexoxyphenyl Propionate plus DMPA for Male Contraception. Unpublished manuscript, 1993.
115. Foegh M: Evaluation of steroids as contraceptives in men. Acta Endocrinol Suppl (Copenh) 260:1–48, 1983.
116. Knuth UA, Yeung CH, Nieschlag E: Combination of 19-nortestosterone hexoxyphenylpropionate (Anadur) and depot medroxyprogesterone acetate (Clinovir) for male contraception. Fertil Steril 51:1011–1018, 1989.
117. Marshall GF, Akhtar FB, Weinbauer GF, Nieschlag E: Gonadotrophin-releasing hormone (GnRH) overcomes GnRH antagonist–induced suppression of LH secretion in primates. J Endocrinol 110:145–150, 1986.
118. Bremner WJ, Bagatell CJ, Steiner RA: Gonadotropin-releasing hormone antagonist plus testosterone: a potential male contraceptive. J Clin Endocrinol Metab 73:465–469, 1991.
119. Weinbauer GF, Surmann FJ, Nieschlag E: Suppression of spermatogenesis in a non-human primate (Macaca fascicularis) by concomitant gonadotrophin-releasing hormone antagonist and testosterone treatment. Acta Endocrinol (Copenh) 114:138–146, 1987.
120. Weinbauer GF, Khurshid S, Findscheidt U, Nieschlag E: Sustained inhibition of sperm production and inhibin secretion by a gonadotrophin-releasing hormone antagonist and delayed testosterone substitution in non-human primates (Macaca fascicularis). Acta Endocrinol (Copenh) 123:303–310, 1989.
121. Tom L, Bhasin S, Salameh W, et al: Induction of azoospermia in normal men with combined Nal-Glu GnRH antagonist and testosterone enanthate. J Clin Endocrinol Metab 75:476–483, 1992.
122. Pavlou SN, Brewer K, Farley MG, et al: Combined administration of a gonadotropin-releasin hormone antagonist and testosterone in men induces reversible azoospermia without loss of libido. J Clin Endocrinol Metab 73:1360–1369, 1991.
122a. Bagatell CJ, Matsumoto AM, Christensen RB, et al: Comparison of a gonadotropin releasing hormone antagonist plus testosterone (T) versus T alone as potential male contraceptive regimens. J Clin Endocrinol Metab 77:427–432, 1993.
123. Giri DK, Jayaraman S, Neelaram GS, et al: Prostatic hypoplasia in bonnet monkeys following active immunization with semisynthetic anti-LHRH vaccine. Exp Mol Pathol 54:255–264, 1991.
124. Talwar GP, Raghupathy R: Anti-fertility vaccines. Vaccine 7:97–101, 1989.
125. Burger HG: Inhibin. Reprod Med Rev 1:1–20, 1992.
126. Wiebe JP, Wood PH: Selective suppression of follicle-stimulating hormone by 3-alpha-hydroxy-4-pregnen-20-one, a steroid found in Sertoli cells. Endocrinology 120:2259–2264, 1987.
127. Moudgal NR: The immunobiology of follicle-stimulating hormone and inhibin: Prospects for a contraceptive vaccine. Curr Opin Immunol 2:736–742, 1989-90.
128. Noort MH-v, Puijk WC, Schaaper WMM, et al: Development of antagonists and agonists of follicle stimulating hormone. In Nieschlag E, Habenicht UF (eds): Spermatogenesis Fertilization Contraception: Molecular, Cellular and Endocrine Events in Male Reproduction. Berlin, Springer-Verlag, 1992, pp 33–55.
129. Matsumoto AM, Karpas AE, Bremner WJ: Chronic human chorionic gonadotropin administration in normal men: Evidence that follicle stimulating hormone is necessary for the maintenance of quantitatively normal spermatogenesis in man. J Clin Endocrinol Metab 62:1184–1192, 1986.
130. Nieschlag E: Reasons for abandoning immunization against FSH as an approach to male fertility regulation. In Zatuchni GI, Goldsmith A, Spieler JM, Sciarra JJ (eds): Male Contraception: Advances and Future Prospects. New York, Harper & Row, 1986, pp 395–400.

138

Endocrinology of the Prostate and of Benign Prostatic Hyperplasia

A. WAYNE MEIKLE

The prostate gland is an accessory organ of reproduction in the male. It incudes glandular, stromal, and muscle tissue. Two well-defined muscular layers are integral structures of the gland.[1-4] One layer consists of both involuntary and striated muscle and extends from the detrusor muscle above to the external sphincter below. A second fibromuscular structure with involuntary muscle fiber encircles the upper half of the urethra that extends through the gland. It is contiguous with the deep trigone and internal sphincter and extends to the level of the verumontanum. This is the preprostatic sphincter, and its closure prevents reflux of the ejaculate by closing the upper prostatic urethra.[1-3]

The glandular structures are both posterior and lateral to the urethra. The glandular elements are separated above the verumontanum by the preprostatic sphincter and lie behind the layer of striated and involuntary muscle encircling the anterior aspect of the gland. This anterior investment of the gland is quite stable throughout life. In contrast, the glandular parenchyma changes during development, maturation, and aging. The preprostatic sphincter is involved in the development of benign prostatic hyperplasia.[1-3, 5, 6]

ORIGIN AND DEVELOPMENT OF THE PROSTATE

The prostate starts as a growth from the urogenital sinus.[4] The prostatic and penile urethra is derived from the urogenital sinus endoderm below the level of the müllerian tubercle. Above the müllerian tubercle there is interaction between the epithelium from the urogenital sinus and the mesonephric and paramesonephric ducts, and it gives rise to the prostatic utricle and primitive ducts.[2]

In postpubertal males, there is branching of ducts, development of new gland buds, followed by acini formation within fibromuscular stroma. The adult gland has several identifiable zones or areas with separate groups of glands: periurethral, central zone, peripheral zone, and transitional zone[2] (Figs. 138–1 and 138–2). The peripheral zone is the largest portion and makes up about 75 per cent of the gland, and the central zone makes up about 25 per cent.[1-3] The peripheral zone is the predominant site for the development of prostatic cancer. The periurethral glands and the transitional zone are small in early adult life. They are the site for the later development of benign prostate hyperplasia (BPH).[1, 2]

The weight of the prostate gland increases rapidly during puberty, as shown in Figure 138–3. It weighs approximately 1 g at birth, increases to 4 g at puberty, and grows to about 20 g by age 20.[7-9] The growth parallels the changes in plasma concentrations of testosterone.[9]

NATURAL HISTORY OF BENIGN PROSTATE HYPERPLASIA (BPH)

The natural history of BPH has been reconstructed from autopsy studies. After reaching a size of about 20 g in association with the growth spurt during puberty because of the rise in androgen secretion, the size of the prostate remains quite constant until about age 45.[4, 7, 9] The renewed growth spurt then begins and results in a mean weight of about 50 g by age 70 in men with BPH.[7-9] The rise in

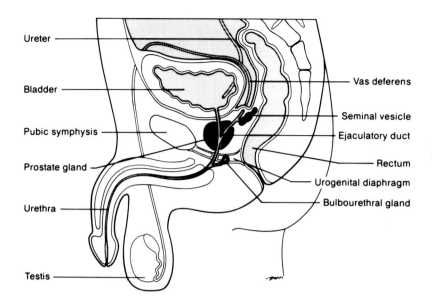

FIGURE 138–1. Normal human anatomy of male reproductive system.

weight with aging is mainly the consequence of growth in the periurethral tissues[4] (Fig. 138–4). There is some discrepancy between the autopsy and clinical incidence of BPH[8–10] (Fig. 138–5). The autopsy incidence of BPH exceeds the clinical incidence by several percentages.[8, 9] There is also a discrepancy between prostatic size and symptoms of urinary obstruction. If tissue in the periurethral area enlarges, it may cause compression of the urethra and surrounding prostate tissue before a striking increase in prostate weight can be documented clinically.

Small nodules that are a "precursor" for clinical BPH are seen by microscopic analysis in prostates of men after age 30.[4] The sites of predilection for these early nodules include only about 2 per cent of the prostate's total mass[4] (Fig. 138–6). The medial transitional zone is the area with most of the early nodules. This area is within or immediately next to the preprostatic sphincter and directly lateral or somewhat ventral to the urethral lumen. The density of the nodules is greater distally near the base of the verumontanum than proximally toward the bladder neck.

Stroma of the periurethral area is the next most common site for early nodule formation. These nodules occur with about equal frequency around the urethral lumen.[4]

In prostates of older men, the BPH nodules are larger and more numerous than in younger men, but the anatomical focus for the nodules is similar between the older and younger age groups.[4] There is a histological difference between nodules developing in the periurethral area and those in the transitional zone.[4, 5] Most nodules in the periurethral area are largely stromal in character and have a few small glands penetrating from the periphery. In contrast, in large nodules, glandular tissue predominates over stroma that consists of mature smooth muscle. The glandular tissue of these nodules is derived from small duct branches that grow into adjacent stroma.[4]

Small glandular and stromal nodules can be seen in the transitional and periurethral zones even in men in the fourth decade but rarely cause symptoms.[4] Their numbers increase in a linear progression with age, and larger nodules are observed in many prostates in the seventh decade.

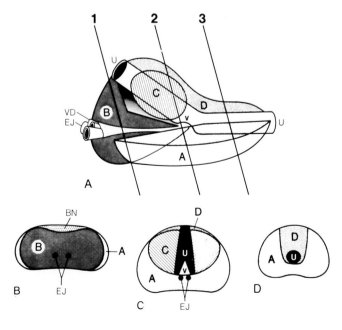

FIGURE 138–2. Schema of areas of the prostate. (A, peripheral zone; B, central zone; C, transitional zone; D, anterior fibromuscular stroma; EJ, ejaculatory ducts; v, verumontanum; VD, vas deferens; U, urethra). (Modified from Stamey TA, Hodge KK: Ultrasound visualization of prostate anatomy and pathology. Monogr Urol 9(3):56, 1988.)

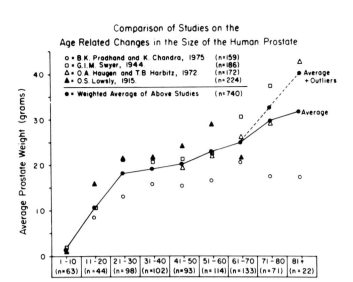

FIGURE 138–3. Age-related changes in prostate size in men. (From Walsh PC: Human benign prostatic hyperplasia: Etiological considerations. Prog Clin Biol Res 145:2, 1984.)

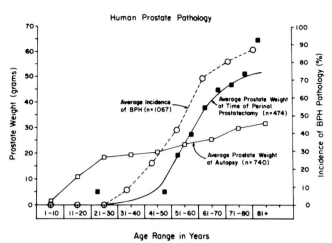

FIGURE 138–5. Age-related incidence of human prostatic hyperplasia. (From Walsh PC: Human benign prostatic hyperplasia: Etiological considerations. Prog Clin Biol Res 145:2, 1984.)

Between the seventh and eighth decades, there is an abrupt increase in the numbers of prostates with large nodules.[4] In the early and late phases of nodule evolution, the glandular nodules are larger than the stromal nodules, and in the later decades of life, this difference becomes accentuated. Prostate-specific antigen (PSA) is synthesized in epithelium of both BPH and prostate cancer.[11-15]

THEORIES OF PATHOGENESIS OF BPH

The pathogenesis of BPH is unknown,[9] but several theories have been proposed. They include roles for sex steroids, growth factors,[16-18] stem cells[19-21] and stromal-epithelial interactions,[22-23] hormonal imprinting,[24] insulin,[25] and prolactin.[26] Our studies[27-29] proved that plasma sex steroids and parameters of androgen action in men are influenced by familial (both genetic and common environmental influences) factors. It is unknown whether some of these factors cause prostate growth and BPH. Men develop BPH

at different ages, and some never develop the disease, suggesting that there are genetic and environmental differences in development of the disease.

Models of BPH

Excessive hormone stimulation by sequential administration of dihydrotestosterone (DHT) or 3α-androstanediol with or without estrogen resulted in a high percentage of BPH in dogs.[30, 31] The mechanism for the development of the neoplastic response to excessive sex steroid stimulation is unknown. Estrogen increases androgen receptor content of the prostate of dogs treated with androgen.[32]

Inhibitors of aromatase reduced estrogen concentrations in sera of humans and experimental animals without altering testosterone and DHT levels.[33] In the dog BPH model, an aromatase inhibitor blocks the hyperplasia produced by treatment with androstenedione. This steroid is an effective precursor for both testosterone and estrone.[34] Androstenedione administration restores prostate growth after castration according to Habenicht and El Etreby[35] (Fig. 138–7). An aromatase inhibitor markedly decreased the stromal growth without affecting overall prostate size. However, the antiandrogen cyproterone acetate markedly decreased prostate size by reducing epithelial cell growth in

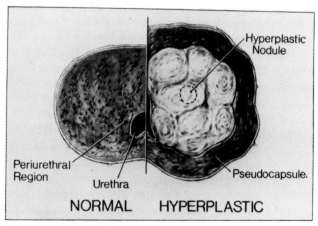

FIGURE 138–4. The periurethral origin of prostatic hyperplasia. (From Wilson JD: The pathogenesis of benign prostatic hyperplasia. Am J Med 68:746, 1980.)

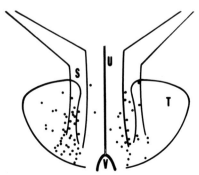

FIGURE 138–6. Periurethral and transitional origin of human BPH nodules. (From McNeal JE: Origin and evolution of benign prostatic enlargements. Invest Urol 15:340, 1978. © by Williams & Wilkins, 1978.)

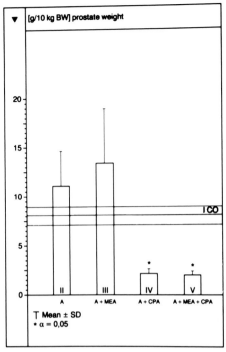

FIGURE 138–7. Androstenedione induction of BPH in dogs (*MEA* = 1-methyl-androsta-1,4-diene-3,17-dione, and *CPA* = cyproterone acetate). (From Habenicht U-F, El Etreby MF: Selective inhibition of androstenedione-induced prostate growth in intact beagle dogs. Prostate 14:309–322, 1989.)

response to androstenedione. These results suggest that androgen controls growth of epithelial tissue and estrogen markedly affects stromal growth. Since some BPH tissue in humans has more stromal than epithelial elements, estrogen may be important in the pathogenesis of BPH in humans. Treatment to reduce estrogen effects may therefore lead to the overall reduction of prostate size in men with BPH.

Prins[36] studied the effects of estrogen administration on adult rat prostate development. Prostate size was reduced in adults treated neonatally with estrogen. This inhibition of adult prostate growth could not be reversed by concomitant administration of androgen. The hypoplastic prostate lobes exhibited a relative increase in stromal tissue. Androgen receptor concentrations also were reduced in the ventral and dorsal prostate lobes by estrogen therapy.

HORMONAL REGULATION OF NORMAL GROWTH OF THE PROSTATE

Androgens secreted by the testes have the most prominent role in differentiation and growth of the prostate throughout life.[7, 10] Other hormones will modify growth of the epithelium and the gland. Estrogen alone causes metaplasia of the epithelium.[5, 6] Prolactin,[37] estrogen,[5, 6, 38, 39] insulin,[25, 40] and perhaps other growth factors[41] may increase the actions of androgens on growth of the gland. Gonadotropins, gonadotropin-releasing hormone, and drugs affecting their normal secretion have a role in modifying normal prostate growth, primarily by controlling androgen secretion by the Leydig cells,[42, 43] but also by direct inhibitory effects on prostate epithelial cells.[44] Adrenal an-

drogens and estrogens produced in peripheral tissues from androgen precursors have only modest effects in stimulating normal growth of the gland.[45]

5α-Reductase localized primarily in the nuclei of the prostate cells transforms testosterone to 5α-dihydrotestosterone (DHT).[46, 47] DHT binds to a nuclear androgen receptor and results in growth of gland tissue.[7] There is indirect evidence in humans that DHT is the major androgen producing normal growth of the prostate.[7] Castration or hypogonadism before puberty prevents secondary growth of the gland, indicating that testicular androgen secretion has a crucial role in the growth spurt.[7, 10] In genetic males with testicular feminization syndrome because of a defect in androgen receptors, the prostate is undeveloped.[48] Patients with 5α-reductase deficiency secrete near-normal quantities of testosterone at puberty but have a marked reduction in tissue formation of DHT.[49] The small prostate glands in these patients suggest that DHT rather than testosterone is the major androgen inducing growth of the gland.[50, 51] Administration of DHT will stimulate growth of the gland in patients with 5α-reductase deficiency. This shows that these patients have normal androgen responsiveness of the gland without an androgen receptor defect. These observations and those on the metabolism of adrenal androgens, such as DHEA and androstanediol to DHT, suggest that the action of androgens on growth of the gland is via their conversion to DHT.[45, 52]

The tissue content of androgens does not parallel the circulating levels of sex steroids.[53, 54] The predominant androgen in normal prostate is DHT, and the intranuclear concentration exceeds the levels observed in other subcellular fractions such as cytosol, microsomes, and mitochondria.[55, 56] There may be two major reasons for the nuclear accumulation of DHT: the localization of 5α-reductase and androgen receptors in nuclei. A regional difference between the periurethral tissue and the peripheral zone was reported by Sitteri et al.,[57] who reported that the periurethral tissue had a two- to three-fold higher concentration of DHT than the peripheral zone.

HORMONAL REGULATION OF BPH

Testicular androgens play an important role in the development of BPH.[7, 10] Early castration prevents the development of BPH.[10] The regression of BPH seen following surgical or medical castration or after antiandrogen therapy[58, 59] supports the hypothesis that endocrine factors participate in the pathogenesis of the disease. It is unclear whether androgens have a causal or permissive role in its occurrence. Testosterone and androstenedione are the major precursors, respectively, for estradiol and estrone that are formed by an aromatase present in many tissues.[60–62] These estrogens may contribute to the overgrowth of stromal elements that compose BPH lesions.[33, 34]

Sex Steroid Abnormalities in BPH

Circulating levels of sex steroids have been compared in men with BPH and younger controls and age-matched control subjects. The effect of aging on sex steroid concentrations makes comparison of data in normal younger men

TABLE 138–1. CORRELATION OF 23 SERUM HORMONAL FACTORS WITH AGE AND BPH VOLUME IN 64 MEN AGES 42–71 YEARS

HORMONAL FACTORS		VS. AGE		VS. BPH VOLUME		VS. BPH VOLUME (AGE CORRECTED)	
	Steroid	R	P	R	P	R	P
C 19	Testosterone	0.09	NS	0.03	NS	−0.02	NS
	Free testosterone	−0.28	0.03	0.03	NS	0.25	0.02
	Dihydrotestosterone	0.09	NS	0.09	NS	0.15	NS
	Androstenedione	−0.45	0.0002	−0.27	0.03	−0.1	NS
	DHA	−0.44	0.0003	−0.20	NS	−0.02	NS
	DHAS	−0.47	0.0001	−0.21	NS	−0.02	NS
	Δ-androstenediol	−0.33	0.0008	−0.11	NS	0.03	NS
	Androstanediol glucuronide	−0.22	NS	−0.11	NS	−0.03	NS
	Etiocholanolone	−0.1	NS	0.008	NS	0.06	NS
C 18	Estrone	−0.22	NS	−0.22	NS	−0.15	NS
	Estradiol	−0.05	NS	0.19	NS	0.24	<0.05
	Estriol	0.03	NS	0.24	0.05	0.26	<0.05
C 21	Cortisol	−0.12	NS	−0.22	NS	0.19	NS
	Progesterone	−0.19	NS	−0.06	NS	0.02	NS
	Pregnenolone	0.06	NS	0.02	NS	0.04	NS
	17-Hydroxyprogesterone	−0.14	NS	−0.08	NS	−0.02	NS
	17-Hydroxypregnenolone	−0.26	0.04	−0.17	NS	−0.07	NS
	Polypeptide						
	SHBG	0.25	0.05	0.04	NS	−0.07	NS
	CBG	0.06	NS	−0.19	NS	−0.24	<0.05
	LH	0.31	0.02	0.09	NS	−0.03	NS
	FSH	0.28	0.03	−0.06	NS	−0.20	NS
	Prolactin	−0.04	NS	−0.09	NS	−0.08	NS
	TSH beta	0.18	NS	0.16	NS	0.09	NS

and older men with BPH a problem.[63–67] Two clinical findings support the role of androgens and estrogens in the development of BPH. One was reported by Partin et al.,[68] who found that patients with larger volumes of BPH tissue, corrected for influences of age, had higher serum free testosterone, estradiol, and estriol concentrations. BPH volume, excised during radical prostatectomy, also correlated positively ($r = 0.42$) with age (Table 138–1). The second is that as men age, prostate size parallels the known increase in the ratio of estrogen to testosterone concentrations.[64–66, 69–72] Free testosterone levels decline, and estrogen levels rise.[68] The alteration in metabolism of testosterone and estrogens as men age could be controlled by both genetic and environmental factors.[27]

The concentrations of DHT have been reported to be normal or elevated in men with BPH as compared with age-matched controls.[73–76] The prostate secretes DHT, but this is apparently not the major source of plasma DHT in men with BPH.[77] The ratio of testosterone to DHT is abnormally low in men with the BPH.[73, 74] Horton and co-workers[78] showed that men with BPH have a reduced conversion of DHT to 3α-androstanediol as the major explanation for the elevation of plasma DHT concentrations.[54] DHT production rates are not elevated. Plasma 3α-androstanediol concentrations have been reported as either normal or elevated in men with BPH.[54, 74, 79]

In patients with BPH, other results of hormone levels also have been reported: Serum testosterone has been reported as increased,[73, 74, 76, 80–82] decreased,[73, 78] or unchanged[74, 81, 83, 84]; free testosterone as increased[76, 80]; DHT levels as elevated[73, 74, 76, 78, 81, 83]; DHEA values as increased[84] or unchanged[81]; estradiol concentrations as elevated,[68] decreased,[83] or unchanged[76, 81, 84]; 17-hydroxyprogesterone as increased,[81] decreased,[83] or unchanged[76]; and follicle-stimulating hormone (FSH) and luteinizing hormone (LH) as unchanged.[74] In addition, an elevated ratio of estradiol to testosterone[82, 85] and of estradiol to free testosterone,[86] higher than normal concentrations of unconjugated androstanediol,[87] and excessive excretion rates of estrogen in the urine have been reported.[88, 89]

Sex Steroid Metabolism in the Prostate

Figure 138–8 shows some pathways of sex steroid metabolism in prostate tissue of humans. In BPH tissue, the reductive pathway for metabolism of androgens predominates over the oxidative. The activity of the 5α-reductase is higher in BPH than in normal tissue of humans, and 3α-oxidoreductase is lower than normal.[90] About 30 years ago, Farnsworth and Brown[91] showed that testosterone was mainly converted to dihydrotestosterone in BPH tissue. 5β-Reductase also has been shown, but its activity is much less than for the 5α-reductase.[46, 90, 92–97] Although there is some controversy about an alteration of enzyme activity in BPH, there is agreement on the distribution of enzyme activity

PATHWAYS OF SEX-STEROID METABOLISM

17 β-Hydroxysteroid Dehydrogenase

Estrone (E₁) ⟷ Estradiol-17β (E₂)

↑   ↑ Aromatase

Δ4 Androstenedione ⟷ Testosterone

↓   ↓ 5α-Reductase

5α-Androstanedione ⟷ Dihydrotestosterone (DHT)

↕   ↕ 3α-Oxidoreductase

Androsterone ⟷ 3α-Androstanediol (3α-diol)

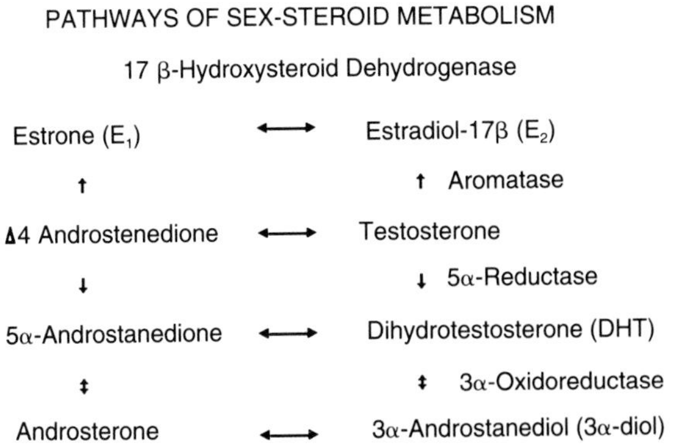

FIGURE 138–8. Pathways of metabolism of sex steroids.

in stromal and epithelial cells. The 5α-reductase activity is higher in stroma than in the epithelium of BPH tissue.

17β-Hydroxysteroid dehydrogenases are oxidoreductases.[93, 96, 98–100] They can interconvert androstenedione and testosterone, 5α-androstanedione and 5α-dihydrotestosterone, and androsterone and 3α-androstanediol, respectively. These enzymes occur in cytosol, microsomes, and mitochondria.[90, 93, 95, 96, 98, 101–103] In BPH and normal prostate compared with prostate cancer, reduced androgens are favored over the oxidized androgens. The high activity of this enzyme and that of the 5α-reductase contribute to the accumulation of DHT in normal and BPH tissue.

The 3α-hydroxysteroid oxidoreductase interconverts dihydrotestosterone and 3α-androstanediol.[104, 105] In BPH tissue as compared with normal prostate, the equilibrium of the enzyme reactions favors the formation of DHT over 3α-androstanediol. The activity of this enzyme also results in accumulation of DHT in BPH tissue compared with normal. This enzyme rapidly converts exogenous 3α-androstanediol to dihydrotestosterone and apparently accounts for the high androgen action of 3α-androstanediol reported in bioassays. Bruchovsky et al.[106] reported that the distribution of 3α(3β)-hydroxysteroid oxidoreductase is almost evenly divided between the stroma and epithelium.[107] No receptor has been identified with a high binding constant for 3α-androstanediol, as has been shown for dihydrotestosterone.

The prostate also has enzymes that can convert dehydroepiandrosterone and Δ5-androstenediol to testosterone, but these steroids are minor precursors for dihydrotestosterone. 3α- and 3β-androstanediols are converted to triols by 6α- and 7α-hydroxylase enzymes.[108] Schweikert[109] also found that fibroblasts cultured from BPH tissue can form estrogen from androstenedione.

Tissue Levels of Sex Steroids in Stroma and Epithelium of BPH

Measurements of hormones within the gland could provide more accurate assessment of the hormonal environment in the gland than circulating levels of hormone. The tissue concentrations of DHT are about 5 ng/g of tissue in both normal and BPH tissue, and its content is higher than testosterone and androstenedione.[57, 110] Nuclei from both normal and BPH tissue have higher concentrations of DHT than cytosol.[55] Although total tissue DHT concentrations may not be elevated in BPH tissue,[110] the nuclear content of DHT is higher in BPH tissue than in normal prostate. Nuclear androgen receptor concentrations are elevated in BPH tissue.[111, 112] Thus DHT may have an important role in the development of BPH.

The interaction between stromal and epithelial elements in the development of BPH growth has been a major focus of research.[89, 113, 114] DHT concentrations are slightly higher in epithelium than stroma in both normal and hyperplastic prostate tissue.[114–117]

In the studies of Bruchovsky et al.[118] in human prostate tissue, no increase was found in DHT concentrations of stroma despite the higher 5α-reductase activity in stroma compared with epithelium. The isoenzymes for the 5α-reductases are different between stroma and epithelium. Thus BPH stromal tissue has higher than normal 5α-reductase activity without excessive accumulation of DHT. When

the plasma concentrations of testosterone, DHT, 3α-androstanediol, and estradiol are expressed as nanomoles per liter and tissue levels of the steroids are expressed in nanomoles per kilogram wet weight, the ratio of tissue to plasma concentrations is less than 1 for testosterone, slightly greater than 1 for 3α-androstanediol and estradiol, and about 10 for DHT[53] (Fig. 138–9). Therefore, testosterone values are higher in plasma than in prostatic tissue, and the reverse is seen for the other three steroids.

In BPH tissue, estrogen is mainly associated with stroma rather than epithelium[92, 119] but there are no observations showing any differences in concentrations of the receptor between normal and BPH tissue. In human BPH tissue, a negative correlation has been observed between DHT or 3α-androstanediol and estradiol. Both estradiol concentrations and receptors correlated significantly with the presence of stromal elements. These observations support the postulate that estradiol may have a role in stromal growth associated with the development of BPH.

Relative Composition of Epithelium and Stroma in BPH

The proportion of epithelial to stromal cells within the prostate varies among species. In the rat and dog, the ratio of epithelium to stroma is high, about 5:1. In primates, the ratio is about equal, but in humans, 70 to 82 per cent of the prostate is composed of stroma, 20 to 30 per cent glandular elements, and less than 10 per cent epithelia and acinar lumina (Fig. 138–10). Androgen deficiency produced by castration leads to a disproportionate reduction in epithelial cells compared with stromal cells in rat prostate.[120, 121] Further, androgen deprivation results in a much greater reduction in distal ductal epithelium than in the proximal epithelium.[122] Thus, after castration, the number of androgen-independent stromal and basal epithelial cells is increased compared with the number of those in the intact male.

The composition of stromal and epithelial cells in hu-

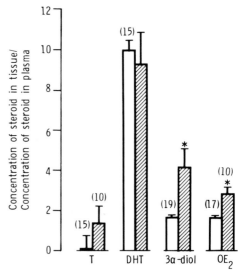

FIGURE 138–9. Relationship between tissue and serum sex steroids in men with BPH. (Reproduced by permission of MTP Press Limited, Lancaster, England, from Chanadian R, Puah CM: The Endocrinology of Prostate Tumours. Boston, MTP Press Ltd., 1983, p 74.)

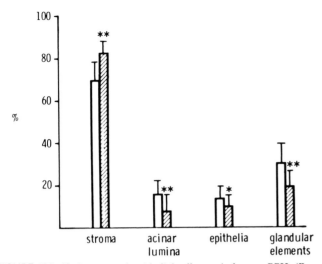

FIGURE 138–10. Stroma and epithelial cell types in human BPH. (Reproduced by permission of MTP Press Limited, Lancaster, England, from Chanadian R, Puah CM: The Endocrinology of Prostate Tumours. Boston, MTP Press Ltd., 1983, p 74.)

man BPH suggests that specimens obtained by transurethral resection (TUR) or retropubic prostatectomy (RPP) are different.[113, 123–127] The procedure used for removal of BPH tissue has a bearing on the type of sample collected for study. TUR usually removes tissue down to the verumontanum, and sometimes 50 per cent of the total BPH tissue may escape resection. With open prostatectomy, most of the adenoma is removed, including that located down to and below the verumontanum. Anatomical differences in specimens may have considerable influence in relation to the biochemical measurements made in specimens.[128] The concentrations of total protein, nucleic acids (DNA and RNA), and water are similar in specimens obtained by TUR and RPP. DHT is higher and estradiol lower in specimens obtained by RPP than in TUR samples[54, 92] because TUR specimens have more stroma and less glandular elements than those collected by RPP.[54]

DEVELOPMENTAL INTERACTIONS BETWEEN MESENCHYMAL AND EPITHELIAL CELLS

Cunha et al.[129, 130] studied the effects of androgens on prostate development in the androgen receptor–deficient murine system. The development of the prostatic epithelium from the urogenital sinus depends on androgen action on mesenchyme[129] (Fig. 138–11). Trophic factors produced in androgen-responsive mesenchyme result in prostatic epithelial morphogenesis, growth, and secretory cytodifferentiation. In their combination studies, epithelium lacking androgen receptors will differentiate provided prostate stroma with androgen receptor is available for the interaction.[129] The reverse recombination will not support the differentiation.

The observation that fetal urogenital mesenchyme (UGM) and not urogenital epithelium (UGE) produced a dose-response overgrowth of adult host prostate is relevant to the pathogenesis of BPH. It is presumed that growth of the adult prostate in men is strongly influenced by stromal growth factors stimulated by androgens. BPH implants into the prostate of the nude mouse failed to stimulate prostate growth of the host. The question of whether BPH tissue causes regenerative growth by producing growth factors is unresolved.

GROWTH FACTORS AND PROSTATE ENLARGEMENT

Several families of growth factors have been identified in prostate tissue of humans: heparin-binding growth factor (HBGF), transforming growth factor β (TGF-β), epidermal growth factor (EGF), and TGF-α. Basic fibroblast growth factor (bFGF), a member of the HBGF family, is several-fold higher than normal in BPH tissue.[131–133] Stroma of prostate is a rich source of bFGF (Story, unpublished data). Prostate epithelial cells also may synthesize bFGF. Levine et al.[134] showed that estrogen had no effect on growth of fibroblasts cultured from fetal and adult prostates (Fig. 138–12), but that bFGF, EGF, and DHT increased fibroblast growth. The results were consistent with an indirect effect of DHT, suggesting that it stimulated another growth factor.

Sherwood et al.[135] studied human BPH tissue in vitro and isolated both stromal and epithelial cells. bFGF analyzed by immunofluorescence was localized mainly in the prostatic stroma. In addition, bFGF was a potent stimulator of stromal cell proliferation in vitro but did not enhance mitogenic activity of cultured epithelial cells (Tables 138–2 and 138–3). Stromal but not epithelial cells also had high-affinity (K_d = 258 pM; 61,400 receptors per cell) bFGF receptors. Although both epithelial and stromal cells produce bFGF, it is largely not secreted. The epithelial cells produce a substance that is mitogenic for stromal cells and is not inhibited by anti-bFGF antibodies, suggesting that a factor separate from bFGF stimulates the stromal cells.

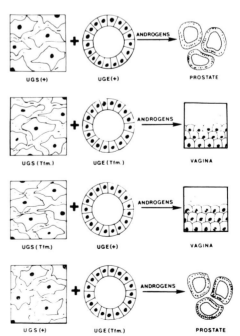

FIGURE 138–11. Mesenchymal and epithelial cell interaction in prostate development (UGE = urogenital epithelium; UGS = urogenital sinus). (From Cunha GR, Chung LW, Shannon JM, Reece BA: Stromal-epithelial interactions in sex differentiation. Biol Reprod 22:19, 1980.)

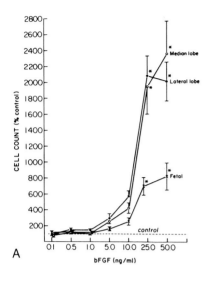
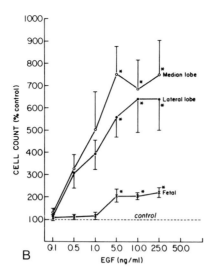

FIGURE 138–12. Mitogenic effects of growth factors on fibroblasts from human adult and fetal prostate. (From Levine AC, Ron M, Huber GK, Kirschenbaum A: The effect of androgen, estrogen and growth factors on the proliferation of cultured fibroblasts derived from human fetal and adult prostates. Endocrinology 130:2413–2419, copyright © 1992, The Endocrine Society.)

TGF-α and EGF were potent mitogens for epithelial cells isolated from BPH tissue,[135] but bFGF, aFGF, and platelet-derived growth factor (PDGF) were poor mitogens. In contrast, growth of isolated prostate stromal cells was enhanced two- to threefold by bFGF, aFGF, PDGF, or EGF, but only 0.7-fold by TGF-α. Thus a growth factor other than bFGF could be made by epithelial cells and stimulate stromal cells. Stromal cells produce a growth factor, possibly keratinocyte growth factor (KGF), that may be a mediator of epithelial mitosis.

EGF is produced and secreted by human prostate. Prostatic fluid has a higher concentration of EGF than any other tissue of humans. Both Habib[136] and Shaikh[137] reported that EGF is significantly higher in BPH tissue than in prostate cancer tissue.

TGF-β1 and TGF-β2 enhance proliferation of fibroblasts in soft agar but inhibit mitosis of epithelial cells. However, Story et al.[138] reported that growth of human prostate fibroblasts was inhibited by TGF-β1. The inhibitory effect of TGF-β1 could be reversed by bFGF but not by EGF, PDGF, insulin-like growth factor I (IGF-I), or insulin. In addition, TGF-β1 enhanced the synthesis of bFGF. Schuurmans et al.[139] reported that TGF-β suppressed the stimulatory effect of EGF on LnCap human prostate cancer cells. TGF-β1 and TGF-β2 transcripts have been identified in BPH and normal prostate tissue.[132] In rat ventral prostate, androgen

withdrawal induces TGF-β gene expression. Thus increased TGF-β might increase bFGF synthesis and inhibit epithelial cell proliferation. Androgens may increase bFGF, EGF, and TGF-α and decrease TGF-β expression and enhance growth of both the stromal and epithelial cells of the prostate. This might lead to an increase in prostate size and contribute to the growth of prostate that causes BPH.

Mori et al.[132] reported elevated TGF-β2 expression in BPH tissue compared with normal tissue. The inhibitory effects of TGF-β on epithelial cell growth may be mediated through the retinoblastoma tumor gene[140–142] suppressor gene product and the proto-oncogene c-myc.

EGF receptors have been identified in membrane fractions of BPH tissue.[143] Lubrano et al.[144] also reported a significant linear relationship between nuclear androgen receptor levels and endogenous immunoreactive EGF (Fig. 138–13). However, the negative correlation between EGF receptor binding and nuclear androgen receptor content observed may have resulted from EGF receptor down-regulation in response to elevated EGF stimulated by androgens. No such relationship was shown between estrogen receptor content and EGF levels. Further, reducing androgens by treatment with GnRH agonists results in higher

TABLE 138–2. GROWTH RESPONSES OF ISOLATED PROSTATIC STROMAL CELLS TO DEFINED GROWTH FACTORS

GROWTH FACTOR	DAYS IN CULTURE (RELATIVE GROWTH)		
	2	4	6
10% FBS	242.7 ± 7.5*	698.2 ± 46.1*	876.2 ± 47.1*
ITS+	100	100	100
bFGF (10 ng/ml)	221.6 ± 23.4*	424.4 ± 65.9*	576.2 ± 31.9*
aFGF (10 ng/ml)	142.3 ± 7.4*	206.2 ± 14.3*	283.3 ± 21.9
PDGF (10 ng/ml)	133.8 ± 28.6	190.3 ± 29.0*	250.4 ± 33.3*
TGF-α (10 ng/ml)	109.7 ± 23.6	125.3 ± 8.9	170.6 ± 24.4*
EGF (10 ng/ml)	78.5 ± 4.3	198.6 ± 47.9*	207.5 ± 18.1*

Stromal cells (1 × 10⁵/flask) were plated in 25-cm² flasks and allowed to adhere for 16 to 8 h. Media were then changed to RPMI-1640 containing 10% fetal bovine serum (positive control), ITS+ (negative control), or ITS+ plus growth factors. Cells were counted on days 2, 4, and 6. The media in remaining flasks were replaced with fresh media containing appropriate additives on days 2 and 4. (n = 6/group).

*Significantly (p < 0.05) greater than ITS+ negative control.

TABLE 138–3. EFFECTS OF SEVERAL DEFINED GROWTH FACTORS ON THE PROLIFERATION OF ISOLATED PROSTATIC EPITHELIAL CELLS

GROWTH FACTOR	DAYS IN CULTURE (RELATIVE PROLIFERATION)		
	2	5	8
Complete WAJC 404	94.4 ± 15.7	329.9 ± 25.5*	1290 ± 192.4*
Basal WAJC 404	100	100	100
bFGF (10 ng/ml)	84.3 ± 14.2	96.3 ± 20.6	123.7 ± 21.5
aFGF (10 ng/ml)	119.6 ± 41	144.1 ± 7.1*	148.4 ± 6.8*
TGF-α (10 ng/ml)	85.0 ± 5.5	255.1 ± 43.9*	688.2 ± 49.5*
EGF (10 ng/ml)	73.2 ± 8.7	272.9 ± 36.4	640.9 ± 65.6*
PDGF (10 ng/ml)	64.6 ± 3.9	88.5 ± 29.9	127.4 ± 20.5

Prostatic epithelial cells (1 × 10⁵/flask) were plated in 25-cm² tissue culture flasks and allowed to adhere for 16 to 18 h. Media were changed to complete WAJC 404 (positive control), basal WAJC 404 (negative control), or basal WAJC 404 plus the designated growth factors. Cells were counted on days 2, 5, and 8. Media were replaced with fresh media containing appropriate additives on days 2 and 5. Values are expressed as the mean ± SE (n = 6/group).

*Significantly (p < 0.05) greater than basal WAJC 404 negative control.

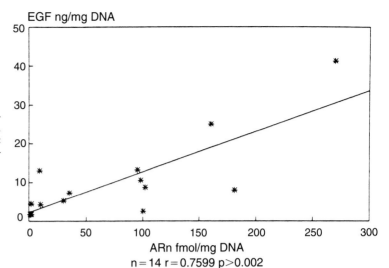

FIGURE 138–13. The relationship between EGF and androgen receptor in human BPH tissue. (From Lubrano C, Sciarra F, Spera G, et al: Immunoreactive EGF in human benign prostatic hyperplasia: Relationships with androgen and estrogen receptors. J Steroid Biochem Mol Biol 41:683–687, 1992.)

EGF receptor content of prostate tissue than observed in BPH tissue from untreated men.[145] These studies in benign tissue suggest that androgens may decrease EGF receptor expression, which contrasts with observations in epithelial prostate cancer cell lines.[139, 146] Liu and Meikle[146] conducted studies in a prostate cancer epithelial cell line that is modestly responsive to androgen. Androgen increased proliferation of the cells' TGF-α and EGF receptor mRNAs. The mitogenic effect of androgen could be inhibited by antibodies to the EGF receptor. These results suggest that in this epithelial cell line androgen stimulates cell mitosis indirectly by increasing a growth factor and EGF receptor concentrations.

In limited studies, low concentrations of IGF-I (insulin-like growth factor) can support proliferation of both normal and tumor-derived prostate epithelium and mesenchymal cells. Higher concentrations of insulin and IGF-II were required to cause proliferation.[147, 148] Androgens elevated IGF-I gene expression in regenerating prostate from rats and rat tumors.[148]

The PDGF family of receptors has not been characterized in prostate tissue. However, PDGF has been shown to stimulate growth of stromal cells isolated from BPH tissue of humans.[135]

THERAPY OF BPH

Hormonal Therapy

Prostatism is a complex of obstructive (hesitancy, decreased urinary stream force, interrupted stream, a sense of incomplete emptying, and terminal dribbling) and irritative (frequency, nocturia, and urgency) symptoms associated with BPH.[149] The definition of BPH has included pathological characteristics, a prostate volume of greater than 25 g, or a prostate size over 20 g with a urine flow rate of less than 15 ml/s.

Now that nonsurgical therapeutic options for symptomatic BPH are available to all physicians, primary care physicians will have an increasing role in management of BPH. Disorders that may mimic BPH as a cause of lower urinary tract symptoms, such as prostate cancer, neurolog-

ical disorders, detrusor dysfunction without BPH, or drugs, must be excluded.[149, 150] Although the digital rectal examination may detect nodules suggestive of prostate cancer, it is inaccurate in estimating prostate size. However, transrectal ultrasound (TRUS) is accurate and is used for guided biopsy of suspicious lesions. A PSA, urinalysis, postvoid residual urine volume, urine flow rates and voiding cystourethrography, and medical treatment may be indicated before referral to a urologist.

PSA (monoclonal assays) values above 10 ng/ml strongly support the diagnosis of prostate cancer rather than BPH, but elevated values between 4 and 9 ng/ml may be observed in both BPH and prostate cancer.[11–15, 151] Lee et al.[152] proposed a TRUS estimated volume correction of PSA for improving the positive predictive value of PSA for the diagnosis of prostate cancer in men who also have BPH.

Limited studies have been conducted to assess the effects of hormonal and nonhormonal therapy in management of BPH.[6, 153–155] However, endocrine therapy for both prevention and treatment of BPH has considerable promise. Controlled studies in which endocrine therapy has been compared with surgical treatment are limited because most symptomatic patients are advised to have surgical treatment. Nevertheless, effective endocrine therapy with a goal to prevention of the disease or treatment of selected symptomatic patients would be highly desirable. Most studies have tried to test the effects of endocrine treatment on size of the prostate, urine flow, and residual volume rather than compare the results of the two types of therapy. The measurements have included (1) changes in maximum urine flow rate, (2) changes in residual urine volume, (3) the ability to void in patients with retention, and (4) prostate size.

Surgical Castration

Surgical castration for management of symptomatic BPH has been satisfactory but is mainly of historical interest. There is regression of prostatic size and improvement in urine flow and residual urine following castration. Any recent studies evaluating castration therapy on BPH have involved patients treated for prostatic cancer. These investigators then assessed the results on BPH. In 1895, White[156] performed castration in 200 men with BPH for treatment of urinary obstruction. In 111 cases where adequate follow-up evaluation could be made, 87 per cent had rapid regression of the prostate enlargement, and 66 per cent had a marked reduction in residual urine volume. A year after White's study, Cabot[157] conducted another study and castrated 61 patients and provided follow-up for several weeks. About 90 per cent had improvement, but 10 per cent did not improve. Huggins and Stevens[158] and Wendel et al.[159] reported atrophic changes in glandular epithelium of the prostate of castrated men. These observations support the postulate that growth of prostatic epithelium in BPH is at least partially changed by androgen secreted by the testes.

Medical Castration

Peters and Walsh[58] treated nine patients with bladder-outlet obstruction caused by BPH with nafarelin acetate, a gonadotropin-releasing hormone (GnRH) agonist, for 6 months. Prostate size determined by TRUS declined from 14 to 48 per cent (24.2 ± 3 per cent, mean ± SE), and the regression reached a trough after about 4 months. Plasma testosterone values were suppressed to castrate concentrations. Histologic analysis of biopsy specimens showed atrophic epithelium during therapy, but regression of stroma was only about 20 per cent compared with 40 per cent for epithelium. Three of the nine patients experienced symptomatic improvement.

Fifteen patients with BPH were treated with leuprolide, a long-acting GnRH analogue, by Gabrilove et al.[59] The average regression of prostate size was about 40 per cent by 4 months of treatment, with minimal additional regression (46 per cent) at 6 months (Fig. 138–14). All 15 patients had improvement in urinary flow rates, but not all had improvement in nocturia and frequency of urination. In this study and the report of Peters and Walsh,[58] prostate size returned to the initial size within about 4 months of discontinuing therapy. A major side effect of this therapy was reduced potency and flushing.

These studies confirm that endocrine factors contribute to prostate growth in men with BPH and that epithelium is more responsive to androgen deprivation than stroma.

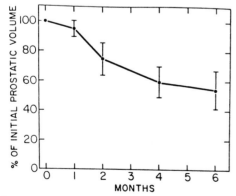

FIGURE 138–14. The effect of leuprolide treatment on volume of human prostate measured by transrectal ultrasound. (From Gabrilove JL, Levine AC, Kirschenbaum A, Droller M: Effect of long-acting gonadotropin-releasing hormone analog (leuprolide) therapy on prostatic size and symptoms in 15 men with benign prostatic hypertrophy. J Clin Endocrinol Metab 69:629–632, 1989, copyright © 1989, The Endocrine Society.)

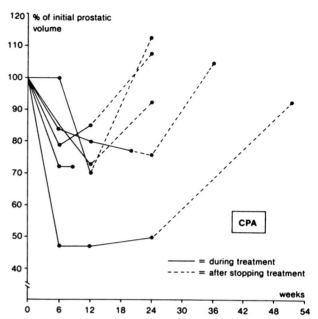

FIGURE 138–15. Human prostate size determined by transrectal ultrasound before and after treatment with cyproterone acetate. (From Bosch RJLH, Griffiths DJ, Blom JHM, Schroeder FH: Treatment of benign prostatic hyperplasia by androgen deprivation: Effects on prostate size and urodynamic parameters. J Urol 141:68–72, 1989.)

Antiandrogens

Administration of antiandrogens has been shown to influence BPH.[160–164] Side effects, which include breast enlargement and tenderness, loss of libido, impotence, and acne, have limited their usefulness. Those antiandrogens derived from 17α-hydroxyprogesterone[165–168] have had equivocal effects on BPH, although subjective improvement has been reported. A reduction in epithelial cell height of BPH tissue has usually been seen.

Cyproterone acetate (CPA) is a synthetic progestogen which suppresses pituitary gonadotropins, decreases serum testosterone, and inhibits binding of DHT to the androgen receptors.[169] CPA treatment of patients with BPH for 12 weeks resulted in 15 to 50 per cent (mean about 30 per cent) reduction in prostate size[170] (Fig. 138–15). Urodynamic parameters also improved with CPA therapy. Both the prostate size and urodynamic parameters reversed after discontinuation of CPA treatment. This reduction in prostate size produced by CPA has been attributed to a fourfold suppression of DHT in total prostate and its subfractions without affecting prostate testosterone or nuclear androgen concentrations. It lowers DHT levels in the prostate by reducing 5α-reductase activity in prostate and suppression of plasma testosterone concentrations.

Antiestrogens

Preliminary results with tamoxifen therapy of BPH suggest that stromal growth and the concentration of nuclear androgen receptors are both reduced.[171, 172] The antiestrogen also has been shown to inhibit protein synthesis in prostate tissue. This effect could inhibit the stromal growth influence of estrogens. Clinical experience with the drug has been mixed. Additional studies are needed to determine whether antiandrogen and/or antiestrogen drugs will be effective in either preventing or treating BPH.

5α-Reductase Inhibition

Finasteride is a 5α-reductase inhibitor that blocks the conversion of testosterone to dihydrotestosterone (DHT). McConnell et al.[173] reported that mean prostate DHT concentrations decreased from 10.3 ± 0.6 nmol/kg on placebo to less than 15 per cent of this concentration after 7 days of treatment with 1 to 100 mg/d finasteride. Tissue testosterone concentrations increased in a reciprocal fashion. Serum concentrations of testosterone were unaffected by finasteride therapy, but serum DHT declined from a mean value of 1.37 ± 0.13 to 0.3 to 0.5 nmol/L with therapy (Fig. 138–16).

Other studies[174–176] showed that finasteride therapy also results in a reduction in prostate size and symptomatic improvement of urethral obstruction. After 12 and 24 weeks of therapy, prostate volume determined by magnetic resonance imaging decreased 9 to 22.8 per cent and 1.1 to 18.5 per cent, respectively. There was no clear dose-response relationship. However, only the mean decreases observed in the 5- and 10-mg groups were significantly different from baseline ($p < 0.01$). Twenty-four weeks after stopping therapy, most patients had a return to baseline volumes of prostate tissue. The mean changes in prostate volume in another group showed decreases in size at 12 weeks from 11.5 to 17.3 per cent. These declines were significantly different from baseline ($p < 0.05$) but not from the placebo group. After 12 additional weeks of therapy, the mean group decreases ranged from 17.9 to 27.7 per cent. These changes were all significantly different from baseline, but not all were significantly different from the placebo. There may be some gradual decline in prostate size from the 12- to 24-week interval of treatment. All patients had significant decreases in PSA over the 12 to 24 weeks of therapy that ranged from 20.4 to 50 per cent. Maximum urinary flow was increased by a mean of 3.7 cc/s in the 1- and 5-mg groups combined ($p < 0.05$). The symptom score also improved significantly ($p < 0.05$). The reduction in tissue DHT is more dramatic than the decrease in prostate size, improvement in urinary flow rates, and symptomatic improvement. Since hormonal therapy lowers PSA, prostate cancer needs to be excluded before beginning therapy. A rise of PSA during therapy would suggest further diagnostic testing for prostate cancer is indicated.

Aromatase Inhibition

El Etreby et al.[33, 177] reviewed the effects of a new aromatase inhibitor, atamestane, for management of BPH in animal models and in humans. This agent is highly effective in inhibiting estrogen-induced fibromuscular stromal hyperplasia of the prostate produced by treatment of dogs and monkeys with androstenedione. In normal men and men with BPH, atamestane decreases both serum and prostate tissue concentrations of estrogen without significantly affecting androgen levels. A combination therapy that suppresses DHT and estrogen concentrations in BPH tissue has theoretical promise.

Non–Sex-Steroid Therapy

Bromocriptine[178, 179] is a dopamine agonist that inhibits the release of prolactin from the pituitary. In vitro studies with human prostate have suggested that bromocriptine may have alpha-adrenergic blocking actions and anticholinergic actions. Data are limited on treatment of BPH, but improvement in symptoms and increased urine flow rate have been reported in patients treated with the drug. It is uncertain whether the benefits were related to its endocrine effects or actions on smooth muscle of the gland.

Phenoxybenzamine,[180–182] an alpha-adrenergic antagonist, has been used in treatment of BPH. Symptoms of hesitancy and slow stream were improved in patients using the drug compared with placebo. Bladder outflow obstruction was improved as the drug apparently decreased the pressure of the proximal urethra. However, dizziness may limit the usefulness of the medication in treatment of BPH in elderly men.

Surgical Treatment

Standard therapy for symptomatic BPH has been transurethral prostatectomy (TURP), and success rates are high (84 to 92 per cent).[149, 183] In addition to the surgical morbidity and recurrence of symptoms in some, the quality of life may not be improved, particularly in the elderly treated with TURP.

Newer surgical options have included transurethral prostatomy (TUIP), transurethral balloon dilatation, prostatic stents, and microwave hyperthermia. Of these surgical methods used to treat symptomatic BPH in patients with glands less than 30 g, only TUIP compares favorably with TURP in success rates. However, complication rates are lower with TUIP than with TURP.

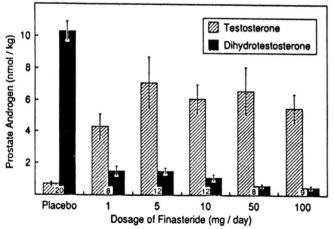

FIGURE 138–16. Human prostate testosterone and DHT concentrations in prostate before and after finasteride therapy. (From McConnell JD, Wilson JD, George FW, et al: Finasteride, an inhibitor of 5α-reductase, suppresses prostatic dihydrotestosterone in men with benign prostatic hyperplasia. J Clin Endocrinol Metab 74:505–508, 1992, copyright ©, The Endocrine Society.)

ACKNOWLEDGMENT: This work was supported in part by United States Public Health Service Grants M01 RR-00064 and DK-43344.

REFERENCES

1. McNeal J: Regional morphology and pathology of the prostate. Am J Clin Pathol 49:347, 1968.
2. McNeal J: The prostate and prostatic urethra: A morphologic synthesis. J Urol 107:1008, 1972.
3. McNeal J: Origin and evolution of benign prostate enlargement. Invest Urol 15:340–345, 1978.
4. McNeal JE: Anatomy of the prostate and morphogenesis of BPH. Prog Clin Biol Res 145:27–53, 1984.
5. Franks LM: Benign nodular hyperplasia of the prostate: A review. Ann R Coll Surg Engl 14:92, 1954.
6. Huggins C, Webster WO: Duality of the human prostate in response to oestrogens. J Urol 59:258, 1948.
7. Wilson JD: The pathogenesis of benign prostatic hyperplasia. Am J Med 68:745–756, 1980.
8. Berry SJ, Coffey DS, Walsh PC, Ewing LL: Development of benign prostatic hyperplasia with age. J Urol 132:474–479, 1984.
9. Walsh PC: Human benign prostatic hyperplasia: etiological considerations. Prog Clin Biol Res 145:1–25, 1984.
10. Moore RA: Benign hypertrophy and carcinoma of the prostate: Occurrence and experimental production in animals. Surgery 16:152–167, 1944.
11. Perrin P, Francois O, Maquet JH, Gringeon G: Circulating prostate cancer specific antigens in benign hypertrophy and localized cancer of the prostate. Presse Med 20:1313–1319, 1991.
12. Drago JR: The role of new modalities in the early detection and diagnosis of prostate cancer. CA 39:326–335, 1991.
13. Brawer MK, Lange PH: Prostate-specific antigen and premalignant change: Implications for early detection. CA 39:361–375, 1991.
14. Stamey TA, Yang N, Hay AR, et al: Prostate specific antigen as a serum marker for adenocarcinoma of the prostate. N Engl J Med 317:909–916, 1987.
15. Cooner WH, Mosley BR, Rutherford CL, et al: Clinical application of transrectal ultrasonography and prostate specific antigen in the search for prostate cancer. J Urol 139:758–761, 1988.
16. Armelin HA: Pituitary extracts and steroid hormones in the control of 3T3 cell growth. Proc Natl Acad Sci USA 70:2702–2706, 1973.
17. Goustin AS, Leof EB, Shipley GD, Moses HL: Growth factors and cancer. Cancer Res 46:1015–1029, 1986.
18. Tachman ML, Guthrie GP Jr: Hypothyroidism: Diversity of presentation. Endocr Rev 5:456–465, 1984.
19. Mackillop WJ, Ciampi A, Till JE, Buick RN: A stem model of human tumor growth: Implications for tumor cell clonogenic assays. J Natl Cancer Inst 70:9–16, 1983.
20. Zondek T, Zondek L: The fetal and neonatal prostate. In Goland M (ed): Normal and Abnormal Growth of the Prostate. Springfield, IL, Charles C Thomas, 1975, pp 5–28.
21. Coffey DS: The biochemistry and physiology of the prostate and seminal vesicles. In Harrison JH, Gittes RF, Perlmutter AD, et al (eds): Campbell's Urology. Philadelphia, WB Saunders Co, 1985, p 248.
22. Chung LWK, Cunha GR: Stromal-epithelial interactions: II. Regulation of prostatic growth by embryonic urogenital sinus mesenchyme. Prostate 4:503–511, 1983.
23. Cunha GR: Prostatic epithelial morphogenesis, grwoth, and secretory cytodifferentiation are elicited via trophic influences from mesenchyme. In Bresciani F, Lippman ME, King RJB, Namer M (eds): Progress in Cancer Research and Therapy. New York, Raven Press, 1984, pp 121–128.
24. Naslund MJ, Coffey DS: The hormonal imprinting of the prostate and the regulation of stem cells in prostatic growth. In Rodgers CH, Coffey DS, Cunha G, et al (eds): Benign Prostatic Hyperplasia, Vol II. Bethesda, National Institutes of Health, 1985, pp 73–83.
25. Johansson R: Effect of prolactin, growth hormone and insulin on the uptake and binding of dihydrotestosterone to the cultured rat ventral prostate. Acta Endocrinol (Copenh) 81:854–864, 1976.
26. Thomas JA, Keenan EJ: Prolactin influences upon androgen action in male accessory sex organs. In Singhal RL, Thomas JA (eds): Advances in Sex Hormone Research. Baltimore, University Park Press, 1976, pp 425–470.
27. Meikle AW, Bishop DT, Stringham JD, West DW: Quantitating genetic and nongenetic factors that determine plasma sex-steroid variation in normal male twins. Metabolism 35:1090–1095, 1986.
28. Bishop DT, Meikle AW, Slattery ML, et al: The effect of nutritional factors on sex hormone levels in male twins. Genet Epidemiol 5:43–59, 1988.
29. Meikle AW, Stringham JD, Bishop DT, West DW: Quantitating genetic and nongenetic factors influencing androgen production and clearance in men. J Clin Endocrinol Metab 67:104–109, 1988.
30. Moore RJ, Gazak JM, Quebbeman JF, Wilson JD: Concentration of dihydrotestosterone and 3α-androstanediol in naturally occurring and androgen-induced prostatic hyperplasia in the dog. J Clin Invest 64:1003–1010, 1979.
31. Trachtenberg J, Hicks LL, Walsh PC: Androgen- and estrogen-receptor content in spontaneous and experimentally induced canine prostatic hyperplasia. J Clin Invest 65:1051–1059, 1980.
32. Moore RJ, Gazak JM, Wilson JD: Regulation of cytoplasmic dihydrotestosterone binding in dog prostate by 17β-estradiol. J Clin Invest 63:351–357, 1979.
33. El Etreby MF, Nishino Y, Habenicht U-F, Henderson D: Atamestane, a new aromatase inhibitor for the management of benign prostatic hyperplasia. J Androl 12:403–414, 1991.
34. Habenicht U-F, El Etreby MF: Rationale for using aromatase inhibitors to manage benign prostatic hyperplasia: Experimental studies. J Androl 12:395–402, 1991.
35. Habenicht U-F, El Etreby MF: Selective inhibition of androstenedione-induced prostate growth in intact beagle dogs by a combined treatment with the antiandrogen cyproterone acetate and the aromatase inhibitor 1-methyl-androsta-1, 4-diene-3, 17-dione (1-methyl-ADD). Prostate 14:309–322, 1989.
36. Prins GS: Neonatal estrogen exposure induces lobe-specific alterations in adult rat prostate androgen receptor expression. Endocrinology 130:2401–2412, 1992.
37. Farnsworth WE, Slaunwhite WR Jr, Sharma M, et al: Interaction of prolactin and testosterone in human prostate. Urol Res 9:79, 1981.
38. Farnsworth WE: A direct effect of oestrogens on prostatic metabolism of testosterone. Invest Urol 6:423, 1969.
39. Mawhinney MG, Belis JA: Androgens and estrogens in prostatic neoplasia. In Singhal RL, Thomas JA (eds): Advances in Sex Hormone Research. Baltimore, University Park Press, 1976, pp 142–209.
40. Dilley WG, Birkhoff JD: Hormone response of benign hyperplastic prostate tissue in organ culture. Invest Urol 15:873–886, 1977.
41. Maehama S, Li D, Nanri H, et al: Purification and partial characterization of prostate derived growth factor. Proc Natl Acad Sci USA 83:8162–8166, 1986.
42. Lipsett MB: Steroid secretion by the human testis. In Resenberg E, Paulsen CA (eds): The Human Testis. New York, Plenum Press, 1977, pp 407–422.
43. Bardin CW: Pituitary-testicular axis. In Yen SSC, Jaffe RB (eds): Reproductive Endocrinology. Philadelphia, WB Saunders Co, 1978, pp 110–125.
44. Rosner W, Hryb DJ, Khan MS, et al: Sex hormone binding globulin binding to cell membranes and generation of a second messenger. J Androl 13:101–106, 1992.
45. Bruchovsky N, Lesser B: Control of proliferative growth in androgen responsive organs and neoplasma. In Singhal RL, Thomas JA (eds): Advances in Sex Hormone Research. Baltimore, University Park Press, 1976, p 1.
46. Habib FK, Beynon L, Chisholm GD, Busuttil A: The distribution of 5α-reductase and 3α(β)-hydroxysteroid dehydrogenase activities in the hyperplastic human prostate gland. Steroids 41:3049–3053, 1983.
47. Houston B, Chisholm GD, Habib FK: Evidence that human prostatic 5α-reductase is located exclusively in the nucleus. FEBS Lett 185:231–235, 1985.
48. Wilson JD, Harrod MJ, Goldstein JL, et al: Familial incomplete male pseudohermaphroditism type 1. N Engl J Med 290:1097–1103, 1974.
49. Walsh PC, Harrod MJ, Goldstein JL, et al: Familial incomplete male pseudohermaphroditism, type 2, decreased dihydrotestosterone formation in pseudovaginal perineoscrotal hypospadias. N Engl J Med 291:944, 1974.
50. Peterson RE, Imperato-Mcginley J, Gautier T, Sturla E: Male pseudohermaphroditism due to steroid 5α-reductase deficiency. Am J Med 62:170–191, 1977.
51. Imperato-McGinley J, Peterson RE, Gantier T, et al: Hormonal evaluation of a large kindred with complete androgen insensitivity: Evidence of a secondary 5 alpha-reductase deficiency. J Clin Endocrinol Metab 54:931–941, 1982.
52. Wilson JD, George FW, Griffin JE: The hormonal control of sexual development. Science 211:1278–1284, 1981.
53. Ghanadian R: Hormonal control and rationale for endocrine therapy of prostatic tumours. In Ghanadian R (ed): The Endocrinology of Prostate Tumours. Lancaster, MTP Press, 1983, pp 59–86.
54. Ghanadian R, Puah CM: Relationships between oestradiol-17β, testosterone, dihydrotestosterone and 5α-androstane-3α, 17β-diol in hu-

man benign hypertrophy and carcinoma of the prostate. J Endocrinol 88:255–262, 1981.

55. Meikle AW, Collier ES, Middleton RG, Fang SM: Supranormal nuclear content of 5α-dihydrotestosterone in benign hyperplastic prostate of humans. J Clin Endocrinol Metab 51:945–947, 1980.

56. Meikle AW, Stringham JD, Olsen DC: Subnormal tissue 3α-androstanediol and androsterone in prostatic hyperplasia. J Clin Endocrinol Metab 47:909–913, 1978.

57. Siiteri PK, Wilson JD, Mayfield J: The formation and content of dihydrotestosterone in the hypertrophic prostate of man. J Clin Invest 49:1737–1745, 1970.

58. Peters CA, Walsh PC: The effect of nafarelin acetate, a luteinizing hormone–releasing hormone agent agonist, on benign prostatic hyperplasia. N Engl J Med 317:599–604, 1987.

59. Gabrilove JL, Levine AC, Kirschenbaum A, Droller M: Effect of long-acting gonadotropin-releasing hormone analog (leuprolide) therapy on prostatic size and symptoms in 15 men with benign prostatic hypertrophy. J Clin Endocrinol Metab 69:629–632, 1989.

60. Longcope C, Kato T, Horton R: Conversion of blood androgens to estrogens in normal adult men and women. J Clin Invest 48:2191–2201, 1969.

61. Siiteri PK, MacDonald PC: Role of estraglandular estrogen in human endocrinology. In Greep RO, Astwood EB, Geiger SR (eds): Handbook of Physiology. Baltimore, Waverly Press, 1973, pp 615–629.

62. MacDonald PC, Madden JD, Brenner PF, et al: Origin of estrogen in normal men and in women with testicular feminization. J Clin Endocrinol Metab 49:905–916, 1979.

63. Kaufman JM, Giri M, Deslypere JP, et al: Influence of age on the responsiveness of the gonadotrophs to luteinizing releasing hormone in males. J Clin Endcrinol Metab 72:1255–1280, 1991.

64. Vermeulen A, Rubens R, Verdonck L: Testosterone secretion and metabolism in male senescence. J Clin Endocrinol Metab 34:730–735, 1972.

65. Baker HW, Burger DM, de Kretser DM, et al: Changes in the pituitary-testicular system with age. Clin Endocrinol (Oxf) 5:349–372, 1976.

66. Deslypere JP, Vermeulen A: Leydig cell function in normal men: Effect of age, life-style, residence, diet, and activity. J Clin Endocrinol Metab 59:955–961, 1984.

67. Ortega E, Ruiz E, Mendoza MC, et al: Plasma steroid and protein hormone concentrations in patients with benign prostate hypertrophy and in normal men. Experientia 35:844–845, 1983.

68. Partin AW, Oesterling JE, Epstein JI, et al: Influence of age and endocrine factors on the volume of benign prostatic hyperplasia. Urology 145:405–409, 1991.

69. Rubens R, Dhont M, Vermeulen A: Further studies on Leydig cell function in old age. J Clin Endocrinol Metab 39:40–45, 1974.

70. Vermeulen A, Verdonck L, Van Der Straeten M, Orie N: Capacity of the testosterone-binding globulin in human plasma and influence of specific binding of testosterone on its metabolic clearance rate. J Clin Endocrinol Metab 29:1470–1480, 1969.

71. Pirke KM, Doerr P: Age-related changes and interrelationships between plasma testosterone and oestradiol and testosterone binding globulin in normal adult males. Acta Endocrinol (Copenh) 74:792–800, 1973.

72. Mirovics JC, Dunlop M, Rennie GC: Changes in the pituitary-testicular system with age. Clin Endocrinol (Oxf) 5:349–372, 1976.

73. Ishimaru T, Pages L, Horton R: Altered metabolism of androgens in elderly men with benign prostatic hyperplasia. J Clin Endocrinol Metab 45:695–701, 1977.

74. Bartsch W, Becker H, Pinkenburg FA, Krierg M: Hormone blood levels and their inter-relationships in normal men with benign prostatic hyperplasia. Acta Endocrinol (Copenh) 90:727, 1979.

75. Ghanadian R, Lewis JG, Chisholm GD, O'Donoghue EPN: Serum dihydrotestosterone in patients with benign prostatic hypertrophy. Br J Urol 49:541, 1977.

76. Vermeulen A, DeSy W: Androgens in patients with benign prostatic hyperplasia before and after prostatectomy. J Clin Endocrinol Metab 43:1250–1254, 1976.

77. Mahoudeau JA, Delassalle A, Bricaire H: Secretion of dihydrotestosterone by human prostate in benign prostatic hypertrophy. Acta Endocrinol (Copenh) 77:401–407, 1974.

78. Horton R, Hsieh P, Barberia J, et al: Altered blood androgens in elderly men with prostate hyperplasia. J Clin Endocrinol Metab 41:793–796, 1975.

79. Ghanadian R, Puah CM, Williams G: Serum 5α-androstane-3α, 17β-diol in patients with prostatic tumours. Br J Cancer 44:308, 1977.

80. Lukkarinen O: Total and SHBG-bound testosterone and 5α-dihydro-

testosterone serum concentrations in normal elderly men and patients with benign prostatic hypertrophy before and after removal of the adenoma. Br J Urol 52:377, 1980.

81. Hammond GL, Kontturi M, Vihko P, Vihko R: Serum steroids in normal males and patients with prostatic diseases. Clin Endocrinol (Oxf) 9:113–121, 1978.

82. Prostate Cancer: A Series of Workshops on the Biology of Human Cancer. Report No 9, Vol 48. Geneva, UICC Technical Report Series, 1979.

83. Drafta D, Proca E, Zamfir V, et al: Plasma steroids in benign prostatic hypertrophy and carcinoma of the prostate. J Steroid Biochem 17:689–693, 1982.

84. Brochu M, Belanger A: Comparative study of plasma steroid and steroid glucuronide levels in normal men and in men with benign prostatic hyperplasia. Prostate 11:33, 1987.

85. Hulka BS, Hammond JE, DiFernando G, et al: Serum hormone levels among patients with prostatic carcinoma or benign prostatic hypertrophy and clinic controls. Prostate 11:171–182, 1987.

86. Rannikko S, Adlercreutz H: Plasma estradiol, free testosterone, sex hormone binding globulin binding capacity, and prolactin in benign prostatic hyperplasia and prostatic cancer. Prostate 4:223–229, 1983.

87. Ghanadian R, Masters JRW, Smith CB: Altered androgen metabolism in carcinoma of the prostate. Eur Urol 7:169, 1981.

88. Skoldefors H, Carlstrom K, Furuhjelm M: Urinary hormone excretion in benign prostatic hyperplasia. J Steroid Biochem 7:477–480, 1986.

89. Seppelt U: Correlation among prostate stroma, plasma estrogen levels, and urinary estrogen excretion in patients with benign prostatic hypertrophy. J Clin Endocrinol Metab 47:1230–1235, 1978.

90. Bruchovsky N, Lieskovsky G: Increased ratio of 5α-reductase: 3α(β)-Hydroxysteroid dehydrogenase activities in the hyperplastic human prostate. J Endocrinol 80:289–301, 1979.

91. Farnsworth WE, Brown JR: Androgen of the human prostate. Endocr Res 3:105–117, 1976.

92. Bashirelahi N, Young JD, Sidh SM, Sanefuji H: Androgen, oestrogen and progestogen and their distribution in epithelial and stromal cells of human prostate. In Schroder FH, DeVoogt HJ (eds): Steroid Receptors, Metabolism and Prostatic Cancer. Amsterdam, Excerpta Medica, 1980, pp 240–256.

93. Becker H, Horst HJ, Krieg M, et al: Uptake metabolism and binding of various androgens in human prostatic tissue: In vivo and in vitro studies. J Steroid Biochem 6:477, 1975.

94. Morfin RF, Stefano SD, Bercovici JP, Floch HH: Comparison of testosterone 5α-dihydrotestosterone and 5α-androstane-3β,17β-diol metabolisms in human normal and hyperplastic prostates. J Steroid Biochem 9:245–252, 1978.

95. Malathi K, Gurpide E: Metabolism of 5α-dihydrotestosterone in human benign hyperplastic prostate. J Steroid Biochem 8:141–145, 1977.

96. Morfin RF, Bercovici JP, Charles JF, Floch HH: Testosterone and progesterone metabolism and their interaction in the human hyperplastic prostate. J Steroid Biochem 6:1347, 1986.

97. Rennie PS, Bruchovsky N, McLoughlin MG, et al: Kinetic analysis of 5α-reductase isoenzymes in benign prostatic hyperplasia (BPH). J Steroid Biochem 25:169–173, 1986.

98. Krieg M, Smith K, Elvers B: Androgen receptor translocation from cytosol of rat heart muscle, bulbocavernosus/levator ani muscle and prostate into heart muscle nuclei. J Steroid Biochem 13:577–587, 1982.

99. Mabin TA, McMahon MJ, Thomas GH: The interconversion of oestrone and oestradiol by human endometrium and human benign prostatic hyperplasia in organ culture. Biochem J 118:8P–9P, 1970.

100. Perel E, Killinger DW: The metabolism of androstenedione and testosterone to C19 metabolites in normal breast, breast carcinoma and benign prostatic hypertrophy tissue. J Steroid Biochem 19:1135–1139, 1983.

101. Bartsch W, Kozak I, Gorenflos P, et al: Concentrations of 3β-hydroxy androgens in epithelium and stroma of benign hyperplastic and normal human prostate. Prostate 8:3–10, 1986.

102. Shida K, Shimazaki J, Ito Y, et al: 3α-Reduction of dihydrotestosterone in human normal and hypertrophic prostatic tissues. Invest Urol 13:241–245, 1975.

103. Jacobi GH, Wilson JD: The formation of 5α-androstane-3α, 17β-diol by dog prostate. Endocrinology 99:602–610, 1976.

104. Walsh PC, Wilson JD: The induction of prostatic hypertrophy in the dog with androstanediol. J Clin Invest 57:1093–1097, 1976.

105. Hudson RW: Comparison of 3α-hydroxysteroid dehydrogenase activities in the microsomal fractions of hyperplastic, malignant and normal human prostatic tissues. J Steroid Biochem 20:829–833, 1984.

106. Bruchovsky N, Rennie PS, Wilkin RP: New aspects of androgen action in prostatic cells: Stromal localization of 5α-reductase, nuclear abundance of androstanolone and binding of receptor to linker deoxyribonucleic acid. *In* Schroder FH, DeVoogt HJ (eds): Steroid Receptors, Metabolism and Prostatic Cancer. Amsterdam, Excerpta Medica, 1980, pp 57–75.

107. Sirett DAN, Cowan SK, Janeczko AE, et al: Prostatic tissue distribution of 17β-hydroxy-5α-androstane-3-one and of androgen receptors in benign hyperplasia. J Steroid Biochem 13:723–728, 1980.

108. Morfin RF, Distefano S, Charles JF, Floch HH: 5α-Androstane-3β-diol and 5α-androstane-3β, 7α, 17β-triol in the hyperplastic prostate. J Steroid Biochem 12:529, 1980.

109. Schweikert HU: Conversion of androstenedione to estrone in human fibroblasts cultured from prostate, genital and nongenital skin. Horm Metab Res 11:635, 1979.

110. Walsh PC, Hutchins GM, Ewing LL: Tissue content of dihydrotestosterone in human prostatic hyperplasia is not supranormal. J Clin Invest 72:1772–1777, 1983.

111. Barrack ER, Bujnovszky P, Walsh PC: Subcellular distribution of androgen receptors in human normal, benign hyperplastic, and malignant prostatic tissues: Characterization of nuclear salt-resistant receptors. Cancer Res 43:1107–1116, 1983.

112. Grimaldo JI, Meikle AW: Increased levels of nuclear androgen receptors in hyperplastic prostate of aging men. J Steroid Biochem 21:147–150, 1984.

113. Puah CM, Ghanadian R: Correlative studies between endogenous steroids and stromal-epithelial composition in human benign hypertrophied prostate. Br J Cancer 44:308, 1981.

114. Bruchovsky N, McLoughlin MG, Rennie PS, To MP: Partial characterization of stromal and epithelial forms of 5α-reductase in human prostate. Prog Clin Biol Res 75A:161–175, 1981.

115. Lahtonen R, Bolton NJ, Lukkarinen O, Vihko R: Androgen concentrations in epithelial and stromal cell nuclei of human benign prostatic hypertrophic tissues. J Endocrinol 99:409–414, 1983.

116. Bolton NJ, Lahtonen R, Hammond GL, Vihko R: Distribution and concentrations of androgens in epithelial and stromal compartments of the human benign hypertrophic prostate. J Endocrinol 90:125–131, 1981.

117. Bartsch W, Krieg M, Becker H, et al: Endogenous androgen levels in epithelium and stroma of human benign prostatic hyperplasia and normal prostate. Acta Endocrinol (Copenh) 100:634–640, 1982.

118. Bruchovsky N, Rennie PS, Batzold FH, et al: Kinetic parameters of 5α-reductase activity in stroma and epithelium of normal, hyperplastic and carcinomatous human prostates. J Clin Endocrinol Metab 67:806–816, 1988.

119. Krieg M, Klotzl G, Kaufmann J, Voigt KD. Stroma of human benign prostatic hyperplasia: Preferential tissue for androgen metabolism and oestrogen binding. Acta Endocrinol (Copenh) 96:422–432, 1981.

120. DeKlerk DP, Coffey DS: Quantitative determination of prostatic epithelial and stromal hyperplasia by a new technique: Biomorphometrics. Invest Urol 16:240, 1978.

121. English HF, Drago JR, Santen RJ: Cellular response to androgen depletion and repletion in the rat ventral prostate, autoradiography and morphometric analysis. Prostate 7:41, 1985.

122. Sugimura Y, Cunha GR, Bigsby RM: Androgenic induction of deoxyribonucleic acid synthesis in prostate glands induced in the urothelium of testicular feminized (Tfm/y) mice. Prostate 9:217–395, 1986.

123. Bartsch G, Muller HR, Oberholzer M, Rohr HP: Light microscopic stereological analysis of the normal human prostate and of benign prostatic hyperplasia. J Urol 122:487, 1979.

124. Bartsch G, Frick J, Rohr HP: Stereology, a new morphological method of study of prostatic function and disease. *In* Marberger H, Haschek H, Schirmer HKA, et al (eds): Progress in Clinical and Biological Research: Prostatic Disease. New York, Alan R Liss, 1976, pp 123–141.

125. Bartsch G, Rohr HP: Ultrastructural stereology: A new approach to the study of prostatic function. Invest Urol 14:310, 1977.

126. DeKlerk DP, Coffey DS: Quantitative determination of prostatic epithelial and stromal hyperplasia by a new technique: Biomorphometrics. Invest Urol 16:240, 1978.

127. Ghanadian R, Puah CM: Biochemical and morphometric evaluation of prostatic epithelial and stromal cells. *In* Ghanadian R (ed): The Endocrinology of Prostate Tumours. Lancaster, MTP Press, 1986, pp 87–112.

128. Shah PJR, Abrams PH, Feneley RCL, Green NA: The influence of prostate anatomy on the differing results of prostatectomy according to the surgical approach. Br J Urol 51:549, 1979.

129. Cunha GR, Donjacour AA, Cooke PS, et al: The endocrinology and developmental biology of the prostate. Endocr Rev 814:338–362, 1987.

130. Cunha GR, Cooke PS, Mee S, et al: Mesenchymal-epithelial interactions in androgen-induced prostatic growth and development. *In* Bresciani F, King RJB, Lippman ME, Raynaud J-P (eds): Progress in Cancer Research and Therapy, Vol 35: Hormones and Cancer 3. New York, Raven Press, 1988, pp 460–473.

131. Story MT, Esch F, Shimasaki S, et al: Amino-terminal sequence of a large form of basic fibroblast growth factor isolated from human benign prostatic hyperplastic tissue. Biochem Biophys Res Commun 142:702–709, 1987.

132. Mori H, Maki M, Oishi K: Increased expression of genes for basic fibroblast growth factor and transforming growth factor type 2 in human benign prostatic hyperplasia. Prostate 16:71–80, 1990.

133. Nishi N, Matuo Y, Kunitomi K: Comparative analysis of growth factors in normal and pathologic human prostates. Prostate 13:39–48, 1988.

134. Levine AC, Ren M, Huber GK, Kirschenbaum A: The effect of androgen, estrogen, and growth factors on the proliferation of cultured fibroblasts derived from human fetal and adult prostates. Endocrinology 130:2413–2419, 1992.

135. Sherwood ER, Fong CJ, Lee C, Kozolowski JM: Basic fibroblast growth factor: A potential mediator of stromal growth in the human prostate. Endocrinology 130:2955–2963, 1992.

136. Habib FK: Peptide growth factors: A new frontier in prostate cancer. Prog Clin Biol Res 357:107–115, 1990.

137. Shaikh N, Lai L, McLoughlin J, et al: Quantitative analysis of epidermal growth factor in human benign prostatic hyperplasia and prostatic carcinoma and its prognostic significance. Anticancer Res 10:873–874, 1990.

138. Story MT, Baeten LA, Molter MA, Lawson RK: Influence of androgen and transforming growth factor beta on basic fibroblast growth factor levels in human prostate-derived fibroblast cell cultures. J Urol 143:241A, 1990.

139. Schuurmans ALG, Bolt J, Mulder E: Androgens stimulate both growth rate and epidermal growth factor receptor activity of the human prostate tumor cell LNCaP. Prostate 12:55–63, 1988.

140. Laiho M, DeCaprio JA, Ludlow JW, et al: Growth inhibition by TGF-beta linked to suppression of retinoblastoma protein phosphorylation. Cell 62:175–185, 1990.

141. Pietenpol JA, Holt JT, Stein RW, Moses HL: Transforming growth factor beta 1 suppression of c-*myc* gene transcription: Role in inhibition of keratinocyte proliferation. Proc Natl Acad Sci USA 87:3758–3762, 1990.

142. Pietenpol JA, Stein RW, Moran E: TGF-beta 1 inhibition of c-*myc* transcription and growth in keratinocytes is abrogated by viral transforming proteins with pRB binding domains. Cell 61:777–785, 1990.

143. Maddy SQ, Chisholm GD, Hawkins RA, Habib FK: Localization of epidermal growth factor receptor in the human prostate by biochemical and immunochemical methods. J Endocrinol 113:147–153, 1987.

144. Lubrano C, Sciarra F, Spera G, et al: Immunoreactive EGF in human benign prostatic hyperplasia: Relationships with androgen and estrogen receptors. J Steroid Biochem Mol Biol 41:683–687, 1992.

145. Fiorelli G, De Bellis A, Longo A, et al: Epidermal growth factor receptors in human hyperplastic prostate tissue and their modulation by chronic treatment with a gonadotropin-releasing hormone analogue. J Clin Endocrinol Metab 68:740–743, 1989.

146. Liu XH, Meikle AW: Androgens regulate growth of human prostate cancer cells in culture by increasing TGFαβ secretion and EGF receptor content. *In* Endocrine Society Meeting Abstract 1992.

147. McKeehan WL, Adams PS, Rosser MP: Direct mitogenic effects of insulin, epidermal growth factor, glucocorticoid, cholera toxin, unknown pituitary factors and possibly prolactin, but not androgen, on normal rat prostate epithelial cells in serum-free, primary cell culture. Cancer Res 44:1998–2010, 1984.

148. McKeehan WL, Kan M, Hou J, et al: Heparin-Binding (Fibroblast) Growth Factor/Receptor Gene Expression in the Prostate. New York, Plenum Press, 1991, pp 115–126.

149. DuBeau CE, Resnick NM: Controversies in diagnosis and management of benign prostatic hypertrophy. Adv Intern Med 37:55–83, 1992.

150. Grayhack JT: Benign prostatic hyperplasia: The scope of the problem. Cancer 70:275–279, 1992.

151. Bostwick DG, Cooner WH, Denis L, et al: The association of benign prostatic hyperplasia and cancer of the prostate. Cancer 70(Suppl):291–301, 1992.

152. Lee F, Littrup PJ, Loft-Christensen L, et al: Predicted prostate specific antigen results using transrectal ultrasound gland volume: Dif-

ferentiation of benign prostatic hyperplasia and prostate cancer. Cancer 70(Suppl):211–220, 1992.

153. Flocks RH: Benign prostatic hypertrophy: its diagnosis and management. Med Times 92:519, 1964.

154. Geller J, Angrist A, Nakao K, Newman H: Therapy with progestational agents in advanced benign prostatic hypertrophy. JAMA 210:1421, 1969.

155. Kaufman JJ, Goodwin WE: Hormonal management of the benign obstructing prostate: The use of combined androgen oestrogen therapy. J Urol 81:165, 1969.

156. White JW: The results of double castration in hypertrophy of the prostate. Ann Surg 22:1, 1895.

157. Cabot AT: The question of castration for enlarged prostate. Ann Surg 24:266, 1896.

158. Huggins C, Stevens RA: The effect of castration on benign hypertrophy of the prostate in man. J Urol 43:705–714, 1940.

159. Wendel EF, Brannen GE, Putong PB, Grayhack JT: The effect of orchidectomy and estrogens on benign prostatic hyperplasia. J Urol 108:116, 1972.

160. Caine M, Perlberg S, Gordon R: The treatment of benign prostatic hypertrophy with Flutamide (SCH13521): A placebo-controlled study. J Urol 114:564, 1975.

161. Ibrahim A, Elnur SH: A clinical trial with nor-progesterone caproate (Primostat) in benign prostatic hyperplasia. East Afr Med J 55:429, 1978.

162. Paulson DF, Kane RD: Medrogestone: A prospective study in the pharmaceutical management of benign prostatic hyperplasia. J Urol 113:811, 1975.

163. Rangno RE, McLeod PJ, Ogilvy RI: Treatment of benign prostatic hypertrophy with Medrogestone. Clin Pharmacol Ther 12:658, 1971.

164. Scott WW, Wade JC: Medical treatment of benign prostatic hyperplasia with cyproterone acetate. J Urol 101:81, 1969.

165. Brooks ME, Braf ZF: Effect of 17α-hydroxy progesterone 17-N-caproate on urine flow. Urology 17:488, 1981.

166. Geller J, Nelson CG, Albert TD, Pratt C: The effect of megestrol acetate on uroflow rates in patients with prostatic hypertrophy. Urology 14:467, 1979.

167. Geller J, Roberts T, Newman H, et al: Treatment of benign prostatic hypertrophy with hydroxy progesterone caproate: The effect on clinical symptoms, morphology and endocrine function. JAMA 193:121, 1965.

168. Gingell JC, Miller IN, Roberts JBN: A clinical trial of gestronol hexanoate (SH582) in benign prostatic hypertrophy. Proc R Acad Med 65:130, 1972.

169. Fishman J, Geller J: The effect of the anti-androgen cyproterone acetate and oestradiol production and metabolism in man. Steroids 16:531, 1970.

170. Bosch RJLH, Griffiths DJ, Blom JHM, Schroeder FH: Treatment of benign prostatic hyperplasia by androgen deprivation: Effects on prostate size and urodynamic parameters. J Urol 141:68–72, 1989.

171. Geller J, Albert JD: BPH and prostate cancer: Results of hormonal manipulation. In Bruchovsky A, Chapdelaine A, Neumann F (eds): Regulation of Androgen Action. West Berlin, Congressdruck R Bruckner, 1985, pp 51–75.

172. Henderson D, Habenicht U-F, Nishino Y, et al: Aromatase inhibitors and benign prostatic hyperplasia. J Steroid Biochem 25:867–876, 1986.

173. McConnell JD, Wilson JD, George FW, et al: Finasteride, an inhibitor of 5α-reductase, suppresses prostatic dihydrotestosterone in men with benign prostatic hyperplasia. J Clin Endocrinol Metab 74:505–508, 1992.

174. Stoner E: The clinical development of a 5 alpha-reductase inhibitor, finasteride. J Steroid Biochem Mol Biol 37:375–378, 1990.

175. The MK-906 (Finasteride) Study Group: One-year experience in the treatment of benign prostatic hyperplasia with finasteride. J Androl 12:372–375, 1991.

176. Gormley GJ, Stoner E, Bruskewitz RC, et al: The effect of Finasteride in men with benign prostatic hyperplasia. N Engl J Med 327:1185–1191, 1992.

177. El Etreby MF, Nishino Y, Habenicht U-F, Henderson D: Atamestane, a new aromatase inhibitor for the management of benign prostatic hyperplasia. J Androl 12:403–414, 1991.

178. Farrar DJ, Pryor JS: The effect of bromocriptine in patients with benign prostatic hypertrophy. Br J Urol 48:73–75, 1976.

179. Shaprio A, Ron M, Caine M, Kramer J: The pharmacological effect of bromocriptine on the human prostate. Urol Res 8:25, 1980.

180. Abrams PM, Shah PJ, Stone R, Choa RG: Bladder outflow obstruction treated with phenoxybenzamine. Br J Urol 54:527–530, 1982.

181. Caine M, Perlberg S, Meretyk S: A placebo-controlled double-blind study of the effect of phenoxybenzamine in benign prostatic obstruction. Br J Urol 50:551, 1978.

182. Lepor H, Soloway MS, Klimerg IW, et al: Long-term safety and efficacy of terazosin, a selective alpha-1 blocker, in patients with benign prostatic hyperplasia (BPH). J Urol 147(Suppl 365A):211–220, 1992.

183. Flood AB, Black NA, McPherson K, et al: Assessing symptom improvement after elective prostatectomy for benign prostatic hypertrophy. Arch Intern Med 152:1507–1512, 1992.

139

Gynecomastia

RICHARD J. SANTEN

During fetal development, epithelial cells from the nipple anlage migrate into the surrounding mesenchymal tissues and form precursors of the ductal system. The ducts differentiate during transient stimulation by maternal hormones during fetal life. After birth, hormonal levels diminish, and mammary tissues remain quiescent during the prepubertal period. Notably, parenchymal and stromal cells with a potential for full breast development are equally present in boys and girls prior to puberty. Thus an appropriate hormonal stimulus can produce breast maturation (gynecomastia) in the male.[1]

Experimental and clinical studies indicate that both stimulatory and inhibitory hormones control the growth and differentiation of breast tissues[2, 3] (Fig. 139–1). Estradiol stimulates the proliferation and differentiation of parenchymal epithelium to form ductal elements. Estrogen receptors are present and are up-regulated by both estradiol and progesterone.[4–9] Some of the estradiol present in the breast may be made locally through conversion of androgens to estrogens via the enzyme aromatase. Prolactin acts on differentiated breast acini to stimulate the synthesis of milk protein. Prolactin receptors are present and are up-regulated by estradiol.[5] Progesterone acts in concert with prolactin to stimulate lobuloalveolar growth.[1] Testosterone exerts a generalized inhibitory action on breast tissue growth and differentiation, perhaps through a specific antiestrogenic action.[3]

The breast requires additional hormones which act in a permissive manner.[1, 10–12] In tissue culture, growth hormone, insulin, insulin-like growth factor I (IGF-I), and cortisol exert no specific effects, but estradiol, progesterone, and prolactin are inactive in the absence of these factors. Certain regulatory hormones also modulate systemic hormonal effects, which, in turn, influence breast growth and differentiation. Thyroxine increases the level of testosterone-estradiol–binding globulin (TeBG) and the serum estradiol concentration and thus exerts indirect effects on the breast. Both cortisol and prolactin lower circulating testosterone levels through hypothalamic and testicular ef-

fects, and thus they diminish inhibitory influences on the breast.

The application of these physiological principles allows gynecomastia to be considered on a pathophysiological basis. A disordered balance between secretion of stimulatory hormones and that of inhibitory hormones underlies the development of the pathological forms of gynecomastia in men. Gynecomastia also may occur as a normal physiological process at various stages of life. Major emphasis has been placed on the balance between estradiol, the major facilitative hormone, and testosterone as an inhibitor in both the physiological and pathological types.

PHYSIOLOGICAL FORMS OF GYNECOMASTIA

Newborn Gynecomastia

The high levels of estradiol and progesterone produced by the mother during fetal life cause stimulation of breast tissue which is present transiently after birth in boys. Secretory function resulting in a minimal breast discharge called "witch's milk" also may be present.

Pubertal Gynecomastia

Beginning at age 11, approximately 30 per cent of boys develop detectable gynecomastia (i.e., glandular tissue > 0.5 cm in diameter); by age 14, gynecomastia is detectable in 65 per cent.[13] Surprisingly, unilateral gynecomastia is common, occurring on the left in 19 per cent and on the right in 29 per cent. Bilateral gynecomastia occurs in 55 per cent of those with palpable breast tissue.[14] Gynecomastia resolves spontaneously in the majority after 1 year. Hormonal alterations in pubertal boys with gynecomastia are not found consistently and are variably reported as low free

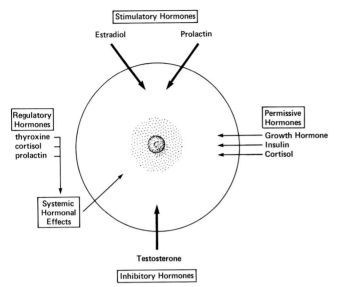

FIGURE 139–1. Diagrammatic representation of the hormones that affect breast tissue growth and differentiation.

testosterone, increased estradiol, elevated estradiol/testosterone ratio, and increased TeBG levels.[14–19]

Adult Gynecomastia

Four studies[20–23] found that gynecomastia was present in hospitalized adults with high prevalence. Patients and physicians, however, were found to have minimal awareness of the existence of the condition. Thirty-three per cent of men in their mid-20's and 57 per cent between ages 45 and 59 had palpable breast tissue that exceeded 2 cm in diameter. These findings do not appear to represent pseudogynecomastia as a result of fat but rather glandular tissue beneath the nipple. Autopsy confirmed the physical findings in 60 consecutive cases in one study[23] and independently detected gynecomastia in another. Two subtypes of gynecomastia can be distinguished histologically.[24, 25] Glandular predominance occurs in 5 to 9 per cent of patients and presumably represents active hormonal stimulation of ductal elements. Stromal tissue predominates in 32 to 48 per cent and probably reflects the aftermath of a process that becomes quiescent.

In 83 per cent of hospitalized men with gynecomastia, the diameter of breast tissue was found to be 5 cm or less.[23]

The etiology of this form of physiological gynecomastia is not clear but is thought to reflect increased aromatase activity in adipose tissue. The percentage of patients with gynecomastia appears to increase as a function of body mass index (Fig. 139–2). Aromatase activity increases as a function of body fat. In support of this theory, the diameter of breast tissue correlated significantly ($r = 0.52$) with body mass index in a group of 214 well-studied men[23] (Fig. 139–3). As a note of caution, the presence of true gynecomastia in these subjects as opposed to fat deposition (pseudogynecomastia) was judged on physical examination only. Although the authors have correlated physical findings with autopsy evidence of gynecomastia in 60 subjects, the issue of true gynecomastia in their patients remains less than completely certain.

PATHOLOGICAL FORMS OF GYNECOMASTIA

Causes of the pathological forms of gynecomastia in adults are multiple. However, the clinician must be concerned only when there is breast tenderness, a progressive increase in breast size, or enlargement beyond the physiological range (2 to 5 cm). Otherwise, the patient probably has a physiological form of adult gynecomastia, which is quite common. A distinction also must be made between pseudogynecomastia—fat tissue present underneath the nipple—stromal or glandular tissue, and gynecomastia. Mammography may be helpful in making this distinction[26] (Fig. 139–4). Ultrasonography can also be used but is not considered as sensitive as mammography.[27]

A logical approach to the differential diagnosis can be based on known physiology (Table 139–1). An excess of breast stimulatory hormones, deficiency of inhibitory ones, a stimulatory/inhibitory imbalance, or abnormalities of the regulatory hormones cause gynecomastia in the majority of patients. The remainder of causes remain largely idiopathic or uncertain. Pathological forms of gynecomastia have been of concern to physicians for many millennia. Interestingly, this condition was detected in ancient times in the pharaohs of Egypt[28] (Fig. 139–5).

Two approaches are useful for the clinician in approaching this problem: consideration of the various disorders on a pathophysiological basis (see Table 139–1) and practical attention to the most frequent causes of this condition (Fig. 139–6). With the first approach, the specific hor-

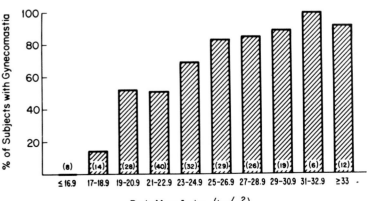

FIGURE 139–2. Correlation of percentage of subjects with gynecomastia and body mass index. (From Niewoehner CB, Nutall FQ: Gynecomastia in a hospitalized male population. Am J Med 77:633, 1984.)

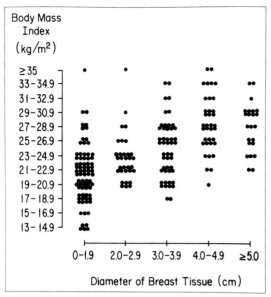

FIGURE 139-3. Correlation of breast tissue diameter with body mass index ($n=214$, $r=0.52$, $p<0.001$). Correlation coefficient was determined by method of least squares. (From Niewoehner CB, Nutall FQ: Gynecomastia in a hospitalized male population. Am J Med 77:633, 1984.)

mones involved in breast glandular development and their potential sources are recalled in relationship to the possible causes of gynecomastia. For testosterone, dihydrotestosterone, prolactin, thyroxine, growth hormone, and insulin, the sources are well understood. For estradiol, approximately 6 µg/d is secreted directly from the testes, 20 µg arises from peripheral aromatization of testicular testosterone to estradiol, and another 20 µg arises from the aromatization of the weak adrenal androgens, androstenedione, and dehydroepiandrosterone (DHEA) or dehydroepiandrosterone sulfate (DHEAS).[29-32] Under conditions of increased luteinizing hormone (LH) secretion, the amount of estradiol secreted by the testes increases.

Using the second approach, Carlson[21] reviewed a consecutive series of patients and found chronic illness and drugs to be the most frequent causes (see Fig. 139-6).

Elevated Estrogen Levels

Several clinical entities result in an increase in estradiol production.[33] Adrenal tumors may be present that result in secretion of several hormones in excess. Adenomas or carcinomas of the adrenal may produce large amounts of estradiol directly. Alternatively, the adrenal tumor secretes androstenedione, DHEA, and DHEAS, which are then aromatized in peripheral tissues to estradiol. These patients generally exhibit a rapid onset of gynecomastia in association with hypertension, elevated ketosteroids, elevated DHEA and DHEAS levels, and an adrenal mass.

Testicular tumors secrete an excess of estrogen through one of three mechanisms: an increase in steroid substrate for aromatization, increased levels of the aromatase enzyme, and increased stimulation of steroidogenesis induced by human chorionic gonadotropin (hCG) secretion

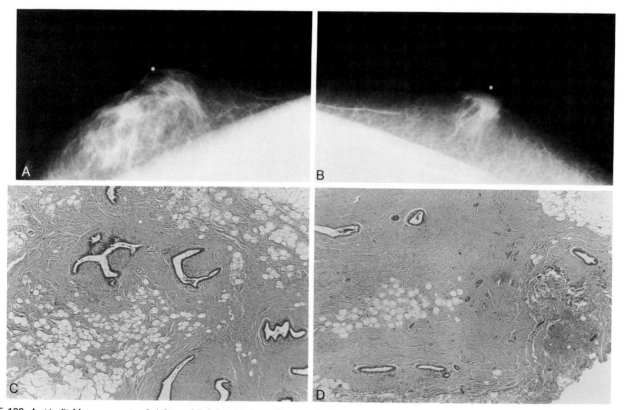

FIGURE 139-4. (A, B) Mammograms of right and left breasts in a 27-year-old male patient with bilateral persistent pubertal gynecomastia. The white circles represent the nipple markers. The glandular elements are apparent as radiopaque areas within the breast tissue. (C, D) Histological appearance of the tissue excised from the right and left breasts during reduction mammoplasty. The left panel illustrates ductal tissue interspersed with stroma and a minimal amount of fat tissue. The right panel contains a predominance of stroma.

TABLE 139–1. CAUSES OF GYNECOMASTIA

Stimulatory hormone excess
  Estradiol
    Adrenal or testicular tumors
    Drug therapy with
      Estrogens
      Estrogen creams
      Embalming cream
      Delousing powder
      Hair oil
      Estrogen analogues: *digitoxin**
      Estrogen precursors: aromatizable androgens
        Testosterone enanthate
        Testosterone propionate
    Increased peripheral aromatase activity due to
      Heredity
      Obesity
  Prolactin
    Pituitary tumor
    Drug therapy with
      Catecholamine antagonists or depleters
        Sulpiride   Phenothiazines
        Metoclopropamide   Reserpine
        Domperidone   Tricyclic antidepressants
        Methyldopa
    Hypothyroidism
Inhibitory hormone deficiency
  Androgen resistance
    Complete testicular feminization
    Partial: Reifenstein, Lubbs, Rosewater, and Dreyfus syndromes
  Androgen antagonist drugs
    Spironolactone   Progestagens
    Cimetidine   Flutamide
    Marijuana
Stimulatory-inhibitory hormone imbalance
  Hypergonadotropic syndromes
    Primary gonadal diseases
    Cytotoxic drug-induced hypogonadism from
      Busulfan   Nitrosourea
      Vincristine Combination chemotherapy
    Steroid synthesis inhibitory drugs
      Ketoconazole   Metronidazole
    Tumor-related: hCG-producing tumors (testis, lung, GI tract, etc.)
      Hepatic tumor with aromatase
    hCG administration
  Hypogonadotropic syndromes
    Isolated gonadotropin deficiency, particularly "fertile eunuch syndrome"
    Panhypopituitarism
  Systemic illnesses
    Renal disease
    Severe liver disease
Miscellaneous endocrine causes
  Hyperthyroidism
  Acromegaly
  Cushing's syndrome
Local trauma
  Hip spica cast
  Chest injury
  Herpes zoster of chest wall
  Post thoracotomy
Primary breast tumor
Uncertain causes
  Refeeding
  Other chronic illnesses
    Pulmonary tuberculosis
    Diabetes mellitus
    Leprosy
  Persistent pubertal macromastia
  Idiopathic
    Familial

*Drugs are listed in italics.

by the tumor. Tumors originate from either Leydig or Sertoli cells and are large enough to be palpated in approximately half of patients.[33–36] hCG administration characteristically produces prolonged and excessive increments in estradiol rather than the usual transient increase for 12 to 24 hours followed by a later increase from 72 to 96 h observed in normal subjects. These tumors may be detected only by testicular ultrasound (Fig. 139–7).

A genetic syndrome has recently been associated with prepubertal gynecomastia. In boys with the Peutz-Jeghers syndrome (pigmented lesions around the oral mucosa and colon cancer), Sertoli cell tumors with very high levels of aromatase result in excessive estradiol production.[37] These tumors are unique in producing large amounts of estrogen even though the levels of precursor substrate testosterone in the testes are low. This results from very high levels of aromatase in the testis. Choriocarcinomas of the testis may produce hCG locally and stimulate production of both estradiol and testosterone.[36]

Estrogen administration for therapy of prostatic carcinoma or for other reasons produces gynecomastia with a very high frequency.[38] Epidemics of gynecomastia have occurred in which an excess of estrogens present in meats was ingested. Regulatory agencies inspect for illegal feeding of diethylstilbestrol (DES) or other estrogens to animals prior to slaughter.[39] However, the practice of estrogen use as an anabolic steroid continues in some areas and can result in gynecomastia if residual estrogens in meat remain sufficiently high. Inadvertent ingestion of oral contraceptives by boys from their mother's medicine bottles can cause gynecomastia. Industrial exposure to oral contraceptives during the manufacturing process also can cause a problem.[40] Administration of aromatizable androgens such as testosterone enanthate or testosterone propionate allows an increase in estradiol to be formed in extraglandular sites, and gynecomastia can result. This is most common in hypogonadal boys during testosterone treatment, but adults receiving these agents for their anabolic effects frequently experience this problem as well. Other drugs such as digitoxin may have intrinsic estrogenic properties and stimulate breast enlargement.[41] Since this drug is administered to patients with severe systemic illnesses and often liver disease, other factors may be involved in the development of gynecomastia. Environmental toxins such as embalming fluid may be estrogenic and produce gynecomastia.[42] Unintended exposure to estrogen can occur from coital exposure to women using vaginal estrogen cream or even from women using estrogen-containing cosmetics.[43, 44] In France, estrogen cream is distributed over large portions of the body as a means of transdermal estrogen delivery. Gynecomastia in their male partners could occur in this instance as well.

Increased estrogen production may result from increases in systemic aromatase activity (as opposed to local testicular aromatase increments). This enzyme is present in testes as well as in muscle, fat, liver, brain, hair follicles, and skin. Bulard et al.[44] suggested that a mild increase in peripheral aromatase activity might be responsible for gynecomastia in subsets of patients with idiopathic gynecomastia. This conclusion was based on cultures of public skin fibroblasts and demonstration of excessive aromatase activity in this tissue.

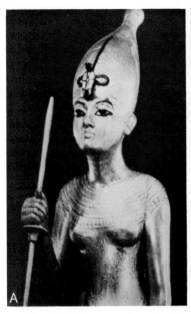
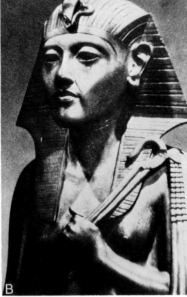

FIGURE 139–5. *(A)* King Tutankhamun. *(B)* His brother Smenkhare. Both are depicted by the artists of the time as having gynecomastia. *(C)* The family tree of the royal dynasty. Amenophis III and Akhenaton are also represented in contemporary art as having gynecomastia.

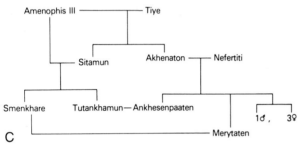

Prolactin

Prolactin secretion is modulated by central aminergic neuronal pathways, particularly of the dopaminergic variety. A wide range of drugs with catecholamine antagonistic or depleting actions can stimulate prolactin release. It is unlikely that prolactin alone causes gynecomastia, since many men with very high prolactin levels lack this finding.[32] Prolactin elevations, however, result in reductions of GnRH, LH, and testosterone and can alter the balance between testosterone and estradiol. It is in this setting that gynecomastia occurs. While these putative mechanisms are not fully substantiated, a number of drugs with catecholamine-related properties are associated with gynecomastia (see Table 139–1). Prolactin-producing pituitary tumors (i.e., prolactinomas) also may cause gynecomastia through similar mechanisms.

Hypothyroidism is another cause of increased prolactin and of gynecomastia. Reductions in serum thyroxine result in an increase in thyrotropin-releasing hormone (TRH) and in thyroid-stimulating hormone (TSH) secretion. If sufficiently high, TRH can stimulate prolactin as well as TSH secretion through its "cross-talk" properties.

Androgen Resistance

A number of disorders and drugs result in a lack of tissue responsiveness to androgen.[45] Since androgens are generally inhibitory to breast development, these conditions are associated with gynecomastia. In the most extreme instance, complete androgen resistance results in the development of normal to greater than normal breast tissue in a genetic male. Since the hypothalamus and pituitary are also resistant to androgens, LH is elevated, as is testosterone, the substrate for aromatization. The combination of estrogen excess and androgen resistance results in the degree of breast development which occurs. In syndromes of partial androgen resistance (Reifenstein, Lubbs, Rosewater, and Dreyfus syndromes),[46] a lesser degree of gynecomastia occurs from similar mechanisms. Cloning and sequencing of the androgen receptor have enabled the detection of specific molecular defects in patients with these disorders.[45]

Several drugs are capable of blocking the tissue effects of androgens by binding to the androgen receptor. These agents also may act in two ways by reducing the inhibitory effects of androgen on breast tissue and by interrupting negative feedback with resulting increments in LH, testosterone, and its aromatized product estradiol. Cimetidine acts in this fashion, as do spironolactone and flutamide.[47–49] Cyproterone acetate acts predominantly as an antiandrogen, since its progestational actions prevent the reflex rise in LH.[50] Marijuana also has been associated with gynecomastia and may act through an antiandrogenic mechanism, although this has not been proved.[51]

Stimulatory/Inhibitory Hormone Imbalance

Primary gonadal disease is associated with a relative deficiency of androgen secretion and reflex rises in LH and

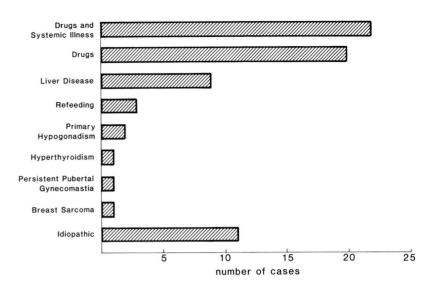

FIGURE 139–6. Frequency of etiologies of gynecomastia in men hospitalized at a Veterans Administration Hospital. The "drugs and systemic illness" category included patients with male climacteric, cirrhosis, hepatitis, hyperthyroidism, refeeding syndrome, and primary hypogonadism. The "drug alone" category included α-methyldopa, phenothiazines, amitriptyline, imipramine, spironolactone, isoniazid, testosterone, narcotics, estradiol, amphetamines, and reserpine. (Reprinted with permission from Carlson HE: Current concepts: Gynecomastia. N Engl J Med 303: 795–799, 1980)

follicle-stimulating hormone (FSH). The hypergonadotropism stimulates the testes to secrete an excess of estradiol. The resulting alteration of the testosterone/estradiol ratio is causative in producing gynecomastia. Klinefelter's syndrome, with an 85 per cent prevalence of gynecomastia, is typical of this condition.[52] These patients exhibit a reduction in total serum testosterone, a further reduction in free testosterone, and increases in plasma estradiol, LH, and FSH. All other forms of primary testicular disease, including mumps orchitis, may be associated with gynecomastia on the same basis.[53]

Cytotoxic chemotherapeutic drugs or irradiation frequently produce transient or permanent testicular dysfunction. Treatment of testicular tumors with these drugs caused gynecomastia in 10 per cent of subjects followed prospectively. Gynecomastia after treatment of Hodgkin's disease, lymphomas, or other cancers with chemotherapeutic drugs also occurs.[54]

Compromise of androgen secretion on an enzymatic basis alters testosterone/estradiol ratios. Patients with congenital deficiency of 17-ketoreductase, C_{21} hydroxylase, or 3β-OL dehydrogenase/Δ_5- to Δ_4-isomerase may experience gynecomastia.[55–57] Drugs inhibiting testosterone biosynthesis such as the $C_{17–20}$ lyase inhibitor ketoconazole also commonly produce gynecomastia.[58]

Malignant neoplasms produce excessive hCG, which stimulates overproduction of estradiol by the testes. For unexplained reasons, but perhaps because of LH receptor down-regulation, testosterone levels are low in this setting. Testicular tumors (choriocarcinoma > embryonal > dysgerminoma > seminoma) as well as lung and gastrointestinal cancers produce gynecomastia through this mechanism.[32, 36] Hepatic tumors and choriocarcinomas also may contain large amounts of aromatase and directly convert testosterone to estradiol in the tumor as another mechanism to produce gynecomastia. hCG given exogenously to hypogonadal patients may be associated with gynecomastia, but usually for a transient period of several months.

Hypogonadotropic syndromes do not usually result in complete gonadotropin deficiency, and FSH secretion may be relatively preserved. Under these circumstances, partial secretion of testosterone and estradiol occurs, and gynecomastia may be present. More commonly, this is observed in the "fertile eunuch syndrome" of incomplete gonadotropin deficiency, but patients with panhypopituitarism also may have gynecomastia.[46]

Several systemic illnesses produce gynecomastia through an endocrine mechanism. Patients with chronic renal failure manifest hypogonadal signs and symptoms. Endocrine evaluation reveals high prolactin levels, moderate elevations of LH and FSH, and reductions in testosterone levels.[59–61] These changes reflect several pathophysiological abnormalities, including delayed peptide hormone clearance, altered gonadotropin negative-feedback setpoint, and perhaps primary gonadal dysfunction. This constellation of abnormalities frequently results in chronic gynecomastia.

Chronic liver disease also produces gynecomastia through a number of mechanisms.[62, 63] Increased aromatization of androgens to estrogens occurs in the liver. Alcohol ingestion damages testicular steroidogenic capacity, and a state of hypergonadotropic hypogonadism can ensue. Acute alterations in nutritional state and ingestion of drugs such as spironolactone can further contribute to the gynecomastia. Even though liver disease is commonly believed to cause gynecomastia, a recent study found gyneco-

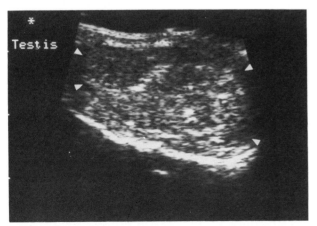

FIGURE 139–7. Testis ultrasound from a patient with Sertoli cell tumor of the testis. Arrowheads define poles (2.9 cm in length). The inhomogeneous texture is markedly abnormal.

mastia as frequently in hospitalized patients without liver disease as in those with severe hepatic dysfunction.[64]

CAUSES

Miscellaneous Endocrine Causes

Hyperthyroidism may present with or be associated with breast tenderness and gynecomastia.[65] Thyroxine stimulates the production of sex hormone–binding globulin (SHBG), which binds plasma estradiol and increases total serum levels. Because the affinity of SHBG for estradiol is less than that for testosterone, increased estradiol may be available to tissue as a cause of gynecomastia in hyperthyroid men. Increased aromatization of androgens to estrogens also accounts for the increased estradiol levels.[66] Increased levels of circulating estradiol in hyperthyroid patients was first described by Chopra et al.[67]

In acromegaly, partial gonadotropin deficiency is frequently present. Increased lactotrophic activity (both from growth hormone itself and from the increase in prolactin which occurs in 50 per cent of patients) may contribute to the presence of gynecomastia.

Cushing's syndrome causes gynecomastia, which is probably mediated by several mechanisms. Glucocorticoids directly interfere with testosterone synthesis and induce a state of relative hypogonadism. The increased adipose mass may cause enhanced aromatase activity. Increased aromatizable substrates from the adrenal also might contribute to an increase in local breast or systemic aromatization.

Local Trauma

Trauma to the chest wall is often considered a cause of gynecomastia. Although an etiological relationship is difficult to prove, in 20 of 21 patients of Greene and Howard, unilateral gynecomastia followed unilateral trauma.[68] Traumatic gynecomastia has been reported following thoracotomy, in army recruits wearing military packs, in patients with hip spica casts irritating the chest wall, following herpes-zoster infection of the chest wall, and following local chest wall irradiation.[69, 70] Neurovascular reflexes have been implicated in the development of this form of gynecomastia, but the exact mechanism for this phenomenon is unknown.[69]

Primary Breast Tumor

Carcinoma of the breast occurs in men with 1/100th the frequency observed in women. The firm, irregular, and unilateral nature of the lesion raises suspicion of this diagnosis. Ultrasonography, mammography, and fine-needle aspiration provide means to make the diagnosis if suspected.

Uncertain Causes

Following World War II, starved prisoners developed gynecomastia upon refeeding. Starvation suppresses gonadotropin production, and refeeding allows return to normal function. The recovery phase mimics the changes that occur during prepuberty. The gynecomastia that ensues is probably also similar to pubertal gynecomastia. This form of gynecomastia is quite frequent and affects patients recovering from chronic illnesses associated with undernutrition. This mechanism is probably responsible for the gynecomastia observed in certain patients with diabetes mellitus, tuberculosis, and perhaps also those with leprosy.[71–73]

Persistent Pubertal Macromastia

The gynecomastia occurring normally at puberty usually resolves spontaneously. However, in boys with a greater than the usual degree of pubertal gynecomastia (i.e., Tanner grades III, IV, and V), this condition persists after puberty. Extensive evaluation reveals no hormonal abnormality, and the only effective therapy is surgical.[74]

Familial

An appreciation of familial gynecomastia emerges from inspection of the statues of King Tutankhamun and his brother Smenkhare dating from approximately 3500 years ago (see Fig. 139–5). Recently, other familial gynecomastia syndromes also have been described.[75, 76] Five males in two generations of a family exhibited gynecomastia and were found to have 10-fold higher levels of peripheral aromatization than normal. The cause for increased expression of aromatase is unknown. However, an animal model of increased skin aromatase activity, the Sebright bantam rooster, is associated with insertion of a retroviral promotor just upstream of the aromatase gene.[77] Familial gynecomastia and mental retardation also have been described recently in a syndrome linked to the DXS255 region of the X chromosome.[78]

Androgen-Induced

A number of drugs are reported to cause gynecomastia.[21, 23, 38, 40, 41, 43, 47, 54, 58, 79–88] Documentation does not always involve drug rechallenge, and the causative nature of these associations is not always valid. This review lists several drugs with known pathophysiological mechanisms (see Table 139–1). In addition, Table 139–2 lists agents reported to cause gynecomastia when the mechanism is not known.

TABLE 139–2. MISCELLANEOUS DRUGS ASSOCIATED WITH GYNECOMASTIA—MECHANISM UNKNOWN

Isoniazid	Amiodarone
Ethionamide	Phenytoin
Thiacetazone	Penicillamine
Griseofulvin	Beta blockers
Omeprazole	Quinidine
Calcium channel blockers	Nitrates
Captopril	Heparin
Narcotic analgesics	Steroids
Diazepam	

Idiopathic

A majority of patients referred to an endocrinologist will fall into the idiopathic category after careful endocrinological evaluation. Whether these patients have increased local aromatization of androgens to estrogens in breast tissue, as suggested by Bulard et al., or other causes is unknown.

EVALUATION

The clinician must decide when to evaluate men with gynecomastia, a condition found in approximately 50 per cent of hospitalized patients.[23] Clear indications for evaluation include breast tenderness, rapid enlargement, and eccentric or hard, irregular masses and lesions greater than 5 cm in diameter. Asymptomatic stable gynecomastia less than 5 cm in diameter, particularly in obese patients, probably requires only a careful history and physical examination for evaluation. In lean subjects, gynecomastia with a breast diameter of 2 to 5 cm should probably be evaluated more extensively.

The appropriate technique for physical examination to detect gynecomastia includes pinching the tissue between thumb and forefinger lateral to the nipple. Ability to "flip an edge" of tissue at the interface of normal and glandular tissue confirms the presence of gynecomastia. Comparison of consistency with that of the fat tissue over the abdomen or along the axillary line is useful. Palpation of tissue with the fingers by pressing over the nipple or lateral to it is an insensitive technique. Mammograms or ultrasound[26, 27] can be used to distinguish the presence of fat (pseudogynecomastia) from glandular tissue (see Fig. 139–4).

After deciding that it is warranted, an evaluation should be initiated (Fig. 139–8), including in all patients (1) a careful drug history, (2) identification of the presence of systemic renal, hepatic, cardiac, or pulmonary disease and particularly previous malnutrition due to other disorders, (3) detection of obvious signs and symptoms of underlying malignancy, especially testicular, and (4) detection of clinically evident syndromes of estradiol, prolactin, growth hormone, cortisol, or thyroxine excess or androgen deficiency.

If the initial evaluation is unrevealing, screening tests to exclude the presence of a neoplasm, including measurement of β-hCG as a tumor marker and a chest x-ray to rule out pulmonary carcinoma, should be performed on all patients. Clinical judgment then dictates whether additional studies such as thyroxine, prolactin, LH, FSH, estradiol, testosterone, and DHEAS concentrations should be obtained. Most commonly, these measurements are ordered to exclude hypogonadism, thyroid dysfunction, and adrenal and testicular tumors. Frequently, the only abnormality found is a mild elevation of plasma estradiol. Testicular ultrasound in such patients is useful, since testicular tumors may not be large enough to palpate but can be detected by ultrasound. Adrenal CT scan is obtained only if DHEAS levels are concomitantly elevated or other reasons for suspicion of adrenal disease exist. Adrenal and testicular vein sampling studies for localization of these tumors have now been largely replaced by the sensitive scanning procedures. After this evaluation, many patients, particularly those referred to an endocrinologist, remain in the idiopathic category.

TREATMENT

Specific therapy for treatable disease should be used when feasible, and offending drugs should be discontinued. Reduction mammoplasty is required under certain clinical circumstances. Persistent pubertal macromastia resistant to medical therapy requires surgical excision.[74] Reduction mammoplasty occasionally is necessary in men with painful or cosmetically disabling lesions. A highly ex-

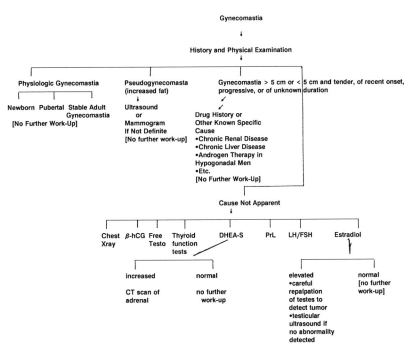

FIGURE 139–8. Algorithim depicting evaluation of patient with gynecomastia.

TABLE 139–3. MEDICAL TREATMENT OF GYNECOMASTIA

MODALITY	MECHANISM	STUDY DESIGN	SUBJECTS	NUMBER	DOSE	RESULTS	COMMENTS	REFERENCE
Tamoxifen	Antiestrogen	Randomized, placebo, cross-over, double-blind	Adults	6	20 mg	5/6 pain reduction, tam. vs. 1/6 placebo Size reduction 3/6 tam. vs. 0/6 placebo	Small study but well conducted	89
Tamoxifen	Antiestrogen	Randomized, placebo, cross-over, double-blind	Adults	10	10 mg	4/4 pain reduction with tam. vs. 0/4 on placebo 7/10 size reduction vs. placebo 1/10	Small study but well conducted	90
Tamoxifen	Antiestrogen	Case report	Adults	1	30 mg	Size reduction	Patient with lung cancer	91
Tamoxifen	Antiestrogen	Uncontrolled	Adults	3	20 mg	3 pain reduction 1 size reduction	Small study	92
Tamoxifen	Antiestrogen	Uncontrolled	Adults	16	20 mg	10/12 pain reduction 4/16 size reduction	Authors concluded treatment beneficial	93
Clomiphene	Antiestrogen	Uncontrolled	Pubertal	19	50 mg	17/19 size reduction >20%	11 underwent surgical reduction after treatment	94
Clomiphene	Antiestrogen	Uncontrolled	Pubertal	12	50 mg	5/12 size reduction >20%	5 underwent surgical reduction after treatment	95
Clomiphene	Antiestrogen	Uncontrolled	Pubertal	22	100 mg	17/22 size reduction >20% 14/22 disappearance of visual tissue	No comment about surgery in any patients	96
Testolactone	Aromatase inhibitor	Uncontrolled	Pubertal	22	450 mg	20/22 breast size reduction—mean 4.4 cm decreasing to 1.7 cm	Authors conclude therapy is effective No comment about surgery in any patients	97
Danazol	Impeded androgen	Randomized, placebo, double-blind	Adults	43	200 mg	5/6 pain reduction, danazol vs. 6/9 placebo Significant improvement (mean 3.70–2.85 cm) in gynecomastia with danazol ($p < 0.05$) but not with placebo	Authors conclude therapy is effective	98
Danazol	Impeded androgen	Uncontrolled	Adults	17	300–600 mg	13/17 marked or moderate reduction in size	Authors conclude therapy is effective	99
			Pubertal	11	200–300 mg	10/11 marked or moderate reduction in size		
Danazol	Impeded androgen	Uncontrolled	Adults	15	Unknown	7/15 had objective response		100
Dihydrotestosterone	Nonaromatizable androgen	Uncontrolled	Pubertal	4	200 mg q4wk IM	4/4 had 67–78% size reduction	Small study	101
Dihydrotestosterone	Nonaromatizable androgen	Uncontrolled	Pubertal	10	125–375 mg	6/10 size reduction	Authors conclude therapy is effective	102
		Uncontrolled	Pubertal	20	Daily on skin	18/20 size reduction		

perienced surgeon should be asked to perform this procedure because of the precise sculpturing necessary to produce the desired cosmetic effects. Boys with pubertal gynecomastia generally can be reassured that regression usually occurs after 1 year and at most after 3 years.[13, 14] Medical therapy has been considered when gynecomastia is severe or of prolonged duration. The use of antiestrogens to block estrogen action, stimulate testosterone secretion, and alter the estrogen-androgen balance has been evaluated. Improvement has been seen in some but not all patients (Table 139–3).[89-96] The administration of nonaromatizable androgens, such as dihydrotestosterone or danazol, which lower estradiol concentration and increase androgen levels, is associated with an improvement in gynecomastia.[97-102] The aromatase inhibitor testolactone also has been used to suppress estradiol but not androgen levels. Each of these medications can be considered and individual responses assessed. Surgical therapy with reduc-

tion mammoplasty is usually required for more severe gynecomastia. Otherwise, a trial of observation without therapy or initiation of a therapeutic trial may be chosen. No comparative trials among medical agents are available, and choices of therapy are based on drug availability, experience of the physician, and cost factors.

REFERENCES

1. Topper YJ, Freeman CS: Multiple hormone interactions in the developmental biology of the mammary gland. Physiol Rev 60:1049–1105, 1980.
2. Casey RW, Wilson JD: Antiestrogenic action of dihydrotestosterone in mouse breast: Competition with estradiol for binding to the estrogen receptor. J Clin Invest 74:2272–2278, 1984.
3. Wilson JD, Aiman J, MacDonald PC: The pathogenesis of gynecomastia. Adv Intern Med 25:1–32, 1980.
4. Wagner RK, Jungblut PW: Oestradiol and dihydrotestosterone recep-

tors in normal and neoplastic human mammary tissue. Acta Endocrinol (Copenh) 82:105–120, 1976.

5. Muldoon TG: Prolactin mediation of estrogen-induced changes in mammary tissue estrogen and progesterone receptors. Endocrinology 121:141–149, 1987.

6. Rajendran KG, Shah PN, Bagli NP, et al: Oestradiol receptors in non-neoplastic gynaecomastic tissue of phenotypic males. Horm Res 7:193–200, 1976.

7. Poulsen HS, Hermansen C, Andersen A, et al: Gynecomasty: Estrogen and androgen receptors. A clinical-pathological investigation. Acta Pathol Microbiol Immunol Scand [A] 93:229–233, 1985.

8. Pacheco MM, Oshima CF, Lopes MP, et al: Steroid hormone receptors in male breast diseases. Anticancer Res 6:1013–1018, 1986.

9. Andersen J, Orntoft TF, Andersen JA, et al: Gynecomastia: Immunohistochemical demonstration of estrogen receptors. Acta Pathol Microbiol Immunol Scand [A] 95:263–267, 1987.

10. Furlanetto RW, DiCarlo JN: Somatomedin-C receptors and growth effects in human breast cells maintained in long-term tissue culture. Cancer Res 44:2122–2128, 1984.

11. Peyrat JP, Bonneterre J, Laurent JC, et al: Presence and characterization of insulin-like growth factor I receptors in human benign breast disease. Eur J Cancer Clin Oncol 24:1425–1431, 1988.

12. Imagawa W, Tomooka Y, Hamamoto S, et al: Stimulation of mammary epithelial cell growth in vitro: Interaction of epidermal growth factor and mammogenic hormones. Endocrinology 116:1514–1524, 1985.

13. Nydick M, Bustos J, Dale JH Jr, Rawson RW: Gynecomastia in adolescent boys. JAMA 178:449–454, 1961.

14. Biro FM, Lucky AW, Huster GA, Morrison JA: Hormonal studies and physical maturation in adolescent gynecomastia. J Pediatr 116:450–455, 1990.

15. Lee PA: The relationship of concentrations of serum hormones to pubertal gynecomastia. J Pediatr 86:212–215, 1975.

16. LaFranchi SH, Parlow AF, Luppe BM, et al: Pubertal gynecomastia and transient elevation of serum estradiol level. Am J Dis Child 129:927–931, 1975.

17. Knorr D, Bidlingmaier F: Gynecomastia in male adolescents. J Clin Endocrinol Metab 4:157–171, 1975.

18. Large DM, Anderson DC: Twenty-four hour profiles of circulating androgens and estrogens in male puberty with and without gynecomastia. Clin Endocrinol (OXF) 11:505–521, 1979.

19. Moore DC, Schlaepfor LV, Paunier L, Sizonenko PC: Hormonal changes during puberty: V. Transient pubertal gynecomastia: Abnormal androgen-estrogen ratios. J Clin Endocrinol Metab 58:492–499, 1984.

20. Nuttal FQ: Gynecomastia as a physical finding in normal men. J Clin Endocrinol Metab 48:338–340, 1979.

21. Carlson HE: Current concepts: Gynecomastia. N Engl J Med 303:795–799, 1980.

22. Ley SB, Mozaffarian GA, Leonard JM, et al: Palpable breast tissue versus gynecomastia as a normal physical finding. Clin Res 28:24A, 1980.

23. Niewoehner CB, Nuttal FQ: Gynecomastia in a hospitalized male population. Am J Med 77:633–638, 1984.

24. Andersen JA, Gram JB: Male breast at autopsy. Acta Pathol Microbiol Immunol Scand [A] 90:191–197, 1982.

25. Sandison AT: An autopsy study of the adult human breast. Natl Cancer Inst Monogr 8:77–80, 1962.

26. Dershaw DD: Male mammography. AJR 146:127–131, 1986.

27. Jackson VP, Gilmore RL: Male breast carcinoma and gynecomastia: Comparison of mammography with sonography. Radiology 149:533–536, 1986.

28. Paulshock BZ: Tutankhamen and his brothers: Familial gynecomastia in the eighteenth dynasty. JAMA 244:160–164, 1980.

29. Weinstein RL, Kelch RP, Jenner MR, et al: Secretion of unconjugated androgens and estrogens by the normal and abnormal human testis before and after human chorionic gonadotropin. J Clin Invest 53:1–6, 1974.

30. Payne AH, Kelch RP, Musich SS, Halpern ME: Intratesticular site of aromatization in the human. J Clin Endocrinol Metab 42:1081–1087, 1976.

31. Kelch RP, Jenner MR, Weiein R, et al: Estradiol and testosterone secretion by human, simian and canine testes in males with hypogonadism and in male pseudohermaphrodites with the feminizing testis syndrome. J Clin Invest 51:824–830, 1972.

32. Frantz AG, Wilson JD: Endocrine disorders of the breast. In Wilson JD, Foster DW (eds): Williams' Textbook of Endocrinology (ed 8). Philadelphia, WB Saunders Co, 1992, pp 953–975.

33. Gabrilove JL, Nicholis GL, Mitty HA, et al: Feminizing interstitial cell tumor of the testis: personal observations and a review of the literature. Cancer 38:1184–1202, 1975.

34. Hendry WS, Garvie WHH, Ah-See AK, et al: Ultrasonic detection of occult testicular neoplasms in patients with gynaecomastia. Br J Radiol 57:571–572, 1984.

35. Kuhn JM, Mahoudeau JA, Billaud L, et al: Evaluation of diagnostic criteria for Leydig cell tumours in adult men revealed by gynaecomastia. Clin Endocrinol (Oxf) 26:407–416, 1987.

36. Whitcomb RW, Schimke RN, Kyner JL, et al: Endocrine studies in a male patient with choriocarcinoma and gynecomastia. Am J Med 81:917–920, 1986.

37. Coen P, Kulin H, Ballantine T, et al: An aromatase-producing sex-cord tumor resulting in prepubertal gynecomastia. N Engl J Med 324:317–322, 1991.

38. Hendrickson DA, Anderson WR: Diethylstilbesterol therapy: Gynecomastia. JAMA 213:468, 1970.

39. Henricks DM, Gray SL, Hoover JLB: Residue levels of endogenous estrogens in beef tissues. J Anim Sci 57:247–255, 1983.

40. Harrington JM, Stein GF, Rivera RO, et al: The occupational hazards of formulating oral contraceptives—a survey of plant employees. Arch Environ Health 33:12–15, 1978.

41. Rifka SM, Pita JC, Vigersky RA, et al: Interaction of digitalis and spironolactone with human sex steroid receptors. J Clin Endocrinol Metab 46:338–344, 1977.

42. Finkelstein JS, McCully WF, MacLaughlin DT, et al: The mortician's mystery: Gynecomastia and reversible hypogonadotropic hypogonadism in an embalmer. N Engl J Med 318:961–965, 1988.

43. DeRaimondo CV, Roach AC, Meador CK: Gynecomastia from exposure to vaginal estrogen cream. N Engl J Med 302:1089–1090, 1980.

44. Bulard J, Mowszkowicz I, Schaison G: Increased aromatase activity in pubic skin fibroblasts from patients with isolated gynecomastia. J Clin Endocrinol Metab 64:618–623, 1987.

45. Griffin JE, Wilson JD: The androgen resistance syndromes: 5α-Reductase deficiency, testicular feminization, and related disorders. In Scriver CR, Beaudet AL, Sly WS, et al (eds): Metabolic Basis of Inherited Disease (ed 6). New York, McGraw-Hill, 1989, pp 1919–1944.

46. Santen RJ: The testis. In Felig P, Baxter JD, Broadus AE, Frohman LA (eds): Endocrinology and Metabolism (ed 3). New York, McGraw-Hill, in press.

47. Jensen RT, Collen MJ, Pandol SJ, et al: Cimetidine-induced impotence and breast changes in patients with gastric hypersecretory states. N Engl J Med 308:883–887, 1983.

48. Caine M, Perlberg S, Gordon R: The treatment of benign prostatic hypertrophy with flutamide (SCH 13521): A placebo controlled study. J Urol 114:564–568, 1975.

49. Caminos-Torres R, Ma L, Snyder PJ: Gynecomastia and semen abnormalities induced by spironolactone in normal men. J Clin Endocrinol Metab 5:255–260, 1977.

50. Geller J, Vazakas G, Fruchtman B, et al: The effect of cyproterone acetate on advanced carcinoma of the prostate. Surg Gynecol Obstet 127:748–758, 1968.

51. Harmon JW, Aliapoulios MA: Marijuana-induced gynecomastia: Clinical and laboratory experience. Surg Forum 25:423–425, 1974.

52. Wang C, Baker HWG, Burger HG, et al: Hormonal studies in Klinefelter's syndrome. Clin Endocrinol (Oxf) 4:399–411, 1975.

53. Aiman J, Brenner PF, MacDonald PC: Androgen and estrogen production in elderly men with gynecomastia and testicular atrophy after mumps orchitis. J Clin Endocrinol Metab 50:380–386, 1980.

54. Saeter G, Fossa DK, Norman N: Gynecomastia following cytotoxic therapy for testicular cancer. Br J Urol 59:348–352, 1987.

55. Maclaren NK, Migeon CJ, Raiti S: Gynecomastia with congenital virilizing adrenal hyperplasia (11β-hydroxylase deficiency). J Pediatr 86:579–581, 1975.

56. Kadair RG, Block MB, Katz FH, et al: "Masked" 21-hydroxylase deficiency of the adrenal presenting with gynecomastia and bilateral testicular masses. Am J Med 62:278–282, 1977.

57. Frank-Raue K, Raue F, Korth-Schutz S, et al: Clinical features and diagnosis of mild 3-beta-hydroxysteroid dehydrogenase deficiency in men. Dtsch Med Wochenschr 114:331–334, 1989.

58. Feldman D: Ketoconazole and other imidazole derivatives as inhibitors of steroidogenesis. Endocr Rev 7:409–420, 1986.

59. Nagel TC, Freinkel N, Bell RH, et al: Gynecomastia, prolactin and other peptide hormones in patients undergoing chronic hemodialysis. J Clin Endocrinol Metab 36:428–432, 1973.

60. Holdsworth S, Atkins RC, de Kretser DM: The pituitary testicular axis in men with chronic renal failure. N Engl J Med 296:1245–1249, 1977.

61. Emmanouel DS, Lindheimer MD, Katz Al: Pathogenesis of endocrine abnormalities in uremia. Endocr Rev 1:28, 1980.
62. Edman DC, Hemsell DL, Brenner PF, et al: Extraglandular estrogen formation in subjects with cirrhosis. Gastroenterology 69:819, 1975.
63. Baker HWG, Burger HG, deKretser DM, et al: A study of the endocrine manifestations of hepatic cirrhosis. Q J Med 45(NS):145–178, 1976.
64. Cavanaugh J, Niewoehner CB, Nuttal FQ: Gynecomastia and cirrhosis of the liver. Arch Intern Med 150:563–565, 1990.
65. Becker KL, Winnacker JL, Matthews MJ, et al: Gynecomastia and hyperthyroidism: An endocrine and histological investigation. J Clin Endocrinol 28:227–285, 1968.
66. Southren AL, Olivo J, Gordon GG, et al: The conversion of androgens to estrogens in hyperthyroidism. J Clin Endocrinol Metab 38:207–214, 1974.
67. Chopra IJ, Abraham GE, Chopra N, et al: Alterations in circulating estradiol-17 in male patients with Graves' disease. N Engl J Med 286:124–129, 1972.
68. Greene WW, Howard NJ: Relationship of trauma to lesions of male breast. Am J Surg 85:431–437, 1953.
69. Field JB, Solis RT, Dear WE: Case report: Unilateral gynecomastia associated with thoracotomy following resection of carcinoma of the lung. Am J Med Sci 298:402–406, 1989.
70. Epstein S. Herpes zoster of the chest wall and gynaecomastia: A case report. S Afr Med J 54:368–369, 1978.
71. Klatskin G, Saltin WT, Humm FD: Gynecomastia due to malnutrition. Am J Med Sci 213:19–30, 1947.
72. Zurbiran S, Gomez-Mont F: Endocrine disturbances in chronic human malnutrition. Vitam Horm 11:97–132, 1953.
73. Morely JE, Distiller LA, Sagel J, et al: Hormonal changes associated with testicular atrophy and gynecomastia in patients with leprosy. Clin Endocrinol (Oxf) 6:299–303, 1977.
74. Eil C, Lippman ME, de Moss EV, Loriaux DL: Androgen receptor characteristics in skin fibroblasts from men with pubertal macromastia. Clin Endocrinol (Oxf) 19:223–230, 1983.
75. Hemsell DL, Edman CD, Marks JF, et al: Massive extraglandular aromatization of plasma androstenedione resulting in feminization of a prepubertal boy. J Clin Invest 60:455–464, 1977.
76. Berkowitz GD, Gerami A, Brown TR, et al: Familial gynecomastia with increased extraglandular aromatization of plasma carbon 19-steroid. J Clin Invest 75:1763–1769, 1985.
77. Wilson JD, Leshin M, George FW: The Sebright bantam chicken and the genetic control of extraglandular aromatase. Endocr Rev 8:363–376, 1987.
78. Wilson M, Mulley J, Gedeon A, et al: New X-linked syndrome of mental retardation, gynecomastia, and obesity is linked to DXS255. Am J Med Gen 40:406–413, 1991.
79. Fagan TC, Johnson DG, Grosso DS: Metronidazole-induced gynecomastia. JAMA 254:3217, 1985.
80. Markusse HM, Meyboom RHB: Gynaecomastia associated with captopril. Br Med J 296:1262–1263, 1988.
81. Bergman D, Futterweit W, Segal R, et al: Increased oestradiol in diazepam related gynecomastia. Lancet 1:1225–1226, 1981.
82. Mendelson JH, Kuehnle J, Ellingboe J, et al: Plasma testosterone levels before, during and after chronic marijuana smoking. N Engl J Med 291:1051–1055, 1974.
83. Pont A, Goldman ES, Sugar AM, et al: Ketoconazole-induced increase in estradiol-testosterone ratio. Arch Intern Med 145:1429–1431, 1985.
84. Monson JP, Scott DF: Gynaecomastia induced by phenytoin in men with epilepsy. Br Med J 294:612, 1987.
85. Markusse HM, Meyboom RHB: Gynaecomastia associated with captopril. Br Med J 296:1262–1263, 1988.
86. deGasparo M, Whitebread SE, Preiswerk G, et al: Antialdosterones: Incidence and prevention of sexual side effects. J Steroid Biochem 32:223–227, 1989.
87. Beas F, Vargas L, Spada RP, et al: Pseudoprecocious puberty in infants caused by a dermal ointment containing estrogens. J Pediatr 75:127–130, 1969.
88. Cicero TJ, Bell RD, Wiest WG, et al: Function of the male sex organs in heroin and methadone users. N Engl J Med 292:882–887, 1975.
89. McDermott MT, Hofeldt FD, Kidd GS: Tamoxifen therapy for painful idiopathic gynecomastia. South Med J 83:1283–1285, 1990.
90. Parker LN, Gray DR, Lai MK, Levin ER: Treatment of gynecomastia with tamoxifen: A double-blind crossover study. Metabolism 35:705–708, 1986.
91. Fairlamb D, Boesen E: Gynaecomastia associated with gonadotropin-secreting carcinoma of the lung. Postgrad Med J 53:269–271, 1977.
92. Jefferys DB: Painful gynaecomastia treated with tamoxifen. Br Med J 1:1119–1120, 1979.
93. Eversmann T, Moito J, von Werder K: Testosteron- und Ostradiolspiegel bei der gynakomastie des mannes. Dtsch Med Wochenschr 109:1678–1682, 1984.
94. Stepanas AV, Burnet RB, Harding PE, Wise PH: Clomiphene in the treatment of pubertal-adolescent gynecomastia: A preliminary report. J Pediatr 90:651–653, 1977.
95. Plourde PV, Kulin HE, Santner SJ: Clomiphene in the treatment of adolescent gynecomastia. Am J Dis Child 137:1080–1082, 1983.
96. LeRoith D, Sobel R, Glick SM: The effect of clomiphene citrate on pubertal gynecomastia. Acta Endocrinol (Copenh) 95:177–180, 1980.
97. Zachmann M, Eiholzer U, Muritano M, et al: Treatment of pubertal gynecomastia with testolactone. Acta Endocrinol (Copenh) 279:218–226, 1986.
98. Jones DJ, Davison DJ, Holt SD, et al: A comparison of danazol and placebo in the treatment of adult idiopathic gynaecomastia: Results of a prospective study in 55 patients. Ann R Coll Surg Engl 72:296–298, 1990.
99. Buckle R: Danazol therapy in gynaecomastia: Recent experience and indications for therapy. Postgrad Med J 55:71–78, 1979.
100. Hughes LE, Mansel RE, Webster DJT: The male breast. In Benign Disorders and Disease of the Breast. London, Bailliere Tindall, 1989, pp 167–174.
101. Eberle AJ, Sparrow JT, Keenan BS: Treatment of persistent pubertal gynecomastia with dihydrotestosterone heptanoate. Adolesc Med 109:144–149, 1986.
102. Kuhn JM, Laudat MH, Roca R, et al: Gynecomasties: Effet due traitement prolonge par la dihydrotestosterone par voie per-cutanee. Presse Med 8:21–25, 1983.

PART XI

INTEGRATED ENDOCRINE SYSTEMS

Endocrine and Other Biological Rhythms

EVE VAN CAUTER
FRED W. TUREK

A prominent feature of the endocrine system is its high degree of temporal organization. Indeed, far from obeying the concept of "constancy of the internal milieu," which was the dogma of early 20th Century endocrinology, circulating hormonal levels undergo pronounced temporal oscillations. Figure 140–1 illustrates as an example the 24-hour profiles of plasma cortisol, thyrotropin-releasing hormone (TSH), prolactin, and growth hormone (GH) observed simultaneously in a young healthy man. As is the case for the majority of hormones, the plasma levels of these four hormones follow a pattern which repeats itself day after day. The nocturnal rise of TSH starts at a time when cortisol secretion is quiescent and ends at the beginning of the sleep period, when GH and prolactin concentrations surge. The early morning period is associated with low TSH, prolactin, and GH concentrations and high cortisol levels.

Thus the release of these four pituitary hormones follows a highly coordinated temporal program which results from the interaction of circadian rhythmicity (i.e., intrinsic effects of time of day, irrespective of the sleep or wake state), sleep (i.e., intrinsic effects of the sleep state, irrespective of the time of day when it occurs), and pulsatile release. This intricate temporal organization provides the endocrine system with remarkable flexibility. Not only can specific physiological processes be turned on and off depending on the presence or absence of a particular hormone, but the precise pattern of hormonal release may provide specific signaling information. Thus a given hormone produced in one temporal pattern may provide a different message to the target tissues than when the same hormone shows a different pattern.

While the profiles shown in Figure 140–1 illustrate hormonal variations in the circadian (i.e., approximately once per 24 hours) and ultradian (i.e., once per 1 to 2 hours) range, the whole spectrum of endocrine rhythms includes both higher- and lower-frequency ranges. Indeed, secretory oscillations with periods in the 5- to 15-minute range have been observed for a number of hormones, including insulin[1, 2] and ACTH.[3] The menstrual cycle and seasonal rhythms belong to the so-called infradian range, corresponding to periods longer than the circadian range. While all endocrine rhythms arise from internal timing systems, only the circadian and seasonal rhythms are synchronized by external environmental factors such as the light-dark (LD) cycle. The remarkable reproducibility of endocrine rhythms, as well as their relative ease of measurement, has resulted in their frequent use as indicators of the status of the neural mechanisms underlying the human circadian system.

The first three sections of this chapter provide an overview of current concepts and recent advances in the fields of circadian rhythms, ultradian oscillations, and seasonal variations. General properties, physiological significance, and medical implications are presented in a broad context. Methodological aspects specific to the study of hormonal rhythms in human subjects are described in the fourth section. The last section summarizes the present state of knowledge on circadian and ultradian endocrine rhythms in health and disease.

CIRCADIAN RHYTHMS

General Characteristics

Endogenous Nature

One of the most obvious characteristics of life on earth is the ability of almost all species to change their behavior on a daily or 24-h basis. Daily changes in lifestyle are, of course, correlated with the pronounced changes which take place in the physical environment due to the rotation of the earth on its axis. While not as readily apparent as the behavioral changes, just about every aspect of the internal environment of the organism also undergoes pronounced fluctuations over the course of the 24-h day.

A remarkable feature of the daily rhythms that are observed in organisms as diverse as algae, fruit flies, and humans is that they are not simply a response to the 24-h changes in the physical environment imposed by the principles of celestial mechanics but instead arise from an internal time-keeping system. Under laboratory conditions devoid of any external time-giving cues, it has been found that just about all diurnal rhythms continue to be expressed. However, under such constant environmental conditions, the period of the rhythm rarely remains exactly 24 hours but instead is "about" 24 hours, and this is why these rhythms are referred to as *circadian*, from the Latin *circa diem*, meaning "around a day." When a circadian rhythm is expressed in the absence of any 24-h signals in the external environment, it is said to be "free-running." Strictly

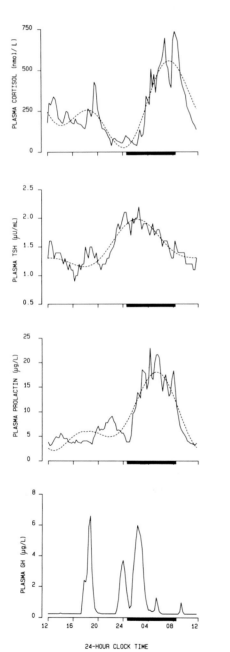

FIGURE 140–1. Twenty-four-hour profiles of plasma cortisol, TSH, prolactin, and GH collected at 15-min intervals in a normal young man. Black bars represent sleep periods. Dashed lines illustrate best-fit curves quantifying the waveshape of the rhythm. (Adapted from van Coevorden A, Mockel J, Laurent E, et al: Neuroendocrine rhythms and sleep in aging. Am J Physiol 260:E651–E661, 1991.)

speaking, a diurnal rhythm should not be referred to as circadian until it has been demonstrated that such a rhythm persists under constant environmental conditions. The purpose of this distinction is to separate out those rhythms which are simply a response to 24-h changes in the physical environment from those which are driven by some internal time-giving system. However, for practical purposes, there is little reason to make a distinction between *diurnal* and *circadian* rhythms, since almost all diurnal rhythms expressed under natural conditions are found to persist under constant environmental conditions in the laboratory. In this chapter we will extend the use of the term *circadian rhythm* to mean all diurnal variations recurring regularly at a time interval of approximately 24 h.

Genetic, physiological, and behavioral experiments have established that the timing system which underlies the generation of circadian rhythms is endogenous to the organism itself. To date, it has not been possible to assay the state of a circadian clock directly in any experimental model. Thus attempts to understand the properties of the circadian clock system focus on the "hands" of the clock, i.e., the expression of overt rhythms regulated by the clock system. While the list of biochemical and physiological processes that show circadian fluctuations is enormous, a few select behavioral rhythms (e.g., locomotor activity, drinking) are most often utilized to characterize the basic features of the clock system in animal studies. Behavioral rhythms are utilized because of their ease of measurement for many cycles without disturbing the animal. Figure 140–2 provides an example of the circadian rhythm of locomotor activity in a male golden hamster held under free-running conditions for 100 days. This rhythm can be monitored via automated systems for essentially the lifetime of the animal without any interference of the sampling procedure on the

rhythm itself. Such long-term continuous sampling of endocrine rhythms is not possible. However, data obtained in mammals indicate that behavioral rhythms represent the hands of the same circadian clock system that underlies most, if not all, endocrine rhythms.

Period, Amplitude, and Phase

An *oscillation* is defined by its *period* (i.e., the time interval after which the waveshape of the oscillation recurs), by its *range* (i.e., the difference between the maximal and minimal values within one period), and by its *mean value* (i.e., the arithmetic mean of all instantaneous values of the oscillating variable within one period). For sinusoidal oscillations such as illustrated in the upper panel of Figure 140–3, half the range of oscillation is called the *amplitude*. Each instantaneous state of an oscillation represents a *phase*. The waveshape of biological oscillations is rarely sinusoidal. Therefore, these definitions have had to be extended, often using best-fit curves to quantify circadian changes independently of more rapid fluctuations. The lower panel of Figure 140–3 shows how period, amplitude, and phase may be defined in the case of the 24-h profile of plasma cortisol. Phase reference points that are commonly used include the timing of the fitted maximum, often referred to as the *acrophase*, and the timing of the fitted minimum, often referred to as the *nadir*.

Not all features of a given overt rhythm represent a property of the circadian pacemaker generating that rhythm. Two properties of circadian rhythms that are considered to be representative of the circadian clock itself are the steady-state phase of the oscillation and its period length under nonentrained conditions.[4] Thus a change in phase or period of an overt rhythm is believed to indicate

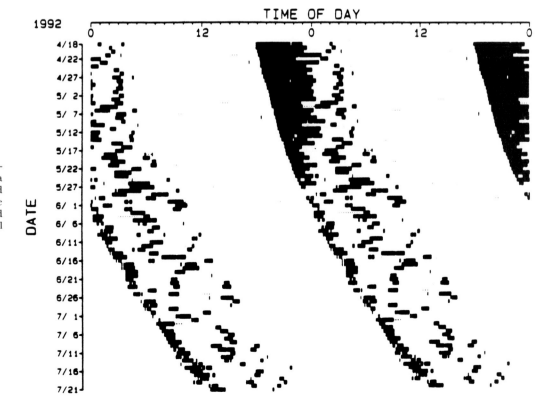

FIGURE 140–2. Continuous record of running-wheel activity in a single golden hamster maintained in constant light for 100 days. The record has been double plotted over a 48-h scale to facilitate visual examination.

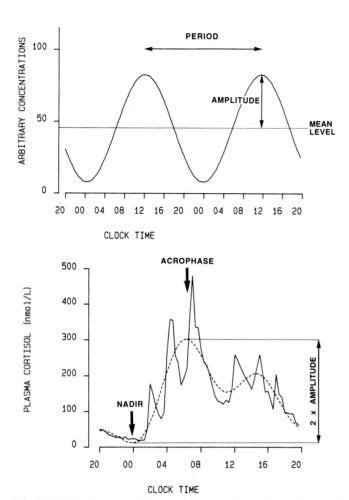

FIGURE 140-3. *Upper panel*, Classical definitions of amplitude, phase, and period of a sinusoidal oscillation. *Lower panel*, 24-Hour profile of plasma cortisol obtained at 15-min intervals in a normal subject and quantified by a best-fit curve shown in dashed lines; the mean cortisol level over the 24-h period is indicated by a thin horizontal line; the period, amplitude, acrophase, and nadir are defined using the best-fit curve rather than the raw data.

that the circadian output from the clock has itself been altered. In contrast, since the amplitude of a rhythm is highly sensitive to factors downstream from the clock, changes in rhythm amplitude are not necessarily due to a change in the centrally generated circadian signal. Perhaps for this reason, in the past, few studies have focused on the modulation of circadian amplitude. However, recently, a series of studies has demonstrated that the amplitude of the central circadian signal is decreased in old age, and this finding has resulted in a growing interest in the regulation of circadian amplitude.

Synchronizing Agents and Entrainment

The fact that the endogenous circadian period observed under constant conditions is not exactly equal to 24 hours implies that changes in the physical environment must synchronize or entrain the internal clock system regulating circadian rhythms. Otherwise, a clock with a period even only a few minutes shorter or longer than 24 hours would soon be totally out of synchrony with the environmental day. Agents that are capable of entraining or synchronizing

circadian rhythms are often called *zeitgebers*, a German neologism meaning "time giver." The focus of this section is on those agents or stimuli which can control the phase of the circadian clock itself rather than on agents or stimuli which might modulate an overt circadian rhythm by influencing a process between the endogenous clock and the peripheral system where the rhythm is observed.

The LD cycle is the primary agent which synchronizes most circadian rhythms to the 24-h environmental cycle. Thus, in the presence of a 24-h LD cycle, the period of circadian rhythms exactly matches the period of the LD cycle, as illustrated in the upper part of Figure 104–4. In addition to establishing "period control," an entraining LD cycle establishes "phase control" such that specific phases of the circadian rhythm occur at the same time in each cycle. For example, in a hamster entrained to a LD 14:10 cycle (i.e., 14 h of light followed by 10 h of darkness every 24 h), the onset of the main bout of daily activity always occurs within a few minutes after lights off, day after day (Fig. 140–4). Following a phase shift in the LD cycle, such as the 5-h delay shown in Figure 140–4, the rhythm re-entrains, although the development of a steady-state phase relationship between the circadian rhythm and the entraining LD cycle often takes several days.

Although circadian rhythms can be entrained to LD cycles that are not exactly 24 h in duration, entrainment is restricted to cycles with periods that are "close" to 24 h in duration. The *range of entrainment* can vary from species to species and is dependent on the experimental conditions

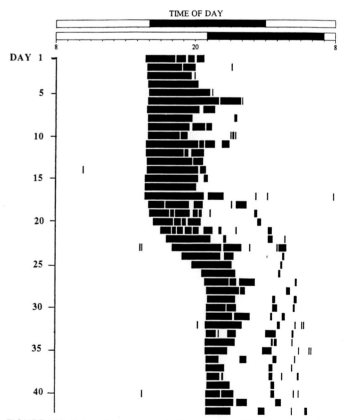

FIGURE 140-4. Continuous record of locomotor activity in a single hamster exposed to a fixed light-dark cyle (LD 14:10) for 17 consecutive days. On the 18th day, the dark period is abruptly delayed by 5 h. The animal takes approximately 10 days to re-entrain to the new LD cycle.

(e.g., intensity of LD cycle, gradual or abrupt modification of LD cycle), but in general, animals do not entrain readily to LD cycles that are more than a few hours shorter or longer than the endogenous circadian period. If the period of the LD cycle is too short or long for entrainment to occur, the circadian rhythm free runs.

One of the most widely used methods to examine how the LD cycle influences the circadian system has been to expose animals maintained in constant darkness (DD) to a brief pulse of light (e.g., 1 to 60 min in duration) and then to return the animals to DD.[4] The effects of the light pulse on a phase reference point of a circadian rhythm (e.g., onset of locomotor activity, minimum of body temperature) in subsequent cycles is then determined. The upper left panel of Figure 140–5 illustrates the phase-advancing effect of a pulse of light given late in the subjective day. This approach has demonstrated that light pulses can induce phase advances or phase delays or have no effect on free-running circadian rhythms. The direction and magnitude of the shifts depend on the circadian time at which the light pulse occurs. A plot of the phase shift induced by an environmental perturbation as a function of the circadian time at which the perturbation is given is called a *phase-response curve* (PRC). The lower panel of Figure 140–5

shows a typical PRC to light pulses obtained in the hamster. The PRC's to light pulses for all organisms share certain characteristics, including the fact that light pulses presented near the onset of the subjective night induce phase delays, while light pulses presented in the late subjective night or early subjective day induce phase advances. In contrast, light pulses presented during most of the subjective day induce no phase shifts. Entrainment of the circadian clock to the LD cycle occurs because each day, light induces phase advances and/or delays that equal the difference between the endogenous period of the clock and the period of the daily LD cycle. It should be noted that while differences in amplitude may exist, the general shape and characteristics of the PRC's to light pulses are similar for all species.

Until relatively recently, a fundamental assumption in circadian rhythm research has been that, except for the LD cycle, endogenous circadian clocks were independent of most changes in the internal and external environments.[4] The early finding that the endogenous period is little influenced by increases or decreases in temperature led to the generalization that to keep accurate time, circadian clocks are buffered from most external and internal factors. Over the past decade, however, a number of inter-

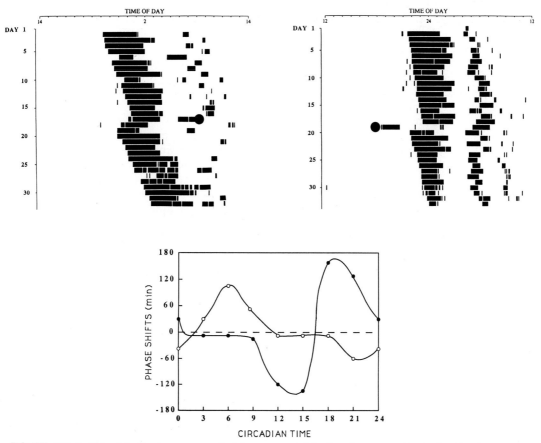

FIGURE 140–5. *Upper left*, Continuous record of locomotor activity in a hamster maintained under free-running conditions for 16 days and exposed to a pulse of bright light indicated by a dark circle at the end of the subjective day, resulting in an advance of about 2 h in the rhythm of locomotor activity. *Upper right*, Continuous record of locomotor activity in a hamster maintained under free-running conditions for 16 days who received an intraperitoneal injection of triazolam (indicated by a dark circle) in the later part of the inactive period. Injection of the benzodiazepine was associated with a bout of activity and an approximately 2-h advance of the rhythm of locomotor activity. *Lower panel*, Typical phase-response curves to light (*closed circles*) and induced activity (*open circles*) in the hamster. Circadian time 12 corresponds to the onset of locomotor activity.

nal and external stimuli other than light have been found to influence the circadian system.[5-7] Although the importance of nonphotic factors in the entrainment of circadian rhythms under natural conditions in mammals is not clear, under laboratory conditions, treatment with hormones of gonadal or pineal origin, changes in ambient temperature, periodic presentation of food, and agents that alter the sleep-wake cycle can all alter the circadian clock system.[4-7] In particular, detailed studies in rats have demonstrated that injections of the pineal hormone melatonin at certain times of the day can phase shift or entrain the circadian rhythm of locomotor activity,[8, 9] and treatment with melatonin has been shown to synchronize human circadian rhythms.[10]

A great deal of attention has recently been focused on the possibility that changes in the activity-rest state can alter the circadian clock system in mammals. The acute presentation of a variety of pharmacological (e.g., benzodiazepine injection) and nonpharmacological stimuli (e.g., exposure to a pulse of darkness on a background of constant light) that induce an acute increase in activity can cause phase advances or phase delays in the circadian rhythms of activity and of other behavioral, physiological, and endocrine variables.[6, 7, 11-14] The upper right panel of Figure 140–5 illustrates the phase-advancing effect of a triazolam injection given at a time when the animal is normally inactive. Note that the benzodiazepine induced a bout of activity shortly after the injection. As shown in the lower panel of Figure 140–5, in the hamster, the PRC's to activity-inducing stimuli are about 12 h out of phase with the PRC's to light pulses. The hypothesis that the increase in locomotor activity is responsible for inducing the phase shifts is supported by recent data demonstrating that these phase shifts can be blocked by restraining the animal following stimulus presentation.[15, 16] Rendering hamsters inactive by immobilizing them at a time when they are normally very active (i.e., during the early part of the subjective night) also can induce phase shifts.[17] Other experiments have demonstrated that induced activity can accelerate the rate of re-entrainment of hamsters following a phase shift in the LD cycle,[18, 19] and the period of the circadian rhythm of locomotor activity in mice, hamsters, and rats may be different when the animal is exposed to a free versus a locked running wheel.[20, 21] Regularly scheduled voluntary exercise can even synchronize the circadian clock of mice maintained in constant darkness.[22] The possible role of activity-modifying stimuli in synchronizing human circadian rhythms is currently under investigation in a number of laboratories.

Functional Significance

The ubiquity of circadian rhythms in all aspects of eukaryotic life emphasizes their evolutionary importance for the survival of the species. The functional significance of circadian rhythms may be viewed in two equally important ways. First, circadian rhythms provide synchronization with the pronounced periodic fluctuations in the external environment. Second, they organize the internal milieu so that there is coordination and synchronization of internal processes.

The predictability of the daily changes in the physical environment has provided natural selection favoring those organisms with an internal temporal program of biological function that is in synchrony with the environmental periodicity. Many behaviors such as feeding, drinking, sleep, exploration, and reproductive activity that change on a daily basis are correlated with the daily changes in the physical environment (e.g., temperature, illumination, humidity) as well as changes in the biological environment (e.g., food availability, presence of predators, parasites, competitors, and reproductive mates). Associated with these behavioral changes are changes in perception, sensation, learning, and performance that occur on a daily basis in many animal species, including humans.[23, 24] Underlying the behavioral adaptations to the daily changes in the external environment are a multitude of metabolic, hormonal, and biochemical rhythms. For example, changes in the digestive system occur before behavioral changes lead to food intake, and the rise in body temperature occurs before animals wake up in anticipation of the increased metabolic demands.[25-27]

External synchronization is of obvious importance for the survival of the species and ensures that the organism does the "right thing" at the right time of day. Of equal but perhaps less appreciated importance is the fact that the circadian clock system provides internal temporal organization. Just as living organisms are organized spatially, they are also organized temporally to ensure that there is *internal synchronization* between the myriad of biochemical and physiological systems in the body. Thus circadian rhythms have specific phase relationships not only with the external environment but also with one another. While lack of synchrony between the organism and the external environment may lead to the immediate demise of the individual (e.g., as would be expected if a nocturnal rodent attempted to navigate the hazards of the diurnal world), lack of synchrony within the internal environment may lead to chronic difficulties with equally severe consequences for the health and well-being of the organism. Indeed, a basic tenet of the field of circadian rhythms is that internal temporal organization is central to the health and well-being of the organism. The physical and mental malaise occurring following rapid travel across time zones (i.e., the "jet lag" phenomenon) and the pathologies associated with long-term shift work are assumed to be due in part to an alteration in the normal phase relationships between various internal rhythms.[28, 29] In addition, it has been speculated that alterations of internal phase relationships between rhythms underlie certain forms of affective illness.[30, 31]

Interactions with Other Biological Rhythms

The circadian clock system plays a fundamental role in the expression of other biological rhythms with periods which are both shorter (*ultradian*) than 24 hours, such as pulsatile hormonal release, and longer (*infradian*) than 24 hours, such as the menstrual cycle and seasonal rhythms.

Ultradian rhythms with periods ranging from a few minutes to several hours have been well documented in many mammalian species.[32-35] There is evidence that the phase, amplitude, and frequency of ultradian oscillations can be modulated by the circadian clock. Perhaps the best examples of the circadian modulation of ultradian rhythms are found in the human endocrine system. Thus the onset of sleep (itself gated by a circadian clock) has a phase-setting effect on the episodic variations of all hormonal secretions influenced by sleep, including prolactin and LGH.[36, 37] The concept of amplitude modulation of ultradian hormonal variations by circadian rhythmicity is also supported by strong experimental evidence. The magnitude of the sleep-associated increase in GH[37] and pubertal luteinizing hormone (LH) release[38] depends on the circadian time at which sleep occurs. Mathematical derivations of cortisol secretory rates from plasma concentrations have suggested that the jagged 24-h profile of plasma cortisol results from a succession of pulses of adrenal secretion in which the magnitude is modulated by a circadian rhythm.[36, 39, 40] There is also evidence to suggest a role for the circadian system in modulating the frequency of ultradian oscillations. Indeed, in women studied at the beginning of the follicular phase, there is a nocturnal slowing of LH pulsatility, indicating that at a specific phase point of the menstrual cycle an interaction between the ultradian rhythm of hormonal release and the circadian sleep-wake cycle occurs.[41, 42]

In mammals, rhythms with periods in the range from a few days to about a month are primarily associated with the female reproductive cycle. While there have been some unusual claims for the appearance of rhythms with a period of about 7 days and even "semiweekly" rhythms,[43, 44] these findings appear to be an artifact of the statistics used to extract such rhythms from the raw data.[45] There are substantial data from different rodent species demonstrating that various estrus-related events are linked to the circadian system. Indeed, in rats, mice, and hamsters, the proestrous surge in pituitary LH release as well as ovulation, the increase in progesterone secretion following ovulation, and the onset of sexual receptivity all occur at specific times of day on the days when they occur.[46, 47] During exposure to constant darkness or constant light, these behavioral and endocrine rhythms continue to occur at specific circadian times. Even though the circadian-timed pre-ovulatory LH surge occurs only once every 4 or 5 days in rats and hamsters, the neural signal for the LH surge can actually be generated every day in ovariectomized estrogen-primed animals, which show a daily release of LH at a time similar to that observed on proestrus in intact animals. There is some evidence to suggest that in women the pre-ovulatory LH surge occurs in the early morning, indicating that circadian involvement in the ovarian cycle may be more widespread than previously thought,[48, 49] although contrary evidence also has been presented.[50]

Since it was first discovered that day length was a primary environmental signal for the regulation of seasonal rhythms, a great deal of attention has been directed toward the question, "How do living organisms measure the length of the day?" Over the years, studies involving light exposure for a short period of time relative to the total amount of darkness, often referred to as "skeleton photoperiods," have led to the conclusion that the circadian clock is involved in photoperiodic time measurement.[47, 51–53] For example, in the Djungarian hamster, a nocturnal species for which long days are stimulatory and short days are inhibitory to testicular function, entrainment of the activity rhythm to the same skeleton photoperiod may be typical of either a short day or a long day, but testicular growth is induced only in the animals showing a long-day entrainment pattern.[53] Thus, depending on the way the circadian clock entrains to a skeleton photoperiod, the same light cycle can be photostimulatory or inhibitory to testicular growth. The results of this and many other studies point to the importance of the phase relationship between the LD cycle and the circadian system in determining whether a given photoperiod will be interpreted as a long or short day. Thus there appears to be a circadian rhythm of sensitivity to light, and the presence or absence of light at critical times will determine whether photoperiodic animals show a "summer" or "winter" response.

The Organization of the Mammalian Circadian System

The Suprachiasmatic Nucleus: A Master Circadian Pacemaker

Many complex behaviors, such as feeding and sleeping, involve a network of brain areas. In contrast, it appears that in mammals a single anatomical locus involving two small bilaterally paired nuclei is responsible for regulating all the diverse 24-h rhythms of the body. The suprachiasmatic nuclei (SCN) are located in the anterior hypothalamus immediately above the optic chiasm and lateral to the third ventricle in all mammals.[54] While each SCN contains only about 8000 neurons in rodents, from both ultrastructural and immunocytochemical studies, the SCN appears to be a complex structure. Extensive lines of evidence, briefly summarized below, have clearly demonstrated that the SCN functions as the master clock in mammals. At the present time, there is no convincing evidence that any other area of the brain can function as a master circadian pacemaker. A milestone in the field of circadian rhythms was achieved in 1972 when the SCN, an area of the brain that had been little studied, was first destroyed in rodent experiments and the observation that circadian rhythmicity was abolished or markedly disrupted was made.[55, 56]

Under both free-running and entrained conditions, destruction of the SCN in a variety of mammalian species, including primates, leads to the abolishment or the severe disruption of many behavioral and physiological rhythms, including those of feeding, drinking, locomotor activity, body temperature, sleep-wake, and cortisol, pineal melatonin, and GH secretion.[5, 57–60] Neonatal ablation of the SCN in rats permanently eliminates the circadian rhythms of locomotor activity and drinking behavior, suggesting that other regions of the brain do not have the capacity to reorganize and take over the function of the SCN.[54] A few controversial studies indicate that some circadian rhythms may persist after SCN lesions,[61] and there is good evidence to suggest that some timing system, which can be entrained by the daily presentation of food at a restricted time, is still present after abolishment of the SCN.[62, 63] The clear role of the SCN as the control center for the circadian system, first suggested by the lesion studies, has been confirmed following transplantation of the SCN from one animal to another. Indeed, circadian rhythmicity can be restored in adult arrhythmic SCN-lesioned rodents by transplanting fetal SCN tissue into the region of the SCN.[64, 65] Furthermore, the discovery of a period mutation in golden hamsters,[66] referred to as the *tau mutant*, in which the free-running period of the activity rhythm is shortened to about 20 h in animals homozygous for the mutation (see below), provided the opportunity to directly demonstrate that the SCN actually contained a circadian clock which itself is driving the expression of overt circadian rhythms. In a series of elegant experiments, Ralph, Menaker, and colleagues[65, 67] performed a number of reciprocal transplants whereby SCN-lesioned arrhythmic wild-type and *tau* mutant animals were implanted with fetal SCN tissue from animals with a different genotype. In all cases in which rhythmicity was restored, the periods of the restored rhythms were always similar to those of the donor genotype, and there was no indication that the host brain significantly affected either the period or the long-term stability of the restored rhythm. While SCN grafts make neural connections with the host brain, it is still not clear if the restored rhythms are due to neural or hormonal circadian outputs from the grafted tissue. Although not a consistent finding between laboratories, it appears that some grafts situated far from the site of the host SCN can restore rhythmicity, suggesting a hormonal signal. To date the rhythms that have been restored following SCN grafting are behavioral ones (e.g., locomotor activity, drinking) which probably involve many different areas of the brain. In contrast, it has not been possible to restore the pineal melatonin rhythm, which depends on specific neural connections between the SCN and the pineal gland.[68]

The SCN itself can express circadian rhythms such as that of glucose utilization.[69] In all species examined to date, whether nocturnal or diurnal, the SCN shows higher metabolic activity during the light phase of the LD cycle. This metabolic rhythm, however, persists under constant lighting conditions. Multiple-unit firing activity is also higher during the light phase, and this rhythm also persists under constant lighting conditions.[70] Importantly, even after surgical isolation of the SCN region from the rest of the brain, a procedure which abolishes the rhythm of locomotor activity and neural firing rhythms in other brain regions, the rhythm in multiple-unit activity persists within the hypothalamic island containing the SCN.[70] It also has been established that there is a rhythm in vasopressin mRNA in the SCN[71, 72] and that the SCN is a major source for vasopressin in the cerebrospinal fluid. Perhaps the most convincing evidence that the SCN contains a circadian clock is the finding that in vitro a number of rhythms persist. In both hypothalamic slice and organ culture preparations, a variety of rhythms have been observed, including those of neural firing, vasopressin release, and glucose metabolism.[73, 74]

Information Flow In and Out of the SCN

The eyes are involved in relaying entraining information from the LD cycle to the circadian timing system in mammals via a unique pathway, separate from the visual system and referred to as the *retinohypothalamic tract* (RHT).[75] At the level of the optic chiasm, retinal projections first enter the brain in the region of the SCN and surrounding hypothalamic areas.[75] If the primary optic tracts are severed posterior to this innervation of the SCN, entrainment of the various circadian rhythms to the LD cycle still occurs, demonstrating that the RHT is sufficient for the entrainment of circadian rhythms. The primary visual centers of the brain and/or the "perception" of light are not necessary for entrainment of circadian rhythms by the LD cycle.

In addition to the RHT, the SCN also receives retinal information indirectly from the lateral geniculate nucleus (LGN), which receives a direct projection from the retina.[75] A geniculohypothalamic tract (GHT) arises from a distinct subdivision of the LGN, referred to as the *intergeniculate leaflet* (IGL), and gives rise to a dense terminal projection which is co-extensive with the termination of the RHT in the SCN. While the GHT projection to the SCN is not necessary for entrainment to the LD cycle, this tract appears to have a functional photic input to the SCN, since destruction of the GHT can modulate the phase angle of entrainment, the circadian period during exposure to constant light, and the rate of re-entrainment following a shift in the timing of the LD cycle.[76]

Early studies suggested that acetylcholine (Ach) may be a neurotransmitter in the circadian system that mediates the effects of light, since the cholinergic agonist carbachol was found to mimic many of the effects of light on the circadian clock.[77] However, the lack of pharmacological and anatomical support for Ach as an active transmitter in the SCN has questioned the validity of this hypothesis.[57, 78] In recent years, more attention has focused on the role of excitatory amino acids, in particular glutamate, in the photic response, but the identification of the neurotransmitter(s) mediating the effects of light on the circadian system is still an open question.

Interestingly, while the neural pathways from the retina to the SCN have been well defined, the identification of the photoreceptors in the eye that are involved in entrainment is still to be established. A substantial body of evidence indicates that circadian photoreceptors may be different from the image-forming rods of the retina. In mutant mice with degenerate retinas, the photosensitivity of the circadian system over a large range of irradiances is not very different from the sensitivity of mice with normal retinas.[79] Studies on the spectral sensitivity of the photoreceptors involved in relaying light to the circadian system as well as the reproductive system in the Djungarian hamster indicate that a short-wavelength cone-like photoreceptor may be the primary receptor relaying non–visual-light information to the brain.[80] It is thus clear that the properties of the response of the mammalian circadian system to light are vastly different from the response of the visual system to light,[81] highlighting the evolutionary divergence of these two systems. This evolutionary divergence is not surprising given the fact that in all nonmammalian vertebrate classes specialized extraretinal photoreceptors mediate the effects of light on the circadian system.[82]

As noted above, nonphotic stimuli also can influence the circadian clock system. How nonphotic information reaches the SCN is still not known, although there is evidence from lesion studies to suggest that the LGN/IGL may be involved in mediating the effects of activity on the clock[76, 83, 84] (Wickland and Turek, unpublished observations). Furthermore, the IGL is the source of the neuropeptide Y (NPY) innervation of the SCN, and the administration of NPY into the SCN area and electrical stimulation of the GHT both induce phase shifts in the hamster locomotor activity rhythm that are similar to those induced by activity-inducing stimuli.[83, 85] The LGN/IGL may be a common pathway by which information about the lighting environment and the activity-rest state reach the circadian clock in the SCN and may be involved in integrating information in the circadian time-keeping system from the external and internal environments. Both the LGN/IGL and the SCN receive a dense serotonergic projection from the midbrain raphe nuclei,[85] and there is now substantial evidence that alterations in serotonergic activity can influence circadian rhythmicity. For example, treatment with fluoxetine, a serotonin reuptake inhibitor, can shorten the circadian period of the activity rhythm in mice, while depletion of brain serotonin levels alters the response of the hamster circadian clock to the phase-shifting effects of light pulses.[86, 87]

Because the physiological nature of the circadian pacemaker within the SCN remains unknown, all studies of circadian outputs have, by necessity, involved the monitoring of some rhythmic variable that is "downstream" from the clock itself. Even circadian rhythms that have been measured within the SCN (e.g., electrical activity or glucose metabolism) may simply represent rhythmic processes that are driven by the clock mechanism, and it has not been demonstrated that these rhythms are involved in the regulation of circadian rhythms outside the SCN. Thus essentially nothing is known about the nature of the neural and/or hormonal signals by which the SCN communicates with the rest of the organism.

Cellular and Molecular Basis for Rhythm Generation and Entrainment

Despite intensive efforts over the past few years, very little is known about the mechanism generating the central circadian signal within the SCN. Models for oscillatory behavior in other physiological systems, such as heart rate and glycolytic oscillations, which have endogenous periods in the range of seconds to minutes, seem to have little relevance to the circadian pacemaker system within the SCN, where the generation of a 24-h period has to be accounted for. Current extrapolations from the field of nonlinear system dynamics indicate that the existence of feedback loops with delays in the range of several hours would be one type of mechanism that could generate oscillatory behavior in the circadian range. Beat phenomena involving coupling of multiple individual oscillators could constitute an alternative circadian clock mechanism.

Two findings suggest that the SCN involves multiple circadian oscillators. First, under certain conditions, behavioral and endocrine rhythms can dissociate or "split" into two distinct components which initially free-run with distinctly different circadian periods resulting in a series of changing phase relationships between the two components.[57, 88] Usually, these components become recoupled some 12 h out of phase with each other and thereafter assume an identical free-running period. Despite the fact that splitting has been consistently observed in a wide variety of vertebrate species,[59, 88] no satisfactory explanation for this intriguing property of the circadian clock has been forthcoming. Lesioning one of the two SCN can abolish splitting.[89] However, it is unlikely that splitting is solely due to each nucleus acting as an independent pacemaker, since the phenomenon has been observed in hamsters with only a single SCN.[90] Splitting appears to be a characteristic of the central pacemaker system in the SCN region, since recent studies indicate that electrical activity within the

SCN obtained from animals showing a split rhythm of activity also shows a bimodal firing frequency in vitro.[91]

A second finding indicating that the SCN itself may be comprised of more than one circadian oscillator is the observation that pieces of the SCN, both in vitro and in vivo, are capable of sustaining circadian oscillations. Thus brain slices containing only a portion of the SCN continue to show rhythmicity in vitro,[74] and following lesions of different regions of the SCN, rhythmicity is maintained in the whole animal.[92] There is also evidence indicating that dispersed SCN cells can still generate circadian signals, suggesting that the ability to generate circadian rhythms does not depend on the structural integrity of the SCN.[64, 93] Taken together with data from nonmammalian circadian pacemakers,[94] it would appear that the ability of the SCN to generate circadian signals is a cellular property and is not dependent on specific neural networks.

Diurnal rhythms in mRNA for various peptides, including vasopressin, gastrin-releasing peptide, and somatostatin, have been observed in the SCN.[85, 95] However, to date, there is no evidence to indicate that any of these gene products plays a fundamental role in the generation of circadian signals. It has been reported recently that in the absence of a LD cycle, there is still a clear circadian rhythm of somatostatin mRNA levels in the SCN, while the rhythm of other peptide mRNA's is no longer present.[95] This finding indicates that certain peptide rhythms in the SCN are a response to the LD cycle, while others depend on the endogenous oscillator.

While no specific gene products that are part of the circadian clock itself have been identified in the SCN, a role for protein synthesis in the generation of circadian rhythms has been established. The acute administration of either of two protein synthesis inhibitors (anisomycin or cycloheximide), with two different mechanisms of action, induces pronounced phase shifts in the circadian clock of hamsters, and the effects of these inhibitors appear to be on cells within the SCN region.[96–98] A number of groups are presently using two-dimensional gel electrophoresis to identify proteins that are unique to the SCN and/or produced at certain times of the circadian cycle when protein synthesis is known to be involved in clock function. One promising lead for the identification of clock-specific proteins is the finding that one of the proteins in the SCN of wild-type hamsters is not present in the SCN of homozygous mutant animals with an abnormally short circadian period.[99]

Molecular and cellular mechanisms underlying entrainment are also poorly defined. Recently, a number of laboratories have demonstrated that light can induce the expression of the proto-oncogene c-fos within the rodent SCN.[100–104] C-fos, as well as other immediate-early gene (IEG) products, appears to function by coupling transient stimuli to the regulation of specific genes in the nucleus. The fos protein dimerizes with products of the Jun family of proteins to form a transcriptional regulatory complex referred to as activating protein 1 (AP-1), and AP-1 can bind to specific regions of the DNA to regulate the transcription of specific genes. Recent studies indicate that light also regulates jun-B activity in the SCN as well.[105] Of particular interest are the findings that the effectiveness of light in inducing c-fos mRNA in the SCN at a particular circadian phase is quantitatively correlated with the magnitude of

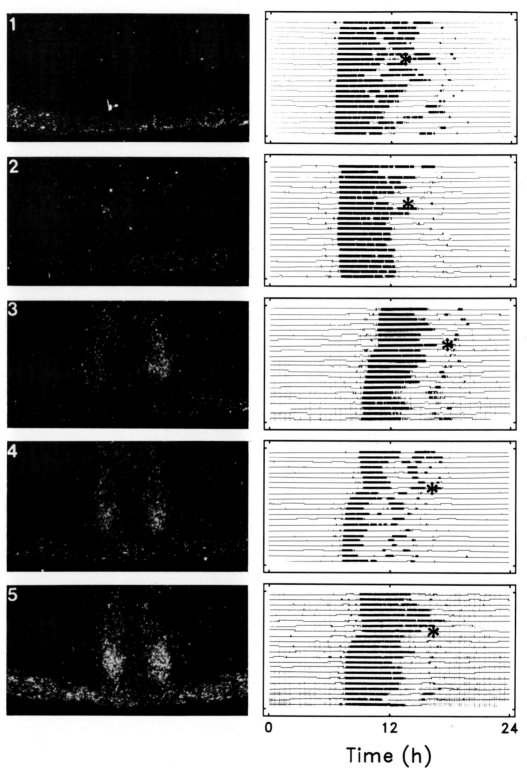

Time (h)

FIGURE 140–6. C-*fos* induction and associated phase-advance shifts. Effects of pulses of light with varying light irradiance on c-*fos* mRNA in the SCN region and the phase of the activity rhythm in hamsters maintained in constant darkness. All light pulses were 5 min in duration and were presented at CT 19. *Left panels,* Following exposure to the light pulse, the animals were returned to constant darkness for 25 min before the brains were prepared for c-*fos* analysis by in situ hybridization procedures. Panel 1 shows c-*fos* levels in an animal receiving no light pulse, while panels 2 to 5 show levels in animals exposed to increasing levels of illumination. *Right panels,* Representative activity records of hamsters exposed to light stimuli of similar irradiance to the corresponding left panels. The asterisks mark the time of the light pulse, after which the animals continued to free run in constant darkness. (From Kornhauser JM, Nelson DE, Mayo KE, Takahashi JS: Photic and circadian regulation of c-*fos* gene expression in the hamster suprachiasmatic nucleus. Neuron 5:127–134, 1990.)

the light-induced phase shifts in the activity rhythm.[102] This is shown in Figure 140–6, where the increase in c-*fos* expression is paralleled by increasing phase advances of the rhythm of locomotor activity. Furthermore, the photic induction of c-*fos* and *jun*-B in the SCN is gated by the circadian clock such that the synthesis of these genes is only induced in response to light pulses presented at circadian phases, where light induces phase shifts in the circadian rhythm of locomotor activity.[102, 105] Figure 140–7 shows that pulses of light induce c-*fos* and *jun*-B expression only when they are presented at circadian times, when a phase shift is induced.

Genetic Basis of Circadian Rhythms

Early studies in various species demonstrated that circadian rhythms were an inherited property of the organism. Circadian rhythms develop normally in diverse species such as fruitflies, lizards, and mice, even if the animals are never exposed to any LD cycles.[106] Indeed, even when mice are raised under LD cycles with periods of 20 or 28 h in

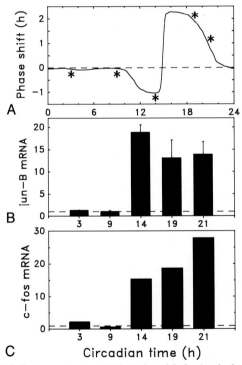

FIGURE 140–7. Dependence of light-induced behavioral phase-shifting and *jun*-B and c-*fos* mRNA levels in the suprachiasmatic nucleus (SCN) region as a function of circadian phase. Hamsters were maintained in constant dark (DD) before being exposed to a 5-min pulse of light. *A*, The asterisks superimposed on the phase-response curve to light pulses denote the time of the pulses in *B* and *C*. *B*, *Jun*-B mRNA in the SCN after pulse presentation at circadian times (CT) 3, 9, 14, 19, and 21. Animals were returned to DD, and brains were prepared for in situ hybridization. Values represent the mean signal in the SCN of light-pulsed hamsters relative to the mean signal at the same CT in animals receiving no light. Hamsters receiving no light exhibited no significant *jun*-B mRNA hybridization in the SCN at all CT examined. *C*, C-*fos* mRNA in the SCN region induced by light following the procedures described in *B*. (From Kornhauser JM, Nelson DE, Mayo KE, Takahashi JS: Regulation of *jun*-B messenger RNA and AP-1 activity by light and a circadian clock. Science 255:1581–1584, 1992. Copyright 1992 by the American Association for the Advancement of Science.)

duration, upon exposure to constant darkness, the period of the free-running rhythm returns immediately to around 24 h.[106]

The first demonstration that specific genes regulate the period of the clock was obtained in the fruitfly *Drosophila*, where mutant alleles inducing very short period, long period, or arrhythmic phenotypes were identified.[107] Mutagenesis has uncovered single-gene mutations in plants and invertebrates that alter such basic clock properties as the period of free-running rhythms, entrainment to LD cycles, and temperature compensation.[108–110] Multiple alleles have been identified at the two most well studied clock genetic loci in *Drosophila* (the *per* gene) and in the fungus *Neurospora* (the *frq* gene), with different alleles inducing a variety of circadian phenotypes.[108–110] Genetic analysis of these mutations has led to the cloning of clock-related genes and the study of their molecular structure and expression.

Unfortunately, no such detailed genetic or molecular studies have been performed on clock-related genes in any vertebrates. Indeed, only recently has a single-gene mutation in a clock-related gene been identified. To date, most genetic studies of circadian rhythms in mammals have focused on the examination of inbred strains. In addition, recent studies on human twins have provided information on the characteristics of certain overt rhythms which are genetically influenced.

Differences in circadian rhythm parameters have been observed between various inbred strains of rodents, indicating that the genetic background influences the expression of circadian rhythms in mammals. Small differences in period, phase angle of entrainment, amplitude of rhythms, and the PRC to light pulses have been noted between various inbred strains of mice, rats, and hamsters.[111–113] In a recent examination of four inbred strains of golden hamsters, it was found that differences in the free-running period of the activity rhythm were correlated with the phase angle of entrainment to the LD cycle (Vitaterna and Turek, unpublished results). In these same strains, there were no apparent differences in the PRC's for light; however, there were clear differences in the PRC's for an activity-inducing stimulus, i.e., triazolam.

The first evidence that the period of a circadian rhythm in mammals could be influenced by a single gene was found in a male hamster from a commercial supplier with a free-running period of 22 h.[66] Subsequent breeding experiments revealed that this animal was heterozygous for a single autosomal mutant gene, which was called *tau*. Further crosses established that the mutant allele was co-dominant and that the homozygote phenotype of the free-running period was about 20 h. Figure 140–8 shows 38 calendar days of recording of the free-running rhythm of locomotor activity of a *tau* mutant hamster. When plotted on a 24-h scale, the rhythm is difficult to observe (left), whereas when plotted on a 20-h scale, a clear free-running rhythm becomes readily apparent. *Tau* is expressed equally in males and females, and the ranges of the circadian periods between the three genotypes do not overlap.[66] In addition to altering the period of the circadian clock, the *tau* mutation also alters the shape of the PRC's to both photic and nonphotic stimuli.[114, 115] Studies involving transplantation of fetal SCN between wild-type and *tau* mutant hamsters have demonstrated that the *tau* mutation acts on circadian timing through a product in the SCN.[65, 67] Exper-

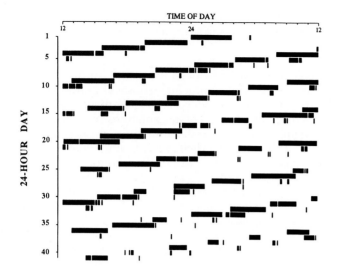

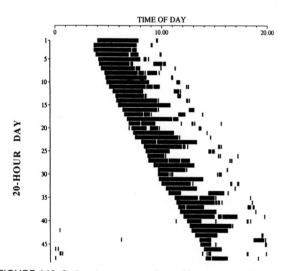

FIGURE 140–8. Continuous recording of locomotor activity in a hamster with the *tau* mutation. On the top, the records are plotted on a 24-h scale, showing 42 calendar days of recording. On the bottom, the records are replotted on a 20-h scale, showing 48 subjective "days," and a clear free-running rhythm emerges.

iments in which donor SCN tissue of one genotype is implanted into an SCN-lesioned host animal of a different genotype have demonstrated conclusively that the restored behavioral rhythms always have the period of the donor tissue. Use of the *tau* mutant for mapping the location and identifying genes that may be involved in the generation of circadian rhythms, however, is unlikely because of the lack of background genetic information in the hamster. Isolation of clock mutants in mice would, in contrast, be important for mapping clock genes, since many genetic markers are available in this species.

Little is known about the contributions of heredity and the environment in the expression of human circadian rhythms. However, in a recent study, a detailed quantitative analysis of the 24-h profile of plasma cortisol in monozygotic and dizygotic pairs of normal male twins under entrained conditions was performed.[116] Figure 140–9 shows the profiles obtained in one pair of monozygotic twins and

one pair of dizygotic twins. Genetic control was demonstrated for the timing of the nocturnal nadir, which is a robust marker of the phase angle of entrainment. Environmental influences were significant for the 24-h mean cortisol level and the timing of the morning acrophase. Although very few studies of this type have been performed, these findings indicate that while some features of overt circadian rhythms are influenced by life habits (e.g., dietary intake, exercise), other features may be under genetic control.

Ontogeny of Circadian Rhythms

Development of Clock and Expression of Rhythms

Four stages in the development of circadian function regulated by the SCN have been defined.[54] First, the SCN cells are formed, grow and mature, and rhythmic function within the nucleus is established well before major synaptic contacts either between SCN cells or with the rest of the brain are established. Second, entrainment pathways, primarily the retinohypothalamic tract, develop, with the resulting ability of the SCN to respond to environmental information. Third, SCN projections appear, resulting in the coupling of the SCN to effector systems, often before those systems can express rhythms. Fourth, the output systems mature to the point where they can now express circadian function.

In several mammalian species, circadian oscillations are present in the SCN during fetal life.[117] In the rat, a circadian rhythm of metabolic activity is apparent within the fetal SCN as early as on day 19 of gestation, and day-night oscillations in vasopressin mRNA levels are present on day 21 of gestation.[117] The fetal SCN is entrained by circadian signals from the mother, and although rhythms develop normally in pups born to SCN-lesioned mothers, fetal SCN rhythms are not entrained without the presence of the maternal SCN.[117] Studies in both rats and hamsters indicate that the fetal SCN can be entrained by the mother approximately at the time of neurogenesis of the SCN.[117, 118] Entrainment may be realized by multiple circadian signals from the mother, including patterns of maternal melatonin and feeding schedules.[117, 119] In rats, the postnatal maternal influence on rhythmicity persists for about a week after birth, when the pups become capable of responding to the entraining effects of the ambient LD cycle.

Despite the early development of circadian rhythms within the SCN, the ability of the SCN to function as a pacemaker for the regulation of overt behavioral and physiological rhythms does not occur until much later. For example, in rats, most behavioral and endocrine rhythms do not appear until the second or third week of life. Thus the circadian clock in the SCN becomes a circadian pacemaker when it develops sufficient afferent, intrinsic, and efferent neural connections to be entrained and to regulate effector systems.[54] However, a series of ingenious experiments[117, 120, 121] has demonstrated that even before specific rhythms are expressed, their eventual phase can already be set.[117, 118]

Recent studies in low-risk preterm infants (29 to 35 weeks) have demonstrated that significant circadian

MONOZYGOTIC TWINS   DIZYGOTIC TWINS

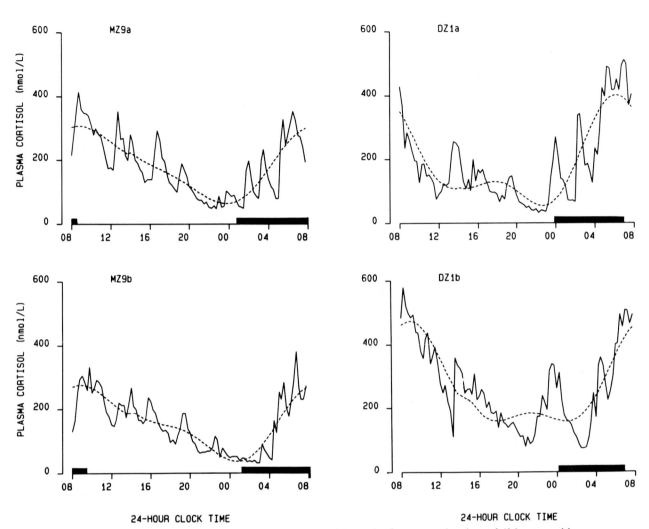

FIGURE 140–9. Twenty-four-hour profiles of plasma cortisol in a pair of monozygotic twins and (*left upper and lower panels*) and in a pair of dizygotic twins (*right upper and lower panels*). The best-fit curve quantifying the circadian waveshape is shown in dashed lines. The black bars represent the sleep period. Note the similarity of circadian waveshape and parallelism of secretory episodes in monozygotic, but not dizygotic, twins. (From Linkowski P, Van Onderbergen A, Kerkhofs M, et al: Twin study of the 24-h cortisol profile: Evidence for genetic control of the human circadian clock. Am J Physiol 264:E173–E181, 1993.)

rhythms were present for both body temperature and heart rate in 50 per cent of the infants.[122] These rhythms were present even though the infants were fed every 2 h intragastrically and maintained in constant light and temperature. The finding that rhythms are present so early in fetal development raises questions about the importance of providing adequate circadian cues to infants who are in need of the best medical care in order to survive.

Aging of the Circadian Clock System

Age-related changes in endocrine, metabolic, and behavioral circadian rhythms have been reported in a variety of species, including humans.[26, 123–127] One of the most prominent changes is a reduction in rhythm amplitude. The overall findings of a study that examined age-related differences in 24-h endocrine rhythms and sleep in healthy sub-

jects are shown in Figure 140–10. A decrease by at least 50 per cent in the nocturnal release of both GH and melatonin was observed in the older volunteers, and slow-wave (SW) sleep was drastically diminished. Other studies have shown that these deficits in the maintenance and depth of nocturnal sleep[128] are paralleled by decreased alertness during the daytime. In both rodents and humans, many circadian rhythms are also phase advanced under entrained conditions such that specific phase points of the rhythms occur earlier than in young animals.[127, 129] Both amplitude reduction and phase advance of the rhythm of body temperature have been observed in elderly subjects, and these alterations in circadian regulation were closely associated with changes in sleep-wake habits, i.e., earlier bedtimes and waketimes.[130]

Age-related changes in the amplitude and/or the phase of circadian rhythms could be due to changes in the circa-

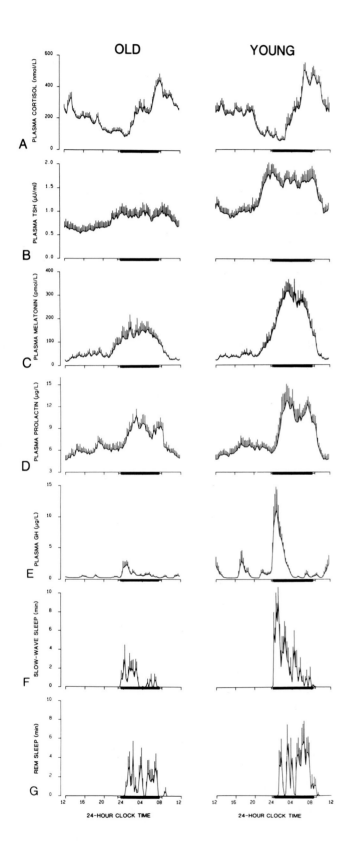

FIGURE 140–10. From *A* to *G,* mean 24-h profiles of plasma cortisol, TSH, melatonin, prolactin, GH levels, and amounts of slow-wave (SW) sleep and rapid-eye-movement (REM) sleep in old (67 to 84 years) and young (20 to 27 years) subjects. Data were sampled at 15-min intervals. At each time point, the vertical line represents the standard error for the group (*n* = 8). The black bars represent the mean sleep period. (From van Coevorden A, Mockel J, Laurent E, et al: Neuroendocrine rhythms and sleep in aging. Am J Physiol 260:E651–E661, 1991.)

dian clock driving these rhythms, to alterations in the input pathways to the clock, or to factors "downstream" between the circadian clock and the system expressing the rhythm. There is convincing evidence indicating that the circadian clock itself is altered in advanced age, since the free-running periods of various rhythms in rodents change systematically with age.[131, 132] While no direct evidence exists for an altered period of human rhythms with advanced age, age-related phase advances of a number of different behavioral and endocrine rhythms are consistent with the hypothesis that the period of the human circadian clock is shorter in the elderly.[26, 127, 130, 133, 134] Recent reports have indicated that both the morphology of the SCN and the biochemical and neuropeptide activity within the SCN are altered in advanced age.[135–138] For example, aging alters the circadian rhythms of glucose utilization and α-adrenergic receptor levels in the SCN, and these changes are correlated with changes in the circadian rhythm of LH release (i.e., the preovulatory LH surge) that are observed with aging in female rats.[136–138] Thus at least some of the age-related changes in rhythmicity appear to be due to alterations in the pacemaker itself.

Studies in rodents indicate that aging is also associated with a decreased responsiveness to the phase-shifting effects of both photic and nonphotic stimuli. Old hamsters show a decreased response to the phase-shifting effects of low-intensity light pulses (Zhang, Takahashi, and Turek, unpublished observations). This observation raises the possibility that in old age there is either decreased signal transmission of light information to the SCN or that the SCN itself is less responsive to photic stimulation. Similarly, while induction of locomotor activity during a time of normal inactivity can induce pronounced phase shifts in the circadian rhythm of locomotor activity in young animals, in old animals the response is greatly diminished or completely abolished.[139] Interestingly, transplantation of fetal SCN tissue into the SCN region of old hamsters with an intact SCN can restore the response to the phase-shifting effects of triazolam on the activity rhythm (Van Reeth, Zhang, and Turek, unpublished results).

Behavioral changes in the elderly also may lead to changes in environmental inputs to the clock. In older adults, exposure to bright light and social cues, both potential entraining agents, is markedly diminished when compared with young adults.[140, 141] Absence of professional constraints, decreased mobility due to illness, and reduced socialization and outdoor activities are all hallmarks of old age. Thus decreased exposure to environmental stimuli that entrain circadian rhythms could contribute to disruptions in circadian rhythmicity. The use of exposure to bright light and "enriched" social schedules to reinforce circadian rhythms in older adults and possibly improve nighttime sleep and daytime alertness is currently being investigated in various gerontology centers.

Human Circadian Rhythms

Observations in Free-Running Conditions

There is virtually neither tissue nor function within the human organism that does not manifest regular changes from day to night. The endogenous nature of human cir-

cadian rhythms has been established by experiments in which subjects were isolated with no access to the natural LD cycle and no time cues. Such experiments were first performed in natural caves, then in underground bunkers, and finally in specially designed windowless soundproof apartments. The results of such an experiment, conducted in an artificial underground unit in Germany, are shown in Figure 140–11.[142–144] The rest-activity cycle of the subject is plotted horizontally, day by day, and the times of occurrence of the daily maximum of the body temperature cycle are indicated by closed triangles. During the first 7 days of the experiment, the door of the isolation unit was left open and the subjects knew the time of day. The average period t of the rest-activity cycle and of the rhythm of body temperature was 24 h. When, thereafter, the subject lived in complete isolation, both rhythms persisted, but with a mean period of about 26 h. The rhythms were free-running as opposed to being synchronized to the environment. The free-running period varies from one individual to another. In humans, the free-running period is usually longer than 24 h, and periods of 24.5 to 26 h have been observed commonly. In the experiment depicted in Figure 140–11, when access to time cues was again allowed, the periodicities in the environment immediately resynchronized the endogenous rhythmicity, resulting in a period of exactly 24 h. The maintenance of circadian rhythms of endocrine release during free-running conditions also has been clearly demonstrated in experiments conducted in isolation units in Germany and the United States.[142, 143, 145]

An immense variety of circadian rhythms has been observed in humans. Only a few examples of circadian variations outside the endocrine system will be mentioned here. These include a wide variety of blood constituents, such as

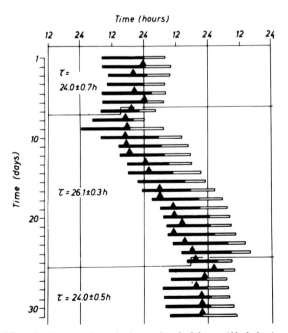

FIGURE 140–11. Circadian rhythms of wakefulness (*black bars*), sleep (*white bars*), and maximum of rectal temperature (*triangles*) in a subject who was exposed to the external synchronizing agents for the first and last 7 days and was isolated from all time cues between days 8 and 24. (From Aschoff J: Circadian rhythms: General features and endocrinological aspects. *In* Krieger DT (ed): Endocrine Rhythms. New York, Raven Press, 1979, pp 1–61.)

white blood cells, amino acids, and phosphorus; innumerable physiological variables, such as body temperature, heart rate, blood pressure, urinary volume, propensity for rapid eye movement (REM) sleep, intraocular pressure, and taste threshold for salt; as well as behavioral parameters, such as time of birth, time of death, mood, reaction time, performance on learning tasks, computation skills, pattern recognition, and relative coordination. There are also rhythms in responsiveness to various challenges such as drugs and stress.

Circadian rhythmicity is maintained when subjects are sleep-deprived, when they are starved, and when they receive equal amounts of food at short intervals over the day. The timing of single meals, however, can have effects on the pattern of at least some variables, including hormones, and the sleep-wake cycle can have phase-setting as well as phase-masking effects on many rhythms, especially those of the endocrine system.

Interactions Between Circadian Rhythmicity and Sleep

There are several features of the interaction between sleep and circadian rhythmicity that appear to be unique to the human species. First, human sleep is generally consolidated in a single 6- to 9-h period, whereas fragmentation of the sleep period in several bouts is the rule in other mammals. Possibly as a result of this consolidation of the sleep period, the wake-sleep transition in humans is associated with physiological changes which are usually more marked than those observed in animals. For example, the secretion of GH in normal adults is tightly associated with the beginning of the sleep period, whereas the relationship between GH secretory pulses and sleep stages is much less evident in rodents, primates, and dogs. Secondly, humans are also unique in their capacity to ignore circadian signals and to maintain wakefulness despite an increased pressure to go to sleep. Finally, approximately 25 per cent of human subjects maintained for prolonged periods of time in temporal isolation have shown behavioral modifications that have not been observed in laboratory animals under constant conditions. These modifications consist of a desynchronization between the sleep-wake cycle and other rhythms, such as those of body temperature and cortisol secretion, which continue to free-run with a circadian period. Under conditions of so-called internal desynchronization, the sleep-wake cycle may be suddenly lengthened to 30 h and more or shortened to less than 22 h, while the rhythm of body temperature continues to free-run with a circadian period.[143, 146] Examples of such spontaneous internal desynchronization are provided in Figure 140–12. Wakefulness may last more than 30 h or be less than 12 h. Remarkably, the subjects are not aware of these drastic changes in their way of living. Instead, most of them believe they are living on a more or less regular 24-h schedule. This can be explained by the observation that time perception is profoundly altered; estimations of 1-h intervals are positively correlated with the duration of wakefulness.[147] Of particular interest is that the subjects continue to have three meals per "day" irrespective of the actual number of hours they are awake.[148] The intervals between meals as well as those between wakeup and breakfast or between dinner and bedtime are stretched or compressed

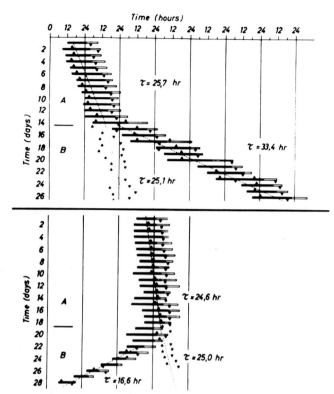

FIGURE 140–12. Free-running circadian rhythms of wakefulness and sleep (*black and white bars*, respectively) and of rectal temperature (*triangles above and below bars* for maxima and minima, respectively) in two subjects who lived alone in an isolation unit. In each record, part A shows internal synchronization and part B shows spontaneous internal desynchronization between the sleep-wake cycle and the rhythm of body temperature. τ is the mean circadian period.

in strong proportionality to the duration of wakefulness.[149] The mechanisms causing spontaneous internal desynchronization are not understood. The observation has been taken to indicate that two central oscillators are involved in the control of circadian rhythms in humans, one characterized by a narrow range of circadian periods and driving autonomous rhythms such as the rhythm of body temperature and the other controlling weaker oscillations of more labile periods such as the sleep-wake cycle.[143, 146, 150, 151] This conceptualization has led to fruitless efforts to anatomically identify a second central circadian pacemaker that would drive the sleep-wake cycle. Several mathematical models describing the interaction between the central circadian clock and the sleep-wake cycle have been developed.[143, 150, 152–155] More recent versions of some of these models also simulate the circadian control of the REM–non REM cycle[156] or the coupling to *zeitgebers*.[157]

Detailed analyses of data obtained during temporal isolation showed indeed that the timing, duration, and architecture of sleep are partially regulated by circadian rhythmicity.[158] Thus the duration of sleep episodes is correlated with the phase of the circadian rhythm of body temperature and not with the duration of prior wakefulness. Short (i.e., 7 to 8 h) sleep episodes occur in free-running conditions when the subject goes to sleep around the minimum of body temperature, whereas long (i.e., 12 to 14 h) sleep episodes occur when sleep starts around the maximum of body temperature. Pronounced circadian variations occur

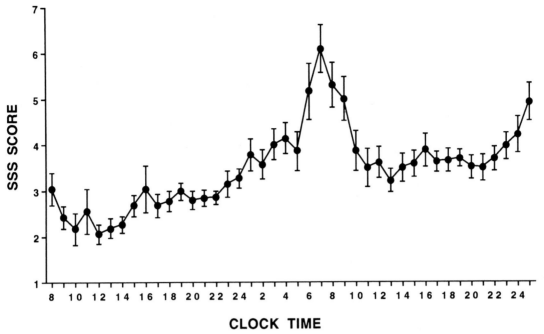

FIGURE 140–13. Mean (± SE) scores on the Stanford sleepiness scale (SSS) obtained at hourly intervals in 11 normal subjects during 40 h of continuous wakefulness in a recumbent position in normal indoor light. Caloric intake was exclusively in the form of a constant glucose infusion. A score of 1 corresponds to full alertness while a score of 7 corresponds to overwhelming sleepiness. (Unpublished observations from E Van Cauter, O Van Reeth, MM Byrne, JD Blackman, J Sturis, and S Refetoff.)

for all objective and subjective measures of sleep tendency.[159, 160] Figure 140–13 shows mean profiles of subjectively rated sleepiness obtained in 11 young men studied during 40 h of continuous wakefulness. Sleepiness scores are highest in the early morning hours, between 6:00 and 9:00, and then decrease despite the persistence of the sleep-deprivation condition. The propensity for REM sleep is also dependent on circadian phase, with a maximum around the minimum of body temperature.[158] In contrast, SW sleep appears to be primarily regulated by a homeostatic process.[161]

Circadian rhythmicity (intrinsic effects of time of day, irrespective of the sleep or waking state) and sleep interact to regulate hormonal secretion. These modulatory effects were long thought to be present only in hormones directly dependent of the hypothalamopituitary axis. However, over the past few years, a number of studies have indicated that modulation by circadian rhythmicity and sleep is also present in other endocrine systems, such as glucose regulation and the renin-angiotensin system.[35, 36, 162]

To delineate the relative roles of circadian and sleep effects in the temporal organization of hormonal secretion, strategies based on the fact that circadian rhythmicity needs several days to adapt to abrupt shifts of the sleep-wake cycle have been used. Thus, by shifting the sleep times by 8 to 12 h, masking effects of sleep on circadian inputs are removed, and the effects of sleep at an abnormal circadian time are revealed.[36] Early studies using this type of experimental design demonstrated that the secretion of some hormones is primarily modulated by circadian rhythmicity (e.g., cortisol, melatonin), while others appeared to be strictly sleep-dependent (e.g., prolactin, GH). Until relatively recently, this classification of temporal hormonal

profiles into "circadian-dependent" or "sleep-related" was seen as a true dichotomy. A number of endocrine rhythms were referred to as sleep-related and assumed to have no intrinsic circadian nature. Conversely, circadian endocrine rhythms were believed to be totally independent of sleep. Over the past few years, this dichotomy of endocrine rhythms was challenged by evidence showing that both sleep effects and circadian effects interact to produce the overall temporal pattern of the majority of hormones.

Examples of 24-h profiles of hormones which are strongly modulated by circadian rhythmicity and sleep are shown in Figure 140–10. The periodicity of cortisol secretion was long considered as a "pure" circadian rhythm, but an inhibitory effect of the first few hours of sleep was later demonstrated.[163] The 24-h profile of thyroid-stimulating hormone (TSH) represents an excellent marker of sleep and circadian interactions. Indeed, the evening rise occurs well prior to sleep onset, reflecting circadian timing. During sleep, an inhibitory influence is exerted on TSH secretion.[164, 165] This inhibitory effect is best demonstrated using the paradigm of sleep deprivation, which shows that the evening rise of TSH is prolonged and enhanced when sleep does not occur. Plasma levels of the pineal hormone melatonin undergo a pronounced diurnal variation, and the onset of the nocturnal rise of melatonin secretion is believed to be an accurate marker of circadian phase.[166, 167] There is evidence showing correlations between endogenous melatonin secretion and measures of sleepiness.[168] Among the hormonal patterns that were long thought to be solely determined by sleep timing is the 24-h profile of GH (middle right panel). In a normal human, a major pulse of GH secretion occurs shortly after sleep onset in association with the first period of SW sleep. Careful analyses indicated, however, that the amplitude of this sleep-related GH pulse is maximal when sleep occurs around the usual bedtime, indicating the existence of a weak circadian modulation.[37, 169] Sleep is also a major physiological stimulus for prolactin release, but as will be shown later, the timing of the nocturnal rise is also partially controlled by circadian rhythmicity.[162]

Hormonal profiles are thus easily measurable reflections of central mechanisms of biological time keeping. In clinical investigations of conditions of abnormal circadian rhythmicity such as "jet lag" and in human studies of the effects of exposure to artificial *zeitgebers*, they are commonly used as markers of the status of the circadian clock and of its interactions with sleep.

Photic Synchronization of Human Rhythms

Until approximately 10 years ago it was thought that, unlike all other mammalian species, the human circadian system was largely insensitive to the LD cycle and that social cues were the primary synchronizing agents.[143] During the past decade a number of detailed studies have demonstrated that light has major synchronizing effects on human rhythms. In particular, appropriately timed exposure to bright light is capable of advancing or delaying circadian rhythms independently of changes in the sleep-wake cycle.[170, 171] Bright light can accelerate adaptation to shifts such as those occurring in "jet lag" and shift work as well as widen the limits of entrainment of the circadian system to periods deviating from 24 h.[28, 172–177] In contrast to previous thinking, human circadian rhythms can rapidly and totally adapt to abrupt shifts of the LD and sleep-wake cycles in the presence of multiple environmental time cues and conflicting social *zeitgebers* when indoor light is increased to 1500 to 2000 lux during the periods of wakefulness.[178]

A recent study has attempted to define the "human" equivalent of the PRC to light using experimental protocols similar to those used in animal species, i.e., when shifts are evaluated after a single exposure to light during free-running conditions.[179] The subjects were exposed to a single 3-h pulse of light of 5000 to 10000 lux intensity, and the rhythm of body temperature was continuously recorded. Confirming previous preliminary findings,[180] phase advances averaging 1 to 2 h were observed when light was applied in the later part of the subjective night, after the time of occurrence of the nocturnal minimum of body temperature. Limited evidence to suggest the occurrence of phase delays when light is given in the early part of the subjective night was obtained. When the subjects are entrained to a 24-h LD cycle, which is the real-life situation, phase advances and delays may be observed on the first day after exposure to a single 3-h light pulse.[181, 182] This is illustrated in Figure 140–14, which shows mean profiles of plasma TSH observed in normal subjects under "constant routine" conditions (i.e., constant wakefulness, constant posture, constant dim light exposure except during stimulus application, constant caloric intake under the form of an intravenous glucose infusion) in baseline studies and in studies where the light pulse was presented either in the early part of the night (i.e., before the minimum of body temperature) or in the later part of the night (i.e., after the minimum of body temperature). As may be seen in

Figure 140–14, the evening rise of TSH was advanced by approximately 1 h when light was presented late in the night and delayed by approximately 1 h when light was administered early in the night. These findings were confirmed by analysis of the simultaneous melatonin profiles. Taken together, these studies indicate that the human circadian clock responds to light in a manner similar to that observed in other mammalian species.

All other human studies which have examined the phase-shifting effects of light pulses have used protocols involving repeated application of the stimulus.[28, 170, 171, 174–177, 183] Generally, phase advances are seen when light is presented in

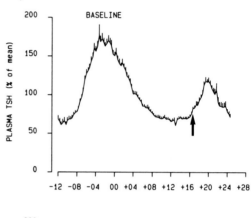

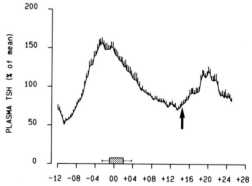

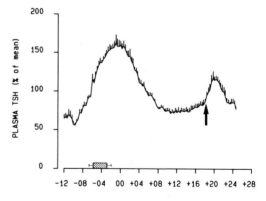

CIRCADIAN TEMPERATURE MINIMUM

FIGURE 140–14. Advance and delay of the evening TSH rise (indicated by the *arrows*) following exposure to light (*shaded area*) in the late (*middle panel*) or early (*lower panel*) part of the night as compared with profiles obtained in the same subjects under continuous dim light. (From Van Cauter E, Sturis J, Byrne MM, et al: Preliminary studies on the immediate phase-shifting effects of light and exercise on the human circadian clock. J Biol Rhythms, in press.)

the later part of the night or in the early morning, and phase delays are observed when light is presented in the evening. For example, the onset of nocturnal melatonin secretion is delayed by approximately 2 h after 1 week of exposure to 2 h of bright light in the evening[175] and is advanced following repeated morning exposure.[176] In another study, evening exposure to a higher-intensity 5-h pulse of light for three consecutive days resulted in phase delays of the temperature rhythm averaging 3 h in magnitude.[171]

To obtain larger phase shifts, Czeisler et al.[177] have developed a different experimental approach involving repeated presentation of the light stimulus during usual sleep times, resulting in a drastic displacement in the timing of sleep and consequently in the timing of exposure to darkness. These investigators have generated a detailed PRC to a stimulus consisting of exposure to 5 h of bright light followed 12 h later by exposure to 7 to 8 h of sleep in total darkness for 3 consecutive days.[177] The PRC to this repeated application of this mixed stimulus indicates that there is a critical time of stimulus presentation when very large (6 to 12 h) phase changes in either direction may occur. Based on a theoretical analysis of these data and on additional observations obtained with a slightly different protocol, the investigators have suggested that the human circadian system may respond to light in a manner different from that known in all other mammalian species in that a single exposure to light may not cause consistent phase shifts but may instead decrease rhythm amplitude, making the system more sensitive to the second and third exposures, which result in large phase shifts.[184] The validity of this interpretation remains to be confirmed. Indeed, the displacement of the sleep-dark episode could play a role in causing the large shifts. Furthermore, the possibility that large phase shifts following repeated exposure may be obtained in the absence of amplitude reduction by additive effects of smaller phase shifts following single exposure on successive days cannot be excluded, despite theoretical evidence to the contrary.

Nonphotic Synchronization of Human Rhythms

The evolution of concepts regarding *zeitgebers* for nonhuman mammalian rhythms has run in many ways opposite to that occurring in the field of human rhythms. Indeed, social and/or behavioral cues were long thought to be ineffective as *zeitgebers* in rodents and other mammals, but as discussed earlier, evidence has accumulated over the past few years to indicate that behavioral changes are indeed capable of inducing shifts in circadian rhythms. Specifically, stimuli that cause an alteration of the rest-activity cycle, either by eliciting activity during the normal rest period or by preventing activity during the normal active period, result in phase shifts of circadian rhythms.[7, 185] So far, there has been no systematic evaluation of the potential phase-shifting effects of enforcing nighttime activity or daytime sleep in human volunteers. Small shifts of the sleep period around the habitual bedtimes and waketimes do not alter the timing of the body temperature and melatonin rhythms.[186] The early work of Aschoff et al.[187] demonstrated that human rhythms in continuous darkness may be entrained by a rigorous schedule of bedtimes, mealtimes, and performance tasks. Similarly, an "information"

zeitgeber, under the form of acoustic signals, has a range of entrainment similar to that of a weak LD cycle.[188] There have been no systematic studies of the potential phase-shifting effects of scheduled physical or mental activity. It should be noted that in human studies it is particularly difficult to totally dissociate effects of the rest-activity cycle from effects of the LD cycle. Indeed, activity at a time of normal sleep will generally involve exposure to light with eyes open, while sleep at a time of normal activity will result in diminished exposure to light (or exposure to dark) with eyes closed. Conversely, the absence of light will generally result in a marked decrease of activity.

Another nonphotic agent that has been shown to induce phase shifts in human circadian rhythms is melatonin.[189] As shown in Figure 140–10, circulating melatonin levels undergo a pronounced diurnal variation. Daytime levels are low or undetectable. The nocturnal rise starts in the early evening, between 20:00 and 22:00, and the maximum occurs around the middle of the sleep period. There is strong evidence demonstrating that the diurnal variation of plasma melatonin levels is driven by the circadian clock, and phase shifts of the central circadian signal induced by changes in the LD cycle will be faithfully reflected in the synchronization of the melatonin rhythm.[190] The only stimulus that consistently exerts a marked effect on melatonin secretion is light exposure.[191, 192] Indeed, exposure to light of sufficient intensity results in an acute dose-dependent inhibition of nocturnal melatonin secretion, with a prompt return to high nighttime levels when darkness resumes.[191, 193] Rapidly accumulating data indicate that the melatonin rhythm feeds back on the clock and exerts synchronizing effects. Indeed, exogenous administration of melatonin has been shown to resynchronize certain overt rhythms in a variety of conditions, including "jet lag."[194–196] Lewy and associates[189] have recently demonstrated the existence of a PRC of the "dim light melatonin onset" to repeated (on 4 consecutive days) oral administration of low-dose melatonin (0.5 mg) in human subjects. In this paradigm, melatonin administration causes phase advances when administered in the afternoon and evening and phase delays when given in the morning. Nocturnal administration does not result in any phase shift. These characteristics are similar to those of the PRC to dark pulses given to rodents free running in constant light which constitutes a mirror image of the shape of the PRC to light.

Conditions of Abnormal Circadian Rhythmicity

Transmeridian Flights (Jet Lag). Subjects who travel rapidly across time zones are confronted with a desynchronization between their internal circadian rhythms and the periodicity of the new external environment. Upon arrival, the timings of the LD cycle, social schedule, and meal schedule are abnormally matched to the phase of the physiological rhythms of the traveler. Associated with this lack of synchronization are symptoms of fatigue, subjective discomfort, sleep disturbances, reduced mental and psychomotor performance, and gastrointestinal tract disorders. The syndrome is commonly referred to as "jet lag." Phase shifts of human circadian rhythms have been studied after actual "jet lag," i.e., transmeridian flights across time zones, as well as after abrupt displacements of the sleep-wake cycle and/or the LD cycle designed to reproduce in the laboratory the desynchrony occurring in "jet lag." Figure 140–15 illustrates the mean 24-h profiles of plasma cortisol and prolactin levels observed in six normal young men studied under baseline conditions and 1, 3, and 5 days after an abrupt 8-h delay shift of the LD and sleep-wake cycle in the laboratory.[178] Examination of these profiles reveals three general characteristics of adaptation of overt circadian rhythms to real or simulated "jet lag": (1) adaptation is not immediate and requires several days, (2) the rate at which re-entrainment occurs differs among variables, with the prolactin rhythm showing adaptation on the third day after the shift, when disturbances of the cortisol rhythm are still evident, and (3) during the period of adaptation, abnormal phase relationships between overt rhythms occur. Thus, under baseline conditions, the nocturnal prolactin rise occurs at a time when cortisol secretion is quiescent, whereas one day after the shift, prolactin rises during a period of elevated cortisol levels. The general feeling of malaise associated with jet lag is likely to be caused not only by the desynchronization between internal and external rhythms but also by the perturbation of internal temporal organization of physiological functions.

The rate of adaptation appears to be generally slower for overt rhythms that are strongly dependent on the circadian system, such as those of cortisol and melatonin secretions, than for those which are markedly modulated by sleep, such as prolactin and GH secretions. Indeed, within 3 to 4 days after the shift, sleep perturbations, while still present, become rather subtle and are therefore not translated into significant abnormalities of sleep-related hormone secretion. In what follows, the overall rate of adaptation is taken to be that of the slowest-adapting component measured in the study. Depending on the strength of the *zeitgebers*, the rate of adaptation can be as low as half an hour a day or as high as 3 h a day. The rate of adaptation is not constant; adaptation to a large shift occurs at a faster rate during the first few days and progresses at a slower pace thereafter.[197] The rate of adaptation is also dependent on the direction of the shift, with adaptation occurring generally faster after a delay (i.e., westward) shift than after an advance (i.e., eastward) shift.[197] This eastward-westward difference in rate of adaptation is generally believed to be due to the fact that the endogenous circadian period of the human is longer than 24 h, and thus adjustments by delays are more easily achieved than adjustments by advances. However, in elderly subjects, the opposite situation may occur because of the tendency for rhythms to be phase-advanced that is characteristic of aging.[198] Usually, all overt rhythms move

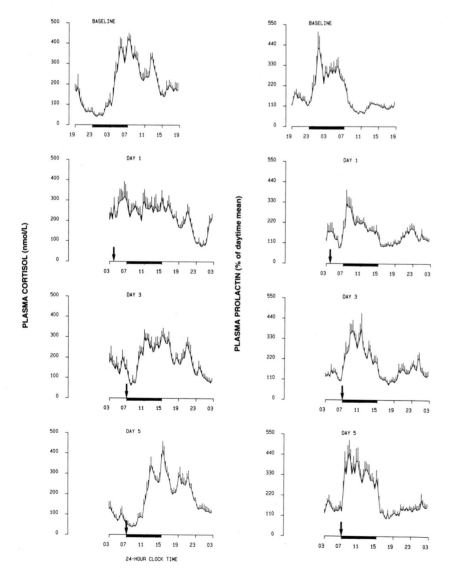

FIGURE 140–15. Twenty-four-hour profiles of plasma cortisol (*left*) and prolactin (*right*) observed in six young men before and 1, 3, and 5 days after an abrupt 8-h delay of the sleep-wake and light-dark cycles. Following the shift, the light intensity during the wake period was 1500 to 2000 lux. Blood samples were collected at 20-min intervals. Bedtimes are indicated by black bars. The vertical lines at each time point represent the SE. (Unpublished data from E Van Cauter, M L'Hermite-Balériaux, D Bosson, A Van Onderbergen, and G Copinschi.)

in the direction of the flight; i.e., an eastbound flight is followed by advance shifts and a westbound flight by delay shifts. However, in the case of large shifts (i.e., 9 h or more), this is not always the case, and some overt rhythms may adapt by delays and others may adapt by advances.[144] Such *re-entrainment by partition*, in which different overt rhythms move in opposite directions, is observed more often after advance rather than delay shifts.[199] Finally, there are also interindividual differences in rate of adaptation which can be attributed to differences in the "rigidity" of the circadian system. As a measure of rigidity, the range of oscillation of the rhythm of body temperature has proven useful. Results from flight experiments and from shift experiments in isolation units demonstrate that the time needed for re-entrainment is positively correlated with the amplitude of the rhythm of body temperature as measured before the flight or shift, respectively.[197, 200] There is strong evidence to suggest that re-entrainment after a transmeridian flight is facilitated by exposure to bright light at appropriate circadian phases.[174] Differential effects of normal and bright light have indeed been shown in experiments simulating a 6-h delay shift of the LD cycle in a laboratory environment.[201] Adaptation to the 6-h shift progressed at an average rate of 1 h per day when normal indoor light intensity was used (i.e., around 300 lux) and at a faster rate of 1.4 h per day when the subjects were exposed to brighter light (i.e., >3000 lux). In the study on adaptation of endocrine rhythms illustrated in Figure 140–15, bright (i.e., 1500 to 2000 lux) light was used during the wakefulness periods, and complete adaptation to the 8-h delay was observed on the fifth day after the shift, corresponding to an average rate of adaptation of at least 1.6 h per day. In contrast, in an earlier study involving a 7-h delay without scheduled exposure to light, adaptation was not complete 10 days after the travel, implying that the overall rate of adaptation was less than 45 min per day.[202] Taken together, these findings suggest that critically timed exposure to bright light is helpful to alleviate jet lag.

An early study indicated that re-entrainment takes longer if the subjects are confined to their hotel rooms rather than exposed to outdoor light and social activities.[203] While this effect may partially reflect increased exposure to light, it also has been interpreted as evidence that adherence to the local social and meal schedule upon arrival will accelerate the adaptation to jet lag. The advice of quickly changing the timing of behavior to match local schedules is commonly given,[204] although supporting data are largely nonexistent. The finding that increased activity is capable of inducing phase shifts in hamster circadian rhythms[18, 19] has elicited claims regarding beneficial effects of physical exercise in promoting adaptation to jet lag,[204] but the effectiveness of exercise as a *zeitgeber* for the human circadian system remains to be demonstrated.

Several studies have shown a beneficial effect of oral administration of the pineal hormone melatonin in alleviating jet lag in both field and laboratory studies.[194–196, 205] While all studies claim that melatonin administration can facilitate adaptation, the findings are somewhat inconsistent. Thus three studies[194–196] report pronounced decreases in subjective ratings of the severity of the jet lag syndrome following melatonin administration, but in another study,[205] where beneficial effects were seen on the adaptation of phase and amplitude of physiological rhythms,

there were no significant changes in subjective ratings and the subjects were unable to correctly guess whether they had taken melatonin or placebo. One study involved both advance and delay shifts,[196] but the schedule of melatonin administration was the same, irrespective of the direction of the shift, and beneficial effects were seen for both eastward and westward travel. These observations would suggest that the beneficial effects of melatonin may have been mediated by facilitating sleep rather than via a direct effect on the circadian pacemaker, since effects on the pacemaker would be expected to be strongly dependent on the timing of administration relative to the direction of the shift. Even low doses of melatonin can induce drowsiness, and higher doses have clear hypnotic effects.[206] The most convincing results regarding a positive influence of melatonin treatment on the adaptation of circadian rhythms were obtained in a placebo-controlled study involving a 9-h advance shift with 3 days of treatment prior to the shift to "preadapt" the subjects before the simulated time zone change. Even so, the authors conclude that "the improvement is not, however, sufficiently great that we can recommend melatonin for the alleviation of jet lag."[205]

A number of studies have indicated that treatment with short-acting benzodiazepine hypnotics may reverse the nocturnal insomnia and daytime sleepiness associated with large abrupt shifts of the sleep-wake cycle.[207–209] The finding that the short-acting benzodiazepine triazolam induces phase shifts of circadian rhythms in hamsters,[210] with the direction and magnitude of the phase shifts being dependent on the time of administration of the drug, has stimulated clinical studies to examine the efficacy of triazolam administration in accelerating the adaptation of human circadian rhythms to jet lag. In hamsters, appropriately timed delivery of the drug may reduce the duration of adaptation to an 8-h shift of the LD cycle by about 50 per cent.[18] In this species, the phase-shifting effects of the drug are mediated by its ability to induce a bout of intense physical activity. In humans, possible beneficial effects of triazolam or other short-acting hypnotics on the resynchronization of circadian rhythms could be mediated by their ability to induce and maintain sleep at an abnormal circadian time. Estimations of amplitude and phase of circadian rhythms during adaptation to an 8-h delay shift treated with triazolam or placebo have indeed shown an accelerated adaptation of the amplitude and phase of the cortisol rhythm.[178]

SHIFT WORK. Shift work, which is voluntarily accepted by millions of workers, is a major health hazard involving an increased risk of cardiovascular illness, gastrointestinal disorders, infertility, and insomnia.[28] The medical consequences of shift work are associated with chronic misalignment of physiological circadian rhythms and the activity-rest cycle. After transmeridian flights or shift experiments in the laboratory, subjects are usually confronted with an unambiguous situation in which all available environmental cues are displaced in the same direction and cooperate to shift the circadian system. In contrast, shift work usually creates conditions in which some *zeitgebers* (e.g., an artificial LD cycle) and additional phase-setting factors such as the rest-activity cycle are displaced while others remain unaltered, e.g., the natural LD cycle and the routines of family life. Shift workers thus live in a situation of conflicting *zeitgebers* that almost never allows a complete alteration of the circadian system. Indeed, several studies have shown that workers on permanent or rotating night shifts do not adapt to these schedules, even after several years.[211, 212] Besides its health implications, this misalignment with the circadian system has important social and economic implications, because night work is associated with substantial decrements in performance and vigilance, resulting in diminished productivity and increased accident rates. The degree of adjustment to shift work shows large interindividual variability and seems related to the rigidity of the circadian system. In accordance with the results obtained in jet lag studies, a negative correlation was found between the range of the oscillation in the rhythm of body temperature and the shift of acrophases during shift work.[144] Of practical relevance is the observation that the tolerance to shift work, as measured by reports on clinical symptoms and sleep disorders, is inversely related to the degree of phase adaptation; subjects with a large amplitude of oscillation, and hence with little adaptation, report fewer complaints than do workers whose rhythms have small amplitudes and adapt faster.

Although shift work has been part of modern life for several decades, few strategies that could improve physiological adaptation to conditions when an enforced activity-rest cycle conflicts with endogenous circadian rhythmicity have been developed. In one study conducted in a Utah factory, workers' satisfaction and productivity were improved by slowing the rotation rate from one shift every week to one shift every 3 weeks.[213] The improvement was attributed to the slower rotation, giving workers more time to adjust, as well as to the fact that at the time of shift rotation the shift consisted of a delay, rather than an advance, of working hours (i.e., from day shift to evening shift to night shift rather than in the opposite direction), a design that allegedly took into account circadian principles. This latter argument was disputed, however, in a later analysis.[214] More recent studies have demonstrated that scheduled exposure to bright light during night work and complete darkness during daytime sleep following night work are capable of accelerating the adjustment to the new schedule.[28, 215, 216] Nighttime alertness and performance are improved in bright ambient light as compared with dim light.[217] The success of these nonpharmacological approaches probably reflects a combination of the powerful synchronizing effects of the enhanced LD cycle and of the improvement and prolongation of sleep in total darkness.[29]

BLINDNESS. Several studies have shown that some totally blind individuals have abnormal sleep-wake cycles and rhythms of melatonin secretion.[218–220] These disturbances are thought to reflect a lack of entrainment to the 24-h environmental periodicity, similar to that seen in sighted people living in isolation units under free-running conditions. Free-running rhythms of body temperature, plasma cortisol, plasma melatonin, and sleep propensity have been demonstrated in blind subjects.[220] Sleep disorders in the blind are thus likely to reflect a condition of abnormal entrainment of circadian rhythms. Figure 140–16 shows the 24-h profiles of plasma levels of melatonin and cortisol measured at approximately 2-week intervals in a 41-year-old totally blind subject who suffered from periodic insomnia. The rhythms free ran with a period of 25.1 h. The abnormalities of endocrine rhythms in blindness may be of practical importance; very low morning levels of cortisol in this condition may reflect a lack of synchronization of the

circadian rhythm rather than a disorder of the pituitary-adrenal axis. For example, in Figure 140–16, cortisol levels at 9:00 were below 100 nmol/L, an abnormal laboratory value at that time of day when levels are normally maximal.

Therapeutic strategies to treat circadian-related insomnias in the blind depend crucially on the development of nonphotic methods for entrainment. Appropriately timed administration of oral melatonin in blind subjects has been reported to restore normal entrainment to a 24-h cycle in several studies.[10, 221]

SLEEP DISORDERS. Certain forms of sleep disorders seem to originate from a disturbance in the circadian system. In addition to the jet lag syndrome and sleep disorders associated with shift work already discussed above, the *International Classification of Sleep Disorders*[222] lists, under the heading "Circadian Rhythm Sleep Disorders," the following conditions: irregular sleep-wake pattern, delayed sleep phase syndrome, advanced sleep phase syndrome, and 24-h sleep-wake disorder.

Subjects with irregular sleep-wake patterns present temporally disorganized and variable episodes of sleep and waking. This condition is frequently seen in elderly institutionalized subjects and probably represents a degeneration of the circadian system. Low-amplitude, markedly attenuated rhythms of physiological functions, particularly body temperature, have been demonstrated in these patients.[223, 224] The decreased exposure to a normal LD cycle and social schedule contributes to the severity of the condition.[140]

Delayed sleep phase insomnia is characterized by a chronic inability to fall asleep at a normal bedtime and to awake in the morning.[225] It has been proposed that the basis of this disorder is an inability to advance the timing of the circadian sleep-wake cycle once it has been delayed to an abnormal phase by late bedtimes during a weekend or after transmeridian travel. Nonpharmacological chronotherapy involving repeated scheduled exposure to bright light is the treatment of choice for this disorder.[222, 226] In contrast, in the advanced sleep phase syndrome, the timing of the major sleep episode is advanced in relation to normal bedtime, resulting in symptoms of extreme evening sleepiness and early morning awakening. A treatment of phase-advance chronotherapy has been proposed for this rare condition.[227]

The non–24-h sleep-wake syndrome refers to the subjects who are free running with a circadian period generally longer than 24 h and are unable to entrain to the external 24-h cycle. As discussed above, this is most commonly seen in totally blind subjects.

AFFECTIVE DISORDERS. Early timing of a number of circadian rhythms, including hormonal rhythms, has been observed in acutely ill patients with endogenous depression. These findings provide the basis for the so-called phase-advance hypothesis for affective illness, which proposes that abnormalities in circadian time keeping are involved in the pathophysiology of depression.[30, 31, 227] Figure 140–17 shows representative examples of 24-h profiles of circulating levels of cortisol, prolactin, and GH in a normal subject and in a patient with unipolar depression studied during the acute phase of the illness.[228–231] The nadir of cortisol secretion, the nocturnal rise of prolactin levels, and the timing of the major nocturnal pulse of GH release are all advanced by 2 to 3 h as compared with the control

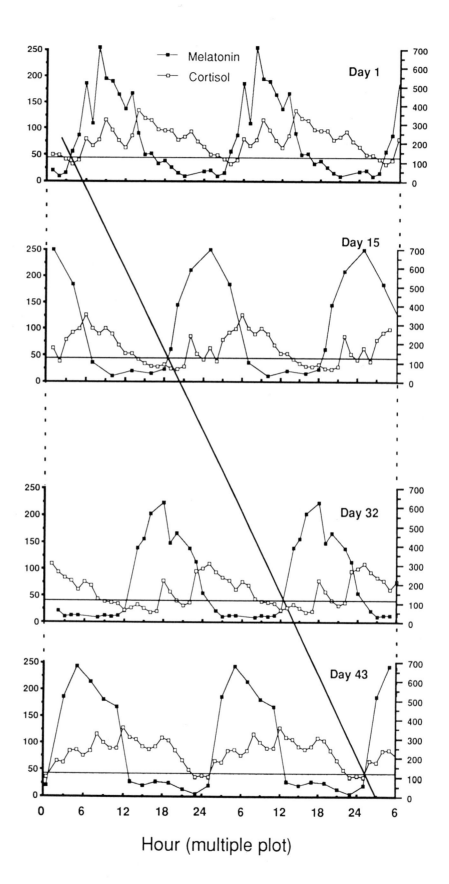

FIGURE 140–16. Free-running circadian rhythms of plasma levels of melatonin (*closed circles*) and cortisol (*open circles*) observed on four consecutive occasions separated by approximately 2 weeks in a totally blind subject. The times of occurrence of successive onsets of melatonin secretion fall on a straight line, indicating an endogenous period of 25.1 h. The data are double-plotted on a 48-h scale to facilitate visual inspection. (From Sack RL, Lewy AJ, Blood ML, et al: Circadian rhythm abnormalities in totally blind people: incidence and clinical significance. J Clin Endocrinol Metab 75:127–134, 1992. © by the Endocrine Society, 1992.)

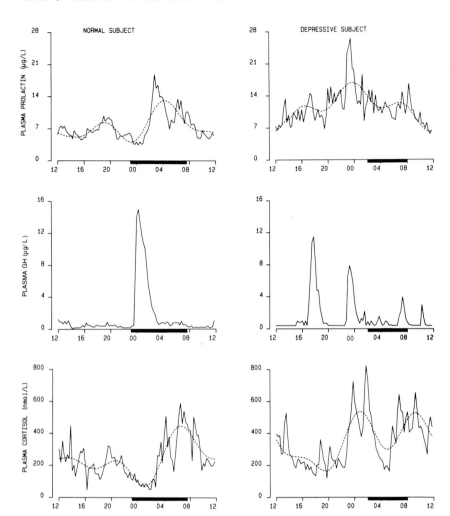

FIGURE 140–17. Representative 24-h profiles of plasma prolactin, GH, and cortisol in an acutely ill patient with unipolar depression (*right*) as compared with an age- and sex-matched healthy subject (*right*). (Data From: 1. Mendlewicz J, Linkowski P, Kerkhofs M, et al: Diurnal hypersecretion of growth hormone in depression. J Clin Endocrinol Metab 60:505–512, 1985; 2. Linkowski P, Mendlewicz J, Leclercq R, et al: The 24-hour profile of adrenocorticotropin and cortisol in major depressive illness. J Clin Endocrinol Metab 61:429–438, 1985; 3. Linkowski P, Van Cauter E, L'Hermite-Balériaux M, et al: The 24-hour profile of plasma prolactin in men with major endogenous depressive illness. Arch Gen Psychiatry 46:813–819, 1989.)

group. Cortisol is hypersecreted throughout the 24-h cycle, whereas excessive GH secretion appears mostly confined to daytime hours. The phase advance of circadian rhythms has been observed in some studies but not in others, so the existence and significance of circadian rhythm abnormalities in depression remains controversial.

Implications of Circadian Rhythms for Clinical Diagnosis and Treatment

Recognition of the existence of circadian rhythms in physiological and endocrine variables has challenged simplistic interpretations of Claude Bernard's concept of the "*constance du milieu intérieur.*" Indeed, because of the wide amplitude of certain circadian oscillations, the estimation of the mean level of a parameter from a single measurement may involve an error exceeding 100 per cent. In many cases, time of day when the sample was obtained has to be taken into account in evaluation of the result. For example, a plasma cortisol level of 15 µg/dl (414 nmol/L) at 8:00 is perfectly normal, while the same value obtained 12 h later is indicative of some form of hypercortisolism. The implications for clinical diagnosis are obvious.

Differentiation between normal and pathological levels may actually be greatly improved by adequately selecting the time of sample collection. Figure 140–18 illustrates this

concept in the case of the diagnosis of Cushing's syndrome. The mean, across individuals, of 56 circadian profiles of plasma cortisol obtained in patients with demonstrated Cushing's syndrome is compared with the mean of 60 profiles obtained in normal subjects. The areas delineated by the standard error above and below the means indicate that overlap between individual values from the two groups of subjects should be expected at all times except in a 4-h interval centered around midnight. In fact, the mean of the cortisol levels measured between 22:00 and 2:00 offers an excellent index of discrimination between normals and patients with hypercortisolism, misclassifying only 2 of the 116 subjects.

Similarly, the demonstration of differences in levels of a given parameter between two groups of subjects may require multiple measurements throughout the 24-h span. For example, Figure 140–19 illustrates data showing clear changes in testosterone levels associated with aging in normal men.[232] Blood was sampled hourly for 24 h. Earlier studies, based on infrequent sampling in the afternoon only, had failed to observe such changes. As a result of the loss of circadian rhythmicity of testosterone in older men, samples obtained in the morning will allow the observation of an age effect, while samples obtained in the afternoon or evening will not.

The circadian time structure is of further significance in

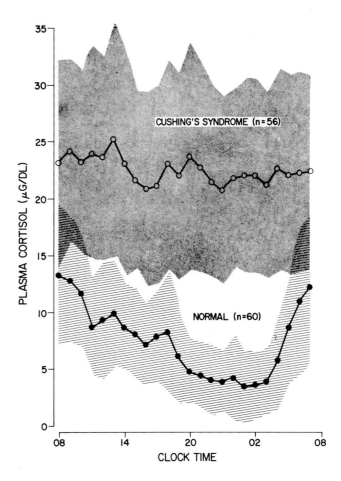

FIGURE 140–18. Mean 24-h profiles of plasma cortisol for 60 normal subjects (*closed circles*) and 56 patients with Cushing's syndrome (*open circles*). The hatched and shaded areas represent one SEM above and below the mean for the normal group and the patient group, respectively.

medicine in so far as the response of the organism to any stimulus may depend on the time at which such a stimulus is applied. This is not surprising in view of the fact that the organism is in a different physicochemical state at each time of the circadian cycle. Rhythms in responsiveness have been described for a large variety of stimuli and provide the theoretical basis for chronopharmacology, i.e., the investigation of drug effects as a function of the timing of their administration, and chronotherapy, i.e., the design of better protocols of treatment taking into account the

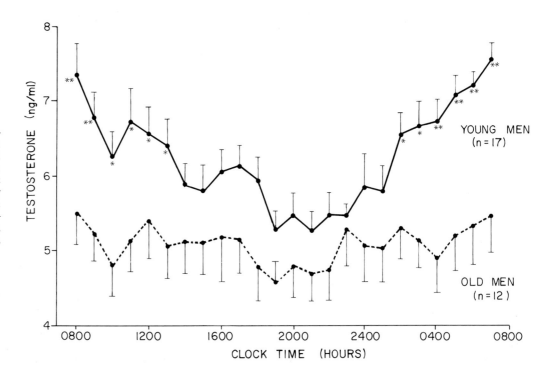

FIGURE 140–19. Hourly testosterone levels (mean ± SEM) in young (*n* = 17, *solid line*) and old (*n* = 12, *dotted line*) men. (From Bremner WJ, Vitiello MV, Prinz PN: Loss of circadian rhythmicity in blood testosterone levels with aging in normal men. J Clin Endocrinol Metab 56:1278–1280, 1983. © by the Endocrine Society, 1983.)

chronobiological characteristics of the system.[151] One of the exciting prospects of this research is that the therapeutic benefits may be maximized and the toxic effects minimized by administering the drug or other forms of treatment at the appropriate time of day. Current concepts and facts in the field of chronopharmacology have been described in recent reviews.[233–235]

ULTRADIAN RHYTHMS

Range of Ultradian Rhythms

In its original definition, the term *ultradian* referred to the entire range of periods shorter than the circadian (i.e., 20 to 28 h) range. Currently, the term *ultradian* is used primarily to designate rhythmicities with periods ranging from fractions of hours to several hours. Ultradian rhythms with a period of around 1 h are often termed *circhoral*. Ultradian oscillations are often less regular and less reproducible than circadian rhythms. In most cases, they appear to represent an optimal functional status within the system where they occur rather than serve the primary function of a "clock," i.e., an accurate time-measuring device. There is a wide variety of ultradian endocrine and nonendocrine rhythms, and many of these rhythms may have little in common in terms of functional significance and causal mechanisms. One of the most prominent is the alternation of rapid eye movement (REM) and non-REM stages in sleep. In the human, the approximately 90-min REM–non-REM cycle is accompanied by similar periodicity of dreaming, penile erections, cardiac irregularity, and breathing. Kleitman[236] has suggested that this ultradian rhythm during sleep is a reflection of a "basic rest-activity cycle" (BRAC), which would occur during wakefulness as well. When various mammalian species are considered, there is an intriguing correlation between the length of the REM–non-REM cycle and the length of the interpulse interval of LH release. This observation has led to the hypothesis of a common mechanism controlling all ultradian oscillations in the 80- to 120-min range.[237] In humans, this range includes the time of recurrence of the episodic pulses of many hormones as well as rhythms in apparently unrelated physiological and behavioral variables, such urine flow, gastric motility, and cognitive style.[33] However, so far there is no strong experimental evidence in favor of a common mechanism underlying diverse ultradian rhythms with a similar period.[238]

In the endocrine system, ultradian variations have been observed for anterior and posterior pituitary hormones, for hormones under direct pituitary control, as well as for other endocrine variables such as parathyroid hormone, norepinephrine, plasma renin activity, and stimulated insulin secretion.

Pulsatile Hormonal Release

Properties and Implications for Diagnostic Procedures

The recognition that a large number of hormones are released in the bloodstream in a pulsatile fashion was made possible by the development of sensitive and precise assays. Repeated measurements showed that the plasma levels of most hormones undergo not only a circadian rhythm but also episodic fluctuations of variable duration and magnitude, generally referred to as secretory *episodes* or *pulses*. The repetition of such episodes, which tend to recur at intervals ranging from 1 to 4 h, may be considered as an ultradian rhythm. The interval of recurrence varies from hormone to hormone and from species to species. In human studies where blood was sampled every 15 minutes, the average number of pulses per 24-h span was 12 for prolactin, 15 for ACTH, 18 for TSH, but only 4 for GH.[34] Examples have been shown in Figure 140–1. In the rat, the ultradian rhythm of LH release has a 20- to 30-min period.[239] In the rhesus monkey, LH pulses recur at intervals of approximately 1 h.[240] When comparing episodic hormonal profiles, one must keep in mind that quantitative characterizations of pulsating activity depend also on the interval of blood sampling and on the precision of the assay.

Whether pulsatile hormonal release is a strictly periodic phenomenon (i.e., generated by an accurate "clock" mechanism) or a pseudoperiodic process with a preferred frequency of recurrence remains to be determined. Generally, episodic variations of plasma concentrations do not appear to be strictly periodic on eyesight examination. However, hormonal profiles obtained in rodents and/or in primates may show a more regular pattern of secretory pulses than those obtained in humans, possibly because laboratory animals are exposed to more constant environments. Moreover, fluctuations in plasma levels not only reflect changes in secretion but also are dependent on the kinetics of dilution, distribution, and degradation. These processes, as well as other modulatory influences, such as circadian rhythmicity and feedback regulation, may obscure a true periodicity inherent to pulsatile hormonal release. The timing of successive pulses and interpulse intervals has been examined in detail in the case of LH release in adult men and in the ram.[241, 242] Both studies have concluded that there is no significant correlation between the durations of successive interpulse intervals, implying that the mechanism underlying the pulsatile LH release is a renewal process, i.e., an oscillator that is reset at each cycle.

Another important property of pulsatile hormonal release is the relative importance of pulsatile or oscillatory secretory activity versus tonic release. This property may differentiate two major subtypes of ultradian oscillations within the endocrine system. In the first type, the secretory activity is entirely pulsatile, with no detectable secretion between pulses. Thus secretion occurs as an on–off process. In normal men, evidence suggestive of intermittent secretion without tonic release has been obtained for LH, follicle-stimulating hormone (FSH), GH, and ACTH-cortisol based on mathematical derivations of the secretory rates from plasma concentrations, a procedure commonly referred to as *deconvolution*.[36, 243, 244] These calculations involve various assumptions on the kinetics of hormonal release, distribution, and degradation, and therefore, their conclusions should be regarded as indicative rather than definitive. An example is shown in the case of cortisol in Figure 140–20, where the middle panel illustrates the 24-h profile of cortisol secretory rates derived from the 24-h profile of plasma concentration (shown in the lower panel)

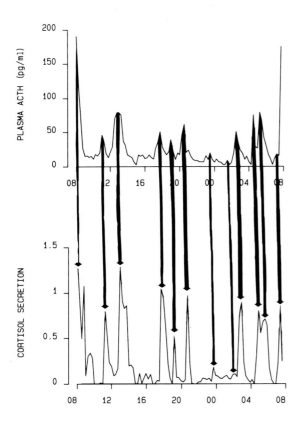

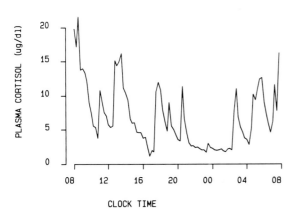

FIGURE 140–20. The 24-h profiles of plasma ACTH (*top*) and cortisol (*bottom*) obtained at 15-min intervals in a normal man. The center panel depicts the cortisol secretory rates derived from the plasma levels by mathematical deconvolution. Note that cortisol secretion is intermittent, without evidence of tonic secretion. The vertical lines associate pulses of plasma ACTH and pulses of cortisol secretion that occur within one sampling interval of each other.

by deconvolution using a two-compartment model for cortisol distribution and degradation. This calculation suggests that within the limits of experimental error and model validity, there is no detectable tonic cortisol secretion between pulses. Similar conclusions have been obtained using different deconvolution procedures. Systems where hormonal secretion is occurring continuously but is increased and decreased in an oscillatory fashion represent a second type of ultradian oscillators within the endocrine system. Pancreatic insulin secretion, which can be derived accurately from peripheral C-peptide levels, is a well-established example of this type of ultradian oscillation.[245–247]

Recent studies also have indicated the existence of tonic secretion for pituitary prolactin and TSH release.[243, 244]

As exemplified in the profiles illustrated in Figure 140–1, the pulsatile nature of hormone release implies that changes well in excess of 100 per cent may occur within less than 1 h. Therefore, it is necessary to obtain multiple samples to estimate the mean circulating level of most hormones. The physiological variability, the precision of the assay, and the accuracy of the estimate needed must be taken into consideration to select an adequate sampling protocol. For many hormones, frequent sampling is also necessary to determine the presence or absence of a circadian rhythm. Measurement of the cortisol level on only two blood samples taken in the morning (i.e., between 8:00 and 10:00) and in the late afternoon (i.e., between 16:00 and 18:00) is routinely used to assess the normality of the diurnal variation and is part of the diagnostic workup of Cushing's syndrome. However, as illustrated in Figure 140–20, this procedure may provide inaccurate results because of the highly pulsatile nature of both ACTH and cortisol secretion. Indeed, in these representative patterns, the cortisol level at 9:00 is only marginally higher than at 18:00, and the ACTH levels between 9:00 and 10:00 are lower than around 18:00, a result that suggests the absence of circadian rhythmicity despite the presence of a normal diurnal variation.

Origin

In discussing the origin of ultradian hormonal fluctuations, one must distinguish two general cases, that of the hormones under direct hypothalamic control and that of hormones that are part of more peripheral endocrine systems. In the first case, periodic release ultimately reflects phasic neural activation, whereas in the second case, oscillatory behavior may be a property of the dynamics of local regulatory networks.

The episodic pulses of anterior pituitary hormones are representative of the first case and have been shown to result from secretion in discrete bursts in response to pulsatile stimulation and/or inhibition by hypothalamic factors. The specific hypothalamic mechanism controlling pulsatile release appears to be different for each hypothalamopituitary axis. However, as discussed under Procedures to Quantify Temporal Associations, common stimuli may operate in different axes.

In the case of the gonadotropins, extensive in vivo and in vitro data have shown that the pulsatile release is caused by intermittent discharges of gonadotropin-releasing hormone (GnRH) into the pituitary portal circulation. The GnRH pulses are obtained by synchronous discharges of GnRH-containing neurons controlled by an ultradian pacemaker. In the rhesus monkey, this circhoral oscillator appears to be located in the arcuate nucleus, a structure in the mediobasal hypothalamus.[248] Sharp increases in the frequency of hypothalamic multiunit electrical activity are associated with each LH pulse measured in the peripheral circulation under a variety of experimental conditions in the monkey[248–250] and in the rat.[251] The recent finding that an immortalized hypothalamic neuronal cell line that expresses prepro-GnRH mRNA continues to secrete GnRH in a pulsatile manner raises the possibility that the GnRH pulse generator is located within the GnRH neuronal network itself.[252]

While the pulsatility of gonadotropin release appears to be controlled primarily by a single hypothalamic factor, the pulsatility of GH secretion is due to a complex interaction between intermittent stimulation by hypothalamic growth-releasing factor (GRF) and inhibition by somatostatin. Studies with direct sampling of the hypophyseal-portal circulation have shown that pulses of somatostatin are released in between pulses of GRF.[253, 254] The dual roles of GRF and somatostatin were further demonstrated in experiments involving passive immunization to block endogenous GRF or somatostatin release. Recent data in the rat have further suggested that the complex temporal pattern of GRF and somatostatin release may reflect a mechanism of GH autofeedback involving increased somatostatin release.[255] In humans, information supporting the concept that pulses of GH secretion occur during withdrawal of tonic somatostatin secretion has been based primarily on observations of pulsatile GH secretion in subjects receiving a continuous intravenous infusion of GRF[256] or in patients with GRF-secreting tumors who have sustained high peripheral levels of GRF.[257]

The control of pulsatile ACTH release also appears to involve two hypothalamic factors, corticotrophin-releasing hormone (CRH) and arginine vasopressin (AVP). Under basal conditions as well as under conditions where ACTH secretion is either increased or decreased, pulses of ACTH in the pituitary venous circulation are coincident with pulses of AVP.[258] CRH is packaged in the same secretory vesicles as AVP, and circhoral pulses of ACTH are believed to be driven by simultaneous pulses of CRH and AVP.[51] However, a study using passive immunoneutralization of CRH has provided evidence for a major role of CRH in the control of ultradian rhythms of ACTH release.[259] The precise control of the temporal pattern of pulsatile ACTH release remains otherwise to be defined.

Much less is known about the hypothalamic control of pulsatile prolactin and TSH release. A dual mechanism involving inhibitory control by dopamine and stimulatory control by thyrotropin-releasing hormone (TRH) has been suggested in the case of prolactin.[51] Dopaminergic mechanisms seem to be involved in the amplitude, but not the frequency, regulation of prolactin pulses.[260] Intermittent intravenous TRH infusions elicit coordinated pulses of prolactin release and are more efficient than continuous infusions in elevating prolactin levels.[261] A primary role for TRH in controlling pulsatile TSH release in humans has been suggested by studies showing that a normal pulsatile pattern of TSH can be restored in patients with hypothalamic destruction by repetitive TRH administration.[262] The frequency of TSH pulses in normal subjects is unaltered by dopamine or somatostatin infusion, suggesting that these inhibitory factors do not play a major role in the generation of pulsatile activity in the thyrotropic axis.[262]

Intermittent stimulation by pituitary hormones is, in turn, responsible for the episodic release of hormones under their control. The example of ACTH and cortisol clearly demonstrates that the pulsatile variations of a stimulating hormone may be reflected in the plasma levels of a hormone secreted in response by its target tissue (see Fig. 140–20). The overall temporal correlation between the major secretory pulses of both hormones is evident. However,

the pulsatile variations of ACTH are not transmitted to cortisol levels without distortion, and there is no direct correspondence in magnitude or duration of ACTH and cortisol pulses.[263] Indeed, when expressed as percentage increase over the preceding trough, the median magnitude of pulses is 128 per cent for ACTH but only 70 per cent for cortisol.[34] Two consecutive ACTH pulses may result in a single cortisol pulse, and an increase in ACTH is not always associated with a rise in cortisol. The lack of one-to-one correlation between ACTH and cortisol pulses could be due to differences in the clearance rate of these hormones, effects of binding proteins in the serum, feedback mechanisms, and possibly, the fact that the adrenal may not be responsive to every pulse of ACTH. The distortion may be much more pronounced, such as in the case of LH and testosterone in the human male, in whom it is often difficult to identify testosterone increases following LH pulses. However, in monkeys and other mammalian species, there is a virtual one-to-one relationship between LH and testosterone peaks.

Generating mechanisms for ultradian oscillations of hormones that are part of more peripheral endocrine systems have been little studied. A notable exception are the ultradian 1- to 2-h oscillations of insulin secretion that may be observed following meal ingestion as well as under conditions of constant glucose infusion or continuous enteral nutrition.[245, 246, 262, 264, 265] Theoretical as well as experimental evidence suggests that, in conditions of normal glucose tolerance, these oscillations arise from the negative-feedback interactions linking insulin and glucose.[247, 266] The alternative hypothesis, i.e., the existence of an intrapancreatic ultradian pacemaker generating insulin oscillations and passively entraining glucose, was not supported by studies showing that complete entrainment of pulsatile insulin secretion occurred during oscillatory infusion of exogenous glucose. This is illustrated in Figure 140–21, in which the patterns of insulin secretion and glucose levels are compared during constant glucose infusion, rapid oscillatory glucose infusion, and very slow oscillatory glucose infusion in the same subject. Note that in all three conditions, no significant pulse of insulin secretion occurred in the absence of a concomitant pulse of plasma glucose.

Physiological Significance and Clinical Implications

The physiological significance of pulsatile hormone secretion was first proven when the essential role of the episodic nature of GnRH release for the normal functioning of the pituitary-ovarian axis was demonstrated.[240] Landmark studies showed that continuous infusions of exogenous GnRH in rhesus monkeys with lesions of the arcuate nucleus, which abolished endogenous GnRH production, inhibited the secretion of LH and FSH. In contrast, the pulsatile administration of the synthetic hypothalamic hormone at a rate of one 6-min pulse per hour restored normal LH and FSH levels.[240] Furthermore, if the rate of pulse delivery was increased to three pulses per hour or decreased to one pulse every 2 h, serum LH and FSH levels were not maintained in the normal range. Further discussions of the physiological and clinical significance of pulse frequency for the reproductive axis may be found in Chapters 13 to 15.

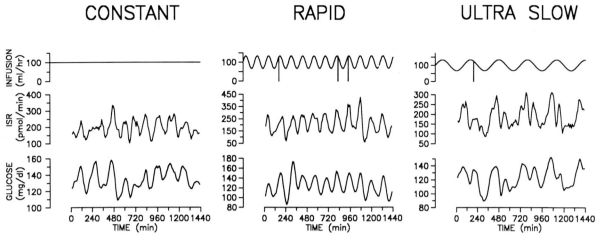

FIGURE 140–21. The 24-h profiles of glucose, plasma insulin, and insulin secretory rate observed in the same subject studied during constant glucose infusion (*left*), rapid oscillatory glucose infusion (*center*; period = 128 min), and ultraslow oscillatory glucose infusion (*right*; period = 320 min). The upper profile in each panel represents the mode of infusion. (Adapted from Sturis J, Van Cauter E, Blackman JD, Polonsky KS: Entrainment of pulsatile insulin secretion by oscillatory glucose infusion. J Clin Invest 87:439–445, 1991, by copyright permission of the American Society for Clinical Investigation.)

The demonstration that the response of the pituitary gland to GnRH is frequency-dependent has led to the search for the cellular mechanisms by which pituitary gonadotrophs can decode changes in GnRH frequency. Studies in both rats and sheep[267–269] have demonstrated that the characteristics of the GnRH pulse signal regulate gonadotropin subunit gene expression. The same dose of GnRH applied at a high pulse frequency to pituitary glands in vitro preferentially stimulates the synthesis of mRNA of LH-β over FSH-β, whereas lower frequencies of GnRH pulse administration forces FSH-β mRNA synthesis.[270] Similarly, the frequency of pulsatile GnRH stimulation in rats can selectively regulate gonadotropin subunit gene transcription, with faster frequencies increasing LH-β (as well as the α gonadotropin subunit) transcription and slower pulses increasing FSH-β transcription.[271] A recent in vitro study has indicated that pulsatile GnRH also exerts its control at the post-transcriptional level.[272] The altered response of the pituitary gland to different GnRH frequencies also may involve pituitary receptors, since GnRH pulse frequency is involved in the regulation of the number of GnRH receptors in the pituitary gland.[273]

As will be detailed later in this chapter under The Gonadotropic Axis: Alterations in Disease States, the findings from the early studies on GnRH pulsatility were rapidly applied to the treatment of a variety of disorders of the pituitary-gonadal axis.[274] Clinical applications are further described in Chapter 15 and in the sections on male and female reproduction.

Advances in the understanding of the physiological importance of pulsatility in the pituitary-gonadal axis have served as a model for investigating the significance and implications of pulsatile release in other endocrine systems. However, because of the differences in mechanisms of central control of pulsatility, which seem to involve only one major hypothalamic factor in the case of the pituitary-gonadal axis but at least two hypothalamic factors in the case of the other pituitary hormones, the physiological importance of pulsatility has been more difficult to demon-

strate, and clinical applications have not yet been developed. However, in the somatotropic axis, studies in hypophysectomized rats have indicated that long-term intravenous pulsatile GH administration is more effective than continuous delivery in promoting body weight gain, longitudinal bone growth, and increases in insulin-like growth factor I (IGF-I) levels.[275, 276] The expression of liver proteins following GH stimulation has been shown to be sensitive to the temporal pattern of the hormone, probably because of a matching program of up-regulation and down-regulation of receptors.[277] Thus, in the rat, sex differences in the pulsatile delivery of GH result in sexually dimorphic expression of hepatic liver genes and are partially responsible for sex differences in somatic growth.[278] Further implications of pulsatility for somatotropic function are described in Chapter 18. Surprisingly, current regimens for GH replacement in GH-deficient adults and children do not take into account the pulsatile nature of physiological GH release or the sexually dimorphic nature of the pattern. It remains to be determined whether there is a relationship between the adverse effects of GH therapy (which is usually administered via subcutaneous injection of recombinant GH, resulting in continuously elevated peripheral GH levels for at least 10 h) and the nonpulsatile, nonphysiological route of delivery.

Modulation of Pulsatility

A number of mechanisms modulating the amplitude and/or frequency of pulsatile or oscillatory hormonal release have been identified. Among the most prominent are modulation by feedback of peripheral hormones and modulation by central signals such as circadian rhythmicity and the alternation of sleep and wake.

The modulation of the frequency and magnitude of the pulsatile release of the gonadotropins by steroid feedback has been well demonstrated. For example, pulses of LH are less frequent and of lesser amplitude in the luteal phase of the menstrual cycle of women, and this reduction in pulse frequency and amplitude is correlated with the duration of exposure of the hypothalamic-pituitary axis to progesterone.[42] Estradiol exerts action on both the amplitude and the frequency of LH pulses.[279] Another example of modulation by steroid feedback is that of ACTH pulsatility. Indeed, high-dose administration of dexamethasone in patients with Cushing's disease suppresses the magnitude, but apparently not the number, of ACTH pulses.[280] Under this condition of a reduced magnitude in ACTH pulsatility, fewer ACTH pulses are able to elicit a detectable cortisol response, and a dramatic decrease in both number and size of episodic cortisol pulses is observed.

The roles of circadian rhythmicity, i.e., intrinsic effects of time of day independent of the sleep or wake state, and sleep, i.e., intrinsic effects of the sleep state irrespective of the time of day when it occurs, on pulsatile neuroendocrine release have long been recognized. The dissociation between circadian effects and sleep effects and the nature of the modulatory mechanisms have been more difficult to establish, however. Theoretically, the modulation of hormonal release by circadian rhythmicity and sleep could be achieved by two distinct types of mechanisms. Circadian modulation could be achieved by modulation of pulse amplitude, with larger or smaller pulses occurring around the daily maximum or minimum, respectively. Alternatively, circadian modulation could be achieved by modulation of pulse frequency, with more pulses occurring around the time of the daily maximum and fewer pulses occurring around the time of the daily minimum. Similarly, modulatory effects of sleep on pulsatile release, whether stimulatory or inhibitory, could be exerted by either amplitude or frequency modulation. Importantly, to distinguish circadian effects from sleep effects, it is necessary to study circadian modulation in the absence of the confounding effects of sleep (i.e., during sleep deprivation) and sleep modulation at abnormal times of day to avoid confounding circadian effects. These issues have only been examined in a handful of studies which used mathematical deconvolution to remove the effects of distribution and degradation on peripheral concentrations to reveal the temporal pattern of secretion. In the case of the corticotropic axis, several studies based on different deconvolution techniques and underlying assumptions for hormonal kinetics have concluded that the pronounced circadian variation of ACTH and cortisol secretion is achieved by modulation of pulse amplitude without changes in pulse frequency.[36, 39, 40] The relative constancy of frequency of ACTH and cortisol pulses throughout the 24-h cycle is indeed apparent in the representative profiles illustrated in Figure 140–20. Similar analyses have been performed to examine the mechanisms involved in the circadian modulation of TSH secretion and have concluded that both amplitude and frequency modulations were implicated.[243] However, sleep, which exerts major inhibitory effects on nocturnal TSH secretion, was not controlled in these studies, and the findings thus need to be replicated in sleep-deprived subjects.

As noted earlier, sleep control of pulsatile hormone release was long thought to be largely limited to the somatotropic and lactotropic axes. In the case of GH secretion, available evidence suggests that sleep exerts some control on pulse frequency, since a pulse of GH release is consistently associated with sleep onset, irrespective of the time

of day.[35, 37, 162] More detailed evaluation of circadian and sleep control of pulsatile GH release will be possible when temporal profiles are obtained using new ultrasensitive assays revealing variations of GH levels occurring in a concentration range below the limit of sensitivity of current procedures. Deconvolution analyses of prolactin profiles, assuming monoexponential disappearance kinetics with a fixed half-life of 25 min, have indicated that the nocturnal rise of plasma prolactin is obtained by increasing both tonic secretion and pulse amplitude.[243] The modulation of LH pulsatility by sleep varies according to the stage of sexual maturation.[35] Early studies showed a sleep-associated increase in LH concentrations in pubertal children which appeared to be realized by an increase of pulse amplitude.[38] In male adults, LH amplitude and frequency do not show any consistent diurnal variations. In normally menstruating women in the early part of the follicular phase, the frequency of LH pulses is markedly decreased during sleep. Figure 140–22 shows data representative of this modulation of LH pulse frequency by sleep from four laboratories.[41, 42, 281, 282] Evidence from sleep-reversal studies has indicated that the slowing of LH pulsatility during sleep is specifically related to SW sleep.[283] Sleep also exerts some control over the frequency of neuroendocrine release in the corticotropic axis, with a clear inhibition of pulsatility during the first few hours after sleep onset.[163]

A number of studies have investigated the possible relationship between pulsatile hormonal release and the most prominent nonendocrine ultradian rhythm, i.e., the alternation of REM and non-REM stages in sleep. The most robust association between pituitary release and sleep stages is observed in the case of GH pulses, which occur preferentially during SW sleep, with a quantitative association between duration of the SW stage and amount of GH secreted.[37] In early studies in pubertal boys, LH levels appear to be elevated during REM sleep as compared with non-REM sleep.[284] A 1974 report[285] found that episodic prolactin secretion during sleep was entrained by the REM–non-REM cycle. However, this result was not confirmed in later studies.[286] A recent analysis of patterns of prolactin, TSH, LH, GH, and ACTH release during polygraphically recorded nocturnal sleep has indicated that REM sleep generally begins when pituitary secretion is decreased, i.e., when plasma levels are at a peak or plateau, when they decline, or when they are at a trough.[287] In contrast, REM sleep was never initiated during active pulsatile release, i.e., ascending portions of pulses. These interesting findings need to be confirmed for daytime sleep periods, i.e., in the absence of masking effects of circadian rhythmicity. Other studies have indicated a stimulatory role of nocturnal awakenings on ACTH-cortisol secretion and an inhibitory role on GH secretion.[36, 288] Remarkably, if GH secretion is stimulated by a GRF injection during sleep and the subject is awakened 30 to 60 min after the injection, the secretory response is immediately interrupted.[288] A close relationship between oscillations of plasma renin activity and the REM–non-REM cycle, with a decline of renin activity at the beginning of each REM phase, has been clearly demonstrated.[289–292] Examples of 24-h profiles of plasma renin activity in subjects studied during normal nocturnal sleep or shifted daytime sleep are shown in Figure 140–23.

Taken together, these findings indicate that sleep exerts profound modulatory effects on endocrine function which are currently underestimated and understudied. In particular, the possibility that endocrine disturbance may be associated with chronic sleep disorders has never been examined. Furthermore, preservation of normal sleep-related endocrine patterns has not so far been incorporated in the design of safe hypnotic agents.

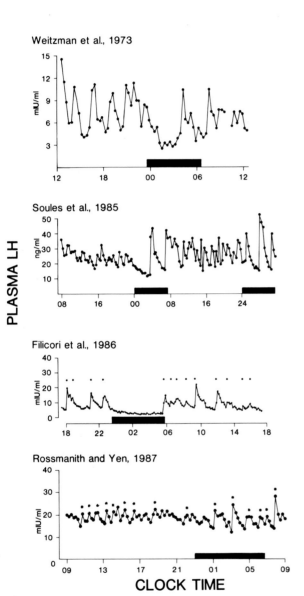

FIGURE 140–22. Representative profiles of plasma LH in normal women studied during the early follicular phase. Black bars represent the sleep period. Asterisks denote statistically significant pulses. Data sources: 1. Soules M, Steiner R, Cohen N, Bremner W, Clifton D: Nocturnal slowing of pulsatile luteinizing hormone secretion in women during the follicular phase of the menstrual cycle. J Clin Endocrinol Metab 61:43–49, 1985; 2. Filicori M, Santoro N, Merriam GR, Crowley WFJ: Characterization of the physiological pattern of episodic gonadotropin secretion throughout the menstrual cycle. J Clin Endocrinol Metab 62:1136–1144, 1986; 3. Weitzman ED. Effect of Sleep-wake Cycle Shifts on Sleep and Neuroendocrine Function. New York, Plenum Press, 1973, pp 93–111; 4. Rossmanith WG, Yen SSC: Sleep-associated decrease in luteinizing hormone pulse frequency during the early follicular phase: Evidence for an opioidergic mechanism. J Clin Endocrinol Metab 65:715–718, 1987. © by the Endocrine Society, 1987.)

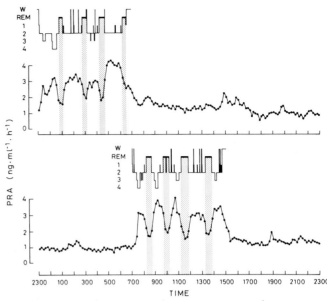

FIGURE 140–23. The 24-h profiles of plasma renin activity (PRA) in two individual subjects who had regular sleep-wake cycle. In the subject shown in the lower panel, sleep times had been shifted from 23:00 to 7:00 to 7:00 to 15:00. The temporal distributions of stages of wake (W), rapid-eye-movement (REM), 1, 2, 3, and 4 are shown above the PRA profiles. The shaded vertical areas show the temporal association of REM stages and declining PRA. (Unpublished data from G Brandenberger, M Follenius, B Goichot, et al.)

Higher-Frequency Oscillations in the Endocrine System

Oscillations at frequencies higher than the hourly (i.e., circhoral) range characterizing pulsatile release have been observed for a variety of hormones. In particular, rapid oscillations of insulin secretion with periods in the 10- to 15-min range have been well characterized in humans,[2, 293, 294] monkeys,[1, 295] and dogs.[296] As shown in Figure 140–24, these rapid pulsations are superimposed on the ultradian 100- to 140-min oscillations. Work on isolated perfused dog pancreas and other in vitro systems has demonstrated that these oscillations are both self-sustained and intrinsic to the pancreas.[297] The fact that pulsatile insulin administration at 13-min intervals to normal subjects has greater hypoglycemic effect than continuous delivery also indicates the physiological importance of these oscillations.[298] Studies with blood sampling at 1- or 2-min intervals have shown that plasma levels of LH and GH undergo high-frequency oscillations of low amplitude which exceed the range compatible with measurement error.[299, 300] These micropulses recurred at irregular 3- to 5-min intervals. The cause and implications of this inherent instability remain to be elucidated. Their biological significance has been questioned.[301] Studies in the rat and humans also have revealed the existence of rapid oscillations of plasma ACTH, with periods around 20 min.[3, 302] Amplitude modulation of these rapid oscillations apparently generates pulsatile ACTH variations with frequencies in the ultradian range of 15 to 20 pulses per 24 h.[259] Immunoneutralization of CRH suppresses the amplitude, but not the frequency, of the rapid pulses and suppresses ultradian fluctuations, suggesting a different origin for the two oscillations.[259]

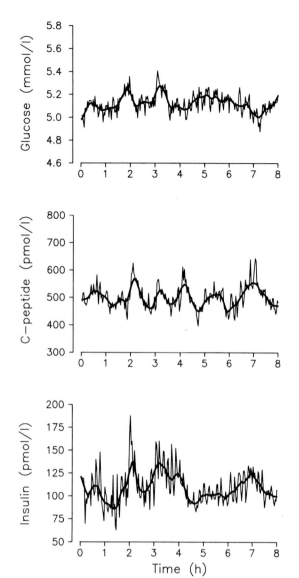

FIGURE 140–24. Profiles of plasma glucose (*top*), plasma C-peptide (*center*), and serum insulin (*bottom*) obtained at 2-min intervals in a fasted normal subject. The smooth regression curve quantifies the ultradian variations. The data were detrended prior to calculating the regression curve. (From Sturis J, Polonsky KS, Shapiro ET, et al: Abnormalities in the ultradian oscillations of insulin secretion and glucose levels in type 2 (non–insulin-dependent) diabetic patients. Diabetologia 35:681–689, 1992.)

SEASONAL RHYTHMS

Circannual Clocks and Photoperiodic Measurement

For a majority of species, a multitude of adaptive mechanisms have evolved to cope with the pronounced changes that occur in the physical environment on an annual basis. Some organisms make use of internal *circannual* clocks, which like circadian clocks, can free run under constant environmental conditions but normally are entrained by periodic signals in the environment.[303, 304] Other species rely exclusively on periodic changes in the physical environment to time their seasonal cycles, and for many species, it is the change in day length that synchronizes seasonal rhythms to the annual environmental changes.[47]

There is presently little evidence to implicate the circadian system in the regulation of endogenous circannual rhythms. Indeed, the circannual rhythm in hibernation in golden mantled ground squirrels persists even after SCN destruction.[304]

Seasonal Rhythms in Reproductive Function

One of the most pronounced seasonal rhythms observed in the majority of vertebrate species inhabiting the temperate zones of the world is the annual rhythm in reproduction.[51, 52, 305] For many species, the young are born during specific times of the year when the probability of survival for both the parents and offspring is maximal. The primary environmental cue for stimulating gonadal activity and reproductive behavior during the appropriate time of the year is the change in day length.[47, 52, 305] Thus, in many rodent species and birds, the long days of spring and summer are stimulatory to reproductive activity, while the short days of fall and winter are inhibitory. The value of using the seasonal change in day length for the timing of the reproductive season is undoubtedly due to its reliability as a marker of the phase of the seasonal environmental cycle. While most studies on seasonal rhythms have focused on reproductive activity, other physiological and behavioral annual cycles have been well documented, including milk production, growth, pelage color, molting, migration, and hibernation. Similar to reproductive cycles, seasonal rhythms in other physiological systems are also often regulated by the seasonal change in day length. For example, the production of insulin-like growth factor I (IGF-I) in reindeer is day length–dependent, and the seasonal growth spurt in this species is preceded by an elevation in plasma IGF-I concentration.[306]

Role of the Circadian System in Photoperiodic Measurement

The circadian system is involved in the timing of seasonal rhythms in many species by way of its central role in measuring the seasonal change in day length. Early studies in the golden hamster demonstrated that bilateral destruction of the SCN abolishes the photoperiodic gonadal response and that lesioned animals are no longer capable of responding to the inhibitory effects of short days on gonadal function.[47] While the role of the SCN in the photoperiodic control of reproduction has been examined in only a few species, in all cases, disruption of SCN function disrupts the effects of day length on reproductive activity. The circadian clock in the SCN mediates the effects of day length on reproductive function, at least in part through its regulation of the diurnal rhythm in pineal melatonin production.[307–309] The synthesis and release of pineal melatonin are tightly coupled to the LD cycle such that circulating melatonin levels are high during the night and low during the day, and if the night is interrupted by even a brief period of light, circulating melatonin levels are rapidly depressed.[308] Studies originally carried out in the Djungarian hamster and sheep have established that it is the duration of the uninterrupted nighttime melatonin release that determines whether the photoperiod will be interpreted as a long or short day.[305, 310]

It should be noted that while a day length consisting of a short night (e.g., LD 16:8), and its associated short period of elevated melatonin levels, is stimulatory to neuroendocrine-gonadal activity in hamsters, the same day length is inhibitory to reproductive function in short-day breeding sheep.[305, 310] At the present time, it is not known how the circadian melatonin signal is decoded by the brain for measuring day length, nor is it known how a melatonin duration signal is transduced into a change in neuroendocrine-gonadal activity. The recent finding that the SCN itself contains melatonin receptors[311] raises the possibility that there is an intricate feedback relationship between the SCN and the pineal gland in the photoperiodic control of seasonal cycles.

Seasonal Variations in Human Endocrine Function

While the human reproductive system is not "turned on and off" on a seasonal basis as it is in many other mammalian species, there is evidence to indicate that seasonal changes can occur in the timing of the preovulatory LH surge,[49] circulating testosterone levels,[312] and semen quality.[313] Whether the change in day length or some other factor in the environment which changes on a seasonal basis is responsible for changes in human reproductive parameters is not known. The study of the potential effects of day length on human physiology is still in its infancy. As noted above, changes in day length can affect a variety of nonreproductive physiological systems in mammals. The recent data obtained by Wehr and co-workers[314, 315] showing that the nocturnal secretory profiles of a series of hormones, including melatonin, cortisol, and prolactin, are modified by exposure to long nights (14 versus 8 h) strongly suggest that humans are also "seasonal animals." Figure 140–25 compares the mean profiles of melatonin, prolactin, and sleep during the two experimental conditions. It is evident that the durations of nocturnal secretion of melatonin and prolactin as well as the sleep period are expanded during the long-night condition. Seasonal changes in the melatonin rhythm and in the timing of sleep in relation to the nocturnal minimum of body temperature have been reported.[316] An influence of season on the peripheral concentrations of GH, cortisol, adrenal androgens, and thyroid hormones also has been noted.[144, 317] These findings have generally been based on a few samples per season or a comparison between summer and winter and await confirmation by longitudinal studies with more frequent sampling. The effects of day length on various endocrine systems could be mediated through the known effects of sunlight on the cutaneous synthesis of vitamin D or could be due to effects that are mediated by the circadian clock system. Seasonal changes in the volume of the human SCN and in the number of vasopressin-immunoreactive neurons within the SCN have recently been observed.[318] The mechanisms, significance, and clinical implications of seasonality in humans represent an understudied area of endocrinology.

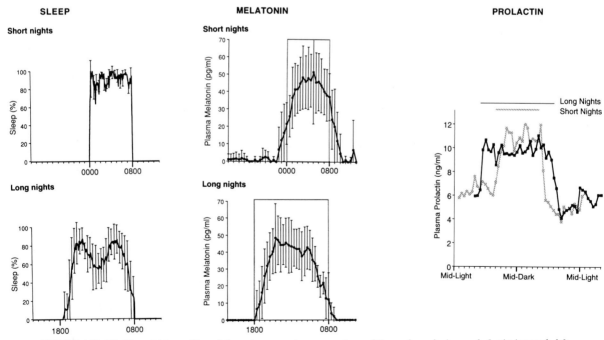

FIGURE 140–25. Mean 24-h profiles of sleep (expressed as percentage of time asleep during each 6-min interval; *left panels*), plasma melatonin (*center panels*), and plasma prolactin (*right panels*) in normal subjects studied following chronic exposure to short (8 h) and long (14 h) nights. Measurements of plasma melatonin were made under constant dim light conditions. The dark phase of the photoperiod schedule that preceded the measurements is indicated by an open rectangle. Vertical lines at each time point in the left and center panels correspond to the standard deviation of the group. For prolactin, the data were referenced to the midpoint of the dark period in both conditions. (Adapted from Wehr TA: The durations of human melatonin secretion and sleep respond to changes in daylength. J Clin Endocrinol Metab 73:1276–1280, 1991; and Wehr TA, Moul DE, Barbato G, et al: Conservation of photoperiod-responsive mechanisms in human beings. Am J Physiol, in press.)

METHODOLOGICAL ASPECTS OF THE STUDY OF ENDOCRINE RHYTHMS

Experimental Protocols to Study Endocrine Rhythms

Studying Circadian Variations

There are, in principle, two ways of studying circadian rhythmicity in human subjects. The first is to study the same individual(s) for a period of time spanning as many 24-h cycles as possible (*longitudinal study*). While such protocols are certainly optimal with respect to evaluation of the presence and reproducibility of circadian variations, their demands on research subjects are often prohibitive. The second is to study a group of individuals for a minimum of one 24-h cycle each, following the same experimental protocol (*transversal study*). The demonstration of circadian rhythmicity is then based on the observation of consistently reproducible characteristics in a set of 24-h profiles. The group of subjects should be as homogeneous as possible not only in terms of physical parameters such as age and sex but also in terms of living habits such as sleep-wake cycles and meal schedules. Prior to the beginning of the experiment, the volunteers should be asked to adhere to a standardized schedule of meals and bedtimes for several days in order to maximize interindividual synchronization. Subjects who have regular social habits and describe themselves as "good sleepers" should be preferred. Shift workers or subjects having made a transmeridian flight less than 2 months before the experiment should be excluded. Most studies of circadian rhythms in endocrinology have been based on transversal rather than longitudinal data sets.

Blood sampling is usually done at regular intervals through a catheter inserted into a forearm vein. Continuous withdrawal systems are less time-consuming but dampen episodic fluctuations, since every sample represents an integrated concentration over the sampling interval rather than an instantaneous level. To avoid disruptions of sleep due to the sampling procedure, the catheter should be connected to tubing extending to an adjoining room during the night. If the quality of sleep is anticipated to play an important role in determining the nocturnal hormonal profile, the subjects should spend 2 to 3 nights of habituation in the study unit prior to the beginning of the investigation. Indeed, the duration of sleep and the total duration of REM stages may be reduced significantly by the presence of the catheter.[319] These alterations of sleep subside as the subject adapts to the experimental procedure. The catheter should be inserted at least 2 h before the collection of the first sample in order to avoid possible artifactual effects related to the venipuncture stress. To obtain valid estimations of the circadian parameters, it is necessary to sample at intervals not exceeding 1 h. Indeed, the pulsatile pattern of hormonal release may bias the estimation of the characteristics of the circadian rhythm if sampling is less frequent.

If hormonal profiles are measured as markers of the output of the central circadian oscillator, as is often the case for the 24-h cortisol profile, direct effects of other factors need to be minimized. Sleep-wake transitions, meals, stressful activity, and postural changes may all be reflected in increases or decreases of hormonal secretion.

To eliminate these "masking" effects, experimental protocols usually referred to as *constant routines* have been developed to reliably derive estimates of circadian amplitude and phase from temporal patterns of peripheral hormones and other physiological variables, such as body temperature.[26] Constant routine conditions generally involve a regimen of continuous wakefulness, constant recumbent posture, constant illumination, and constant caloric intake either in the form of hourly identical aliquots of liquid diet or solid food or in the form of a constant glucose infusion. Such conditions are generally maintained for 30 to 40 h. Figure 140–26 compares mean cortisol and TSH profiles obtained under the two conditions. As may be seen, the absence of sleep-wake transitions results in an earlier and higher nadir of cortisol secretion and in a slightly lower morning acrophase. The sleep deprivation imposed by the experimental conditions results, however, in a marked elevation of nocturnal TSH levels.

While constant routine conditions are quasi-universally employed in basic studies of human circadian rhythmicity, they have obvious limitations. Sleep deprivation is a stressful condition, and while the effects of sleep-wake transitions are removed in this protocol, other possibly confounding factors, such as the amplification of the circadian variation of sleepiness (see Fig. 140–15) and the marked elevation of TSH levels (as shown in Fig. 140–33), are added. The use of circadian markers that are not masked by sleep, meals, and other factors has therefore been advocated. In particular, the measurement of the 24-h profile of melatonin secretion under dim light conditions, which appears unaffected by the sleep or wake condition, posture, and food intake, has been shown to provide estimations of circadian phase and amplitude highly correlated with those derived from the temperature rhythm and the cortisol rhythm observed under constant routine conditions.

Studying Pulsatile Variations

Sampling rates from 1 to 20 min and lengths of sampling ranging from 1 to 24 h have been used to characterize episodic hormonal fluctuations. Not surprisingly, widely different results have been obtained for the same hormone depending on the sampling protocol chosen. Considerations of the total amount of blood withdrawn and of the amount of plasma needed to assay the hormones under study are obviously essential to the definition of an adequate sampling protocol. The intuitive notion that more frequent sampling will unmask more rapid episodic fluctuations has been shown to hold true for hormones such as ACTH, GH, LH, and insulin.[2, 299, 300, 302] However, the very rapid, low-amplitude pulses uncovered by sampling rates of 1 to 4 min probably have a different origin and physiological significance than the large secretory ultradian oscillations. The definition of an optimal sampling protocol depends thus on the type of phenomenon under study. At the present time, sampling at 1-min intervals probably represents the fastest rate technically achievable with reasonable precision. Sampling rates of 1 and 2 min will uncover high-frequency, low-amplitude episodic variations superimposed on the slower pulsatile release at intervals of 1 to 2 h. These intensified rates of venous sampling may not allow for estimation of the characteristics of major secre-

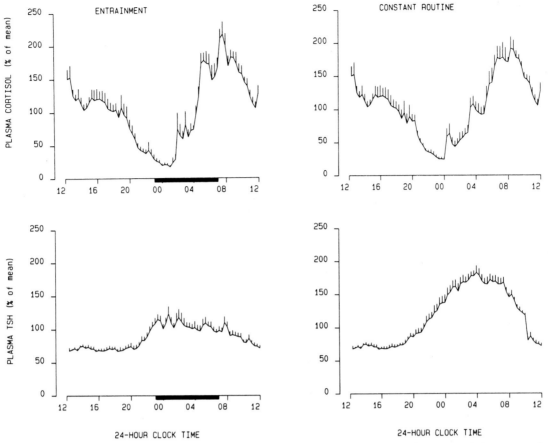

FIGURE 140–26. Mean profiles of plasma cortisol (*top*) and TSH (*bottom*) observed at 15-min intervals in a group of 8 normal subjects studied during entrainment (*left*) and during ''constant routine'' conditions (*right*). The vertical bars at each time point represent the SEM. The black bar represents the mean sleep period. For each subject, the data were expressed as a percentage of the 24-h mean prior to calculating group values.

tory bursts, since the total duration of sampling compatible with this rate of blood withdrawal limits the observed number of large peaks to a few units. Sampling rates of 20 and 30 min will only detect major pulses lasting more than 1 h. De Nicolao et al.[320] have proposed a method based on a mathematical modeling of the secretory pattern to estimate the relationship between the sampling interval and the visible frequency of pulses.

Procedures to Quantify Circadian Variations

To determine rhythm parameters in biological time series, fairly laborious mathematical procedures are often unavoidable. Among the methods proposed for and applied to 24-h profiles of blood components, the Cosinor test developed by Halberg was both the first and the most widely used.[321] The major disadvantage of the Cosinor test and of its derivatives is its assumption that the observed profile may be described adequately by a single sinusoidal curve. This assumption is practically never met for biological rhythms which are asymmetrical in nature (e.g., the sleep-wake cycle is an 8:16 alternation, not 12:12). Therefore, the Cosinor test generally provides unreliable estimations of rhythm parameters.

Other procedures for the detection and estimation of circadian variation have been based on periodogram calculations or on nonlinear regression procedures.[322–324] As shown in Figure 140–3, these methods provide an adequate description of asymmetrical waveshapes. The times of occurrence of the maximum and the minimum of the best-fit curve are often referred to as the *acrophase* and the *nadir*, respectively. The amplitude of the rhythm may be estimated as 50 per cent of the difference between the maximum and the minimum of the best-fit curve. With the periodogram procedure, confidence intervals for the amplitude, acrophase, and nadirs may be calculated.

When comparing 24-h hormonal profiles from different subjects, it may be advantageous to reference the data according to sleep onset rather than according to clock time. It should be noted that for many variables it is not so much the sleep time on the day of experimentation but the habitual sleep schedule prior to the experiment that mainly determines circadian phase.

Procedures to Quantify Pulsatile Hormonal Secretion

The analysis of pulsatile variations may be considered at two levels. One may wish to define and characterize significant variations in peripheral levels, based on estimations of the size of measurement error (i.e., primarily assay error). However, under certain circumstances, it is possible to mathematically derive secretory rates from the peripheral concentrations. This procedure, also referred to as deconvolution, often will reveal more pulses of secretion than the analysis of peripheral concentrations. It also will more accurately define the temporal limits of each pulse. However, deconvolution involves an amplification of measurement error, with increased risk of false-positive error. Whether examining peripheral concentrations or secretory rates, there are two major approaches to analyzing the episodic fluctuations. The first, and most commonly used, is the *time-domain analysis*, in which the data are plotted against time and pulses are detected and identified. The second is the *frequency-domain analysis*, in which amplitude is plotted against frequency or period. These two approaches differ fundamentally both in the mathematical treatment of the data and in the questions they may help to resolve and should therefore be viewed as complementary.

Time-Domain Analysis of Pulses of Plasma Concentrations

Since the pioneering approach proposed by Santen and Bardin[325] in their classic article describing pulsatile LH release in the woman, a number of computer algorithms for identification of pulses of hormonal concentration have been proposed. A detailed presentation of the operating principles of each of these procedures is beyond the scope of this chapter. Recent review articles[326–328] have provided comparisons of performance of several pulse-detection algorithms, including Ultra,[324, 329] Pulsar,[330] Cycle Detector,[331] Cluster,[332] and Detect.[333] A comparative study of the performance of various pulse-detection algorithms on experimental series conducted by Urban et al.[334] indicated that Ultra, Cluster, and Detect perform similarly when used with appropriate choices of parameters. Objective assessment of the performance of a pulse-detection program may be by testing computer-generated profiles including both pulses and "noise" and examining false-positive and false-negative errors. This approach has been used by the authors of Ultra, Cluster, and Detect.[329, 335–337] A more recent procedure (PulseFit[338]) for hormonal pulse detection is based on a statistical model for the underlying processes of pulsatile release, distribution, and degradation. We will briefly describe below the major operating principles of the frequently used algorithms.

Ultra, which predates all the other algorithms, has the following characteristics: (1) it takes into account both the increasing limb and the declining limb in determining the significance of a pulse, (2) it allows for variable precision of the assay in various concentration ranges, (3) the significance of a pulse is evaluated independently of its width, and (4) its performance is not affected by the existence of a fluctuating baseline, as may be caused by circadian variation. In summary, a pulse is considered significant if both its increment and its decline exceed, in relative terms, a threshold expressed in multiples of the intra-assay coefficient of variation in the relevant range of concentration. All changes in concentration which do not meet the criteria for significance are eliminated by an iterative process,

providing a "clean" profile as an output. Figure 140–27 illustrates the performance of Ultra on a 24-h profile of plasma C-peptide obtained in a normal volunteer under constant glucose infusion. The coefficient of variation of the assay averaged 4 per cent throughout the relevant range of concentrations. A threshold of 2 coefficients of variation (CV's) was used. To test Ultra for false-positive and false-negative errors,[329] the program was applied to a large set of computer-generated series including both signal (i.e., pulses) and noise (i.e., measurement error). These simulation studies indicated that for series with a medium to high signal-to-noise ratio (i.e., large and frequent pulses), a threshold of 2 local intra-assay CV's minimizes both false-positive and false-negative errors. For series with low signal-to-noise ratios (i.e., low pulse amplitude and/or frequency), a threshold of 3 CV's is preferable.

In program Pulsar,[330] a smoothing procedure is used to obtain a baseline, which is then subtracted from the data. The significance of the pulses is examined in the residual

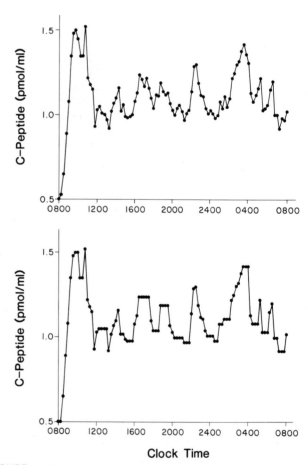

FIGURE 140–27. Representative analysis of ultradian oscillations of plasma C-peptide levels (observed at 15-min intervals in a normal subject receiving a constant glucose infusion) using the computer algorithm for pulse identification Ultra. The upper panel shows the raw data. The lower panel shows the profile obtained after eliminating all the variations which did not exceed in relative terms twice the intra-assay coefficient of variation in the relevant range of concentration. (From Van Cauter E: Computer-assisted analysis of endocrine rhythms. *In* Rodbard D, Forti G (eds): Computers in Endocrinology. New York, Raven Press, 1990, pp 59–70. Data from: Shapiro ET, Tillil H, Polonsky KS, et al: Oscillations in insulin secretion during constant glucose infusion in normal man: relationship to changes in plasma glucose. J Clin Endocrinol Metab 67:307–314, 1988. © by the Endocrine Society, 1988.)

series. In this algorithm, both the height and the width of the pulses are taken into account so that narrow, high pulses as well as broader peaks may be detected. However, when it is known a priori that the profile does not include a detectable baseline trend, the estimation and subsequent removal of a baseline, such as performed by Pulsar, may bias the identification and characterization of pulses.

The Cycle Detector[331] assumes that a cyclical component of fairly stable amplitude underlies the data and provides an estimation of the number of such cycles present in the series instead of a pulse-by-pulse identification of significant secretory pulses. This method is poorly suited to the analysis of profiles in which pulse amplitudes vary with time of day, such as that of cortisol.

The Cluster[332] algorithm derives its name from the fact that the user has the option to define peaks and troughs of plasma concentration as "clusters" of two, three, or more data points rather than as isolated time points. The general principle of the Cluster program is the comparison by standard t tests of replicate measurements at the peak and the preceding and following nadir. In some cases, the performance of Cluster may be crucially dependent on the choice of cluster sizes. It has been suggested that to optimize its performance, several cluster sizes should be tested on synthetic data simulating the putative characteristics of the hormonal signal under study.[335, 338]

Detect identifies significant pulses by combining two different strategies, one based on the analysis of first derivatives to detect rapid changes and one based on the fitting of linear segments to detect slow changes. It has been tested for both false-positive and false-negative errors and was found to have excellent sensitivity.[335]

From this brief description of some of the currently available procedures for pulse analysis, it is obvious that there is no universal ready-to-use recipe applicable to all types of data. The investigator must choose the procedure whose underlying assumptions best match the data in hand and repeat the analysis with various choices of entry parameters to evaluate the sensitivity of the results with respect to parameter selection. Comparisons of the performances of several procedures are often very informative.

Time-Domain Analysis of Profiles of Secretory Rates

When the clearance kinetics of the hormone under study are known with reasonable accuracy, secretory rates can be derived from plasma levels by calculation using a mathematical model to remove the effects of hormonal distribution and degradation. This procedure, commonly referred to as deconvolution, may be based on a one-compartment model, i.e., single exponential decay, or a two-compartment model, i.e., double exponential decay. The advantage of examining secretory rates rather than peripheral concentrations are obvious.[339] Indeed, the dynamic nature of the secretory process, e.g., entirely pulsatile or involving both tonic and intermittent secretion, is revealed, and the mechanisms underlying modulatory influences such as those of circadian rhythmicity or sleep can be analyzed. Moreover, deconvolution provides a more accurate estimation of the temporal limits of the secretory process than peripheral concentrations and allows therefore for more precise evaluation of temporal concordance between dif-

ferent endocrine and/or nonendocrine events. An example was shown in Figure 140–20, where the association between pulsatile ACTH and cortisol release became more clearly apparent when cortisol secretory rates, rather than plasma levels, were examined.

Several deconvolution procedures have been proposed for hormonal data. The earliest, simplest, and most widely used approaches involve calculating the amount of hormone secreted between successive sampling times by solving the corresponding linear differential equations without postulating an underlying model for the waveshape of pulsatile release. The kinetics of hormonal clearance need to be known with good accuracy. The first use of *waveform-independent deconvolution*[339] in hormone research has been to estimate the secretion rate of insulin from the plasma levels of C-peptide.[340–342] This procedure was subsequently used in numerous clinical studies in which the clearance kinetics of C-peptide were derived experimentally in each research volunteer.[342, 343] While such straightforward approaches are attractive because of their relative simplicity, they also may provide absurd results, such as negative secretory rates, and involve a large false-positive error in the estimation of the number of secretory pulses. Negative secretory rates will be found if the kinetic model is inadequate (the number of compartments is incorrect and/or wrong estimations for the values of the kinetic parameters have been used) or if there was a drop in concentration due to dilution rather than decreasing or interrupted secretion. Even if none of these problems exists, negative secretory rates may still occur because deconvolution involves amplification of measurement error, particularly when secretory rates are low. However, if one assumes that the measurement errors on the concentrations are normally distributed, statistical errors on the calculated secretory rates can be estimated, and secretory rates which are significantly negative can be identified.[344] The other problem with straightforward deconvolution is the fact that errors on the secretory rates increase when the sampling interval decreases. This paradoxical phenomenon reflects the fact that the secretory rate is estimated separately in each sampling interval. Smoothing of the raw concentration data prior to deconvolution has been used to remedy this problem.[341] To identify significant pulses of secretory rates, pulse analysis may be repeated using a modified version of the pulse-detection algorithm where the thresholds for pulse detection are based on the calculated errors on the instantaneous secretory rates.[344] A number of computerized algorithms for waveform-independent deconvolution have been proposed recently, with increasingly complex mathematical procedures to attempt to circumvent some of the above-mentioned difficulties.[243, 345] In all cases, it is essential that the clearance kinetics of the hormone under consideration be well defined to obtain reliable conclusions. Other approaches to hormonal deconvolution have been made model-based or waveform-specific.[339, 346, 347] In *model-based methods*, the waveshapes of underlying pulses are postulated, and the number of pulses, their location and amplitudes, and the half-life of the hormone are estimated by multiparameter optimization techniques.

Frequency-Domain Analysis

The time-domain analysis will provide an estimation of pulse frequency, calculated as the total number of pulses

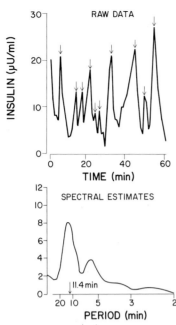

FIGURE 140–28. Analysis of pulsatile variations of insulin levels measured at 2-min intervals in the portal vein in a conscious dog. The top panel shows the raw data, with significant pulses indicated by arrows. The frequency of pulses (i.e., 10 in 60 min) suggests an average periodicity of 6 min. The lower panel shows the spectral estimations revealing a dominant 11.4-min periodicity. (Adapted from Jaspan JB, Lever E, Polonsky KS, Van Cauter E: In vivo pulsatility of pancreatic islet peptides. Am J Physiol 251:E215–E226, 1986.)

detected divided by the duration of the study period. However, little information about the pattern of pulse recurrence will be gained. Analysis in the frequency domain may indicate whether the underlying process is periodic, quasiperiodic, or random.[348, 349] Descriptions of the principles and applications of spectral analysis are outside of the scope of this chapter. Figure 140–28 illustrates an example of spectral analysis of hormonal data in the case of rapid insulin oscillations observed at 1-min intervals in the portal vein in the dog.[296] Nine pulses were found significant by analysis in the time domain using the Ultra algorithm, corresponding to an average pulse frequency of one pulse per 6.7 min. However, spectral analysis reveals that the dominant frequency of pulse recurrence is 11.4 min, i.e., similar to what has been observed in the monkey and in the human.[1, 293, 294] Analyses in the frequency domain have been used in several recent studies of endocrine oscillations.[350–352]

Procedures to Quantify Temporal Associations

Over the past few years, a number of investigators have addressed the issue of temporal concordance between pulses or oscillations of different hormones and/or metabolites. Similar methodological questions underly the study of interactions between rhythms of endocrine release and oscillations in other physiological systems, such as the alternation of REM and non-REM stages during sleep or rapid changes in blood pressure and heart rate.

There have been two general types of studies involving attempts to quantify temporal associations between hormonal pulses or oscillations. In the first type, the existence of a strong relationship between the variables under consideration was well-established and the aim of the study was to further quantify this relationship in normal or abnormal conditions. Typical examples are the study of the concomitance between oscillations of insulin secretion and glucose levels, of the temporal concordance of pulses of LH, FSH, and α subunit, and of the relationship between pulses of plasma ACTH and pulses of cortisol secretion. In the second type of study, the analysis of temporal associations has the primary goal of obtaining evidence for a putative common influence on the various processes under consideration. The possible existence of a temporal coupling between pulses of LH and pulses of prolactin[353] or TSH[354] and between pulses of corticotropin activity and pulses of testosterone[355] justifies this type of approach.

Methods for analyzing and quantifying temporal concordance also fall in two categories: cross-correlation analysis, which provides a global description of the relationship between the two oscillatory processes, and assessment of coincidence of individual secretory pulses in two or more endocrine profiles.[356–359] Calculations of cross-correlations will provide an overall estimation of the strength and significance of the linkage as well as of the possible time lag between the two pulsating or oscillatory patterns. However, analysis of ultradian variations by cross-correlation requires the removal of longer-term trends, such as circadian rhythmicity, prior to calculation, because otherwise the result would reflect the combined effects of the two period ranges. Furthermore, these calculations are sensitive to differences in amplitude of the pulses (e.g., a large pulse in one of the hormones is coincident with a small pulse in the other, or vice versa), even when their timing is highly concordant. Examples of the use of cross-correlation to analyze coupling between hormonal profiles can be found in studies of temporal linkage of pituitary hormones[353] and in studies of ultradian glucose and insulin oscillations.[350, 360] Various procedures to quantify the concordance of secretory pulses in hormonal profiles have been proposed.[356–359, 361] All involve computer-assisted detection of statistically significant pulses in the two profiles as a first step. The second step is then to identify concordant events. Generally, a temporal window of one or two sampling intervals around the peak time is allowed to count simultaneous and near-simultaneous events. The last, and perhaps the most difficult step, is to determine whether the observed concordance rates significantly exceed those which could have occurred by chance. Approaches that have been proposed and applied have involved estimations of probability levels from observed frequencies[34] and from computer simulations of hormonal profiles pulsating independently at known frequencies,[357, 361] as well as testing the observed concordance rate against the concordance rate in "mismatched" (i.e., series originating from two different subjects) or "scrambled" profiles (i.e., profiles in which the order of the pulses is deliberately modified).[356] The most recent procedures have combined combinatorial algebra with computer simulations.[358, 359] The relative merits of all these methods need further evaluation. Not surprisingly, divergent findings regarding putative temporal coupling of pulsatility in different pituitary axes (i.e., gonadotropic and lactotropic) have been reported, based on the use of different algorithms.[359, 362]

Two problems which can complicate the analysis of temporal coincidence or even invalidate the conclusions are worth mentioning. First, the two hormones under study may have different clearance kinetics and different levels of assay precision. Ideally, examination of temporal concordance should be performed on secretory rates, not peripheral levels, and take into account measurement error in each series. Second, some degree of temporal coincidence may reflect simultaneous effects of a common stimulus on two different endocrine axes. For example, meal intake can evoke significant rises of both cortisol[363, 364] and prolactin[365] levels. Any estimation of the concordance of cortisol and prolactin pulsatility would therefore need to take into account the effect of these "external" stimuli, preferably by studying the subject during a prolonged fast or during constant glucose infusion or enteral nutrition. Similarly, sleep onset exerts phase-setting effects on the pulsatility of essentially all endocrine axes and will therefore result in a certain degree of temporal coincidence (or inhibition of temporal coincidence) which will influence the estimations of overall concordance rates. Interestingly, none of the studies which have examined a putative copulsatility of LH and prolactin has taken into account the major stimulatory effect of sleep onset on pulsatile prolactin secretion.[353, 356, 357, 359, 361, 362] Thus, while analyses of temporal associations hold promises of increased understanding of the temporal organization of the endocrine system, methodological refinements are still needed to further validate this approach.

ENDOCRINE RHYTHMS IN HEALTH AND DISEASE

Diurnal and/or ultradian oscillations have been observed in essentially all endocrine systems. An exhaustive review of all such observations is not possible. The following summary of the findings will therefore be limited to the various hypothalamopituitary axes, glucose regulation, and pineal function. The reader should be aware, however, that there are also prominent rhythms in the parathyroid system, the renin-angiotensin system, and neurotransmitter concentrations and that these rhythms are likely to have important medical implications.

The Corticotropic Axis

Rhythms of ACTH and Adrenal Secretions in Normal Subjects

Among all endocrine circadian rhythms known to occur in normal humans, the 24-h periodicity of pituitary-adrenal secretion has been studied most extensively. It is endogenous in nature, largely unaffected by short-term manipulations of the sleep-wake cycle, such as abrupt changes in sleep times and total sleep deprivation, and it persists during complete fast or continuous feeding. To cause a rapid (i.e., within 3 to 5 days, as seen in Fig. 140–18) shift in the rhythm, crucially timed exposure to bright light is necessary. Transient evoked responses may affect the waveshape

of the cortisol rhythm. In particular, the first few hours of sleep have a modest inhibitory effect on cortisol secretion,[163] brief elevations of plasma levels are associated with meals,[363, 364] and stressful events such as venipuncture[34] may cause a 1- to 2-h secretory episode. Twenty-hour profiles of ACTH and cortisol typical of normal young adults are illustrated in Figure 140–20. Changes in plasma cortisol occur in parallel with those in ACTH. Their pattern shows an early morning maximum, declining levels throughout daytime, a quiescent period of minimal secretory activity centered around midnight, and an abrupt elevation during late sleep. This circadian profile is produced by modulation of the height of successive secretory pulses.[36, 39, 40] When a smooth curve is fitted to the data to estimate the parameters of the circadian rhythm (as shown in Fig. 140–3), the amplitude of the cortisol rhythm averages 75 per cent of the 24-h mean. Estimations of the amplitude of the circadian rhythm of ACTH are more variable due to the highly pulsatile nature of the pattern. In normal conditions, the acrophase of the pituitary-adrenal periodicity occurs between 6:00 and 10:00. The quiescent period typically extends from 22:00 to 2:00. With a 15-min sampling interval, 15 to 18 significant pulses of plasma ACTH and cortisol per 24-h span can be detected.[34, 202, 229]

Studies on the adaptation of the 24-h cortisol profile to abrupt shifts of the sleep-wake cycle have demonstrated that the timing of the morning acrophase, on the one hand, and the timing of the nocturnal quiescent period, on the other hand, are controlled by different mechanisms.[169] The nadir and the end of the quiescent period take longer to adjust to a change in schedule and appear to be robust markers of circadian timing. Twin studies have demonstrated that the timing of the nadir is genetically controlled[116] (see Fig. 140–9). The timing of the acrophase is more labile, and its adaptation can be accelerated by appropriately timed meal ingestion.

The 24-h rhythm of adrenal secretion is primarily dependent on the circadian pattern of ACTH release, which is amplified by a daily variation in adrenal responsiveness to ACTH. The rhythm in ACTH release results, in turn, from periodic changes in level of stimulation by corticotropin-releasing hormone (CRH). A circadian variation parallel to that of cortisol has been demonstrated for the plasma levels of adrenal steroids.[355] Figure 140–29 shows the mean 24-h profiles of cortisol, 11-hydroxyandrostenedione (11-OAD), dehydroepiandrosterone (DHEA), and androstenedione (AD) from 10 normal young men. The amplitude of the circadian variation in 11-OAD levels, a steroid derived from adrenal AD, is essentially similar to that of cortisol, whereas the amplitude of the variation in DHEA and AD levels, two steroids partially of gonadal origin, is much lower.[355] Pulses of plasma concentration of adrenal steroids occur in remarkable synchrony with bursts of cortisol secretion.

A distinct circadian rhythm of serum cortisol levels emerges at approximately 6 months of age.[366] Once this periodicity has been established, it persists throughout adulthood and has been observed through the ninth decade.[127] As shown in Figure 140–10, the overall pattern of the rhythm remains unchanged, but in older subjects, the nadir is advanced by 1 to 2 h and the amplitude is decreased.[127] In humans, the 24-h profile of cortisol appears to be similar for both sexes. In females, oral contraceptive

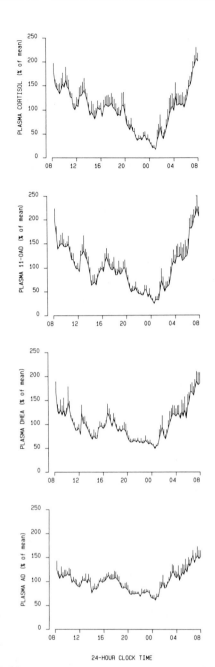

FIGURE 140–29. Mean 24-h profiles of plasma cortisol, 11-hydroxyandrostenedione (11-OAD), dehydroepiandrosterone (DHEA), and androstenedione (AD) obtained at 15-min intervals in 10 normal young men. For each subject and each hormone, the data were expressed as a percentage of the individual 24-h mean prior to calculating group values. The vertical bars at each time point represent the SEM. (Data from: Lejeune-Lenain C, Van Cauter E, Desir D, et al: Control of circadian and episodic variations of adrenal androgen secretion in man. J Endocrinol Invest 10:267–276, 1987.)

therapy results in a large increase of the mean cortisol level and of the amplitude of the rhythm resulting from an estrogen-induced elevation of transcortin-binding capacity.[367] Thus, when hypercortisolism is suspected in a female patient, it is essential to know whether the patient is under estrogen treatment. In pregnancy, total and, to a much lesser extent, free cortisol levels are elevated, but the circadian pattern of secretion persists, albeit set at a higher level.[368] Preoperative anxiety does not affect the circadian and episodic pattern of cortisol secretion, but following surgery, the mean plasma cortisol level is elevated for at least 48 h.[144]

Alterations in Disease States

The 24-h profile of pituitary-adrenal secretion remains unaltered in a wide variety of pathological states. Disease states in which alterations of the cortisol rhythm have been observed include primarily (1) disorders involving abnormalities in binding and/or metabolism of cortisol, (2) the various forms of Cushing's syndrome, and (3) affective illness (i.e., depression).

The relative amplitude of the circadian rhythm and of the episodic fluctuations of cortisol is blunted in patients with liver disease[369] and in patients with anorexia nervosa,[370] primarily because of the decreased metabolic clearance of cortisol. In contrast, in hyperthyroidism, where cortisol production and peripheral metabolism are increased, episodic pulses are enhanced.[371] In hypothyroid patients, the mean level is markedly elevated, and the relative amplitude of the rhythm is therefore dampened.[372] These alterations are thought to be due to both diminished clearance and decreased efficiency of the feedback control.

Figure 140–30 illustrates the alterations in the 24-h pattern of plasma cortisol which characterize pituitary Cushing's disease and major endogenous depression. The upper panels represent individual profiles obtained in representative subjects, whereas the lower panels show mean profiles obtained in groups of 8 to 12 subjects in each category. In patients with Cushing's syndrome secondary to adrenal adenoma or ectopic ACTH secretion, the circadian variation of plasma cortisol is invariably absent.[280] However, in pituitary-dependent Cushing's disease, a low-amplitude circadian variation may persist, suggesting that there is no defect in the neural clock generating the periodicity.[280] Cortisol pulsatility is blunted in about 70 per cent of patients with Cushing's disease, suggesting autonomous tonic secretion of ACTH by a pituitary tumor.[373] However, in about 30 per cent of these patients, the magnitude of the pulses is instead enhanced.[373] These "hyperpulsatile" patterns could be caused by enhanced hypothalamic release of CRH or persistent pituitary responsiveness to CRH.

Hypercortisolism with persistent circadian rhythmicity and increased pulsatility is found in a majority of acutely depressed patients.[229, 374–377] In these patients, who do not develop the clinical signs of Cushing's syndrome despite the high circulating cortisol levels, the quiescent period of cortisol secretion often occurs earlier than in normal subjects of comparable age (compare in Fig. 140–37 the positions of the nadir in normal subjects around 1:00 and in depressed patients around 21:00). As discussed earlier, this phase advance could reflect a decrease in the endogenous period of the circadian pacemaker. Interestingly, similar alterations of the cortisol rhythm are observed in the manic state[378] and in alcoholic subjects during acute abstinence.[379] When a clinical remission of the depressed state is obtained, the hypercortisolism and the abnormal timing of the quiescent period disappear, indicating that these disturbances are "state" rather than "trait" dependent.[230] Similarly, alterations associated with acute alcohol withdrawal are also reversed by sustained abstinence.[379] Abnormalities in the circadian regulation of cortisol appear to be somewhat specific to the depressed state, since normal profiles are observed in schizophrenics.[380]

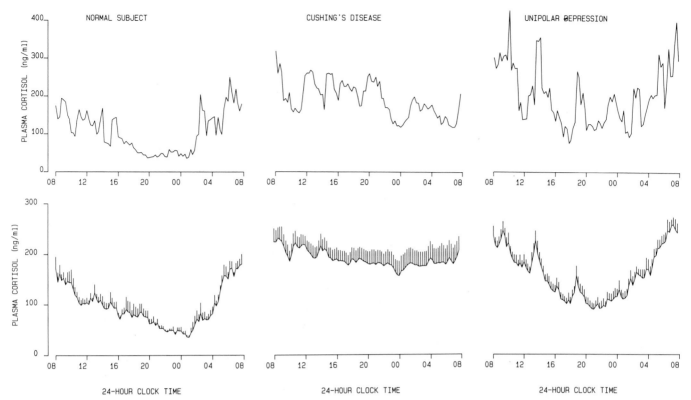

FIGURE 140–30. The 24-h profiles of plasma cortisol in normal subjects (*left*), patients with pituitary Cushing's disease (*middle*), and patients with major endogenous depression of the unipolar subtype (*right*). For each condition, a representative example is shown in the top panel, and mean profiles from 8 to 10 subjects are shown in the lower panel. In the lower panels, the vertical bars at each time point represent the SEM. (From Van Cauter E: Physiology and pathology of circadian rhythms. *In* Edwards CW, Lincoln DW (eds): Recent Advances in Endocrinology and Metabolism. Edinburgh, Churchill Livingstone, 1989, pp 109–134.)

The Somatotropic Axis

The 24-Hour Profile of GH in Normal Subjects

In normal adult subjects, the 24-h profile of plasma GH levels consists of stable low levels abruptly interrupted by bursts of secretion. The most reproducible pulse occurs shortly after sleep onset, in association with the first phase of SW sleep. Other pulses may occur in later sleep and during wakefulness, in the absence of any identifiable stimulus. In men, the sleep-onset GH pulse is generally the largest and often the only pulse observed over the 24-h span. Typical examples are shown in Figures 140–1, 140–10, and 140–17. In women, daytime GH pulses are more frequent, and the sleep-associated pulse, while still present in most cases, does not generally account for the majority of the 24-h GH release. Circulating estradiol concentrations play an important role in determining overall levels of spontaneous GH secretion.[381] The recent development of ultrasensitive GH assays will permit a more detailed definition of the physiological pattern of human GH release in the near future and may demonstrate that in humans as well as in other mammals there is an endogenous ultradian rhythm of GH release which is modulated by the circadian sleep-wake cycle.

Sleep onset will elicit a pulse in GH secretion whether sleep is advanced, delayed, interrupted, or fragmented. Delta wave electroencephalographic activity consistently precedes the elevation in plasma GH levels. A study using blood sampling at 30-sec intervals during sleep has shown that maximal GH release occurs within minutes of the onset of SW sleep.[383] The analysis of the relationship between sleep stages and GH release is more accurate when GH secretory rates, rather than peripheral concentrations, are examined. This is exemplified in Figure 140–31, where the association between pulsatile GH secretion and sleep stages is studied in a single subject.[35, 37, 344] The profile shown on the top represents the plasma levels of GH measured at 15-min intervals. Three pulses of plasma concentration were found significant using a computerized pulse-detection algorithm (Ultra[329]). The corresponding profile of GH secretory rates calculated by deconvolution is shown in the second profile from the top. These secretory rates were derived from the plasma levels using a single compartment model for GH disappearance with a half-life of 19 minutes and a volume of distribution of 7 per cent of body weight. Pulse analysis of the secretory rates now reveals the occurrence of three additional pulses of GH secretion. The three lower profiles illustrate the percentages of each 15-min interval between blood samplings spent in stages wake, slow-wave (SW: III + IV), and REM, respectively. When the profile of plasma concentration is compared with the SW profile, it appears that subsequent to its initiation in concomitance with the beginning of the first SW period, the sleep-onset GH pulse spanned the first 3 h of sleep, without apparent modulation by the succession of non-REM and REM stages. However, the profile of secretory rates clearly reveals that GH was preferentially secreted

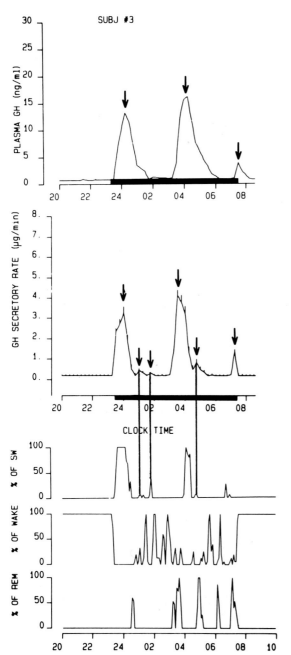

FIGURE 140–31. Temporal profile of plasma GH (*top*) sampled at 15-min intervals in a normal man. The black bar indicates the period of polygraphically recorded sleep. The second panel from the top shows the profile of GH secretory rates derived by deconvolution from the profile of peripheral concentrations. Significant pulses of plasma levels and secretory rates are indicated by arrows. The three lower panels represent the temporal distribution of SW stages (III + IV), wake, and REM during sleep. Vertical lines indicate the temporal association between pulses of GH secretion evidenced by deconvolution and SW stages. (From Van Cauter E: Computer-assisted analysis of endocrine rhythms. *In* Rodbard D, Forti G (eds): Computers in Endocrinology. New York, Raven Press, 1990, pp 59–70.)

during SW stage, with interruptions of secretory activity coinciding with the intervening REM or wake stages. Thus deconvolution provided a closer association between SW stages and active GH secretion than the analysis of plasma concentration because the temporal limits of each pulse were more accurately defined and additional pulses were revealed.[37] Based on a pulse-by-pulse analysis of nocturnal

profiles of GH secretory rates, we have recently shown that approximately 70 per cent of GH pulses during sleep are correlated with SW stages and that the amount of GH secreted in SW-associated pulses is correlated with the amount of SW occurring during the pulse.[37] While SW sleep is clearly a major determinant of the 24-h profile of GH secretion in humans, there is also evidence for the existence of a circadian modulation.[169] In a recent study where the nocturnal profile of GH was observed following a 5-h delay of bedtimes in normal young men, a GH pulse occurred during wakefulness within 1 h of the usual bedtime in 12 of 16 nights. It is likely that the use of ultrasensitive GH assays will further reveal the existence of a sleep-independent circadian rhythm of GH release.

Various studies have indicated that sleep-related GH release is partially regulated by GRF stimulation. In addition, effects of GRF on sleep have been demonstrated, and it has been suggested that GH secretion and sleep may share common regulatory mechanisms.[384] Intracerebroventricular injections of GRF in rats and rabbits increase both REM and non-REM sleep.[385, 386] Inhibition of endogenous GRF, either by administration of a competitive antagonist or by immunoneutralization, inhibits sleep.[384] While intravenous administration of synthetic GRF during the daytime does not modify sleep in normal young men,[387] we and others have recently shown that administration of GRF during sleep may decrease the amount of wake and increase the amount of SW sleep.[388] Whether or not GRF can cross the blood-brain barrier is a matter of controversy. The somnogenic effects of GRF could be mediated by GH. This hypothesis is not supported by the finding of a significant decrease in stage 3 sleep following GH therapy in GH-deficient children.[389] Furthermore, injections of pharmacological doses of GH in normal subjects have been reported to increase REM rather than SW sleep.[390] In support of the link between activity of the somatotropic axis and sleep regulation are the observations that subjects with congenital isolated GH deficiency have a significant decrease in power of delta sleep as compared with normal controls.[391] Furthermore, REM and delta sleep energy are elevated in acromegalic patients and return to normal following successful adenomectomy.[392] The association of elevated levels of GH secretion with an increased need for sleep in adolescents is also consistent with a functional relationship between GH secretion and sleep. Short stature and poor weight gain have been described in children with obstructive sleep apnea, and therapeutic tracheostomy may lead to a sustained increase in growth rate.[393]

The total amount and the temporal distribution of GH release is strongly dependent on age. Spontaneous GH secretion is detectable in term infants, who appear to have a high level of tonic secretion.[394] As the infant matures, GH pulse frequency and pulse amplitude decrease, and tonic secretion diminishes.[394] A pulsatile pattern of GH release, with increased pulse amplitude during sleep, is present in prepubertal boys and girls.[395] During puberty, the amplitude of the pulses, but not the frequency, is increased, particularly at night.[396, 397] Maximal overall GH concentrations are reached in early puberty in girls and in late puberty in boys.[397] Age-related decreases in GH secretion have been well documented in both men and women.[127, 381, 398–400] As illustrated in Figure 140–10, in healthy elderly men aged 67 to 84 years, the total amount of GH secreted over the 24-h span averaged one third of the daily output of young men aged 20 to 27 years.[127] Similarly, the amount of SW sleep in the elderly was reduced threefold as compared with the young. Studies using standard GH assays have indicated that this decline in overall GH secretion appears to be achieved primarily by a decrease in amplitude rather than frequency of GH pulses. Since in adult subjects the sleep-onset GH pulse often constitutes the major secretory output, age-related decrements in GH secretion are particularly prominent at that time of day. Although early studies had generally concluded that sleep-related GH pulses were absent in the elderly, the findings of more recent studies are concordant in showing persistent but reduced GH secretion during sleep.[127, 381, 400]

Basal GH secretion as well as responsiveness are higher in premenopausal women than in age-matched men.[381, 401] Well-documented studies have demonstrated that the daily GH output as well as the magnitude of the GH response to GRF stimulation in women is correlated with the circulating level of estradiol.[381, 401] In old age, these sex differences are abolished.

Alterations in Disease States

Abnormalities in the 24-h profile of plasma GH have been reported in a variety of metabolic, endocrine, neurological, and psychiatric conditions. We will briefly describe the major alterations found in those conditions for which the temporal pattern has been defined in detail. Chapters 19 and 20 provide clinical descriptions of the various conditions of hypo- and hypersomatotropism.

There is an inverse relationship between adiposity and GH release which results in a marked suppression of GH levels throughout the 24-h span in obese subjects. A reduction in pulse frequency as well as a decrease in GH half-life has been suggested to underlie the hyposomatotropism of obesity.[402] A normal pattern can be restored after prolonged fasting.[403] In normal-weight subjects, fasting, even for only 1 day, enhances GH secretion via an increase in both pulse amplitude and pulse frequency.[404, 405] Nonobese juvenile or maturity-onset diabetics hypersecrete GH during wakefulness as well as during sleep, primarily because of an increase in amplitude of pulses.[406] This abnormality may disappear when glycemia is strictly controlled.

In acromegaly, GH is hypersecreted throughout the 24-h span, with a pulsatile pattern superimposed on elevated basal levels, indicative of the presence of tonic secretion.[407–409] Some studies,[407, 409] but not others,[408] have observed the persistence of elevated levels during sleep. After transsphenoidal surgery, a normal circadian pattern of GH release can be restored.[409, 410] In contrast, bromocriptine therapy lowers the overall GH secretion but does not lead to the resumption of normal 24-h profiles.[410] Diurnal and nocturnal episodes of GH secretion are more frequent and of higher amplitude in adult subjects with hyperthyroidism, who have an overall daily GH production rate fourfold above normal.[411] Patients with major endogenous depression, especially those suffering from unipolar illness, have an increased number of GH pulses during the daytime.[228] The early sleep GH peak is generally absent in these patients, who frequently have a burst of GH release before, rather than after, sleep onset (exemplified in Fig. 140–17).

The Lactotropic Axis

The 24-Hour Profile of Prolactin in Normal Subjects

Under normal conditions, the 24-h profile of prolactin levels follows a bimodal pattern, with minimal concentrations around noon, an afternoon phase of slightly augmented secretion, and a major nocturnal elevation starting shortly after sleep onset and culminating around midsleep. Examples have been shown in Figures 140–1, 140–10, 140–15, and 140–17. In men, the range of the variation corresponds to an average increase of more than 250 per cent above the minimum noon level. Pulses occur during daytime as well as during the night.[353, 412] Their number appears to be a reproducible individual characteristic, ranging between 7 and 22 per 24-h span.[412] Deconvolution analysis has indicated that the prolactin profile reflects both tonic and intermittent release.[243] Food intake, especially at lunch time, may trigger an elevation of plasma prolactin levels.[365]

Studies of prolactin levels during daytime naps or after shifts of the normal sleep period have consistently demonstrated increased prolactin secretion associated with sleep onset.[169] Based on pharmacological studies, dopaminergic as well as serotoninergic mechanisms seem to be implicated in this sleep-related elevation of secretion. While early reports described the 24-h rhythm of plasma prolactin as "entirely dependent on sleep," the existence of a circadian component in the secretory pattern of prolactin is now well recognized. Studies involving abrupt shifts of the sleep-wake cycle during real or simulated jet lag have indeed revealed the existence of a sleep-independent secretory rise.[169, 178, 413] Under normal conditions, this circadian rise is synchronized with the early part of sleep, and both circadian and sleep effects are superimposed. This circadian component is apparent in the profiles of plasma prolactin observed during adaptation to an 8-h delay of the sleep-wake and LD cycles[178] shown in Figure 140–15. On day 1 after the shift, an elevation of prolactin occurred immediately after sleep onset but was not maintained throughout the night, and an "anamnestic" elevation was observed around the time of usual sleep onset before the shift (i.e., 23:00). A recent study[315] involving prolonged exposure to long nights (i.e., 14 h of recumbency in total darkness) has shown that prolactin levels rise shortly after lights off, even though the subjects are still awake (data shown in Fig. 140–30), further confirming that the nocturnal rise is not solely sleep-dependent.

As indicated earlier in the section entitled Modulation of Pulsatility, a number of studies have examined the relationship between sleep stages, i.e., the alteration of REM and non-REM stages, and pulsatile variations of prolactin. No clear relationship has so far emerged. However, prolonged awakenings interrupting sleep are often associated with decreasing prolactin concentrations, suggesting that fragmented sleep may result in lower nocturnal prolactin levels. This is indeed what is observed in elderly subjects,[127] who have an increased number of awakenings and decreased amounts of non-REM stages and in whom a dampening of the nocturnal rise is evident (see Fig. 140–10). This diminished nocturnal rise in aging is associated with a decrease in the amplitude of the secretory pulses.[260] Benzodiazepine hypnotics taken at bedtime may cause an increase in the prolactin rise, resulting transiently in concentrations in the pathological range.[414] Current data indicate that the day-night difference in prolactin levels is present in newborns and persists into the ninth decade. During pregnancy, serum prolactin levels rise, but the 24-h pattern of secretion is maintained, albeit at a higher level.[415] The nocturnal rise is also maintained throughout the postpartum period.[416]

Alterations in Disease States

Absence or blunting of the nocturnal increase of plasma prolactin has been reported in a variety of pathological states, including uremia and breast cancer in postmenopausal women. In Cushing's disease, prolactin levels are elevated throughout the nycthemere, and the relative amplitude of the nighttime rise is reduced.[417] In subjects with insulin-dependent diabetes, the circadian and sleep modulation of prolactin secretion is preserved, but overall levels are markedly diminished.[418]

In hyperprolactinemia associated with prolactinomas, the nocturnal elevation of prolactin is preserved in patients with microadenomas but altered in patients with macroadenomas.[419, 420] The persistence of a normal nocturnal profile in subjects with microadenomas suggests that there is no defect in the CNS mechanism governing the temporal program of prolactin release. This hypothesis is further supported by the fact that selective removal of prolactin-secreting adenomas can result in the normalization of the prolactin pattern.

Abnormal prolactin profiles also have been reported in a variety of neurological and psychiatric disorders. In narcoleptic patients, the nocturnal rise is blunted rather than abolished.[421] It is conceivable that this blunting reflects the persistence of a circadian rise without normal sleep-related elevation. Circadian rhythmicity is indeed preserved in these patients who have normal cortisol profiles.[421] In some patients with endogenous depression, a surge of prolactin levels occurs before sleep onset.[231, 422] An example is shown in Figure 140–17. This early timing of the nocturnal prolactin rise may characterize a subset of depressed patients for whom the illness may involve a disorder of time keeping with a phase advance of various circadian rhythms. In drug-free schizophrenic patients, the nighttime rise of prolactin is markedly enhanced.[380]

The Gonadotropic Axis

The 24-Hour Profiles of LH, FSH, and Sex Steroids in Normal Subjects

Rhythms in the gonadotropic axis cover a wide range of frequencies, from ultrafast oscillations of plasma LH levels recurring at intervals of a few minutes, to episodic release in the circhoral range, to diurnal rhythmicity, and finally, to monthly and seasonal cycles. These various rhythms interact to provide a coordinated temporal program governing the development of the reproductive axis and its operation at every stage of maturation. In the early seventies, the finding that changes in the diurnal and episodic pat-

terns of LH and FSH release were associated with various stages of sexual maturation provided the first demonstration of the physiological significance of the temporal organization of endocrine secretions.[423] It is therefore not surprising that the modulation and the interactions of ultradian, circadian, and infradian rhythms have been studied more extensively in the gonadotropic axis than in other endocrine systems. The following description of the current state of knowledge in this area will be centered on 24-h rhythms and their interaction with pulsatile release at the various stages of maturation of the reproductive system.

Prior to puberty, LH levels are very low, and findings regarding the temporal pattern of release have been somewhat divergent, depending on the nature of the assay procedure, i.e., RIA methods, monoclonal antibody-based immunoradiometric assay (IRMA) methods, and ultrasensitive time-resolved immunofluorometric methods. The most recent studies generally agree in indicating that both LH and FSH are secreted in a pulsatile pattern and that an augmentation of pulsatile activity is associated with sleep onset in a majority of both girls and boys.[424–427] Some studies have found an increase in both frequency and amplitude of pulses during the late prepubertal stages.[425–427] In pubertal children, the magnitude of the nocturnal pulses of LH and FSH is consistently increased during sleep. As the pubescent child enters adulthood, the daytime pulse amplitude increases as well, eliminating or diminishing the diurnal rhythm. Based on an early study showing that during reversal of the sleep-wake cycle of pubertal boys LH augmentation occurred during the daytime sleep period, the nocturnal increase in overall LH levels during puberty has been attributed primarily to some state-dependent change occurring during sleep rather than to a circadian effect[38] (Fig. 140–32). However, as is evident in Figure 140–32, although LH secretion increased during the daytime sleep period, there also was an elevation in LH concentrations at the time when sleep occurred under basal conditions, indicating the presence of an inherent circadian component. In pubertal girls, a diurnal variation of circulating estradiol levels, with higher concentrations during the daytime instead of the nighttime, appears.[423] It has been suggested that the lack of parallelism between gonadotropin and estradiol levels reflects an approximate 10-h delay between gonadotropin stimulation and the subsequent ovarian response. In pubertal boys, the nocturnal rise of testosterone coincides with the elevation of gonadotropins.[423] Interestingly, a recent study in hypogonadal men reported that the diurnal LH rhythm characteristic of pubertal boys is observed in adult men with hyperprolactinemia and gonadotropin insufficiency.[428]

Patterns of LH release in adult men exhibit large interindividual variability.[429] The diurnal variation is dampened and may become undetectable. A number of studies, however, have observed modest elevations of nocturnal LH, and possibly FSH, levels in young adult men,[243, 429, 430] and a recent report noted a sleep-associated augmentation with a coupling of LH pulses to the REM–non-REM cycle.[431] A marked diurnal rhythm in circulating testosterone levels in young adults, with minimal levels in the late evening and maximal levels in the early morning, has been well demonstrated and has been illustrated in Figure 140–19.[232, 355, 429, 432] In young male adults, the amplitude of the circadian variation averages 25 per cent of the 24-h mean.[355] With a

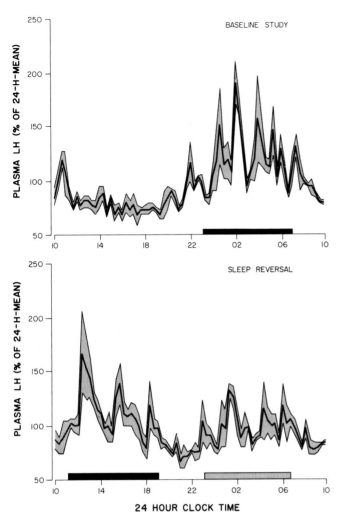

FIGURE 140–32. Mean 24-h plasma LH profiles in pubertal boys studied during a normal sleep-wake cycle (*top panel*) and after a reversal of the sleep-wake cycle (*bottom panel*). The shaded area represents one SEM above and below the mean. Sleep periods are indicated by black bars. The nocturnal period of sleep deprivation is indicated by a gray bar. Note that there is an augmentation of LH during sleep under both conditions. However, following reversal of the sleep-wake cycle, there is a significant augmentation of LH release during the nocturnal wake period that is unrelated to sleep. (Data from: Kapen S, Boyar RM, Finkelstein JW, et al: Effect of sleep-wake cycle reversal on luteinizing hormone pattern in puberty. J Clin Endocrinol Metab 39:293–299, 1974, copyright ©, The Endocrine Society.)

15-min sampling interval, 17 to 18 testosterone pulses per 24-h span can be detected.[355] Since, as mentioned above, 24-h LH patterns in normal men are very variable and the nocturnal increase in peripheral LH concentrations is relatively inconsistent and of modest magnitude, the robust circadian rhythm of plasma testosterone may be partially controlled by other factors such as sleep-associated variations in testicular blood flow, diurnal changes in Leydig cell response to LH, and/or circadian fluctuations in other hormones. In this respect, the remarkable parallelism between the prolonged decline of cortisol and testosterone concentrations during daytime hours and the temporal coincidence of the morning maximum deserves further examination. An earlier study has indicated that as is the case for cortisol, nighttime elevations in testosterone levels in adult men appear to be driven by a circadian clock and are

not simply a response to sleep or any stage of sleep.[432] In one study, the morning maximum of testosterone was found to be paralleled by peak inhibin levels,[433] but in another, the daily maximum of inhibin levels occurred more than 7 h later than the testosterone acrophase.[434] These contradicting findings probably reflect the known difficulties in measuring accurately peripheral inhibin levels in normal subjects.

In older men, the frequency of LH release has been variably described as unchanged,[430] increased,[435] or decreased.[436] These discrepancies may be due to differences in methods of analysis, particularly in the detection of small-amplitude pulses. Findings have been more concordant in describing an age-related decrease in pulse amplitude.[435, 436] No significant diurnal pattern can be detected.[430] However, the testosterone rhythm persists, although markedly dampened.[232, 430]

In adult women, the 24-h variation in plasma LH is markedly modulated by the menstrual cycle.[42, 437] In the early follicular phase (EFP), LH pulses are large and infrequent, and a slowing of the frequency of secretory pulses occurs during sleep. In the midfollicular phase (MFP), pulse amplitude is decreased, pulse frequency increased, and the frequency modulation of LH pulsatility by sleep is less apparent. Pulse amplitude increases again by the late follicular phase (LFP). No modulation by sleep is apparent until the early luteal phase, when nocturnal slowing of pulsatility is again evident. During the luteal-follicular transition, there is a four- to fivefold increase in LH pulse frequency, which accompanies the selective FSH rise necessary for normal folliculogenesis.[438] The apparent inhibitory effect of sleep during the EFP is particularly intriguing, since this effect is in the opposite direction from that observed in pubertal girls, in whom the sleep period is associated with an increase in LH pulse amplitude and an elevation of overall LH levels. The findings have been quite consistent across laboratories,[41, 42, 281, 282] as illustrated in Figure 140–22. Toward menopause, gonadotropin levels are elevated but show no consistent circadian pattern.[423]

An interaction between the menstrual cycle and circadian rhythmicity is involved in the timing of the preovulatory LH surge. In normal women, the onset of the LH surge occurs most often in late sleep or early morning.[48, 49] Moreover, a seasonal variation of this circadian timing has been reported, consisting of the appearance of a biphasic pattern of occurrence in spring only.[49]

Alterations in Disease States

The therapeutic implications of the pulsatile nature of GnRH secretion were rapidly recognized, and treatments with specific temporal patterns of hormone administration were developed.[274] As reviewed by Conn and Crowley,[274] the pulsatile administration of GnRH is an effective treatment of hypothalamic amenorrhea, idiopathic hypogonadotropic hypogonadism, and other conditions characterized by an insufficient production of endogenous GnRH. Conversely, the therapeutic use of pituitary desensitization with long-acting GnRH agonists has been recommended for the treatment of precocious puberty and offers promise for prostatic cancer, uterine fibroids, endometriosis, and polycystic ovary syndrome. Abnormal ultradian and/or circadian hormonal profiles have been found in a number of reproductive disorders. While a description of all these conditions is outside of the scope of this chapter, we will briefly review the findings pertaining to disorders of female and male reproduction in which an abnormal function of the hypothalamic pulse generator and/or its modulation by diurnal rhythmicity seem to be primarily involved.

Early studies on the 24-h profile of plasma LH in anorexia nervosa have established the importance of an adequate temporal secretory program in the maintenance of normal reproductive function, indicating that in women with amenorrhea secondary to anorexia nervosa, the secretory pattern of LH regresses to the pubertal or prepubertal pattern, with low daytime pulsatility and increased secretion at night.[47] More recent studies have confirmed that pulsatile release during the daytime is still present, but with an increased frequency and a decreased amplitude.[439] Following weight gain and clinical remission, normal secretory profiles of LH are usually observed. Twenty-four-hour profiles of plasma LH and FSH with augmented nocturnal release characteristic of pubertal subjects also may occur in various forms of sexual precocity.[47]

The slowing or absence of pulsatile hypothalamic GnRH release is the underlying cause of ovarian acyclicity in women with functional hypothalamic amenorrhea (FHA).[47, 440] The reduction appears more marked during the daytime than during sleep, suggesting that the mechanisms involved in this pathological suppression of pulsatile GnRH release are partially inhibited during sleep.[440] It appears that the 24-h secretory patterns of LH, FSH, cortisol, GH, and prolactin are all altered in women with FHA. Women afflicted with FHA show a 53 per cent reduction in LH pulse frequency and an increase in the LH pulse interval, while the integrated plasma LH and FSH concentrations are reduced by 30 per cent.[441] Replacement of pulsatile GnRH by intravenous administration via a pump is maximally efficient, with achievement of ovulation in essentially all subjects when the frequency of pulses is one per hour.[442] However, if the frequency of exogenous pulsatile administration is reduced to one pulse every 2 h, the midcycle gonadotropin surge is blunted, FSH levels do not increase, and a reduced rate of ovulation is obtained.[442] Decreased LH pulse frequency and amplitude also may be observed in women runners who are normally menstruating,[443] suggesting that exercise-associated amenorrhea is a further development of the alterations in the pattern of GnRH activity seen in eumenorrheic women runners. Similar defects in pulse amplitude and frequency are seen in women with pseudocyesis.[444]

Different forms of abnormal temporal organization of the GnRH signal seem involved in the polycystic ovary syndrome (PCO). In an early study in pubertal girls with recent-onset PCO,[445] the circadian rhythm of LH secretion was found to be out of phase with the sleep-wake cycle so that in normal pubertal children LH increased during the night, whereas in PCO patients the LH augmentation occurred during the day. The authors speculate that the abnormal circadian timing of the LH rhythm during puberty in PCO patients might not allow normal ovulatory cycles to develop. More recent studies in adult patients have concurred in indicating an increase in pulse amplitude in PCO.[446, 447] In one study employing 10-min sampling throughout the 24-h cycle,[447] the frequency of pulses also was clearly increased, and overall levels of FSH were de-

pressed, suggesting that the excessively rapid GnRH pulsations selectively suppressed FSH secretion, as has been shown to occur in animal models.[240] A similar defect of abnormally high GnRH frequency seems to underlie luteal phase deficiency. Indeed, in a series of studies (reviewed in ref. 448), Soules and coworkers have shown that LH pulse frequency is increased during the follicular phase and have provided evidence indicating that this temporal alteration is implicated in the etiology of the condition.

Increased LH pulse frequency and decreased pulse amplitude also have been observed in patients suffering from the premenstrual syndrome (PMS), and these findings have suggested the possible involvement of opioidergic dysfunction in this condition.[449] Alterations in circadian rhythmicity, consisting of advances in circadian rhythms relative to the timing of the sleep-wake cycle, as well as reduced melatonin levels, also have been found in PMS patients.[450] These abnormalities may contribute to pathologies associated with PMS, and correcting such circadian disturbances may lead to clinical remission.[450] Patients with late luteal phase dysphoric disorders have abnormally phase-advanced rhythms, and exposure to bright light in the evening but not in the morning was effective in inducing a significant reduction in the depression score.[450] Since evening bright light can cause phase delays of circadian rhythms, these results raise the possibility that circadian dysregulation, whether induced by lifestyle, the environment, or the reproductive system itself, may be a common pathogenetic factor in mood disorders observed in women.[450]

In the majority of men with idiopathic hypogonadotropic hypogonadism, LH pulses are undetectable.[426, 451] Puberty may be induced by pulsatile GnRH administration.[274] In a small number of patients, an early pubertal pattern with enhanced pulse amplitude during the nighttime may be observed.[451] States of hyperprolactinemia are also associated with suppression of LH pulse amplitude and frequency.[452] Studies in women indicate that these defects may be reversed by treatment, whether pharmacological[453] or surgical.[454]

The Thyrotropic Axis

The 24-Hour Profile of TSH in Normal Subjects

In normal adult men and women, TSH levels are low throughout the daytime and begin to increase in the late afternoon or early evening. Maximal levels occur shortly before sleep.[164, 455, 456] During sleep, TSH levels generally decline slowly. A sharp decrease occurs in the morning hours. Representative profiles have been shown in Figures 140–1, 140–10, and 140–14. Studies involving sleep deprivation and shifts of the sleep-wake cycle have consistently indicated that an inhibitory influence is exerted on TSH secretion during sleep.[164, 165] The pronounced enhancing effect of sleep deprivation on the nighttime TSH rise is illustrated in Figure 140–26. The timing of the evening rise seems to be controlled by circadian rhythmicity. The temporal pattern of TSH secretion seems to reflect both tonic and pulsatile release, with both the frequency and the amplitude of the pulses increasing during the nighttime.[243, 456, 457] Pulses of TSH secretion persist under both somatostatin and dopamine treatment, suggesting that the control of pulsatility is largely TRH-dependent.[262] When the depth of sleep is increased by prior sleep deprivation, the nocturnal TSH rise is markedly decreased, suggesting that SW sleep is probably the primary determinant of the sleep-associated fall.[456] Indeed, an analysis of TSH profiles and sleep stages has revealed a consistent association between descending slopes of TSH and SW stages.[458]

Because T_3 and T_4 are largely bound to serum protein, the existence of a circadian variation of thyroid hormone secretion, independent of the diurnal variation in hemodilution caused by postural changes, has been difficult to establish. Studies measuring free T_3 or the ratio T_3/T_4 have shown, however, that changes in thyroid hormone secretion occur in parallel with those of plasma TSH, but the amplitude of this rhythm is very modest, averaging less than 10 per cent (reviewed in ref. 162). However, under conditions of sleep deprivation, the increased amplitude of the TSH rhythm results in an increased amplitude of the T_3 rhythm, which becomes clearly apparent. This is illustrated in Figure 140–33, where the patterns of plasma TSH and T_3 in a normal young man are observed at 20-min intervals during a 32-h period of sleep deprivation, followed by recovery sleep. There is a remarkable parallelism between the nocturnal rise of TSH and T_3 on the first night. Presumably because of the prolonged half-life of the hormone, T_3 levels do not return to baseline in the morning, probably limiting the subsequent TSH rise at the beginning of the next nighttime period. However, both TSH and T_3 decline abruptly after the onset of recovery sleep.

The diurnal rhythmicity of plasma TSH levels is not apparent until the second month of life[459] but then seems to remain stable throughout childhood, without notable changes at the time of puberty.[460] There do not seem to be consistent sex differences in the diurnal pattern, whether in childhood or adulthood. In elderly men, there is an overall decrease of TSH levels (see Fig. 140–12), but the rhythm persists, albeit slightly dampened and with an earlier evening rise than in younger adults.[125] Fasting decreases overall TSH levels by decreasing pulse amplitude, resulting in a dampening of the nocturnal surge.[461] Thyroxine concentrations remain unchanged.[461]

Alterations in Disease States

Decreased or absent nocturnal rise of TSH has been observed in a variety of nonthyroidal illnesses,[462] therefore suggesting that hypothalamic dysregulation will generally affect the circadian TSH surge. This is in contrast to the circadian variation of plasma cortisol, which persists in a wide variety of disease states. The nocturnal TSH surge is diminished or absent in hyperthyroidism, central hypothyroidism,[463, 464] and conditions of hypercortisolism,[465, 466] whether associated with pituitary and nonpituitary Cushing's syndrome, with surgical stress, or with a depressive state.[467] In poorly controlled diabetic states, whether insulin-dependent or non–insulin-dependent, the surge also disappears.[468] Correction of hyperglycemia is associated with a reappearance of the nocturnal elevation.[468] Interestingly, morning TSH values in the hyperglycemic patients do not differ from those of control subjects, and the TSH response to TRH is only marginally reduced.[468] The lack of

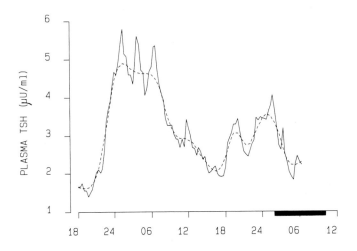

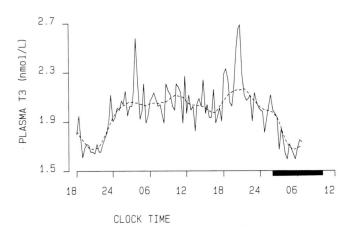

FIGURE 140–33. Temporal profiles of plasma levels of TSH (*top*) and T_3 (*bottom*) observed in a single male subject studied during a 38-h period including 32 h of sleep deprivation. Blood was sampled at 20-min intervals. The black bar represents the period of recovery sleep. The dashed line represents a best-fit curve obtained by a regression procedure. (Unpublished observations from E Van Cauter, O Van Reeth, MM Byrne, JD Blackman, J Sturis, and S Refetoff.)

normal nocturnal elevation of TSH levels appears also to be a sensitive index of preclinical hyperthyroidism.[469]

Glucose Tolerance and Insulin Secretion

Diurnal and Ultradian Variations in Normal Subjects

In normal humans, glucose tolerance varies with the time of day. Plasma glucose responses to oral glucose, intravenous glucose, or meals are markedly higher in the evening than in the morning.[364, 470–472] Figure 140–34 shows the mean 24-h profiles of glucose and insulin secretion from normal subjects who received identical meals at 8:00, 14:00, and 20:00, i.e., at 6-h intervals. The glucose response, as quantified by the area under the curve, was approximately twofold larger in the evening than in the morning, and the insulin secretory response was almost 50

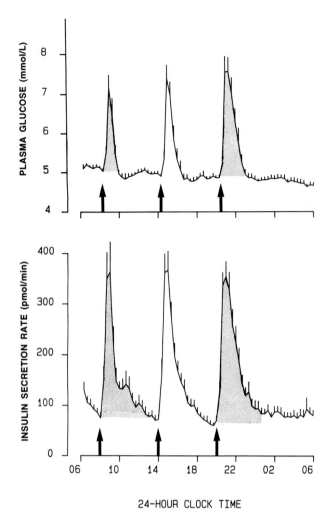

FIGURE 140–34. Mean 24-h profile of plasma glucose (*top*) and insulin secretion rates (*bottom*) observed in 8 normal subjects who received three identical meals at 8:00, 14:00, and 20:00 (indicated by *arrows*). The vertical lines at each time point represent the SEM. Note the morning versus evening difference in duration of the meal response, as estimated by the area under the curve during the first 4 h following the meal (shown as a *shaded area*). Peak glucose levels after the evening meal were significantly higher than after the morning meal. (Adapted from Van Cauter E, Shapiro ET, Tillil H, Polonsky KS: Circadian modulation of glucose and insulin responses to meals: Relationship to cortisol rhythm. Am J Physiol 262:E467–E475, 1992.)

per cent larger in the evening.[364] Diminished insulin sensitivity and decreased insulin secretion in relation to elevated glucose levels are both involved in causing reduced glucose tolerance later in the day.[471, 473, 474] Using experimental protocols involving intravenous glucose infusion at a constant rate for 24 to 30 h, it has been shown that glucose tolerance further deteriorates as the evening progresses, reaching a minimum around the middle of the night.[360, 475] This diurnal variation is not caused by changes in activity level, since it persists during continuous bed rest.[360] A mean profile of plasma glucose in recumbent fasted subjects receiving a constant glucose infusion is shown in Figure 140–35. Since glucose concentrations begin to increase in the late afternoon or early evening, well before bedtime, and continue to rise until approximately the middle of the night, both sleep-independent effects, reflecting circadian rhythmicity, and sleep-dependent effects could be involved in

producing this overall 24-h pattern. To differentiate between the effects of circadian rhythmicity and those of sleep, an experimental protocol involving a 12-h delay of the sleep period has been used to allow the effects of time of day to be observed in the absence of sleep and the effects of sleep to be observed at an abnormal circadian time.[476] Glucose was infused at a constant rate throughout the study. Figure 140–36 shows representative profiles of plasma glucose, insulin secretion rate, serum insulin levels, plasma cortisol levels, and plasma GH levels during the 53-h study period, which included 8 h of nocturnal sleep, 28 h of continuous wakefulness, and 8 h of daytime sleep. During nocturnal sleep, levels of glucose and insulin secretion increased by approximately 30 and 60 per cent, respectively, and returned to baseline in the morning. During sleep deprivation, glucose levels and insulin secretion rose again to reach a maximum at a time corresponding to the beginning of the habitual sleep period, indicating the existence of an intrinsic circadian modulation of glucose regulation. The magnitude of the rise above morning levels was less than during nocturnal sleep. Serum insulin levels did not parallel the circadian variation in insulin secretion, suggesting the existence of a nighttime increase in insulin clearance. Daytime sleep was associated with marked elevations of glucose levels, insulin secretion, and serum insulin,[476] indicating that the sleep condition per se, irrespective of the time of day when sleep does occur, exerts modulatory influences on glucose regulation. Examination of correlations with the variations of the counterregulatory hormones cortisol and GH indicated that the diurnal variation in insulin secretion was inversely related to the cortisol rhythm, with a significant correlation of the magnitudes of their morning to evening excursions. Sleep-associated rises in glucose correlated with the amount of concomitant GH secreted. These studies show that glucose regulation is markedly influenced by circadian rhythmicity and sleep and suggest that these effects could be partially mediated by cortisol and GH.

Rhythms in insulin secretion also have been found outside the circadian range. A number of studies have indeed demonstrated that human insulin secretion is a complex

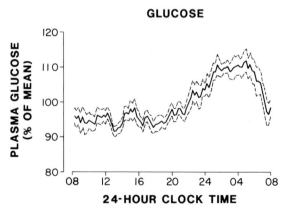

GLUCOSE

FIGURE 140–35. Mean (± SEM) blood glucose levels from 14 normal subjects studied during constant glucose infusion. For each subject, glucose levels were expressed as a percentage of the individual 24-h mean prior to group averaging. (Data from: Van Cauter E, Desir D, Decoster C, et al: Nocturnal decrease of glucose tolerance during constant glucose infusion. J Clin Endocrinol Metab 69:604–611, 1989. Adapted from Van Cauter E: Diurnal and ultradian rhythms in human endocrine function: A mini-review. Horm Res 34:45–53, 1990.)

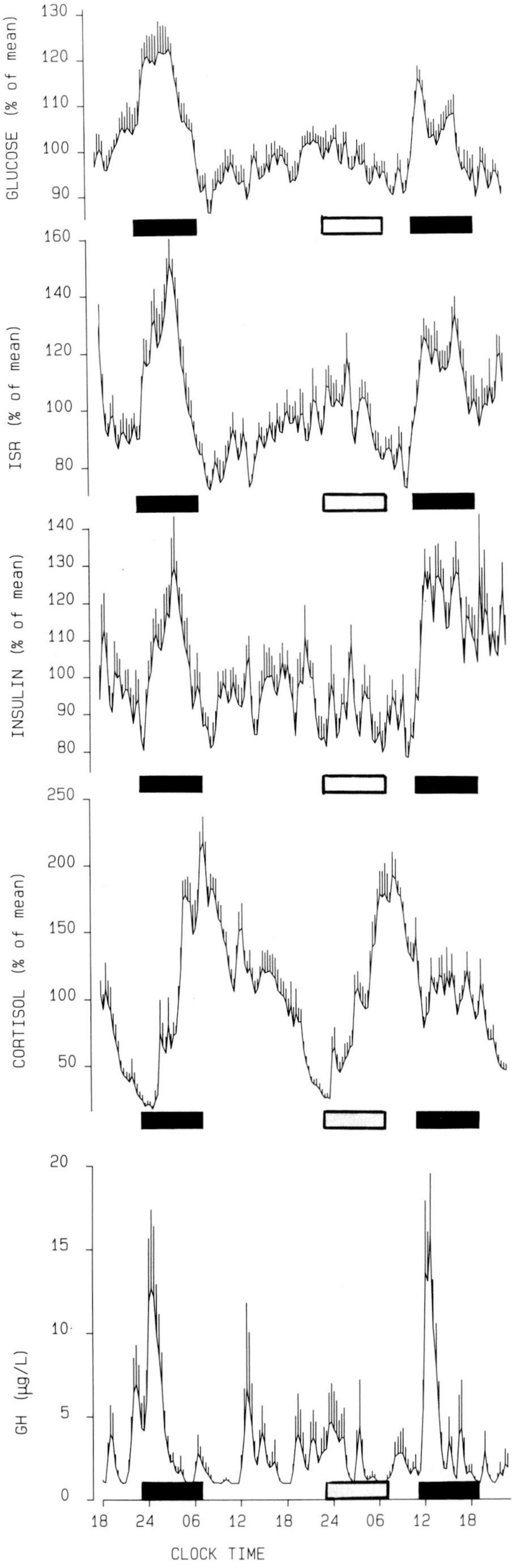

FIGURE 140–36. Mean profiles of plasma glucose, serum insulin, insulin secretion rates (ISR), cortisol, and growth hormone (GH) concentrations observed in a group of 8 subjects studied during a 53-h period, including 8 h of nocturnal sleep, 28 h of sleep deprivation, and 8 h of daytime sleep. The vertical bars at each time point represent the SEM. To eliminate the effects of interindividual variations in mean glucose, insulin, ISR, and cortisol level on the group pattern, the individual values were expressed as percentages of the mean. The black bars represent the sleep periods. The shaded bar represents the period of nocturnal sleep deprivation. (Reproduced from Van Cauter E, Blackman JD, Roland D, et al: Modulation of glucose regulation and insulin secretion by circadian rhythmicity and sleep. J Clin Invest 88:934–942, 1991, by copyright permission of the American Society for Clinical Investigation.)

oscillatory process including rapid pulses recurring every 10 to 15 min[2, 293, 477–479] superimposed on slower, ultradian oscillations with periods in the range of 90 to 120 min.[245, 246, 264, 265] Examples of ultradian oscillations have been illustrated in Figures 140–21 and 140–24. The superimposition of rapid pulses on the ultradian oscillations was shown in Figure 140–24. The ultradian oscillations are tightly coupled to glucose, with a high degree of concomitance between pulses of insulin secretion and pulses of glucose levels. Moreover, as shown in Figure 140–21, the periodicity of the insulin secretory oscillations can be entrained to the period of an oscillatory glucose infusion.[247] When glucose levels are increased, the amplitude, but not the frequency, of the oscillations of insulin secretion is enhanced.[480] These findings are entirely compatible with the concept that these ultradian oscillations are generated by the glucose-insulin feedback mechanism.[266] The rapid 10- to 15-min pulsations seem to have a different origin than the ultradian oscillations. Indeed, they may appear independently of glucose, since they were observed in the isolated perfused pancreas and in isolated islets.[297, 480, 481] Thus the existence of an intrapancreatic pacemaker generating rapid oscillations has been postulated. In contrast to what was found for the ultradian oscillations, the relative amplitude of the rapid pulses decreases rather than increases during glucose stimulation.[480] Because of their small amplitude, the detection of these rapid pulses of insulin levels necessitates multiple assay determinations at each time point and detailed statistical analyses.[2]

Alterations in Conditions of Impaired Glucose Tolerance

Early observations have indicated that the morning versus evening difference in glucose tolerance observed in normal subjects was abolished in obese subjects and reversed in diabetic subjects who have instead higher glucose responses in the morning than in the evening.[471] These findings are consistent with the observation of the "dawn phenomenon" in diabetic patients, i.e., an increase in glucose levels and/or insulin requirements in a prebreakfast period ranging from 5:00 to 9:00.[482] The existence of a dawn phenomenon in patients with either insulin-dependent diabetes mellitus (IDDM) or non–insulin-dependent diabetes mellitus (NIDDM) was clearly evident in subjects receiving closed-loop insulin infusions.[482–485] A role for nocturnal GH secretion in the pathogenesis of the dawn phenomenon was demonstrated in some studies,[486, 487] but evidence to the contrary was obtained in others.[488] In the absence of exogenous insulin infusion, the occurrence of a dawn phenomenon in NIDDM patients under normal dietary conditions has been less consistent, with both positive[489, 490] and negative[491, 492] findings. Evidence was obtained suggesting that the occurrence of an early morning rise in glucose levels in patients with NIDDM may be dependent on the size and timing of the last meal on the previous day.[490] Prominent diurnal variations in glucose levels and insulin secretion in both normal subjects and diabetic patients become apparent during prolonged fasting.[475] Figure 140–37 illustrates these variations in diabetic patients and age-, sex-, and weight-matched controls studied during a 24-h fast following an overnight fast.[475] Mean profiles of glucose, insulin secretion, cortisol, and GH are shown for both groups of subjects. As expected, glucose levels (top panels) initially declined as a result of the fasting condition but started rising again in the late evening to reach a morning maximum. Note that in normal subjects, but not in diabetic patients, the pattern of insulin secretion paralleled glucose changes. Cortisol levels were elevated in the fasting diabetic subjects, and in both groups of subjects, the nighttime glucose elevation was temporally and quantitatively correlated with the circadian cortisol rise. In NIDDM subjects, but not in controls, the size of the morning glucose rise also correlated with the increase in GH secretion in the evening period. Interestingly, the timing of the glucose rise in these fasted subjects is similar to that of the rise during constant glucose infusion (compare Figs. 140–35 and 140–37). The nocturnal rise of glucose during prolonged fasting could thus represent a normal diurnal variation in the setpoint of glucose regulation amplified by counterregulatory mechanisms activated by the fasting condition.[475]

The rapid and ultradian oscillations of insulin secretion are perturbed in NIDDM and impaired glucose tolerance without hyperglycemia. The rapid pulses appear to be less regular and of shorter duration than in normal subjects.[294, 493] The ultradian oscillations, which have an exaggerated amplitude in obese subjects without apparent changes in frequency or pattern of recurrence, are also more irregular in subjects with established NIDDM.[494] In addition, in NIDDM, the ultradian oscillations in insulin secretion are dampened and their association with similar changes in glucose levels is markedly diminished.[350, 494, 495] These latter observations could reflect a disruption of a specific dynamic property of the insulin-glucose feedback loop, which is already present before the development of overt diabetes. Recently demonstrated disturbances in the pattern of entrainment of insulin secretion to oscillatory glucose infusions further support this concept.[350]

The Pineal Gland

The 24-h profile of plasma melatonin is a robust marker of the human circadian clock.[167] As may be seen in the examples shown in Figures 140–10, 140–16, and 140–25, daytime levels are low or undetectable. The nocturnal rise starts in the early evening, between 20:00 and 22:00, and the maximum occurs around the middle of the sleep period. The melatonin rhythm and the rhythm of body temperature undergo equivalent phase shifts following a regimen of scheduled exposures to bright light and darkness,[190] supporting the concept that both rhythms are controlled by the central circadian pacemaker. Recent studies have indicated that nocturnal melatonin secretion may contribute to the circadian regulation of body temperature.[496] Exposure to light of sufficient intensity (>500 lux) results in an acute dose-dependent inhibition of nocturnal melatonin secretion, with a rapid return to high nighttime levels when darkness resumes.[191] The melatonin rhythm appears to be largely insensitive to stimuli other than light, such as sleep and food intake.

The functional significance of the melatonin rhythm has been well established for a wide variety of seasonal vertebrate species.[206] Indeed, changes in day length are perceived via the duration of elevated nocturnal melatonin

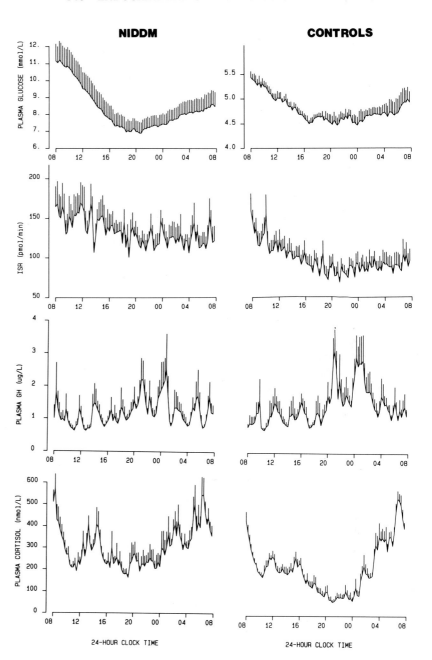

FIGURE 140–37. Mean profiles of glucose, insulin secretion, GH, and cortisol from a group of 7 patients with NIDDM (*left*) and 7 nondiabetic controls (*right*). The vertical lines at each time point represent the SEM. Note that a different scale was used to represent the mean glucose profile in NIDDM and control subjects, respectively. (Adapted from Shapiro ET, Polonsky KS, Copinschi G, et al: Nocturnal elevation of glucose levels during fasting in noninsulin-dependent diabetes. J Clin Endocrinol Metab 72:444–454, 1991. © by the Endocrine Society, 1991.)

levels. In the human, this relationship between duration of melatonin secretion and length of the photoperiod has only recently been firmly established,[314] raising the possibility that seasonal changes in melatonin production could influence human physiology. Although there is little indication that day length affects human reproduction, two early observations have stimulated studies on melatonin secretion in human puberty.[497] First, children with pinealomas may have either precocious or delayed puberty. Second, the onset of human puberty seems to occur preferentially during months with increased daylight duration. Analogy with findings in other mammals suggested that pineal function might be involved in the timing of puberty. The initial efforts to examine this hypothesis in humans were often confounded by the lack of availability of specific and sensitive assays applicable to studies involving frequent sampling over prolonged periods of time. Recently, nocturnal melatonin levels in central sexual precocity have been

found to be significantly lower than in age-matched normal children, even when differences in body weight are controlled for.[498] The cause for this abnormality in melatonin secretion in precocious puberty does not appear to be directly related to the ambient gonadotropin or steroid levels, since treatment with a GnRH analogue failed to restore higher nocturnal melatonin levels.[498] During puberty itself, several studies have reported a decrease in nocturnal melatonin levels.[497, 499] During the normal menstrual cycle, the circadian rhythm of melatonin remains unaltered. However, in women with hypothalamic amenorrhea[500] or in women with anorexia nervosa,[501] the 24-h pattern of melatonin reverts to a "younger" stage, since the nocturnal elevation is markedly amplified. Similarly, amenorrheic athletes also present a marked augmentation of nocturnal melatonin levels.[502] Neither opioidergic nor dopaminergic pathways seem to be involved in this abnormality.[502] Interestingly, daytime treatment of normal women with melatonin in the early part of the follicular phase appears associated with an increased amplitude of LH pulses,[503] as seen during the nighttime period in pubertal subjects. Taken together, these recent findings have pointed at a possible role for the melatonin rhythm in the development of reproductive function.

There is growing evidence (reviewed in refs. 9, 504, and 505) to indicate that while the rhythm of melatonin secretion is driven by the circadian pacemaker, this rhythm also feeds back on the clock. Indeed, exogenous administration of melatonin has been shown to resynchronize certain overt rhythms, and in particular the sleep-wake cycle, in a variety of conditions, including, as reviewed earlier, "jet lag" and free-running rhythms in blind subjects. Lewy and associates[189] have recently demonstrated the existence of a phase-response curve of the "dim light melatonin onset" to four consecutive oral administrations of low-dose melatonin (0.5 mg) in humans. Melatonin administration caused phase advances when administered in the afternoon and evening and phase delays when given in the morning. Nocturnal administration did not result in any phase shift. These characteristics are similar to those of the phase-response curve to dark pulses given to animals free running in constant light which constitutes a mirror image of the phase-response curve to light. These human data have been interpreted as indicative of a role for melatonin as an internal *zeitgeber*.

A number of studies have described a marked decrease in nocturnal melatonin levels from early childhood (1 to 3 years) through the prepubertal and pubertal periods.[499, 506, 507] Adult levels are attained in early adolescence (15 to 18 years). The chronology of the melatonin decline in childhood occurs in a mirror image with the increase in body weight.[499] This could suggest that the decline is due to a constant production by the pineal, which is distributed in a larger volume over time. As illustrated in Figure 140–10, in adults, there is a pronounced decrease in melatonin secretion with advancing age. A dampening of the circadian amplitude, with lower nighttime levels, has been consistently reported.[123, 127] The rising phase of nocturnal melatonin levels also appears advanced by approximately 1½ h in elderly men as compared with young men.[127]

CONCLUSION

In conclusion, oscillatory behavior appears to be the rule rather than the exception throughout the endocrine system. As more precise procedures for hormone sampling and assay become available, an increasing number of complex oscillatory patterns, covering multiple frequencies, unravel. Current research efforts are reaching beyond the descriptive stage to address the issue of the physiological importance and clinical relevance of endocrine rhythms.

ACKNOWLEDGMENTS: We wish to thank Ms. Rachel Leproult for expert assistance with the use of word-processing, graphics, and bibliography softwares. This work was supported by NIH Grant HD-09885, by a Senior Fogarty International Fellowship, and by a Guggenheim Memorial Fellowship to Fred W. Turek. Partial support also was obtained from Grants DK-41814 (NIH) and AFOSR 90-0222 (Air Force Office of Scientific Research) to Eve Van Cauter.

REFERENCES

1. Goodner C, Walike B, Koerker D, et al: Insulin, glucagon, and glucose exhibit synchronous, sustained oscillations in fasting monkeys. Science. 195:177–179, 1977.
2. O'Meara NM, Sturis J, Blackman JD, et al: Analytical problems in detecting rapid insulin secretory pulses in normal humans. J Clin Endocrinol Metab 27:231–238, 1993.
3. Carnes M, Lent S, Feyzi J, Hazel D: Plasma adrenocorticotropic hormone in the rat demonstrates three different rhythms within 24 h. Neuroendocrinology 50:17–25, 1989.
4. Turek FW: Pharmacological probes of the mammalian circadian clock: Use of the phase response curve approach. Trends Pharmacol Sci 8:212–217, 1987.
5. Mistlberger R, Rusak B: Mechanisms and models of the circadian timekeeping system. In Kryger MH, Roth T, Dement WC (eds): Principles and Practice of Sleep Medicine. Philadelphia, WB Saunders Co, 1989, pp 141–152.
6. Mrosovsky N: Phase response curves for social entrainment. J Comp Physiol [A] 162:35–46, 1988.
7. Turek FW: Effects of stimulated physical activity on the circadian pacemaker of vertebrates. J Biol Rhythms 4:135–148, 1989.
8. Cassone VM: Melatonin and suprachiasmatic nucleus. In Klein DC, Moore RY, Reppert SM (eds): Suprachiasmatic Nucleus: The Mind's Clock. New York, Oxford University Press, 1991, pp 309–323.
9. Armstrong SM: Melatonin and circadian control in mammals. Experientia 45:932–938, 1989.
10. Sack RL, Lewy AJ, Blood ML, Stevenson J: Melatonin administration to blind people: Phase advances and entrainment. J Biol Rhythms 6:249–261, 1991.
11. Reebs S, Mrosovsky N: Effects of induced wheel running on the circadian activity rhythms of Syrian hamsters: Entrainment and phase response curve. J Biol Rhythms 4:39–48, 1989.
12. Wickland C, Turek FW: Phase-shifting effects of acute increases in activity on circadian locomotor rhythms in hamsters. Am J Physiol 261:R1109–R1117, 1991.
13. Wickland C, Turek FW: Phase-shifting effect of triazolam on the hamster's circadian rhythm of activity is not mediated by a change in body temperature. Brain Res 560:12–16, 1991.
14. Turek FW, Losee-Olson S: The circadian rhythm of LH release can be shifted by injections of a benzodiazepine in female golden hamsters. Endocrinology 122:756–758, 1988.
15. Reebs S, Mrosovsky N: Running activity mediates the phase-advancing effects of dark pulses on hamster circadian rhythms. J Comp Physiol [A] 165:811–818, 1989.
16. Van Reeth O, Turek FW: Stimulated activity mediates phase shifts in the hamster circadian clock induced by dark pulses or benzodiazepines. Nature 339:49–51, 1989.
17. Van Reeth O, Hinch D, Tecco JM, Turek FW: The effects of short periods of immobilization on the hamster circadian clock. Brain Res 545:208–214, 1991.
18. Van Reeth O, Turek FW: Adaptation of circadian rhythmicity to a shift in the light-dark cycle can be accelerated by a benzodiazepine. Am J Physiol 253:R204–R207, 1987.
19. Mrosovsky N, Salmon PA: A behavioral method for accelerating re-entrainment of rhythms to new light-dark cycles. Nature 330:372–373, 1987.
20. Edgar DM, Kilduff TS, Martin CE, Dement WC: Influence of running wheel activity on free-running sleep/wake and drinking circadian rhythms in mice. Physiol Behav 50:373–378, 1991.
21. Yamada N, Shimoda K, Ohi K, et al: Free-access to a running wheel shortens the period of the free-running rhythm in blinded rats. Physiol Behav 42:87–91, 1988.
22. Edgar DM, Dement WC: Regularly scheduled voluntary exercise synchronizes the mouse circadian clock. Am J Physiol 261:R928–R933, 1991.
23. Monk TH, Fookson JE, Moline ML, Pollak CP: Diurnal variation in mood and performance in a time-isolated environment. Chronobiol Int 2:185–193, 1985.
24. Daan S: Adaptive daily strategies in behavior. In Aschoff J (eds): Biological Rhythms. New York, Plenum Press, 1981, pp 275–298.
25. Comperatore CA, Stephan FK: Entrainment of duodenal activity to periodic feeding. J Biol Rhythms 2:227–242, 1987.
26. Czeisler CA, Chiasera AJ, Duffy JF: Research on sleep, circadian rhythms and aging: Applications to manned spaceflight. Exp Gerontol 26:217–232, 1991.

27. Monk TH: Sleep and circadian rhythms. Exp Gerontol 26:233–243, 1991.
28. Czeisler CA, Johnson MP, Duffy JF, et al: Exposure to bright light and darkness to treat physiologic maladaptation to night work. N Engl J Med 322:1253–1259, 1990.
29. Van Cauter E, Turek FW: Strategies for resetting the human circadian clock. N Engl J Med 322:1306–1308, 1990.
30. Wehr TA, Goodwin FK: Biological rhythms in manic-depressive illness. *In* Wehr TA, Goodwin FK (eds): Circadian Rhythms in Psychiatry. Pacific Grove, Boxwood Press, 1983, pp 129–184.
31. Van Cauter E, Turek FW: Depression: A disorder of timekeeping? Perspect Biol Med 29:510–519, 1986.
32. Daan S, Aschoff J: Short-term rhythms in activity. *In* Aschoff J (ed): Biological Rhythms. New York, Plenum Press, 1981, pp 491–498.
33. Schulz H, Lavie P. Ultradian Rhythms in Physiology and Behavior. Berlin: Springer-Verlag, 1985.
34. Van Cauter E, Honinckx E: Pulsatility of pituitary hormones. Exp Brain Res Suppl 12:41–60, 1985.
35. Van Cauter E: Diurnal and ultradian rhythms in human endocrine function: A minireview. Horm Res 34:45–53, 1990.
36. Van Cauter E, van Coevorden A, Blackman JD: Modulation of neuroendocrine release by sleep and circadian rhythmicity. *In* Yen SSC, Vale WW (eds): Advances in Neuroendocrine Regulation of Reproduction. Norwell, Serono Symposia USA, 1990, pp 113–122.
37. Van Cauter E, Kerkhofs M, Caufriez A, et al: A quantitative estimation of GH secretion in normal man: Reproducibility and relation to sleep and time of day. J Clin Endocrinol Metab 74:1441–1450, 1992.
38. Kapen S, Boyar RM, Finkelstein JW, et al: Effect of sleep-wake cycle reversal on luteinizing hormone pattern in puberty. J Clin Endocrinol Metab 39:293–299, 1974.
39. Veldhuis J, Iranmanesh A, Lizarralde G, Johnson M: Amplitude modulation of a burstlike mode of cortisol secretion subserves the circadian glucocorticoid rhythm. Am J Physiol 257:E6–E14, 1989.
40. Veldhuis JD, Iranmanesh A, Johnson ML, Lizarralde G: Amplitude, but not frequency, modulation of adrenocorticotropin secretory bursts gives rise to the nyctohemeral rhythm of the corticotropic axis in man. J Clin Endocrinol Metab 71:452–463, 1989.
41. Soules M, Steiner R, Cohen N, et al: Nocturnal slowing of pulsatile luteinizing hormone secretion in women during the follicular phase of the menstrual cycle. J Clin Endocrinol Metab 61:43–49, 1985.
42. Filicori M, Santoro N, Merriam GR, Crowley WFJ: Characterization of the physiological pattern of episodic gonadotropin secretion throughout the menstrual cycle. J Clin Endocrinol Metab 62:1136–1144, 1986.
43. Halberg F, et al: Circaseptan (about 7-day) and circasemiseptan (about 3.5-day) rhythms and contributions by Ladislav Derer: 2. Examples from botany, zoology and medicine. Biologia (Bratislava) 41:233–252, 1986.
44. Schweiger H-G, Berger S, Kretschmer H, et al: Evidence for a circaseptan and a circasemiseptan growth response to light/dark cycle shifts in nucleated and enucleated acetabularia cells, respectively. Proc Natl Acad Sci USA 83:8619–8623, 1989.
45. Enright JT: The parallactic view, statistical testing, and circular reasoning. J Biol Rhythms 4:295–304, 1989.
46. Campbell CS, Turek FW: Cyclic function in the mammalian ovary. *In* Aschoff J (ed): Biological Rhythms. New York, Plenum Press, 1981, pp 523–545.
47. Turek FW, Van Cauter E: Rhythms in reproduction. *In* Knobil E, Neill J (eds): The Physiology of Reproduction. New York, Raven Press, 1988, pp 1789–1830.
48. Seibel MM, Shine W, Smith DM, Taymor ML: Biological rhythm of the luteinizing hormone surge. Fertil Steril 37:709–711, 1982.
49. Testart J, Frydman R, Roger M: Seasonal influence of diurnal rhythms in the onset of the plasma luteinizing hormone surge in women. J Clin Endocrinol Metab 55:374–377, 1982.
50. Hoff JD, Quigley ME, Yen SSC: Hormonal dynamics at midcycle: A reevaluation. J Clin Endocrinol Metab 57:792–796, 1983.
51. Hastings MH: Neuroendocrine rhythms. Pharmacol Ther 50:35–71, 1991.
52. Follett BK, Follett DE. Biological Clocks in Seasonal Reproductive Cycles. Bristol: Wright, 1981.
53. Milette JJ, Turek FW: Circadian and photoperiodic effects of brief light pulses in male Djungarian hamsters. Biol Reprod 35:327–335, 1986.
54. Moore RY: Development of the suprachiasmatic nucleus. *In* Klein DC, Moore RY, Reppert SM (eds): Suprachiasmatic Nucleus: The Mind's Clock. New York, Oxford University Press, 1991, pp 391–404.
55. Moore RY, Eichler VB: Loss of a circadian adrenal corticosterone rhythm following suprachiasmatic lesions in the rat. Brain Res 42:201–206, 1972.
56. Stephan FK, Zucker I: Circadian rhythm in drinking behavior and locomotor activity of rats are eliminated by hypothalamic lesions. Proc Natl Acad Sci USA 69:1583–1586, 1972.
57. Meijer JH, Rietveld WJ: Neurophysiology of the suprachiasmatic circadian pacemaker in rodents. Physiol Rev 69:671–707, 1989.
58. Moore RY: Organization and function of a central nervous system circadian oscillator: The suprachiasmatic hypothalamic nucleus. Fed Proc 42:2783–2789, 1983.
59. Rosenwasser AM, Adler NT: Structure and function in circadian timing systems: Evidence for multiple coupled circadian oscillators. Neurosci Behav Rev 10:431–448, 1986.
60. Turek FW: Circadian neural rhythms in mammals. Annu Rev Physiol 47:49–64, 1985.
61. Kittrell EMW: The suprachiasmatic nucleus and temperature rhythms. *In* Klein DC, Moore RY, Reppert SM (eds): Suprachiasmatic Nucleus: The Mind's Clock. New York, Oxford University Press, 1991, pp 233–245.
62. Stephan FK, Swann JM, Sisk CL: Anticipation of 24-h feeding schedules in rats with lesions of the suprachiasmatic nucleus. Behav Biol 25:346–363, 1979.
63. Stephan FK: Forced dissociation of activity entrained to T cycles of food access in rats with suprachiasmatic lesions. J Biol Rhythms 4:467–480, 1989.
64. Lehman MN, Silver R, Bittman EL: Anatomy of suprachiasmatic nucleus grafts. *In* Klein DC, Moore RY, Reppert SM (eds): Suprachiasmatic Nucleus: The Mind's Clock. New York, Oxford University Press, 1991, pp 349–374.
65. Ralph MR: Suprachiasmatic nucleus transplant studies using the tau mutation in golden hamsters. *In* Klein DC, Moore RY, Reppert SM (eds): Suprachiasmatic Nucleus: The Mind's Clock. New York, Oxford University Press, 1991, pp 341–348.
66. Ralph MR, Menaker M: A mutation in the circadian system of the golden hamster. Science 241:1225–1227, 1988.
67. Ralph M, Foster RG, Davis FC, Menaker M: Transplanted suprachiasmatic nucleus determines circadian period. Science 247:975–978, 1990.
68. Lehman MN, Silver R, Gladstone WR, et al: Circadian rhythmicity restored by neural transplant: Immunocytochemical characterization of the graft and its integration with the host brain. J Neurosci 7:1626–1638, 1987.
69. Schwartz WJ: SCN metabolic activity in vivo. *In* Klein DC, Moore RY, Reppert SM (eds): Suprachiasmatic Nucleus: The Mind's Clock. New York, Oxford University Press, 1991, pp 144–156.
70. Inouye ST, Kawamura H: Persistence of circadian rhythmicity in a mammalian hypothalamic island containing the suprachiasmatic nucleus. Proc Natl Acad Sci USA 76:5962–5966, 1979.
71. Majzoub JA, Robinson BG, Emanuel RL: Suprachiasmatic nuclear rhythms of vasopressin mRNA in vivo. *In* Klein DC, Moore RY, Reppert SM (eds): Suprachiasmatic Nucleus: The Mind's Clock. New York, Oxford University Press, 1991, pp 177–190.
72. Uhl GR, Reppert SM: Suprachiasmatic nucleus vasopressin messenger RNA: Circadian variation in normal and Brattleboro rats. Science 232:390–393, 1986.
73. Earnest DJ, Sladek CD: Circadian vasopressin release from perfused rat suprachiasmatic explants in vitro: effects of acute stimulation. Brain Res 422:398–402, 1987.
74. Gillette MU: SCN electrophysiology in vitro: Rhythmic activity and endogenous clock properties. In Klein DC, Moore RY, Reppert SM (eds): Suprachiasmatic Nucleus: The Mind's Clock. New York, Oxford University Press, 1991.
75. Card JP, Moore RY: The organization of visual circuits influencing the circadian activity of suprachiasmatic nucleus. *In* Klein DC, Moore RY, Reppert SM (eds): Suprachiasmatic Nucleus: The Mind's Clock. New York, Oxford University Press, 1991, pp 51–76.
76. Morin LP, Michels KM, Smale L, Moore RY: Serotonin regulation of circadian rhythmicity. Ann NY Acad Sci 600:418–426, 1990.
77. Earnest DJ, Turek FW: Neurochemical basis for the photic control of circadian rhythms and seasonal reproductive cycles: Role for acetylcholine. Proc Natl Acad Sci USA 82:4277–4281, 1985.
78. Rusak B, Bina KG: Neurotransmitters in the mammalian circadian system. Annu Rev Neurosci 13:387–401, 1990.
79. Foster RG, Provencio I, Hudson D, et al: Circadian photoreception in the retinally degenerate mouse (rd/rd). J Comp Physiol [A] 169:39–50, 1991.

80. Hotz MM, Milette JJ, Takahashi JS, Turek FW: Spectral sensitivity of the circadian clock's response to light in Djungarian hamsters. Soc Res Biol Rhythms Abstr 1:18, 1990.
81. Nelson DE, Takahashi JS: Sensitivity and integration in a visual pathway for circadian entrainment in the hamster (*Mesocricetus auratus*). J Physiol 439:1991.
82. Menaker M: Extraretinal photoreception. *In* Smith K (ed): The Science of Photobiology. New York, Plenum Press, 1989, chap 8.
83. Morin LP: Neural control of circadian rhythms as revealed through the use of benzodiazepines. *In* Klein DC, Moore RY, Reppert SM (eds): Suprachiasmatic Nucleus: The Mind's Clock. New York, Oxford University Press, 1991, pp 324–338.
84. Johnson R, Smale L, Moore RY, Morin LP: Lateral geniculate lesions block circadian phase shift responses to a benzodiazepine. Proc Natl Acad Sci USA 85:5301–5304, 1988.
85. Albers HE, Liou S-Y, Ferris CF, et al: Neurochemistry of circadian timing. *In* Klein DC, Moore RY, Reppert SM (eds): Suprachiasmatic Nucleus: The Mind's Clock. New York, Oxford University Press, 1991, pp 263–288.
86. Possidente B, Lumia AR, McEldowney A, Rapp M: Fluoxetine shortens circadian period for wheel-running activity in mice. Brain Res Bull 28:629–631, 1992.
87. Morin LP, Blanchard J: Depletion of brain serotonin by 5,7-DHT modifies hamster circadian rhythm response to light. Brain Res 566:173–185, 1991.
88. Swann JM, Turek FW: Multiple circadian oscillators regulate the timing of behavioral and endocrine rhythms in female golden hamsters. Science 228:898–900, 1985.
89. Pickard GE, Turek FW: Splitting of the circadian rhythm of activity is abolished by unilateral lesions of the suprachiasmatic nuclei. Science 215:1119–1121, 1982.
90. Davis FC, Gorski RA: Unilateral lesions of the hamster suprachiasmatic nuclei: Evidence for redundant control of circadian rhythms. J Comp Physiol 154:221–232, 1984.
91. Zlomanczuk P, Margraf RR, Lynch GR: In vitro electrical activity in the suprachiasmatic nucleus following splitting and masking of wheel-running behavior. Brain Res 559:94–99, 1991.
92. Pickard GE, Turek FW: The suprachiasmatic nuclei: Two circadian clocks? Brain Res 268:201–210, 1983.
93. Murakami N: Long-term cultured neurons from rat SCN retain the capacity for circadian oscillation of vasopressin release. Brain Res 545:347–350, 1991.
94. Takahashi JS, Murakami N, Nikaido SS, et al: The avian pineal, a vertebrate model system of the circadian oscillator: Cellular regulation of circadian rhythms by light, second messengers, and macromolecular synthesis. Rec Prog Horm Res 45:279–352, 1989.
95. Takeuchi J, Nagasake H, Shinohara K, Inouye ST: A circadian rhythm of somatostatin messenger RNA levels, but not vasoactive intestinal polypeptide/peptide histidine isoleucine messenger RNA levels in rat suprachiasmatic nucleus. Mol Cell Neurosci 3:29–35, 1992.
96. Inouye SIT, Takahashi JS, Wollnik F, Turek FW: Inhibitor of protein synthesis phase shifts a circadian pacemaker in the mammalian SCN. Am J Physiol 255:R1055–R1058, 1988.
97. Takahashi JS, Turek FW: Anisomycin, an inhibitor of protein synthesis, perturbs the phase of a mammalian circadian pacemaker. Brain Res 405:199–203, 1987.
98. Wollnik F, Turek FW, Majewski P, Takahashi JS: Phase shifting the circadian clock with cycloheximide: Response of hamsters with an intact or split rhythm of locomotor activity. Brain Res 496:82–88, 1989.
99. Joy JE, Johnson GS, Lazar T, et al: Protein differences in tau mutant hamsters: Candidate clock proteins. Mol Brain Res 14:8–14, 1992.
100. Aronin N, Sagar SM, Sharp FR, Schwartz WJ: Light regulates expression of a *Fos*-related protein in rat suprachiasmatic nuclei. Proc Natl Acad Sci USA 87:5959–5962, 1990.
101. Earnest DJ, Iadarola M, Yeh HH, Olschowka JA: Photic regulation of c-*fos* expression in neural components governing the entrainment of circadian rhythms. Exp Neurol 109:353–361, 1990.
102. Kornhauser JM, Nelson DE, Mayo KE, Takahashi JS: Photic and circadian regulation of c-*Fos* gene expression in the hamster suprachiasmatic nucleus. Neuron 5:127–134, 1990.
103. Rea MA: Light increases fos-related protein immunoreactivity in the rat suprachiasmatic nuclei. Brain Res 23:577–581, 1989.
104. Rusak B, Robertson HA, Wisden W, Hunt SP: Light pulses that shift rhythms induce gene expression in the suprachiasmatic nucleus. Science 248:1237–1240, 1990.
105. Kornhauser JM, Nelson DE, Mayo KE, Takahashi JS: Regulation of *jun*-B messenger RNA and AP-1 activity by light and a circadian clock. Science 255:1581–1584, 1992.
106. Davis FC, Menaker M: Development of the mouse circadian pacemaker: independence from environmental cycles. J Comp Physiol 143:527–539, 1981.
107. Konopka RJ, Benzer S: Clock mutants of Drosophila melanogaster. Proc Natl Acad Sci USA 68:2116–2116, 1971.
108. Dunlap JC: Closely watched clocks. Trends Genet 6:135–143, 1990.
109. Hall JC: Genetics of circadian rhythms. Annu Rev Genet 24:659–697, 1990.
110. Young MW, Bargiello TA, Baylies MK, et al: Molecular biology of the *Drosophila* clock. *In* Jacklet JW (ed): Neuronal and Cellular Oscillators. New York, Dekker, 1989, pp 529–542.
111. Büttner D, Wollnik F: Strain-differentiated circadian and ultradian rhythms in locomotor activity of the laboratory rat. Behav Genet 14:137–152, 1984.
112. Hotz MM, Connolly MS, Lynch CB: Adaptation to daily meal-timing and its effect on circadian temperature rhythms in two inbred strain of mice. Behav Genet 17:37–51, 1987.
113. Schwartz WJ, Zimmerman P: Circadian timekeeping in BALB/c and C57 BL/6 inbred mouse strains. J Neurosci 10:3685–3694, 1990.
114. Menaker M, Refinetti R: The tau mutation in golden hamsters. *In* Young M (ed): Molecular Genetics of Biological Rhythms. New York, Marcel-Dekker, 1992.
115. Mrosovsky N, Salmon PA, Menaker M, Ralph MR: Non-photic phase-shifting in hamster clock mutants. J Biol Rhythms 7:41–49, 1992.
116. Linkowski P, Van Onderbergen A, Kerkhofs M, et al: Twin study of the 24-h cortisol profile: Evidence for genetic control of the human circadian clock. Am J Physiol 264:E173–E181, 1993.
117. Reppert SM, Weaver DR: A biological clock is oscillating in the fetal suprachiasmatic nuclei. *In* Klein DC, Moore RY, Reppert SM (eds): Suprachiasmatic Nucleus: The Mind's Clock. New York, Oxford University Press, 1991, pp 405–418.
118. Davis FC, Gorski RA: Development of hamster circadian rhythms: Role of the maternal suprachiasmatic nucleus. J Comp Physiol 162:601–610, 1988.
119. Davis FC, Mannion J: Entrainment of hamster pup circadian rhythms by prenatal melatonin injections to the mother. Am J Physiol 255:R439–R448, 1988.
120. Deguchi T: Ontogenesis of a biological clock for serotonin acetyl coenzyme A N-acetyltransferase in pineal gland of rat. Proc Natl Acad Sci USA 72:2814–2818, 1975.
121. Davis FC: Use of postnatal behavioral rhythms to monitor prenatal circadian function. *In* Reppert SM (ed): Development of Circadian Rhythmicity and Photoperiodism in Mammals. New York, Perinatology Press, 1989, pp 45–65.
122. Mirmiran M, Kok JH: Circadian rhythms in early human development. Early Hum Dev 26:121–128, 1991.
123. Sharma M, Palacios-Bois J, Schwartz G, et al: Circadian rhythms of melatonin and cortisol in aging. Biol Psychiatry 25:305–319, 1989.
124. McGinty D, Stern N: Circadian and sleep-related modulation of hormone levels: Changes with Aging. *In* Sowers JR, Felicetta JV (eds): Endocrinology of Aging. New York, Raven Press, 1988, pp 75–111.
125. van Coevorden A, Laurent E, Decoster C, et al: Decreased basal and stimulated thyrotropin secretion in healthy elderly men. J Clin Endocrinol Metab 69:177–185, 1989.
126. Brock MA: Chronobiology and aging. JAGS 39:74–91, 1991.
127. van Coevorden A, Mockel J, Laurent E, et al: Neuroendocrine rhythms and sleep in aging. Am J Physiol 260:E651–E661, 1991.
128. Prinz PN, Halter JB: Sleep disturbances in the elderly: Neurohormonal correlates. *In* Chase MH, Weitzman ED (eds): Sleep Disorders: Basic and Clinical Research. Jamaica, NY, Spectrum Publications, 1983, pp 463–488.
129. Zee PC, Rosenberg RS, Turek FW: Effects of aging on entrainment and rate of resynchronization of the circadian locomotor activity. Am J Physiol 263:1099–1103, 1992.
130. Czeisler CA, Dumont M, Duffy JF, et al: Association of sleep-wake habits in older people with changes in output of circadian pacemaker. Lancet 340:933–936, 1992.
131. Pittendrigh CS, Daan S: Circadian oscillations in rodents: A systematic increase of their frequency with age. Science 186:548–550, 1974.
132. Morin LP: Age-related changes in hamster circadian period, entrainment and rhythm splitting. J Biol Rhythms 3:237–248, 1988.
133. Lieberman HB, Wurtman JJ, Teicher MH: Circadian rhythms of activity in healthy young and elderly humans. Neurobiol Aging 10:259–265, 1989.

134. Weitzman ED, Moline ML, Czeisler CA, Zimmerman JC: Chronobiology of aging: Temperature, sleep-wake cycle rhythms and entrainment. Neurobiol Aging 3:299–309, 1982.

135. Swaab DF, Fisser B, Kamphorst W, Troost D: The human suprachiasmatic nucleus: Neuropeptide changes in senium and Alzheimer's disease. Bas Appl Histochem 32:43–54, 1988.

136. Wise PM, Walovitch RC, Cohen IR, et al: Diurnal rhythmicity and hypothalamic deficits in glucose utilization in aged ovariectomized rats. J Neurosci 7:3469–3473, 1987.

137. Wise PM, Cohen IR, Weiland NG, London DE: Aging alters the circadian rhythm of glucose utilization in the suprachiasmatic nucleus. Proc Natl Acad Sci USA 85:5305–5309, 1988.

138. Weiland NG, Wise PM: Aging progressively decreases the densities and alters the diurnal rhythms of alpha-1 adrenergic receptors in selected hypothalamic regions. Endocrinology 126:2392–2397, 1990.

139. Van Reeth O, Zhang Y, Zee PC, Turek FW: Aging alters feedback effects of the activity-rest cycle on the circadian clock. Am J Physiol 263:R981–986, 1992.

140. Campbell SS, Kripke DF, Gillin JC, Hrubovcak JC: Exposure to light in healthy elderly subjects and Alzheimer's patients. Physiol Behav 42:141–144, 1988.

141. Ehlers CL, Frank E, Kupfer DJ: Social zeitgebers and biological rhythms. Arch Gen Psychiatry 45:948–952, 1988.

142. Aschoff J: Circadian rhythms: General features and endocrinological aspects. In Krieger DT (ed): Endocrine Rhythms. New York, Raven Press, 1979, pp 1–61.

143. Wever RA. The Circadian System of Man: Results of Experiments under Temporal Isolation. New York, Springer-Verlag, 1979.

144. Van Cauter E, Aschoff J: Endocrine and other biological rhythms. In DeGroot LJ (ed): Endocrinology. Philadelphia, WB Saunders Co, 1989, pp 2658–2705.

145. Weitzman ED, Czeisler CA, Moore-Ede MC: Sleep-wake, neuroendocrine and body temperature rhythms under entrained and non-entrained (free-running) conditions in man. In Suda M, Hayaishi O, Nagakawa H (eds): Biological Rhythms and their Central Mechanisms. Amsterdam, Elsevier–North Holland, 1979, pp 199–231.

146. Aschoff J, Wever R: Human circadian rhythms: A multi-oscillator system. Fed Proc 35:2326–2332, 1976.

147. Aschoff J: On the perception of time during prolonged temporal isolation. Hum Neurobiol 4:41–52, 1985.

148. Aschoff J, von Goetz C, Wildgruber C, Wever RA: Meal timing in humans during isolation without time cues. J Biol Rhythms 1:151–162, 1986.

149. Aschoff J: On the dilatability of subjective time. Perspect Biol Med 35:276–280, 1992.

150. Kronauer RE, Czeisler CA, Pilato SF, et al: Mathematical model of the human circadian system with two interacting oscillators. Am J Physiol 242:R3–R17, 1982.

151. Moore-Ede MC. The Clocks that Time Us. Cambridge, Mass, Harvard University Press, 1982.

152. Daan S, Beersma DGM, Borbély AA: Timing of human sleep: recovery process gated by a circadian pacemaker. Am J Physiol 246:R161–R178, 1984.

153. Borbély AA: A two process model of sleep regulation. Hum Neurobiol 1:195–204, 1982.

154. Wever RA: Toward a mathematical model of circadian rhythmicity. In Moore-Ede MC, Czeisler CA (eds): Mathematical Models of the Sleep-Wake Cycle. New York, Raven Press, 1984, pp 17–29.

155. Strogatz SH. The Mathematical Structure of the Human Sleep-Wake Cycle. Berlin, Springer-Verlag, 1986.

156. Achermann P, Borbély AA: Simulation of human sleep: Ultradian dynamics of electroencephalographic slow-wave activity. J Biol Rhythms 5:141–157, 1990.

157. Gander PH, Kronauer RE, Czeisler CA, Moore-Ede MC: Simulating the action of zeitgebers on a coupled two-oscillator model of the human circadian system. Am J Physiol 247:R418–R426, 1984.

158. Czeisler CA, Weitzman ED, Moore-Ede MC, et al: Human sleep: Its duration and organization depends on its circadian phase. Science 210:1264–1267, 1980.

159. Akerstedt A, Gillberg M: The circadian variation of experimentally displaced sleep. Sleep 4:159–169, 1981.

160. Carskadon MA, Dement WC: Multiple sleep latency tests during the constant routine. Sleep 15:396–399, 1992.

161. Dijk D-J, Brunner DP, Beersma DGM, Borbély AA: Electroencephalogram power density and slow wave sleep as a function of prior waking and circadian phase. Sleep 13:430–440, 1990.

162. Van Cauter E: Physiology and pathology of circadian rhythms. In Edwards CW, Lincoln DW (eds): Recent Advances in Endocrinology and Metabolism. Edinburgh, Churchill Livingstone, 1989, pp 109–134.

163. Weitzman ED, Zimmerman JC, Czeisler CA, Ronda JM: Cortisol secretion is inhibited during sleep in normal man. J Clin Endocrinol Metab 56:352–358, 1983.

164. Parker DC, Pekary AE, Hershman JM: Effect of normal and reversed sleep-wake cycles upon nyctohemeral rhythmicity of thyrotropin (TSH): Evidence suggestive of an inhibitory influence in sleep. J Clin Endocrinol Metab 43:315–322, 1976.

165. Parker DC, Rossman LG, Pekary AE, Hershman JM: Effect of 64-hour sleep deprivation on the circadian waveform of thyrotropin (TSH): Further evidence of sleep-related inhibition of TSH release. J Clin Endocrinol Metab 64:157–161, 1987.

166. Lewy AJ, Sack RL: The dim light melatonin onset as a marker for circadian phase position. Chronobiol Int 6:93–102, 1989.

167. Rosenthal NE: Plasma melatonin as a measure of the human clock. J Clin Endocrinol Metab 73:225–226, 1991.

168. Akerstedt T, Giliberg M, Wetterberg L: The circadian covariation of fatigue and urinary melatonin. Biol Psychiatry 17:547–554, 1982.

169. Van Cauter E, Refetoff S: Multifactorial control of the 24-hour secretory profiles of pituitary hormones. J Endocrinol Invest 8:381–391, 1985.

170. Czeisler CA, Allan JS, Strogatz SH, et al: Bright light resets the human circadian pacemaker independent of the timing of the sleep-wake cycle. Science 233:667–671, 1986.

171. Drennan M, Kripke DF, Gillin JC: Bright light can delay human temperature rhythm independent of sleep. Am J Physiol 257:R136–R141, 1989.

172. Wever RA: Bright light affects human circadian rhythms. Pflugers Arch 396:85–87, 1983.

173. Czeisler CA, Richardson GS, Zimmerman JC, et al: Entrainment of human circadian rhythms by light-dark cycles: A reassessment. Photochem Photobiol 34:239–247, 1981.

174. Daan S, Lewy AJ: Scheduled exposure to daylight: a potential strategy to reduce "jet lag" following transmeridian flight. Psychopharmacol Bull 20:566–568, 1984.

175. Lewy AJ, Sack RL, Miller LS, Hoban TM: Antidepressant and circadian phase-shifting effects of light. Science 235:352–354, 1987.

176. Dijk DJ, Beersma DGM, Daan S, Lewy AJ: Bright morning light advances the human circadian system without affecting NREM sleep homeostasis. Am J Physiol 256:R106–R111, 1989.

177. Czeisler CA, Kronauer RE, Allan JS, et al: Bright light induction of strong (type O) resetting of the human circadian pacemaker. Science 244:1328–1333, 1989.

178. Van Cauter E, Van Onderbergen A, Bosson D, et al: Effect of triazolam on the adaptation of the circadian rhythms of cortisol, melatonin and REM propensity to an 8-hour delay of the sleep-wake cycle in man. First Meeting of the Society for Research on Biological Rhythms, 1988, abstract 18.

179. Minors DS, Waterhouse JM, Wirz-Justice A: A human phase-response curve to light. Neurosci Lett 13:36–40, 1991.

180. Honma K, Honma S, Wada T: Phase-dependent shift of free-running human circadian rhythms in response to bright light pulse. Experientia 43:1205–1207, 1987.

181. Buresova M, Dvorakova M, Zvolsky P, Illnerova H: Early morning bright light phase advances the human circadian pacemaker within one day. Neurosci Lett 121:47–50, 1991.

182. Van Cauter E, Sturis J, Byrne MM, et al: Preliminary studies on the immediate phase-shifting effects of light and exercise on the human circadian clock. J Biol Rhythms (in press).

183. Broadway J, Arendt J, Folkard S: Bright light phase-shifts the human melatonin rhythm during the Antarctic winter. Neurosci Lett 79:185–189, 1987.

184. Jewett M, Kronauer RE, Czeisler CA: Light-induced suppression of endogenous circadian amplitude in humans. Nature 350:59–62, 1991.

185. Mrosovsky N, Reebs SG, Honrado GI, Salmon PA: Behavioral entrainment of circadian rhythms. Experientia 45:696–702, 1989.

186. Hoban TM, Lewy AJ, Sack RL, Singer CM: The effects of shifting sleep two hours within a fixed photoperiod. J Neurol Transm 85:61–68, 1991.

187. Aschoff J, Fatranska M, Giedke H, et al: Human circadian rhythms in continuous darkness: Entrainment by social cues. Science 171:213–215, 1971.

188. Wever RA: Light effects on human circadian rhythms: A review of recent Andechs experiments. J Biol Rhythms 4:161–185, 1989.

189. Lewy AL, Ahmed S, Jackson JML, Sack RL: Melatonin shifts human circadian rhythms according to a phase-response curve. Chronobiol Int 9:380–392, 1992.

190. Shanahan TL, Czeisler CA: Light exposure induces equivalent phase shifts of the endogenous circadian rhythms of circulating plasma melatonin and core body temperature in men. J Clin Endocrinol Metab 73:227–235, 1991.

191. Lewy AJ, Wehr TA, Goodwin FK, et al: Light suppresses melatonin secretion in humans. Science 210:1267–1269, 1980.

192. Lewy AJ, Sack RL, Singer CM: Melatonin, light and chronobiological disorders. In Evered D, Clark S (eds): Photoperiodism, Melatonin and the Pineal. London, Pitman, 1985, pp 231–252.

193. McIntyre IM, Norman TR, Burrows GD, Armstrong SM: Human melatonin suppression by light is intensity-dependent. J Pineal Res 1988.

194. Arendt J, Aldhous M, English J, et al: Some effects of jet-lag and their alleviation by melatonin. Ergonomics 9:1379–1393, 1987.

195. Claustrat B, Brun J, David M, et al: Melatonin and jet lag: Confirmatory result using a simplified protocol. Biol Psychiatry 32:705–711, 1992.

196. Petrie K, Conaglen JV, Thompson L, Chamberlain K: Effect of melatonin on jet lag after long haul flights. Br Med J 298:705–707, 1989.

197. Aschoff J, Hoffman K, Pohl H, Wever RA: Re-entrainment of circadian rhythms after phase shifts of the zeitgeber. Chronobiologia 28:119–133, 1975.

198. Monk TH, Buysse DJ, Reynolds CFI, Kupfer DJ: Inducing jet lag in older people: adjusting to a 6-hour phase advance in routine. Exp Gerontol 28:119–133, 1993.

199. Mills JN, Minors DS, Waterhouse JM: Adaptation to abrupt time shifts of the oscillators controlling human circadian rhythms. J Physiol 285:455–470, 1978.

200. Wever R: Phase shifts of human circadian rhythms due to shifts of artificial zeitgebers. Chronobiologia 7:303–327, 1980.

201. Wever RA: Use of bright light to treat jet lag: Differential effects of normal and bright artificial light on human circadian rhythms. Ann NY Acad Sci 453:282–304, 1986.

202. Desir D, Van Cauter E, Fang V, et al: Effects of "jet lag" on hormonal patterns: I. Procedures, variations in total plasma proteins, and disruption of adrenocorticotropin-cortisol periodicity. J Clin Endocrinol Metab 52:628–641, 1981.

203. Klein KE, Wegmann HM: The resynchronisation of human circadian rhythms after transmeridian flights as a result of flight direction and mode of activity. In Scheving LE, Halberg F, Pauly JE (eds): Chronobiology. Tokyo, Igaku Shoin, 1974, pp 564–570.

204. Comperatore CA, Krueger GP: Circadian rhythm desynchronosis, jet lag, shift lag, and coping strategies. Occup Med 5:323–341, 1990.

205. Samel A, Wegmann H-M, Vejvoda M, et al: Influence of melatonin treatment on human circadian rhythmicity before and after a simulated 9-hr time shift. J Biol Rhythms 6:235–248, 1991.

206. Arendt J: Melatonin. Clin Endocrinol 29:205–229, 1988.

207. Seidel WF, Roth T, Roehrs T, et al: Treatment of a 12-hour shift of sleep schedule with benzodiazepines. Science 224:1262–1264, 1984.

208. Seidel WF, Cohen SA, Bliwise NG, et al: Dose-related effects of triazolam and flurazepam on a circadian rhythm insomnia. Clin Pharmacol Ther 40:314–320, 1986.

209. Walsh JK, Schweitzer PK, Anch AM, et al: Sleepiness/alertness on a simulated night shift following sleep at home with triazolam. Sleep 14:140–146, 1991.

210. Turek FW, Losee-Olson S: A benzodiazepine used in the treatment of insomnia phase-shifts the mammalian circadian clock. Nature 321:167–168, 1986.

211. Roden M, Koller M, Pirich K, et al: The circadian melatonin and cortisol secretion pattern in permanent night shift workers. Am J Physiol 1992.

212. Folkard S, Minors DS, Waterhouse JM: Chronobiology and shift work: Current issues and trends. Chronobiologia 12:31–54, 1985.

213. Czeisler CA, Moore-Ede MC, Colemna RM: Rotating shift work schedules that disrupt sleep are improved by applying circadian principles. Science 217:460–463, 1982.

214. Turek FW: Circadian principles and design of rotating shift work schedules. Am J Physiol 251:R636–R638, 1986.

215. Dawson D, Campbell SS: Timed exposure to bright light improves sleep and alertness during simulated night shifts. Sleep 14:511–516, 1991.

216. Eastman CI: High-intensity light for circadian adaptation to a 12-h shift of the sleep schedule. Am J Physiol 263:R428–R436, 1992.

217. Campbell SS, Dawson D: Enhancement of nighttime alertness and performance with bright ambient light. Physiol Behav 48:317–320, 1990.

218. Miles LEM, Raynal DM, Wilson MA: Blind man living in normal society has circadian rhythms of 24.9 hours. Science 198:421–423, 1977.

219. Lewy FJ, Newsome DA: Different types of melatonin circadian secretory rhythms in some blind subjects. J Clin Endocrinol Metab 56:1103–1107, 1983.

220. Sack RL, Lewy AJ, Blood ML, et al: Circadian rhythm abnormalities in totally blind people: Incidence and clinical significance. J Clin Endocrinol Metab 75:127–134, 1992.

221. Arendt J, Aldhous M, Wright J: Synchronization of a disturbed sleep-wake cycle in a blind man by melatonin treatment. Lancet 1:772–773, 1988.

222. American Sleep Disorders Association (ASD). The International Classification of Sleep Disorders. Lawrence, Kansas, Allen Press, Inc., 1990.

223. Vitiello MV, Smallwood RG, Avery DH, et al: Circadian temperature rhythms in young adults and aged men. Neurobiol Aging 7:97–100, 1986.

224. Campbell SS, Gillin JC, Kripke DF, et al: Gender differences in the circadian temperature rhythms of healthy elderly subjects: relationships to sleep quality. Sleep 12:529–536, 1989.

225. Weitzman ED, Czeisler CA, Coleman RM, et al: Delayed sleep phase insomnia: A chronobiologic disorder associated with sleep onset insomnia. Arch Gen Psychiatry 38:737–746, 1981.

226. Rosenthal RE, Vanderpool JRJ, Levendosky AA, et al: Phase-shifting effects of bright morning light as treatment for delayed sleep phase syndrome. Sleep 13:354–361, 1990.

227. Modolfsky H, Musisi S, Phillipson EA: Treatment of advance sleep phase syndrome by phase advance chronotherapy. Sleep 9:61–65, 1986.

228. Mendlewicz J, Linkowski P, Kerkhofs M, et al: Diurnal hypersecretion of growth hormone in depression. J Clin Endocrinol Metab 60:505–512, 1985.

229. Linkowski P, Mendlewicz J, Leclercq R, et al: The 24-hour profile of adrenocorticotropin and cortisol in major depressive illness. J Clin Endocrinol Metab 61:429–438, 1985.

230. Linkowski P, Mendlewicz J, Kerkhofs M, et al: 24-Hour profiles of adrenocorticotropin, cortisol, and growth hormone in major depressive illness: Effect of antidepressant treatment. J Clin Endocrinol Metab 65:141–152, 1987.

231. Linkowski P, Van Cauter E, L'Hermite-Balériaux M, et al: The 24-hour profile of plasma prolactin in men with major endogenous depressive illness. Arch Gen Psychiatry 46:813–819, 1989.

232. Bremner WJ, Vitiello MV, Prinz PN: Loss of circadian rhythmicity in blood testosterone levels with aging in normal men. J Clin Endocrinol Metab 56:1278–1280, 1983.

233. Hrushevsky WJM, Roemeling RV, Sothern RB: Preclinical and clinical cancer chronotherapy. In Arendt J, Minors DS, Waterhouse JM (eds): Biological Rhythms in Clinical Practice. London, Wright, 1989, pp 225–252.

234. Reinberg AE: Concepts in chronopharmacology. Annu Rev Pharmacol Toxicol 32:51–66, 1992.

235. Labrecque G, Bélanger PM: Biological rhythms in the absorption, distribution, metabolism and excretion of drugs. Pharmacol Ther 52:95–107, 1991.

236. Kleitman N: Basic rest activity cycle: 22 years later. Sleep 5:311–317, 1982.

237. Rasmussen DD: Physiological interactions of the basic rest-activity cycle of the brain: Pulsatile luteinizing hormone secretion as a model. Psychoneuroendocrinology 11:389–405, 1986.

238. Brandenberger G, Simon C, Follenius M: Ultradian endocrine rhythms: A multioscillatory system. J Interdis Cycle Res 18:307–315, 1987.

239. Gallo VR: Neuroendocrine regulation of pulsatile luteinizing hormone release in the rat. Neuroendocrinology 30:122–131, 1980.

240. Pohl CR, Knobil E: The role of the central nervous system in the control of ovarian function in higher primates. Annu Rev Physiol 44:583–593, 1982.

241. Butler JP, Spratt DI, O'Dea LSL, Crowley WFJ: Interpulse interval sequence of LH in normal men essentially constitutes a renewal process. Am J Physiol 250:338–340, 1986.

242. Laurentie MP, Garcia-Villar R, Toutain PL, Pelletier J: Pulsatile secretion of LH in the ram: A re-evaluation using a discrete deconvolution analysis. J Endocrinol 133:75–85, 1992.

243. Veldhuis JD, Johnson ML, Lizarralde G, Iranmanesh A: Rhythmic

and nonrhythmic modes of anterior pituitary gland secretion. Chronobiol Int 9:371–379, 1992.

244. Veldhuis JD, Iranmanesh A, Johnson ML, Lizarralde G: Twenty-four-hour rhythms in plasma concentrations of adenohypophyseal hormones are generated by distinct amplitude and/or frequency modulation of underlying pituitary secretory bursts. J Clin Endocrinol Metab 71:1616–1623, 1990.

245. Simon C, Brandenberger G, Follenius M: Ultradian oscillations of plasma glucose, insulin, and C-peptide in man during continuous enteral nutrition. J Clin Endocrinol Metab 64:669–674, 1987.

246. Shapiro ET, Tillil H, Polonsky KS, et al: Oscillations in insulin secretion during constant glucose infusion in normal man: relationship to changes in plasma glucose. J Clin Endocrinol Metab 67:307–314, 1988.

247. Sturis J, Van Cauter E, Blackman JD, Polonsky KS: Entrainment of pulsatile insulin secretion by oscillatory glucose infusion. J Clin Invest 87:439–445, 1991.

248. Knobil E, Hotchkiss J: The menstrual cycle and its neuroendocrine control. In Knobil E, Neill JD (eds): The Physiology of Reproduction. New York, Raven Press, 1988, pp 1971–1994.

249. Williams CL, Thalabard JC, O'Byrne KT, et al: Duration of phasic electrical activity of the hypothalamic gonadotropin-releasing hormone pulse generator and dynamics of luteinizing hormone pulses in the rhesus monkey. Proc Natl Acad Sci USA 87:8580–8582, 1990.

250. O'Byrne KT, Thalabard JC, Grosser PM, et al: Radiotelemetric monitoring of hypothalamic gonadotropin-releasing hormone pulse generator activity throughout the menstrual cycle of the rhesus monkey. Endocrinology 129:1207–1214, 1991.

251. Hiruma H, Nishihara M, Kimura F: Hypothalamic electrical activity that relates to the pulsatile release of luteinizing hormone exhibits diurnal variation in ovariectomized rats. Brain Res 582:119–122, 1992.

252. Wetsel WC, Valenca MM, Merchenthaler I, et al: Intrinsic pulsatile secretory activity of immortalized luteinizing hormone-releasing hormone-secreting neurons. Proc Natl Acad Sci USA 89:4149–4153, 1992.

253. Frohman LA, Downs TR, Clarke IJ, Thomas GB: Measurement of GH-releasing hormone in hypothalamic-portal plasma of unanesthetized sheep: Spontaneous secretion and response to insulin-induced hypoglycemia. J Clin Invest 86:17–24, 1990.

254. Plotsky PM, Vale W: Patterns of growth hormone-releasing factor and somatostatin secretion into the hypophysial-portal circulation of the rat. Science 230:461–463, 1985.

255. Lanzi R, Tannenbaum GS: Time-dependent reduction and potentiation of growth hormone (GH) responsiveness to GH-releasing factor induced by exogenous GH: Role for somatostatin. Endocrinology 130:1822–1828, 1992.

256. Vance ML, Kaiser DL, Evans WS, et al: Pulsatile growth hormone secretion in normal man during a continuous infusion of human growth hormone releasing factor (1–40): Evidence for intermittent somatostatin secretion. J Clin Invest 75:1584–1590, 1985.

257. Thorner MO, Vance ML, Hartman ML, et al: Physiological role of somatostatin in growth hormone regulation in humans. Metabolism 39:40–42, 1990.

258. Redekopp C, Irvine CHG, Donald RA, et al: Spontaneous and stimulated adrenocorticotropin and vasopressin pulsatile secretion in the pituitary venous effluent of the horse. Endocrinology 118:1410–1416, 1986.

259. Carnes M, Lent SJ, Goodman B, Mueller C, et al: Effects of immunoneutralization of corticotropin-releasing hormone on ultradian rhythms of plasma adrenocorticotropin. Endocrinology 126:1904–1913, 1990.

260. Greenspan SL, Klibanski A, Rowe JW, Elahi D: Age alters pulsatile prolactin release: Influence of dopaminergic inhibition. Am J Physiol 258:E799–E804, 1990.

261. Pavasuthipaisit K, Norman RL, Ellinwood WE, et al: Different prolactin, thyrotropin, and thyroxine responses after prolonged intermittent or continuous infusions of thyrotropin-releasing hormone in rhesus monkeys. J Clin Endocrinol Metab 56:541–548, 1983.

262. Brabant G, Prank K, Hoang-Vu C, et al: Hypothalamic regulation of pulsatile thyrotropin secretion. J Clin Endocrinol Metab 72:145–150, 1991.

263. Follenius M, Simon C, Brandenberger G, Lenzi P: Ultradian plasma corticotropin and cortisol rhythms: Time-series analyses. J Endocrinol Invest 10:261–266, 1987.

264. Polonsky KS, Given BD, Van Cauter E: Twenty-four-hour profiles and pulsatile patterns of insulin secretion in normal and obese subjects. J Clin Invest 81:442–448, 1988.

265. Simon C, Follenius M, Brandenberger G: Postprandial oscillations of plasma glucose, insulin and C-peptide in man. Diabetologia 30:769–773, 1987.

266. Sturis J, Polonsky KS, Mosekilde E, Van Cauter E: Computer model for mechanisms underlying ultradian oscillations of insulin and glucose. Am J Physiol 260:E801–E809, 1991.

267. Haisenleder DJ, Khoury S, Zmeili SM, et al: The frequency of GnRH secretion regulates expression of alpha- and beta-LH-subunit mRNAs in male rats. Mol Endocrinol 1:834–838, 1987.

268. Dalkin AC, Haisenleder DJ, Ortolano GA, et al: The frequency of GnRH stimulation differentially regulates gonadotropin subunit mRNA expression. Endocrinology 125:917–924, 1989.

269. Leung K, Kaynard AH, Negrini BP, et al: Regulation of gonadotropin subunit mRNAs by GnRH pulse frequency in ewes. Mol Endocrinol 1:724–728, 1987.

270. Shupnik MA: GnRH effects on rat gonadotropin gene transcription in vitro: Requirement for pulsatile administration for LH-beta gene stimulation. Mol Endocrinol 4:1444–1450, 1990.

271. Haisenleder DJ, Dalkin AC, Ortolano GA, et al: A pulsatile gonadotropin-releasing hormone stimulus is required to increase transcription of the gonadotropin subunit genes: Evidence for differential regulation by pulse frequency in vivo. Endocrinology 128:509–517, 1991.

272. Weiss J, Crowley WFJ, Jameson JL: Pulsatile gonadotropin-releasing hormone modifies polyadenylation of gonadotropin subunit messenger ribonucleic acids. Endocrinology 130:415–420, 1992.

273. Katt JA, Duncan JA, Herbon L, et al: The frequency of gonadotropin-releasing hormone stimulation determines the number of pituitary gonadotropin hormone receptors. Endocrinology 116:2113–2115, 1985.

274. Conn PM, Crowley WF: Gonadotropin-releasing hormone and its analogues. N Engl J Med 324:93–103, 1991.

275. Maiter D, Underwood LE, Maes M, et al: Different effects of intermittent and continuous growth hormone administration on serum somatomedin/insulin-like growth factor I and liver GH receptors in hypophysectomized rats. Endocrinology 123:1053–1059, 1988.

276. Clark RG, Jansson JO, Isaksson OGP, Robinson ICAF: Intravenous growth hormone: Growth responses to patterned infusions in hypophysectomized rats. J Endocrinol 104:53–61, 1985.

277. Bick T, Youdim MBH, Hochberg Z: Adaptation of liver membrane somatogenic and lactogenic growth hormone (GH) binding to the spontaneous pulsation of GH secretion in the male rat. Endocrinology 125:1711–1717, 1989.

278. Waxman DJ, Pampori NA, Ram PA, et al: Interpulse interval in circulating growth hormone patterns regulates sexually dimorphic expression of hepatic cytochrome P450. Proc Natl Acad Sci USA 88:6868–6872, 1991.

279. Veldhuis JD, Dufau ML: Estradiol modulates the pulsatile secretion of biologically active luteinizing hormone in man. J Clin Invest 80:631–638, 1987.

280. Refetoff S, Van Cauter E, Fang V, et al: The effect of dexamethasone on the 24-hour profiles of adrenocorticotropin and cortisol in Cushing's syndrome. J Clin Endocrinol Metab 60:527–535, 1985.

281. Weitzman ED: Effect of Sleep-Wake Cycle Shifts on Sleep and Neuroendocrine Function. New York, Plenum Press, 1973, pp 93–111.

282. Rossmanith WG, Yen SSC: Sleep-associated decrease in luteinizing hormone pulse frequency during the early follicular phase: Evidence for an opioidergic mechanism. J Clin Endocrinol Metab 65:715–718, 1987.

283. Hall JE, Richardson GS, Sullivan JP, et al: Nocturnal slowing of GnRH secretion in the early follicular phase is specifically related to slow wave sleep: Evidence from sleep-reversal studies. 74th Annual Meeting of the Endocrine Society, San Antonio, Texas, 1992.

284. Boyar R, Finkelstein J, Roffwarg H, et al: Synchronization of augmented luteinizing hormone secretion with sleep during puberty. N Engl J Med 287:582–586, 1972.

285. Parker DC, Rossman LG, Vanderlaan EF: Relation of sleep-entrained human prolactin release to REM–non-REM cycles. J Clin Endocrinol Metab 38:646–651, 1974.

286. Van Cauter E, Desir D, Refetoff S, et al: The relationship between episodic variations of plasma prolactin and REM–non-REM cyclicity is an artifact. J Clin Endocrinol Metab 54:70–75, 1982.

287. Follenius M, Brandenberger G, Simon C, Schlienger JL: REM sleep in humans begins during decreased secretory activity of the anterior pituitary. Sleep 11:546–555, 1988.

288. Van Cauter E, Caufriez A, Kerkhofs M, et al: Sleep, awakenings and insulin-like growth factor I modulate the growth hormone secretory response to growth hormone-releasing hormone. J Clin Endocrinol Metab 74:1451–1459, 1992.

289. Brandenberger G, Follenius M, Muzet A, et al: Ultradian oscillations in plasma renin activity: Their relationship to meals and sleep stages. J Clin Endocrinol Metab 61:280–284, 1985.

290. Brandenberger G, Follenius M, Simon C, et al: Nocturnal oscillations in plasma renin activity and REM-NREM sleep cycles in man: A common regulatory mechanism? Sleep 11:242–250, 1988.

291. Brandenberger G, Krauth MO, Ehrhart J, et al: Modulation of episodic renin release during sleep in humans. Hypertension 15:370–375, 1990.

292. Brandenberger G, Follenius M, Goichot B, et al: 24-Hour profiles of plasma renin activity in relation to the sleep-wake cycle. 1992.

293. Lang DA, Matthews DR, Phil D, et al: Cyclic oscillations of basal plasma glucose and insulin concentrations in human beings. N Engl J Med 301:1023–1027, 1979.

294. Lang DA, Matthews DR, Burnett M, Turner RC: Brief, irregular oscillations of basal plasma insulin and glucose concentrations in diabetic man. Diabetes 30:435–439, 1981.

295. Goodner C, Hom F, Koerker D: Hepatic glucose production oscillates in synchrony with the islet secretory cycle in fasting rhesus monkeys. Science 215:1257–1260, 1982.

296. Jaspan JB, Lever E, Polonsky KS, Van Cauter E: In vivo pulsatility of pancreatic islet peptides. Am J Physiol 251:E215–E226, 1986.

297. Stagner JI: Pulsatile secretion from the endocrine pancreas: Metabolic, hormonal, and neural modulation. In Samols E (ed): The Endocrine Pancreas. New York, Raven Press, 1991, pp 283–302.

298. Paolisso G, Scheen AJ, Giugliano D, et al: Pulsatile insulin delivery has greater metabolic effects than continuous hormone administration in man: Importance of pulse frequency. J Clin Endocrinol Metab 72:607–615, 1991.

299. Evans WS, Faria ACS, Christiansen E, et al: Impact of intensive venous sampling on characterization of pulsatile GH release. Am J Physiol 252:E549–E556, 1987.

300. Veldhuis JD, Evans WS, Rogol AD, et al: Intensified rate of venous blood sampling unmask the presence of spontaneous, high frequency pulsations of luteinizing hormone in man. J Clin Endocrinol Metab 59:96–102, 1986.

301. Scheele F, Lambalk CB, Schoemaker J, et al: Patterns of LH and FSH in men during high frequency blood sampling. J Endocrinol 114:153–160, 1987.

302. Iranmanesh A, Lizarralde G, Short D, Veldhuis JD: Intensive venous sampling paradigms disclose high frequency adrenocorticotropin release episodes in normal men. J Clin Endocrinol Metab 71:1276–1283, 1990.

303. Gwinner E: Photoperiod as a modifying and limiting factor in the expression of avian circannual rhythms. J Biol Rhythms 4:237–266, 1989.

304. Zucker I, Lee TM, Dark J: The suprachiasmatic nucleus and annual rhythms of mammals. In Klein DC, Moore RY, Reppert SM (eds): Suprachiasmatic Nucleus: The Mind's Clock. New York, Oxford University Press, 1991, pp 246–260.

305. Goldman BD, Elliott JA: Photoperiodism and seasonality in hamsters: role of the pineal gland. In Stetson MH (ed): Processing of Environmental Information in Vertebrates. New York, Springer-Verlag, 1988, pp 203–218.

306. Suttie JM, White RG, Breier BH, Gluckman PD: Photoperiod associated changes in insulin-like growth factor-I in reindeer. Endocrinology 129:679–682, 1991.

307. Stetson MH, Watson-Whitmyre M: Physiology of the pineal and its hormone melatonin in annual reproduction in rodents. In Reiter RJ (ed): The Pineal Gland. New York, Raven Press, 1984, pp 109–154.

308. Illnerova H: The suprachiasmatic nucleus and rhythmic pineal melatonin production. In Klein DC, Moore RY, Reppert SM (eds): Suprachiasmatic Nucleus: The Mind's Clock. New York, Oxford University Press, 1991, pp 197–216.

309. Reiter RJ: Pineal melatonin: Cell biology of its synthesis and of its physiological interactions. Endocr Rev 12:151–180, 1991.

310. Karsch FJ, Woodfill CJI, Malpaux B, et al: Melatonin and mammalian photoperiodism: Synchronization of annual reproductive cycles. In Klein DC, Moore RY, Reppert SM (eds): Suprachiasmatic Nucleus: The Mind's Clock. New York, Oxford University Press, 1991, pp 217–232.

311. Weaver DR, Rivkees SA, Carlson LL, Reppert SM: Localization of melatonin receptors in mammalian brain. In Klein DC, Moore RY,

Reppert SM (eds): Suprachiasmatic Nucleus: The Mind's Clock. New York, Oxford University Press, 1991, pp 289–308.

312. Dabbs JMJ: Age and seasonal variation in serum testosterone concentration among men. Chronobiol Int 7:245–249, 1990.

313. Levine RJ, Mathew RM, Chenault CB, et al: Differences in the quality of semen in outdoor workers during summer and winter. N Engl J Med 323:12–16, 1990.

314. Wehr TA: The durations of human melatonin secretion and sleep respond to changes in daylength. J Clin Endocrinol Metab 73:1276–1280, 1991.

315. Wehr TA, Moul DE, Barbato G, et al: Conservation of photoperiod-responsive mechanisms in human beings. Am J Physiol (in press).

316. Honma K, Honma S, Kohsaka M, Fukuda N: Seasonal variation in the human circadian rhythm: dissociation between sleep and temperature rhythm. Am J Physiol 262:R885–R891, 1992.

317. Malarkey WB, Hall JC, Pearl DK, et al: The influence of academic stress and season on 24-hour concentrations of growth hormone and prolactin. J Clin Endocrinol Metab 73:1089–1092, 1991.

318. Hofman MA, Swaab DF: Seasonal changes in the suprachiasmatic nucleus of man. Neurosci Lett 139:257–260, 1992.

319. Kerkhofs M, Linkowski P, Mendlewicz J: Effects of intravenous catheter on sleep in healthy men and in depressed patients. Sleep 12:113–119, 1989.

320. De Nicolao G, Guardabasso V, Rocchetti M: The relationship between rate of venous sampling and visible frequency of hormone pulses. Comput Methods Programs Biomed 33:145–157, 1990.

321. Halberg F, Tong YL, Johnson EA: Circadian system phase: an aspect of temporal morphology: Procedures and illustrative examples. In Cellular Aspects of Biorhythms. Berlin, Springer-Verlag, 1967, pp 20–48.

322. Cleveland WS: Robust locally weighted regression and smoothing scatterplots. J Am Stat Assoc 74:829–836, 1979.

323. Van Cauter E: Method for characterization of 24-h temporal variation of blood constituents. Am J Physiol 237:E255–E264, 1979.

324. Van Cauter E: Quantitative methods for the analysis of circadian and episodic hormone fluctuations. In Van Cauter E, Copinschi G (eds): Human Pituitary Hormones: Circadian and Episodic Variations. The Hague, Martinus Nijhoff, 1981, pp 1–25.

325. Santen RJ, Bardin CW: Episodic luteinizing hormone secretion in man: Pulse analysis, clinical interpretation, physiologic mechanisms. J Clin Invest 52:2617–2628, 1973.

326. Royston JP: The statistical analysis of pulsatile hormone secretion data. Clin Endocrinol 30:201–210, 1989.

327. Urban RJ, Evans WS, Rogol AD, et al: Contemporary aspects of discrete peak-detection algorithms: I. The paradigm of the luteinizing hormone pulse signal in men. Endocr Rev 9:3–37, 1988.

328. Evans WS, Sollenberger MJ, Booth RAJ, et al: Contemporary aspects of discrete peak-detection algorithms: II. The paradigm of the luteinizing hormone signal in women. Endocr Rev 13:81–104, 1992.

329. Van Cauter E: Estimating false-positive and false-negative errors in analyses of hormonal pulsatility. Am J Physiol 254:E786–E794, 1988.

330. Merriam GR, Wachter KW: Algorithms for the study of episodic hormone secretion. Am J Physiol 243:E310–E318, 1982.

331. Clifton DK, Steiner RA: Cycle detection: A technique for estimating the frequency and amplitude of episodic fluctuations in blood hormone and substrate concentrations. Endocrinology 112:1057–1064, 1983.

332. Veldhuis JD, Johnson ML: Cluster analysis: A simple, versatile, and robust algorithm for endocrine pulse detection. Am J Physiol 250:E486–E493, 1986.

333. Oerter KE, Guardabasso V, Rodbard D: Detection and characterization of peaks and estimation of instantaneous secretory rate for episodic pulsatile hormone secretion. Comput Biomed Res 19:170–191, 1986.

334. Urban RJ, Kaiser DL, Van Cauter E, et al: Comparative assessment of objective pulse detection algorithms: II. Studies in men. Am J Physiol 254:E113–E119, 1988.

335. Genazzani AD, Rodbard D: Use of the receiver operating characteristics curve to evaluate sensitivity, specificity, and accuracy of methods for detection of peaks on hormonal series. Acta Endocrinol (Copenh) 124:295–306, 1991.

336. Urban RJ, Johnson ML, Veldhuis JD: Biophysical modeling of sensitivity and positive accuracy of detecting episodic endocrine signals. Am J Physiol 257:E88–E94, 1989.

337. Guardabasso V, De Nicolao G, Rochetti M, Rodbard D: Evaluation of pulse-detection algorithms by computer simulation of hormone secretion. Am J Physiol 255:E775–E784, 1988.

338. Kushler RH, Brown MB: A model for the identification of hormone pulses. Stat Med 10:329–340, 1991.

339. Veldhuis JD, Johnson ML: A review and appraisal of deconvolution methods to evaluate in vivo neuroendocrine secretory events. J Neuroendocrinol 2:755–771, 1990.

340. Eaton RP, Allen RC, Schade DS, et al: Prehepatic insulin production in man: Kinetic analysis using peripheral connecting peptide behavior. J Clin Endocrinol Metab 51:520–528, 1980.

341. Pilo A, Ferrannini E, Navalesi R: Measurement of glucose-induced insulin delivery rate in man by deconvolution analysis. Am J Physiol 233:E500–E508, 1977.

342. Polonsky KS, Licinio-Paixao J, Given BD, et al: Use of biosynthetic human C-peptide in the measurement of insulin secretion rates in normal volunteers and type I diabetic patients. J Clin Invest 77:98–105, 1986.

343. Van Cauter E, Mestrez F, Sturis J, Polonsky KS: Estimation of insulin secretion rates from C-peptide levels: Comparison of individual and standard kinetic parameters for C-peptide clearance. Diabetes 41:368–377, 1992.

344. Van Cauter E: Computer-assisted analysis of endocrine rhythms. In Rodbard D, Forti G (eds): Computers in Endocrinology. New York, Raven Press, 1990, pp 59–70.

345. De Nicolao G, Rocchetti M: Stable and efficient techniques for the deconvolution of hormone time series. In Rodbard D, Forti G (eds): Computers in Endocrinology. New York, Raven Press, 1990, pp 83–91.

346. O'Sullivan F, O'Sullivan J: Deconvolution of episodic hormone data: an analysis of the role of season in the onset of puberty in cows. Biometrics 44:339–353, 1988.

347. Veldhuis JD, Carlson ML, Johnson ML: The pituitary gland secretes in bursts: Appraising the nature of glandular secretory impulses by simultaneous multiple-parameter deconvolution of plasma hormone concentrations. Proc Natl Acad Sci USA 84:7686–7690, 1987.

348. Van Cauter E: Time series analysis in pulse detection techniques. In Wagner TOF, Filicori M (eds): Episodic Hormone Secretion: From Basic Science to Clinical Application. Hameln, TM-Verlag, 1987, pp 51–60.

349. Matthews DR: Time series analysis in endocrinology. Acta Paediatr Scand Suppl 347:55–62, 1988.

350. O'Meara NM, Sturis J, Van Cauter E, Polonsky KS: Lack of control by glucose of ultradian insulin secretory oscillations in impaired glucose tolerance and in NIDDM. J Clin Invest (in press).

351. McLeod BJ, Craigon J: Time series analysis of plasma LH and FSH concentrations as a method of assessing episodic secretion. J Reprod Fertil 74:575–587, 1985.

352. Sturis J, Polonsky KS, Shapiro ET, et al: Abnormalities in the ultradian oscillations of insulin secretion and glucose levels in type 2 (non-insulin-dependent) diabetic patients. Diabetologia 35:681–689, 1992.

353. Veldhuis JD, Johnson ML: Operating characteristics of the hypothalamo-pituitary-gonadal axis in men: circadian, ultradian, and pulsatile release of prolactin and its temporal coupling with luteinizing hormone. J Clin Endocrinol Metab 67:116–123, 1988.

354. Samuels MH, Veldhuis JD, Henry P, Ridgway EC: Pathophysiology of pulsatile and copulsatile release of thyroid-stimulating hormone, luteinizing hormone, follicle-stimulating hormone, and alpha-subunit. J Clin Endocrinol Metab 71:425–432, 1990.

355. Lejeune-Lenain C, Van Cauter E, Desir D, et al: Control of circadian and episodic variations of adrenal androgen secretion in man. J Endocrinol Invest 10:267–276, 1987.

356. Merriam GR, Ma N, Liu L, et al: Methods for assessing the linkage between pulsatile hormone profiles. Acta Paediatr Scand Suppl 349:167–172, 1989.

357. Clifton DK, Aksel S, Bremner WJ, et al: Statistical evaluation of coincident prolactin and luteinizing hormone pulses during the normal menstrual cycle. J Clin Endocrinol Metab 67:832–838, 1988.

358. Guardabasso V, Genazzani AD, Veldhuis JD, Rodbard D: Objective assessment of concordance of secretory events in two endocrine time series. Acta Endocrinol (Copenh) 124:208–218, 1991.

359. Veldhuis JD, Johnson ML, Seneta E: Analysis of the copulsatility of anterior pituitary hormones. J Clin Endocrinol Metab 73:569–576, 1991.

360. Van Cauter E, Desir D, Decoster C, et al: Nocturnal decrease of glucose tolerance during constant glucose infusion. J Clin Endocrinol Metab 69:604–611, 1989.

361. Veldhuis JD, Iranmanesh A, Clarke I, et al: Random and non-random coincidence between luteinizing hormone peaks and follicle-stimulating hormone, alpha subunit, prolactin and gonadotropin-releasing hormone pulsations. J Neuroendocrinol 1:185–194, 1989.

362. Genazzani AD, Forti G, Guardabasso V, et al: Frequency of prolactin pulsatile release in normal men and in agonadal patients is neither coupled to LH release nor influenced by androgen modulation. Clin Endocrinol 37:65–71, 1992.

363. Follenius M, Brandenberger G, Hietter B, et al: Diurnal cortisol peaks and their relationship to meals. J Clin Endocrinol Metab 55:757–761, 1982.

364. Van Cauter E, Shapiro ET, Tillil H, Polonsky KS: Circadian modulation of glucose and insulin responses to meals: Relationship to cortisol rhythm. Am J Physiol 262:E467–E475, 1992.

365. Quigley ME, Ropert JF, Yen SSC: Acute prolactin release triggered by feeding. J Clin Endocrinol Metab 52:1043–1045, 1981.

366. Onishi S, Miyazawa G, Nishimura Y, et al: Postnatal development of circadian rhythm in serum cortisol levels in children. Pediatrics 72:399–404, 1983.

367. Van Cauter E, Golstein J, Vanhaelst L, Leclercq R: Effects of oral contraceptive therapy on the circadian pattern of cortisol and thyrotropin. Eur J Clin Invest 5:115–121, 1975.

368. Nolten WE, Lindheimer MD, Rueckert PA, et al: Diurnal patterns and regulation of cortisol secretion in pregnancy. J Clin Endocrinol Metab 51:466–472, 1980.

369. Rosman PM, Farag A, Benn R, et al: Modulation of pituitary-adrenal function: Decreased secretory episodes and blunted circadian rhythmicity in patients with alcoholic liver disease. J Clin Endocrinol Metab 53:709–717, 1981.

370. Boyar RM, Hellman LD, Roffwarg H, et al: Cortisol secretion and metabolism in anorexia nervosa. N Engl J Med 296:190–193, 1977.

371. Gallagher TF, Hellman L, Finkelstein J, et al: Hyperthyroidism and cortisol secretion in man. J Clin Endocrinol Metab 34:919–927, 1972.

372. Iranmanesh A, Lizarralde G, Johnson ML, Veldhuis JD: Dynamics of 24-hour endogenous cortisol secretion and clearance in primary hypothyroidism assessed before and after partial thyroid hormone replacement. J Clin Endocrinol Metab 70:155–161, 1990.

373. Van Cauter E, Refetoff S: Evidence for two subtypes of Cushing's disease based on the analysis of episodic cortisol secretion. N Engl J Med 312:1343–1344, 1985.

374. Halbreich U, Asnis G, Shindledecker R, et al: Cortisol secretion in endogenous depression. Arch Gen Psychiatry 42:909–914, 1985.

375. Rubin RT, Poland RE, Lesser IM, et al: Neuroendocrine aspects of primary endogenous depression: I. Cortisol secretory dynamics in patients and matched controls. Arch Gen Psychiatry 44:328–336, 1987.

376. Sachar ED. Twenty-Four-Hour Cortisol Secretory Patterns in Depressed and Manic Patients. Amsterdam, Elsevier, 1975, pp 81–91.

377. Pfohl B, Sherman B, Schlechte J, Stone R: Pituitary-adrenal axis rhythm disturbances in psychiatric depression. Arch Gen Psychiatry 42:897–903, 1985.

378. Linkowski P, Kerkhofs M, Van Onderbergen A, et al: The 24-hour profiles of cortisol, prolactin and growth hormone in mania. Arch Gen Psychiatry (in press).

379. Iranmanesh A, Veldhuis JD, Johnson ML, Lizarralde G: 24-Hour pulsatile and circadian patterns of cortisol secretion in alcoholic men. J Androl 10:54–63, 1989.

380. Van Cauter E, Linkowski P, Kerkhofs M, et al: Circadian and sleep-related endocrine rhythms in schizophrenia. Arch Gen Psychiatry 48:348–356, 1991.

381. Ho KY, Evans WS, Blizzard RM, et al: Effects of sex and age on the 24-hour profile of growth hormone secretion in man: Importance of endogenous estradiol concentrations. J Clin Endocrinol Metab 64:51–58, 1987.

382. Winer LM, Shaw MA, Baumann G: Basal plasma growth hormone levels in man: New evidence for rhythmicity of growth hormone secretion. J Clin Endocrinol Metab 70:1678–1686, 1990.

383. Holl RW, Hartmann ML, Veldhuis JD, et al: Thirty-second sampling of plasma growth hormone in man: Correlation with sleep stages. J Clin Endocrinol Metab 72:854–861, 1991.

384. Obál FJ, Payne L, Kapás L, et al: Inhibition of growth hormone-releasing factor suppresses both sleep and growth hormone secretion in the rat. Brain Res 557:149–153, 1991.

385. Obál FJ, Alfödi P, Cady AP, et al: Growth hormone-releasing factor enhances sleep in rats and rabbits. Am J Physiol 255:R310–R316, 1988.

386. Ehlers CL, Reed TK, Henriksen SJ: Effects of corticotropin-releasing factor and growth hormone-releasing factor on sleep and activity in rats. Neuroendocrinology 42:467–474, 1986.

387. Garry P, Roussel B, Cohen R, et al: Diurnal administration of human growth hormone-releasing factor does not modify sleep and sleep-related growth hormone secretion in normal young men. Acta Endocrinol (Copenh) 110:158–163, 1985.

388. Kerkhofs M, Van Cauter E, Van Onderbergen A, et al: Sleep-promoting effects of growth hormone-releasing hormone in normal men. Am J Physiol 264:E594–E598, 1993.

389. Wu RH, Thorpy MJ: Effect of growth hormone treatment on sleep EEGs in growth hormone-deficient children. Sleep 11:425–429, 1988.

390. Mendelson WB, Slater S, Gold P, Gillin JC: The effect of growth hormone administration on human sleep: A dose-response study. Biol Psychiatry 15:613–618, 1980.

391. Aström C, Lindholm J: Growth hormone deficient young adults have decreased deep sleep. Neuroendocrinology 51:82–84, 1990.

392. Aström C, Trojaborg W: Effect of growth hormone on human sleep energy. Clin Endocrinol 36:241–245, 1991.

393. Goldstein SJ, Wu RHK, Thorpy MJ, et al: Reversibility of deficient sleep entrained growth hormone secretion in a boy with achondroplasia and obstructive sleep apnea. Acta Endocrinol (Copenh) 116:95–101, 1987.

394. Miller JD, Esparza A, Wright NM, et al: Spontaneous growth hormone release in term infants: changes during the first four days of life. J Clin Endocrinol Metab 76:1058–1062, 1993.

395. Costin G, Ratner-Kaufman F, Brasel JA: Growth hormone secretory dynamics in subjects with normal stature. J Pediatr 115:537–544, 1989.

396. Mauras N, Blizzard RM, Link K, et al: Augmentation of growth hormone secretion during puberty: Evidence for a pulse amplitude-modulated phenomenon. J Clin Endocrinol Metab 64:596–601, 1987.

397. Rose SR, Municchi G, Barnes KM, et al: Spontaneous growth hormone secretion increases during puberty in normal girls and boys. J Clin Endocrinol Metab 73:428–435, 1991.

398. Finkelstein JW, Roffwarg HP, Boyar RM, et al: Age-related change in the twenty-four-hour spontaneous secretion of growth hormone. J Clin Endocrinol Metab 35:665–670, 1972.

399. Iranmanesh A, Lizarralde G, Veldhuis JD: Age and relative adiposity are specific negative determinants of the frequency and amplitude of growth hormone (GH) secretory bursts and the half-life of endogenous GH in healthy men. J Clin Endocrinol Metab 73:1081–1088, 1991.

400. Vermeulen A: Nyctohemeral growth hormone profiles in young and aged men: Correlation with somatomedin-C levels. J Clin Endocrinol Metab 64:884–888, 1987.

401. Lang I, Schernthaner G, Pietschmann P, et al: Effects of sex and age on growth hormone response to growth hormone-releasing hormone in healthy individuals. J Clin Endocrinol Metab 65:535–540, 1987.

402. Veldhuis JD, Iranmanesh A, Ho KKY, et al: Dual defects in pulsatile growth hormone secretion and clearance subserve the hyposomatotropism of obesity in man. J Clin Endocrinol Metab 72:51–59, 1991.

403. Copinschi G, De Laet MH, Brion JP, et al: Simultaneous study of cortisol, GH and PRL circadian variations of hourly integrated concentrations in normal and obese subjects. Clin Endocrinol 9:15–26, 1978.

404. Ho KY, Veldhuis JD, Johnson ML, et al: Fasting enhances growth hormone secretion and amplifies the complex rhythms of growth hormone secretion in man. J Clin Invest 81:968–975, 1988.

405. Hartman ML, Veldhuis JD, Johnson ML, et al: Augmented growth hormone (GH) secretory burst frequency and amplitude mediate enhanced GH secretion during a two-day fast in normal men. J Clin Endocrinol Metab 74:757–765, 1992.

406. Edge JA, Dunger DB, Matthews DR, et al: Increased overnight growth hormone concentrations in diabetic compared with normal adolescents. J Clin Endocrinol Metab 71:1356–1362, 1990.

407. Christensen SE, Weeke J, Orskow H, et al: Plasma growth hormone in acromegalic patients. Acta Endocrinol (Copenh) 116:49–52, 1987.

408. Gelato MC, Oldfield E, Loriaux DL, Merriam GR: Pulsatile growth hormone secretion in patients with acromegaly and normal men: The effects of growth hormone-releasing hormone infusion. J Clin Endocrinol Metab 71:585–590, 1990.

409. Hartman ML, Veldhuis JD, Vance ML, et al: Somatotropin pulse frequency and basal concentrations are increased in acromegaly and are reduced by successful therapy. J Clin Endocrinol Metab 70:1375–1384, 1990.

410. Jaquet P, Guibout M, Jaquet C, et al: Circadian regulation of growth hormone secretion after treatment in acromegaly. J Clin Endocrinol Metab 50:322–328, 1980.

411. Iranmanesh A, Lizarralde G, Johnson ML, Veldhuis JD: Nature of altered growth hormone secretion in hyperthyroidism. J Clin Endocrinol Metab 72:108–115, 1991.

412. Van Cauter E, L'Hermite-Balériaux M, Copinschi G, et al: Quantitative analysis of spontaneous variations of plasma prolactin in normal man. Am J Physiol 241:E355–E363, 1981.

413. Desir D, Van Cauter E, L'Hermite-Balériaux M, et al: Effects of "jet lag" on hormonal patterns: III. Demonstration of an intrinsic circadian rhythmicity in plasma prolactin. J Clin Endocrinol Metab 55:849–857, 1982.

414. Copinschi G, Van Onderbergen A, L'Hermite-Balériaux M, et al: Effects of the short-acting benzodiazepine triazolam, taken at bedtime, on circadian and sleep-related hormonal profiles in normal men. Sleep 13:232–244, 1990.

415. Quigley ME, Ishizuka B, Ropert JF, Yen SSC: The food-entrained prolactin and cortisol release in late pregnancy and prolactinoma patients. J Clin Endocrinol Metab 54:1109–1112, 1982.

416. Diaz S, Seron-Ferre M, Cardenas H, et al: Circadian variation of basal plasma prolactin, prolactin response to suckling, and length of amenorrhea in nursing women. J Clin Endocrinol Metab 68:946–955, 1989.

417. Caufriez A, Desir D, Szyper M, et al: Prolactin secretion in Cushing's disease. J Clin Endocrinol Metab 53:843–846, 1981.

418. Iranmanesh A, Veldhuis JD, Carlsen EC, et al: Attenuated pulsatile release of prolactin in men with insulin-dependent diabetes mellitus. J Clin Endocrinol Metab 71:73–78, 1990.

419. Boyar RM, Kapen S, Finkelstein JW, et al: Hypothalamic-pituitary function in diverse hyperprolactinemic states. J Clin Invest 53:1588–1598, 1974.

420. Seki K, Uesato T, Kato K, Shima K: Twenty-four-hour secretory pattern of prolactin in hyperprolactinaemic patients with pituitary micro- and macroadenomas. Acta Endocrinol (Copenh) 106:433–436, 1984.

421. Higuchi T, Takahashi Y, Takahashi K, et al: Twenty-four-hour secretory patterns of growth hormone, prolactin, and cortisol in narcolepsy. J Clin Endocrinol Metab 49:197–204, 1979.

422. Halbreich U, Grunhaus L, Ben-David M: Twenty-four-hour rhythm of prolactin in depressive patients. Arch Gen Psychiatry 36:1183–1186, 1979.

423. Turek FW, Van Cauter E: Rhythms in reproduction. In Knobil E, Nea J (eds): The Physiology of Reproduction. New York, Raven Press, 1993, pp 1789–1830.

424. Jakacki RI, Kelch RP, Sauder SE, et al: Pulsatile secretion of luteinizing hormone in children. J Clin Endocrinol Metab 55:453–458, 1982.

425. Dunkel L, Alfthan H, Stenman UH, et al: Developmental changes in 24-hour profiles of luteinizing hormone and follicle-stimulating hormone from prepuberty to midstages of puberty. J Clin Endocrinol Metab 74:890–897, 1992.

426. Wu FCW, Butler GE, Kelnar CJH, et al: Patterns of pulsatile luteinizing hormone and follicle-stimulating hormone secretion in prepubertal (midchildhood) boys and girls and patients with idiopathic hypogonadotropic hypogonadism (Kallman's syndrome): A study using an ultrasensitive time-resolved immunofluorometric assay. J Clin Endocrinol Metab 72:1229–1237, 1991.

427. Apter D, Bützow TL, Laughlin GA, Yen SSC: Gonadotropin-releasing hormone pulse generator activity during pubertal transition in girls: Pulsatile and diurnal patterns of circulating gonadotropins. J Clin Endocrinol Metab 76:940–949, 1993.

428. Winters SJ: Diurnal rhythm of testosterone and luteinizing hormone in hypogonadal men. J Androl 12:185–190, 1991.

429. Spratt DI, O'Dea LL, Schoenfeld D, et al: Neuroendocrine-gonadal axis in men: Frequent sampling of LH, FSH and testosterone. Am J Physiol 254:E658–E666, 1988.

430. Tenover JS, Matsumoto AM, Clifton DK, Bremner WJ: Age-related alterations in the circadian rhythms of pulsatile luteinizing hormone and testosterone secretion in healthy men. J Gerontol 43:M163–169, 1988.

431. Fehm HL, Clausing J, Kern W, et al: Sleep-associated augmentation and synchronization of luteinizing hormone pulses in adult men. Neuroendocrinology 54:192–195, 1991.

432. Miyatake A, Morimoto Y, Oishi T, et al: Circadian rhythm of serum testosterone and its relationship to sleep: Comparison with the variations in serum luteinizing hormone, prolactin, and cortisol in normal men. J Clin Endocrinol Metab 51:1365–1371, 1980.

433. Yamaguchi MA, Nizunuma H, Miyamoto K, et al: Immunoreactive

inhibin concentrations in adult men: presence of a circadian rhythm. J Clin Endocrinol Metab 72:554–559, 1991.

434. Tenover JS, Bremner WJ: Circadian rhythm of serum immunoreactive inhibin in young and elderly men. J Gerontol 46:M181–184, 1991.

435. Veldhuis JD, Urban RJ, Lizarralde G, et al: Attenuation of luteinizing hormone secretory burst amplitude as a proximate basis for the hypoandrogenism of healthy aging in men. J Clin Endocrinol Metab 75:52–58, 1992.

436. Vermeulen A, Deslypere JP, Kaukman JM: Influence of antiopioids on luteinizing hormone pulsatility in aging men. J Clin Endocrinol Metab 68:68–72, 1989.

437. Reame N, Sauder SE, Kelch RP, Marshall JC: Pulsatile gonadotropin secretion during the human menstrual cycle: Evidence for altered frequency of gonadotropin-releasing hormone secretion. J Clin Endocrinol Metab 59:328–337, 1984.

438. Hall JE, Schoenfeld DA, Martin KA, Crowley WFJ: Hypothalamic gonadotropin-releasing hormone secretion and follicle-stimulating hormone dynamics during the luteal-follicular transition. J Clin Endocrinol Metab 74:600–607, 1992.

439. Genazzani AD, Pentraglia F, Fabbri G, et al: Evidence of luteinizing hormone secretion in hypothalamic amenorrhea associated with weight loss. Fertil Steril 54:222–226, 1990.

440. Khoury SA, Reame NE, Kelch RP, Marshall JC: Diurnal patterns of pulsatile luteinizing hormone secretion in hypothalamic amenorrhea: Reproducibility and responses to opiate blockade and an alpha-adrenergic agonist. J Clin Endocrinol Metab 64:755–762, 1987.

441. Berga SL, Mortola JF, Girton L, et al: Neuroendocrine aberrations in women with functional hypothalamic amenorrhea. J Clin Endocrinol Metab 68:301–308, 1989.

442. Filicori M, Flamigni C, Campaniello E, et al: Evidence for a specific role of GnRH pulse frequency in the control of the human menstrual cycle. Am J Physiol 257:930–936, 1989.

443. Fumming DC, Vickovic MM, Fluker MR: Defects in pulsatile LH release in normally menstruating runners. J Clin Endocrinol Metab 60:810–812, 1985.

444. Bray MA, Muneyyirci-Delale O, Kofinas GD, Reyes FI: Circadian, ultradian, and episodic gonadotropin and prolactin secretion in human pseudocyesis. Acta Endocrinol (Copenh) 124:501–509, 1991.

445. Zumoff B, Freeman R, Coupey S, et al: A chronobiologic abnormality in luteinizing secretion in teenage girls with the polycystic-ovary syndrome. N Engl J Med 309:1206–1209, 1983.

446. Venturoli S, Porcu E, Fabbri R, et al: Episodic pulsatile secretion of FSH, prolactin, oestradiol, oestrone, and LH circadian variations in polycystic ovary syndrome. Clin Endocrinol 28:93–107, 1988.

447. Waldstreicher J, Santoro NF, Hall JE, et al: Hyperfunction of the hypothalamo-pituitary axis in women with polycystic ovarian disease: Indirect evidence for partial gonadotroph desensitization. J Clin Endocrinol Metab 66:165–172, 1988.

448. Blomquist CH, Holt JPJ: Chronobiology of the hypothalamo-pituitary-gonadal axis in men and women. In Touitou Y, Haus E (eds): Biological Rhythms in Clinical and Laboratory Medicine. Berlin, Springer-Verlag, 1992, pp 315–329.

449. Fachinetti F, Genazzani AD, Martignoni E, et al: Neuroendocrine correlates of premenstrual syndrome: Changes in the pulsatile pattern of plasma LH. Psychoneuroendocrinology 15:269–277, 1990.

450. Parry BL: Sleep, mood, and the menstrual cycle. Semin Reprod Med 8:81–88, 1990.

451. Spratt DI, Carr DB, Merriam GR, et al: The spectrum of abnormal patterns of gonadotropin-releasing hormone secretion in men with idiopathic hypogonadotropic hypogonadism: Clinical and laboratory correlations. J Clin Endocrinol Metab 64:283–291, 1987.

452. Winters SJ, Troen P: Testosterone and estradiol are co-secreted episodically by the human testes. J Clin Invest 78:870–873, 1986.

453. Klibanski A, Beitins IZ, Merriam GR, et al: Gonadotropin and prolactin pulsations in hyperprolactinemic women before and during bromocriptine therapy. J Clin Endocrinol Metab 58:1141–1147, 1984.

454. Stevenaert A, Beckers A, Vandalem JL, Hennen G: Early normalization of luteinizing hormone pulsatility after successful transsphenoidal surgery in women with hyperprolactinomas. J Clin Endocrinol Metab 62:1044–1047, 1986.

455. Brabant G, Brabant A, Ranft U, et al: Circadian and pulsatile thyrotropin secretion in euthyroid man under influence of thyroid hormone and glucocorticoid administration. J Clin Endocrinol Metab 65:83–88, 1987.

456. Brabant G, Prank K, Ranft U, et al: Physiological regulation of circa-

dian and pulsatile thyrotropin secretion in normal man and woman. J Clin Endocrinol Metab 70:403–409, 1990.

457. Greenspan SL, Klibanski A, Schoenfeld D, Ridgway EC: Pulsatile secretion of thyrotropin in man. J Clin Endocrinol Metab 63:661–668, 1986.

458. Goichot B, Brandenberger G, Sainio J, et al: Nocturnal plasma thyrotropin variations are related to slow-wave sleep. J Sleep Res 1:186–190, 1992.

459. Mantagos S, Koulouris A, Makri M, Vagenakis AG: Development of thyrotropin circadian rhythm in infancy. J Clin Endocrinol Metab 74:71–74, 1992.

460. Rose SR, Nisula BC: Circadian variation of thyrotropin in childhood. J Clin Endocrinol Metab 68:1086–1090, 1989.

461. Romijn JA, Adriaanse R, Brabant G, et al: Pulsatile secretion of thyrotropin during fasting: A decrease of thyrotropin pulse amplitude. J Clin Endocrinol Metab 70:1631–1636, 1990.

462. Romijn JA, Wiersinga WM: Decreased nocturnal surge of thyrotropin in nonthyroidal illness. J Clin Endocrinol Metab 70:35–42, 1990.

463. Caron PJ, Nieman LK, Rose SR, Nisula BC: Deficient nocturnal surge of thyrotropin in central hypothyroidism. J Clin Endocrinol Metab 62:960–964, 1986.

464. Samuels MH, Lillehei K, Kleinschmidt-Demasters BK, et al: Patterns of pulsatile pituitary glycoprotein secretion in central hypothyroidism and hypogonadism. J Clin Endocrinol Metab 70:391–395, 1990.

465. Bartalena F, Martino E, Petrini L, et al: The nocturnal serum thyrotropin surge is abolished in patients with ACTH-dependent or ACTH-independent Cushing's syndrome. J Clin Endocrinol Metab 72:1195–1199, 1991.

466. Bartalena L, Martino E, Brandi LS, et al: Lack of nocturnal serum thyrotropin surge after surgery. J Clin Endocrinol Metab 70:293–296, 1990.

467. Bartalena L, Placidi GF, Martino E, et al: Nocturnal serum thyrotropin (TSH) surge and the TSH response to TSH-releasing hormone: Dissociated behavior in untreated depressives. J Clin Endocrinol Metab 71:650–655, 1990.

468. Bartalena L, Cossu E, Grasso L, et al: Relationship between nocturnal serum thyrotropin peak and metabolic control in diabetic patients. J Clin Endocrinol Metab 76:983–987, 1993.

469. Bartalena L, Martino E, Velluzzi F, et al: The lack of nocturnal serum thyrotropin surge in patients with non-toxic nodular goiter may predict the subsequent occurrence of hyperthyroidism. J Clin Endocrinol Metab 73:604–608, 1991.

470. Carroll K, Nestel P: Diurnal variation in glucose tolerance and in insulin secretion in man. Diabetes 22:333–348, 1973.

471. Jarrett RJ: Rhythms in insulin and glucose. In Krieger D (ed): Endocrine Rhythms. New York, Raven Press, 1979, pp 247–258.

472. Service FJ, Hall LD, Westland RE, et al: Effects of size, time of day and sequence of meal ingestion on carbohydrate tolerance in normal subjects. Diabetologia 25:316–321, 1983.

473. Verrillo A, De Teresa A, Martino C, et al: Differential roles of splanchnic and peripheral tissues in determining diurnal fluctuation of glucose tolerance. Am J Physiol 257:E459–E465, 1989.

474. Lee A, Agajanian T, Bray GA: Diurnal variation in insulin sensitivity exists in normal subjects, but not in obese subjects. Diabetes 34:125a, 1985.

475. Shapiro ET, Polonsky KS, Copinschi G, et al: Nocturnal elevation of glucose levels during fasting in noninsulin-dependent diabetes. J Clin Endocrinol Metab 72:444–454, 1991.

476. Van Cauter E, Blackman JD, Roland D, et al: Modulation of glucose regulation and insulin secretion by circadian rhythmicity and sleep. J Clin Invest 88:934–942, 1991.

477. Lang D, Matthews D, Burnett M, et al: Pulsatile, synchronous basal insulin and glucagon secretion in man. Diabetes 31:22–26, 1982.

478. Hansen BC, Jen KL, Pek SB, Wolfe RA: Rapid oscillations in plasma insulin, glucagon, and glucose in obese and normal weight humans. J Clin Endocrinol Metab 54:785–792, 1982.

479. Matthews D, Lang D, Burnett M, Turner R: Control of pulsatile insulin secretion in man. Diabetologia 24:231–237, 1983.

480. Sturis J, O'Meara NM, Shapiro ET, et al: Differential effects of glucose stimulation upon rapid pulses and ultradian oscillations of insulin secretion. J Clin Endocrinol Metab 76:895–901, 1993.

481. Chou HF, Ipp E: Pulsatile insulin secretion in isolated rat islets. Diabetes 39:112–117, 1990.

482. Bolli G, Gerich J: The "dawn phenomenon"—A common occurrence in both non-insulin-dependent and insulin-dependent diabetes mellitus. N Engl J Med 310:746–750, 1984.

483. Clarke W, Haymond M, Santiago J: Overnight basal insulin requirements in fasting insulin-dependent diabetics. Diabetes 29:78–80, 1980.
484. Bright G, Melton T, Rogol A, Clarke W: Failure of cortisol blockade to inhibit early morning increases in basal insulin requirements in fasting insulin-dependent diabetics. Diabetes 29:662–664, 1980.
485. Schmidt M, Hadji-Georgopoulos A, Rendell M, et al: The dawn phenomenon, an early morning glucose rise: Implications for diabetic intraday blood glucose variation. Diabetes Care 4:579–585, 1981.
486. Campbell P, Bolli G, Cryer P, Gerich J: Pathogenesis of the dawn phenomenon in patients with insulin-dependent diabetes mellitus. N Engl J Med 312:1473–1479, 1985.
487. Davidson M, Harris M, Ziel F, Rosenberg C: Suppression of sleep-induced growth hormone secretion by anticholinergic agent abolishes dawn phenomenon. Diabetes 37:166–171, 1988.
488. Beaufrere B, Beylot M, Metz C, et al: Dawn phenomenon in type 1 (insulin-dependent) diabetic adolescents: Influence of nocturnal growth hormone secretion. Diabetologia 31:607–611, 1988.
489. Altiea JA, Ryder RRJ, Vora J, et al: Dawn phenomenon: Its frequency in non-insulin-dependent diabetic patients on conventional therapy. Diabetes Care 10:461–465, 1987.
490. Beebe CA, Van Cauter E, Shapiro ET, et al: Effect of temporal distribution of calories on the diurnal patterns of glucose levels and insulin secretion in NIDDM. Diabetes Care 13:748–755, 1990.
491. Reaven G, Hollenbeck C, Jeng C-Y, et al: Measurement of plasma glucose free fatty acid, lactate, and insulin for 24 h in patients with NIDDM. Diabetes 37:1020–1024, 1988.
492. Chen YDI, Jeng CY, Hollenbeck CB, et al: Relationship between plasma glucose and insulin concentration, glucose production, and glucose disposal in normal subjects and patients with non-insulin-dependent diabetes. J Clin Invest 82:21–25, 1988.
493. O'Rahilly S, Turner R, Matthews D: Impaired pulsatile secretion of insulin in relatives of patients with non-insulin-dependent diabetes. N Engl J Med 318:1225–1230, 1988.
494. Polonsky KS, Given BD, Hirsch LJ, et al: Abnormal patterns of insulin secretion in non-insulin-dependent diabetes mellitus. N Engl J Med 318:1231–1239, 1988.
495. Simon C, Brandenberger G, Follenius M, Schlienger JL: Alteration in the temporal organisation of insulin secretion in type 2 (non-insulin-dependent) diabetic patients under continuous enteral nutrition. Diabetologia 34:435–440, 1991.
496. Cagnacci A, Elliott JA, Yen SSC: Melatonin: A major regulator of the circadian rhythm of core temperature in humans. J Clin Endocrinol Metab 75:447–452, 1992.
497. Cardinali DP, Vacas MI: Pineal gland, photoperiodic responses, and puberty. J Endocrinol Invest 7:157–165, 1984.
498. Waldhauser F, Boepple PA, Schemper M, et al: Serum melatonin in central precocious puberty is lower than in age-matched prepubertal children. J Clin Endocrinol Metab 73:793–796, 1991.
499. Waldhauser F, Weiszenbacher G, Tatzer E, et al: Alterations in nocturnal serum melatonin levels in humans with growth and aging. J Clin Endocrinol Metab 66:648–652, 1988.
500. Berga SL, Mortola JF, Yen SSC: Amplification of nocturnal melatonin secretion in women with functional hypothalamic amenorrhea. J Clin Endocrinol Metab 66:242–244, 1988.
501. Tortosa F, Puig-Domingo M, Peinado MA, et al: Enhanced circadian rhythm of melatonin in anorexia nervosa. Acta Endocrinol (Copenh) 120:574–578, 1989.
502. Laughlin GA, Loucks AB, Yen SSC: Marked augmentation of nocturnal melatonin secretion in amenorrheic athletes, but not in cycling athletes: unaltered by opioidergic or dopaminergic blockade. J Clin Endocrinol Metab 73:1321–1326, 1991.
503. Cagnacci A, Elliott JA, Yen SSC: Amplification of pulsatile LH secretion by exogenous melatonin in women. J Clin Endocrinol Metab 73:210–212, 1991.
504. Armstrong SM: Melatonin: A chronobiotic with anti-aging properties? Med Hypotheses 34:300–309, 1991.
505. Cassone VM: Effects of melatonin on vertebrate circadian systems. TINS 13:457–464, 1990.
506. Waldhauser F, Weiszenbacher G, Frisch H, et al: Fall in nocturnal serum melatonin during prepuberty and pubescence. Lancet 1:362–365, 1984.
507. Attanasio A, Borrelli P, Gupta D: Circadian rhythms in serum melatonin from infancy to adolescence. J Clin Endocrinol Metab 61:388–390, 1985.

Somatic Growth and Maturation

ROBERT L. ROSENFIELD
JOSÉ F. CARA

Growth is an inherent property of life. Normal somatic growth requires the integrated function of many of the hormonal, metabolic, and other growth factors discussed in preceding chapters. This chapter will first briefly review the determinants of growth. Then it will deal in detail with the overall result of these processes—normal growth patterns. Finally, the differential diagnosis and management of disorders of growth will be discussed.

DETERMINANTS OF GROWTH: BIOLOGICAL, BIOCHEMICAL, AND ENDOCRINOLOGICAL

Cellular Growth

The body grows primarily through proliferation of cells by mitosis.[1, 2] Increase in cell size generally plays more of a role in organ growth as development approaches completion. The ratio of increment in cell number to increment in cell size changes during life. It is highest during the period of differentiation, the diversification of structure and function that occurs during the first 16 weeks of gestation in humans. The entire growth process requires an intrinsically normal cell that is nourished by an optimal milieu (with respect to pH, trace minerals, and substrates for structural and energy purposes) and that is exposed to the necessary growth factors. Cell growth during differentiation and development is regulated by the same mechanisms that determine physiological responses in the mature cell.

Cells replicate by a complicated series of events collectively known as the *cell cycle*. There are two main steps in the cell cycle, interphase and mitosis.[3–5] Cell proliferation requires extracellular signals to move the cell from the resting state (G_0) into the first phase of growth (G_1). Growth is initiated by peptides that interact with cell surface receptors which trigger intracellular second messenger systems. These include cyclic nucleotides, Ca^{2+}, inositol phosphates, and polyamines. *Proto-oncogene* products such as *fos* and *jun* appear early and are thought to activate transcription of genes important for later steps of the cycle. The cell cycle is believed to be regulated by "competence" and "progression" factors. The first subphase of G_1 requires competence factors that induce the potential competence to synthesize DNA.[7] Platelet-derived growth factor and fibroblast growth factor exemplify competence factors specific for mesenchymal cells. After achieving competence, cells require essential amino acids to progress to a checkpoint in the cycle at which progression factors can induce competent cells to complete G_1. Such factors are exemplified by epidermal growth factor, insulin, insulin-like growth factor I (IGF-I), thyroxine, and hydrocortisone.[6–8] Cells are held at a checkpoint at the end of G_1 by the action of p53 protein, a *tumor suppressor*.[9] Cytoplasmic signals then initiate the phase of DNA synthesis (S phase). Processes beyond this point in the cell cycle depend on intracellularly triggered controls. The entire genome must be duplicated with extreme rapidity and precision during this phase.[10] Failure to complete replication within S phase leads to chromosomal breakage. During the phase after completion of DNA synthesis (G_2), the individual cell doubles its entire contents. G_2 is characterized by accumulation of mitosis-specific protein kinases associated with *cyclins*. Cyclins and a cell division cycle protein, p34, comprise maturation-promoting factor (MPF), which, when activated,[6] triggers mitosis (M phase of cycle).[11]

Somatic Growth

Skeletal differentiation occurs concomitantly with rapid growth during the first trimester.[12] Linear growth occurs primarily by endochondral bone formation.[13] The chondrocytes of the epiphysis lay down an orderly cartilage template. The cartilage becomes calcified, chondrocyte degeneration occurs, and the cartilage cross-bands are lysed. This leaves longitudinal spicules extending into the metaphysis. Mesenchymal progenitor cells then differentiate into osteoblasts, which deposit osteoid onto this template. The specific bone matrix protein osteocalcin appears to index this osteoblastic activity.[14] Bone is formed by calcification of osteoid. This primary spongiosa is remodeled by osteoclasts, according to the demands of physical stress. Bone remodeling is tightly coupled via growth factors to bone formation. The cycle of bone cell differentiation for structural purposes is closely linked to the overall metabolic needs for calcium and phosphorus homeostatis by the actions of parathormone, calciferol, and calcitonin.

Good *nutrition* is essential for optimal growth and maturation.[15-17] Multiple factors are involved. Energy sources, calories, and oxygen seem particularly critical for cell multiplication. Between about 2 and 13 per cent of normal energy consumption goes into promoting growth.[1, 18] Oxygen consumption and metabolic rate per gram fall with age.[18-20] Protein intake is relatively important for normal growth in cellular size. Protein intake must be adequate with respect to both amount and provision of essential amino acids or their ketoanalogues, or nitrogen accretion and growth cannot occur.[21-23] Essential fatty acids are necessary for normal growth in lower animals, but this may not hold true for primates.[24] Vitamins A and D are important for normal growth.[1, 25] Trace metals, such as zinc, are probably essential for normal growth and sexual maturation[26-29] because of their role as co-factors for enzyme function. In this regard, the pH must be maintained at optimal levels to conserve mineral homeostasis.[30] The general level of activity seems to promote body growth, just as normal muscular activity is necessary for limb growth. Viteri[31] has reported decreased efficiency of nitrogen accretion and growth in inactive rats.

Hormones are essential catalysts of growth. Yet, as can be seen from the preceding discussion, they are not the only growth-promoting factors. Hormones bring about specific patterns of cell growth.[1] Growth hormone (GH) and thyroid hormones are especially important for cell multiplication. Thyroid hormone has more noticeable effects on cell size than growth hormone. However, these effects of thyroid hormones seem paradoxical, cell size being small in congenital hypothyroidism and large in acquired hypothyroidism. Sex steroids are capable of stimulating both hyperplasia and hypertrophy in target organs to an extent that is organ-specific and may be sex- and steroid-specific.[32] There is evidence that estrogens inhibit cell multiplication in muscle[1] while promoting it in the cartilage of females.[33]

GH secretion is normally mainly controlled by the balance between hypothalamic secretion of growth hormone–releasing factor (GRF) and somatostatin, which is, in turn, subject to periodic regulation by higher cerebral centers[34-37] (Fig. 141–1). GH secretion rises during puberty.[37] Serum GH is approximately 50 per cent bound to GH binding protein, which rises through childhood.[38] This binding protein appears to be an alternatively spliced form of the extracellular domain of the GH receptor. Evidence is emerging that GH receptors and GH binding protein are differentially regulated, however.[39] It has been suggested that continuous exposure to GH is required for up-regula-

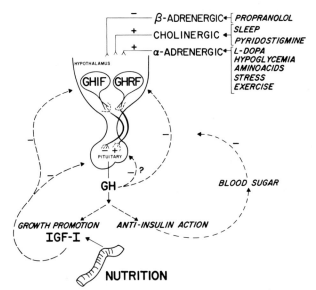

FIGURE 141–1. Major factors in regulation of growth hormone (GH) secretion (+ = stimulators of GH release; − = inhibitors of GH release). GH secretion is stimulated primarily by hypothalamic GH-releasing factor (GHRF) and inhibited by hypothalamic somatostatin (GHIF) neuronal secretion. GH is secreted after integration of diverse hypothalamic stimuli. Secretion of GH is facilitated by α-adrenergic, dopaminergic, and cholinergic neurons to the hypothalamus. It is inhibited by β-adrenergic tracts. GH directly exerts negative feedback at the level of the hypothalamus and possibly at the pituitary gland. GH secretion is also inhibited by insulin-like growth factor I (IGF-I), which appears to inhibit GH secretion directly at the pituitary gland and indirectly through stimulation of somatostatin release. (Modified from Schaff-Blass E, Burstein S, Rosenfield RL: Advances in diagnosis and treatment of short stature, with special reference to the role of growth hormone. J Pediatr 104:801, 1984.)

tion of liver GH receptors, but that GH pulsatility is crucial for maximal stimulation of growth and IGF-I.[40] GH appears to stimulate growth through dual effects. It induces the formation of chondrocyte colonies directly and makes them responsive to the growth-promoting effect of somatomedins (insulin-like growth factors, IGF's) produced both elsewhere and locally in response to GH.[41]

IGF-I (somatomedin-C) production is more indicative of GH status than that of other IGF's.[41] GH stimulates both hepatic and target cell IGF-I generation. IGF-I produced in growing cells acts through autocrine or paracrine mechanisms, having its biological actions at or near sites of origin. Plasma IGF-I rises throughout the prepubertal years and then increases further during puberty (Table 141–1). The prepubertal rise correlates with the rising level of the GH-dependent, most abundant high-affinity IGF binding protein, IGFBP-3.[42] The pubertal increase in IGF-I is mediated primarily by sex hormone stimulation of GH secretion.[43]

Factors other than GH regulate plasma IGF-I concentrations. The nutritional state is a major independent determinant. Severe malnutrition decreases plasma IGF-I levels despite normal or elevated GH concentrations. IGF-I levels and somatomedin activity rise during the prepubertal years[44] without any change in GH. Prolactin appears to have a slight effect, and small amounts of thyroid hormone and cortisol are necessary.[45] Insulin is synergistic with small amounts of GH in hypopituitary rats.[46]

The relationship of plasma IGF-I levels to normal growth is poorly understood. IGF-I levels rise during compensatory

TABLE 141–1. TYPICAL NORMAL PLASMA IGF-I CONCENTRATIONS

AGE	MALES (NG/ML)		FEMALES (NG/ML)	
	Mean	Range	Mean	Range
0–2 years	42	14–98	56	14–238
3–5 years	56	59–210	84	21–322
6–10 years	98	28–308	182	56–364
Prepubertal > 10 years	126	84–182	182	70–280
Early pubertal	210	140–420	224	84–392
Midpubertal	266	168–392	434	154–644
Late pubertal	364	224–462	434	224–686
Adults > 23 years	112	42–266	140	56–308

Exact results may vary with particular assay system and standard. To convert these data to units, divide by 140.

From Schaff-Blass E, Burstein S, Rosenfield RL: Advances in diagnosis and treatment of short stature, with special reference to the role of growth hormone. J Pediatr 104:801, 1984.

growth of the kidney even in hypophysectomized rats.[47] Peripheral responsiveness to IGF-I decreases with age.[48] Plasma IGF-I levels do not correlate with growth rate in childhood except during the pubertal growth spurt.[34] IGF binding proteins hinder IGF-I bioavailability under some circumstances[49] but not others.[42] IGF bioactivity is also influenced by somatomedin inhibitory factors present in serum. Examples of such inhibitors are peptides and glucocorticoids.[50, 51]

IGF-I levels and growth may be normal with subnormal plasma GH levels in two pathological conditions. The first of these is obesity.[44, 52] Hypernutrition itself may be the stimulus to growth. It is doubtful whether this situation is entirely due to the accompanying change in insulin secretion, although insulin is a growth-promoting hormone,[53] because the blood insulin level achieved in obese humans is probably too low to have IGF-I activity. The second condition occurs in hypopituitary patients who have the *growth without growth hormone syndrome*.[54] Most often this syndrome has been identified after treatment for pituitary tumors, but the syndrome has been recognized occasionally in congenital or idiopathic hypopituitarism. Most such patients have obesity and diabetes insipidus; hyperprolactinemia is seldom found. Recent evidence suggests that growth results from secretion of a non-GH growth factor by pituitary tissue.[55, 56] Other theories include production of a variant form of GH[57] or residual production of IGF-II.[40]

Glucocorticoids in above-normal amounts are inhibitors of linear growth.[57, 58] The smallest dose of cortisone that is crucial for growth inhibition averages approximately 15 mg/m²/day. Corticoids have effects on GH secretion that are just now becoming clear. Glucocorticoid in small amounts is necessary for GH secretion, and dexamethasone administration acutely promotes GH secretion; however, prolonged or large glucocorticoid doses clearly suppress the GH response to GRF and 24-h integrated GH levels.[35, 59, 60] Corticoids also inhibit IGF action,[44] while IGF-I plasma levels are normal. Since glucocorticoids inhibit bone formation, they may antagonize bone growth at a site distal to IGF-I action. Such effects may be counteracted by androgen[61] and to a lesser extent by GH. Clues are beginning to emerge regarding the molecular mechanism of action of glucocorticoid growth inhibition. The glucocorticoid-receptor complex suppresses the activity of the transcription factor AP-1.[62, 63] AP-1 is involved in mediating both proliferative responses to growth factors and collagenase synthesis in response to phorbol esters, and its subunits are coded for by the proto-oncogenes c-*jun* and c-*fos*. Its activity is inhibited by glucocorticoid doses one order of magnitude below those required for gene activation.

Increased secretion of sex hormones clearly initiates the pubertal growth spurt. The limited data available indicate that the peak growth velocity of boys normally occurs at a testosterone production rate of 50 to 100 mg/m²/month.[64] Physiological levels of estrogen contribute to the pubertal growth spurt of girls, in contrast to the inhibitory effect of high doses of estrogen.[65] Sex hormones also may play a subtle role in normal fetal and prepubertal growth. Plasma testosterone, estradiol, and dehydroepiandrosterone levels of the fetus are equal to or greater than those of the pubertal male.[65–67] The effects of sex hormones on fetoplacental growth are complex and poorly understood. For example, estrogen promotes fetal bone development, yet some evidence suggests that estrogen inhibits placental and fetal growth. Boys have higher plasma testosterone levels[68] and a slightly greater growth rate in early infancy than girls. Evidence is emerging that prepubertal girls normally produce estrogen.[67] Adrenocortical production of 17-ketosteroids begins to increase at about 6 years of age. It has been reported that dehydroepiandrosterone sulfate promotes calcification of cartilage and that subandrogenic doses of androstenedione promote growth.[67]

Fetal Growth

Fetal and postnatal requirements for growth differ in several respects. Growth in utero seems relatively free from some of the hormonal controls so important in extrauterine life. GH and thyroxine do not seem to play important roles in fetal somatic growth, as indicated by the following evidence. The congenitally hyposomatotropic or hypothyroid human is often of normal size at birth, although neither hormone crosses the placenta well.[69, 70] Fetal hypophysectomy by means of decapitation or thyroid ablation of the experimental animal does not necessarily prevent attainment of normal fetal size.[71] However, about 50 per cent of congenitally GH-deficient or GH-resistant patients are short at birth.[72] Furthermore, body size and organ cellularity of anencephalic infants can be correlated with the amount of pituitary tissue. Maternal T₄ contributes to about one third of the fetus's blood level and so may contribute to growth.[73] Furthermore, bone maturation of the congenitally hypothyroid fetus becomes impaired during the last trimester.[74]

Fetal growth depends on placental growth, which, in turn, has multiple determinants, such as maternal nutrition and uteroplacental blood flow. Placental growth influences fetal growth through diverse mechanisms, such as nutrition, oxygenation, and perhaps placental hormones. Human placental lactogen (chorionic somatomammotropin, hCS) may contribute to the growth of the placenta. The placental concentration of this hormone correlates with placental size as well as birth size of twins[75] and fetal IGF levels.[76] However, the isolated absence of human placental lactogen is of no biological consequence.[77] Novel peptides in the prolactin-GH family have been identified in rat placenta.[78] A placental GRF system has been identified recently.[79]

Serum IGF levels rise during gestation and correlate with size at birth.[76, 80] IGF-II seems to be the major somatomedin in the fetus, and its tissue levels are regulated independently of GH.[76, 81] Although IGF-I levels are lower than those of IGF-II in fetal blood, they are significantly related to birth size.[72] The rise in IGF-I levels during fetal life is accompanied by a distribution of IGF binding proteins resembling that of hyposomatotropic subjects. Fetal rat cartilage has been reported to be resistant to IGF action.[48] Although prolactin probably has only about 5 per cent the anabolic potency of GH,[82] it may contribute to nitrogen retention in the fetus, in which levels are quite high. Insulin itself has been postulated to contribute to normal intrauterine growth.[83]

PATTERNS OF NORMAL SOMATIC GROWTH

Intrauterine Growth

The most rapid relative increase in growth occurs in the first trimester[12] (Table 141–2). The normal rate of third-trimester fetal somatic growth has been estimated from cross-sectional data regarding size attained by live-born babies of various gestational ages. The standards for intrauterine growth collected between 1959 and 1966 by the National Institute of Neurological and Communicative Disorders and Stroke are shown in Figure 141–2.[84] The data are representative of the general population in the United States. Nevertheless, they share some deficiencies common to all such studies—namely, that it is difficult to estimate gestational age accurately and that it is possible that prematurity may represent the consequences of an unidentified unphysiological state that has retarded growth. The tenth percentile of the original standards (Lubchenco), collected earlier in a medically indigent population at an altitude of about 1 mile,[85] is about 200 g less at 28 weeks and 100 g less at 40 weeks with respect to weight and about 4 cm less at 28 weeks and 1.5 cm less at 40 weeks with respect to length. It is not clear whether there are any systematic differences between the intrauterine growth of blacks and whites.[86, 87] The overall pattern of fetal growth shown by all workers indicates that the rate of weight gain is fastest during the early portion of the third trimester in parallel with growth of subcutaneous fat and muscle. Lin-

TABLE 141–2. CROWN–HEEL LENGTH AND WEIGHT OF HUMAN EMBRYOS AND IMMATURE FETUSES

GESTATIONAL AGE (WK)	LENGTH (MM)	WEIGHT (G)
1	0.1	—
2	0.2	—
7	19	—
8	30	1
12	73	14
16	157	105
20	239	310
24	296	640
28	355	1080

From Arey LB: Developmental Anatomy (ed 6). Philadelphia, WB Saunders Co, 1954.

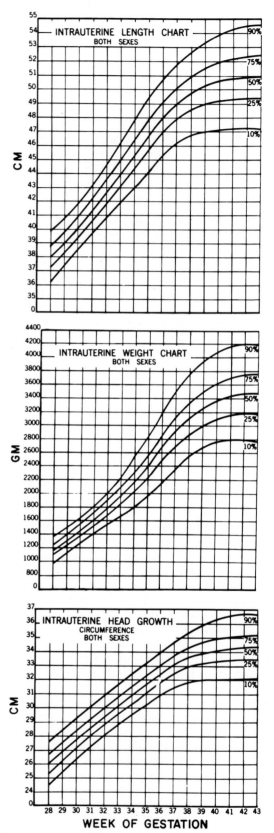

FIGURE 141–2. Intrauterine growth chart. (From Naeye RL, Dixon JB: Distortions in fetal growth standards. Pediatr Res 12:987, 1978.)

ear growth, on the other hand, begins to slow at about 36 weeks. Head circumference reflects brain growth to a great extent. Secondary ossification centers appear radiographically in fetal endochondral bone in the following order:

calcaneus, talus, distal femoral epiphysis, proximal tibial epiphysis, and cuboid.[88] The gestational age by which each of these centers appears in about 50 per cent of the population is 24, 28, 36, 38, and 42 weeks, respectively.

Healthy infants born prematurely continue to grow in length at the same rate they would have grown in utero.[89-91] Consequently, small differences are found between the lengths of preterm and full-term infants when followed up at 1 to 5 years of age. The weights of premature infants tend to increase along the fetal weight percentile into which they dip in the first few days of life. Weight seems appropriate for height once these measurements can be plotted on the postnatal standards used for full-term infants.[91]

Several major common family and environmental (uteroplacental) variables affect birth size independently of gestational age.[85, 92-95] Genetic factors include (1) fetal sex (male infant average is 150 g larger than female infant average by 38 weeks' gestation), (2) sibling birth weight (the prediction of size at birth is about one third more accurate when sibling birth weight is taken into account), and (3) maternal size (each 10 kg by which a mother's midpregnancy weight differs from the average is correlated with a 150-g difference from average birth weight; maternal height has relatively less influence except when it is less than 150 cm). Fetal hypoxia inhibits intrauterine growth.[96, 97] Parity and multiparity alter fetal growth, seemingly via uteroplacental factors. Later babies tend to be 100 g heavier than the first after 32 weeks' gestation, an effect that has been ascribed to more efficient uterine blood flow. Growth is unaffected by the number of fetuses until about 30 weeks.[98] Subsequently, the rate of weight gain slows, such that twins, for example, each average about 700 g less than singletons at term. Monozygotic twins, especially monochorionic, are more discordant in size (and anomalies) than dizygotic.[99] This discrepancy may be related to unequal distribution of blood flow, placental arteriovenous anastomoses between monozygotic twins being somewhat more frequent. Growth can be monitored longitudinally in utero and related to centiles adjusted for these variables.[95]

Postnatal Growth

Linear growth standards are shown in Figure 141–3.[100] Linear growth velocity is most rapid in infancy and decreases geometrically during this period, unlike the situation thereafter. Clear shifts in linear growth percentile rank occur in two thirds of normal infants. Furthermore, the body segments of infants do not necessarily grow in proportion to one another, as in the remainder of the prepubertal period.[101] A stable linear growth channel is typically established by 2 to 3 years of age.[102] The factors regulating growth during about the first 2 years of life are not well understood. Birth size correlates loosely with subsequent early childhood growth.[103] Infants congenitally deficient in GH or thyroid hormone grow more rapidly in the neonatal period than in later childhood (see below).[104] Therefore, it seems as if the growth curve of infants is the result of an initial vector that is produced by the factors uniquely affecting intrauterine growth (e.g., uteroplacental function and GH-independent cell proliferation) superimposed on a vector that represents the factors that determine subsequent growth during childhood (e.g., genetic, endocrine, and other systemic factors discussed below).

Normal prepubertal children after 2 to 3 years of age have a strong tendency to grow along a predictable channel that corresponds to a given height-attained percentile.[100] Figure 141–3 shows current cross-sectional growth standards and percentiles in the United States. There is a "secular trend" toward increasing height of the population with time; the mean height of American 18-year-olds in 1963 to 1975 exceeded that in 1930 to 1945 by about 2.3 cm. Linear growth occurs at a relatively constant rate of about 6 cm/year during midchildhood. The height-attained channel can be expressed mathematically as a triple logistic function of age and growth velocity after 1 year of age[105]; this consists of early childhood, midchildhood, and pubertal components. However, spontaneous long-term drifts in the statural growth track may occur in normal children. On rare occasions, a gradual change of as much as 40 percentile positions in height attained may occur over a period of several years.[106]

Children cross height-velocity percentiles (Fig. 141–4) to maintain their "distance" channel.[107, 108] Growth consistently along the third percentile for height velocity will lead to a subnormal height. Deflections from an individual's growth channel are firmly resisted, as if growth is being channeled to reach a genetically predetermined target size. This *developmental channelization* of growth occurs in humans, as it does in lower organisms.[109] The mechanisms by which the growth channel is maintained are unknown. The factors involved may be inherent, analogous to those determining cell density in tissue culture.[110] Healthy children maintain their percentile position with respect to height attained by means of short-term fluctuations in growth velocity.[107, 111] These oscillations may be marked, growth sometimes seeming nil over 3-month periods. It is suspected that these changes are related to minor intercurrent illness, although this has not been proved.[112] The variations tend to be seasonal, a "blooming" trend most often occurring in the spring and summer.

An individual's growth channel has genetic origins. The genetic target height is obtained by calculating the midparent height (the average of the parents' heights) and adding 6.5 cm for boys or subtracting 6.5 cm for girls. Parental height correlates with child height by 2 years ($r = 0.5$).[102, 113] Some of the determinants for bone-growth proportions reside on the sex chromosomes. On the basis of studies in men with two Y chromosomes, it seems as if this chromosome may enhance stature commencing in antenatal life.[114, 115] Studies of prepubertal patients with Klinefelter's syndrome have led to the conclusion that their extra X chromosome is responsible for their eunuchoid proportions.[116] The distal short arm of the X chromosome also clearly carries genetic determinants for bone growth; this set of genes is not subject to X inactivation. A variety of evidence from pathological states indicates that other genetic determinants of growth lie on the autosomes.

Catch-up growth occurs upon relief from a chronic illness that has retarded growth. Such compensatory changes may completely preserve the child's height potential. During the period of recovery, the growth-velocity deficit that has been incurred is matched by an equal velocity excess.[117] The rate of compensatory growth exceeds that expected for the age at which growth had been arrested. Catch-up

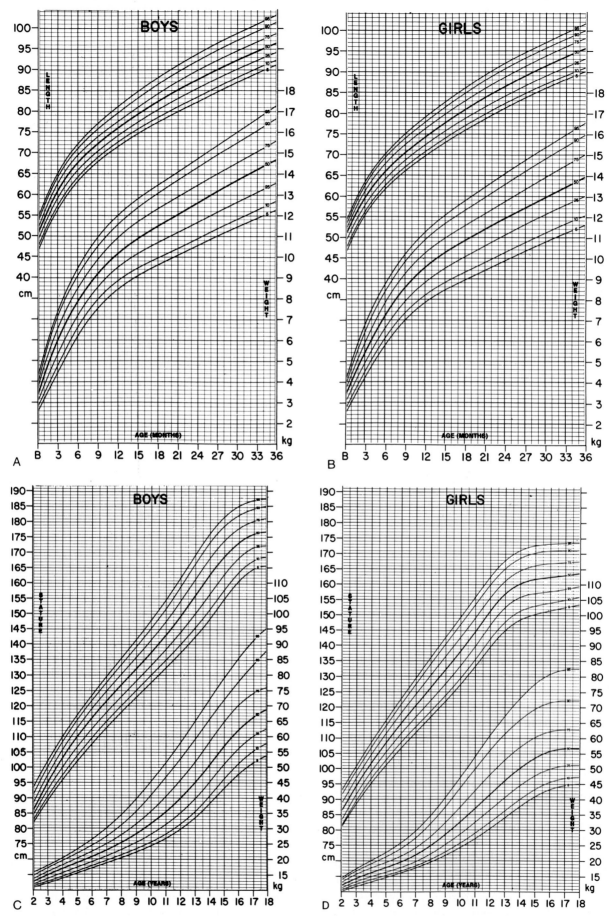

FIGURE 141–3. Current standards for height and weight of normal children in the United States. Smoothed percentiles from 5th to 95th are shown; the data are not normally distributed. *A,B,* Infant growth charts for length and weight from Fels Research Institute. *C,D,* Older children's growth charts for standing height and weight from National Health Examination Survey, 1963–1975.

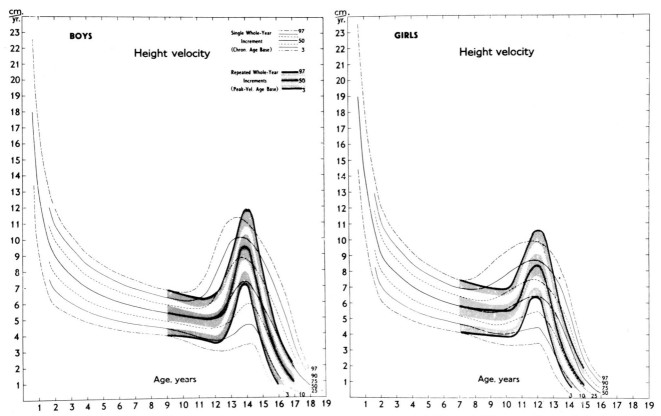

FIGURE 141–4. Growth velocity charts modified from Tanner to emphasize 3rd, 50th, and 97th percentiles based on years before and after age of pubertal peak height velocity. Peak height velocity in North American children currently occurs between 11.5 and 15.2 years of age in boys and 9.6 and 13.2 years of age in girls. (Modified from Tanner JM, Whitehouse RH, Takaishi M: Standards from birth to maturity for height, weight, height velocity, and weight velocity: British children, 1965. Arch Dis Child 41:454, 613, 1966.)

growth has been documented following successful treatment of hypothyroidism, renal acidosis, malnutrition, and Cushing's syndrome.[109, 117] A different kind of catch-up growth (type 2) occurs following adequate therapy of sexual precocity.[118, 119] In this situation, restoration of height potential occurs because restitutional linear growth proceeds without bone maturation advancement; i.e., "height age" catches up to "bone age." Complete compensation for growth failure cannot occur in either growth-retarded or growth-accelerated patients if the growth disorder is of many years' duration and extends to within 3 to 4 years of the onset of normal puberty.[120] The possibility that subtle changes in hormone dynamics may mediate compensatory growth seems likely. Spontaneous GH secretion and IGF-I levels rise during the catch-up growth of hypothyroid patients induced by replacement therapy.[121] Our experience with children partially deficient in GH and thyrotropin (TSH) indicates that more GH is required for catch-up than for normal growth. In response to thyroid hormone replacement, growth rate normalizes, but catch-up growth does not occur until GH is added.

Growth of bone mass can now be measured in populations. Age, sex, body weight, and race account for about half the variance.[122, 123]

The timing of the onset of the adolescent growth spurt is to some extent a determinant of mature height. Some of the greater ultimate height of boys compared with girls results from their longer period of prepubertal growth.[105]

Boys also have a greater peak linear growth velocity than girls.[108] During the course of sexual maturation, the epiphyseal cartilage plates become progressively obliterated, with resultant fusion of the shafts and epiphyseal ossification centers, at which time linear growth ceases. Because the pubertal spurts of individuals occur out of phase, the magnitude of this pubertal growth spurt is not apparent from cross-sectional data. The normal child may transiently dip below the third percentile of standard height-attained graphs if puberty occurs at a later than average age. In order to appreciate the normal pattern of growth during adolescence, one must turn to growth-velocity standards based on longitudinal data. The lower percentiles on height-velocity charts based on cross-sectional data are misleadingly wide. Height-velocity standards are meaningful for teenagers only when interpreted in terms of pubertal events, such as the age at which peak height velocity (see Fig. 141–4) or age of menarche (Fig. 141–5) occurs.[124] Peak growth velocity follows the onset of sexual maturation. Height-velocity standards based on longitudinal data show that the third percentile for linear growth ranges from 3.7 cm/year prepubertally to 7.2 cm/year at the time of peak pubertal growth in boys. The respective figures are 4.1 and 6.2 cm/year for girls.[108]

Early maturers have more brisk pubertal growth than late maturers. For example, boys entering puberty 2 years earlier than average follow percentiles that peak 1.4 cm/year greater than those of boys entering at an average

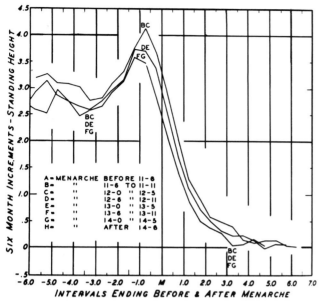

FIGURE 141-5. Growth increments (cm) in years before and after menarche. Groups of cases menstruating at different ages are arranged so that points corresponding to the advent of menarche are in the same vertical line. (Modified from Shuttleworth FK: Sexual maturation and physical growth of girls age six to nineteen. Monogr Soc Res Child Dev 2:5, 1937.)

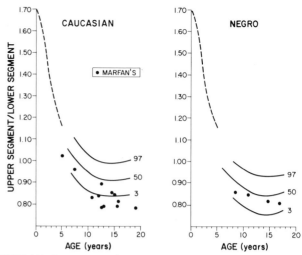

FIGURE 141-6. Normal standards for the ratio of upper segment to lower segment of the body. Lower segment is the measurement from the top of the symphysis pubis to the heel; upper segment is computed by subtracting the lower segment from height. Dotted line shows the average for young children in 1932. (Percentile and Marfan data from McKusick VA: Heritable Disorders of Connective Tissue (ed 4). St. Louis, CV Mosby, 1972. Reproduced with permission.)

age. Late-maturing boys grow less than average by a comparable amount; this phenomenon is less pronounced in girls.[108] This tendency occurs at comparable levels of bone maturation.[125] In late puberty, deceleration of growth occurs. In girls, this slowing usually begins shortly prior to the onset of menses; hence girls generally achieve only 7 cm further growth subsequent to menarche. Only about 1 cm of growth occurs after fusion is complete in the femur and tibia. Statural growth ceases at the median ages of 17 years in girls and 18 years in boys.[125] Growth of nonwhite American children differs from that of whites in some particulars. Black children from 5 to 12 years of age are approximately 7 cm taller than white children matched for family income, but puberty occurs about 0.28 year earlier than in whites, so after 14 years the size of blacks and whites is virtually identical.[126, 127] Median heights of Oriental-American boys are less than those of whites by about 5 cm during the prepubertal years, but they undergo a later growth spurt to catch up in height by 14 years. However, the statural differences between Oriental and white girls are not resolved by 14 years of age and seem to be inherent. The prepubertal growth rate of all these groups is similar. Immigrant children go into a phase of catch-up growth in an optimal nutritional environment.[127]

Body proportions change in concert with growth. The limbs are relatively short in infancy. By about 12 years of age, adult proportions are reached. The ratio of upper segment to lower segment averages 1.5:1 at birth and then falls[128, 129] (Fig. 141-6). Data for span relative to height (Fig. 141-7) are only approximations; they were published in 1932.[129] Occasional marked changes in segmental proportions appear during puberty.[102] Facial configuration matures as well. The change in the nasal root can be documented by measurement of the intercanthal and interorbital distances.[130]

Head circumference increases most rapidly during the first

year[131] (Fig. 141-8). It is related to both skeletal and brain growth, and about half the variation is familial.[132] Consequently, the relationship of head circumference to height is not a simple one and has been a subject of controversy.[133–134] It seems appropriate to plot the head circumference of GH-deficient children versus height age rather than chronological age. The head size of hypothyroid children is normal for age, however.[135] The anterior fontanel normally closes by about 15 months of age; abnormal fontanel size for age may indicate disorders of somatic growth.[136]

Weight is a labile parameter relative to height, being sensitive to acute illnesses and short-term changes in feeding and activity patterns. Whether nutrition is appropriate is generally assessed by comparing a child's percentile position for weight with that for height. Percentile standards for fatness are now available for infants and children[100] and at menarche and maturity in women[137] (Fig. 141-9). Fat

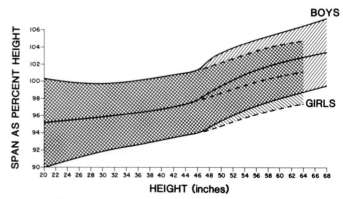

FIGURE 141-7. Standards for arm span as a percentage of height. Shaded area represents the normal range, smoothed. (Data from Engelbach W: Endocrine Medicine, Vol 1. Springfield, IL, Charles C Thomas, 1932, p 261).

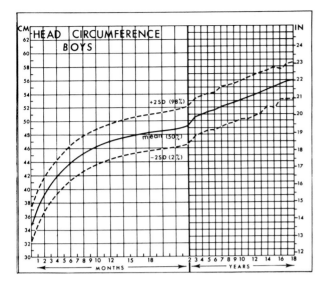

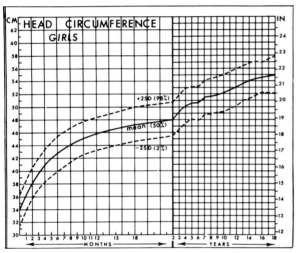

FIGURE 141–8. Interracial standards for maximal fronto-occipital head circumference. Boys' measurements are about 1 cm greater than those of girls at all ages. (From Nellhaus G: Head circumference from birth to eighteen years. Pediatrics 41:106, 1968.)

stores increase markedly during the first 9 months of life. Subcutaneous fat thickness subsequently decreases until about 7 years of age and then begins to rise during preadolescence.[112, 138] During puberty, fat stores tend to increase slightly in girls and decrease in boys. The waist/hip ratio decreases during adolescence in girls due to a relatively great increase in hip circumference.[139]

Bone Age and Prediction of Adult Height and Age of Puberty

Bone growth is normally accompanied by a predictable sequence, rate, and morphology of bone maturation. Figures 141–10 and 141–11 show schematically the roentgenographic standards for bone development reported by Gruelich and Pyle.[125, 140] These are anteroposterior roentgenograms of the left hand and wrist. Epiphyseal ossification centers first appear, then undergo modeling in shape, and finally go through fusion with the shaft. Skeletal ma-

turity is expressed as *bone age* (BA) or *skeletal age*. The BA is the age at which the observed degree of bone maturation would be typical. The evaluation is most reliable if BA is assigned to each bone of the hand film and the average is calculated.[141] Other atlas methods are available for assessing bone maturation.[142] The major drawbacks of hand atlases are the paucity of centers in early childhood and the subjective nature of the assessment of modeling. These difficulties contribute to the relatively wide coefficients of variation before puberty. During puberty, as epiphyseal fusion commences, fewer indicators become available in the hand films from which to assess the skeletal age precisely. The asymmetries and variations in sequence of ossification observed in wrist radiographs in normal children are within the variability of the initiation of ossification.[143] Skeletal development of young black children is about 0.67 standard deviation (SD) advanced over whites of comparable economic status.[144]

BA correlates better with age of peak height velocity and menarche than does chronological age, height, or weight.[145] Peak height-velocity phase differences are 25 per cent less when plotted against skeletal age instead of chronological age.[107] Performance in sporting events is similarly related best to BA.[146] The specifics of the relationship between sex hormones and BA have not been well defined.

The most widely used method of predicting the mature height of a normal child from the preadolescent height is that devised by Bayley and Pinneau,[125] which involves the use of the BA (Table 141–3). The statistical error inherent in this method is given in Table 141–4. One also can predict the amount of growth remaining in body segments from the BA (Table 141–5).[147] The principle is that the degree of bone maturation is inversely proportional to the amount of epiphyseal cartilage growth remaining. It follows that if a child's BA and height age (defined similar to BA; see next section) are equal, he or she has the potential to reach an average adult height. The Bayley-Pinneau tables show the percentage of mature height that has been achieved at skeletal ages of 6 years or more; different figures apply if the skeletal age differs by over 1 year from the average. Spontaneous shifts by as much as 5 inches in predicted height may occur in 3 per cent of the population for reasons that are unclear.[148] The error is not reduced by serial readings.[141]

In order to reduce the error in height prediction, elaborate tables have been devised that empirically take into consideration not only a child's BA and height but also the genetic target height and weight.[149] Genetic influences on height predicted from bone age can be roughly accounted for by adding one third the amount that the midparent height differs from the average.[150]

Frisch and associates have hypothesized that the critical weight for puberty represents a critical body composition with respect to fatness. At peak growth velocity and menarche, the average height of early- and late-maturing girls differs, but not their average weight.[151] The same is true of boys with respect to peak growth velocity, except for the very latest maturing boys. One can predict the age of menarche for prepubertal girls better by using percentiles of fatness than by using percentiles of height, weight, weight for height, or pubertal stage.[152] Percentiles of fatness at menarche for girls of various heights and weights are given in Figure 141–9.[138] Though there is a statistical relationship

TABLE 141–3. PERCENTAGE OF MATURE HEIGHT ACHIEVED AT A GIVEN BONE AGE

	SKELETAL AGE (YEARS)												
	6.0	6.5	7.0	7.5	8.0	8.5	9.0	9.5	10.0	10.5	11.0	11.5	12.0
Percentage of Mature Height													
Boys													
Average*	—	—	69.5	70.9	72.3	73.9	75.2	76.9	78.4	79.5	80.4	81.8	83.4
Accelerated*	—	—	67.0	68.3	69.6	70.9	72.0	73.4	74.7	75.8	76.7	78.6	80.9
Retarded*	68.0	70.0	71.8	73.8	75.6	77.3	78.6	80.0	81.2	81.9	82.3	83.2	84.5
Girls													
Average	72.0	73.8	75.7	77.2	79.0	81.0	82.7	84.4	86.2	88.4	90.6	91.4	92.2
Accelerated	—	—	71.2	73.2	75.0	77.1	79.0	80.9	82.8	85.6	88.3	89.1	90.1
Retarded	73.3	75.1	77.0	78.8	80.4	82.3	84.1	85.8	87.4	89.6	91.8	92.6	93.2

*With respect to whether the bone age is within 1 year of chronological age.
From Gruelich WW, Pyle SI: Radiographic Atlas of Skeletal Development of the Hand and Wrist. Palo Alto, CA, Stanford University Press, 1959.

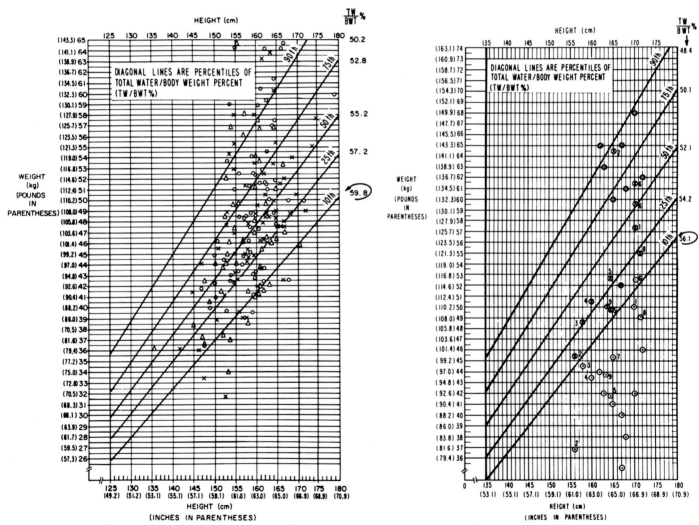

FIGURE 141–9. Percentile of fatness for Caucasian girls at menarche *(left)* and after menarche *(right)* equated with computed percentiles of total water as a percentile of body weight. The percentiles are diagonal lines. The minimal weight necessary at a particular height for the onset *(left)* or maintenance *(right)* of menses is very close to the 10th percentile of fatness. The latter is 59.8 and 56.1 per cent total-body water/body weight for menarcheal *(left)* and postmenarcheal *(right)* females. Data for anorexia nervosa cases are shown on the right panel: open circle with dot = time of presentation; open circle with X = resumption of menses. (Reproduced with permission from Frisch RE, McArthur JW: Menstrual cycles as a determinant of minimum weight for height necessary for their maintenance or onset. Science 185:949, 1974. Copyright 1974 by the American Association for the Advancement of Science.)

TABLE 141–3. PERCENTAGE OF MATURE HEIGHT ACHIEVED AT A GIVEN BONE AGE *Continued*

	SKELETAL AGE (YEARS)												
	12.5	13.0	13.5	14.0	14.5	15.0	15.5	16.0	16.5	17.0	17.5	18.0	18.5
Percentage of Mature Height													
Boys													
Average	85.3	87.6	90.2	92.7	94.8	96.8	97.6	98.2	98.7	99.1	99.4	99.6	100.0
Accelerated	82.6	85.0	87.5	90.5	93.0	95.8	97.1	98.0	98.5	99.0	—	—	—
Retarded	86.0	88.0	—	—	—	—	—	—	—	—	—	—	—
Girls													
Average	94.1	95.8	97.4	98.0	98.6	99.0	99.3	99.6	99.7	99.9	99.95	100	
Accelerated	92.4	94.5	96.3	97.2	98.0	98.6	99.0	99.3	99.5	99.8	—	—	
Retarded	94.9	96.4	97.7	98.3	98.9	99.4	99.6	99.8	99.9	100.0	—	—	

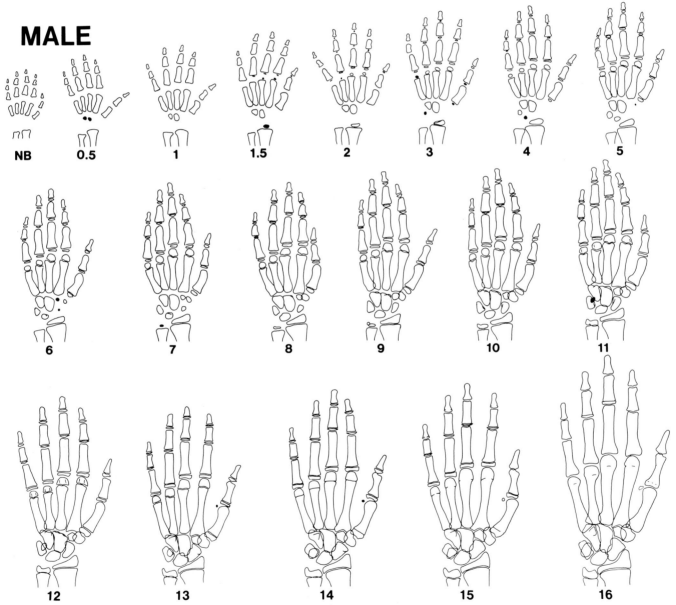

FIGURE 141–10. Progression of ossification of the hand and wrist in boys. Tracings modified from the standards of Gruelich and Pyle[125] according to the manner of Wilkins.[140] Newly apparent ossification centers are shown in black. Late prefusion is depicted as a single line at the junction of epiphysis and shaft. Bony projections, which appear as a double contour within the outlines of a center, are not illustrated after their appearance has matured.

FEMALE

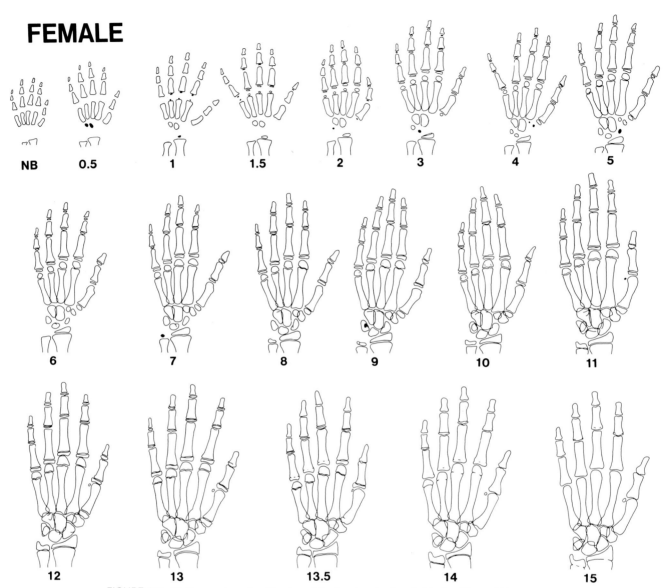

FIGURE 141–11. Progression of ossification of the hand and wrist of girls. See Figure 141–10.

TABLE 141–4. STANDARD DEVIATIONS FOR BONE AGE AND HEIGHT PREDICTION ACCORDING TO CHRONOLOGICAL AGE

	CHRONOLOGICAL AGE (YEARS)																
	1.0	2.0	3.0	4.0	5.0	6.0	7.0	8.0	9.0	10.0	11.0	12.0	13.0	14.0	15.0	16.0	17.0
Bone age (months)																	
Boys	2.1	4.0	6.0	7.0	8.4	9.3	10.1	10.8	11.0	11.4	10.5	10.4	11.1	12.0	14.2	15.1	15.4
Girls	2.7	4.0	5.6	7.2	8.6	9.0	8.3	8.8	9.3	10.8	12.3	14.0	14.6	12.6	11.2	—	—
Height prediction (inches)*																	
Boys								1.47	1.27	1.33	1.14	1.09	1.21	1.21	0.88	0.49	0.41
Girls								1.73	1.46	1.37	1.15	1.06	0.62	0.42	0.38	0.26	0.20

*Validating sample.
From Gruelich WW, Pyle SI: Radiographic Atlas of Skeletal Development of the Hand and Wrist. Palo Alto, CA, Stanford University Press, 1959.

TABLE 141–5. PERCENTAGE OF ULTIMATE LENGTH OF FEMUR AND TIBIA THAT IS ATTAINED AT A GIVEN SKELETAL AGE

	SKELETAL AGE (YEARS)										
	8.0	**9.0**	**10.0**	**11.0**	**12.0**	**13.0**	**14.0**	**15.0**	**16.0**	**17.0**	**18.0**
Percentage of Final Length											
Boys	70	74	77	81	85	90	94	97	99	99	100
Girls	78	81	85	90	93	96	98	99	99	100	100

Calculated from data of Aanderson M, Green WT, Messner MB: Growth and predictions of growth in the lower extremities. J Bone Joint Surg 45A:1, 1961. Based on measurements of orthoroentgenograms that include both proximal and distal epiphyses. An average of 71 per cent of femoral growth occurs at its lower end, and 57 per cent of tibial growth occurs at its upper end. Note correspondence of percentage of long-bone growth to percentage of whole-body growth at a given bone age (Table 141–3).

between a critical weight and menarche, this cannot be relied on to predict the onset of menses in the individual child.[153] For example, fatness cannot be used to predict menarche in the prepubertal or early pubertal obese girl. Weight and age seem independently related to menarcheal status.[154] Menarche, in turn, is a predictor of ultimate height.[150, 155]

It seems as if bone and neuroendocrine maturation have common determinants, which include age and nutrition. Consequently, the BA is, in most circumstances, the single best available predictor of pubertal events. In girls, menarche has been demonstrated to occur at a mean skeletal age of approximately 13 years.[125, 156] By extrapolation, a BA of about 10.75 years is expected at the onset of breast development in girls and 11.5 at the onset of testicular enlargement and 13 at the onset of sexual pubic hair appearance in boys.

CONCOMITANTS OF SOMATIC GROWTH

Brain growth is probably nearly complete with respect to neuronal number by midpregnancy.[157] The major portion of the spurt in brain weight and cell number that commences in midpregnancy and continues postnatally is due to glial multiplication and myelination. It is during this time that dendritic branching and synapsing occur. Cerebellar development begins several weeks later than cerebral development and ends earlier. The development of posture and reflexes is used widely to estimate gestational age.[158, 159]

Normal fetal maturation has various endocrinological and metabolic concomitants that have proved useful in estimating fetal well-being antenatally and gestational age. The fetoplacental unit is responsible for the normal increase in the mother's estrogen levels throughout pregnancy.[160] Placental lactogen production generally parallels the changes in estrone levels.[160] Total cortisol and lecithin/sphingomyelin ratios in amniotic fluid increase sharply after 34 weeks' gestation.[161] Palpable breast tissue appears at 36 weeks. The testes are found in the inguinal canal in small premature infants and do not come to lie in the scrotum until about 36 weeks after conception. It is of interest that the energy metabolism and RNA polymerase activity of maternal leukocytes are correlated with fetal growth.[162] Frank peripheral edema is present in the young premature infant and disappears by approximately 32 weeks' gestation. About 5 per cent of the weight of the term newborn seems attributable to sodium and water retention and is lost in the first few days of extrauterine life.[91]

Therefore, salt and water requirements in the first few days of life are 50 and 75 per cent, respectively, of those thereafter.

Postnatal organ and tissue growth occur in characteristic patterns.[112, 163] The growth of most organs follows the general somatic model: respiratory and digestive organs, kidneys, cardiovascular system, spleen, liver, and musculature as a whole. Consequently, blood volume closely approximates 7 per cent of body weight throughout life. The neuronal growth pattern differs: 50 per cent of adult brain weight is achieved at 1 year and nearly 100 per cent by about 8 years of age. Bursal lymphoid tissue mass grows to exceed adult levels in individuals between 8 and 18 years of age, the peak occurring at 11 to 12 years. Thymic size is two thirds of the maximum in infancy, is maximal in the preadolescent, and then regresses during puberty. Growth of the reproductive organs is relatively slow until about a year before the appearance of secondary sex characteristics.

Infants are hypermetabolic compared with adults because of the great size of the high-energy-consuming organs (such as brain, heart, liver, and kidney) relative to somatic size.[19, 20] Water requirements change in proportion to calorie requirements (Table 141–6). Salt, hormone, and drug dosage change in proportion to water requirements. Two schemes for calculating average water needs are given in Table 141–6, one based on surface area and another empirically based on weight.[164, 165] One hundred ml of water are required per 100 calories. Normal sodium and potassium requirements average 40 and 30 mEq/L water,

TABLE 141–6. CHANGES IN AVERAGE DAILY WATER REQUIREMENT WITH GROWTH*

AGE	AVERAGE WEIGHT (KG)	SURFACE AREA (M²)	PREDICTED WATER NEED† (ML/DAY)	
			By Surface Area‡	*By Weight§*
1.0 wk	3.0	0.2	286	300
5.0 mos	6.0	0.3	428	600
1.0 yr	10.0	0.45	642	1000
5.5 yrs	20.0	0.80	1140	1500
9.0 yrs	30.0	1.00	1430	1700
14.5 yrs	50.0	1.50	2140	2100
Adult	70.0	1.75	2500	2500

*Data for males.

†The water requirements given are approximately 50 per cent above basal.

‡Calculated on the assumption of 2500 ml total requirements in an adult whose surface area is 1.75 m².

§Calculated as 100 ml/kg up to 10 kg body weight; 1000 ml + 50 ml/kg from 10 to 20 kg; 1500 ml + 20 ml/kg over 20 kg.

respectively. The extracellular compartment is relatively larger in children than in adults, falling from about 40 per cent at 1 week to 30 per cent at 3 to 6 months to 20 per cent of body weight at maturity. Striking changes in the levels of serum phosphorus and alkaline phosphatase occur commensurate with bone growth.[166] The concentration of serum phosphorus falls steadily from a range of about 5 to 7.5 mg/dl in infancy to 3 to 5 mg/dl in the adult. Serum alkaline phosphatase falls from 40 to 140 IU/L in infancy to 20 to 40 IU/L in adults; the decline is interrupted by a secondary peak during the late preadolescent and adolescent years. The bone isozyme accounts for the difference in phosphatase levels between children and adults, reflecting osteoblastic activity. A downward trend in serum calcium and parathormone levels is observed with growth, but it is not prominent; for practical purposes, the plasma levels of these substances can be considered stable at adult levels.

Primary teeth begin to calcify before birth. The timing of calcification and eruption of the permanent teeth follows a consistent pattern (Table 141–7) and is dependent on many of the nutritional and hormonal factors that determine somatic growth.[167] Nevertheless, the correlation between dental and bone maturation is not a good one.

Plasma hormone concentrations are, in general, similar in children and adults. In the case of some hormones—e.g., cortisol—this signifies that the secretion rate changes in proportion to surface area.[168] Exceptions to this general rule are free thyroid hormone levels (up to 25 per cent higher during infancy), renin and aldosterone (falling progressively throughout childhood, apparently to compensate for functional immaturity of the kidney),[169] and of course sex steroid, luteinizing hormone (LH), and follicle-stimulating hormone (FSH) levels.

GROWTH DISORDERS

Classification of Growth Disorders

Growth disturbances are caused by a myriad of disorders. The physician is faced with an awesomely long differential diagnosis. In addition, he or she must keep in mind that most children whose size is outside the 3rd to 97th percentiles have a growth pattern that is a variation of normal.

Growth derangements can be classified according to the relationships among chronological age (CA), height age (HA), weight age (WA), bone age (BA), and growth rate. The HA is the age for which a child's height would be average (i.e., at the 50th percentile). The WA and BA are similarly defined. For example, a subject with the height and bone development of an average 6-year-old child has an HA and BA of 6, regardless of the CA. The proper evaluation of the growth rate (height velocity) and bone development is essential to the clinical assessment of patients with disturbances of linear growth. The most common error in the diagnosis of growth disorders is the physician's reliance on "routine" height measurements that have been taken inaccurately. Height can be measured reproducibly with less than 0.4 cm error if taken and rechecked in standard fashion: without shoes and with correct posture (standing "at attention": heels together; heels, buttocks, shoulders, and occiput touching the vertical plane; abdominal muscles tensed; and the lower margin of the orbits held in the horizontal plane, which includes the external auditory meatus). Length (supine) is greater than height and is a more reproducible measure in infants (see Fig. 141–3). Measurements should be made at approximately the same time of day to avoid the effect of the diurnal variation that seems to result from changes in postural tone. This decrease in height between the early morning and late afternoon averages 1.54 cm.[170] The longitudinal growth rate cannot be accurately evaluated over periods of less than 6 to 12 months because of the short-term fluctuations that sometimes occur.[111]

For growth diagnosis, the BA roentgenograph (see Figs. 141–10 and 141–11) should be assigned a precise BA. A statement that the BA is "significantly retarded" is hardly more helpful in the differential diagnosis than to say that the child is short. The limitations of the determination of skeletal age should be kept in mind, however. A disturbed BA may be one manifestation of a bone dystrophy—it may be delayed (as in trichorhinophalangeal syndrome, Fig. 141–12) or advanced (as in the Weaver-Smith syndrome[171]) in association with subtle disturbances of bone modeling. The normal variations and asymmetries may be exaggerated in a variety of growth disorders, whether growth is altered generally (Fig. 141–13) or locally.[172] In cases where body proportions are altered, a skeletal survey is indicated, since the hand-wrist radiograph is not altered in some dysplasias. On the other hand, the film may reveal the unexpected presence of a bone dystrophy (see Fig. 141–12) or ossification disturbance.

Diagnostic decisions are simplified by first categorizing the disorder of growth with regard to whether it is a primary disturbance of height or weight by the relationship between HA and WA. A child with a primary disorder of linear growth usually has a weight that is normal for his or her length (WA = HA). A child with a primary nutritional disorder typically has a height that is considerably closer to the norm than the weight (i.e., WA<HA).

Primary disturbances of linear growth result from inherent aberrations of bone growth or of the extrinsic factors

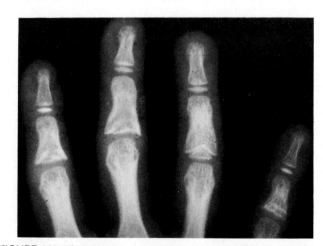

FIGURE 141–12. Detail from x-ray taken for determination of bone age of a 10.8-year-old girl whose height age was 5.5 years. Note the cone-shaped epiphyses in various stages of prefusion and premature fusion. This is characteristic of trichorhinophalangeal syndrome. Without consideration of the significance of the abnormal epiphyseal shape, the overall retardation of bone age (otherwise 5.4 years) would lead to overestimation of this person's predicted adult height.

TABLE 141–7. CHRONOLOGY OF HUMAN DENTITION

TOOTH		CALCIFICATION BEGINS	CROWN COMPLETED	ERUPTION	ROOT COMPLETED	ROOT RESORPTION BEGINS
Primary	I	14 wks	4 mos	6–18 mos	1½–2 yrs	5–6 yrs
	II	16 wks	5 mos	8–10 mos	1½–2 yrs	5–6 yrs
	III	17 wks	9 mos	16–20 mos	2½–3 yrs	6–7 yrs
	IV	15½ wks	6 mos	12–16 mos	2–2½ yrs	4–5 yrs
	V	18–19 wks	10–12 mos	20–30 mos	3 yrs	4–5 yrs
Upper permanent	1	3–4 mos	4–5 yrs	7–8 yrs	10 yrs	
	2	1 yr	4–5 yrs	8–9 yrs	11 yrs	
	3	4–5 mos	6–7 yrs	11–12 yrs	13–15 yrs	
	4	1½–1¾ yrs	5–6 yrs	10–11 yrs	12–13 yrs	
	5	2–2½ yrs	6–7 yrs	10–12 yrs	12–14 yrs	
	6	8 mos	2½–3 yrs	6–7 yrs	9–10 yrs	
	7	2½–3 yrs	7–8 yrs	12–14 yrs	14–16 yrs	
	8	7–9 yrs	12–16 yrs	17–30 yrs	18–25 yrs	
Lower permanent	1	3–4 mos	4–5 yrs	6–7 yrs	9 yrs	
	2	3–4 mos	4–5 yrs	7–8 yrs	10 yrs	
	3	4–5 mos	6–7 yrs	10–11 yrs	12–14 yrs	
	4	1¾–2 yrs	5–6 yrs	10–12 yrs	12–13 yrs	
	5	2¼–2½ yrs	6–7 yrs	11–12 yrs	13–14 yrs	
	6	8 mos	2½–3 yrs	6–7 yrs	9–10 yrs	
	7	2½–3 yrs	7–8 yrs	12–13 yrs	14–15 yrs	
	8	8–10 yrs	12–16 yrs	17–30 yrs	18–25 yrs.	

From Rosenstein SN: The teeth. *In* Barnett H (ed): Pediatrics (ed 16). New York, Appleton-Century-Crofts, 1977.

that affect the rate of bone growth. Disturbances of linear growth may be understood on the basis of two general principles. First, *normal linear growth during childhood proceeds in a predictable channel and is accompanied by a predictable rate of advance of BA.* Two corollaries of this proposition are (1) all correctable diseases that interfere with growth do so by interfering with the progression of bone growth, hence BA, and conversely, (2) if a child's BA is normal, there is no correctable disease underlying his or her height abnormality. Second, *children normally enter puberty at a pubertal BA independent of chronological age.* Thus disorders of linear growth can be approached in a discriminatory manner based on the relationships among CA, HA, BA, and growth rate.

Short stature results from three types of growth patterns:

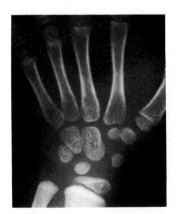
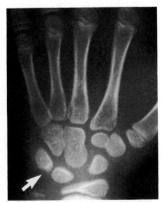

FIGURE 141–13. Details from x-rays taken for determination of bone age of a girl with premature breast development. *(Left)* At time of presentation at 4.8 years of age. Bone age 5.0 years. *(Right)* Three months later at time of removal of a feminizing tumor. Bone age averaged 7.5 years; however, the ossification of the distal ulnar and pisiform *(arrow)* centers has rapidly advanced to the 8- and 9-year levels, respectively.

intrinsic shortness, delayed growth, or attenuated growth[34] (Table 141–8). For example, a 9-year-old child with an HA of 6.5 and a BA of 9 will be small as an adult, i.e., *intrinsically* short. Since the BA is normal, linear growth has almost certainly occurred at a normal rate. On the other hand, a 9-year-old of the same size (HA = 6.5) with a BA of 6.5 typically has a normal growth potential. If such a child is growing at a normal rate, he or she is following a *delayed* growth pattern. If such a child has a growth rate less than normal, growth has been *attenuated* by endocrine, metabolic, or systemic disease until proved otherwise.

Tall stature results from three analogous growth patterns (Table 141–9): intrinsic tallness, advanced growth, and accelerated growth. The terminology used here is chosen to clarify and simplify the nomenclature that has confused many physicians. Most confusion revolves around the application of the terms *familial* and *constitutional* to the most common normal variant forms of childhood short stature. The term *familial* without further qualification is misleading because either the intrinsically short/tall or the delayed/advanced growth patterns may have a familial basis. The term *constitutional* alone conveys no clear meaning. In the terminology used here *familial intrinsic shortness* is a form of short stature in which a normal child's growth potential approximates that of the short parents, and *constitutionally delayed shortness* is a form of the delayed growth pattern in which a healthy child spontaneously achieves a normal growth potential at a later than average age, possibly on the basis of a familial pattern.

As a further comment on the subject of terminology, *dwarfism* means marked, permanent shortness, and the term should be applied only if predicted adult height (see above) or the child's height is less than 4 standard deviations from the mean. The expression carries distasteful implications of deformity to lay persons. Actually, only some dwarfs are disproportionate (*imperfect*); many are proportionate (*perfect* or *ateliotic* dwarfs, *midgets*).

TABLE 141–8. CLASSIFICATION OF CAUSES OF SHORT STATURE

TYPE OF GROWTH PATTERN	BONE AGE APPROXIMATES*	GROWTH RATE	ABBREVIATED DIFFERENTIAL DIAGNOSIS

Intrinsic shortness	Chronological age (BA = CA > HA)	Usually normal	Familial normal variant
			Genetic syndromes
			    Chromosomal anomalies
			    Bone dysplasia
			    Dysmorphic syndromes
			Intrauterine growth retardation, other
			Acquired

Delayed growth	Height age (BA = CA < HA)	Usually normal	"Constitutional" normal variant Undernutrition

Attenuated growth	Height age (BA = CA < HA)	Subnormal	Endocrinopathies
			    GH deficiency–related
			    Hypothyroidism
			    Cushing's syndrome
			    Hypogonadism after 10–12 years of age
			Acid–base disturbances
			Chronic disease, severe (e.g., Crohn's disease)
			Malnutrition

*BA = bone age; CA = chronological age; HA = height age.

Disorders of Intrauterine Growth

Intrauterine Growth Retardation (IUGR)

Intrauterine growth retardation (IUGR) is defined as birth size inappropriately small for gestational age[173] and is commonly equated with sizes below the 10th percentile. Clinically, IUGR can be subdivided into disorders that primarily retard linear growth and those that primarily hinder fetal "nutrition." Several conditions falling into the former group are known to be characterized by a decrease in cell number in various organs—e.g., congenital rubella, certain cases of primordial dwarfism, some congenital malformations of the heart, and hypoxia.[1, 174] This finding suggests that bone, too, is endowed with a subnormal population of cells in these disorders.

The distinction between retardation of linear growth and undernutrition is not as clear in disorders of prenatal growth as it is in disorders of postnatal growth. Infants with fetal malnutrition tend to be short for gestational age if the insult begins early and is of long duration,[175] and bone maturation is retarded in most cases.[88, 176] This retardation of linear growth may be related to the evidence that fetal malnutrition retards growth in both cell number and cell

size.[2, 177] Cell number is particularly vulnerable to insult relatively early in the critical period of organ development. The extent to which subnormal endowment in cell number is necessarily lasting and limits the capacity for catch-up growth is unknown.

PRIMORDIAL (CONGENITAL) DWARFS PRESENTING WITH IUGR. Disorders of fetal linear growth result from genetic, chromosomal, infectious, drug-induced, and unknown causes. They are sometimes associated with skeletal disproportions or multiple nonskeletal anomalies, which are, in turn, important clues to the presence of true dwarfism.[178–182]

Disproportionate IUGR indicates that one is dealing with osteochondrodysplasia (bone dysplasia) as the cause of an intrinsic growth disorder. These generalized disturbances of bone and cartilage growth result in permanent dwarfism. The terminology underwent a change in 1977.

Many of these dystrophies are manifest at birth. Achondroplasia is the most frequent of these disorders. It is characterized by short-limbed dwarfism with normal head size. Standard growth curves are available for achondroplastic individuals; the average adult height is about 125 cm in females and 131 cm in males.[181] A phenotypically mild allelic variant is hypochondroplasia.[183] A constant finding

TABLE 141–9. CLASSIFICATION OF CAUSES OF EXCESSIVE HEIGHT

TYPE OF GROWTH PATTERN	BONE AGE RELATIONSHIP TO CA AND HA*	GROWTH RATE	ABBREVIATED DIFFERENTIAL DIAGNOSIS
Intrinsic tallness	= Chronological age (BA = CA < HA)	Usually normal	Familial tallness Marfanoid syndromes
Advanced growth	= Height age (BA = HA > CA)	Usually normal	"Constitutional" normal variant Obesity Hyperthyroidism Infant giants Lipodystrophy
Accelerated growth	≤ Height age (BA ≤ HA > CA)	Supranormal	GH excess
	> Height age (BA > HA > CA)	Supranormal	Sexual precocity

*BA = bone age; CA = chronological age; HA = height age.

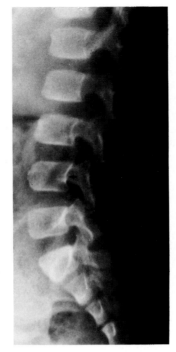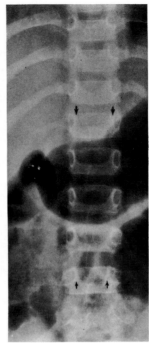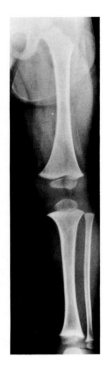

FIGURE 141–14. Radiographic appearance of skeleton in hypochondroplasia, an allelic variant of achondroplasia. Despite the characteristic clinical finding of short limbs, the most objective radiographic findings are in the spine. Note the characteristic narrowing of interpedicular distance *(center, arrows)* between L1 and L5. Other radiographic findings are more subtle, e.g., scalloping of vertebral pedicles *(left, arrows)* and a relatively short tibia compared to the fibula *(right)*.

is narrowing of the spinal canal on anteroposterior roentgenograms (Fig. 141–14). Achondrogenesis and thanatophoric dysplasia are lethal disorders. Other dystrophies recognizable at birth include chondrodysplasia punctata (congenital stippled epiphyses) of the autosomal recessive and warfarin (Coumadin)–induced types, metatrophic dysplasia (in which body proportions change with development), diastrophic dysplasia (''twisted,'' in reference to the multiple joint contractures), chondroectodermal dysplasia (Ellis–van Creveld syndrome), some other forms of mesomelic dysplasia, asphyxiating thoracic dysplasia, spondyloepiphyseal dysplasia, spondylometaphyseal dysplasia, cleidocranial dysplasia (formerly termed a dysostosis until it was recognized that generalized bone changes develop with time), camptomelic (''bent'') dysplasia, and short-rib polydactyly syndromes. Metabolic bone disease, such as hypophosphatasia, may cause IUGR with deformities. The reader is referred to the referenced reviews, atlases, and books for comprehensive discussions of these disorders. Most of these disorders have a characteristic hereditary pattern, and families should be counseled appropriately.

Proportionate IUGR is also compatible with an intrinsic generalized growth disorder. This may be the case with few, if any, obvious stigmata. Bone dysplasia may appear in this fashion—e.g., tubular stenosis (Kenny's syndrome). This syndrome may sometimes be a manifestation of congenital hypoparathyroidism.[184] Facial disproportion in a small newborn may be the only evidence of congenital defect that will result in dwarfism. A facies characterized by upturned nostrils and upper lip suggests Cornelia de Lange's syndrome if associated with confluent eyebrows. Williams' syndrome is characterized by an ''elfin facies''; there is a predisposition to hypercalcemia if associated with aortic stenosis.[25, 185, 186] Micrognathia with microcephaly suggests Virchow-Seckel (bird-headed) dwarfism.[187] IUGR with pseudohydrocephalus (relatively normal-sized head with small face) is known as Russell's syndrome or, if asymmetry is present in addition, Silver's syndrome.[188, 189]

An intrinsic generalized growth disorder is likely when multiple congenital defects are associated with proportionate IUGR[181] (Table 141–10). Such syndromes may result from chromosomal abnormalities, genetic disorders, congenital infection, or exposure to teratogenic drugs. Improvements in chromosomal banding techniques are leading to the documentation of the basis of previously unrecognized birth defect syndromes.[190] In Bloom's syndrome, a defect has been identified in chromosomal repli-

TABLE 141–10. EXAMPLES OF MULTIPLE CONGENITAL BIRTH DEFECT SYNDROMES WITH PROPORTIONATE IUGR AND SUBSEQUENT INTRINSIC GROWTH FAILURE[181]

ETIOLOGY	COMMON FEATURES
Autosomal Trisomy	
D	Mental retardation, congenital heart disease, third branchial arch syndrome, foot and hand deformities, bilateral cleft palate and lip, microphthalmia, colobomata, holoprosencephaly
E	Mental retardation, congenital heart disease, foot and hand deformities, third branchial arch anomaly
Genetic	
Bloom's syndrome	Photosensitive dermatitis with telangiectatic erythema, malar hypoplasia, small nose
Leprechaunism	Congenital lipodystrophy, ''puckish'' facies
Congenital Infection	
Rubella	Hepatosplenomegaly, thrombocytopenia, anemia, patent ductus arteriosus, cataract, deafness
Drugs	
Ethanol	Characteristic facies (short palpebral fissures, hypoplastic philtrum, thinned upper vermilion, indistinct philtrum), microcephaly, mental retardation
Hydantoin	Hypertelorism, terminal digit hypoplasia, mental retardation, seizures

cation: a high frequency of chromosome breakage and chromatid exchange, which suggests abnormal regulation of the cell cycle.[191] A similar syndrome results from mutation of the DNA ligase I gene.[192] Donohue's syndrome ("leprechaunism") is characterized by resistance to insulin and insulin-like growth factors and other growth factors.

Congenital rubella often leads to permanent growth retardation; about 50 per cent of patients are below the 10th percentile in adulthood.[193] The severity of the growth failure in congenital rubella seems to correlate with onset of infection in very early gestation and persistence of infection postnatally. Congenital infection with cytomegalovirus may stunt growth. Intrauterine growth retardation occurs in the case of maternal addiction to heroin.[194] Permanent short stature might be suspected on the basis of the finding of subnormal cell numbers in several organs. Whether the shortness of stature at birth which is associated with maternal cocaine use persists is unknown.[195] The isolated retardation of linear growth resulting from tetracycline exposure is temporary.[196, 197]

Two or more minor malformations are sometimes clues to an occult major malformation. Although 14 per cent of newborns have a single minor anomaly, only 0.8 per cent have two minor malformations, and the latter group has a fivefold increased incidence of a major defect.[181] Three or more minor malformations confer a 20 per cent risk.[198] Smith has illustrated the most important of the minor defects: (1) eyes: epicanthal folds, slanting palpebral fissures, hypertelorism; (2) ears: auricular malformation, low set, and slanted; (3) hands and feet: abnormal creases, dermatoglyphics, nail shape, and digit formation; (4) skin, hair, and teeth dysplasias; (5) mouth: frenulum and palatal arch abnormalities; and (6) genitalia: "saddle" scrotum or hypoplasia of labia majora. Hypertelorism, dermatoglyphics, and the abnormal ear position are quantifiable; the diagnostic value of intercanthal distance may be improved if head circumference is taken into account.[130] A single or absent umbilical artery also has been claimed to be a clue to serious congenital anomalies.[199]

One must not prognosticate future dwarfism on the basis of criteria that are not clear-cut. The prognosis for postnatal growth depends on the specific diagnosis. The various atlases referenced at the beginning of this section are invaluable in this regard. However, they will never be all-inclusive, since new syndromes are delineated with regularity and many dystrophies are still unclassified.[199, 200] The difficulty in making an exact diagnosis in many infants with IUGR is reminiscent of the midcentury dialectic with respect to the diagnosis of Down syndrome. There was considerable dispute over which physical findings were the most reliable diagnostic signs: simian creases, epicanthal folds, and so forth. These disputes were laid to rest with the discovery that chromosome 21 excess was constant and that the phenotypic expression of the trisomy varied. Similarly, many atypical malformation syndromes may prove to represent the partial expression of some single genetic defect.[202]

It is important to remember that in some infants with multiple malformations, particularly those with midline craniofacial anomalies, postnatal growth failure may not be due to an intrinsic defect in skeletal growth but may be mediated by GH deficiency.

Management requires attention to the basic underlying disorder. Prophylaxis is possible with respect to certain of these disorders—e.g., interdiction of teratogenic drugs, active immunization to prevent congenital rubella, and amniocentesis or chorionic villus sampling in women at risk to permit abortion of fetuses afflicted with major anomalies. Treatment is often only expectant and supportive. Limb-lengthening operations have received attention, but the time and discomfort make them impractical for most.[182] Genetic counseling should not be overlooked. Guidance and advice with respect to handling congenital malformations or the mental retardation so frequently associated are important aspects of care.

FETAL MALNUTRITION. Fetal malnutrition results from maternal, fetal, and placental disturbances. Fetal factors include multiple fetuses and hypoxia.[96–99] Evidence for malnutrition of twins is most clear in those sets in which there is marked discrepancy of size. This situation arises because of placental arteriovenous anastomoses. The smaller (donor) twin of such a parabiotic set has organ abnormalities characteristic of malnutrition.[99, 203] Placental insufficiency and postmaturity are associated with fetal undernutrition. Maternal disorders resulting in fetal malnutrition include vascular disease, undernutrition, drug addiction, heavy cigarette smoking, and various chronic diseases, including neuropsychiatric disorders.[177, 204–208] Diabetes mellitus of neonatal onset is associated with proportionate retardation of intrauterine weight and length.[83, 208, 209] Fetal hypoinsulinism has been postulated to contribute to the growth failure of these diabetic infants.

Serum IGF-I levels and bioactivity are low in IUGR.[77] However, the pathogenesis of fetal undergrowth in the diverse causes of IUGR may prove to be quite different. The IUGR of heroin addicts' babies cannot always be attributed to co-incident undernutrition.[194] The poor uterine perfusion in toxemia is often assumed to stunt the fetus simply by limiting the supply of protein and calories. However, metabolic differences are reported between rats whose intrauterine growth is stunted by different mechanisms. Insulin levels were inappropriately high in hypoglycemic pups born after maternal uterine vascular insufficiency, in contrast to those born of hypoglycemic, malnourished mothers.[211]

Data regarding the prognosis for growth of IUGR infants are meager.[89, 91, 94, 175, 176, 212] The mean growth of these infants in length and weight is inclined to proceed appropriately for their gestational age. Bone growth velocity is usually normal, too. Consequently, their length is less than that of truly premature infants of comparable birth weight at 1 year, a tendency that persists at 10 years of age. Since bone maturation of IUGR babies is retarded somewhat, one would expect them to tend to follow a "delayed" growth pattern and have the potential to reach a normal adult height (see below). It is interesting that about 40 per cent of the very small IUGR newborns have a supranormal rate of linear growth within the first 6 months of life; however, one cannot predict which infants will "catch up" in this manner. It has been suggested that insulin is involved in this catch-up growth.[213]

A high neonatal mortality rate is found in infants with IUGR.[214, 215] To some extent, this is due to associated serious congenital anomalies. Hypoglycemia and hypothyroidism, for which fetal malnutrition is an important predisposing element, are other factors.[216, 217] There is considerable interest in the possibility that fetal malnutrition may impair subsequent intellectual development irreparably.[157] A 300-g discrepancy in the birth weight of monozygotic twins reportedly leads to a significant 5-point disparity in intelligence quotient (IQ) scores.[219] Placental insufficiency is clearly associated with a high incidence of subsequent frank neurological abnormalities in the affected infants.[220]

The treatment of fetal malnutrition is preventive with respect to maternal health care. This requires optimal nutritional provisions and attention to proper treatment of underlying maternal disease. The infant born small for gestational age should likewise be provided with an optimal diet. If hypoglycemia occurs, it must be treated promptly. It is important not to mislabel the IUGR infants as "dwarfed" because of an unusual facies or head size. About half the IUGR infants who follow a delayed growth pattern postnatally respond to GH therapy in replacement doses despite seemingly normal GH reserve.[221] The positive responses are generally not as great or sustained as those of hyposomatotropic dwarfs. There are currently no means of predicting which patients will benefit.

Fetal Overgrowth

Hyperinsulinism is characteristic of most infant giant syndromes. Infants of diabetic mothers become overweight unless there is placental insufficiency.[222, 223] This occurs because of increased adiposity and enlargement of certain organs, particularly the liver and heart, where cell hypertrophy predominates over hyperplasia. Length is increased to a lesser extent than weight. Brain growth is usually normal. Infants of mothers with impaired glucose tolerance are similarly affected but usually less severely.

Infants with the Beckwith-Wiedemann syndrome resemble the overgrown infants of diabetic mothers in general appearance, but they have characteristic congenital anomalies.[181, 223–227] This is a syndrome of infant gigantism (not necessarily present at birth). The most consistent external features are macroglossia and umbilical abnormalities (ranging from hernia to omphalocele). Occasionally, there is hemihypertrophy. Hypoglycemia is typical and usually results from hyperinsulinism; glucagon deficiency has been suspected on occasion.[228, 229] Hyperplasia of various visceral (kidney) and endocrine organs (pancreatic beta cells, adrenal fetal cortex and medulla, pituitary amphophils, and gonadal interstitial cells) is the rule, and there is a high incidence of postnatal intra-abdominal tumor development. Incomplete variants of the syndrome occur. Increased somatomedin activity has been described. The disorder is associated with loss of heterozygosity at chromosomal locus 11p15.5 due to duplications, trisomy, or disomy for the paternal allele.[230] This is a chromosomal area that contains the genes for insulin, IGF-II, and a tumor suppressor gene. Growth during childhood is usually rapid and accompanied by an accelerated BA. In treating these patients, a major effort must be directed toward detection and vigorous treatment of hypoglycemia; the hypoglycemic tendency usually regresses within 4 months. Surgery may be required for the umbilical abnormality or macroglossia. Recognition of variants of the syndrome is important because of the potential for the development of neoplasia.

Infants with erythroblastosis fetalis are also hyperinsulinemic. It has been suggested that beta cells become hyperplastic in response to inactivation of insulin by the placenta[231] or by-products of hemolysis.[232] Hyperinsulinism and hypoglycemia correlate with severity of the anemia. However, the increased weight of the fetuses with erythroblastosis is mostly attributable to the development of edema. Treatment is directed not only at the hypoglycemia, as for infants of diabetic mothers, but also toward alleviating the perinatal hyperbilirubinemia and anemia.

Cerebral gigantism (Sotos' syndrome) is characterized by the presence of acromegalic features and cerebral dysfunction (usually mild mental retardation with a dilated ventricular system) but normal GH levels and GH dynamics.[181, 233] Most affected infants are large at birth, all grow rapidly in early childhood, though BA is normal, yet only a few achieve an excessive adult height. High plasma levels of branched-chain amino acids have been reported.[234] Fragile X syndrome can present similarly.[235] Management is confined to supportive counseling.

The Weaver-Marshall-Smith syndrome is an infant overgrowth syndrome with accelerated skeletal maturation and unusual facies.[171, 181] Some affected infants had relatively poor weight gain. Weaver's cases involved infants with multiple contractures and high amino acid levels.

The neonatal mortality of babies inappropriately large for gestational age is quite high. This is probably mostly because this group includes infants of diabetic mothers and infants with severe hemolytic disease of the newborn. When these disorders are excluded from consideration, the risks to the overweight baby are increased only moderately.

Disorders of Postnatal Growth

Disturbances of Generalized Linear Growth

LINEAR GROWTH RETARDATION. The three growth patterns causing short stature (see Table 141–8) are illustrated in Figure 141–15. *Intrinsic shortness* is characterized by inherent limitation of bone growth that destines affected children to be short adults. Birth size may or may not be normal. Growth curves in these children are below but approximately parallel to normal percentiles, and the growth velocity is usually within normal limits. The BA typically approximates the chronological age except in some IUGR and bone dysplasia syndromes.

A *delayed growth pattern* is characterized by delayed puberty. Children in this category continue to grow for longer than their peers and thus reach normal adult height. The characteristic growth curve is below but parallel to the normal growth channels, the growth velocity is usually normal, and the BA approximates the HA.

Children with an *attenuated growth pattern* have a sufficiently subnormal growth rate that their height progressively deviates from standard growth channels. Their BA is approximately equal to HA; consequently, adult height potential is normal. However, this growth pattern virtually always has a pathological basis that, unless optimally treated, precludes achievement of this potential.

Intrinsic Shortness. Intrinsic shortness is most commonly a familial normal variant that has a polygenic nonpathological basis. This growth pattern also can result from a variety of more serious congenital disorders, some of which present with IUGR (see Table 141–7) and some of which do

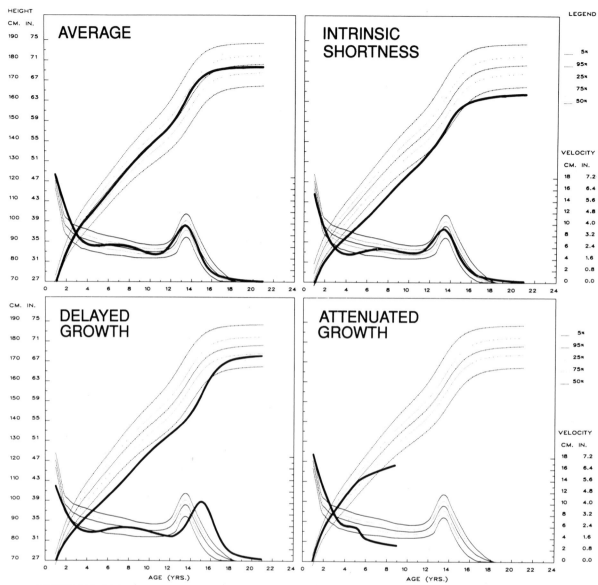

FIGURE 141–15. Linear growth curves in children with various types of growth patterns. Note that three prepubertal children of similar short stature at 9 years of age have different prognoses for growth. Growth curve of an average size child is shown for comparison. On each chart, upper scale shows height attained, lower scale shows height velocity. Normal percentiles from National Center for Health Statistics.[100] Growth curves generated by the TRIFOUR program of Bock et al. (Bock RD, du Toit SHC, Thissen D: A.U.X.A.L.: Auxological Analysis of Longitudinal Data. Chicago, Scientific Software, Inc., 1993).

not (see Table 141–9). Chromosomal disorders, bone dysplasias, and dysmorphic syndromes are the major secondary considerations.

Stunting of growth and cerebral dysfunction are virtually uniform features of autosomal aneuploidy. Down syndrome (trisomy 21 and variants thereof) is the most common multiple malformation syndrome in humans. Adult height averages 155 cm in affected males and 145 cm in females.[236] Thyroid autoimmunity has been reported to be a factor associated with the chromosomal nondisjunction causing aneuploidy.[237]

All girls with intrinsic short stature must be considered to have Turner's syndrome or a variant thereof until proved otherwise. It is the most common pathological cause of short stature in girls, with an incidence of about 1 in 5000 newborns. The most characteristic features of Turner's syndrome are short stature and gonadal dysgenesis[181, 238–243] (Table 141–11). Shortness is a more consistent finding in those patients who partially lack genetic material on the distal short arm of the X chromosome than is gonadal failure.[244] However, the Turner phenotype occurs on rare occasions in XY females with deletions of portions of Yp which are homologous with Xq.[245] This is compatible with the proposal that gene(s) are located on Xq that prevent short stature and that these escape X inactivation on intact X chromosomes but are prone to X inactivation on structurally abnormal ones. A normal buccal smear is not adequate to rule out Turner's syndrome. Since the average birth size of these children is at the lower end of the normal range, mild IUGR occurs sometimes. Linear growth and BA typically drop so as to parallel the 3rd percentile during childhood.[246] Growth

TABLE 141–11. ESTIMATED INCIDENCE OF SOMATIC
ABNORMALITIES IN TURNER'S AND NOONAN'S SYNDROMES[a]

ABNORMALITY	TURNER'S SYNDROME[181, 238–243] (%)	NOONAN'S SYNDROME[181, 238–243] (%)
Short stature (<10%)	100/80?[b]	90/90
Gonadal failure	99/85?	≤10/≤10[c]
Cryptorchidism	NA/33[d]	NA/75
Hypertelorism	<25	100
High palate	80	75
Neck webbed	50	10
Neck short	68	100
Cubitus valgus	68	30
Chest deformity[e]	50	50
Coarctation of aorta	20	<1
Pulmonic stenosis	10	50[f]
Mental retardation	10[g]	25
Pigmented moles, multiple	50	<10

[a]Defined on the basis of presence (Turner) or absence (Noonan) of sex chromosome abnormality. Turner's syndrome in the female results from the deletion of genetic material on the X chromosome. Various sex chromosomal abnormalities have been reported in Turner's syndrome in the male—e.g., XO, XXY, XO/XY, XO/XY/XYY, XX/XXY.

[b]Female/male.

[c]The distinction between delayed puberty and hypogonadisim has seldom been made.

[d]NA = not applicable.

[e]Chest deformity: pectus or apparent increase in internipple distance

[f]The high incidence of congenital heart disease in Noonan's syndrome may be due to ascertainment, Dr. Noonan being a cardiologist. A variety of other congenital heart defects have been reported in both syndromes.

[g]Males seem to have a greater incidence of mental retardation, though this may be a matter of ascertainment.

then becomes attenuated in the teenage years owing to hypogonadism. Sex hormone replacement therapy increases endogenous GH production but not final height.[247] Final height averages only 56.5 inches without GH therapy[248] (Fig. 141–16).

One of the most perplexing problems in the classification of syndromes of intrinsic short stature is that of *Noonan's syndrome*. This term has been used interchangeably with *male Turner's syndrome*. However, the term *Noonan's syndrome* is now applied to those patients of either sex with normal external genitalia who have a Turner-like phenotype but whose sex chromosomes are normal. *Turner's syndrome* is thus reserved for those individuals with abnormal sex chromosomes.[238, 243] Probably fewer than 20 per cent of males with the Turner phenotype have a sex chromosomal abnormality.[239, 240] Noonan's syndrome may be transmitted as an autosomal dominant disorder; partial deletion of a 6–12 autosome has been reported.[242, 243] Although the anomalies may be identical in many patients with these syndromes, and although chromosomal mosaicism has not been thoroughly ruled out in most patients with Noonan's syndrome, the overall incidence of certain malformations is different (Table 141–11). Patients with Noonan's syndrome have a better prognosis for gonadal function and height than those with Turner's syndrome. Noonan's syndrome patients are at greater risk for malignant hyperpyrexia[249] and coagulation defect.[243]

Other endocrine disorders may be associated with intrinsic short stature. Hypocalcemia is associated with inherent short stature in pseudohypoparathyroidism. Male genital abnormalities are accompanied by the development of short stature, which is sometimes manifest as mild IUGR, in the syndromes of Robinow, Smith-Lemli-Opitz, and Aar-

skog, as well as with aneuploidy of certain autosomes.[181] In Robinow's syndrome, although the mesomelia is present at birth, overall length may be within normal limits.

In some types of osteochondrodystrophies, stunting of growth is of postnatal onset. Some individuals with bone dystrophies have only subtle deformity (e.g., dyschondrosteosis), or the skeletal abnormality or malformation makes its appearance only very gradually (e.g., spondyloepiphyseal dysplasia tarda and trichorhinophalangeal syndrome). The Weismann-Netter syndrome is an autosomal dominant dysplasia with asymptomatic bowing of the legs and short stature resembling Blount's disease.[250] The mucopolysaccharide storage diseases are characterized by various combinations of skeletal deformity, joint deformity, mental deterioration, corneal clouding, deafness, and hepatosplenomegaly. It has been estimated that in only about half the patients with multiple defects has a pattern or cause been discerned; "new" disorders are being delineated continually.[251, 252] The dysostoses (malformations of single bones, singly or in combination) are not usually accompanied by intrinsic short stature. However, there are exceptions to this generalization, as in the brachydactyly type E and Weill-Marchesani and Rubinstein-Taybi syndromes. In some malformation syndromes, insufficient data are available to deduce whether the short stature is intrinsic or has an endocrine basis—e.g., GH deficiency has been described in Fanconi's anemia.[253, 254]

Abnormalities of cellular growth in vitro have been noted in some types of primordial dwarfs, particularly those characterized by a prematurely senile appearance. The decreased growth of isolated cells from patients with progeria may be attributable to deficient repair of DNA chains.[255, 256] In Cockayne's syndrome, there is depressed recovery of DNA and RNA synthesis in response to ultraviolet light.[257] A decreased rate of mitotic division of fibroblasts from patients with Werner's syndrome also has been noted.[258]

The development of skin, hair, or joint abnormalities is common to several of the congenital syndromes of intrinsic growth failure in the absence of skeletal dysplasia[259] (Table 141–12). In addition, defects of these structures may occur in association with dystrophic disorders of bone (e.g., McKusick's metaphyseal chondrodysplasia).

The proper management of intrinsic growth disorders includes genetic counseling when a specific diagnosis can be made. The various atlases referenced are invaluable in this regard. Guidance must be given in the management of associated abnormalities and psychosocial problems. Attention must be directed toward treatment of associated endocrine or metabolic disease. Frankness regarding the prognosis for ultimate height is best. Dwarfed children tend to be treated as babies or "mascots." These children need advice on ways they can project their age and maturity.[260] Support groups have been formed for affected children by Little People of America (Box 126, Owatonna, MN 55060) and the Human Growth Foundation (7777 Leesburg Pike, Suite 202–5, P.O. Box 3090, Falls Church, VA 22043). There is no therapy that will clearly increase the ultimate height of children with intrinsic growth disorders.

There is considerable interest in the use of human recombinant GH in current replacement doses (about 0.15 mg/kg/week administered subcutaneously) to increase growth of nonhypopituitary dwarfs.[183] GH therapy increases

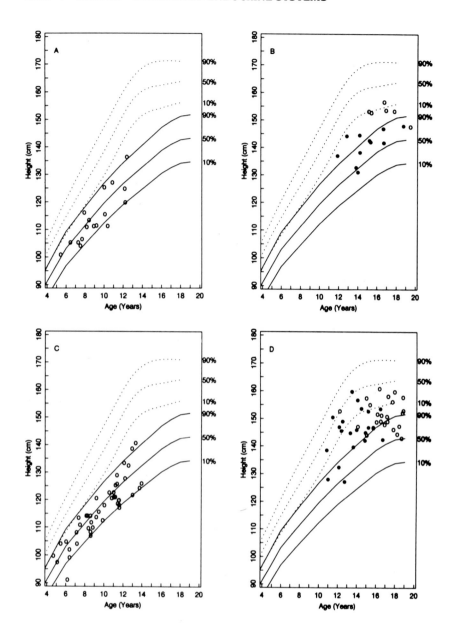

FIGURE 141–16. Growth in Turner's syndrome in response to 6 years of GH treatment, alone or in combination with oxandrolone. Normal female growth percentiles from the National Center for Health Statistics *(dotted lines)* and Turner's syndrome growth curves *(solid lines)*. A, Recipients of GH alone, before treatment. B, Recipients of GH alone, during or after treatment. C, Recipients of combination therapy, before treatment. D, Recipients of combination therapy, during or after treatment (○ = Before treatment or after cessation of therapy; ● = during treatment). (Reproduced with permission from Rosenfeld RG, Frane J, Attie KM, et al: Six-year results of a randomized prospective trial of human growth hormone and oxandrolone in Turner syndrome. J Pediatr 121:49, 1992).

the adult height of patients with Turner's syndrome[248] (see Fig. 141–16). This is possibly because the period of growth is prolonged by the concomitant hypogonadism. Growth seems proportionate, but patients must be observed for possible glucose intolerance. Treatment with the anabolic steroid oxandrolone (2-oxo-17-α-methyldihydrotestosterone), 0.05 mg/kg/day, may be a useful ancillary measure with GH in the prepubertal years. Sex steroids in replacement dosage or anabolic steroids alone improve growth rate and permit attainment of predicted adult height but do not improve on it.[261, 262] The optimal timing and dosage for use of estrogen with GH in Turner's syndrome remain to be established. Although GH therapy frequently improves growth velocity, the evidence is not convincing that GH therapy improves adult height in dwarfing syndromes other than Turner's syndrome. Off-label therapeutic uses of GH are discussed further under GH deficiency.

Delayed Growth and Development. This growth pattern usually occurs as a variation of normal but may result from ongoing health disturbances. It is postulated that disease may lead to this mode of growth in various ways. First, an early and sustained 10 per cent disturbance of linear growth rate can be calculated to lead to nearly 5 cm of growth retardation within the first 3 years of life but only about 2.5 cm of deviation from normal over the next 5 years. Alternatively, undernutrition or unknown factors may prevent catch-up growth after alleviation of an insult to growth in early childhood. The possibility also exists that variations in overall GH secretion among individuals underlie some of the variability in growth rate within the population. This concept is supported by some studies of IGF-I levels and GH dynamics and efficacy in children with constitutionally delayed growth.[263, 264]

A "constitutional" variation of normal is by far the most common cause of this growth pattern (see Fig. 141–15). There is often a parent or close relative with a similar growth pattern. The typical patient is male, perfectly healthy, and of normal birth size. Linear growth and bone maturation are proportionately retarded in infancy such that length deviates into a growth channel below the 5th percentile on distance standards beginning by 2 years of age[265]; HA and BA then typically advance at a normal rate

TABLE 141–12. Examples of Multisystem Disorders Giving Rise to Intrinsic Shortness of Postnatal Onset[181]

SYNDROMES	COMMON ASSOCIATED FEATURES
Chromosomal	
Trisomy 21 (Down)	Characteristic facies, hypotonia, mental retardation
Turner	High palate, gonadal dysgenesis
Calcium Disturbance	
Pseudohypoparathyroidism	Mental retardation, brachydactyly
Genital Abnormalities	
Smith-Lemli-Opitz	Male pseudohermaphroditism, microcephaly, characteristic facies, syndactyly
Aarskog	Scrotal anomalies, cryptorchidism, characteristic facies, hand webbing
Robinow	Mesomelia, hemivertebrae
Mucopolysaccharidoses	See text
Osteochondrodystophies and Dysostoses	See text
Premature senility	
Progeria (Hutchinson-Gilford)	Onset in infancy, characteristic facies, arteriosclerosis, lipodystrophy, mental retardation
Cockayne	Onset in early childhood, lipodystrophy, retinitis pigmentosa, photosensitivity, mental retardation, microcephaly
Werner	Onset in late childhood, characteristic facies, atherosclerosis, cataract
Skin and Hair Defects	
Poikiloderma congenita (Rothmund-Thomson)	
Sjögren-Larsson	Ichthyosis, spasticity
Contractures	
Freeman-Sheldon	"Whistling face," finger contractures, clubfeet
Moore-Federman	Joint limitation, short limbs

so that height is below, but parallel to, the 5th percentile by 3 years of age through the prepubertal years. There is delay of puberty until the child reaches a pubertal BA. A normal pubertal growth spurt subsequently culminates in a normal adult height.

Prolonged undernutrition is associated with a delayed growth pattern. Although zinc deficiency causes short stature, among 12 children with constitutional delay in growth as a normal variant, we have not found zinc deficiency.[266] A study of monozygotic twins discordant for diabetes mellitus has revealed a growth-retarding effect of this disease.[267] Growth, IGF levels, and IGF activity are probably dependent on metabolic control.[268, 269]

Tissue hypoxia causes a delayed growth pattern. This is the case in chronic anemia[154] and congenital heart disease.[270–272] Whether poor tissue perfusion mediates the growth retardation of patients with left-to-right shunts is unknown; correction of the shunt before 8 years of age results in catch-up growth if there are no complicating factors. Intrinsic intrauterine dwarfism and malnutrition are other factors implicated in the growth retardation of children with congenital heart disease.

Rickets causes a delayed growth pattern.[273, 274] Calcitriol therapy with phosphate supplementation heals resistant rickets and improves adult stature. Phosphate therapy should be monitored closely after growth is achieved because of its role in the pathogenesis of nephrocalcinosis. On the other hand, phosphate restriction improves growth in patients with renal osteodystrophy.[275]

Chronic illness of a variety of organ systems may cause growth retardation, particularly among those who are socioeconomically disadvantaged.[112] The mechanisms of growth failure in these circumstances are not clear. Although prolonged use of stimulant drugs in high dosage

(e.g., methylphenidate over 20 mg/day) for the therapy of hyperactive children has reportedly been associated with reversible retardation of growth,[276] the height measurements in these studies have not been properly controlled. The average size of mentally defective children is moderately less than normal.[277] The possibility is great that this observation is due to inclusion of patients with unrecognized chromosomal, endocrine, metabolic, and nutritional disorders.

Constitutional delay is a diagnosis of exclusion and in extreme cases is difficult, if not impossible, to distinguish from subtle deficits of GH (Figs. 141–17 and 141–18). The diagnosis of constitutionally delayed growth is made if careful medical history and examination—including careful determination of the growth rate—as well as screening tests (complete blood count, erythrocyte sedimentation rate, urinalysis, and serum electrolytes, calcium, phosphorus, urea nitrogen, and proteins) are nonrevealing.[64] The plasma IGF-I level tends to be low in such children until sexual maturation begins. After the skeletal age has reached 10 to 11 years, gonadotropin levels should be checked to determine if the patient's delayed puberty is due to primary hypogonadism. The distinction of organic hypogonadotropism from delayed puberty usually can be made by determination of gonadotropin levels during sleep or in response to a gonadotropin-releasing hormone agonist test by 14 years of age. A family history of constitutional delay in puberty is useful in helping the child's psychological outlook but should not be relied on to make a diagnosis. From the BA, prediction can be made regarding the approximate potential for adult height and the approximate time of onset of puberty (in the most severely delayed cases, height-prediction tables are, unfortunately, likely to overestimate adult height because puberty occurs

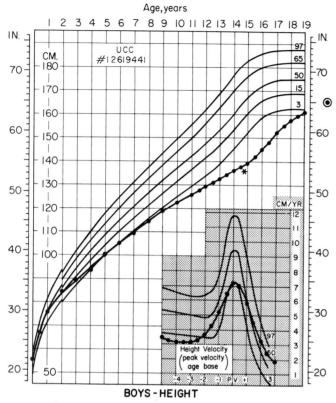

BOYS - HEIGHT

*testes 2.4 cm, pH III, BA II.25 yr.

FIGURE 141–17. Linear growth curve in a boy with unusual growth pattern as an apparent variation of normal. Parental heights, 40th to 50th percentile. Patient had a history of mild asthma. Endocrine evaluation in 1974 at 10.5 years of age, when growth rate was 3.7 cm/year, revealed normal findings. Peak serum GH levels in response to insulin, L-dopa, and estrogen-primed L-dopa tests were 3, 7, and 8 ng/ml, respectively. These results were interpreted at that time to be within normal limits. Puberty began at 14.8 years of age (*) and progressed normally. At 18.5 years of age, height was 159.7 cm, weight 53.2 kg, bone age 15.5 years, and the plasma somatomedin-C value 0.9 U/ml. Adult height is predicted to be 165 cm. Although this boy might now be considered to have a partial deficit in GH, he is achieving normal adult height. (Reproduced with permission from Schaff-Blass E, Burstein S, Rosenfield RL: Advances in diagnosis and treatment of short stature, with special reference to the role of growth hormone. J Pediatr 104:801, 1984.)

at an earlier than average BA[278]). If the test results are within the normal prepubertal range and the expectations for continued normal linear growth and pubertal development are not fulfilled, the child should be reevaluated.

The first step in managing a patient with constitutionally delayed development is to reassure him or her regarding probable normality. The patient also should be assured that a pubertal growth spurt will surely occur, probably spontaneously. The wide normal variation in the pattern and timing of the pubertal spurt should be explained in detail, and the patient should be informed of the predicted ultimate height. Meanwhile, the psychological state of the child should be considered. Amazingly, the majority of children with delayed puberty do not have overt psychological symptoms. Obviously, complex compensations and sublimations occur. However, peer group pressure may make adjustment to shortness and sexual infantilism especially difficult for some by the time they start high school at about 14 years. A poor self-image may lead to social

withdrawal and feelings of hopelessness in such children. Physical immaturity may prolong psychological immaturity. A short course of sex hormone therapy may alleviate these anxieties. If puberty is delayed beyond 13 or 14 years of age, the age at which 90 per cent of girls and boys, respectively, have begun to mature, cautious sex hormone therapy may be considered. Before undertaking the induction of puberty, the child and family must be advised with regard to the normality of the child's condition and the unknown factors (though therapy seems safe, no long-term follow-up studies have been reported; errors are inherent in height predictions). Those children who are more concerned with eventual height than immediate gains often choose to forego medical intervention at this point.

In order to minimize the possibility of loss of growth potential, we recommend that the initial course of therapy or the induction of sexual development consist of monthly injections for 6 months of 50 mg/m² repository testosterone in boys and 0.5 mg depot estradiol in girls.[64] Such a course of therapy has no deleterious effect on height po-

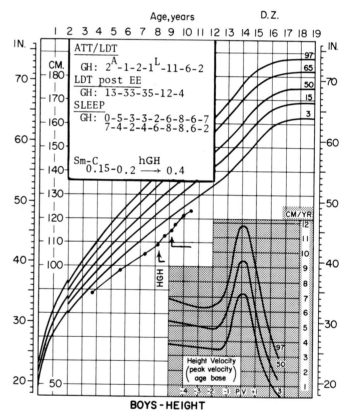

BOYS - HEIGHT

FIGURE 141–18. Growth pattern of a patient with a delayed growth pattern as an unexplained, apparently constitutional variation of normal. Family history revealed his mother to be 157 cm and father 191 cm in height. At the chronological age of 9.1 years, bone age was 6.2 years, and growth rate was marginally subnormal at 5.6 cm/year. GH levels (see inset, including ATT, LDT, and sleep GH every 30 min) were normal; the plasma somatomedin-C concentration was compatible with hyposomatotropism, although normal for bone age, and rose with GH 0.1 U/kg daily × 4. The growth rate improved 50 per cent during a 6-month course of GH, 0.1 U/kg 3 times weekly, and subsequently reverted to the pretreatment rate. A 1.5-year course of GH therapy led to an initial improvement in growth rate followed by waning of responsiveness to 5.5 cm/year. Upon subsequent discontinuation of GH, the growth rate fell further to 3.2 cm/year. After 2 years, the child's height is about 3 cm greater than would have been projected. However, predicted adult height is unimproved at 156.5 cm.

tential and has clearly positive effects on self-image. The patient's growth, development, and predicted height should be carefully re-evaluated immediately upon completion of the therapeutic regimen and again 6 months later before undertaking a second course of therapy. Depot testosterone, 100 mg/m²/month, and depot estradiol, 1.0 mg/month, closely approximate midpubertal sex hormone production in boys and girls, respectively. We prefer administering injections of repository forms of sex hormones to avoid the occasional side effects of 17-alkylated steroid analogues. However, the anabolic steroid oxandrolone, 0.1 mg/kg/day for 3 to 6 months, has been used without compromising final height.[279] We also prefer to avoid the frequent injections necessary if chorionic gonadotropin is used for puberty induction. Premature use of adult replacement doses of androgen or estrogen (about two-fold greater than the midpubertal doses) will cause a disproportionate advance of BA relative to linear growth. Thyroid hormone is a controversial, though relatively benign, mode of treatment of constitutionally delayed growth.[280] If treatment is to be undertaken, the following precautions seem necessary to avoid prolonged unnecessary dependence on the hormone: (1) control observations for two consecutive 6-month periods and (2) observation for the height acceleration and transient weight loss characteristic of the juvenile hypothyroidal patient's response to replacement therapy 3 and 6 months after treatment is begun.

GH therapy occasionally seems efficacious in patients

TABLE 141–13. PRIMARY GH-RELATED GROWTH FAILURE

MECHANISM	GH LEVEL*	IGF-I LEVEL
GH deficiency		
Profound	Low	Low
Incomplete	Variable	Variable
Partial		
Neurosecretory defect		
Transient		
Bioinactive GH	Variable	Low
GH resistance		
GH action (Laron's syndrome)	High	Low
IGF-I Sm-C deficiency (pygmy syndrome)	Normal	Low
IGF-I Sm-C resistance	Normal	High

*Overall secretory dynamics, considering spontaneous and stimulated flux.
From Schaff-Blass E, Burstein S, Rosenfield RL: Advances in diagnosis and treatment of short stature, with special reference to the role of growth hormone. J Pediatr 104:801, 1984.

with a constitutionally delayed growth pattern (see Fig. 141–18). About one third of children with unexplained short stature respond with an increased growth rate to replacement doses of GH[263, 264, 281, 282] (Fig. 141–19). The use of GH as therapy for nonstandard as well as standard indications is discussed in detail in the next section.

Attenuated Growth Pattern. This growth pattern is characterized by a sustained subnormal growth rate. This causes the child to cross percentiles on growth charts (see Fig. 141–15). It is clearly abnormal. It can almost always be proved to result from endocrine, metabolic, or severe systemic disease.[34] The differential diagnosis is given in Table 141–8.

GH-related growth failure is the most subtle cause of growth failure because the child may be normal in every respect but growth. GH-related growth failure results from specific alterations in the chain of events from GH synthesis to its growth-promoting action (see Fig. 141–1). Primary GH-related growth failure can result from deficient secretion of GH (which may be complete or incomplete), secretion of a bioinactive GH, or resistance to GH action (Table 141–13).

GH deficiency is the most common of these disorders. It can be congenital or acquired; isolated or associated with other pituitary hormone deficiencies; idiopathic or secondary to either destructive lesions of the hypothalamic-pituitary axis or emotional disturbances.

Congenital GH deficiency may have a genetic basis, which accounts for 5 to 35 per cent of cases.[283] The human GH gene cluster consists of five similar hGH and hCS genes all located on the long arm of chromosome 17 at bands q22–24.[284] These include hGH-1, the gene that encodes the hGH peptide synthesized by the somatotropic cells of the anterior pituitary, hGH-2, hCS-L, and hCS-B. Based on the genetic and clinical characteristics, four distinct types of familial isolated GH deficiency have been described.[285] Isolated GH deficiency type IA results from a GH-1 gene deletion and is characterized by severe GH deficiency presenting by 6 months of age and frequent development of anti-GH antibodies during the course of exogenous GH treatment in a titer sufficient to produce growth arrest. Isolated GH deficiency type IB is not associated with GH-1 gene deletions and is autosomal recessive

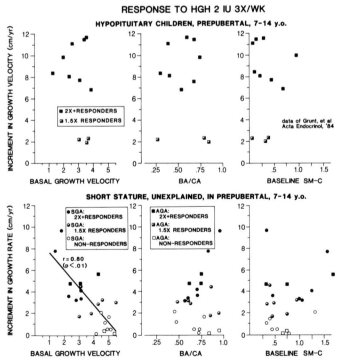

FIGURE 141–19. Response to GH therapy of short children with *(top)* and without *(bottom)* apparent GH deficiency. Many apparently normal short children experience a 50 per cent or greater increase in growth rate, whether born of appropriate size or small for gestational age (AGA or SGA, respectively). Among such children, the best predictor of response was the pretreatment growth rate *(lower left)*. Most, but not all, responders have a bone age that is 75 per cent or more retarded. (Data of Grunt et al.[281])

in nature. Isolated GH deficiency type II is autosomal dominant, while isolated GH deficiency type III is X-linked; both of these have characteristics similar to those of type IB. Familial TSH and GH deficiency may be due to mutations of the pit-1 gene.[286] Congenital GH deficiency also can occur as part of familial congenital malformation syndromes associated with midline facial and central nervous system (CNS) defects (cleft lip, cleft palate,[287, 288] dental anomalies,[289] optic dysplasia,[290, 291] absence of septum pellucidum, holoprosencephaly[292]) or limb abnormalities (radial aplasia, polydactyly).[293]

Acquired GH deficiency can occur as the result of any insult to the hypothalamus or pituitary. It is seen with tumors of the sellar or suprasellar[294] region, including craniopharyngiomas,[295] hamartomas of the third ventricle, and germinomas.[296] Hypothalamic injury also can occur as the result of ionizing radiation.[297] The onset of hypothalamic dysfunction is often gradual and is directly related to the dose of radiation; while hypothalamic dysfunction rarely occurs with low radiation doses (i.e., 1200 rads), it occurs in approximately 15 per cent of patients receiving 2400 rads and half of patients receiving 5000 rads.[298] Other rare causes of acquired GH deficiency include cerebrovascular malformations, infections of the CNS,[299] hemosiderosis,[300] and trauma.[301]

Isolated GH deficiency is usually idiopathic. This occurs in about 1 child in 5000.[302, 303] These patients, as a group, have a higher incidence of breech presentations and difficult deliveries as well as an "ectopic posterior pituitary gland" visualizable by MRI, suggesting that birth trauma may play a role in the development of GH deficiency.[304, 304a] Most often, the defect is the result of deficient secretion of hypothalamic GRF rather than of pituitary GH itself.[305, 306]

Abnormal neural control of GH secretion (*neurosecretory defect*) may be a common cause of GH deficiency.[307] Cranial irradiation has been discovered to be a model for neurosecretory defect.[308, 309] GH responses to insulin, arginine, or L-dopa testing are clearly normal (greater than 10 ng/ml) in about one third of these cases, although there is a marked blunting in spontaneous pulsatile GH secretion, and the abnormal growth rate is normalized by GH replacement therapy. The blunting of GH secretion appears to be due to GRF deficit,[310] GRF being relatively vulnerable because of the paucity of GRF neurons.[311] The abnormalities of GH release observed in patients with congenital brain dysfunction and growth failure[312] may signify that a neurosecretory defect is the cause of their growth failure.

Functional GH deficiency occurs in children who have been emotionally deprived.[313–315] This *deprivational dwarfism* may be seen in children who may or may not be overtly disturbed but who typically show abnormal behavior patterns, including hoarding food, drinking from toilets or puddles, and sleepwalking.[316] The basis of their growth failure is not clear but may be related, in part, to nutritional factors.[317, 318] The diagnosis of deprivational dwarfism is often difficult because the patient's appearance may belie undernutrition. GH deficiency may disappear within days of hospitalization or require several weeks to resolve.[319] ACTH and TSH deficiency sometimes coexist. These children are often mistakenly labeled as having hypopituitarism and treated with exogenous GH or thyroid hormone without significant improvement.[320] Their biochemical abnormalities and abnormal growth improve only after they

have been removed from the home and placed in a favorable psychosocial environment.

The secretion of a structurally abnormal GH molecule may result in GH-related growth failure. Kowarski and co-workers[321] have postulated that some children with typical characteristics of GH deficiency but normal GH responses to provocative testing produce an immunoassayable GH that is biologically inactive. Whereas these investigators were able to show a low ratio of radioreceptor-assayable to radioimmunoassayable GH in their subjects, the existence of mutant GH molecules which might account for these findings remains to be proven. The application of newly available molecular biology techniques to these issues should help delineate the bioinactive GH syndromes and establish the molecular basis of the defects.

Peripheral resistance to the actions of GH may result from a variety of causes. Laron-type dwarfism, the most common form of primary GH resistance, results from abnormalities of the GH receptor gene.[322, 323] These subjects typically have high GH levels, low IGF-I levels, and low or undetectable levels of GH binding protein, the truncated, circulating form of the GH receptor.[324, 325] This disorder responds to IGF-I treatment.[326] A similar defect probably is responsible for the occurrence of pygmies, although there is controversy about this.[327, 328]

In other cases of GH resistance, the defect appears to reside in the actions of IGF-I; Heath-Monnig et al.[329] reported on a subject with unexplained growth failure and high IGF-I levels, suggesting primary tissue unresponsiveness to IGF-I. More commonly, however, the resistance to IGF-I is the result of IGF inhibitors, some of which have been shown to have structural homology with IGF binding proteins.[330, 331] Secondary resistance to the actions of GH with deficient IGF-I generation may occur in several systemic illnesses, such as malnutrition (including anorexia nervosa),[332] poorly controlled diabetes, liver disease,[333] and chronic renal insufficiency.[330, 331]

A GH-related disorder must be suspected in any child with a subnormal rate of growth, regardless of stature, or in any child with unexplained severe short stature, especially when accompanied by a significant delay in BA maturation.[34] Because of their GH dependency, IGF-I and IGF-II measurements may prove helpful in screening for possible GH deficiency.[334] However, only a high-normal IGF-I concentration excludes GH deficiency, and a low level is not diagnostic because IGF-I levels may be in the hyposomatotrophic range in very young normal children or in malnutrition and other chronic systemic illnesses.[335] Recent data suggest that determinations of IGFBP-3 levels may prove helpful in screening for GH deficiency.[336]

The diagnosis of GH deficiency is based on finding evidence of low GH secretion. However, there is uncertainty about the best methods for documenting GH deficiency and for quantitating serum GH levels. Because GH secretion occurs only in a few pulses a day, most of which occur during sleep, and because serum concentrations fall to nearly undetectable levels between secretory bursts, GH sufficiency (or deficiency) traditionally has been established by measuring GH concentrations after pharmacological stimulation.[337] The situation is complicated by the fact that GH assays using monoclonal antibodies yield values that are about one half the values of assays using polyclonal antisera.[338]

TABLE 141–14. COMMONLY EMPLOYED TESTS OF GROWTH HORMONE SECRETORY CAPACITY

TYPE OF TEST	CONDITIONS	COMMENTS
Physiological tests		
Exercises	15 min of moderate exercise followed by 5 min of vigorous exercise	Lack of standardization, frequent findings of low responses in normals
Sleep	Deep sleep (EEG stages 3–4) Diurnal secretory studies	Best utilized in association with EEG Lack of reliable normative data, high variability, requires skilled nursing
Pharmacological tests		
Insulin tolerance test	Regular insulin 0.05 to 1.0 U/kg IV push	Severe hypoglycemia, seizures
Arginine	0.5 g/kg IV over 30 min	Nausea, vomiting, hypoglycemia, local irritation, numbness
Levodopa	0.5 g/m² orally	Nausea, vomiting, cardiac and BP changes
Glucagon	0.03 mg/kg IM up to 0.5 mg	Nausea, vomiting
Propranolol	1.0 mg/kg up to 40 mg (can be used to augment responses to primary stimulation test, such as with glucagon; must be given 2 h before stimuli)	Changes in heart rate, BP, hypoglycemia
Clonidine	150 μg/m² orally	Severe somnolence, cardiac and BP changes

GH deficiency classically has been defined as a lack of an increase in serum GH to 7 ng/ml or more in response to two pharmacological stimulation tests in a child growing at a subnormal rate.[34, 263, 337] Responses consistently between 7 and 10 ng/ml by a polyclonal radioimmunoassay are interpreted by most endocrinologists as compatible with partial GH deficiency.[263] Whereas there are a variety of stimulation tests available (Table 141–14), it is our impression that the insulin tolerance test (ITT), arginine infusion test (AIT), and levodopa stimulation test (LST) are the most reliable. Further, two pharmacological tests are used because 10 to 20 per cent of apparently normal children have a blunted response to any given single test, whereas this occurs only rarely (<5 per cent) when at least two tests are employed.[34, 263, 337] The GH response to a test may be depressed by glucose, obesity, hypothyroidism, or a variety of drugs that affect neurotransmission.[34, 337] Poor GH release during the ITT cannot be interpreted if the blood glucose level falls less than 40 to 50 per cent. Glucose administration blocks the response to insulin and to L-dopa.[339]

In the case of discordant GH responses to the two pharmacological studies or presumed partial GH deficiency, we rely on either sex hormone priming or a spontaneous GH secretory study as an additional means of defining the GH sufficiency of the subject. One to two bedtime 10-μg doses of ethinyl estradiol normalize GH responses in patients with delayed puberty.[340] In our hands, using a polyclonal assay, a mean nighttime GH of 1.5 ng/ml or less or peak nighttime GH values of 6 ng/ml or less are considered abnormal.[341]

Although it has been proposed that measurement of integrated GH levels over a 12- to 24-h period permits the diagnosis of GH deficiency,[263] the reliability of this test has been questioned recently. Rose et al.[342] assessed the clinical utility of measuring spontaneous GH secretion in short children with and without GH deficiency. Whereas GH-deficient children, classically defined, had low mean 24-h GH levels as a group, 43 per cent had mean 24-h GH levels that were within the normal range. On the other hand, all short normal children had both normal responses to provocative stimulation tests and normal mean 24-h GH levels. Further, studies by Costin et al.[343] and Lin et al.[344] indicate that overnight GH secretory profiles have considerable var-

iation, with substantial overlap between normal and hypopituitary children. Taken together, these studies suggest that spontaneous GH secretory studies occupy an ancillary position in our diagnostic armamentarium.

Pituitary GH was first shown to be an effective treatment for GH deficiency in the late 1950's.[345] Only human GH is efficacious in GH deficiency due to the species specificity of the hormone.[82] Because of the association of human cadaveric pituitary GH with Creutzfeldt-Jakob disease, a progressive form of dementia presumably caused by an infectious agent known as a *prion*,[346] only recombinant DNA–derived hormone has been available for the treatment of GH deficiency in the United States since 1985. Replacement therapy with GH can be expected to normalize carbohydrate and fat metabolism as well as growth.[347] It also potentiates the effect of sex hormones.[348] GRF would seem to be a physiological form of therapy for many, but the requirement for multiple daily injections to give a response equivalent to GH therapy makes it impractical.[349] Dopaminergic agents have been reported to be effective in certain circumstances, but their role is uncertain.[350]

The optimal dosage regimen for GH administration is not known.[345] The dosage regimens currently used reflect, to some extent, criteria developed at a time when the quantity of the hormone was limited and insufficient to meet the needs for adequate treatment of all GH-deficient patients. It should be kept in mind that GH-deficient patients with the growth without GH syndrome will grow normally without GH treatment.[54–56, 291]

GH is administered parenterally (preferably by the subcutaneous route) in multiple weekly doses.[345] The usual starting dose is 0.05 mg/kg (0.1 U/kg) given three times a week. Occasionally, daily GH administration is necessary to prevent hypoglycemia.[351] The vast majority of children with GH deficiency will have at least a 50 per cent improvement in growth rate after the initiation of GH therapy. The growth is proportionate (Fig. 141–20). The increase in growth rate is greatest during the first year of therapy, averaging 9 to 11 cm/year, but then typically declines to lower levels during subsequent years of treatment. The cause of this waning effect is not known but may represent, in part, normalization of the growth rate once children begin to reach their preestablished growth channels.[109] Other factors which tend to prognosticate excellent growth

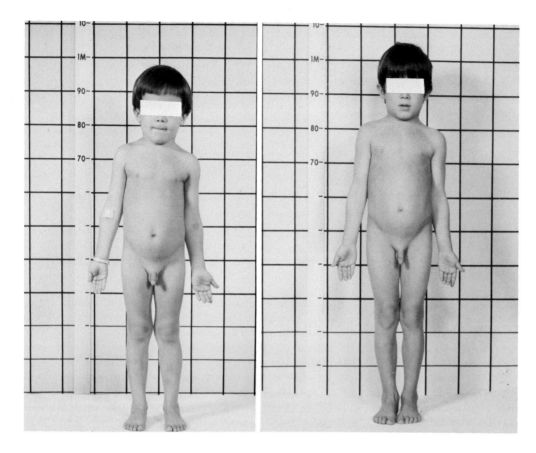

FIGURE 141–20. GH-deficient patient before *(left)* and after *(right)* treatment with GH for 1 year. Note that the growth spurt is accompanied by normal maturation of body proportions.

response include younger chronological age, younger bone age, shorter height at initiation of therapy, and idiopathic versus organic GH deficiency.[352–354] Emerging data suggest that daily GH treatment (using the same total weekly dose but divided into daily doses) results in a slightly greater increase in initial growth rate with a less pronounced waning effect in the subsequent years of therapy.[355]

Treatment should be monitored by measurement of linear growth and plasma IGF-I levels. Poor response to treatment may be due to poor compliance with therapy, undernutrition,[320] or other causes. Antibodies against GH have been detected in approximately 5 to 30 per cent of GH-deficient patients who have received human GH, but rarely have these resulted in blunting of the growth response.[356] Hypothyroidism due to development of TSH deficiency[357] should be treated. Glucocorticoid therapy may interfere with the response to GH.[358] Hyposomatotropic children are unusually sensitive to the growth-inhibiting effects of glucosteroids. Therefore, these hormones should be replaced only if there are clinical symptoms or signs of glucocorticoid deficiency, such as lethargy, cachexia, or hypoglycemia. If necessary, cortisol should be given in the lowest maintenance dose that will restore health, 5 to 20 mg/m²/day in three divided doses. Unexplained refractoriness to GH may be overcome by increasing the dose.[359] Anabolic steroids may enhance the effectiveness of GH.[360]

Reports on the long-term results and final adult heights attained by GH-deficient children treated with pituitary human GH have been few and generally disappointing (Fig. 141–21). Burns et al.[352] reported final heights ranging from 158.1 to 168.1 cm (62.2 to 66.2 in) in boys and 142.5 to 154.4 cm (56.1 to 60.8 in) in girls with idiopathic GH

deficiency. Boys and girls with organic GH deficiency due to craniopharyngioma had average final heights of 167.5 cm (65.9 in) and 153.5 cm (60.4 in), respectively.[353] Similar results were reported by Hibi et al.[354] Interestingly, Hibi et al. noted that children with associated hypogonadotropism who required exogenous induction of puberty had somewhat better final heights (163.7 ± 3.9 cm in boys and 151.0 ± 5.1 cm in girls), implying that delay in pubertal development may be associated with a better final height prognosis.[354]

The overall poor final height prognosis described in these reports may be related, in part, to frequent interruptions in pituitary GH therapy due to its unavailability, delays in diagnosis and therapy, lack of compliance with the administration of GH, concomitant therapy with glucocorticoids, and mandatory discontinuation of drug with attainment of a height of 5 ft, 5 in in boys and 5 ft in girls because of the scarcity of pituitary GH. It is likely that greater availability of recombinant DNA–derived GH, further optimization of therapy, and earlier diagnosis and initiation of treatment will contribute to an improved final height prognosis in GH-deficient patients.

GH therapy is generally well tolerated and rarely associated with significant side effects.[345] However, there may be mild local pain, irritation, swelling, or redness where the GH injection is given. Slipped capital femoral epiphyses have been reported in a small number of children receiving GH treatment and should be suspected if the child complains of leg pain or limp. The development of glucose intolerance is rare but may be anticipated with the use of higher doses of the drug. Reversible benign intracranial hypertension occurs on rare occasions mostly within the first few months of therapy.[345a]

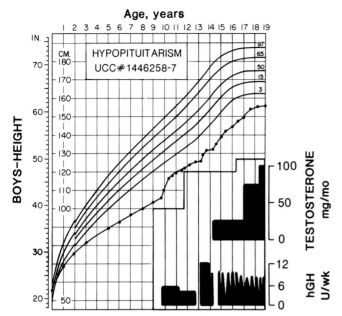

Age, years

BOYS-HEIGHT

HYPOPITUITARISM
UCC#1446258-7

TESTOSTERONE mg/mo

hGH U/wk

FIGURE 141–21. Growth record of TR, a child with congenital hyposomatotropism. He was born with cleft palate, bilaterally cleft lip, and a small penis. The diagnosis of GH deficit was not suspected until a newborn sibling who had a cleft palate, cleft lip, and congenital heart disease died and at autopsy no pituitary gland was found. Although TR grew in infancy, his growth was subnormal and eventually clearly attenuated. He had a typical response to the initiation of GH therapy, transient catch-up growth followed by change to a delayed growth pattern. Therapy was discontinued for a few months at 12.8 years of age because of a short supply of GH. Resumption of GH therapy at 13.1 years of age was followed by a second period of catch-up. However, growth failure quickly ensued which proved to be due to poor compliance with GH (interruptions of GH dose in inset). Normal final height was not attained despite numerous admonitions to take GH as prescribed.

There has been concern about the possible association of GH therapy with leukemia in GH-deficient children.[361] A workshop organized by the Human Growth Foundation and the Lawson Wilkins Pediatric Endocrine Society[362] concluded that there was a possible increased risk of leukemia in GH-deficient patients treated with GH but that it could not be concluded that GH treatment was responsible for this increase. Further, they suggested that if a risk does exist, it is believed to be small. There is no evidence that enlargement of preexisting tumors can be attributed to GH therapy.

Short-term studies have shown that GH treatment improves the growth rates of some short children who are not deficient in GH.[263] However, the results have been somewhat disparate due to the small numbers of patients studied, the heterogeneity of patient selection criteria (especially with regard to growth rates and sexual developmental status), the variable doses of GH used, and the variations in the length of GH treatment. In these studies, the best responders tend to have the lowest pretreatment growth rates and a tendency to retardation of bone age, thus resembling GH-deficient patients (see Fig. 141–19). However, there were no clinical or biochemical determinants that reliably predicted the individual response to GH treatment. Whereas Rudman et al.[363] suggested that IGF-I responses to short-term GH administration correlated with the subsequent response to GH therapy, subsequent reports have not borne this out.[364, 365] In addition, while it has

been proposed that children with lower indices of GH secretion will have a better response to GH therapy, integrated GH concentrations have not proved to be reliable predictors of the response to treatment primarily because of their high variability.[343, 344] Because of the lack of reliable therapeutic predictors, some investigators have suggested using a 6-month trial of GH to identify those subjects who will have an enhanced growth response to GH treatment.[366] This approach is not shared by all pediatric endocrinologists because of the lack of information regarding the efficacy of such a trial in predicting whether long-term therapy will improve adult height.

Despite this increasing body of information on the short-term growth response of short-normal children to GH therapy, there have been few data on the impact of this treatment on final adult heights. Kaplan and Grumbach[367] recently reported on the long-term results of GH treatment of children with isolated short stature and subnormal growth rates. About 80 per cent of children had an improvement in the rate of growth with GH treatment; however, only 30 per cent had an increase in height prediction of 3.0 cm or more. Further, other reports have indicated that short children may have a compensatory deceleration of growth rate once GH treatment is discontinued.[368] Others have suggested that GH may increase the rate of pubertal maturation, possibly accelerating epiphyseal fusion and blunting the long-term response to therapy.[369] Thus short-term gains in height may not necessarily predict long-term improvements in stature. Until more information is available on the long-term response of short-normal children to GH therapy and the side effects of long-term GH therapy in short, otherwise normal children, it seems best to adopt a conservative approach and "not fix what isn't broken."[370]

Hypothyroidism causes retardation of linear growth and bone maturation. Catch-up growth is to be expected after treatment of long-standing juvenile hypothyroidism, as discussed above.[109, 117, 120] The differential diagnosis and management of hypothyroidism are discussed in detail elsewhere (Ch. 45). The replacement dose of thyroid hormone in children averages 100 μg/m²/day.[371] Dosage should be individualized according to the serum T_4 and TSH level achieved.

Glucocorticoid excess, whether due to spontaneous Cushing's syndrome or to therapeutic glucocorticoids, results in linear growth failure. Growth is the most sensitive indicator of corticoid excess, and growth arrest may be the only clear clinical sign of Cushing's syndrome.[372] Pseudo-Cushing's syndrome in an infant has been reported to be caused by ethanol in breast milk[373]; the growth failure in this syndrome may result from inhibition of GRF release by ethanol.[373a] Diagnostic and therapeutic approaches to Cushing's syndrome are discussed in Chapter 100. Catch-up growth may occur after alleviation of the hypercortisolism.[109, 374–376] The cause for poor catch-up growth in some cases is unclear. It has been proposed that this is due to a subtle destructive effect of corticoids on the growth plate, which becomes more noticeable with duration and intensity of glucocorticoid exposure. However, the failure of catch-up growth seems more likely to be noticeable when the glucocorticoid excess is not relieved well before puberty. The potential for further growth and pubertal development if hypothalamic-pituitary function is preserved must be kept in mind when advising therapy for children with Cushing's syndrome due to bilateral adrenal hyperplasia. A trial of cyproheptadine therapy may bring about remission.[376] In children and adolescents, transsphenoidal microadenomectomy in experienced hands appears to be the treatment of choice, even if no adenoma is detected by computed tomography.[377] Subsequent normal growth and few sequelae are reported; however, very few cases have been followed long term. Irradiation therapy of Cushing's disease with about 4000 rad results in a 75 per cent remission rate but a 40 per cent incidence of low GH responses (<7 ng/ml) to hypoglycemia.[378] Not only does bilateral adrenalectomy result in permanent hypoadrenalism, but many patients also develop evidence of a pituitary tumor eventually.[375]

In cases in which growth failure accompanies glucocorticoid therapy of serious nonendocrine disease, it may be difficult to decide whether the growth problem is due to the disease or to the steroid. Prednisone doses of approximately 5 mg/m²/day typically inhibit growth.[57] The decision about steroid dose is particularly difficult, since the amount of steroid analogue that suppresses inflammation does not seem to be proportionate to the amount that inhibits growth and ACTH release. For example, prednisone and dexamethasone are two- and fourfold, respectively, as potent in suppressing growth and ACTH release as they are in suppressing inflammation.[379] Furthermore, there are individual differences in steroid metabolism that influence the extent of steroid side effects.[380] If it is necessary to document the fact that the patient's steroid dose is excessive, it is our practice to determine the plasma dehydroepiandrosterone sulfate level (if the child is postadrenarchal) and/or the ACTH and corticol responses to corticotropin-releasing hormone.

In cases in which growth inhibition is attributable to glucocorticoid treatment of nonendocrine disease, there are four possible alternatives: (1) use another form of therapy, (2) lower the daily steroid dose if the underlying disease can be so controlled, (3) switch the patient to alternate-morning prednisone therapy,[381] or (4) switch the patient to topical (e.g., inhaled) steroid therapy.[382] Alternate-day "pulses" of prednisone or topical administration often result in preservation of the desired therapeutic effect while avoiding the unwanted cushingoid changes, but neither is a certain solution to the dilemma.

Metabolic disturbances or *generalized disease* often attenuates growth. Any chronic disturbance of pH does so. Alkalosis arrests growth unless well controlled with potassium chloride plus possibly spironolactone or triamterene.[383] Acidosis, such as that resulting from renal failure, renal tubular disease, disturbed amino acid or lactate metabolism, and glycogen storage disease, causes growth retardation.[30] Acidosis should be treated with sodium bicarbonate and/or potassium citrate solutions.

Growth attenuation is a major problem in chronic renal failure. The causes are complex and include (1) chronic acidosis, (2) osteodystrophy due to acidosis, hyperphosphatemia with secondary hyperparathyroidism, and deficient vitamin D action, (3) poor nutritional status associated with negative caloric balance, (4) functional abnormalities in the GH axis, and (5) glucocorticoid therapy in the posttransplantation patient.[263, 384, 385] GH treatment improves height velocity, decreases IGFBP-1, and raises IGFBP-3, al-

though not in proportion to the rise in IGF-I levels.[386] Renal transplantation does not consistently improve growth; this is, at least in part, related to glucocorticoid dosage. GH administration appears to improve growth velocity in this setting, too, although there is concern that it may deleteriously affect function of the transplanted kidney.[387, 388] Calcitriol, 0.125 to 0.5 µg/day, is used with phosphate restriction to treat renal osteodystrophy.

Hypoalbuminemia is a common thread in several diseases causing linear growth failure, such as regional enteritis, nephrosis, and liver disease.[112, 333, 389] However, hypoalbuminemia may be only a marker because available data suggest that hereditary analbuminemia is not characterized by growth failure.[390] Regional enteritis is the most common nonendocrine disorder encountered in our clinic as a cause of primary growth failure. It mimics GH deficiency because patients sometimes present with growth failure without bowel symptoms or obvious malnutrition (Fig. 141–22). In our experience, four or five such patients have a low serum albumin level, low hemoglobin level, or high erythrocyte sedimentation rate. Control of inflammation and increase in caloric intake improve growth.[389] Growth failure has just as mysteriously been reported on occasion to be the primary manifestation of celiac disease[391] or hereditary fructose intolerance.[392] The growth failure of chil-

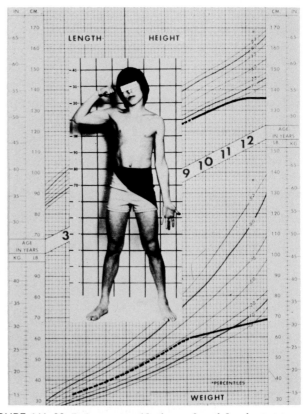

FIGURE 141–22. Patient at age 13 when referred for short stature and delayed puberty. Growth records show plateauing of weight commencing around 9 years of age, of height 1 to 2 years later. The data are plotted on the standards of Stuart and Meredith. The history was unremarkable except for some vague abdominal cramps and loose stools. The photograph shows his seemingly good health, nutritional status, and excellent musculature, in keeping with his interest in competitive swimming. Examination revealed no clear-cut findings. Serum albumin was 3.05 g/dl, globulin 3.65 g/dl. He was found to have regional enteritis.

dren with chronic liver failure is associated with resistance to the effects of their elevated endogenous GH production[333] and improves after liver transplantation.[393] There is increasing evidence that growth after bone marrow transplantation depends in part on the regimen of cytotoxic drugs employed.[394]

Malnutrition which is severe, as in kwashiorkor and marasmus, and deficiency of an essential amino acid (as discussed above) clearly diminish growth velocity. Reduction of caloric intake to 82 to 91 per cent of recommended will arrest growth.[318] The mechanism whereby growth failure comes about in starvation seems to be complex; not only does energy balance seem critical, but somatomedin generation, triiodothyronine production, vitamin and mineral balance, and insulin production are also low. Congenital copper deficiency causes failure to thrive, mental deterioration, kinky hair, and bone changes.[29] Poor control of diabetes mellitus may result in attenuation of growth; the association of diabetic dwarfing with hepatomegaly is termed *Mauriac's syndrome*.[268] Severe chronic disease, such as juvenile rheumatoid arthritis, may halt growth through many mechanisms.[395] It has been difficult to judge whether GH therapy is responsible for the occasional beneficial effects sometimes observed.

Hypogonadism results in attenuation of linear growth once the BA reaches about 10 to 12 years, unless sex hormones are administered. On some occasions, preadolescent growth deceleration may be the first indication of an intrinsic growth disorder such as Turner's syndrome[396] or spondyloepiphyseal dysplasia tarda. Determination of the BA will usually permit recognition of the intrinsic nature of these problems; this criterion becomes more reliable in the second decade. On the other hand, growth arrest may result from disorders that usually manifest as delays in growth, as in hypophosphatemia.

With the exception of hyposomatotropism, the nature of the disorder causing arrested growth will usually be obvious from a carefully taken medical history and thorough examination and/or determination of routine laboratory tests: serum T_4 and cortisol, electrolytes, calcium, phosphorus, urea nitrogen, albumin, complete blood count, erythrocyte sedimentation rate, and urinalysis. Once systemic and metabolic disturbances have been excluded, evaluation for GH deficiency is imperative. Treatment must be directed toward the underlying disease. The prognosis depends on the basic disease and the degree of undernutrition.

EXCESSIVE LINEAR GROWTH. Supranormal height occurs because of either inherent endowment or an excessive stimulation of the rate of bone growth. The diagnostic approach to a child with supranormal height is similar to that used for a child who is short. The first step toward reaching a proper diagnosis is to examine the relationship among CA, HA, BA, and growth rate (see Table 141–9). *Intrinsic tallness* (Fig. 141–23) is characterized by a normal BA. Intrinsically tall people are literally "long boned." The height-attained plot of these children approximately parallels the 95th percentile but is above it. *Advanced growth* (see Fig. 141–23) is the term applied here to the growth pattern in which the linear growth channel during childhood is normal—above, but parallel to, the 95th percentile on height-attained curves—and is accompanied by a proportionately advanced skeletal age. Subjects with this growth pattern have normal predicted adult height because puberty usually occurs at an early age. *Accelerated growth* refers to that pattern in which the growth rate is excessive and adult height will be abnormal unless the underlying disorder is corrected. It is accompanied by a rate of bone maturation that is greater than normal and may advance out of proportion to BA. Thus the predicted adult height in most affected patients is not great and may in fact be subnormal.

Intrinsic Tallness. This growth pattern usually occurs as a familial variation of normal in families of above-average stature. Size is typically normal at birth, but a normal

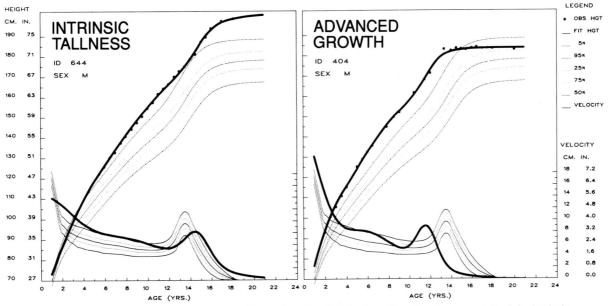

FIGURE 141–23. Growth patterns of two tall boys from the Fels Institute files. One became a tall adult (intrinsic tallness); the other grew to be of normal adult height after undergoing an early pubertal growth spurt (advanced growth). (Courtesy of RD Bock.)

growth channel is established at excessive size by 3 years of age. This growth pattern may result from a benign familial tendency to secrete GH excessively during puberty, since high plasma somatomedin-C levels and paradoxical GH responses to glucose and thyrotropin-releasing hormone have been reported.[397]

The differential diagnosis of inherent tallness includes the marfanoid syndromes (long extremities, tendency toward scoliosis): Marfan's syndrome proper, homocystinuria, and the type 2 polyendocrine syndrome. The McKusick criteria for the diagnosis of true Marfan's syndrome are the presence of two of the following four abnormalities: characteristic musculoskeletal signs (such as arachnodactyly), cardiovascular findings (such as aortic aneurysm), ocular signs (such as ectopia lentis), and autosomal dominant heredity.[128] Arachnodactyly can be quantitated from either the body proportions (see Fig. 141–6) or the metacarpal index (ratio of length to midshaft breadth of metacarpals 2 through 5; normal: male < 8.0:1, female < 8.7:1) on a BA film. Genetic diagnosis of Marfan's syndrome is becoming feasible now that it is linked to the fibrillin gene on chromosome 15.[398] Mental retardation, joint contractures, and tendency to thromboembolism are clinical features unique to homocystinuria, permitting its differentiation from Marfan's syndrome. A marfanoid habitus may be a clue to Sipple's syndrome: mucosal neuromata, familial medullary carcinoma of the thyroid, pheochromocytoma, and parathyroid adenoma or hyperplasia.[399]

An above-average height is often a social disadvantage for girls but seldom one for boys. Consequently, females frequently present to endocrinologists seeking treatment for what they consider to be "excessive" height. The medical evaluation should include judgment of the patient's personality, psychosocial status, posture, outlook if nature is allowed to take its course, and expectations of therapy. In some cases, inordinate concerns about height may be but one aspect of a major adolescent adjustment reaction. From determination of BA, one can get considerable diagnostic information and predict adult height. Many tall girls will not wish to undertake treatment when they find out their ultimate height will be "only" 6 ft. It is our policy to consider the possibility of therapy for girls whose predicted adult height is in the range of 6 ft or more. The usual therapy is high-dose estrogen, which produces premature epiphyseal closure and a drop in plasma somatomedin-C levels. The pros and cons of treatment are discussed frankly. Therapy induces rapid feminization and an early acceleration of growth. The therapeutic regimen outlined below is reported to reduce ultimate height by 3 to 6.5 in if the girl's BA is 11 years.[400] Others report less height reduction in such patients.[401] Whether this discrepancy is due to differences in estrogen dosage or differences in BA interpretation is unknown. Later institution of treatment leads to less striking results. No significant effect is demonstrable once the skeletal age is over 13 years. The risks are the inherent imprecision in predicting height (see Table 141–4), the known exceptional complications of large doses of estrogen (thrombophlebitis, jaundice, and so on), and the unknown possible complications. Regarding the last-named, it must be kept in mind that there are no large follow-up studies of the incidence of ovarian cysts, "postpill amenorrhea," vaginal cancer, and so on in girls so treated.[401] Treatment consists of high-dose estrogen (e.g.,

10 to 15 mg Premarin) *daily and continuously* until epiphyseal fusion is complete. It is best to acclimate the patient to the estrogen by commencing with one quarter to one sixth of the full dose and increasing this gradually over a 4- to 6-week period. A progestin is added cyclically to normalize the endometrial cycle; 10 mg medroxyprogesterone acetate for 5 days monthly brings about withdrawal bleeding in the presence of continuous estrogen administration. Boys have been treated for "excessive" height with repository testosterone in doses of 500 mg every 2 weeks.[402] Bromoergocryptine reduction of predicted height in patients with hyperresponsive GH dynamics has been disputed.[403]

Advanced Growth. Such a pattern occurs most often as a "constitutional" variation of normal. In other words, it usually occurs with some family precedent. These children have a height above, but approximately parallel to, the 95th percentile during the preadolescent years. Occasionally, there is a slightly increased height velocity. The BA is proportional to HA. These children then enter puberty and the pubertal growth spurt earlier than their peers. However, their predicted adult height is normal, since they cease to grow earlier than their classmates. Explanation of the normality of this growth pattern usually is sufficient to allay any anxieties that the children might have.

This growth pattern also arises as a complication of severe, developmental obesity. Various disorders also cause this growth pattern. Most infant giants follow this growth pattern. Hyperthyroidism tends to slightly accelerate linear growth and bone maturation proportionately, and predicted ultimate height is not affected.[404] Craniostenosis is a common feature of thyrotoxicosis in young children.[405] Congenital lipodystrophy causes advanced growth. This diagnosis must be based on clinical findings.[406, 407] Poor fat stores are present at birth. The absence of fat is so profound that muscle insertions are very prominent, giving the impression of muscular hypertrophy. Fatty liver, hyperlipemia, acromegaloid features, and a growth spurt tend to become apparent in infancy. Linear growth acceleration is proportionate to BA advance during the first few years of life and then wanes in later childhood. The age of onset of puberty and adult height are normal. About half the patients are mentally retarded. Acanthosis nigricans and insulin-resistant diabetes mellitus tend to appear eventually, the latter not becoming manifest until the patient is about 12 years of age. Soft-tissue roentgenograms characteristically demonstrate the lack of fat-muscle interface. Hypermetabolism is frequently demonstrable. Variable disturbances of GH and ACTH release have been found. The etiology of the disorder is unclear. Many cases seem to have an autosomal recessive basis. The postulates regarding the mechanism of lipodystrophy range from diencephalic overproduction of lipolytic hormones[407] to a primary defect in fat cells.[8, 408] Pituitary irradiation and hypophysectomy have not proved to be successful forms of therapy.

Accelerated Growth. Hypersecretion of GH is well known to accelerate growth in pituitary gigantism. In many cases, the children have some acromegalic features.[409–412] In most cases, HA advances out of proportion to skeletal age. However, information about the effect of *isolated* GH excess on relationships between HA and BA in young children is scanty. There is a strong association with McCune-Albright syndrome. The diagnosis and therapy of acromegaly are discussed in Chapter 19.

Sexual precocity may cause an excessive growth velocity and advance BA markedly out of proportion to height.[119] The degree of disproportion between BA and HA depends on the duration and amount of sex hormone production.[413] The advance in BA may not be apparent within the first few months of onset (see Fig. 141–13). Sustained, rapidly progressive precocity is characterized by a ratio of BA to HA of 1.2 or more. Unless the disorder is arrested, epiphyseal fusion may occur prematurely, and growth ceases at an early age. The diagnosis and therapy of precocious puberty are discussed in Chapter 111.

Disturbances of Nutrition

PEDIATRIC ASPECTS OF MALNUTRITION. Primary disturbances of nutrition retard weight gain more than linear growth. The linear growth pattern of mildly undernourished children is not strikingly abnormal; it resembles that of normal children who have a constitutionally delayed growth pattern except that they are short as adults if undernutrition persists throughout puberty. Linear growth is retarded by undernutrition sufficient to cause a deficit of weight for height more than about 8 per cent.[318] Depending on the degree of reversal of malnutrition, children may catch up in height or follow a delayed growth pattern.[15, 414] Malnutrition, starvation, marasmus, and kwashiorkor are discussed elsewhere (Ch. 144). Anorexia nervosa on rare occasions is associated with GH deficiency, as noted above,[332] and is also discussed elsewhere (Ch. 145).

A unique cause of malnutrition in infants is the diencephalic syndrome. This is characterized by a paucity of body fat, similar to that in lipodystrophy, in a hyperalert, otherwise healthy child. Radiosensitive brain tumors in the anterior hypothalamic area are the usual cause. Disturbance of the regulation of appetite, the secretion of pituitary lipotrophic hormones such as GH, or increased energy expenditure has been postulated as the mechanism.[415, 415a]

PEDIATRIC ASPECTS OF OBESITY. Obesity is discussed in detail in Chapter 143. Obesity in adolescence is a more powerful predictor of long-term morbidity than obesity in adulthood.[415b] Childhood obesity can lead to localized disturbances of epiphyseal growth.[415c] As in adults, the vast majority of obesity in children seems to have a functional basis, arising from excessive intake of calories relative to energy expenditure (exogenous or regulatory obesity).[138] About one third of obese children have developmental obesity: a history of weight gain since early infancy, a tendency toward an increase in lean body mass, and an advanced growth pattern.[416, 417] Other obese children have reactive obesity: a later onset of obesity, seemingly in response to emotional stresses (which are often not easily identified), and normal lean body mass and growth.

The differential diagnosis of obesity in children is greatly simplified by the fact that linear growth arrest is the most consistent finding in Cushing's syndrome and hypothyroidism. Consequently, a normal linear growth rate effectively rules out these disorders; only when frank virilization coexists with glucocorticoid excess might there be an exception to this rule.[57] Furthermore, plasma cortisol levels are usually below 10 µg/dl in childhood obesity.[418] Hypothalamic obesity can be congenital. Prader-Willi syndrome, the most common of these disorders, is characterized by profoundly poor feeding and hypotonia in the neonatal period.[181, 223, 418a] Mild mental retardation and hypothalamic dysfunction, including short stature that may be due to GH neurosecretory defect,[419] are common. The genetic basis of the disorder can be identified in up to 95 per cent of cases; two thirds have a deletion of the paternally derived chromosome 15q11q13 region, and most of the remainder have maternal uniparental disomy for this chromosome.[420] The new cytogenetic and molecular techniques can be expected to improve understanding of variants of this disorder.[421] The cardinal manifestations of another hereditary form of obesity, the Laurence-Moon-Bardet-Biedl syndrome, have been determined to be retinitis pigmentosa, dysmorphic extremities (broad short feet or brachydactyly), and renal abnormalities.[422] Although it has been assumed that this is a hypothalamic disorder, there is little evidence for hypothalamic-pituitary dysfunction; even the hypogonadism in affected males is primary. The most common endocrinopathy associated with obesity in adolescence is polycystic ovary syndrome and its variants (Ch. 120).

There are two special considerations in the management of exogenous obesity in children. First, stringent dietary restriction for the purpose of bringing about marked weight loss is to be avoided in the growing child. Nitrogen retention, essential for well-being and maturation, is relatively sensitive to caloric restriction during the period of rapid growth.[424] Second, psychological immaturity prevents all young children and many teenagers from complying with a long-term program for weight reduction. For these reasons, the first step in management of the obese child is to aim to modify psychological factors and dietary activity with the goal of maintaining weight so that the child will "grow into it."

Localized Disturbances of Somatic Growth

Local growth may be abnormal in an isolated or multifocal pattern without a disturbance of overall growth. Those aspects of localized growth disturbances that are of endocrinological interest are noted here.

Congenital

Hormone administration or hormonal disturbances at critical periods of development have been associated with localized somatic malformations: cortisone and cleft palate,[424] estrogen-progestin contraceptives and vascular–tracheoesophageal–limb-reduction anomalies (VATER association),[181, 425] and diabetes mellitus and sacral, palatal, neurologic, and cardiac anomalies.[181, 426]

Congenital hemihypertrophy is linked with endocrine disorders and neoplasia.[227] WAGR is one such syndrome: Wilms' tumor, aniridia, genitourinary anomalies, and mental retardation.[428] Adrenal carcinoma occurs more frequently in these patients and their families than is expected by chance. Wilms' tumor also occurs in association with other genitourinary abnormalities, including pseudohermaphroditism and renal dysplasia, the Denys-Drash syndrome.[429] These syndromes result from distinct mutations or deletions affecting chromosome 11p13. Hemihypertrophy is also linked with endocrine dysfunction and neoplasia in von Recklinghausen's neurofibromatosis (endocrine abnormalities can result from adrenal carcinoma or CNS tumors) and the Beckwith-Wiedemann syndrome.[181] The neurofibromatosis I gene on chromosome 17 appears to code for a protein that is particularly important for differentiation of neural crest derivatives and that also acts as a tumor suppressor.[9, 243] The topic of congenital malformations of somatic, endocrine, and other organs is discussed more comprehensively elsewhere.[181]

Acquired

The deleterious effects of a variety of disorders affecting limb growth may be mediated by alterations in blood circulation. The result of occlusion of the arterial flow to a limb is the most obvious instance. It has been shown that longitudinal growth of the arm is retarded out of proportion to bone maturation after sacrifice of the subclavian artery.[430] Growth of an entire limb is well known to be stunted in children paralyzed from any lesion, whether it be of the lower motor neuron, as in poliomyelitis, or of the upper motor neuron, as in cerebral vascular accidents. It is unknown whether growth is affected because of a direct "tropic" effect of innervation or whether activity of the limb somehow promotes normal growth, possibly by promoting the circulation. Local inflammatory disease about a joint may accelerate epiphyseal maturation and lead to premature epiphyseal fusion and cessation of growth.[431] Trauma to the epiphyseal plate will result in growth arrest unless circulation is intact and the anatomy is restored. Epiphyseal growth also will be arrested by irradiation in high, tumoricidal doses. The exact dose-response relationship between radiation dose and the rate of bone growth has not been established in humans for therapy with either x-ray alone or x-ray in combination with such potentiating agents as actinomycin D, nor is there information about the relative sensitivity to x-ray of the various physeal centers. Vertebral growth may be affected by doses of around 4000 rad.[432] After extensive vertebral irradiation for treatment of malignant tumors, significant reductions in upper segment linear growth velocity, with consequent short stature, can be expected in surviving patients.

REFERENCES

1. Cheek DB (ed): Human Growth. Philadelphia, Lea & Febiger, 1968.
2. Winick M, Noble A: Quantitative changes in DNA, RNA, and protein during prenatal and postnatal growth in the rat. Dev Biol 12:451, 1965.
3. Pardee AB: G_1 events and regulation of cell proliferation. Science 246:603–608, 1989.
4. Murray AW, Kirschner MW: What controls the cell cycle? Sci Am 264:56–63, 1991.
5. Murray AW, Kirschner MW: Dominoes and clocks: The union of two views of the cell cycle. Science 246:614–621, 1989.
6. Stiles CD, Capone GT, Scher CD, et al: Dual control of cell growth by somatomedins and platelet-derived growth factor. Proc Natl Acad Sci USA 76:1279, 1979.
7. Clemmons DA: Multiple hormones stimulate the production of somatomedin by cultured human fibroblasts. J Clin Endocrinol Metab 58:850, 1984.
8. Straus DS: Growth-stimulatory actions of insulin in vitro and vivo. Endocri Rev 5:356, 1984.
9. Weinberg RA: Tumor-suppressor genes. Science 254:1138, 1991.
10. Laskey RA, Fairman MP, Blow JJ: S phase of the cell cycle. Science 246:609–613, 1989.
11. McIntosh JR, Koonce MP: Mitosis. Science 246:622–628, 1989.
12. Arey LB: Developmental Anatomy (ed 6). Philadelphia, WB Saunders Co, 1954.
13. Favus M, Haddad JJ Jr, Rodan GA (eds): Primer on Metabolic Bone Diseases and Disorders of Mineral Metabolism. Richmond, VA, William Byrd Press, 1990, pp 3–26.
14. Demiaux B, Arlot ME, Chapuy M-C, et al: Serum osteocalcin is increased in patients with osteomalacia: Correlations with biochemical and histomorphometric findings. J Clin Endocrinol Metab 74:1146–1151, 1992.
15. McCance RA, Widdowson EM: Nutrition and growth. Proc R Soc Lond 156:326, 1962.
16. Caller JR, Ramsey F, Solimano G: A follow-up study of the effects of early malnutrition on subsequent development: 1. Physical growth and sexual maturation during adolescence. Pediatr Res 19:518, 1985.
17. Grantham-McGregor SM, Powell CA, Walker SP, Himes JH: Nutritional supplementation, psychosocial stimulation, and mental development of stunted children: The Jamaican study. Lancet 338:1–5, 1991.
18. Hommes FA, Drost YM, Geraets WXM, Reijenga, MAA: The energy requirement for growth: An application of Atkinson's metabolic price system. Pediatr Res 9:51, 1975.
19. Holliday MA: Metabolic rate and organ size during growth from infancy to maturity and during late gestation and early infancy. Pediatrics 47:169, 1971.
20. Sinclair JC, Silverman WA: Intrauterine growth in active tissue mass of the human fetus, with particular reference to the undergrown baby. Pediatrics 38:48, 1966.
21. Holt LE Jr: Some problems in dietary amino acid requirements. Am J Clin Nutr 21:367, 1968.
22. Fisch RO, Graverm HJ, Feinberg SB: Growth and bone characteristics of phenylketonurics. Am J Dis Child 112:3, 1966.
23. Cahill GF Jr: Nitrogen versatility in bats, bears, and man. N Engl J Med 290:686, 1974.
24. Holman RT: Essential fatty acid deficiency. Prog Chem Fats Lipids 9:275, 1968.
25. Chesney RW: Requirements and upper limits of vitamin D intake in the term neonate, infant, and older child. J Pediatr 116:159–166, 1990.
26. Clement DH, Fomon SJ, Forbes GB, et al: Trace elements in infant nutrition. Pediatrics 26:715, 1960.
27. Ulmer DD: Trace elements. N Engl J Med 297:318, 1977.
28. Nakamura T, Nishiyama S, Futagoishi-Suginohara Y, et al: Mild to moderate zinc deficiency in short children: effect of zinc supplementation on linear growth velocity. J Pediat 123:65, 1993.
29. Danks DM, Stevens BJ, Campbell PE, et al: Menkes kinky-hair syndrome. Lancet 1:1100, 1972.
30. Cooke RE, Boyden DG, Haller E: The relationship of acidosis and growth retardation. J Pediatr 57:326, 1960.
31. Viteri FE: The effect of inactivity on the growth of rats fed diets adequate or restricted with respect to normal caloric intake. *In* New Concepts about Old Aspects of Malnutrition. Mexico, Fondo Editorial Nestle de la Academia Mexicana de Pediatria, 1973 (in Spanish).
32. Baulieu EE, Lasnitzki I, Robel P: Metabolism of testosterone and action of metabolites on prostate glands grown in organ culture. Nature 219:1155, 1968.
33. Somjen D, Weisman Y, Mor Z, et al: Regulation of proliferation of rat cartilage and bone by sex steroids. J Steroid Biochem 40:717, 1991.
34. Schaff-Blass E, Burstein S, Rosenfield RL: Advances in diagnosis and treatment of short stature, with special reference to the role of growth hormone. J Pediatr 104:801, 1984.
35. Devesa J, Lima L, Tresguerres JAF: Neuroendocrine control of growth hormone secretion in humans. Trends Endocrinol Metab 3:175, 1992.
36. McCracken JT, Poland RE, Rubin RT, Tondo L: Dose-dependent effects of scopolamine on nocturnal growth hormone secretion in normal adult men: Relation to d-sleep changes. J Clin Endocrinol Metab 72:90–95, 1990.
37. Kerrigan JR, Rogol AD: The impact of gonadal steroid hormone action on growth hormone secretion during childhood and adolescence. Endocr Rev 13:309, 1992.
38. Wallis M: Growth hormone–binding proteins. Clin Endocrinol 35:291–293, 1991.

39. Walker JL, Moats-Staats BM, Stiles AD, Underwood LE: Tissue-specific developmental regulation of the messenger ribonucleic acids encoding the growth hormone receptor and the growth hormone binding protein in rat fetal and postnatal tissues. Pediatr Res 31:335–339, 1992.
40. Maiter D, Underwood LE, Maes M, et al: Different effects of intermittent and continuous growth hormone (GH) administration on serum somatomedin-C/insulin-like growth factor I and liver GH receptors in hypophysectomized rats. Endocrinology 123:1053–1059, 1988.
41. Daughaday WH, Rotwein P: Insulin-like growth factors I and II: Peptide, messenger ribonucleic acid and gene structures, serum, and tissue concentrations. Endocr Rev 10:68–91, 1989.
42. Hintz RL: Role of growth-hormone and insulin-like growth-factor binding proteins. Horm Res 33:105, 1990.
43. Rosenfield RL, Furlanetto R: Physiologic testosterone or estradiol induction of puberty increases plasma somatomedin-C. J Pediatr 107:415, 1985.
44. Van Den Brande JL, DeCaju MVL: Plasma somatomedin activity in children with growth disturbances. In Raiti S (ed): Advances in Human Growth Hormone Research. Washington, US Government Printing Office, 1974, p 98.
45. Schalch DS, Heinrich UE, Draznin B, et al: Role of the liver in regulating somatomedin activity: Hormonal effects on the synthesis and release of insulin-like growth factor and its carrier protein by the isolated perfused rat liver. Endocrinology 104:1044, 1979.
46. Daughaday WH, Phillips LS, Mueller MC: The effects of insulin and growth hormone on the release of somatomedin by the isolated rat liver. Endocrinology 98:1214, 1976.
47. Mulroney SE, Lumpkin MD, Roberts C Jr, et al: Effect of a growth hormone–releasing factor antagonist on compensatory renal growth, insulin-like growth factor-I (IGF-I), and IGF-I receptor gene expression after unilateral nephrectomy in immature rats. Endocrinology 130:2697–2702, 1992.
48. Heins JN, Carland JI, Daughaday WH: Incorporation of ^{35}S-sulfate into rat cartilage explants in vitro: Effects of aging on responsiveness to stimulation by sulfation factor. Endocrinology 87:688, 1970.
49. Cohen P, Lamson G, Okajima T, Rosenfeld RG: Transfection of the human insulin–like growth factor binding protein-3 gene into Balb/c fibroblasts inhibits cellular growth. Molec Endocr 7:380, 1993.
50. Bomboy JD Jr, Burkhalter VJ, Nicholson WE, Salmon WD Jr: Similarity of somatomedin inhibitor in sera from starved, hypophysectomized, and diabetic rats: Distinction from a heat-stable inhibitor of rat cartilage metabolism. Endocrinology 112:371, 1983.
51. Phillips LS, Fusco AC. Unterman TC, del Creco F: Somatomedin inhibitor in uremia. J Clin Endocrinol Metab 59:764, 1984.
52. Bowers CY: Editorial: a new dimension on the induced release of growth hormone in obese subjects. J Clin Endocrinol Metab 76:817, 1993.
53. Salter J, Best EH: Insulin as a growth hormone. Br Med J 2:353, 1953.
54. Geffner ME, Bersch N, Kaplan SA, et al: Growth without growth hormone: Evidence for a potent circulating human growth factor. Lancet 1:343, 1986.
55. Kasper S, Friesen HC: Human pituitary tissue secretes a potent growth factor for chondrocyte proliferation. J Clin Endocrinol Metab 42:370, 1976.
56. Bistritzer T, Lovchik JC, Cahlew SA, Kowarski AA: Growth without growth hormone: The "invisible" GH syndrome. Lancet 1:321–323, 1988.
57. Loeb JN: Corticosteroids and growth. N Engl J Med 295:547, 1976.
58. Hyams JS, Carey DE: Corticosteroids and growth. J Pediatr 113:249–253, 1988.
59. Miell JF, Corder R, Pralong FP, Gaillard RC: Effects of dexamethasone on growth hormone (GH)–releasing hormone, arginine and dopaminergic stimulated GH secretion, and total plasma insulin-like growth factor I concentrations in normal male volunteers. J Clin Endocrinol Metab 72:675–681, 1991.
60. Giustina A, Simonetta B, Bodini C, et al: Arginine normalizes the growth hormone (GH) response to GH-releasing hormone in adult patients receiving chronic daily immunosuppressive glucocorticoid therapy. J Clin Endocrinol Metab 74:1301–1305, 1992.
61. Shahidi NT, Crigler JF Jr: Evaluation of growth and/or endocrine systems in testosterone-corticosteroid-treated patients with aplastic anemia. J Pediatr 70:233, 1967.
62. Jonat C, Rahmsdorf HJ, Park K-K, et al: Antitumor promotion and antiinflammation: Down-modulation of AP-1 (Fos/Jun) activity by glucocorticoid hormone. Cell 62:1189–1204, 1990.
63. Schüle R, Rangaarajan P, Kliewer S, et al: Functional antagonism between oncoprotein c-Jun and the glucocorticoid receptor. Cell 62:1217–1226, 1990.
64. Rosenfield RL: Diagnosis and management of delayed puberty. J Clin Endocrinol Metab 70:559–562, 1990.
65. Rosenfield RL: The ovary and female sexual maturation. In Kaplan SL (ed), Clinical Pediatric Endocrinology. Philadelphia, WB Saunders Co, 1989, pp 259–323.
66. Winter JSD, Hughes JA, Reyes FL, et al: Pituitary-gonadal relations in infancy: 2. Patterns of serum gonadal steroid concentrations in man from birth to two years of age. J Clin Endocrinol Metab 42:679, 1978.
67. Rosenfield RL: Role of androgens in growth and development of the fetus, child and adolescent. Adv Pediatr 19:171–213, 1972.
68. Forest MG, Cathiard AM, Bertrand JA: Evidence of testicular activity in early infancy. J Clin Endocrinol Metab 37:148, 1973.
69. Naeye RL, Blanc WA: Organ and body growth in anencephaly. Arch Pathol 91:140, 1971.
70. King KC, Adam PAJ, Schwartz R, Terano K: Human placental transfer of human growth hormone. Pediatrics 48:534, 1971.
71. Jost A: Hormonal factors in development of the fetus. Cold Spring Harbor Symp 19:167, 1954.
72. Gluckman PD, Gunn AJ, Wray A, et al: Congenital idiopathic growth hormone deficiency associated with prenatal and early post-natal growth failure. J Pediat 121:920, 1992.
73. Vulsma T, Gons MH, de Vijlder JJM: Maternal-fetal transfer of thyroxine in congenital hypothyroidism due to a total organification defect or thyroid agenesis. N Engl J Med 321:13, 1989.
74. Smith DW, Popick C: Large fontanels in congenital hypothyroidism: A potential clue toward earlier recognition. J Pediatr 80:753, 1972.
75. MacMillan DR, Hawkins R, Collier RN: Chorionic somatomammotrophin as index of fetal growth. Arch Dis Child 51:120, 1976.
76. Lassarre C, Hardouin S, Daffos F, et al: Serum insulin-like growth factors and insulin-like growth factor binding proteins in the human fetus: Relationships with growth in normal subjects and in subjects with intrauterine growth retardation. Pediatr Res 29:219, 1991.
77. Phillips JA III: Genetic diagnosis: Differentiating growth disorders. Hosp Pract 20:85, 1985.
78. Ogilvie S, Buhl WC, Olson JA, Shiverick KT: Identification of a novel family of growth hormone-related proteins secreted by rat placenta. Endocrinology 126:3271, 1990.
79. Spatola E, Pescovitz OH, Marsh K, et al: Interaction of growth hormone–releasing hormone with the insulin-like growth factors during prenatal development in the rat. Endocrinology 129:1193–1200, 1991.
80. Drop SLS, Kortleve DJ, Guyda HJ, Posner BI: Immunoassay of a somatomedin-C binding protein from human amniotic fluid: Levels in fetal, neonatal, and adult sera. J Clin Endocrinol Metab 59:908, 1984.
81. Schofield PN, Tate VE: Regulation of human IGF-II transcription in fetal and adult tissues. Development 101:793, 1987.
82. Blizzard RM, Drash AL, Jenkins ME, et al: Comparative effects of animal prolactins and human growth hormone (GH) in hypopituitary children. J Clin Endocrinol Metab 26:852, 1966.
83. MacDonald MJ: Neonatal diabetes. Lancet 1:737, 1974.
84. Naeye RL, Dixon JB: Distortions in fetal growth standards. Pediatr Res 12:987, 1978.
85. Lubchenco LO, Hansman C, Dressler M, Boyd E: Intrauteine growth as estimated from liveborn birth-weight data at 24 to 42 weeks of gestation. Pediatrics 32:793, 1963.
86. Scott RB, Hiatt HH, Clark BC, et al: IX. Growth and development of Negro infants. Pediatrics 29:65, 1962.
87. Freeman MG. Graves WL, Thompson RL: Indigent Negro and Caucasian birth weight–gestational age tables. Pediatrics 46:91, 1970.
88. Pryse-Davies J, Smithan JH, Napier KA: Factors influencing development of secondary ossification centres in the fetus and newborn. Arch Dis Child 59:425, 1974.
89. Cruise MO: I. A longitudinal study of the growth of low birth weight infants. Pediatrics 51:620, 1973.
90. Wingerd J, Schoen EJ, Solomon IL: Growth standards in the first two years of life based on measurements of white and black children in a prepaid health care program. Pediatrics 47:818, 1971.
91. Shaffer SG, Quimiro CL, Anderson JV, Hall RT: Postnatal weight changes in low birth weight babies. Pediatrics 79:702, 1983.
92. Thomson AM, Billewicz WZ, Hytten FE: The assessment of fetal growth. J Obstet Gynaecol Br Comm 75:90, 1968.
93. Wingerd V, Schoen EJ: Factors influencing length at birth and height at five years. Pediatrics 53:737, 1974.

94. Beck GJ, van der Berg BJ: The relationship of the rate of intrauterine growth of low-birth-weight infants to later growth. J Pediatr 86:504, 1975.

95. Gardoni J, Chang A, Kalyan B, et al: Customized antenatal growth charts. Lancet 339:283–287, 1991.

96. Soothill P, Nicolaides KH, Bilardo CM, Campbell S: Relation of fetal hypoxia in growth retardation to mean blood velocity in the fetal aorta. Lancet 2:1118, 1986.

97. Yip R, Binkin NJ, Trowbridge FL: Altitude and childhood growth. J Pediatr 113:486–489, 1988.

98. Naeye RL, Benirschke K, Hagstrom JWC, Marcus CC: Intrauterine growth of twins as estimated from liveborn birth-weight data. Pediatrics 37:409, 1966.

99. Schinzel AGI, Smith DW, Miller JR: Monozygotic twinning and structural defects. J Pediatr 95:921, 1979.

100. Hamill PVV, Drizd TA, Johnson CL, et al: Physical growth: National Center for Health Statistics percentiles. Am J Clin Nutr 32:607, 1979.

101. Maresh MM: Linear growth of long bones of extremities from infancy through adolescence. Am J Dis Child 89:725, 1955.

102. Smith DW, Truog W, Rogers JE, et al: Shifting linear growth during infancy. J Pediatr 89:225, 1976.

103. Garn SM, Shaw HA: Birth size and growth appraisal. J Pediatr 90:1049, 1977.

104. Lovinger RD, Kaplan SL, Grumbach MM: Congenital hypopituitarism associated with neonatal hypoglycemia and microphallus: Four cases secondary to hypothalamic hormone deficiencies. J Pediatr 87:1171, 1975.

105. Bock RD, Thissen D: Statistical problems of fitting individual growth curves. In Johnson F, Roche A, Susanne C (eds): Human Physical Growth and Maturation. New York, Plenum Press, 1980, p 265.

106. Reed RB, Stuart HC: Patterns of growth in height and weight from birth to eighteen years of age. Pediatrics 24:904, 1959.

107. Tanner JM, Whitehouse RH, Takaishi M: Standards from birth to maturity for height, weight, height velocity, and weight velocity: British children, 1965. Arch Dis Child 41:454, 613, 1966.

108. Tanner JM, Davies PSW: Clinical longitudinal standards for height and height velocity for North American children. J Pediatr 107:317, 1985.

109. Prader A, Tanner JM, Von Harnack GA: Catch-up growth following illness or starvation. J Pediatr 62:646, 1963.

110. Glinos AD: Density dependent regulation of growth and differentiated function in suspension cultures of mouse fibroblasts. In Kulonen E, Pikkarainen J (eds): Biology of Fibroblast. New York, Academic Press, 1973, p 155.

111. Marshall WA: Evaluation of growth rate in height over periods of less than one year. Arch Dis Child 46:414, 1971.

112. Tanner JM: Growth at Adolescence. London, Blackwell, 1962, p 130.

113. Wingerd J, Solomon IL, Schoen EJ: Parent-specific height standards for preadolescent children of three racial groups, with method for rapid determination. Pediatrics 52:555, 1973.

114. Santen RJ, DeKretser DM, Paulsen CA, Vorhees J: Gonadotrophins and testosterone in the XYY syndrome. Lancet 2:371, 1970.

115. Ounsted C, Ounsted M: Effect of Y chromosome on fetal growth rate. Lancet 2:857, 1970.

116. Caldwell PD, Smith DW: The XXY (Klinefelter's) syndrome in childhood: Detection and treatment. J Pediatr 80:250, 1972.

117. Forbes GB: A note on the mathematics of "catchup" growth. Pediatr Res 8:929, 1974.

118. Bongiovanni AM, Moshang T Jr, Parks JS: Maturational deceleration after treatment of congenital adrenal hyperplasia. Helv Paediatr Acta 28:127, 1973.

119. Oerter KE, Manasco P, Barnes KM, et al: Adult height in precocious puberty after long-term treatment with deslorelin. J Clin Endocrinol Metab 73:1235–1240, 1991.

120. Rivkees SA, Bode HH, Crawford JD: Long-term growth in juvenile acquired hypothyroidism: The failure to achieve normal adult stature. N Engl J Med 318:599–602, 1988.

121. Chernausek SD, Turner R: Attenuation of spontaneous, nocturnal growth hormone secretion in children with hypothyroidism and its correlation with plasma insulin-like growth factor I concentrations. J Pediatr 114:968, 1989.

122. Bell NH, Shary J, Stevens J, et al: Demonstration that bone mass is greater in black than in white children. J Bone Miner Res 6:719–723, 1991.

123. Patel DN, Pettifor JM, Becker PJ, et al: The effect of ethnic group on appendicular bone mass in children. J Bone Miner Res 7:263–272, 1992.

124. Shuttleworth FK: Sexual maturation and physical growth of girls age six to nineteen. Monogr Soc Res Child Dev 2:5, 1937.

125. Gruelich WW, Pyle SI: Radiographic Atlas of Skeletal Development of the Hand and Wrist. Palo Alto, CA, Stanford University Press, 1959.

126. Barr GD, Allen CM, Shinefield HR: Height and weight of 7500 children of three skin colors. Am J Dis Child 124:866, 1972.

127. Schumacher LB, Pawson IG, Kretchmer N: Growth of immigrant children in newcomer schools of San Francisco. Pediatrics 80:861, 1987.

128. McKusick VA: Heritable Disorders of Connective Tissue (ed 4). St. Louis, CV Mosby, 1972.

129. Engelbach W: Endocrine Medicine, vol 1. Springfield, IL, Charles C Thomas, 1932, p 261.

130. Mehes K, Kitzveger E: Inner canthal and intermammillary indices in the newborn infant. J Pediatr 85:90, 1974.

131. Nellhaus G: Head circumference from birth to eighteen years. Pediatrics 41:106, 1968.

132. Weaver DD, Christian JC: Familial variation of head size and adjustment for parental head circumference. J Pediatr 96:990–994, 1980.

133. Krieger I: Head circumference, mental retardation and growth failure. Pediatrics 37:384, 1966.

134. Cloutier MD, Stickler GB: Head circumference in children with idiopathic hypopituitarism. Pediatrics 42:209, 1968.

135. Burt L, Kulin HE: Head circumference in children with short stature secondary to primary hypothyroidism. Pediatrics 59:628, 1977.

136. Popich GA, Smith DW: Fontanels: Range of normal size. J Pediatr 80:749, 1972.

137. Frisch RE, McArthur JW: Menstrual cycles as a determinant of minimum weight for height necessary for their maintenance or onset. Science 185:949, 1974.

138. Poissonnet CM, LaVelle M, Burdi AR: Growth and development of adipose tissue. J Pediatr 113:1–8, 1988.

139. Hammer LD, Wilson DM, Litt IF, et al: Impact of pubertal development on body fat distribution among white, Hispanic, and Asian female adolescents. J Pediatr 118:975–980, 1991.

140. Wilkins L: The Diagnosis and Treatment of Endocrine Disorders in Childhood and Adolescence (ed 3). Springfield, IL, Charles C Thomas, 1965.

141. Roche AF, Eyman SL, Davila GH: Skeletal age prediction. J Pediatr 78:997, 1971.

142. Tanner JM, Whitehouse RH, Marshall WM, et al: Assessment of Skeletal Maturity Adult Height (TW 2 Method). New York, Academic Press, 1975.

143. Baer MJ, Durkatz J: Bilateral asymmetry in skeletal maturation of the hand and wrist. Am J Phys Anthropol 15:180, 1957.

144. Garn SM, Sandusky ST, Nagy JM, McCann MB: Advanced skeletal development in low-income Negro children. J Pediatr 80:965, 1972.

145. Donovan BT, Van der Werff ten Bosch JJ: Physiology of Puberty. London, Arnold, 1965.

146. Cumming GR, Garand T, Borysyk L: Correlation of performance in track and field events with bone age. J Pediatr 80:970, 1972.

147. Aanderson M, Green WT, Messner MB: Growth and predictions of growth in the lower extremities. J Bone Joint Surg 45A:1, 1963.

148. Bayer LM, Bayley N: Growth pattern shifts in healthy children: Spontaneous and induced. J Pediatr 62:631, 1963.

149. Roche A, Wainer H, Thissen D: The RWT method for the prediction of adult stature. Pediatrics 56:1026, 1975.

150. Tanner JM, Whitehouse RH, Marshall WA, Carter BS: Prediction of adult height, bone age, and occurrence of menarche, at age 4 to 16 with allowance for midparent height. Arch Dis Child 50:14, 1975.

151. Frisch RE: Critical weight at menarche, initiation of the adolescent growth spurt, and control of puberty. In Grumbach MM, Grave GD, Mayer FE (eds): Control of the Onset of Puberty. New York, John Wiley & Sons, 1974, p 403.

152. Frisch RE: A method of prediction of age of menarche from height and weight at age 9 through 13 years. Pediatrics 53:384, 1974.

153. Johnston FE, Roche AF, Schell LM, Wettenhall NB: Critical weight at menarche. Am J Dis Child 129:19, 1975.

154. Platt OS, Rosenstock W, Espeland MA: Influence of sickle hemoglobinopathies on growth and development. N Engl J Med 311:7, 1984.

155. Frisch RE, Nagal JS: Prediction of adult height of girls from age of menarche. Am J Dis Child 129:19, 1975.

156. Frisancho AR, Garn SM, Rohmann CG: Age at menarche: A new method of prediction and retrospective assessment based on hand x-rays. Hum Biol 41:42, 1969.

157. Dobbins J: The later growth of the brain and its vulnerability. Pediatrics 53:2, 1974.
158. Dubowitz LMS, Dubowitz V, Goldberd C: Clinical assessment of gestational age in the newborn infant. J Pediatr 77:1, 1970.
159. Finnstrom O: Studies on maturity in newborn infants: VI. Acta Paediatr Scand 61:33, 1972.
160. DeHertogh R, Thomas K, Bietlot Y, et al: Plasma levels of unconjugated estrone, estradiol, and estriol and of HCS throughout pregnancy in normal women. J Clin Endocrinol Metab 40:93, 1975.
161. Fencl M, Tulchinsky D: Total cortisol in amniotic fluid and fetal lung maturation. N Engl J Med 292:133, 1975.
162. Metcoff J, Wikman-Coffelt J, Yoshida T, et al: Energy metabolism and protein synthesis in human leukocytes during pregnancy and in placenta related to fetal growth. Pediatrics 51:866, 1973.
163. Children Are Different. Columbus, OH, Ross Laboratories, 1970.
164. Holliday MA: Fluid and electrolyte disturbances in Pediatr. In Maxwell MH, Kleeman CR (eds): Clinical Disorders of Fluid and Electrolyte Metabolism (ed 1). New York, McGraw-Hill, 1962.
165. Butler AM, Richie RH: Simplification and improvement in estimating drug dosage and fluid and dietary allowances for patients of varying sizes. N Engl J Med 262:903, 1960.
166. Arnaud SB, Goldsmith RE, Stickler GB, et al: Serum parathyroid hormone and blood minerals: Interrelationships in normal children. Pediatr Res 7:485, 1973.
167. Rosenstein SN: The teeth. In Barnett H (ed): Pediatrics (ed 16). New York, Appleton-Century-Crofts, 1977, p 931.
168. Kenny FM, Preeyasombat C, Migeon CJ: II. Cortisol production rate. Pediatrics 37:35, 1966.
169. Sippell WG, Dorr HG, Bidlingmaier F, Knorr D: Plasma levels of aldosterone, corticosterone, 11-deoxycorticosterone, progesterone, 17-hydroxyprogesterone cortisol, and cortisone during infancy and childhood. Pediatr Res 14:39, 1980.
170. Strickland AL, Shearin RB: Diurnal height variation in children. J Pediatr 80:1023, 1972.
171. Shimura T, Utsumi Y, Fujikawa S, et al: Marshall-Smith syndrome with large bifrontal diameter, broad distal femora, camptodactyly, and without broad middle phalanges. J Pediatr 94:93, 1979.
172. Poznanski AK, Garn SM, Kuhns LR, Sandusky ST: Dysharmonic maturation of the hand in congenital malformation syndromes. Am J Phys Anthropol 35:417, 1971.
173. Warkany J, Monroe BB, Sutherland BS: Intrauterine growth retardation. Am J Dis Child 102:127, 1961.
174. Medovy H: New parameters in neonatal growth—Cell number and cell size. J Pediatr 71:459, 1967.
175. Fitzhardinge PM, Steven EM: The small-for-date infant: I. Later growth patterns. Pediatrics 49:671, 1972.
176. Philip ACS: Fetal growth retardation: Femurs, fontanels, and follow-up. Pediatrics 62:446, 1978.
177. Naeye RL: Malnutrition: Probable cause of fetal growth retardation. Arch Pathol 79:284, 1965.
178. Bergsma D (ed): Birth Defect Atlas and Compendium. Baltimore, National Foundation, 1973.
179. McKusick VA: Mendelian Inheritance in Man (ed 2). Baltimore, Johns Hopkins University Press, 1968.
180. Silverman RN (ed): Caffey's Pediatric X-Ray Diagnosis, vol 1 (ed 8). Chicago, Year Book Medical Publishers, 1985, p 520.
181. Jones KL: Smith's Recognizable Patterns of Human Malformation. Philadelphia, WB Saunders Co, 1988.
182. Shapiro F: Epiphyseal disorders. N Engl J Med 317:1702–1710, 1987.
183. Mullis PE, Patel MS, Brickett PM, et al: Growth characteristics and response to growth hormone therapy in patients with hypochondroplasia: Genetic linkage of the insulin-like growth factor I gene at chromosome 12q23 to the disease in a subgroup of these patients. Clin Endocrinol 34:265–274, 1991.
184. Fanconi S, Fischer JA, Wieland P, et al: Kenny syndrome: Evidence for idiopathic hypoparathyroidism in two patients and for abnormal parathyroid hormone in one. J Pediatr 109:469, 1986.
185. Anonymous. Williams syndrome—The enigma continues. Lancet 2:490, 1988.
186. Morris CA, Demsey SA, Leonard CO, et al: Natural history of Williams syndrome: Physical characteristics. J Pediatr 113:318–326, 1988.
187. Majewski F, Goecke T: Studies of microcephalic primordial dwarfism: I. Approach to a delineation of Seckel syndrome. Am J Med Genet 12:7, 1982.
188. Saal HM, Pagon RM, Pepin MG: Reevaluation of Russell-Silver syndrome. J Pediatr 107:733, 1985.
189. Davies P, Valley R, Preece M: Adolescent growth and pubertal progression in the Silver-Russell syndrome. Arch Dis Child 63:130, 1988.
190. Lewandowski RC, Yunis JJ: New chromosomal syndromes. Am J Dis Child 129:515, 1975.
191. Langlois RG, Bigbee WL, Jensen RH, German J: Evidence for increased in vivo mutation and somatic recombination in Bloom's syndrome. Proc Nat Acad Sci USA 86:670–674, 1989.
192. Webster ADB, Barnes DE, Arlett CF, et al: Growth retardation and immunodeficiency in a patient with mutations in the DNA ligase I gene. Lancet 339:1508–1509, 1992.
193. Chiriboga-Klein S, Oberfield SE, Casullo AM, et al: Growth in congenital rubella syndrome and correlation with clinical manifestations. J Pediatr 115:251–255, 1989.
194. Kandall SR, Albin S, Lowinson J, et al: Differential effects of maternal heroin and methadone use on birthweight. Pediatrics 58:681, 1976.
195. Frank DA, Bauchner H, Parker S, et al: Neonatal body proportionality and body composition after in utero exposure to cocaine and marijuana. Pediatrics 117:622–626, 1990.
196. Cohlan SQ, Bevelander C, Tiamsic T: Growth inhibition of prematures receiving tetracycline: Clinical and laboratory investigation of tetracycline-induced bone fluorescence. Am J Dis Child 105:453, 1963.
197. Demers P, Fraser D, Goldbloom RB, et al: Effects of tetracyclines on skeletal growth and dentition. Can Med Assoc J 99:849, 1968.
198. Leppig KA, Werler MM, Cann CI, et al: Predictive value of minor anomalies. J Pediatr 110:531, 1987.
199. Feingold M, Fine RN, Ingall D: Intravenous pyelography in infants with single umbilical artery. N Engl J Med 270:1178, 1964.
200. Mietens C, Weber H: A syndrome characterized by corneal opacity, nystagmus, flexion contracture of the elbows, growth failure and mental retardation. J Pediatr 60:624, 1966.
201. Pena SDJ, Shokeir MHK: Syndrome of camptodactyly, multiple ankyloses, facial anomalies, and pulmonary hypoplasia: A lethal condition. J Pediatr 885:373, 1974.
202. Pinsky L, Fraser FC: Atypical malformation syndromes. J Pediatr 80:141, 1972.
203. Naeye R: Organ abnormalities in a human parabiotic syndrome. Am J Pathol 46:299, 1965.
204. Bergner L, Susser MW: Low birth weight and prenatal nutrition: An interpretive review. Pediatrics 46:946, 1970.
205. Stein Z, Susser M: II. The Dutch famine, 1944–1945, and the reproductive process. Pediatr Res 9:76, 1975.
206. Naeye R, Blanc W, Paul C: Effects of maternal nutrition on the human fetus. Pediatrics 52:494, 1973.
207. Miller HC, Hassanein K: Fetal malnutrition in white newborn infants: Maternal factors. Pediatrics 52:504, 1973.
208. Bassi JA, Rosso P, Moessinger AC, et al: Fetal growth retardation due to maternal tobacco smoke exposure in the rat. Pediatr Res 18:127, 1984.
209. Schiff D, Colle E, Stern L: Metabolic and growth patterns in transient neonatal diabetes. N Engl J Med 787:119, 1972.
210. Pagliara AS, Karl E, Kipnis DB: Transient neonatal diabetes: Delayed maturation of the pancreatic beta cell. J Pediatr 82:97, 1973.
211. Levitsky L, Speck S, Shulman S: Metabolic response to fasting in experimental intrauterine growth retardation. Biol Neonate 30:11, 1976.
212. Wilson MC, Meyers HI, Peters SH: Postnatal bone growth of infants with fetal growth retardation. Pediatrics 40:213, 1967.
213. Colle E, Schill D, Andrew C, et al: Insulin reponses during catchup growth of infants who were small for gestational age. Pediatrics 57:363, 1976.
214. Lubchenco LO, Searls DT, Brazie JV: Neonatal mortality rate: Relationship to birth weight and gestational age. J Pediatr 81:814, 1972.
215. Patterson RM, Pouliot MR: Neonatal morphometrics and perinatal outcome. Am J Obstet Gynecol 159:691, 1987.
216. Lubchenco L, Bard H: Incidence of hypoglycemia in newborn infants classified by birth weight and gestational age. Pediatrics 47:831, 1971.
217. Uhrmann S, Mark KH, Maisels MJ, et al: Thyroid function in the preterm infant: A longitudinal assessment. J Pediatr 92:968, 1978.
219. Babson SC, Phillips DS: Growth and development of twins dissimilar in size at birth. N Engl J Med 289:938, 1973.
220. Wallace SJ, Michie EA: A follow-up study of infants born to mothers with low estriol excretion during pregnancy. Lancet 2:560, 1966.
221. Foley TP Jr, Thompson RC, Shaw M, et al: Growth responses to human growth hormone in patients with intrauterine growth retardation. J Pediatr 81:635, 1974.

222. Naeye RL: Infants of diabetic mothers: A quantitative morphologic study. Pediatrics 35:980, 1965.
223. Stevenson DK, Hopper AO. Cohen RS, et al: Macrosomia: Causes and consequences. J Pediatr 100:515, 1982.
224. Pettenati MJ, Haines JL, Higgins RR, et al: Wiedemann-Beckwith syndrome: Presentation of clinical and cytogenetic data on 22 new cases and review of the literature. Hum Genet 74:143, 1986.
225. Filippi C, McKusick VA: The Beckwith-Wiedemann syndrome. Medicine 49:279, 1970.
226. Sotelo-Avila C, Gonzalez-Crussi F, Fowler JW: Complete and incomplete forms of Beckwith-Wiedemann syndrome: Their oncogenic potential. J Pediatr 96:47, 1980.
227. Drummond IA, Sukhatme VP: Molecular biology of Wilms tumor. In Feldman A, Van Dang C (eds): Molecular Basis of Medicine. St Louis, Mosby–Year Book, 1993.
228. Schiff D, Colle E, Wells D, Stern L: Metabolic aspects of the Beckwith-Wiedemann syndrome. J Pediatr 82:258, 1973.
229. Cotlin RW, Silver HK: Neonatal hypoglycemia, hyperinsulinism, and absence of pancreatic alpha-cells. Lancet 1:1346, 1970.
230. Brown KW, Williams JC, Maitland NJ, Mott MG: Genomic imprinting and Beckwith-Wiedemann syndrome. Am J Hum Genet 46:1000, 1990.
231. Schiff D, Lowy C: Hypoglycemia and secretion of insulin in urine in hemolytic disease of the new-born. Pediatr Res 4:280, 1970.
232. Cries FA, Driscoll SC: In vitro studies of insulin inactivation with reference to erythroblastosis fetalis. Blood 30:359, 1967.
233. Hook EB, Reynolds JW: Cerebral gigantism: Endocrinological and clinical observations of six patients including a congenital giant concordant monozygotic twins, and a child who achieved adult gigantic size. J Pediatr 70:900, 1967.
234. Bejar RL, Smith CF, Park S, et al: Cerebral gigantism: Concentrations of amino acids in plasma and muscle. J Pediatr 76:105, 1970.
235. Verloes A, Sacre J-P, Geubelle F: Sotos syndrome and fragile X chromosomes. Lancet 2:329, 1987.
236. Cronk C, Crocker AC, Pueschel SM, et al: Growth charts for children with Down syndrome: 1 month to 18 years of age. Pediatrics 81:102–110, 1988.
237. Failkow PJ: Autoimmunity and chromosomal aberrations. Am J Hum Genet 18:93, 1966.
238. Summitt RL: Turner syndrome and Noonan's syndrome. J Pediatr 74:155, 1969.
239. Carballo EC: Turner's syndrome and Noonan's syndrome. J Pediatr 75:729, 1969.
240. Curts FL, Pucci E, Scappaticci S, et al: XO and male phenotype. Am J Dis Child 128:90, 1974.
241. Wilson JG: Comment on internipple distance. J Pediatr 85:148, 1974.
242. Heller RH: The Turner phenotype in the male. J Pediatr 66:48, 1965.
243. Anonymous. Noonan's syndrome. Lancet 340:22, 1992.
244. Razdan AK, Rosenfield RL, Kim MH: Endocrinologic characteristics of partial ovarian failure. J Clin Endocrinol Metab 43:449, 1976.
245. Fisher EMC, Beer-Romero P, Brown LG, et al: Homologous ribosomal protein genes on the human X and Y chromosomes: Escape from X inactivation and implications for Turner syndrome. Cell 63:1205, 1990.
246. Lyon AL, Preece MA, Grant DB: Growth curve for girls with Turner syndrome. Arch Dis Child 60:932, 1985.
247. Mauras N, Rogol AD, Veldhuis JD: Increased GH production rate after low-dose estrogen therapy in prepubertal girls with Turner's syndrome. Pediatr Res 28:626–630, 1990.
248. Rosenfeld RG, Frane F, Attie KM, et al: Six-year results of a randomized, prospective trial of human growth hormone and oxandrolone in Turner syndrome. J Pediatr 121:49–55, 1992.
249. Pinsky L, Levy EP: Malignant hyperpyrexia or the XX–XY Turner phenotype. J Pediatr 83:896, 1973.
250. Francis GL: The Weismann-Netter syndrome: A cause of bowed legs in childhood. Pediatrics 88:334, 1991.
251. Passwell J, Zipperkowski L, Katnelson D, et al: A syndrome characterized by congenital ichthyosis with atrophy, mental retardation, dwarfism, and generalized aminoaciduria. J Pediatr 82:466, 1973.
252. Niikawa N, Matsurra N, Fukushima Y, et al: Kabuki make-up syndrome. J Pediatr 99:565, 1981.
253. Pochedly C, Collipp PJ, Wolman SR, et al: Fanconi's anemia with growth hormone deficiency. J Pediatr 79:93, 1971.
254. Zachmann M, Illig R, Prader A: Fanconi's anemia with isolated growth hormone deficiency. J Pediatr 80:159, 1972.
255. Epstein J, Williams JR, Little JB: Deficient DNA repair in human progeroid cells. Proc Natl Acad Sci USA 70:977, 1973.
256. Regan JD, Setlow RB: DNA repair in human progeroid cells. Biochem Biophys Res Commun 59:858, 1974.
257. Sugita K, Suzuki N, Kojima T, et al: Cockayne syndrome with delayed recovery of RNA synthesis after ultraviolet irradiation but normal ultraviolet survival. Pediatr Res 21:34–37, 1986.
258. Epstein CJ, Martin GM, Schultz SL, Motulsky AG: Werner's syndrome. Medicine 45:177, 1966.
259. Hollister DW, Rimoin DL, Lachman RS, et al: The Winchester syndrome: A nonlysosomal connective tissue disease. J Pediatr 84:701, 1974.
260. Money J: Dwarfism: Questions and answers in counselling. Rehabil Lit 28:134, 1967.
261. Rosenfield RL: Spontaneous puberty and fertility in Turner syndrome. In Rosenfeld RG, Grumbach MM (eds): Turner Syndrome. New York, Marcel Dekker, 1990, pp 131–148.
262. Ross JL, Long LM, Skerda M, et al: The effect of low dose ethinyl estradiol on six-month growth rates and predicted height in patients with Turner syndrome. J Pediatr 109:950, 1986.
263. Cara JF, Johanson AJ: Growth hormone for short stature not due to classic growth hormone deficiency. Pediatr Clin North Am 37:1229–1254, 1990.
264. Zadik Z, Landau H, Limoni Y, Lieberman E: Predictors of growth response to growth hormone in otherwise normal short children. J Pediatr 121:144–148, 1992.
265. Horner JM, Thorsson AV, Hintz RL: Growth deceleration patterns in children with constitutional short stature: An aid to diagnosis, Pediatrics 62:529, 1978.
266. Solomon NW, Rosenfield RL, Jacob RA, Sandstead HH: Growth retardation and zinc nutrition. Pediatr Res 10:923–927, 1976.
267. Tattersall RB, Pyke DA: Growth in diabetic children. Lancet 2:1105, 1973.
268. Winter RJ, Phillips LS, Green OC, Traisman HS: Somatomedin activity in the Mauriac syndrome. J Pediatr 22:598, 1980.
269. Taylor AM, Sharma AK, Avastly N, et al: Inhibition of somatomedin-like activity by serum from streptozotocin-diabetic rats. Endocrinology 121:1360, 1987.
270. Linde LM, Dunn OJ, Schireson R, Rasof B: Growth in children with congenital heart disease. J Pediatr 70:413, 1967.
271. Naeye RL: Anatomic features of growth failure in congenital heart disease. Pediatrics 39:433, 1967.
272. Umansky R, Hauck AJ: Factors in the growth of children with patent ductus arteriosus. Pediatrics 30:540, 1962.
273. Glorieux FH: Rickets, the continuing challenge. N Engl J Med 325:1875, 1991.
274. Alon U, Donaldson DL, Hellerstein S, et al: Metabolic and histologic investigation of the nature of nephrocalcinosis in children with hypophosphatemic rickets and in the Hyp mouse. J Pediatr 120:899–905, 1991.
275. McCrory WW, Gertner JM, Burke FM, et al: Effects of dietary phosphate restriction in children with chronic renal failure. J Pediatr 111:410, 1987.
276. Safer DJ, Allen RP: Factors influencing the suppressant effects of two stimulant drugs on the growth of hyperactive children. Pediatrics 51:660, 1973.
277. Mosier HD, Grossman HJ, Dingman HF: Physical growth in mental defectives. Pediatrics 36:465, 1965.
278. Blethen SL, Gaines S, Weldon V: Comparison of predicted and adult heights in short boys: Effect of androgen therapy. Pediatr Res 18:467, 1984.
279. Tse W-Y, Buyukgebiz A, Hindmarsh PC, et al: Long-term outcome of oxandrolone treatment in boys with constitutional delay of growth and puberty. J Pediatr 117:588, 1990.
280. Hermosa BD, Sobel EH: Thyroid in the treatment of short stature. J Pediatr 80:988, 1972.
281. Grunt JA, Howard CP, Daughaday WH: Comparison of growth and somatomedin C responses following growth hormone treatment in children with small-for-date short stature, significant idiopathic short stature and hypopituitarism. Acta Endocrinol 106:168, 1984.
282. Moore WV, Moore KC, Gifford R, et al: Long-term treatment with growth hormone of children with short stature and normal growth hormone secretion. J Pediatr 120:702–708, 1992.
283. Mullis PE, Akinci A, Kanaka CH, et al: Prevalence of human growth hormone-I gene deletions among patients with isolated growth hormone deficiency from different populations. Pediatr Res 31:532, 1992.
284. Chen EY, Liao YC, Smith DG, et al: The human growth hormone

locus: Nucleotide sequence, biology and evolution. Genomics 4:479, 1989.

285. Phillips IA III: The growth hormone (hGH) genes and human disease. *In* Caskey CT, White R (eds): Banbury Report 14: Recombinant DNA: Applications to Human Disease. Cold Spring Harbor, NY, Cold Spring Harbor, 1983, pp 305–315.

286. Tatsumi K, Miyai K, Notomi T, et al: Cretinism with combined hormone deficiency caused by a mutation in the *Pit*-1 gene. Nature Genet 1:56, 1992.

287. Rudman D, Davis GT, Priest JH, et al: Prevalence of growth hormone deficiency in children with cleft lip or palate. J Pediatr 93:378, 1978.

288. Berry SA, Pierpont ME, Gorlin RJ: Single central incisor in familial holoprosencephaly. J Pediatr 104:877, 1984.

289. Rappaport EB, Vestrom RS, Gorlin RJ, et al: Solitary maxillary central incisor and short stature. J Pediatr 91:924, 1977.

290. Sadeghi-Nejad A, Senior B: Autosomal dominant transmission of isolated growth hormone deficiency in iris-dental dysplasia (Rieger's syndrome). J Pediatr 85:644, 1974.

291. Costin G, Murphree AL: Hypothalamic-pituitary function in children with optic nerve hypoplasia. Am J Dis Child 139:249, 1985.

292. Ellenberger C, Runyan TE: Holoprosencephaly with hypoplasia of the optic nerve, dwarfism and agenesis of the septum pellucidum. Am J Ophthalmol 70:960, 1970.

293. Culler FL, Jones KL: Hypopituitarism in association with postaxial polydactyly. J Pediatr 104:881, 1984.

294. Newman CB, Levine LS, New MI: Endocrine function in children with intrasellar and suprasellar neoplasma. Am J Dis Child 135:259, 1981.

295. Thomsett MJ, Conte FA, Kaplan SL, Grumbach MM: Endocrine and neurologic outcome in childhood craniopharyngioma: Review of effect of treatment in 42 patients. J Pediatr 97:728, 1980.

296. Sklar CA, Grumbach MM, Kaplan SL, Conte FA: Hormonal and metabolic abnormalities associated with central nervous system germinoma in children and adolescents and the effect of therapy: Report of 10 patients. J Clin Endocrinol Metab 52:9, 1981.

297. Shalet SM: Radiation and pituitary dysfunction. N Engl J Med 328:131, 1993.

298. Clayton PE, Shalet SM: Dose dependency of time of onset of radiation-induced growth hormone deficiency. J Pediatr 118:226, 1991.

299. Russell JD, Wise PH, Rischbieth HG: Vascular malformation of hypothalamus: A cause of isolated growth hormone deficiency. Pediatrics 66:306, 1980.

300. Pintor C, Cella G, Manso P, et al: Impaired growth hormone (GH) response to GH-releasing hormone in thalassemia major. J Clin Endocrinol Metab 62:263, 1986.

301. Miller WL, Kaplan SL, Grumbach MM: Child abuse as a cause of post-traumatic hypopituitarism. N Engl J Med 302:724, 1980.

302. Vimpani GV, Vimpani AF, Lidgard GP, et al: Prevalence of severe growth hormone deficiency. Br Med J 2:427, 1977.

303. Rona RJ, Tanner IM: Aetiology of idiopathic growth hormone deficiency in England and Wales. Arch Dis Child 52:197, 1977.

304. Van-den-Broeck J, Vandershueren-Lodeweyckx M, Malvaux P, et al: Growth hormone deficiency: A hidden obstetrical trauma? Eur J Obstet Gynecol Reprod Biol 26:329, 1987.

304a. Root AW: Magnetic resonance imaging in hypopituitarism. J Clin Endocrinol Metab 72:10–11, 1991.

305. Schriock EA, Lustig RH, Rosenthal SM, et al: Effect of growth hormone (GH)–releasing hormone (GRH) on plasma GH in relation to magnitude and duration of GH deficiency in 26 children and adults with isolated GH deficiency or multiple pituitary hormone deficiencies: Evidence for hypothalamic GRH deficiency. J Clin Endocrinol Metab 58:1043, 1984.

306. Gelato MC, Ross JL, Malozowski S, et al: Effects of pulsatile administration of growth hormone (GH)–releasing hormone on short-term linear growth in children with GH deficiency. J Clin Endocrinol Metab 61:444, 1985.

307. Spiliotis BE, August GP, Hung W, et al: Growth hormone neurosecretory dysfunction. JAMA 251:2223, 1984.

308. Blatt J, Bercu BB, Gillin JC, et al: Reduced pulsatile growth hormone secretion in children after therapy for acute lymphoblastic leukemia. J Pediatr 104:182, 1984.

309. Romshe CA, Zipf WB, Miser A, et al: Evaluation of growth hormone release and human growth hormone treatment in children with cranial irradiation-associated short stature. J Pediatr 104:177, 1984.

310. Lustig RH, Schriock EA, Kaplan SL, Grumbach MM: Effect of growth hormone–releasing factor on growth hormone release in children

with radiation-induced growth hormone deficiency. Pediatrics 76:274, 1985.

311. Kita T, Chihara K, Abe H, et al: Regional distribution of human growth hormone-releasing hormone in the human hypothalamus. J Clin Endocrinol Metab 62:372, 1986.

312. Dacou-Voutetakis C, Karpathios T, Logothetis N, et al: Defective growth hormone secretion in primary microcephaly. J Pediatr 85:498, 1974.

313. Silver HK, Finkelstein M: Deprivation dwarfism. J Pediatr 70:317, 1967.

314. Powell GF, Brasel JA, Raiti S, Blizzard RM: II. Emotional deprivation and growth retardation stimulating idiopathic hypopituitarism. N Engl J Med 276:1271, 1967.

315. Krieger I, Mellinger RC: Pituitary function in the deprivation syndrome. J Pediatr 79:216, 1971.

316. Brasel JA: Review of findings in patients with emotional deprivation. *In* Endocrine Aspects of Malnutrition. Santa Barbara, CA, Kroc Foundation Symposium, 1973, p 115.

317. Whitten CF, Pettit MG, Fischhoff J: Evidence that growth failure from maternal deprivation is secondary to undereating. JAMA 209:1675, 1969.

318. Sandberg DE, Smith MM, Fornari V, et al: Nutritional dwarfing: Is it a consequence of disturbed psychosocial functioning? Pediatrics 88:926–933, 1991.

319. Guilhaume A, Benoit O, Gourmelen M, Richardet JM: Relationship between sleep stage IV deficit and reversible HGH deficiency in psychosocial dwarfism. Pediatr Res 16:299, 1982.

320. Frasier SD, Rallison ML: Growth retardation and emotional deprivation: Relative resistance to treatment with human growth hormone. J Pediatr 80:603, 1972.

321. Kowarski AA, Schneider J, Ben Galim E, et al: Growth failure with normal serum RIA-GH and low somatomedin activity: Somatomedin restoration and growth acceleration after exogenous GH. J Clin Endocrinol Metab 47:461, 1978.

322. Laron Z, Pertzelan A, Karp M, et al: Administration of growth hormone to patients with familial dwarfism with high plasma immunoreactive growth hormone: Measurement of sulfation factor, metabolic, and linear growth responses. J Clin Endocrinol Metab 33:332, 1971.

323. Godowski PJ, Leung DW, Meacham LR, et al: Characterization of the human growth hormone receptor gene and demonstration of a partial gene deletion in two patients with Laron-type dwarfism. Proc Natl Acad Sci USA 86:8083, 1989.

324. Leung DW, Spencer SA, Cachianes G, et al: Growth hormone receptor and serum binding protein: Purification, cloning, and expression. Nature 330:537, 1987.

325. Daughaday WH, Trivedi B: Absence of serum growth hormone binding protein in patients with growth hormone receptor deficiency (Laron dwarfism). Proc Natl Acad Sci USA 84:4636, 1987.

326. Walker JL, Ginalska-Malinowska M, Romer TE, et al: Effects of the infusion of insulin-like growth factor-I in a child with growth hormone insensitivity syndrome. N Engl J Med 324:1483, 1991.

327. Baumann G, Shaw MA, Brumbaugh RC, Schwartz J: Short stature and decreased serum growth hormone binding protein in the mountain Ok people of Papua New Guinea. J Clin Endocrinol Metab 72:1346, 1991.

328. Merimee TJ, Hewlett B, Cavalli-Sforza LL, Zapf J: The riddle of pygmy stature. N Engl J Med 317:710, 1987.

329. Heath-Monnig E, Wohltmann HJ, Mills-Dunlap B, Daughaday WH: Measurement of insulin-like growth factor-I (IGF-I) responsiveness of fibroblasts of children with short stature: Identification of a patient with IGF-I resistance. J Clin Endocrinol Metab 64:501, 1987.

330. Lee PDK, Hintz RL, Sperry JB, et al: IGF binding proteins in growth-retarded children with chronic renal failure. Pediatr Res 26:308, 1989.

331. Ooi GT, Herington AC: Recognition of insulin-like growth factor (IGF) serum binding proteins by an antibody raised against a specific IGF inhibitor. Biochem Biophys Res Commun 156:783, 1988.

332. Huseman C, Johanson A: Growth hormone deficiency in anorexia nervosa. J Pediatr 87:946, 1975.

333. Bucuvalas JC, Cutfield W, Horn J, et al: Resistance to the growth-promoting and metabolic effects of growth hormone in children with chronic liver disease. J Pediatr 117:397, 1990.

334. Rosenfeld RG, Wilson M, Lee PD, Hintz RL: Insulin-like growth factors I and II in evaluation of growth retardation. J Pediatr 109:428, 1986.

335. Furlanetto RW: Insulin-like growth factor-I measurements in the evaluation of growth hormone secretion. Horm Res 33(Suppl 4):25, 1990.

336. Blum WF, Rainke MB: Use of insulin-like growth factor-binding protein 3 for the evaluation of growth disorders. Horm Res 33(Suppl):31, 1990.

337. Frasier SD: A review of growth hormone stimulation tests in children. Pediatrics 53:979, 1974.

338. Blethen SL, Chasalow FI: Use of a two-site immunonoradiometric assay for growth hormone (GH) in identifying children with GH-dependent growth failure. J Clin Endocrinol Metab 57:1031, 1983.

339. Mims RB, Scott CL, Modebe OM, Bethune JE: Prevention of L-dopa-induced growth hormone stimulation by hyperglycemia. J Clin Endocrinol Metab 37:660, 1973.

340. Moll GW Jr, Rosenfield RL, Fang VS: Administration of low-dose estrogen rapidly and directly stimulates growth hormone production. Am J Dis Child 140:124–127, 1986.

341. Cara JF, Burstein S, Cuttler L, et al: Growth hormone deficiency impedes the rise in plasma insulin-like growth factor-I levels associated with precocious puberty. J Pediatr 115:64, 1989.

342. Rose SR, Ross JL, Uriate M, et al: The advantage of measuring stimulated as compared with spontaneous growth hormone levels in the diagnosis of growth hormone deficiency. N Engl J Med 319:201, 1988.

343. Costin G, Kaufman FR, Brasel JA: Growth hormone secretory dynamics in subjects with normal stature. J Pediatr 115:537, 1989.

344. Lin TH, Kirkland RT, Sherman BM, et al: Growth hormone testing in short children and their response to growth hormone therapy. J Pediatr 115:57, 1989.

345. Frasier SD: Human pituitary growth hormone (hGH) therapy in growth hormone deficiency. Endocr Rev 4:155, 1983.

345a. Malozowski S, Tanner LA, Wysowski D, Fleming GA: Growth hormone, insulin-like growth factor I, and benign intracranial hypertension. N Engl J Med 329:665, 1993.

346. Brown P, Gajdusek C, Gibbs CJ Jr, Asher DM: Potential epidemic of Creutzfeldt-Jakob disease from human growth hormone therapy. N Engl J Med 313:728, 1985.

347. Zachman MM, Prader A: Anabolic and androgenic effect of testosterone on sexually immature boys and its dependency on growth hormone. J Clin Endocrinol Metab 30:85, 1970.

348. Lippe BM, Kaplan SA, Golden MP, et al: Carbohydrate tolerance and insulin receptor binding in children with hypopituitarism: Responses after acute and chronic human growth hormone administration. J Clin Endocrinol Metab 53:507, 1981.

349. Smith PJ, Brook CGD: Growth hormone releasing hormone or growth hormone treatment in growth hormone insufficiency? Arch Dis Child 63:629, 1988.

350. Huseman CA, Hassing JM: Evidence for dopaminergic stimulation of growth velocity in some hypopituitary children. J Clin Endocrinol Metab 58:419, 1984.

351. Press M, Notarfrancesco A, Genel M: Risk of hypoglycaemia with alternate-day growth hormone injections. Lancet 1:1002, 1987.

352. Burns EC, Tanner JM, Preece MA, et al: Final height and pubertal development in 55 children with idiopathic growth hormone deficiency, treated for between 2 and 15 years with human growth hormone. Eur J Pediatr 137:155, 1981.

353. Burns EC, Tanner JM, Preese MA, et al: Growth hormone treatment in children with craniopharyngioma: Final growth status. Clin Endocrinol 14:587, 1981.

354. Hibi I, Tanaka T: Final height of patients with idiopathic growth hormone deficiency after long-term growth hormone treatment. Acta Endocrinol (Copenh) 120:409, 1989.

355. Albertsson-Wikland K, Isaksson O, Rosberg S, et al: Frequency and mode of growth hormone administration—Relationship to growth in prepubertal children. Acta Endocrinol Suppl (Copenh) 103:215, 1983.

356. Kaplan SL, Savage DCL, Suter S, et al: Antibodies to human growth hormone arising in patients treated with human growth hormone: Incidence, characteristics, and effects on growth. In Raiti S (ed): Advances in Human Growth Hormone Research. Washington, US Government Printing Office, 1974, p 725.

357. Lippe BM, Van Herle AJ, La Franchi SH, et al: Reversible hypothyroidism in growth hormone-deficient children treated with human growth hormone. J Clin Endocrinol Metab 40:612, 1975.

358. Van den Brande JL, Van Wyk JJ, French FS, et al: Advancement of skeletal age of hypopituitary children treated with thyroid hormone plus cortisone. J Pediatr 82:22, 1983.

359. Winterer J, Chrousos C, Cassorla F, Loriaux L: Acquired refractoriness to growth hormone in a patient with isolated growth hormone deficiency: Growth and plasma somatomedin-C response to high-dose growth hormone therapy. J Pediatr 104:908, 1984.

360. Romshe CA, Sotos JF: The combined effect of growth hormone and oxandrolone in patients with growth hormone deficiency. J Pediatr 96:127, 1980.

361. Watanabe S, Tsunematsu Y, Fujimoto J, Komiyama A: Leukemia in patients treated with growth hormone. Lancet 1:1159, 1988.

362. Report of the International Workshop on Growth Hormone and Leukemia, May 5, 1988.

363. Rudman D, Kutner MH, Blackston RD, et al: Children with normal-variant short stature: Treatment with human growth hormone for six months. N Engl J Med 305:123, 1983.

364. Rosenfeld RG, Kemp SF, Hintz RL: Constancy of somatomedin response to growth hormone treatment of hypopituitary dwarfism, and lack of correlation with growth rate. J Clin Endocrinol Metab 53:611, 1981.

365. Plotnick LP, Van Meter QL, Kowarski AA: Human growth hormone treatment of children with growth failure and normal growth hormone levels by immunoassay: Lack of correlation with somatomedin generation. Pediatrics 71:324, 1983.

366. Allen D, Fost N: Growth hormone therapy for short stature: Panacea or Pandora's box? J Pediatr 117:16, 1990.

367. Kaplan SL, Grumbach MM: Long-term treatment with growth hormone of children with non-growth hormone deficient short stature. In Isaksson O, Binder C, Hall K, et al (eds): Growth Hormone: Basic and Clinical Aspects. Amsterdam, Excerpta Medica, 1987, pp 197–204.

368. Gertner JM, Genel M, Gianfredi SP, et al: Prospective clinical trial of human growth hormone in short children without growth hormone deficiency. J Pediatr 104:172, 1984.

369. Darendeliler F, Hindmarsh PC, Preece MA, et al: Growth hormone increases rate of pubertal maturation. Acta Endocrinol (Copenh) 122:414, 1990.

370. Underwood LE: Growth hormone treatment for short children. Pediatrics 104:237, 1984.

371. Rezvani I, DiGeorge AM: Reassessment of the daily dose of oral thyroxine for replacement therapy in hypothyroid children. J Pediatr 90:291, 1977.

372. Lee PA, Weldon W, Migeon CV: Short stature as the only clinical sign of Cushing's syndrome. J Pediatr 86:89, 1975.

373. Binkiewicz A, Robinson M, Senior B: Pseudo-Cushing syndrome caused by alcohol in breast milk. J Pediatr 93:965, 1978.

373a. Soszynski PA, Frohman LA: Inhibitory effects of ethanol on the growth hormone (GH)-releasing hormone–GH-insulin-like growth factor-I axis in the rat. Endocrinology 131:2603, 1992.

374. Strickland AL, Underwood LE, Voina SJ, et al: Growth retardation in Cushing's syndrome. Am J Dis Child 123:207, 1972.

375. McArthur RG, Hayles AB, Salassa RM: Growth retardation in Cushing disease. J Pediatr 96:783, 1979.

376. Couch RM, Smail RJ, Dean HJ, Winter JSD: Prolonged remission of Cushing disease after treatment with cyproheptadine. J Pediatr 104:906, 1984.

377. Styne DM, Grumbach MM, Kaplan SL, et al: Treatment of Cushing's disease in childhood and adolescence by transsphenoidal microadenomectomy. N Engl J Med 310:889, 1984.

378. Jennings AS, Liddle CW, Orth DN: Results of treating childhood Cushing's disease with pituitary irradiation. N Engl J Med 297:213, 1977.

379. Hansen JW, Loriaux DL: Variable efficacy of glucocorticoids in congenital adrenal hyperplasia. Pediatrics 57:942, 1976.

380. Kozower M, Veatch L, Kaplan MM: Decreased clearance of prednisolone, a factor in the development of corticosteroid side effects. J Clin Endocrinol Metab 38:407, 1974.

381. Soyka LF: Alternate-day corticosteroid therapy. Adv Pediatr 19:47, 1972.

382. Hollman GA, Allen DB: Overt glucocorticoid excess due to inhaled corticosteroid therapy. Pediatrics 81:452, 1988.

383. Simopoulos AP, Bartter FC: Growth characteristics and factors influencing growth in Bartter's syndrome. J Pediatr 81:56, 1972.

384. Simmons JM, Wilson CJ, Potter DE, Holliday MA: Relation of calorie deficiency to growth failure in children on hemodialysis and the growth response to calorie supplementation. N Engl J Med 285:642, 1974.

385. Schaefer F, Hamill G, Stanhope R, et al: Pulsatile growth hormone

secretion in peripubertal patients with chronic renal failure. J Pediatr 119:568–577, 1991.

386. Hokken-Koelega ACS, Stijnen T, Keizer-Schrama SMPF deM, et al: Placebo-controlled, double-blind, cross-over trial of growth hormone treatment in prepubertal children with chronic renal failure. Lancet 338:585–590, 1991.

387. Bartosh S, Kaiser B, Rezvani I, et al: Effects of growth hormone administration in pediatric renal allograft recipients. Pediatr Nephrol 6:68–73, 1992.

388. Van Dop C, Jabs KL, Donohue PA, et al: Accelerated growth rates in children treated with growth hormone after renal transplantation. J Pediatr 120:244–250, 1992.

389. Kirschner BS: Growth retardation in juvenile Crohn's disease. Clin Nutr 2:26, 1983.

390. Waldmann TA, Gordon RS Jr, Rosse W: Studies on the metabolism of the serum proteins and lipids in a patient with analbuminemia. Am J Med 37:960, 1964.

391. Cacciari E, Salardi S, Volta U, et al: Can antigliadin antibody detect symptomless coeliac disease in children with short stature. Lancet 1:1469, 1985.

392. Mock DM, Perman JA, Thaler M, Morris RC: Chronic fructose intoxication after infancy in children with hereditary fructose intolerance. N Engl J Med 309:764, 1983.

393. Spolidoro JVN, Berquist WE, Pehlivanoglu E, et al: Growth acceleration in children after orthotopic liver transplantation. J Pediatr 112:41–44, 1988.

394. Willi SM, Cooke K, Goldwein J, et al: Growth in children after bone marrow transplantation for advanced neuroblastoma compared with growth after transplantation for leukemia or aplastic anemia. J Pediatr 120:726–732, 1992.

395. Butenandt O: Rheumatoid arthritis and growth retardation in children: Treatment with human growth hormone. Eur J Pediatr 130:15, 1979.

396. Hsu LYF, Hirschhorn K: Unusual Turner mosaicism (45,X/47,XXX; 45,X/46,XX; 45,X/46,XX): Detection through deceleration from normal linear growth or secondary amenorrhea. J Pediatr 79:276, 1971.

397. Gourmelen M, le Bouc Y, Girard F, Binoux M: Serum levels of insulin-like growth factor (IGF) and IGF binding protein in constitutionally tall children and adolescents. J Clin Endocrinol Metab 59:1197, 1984.

398. Tsipouras P, Mastro RD, Sarfarazi M, et al: Genetic linkage of the Marfan syndrome, ectopia lentis, and congenital contractural arachnodactyly to the fibrillin genes on chromosomes 15 and 5. N Engl J Med 326:905–909, 1992.

399. Schimke RN: Phenotype of malignancy: The mucosal neuroma syndrome. Pediatrics 52:283, 1973.

400. Greenblatt RB, McDonough PC, Mahesh VB: Projection of growth. J Clin Endocrinol Metab 27:1761, 1967.

401. Wettenhall HNB, Cahill C, Roche AF: Tall girls: A survey of 15 years of management and treatment. J Pediatr 86:602, 1975.

402. Zachmann M, Ferrandez A, Murset G, et al: Testosterone treatment of excessively tall boys. J Pediatr 88:116, 1975.

403. Schoenle EJ, Theintz C, Torresani T, et al: Lack of bromocriptine induced reduction of predicted height in tall adolescents. J Clin Endocrinol Metab 65:355, 1987.

404. Schlesinger S, MacGillivray MH, Manschauer RW: Acceleration of growth and bone maturation in childhood thyrotoxicosis. J Pediatr 83:233, 1973.

405. Wilroy RS Jr, Etteldorf JN: Familial hyperthyroidism including two siblings with neonatal Graves disease. J Pediatr 78:625, 1971.

406. Seip M: Generalized lipodystrophy. Ergeb Inn Med Kinderheilkd 31:65, 1971.

407. Mabry CC, Hollingsorth DR, Upton CV, Corbin A: Pituitary-hypothalamic dysfunction in generalized lipodystrophy. J Pediatr 82:625, 1973.

408. Senior B, Loridan LL: Fat cell function and insulin in a patient with generalized lipodystrophy. J Pediatr 74:972, 1969.

409. AvRuskin TW, Sau K, Tang S, Juan C: Childhood acromegaly: Successful therapy with conventional radiation and effects of chlorprom-

azine on growth hormone and prolactin secretions. J Clin Endocrinol Metab 37:380, 1973.

410. Blumberg DL, Sklar CA, David R, Rothenberg S, Bell J: Acromegaly in an infant. Pediatrics 83:998–1002, 1989.

411. Gelber SJ, Haffez DS, Donohue PA: Pituitary gigantism caused by growth hormone excess from infancy. J Pediatr 120:931–934, 1992.

412. Zimmerman D, Young WF Jr, Ebersold MJ, et al: Congenital gigantism due to growth hormone-releasing hormone excess and pituitary hyperplasia with adenomatous transformation. J Clin Endocrinol Metab 76:216, 1993.

413. Kreiter M, Burstein S, Rosenfield RL, et al: Preserving adult height potential in girls with idiopathic true precocious puberty. J Pediatr 117:364–370, 1990.

414. Hansen JDL, Freesemann C, Moodie AD, Evans DE: What does nutritional growth retardation imply? Pediatrics 47:299, 1971.

415. Addy DP, Hudson FP: Diencephalic syndrome of infantile emaciation. Arch Dis Child 47:338, 1972.

415a. Vlachopapadopoulou E, Tracey KJ, Capella M, et al: Increased energy expenditure in a patient with diencephalic syndrome. J Pediatr 122:922, 1993.

415b. Must A, Jacques P, Dallas GE, et al: Long-term morbidity and mortality of overweight adolescents. N Engl J Med 327:1350, 1992.

415c. Henderson RC: Tibia vara: a complication of adolescent obesity. J Pediatr 121:482, 1992.

416. Forbes CB: Lean body mass and fat in obese children. Pediatrics 34:308, 1964.

417. Cheek DB, Schultz RB, Parra A, Reba RC: Overgrowth of lean and adipose tissue in adolescent obesity. Pediatr Res 4:268, 1970.

418. Chalew SA, Lozano RA, Armour KM, et al: Reduction of plasma cortisol levels in childhood obesity. J Pediatr 119:778–780, 1991.

418a. Holm VA, Cassidy SB, Butler MG, et al: Prader-Willi syndrome: consensus diagnostic criteria. Pediatrics 91:398, 1993.

419. Lee DK, Wilson DM, Rountree L, et al: Linear growth response to exogenous growth hormone in Prader-Willi syndrome. Am J Med Genet 28:865–871, 1987.

420. Mascari MJ, Gottlieb W, Rogan PK, et al: The frequency of uniparental disomy in Prader-Willi syndrome. N Engl J Med 326:1599–1607, 1992.

421. Carey JC, Hall BD: Confirmation of the Cohen syndrome. J Pediatr 93:239, 1978.

422. Green JS, Parfrey PS, Harnett JD, et al: The cardinal manifestations of Bardet-Biedl syndrome, a form of Laurence-Moon-Biedl syndrome. N Engl J Med 321:11002–11009, 1989.

423. Heald FP, Hunt SM: Caloric dependency in obese adolescents as affected by degree of maturation. J Pediatr 66:1035, 1965.

424. Warkany J, Kalter H: Congenital malformations. N Engl J Med 265:993, 1961.

425. Nora JJ, Nora AH: Can the pill cause birth defects? N Engl J Med 291:731, 1974.

426. Goldman AS, Baker L, Piddington R, et al: Hyperglycemia-induced teratogenesis is mediated by a functional deficiency of arachidonic acid. Proc Natl Acad Sci USA 82:8227–8231, 1985.

427. Meadows AT, Lichtenfeld JL, Koop CE: Wilms' tumor in three children of a woman with congenital hemihypertrophy. N Engl J Med 291:23, 1974.

428. Davis LM, Stallard R, Thomas GH, et al: Two anonymous DNA segments distinguish the Wilm's tumor and aniridia loci. Science 241:840–842, 1988.

429. Pelletier J, Bruening W, Kashtan CE, et al: Germline mutations in the Wilm's tumor suppressor gene are associated with abnormal urogenital development in Denys-Drash syndrome. Cell 67:437–447, 1991.

430. Currarino G, Engle MA: The effects of ligation of the subclavian artery on the bones and soft tissues of the arms. J Pediatr 67:808, 1965.

431. Ansell BM, Bywaters EGL: Growth in Stills' disease. Ann Rheum Dis 15:292, 1956.

432. Young RC, De Vita VT, Johnson RE: Hodgkin's disease in childhood. Blood 42:163, 1973.

142

Peptide Growth Factors

WILLIAM E. RUSSELL
JUDSON J. VAN WYK

GENERAL CONSIDERATIONS

Relationships Between Peptide Growth Factors, Cytokines, and Other Hormones of the Endocrine System

The term *growth factor* encompasses not only those peptides that stimulate or inhibit cell division, but also others, such as nerve growth factor, that have no effect on mitotic events but stimulate growth by inducing differentiation and cellular hypertrophy. During the past several decades dozens of peptide growth factors have been described in blood, tissue extracts, or conditioned media from cell or organ cultures. Although by definition all growth factors are cytokines, the term *cytokine* is usually reserved for growth and differentiation factors produced by inflammatory cells.

Whether or not growth factors and cytokines should be considered true hormones depends on how rigidly this term is defined. When Starling[1] first used the term *hormone* in 1905, he divided chemical regulators into two categories: those that increase the "growth" of a tissue or organ, and those that cause "increased activity of an organ." He further postulated that "all organs of the body are regulated in their growth and activity by chemical mechanisms." Although Starling used the term *hormone* as a generic designation for chemical mediators, soon thereafter endocrinologists and textbook writers began to restrict this term so that it included only those chemical regulators that are made in the seven or so authentic glands of internal secretion. This restricted view of the endocrine system was not significantly revised until it was recognized that many growth-regulating hormones originate in multiple tissues outside of the glands of internal secretion, and that hormones originating in highly specialized tissues, such as the gut, may also be powerful mitogens for certain cell types

Supported by research grant 5 RO1 DK 01022 from NIDDK to JJVW, and grant RO1 DK 44557 from NIDDK to WER.

and are also found in the brain, where they may function as neurotransmitters.

In most respects peptide growth factors, gastrointestinal hormones, neurotransmitters, and cytokines resemble the more traditional hormones in their behavior: They act through specific receptors, are subject to physiological regulation, and utilize similar mechanisms of signal transduction to produce their biological effects in target tissues. Because of these changing perceptions, the terms *hormone* and *growth factor* are now being interchangeably applied to a variety of extracellular regulators of cell growth and function regardless of their origin. This trend signals a return to the original concepts that Starling and his contemporaries proposed nearly a century ago.

Evolution of Superfamilies of Growth Factors and Their Receptors

Because all life depends on cellular proliferation, it seems on a priori grounds that the evolution of peptides that regulate cell proliferation should have preceded the evolution of hormones that regulate more specialized functions (see Ch. 2). Niall[2] has suggested that duplication of the genes encoding the more primitive mitogens permitted families of structurally related growth factors and hormones to evolve without losing more basic functions. Parallel evolution of their respective receptors, when it occurs, further increases the functional heterogeneity within the growing superfamily. Evolution from stem mitogens and their receptors explains why so many growth factors and their receptors are clustered into structurally homologous superfamilies in which the individual members exhibit considerable functional diversity.

Although the *paterfamilias* of most superfamilies cannot be identified with certainty, in the case of the insulin-like family of peptides and receptors, for example, it may be surmised that one of the insulin-like growth factors (IGF-I or IGF-II) preceded the emergence of the homologous hormone proinsulin. IGF's are essential for the replication of most cell lines, whereas insulin assumes its most critical role in complex organisms with episodic periods of food intake. Similarly, it may be inferred that the insulin receptor evolved from the homologous type I IGF receptor.

In recent years, many new members of the various superfamilies have been discovered by molecular screening of appropriate libraries with probes based on the most conserved nucleotide sequences of other family members. The function of peptides discovered by such molecular fishing expeditions is often obscure.

Local Modalities of Growth Factor Action

The most striking difference between peptide growth factors and classic hormones is that growth factors originate in many different sites in the body and appear to act primarily upon neighboring tissues (paracrine modality of action) or even on their own cells of origin (autocrine modality of action) rather than on distant tissues that can be accessed only via the blood stream (endocrine modality of action) (Fig. 142–1). These modes of action are not mutually exclusive, however, because a given hormone may

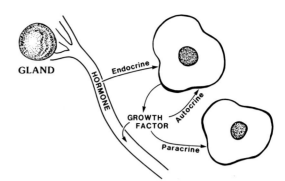

FIGURE 142–1. **Mechanisms of hormone/growth factor action.** In the classic endocrine modalities of hormone action, hormones are produced by specialized glands and transported in the blood or other body fluids to distant target tissues. It is now recognized that all cells are capable of elaborating hormones that can interact with receptors on nearby cells (paracrine mode of action) or with receptors on the cell of origin (autocrine control). (From Russell WE, Underwood LE: Nutrition and the humoral regulation of growth. *In* Walker WA, Watkins JB (eds): Nutrition in Pediatrics: Basic Science and Clinical Application. Boston, Little, Brown and Company, 1985, pp 279–299.)

act by different modalities in different tissues and may even produce biologic effects in distal tissues through the classic endocrine modality of distribution.

Paracrine

The term *paracrine* was proposed by Feyrter[3] in the 1930's to describe a network of epithelial clear cells distributed throughout the gut and other organs in close proximity to nerve endings and blood vessels. He postulated that these cells were "peripheral endocrine glands" and speculated that in addition to actions on distant tissues, these cells might have local "paracrine" effects in the regulation of gut function. By the 1970's many of the so-called gut hormones had also been found in the CNS, thus linking hormones, growth factors, and neurotransmitters within the overall scheme of humoral regulation.[4]

Autocrine

In 1980 Sporn and Todaro[5] added the concept of autocrine secretion to explain the endogenous production of autostimulatory "transforming" growth factors by transformed cells. Although Todaro postulated that autocrine production of such "transforming growth factors" plays a causative role in malignant transformation of cells, it has since become apparent that all growth factors, including the so-called transforming growth factors, are produced by normal growing cells and that autocrine modes of action are a central feature of normal cell biology rather than an aberration limited to malignant cells. Direct evidence that endogenously produced growth factors are necessary for the growth of normal cells was provided by demonstrations that the growth of normal cells can be inhibited by monoclonal antibodies directed at specific growth factors that were originally present in the media in which the cells were grown.[6, 7]

Juxtacrine

"Juxtacrine" control refers to biological actions by growth factors still anchored to the plasma membranes of the cells that produced them.[8] Juxtacrine control differs from autocrine and paracrine modes in that it requires cell contact to bring the receptors into proximity with their membrane-anchored ligands. Many growth factors, notably those belonging to the epidermal growth factor (EGF) superfamily, but also including colony stimulating factor (CSF-1) and tumor necrosis factor (TNF-α), are synthesized embedded within larger, membrane-spanning precursor proteins that structurally resemble receptors but have no known signaling mechanisms. Although membrane-anchored growth factor precursors were initially considered to be inactive substrates that require further processing to release active molecules, some growth factors retain biological activity within their precursors and are capable of inducing a signal through receptors on contiguous cells. For example, Wong et al.[9] transfected cells with a TGF-α construct in which amino acid substitutions at proteolytic cleavage sites prevented release of soluble TGF-α. The transfected cells displaying membrane-anchored TGF-α precursor were able to activate EGF/TGF-α receptors in adjacent cells, as demonstrated by receptor autophosphorylation and calcium fluxes.

Evidence exists for the importance of juxtacrine control in vivo as well. A naturally occurring mutation of the mouse hematopoietic and germ cell growth factors KL-1 and KL-2 prevents them from anchoring in plasma membranes and results in their secretion into the extracellular fluid. Despite the fact that the membrane-anchored and soluble forms of these peptides have comparable biologic potency in vitro, affected mice exhibit sterility and anemia.[10] Juxtacrine interactions between cell-immobilized growth factors and receptors on neighboring cells have also been implicated in cell-cell adhesion and in embryonic induction.[8]

A form of juxtacrine control is exerted by growth factors with strong affinity for extracellular matrix. For example, the heparin-binding growth factors such as the fibroblast growth factors (FGF's, discussed below) can induce responses in cells that contact them in the matrix.

Growth factor precursors, like other cell surface proteins, such as growth factor receptors, can be converted into soluble forms by regulated proteolysis.[11] Cleavage of the extracellular domains of growth factor precursors appears to be a regulated process that is controlled by serum factors, activators of protein kinase C, and mobilization of intracellular calcium.[12] Thus, membrane-anchored and matrix-immobilized juxtacrine growth factors can also serve as reservoirs of soluble ligand to act in autocrine, paracrine, or endocrine modes.

Intracrine

O'Malley[13] has postulated that many of the orphan zinc finger DNA-binding proteins that have been identified by gene cloning may actually serve as receptors for ligands that are synthesized within the same cell and that are transported to the nucleus without first being secreted. One such orphan receptor proved to be a transcription factor (COUP) that binds to the upstream promotor for the chicken ovalbumin gene. Other known growth factors and ligands such as angiotensin II may act in a similar manner by transport to nuclear binding sites without being secreted outside of the cell.[14]

Effects of Growth Factors on Differentiated Cellular Functions Versus Their Effects on Cell Proliferation

Distinctions between mitogens and differentiating agents are somewhat artificial, and the effects of growth factors on cytodifferentiation are often overlooked. Most hormones and growth factors are capable of stimulating either a mitogenic response or the induction of differentiated cell functions, depending on cell type, developmental stage, the hormonal milieu, and other environmental circumstances. For example, IGF-I stimulates a proliferative response in chondrocytes populating the proliferative zone of the growth plate, whereas in the hypertrophic zone it stimulates the synthesis of proteoglycans. Some growth factors, such as TGF-β, are bifunctional and capable of either stimulating or reversibly inhibiting growth. The nature of the cellular response to hormones and growth factors is thus due less to the intrinsic properties of the chemical messengers than to the context in which they act. This was well stated by Sporn and Roberts,[15] who view growth factors as:

> part of a complex cellular signalling language, in which the individual peptides are the equivalent of characters of an alphabet code. . . . It is not surprising that meaning in this cellular language is contextual, because that is the case for all languages or codes.

Classification of Peptide Growth Factors: Problems of Nomenclature

The naming of growth factors has followed no consistent pattern: Some were named after some specialized property, others were assigned names corresponding to the tissue or cell type from which they were first isolated, and yet others were named according to the tissue on which they were presumed to act. Thus, such terms as *endothelial growth factor* might signify a mitogenic peptide isolated from endothelial cells or a peptide from some other source that acted primarily on endothelial cells. Similarly, *keratinocyte growth factor* (KGF) is a member of the fibroblast growth factor superfamily that was initially isolated from cultures of mesenchymal cells on the basis of its mitogenicity for keratinocytes,[16] whereas the *keratinocyte-derived autocrine factor* (KAF) is a member of the EGF superfamily (amphiregulin) that is both secreted by and is mitogenic for its cell of origin.[17] Designations such as *platelet-derived growth factor* led to even more confusion when it was recognized that platelets are a highly enriched source of at least four different growth factors.[18]

Further chaos has resulted from the fact that most growth factors have been isolated by different investigators, either from different sources or on the basis of different properties, and therefore have been reported under a variety of different names. The best example of this is fibroblast growth factor (FGF), a substance that was originally isolated from bovine pituitary glands and brain as a highly basic mitogen for fibroblasts. Basic FGF was found to be widely distributed in many normal tissues derived from mesoderm and neuroectoderm. It is thus not surprising that FGF has been discovered and rediscovered under more than 30 different names.

In this chapter we have grouped currently recognized growth factors as members of five structurally related superfamilies, and the remainder into groupings that are based either on the organ systems that they regulate or on similarities in their effects (Table 142–1).

THE MAJOR SUPERFAMILIES OF PEPTIDE GROWTH FACTORS

Somatomedins (Insulin-like Growth Factors)

History and Nomenclature

In 1957 Salmon and Daughaday[19] proposed that the growth-promoting effects of growth hormone (GH) in vivo are not direct, but instead are mediated by peptide growth factors that came to be known as somatomedins.[20] It now

TABLE 142–1. THE MAJOR MAMMALIAN GROWTH FACTOR SUPERFAMILIES

GROWTH FACTOR FAMILY/ MEMBERS	SYNONYMS/HOMOLOGUES
Somatomedins	
Insulin-like growth factor-I	IGF I; somatomedin C
Insulin-like growth factor-II	IGF II; MSA; skeletal GF
Proinsulin	
Epidermal Growth Factors	
Epidermal growth factor	EGF; urogastrone; hEGF
Transforming growth factor-α	TGF-α; sarcoma GF
Amphiregulin	Keratinocyte autocrine factor (KAF)
	Schwannoma-derived GF
	Colorectum cell–derived GF (CRDGF)
Heparin-binding EGF	HB-EGF
Cripto	
Betacellulin	
Transforming growth factors-β	
Transforming growth factor-β's	TGF-β1 (cartilage inducing factor-A)
	TGF-β2 (BSC-1 growth inhibitor; polyergin)
	TGF-β3
Activins	Activin-AA; -AB; -BB
Inhibins	Inhibin-A; Inhibin-B
Müllerian-inhibiting substance	MIS; Antimüllerian hormone; AMH
Bone morphogenetic proteins	BMP-2A; BMP-2B; BMP-3
Vgr-1	
Platelet-Derived Growth Factors	
Platelet-derived growth factor	PDGF-AA; PDGF-AB; PDGF-BB
Osteosarcoma cell growth factor	PDGF-AA
p28*sis*	PDGF-BB
Fibroblast Growth Factors (Heparin-binding Growth Factors)	
Acidic FGF	aFGF
Basic FGF	bFGF
*int*2	
FGF-4	*hst*-1; Kaposi's sarcoma growth factor (kFGF)
FGF-5	
FGF-6	
FGF-7	Keratinocyte growth factor (KGF)
Nerve Growth Factors	
Nerve growth factor	NGF
Brain-derived neurotrophic factor	BDNF
Neurotropin-3	NT-3
Ciliary neurotrophic factor	CNTF

appears that essentially all of the biological activities that have been attributed to these factors can be accounted for by two distinct peptides. The somatomedin with the greater GH dependency was independently isolated and sequenced under the names IGF-I[21] and somatomedin-C (Sm-C).[22] The other somatomedin, IGF-II, is similar in structure to IGF-I but is less GH dependent and more potent in assays for insulin-like activity.[23, 24] In this chapter we follow the current consensus by using the term "somatomedin" only when referring to these peptides in a generic sense and use the terms IGF-I and IGF-II when referring to the specific peptides.[25]

IGF-I is a 70-amino-acid residue straight-chain basic (pI 8.1–8.5) peptide containing three intrachain disulfide bridges. IGF-II is a 67-residue neutral peptide that is similar in structure to IGF-I. Both IGF-I and IGF-II are highly homologous with human proinsulin in the domains comparable to the A and B chains of insulin, whereas the C domains are shorter and quite different from the C peptide of proinsulin. Also IGF-I and IGF-II have unique extensions (D domains) at their carboxy-termini (Fig. 142–2).

IGF-I and IGF-II are synthesized like other secreted proteins with leader sequences of 25 and 24 amino acids, respectively, at their amino-termini. In addition, the prohormone for IGF-I has an extension of 35 amino acid residues and that for IGF-II an extension of 89 residues (E domain) at their respective carboxy-termini.[26–29] Thus the prepro- forms of the hormones require post-translational processing to arrive at their mature forms.

IGF Genes and Regulation of Gene Expression

GENE STRUCTURE. Both of the somatomedins are single-copy genes, with the gene for prepro-IGF-I localized to the short arm of chromosome 12 and the gene for prepro-IGF-II localized in close proximity to the proinsulin gene on the short arm of chromosome 11.[30] The somatomedin locus on each chromosome is also very close to proto-oncogenes of the c-*ras* family. It is believed that chromosomes 11 and 12 have a common ancestry and that the close linkage of genes for members of the insulin-like family with these cellular oncogenes is of evolutionary and possibly functional significance.[30]

The IGF-I and IGF-II precursors, as deduced from cDNA sequences, are highly conserved across species, with the greatest conservation in the mature peptides. The coding regions for the mature peptides are flanked by 3′ and 5′ extensions that account for considerable heterogeneity in transcripts. In the case of rat IGF-I, transcripts ranging in size from 7.5 to 0.8 kb are due to two different classes of untranslated sequences at the 5′ end, and by two variants at the carboxy-terminal of rat IGF-I (termed IA and IB type E domains) that are generated by alternate splicing. The size of the transcripts depends primarily on the locus of the polyadenylation site in the long 3′ untranslated region.[31] The nature of the IGF-I mRNA's expressed in the rat is highly dependent on the organ in which they are expressed and the developmental stage of the animal, although the physiological significance of this heterogeneity is not yet known.[32, 33]

GENETIC IMPRINTING. The genes encoding IGF-II and its receptor are "imprinted" in the early embryo, and their

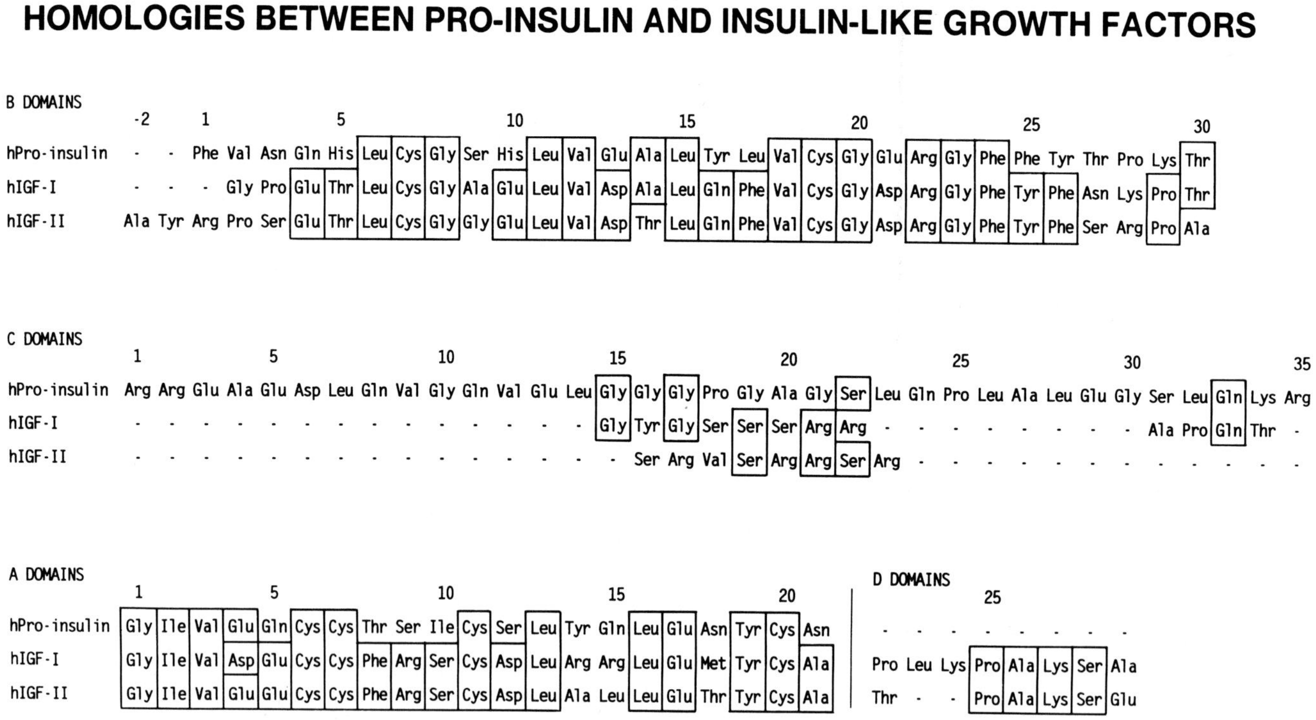

HOMOLOGIES BETWEEN PRO-INSULIN AND INSULIN-LIKE GROWTH FACTORS

B DOMAINS

	-2		1				5					10					15					20					25					30
hPro-insulin	-	-	Phe	Val	Asn	Gln	His	Leu	Cys	Gly	Ser	His	Leu	Val	Glu	Ala	Leu	Tyr	Leu	Val	Cys	Gly	Glu	Arg	Gly	Phe	Phe	Tyr	Thr	Pro	Lys	Thr
hIGF-I	-	-	-	Gly	Pro	Glu	Thr	Leu	Cys	Gly	Ala	Glu	Leu	Val	Asp	Ala	Leu	Gln	Phe	Val	Cys	Gly	Asp	Arg	Gly	Phe	Tyr	Phe	Asn	Lys	Pro	Thr
hIGF-II	Ala	Tyr	Arg	Pro	Ser	Glu	Thr	Leu	Cys	Gly	Gly	Glu	Leu	Val	Asp	Thr	Leu	Gln	Phe	Val	Cys	Gly	Asp	Arg	Gly	Phe	Tyr	Phe	Ser	Arg	Pro	Ala

C DOMAINS

	1			5					10					15					20					25					30					35
hPro-insulin	Arg	Arg	Glu	Ala	Glu	Asp	Leu	Gln	Val	Gly	Gln	Val	Glu	Leu	Gly	Gly	Gly	Pro	Gly	Ala	Gly	Ser	Leu	Gln	Pro	Leu	Ala	Leu	Glu	Gly	Ser	Leu	Gln	Lys	Arg
hIGF-I	.	.	.	.	.	.	.	.	.	.	.	.	.	Gly	Tyr	Gly	Ser	Ser	Ser	Arg	Arg	.	.	.	.	.	.	.	Ala	Pro	Gln	Thr	.		
hIGF-II	.	.	.	.	.	.	.	.	.	.	.	.	.	Ser	Arg	Val	Ser	Arg	Arg	Ser	Arg	.	.	.	.	.	.	.	.	.	.	.			

A DOMAINS

	1				5					10					15					20	
hPro-insulin	Gly	Ile	Val	Glu	Gln	Cys	Cys	Thr	Ser	Ile	Cys	Ser	Leu	Tyr	Gln	Leu	Glu	Asn	Tyr	Cys	Asn
hIGF-I	Gly	Ile	Val	Asp	Glu	Cys	Cys	Phe	Arg	Ser	Cys	Asp	Leu	Arg	Arg	Leu	Glu	Met	Tyr	Cys	Ala
hIGF-II	Gly	Ile	Val	Glu	Glu	Cys	Cys	Phe	Arg	Ser	Cys	Asp	Leu	Ala	Leu	Leu	Glu	Thr	Tyr	Cys	Ala

D DOMAINS

		25				
hPro-insulin	.	.	.	.	.	.
hIGF-I	Pro	Leu	Lys	Pro	Ala	Lys	Ser	Ala
hIGF-II	Thr	-	-	Pro	Ala	Lys	Ser	Glu

FIGURE 142–2. **Primary structure of somatomedin-C/insulin-like growth factor-I (IGF-I).** The residues enclosed in boxes in the A and B domains of IGF-I are identical to the amino acids in corresponding positions in human proinsulin. The C-peptides of the somatomedins, however, are much shorter than the C-peptide of proinsulin and exhibit no homology. The D domain is an 8-residue extension at the carboxy-terminus that does not exist in proinsulin. The B and A domains of IGF-II are about 70 per cent identical to similar regions in IGF-I. The C domain of IGF-II is composed of 8 amino acid residues that are not homologous with the 12 in IGF-I. The D domain of IGF-II is also 2 residues shorter than and not homologous with the D domain of IGF-I. The prohormones for IGF-I and IGF-II have additional E domains that consist of 35-residue and 89-residue extensions, respectively, at the COOH termini.[101] (From Underwood LE, Van Wyk JJ: Role of hormones in normal and aberrant growth. *In* Wilson J, Foster D (eds): Williams Textbook of Endocrinology (ed 8). Philadelphia, WB Saunders, 1992.)

subsequent expression depends upon whether the gene was inherited from the mother or father. IGF-II is produced only from the paternal allele, and the maternal IGF-II allele is inactivated. Conversely, the IGF-II receptor is derived only from the maternal allele, and the paternal IGF-II receptor allele is suppressed.[34, 35]

Evidence is mounting that the IGF-II gene is frequently overexpressed in Wilms' embryonic kidney tumors. Several mechanisms exist for this overexpression: In children with Beckwith-Wiedemann syndrome, for example, disomy of the paternal IGF-II locus on chromosome 11 leads to overexpression of IGF-II with resultant overgrowth, tendency toward hypoglycemia, and susceptibility for Wilms' tumors.[36] It has more recently been reported that genetic imprinting may be suppressed in some Wilms' tumors so that both the maternal and the paternal alleles are expressed.[37, 38]

REGULATION OF IGF GENE EXPRESSION. Although IGF genes are expressed in many tissues, most of the IGF's that circulate in blood arise in the liver. IGF's are not stored in any tissue, however, and concentrations of IGF in liver and other tissues are considerably lower than in blood. Tissues from hypophysectomized rats contain less than 30 per cent of the IGF-I extractable from normal tissues[39] (Table 142–2).

In the fetus, transcripts for IGF-II are more abundant than those for IGF-I, whereas IGF-I predominates postnatally.[40] By Northern analysis, mRNA's for IGF-I are mark-edly reduced in the livers of hypophysectomized rats and normalized within four hours after the administration of growth hormone.[41] In contrast, IGF-II transcripts are hardly discernible in most tissues of the postnatal rat, and no clear change follows hypophysectomy or growth hormone administration. A striking exception to this developmental pattern is in the brain, in which IGF-II mRNA's predominate over those for IGF-I.[42, 43] Similarly, IGF-II has proven to be identical to the "skeletal growth factor" isolated from decalcified femora of adult patients following hip replacement procedures.[44, 45]

Although GH controls production of IGF-I in liver and most other tissues, estrogen controls IGF-I production in the endometrium, a tissue in which growth hormone has no effect on IGF-I production.[46] Similarly, IGF-I production is stimulated by ACTH, angiotensin II, and FGF in the adrenal[47] and by gonadotropins in the gonads.[48] Expression of IGF genes is also regulated by other growth factors, nutritional state, and injury.

In situ hybridization studies in human fetal tissues revealed that expression of IGF genes is uniformly greater in connective tissue and other tissues of mesenchymal origin than in epithelial cells.[49] This distribution is quite different from the pattern of IGF distribution disclosed by immunocytochemistry, in which the peptides stain strongly in parenchymal cells.[50] This discrepancy suggests that IGF's are synthesized in cells lacking the capacity for storage in secretory granules and are then rapidly exported to the extra-

TABLE 142–2. EXTRACTABLE IGF I IN ORGANS OF MALE RATS

	UNITS/G WET WEIGHT*		
	Normal	Hypophysectomized	Per Cent Normal
Serum	28.7 ± 0.98	0.74 ± 0.12	2.6
Liver	1.91 ± 0.23	0.23 ± 0.08	12
Lung	2.04 ± 0.86	0.57 ± 0.13	27.9
Kidney	2.59 ± 0.80	0.77 ± 0.29	29.7
Heart	0.92 ± 0.33	0.48 ± 0.14	52.2
Muscle	0.42 ± 0.05	<0.08	<19.1
Testes	1.88 ± 0.42	0.52 ± 0.32	27.7
Prostate	1.06 (pooled)	0.40 (pooled)	37
Submaxillary gland	1.73 (pooled)	0.78 (pooled)	45
Brain	0.26 ± 0.09	0.28 ± 0.04	107.7

*Content of extractable Sm-C/IGF-I in organs from normal and hypophysectomized rats. Male rats were hypophysectomized when they weighed approximately 100 g and sacrificed when they were 48 to 50 days old. Normal controls were the same age at the time of sacrifice and weighed approximately 250 g. There were six or seven rats per group except for the pools as designated. Concentrations of IGF I, as determined by RIA in tissue extracts, are corrected for contamination by residual blood. In this assay 1 "unit" is equivalent to the IGF-I content in 1 ml of a pool of plasma from normal human adults. Note that the content of IGF-I in rat serum is much higher than in human serum. (From D'Ercole AJ, Stiles AD, Underwood LE: Tissue concentrations of somatomedin-C. Further evidence for multiple sites of synthesis and paracrine or autocrine mechanisms of action. Proc Natl Acad Sci USA 81:935–939, 1984.)

cellular fluid and taken up by receptors on neighboring cells in a typical paracrine manner.

INFLUENCE OF AGE. Many influences other than GH regulate somatomedin concentrations in serum. Although in normal adults the concentration of IGF-II is higher (about 650 ng/ml) than that of IGF-I (about 180 ng/ml), the concentrations of IGF-I are much more responsive to hormonal and nutritional changes than are the concentrations of IGF-II.[51] Both IGF-I and IGF-II are very low in fetal and cord blood and rise slowly during childhood so that the concentrations just before the onset of puberty are similar to mean values in adults. There is a dramatic increase of IGF-I during puberty so that at midpuberty the concentrations are between 2.5 and 3 times higher than mean adult values and often are as high as those observed in patients with active acromegaly (Fig. 142–3). Adults show an age-dependent downward trend.[52] The values of IGF-II are lower during the first year of life than in later childhood, but no rise occurs during adolescence.[51]

INFLUENCE OF GROWTH HORMONE STATUS. IGF-I concentrations are uniformly elevated in the plasma of patients with acromegaly,[53] and are low in children with GH deficiency. IGF-I levels rise following the administration of hGH. A low value of IGF-I in a growth-retarded child is not diagnostic of hypopituitarism, however, because malnutrition and hypothyroidism are also frequent causes of subnormal IGF-I levels.

EFFECT OF NUTRITIONAL STATUS. In severe protein-calorie malnutrition, a striking dissociation occurs between GH and IGF-I levels so that GH levels may rise to acromegalic levels or higher at a time when IGF-I levels are unmeasurable. There is great survival value in a mechanism that increases the direct lipolytic, protein-sparing actions of GH (anti-insulin effects) while at the same time preventing the squandering of protein in growth. Merimee et al.[54] showed that after only a three-day fast the IGF-I levels become unresponsive to hGH administration. Clemmons et al.[55] found that plasma IGF-I fell by approximately 75 per cent in moderately obese subjects during a 10-day fast and increased promptly during refeeding. This and subsequent studies showed an impressive correlation between the changes in IGF-I during fasting and changes in nitrogen

balance. For this reason, measurement of plasma IGF-I may find its most important use as an index of optimal nutritional repletion. Following the institution of parenteral alimentation in cachectic patients, the rise in serum concentrations of IGF-I correlated well with nitrogen retention and preceded elevations in serum transferrin, prealbumin, and other traditional markers of nutritional improvement.[56]

The Somatomedin Receptors and Binding Proteins

TYPE I AND TYPE II RECEPTORS. The overlapping biological effects of IGF's and insulin were initially attributed to the structural homologies between the peptides themselves,[57] but this interpretation proved overly simplistic when it was shown that the receptors for insulin and IGF-I are likewise homologous.[58] The Type I receptor has a subunit structure similar to the heterotetrameric structure of the insulin receptor, with two disulfide-linked extracellular α-subunits of about 130-kDa and two 90-kDa β subunits that contain the transmembrane and cytosolic domains (Fig. 142–4). Although the Type I receptor binds IGF-I preferentially, it also has high-affinity binding sites for IGF-II and, to a lesser extent, insulin. There is evidence, however, that IGF-I and IGF-II bind to different binding sites on the same receptor.[59] To complicate matters, chimeric receptors have been encountered in which an αβ subunit of the Type I IGF receptor is covalently linked with an αβ subunit of the insulin receptor.[60]

The β subunits of both the IGF Type I receptor and the insulin receptor contain a tyrosine kinase domain. Binding of ligand to the receptor swiftly activates the tyrosine kinase with resulting autophosphorylation of tyrosine residues on the receptor itself and tyrosine phosphorylation of other substrates. These phosphorylations are essential for the growth-promoting actions of the respective ligands.[61]

Type I IGF receptors are present in most tissues, where their abundance on target cells is regulated in part by hormones that act in concert with IGF's in eliciting biological responses. Thus PDGF stimulates an increase in IGF-I binding in BALB/c 3T3 cells,[62] gonadotropins increase

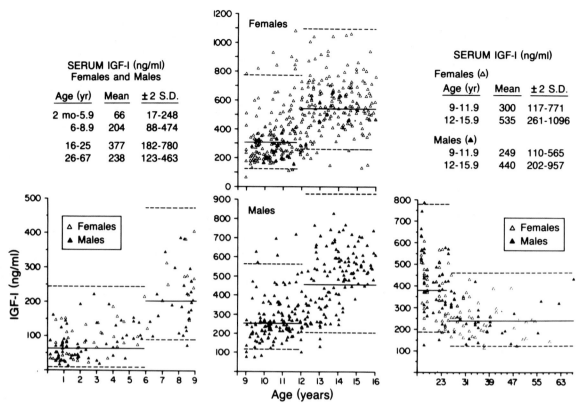

FIGURE 142–3. **Serum concentrations of IGF-I in 944 healthy volunteers, ages 2 months to 68 years.** Males are indicated by closed triangles and females by open triangles. Group means and 2 SD values are indicated in each panel, and numerical values are given above the left and right panels. IGF-I was determined after serum samples were subjected to acid-ethanol extraction for removal of IGF-binding proteins. (Data courtesy of Nichols Institute, San Juan Capistrano, CA.)

IGF-I binding in the testis and ovary,[63] and ACTH increases IGF-I binding in the adrenal.[47] Type I receptors are subject to down-regulation in the same manner as other peptide hormone receptors, and expression of the Type I receptor gene appears to vary inversely with serum levels of IGF-I.[64]

IGF-II preferentially binds to a Type II receptor that has no dissociable subunits and no tyrosine kinase activity and bears little resemblance to either the insulin or the Type I IGF receptor. The Type II receptor binds IGF-I with far lower affinity than does the Type I receptor, and it does not bind insulin at all.

Controversies over the biological role of the Type II receptor took a surprising turn with the discovery that the amino acid composition of the Type II receptor is identical to that of the cation-independent mannose-6-phosphate receptor.[65] The mannose-6-phosphate/IGF-II (M6P/IGF-II) receptor is a single-chain glycosylated transmembrane protein, the nonglycosylated form having a molecular weight of 270 kDa. This receptor has separate binding domains for IGF-II and mannose-6-phosphate.[65] At least one function of the M6P/IGF-II receptor is to act as an intracellular shuttle by transporting acid hydrolases and other mannosylated proteins to the lysosomal compartment, with the unoccupied receptor then being recycled.[66] Approximately 80 per cent of M6P/IGF-II receptors reside on intracellular membranes, although they are in equilibrium with those on the plasma membrane. The M6P binding site mediates a variety of growth factor actions such as processing the mannosylated precursor of TGF-β into its active form.[67] The M6P binding site also serves as the receptor for proli-

ferin, a prolactin-like molecule that is produced in mouse fibroblasts (BALB/c 3T3 cells) in response to mitogenic signals.[68]

Although most of the biological effects of IGF-II are believed to be mediated through the Type I or insulin receptors, Nishimoto et al.[69, 70] have found that a 14-amino-acid sequence in the cytoplasmic portion of the IGF-II receptor interacts with the specific membrane-bound GTP-binding protein (G_{i-2}) that mediates the influx of extracellular calcium into the cell. This effect is triggered by interaction of IGF-II with the Type II IGF receptor and cannot be duplicated by substances that interact with the M6P binding site.

THE SOMATOMEDIN-BINDING PROTEINS. A distinctive feature of the somatomedins is that they are complexed to binding proteins (BP's) both in serum and in other extracellular fluids. Synthesis of one or more IGFBP's parallels the synthesis of IGF's in most if not all tissues in which IGF's are made. Because virtually all of the somatomedins in blood are complexed to binding proteins, concentrations of somatomedin in serum are higher and more stable than those of most peptide hormones. Because of their long half-life in blood and relative immunity from short-term influences, the somatomedin status of an individual can usually be established by measuring the concentration in a single blood specimen.

In humans, six distinct IGFBP's (IGFBP-1 to IGFBP-6) have been chemically characterized and localized to specific genes.[71, 72] Human IGFBP's contain between 216 amino acid residues (BP-6) and 289 residues (BP-2) and

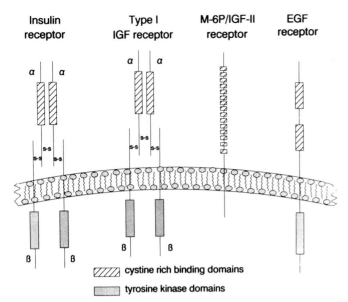

Insulin receptor   Type I IGF receptor   M-6P/IGF-II receptor   EGF receptor

α   α   α   α

β   β   β   β

///// cystine rich binding domains

▓▓ tyrosine kinase domains

FIGURE 142–4. **Structural organization of receptors for insulin, insulin-like growth factors (IGF), and epidermal growth factor.** The insulin receptor and Type 1 IGF receptor are heterotetramers with striking structural similarities and cross-reactivities, as summarized in Table 142–6. The α subunits, which constitute the extracellular binding domains, are rich in tertiary structure owing to their high cysteine content. The β subunits contain an extracellular domain, a transmembrane domain, and a cytosolic domain with intrinsic tyrosine kinase activity. The mannose-6-phosphate/IGF-II receptor contains separate binding regions for IGF-II and proteins that are complexed with mannose-6-phosphate. The circles represent extracellular regions with repeating sequences. The IGF-II/mannose-6-phosphate receptor has 15 such cysteine-rich repeating units. Boxes with diagonal lines show tyrosine kinase domains. The mannose-6-phosphate/IGF-II receptor has no tyrosine kinase activity. The EGF receptor is a single-chain protein with two cysteine-rich binding domains and a cytoplasmic tyrosine kinase domain. (From Underwood LE, Van Wyk JJ: Role of hormones in normal and aberrant growth. *In* Wilson J, Foster D (eds): Williams Textbook of Endocrinology (ed 8). Philadelphia, WB Saunders, 1992.)

exhibit considerable structural similarities in that each possesses 18 cysteine residues (16 in BP-6) that reside in two clusters at each end of their respective molecules. The amino acid sequences in the area of high cysteine density are responsible for binding activity.[72] IGFBP's-3, 4, 5, and 6 exhibit a variable degree of glycosylation, whereas IGFBP's-1 and 2 are not glycosylated. The carboxy-termini of IGFBP's-1 and 2 contain arg-gly-asp sequences that may bind to integrin receptors on cell surfaces.

The production of the different BP's follows a different pattern in different tissues and under different physiological circumstances, thus adding a highly complex degree of specificity to the actions of the IGF's. The BP's modify IGF actions in a variety of ways: They transport IGF's across vessel walls and capillary membranes, they regulate the concentration of IGF's in the vicinities of specific tissues and cell types, they control IGF interaction with cell surface receptors, and they may either directly stimulate or inhibit the biological activity of IGF's by mechanisms that are poorly understood.[73, 74] Most studies of the actions of IGFBP's have suggested that they inhibit binding of IGF's to target cells and thereby attenuate IGF actions.[75] In other studies, however, the addition of purified IGFBP-1 or IGFBP-3 to cell cultures has resulted in increased IGF binding and action.[76] Jones et al.[77] have demonstrated that whether IGFBP-1 inhibits or enhances IGF's mitogenic ac-

tion in fibroblasts depends on its degree of phosphorylation and in turn its binding affinity for IGF-I.

Modification of the somatomedin-binding protein complexes in blood by serum endoproteases and subsequent exposure to heparin-like substances have been shown to liberate free somatomedins from their BP's.[78, 79] Thus, the increased concentrations of proteolytic enzymes and heparin-like substances that occur in the vicinity of wounds may serve to dissociate free ligands from their carrier proteins and facilitate their entry into extravascular spaces.

IGFBP-1 is a 25,272-Da protein that was initially purified from amniotic fluid.[75] In vivo, its major sites of production are the liver, kidney, and reproductive tissues such as prostate, uterus, and decidua. IGFBP-1 is not GH-dependent, and its serum concentrations are increased by conditions in which insulin secretion or insulin sensitivity is diminished. These include fasting, diabetes, insulin resistance, pregnancy, and hypopituitarism. Values are reduced by hyperinsulinism, whether caused by feeding, glucose infusion, GH, or glucocorticoids. Hepatic IGFBP-1 mRNA levels rise promptly after partial hepatectomy and under this circumstance may function as one of the immediate early genes involved in cellular proliferation.

IGFBP-2 was initially purified from Buffalo rat liver cell conditioned media. Its expression is particularly high in tissues of the rat fetus and declines rapidly after birth.[80] Serum IGFBP-2 concentrations are increased by hypophysectomy and decreased by GH and glucocorticoid administration. IGFBP-2 is abundant in the CNS and is the principal BP in human CSF. Like IGFBP-1, IGFBP-2 seems to be suppressed by insulin, because levels in diabetic liver are increased and suppressed by insulin injections.[81]

The concentrations of IGFBP's-1 and 2 are higher in lymph than in serum, and it has been suggested that these proteins play a role in transporting IGF's out of the vascular space. Supporting this is the observation that IGFBP-1 is able to cross the intact vascular endothelium.[82]

IGFBP-3: Over 70 per cent of IGF's in serum circulate as part of a 150-kDa trimeric complex in which either IGF-I or IGF-II is linked to two other subunits, one of which is IGFBP-3. IGFBP-3 is an acid stable protein of 29,480 Da (or approximately 54,000 Da when fully glycosylated). The third subunit of this complex is acid labile with a molecular weight of 88,000.[83] The tethering of IGF's to the 150-kDa complex serves to prevent their egress from the intravascular compartment.

IGFBP-3 levels in serum (and thus total IGF-I levels as well) are highly dependent on GH and nutritional status. These levels are reduced in states of GH deficiency, restored by GH injections, and elevated in acromegaly and adolescence. IGFBP-3 is also induced by the infusion of IGF-I,[84] suggesting that IGF-I mediates the effect of GH on the induction of IGFBP-3. However, the administration of IGF-I to patients with GH insensitivity fails to raise IGFBP-3 levels. IGFBP-3 production is also stimulated in vitro by various growth factors, whereas its production is inhibited by agents that stimulate cAMP. The concentrations of IGFBP-3 are severely reduced when nutrients are restricted and are restored by feeding.[85] A radioimmunoassay for IGFBP-3 has proved to be a useful supplement to the RIA for IGF-I itself in diagnosing GH deficiency.[86]

IGFBP-4 was originally isolated from media conditioned by a human osteosarcoma cell line[87] and later from plasma of humans and rats. It binds both IGF-I and IGF-II with equally high affinity. Unlike IGFBP-3, IGFBP-4 is stimulated by cAMP and by agents that elevate intracellular cAMP levels. IGFBP-4 has been reported to block the effects of exogenous IGF-I when added to cultured cells.

Hepatic tissue contains the greatest abundance of IGFBP-4 mRNA and is probably the source of blood-borne IGFBP-4. However, the IGFBP-4 gene is expressed in many other organs, ranging from the brain to the ovaries. Brar and Chernausek[88] have suggested that IGFBP-4 may modulate the effect of IGF's in the CNS because the IGFBP-4 gene is expressed in areas contiguous with regions that express IGF-I or the Type I receptor.

IGFBP-5 was initially isolated from rat serum and its gene cloned from libraries of rat ovary or human placenta. It has been identified in most tissues, with particular preponderance in kidney, bone, and endocrine tissues. IGFBP-5 is the only IGF-binding protein identified in the rat thyroid FRTL-5 cell line, where the expression of its gene is triggered by interaction of IGF-I with the Type I IGF receptor.[89] IGFBP-5 is more strongly bound to extracellular matrix than the other IGFBP's and thus may serve as a reservoir of IGF's. Furthermore, it has been shown that when associated with extracellular matrix, IGFBP-5 potentiates the mitogenic effect of IGF-I.[90]

IGFBP-6 was initially identified in human CSF. The N-terminal amino acid sequence contains fewer cysteine residues than the other IGFBP's, and IGFBP-6 has a 10-fold higher affinity for IGF-II than for IGF-I. IGFBP-6 has been identified by Northern analysis in virtually all human and rat tissues, in osteosarcomas, and in other transformed cell lines. Blood levels are low in acromegaly, suggesting that its regulation is more like that of IGFBP-1 and IGFBP-2 than IGFBP-3.

Actions of the Somatomedins

Although somatomedins were first described as mediators of the growth-promoting effect of GH and as insulin-like substances in fat and muscle, it is now apparent that they play an essential role in the proliferation and cytodifferentiation of most, if not all, eukaryotic cells. The multitude and diversity of biological systems that are influenced by the somatomedins have made it difficult to define any basic action of the somatomedins that is common to all of their effects.

ROLE IN ACTIONS OF GROWTH HORMONE. As diagrammed in Figure 142–5, the direct actions of GH are those on lipid and fat metabolism and are synergistic with cortisol and opposite to the actions of insulin and the somatomedins. The anabolic and growth-promoting effects of GH are mediated by IGF-I and include cell proliferation and protein synthesis in both skeletal and nonskeletal tissue. In contrast to the direct actions of GH, these growth-promoting actions are insulin-like and opposed by cortisol.

IGF-I participates in a classic negative feedback loop in the regulation of GH secretion. At least two mechanisms appear to account for this effect: IGF-I stimulates the production of somatostatin in hypothalamic remnants,[91] and directly inhibits expression of the GH gene in the pituitary in response to GRH.[92]

Opposing views of the relative roles of GH and somatomedins on skeletal growth have become reconciled with the recognition that both immunoreactive IGF-I and mRNA's for IGF-I increase locally in the epiphysial growth plate in response to GH administration.[93] IGF-I mimics the action of GH on skeletal growth when it is administered parenterally to hypophysectomized rats[94, 95] or to children with genetic forms of resistance to hGH.[96]

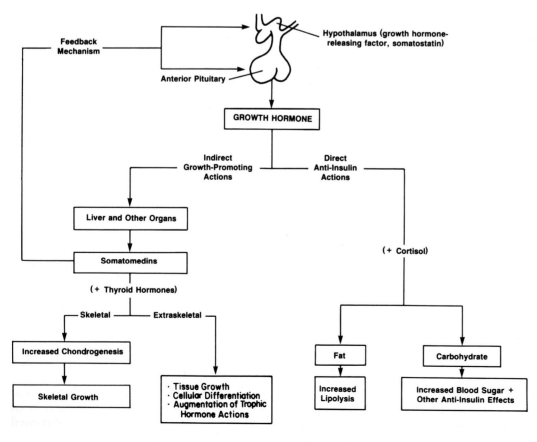

FIGURE 142–5. **The somatomedin hypothesis of growth hormone (GH) action.** The direct actions of GH include diabetogenic and lipolytic actions and stimulatory action on several hepatic enzymes. These direct actions are antagonistic to insulin and often synergistic with cortisol. The anabolic and growth-promoting actions of GH are mediated through the somatomedins. IGF-I participates in the negative feedback on GH secretion at the hypothalamic level by stimulating somatostatin production, and at the pituitary level by directly blocking the effect of GH-releasing hormone on the expression of the GH gene. (From Underwood LE, Van Wyk JJ: Role of hormones in normal and aberrant growth. *In* Wilson J, Foster D (eds): Williams Textbook of Endocrinology (ed 8). Philadelphia, WB Saunders, 1992.)

ROLE IN CELL PROLIFERATION. Very few cell types proliferate under serum-free conditions unless the medium contains either nanogram concentrations of a somatomedin or, more frequently, microgram concentrations of insulin. At these unphysiological concentrations, insulin can serve as a surrogate somatomedin by cross-reacting with the Type I receptor.[97] Some cell types that do not appear to require somatomedins for growth, such as human fibroblasts, have been found to produce their own somatomedin-like substances, thus obviating the requirement for exogenous somatomedins. In such cells, DNA synthesis is often inhibited by a monoclonal antibody to IGF-I.[6, 7]

The pivotal role of IGF-I in cell proliferation and its interaction with other growth factors has been studied most extensively in the mouse BALB/c 3T3 fibroblast cell line. Density-arrested cultures of these cells re-enter the cell cycle if they are transiently exposed to PDGF followed by incubation in either platelet-poor plasma or in a combination of IGF-I and EGF.[98, 99] IGF-I is an essential component of the mitogenic activity of normal plasma because platelet-poor plasma from normal donors loses its mitogenicity in the presence of a neutralizing monoclonal antibody raised against IGF-I.[100] Based on studies in BALB/c 3T3 cells transfected with plasmids constitutively expressing the IGF-I Type I receptor, Pietrzkowski and his colleagues[101] concluded that the role of EGF is to enhance the production of both IGF-I and IGF-I receptors, thus participating in an IGF-I:IGF-I receptor autocrine loop. Transfection of cells so that both IGF-I and the IGF-I receptor were constitutively expressed abrogated all requirements for exogenous growth factors.[102]

In comparison with other peptide growth factors, the biological effects of IGF-I or IGF-II, when added by themselves in vitro to cell or organ cultures, are often quite weak and cannot always be demonstrated except in the presence of other hormones. In a thyroid cell line, for example, the effect of IGF-I on total DNA synthesis is increased over 30-fold in the presence of TSH. TSH also increases the sensitivity of the cells to IGF-I as documented by a 30-fold decrease in the EC_{50} of IGF-I in the presence of TSH or by any agent that increases intracellular cAMP levels.[103] In this example, the increase of intracellular cAMP induced by TSH greatly potentiates the tyrosine phosphorylation mediated through the Type I IGF receptor[104] (Fig. 142–6).

ROLE IN DIFFERENTIATED CELL FUNCTIONS. The somatomedins often have as profound an effect on highly differentiated cell functions as they do on cell proliferation. In cultured myoblasts, for example, Ewton and Florini[105] found that somatomedins stimulate both the proliferation of cultured myoblasts and their differentiation into myotubes. The two effects appear not to be linked because myotube formation can still occur when DNA synthesis is blocked by cytosine arabinoside.[106] In this example IGF's appear to act as a promoter for myogenin, a more proximal effector in muscle differentiation.[107, 108]

In rat granulosa cells IGF-I causes up to a 10-fold increase in the effects of FSH on such cyclic nucleotide–mediated events as synthesis of progesterone and induction of aromatase activity.[109] In rat theca-interstitial cells and in Leydig cells, IGF-I potentiates in a similar manner the action of LH on the biosynthesis of androgen. These actions appear, at least in part, to result from the ability of IGF's to potentiate the formation of cAMP in response to

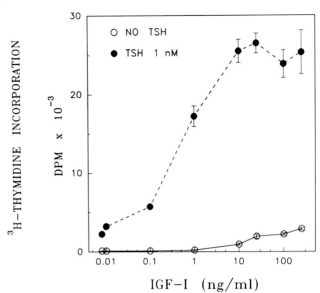

FIGURE 142–6. The effect of IGF-I and TSH on rat thyroid (FRTL-5) cells. FRTL-5 cells (5×10^{-4} cells/ml) were incubated for 48 hours with increasing concentrations of IGF-I in the presence or absence of bovine TSH (1 nM). [^{3}H]-Thymidine (1 μCi) was added to each well four hours before the experiment was terminated. TSH potentiated the mitogenic effects of IGF-I both by increasing the amount of [^{3}H]-thymidine incorporated into the cells (an effect that might be explained by recruitment of additional quiescent cells into the cell cycle) and by sensitizing the cells to the mitogenic effects of IGF-I, as evidenced by a significant reduction of the EC_{50} to IGF-I. (From Takahashi SI, Conti M, Van Wyk JJ: Thyrotropin potentiation of insulin-like growth factor-I dependent deoxyribonucleic acid synthesis in FRTL-5 cells: Mediation by an autocrine amplification factor(s). Endocrinology 126:736–745, © 1990 by the Endocrine Society.)

stimulation by gonadotropic hormones. In the absence of gonadotropin, IGF has little or no effect on these enzymatic activities.

IN VIVO EFFECTS. IGF-I produces a marked nitrogen-sparing effect when given in vivo and causes a lowering of blood glucose. Administration of IGF-I also causes a prompt reduction in serum insulin and C-peptide concentrations, perhaps by a direct effect on the pancreatic cells.[110] The hypoglycemic effect of IGF-I has suggested its possible use in the treatment of insulin-resistant diabetes mellitus. IGF's may be particularly useful in this circumstance because they are not lipogenic.[111]

IGF-I and hGH have opposite effects on carbohydrate metabolism. GH causes insulin resistance and increases insulin secretion, whereas IGF-I causes hypoglycemia and inhibition of insulin secretion. This has provided the rationale for administering GH and IGF-I concurrently in the hope that these opposing effects would cancel each other out. In human volunteers given a hypocaloric diet, the simultaneous administration of IGF-I plus hGH caused a markedly positive nitrogen balance, whereas under the same experimental circumstances GH and IGF-I given individually in the same dosages were much less efficacious.[112]

The most clear-cut indication for the therapeutic use of IGF-I is in children with genetic forms of GH resistance, most commonly due to absence or mutations of the GH receptor. In such children IGF-I causes virtually all of the metabolic effects caused by GH[110] and has permitted sustained linear growth.[96] In one such patient, continuous treatment for over two years has resulted in sustained "catch-up" growth with no recognized side effects. Adults treated with higher doses have experienced fluid retention and painful enlargement of the parotid glands.

Epidermal Growth Factor/Transforming Growth Factor-α Family

History and Nomenclature

EPIDERMAL GROWTH FACTOR (EGF)/UROGASTRONE (hEGF). EGF is a potent mitogen for cells of mesodermal and ectodermal origin. In the process of purifying a nerve growth–promoting activity from mouse submaxillary glands, Cohen[113] observed that injections of certain purified fractions accelerated eyelid opening and incisor tooth eruption when injected into newborn mice. In a series of now classic studies, Cohen and his colleagues then proceeded to isolate and characterize mouse EGF, a 53-amino acid peptide, delineate its interaction with receptors, and describe many of its biological effects.[114-116] For these contributions Cohen was awarded the Nobel Prize in 1987. EGF is the prototype of a large and ever-expanding superfamily of ligands that signal through a family of related receptors.

Gregory[117] isolated the human homologue of mouse EGF from human urine on the basis of its ability to inhibit acid release from gastric mucosa. Although initially named urogastrone, this peptide is now designated hEGF because it was shown to have all of the biological properties of mouse EGF and to be identical in 37 of its 53 amino acid residues. The mouse and human peptides signal through the same receptors but differ considerably in their immunological cross-reactivities.[117]

TRANSFORMING GROWTH FACTOR-α (TGF-α). Malignant transformation in cultured cells is characterized by distinctive morphological changes, loss of contact inhibition at confluence,[118] and loss of anchorage dependance, which results in the ability to grow in soft agar.[119, 120] Because transformed cells in culture have a much lower requirement than normal cells for serum or other exogenous growth factors,[121] Todaro and DeLarco[122] postulated that transformed cells become independent of exogenous stimulation by producing their own growth factors. The term *transforming growth factor* was used to describe tumor-derived polypeptides capable of conferring the transformed phenotype on normal cells. Those same authors identified a transforming activity, sarcoma growth factor (SGF), in the culture medium of murine sarcoma virus–transformed rat kidney (NRK) cells.[123]

Early studies had shown that transformation of NRK cells by a variety of tumor viruses leads to almost complete down-regulation of EGF receptors[124] and that there is a good correlation between the loss of EGF receptors in the transformed cells and the presence of SGF activity in the medium. It was subsequently shown by Roberts et al.[125] that crude preparations of SGF could be purified into two components. Neither component had strong ability to transform alone, but one had EGF-like characteristics. The EGF-like component was subsequently designated TGF-α and the other factor TGF-β. Purification and cloning of human TGF-α showed it to consist of 50 amino acids with 33 per cent amino acid sequence homology with mouse EGF and

44 per cent homology with human EGF and to signal through the EGF receptor (EGFR).[126-128]

AMPHIREGULIN (AR). This 84-amino-acid EGF-like peptide was isolated from the medium of phorbol ester–treated breast carcinoma cells.[129] It differs from EGF by the presence of a hydrophilic 43-amino acid extension at its N-terminus that may help it target to the nucleus.[130] It derives its name from opposing biological actions in different cell types: Amphiregulin inhibits the growth of several breast carcinoma lines and stimulates the proliferation of normal fibroblasts and keratinocytes. AR co-purifies with a 123-amino acid AR-associated protein,[131] and its stimulatory effects on keratinocytes are inhibited by heparin.[132] AR is identical to the keratinocyte-derived autocrine factor (KAF)[133] and to the colorectum cell–derived growth factor (CRDGF)[134] and is probably the human homologue of the rat schwannoma-derived growth factor.[135] The growth-inhibitory peptide TGF-β (see below) inhibits the expression of AR mRNA in A549 human lung adenocarcinomas.[136]

HEPARIN-BINDING EGF (HB-EGF). This substance was isolated from medium conditioned by a phorbol-stimulated human lymphoma cell line.[137] It consists of 208 amino acids and resembles amphiregulin with the presence of a hydrophilic extension. HB-EGF appears to act through the EGFR, although it is a more potent mitogen for smooth muscle cells than is EGF or TGF-α.

CRIPTO. The gene for this peptide was cloned from human and mouse teratocarcinoma cells and encodes a 188-amino acid peptide that lacks the initial cysteine-determined loop that is characteristic of the EGF family consensus sequence.[138] A second copy of the cripto gene with numerous substitutions in the coding region has been detected. The signal-transducing receptor(s) for cripto has not been determined.

BETACELLULIN. The newest member of the EGF family was isolated in the conditioned medium of pancreatic β cell carcinomas from mice carrying a hybrid oncogene composed of the insulin gene regulatory region coupled to SV40 T antigen.[139] Mature betacellulin, which is composed of 80 amino acids containing the EGF family motif, is derived from a larger precursor and is 50 per cent homologous to TGF-α. Consistent with these findings, betacellulin competes at reduced affinity with EGF for binding to the EGFR and stimulates tyrosine phosphorylation. A physiological role remains to be determined.

POX VIRUS GROWTH FACTORS. The initial cloning of the EGF gene revealed similarity to sequences in vaccinia and several related poxviruses such as molluscum contagiosum.[140] Vaccinia-infected cells secrete a 77-amino acid peptide, vaccinia virus growth factor (VGF), which is 37 per cent homologous with EGF, 30 per cent with TGF-α, and is capable of stimulating proliferation of fibroblasts by binding to the EGFR. In some cell lines, VGF binds avidly to the EGFR and blocks EGF-stimulated mitogenesis. It is unclear to what extent this factor is important in viral proliferation or disease states.

EGF Genes, Precursors, and Processing

All members of the EGF family of mitogens share two structural features. All contain a highly conserved 36- to 40-amino acid motif, containing six cysteines that link internally to produce three peptide loops[141] (Fig. 142–7). In

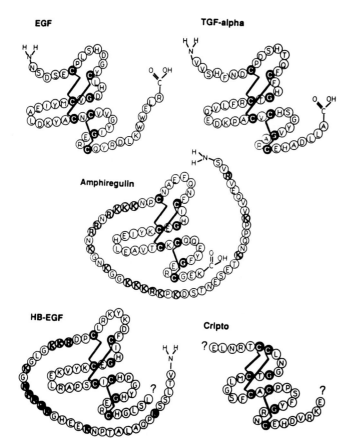

FIGURE 142–7. Members of the EGF superfamily. Cystine bridges are indicated by solid black lines. Conserved amino acids are shown in black, and positively charged residues in the N-terminal extensions of HB-EGF and amphiregulin are indicated by shaded circles. All members of the EGF family of mitogens contain a highly conserved 36- to 40-amino-acid motif, containing six cysteines that link internally to produce three peptide loops.[141] In addition, all members of the family are synthesized embedded within larger precursor proteins. All three forms of TGF-α are capable of activating EGF/TGF-α receptors. (From Prigent SA, Lemoine NR: The type 1 (EGFR-related) family of growth factor receptors and their ligands. Prog Growth Factor Res 4:1–24, 1992.)

addition, all members of the family are synthesized embedded within larger precursor proteins. EGF family precursors resemble receptors in that they contain midmolecule hydrophobic regions that anchor them in membranes. Soluble, "mature" forms of the growth factors result from proteolytic cleavage of the precursors, although the extent of processing may be cell- and tissue-specific, allowing for a possible biological role of membrane-anchored precursors (see the discussion of juxtacrine modalities of growth factor action above).

The 4.9-kb mRNA for hEGF is derived from a 110-kb gene located on chromosome 4q and encodes a 1217-amino acid precursor.[141] Contained within the EGF precursor are eight additional sequences with EGF homology. The EGF precursor appears to be differentially processed in various tissues, and almost certainly has wider functions than as a source of mature EGF. The distal tubule of the mouse kidney, for example, contains almost as much pre-pro-EGF as the male submaxillary gland, although it is not further processed to EGF, suggesting that it may serve a juxtacrine role in cell-cell interaction.[142] Indeed, an extensive compilation of nonmitogenic proteins that contain EGF-like repeats includes blood clotting factors and other

serine proteases, immunomodulators, extracellular matrix proteins, cell adhesion molecules, receptors for LDL and other substances, and molecules important in development.[141] It has been proposed that EGF-like molecules evolved from a primitive transmembrane protein originally involved in cellular communication.[143] Curiously, the transmembrane precursor for HB-EGF appears to function as the receptor by which diphtheria toxin enters cells.[144]

The mechanisms that regulate processing of EGF family precursors are not well understood. Mature TGF-α is flanked within its glycosylated precursor on both its N- and C-termini by sequences of alanine, valine, and leucine that are substrates for elastase-like enzymes (Fig. 142–8). Processing of TGF-α precursor begins only after the molecule reaches the cell surface, and then the N-terminal fragment of the precursor is rapidly cleaved, leaving the mature peptide anchored to the membrane through its C-terminus.[12] The cleavage of the membrane-anchored precursor to yield soluble TGF-α in vitro is regulated by phorbol ester tumor promoters (PMA's) and by factors in serum that act through protein kinase C- and Ca-dependent mechanisms.[12] A membrane-associated serine protease has been implicated in the PMA-stimulated cleavage of the extracellular domain,[145] and the carboxy-terminal valine of the intracytoplasmic tail of the TGF-α precursor is critical for this process. This suggests that intracytoplasmic determinants regulate processing of the ectodomain.

Mutation of the TGF-α precursor to an uncleavable form results in preservation of TGF-α in its membrane-anchored form, which can bind to the EGFR on adjacent cells to generate a mitogenic signal[146] and promote adhesion of adjacent cells.[147] Thus, major questions remain regarding the functions of TGF-α in its various forms: whether processing to the mature peptide is required to change a membrane-anchored (juxtacrine) mitogen to a soluble (auto-

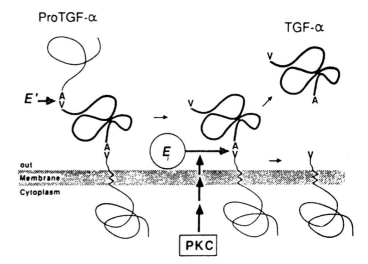

FIGURE 142–8. The two-step cleavage sequence that liberates mature transforming growth factor (TGF)-α from the TGF-α precursor. From left to right are depicted the TGF-α precursor protein (ProTGF-α) anchored in the cell membrane; rapid enzymatic cleavage at the N-terminal end of TGF-α; cleavage of the C-terminal end of mature TGF-α under the influence of protein kinase C-dependent and independent mechanisms to yield soluble TGF-α; E′, enzymatic cleavage event at the N-terminus of TGF-α; E, enzymatic cleavage event at the C-terminus of TGF-α; PKC, protein kinase C; A, alanine; V, valine. (From Pandiella A, Massagué J: Cleavage of the membrane precursor for transforming growth factor α is a regulated process. Proc Natl Acad Sci USA 88:1726–1730, 1991.)

crine/paracrine) one, and whether the two forms have altogether different functions.

EGF Receptors and Signaling

EGF RECEPTOR (EGFR, HER-1). The EGFR was initially isolated from the A431 human squamous carcinoma line and is located on chromosome 7p.[148] It is a single-chain transmembrane glycoprotein of 170 kDa (see Fig. 142–4). Similar to other peptide growth factor receptors, EGF binding leads to receptor aggregation and enhanced receptor autophosphorylation on at least three tyrosine residues at the cytoplasmic C terminus.[149]

Signal transduction continues when the phosphorylated EGFR tyrosine kinase phosphorylates a number of intracellular substrates, including phospholipase C-γ (PLC-γ), MAP kinase, the GTPase-activating protein of the *ras* proto-oncogene (GAP), and lipocortin I (also called calpactin II).[150–152] Many of these proteins interact with the activated EGFR through amino acid sequences that specifically recognize phosphotyrosines.[153] These phosphotyrosine recognition sequences, which were originally identified in the *src* oncogene, are known as SH, or *src* homology, domains.[154] Binding of PLC-γ to the phosphorylated EGFR tethers the enzyme to the plasma membrane and increases its enzymatic activity.

PLC-γ has received considerable attention as a critical link in the EGFR signaling pathway because of its role in the generation of two subsequent intracellular signals. It hydrolyzes phosphatidylinositides to form inositol 1,4,5-triphosphate (IP$_3$) and diacylglycerol (DAG). IP$_3$ releases calcium from intracellular storage compartments, while DAG activates protein kinase C (see Ch. 4). Activation of the EGFR leads to the induction of a number of growth-regulatory genes, many of which are induced rapidly (within minutes) and do not require new protein synthesis, so-called *immediate early* genes. Among these genes are "zinc finger" DNA-binding proteins, β-actin, calcium-binding proteins, and the nuclear proteins c-*jun*, c-*fos*, and c-*myc*.[141] In addition, EGFR is linked to the rapid induction of other genes that appear to have no relationship to mitosis, such as that for prolactin in pituitary tumor cell lines[155] and tyrosine hydroxylase in pheochromocytomas.[156]

Termination of the EGFR signal appears to require endocytic internalization of the ligand-receptor complex and degradation in lysosomes. This results in loss of EGFR from the cell surface, or down-regulation. Differential processing of the internalized EGFR complex may explain why TGF-α appears to be more potent than EGF in some functional assays but not in others.[157] Although both EGF and TGF-α share the EGFR for signal transduction, and both bind with comparable affinity, TGF-α dissociates from the internalized receptor-ligand complex at a higher pH and the receptor is returned to the cell surface largely intact.[157] The EGF-EGFR complex, in contrast, remains stable and is targeted to lysosomes for degradation. As a consequence, TGF-α does not induce EGFR down-regulation at the cell surface to the same extent as EGF, and the "refractory period," or time to recovery of baseline EGFR at the cell surface, is half as long in TGF-α as in EGF-stimulated cells. The EGFR is also inactivated by phosphorylation of its threonine residues, which prevents tyrosine autophosphorylation.[158]

c-*erb*B-2 PROTO-ONCOGENE. The cytosolic portion of the human EGFR has an amino acid structure that is similar to the protein encoded by the v-*erb*B oncogene of avian erythroblastosis virus, and it appears that the virus has transduced the signaling domain of the chicken EGFR.[159] The human cellular counterpart to this oncogene, c-*erb*B-2, which is also known as HER-2, encodes a 185-kDa protein that appears to be involved in signal transduction. Fusion proteins that link the ligand-binding region of EGFR to the cytoplasmic sequence of HER-2/c-*erb*B-2 lead to mitosis and other consequences of EGFR activation when activated by EGF.[160]

Binding of EGF to the EGFR can result in heterodimerization of the EGFR with c-*erb*B-2 and cross-phosphorylation.[161] EGFR/c-*erb*B-2 interactions are likely to be important in normal physiology because the latter molecule is expressed in a variety of normal tissues.[162, 163] Overexpression of the c-*erb*B-2 gene is seen in a sizable fraction of breast, stomach, pancreatic, bladder, ovarian, and lung cancers. A mutation of c-*erb*B-2 known as *neu*, which enhances receptor dimerization to an active state, is seen in CNS tumors.[164]

A single gene has recently been described that encodes multiple ligands for c-*erb*B-2 via alternative splicing. Several of these peptides are *glial cell growth factors* (GGF's),[165] and others, called *ARIA*, or *acetylcholine receptor–inducing activity*, regulate the expression of the acetycholine receptor during muscle differentiation.[166] This gene is expressed in motor neurons in the early stages of embryonic neural development and suggests that natural ligands of c-*erb*B-2 may, among other functions, mediate the trophic effects of neurons on muscle development. In addition, this remarkable gene codes for *heregulins*, EGF consensus–containing peptides that were originally isolated from breast carcinoma cells.[167] Heregulin-α binds to c-*erb*B-2 with high affinity, but not to the EGFR, and its mRNA is found in a number of normal tissues as well as tumors.

c-*erb*B-3 PROTO-ONCOGENE. A tyrosine kinase of 160 kDa that is related to c-*erb*B-2 was identified in normal human genomic DNA.[168] c-*erb*B-3 shares high homology with EGFR and c-*erb*B-2 in its tyrosine kinase domain and appears to be localized to cells of epithelial or neuroectodermal origin.[169] Natural ligands are not known.

Biological Actions and Regulation

EGF/UROGASTRONE. Because of EGF's historical priority and relatively easy purification, the bulk of information regarding biological activity of the EGF superfamily comes from studies on EGF itself. Many of the biological effects of EGF stem from its ability to stimulate proliferation in the basal cell layers of ectodermally derived epithelia. EGF is present in amniotic fluid,[170] and there is considerable evidence that it or TGF-α is an important regulator of fetal development. Although the two substances had previously been thought to have roughly comparable activities, it is clear that EGF and TGF-α are differentially expressed in different tissues and during ontogeny and that the two peptides can have qualitatively and quantitatively different actions (see EGF Receptors and Signaling above).

When administered in utero to fetal lambs, EGF induces maturation of airway epithelium and may protect against hyaline membrane disease.[171, 172] When administered to fetal lambs between 110 and 125 days of gestation, EGF also causes an increase in skin wrinkling and shedding of wool fibers; indeed, the administration of EGF is used as an alternative to the shearing of sheep.

EGF has potent effects on a variety of other developmental and proliferative processes. In the rat it appears to be essential for closure of the palate,[173] and EGF antisense oligonucleotides block odontogenesis in vitro.[174] Significant quantities of EGF are present in human breast milk, and its concentration in human colostrum exceeds 300 ng/ml. It has been postulated that colostral EGF is critical to the maturation of the brush border and other gut functions in neonatal life.[175] EGF has trophic effects on the growth of intestinal epithelium in rats maintained on total parenteral nutrition.[176] Consonant with its role as a "urogastrone," EGF inhibits gastric acid secretion and protects the gastric mucosa from cysteamine-induced damage.[177]

EGF concentrations in salivary glands are highly androgen dependent: male submaxillary glands contain 15-fold more EGF than those from females.[178] The EGF content of salivary glands from females and castrate males is increased following the administration of androgens. Despite these pronounced sex-related differences, serum concentrations of EGF are comparable in male and female mice. In the skin, mEGF concentrations are regulated by thyroid hormones, especially in the first five days of life.[179] Indeed, the accelerating effect of thyroid hormone administration on eyelid opening and tooth eruption in the neonatal mouse is probably mediated through EGF.

TGF-α. Exogenous TGF-α mimics the effects of EGF in most systems. Some unique functions of TGF-α are beginning to evolve: Its mRNA is found in preimplantation mouse embryos[180] and in a number of fetal tissues before that for EGF,[181] leading to the suggestion that TGF-α is the fetal ligand for the EGFR. Protein levels of TGF-α in different fetal tissues show different developmental patterns.[182] TGF-α mRNA has been localized to the anterior pituitary (recall the role of EGF in stimulating prolactin secretion)[183] and in numerous epithelial tissues.[184] It has been implicated in wound healing,[185] angiogenesis,[186] and bone remodeling.[187] TGF-α is expressed in keratinocytes and is overexpressed in psoriatic skin.[188] Locally produced TGF-α appears to be a cytoprotective agent in the stomach: taurocholate injury to the gastric mucosa results in increased TGF-α mRNA and protein and protein production, with no detectable increase in EGF mRNA.[189] Local overexpression of TGF-α is also associated with the gastric mucosal hyperproliferation and hypochlorhydria of Ménétrier's disease.[190]

Consonant with its original identification in the medium of transformed cells, TGF-α is expressed in a number of cancers.[169] In transgenic mice, overexpression of TGF-α results in neoplasia and abnormal development of various epithelial tissues such as liver, pancreas, and breast.[191–193]

AMPHIREGULIN/CRIPTO. Much less information is available regarding the biology of the other members of the EGF superfamily. Because most were derived from transformed cells, the bulk of information is centered on their roles in neoplasia. Amphiregulin is expressed in normal placenta, as well as in gonads.[194] Both AR and cripto mRNA's are elevated in gastrointestinal cancers, especially of the colon, rectum, and stomach.[195, 196] AR appears to be important in normal keratinocyte biology.[133] Its mRNA is markedly elevated in psoriatic lesions.[195]

Transforming Growth Factor-β (TGF-β) Family

History and Nomenclature

TGF-β, the prototype of this growth factor family, was isolated as a growth stimulator associated with cellular transformation, although it is now clear that TGF-β can act as a growth stimulator, a growth inhibitor, and a regulator of differentiated cellular functions that have nothing to do with proliferation.[197–199] The response of a given cell to TGF-β is dictated by its histogenetic type and by the hormone/growth factor milieu.

TGF-β was originally identified as a peptide capable of inducing a transformed phenotype and anchorage-independent growth in cultured embryo–derived (AKR-2B) fibroblasts[200] and in rat kidney–derived (NRK) fibroblastic cells.[201] The historical evolution of our understanding of the roles played by "transforming" growth factors in neoplasia and normal cellular growth control was discussed previously with regard to the EGF/TGF-α superfamily. Roberts and colleagues[202] showed that the ability of a crude preparation of "sarcoma growth factor" to induce anchorage-independent growth of NRK cells actually derived from the coordinate actions of two unrelated peptides, TGF-α and TGF-β, both of which were secreted by murine sarcoma virus–transformed cells.

Purification and cloning of TGF-β revealed three mammalian isoforms (TGF-β1–3), a related form in chickens (TGF-β4), and in frog oocytes (TGF-β5), and a heterogeneous group of more distantly related growth factors with roles in hormonal regulation, sexual differentiation, bone and cartilage development, and embryogenesis. All members of this superfamily share varying degrees of sequence homology, especially with conservation of seven of the nine cysteine residues of TGF-β1, and a similar proteolytic derivation from the C-terminus of variably sized precursor molecules. The different family members act through distinct, but in some cases homologous, receptors.

TGF-β(1–3). After its initial purification from transformed cells, TGF-β was subsequently isolated from a number of normal tissues.[203] The α granules of platelets proved to be the most concentrated source of TGF-β,[204] but in contrast to human platelets, porcine platelets were found to contain a second isoform of TGF-β, called TGF-β2.[205] TGF-β2, which has comparable biological activities to TGF-β1, proved identical to the BSC-1 growth inhibitor previously isolated by Holley et al.[206] in 1978 from the medium of confluent African green monkey (BSC-1) cells. This reversible inhibitor was proposed to be a mechanism by which density-dependent growth inhibition is regulated in vitro. Given its diverse actions, the name "polyergin" was subsequently proposed for TGF-β2.[207]

Based on sequence homology with TGF-β1 and TGF-β2, TGF-β3 was cloned from cDNA isolated from chicken and mouse tissues.[199] All three TGF-β isoforms are found in mammals and are secreted as precursor peptides that dimerize before being proteolytically cleaved to disulfide-linked homodimers of about 25 kDa (Fig. 142–9). The crystalline structure of TGF-β2 has revealed that hydrophobic sequences in each monomer serve as contact points for dimerization, while the center of the dimer is a water-filled pocket rather than a hydrophobic core.[208, 209]

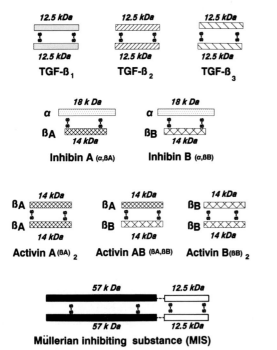

FIGURE 142–9. Structural relationships between members of the transforming growth factor-β (TGF-β) family. TGF-β$_{1-3}$ are homodimers with different subunits. The homology between the subunits is greater than 80 per cent.

The α subunits of inhibins and activins are unlike any other structures in the TGF-β family. The β subunits of inhibin A and inhibin B (designated β$_A$ and β$_B$) are approximately 30 per cent homologous to TGF-β subunits. The activins consist of either homodimers or heterodimers of the β$_A$ and/or β$_B$ subunits.

Members of this family were isolated from intact cells and tissues as larger prohormones, which, in the case of the three patriarchal TGF-β's, remain inactive until the mature dimers shown are liberated from their latent form by exposure to acid conditions or proteases. An exception to this is the müllerian inhibiting substance (MIS), which was isolated as a much larger active dimer, each element of which is 70 kDa. The smaller homodimer, consisting of identical 12.5-Da subunits, is cleaved from the precursor by plasmin digestion and found to retain the same biological activity as the larger form of MIS. (Modified from Underwood LE, Van Wyk JJ: Role of hormones in normal and aberrant growth. *In* Wilson J, Foster D (eds): Williams Textbook of Endocrinology (ed 8). Philadelphia, WB Saunders, 1992.)

INHIBINS AND ACTIVINS. The existence of inhibin, a nonsteroid gonad-derived inhibitor of pituitary FSH secretion, had long been postulated. With the development of in vitro assays of FSH regulation, a glycoprotein inhibitor of pituitary FSH secretion was isolated from ovarian follicular fluid[210] and later from testis.[211] Inhibin is a heterodimer between a common α subunit and one of two β subunits (β$_A$ or β$_B$), yielding two inhibin isoforms: inhibin A (α, β$_A$) and inhibin B (α, β$_B$) (see Ch. 114).

Other fractions of the inhibin purification process were found to stimulate pituitary FSH secretion, and from these "activin" was isolated.[212, 213] Surprisingly, activin was found to be a dimer of two inhibin β subunits and is designated as either activin-AA (β$_A$, β$_A$), activin-AB (β$_A$, β$_B$), or activin-BB (β$_B$, β$_B$) (Fig. 142–9). Both the α- and β-subunits of the activin/inhibin proteins and TGF-β1 share a similar distribution of their nine cysteine residues and are likely to have resulted from a common ancestral gene.[210]

Activin and inhibin have opposite actions in the pituitary and ovaries: In the pituitary, FSH secretion is inhibited by

inhibin and stimulated by activin, whereas in the gonads, gonadotropin-dependent steroidogenesis and cell proliferation are potentiated by inhibin and inhibited by activin.[214, 215]

The range of biological effects of activin/inhibin extends well beyond the pituitary-gonadal axis. Activin induces hemoglobin accumulation and the proliferation of erythroid progenitor cells in a human erythroleukemia cell line and in normal bone marrow with little or no effect on white blood cell differentiation and growth.[216, 217] Activin has also been identified as the factor (XTC-MIF) that is responsible for inducing the formation of mesoderm early in amphibian development.[218, 219]

MÜLLERIAN INHIBITORY SUBSTANCE (MIS). This glycoprotein inducer of müllerian duct regression in the male fetus was originally postulated to explain the phenomenon of the freemartin calf, in which proximity to the male fetus in male-female twins results in müllerian duct regression in the female.[220] The studies of Jost et al[221] demonstrated that this function was performed by a nonsteroidal secretory product of the testis that was later shown to be a heavily glycosylated disulfide-linked dimer with a molecular weight of about 140 kDa.[222] Cloning of the MIS gene showed a homology with TGF-β and the β chains of inhibin, although more distant than that among the TGF-β's and the inhibin subunits.[223] Recent studies indicate that proteolyic cleavage of both chains of the MIS dimer produces a 25-kDa C-terminal fragment that retains full biological potency.[224] Target tissues, such as the male urogenital ridge, appear to be capable of cleaving intact MIS to biologically active forms.[225]

Consonant with its role as a fetal regressor, circulating blood levels of MIS in boys are highest in the earliest months of life, but significant levels persist throughout childhood.[226] The functional significance of this peptide postnatally is unknown. MIS is also present in the fetal ovary, and postnatally in the mature graafian follicle. In girls, one of the functions of MIS is to inhibit meiosis of oocytes, and one possible mechanism for this is inhibition of phosphorylation of the EGF receptor in response to EGF. The inhibitory effect of MIS on meiosis as well as growth in a number of other systems can be counteracted by co-incubation with EGF.[227]

BONE MORPHOGENETIC PROTEIN. These proteins were isolated from efforts to understand the mechanism by which demineralized bone can induce new bone formation when implanted into ectopic sites.[228] With the discovery that many well-characterized growth factors, such as IGF-II, FGF, TGF-β, and PDGF, are found in bone and can influence cartilage and bone formation, the notion of a single bone morphogenetic protein (BMP) required modification.[229] Four bone-derived proteins are now designated BMP's: BMP-1, BMP-2A, BMP-2B, and BMP-3. cDNA sequencing revealed BMP-2A, 2B, and 3 to be members of the TGF-β family, whereas BMP-1 is unrelated.[230]

Vg1 AND Vgr-1. Isolation of Vg1 resulted from studies on the functions of maternal mRNA's that localize to the vegetal pole of *Xenopus* oocytes. Mesoderm is induced in animal pole cells by a signal from the vegetal cells of *Xenopus* oocytes. Vg1 mRNA, which becomes localized to the vegetal cortex of late oocytes, and can induce mesoderm in isolated animal poles, was found to encode a peptide with greater than 40 per cent homology to the C-terminal 120 amino acids of inhibin β$_A$.[231]

A mammalian homologue of Vg1, called Vgr-1, was isolated from mouse tissues.[232] In contrast to Vg1 mRNA in *Xenopus*, which declines after gastrulation, mouse Vgr-1 mRNA is present in multiple embryonic, neonatal, and adult tissues, but its role in development remains to be determined.

DPP-C. The decapentaplegic gene complex (DPP-C) is important in dorsal-ventral specification in *Drosophila* development. The C-terminus of the protein product of this gene shares 25 to 38 per cent amino acid homology with TGF-β family members.[233]

Genes, Precursors, and Processing

The genes for TGF-β1, β2, and β3 have been localized in humans to chromosomes 19, 1, and 14, respectively,[198] although it has been suggested that the various isoforms originated from a common ancestral gene.[199] The TGF-β precursor protein is encoded on seven exons, with the intron/exon junctions largely conserved among the three isoforms.[234] The three mammalian TGF-β isoforms, which show 64 to 82 per cent amino acid homology, are first synthesized as larger, biologically inactive precursor polypeptides that differ markedly in sequence outside of the C-terminal TGF-β motif. Biologically active TGF-β's are 25-kDa homodimers of disulfide-linked, 112-amino acid, 12.5-kDa peptides.[198] The initially translated 390- to 412-amino acid TGF-β precursor proteins become glycosylated, mannose-6-phosphorylated, and then dimerized to form a 110-kDa precursor protein that is biologically inactive.

As initially secreted from cells, the TGF-β's are in a latent form that does not bind to TGF-β receptors and must be activated to become biologically active.[235] Even after proteolytic cleavage of mature TGF-β, it may remain noncovalently associated with the remainder of its precursor, referred to as *latency associated peptide*, or LAP.[236] In platelet α granules, latent TGF-β is also noncovalently associated with a 135-kDa binding protein, called TGF-β1-BP, which contains a sequence of 16 EGF-like repeats.[237] Larger forms of TGF-β1-BP have been isolated from other cell types, suggesting cell-specific proteolysis of the protein or alternative splicing of the TGF-β1-BP gene. The role for these TGF-β binding proteins remains unclear.

Mature TGF-β circulates in the serum complexed with α2-macroglobulin, which helps target the peptide to liver, where it is cleared within minutes and excreted in bile.[238] In contrast, TGF-β1 in the latent complex has a greatly extended plasma half-life, which is largely dependent on the degree of sialation of the complex.[236]

The conditions that cleave and activate latent TGF-β under physiological circumstances are not clear, but transient acidification below pH 4 and treatment with proteases such as plasmin and cathepsin D activate latent TGF-β.[239, 240] Indeed, plasmin inhibitors have been found to block some of the paracrine actions mediated by the secretion of TGF-β.[241] It has been proposed that activation of latent TGF-β requires binding to the cation-dependent M6P/IGF-II receptor through M6P groups on the TGF-β precursor. Both M6P and anti–M6P-receptor antibodies prevent the activation of latent TGF-β by co-cultures of aortic endothelial and smooth muscle cell cultures.[242] Latent TGFβ bound to the M6P/IGF-II receptor might be made more accessible

to proteases at the cell surface or be endocytosed to be activated in the acid environment of lysosomes.

Inasmuch as latent forms of TGF-β are secreted by nearly all cultured cell types, the chemical mechanisms responsible for the latency and activation phenomena are certain to prove central to our understanding of the regulation and biological roles of these peptides in vivo as well as the potentially confounding effect of these substances in models of autocrine and paracrine regulation in vitro.

Receptors and Signaling

Almost all cell types have been shown to bind TGF-β with comparable affinity.[235] Three distinct cell surface–binding proteins are detected when ^{125}I-TGF-β is cross-linked to cell membranes.[205] The largest, the Type III binding site, is a proteoglycan that forms a 280- to 330-kDa complex with TGF-β, and consists of nearly 50 per cent heparan sulfate and chondroitin sulfate.[243] This binding protein has been cloned and contains no obvious intracellular signaling motif.[244] Its function is unknown but may regulate ligand accessibility to other TGF-β binding sites. The Type II TGF-β receptor,[245] which forms a 115- to 140-kDa complex with TGF-β, and a Type I receptor,[246] which forms a 50- to 80-kDa complex with TGF-β, have also been cloned. Both contain an intracellular serine/threonine kinase domain and conserved extracellular domains. Heteromeric complexes of the Type I and II receptors appear to be crucial for TGF-β binding and for signal transduction.[247] As the physical interactions of the TGFβ receptors are determined and their postreceptor signaling pathways elucidated, many of the diverse biological actions of TGF-β are likely to be explained.[248]

Although originally isolated on the basis of their ability to induce anchorage-independent growth on certain mesenchymal cells, their predominant effect is to inhibit cell growth. When elucidated, stimulatory effects of TGF-β are indirect, mediated through the autocrine production of other growth factors. Leof et al.[249] demonstrated that TGF-β induced c-sis mRNA (which encodes the PDGF-B chain, see below) in AKR-2B cells in addition to stimulating the secretion of PDGF-like peptides. In fibroblasts and chondrocytes, TGF-β was shown at low concentrations to stimulate the secretion of PDGF-AA, and the proliferative response to TGF-β could be blocked by anti-PDGF antibodies. At high concentrations, however, TGF-β decreased the expression of α-subunits of the PDGF receptor and growth was inhibited.

The mechanism of TGF-β–induced growth inhibition may be more direct. Its effects are generally reversible, and it appears to inhibit cells in the G1 phase of the cell cycle.[250] In a number of systems, TGF-β does not interfere with the binding or signaling of growth stimulators such as EGF.[251] Recent evidence suggests that inhibition of the cellular proto-oncogene c-myc is associated with the inhibition of proliferation in keratinocytes. Unlike other immediate-early genes, c-myc mRNA remains elevated throughout the G1 and S phases of the cell cycle, and the inhibition of myc protein synthesis with antisense oligonucleotides results in inhibition of keratinocyte growth. Growth inhibition of these cells by TGF-β is associated with an inhibition of the c-myc response to mitogens due to a block in transcriptional activation. A segment of DNA located 5' to the c-myc coding sequence and termed the *TGF-β control element,* or TCE, has been identified,[252] as well as a 106-kDa protein that may be a positive transcription factor for c-*myc* acting via the TCE. The c-*myc* inhibitory effect of TGF-β is also known to require the presence of the protein product of the retinoblastoma gene, pRB. TGF-β is unable to inhibit DNA synthesis in cells transformed with various DNA tumor viruses that are known to bind cellular pRB.[253] Moses and colleagues[252] have proposed a model in which TGF-β acts in concert with proteins such as pRB to inhibit the actions of this proposed transcription activator of c-*myc.* The extent to which c-*myc* inhibition is common to other situations of growth inhibition by TGF-β remains to be determined.

In some circumstances, the inhibitory effects of TGF-β on cell proliferation may not be reversible. In some tissues that typically undergo constant cell renewal, TGF-β has been shown to induce evidence of *apoptosis,* a noninflammatory form of cell death that is initiated by the activation of DNA-degrading endonucleases.[254] A role for TGF-β has been suggested in the apoptosis documented in the regression of tumor and drug-induced liver hypertrophy.[255, 256]

Biological Actions

The actions of the activins, inhibins, and MIS have been outlined above and are covered in other chapters (see Chs. 107 and 114). This section briefly reviews the major biological actions of the mammalian TGF-β's.

GROWTH INHIBITION. TGF-β is the most potent peptide growth inhibitor known, and its spectrum of target cells includes epithelial cells, endothelial cells, lymphoid cells, and myeloid cells. Several good correlations exist between growth inhibition by TGF-β in vitro and significant biologic effects in vivo. For example, TGF-β is a potent inhibitor of DNA synthesis in cultured hepatocytes, the epithelial parenchymal cell of the liver.[251, 257, 258] When injected into rats just prior to the onset of DNA synthesis, 11 hours after partial hepatectomy, TGF-β1 or β2 inhibits the major wave of hepatocyte labeling at 22 hours, but not when injected at the time of partial hepatectomy,[259] suggesting a TGF-β–sensitive restriction point late in the G_1 phase of the cell cycle. Inhibition of DNA synthesis is transient, and continued administration of TGF-β for 48 hours does not prevent ultimate restoration of liver mass. Similar findings have been obtained with parenteral administration of TGF-β encapsulated in liposomes.[260] TGF-β is also inhibitory for mammary cells in culture,[261] and for mammary epithelium in vivo,[262] as well as for keratinocytes, endothelium, and lymphoid cells.[197]

PRODUCTION OF EXTRACELLULAR MATRIX (ECM). TGF-β stimulates the synthesis of Type I collagen (by acting directly on the α2[I] collagen promoter), fibronectin, and other matrix components and is an inhibitor of matrix degradation.[263–265] TGF-β also stimulates the expression of cell membrane adhesion proteins, called integrins, which link the ECM to the cytoskeletal elements of the cell.[266] The direct application of TGF-β has been shown to accelerate wound healing in rats[267] and has also been implicated in the development of hepatic cirrhosis and in proliferative vitreoretinopathy.

IMMUNE MODULATION. TGF-β inhibits the proliferation of both T and B cells and antagonizes the actions of several interleukins and other immunoregulatory agents such as interferon and TNF. It inhibits the secretion of IgG and IgM by B cells.[268] Certain clinical conditions associated with immunosuppression may involve the actions of TGF-β. Glioblastoma is often associated with an immunosuppressed state, and purification of an immunosuppressive factor from glioblastoma cells showed it to be TGF-β2.[269] TGF-β also has profound effects on the growth and differentiation of stem cells in the bone marrow.

DEVELOPMENT. TGF-β mRNA is found in placenta and early embryos, and its functions as a mitogen, growth inhibitor, and matrix regulator all contribute to an important role in development. There is evidence for important roles in embryonic hematopoiesis, angiogenesis, and skeletal development (in addition to the BMP's).[270] All three TGF-β isoforms have been implicated in the formation of the palate[271] and in development of the eye, nervous system, and adrenal cortex.[272]

Platelet-Derived Growth Factor Family

History and Nomenclature

The presence of mitogens in platelets was first suggested by Balk[273] in 1971 when he observed that serum-supplemented culture medium supports the proliferation of chicken fibroblasts better than plasma-supplemented medium. To account for the difference in potency between serum and plasma, he postulated that the clotting of whole blood to produce serum results in the release of mitogens contained in platelets. Further studies confirmed Balk's hypothesis by demonstrating that the addition of platelet extracts to plasma-derived serum restored its mitogenic potency.[274] It is now known that the α granules of human platelets are a rich source of many mitogenic substances, including TGF-β,[275] EGF,[276] and endothelial cell growth factor. Rat platelets were the original source for the purification of hepatocyte growth factor (HGF) (see below),[277–279] which, although expressed in human tissues, is not found in human platelets.

PDGF-AA, PDGF-AB, PDGF-BB. In its unreduced state, PDGF is a highly basic (pI 9.8 to 10.2) dimeric peptide. Its molecular weight is between 28 and 35 kDa, and upon reduction, PDGF dissociates into an A and a B chain of 12 and 18 kDa, respectively.[280–282] Each of the three possible isoforms of PDGF (AA, AB, and BB) has been isolated from natural sources, including human platelets, which contain all three isoforms.[283]

OSTEOSARCOMA CELL–DERIVED GROWTH FACTOR (ODGF). Heldin et al.[284] demonstrated that cultured human osteosarcoma cells secrete an autocrine growth factor, which on purification and sequencing was found to be a homodimer of the PDGF A chain (PDGF-AA).

p28^{sis}. Simian sarcoma virus–transfected cells were known to secrete a growth factor of 28 kDa that was immunologically related to PDGF. Cloning of the v-*sis* oncogene showed it to be the PDGF-B gene containing the entire region encoding pro-PDGF-B[285, 286] and p28^{sis} to be PDGF-BB. V-*sis* and similar genes as well as PDGF receptors have been encountered in human sarcomas and glioma cell lines, suggesting that autocrine secretion of PDGF-like proteins may have a role in the genesis of certain human tumors.

PDGF Genes, Precursors, and Processing

The A and B chains of PDGF, which exhibit approximately 60 per cent sequence identity, are encoded on separate genes with similar structural organization on chromosomes 7 and 22, respectively.[287, 288] The PDGF precursors undergo both C- and N-terminal processing to yield PDGF-A and PDGF-B chains. Studies on cells co-transfected with genes for both PDGF-A and PDGF-B demonstrated that heterodimer assembly is largely a random process.[289]

Whereas PDGF-AA is largely secreted, PDGF-BB (as produced by simian sarcoma virus–transformed cells) remains cell associated in the endoplasmic reticulum and Golgi complex owing to the presence of a sequence of basic amino acids in the C-terminus.[290] This C-terminal basic sequence is also involved in promoting interaction between PDGF and components of the extracellular matrix.[291] The gene for the A-chain of PDGF undergoes differential splicing to yield two peptide variants of different lengths. The larger A-chain variant contains a basic C-terminal domain similar to that in the PDGF-B precursor and, as a consequence, remains cell associated like the B chain.[292]

PDGF Receptors and Signaling

Saturable high-affinity specific PDGF receptors of about 170 kDa have been identified in a broad range of cells, largely of mesenchymal origin.[293, 294] Evidence suggests that both PDGF and its receptor have been highly conserved throughout a significant portion of animal evolution.[295]

As with the two chains of PDGF itself, there are two homologous PDGF receptors, α and β, which are encoded on separate genes. The PDGF α and β receptors are structurally similar and bear some similarity to the receptor for colony stimulating factor (CSF-1) and the protein product of the c-*kit* proto-oncogene, the receptor for stem-cell factor[296] (see Ch. 157). Both PDGF receptors contain five immunoglobulin-like repeats in their extracellular domains and intracellular tyrosine kinase domains that are interrupted in their midportions by poorly conserved sequences of about 100 amino acids.

The binding of dimeric PDGF to a receptor facilitates the noncovalent association of two PDGF receptors to form a receptor dimer. Dimerization of PDGF receptors activates the signal-transducing mechanism, and in the absence of ligand, other agents that promote receptor aggregation, such as antibodies, can induce receptor autophosphorylation.[297]

The two PDGF receptors have differing affinity for the A and B chains of PDGF: the α receptor binds both the A and B chains of PDGF, while the β receptor binds only the B chain.[298] Thus, different PDGF isoforms bind to different homo- and heterodimers of the PDGF receptor: PDGF-AA to αα receptor dimers, PDGF-AB to αα or αβ dimers, and PDGF-BB to either αα, αβ, or ββ dimers[297, 299] (Fig. 142–10).

Functional specificity of the various PDGF heterodimers and homodimers appears to be largely determined by the type of receptor dimers that are induced.[300] While both α and β receptor monomers are capable of transducing a mitogenic signal, only the β receptor mediates chemotaxis and membrane ruffling.[301]

Following PDGF binding, the receptor:ligand complex is

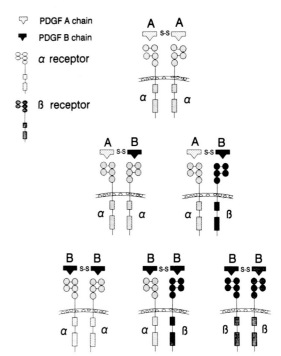

FIGURE 142–10. **Schematic illustrations of the abilities of the three isoforms of the PDGF dimer to bind to dimers composed of the α and β PDGF receptor.** The model is based on the supposition that the PDGF A chain subunit binds only to α receptors, whereas the B chain subunit of PDGF binds to both α and β receptors. The receptors are drawn to indicate that they are each composed of five extracellular immunoglobulin-like domains and a split cytoplasmic tyrosine kinase domain. (From Underwood LE, Van Wyk JJ: Role of hormones in normal and aberrant growth. *In* Wilson J, Foster D (eds): Williams Textbook of Endocrinology (ed 8). Philadelphia, WB Saunders, 1992.)

rapidly internalized and degraded. Both PDGF receptors contain SH-2 domains and may involve some of the same intracytoplasmic second messengers as does the EGF receptor (see above). PDGF stimulates the expression of a number of "immediate early" or "early growth response" genes such as c-*fos* and c-*myc*.[302, 303] Marked changes in the cytoskeletal architecture occur within minutes after exposure to PDGF with translocation of vinculin from adhesion plaques to a perinuclear location and disruption of actin-containing stress fibers.[304] Other early effects include accelerated phosphoinositol turnover, an increase in the density of cellular LDL receptors, increased uptake and synthesis of cholesterol, and prostaglandin release.[305]

Biological Actions

The most prominent activity of PDGF in biological systems is to stimulate proliferation. The role of PDGF in the cell cycle has been extensively studied by Pledger, Stiles, and colleagues, who documented the complex interactions that occur among growth factors in the promotion of cell division. Transient exposure of BALB/c 3T3 cells to PDGF induces a state of *competence* to undergo DNA synthesis, while IGF's, EGF, and other substances that are present in plasma permit *progression* through the G_1 phase of the cell cycle to enter into DNA synthesis. Categorizing growth factors as acting primarily to induce either competence or progression has been useful in establishing their roles in the cascade of events that are required for the transition from a quiescent state (G₀), through G₁, and into S to complete a cell cycle.[296]

PDGF also functions as a potent chemoattractant for smooth muscle cells and fibroblasts,[300] but the mechanism for chemotaxis differs from that for mitogenicity in that it does not require the presence of progression factors. It stimulates the synthesis of connective tissue matrix, including collagen, proteoglycans, and glycosaminoglycans.

Platelet aggregation and degranulation are initiated by injury to blood vessels and other structures. Much research has therefore centered on the role of PDGF as a wound-healing substance. PDGF recruits macrophages into wounds; furthermore, fibroblasts and endothelial cells are very sensitive to the proliferative effects of PDGF, and replication of these cell types would seem essential to normal wound healing. Some of these responses to tissue injury are outlined in Figure 142–11.

Of equally great importance from the standpoint of human pathophysiology is the possible role of PDGF in stimulating the proliferative changes that are invariably associated with atherosclerotic plaques. Ross and Glomset[306] have

outlined a sequence of events beginning with intimal injury that leads to platelet aggregation and degranulation, the release of PDGF, and the consequent migration of smooth muscle cells and their accumulation of lipids. Agents that inhibit the degranulation of platelets have been shown to diminish the atherosclerotic changes induced by homocystine administration in the rabbit.

In addition to roles in atherogenesis and wound healing, PDGF has also been implicated in mammalian embryogenesis, osteogenesis, and fibrosis.[307]

Fibroblast Growth Factor Family[308]

Historical Background and Members of the FGF Family

Gospodarowicz[309, 310] found that pituitary and brain extracts contain "fibroblast growth factors" (FGF's) that can stimulate the proliferation of many cell lines of mesodermal and neuroectodermal origin. Two separate gene products proved responsible for these mitogenic effects: basic FGF (bFGF) and acidic FGF (aFGF). These and newer members of the FGF superfamily subsequently proved to be powerful stimulators of angiogenesis, facilitators of wound healing, and promoters of embryonic differentiation. As pointed out in a previous section, members of this superfamily have been isolated from many tissues under at least 35 different names.

The currently recognized members of the FGF superfamily are the products of at least seven closely related genes.[311] Most of these were identified as members of the FGF superfamily because of their structural homologies to bFGF and aFGF. int-2 was first identified in the normal mouse genome by its proximity to a preferred "integration" site of proviral DNA in breast cancers induced by mouse mammary tumor virus.[312] The int-2 gene is also expressed in the embryo, where its gene product can function as a mesoderm-differentiating factor.[313, 314] It is apparently not expressed postnatally under normal circumstances.

FGF-4, FGF-5, and FGF-6 were also originally isolated as oncogenes. FGF-4 was isolated from a human stomach tumor as hst-1, and from a Kaposi's sarcoma as k-FGF.[315] In the human, int-2 and FGF-4 (k-FGF) are situated in close proximity on the short arm of chromosome 11 and in certain types of tumors both genes are amplified in concert.

FGF-5 is a human oncogene that was isolated from a human bladder tumor, and FGF-6 was identified by systematically screening a mouse cosmid library with a human hst probe.[316]

The keratinocyte growth factor (KGF) was initially isolated from the conditioned medium of a human embryonic lung fibroblast cell line on the basis of its mitogenicity for keratinocytes.[16] Only after determining the sequence of its cDNA was it found to be homologous with other members of the FGF superfamily. Unlike other FGF's, KGF is a highly specific mitogen for epithelial cells and has no effect on the multiplication of fibroblasts or endothelial cells.[317]

Chemical Characteristics and Genes

bFGF is an acid-labile, single-chain nonglycosylated peptide of 146 amino acids (MW 16 kDa, pI 9.6).[318] The acidic

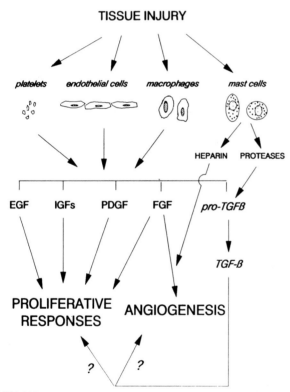

FIGURE 142–11. **Sources of the growth factors that are produced locally at sites of tissue injury and the important role that these factors play in the healing process.** Aggregation and lysis of platelets leads to the release of PDGF, TGF-β, and other growth factors. Endothelial cells release FGF and other growth factors along with plasmin, which activates TGF-β by releasing the active dimer from its latent precursor. TGF-β is a powerful chemotactic agent that recruits macrophages into wounds, following which the macrophages become a further source of proteases and a variety of growth factors including interleukins, tumor necrosis factor, and other cytokines that are not shown. Heparin, released from mast cells, acts synergistically with FGF to stimulate neovascularization. Because TGF-β can act as a mitogen under some circumstances and as a growth inhibitor under other circumstances, its most important role following injury may be to limit the proliferative response to tissue injury. (From Underwood LE, Van Wyk JJ: Role of hormones in normal and aberrant growth. *In* Wilson J, Foster D (eds): Williams Textbook of Endocrinology (ed 8). Philadelphia, WB Saunders, 1992.)

form of FGF (MW 15 kDa, pI 4.5) shares 55 per cent sequence homology with bFGF. The basic form is found in many tissues derived from mesoderm and neuroectoderm, whereas acidic FGF is less widely distributed and is confined mostly to nervous tissues and retina. The other peptides that make up this family are 35 to 55 per cent identical in their amino acid sequences, and their genes have similar exon-intron structures. A unique property of the FGF's (with the exception of int-2) is their strong affinity for heparin, and heparin binding growth factors have been isolated from a wide variety of cultured cells, organ extracts, and tumors.[318, 319] Heparin increases the stability of FGF's and enhances their biological activity.

A curious feature of the bFGF and aFGF genes is the absence of the classic signal sequences at their 5' ends, and for this reason it is unclear how they exit from their cells of origin. Although they are not secreted by the usual secretory pathways, aFGF and bFGF can be identified in the extracellular matrix of their cells of origin, where they bind with high affinity to heparan sulfate and other heparin-like mucopolysaccharides. Mignatti and Rifkin have shown that bFGF is extruded from the cell of origin by calcium-dependent exocytosis independent of the endoplasmic reticulum–Golgi pathway.[320] Following extrusion, bFGF remains bound to negatively charged proteoglycans in the extracellular matrix until liberated by heparinase or plasmin. It is therefore of interest that both tissue plasminogen activator and urokinase plasminogen activator are stimulated by FGF, and this effect is neutralized by TGF-β.[308, 321] However, even in tissues in which relatively high concentrations of FGF-like material are detected by RIA, it is frequently difficult or impossible to detect the presence of mRNA's for one of the known FGF's. Thus, cationic substances in extracellular matrix provide a widely distributed reservoir of FGF that can be released under special circumstances without requiring de novo gene transcription. Unlike aFGF and bFGF, the FGF's isolated as oncogenes contain signal sequences at their 5' ends and hence can be secreted by more traditional mechanisms.

The FGF Receptors and Their Genes

The strong binding of FGF's to the cationic mucopolysaccharides in the extracellular matrix has complicated the delineation of their true receptors. Dionne et al.[322] cloned two FGF receptors from human endothelial cells on the basis of their homologies to receptors termed *flg* and *bek*, which had previously been characterized in chicken and mouse cells, respectively. Both receptors contained three immunoglobulin-like regions in their extracellular domains, single-transmembrane domains, and cytoplasmic portions containing a split tyrosine kinase domain. Both receptors bound either aFGF or bFGF with equally high affinity (2 to 15 × 10^{-11} M). The immunoglobulin-like extracellular domains are similar to those in the PDGF and CSF-1 receptors, although the latter contain five immunoglobulin-like regions.

It is unlikely that all members of the FGF superfamily produce their biological effects through the *flg* and *bek* receptors. Xu et al.[323] have shown that the FGF receptor family is composed of at least 16 different isoforms resulting from splice variants of four different genes that encode FGF receptors. The keratinocyte growth factor, which is mitogenic only for epithelial cells, reportedly binds with high affinity to unique 115- and 140-KDa tyrosine kinase receptors on keratinocytes. These receptors also bind aFGF with high affinity, but the affinity of the receptors for bFGF is 20-fold less.[324]

Biological Actions of FGF

In a functional sense FGF's resemble PDGF in that they also render quiescent BALB/c 3T3 cells competent to respond to platelet-poor plasma (or a combination of IGF's and EGF).[325] As with PDGF, FGF stimulates a host of biochemical processes within its target tissues, including phosphorylation of intracytoplasmic proteins and induction of new protein synthesis.

Gospodarowicz and Mescher[326] showed that bFGF induces mitosis in blastemal cells and can stimulate limb regeneration in amphibia after amputation. FGF's also appear to play key roles in embryonic differentiation. In the mouse embryo, limb development depends on paracrine interactions between specialized epithelial cells at the limb tip with underlying mesenchymal elements. Concurrent with outgrowth of the limb bud, the epithelial cells express the genes for FGF-4 and the bone morphogenic protein (BMP-2), with FGF-4 serving as the major stimulant to mesenchymal differentiation.[314]

FGF delays the senescence of cells maintained in culture, extending the life span of granulosa cells by 10 to 60 generations[327] and of corneal endothelial cells by up to 10-fold.[328] FGF also appears to play a novel role in modulating the secretion of TSH and prolactin by cultured pituitary cells in response to TRH.

Folkman[329] and Shing et al.[330] have drawn attention to the essential role of neovascularization in the growth of embryos, repair of wounds, and growth of tumors. FGF is a potent mitogen for vascular endothelial cells and now appears to account for most of the "angiogenesis factor" activities described by Folkman and other workers. FGF is a potent mitogen for vascular endothelial cells and is very active in biological assays for "angiogenesis factor" activity (Fig. 142–12).

Clinical Effects

Folkman and his colleagues have found that although no FGF can be measured by RIA in human serum under most circumstances, levels become detectable in blood and urine under certain circumstances associated with neovascularization. These include aggressive hemangiomas of the newborn and in metastatic dissemination of prostatic and other human cancers. Indeed, early results suggest that measurement of urinary FGF levels may be one of the best markers of tumor aggressiveness. The search for agents that inhibit the angiogenic activity of the various FGF's offers an important new direction in cancer research.

The clinical utility of heparin-binding growth factors as therapeutic agents in wound healing and in other clinical disorders is similarly under active investigation.[331]

Nerve Growth Factors

History

In 1951, Levi-Montalcini and Hamburger[332] suggested that a diffusible neurotrophic substance was responsible

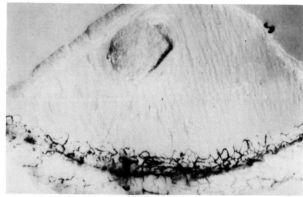
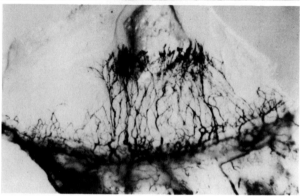

FIGURE 142–12. Stimulation of angiogenesis by basic FGF in rat cornea. Basic FGF (isolated from a rat chondrosarcoma) was incorporated into an ethylene-vinyl acetate polymer and then implanted by microsurgery into rat corneas. Control rats were implanted with polymer containing FGF that had been inactivated by boiling for 15 minutes. After six days the carotid arteries were injected with India ink and the corneas photographed. Note that the implant containing the active growth factor *(lower panel)* attracted neovascularization by blood vessels originating from the limbus, whereas neovascularization is not seen in animals injected with polymer containing inactivated angiogenesis factor *(upper panel).* (From Shing Y, Folkman J, Haudenschild C, et al: Angiogenesis is stimulated by a tumor-derived endothelial cell growth factor. J Cell Biochem 29:275–287, 1985.)

for the growth of dorsal root and sympathetic ganglia in chick embryos that had been implanted with mouse sarcoma tissue. Like EGF, nerve growth factor (NGF) is found in large amounts in the male mouse submaxillary gland, a feature not shared with humans. It was, in fact, while studying the biological effects of NGF in crude submaxillary gland extracts that Stanley Cohen made the observations that led to his discovery of EGF.[333]

As secreted by mouse submaxillary glands, NGF is one component of a biologically inactive 7S complex with a molecular weight of 140 kDa. Active NGF, which is the β subunit of this complex, is a basically charged peptide with a molecular weight of 13,259 Da.[334] β-NGF exhibits about 25 per cent homology with the A and B chains of human insulin.[335] Two β subunits are associated with two α and two γ subunits, and the entire complex is stabilized by two atoms of zinc. The γ subunit is an arginine esterase that is analogous to the EGF-binding protein.[336]

Biological Effects of NGF

The predominant effects of NGF appear to be in promoting the survival, differentiation, and axonal outgrowth of sensory and sympathetic ganglia. Because neurons are end cells that do not replicate, most observers believe that NGF serves no role as a mitogen. Animals injected with neutralizing antibodies to NGF undergo degeneration of their dorsal root and sympathetic ganglia,[337] whereas the injection of NGF into chick embryos prevents the preprogrammed cell death (apoptosis) that characterizes the normal development of these neurons.[338] The effects of NGF on neuron survival appear to be developmentally regulated: The injection of blocking antibodies to NGF produces the expected neuronal degeneration in fetal guinea pigs, but in adult animals the sensory neurons no longer require NGF for survival.[339]

In addition to promoting the survival of this select population of developing neurons, NGF accelerates the biochemical and morphological differentiation of stem cells into sympathetic and sensory neurons.[340] A line of cells derived from a rat pheochromocytoma, PC-12, is induced by NGF to differentiate both morphologically and biochemically into sympathetic neurons. This biochemical differentiation is marked by the synthesis of adrenergic and peptide neurotransmitters that are characteristic of sensory neurons.[340]

A further component of NGF action on the developing nervous system is its ability to induce a chemotropic effect on target neurons. NGF released from a fine pipette causes the axons of cultured neurons to grow toward it.[341] It is believed that the peripheral tissues innervated by sensory and sympathetic neurons produce the NGF that regulates the neuronal outgrowth from their respective ganglia. NGF so produced attracts the neurites of the appropriate sensory and sympathetic neurons along a chemotactic NGF gradient, resulting in selective tissue innervation. Nerve growth factor is then transported in a retrograde fashion to its target ganglia, where it is concentrated.[341] Relatively small amounts of NGF mRNA can be detected in the ganglia themselves.[342]

A growing body of data suggests that NGF may also play some role in inflammatory and immune responses: NGF is a chemoattractant for neutrophilic leukocytes,[343] and the administration of bNGF to neonatal animals leads to an increased number of mast cells in a number of organs and peripheral tissues.[344] NGF stimulates receptors for interleukin-2 on cultured human lymphocytes,[345] and low-affinity receptors for NGF are present on rat splenic mononuclear cells. NGF is a weak mitogen in mixed cultures of spleen mononuclear cells and potentiates the synthesis of DNA in response to several T-cell and B-cell mitogens.[346]

Other Nerve Growth Factors

It has long been speculated that NGF itself is but one member of a family of NGF's, each promoting the survival and tissue innervation of unique neuronal cell types.[347] For several decades little progress was made in the search for additional NGF's, principally because specific bioassays were lacking. Recently, however, several distinct neurotrophins have been described that are homologous with the original NGF: two of these are brain-derived neurotrophic factor (BDNF) and neurotrophin-3 (NT-3). Neurotrophins 4 and 5 have also been described but are less well characterized. In the human, NGF is encoded on human chromosome 1, BDNF on chromosome 11, and NT-3 on chromosome 12. An additional neurotrophin known as the "ciliary neurotrophic factor" (CNFT) is structurally and functionally different from the other nerve growth factors and is discussed below in a separate section.

NGF Receptors

Two distinct types of receptor for NGF have been described in neural cells: a high-affinity, low-capacity receptor with MW between 75 and 80 kDa, and a low-affinity, high-capacity receptor. Lymphocytes and macrophages contain only the low-affinity receptor. Both the high- and low-affinity forms of the NGF receptor are believed to be derived from a single gene on human chromosome 17.[351] More recently, a unique tyrosine kinase receptor for neurotrophic peptides *(trk)* that is found only in neural tissue has been described.[352] Although originally described as a receptor for NF-3, the *trk* receptor also binds NGF and BDNF.[353, 354]

NGF in Human Disease

Walker et al.[355, 356] have noted that the concentration of NGF in the brain of both adult and fetal mice is regulated by thyroxine and have postulated that some of the clinically important effects of thyroid hormones on brain development, especially the devastating effects of hypothyroidism in the first years of life, might result from alterations in NGF concentrations.

Increased amounts of NGF have been found in the serum of patients with the peripheral form of neurofibromatosis[357] and in patients with multiple endocrine neoplasia type III.[358] The latter disorder is characterized by the growth of ganglioneuromas on the lips and throughout the alimentary tract and by a high incidence of medullary thyroid carcinoma and pheochromocytoma. Presumably additional crucial roles will be found for the newer neurotrophins.

Ciliary Neurotrophic Factor (CNTF)

CNTF was originally identified, purified, and cloned as a survival factor for parasympathetic neurons in chick ciliary ganglia.[358a] CNTF is a 200-amino acid residue protein that is structurally distinct from the neurotrophins just discussed. It is encoded on human chromosome 11q12,[358b] and, unlike the other neurotrophins, CNTF lacks a consensus signal peptide. CNTF is widely expressed throughout the central and peripheral nervous systems and promotes the survival of neurons of the peripheral sensory, sympathetic, and ciliary ganglia at various stages in their development.[358c] CNTF also induces the expression of choline acetyltransferase in sympathetic and retinal neurons and vasoactive intestinal peptide in embryonic sympathetic neurons.[358c] CNTF prevents cell death of motor neurons both in vitro and in vivo, a unique property that might prove useful in degenerative diseases of the nervous system.[358d]

CNTF is often referred to as a "neural cytokine" because of its close relationship to some of the hematopoietic cytokines, including the leukemia inhibitory factor (LIF), interleukin-6 (Il-6), oncostatin M (OSM), the granulocyte colony–stimulating factor (G-CSF), and interleukin-11 (Il-11).[358e, 358f] These peptides share certain similarities in their amino acid sequences, in their secondary architectures, and in their gene structures. CNTF is more remotely related to growth hormone and prolactin. More impressive than the structural homologies of the peptides themselves are their similarities in receptor interactions and signaling pathways. Each of these peptides transmits its signals through a homodimeric or heterodimeric transmembrane receptor, the subunits of which are often identical in receptors of the other family members[358g] (Fig. 142–13). These receptors are members of the larger class of prolactin/growth hormone/cytokine receptors.[358h] In addition to sharing a number of structural motifs, the postreceptor signaling mechanisms within this family are similar in their respective target cells. Exposure to ligand is promptly followed by tyrosine phosphorylation of several cytoplasmic proteins, including the β subunits themselves.[358e]

The initial binding of each ligand is to a low-affinity binding site, an event that triggers dimerization of the two β transmembrane subunits and the creation of high-affinity binding sites. Acquisition of high-affinity binding may result from association of WSxWS (tryptophan-serine–any amino acid–tryptophan-serine) motifs in the β subunits with ligand-binding proteoglycans in the cell membrane.[358h] Such a mechanism for generating high-affinity binding sites has been well documented for TGF-β.[358i]

Although the low-affinity binding is by itself insufficient to propagate a signaling sequence, it is the low-affinity binding site that determines the tissue specificity of the several ligands composing this family. As an example, although the receptors for CNTF and LIF share identical β

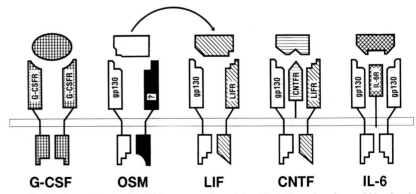

FIGURE 142–13. **Diagram to illustrate similarities between the ligand:receptor complexes of the ciliary neurotrophic factor (CNTF) and related cytokines.** G-CSF, Granulocyte colony–stimulating factor; OSM, oncostatin M; LIF, leukemia inhibitory factor; and Il-6, interleukin-6. The initial step in signal transduction is binding of the respective ligands to a low-affinity binding site, the expression of which determines cellular specificity. The low-affinity binding sites for the CNTF and Il-6 receptors are soluble extracellular α subunits that attach to the cell membrane through glycosophosphatidylinositol (GPI) linkages. A similar α subunit has not been identified for LIF, OSM, and G-CSF, and the initial low-affinity binding is thought to be to one of the transmembrane subunits. Initial binding of the ligand is rapidly followed by dimerization of two transmembrane β subunits. Dimerization creates high binding sites for their respective ligands and permits signal transduction. The binding subunit of OSM has not yet been identified. Note that the gp-130 subunit is utilized by CNTF, Il-6, LIF, and OSM, whereas the subunit initially described as the LIF receptor (LIFR) is shared with CNTF. The arrow signifies that OSM can also bind to the LIF receptor. (From Bruce AG, Linsley PS, Rose TM: in Prog Growth Factor Res 4:165, 1992.)

subunits (gp130 and LIFR), the initial binding of CNFR is to a unique soluble extracellular α subunit that is anchored to the plasma membrane, whereas LIF binds to the LIFR β subunit. Ip et al. found that lymphocytes that are normally responsive to LIP but not CNTF yielded LIF-like responses to CNTF when exposed to CNTF together with the soluble form of CNTFα.[358e, 358f, 358g] Similarly, it is not surprising that LIF has neurotrophic actions in the nervous system and in certain contexts is known as the "cholinergic differentiation factor."[358j]

Studies of CNTF are providing another important link between the nervous system and the immune system and shedding considerable light on the evolutionary interrelationships among hormones, growth factors, and cytokines. They are also adding a new dimension to our understanding of the relationships between the structure and function of receptors and mechanisms of signal transduction.[358g, 358k, 358l]

FAMILIES OF GROWTH FACTORS THAT ARE TISSUE SPECIFIC

Hematopoietic Growth Factors and Cytokines of the Immune System

In contrast to the superfamilies of growth factors discussed above, numerous other growth factors are less easily classified. At present the hematopoietic growth factors and cytokines of the immune system are most easily grouped into families according to their tissue specificities. Most of these substances are differentiating agents in maturing cells and are believed to be mitogenic only for undifferentiated stem cells. We do not discuss hematopoietic growth factors in this chapter because they are thoroughly discussed in Chapter 157. Similarly, we do not discuss the interleukins, interferons, and the tumor necrosis factor because these substances are discussed in Chapter 158.

Unclassified Growth Factors

The intense interest in autocrine and paracrine modes of regulation has resulted in the identification of scores of additional regulatory peptides whose actions appear to be confined to specific tissues. Many such substances do not fit readily into any of the classifications discussed above, even though they fulfill all the criteria for peptide growth factors. Many such growth factors have been identified in the course of systematic studies to optimize the growth of different cell types in defined media. The variety of such mitogens suggests that most biologically active peptides will be found to influence cellular proliferation under certain circumstances.[359] In the following section we will confine our discussion to two such factors, the hepatic growth factor and bombesin, to illustrate the diversity of peptide growth factors and some of the features that they share in common.

Bombesin (Gastrin-Releasing Peptide) and Other Gastrointestinal Hormones

This tetradecapeptide illustrates the functional diversity of substances that on other grounds are authentic peptide growth factors. Bombesin was first isolated from frog skin but is now known to belong to a highly conserved family of brain and gut peptides that regulate a number of neural and gastrointestinal functions in addition to stimulating cell proliferation[360] (see Ch. 153). The mammalian homologue of bombesin is gastrin-releasing peptide (GRP), a 27-amino-acid peptide, in which the terminal seven amino acids at the carboxy-terminus are identical with those of bombesin. Spindel and associates have cloned the bombesin/GRP receptor and shown that it has seven transmembrane-spanning domains.[361, 362] GRP stimulates gallbladder contraction, intestinal peristalsis, and the secretion of gastric acid, pancreatic enzymes, and other gut peptides.[363, 364] Bombesin-like immunoreactivity is also found in the mammalian brain. The intraventricular or intraperitoneal infusion of bombesin in animals suppresses feeding and induces analgesia, increased locomotor activity, hypothermia, hyperglycemia, and the secretion of GH and prolactin.[365]

In addition to these diverse biological effects, bombesin/GRP has been shown to be a potent mitogen for fibroblasts and pneumatocytes. It is present in fetal lung tissue and may play an important role in the development of the respiratory tract. It reaches its highest concentrations in human fetal lung tissue around the time of birth, after which it begins to disappear.[366]

Bombesin/GRP may also play a key role in the initiation or maintenance of small cell carcinomas of the lung.[367] When grown in soft agar, some of these tumors secrete significant amounts of this peptide, which then stimulates the growth of these cells in an autocrine manner. Cuttitta et al.[368] found that a monoclonal antibody directed against the carboxy-terminus of bombesin inhibited the growth of these malignant cells in culture. Even more dramatic was their demonstration that intraperitoneal administration of the antibody caused regression of these tumors in nude mice. Such findings prompted the initiation of clinical trials to determine the possible efficacy of monoclonal antibodies raised against bombesin and other growth factors in patients with tumors of the lung and other organs.[369]

Hepatocyte Growth Factor (HGF)

Originally thought to be a liver-specific growth factor and a good candidate to be the initiator of the dramatic proliferative response of liver to partial hepatectomy, HGF is now known to have a broad spectrum of actions and target tissues. Three lines of investigation led to the isolation and cloning of HGF. It was initially identified in rat platelets as a growth stimulator for cultured hepatocytes[277, 278] and in the serum of partially hepatectomized rats.[370] It was shown to be identical to the liver growth factor, hepatopoietin A, identified in rat plasma[371] and to a hepatostimulatory factor purified from the serum of patients in fulminant hepatic failure.[372] HGF was subsequently shown to be identical to two other substances: scatter factor, a motility- and conformation-altering substance first identified in canine cells,[373] and a tumor cytotoxic factor.[374]

HGF is synthesized as a single 85-kDa precursor protein, which is then cleaved to a disulfide-linked heterodimer consisting of 69-kDa α and 34-kDa β subunits.[375] The HGF precursor protein contains four double-loop structures known as kringle domains, which are common to members of the plasminogen, prothrombin, and Factor XII family of proteases (Fig. 142–14), although HGF itself has not been shown to have protease activity. Tissue plasminogen activator (TPA) may, however, be an important regulator of the production of heterodimeric HGF, because the cleavage site that yields the α and β subunits from the HGF precursor is identical to the site in plasminogen that yields plasmin by the action of TPA.[375] The need for proteolytic processing of HGF precursor is currently unclear because the intact HGF precursor and heterodimeric forms have comparable biological activity.

The receptor for HGF is the protein product of the c-*met* proto-oncogene, a heterodimeric transmembrane protein with tyrosine kinase activity localized to its intracytoplasmic β chain.[376, 377] C-*met* has a wide tissue distribution that includes liver, but also brain, kidney, lung, and skin.[377] The ubiquity of the receptor is in keeping with the diverse range of target tissues for HGF, which stimulates growth in keratinocytes, melanocytes, melanoma cells, proximal renal tubule cells, and breast epithelium, as well as hepatocytes.[378] HGF gene expression is found in placenta, lung, brain, kidney, thymus, and submandibular gland, as well as in liver.[379] Nonparenchymal cells, probably the lipid-storing Ito cells, are the major site of HGF gene expression in the liver.[380, 381]

The role of HGF in liver regeneration is far from clear. It is the most potent known growth stimulator of hepatocytes in vitro, although they remain sensitive to the growth inhibitory actions of TGF-β in the presence of HGF.[382] After partial hepatectomy, there is an immediate increase in serum concentrations of HGF, well before any documented increased tissue transcription of the HGF gene. Within one hour there is a 15-fold increase in HGF in serum,[383, 384] while liver mRNA expression is first detected three hours after partial hepatectomy.[385, 386] These observations suggest two different modes of HGF action after partial hepatectomy. The most immediate role for HGF may be an endocrine one that signals the liver and other organs of the impending need for a proliferative response, while the subsequent onset of HGF production in liver nonparenchymal cells suggests a later paracrine role for HGF in sustaining hepatocyte proliferation.

The experimental support for this model is not complete. Following a partial hepatectomy, a simultaneous increase in HGF mRNA occurs in a variety of nonhepatic tissues, including lung, kidney, and spleen, even though the growth response is confined to the liver.[387] The multiple tissues that express the c-*met* proto-oncogene product are potentially sensitive to HGF. Quite probably, then, the mitogenic effects of HGF in liver require the presence of other factors or else mechanisms exist to inhibit the response of nonhepatic tissues to HGF. One mechanism by which the proliferative signal of HGF might be abrogated in tissues that are not intended as targets may be the proteolytic truncation of the C-terminus of the c-*met* protein, resulting in loss of its signaling mechanism. Physiological roles for HGF have been suggested in other processes, such as the renal response to unilateral nephrectomy.[388]

GROWTH FACTORS, CELLULAR TRANSFORMATION, AND ONCOGENESIS

The finding that oncogenes code for normal cell products has led to an explosion of research to determine the mechanisms of malignant transformation. A complete review of oncogenes is beyond the scope of this chapter, but an overview of growth factors would be incomplete without briefly summarizing the interface between oncogenes and growth factors. Although some proto-oncogenes were found to encode peptide growth factors or growth factor receptors, most code for proteins involved in the postreceptor transduction of signals leading to cell differentiation or replication.[389] Studies of the mechanisms by which oncogenes cause malignant transformation are now providing some of our most important insights on the mechanisms that regulate normal growth.[314, 390] The powerful tools of molecular biology have, in recent years, resulted in rapid escalation in the identification of new oncogenes, and that number is now rapidly approaching 100 well-documented viral oncogenes. Examples of the various types of oncogenes that have been described are shown in Table 142–3.

Oncogenes Encoding Growth Factors and Growth Factor Receptors

The first association of an oncogene with a peptide growth factor was established when the v-*sis* gene (simian sarcoma virus from the wooly monkey) was found to have a nucleotide sequence that codes for a protein that is almost identical to the N-terminal 109 amino acids of the B-

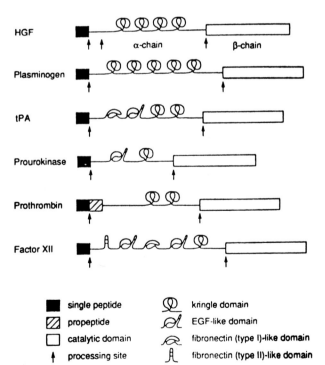

FIGURE 142–14. **The structures of the HGF precursor protein and those of proteins involved in blood coagulation and fibrinolysis.** Sites of proteolytic cleavage are indicated by arrows. HGF is synthesized as a single 85-kDa precursor protein, which is then cleaved to a disulfide-linked heterodimer consisting of a 69-kDa α- and 34-kDa β subunit. The HGF precursor protein contains four double-loop structures known as kringle domains, which are common to members of the plasminogen, prothrombin, and Factor XII family of proteases. (From Matsumoto K, Nakamura T: Molecular structure, roles in liver regeneration, and other biological functions. Crit Rev Oncogen 3:27–54, 1992.)

TABLE 142–3. SOME ONCOGENES RELATED TO NORMAL GROWTH PROCESSES*

ONCOGENE	HOMOLOGUES OR PRODUCTS
Growth factors	
sis	PDGF-β chain
hst; int₂	FGF
vq	TGF-β
Growth factor receptors	
erb-B	Truncated EGF receptor
erb-A	Steroid and thyroxine receptors
kit; fms	PDGF and CSF-1 receptors
Tyrosine-specific protein kinases	
src	Tyrosine-specific protein kinases
abl	
Ser/Thr-specific protein kinases	
mos	Substrates for growth factor
raf	dependent tyrosine kinases (c-*mos* expressed primarily in gonads)
Signal transducers	
ras	GTP/GDP-binding protein (activates GTPase)
Nuclear oncogenes	
myc	Encode phosphoproteins that
myb	regulate gene transcription.
fos	Bind to DNA through leucine
jun	zipper motif. c-*jun* is transcription factor AP-1 (binds to *fos*)

*Examples of genes that were initially identified as the oncogenic moiety of tumor viruses and later were shown to encode proteins that are homologous with proteins in normal cells that play important roles in growth regulation.

chain of human PDGF.[285, 286] Soon thereafter, the v-*erbb* gene, obtained from an avian erythroblastosis virus, was found to code for a protein similar to a truncated portion of the EGF receptor and containing its tyrosine kinase.[159] The *erba* oncogene was then found to be homologous with portions of the genes coding for the DNA-binding regions of the steroid hormone and thyroxine receptors.[391]

Oncogenes Encoding Protein Kinases

Several oncogenes such as *src* and *abl* code for cellular proteins that either are tyrosine kinases or stimulate tyrosine kinase activity.[392] Phosphorylation of tyrosine residues on specific proteins is of prime importance in the mitogenic actions of most if not all growth factors. Some tyrosine kinases, such as *src* and *abl*, have no known functions apart from their kinase activity, whereas other tyrosine kinases such as the *erbb* gene product are embedded within the cytosolic portions of growth factor receptors. The receptor tyrosine kinase of growth factor receptors is essential for the mitogenic effects of the corresponding growth factors.[61] The γ-subunit of phospholipase C is a specific substrate for the tyrosine kinase of several growth factor receptors.[393]

In addition to tyrosine-specific kinases, several oncogenes such as c-*mos* and c-*raf* encode kinases that preferentially phosphorylate serine and threonine residues. Gene expression of c-*mos* is much higher in the gonads than in any other tissue,[394] although the significance of this finding is unknown. c-*raf* is one of the primary substrates for tyrosine phosphorylation in response to PDGF and certain other growth factors.[395]

ras Oncogenes

Eukaryotic cells from yeast to man contain a highly conserved gene family encoding 21-kDa proteins that are intimately involved in growth control (see also Ch. 7). The family of *ras* oncogenes play a crucial role in cell proliferation, and excessive expression or mutant forms of these genes are found in 10 to 40 per cent of human tumors.[396] The importance of *ras* in growth control is underscored by observations that *ras* function is required for the mitogenic effects of many growth-promoting substances.[397] The *ras* proteins, together with the GTPase-activating protein (GAP), function as regulators of the conversion of GTP to GDP in the cell membrane. Mutations that impair GTP hydrolysis cause constitutive activation of *ras*.

Oncogenes Encoding Nuclear Proteins

The nuclear oncogenes c-*myc*, c-*fos*, and c-*jun* regulate gene transcription and are among the earliest genes transcribed after exposure of cells to growth factors. These nuclear oncogenes encode phosphoproteins that dimerize through their "leucine zipper" backbones and bind to DNA to alter gene transcription (see Ch. 5B). In this regard, the *fos* and *jun* proteins act cooperatively: c-*jun* encodes the transcription factor AP-1, which binds tightly through its "leucine zipper" region to specific DNA response elements. The *fos* gene encodes a protein that itself binds only weakly to DNA but forms a heterodimer with the *jun* protein, which has greater affinity for DNA than either protein alone.[398]

Interactions between growth factors and nuclear oncogenes were first brought to light with the discovery that PDGF stimulates in BALB/c 3T3 cells up to 40-fold increases in the mRNA corresponding to c-*myc*, an oncogene that was originally found in avian myelocytomatosis virus.[302] Microinjection of this protein into BALB/c 3T3 cells bypassed their need for PDGF in traversing the G₁ phase of the cell cycle.[303] Expression of c-*myc* and other nuclear oncogenes is not, however, sufficient for growth to occur, and in some particular instances not even necessary.[399] In summary, the great interest in the role of nuclear oncogenes in the control of growth is that these are among the few known genes that are expressed early in the passage through the cell cycle and that may therefore hold a key to the cascade of cellular events that eventuate in cell division.

FRONTIERS OF GROWTH FACTOR RESEARCH

Although knowledge of the function of cellular oncogenes is expanding in too explosive a manner to predict how all of this new information will ultimately fit together, it is clear that the large number of growth factors and products of oncogenes constitute a major physiological growth-regulating system. These peptides operate by autocrine, paracrine, and even endocrine mechanisms to regulate processes as diverse as embryonic differentiation, aging, organ regeneration, and wound repair, as well as normal growth and development. This new knowledge is of potential importance in understanding the pathophysiology of many diseases that are not currently considered within the scope of endocrinology.[400] Indeed, very little of the rapidly accumulating information on these growth-regulating peptides has as yet been incorporated into the fabric of classic endocrinology, and, except for the somatomedins, measurements of these substances have not been used diagnostically.

Now that recombinant DNA technology is capable of providing much larger supplies of these growth-regulating substances to physiologists and clinical investigators, it may be possible to develop strategies to selectively manipulate the growth and differentiation of specific tissues and cell types. This, in turn, should facilitate the emergence of new therapies with specificity comparable to that of erythropoietin in treating the anemia of end-stage renal disease. Whether or not these possibilities are realized, the explosion of knowledge concerning the mechanisms by which growth is regulated at the cellular level is extending the purview of endocrinology far beyond its traditional boundaries.

REFERENCES

1. Starling EH: The Croonian Lectures on the chemical correlation of the functions of the body. Lancet 2:579–583, 1905.
2. Niall HD: The evolution of peptide hormones. Ann Rev Physiol 44:615–624, 1982.
3. Feyrter F: Ueber die These von den peripheren endokrinen Druesen. Wien Z Inn Med 27:9–38, 1946.
4. Dockray GJ: Evolutionary relationships of the gut hormones. Fed Proc 38:2295–2301, 1979.
5. Sporn MB, Todaro GJ: Autocrine secretion and malignant transformation of cells. N Engl J Med 303:878–880, 1980.
6. Clemmons DR, Van Wyk JJ: Evidence for a functional role of endogenously produced somatomedin-like peptides in the stimulation of human fibroblast and porcine smooth muscle cell DNA synthesis. J Clin Invest 75:1914–1918, 1985.
7. Balk SP, Morisi A, Gunther HS, et al: Somatomedin (insulin-like growth factor), but not growth hormone, are mitogenic for chicken heart mesenchymal cells and act synergistically with epidermal growth factor and brain fibroblast growth factor. Life Sci 35:335–346, 1984.
8. Anklesaria P, Teixido J, Laiho M, et al: Cell-cell adhesion mediated by binding of membrane-anchored transforming growth factor alpha to epidermal growth factor receptors promotes cell proliferation. Proc Natl Acad Sci USA 87:3289–3293, 1990.
9. Wong ST, Winchell LF, McCune BK, et al: The TGF-alpha precursor expressed on the cell surface binds to the EGF receptor on adjacent cells, leading to signal transduction. Cell 56:495–506, 1989.
10. Flanagan JG, Chen DC, Leder P: Transmembrane form of the kit ligand growth factor is determined by alternative splicing and is deleted in the Sld mutant. Cell 64:1025–1035, 1991.
11. Savage CR Jr, Inagami T, Cohen S: The primary structure of epidermal growth factor. J Biol Chem 247:7612–7621, 1972.
12. Pandiella A, Massagué J: Cleavage of the membrane precursor for transforming growth factor α is a regulated process. Proc Natl Acad Sci USA 88:1726–1730, 1991.
13. O'Malley BW: Did eucaryotic steroid receptors evolve from intracrine gene regulators? [editorial] Endocrinology 125:119–120, 1989.
14. Re RN: The cellular biology of angiotensin: Paracrine, autocrine, and intracrine actions in cardiovascular tissues. J Mol Cell Cardiol 21:63–69, 1989.
15. Sporn MB, Roberts AB: Peptide growth factors are multifunctional. Nature 332:217–218, 1988.
16. Finch PW, Rubin JS, Miki T, et al: Human KGF is FGF-related with properties of a paracrine effector of epithelial cell growth. Science 245:752–755, 1989.
17. Plowman GD, Whitney GS, Neubauer MG, et al: Molecular cloning and expression of an additional epidermal growth factor receptor-related gene. Proc Natl Acad Sci USA 87:4905–4909, 1990.
18. Miyazono K, Heldin C-H: High-yield purification of platelet-derived endothelial cell growth factor: Structural characterization and establishment of a specific antiserum. Biochemistry 28:1704–1710, 1989.
19. Salmon WD Jr, Daughaday WH: A hormonally controlled serum factor which stimulates sulfate incorporation by cartilage in vitro. J Lab Clin Med 49:825–836, 1957.
20. Daughaday WH, Hall K, Raben MS, et al: Somatomedin: Proposed designation of sulphation factor. Nature 235:107, 1972.
21. Rinderknecht E, Humbel RE: The amino acid sequence of human insulin-like growth factor I and its structural homology with proinsulin. J Biol Chem 253:2769–2776, 1978.
22. Klapper DG, Svoboda ME, Van Wyk JJ: Sequence analysis of somatomedin-C: Confirmation of identity with insulin-like growth factor I. Endocrinology 112:2215–2217, 1983.
23. Rinderknecht E, Humbel RE: Primary structure of human insulin-like growth factor II. FEBS Lett 89:283–286, 1978.
24. Zapf J, Froesch ER, Humbel RE: The insulin-like growth factors (IGF) of human serum: Chemical and biological characterization and aspects of their possible physiological role. Curr Top Cell Regul 19:257–309, 1981.
25. Daughaday WH, Hall K, Salmon WD Jr, et al: On the nomenclature of the somatomedins and insulin-like growth factors. J Clin Endocrinol Metab 65:1075–1076, 1987.
26. Jansen M, van Schaik FMA, Ricker AT, et al: Sequence of cDNA encoding human insulin-like growth factor I precursor. Nature 306:609–611, 1983.
27. Bell GI, Merryweather JP, Sanchez-Pescador R, et al: Sequence of a cDNA clone encoding human preproinsulin–like growth factor II. Nature 310:775–777, 1984.
28. Dull TJ, Gray A, Hayflick JS, Ullrich A: Insulin-like growth factor II precursor gene organization in relation to insulin gene family. Nature 310:777–781, 1984.
29. Jansen M, van Schaik FMA, van Tol H, et al: Nucleotide sequences of cDNAs encoding precursors of human insulin-like growth factor II (IGF-II) and an IGF-II variant. FEBS Lett 179:243–246, 1985.
30. Brissenden JE, Ullrich A, Francke U: Human chromosomal mapping of genes for insulin-like growth factors I and II and epidermal growth factor. Nature 310:781–784, 1984.
31. Lund PK, Hoyt EC, Van Wyk JJ: The size heterogeneity of rat insulin-like growth factor-I mRNAs due primarily to differences in the length of 3′-untranslated sequence. Mol Endocrinol 3:2054–2061, 1989.
32. Hoyt EC, Van Wyk JJ, Lund PK: Tissue and development specific regulation of a complex family of rat insulin-like growth factor I messenger ribonucleic acids. Mol Endocrinol 2:1077–1086, 1988.
33. Lund PK, Hoyt EC, Van Wyk JJ: Structural and functional characterization of IGF-I RNA 3′ variants. Adv Exp Med Biol 293:15–21, 1991.
34. Haig D, Graham C: Genomic imprinting and the strange case of the insulin-like growth factor II receptor. Cell 64:1045–1046, 1991.
35. DeChiara TM, Robertson EJ, Efstratiadis A: Parental imprinting of the mouse insulin-like growth factor II gene. Cell 64:849–859, 1991.
36. Henry I, Bonaiti-Pellie C, Chehensse V, et al: Uniparental paternal disomy in a genetic cancer-predisposing syndrome. Nature 358:609–610, 1991.
37. Ranier S, Johnson LA, Dobry CJ, et al: Relaxation of imprinted genes in human cancer. Nature 362:747–749, 1993.
38. Ogawa O, Eccles MR, Szeto J, et al: Relaxation of insulin-like growth factor II gene imprinting implicated in Wilms' tumor. Nature 362:749–751, 1993.
39. D'Ercole AJ, Stiles AD, Underwood LE: Tissue concentrations of somatomedin C: Further evidence for multiple sites of synthesis and paracrine or autocrine mechanisms of action. Proc Natl Acad Sci USA 81:935–939, 1984.
40. Lunk PK, Moats-Staats BM, Hynes MA, et al: Somatomedin-C/insulin-like growth factor-I and insulin-like growth factor-II mRNAs in rat fetal and adult tissues. J Biol Chem 261:14539–14544, 1986.
41. Hynes MA, Van Wyk JJ, Brooks PJ, et al: Growth hormone dependence of somatomedin-C/insulin-like growth factor-I and insulin-like growth factor-II messenger ribonucleic acids. Mol Endocrinol 1:233–242, 1987.
42. Hynes MA, Brooks PJ, Van Wyk JJ, et al: Insulin-like growth factor II messenger ribonucleic acids are synthesized in the choroid plexus of the rat brain. Mol Endocrinol 2:47–54, 1988.
43. Schoenle EJ, Haselbacher GK, Briner J, et al: Elevated concentration of IGF-II in brain tissue from an infant with macroencephaly. J Pediatr 108:737–740, 1986.
44. Mohan S, Jennings JC, Linkhart TA, et al: Primary structure of human skeletal growth factor: Homology with human insulin-like growth factor II. Biochim Biophys Acta 961:44–55, 1988.

45. Frolik CA, Ellis EF, Williams DC: Isolation and characterization of insulin-like growth factor II from human bone. Biochem Biophys Res Commun 151:1011–1018, 1988.

46. Murphy LJ, Friesen HG: Differential effects of estrogen and growth hormone on uterine and hepatic insulin-like growth factor I gene expression in the ovariectomized hypophysectomized rat. Endocrinology 122:325–332, 1988.

47. Penhoat A, Naville D, Jaillard C, et al: Hormonal regulation of insulin-like growth factor I secretion by bovine adrenal cells. J Biol Chem 264:6858–6862, 1989.

48. Oliver JE, Aitman TJ, Powell JF, et al: Insulin-like growth factor I gene expression in the rat ovary is confined to the granulosa cells of developing follicles. Endocrinology 124:2671–2679, 1989.

49. Han VK, D'Ercole AJ, Lund PK: Cellular localization of somatomedin (insulin-like growth factor) messenger RNA in the human fetus. Science 236:193–197, 1987.

50. Han VKM, Hill DJ, Strain AJ, et al: Identification of somatomedin/insulin like growth factor immunoreactive cells in the human fetus. Pediatr Res 22:245–249, 1987.

51. Zapf J, Walter H, Froesch ER: Radioimmunological determination of insulin-like growth factors I and II in normal subjects and in patients with growth disorders and extrapancreatic tumor hypoglycemia. J Clin Invest 68:1321–1330, 1981.

52. Underwood LE, Van Wyk JJ: Normal and aberrant growth. *In* Wilson JD, Foster DW (eds): Williams Textbook of Endocrinology (ed 8). Philadelphia, WB Saunders, 1991, pp 1079–1138.

53. Clemmons DR, Van Wyk JJ, Ridgway EC, et al: Evaluation of acromegaly by radioimmunoassay of somatomedin-C. N Engl J Med 301:1138–1142, 1979.

54. Merimee TJ, Zapf J, Froesch ER: Insulin-like growth factors in the fed and fasted states. J Clin Endocrinol Metab 55:99–102, 1982.

55. Clemmons DR, Klibanski A, Underwood LE, et al: Reduction of immunoreactive somatomedin-C during fasting in humans. J Clin Endocrinol Metab 53:1247–1250, 1981.

56. Clemmons DR, Underwood LE, Dickerson RN, et al: Use of plasma somatomedin-C/insulin-like growth factor I response to nutritional repletion in malnourished patients. Am J Clin Nutr 41:191–198, 1985.

57. Van Wyk JJ, Underwood LE, Hintz RL, et al: The somatomedins: A family of insulin-like peptides under growth hormone control. Recent Prog Horm Res 30:259–318, 1974.

58. Chernausek SD, Jacobs S, Van Wyk JJ: Structural similarities between human receptors for somatomedin C and insulin: Analysis by affinity labeling. Biochemistry 20:7345–7350, 1981.

59. Casella SJ, Han VK, D'Ercole AJ, et al: Insulin-like growth factor binding to the type I somatomedin receptor: Evidence for two high affinity binding sites. J Biol Chem 261:9268–9273, 1986.

60. Moxham CP, Duronio V, Jacobs S: Insulin-like growth factor I receptor beta-subunit heterogeneity: Evidence for hybrid tetramers composed of insulin-like growth factor I and insulin receptor heterodimers. J Biol Chem 264:13238–13244, 1989.

61. Ullrich A, Schlessinger J: Signal transduction by receptors with tyrosine kinase activity. Cell 61:203–212, 1990.

62. Clemmons DR, Van Wyk JJ, Pledger WJ: Sequential addition of platelet factor and plasma to BALB/c 3T3 fibroblast cultures stimulates somatomedin-C binding early in the cell cycle. Proc Natl Acad Sci USA 77:6644–6648, 1980.

63. Adashi EY, Resnick CE, Svoboda ME, Van Wyk JJ: Follicle-stimulating hormone enhances somatomedin-C binding to cultured rat granulosa cells. J Biol Chem 261:3923–3926, 1986.

64. Lowe WJ Jr, Adamo M, Werner H, et al: Regulation by fasting of rat insulin-like growth factor I and its receptor: Effects on gene expression and binding. J Clin Invest 84:619–626, 1989.

65. Oshima A, Nolan CM, Kyle JW, et al: The human action-independent mannose 6-phosphate receptor: Cloning and sequence of the full-length cDNA and expression of functional receptor in cos cells. J Biol Chem 263:2553, 1988.

66. Kornfeld S: Trafficking of lysosomal enzymes. FASEB J 1:462, 1987.

67. Kovacina KS, Steele-Perkins G, Purchio AF, et al: Interactions of recombinant and platelet transforming growth factor-B1 precursor with the insulin-like growth factor II/mannose 6-phosphate receptor. Biochem Biophys Res Commun 160:393, 1989.

68. Lee SJ, Nathans D: Proliferin secreted by cultured cells binds to mannose 6-phosphate receptors. J Biol Chem 263:3521, 1988.

69. Okamoto T, Katada T, Murayama Y, et al: A simple structure encodes G protein-activating function of the IGF-II/mannose 6-phosphate receptor. Cell 62:709–717, 1990.

70. Okamoto T, Nishimoto I, Murayama Y, et al: Insulin-like growth factor II/mannose 6-phosphate receptor is incapable of activating GTP-binding proteins in response to mannose 6-phosphate, but capable in response to insulin-like growth factor II. Biochem Biophys Res Commun 168:1201–1210, 1990.

71. Drop SLS: Report on the nomenclature of the IGF binding proteins. Endocrinology 130:1736–1737, 1992.

72. Shimasaki S, Ling N: Identification and molecular characterization of insulin-like growth factor binding proteins (IGFBP-1, -2, -3, -4, -5, and -6). Prog Growth Factor Res 3:243–266, 1992.

73. Clemmons DR: Insulin-like growth factor binding protein control secretion and mechanisms of action. Adv Exp Med Biol 293:113–123, 1991.

74. Clemmons DR: Insulin-like growth factor binding proteins: Roles in regulating IGF physiology. J Dev Physiol 15:105–110, 1991.

75. Drop SLS, Valiquette G, Guyda HJ, et al: Partial purification and characterization of a binding protein for insulin-like activity (ILas) in human amniotic fluid: A possible inhibitor of insulin-like activity. Acta Endocrinol (Copenh) 90:505–518, 1979.

76. Elgin RC, Busby WH, Clemmons DR: An insulin-like growth factor binding protein enhances the biological response to IGF-I. Proc Natl Acad Sci USA 84:3254–3258, 1987.

77. Jones JI, D'Ercole AJ, Camacho-Hübner C, Clemmons DR: Phosphorylation of insulin-like growth factor binding protein 1 in cell culture and in vivo: Effects on affinity for IGF. Proc Natl Acad Sci USA 88:7481–7485, 1991.

78. Chatelain PG, Van Wyk JJ, Copeland KC, et al: Effect of in vitro action of serum proteases or exposure to acid on measurable immunoreactive somatomedin-C in serum. J Clin Endocrinol Metab 56:376–383, 1983.

79. Clemmons DR, Underwood LE, Chatelain PG, Van Wyk JJ: Liberation of immunoreactive somatomedin-C from its binding proteins by proteolytic enzymes and heparin. J Clin Endocrinol Metab 56:384–389, 1983.

80. Brown AL, Chariotti L, Orlowski CC, et al: Nucleotide sequences and expression of a cDNA clone encoding a fetal rat binding protein for insulin-like growth factors. J Biol Chem 264:5148–5154, 1989.

81. Ooi GT, Orlowski CC, Brown AL, et al: Different tissue distribution and hormonal regulation of mRNAs encoding rat insulin-like growth factor binding proteins (IGFBP-1 and IGFBP-2). Mol Endocrinol 4:321–328, 1990.

82. Bar RS, Clemmons DR, Boes M, et al: Transcapillary permeability and subendothelial distribution of endothelial and amniotic fluid IGF binding proteins in rat heart. Endocrinology 127:1078–1086, 1990.

83. Furlanetto RW: Somatomedin-C binding protein: Evidence for a heterologous subunit structure. J Clin Endocrinol Metab 51:12–19, 1980.

84. Clemmons DR, Thissen JP, Maes M, et al: Insulin-like growth factor I (IGF-I) infusion into hypophysectomized or protein-deprived rats induces specific IGF-binding proteins in serum. Endocrinology 125:2967–2972, 1989.

85. Clemmons DR, Thissen JP, Maes M, et al: Insulin-like growth factor-I (IGF-I) infusion into hypophysectomized or protein-deprived rats induces specific IGF-binding proteins in serum. Endocrinology 125:2967–2972, 1993.

86. Blum WF, Ranke MB, Kietzmann K, et al: A specific radioimmunoassay for the growth hormone (GH)-dependent somatomedin-binding protein: Its use for the diagnosis of GH deficiency. J Clin Endocrinol Metab 70:1292–1298, 1990.

87. Mohan S, Bautista CM, Wergedal J, Baylink DJ: Isolation of an inhibitory insulin-like growth factor (IGF) binding protein from bone cell-conditioned medium: A potential local regulator of IGF action. Proc Natl Acad Sci USA 86:8338–8342, 1989.

88. Brar AK, Chernausek SD: Localization of IGF binding protein-4 expression in the developing and adult rat brain: Analysis by in situ hybridization. J Neurosci Res 35:103–114, 1993.

89. Backeljauw PF, Zonghan D, Clemmons DR, D'Ercole AJ: Synthesis and regulation of insulin-like growth factor binding protein-5 in FRTL-5 cells. Endocrinology 132:1677–1681, 1993.

90. Jones JI, Gockerman A, Busby WH, et al: Extracellular matrix contains insulin-like growth factor binding protein-5: Potentiation of the effects of IGF-I. J Cell Biol 121:679–687, 1993.

91. Berelowitz M, Szabo M, Frohman LA, et al: Somatomedin-C mediates growth hormone negative feedback by effects on both the hypothalamus and the pituitary. Science 212:1279–1281, 1981.

92. Yamashita S, Melmed S: Insulin-like growth factor I action on rat anterior pituitary cells: Suppression of growth hormone secretion and messenger ribonucleic acid levels. Endocrinology 118:176, 1986.

93. Nilsson A, Carlsson B, Isgaard J, et al: Regulation by GH of insulin-like growth factor I mRNA expression in rat epiphyseal growth plate as studied with in-situ hybridization. J Endocrinol 125:67–74, 1990.

94. Schoenle E, Zapf J, Humbel RE, Froesch ER: Insulin-like growth factor I stimulates growth in hypophysectomized rats. Nature 296:252–256, 1982.

95. Schoenle E, Zapf J, Froesch ER: Insulin-like growth factors I and II stimulate growth of hypophysectomized rats. Diabetologia 23:199, 1982.

96. Walker JL, Van Wyk JJ, Underwood LE: Stimulation of statural growth by recombinant insulin-like growth factor I in a child with growth hormone insensitivity syndrome (Laron type). J Pediatr 121:641–646, 1992.

97. Van Wyk JJ, Casella SJ, Graves DR, Jacobs S: Evidence from monoclonal antibody studies that insulin stimulates deoxyribonucleic acid synthesis through the type I somatomedin receptor. J Clin Endocrinol Metab 61:639–643, 1985.

98. Pledger WJ, Leof EB, Chou BB, et al: Initiation of cell-cycle traverse by serum-derived growth factors. In Sato GH, Pardee AB, Sirbasku DA (eds): Growth of Cells in Hormonally Defined Media. Cold Spring Harbor Conferences on Cell Proliferation 9:259–273, 1982.

99. Leof EB, Wharton WR, Van Wyk JJ, Pledger WJ: Epidermal growth factor and somatomedin-c regulate G1 progression in competent BALB/c 3T3 cells. Exp Cell Res 141:107–115, 1982.

100. Russell WE, Pledger WJ, Van Wyk JJ: Inhibition of the mitogenic effects of plasma by a monoclonal antibody to somatomedin-C. Proc Natl Acad Sci USA 81:935–939, 1984.

101. Pietrzkowski Z, Sell C, Lammers R, et al: Roles of insulinlike growth factor I (IGF-I) and the IGF-I receptor in epidermal growth factor-stimulated growth of 3T3 cells. Mol Cell Biol 12:3883–3889, 1992.

102. Pietrzkowski Z, Lammers R, Carpenter G, et al: Constitutive expression of IGF-I and IGF-I receptor abrogates all requirements for exogeneous growth factors. Cell Growth Differ 3:199–205, 1992.

103. Takahashi SI, Conti M, Van Wyk JJ: Thyrotropin potentiation of insulin-like growth factor-I dependent deoxyribonucleic acid synthesis in FRTL-5 cells: Mediation by an autocrine amplification factor(s). Endocrinology 126:736–745, 1990.

104. Takahashi SI, Conti M, Prokop C, et al: Thyrotropin and insulin-like growth factor-I regulation of tyrosine phosphorylation in FRTL-5 cells: Interaction between cAMP-dependent and growth factor signal transduction. J Biol Chem 266:7834–7841, 1991.

105. Ewton DZ, Florini JR: Effects of the somatomedins and insulin on myoblast differentiation in vitro. Dev Biol 86:31–39, 1981.

106. Turo KA, Florini JR: Hormonal stimulation of myoblast differentiation in the absence of DNA synthesis. Am J Physiol 243:278–284, 1982.

107. Florini JR, Ewton DZ, Roof SL: Insulin-like growth factor-I stimulates terminal myogenic differentiation by induction of myogenin gene expression. Mol Endocrinol 5:718–724, 1991.

108. Florini JR, Ewton DZ: Highly specific inhibition of IGF-I–stimulated differentiation by an antisense oligodeoxyribonucleotide to myogenin mRNA: No effects on other actions of IGF-I. J Biol Chem 265:13435–13437, 1990.

109. Adashi EY, Resnick CE, Svoboda ME, Van Wyk JJ: A novel role for somatomedin-C in the cytodifferentiation of the ovarian granulosa cell. Endocrinology 155:1227–1229, 1984.

110. Walker JL, Ginalska-Malinowska M, Romer TE, et al: Effects of the infusion of insulin-like growth factor-I in a child with growth hormone insensitivity syndrome (Laron dwarfism). N Engl J Med 21:1483–1488, 1991.

111. Usala A-L, Madigan T, Burguera B, et al: Treatment of insulin-resistant diabetic ketoacidosis with insulin-like growth factor I in an adolescent with insulin dependent diabetes. N Engl J Med 327:853–857, 1992.

112. Kupfer SR, Underwood LE, Baxter RC: Enhancement of the anabolic effects of growth hormone and insulin-like growth factor I by use of both agents simultaneously. J Clin Invest 91:391–396, 1993.

113. Cohen S: Isolation of a mouse submaxillary gland protein accelerating incisor eruption and eyelid opening in the newborn animal. J Biol Chem 237:1555–1562, 1962.

114. Cohen S, Taylor JM: Part I. Epidermal growth factor: Chemical and biological characterization. Recent Prog Horm Res 30:533–550, 1974.

115. Cohen S, Savage CR Jr: Part II. Recent studies of the chemistry and biology of epidermal growth factor. Recent Prog Horm Res 30:551–574, 1974.

116. Carpenter G, Cohen S: Epidermal growth factor. Annu Rev Biochem 48:193–216, 1979.

117. Gregory H: Isolation and structure of urogastrone and its relationship to epidermal growth factor. Nature 257:325–327, 1975.

118. Todaro GJ, Green H: An assay for cellular transformation by SV40. Virology 23:117–119, 1964.

119. Temin HM, Rubin H: Characteristics of an assay for Rous sarcoma virus and Rous sarcoma cells in tissue culture. Virology 6:669–688, 1958.

120. Macpherson I, Montagnier L: Agar suspension culture for the selective assay of cells transformed by polyoma virus. Virology 23:291–294, 1974.

121. Holley RW: Control of growth of kidney epithelial cells in culture. Nature 258:487–490, 1975.

122. Todaro GJ, De Larco JE: Growth factors produced by sarcoma virus-transformed cells. Cancer Res 38:4147–4154, 1978.

123. De Larco JE, Todaro GJ: Growth factors from murine sarcoma virus-transformed cells. Proc Natl Acad Sci USA 75:4001–4005, 1978.

124. Todaro GJ, De Larco JE, Fryling CM: Sarcoma growth factor and other transforming peptides produced by human cells: Interactions with membrane receptors. Fed Proc 41:2996–3003, 1982.

125. Roberts AB, Frolik CA, Anzano MA, Sporn MB: Transforming growth factors from neoplastic and nonneoplastic tissues. Fed Proc 42:2621–2626, 1983.

126. Marquardt H, Hunkapiller MW, Hood LE, Todaro GJ: Rat transforming growth factor type I: Structure and relation to epidermal growth factor. Science 223:1079–1082, 1984.

127. Marquardt H, Hunkapiller MW, Hood LE, et al: Transforming growth factors produced by retrovirus-transformed rodent fibroblasts and human melanoma cells: Amino acid sequence homology with epidermal growth factor. Proc Natl Acad Sci USA 80:4684–4688, 1983.

128. Massagué J: Epidermal growth factor-like transforming growth factor: 1. Isolation, chemical characterization and potentiation by other transforming growth factors from feline sarcoma virus–transformed rat cells. J Biol Chem 258:13607–13613, 1983.

129. Shoyab M, Plowman GD: Purification of amphiregulin from serum-free conditioned medium of 12-O-tetradecanoylphorbol-13-acetate-treated cell lines. Methods Enzymol 198:213–221, 1991.

130. Ciardiello F, Kim N, Saeki T, et al: Differential expression of epidermal growth factor-related proteins in human colorectal tumors. Proc Natl Acad Sci USA 88:7792–7796, 1991.

131. Shoyab M, McDonald VL, Dick K, et al: Amphiregulin-associated protein: Complete amino acid sequence of a protein produced by the 12-O-tetradecanoylphorbol-13-acetate-treated human breast adenocarcinoma cell line MCF-7. Biochem Biophys Res Commun 179:572–578, 1991.

132. Cook PW, Mattox PA, Keeble WW, Shipley GD: Inhibition of autonomous human keratinocyte proliferation and amphiregulin mitogenic activity by sulfated polysaccharides. In Vitro Cell Dev Biol 28A:218–222, 1992.

133. Cook PW, Mattox PA, Keeble WW, et al: A heparin sulfate-regulated human keratinocyte autocrine factor is similar or identical to amphiregulin. Mol Cell Biol 11:2547–2557, 1991.

134. Culouscou JM, Remacle Bonnet M, Carlton GW, et al: Colorectum cell-derived growth factor (CRDGF) is homologous to amphiregulin, a member of the epidermal growth factor family. Growth Factors 7:195–205, 1992.

135. Kimura H, Fischer WH, Schubert D: Structure, expression and function of schwannoma-derived growth factor. Nature 348:257–260, 1990.

136. Bennett KL, Plowman GD, Buckley SD, et al: Regulation of amphiregulin mRNA by TGF-beta in the human lung adenocarcinoma cell line A549. Growth Factors 7:207–213, 1992.

137. Higashiyama S, Abraham JA, Miller J, et al: A heparin-binding growth factor secreted by macrophage-like cells that is related to EGF. Science 251:936–939, 1991.

138. Dono R, Montuori N, Rocchi M, et al: Isolation and characterization of the CRIPTO autosomal gene and its X-linked related sequence. Am J Hum Genet 49:555–565, 1991.

139. Shing Y, Christofori G, Hanahan D, et al: Betacellulin: A novel mitogen from pancreatic β tumor cells. Science 259:1604–1607, 1993.

140. Reisner AH: Similarity between vaccinia virus 19K early protein and epidermal growth factor. Nature 313:801–803, 1985.

141. Carpenter G, Wahl MI: The epidermal growth factor family. In Sporn MB, Roberts AB (eds): Handbook of Experimental Pharmacology, Peptide Growth Factors and Their Receptors. I. Berlin, Springer-Verlag, 1990, pp 69–171.

142. Rall LB, Scott J, Bell GI, et al: Mouse prepro-epidermal growth factor synthesis by the kidney and other tissues. Nature 313:228–231, 1985.

143. Pfeffer S, Ullrich A: Epidermal growth factor: Is the precursor a receptor? Nature 313:184, 1985.

144. Naglich JG, Metherall JE, Russell DW, Eidels L: Expression cloning of a diphtheria toxin receptor: Identity with a heparin-binding EGF-like growth factor precursor. Cell 69:1051–1061, 1992.

145. Bosenberg MW, Pandiella A, Massagué J: The cytoplasmic carboxy-terminal amino acid specifies cleavage of membrane TGF-α into soluble growth factor. Cell 71:1157–1165, 1992.

146. Brachmann R, Lindquist PB, Nagashima M, et al: Transmembrane TGF-alpha precursors activate EGF/TGF-alpha receptors. Cell 56:691–700, 1989.

147. Aklesaria P, Teixidó J, Laiho M, et al: Cell-cell adhesion mediated by binding of membrane-anchored transforming growth factor α to epidermal growth factor receptors promotes cell proliferation. Proc Natl Acad Sci USA 87:3289–3293, 1990.

148. Cohen S, Ushiro H, Stoscheck C, Chinkers M: A native 170,000 epidermal growth factor receptor-kinase complex from shed plasma membrane vesicles. J Biol Chem 257:1523–1531, 1982.

149. Yarden Y, Schlessinger J: Epidermal growth factor induces rapid, reversible aggregation of the purified epidermal growth factor receptor. Biochemistry 26:1443–1451, 1987.

150. Wahl M, Nishibe S, Suh PG, et al: Epidermal growth factor stimulates tyrosine phosphorylation of phospholipase C-II independently of receptor internalization and extracellular calcium. Proc Natl Acad Sci USA 86:1568–1572, 1989.

151. Ellis C, Moran M, McCormick F, Pawson T: Phosphorylation of GAP and GAP-associated proteins by transforming and mitogenic tyrosine kinases. Nature 343:377–381, 1990.

152. Margolis B, Rhee SG, Felder S, et al: EGF induces tyrosine phosphorylation of phospholipase C-II: A potential mechanism for receptor signalling. Cell 57:1101–1107, 1989.

153. Waksman G, Kominos D, Robertson SC, et al: Crystal structure of the phosphotyrosine recognition domain SH2 of v-src complexed with tyrosine-phosphorylated peptides. Nature 358:646–653, 1992.

154. Petsko GA: Fishing in Src-infested waters. Nature 358:625–626, 1992.

155. Murdoch GH, Potter E, Nicolaisen AK, et al: Epidermal growth factor rapidly stimulates prolactin gene transcription. Nature 300:192–194, 1982.

156. Goodman R, Slater E, Herschman HR: Epidermal growth factor induces tyrosine hydroxylase in a clonal pheochromocytoma cell line, PC-G2. J Cell Biol 84:495–500, 1980.

157. Ebner R, Derynck R: Epidermal growth factor and transforming growth factor-α: Differential intracellular routing and processing of ligand-receptor complexes. Cell Regul 2:599–612, 1991.

158. Countaway JL, McQuilkin P, Girones N, Davis RJ: Multisine phosphorylation of the epidermal growth factor receptor. J Biol Chem 265:3407–3416, 1990.

159. Downward J, Yarden Y, Mayes E, et al: Close similarity of epidermal growth factor receptor and v-erb-B oncogene protein sequences. Nature 307:521–527, 1984.

160. Sistonen L, Holtta E, Lehvaslaiho H, et al: Activation of the neu tyrosine kinase induces the Fos/Jun transcription factor complex, the glucose transporter and ornithine decarboxylase. J Cell Biol 109:1911–1919, 1989.

161. King CR, Borrello I, Bellot F, et al: EGF binding to its receptor triggers a rapid tyrosine phosphorylation of the erB-2 protein in the mammary tumour cell line SK-BR-3. EMBO J 7:1647–1651, 1988.

162. Gullick WJ, Berger MS, Bennett PL, et al: Expression of the c-erb-2 protein in normal and transformed cells. Int J Cancer 40:246–254, 1987.

163. Quirke P, Pickles A, Tuzi NL, et al: Pattern of expression of c-erbB-2 oncoprotein in human fetuses. Br J Cancer 60:64–69, 1989.

164. Weiner DB, Liu J, Cohen JA, et al: A point mutation in the neu oncogene mimics ligand induction of receptor aggregation. Nature 339:230–231, 1989.

165. Marchionni MA, Goodearl ADJ, Chen MS, et al: Glial growth factors are alternatively spliced erbB2 ligands expressed in the nervous system. Nature 362:312–318, 1993.

166. Falls DL, Rosen KM, Corfas G, et al: ARIA, a protein that simulates acetylcholine receptor synthesis, is a member of the neu ligand family. Cell 72:801–815, 1993.

167. Holmes WE, Sliwkowski MX, Akita RW, et al: Identification of Heregulin, a specific activator of p185erbB2. Science 256:1205–1210, 1992.

168. Kraus MH, Issing W, Miki T, et al: Isolation and characterisation of EFBB3, a third member of the ERBB/epidermal growth factor receptor family: Evidence for overexpression in a subset of human mammary tumors. Proc Natl Acad Sci USA 86:9193–9197, 1989.

169. Shoyab M, Plowman GD, McDonald VL, et al: Structure and function of human amphiregulin: A member of the epidermal growth factor family. Science 243:1074–1076, 1989.

170. Barka T, van der Noen H, Greski EW, Kerenyi T: Immunoreactive epidermal growth factor in human amniotic fluid. Mt Sinai J Med 45:679–684, 1978.

171. Sundell H, Serenius RS, Barthe PL, et al: Effect of EGF on fetal lamb lung maturation. Pediatr Res 9:371–376, 1975.

172. Catterton WZ, Escobedo MB, Sexson WR, et al: Effect of epidermal growth factor on lung maturation in fetal rabbits. Pediatr Res 13:104–108, 1979.

173. Pratt RM, Yoneda T, Silver MH, Solomon DS: Involvement of glucocorticoids and EGF in secondary palate development. In Pratt RM, Christiansen RL (eds): Current Research Trends in Prenatal Craniofacial Development. New York, Elsevier/North Holland, 1980, pp 235–252.

174. Kronmiller JE, Upholt WB, Kollar EJ: EGF antisense oligonucleotides block murine odontogenesis in vitro. Dev Biol 147:485–488, 1991.

175. Read LC, Upton FM, Francis GL, et al: Changes in the growth-promoting activity of human milk during lactation. Pediatr Res 18:133–139, 1984.

176. Goodlad RA, Wilson TGJ, Lenton W, et al: Proliferative effects of urogastrone-EGF on the intestinal epithelium. Gut 28:37–43, 1987.

177. Kirkegaard P, Olsen PS, Poulsen SS, Nexo E: Epidermal growth factor inhibits cysteamine-induced duodenal ulcers. Gastroenterology 85:1277–1283, 1983.

178. Barthe PL, Bullock LP, Monszowicz I, et al: Submaxillary gland epidermal growth factor: A sensitive index of biologic androgen activity. Endocrinology 95:1019–1025, 1974.

179. Hoath SB, Lakshmanan J, Scott SM, Fisher DA: Effect of thyroid hormones on epidermal growth concentration in neonatal mouse skin. Endocrinology 112:308–314, 1983.

180. Rappolee DA, Brenner CA, Schultz R, et al: Developmental expression of PDGF, TGF-a genes in preimplantation mouse embryos. Science 241:1823–1825, 1988.

181. Lee DC, Rochford R, Todaro GJ, Villarreal LP: Developmental expression of rat transforming growth factor-α mRNA. Mol Cell Biol 5:3644–3646, 1985.

182. Brown PI, Lam R, Lakshmanan J, Fisher DA: Transforming growth factor alpha in developing rats. Am J Physiol 259:E256–E260, 1990.

183. Samsoondar J, Kobrin JS, Kudlow JE: Alpha transforming growth factor secreted by untransformed bovine anterior pituitary cells in culture. Int J Biochem 261:14408–14413, 1986.

184. Kommos F, Wintzer HO, Von Kleist S, et al: In situ distribution of transforming growth factor alpha in normal tissues and in malignant tumours of the ovary. J Pathol 162:223–230, 1990.

185. Schultz GS, White M, Mitchell R, et al: Epithelial wound healing enhanced by transforming growth factor-alpha and vaccinia growth factor. Science 235:350–352, 1987.

186. Schreiber AB, Winkler ME, Derynck R: Transforming growth factor-α: A more potent angiogenic mediator than epidermal growth factor. Science 232:1250–1253, 1986.

187. Ibbotson KJ, Harrod J, Gowen M, et al: Human recombinant transforming growth factor-alpha stimulates bone resorption and inhibits formation in vitro. Proc Natl Acad Sci USA 75:4001–4005, 1978.

188. Elder JT, Fisher GJ, Lindquist PB, et al: Overexpression of transforming growth factor alpha in psoriatic epidermis. Science 243:811–813, 1989.

189. Polk WH, Dempsey PJ, Russell WE, et al: Increased production of transforming growth factor alpha following acute gastric mucosal injury. Gastroenterology 102:1467–1474, 1992.

190. Dempsey PJ, Goldenring JR, Soroka CJ, et al: Possible role of transforming growth factor α in the pathogenesis of Ménétrier's disease: Supportive evidence from humans and transgenic mice. Gastroenterology 103:1950–1963, 1992.

191. Matsui Y, Halter SA, Holt JT, et al: Development of mammary hyperplasia and neoplasia in MMTV-TGFα transgenic mice. Cell 61:1147–1155, 1990.

192. Jhappan C, Stahle C, Harkins RN, et al: TFGα overexpression in transgenic mice induces liver neoplasia and abnormal development of the mammary gland and pancreas. Cell 61:1137–1146, 1990.

193. Sandgren EP, Luetteke NC, Palmiter RD, et al: Overexpression of TGFα in transgenic mice: Induction of epithelial hyperplasia, pancreatic metaplasia, and carcinoma of the breast. Cell 61:1121–1135, 1990.

194. Plowman GD, Green JM, McDonald VL, et al: The amphiregulin gene encodes a novel epidermal growth factor–related protein with tumor-inhibitory activity. Mol Cell Biol 10:1969–1981, 1990.

195. Cook PW, Pittelkow MR, Keeble WW, et al: Amphiregulin messenger RNA is elevated in psoriatic epidermis and gastrointestinal carcinomas. Cancer Res 52:3224–3227, 1992.

196. Saeki T, Stromberg K, Qi CF, et al: Differential immunohistochemical detection of amphiregulin and cripto in human normal colon and colorectal tumors. Cancer Res 52:3467–3473, 1992.

197. Roberts AB, Sporn MB: The transforming growth factor-betas. In Sporn MB, Roberts AB (eds): Peptide Growth Factors and Their Receptors. Berlin, Springer-Verlag, 1990, pp 419–472.

198. Barnard JA, Lyons RM, Moses HL: The cell biology of transforming-growth factor β. Biochim Biophys Acta 1032:79–87, 1990.

199. Derynck R, Lindquist PB, Lee A, et al: A new type of transforming growth factor-beta, TGF-beta 3. EMBO J 7:3737–3743, 1988.

200. Moses HL, Branum EB, Proper JA, Robinson RA: Transforming growth factor production by chemically transformed cells. Cancer Res 41:2842–2848, 1981.

201. Roberts AB, Anzano MA, Lamb LC, et al: New class of transforming growth factors potentiated by epidermal growth factor: Isolation from non-neoplastic tissues. Proc Natl Acad Sci USA 78:5339–5343, 1981.

202. Roberts AB, Anzano MA, Lamb LC, et al: Isolation from murine sarcoma cells of novel transforming growth factors potentiated by EGF. Nature 295:417–419, 1982.

203. Roberts AB, Frolik CA, Anzano MA, Sporn MB: Transforming growth factors from neoplastic and nonneoplastic tissues. Fed Proc 42:2621–2626, 1983.

204. Childs CB, Proper JA, Tucker RF, Moses HL: Serum contains a platelet-derived transforming growth factor. Proc Natl Acad Sci USA 79:5312–5316, 1982.

205. Cheifetz S, Weatherbee JA, Tsang ML, et al: The transforming growth factor-beta system, a complex pattern of cross-reactive ligands and receptors. Cell 48:409–415, 1987.

206. Holley RW, Armour R, Baldwin JH: Density-dependent regulation of growth of BSC-1 cells in cell culture: Growth inhibitors formed by the cells. Proc Natl Acad Sci USA 75:1864–1866, 1978.

207. Hanks SK, Armour R, Baldwin JH, et al: Amino acid sequence of the BSC-1 cell growth inhibitor (polyergin) deduced from the nucleotide sequence of the cDNA. Proc Natl Acad Sci USA 85:79–82, 1988.

208. Schlunegger MP, Grütter MG: An unusual feature revealed by the crystal structure at 2.2Å resolution of human transforming growth factor-β2. Nature 358:430–434, 1992.

209. Daopin S, Piez KA, Ogawa Y, Davies DR: Crystal structure of transforming growth factor-β2: An unusual fold for the superfamily. Science 257:369–373, 1992.

210. Mason AJ, Hayflick JS, Ling N, et al: Complementary DNA sequences of ovarian follicular fluid inhibin show precursor structure and homology with transforming growth factor-β. Nature 318:659–663, 1985.

211. McLachlan RI, Robertson DM, DeKretser DM, Burger HG: Advances in the physiology of inhibin and inhibin-related peptides. Clin Endocrinol 29:77–114, 1988.

212. Vale W, Rivier J, Vaughan J, et al: Purification and characterization of an FSH releasing protein from porcine ovarian follicular fluid. Nature 321:776–779, 1986.

213. Ling N, Ying S, Ueno N, et al: Pituitary FSH is released by a heterodimer of the B-subunits from the two forms of inhibin. Nature 321:779–782, 1986.

214. Lin T, Calkins JH, Morris PL, et al: Regulation of Leydig cell function in primary culture by inhibin and activin. Endocrinology 125:2134–2140, 1989.

215. Gonzalez-Manchon C, Vale W: Activin-A, inhibin and transforming growth factor-beta modulate growth of two gonadal cell lines. Endocrinology 125:1666–1672, 1989.

216. Yu J, Shao L, Vaughn J, et al: Characterization of the potentiation effect of activin on human erythroid colony formation in vitro. Blood 73:952–960, 1989.

217. Vale W, Rivier C, Hsueh A, et al: Chemical and biological characterization of the inhibin family of protein hormones. Recent Prog Horm Res 44:1–34, 1988.

218. Smith JC, Price BMJ, Van Nimmen K, et al: Identification of a potent Xenopus mesoderm-inducing factor as a homologue of activin A. Nature 345:729–731, 1990.

219. Van den Eiden-Van Raaij AJM, Van Zoelent JJ, Van Nimmen K, et al: Activin-like factor from a Xenopus laevis cell line responsible for mesoderm induction. Nature 345:732–734, 1990.

220. Lillie F: Theory of the freemartin. Science 43:611–613, 1916.

221. Jost A, Vigier B, Prepin J, Perchellet JP: Studies on sex differentiation in mammals. Recent Prog Horm Res 29:1–41, 1973.

222. Picard JY, Josso N: Anti-müllerian hormone: Estimation of molecular weight by gel filtration. Biomedicine 25:147–150, 1976.

223. Cate RL, Mattaliano RJ, Hession C, et al: Isolation of the bovine and human genes for müllerian inhibiting substance and expression of the human gene in animal cells. Cell 45:685–698, 1986.

224. Pepinsky RB, Sinclair LK, Chow EP, et al: Proteolytic processing of müllerian inhibiting substance produces a transforming growth factor-β–like fragment. J Biol Chem 263:18961–18964, 1988.

225. MacLaughlin DT, Hudson PL, Graciano AL, et al: Müllerian duct regression and antiproliferative bioactivities of müllerian inhibiting substance reside in its carboxy-terminal domain. Endocrinology 131:291–296, 1992.

226. Baker ML, Metcalfe SA, Hutson JM: Serum levels of müllerian inhibiting substance in boys from birth to 18 years, as determined by enzyme immunoassay. J Clin Endocrinol Metab 70:11–15, 1990.

227. Coughlin JP, Donahoe PK, Budzik GP, MacLaughlin DT: Müllerian inhibiting substance blocks autophosphorylation of the EGF receptor by inhibiting tyrosine kinase. Mol Cell Biol 49:75–86, 1987.

228. Urist MR: Bone: Formation by autoinduction. Science 150:893–899, 1965.

229. Urist MR, Mikulski A, Lietze A: Solubilized and insolubilized bone morphogenetic protein. Proc Natl Acad Sci USA 76:1828–1832, 1979.

230. Wozney JM, Rosen V, Celeste AJ, et al: Novel regulators of bone formation: Molecular clones and activities. Science 242:1528–1533, 1988.

231. Weeks DL, Melton DA: A maternal mRNA localized to the vegetal hemisphere in xenopus eggs codes for a growth factor related to TGF-beta. Cell 51:861–867, 1987.

232. Lyons K, Graycar JL, Lee A, et al: Vgr-1, a mammalian gene related to Xenopus Vg-1, is a member of the transforming growth factor bete gene superfamily. Proc Natl Acad Sci USA 86:4554–4558, 1989.

233. Padgett RW, St Johnston RD, Gelbart WM: A transcript from a Drosophila pattern gene predicts a protein homologous to the transforming growth factor-β family. Nature 325:81–84, 1987.

234. Derynck R, Rhee L, Chen EY, VanTilburg A: Intron-exon structure of the human transforming growth factor beta precursor gene. Nucleic Acids Res 15:3188–3189, 1987.

235. Wakefield LM, Smith DM, Masui T, et al: Distribution and modulation of the cellular receptor for transforming growth factor-beta. J Cell Biol 105:965–975, 1987.

236. Wakefield LM, Winokur TS, Hollands RS, et al: Recombinant latent transforming growth factor β1 has a longer plasma half-life in rats than active transforming growth factor β1, and a different tissue distribution. J Clin Invest 86:1976–1984, 1990.

237. Kanzaki T, Olofsson A, Moren A, et al: TGF-β1 binding protein: A component of the large latent complex of TGF-β1 with multiple repeat sequences. Cell 61:1051–1061, 1990.

238. O'Connor-McCourt MD, Wakefield LM: Latent transforming growth factor-beta in serum: A specific complex with alpha-2-macroglobulin. J Biol Chem 262:14090–14099, 1987.

239. Pircher R, Jullien P, Lawrence DA: β-Transforming growth factor is stored in human blood platelets as a latent high molecular weight complex. Biochem Biophys Res Commun 136:30–37, 1986.

240. Lyons RM, Keski-Oja J, Moses HL: Proteolytic activation of latent transforming growth factor-beta from fibroblast-conditioned medium. J Cell Biol 106:1659–1665, 1988.

241. Sato Y, Rifkin DB: Inhibition of endothelial cell movement by pericytes and smooth muscle cells: Activation of a latent transforming growth factor beta-1 like molecule by plasmin during co-culture. J Cell Biol 109:309–315, 1989.

242. Dennis PA, Rifkin DB: Cellular activation of latent transforming growth factor β requires binding to the cation-independent mannose 6-phosphate/insulin-like growth factor type II receptor. Proc Natl Acad Sci USA 88:580–584, 1991.

243. Segarini PR, Seyedin SM: The high molecular weight receptor to transforming growth factor-beta contains glycosaminoglycan chains. J Biol Chem 263:8366–8370, 1988.

244. Wang XF, Lin HY, Ng-Eaton E, et al: Expression cloning and characterization of the TGF-β type III receptor. Cell 67:797–805, 1991.

245. Lin HY, Wang XF, Ng-Eaton E, et al: Expression cloning of the TGF-β type II receptor, a functional transmembrane serine/threonine kinase. Cell 68:775–785, 1992.

246. Ebner R, Chen R-H, Shum L, et al: Cloning of a type I TGF-β receptor and its effect on TGF-β binding to the type II receptor. Science 260:1344–1348, 1993.

247. Wrana JL, Attisano L, Cárcamo J, et al: TGFβ signals through a heteromeric protein kinase receptor complex. Cell 71:1003–1014, 1992.

248. Chen R-H, Ebner R, Derynck R: Inactivation of the type II receptor reveals two receptor pathways for the diverse TGF-β activities. Science 260:1335–1338, 1993.

249. Leof EB, Proper JA, Goustin AS, et al: Induction of c-sis mRNA and activity similar to platelet-derived growth factor by transforming growth factor beta: A proposed model for indirect mitogenesis involving autocrine activity. Proc Natl Acad Sci USA 83:2453–2457, 1986.

250. Shipley GD, Pittelkow MR, Willie JJ Jr, et al: Reversible inhibition of normal human prokeratinocyte proliferation by type beta transforming growth factor-growth inhibitor in serum-free medium. Cancer Res 46:2068–2071, 1986.

251. Russell WE: Transforming growth factor beta (TGF-B) inhibits hepatocyte DNA synthesis independently of EGF binding and EGF receptor autophosphorylation. J Cell Physiol 135:253–261, 1988.

252. Moses HL, Pietenpol JA, Münger K, et al: TGFβ regulation of epithelial cell proliferation: Role of tumor suppressor genes. In Harris CC, et al (eds): Multistage Carcinogenesis. Tokyo, Japan Sci Soc Press/CRC Press, 1992, pp 183–195.

253. Pietenpol JA, Stein RW, Moran E, et al: TGF-β1 inhibition of c-myc transcription and growth in keratinocytes is abrogated by viral transforming proteins with pRB binding domains. Cell 61:777–785, 1990.

254. Gerschenson LE, Rotello RJ: Apoptosis: A different type of cell death. FASEB J 6:2450–2455, 1992.

255. Bursch W, Lauer B, Timmermann-Trosiener I, et al: Controlled cell death (apoptosis) of normal and putative preneoplastic cells in rat liver following withdrawal of tumor promoters. Carcinogenesis (Lond) 5:453–458, 1984.

256. Oberhammer FA, Pavelka M, Sharma S, et al: Induction of apoptosis in cultured hepatocytes and in regressing liver by transforming growth factor β1. Proc Natl Acad Sci USA 89:5408–5412, 1992.

257. Carr BI, Hayashi I, Branum EL, Moses HL: Inhibition of DNA synthesis in rat hepatocytes by platelet-derived type B transforming growth factor. Cancer Res 46:2330–2334, 1986.

258. McMahon JB, Richards WL, del Campo AA, et al: Differential effects of transforming growth factor-B on proliferation of normal and malignant rat liver epithelial cells in culture. Cancer Res 46:4665–4671, 1986.

259. Russell WE, Coffey RJ Jr, Ouellette AJ, Moses HL: Type β transforming growth factor reversibly inhibits the early proliferative response to partial hepatectomy in the rat. Proc Natl Acad Sci USA 85:5126–5130, 1988.

260. Schackert HK, Fand D, Fidler IJ: Transient inhibition of liver regeneration in mice by transforming growth factor-beta I encapsulated in liposomes. Cancer Commun 2:165–171, 1990.

261. Lippman ME, Dickson RB, Gelmann EP, et al: Growth regulation of human breast carcinoma occurs through regulated growth factor secretion. J Cell Biochem 35:1–16, 1987.

262. Silberstein GB, Daniel CW: Reversible inhibition of mammary gland growth by transforming growth factor-B. Science 237:291–293, 1987.

263. Raghow R, Postlethwaite AE, Keski-Oja J, et al: Transforming growth factor-beta increases steady state levels of type I procollagen and fibronectin messenger RNAs. J Clin Invest 79:1285–1288, 1987.

264. Matrisian LM, Hogan BLM: Growth factor-regulated proteases and extracellular matrix remodeling during mammalian development. Curr Top Dev Biol 24:219–259, 1990.

265. Keski-Oja J, Raghow R, Sawdey M, et al: Regulation of mRNAs for type-1 plasminogen activator inhibitor, fibronectin, and type I procollagen by transforming growth factor-beta: Divergent responses in lung fibroblasts and carcinoma cells. J Biol Chem 263:3111–3115, 1988.

266. Ignotz RA, Heino J, Massagué J: Regulation of cell adhesion receptors by transforming growth factor-beta: Regulation of vitronectin receptor and LFA-1. J Biol Chem 264:389–392, 1989.

267. Tucker RF, Volkenant ME, Branum EL, Moses HL: Comparison of intra- and extracellular transforming growth factors from nontransformed and chemically transformed mouse embryo cells. Cancer Res 43:1581–1586, 1983.

268. Kehrl JH, Wakefield LM, Roberts AB, et al: Production of transforming growth factor beta by human T lymphocytes and its potential role in the regulation of T cell growth. J Exp Med 163:1037–1050, 1986.

269. de Martin R, Haendler B, Hofer-Warbinek R, et al: Complementary DNA for human glioblastoma-derived T cell suppressor factor, a novel member of the transforming growth factor-beta gene family. EMBO J 6:3673–3677, 1987.

270. Akhurst RJ, FitzPatrick DR, Gatherer D, et al: Transforming growth factor betas in mammalian embryogenesis. Prog Growth Factor Res 2:153–168, 1990.

271. Pelton RW, Hogan BLM, Miller DA, Moses HL: Differential expression of genes encoding TGFs β1, β2, and β3 during murine palate formation. Dev Biol 141:456–460, 1990.

272. Pelton RW, Saxena B, Jones M, et al: Immunohistochemical localization of TGF-β1, TGF-β2, and TGF-β3 in the mouse embryo: Expression patterns suggest multiple roles during embryonic development. J Cell Biol 115:1091–1105, 1991.

273. Balk SD: Calcium as a regulator of the proliferation of normal, but not transformed, chicken fibroblasts in plasma-containing medium. Proc Natl Acad Sci USA 68:271–275, 1971.

274. Ross R, Glomset J, Kariya B, Harker L: Platelet-dependent serum factor that stimulates the proliferation of arterial smooth muscle cells in vitro. Proc Natl Acad Sci USA 71:1207–1210, 1974.

275. Assoian RK, Komoriya A, Meyers CA, et al: Transforming growth factor-beta in human platelets: Identification of a major storage site, purification, and characterization. J Biol Chem 258:7155–7160, 1983.

276. Childs BJ, Proper JA, Tucker RF, Moses HL: Serum contains a platelet-derived transforming growth factor. Proc Natl Acad Sci USA 79:5312–5316, 1982.

277. Russell WE, McGowan JA, Bucher NLR: Partial characterization of a hepatocyte growth factor from rat platelets. J Cell Physiol 119:183–192, 1984.

278. Russell WE, McGowan JA, Bucher NLR: Biological properties of a hepatocyte growth factor from rat platelets. J Cell Physiol 119:193–197, 1984.

279. Nakamura T, Nawa K, Ichihara A, et al: Purification and subunit structure of hepatocyte growth factor from rat platelets. FEBS Lett 224:311–316, 1987.

280. Heldin C-H, Westermark B, Wasteson A: Platelet-derived growth factor: Purification and partial characterization. Proc Natl Acad Sci USA 76:3722–3726, 1979.

281. Antoniades HN: Human platelet-derived growth factor (PDGF): Purification of PDGF-I and PDGF-II and separation of their reduced subunits. Proc Natl Acad Sci USA 78:7314–7317, 1981.

282. Deuel TF, Huang JS, Proffitt RT, et al: Human platelet-derived growth factor—purification and resolution into two active protein fractions. J Biol Chem 256:8896–8899, 1981.

283. Hart CE, Bailey M, Curtis DA, et al: Purification of PDGF-AB and PDGF-BB from human platelet extracts and identification of all three PDGF dimers in human platelets. Biochemistry 29:166–172, 1990.

284. Heldin C-H, Johnsson AB, Wennegren S, et al: A human osteosarcoma cell line secretes a growth factor structurally related to a homodimer of PDGF A-chains. Nature 319:511–514, 1986.

285. Doolittle RF, Hunkapillar MW, Hood LE, et al: Simian sarcoma virus oncogene, v-sis, is derived from the gene (or genes) encoding a platelet-derived growth factor. Science 221:275–277, 1983.

286. Waterfield MD, Scrace GT, Whittle N, et al: Platelet-derived growth factor is structurally related to the putative transforming protein p28sis of simian sarcoma virus. Nature 304:35–39, 1983.

287. Doolittle RF, Hunkapiller MW, Hood LE, et al: Simian sarcoma virus oncogene, v-sis, is derived from the gene (or genes) encoding a platelet-derived growth factor. Science 221:275–277, 1983.

288. Betscholtz C, Johnson A, Heldin C-H, et al: cDNA sequence and chromosomal localization of human platelet-derived growth factor A-chain and its expression in tumor cell lines. Nature 320:695–699, 1986.

289. Östman A, Rall L, Hammacher A, et al: Synthesis and assembly of a functionally active recombinant platelet-derived growth factor AB heterodimer. J Biol Chem 263:16202–16208, 1988.

290. Thyberg J, Östman A, Bäckström G, et al: Localization of platelet-derived growth factor (PDGF) in CHO cells transfected with A- or B-chain cDNA: Retention of PDGF-BB in the endoplasmic reticulum and Golgi complex. J Cell Sci 97:219–229, 1990.

291. Raines EW, Ross R: Compartment of PDGF on extracellular binding sites dependent on exon-6-encoded sequences. J Cell Biol 116:533–543, 1992.

292. Östman A, Andersson M, Betsholtz C, et al: Identification of a cell retention signal in the B-chain of platelet-derived growth factor and in the long splice version of the A-chain. Cell Regul 2:503–512, 1991.

293. Heldin C-H, Westermark B, Wasteson A: Specific receptors for platelet-derived growth factor on cells derived from connective tissue and glia. Proc Natl Acad Sci USA 78:3664–3668, 1981.

294. Glenn K, Bowen-Pope DF, Ross R: Platelet-derived growth factor: 3. Identification of a platelet-derived growth factor receptor by affinity labeling. J Biol Chem 257:5172–5176, 1982.

295. Singh JP, Chaikin MA, Stiles CD: Phylogenetic analysis of platelet-derived growth factor by radioreceptor assay. J Cell Biol 95:667–671, 1982.

296. Olashaw NE, Olson JE, Drozdoff V, Pledger WJ: Growth factors: Their role in the control of cell proliferation. *In* Molecular and Cellular Approaches to the Control of Proliferation and Differentiation. New York, Academic Press, 1992, pp 3–27.

297. Heldin C-H, Ernlund A, Rorsman C, Ronnstrand L: Dimerization of B-type platelet-derived growth factor receptor occurs after ligand binding and is closely associated with receptor kinase activation. J Biol Chem 264:8905–8912, 1989.

298. Heldin C-H, Bäckström G, Östman A, et al: Binding of different dimeric forms of PDGF to human fibroblasts: Evidence for two separate receptor types. EMBO J 7:1387–1393, 1988.

299. Hart CE, Forstrom JW, Kelly JD, Seifert RA, et al: Two classes of pDGF receptor recognize different isoforms of pDGF. Science 240:1529–1531, 1988.

300. Hosang M, Rouge M, Wipf B, et al: Both homodimeric isoforms of PDGF (AA and BB) have mitogenic and chemotactic activity and stimulate phosphoinositol turnover. J Cell Physiol 140:558–564, 1989.

301. Nistér M, Hammacher A, Mellström K, et al: A glioma-derived PDGF A chain homodimer has different functional activities from a PDGF AB heterodimer purified from human platelets. Cell 52:791–799, 1988.

302. Armelin HA, Armelin MC, Kelly K, et al: Functional role for c-myc in mitogenic response to platelet-derived growth factor. Nature 310:655–660, 1984.

303. Kaczmarek L, Hyland JK, Watt R, et al: Microinjected c-myc as a competence factor. Science 228:1313–1316, 1985.

304. Herman B, Pledger WJ: Platelet-derived growth factor-induced alterations in vinculin and actin distribution in BALB/c-3t3. J Cell Biol 100:1031–1041, 1985.

305. Habenicht AJR, Glomset JA, King WC, et al: Early changes in phosphatidylinositol and arachidonic acid metabolism in quiescent Swiss 3t3 cells stimulated by platelet-derived growth factor. J Biol Chem 256:12329–12335, 1981.

306. Ross R, Glomset JA: The pathogenesis of atherosclerosis. N Engl J Med 295:369–377, 1976.

307. Antoniades HN: PDGF: A multifunctional growth factor. Baillière's Clin Endocrinol Metab 5:595–613, 1991.

308. Baird A, Walicke PA: Fibroblast growth factors. Br Med Bull 45:438–452, 1989.

309. Gospodarowicz D, Bialecki H, Greenburg G: Purification of the fibroblast growth factor activity from bovine brain. J Biol Chem 253:3736–3743, 1978.

310. Gospodarowicz D: Purification of a fibroblast growth factor from bovine pituitary. J Biol Chem 250:2515–2520, 1975.

311. Benharroch D, Birnbaum D: Biology of the fibroblast growth factor gene family. Isr J Med Sci 26:212–219, 1990.

312. Dickson C, Deed R, Dixon M, Peters G: The structure and function of the Int-2 oncogene. Prog Growth Factor Res 1:123–132, 1989.

313. Paterno GD, Gillespie LL: Fibroblast growth factor and transforming growth factor beta in early embryonic development. Prog Growth Factor Res 1:79–88, 1989.

314. Niswander L, Martin GR: FGF-4 and BMP-2 have opposite effects on limb growth. Nature 361:68–71, 1993.

315. Delli-Bovi P, Curatola AM, Newman KM, et al: Processing, secretion, and biological properties of a novel growth factor of the fibroblast growth factor family with oncogenic potential. Mol Cell Biol 8:2933–2941, 1988.

316. Quarto N, Talarico D, Sommer A, et al: Transformation by basic fibroblast growth factor requires high levels of expression: Comparison with transformation by hst/K-fgf. Oncogene Res 5:101–110, 1989.

317. Rubin JS, Osada H, Finch PW, et al: Purification and characterization of a newly identified growth factor specific for epithelial cells. Proc Natl Acad Sci USA 86:802–806, 1989.

318. Boehlen P, Baird A, Esch F, et al: Isolation and partial molecular characterization of pituitary fibroblast growth factor. Proc Natl Acad Sci USA 81:5364–5368, 1984.

319. Burgess WH, Maciag T: The heparin-binding (fibroblast) growth factor family of proteins. Annu Rev Biochem 58:575–606, 1989.

320. Mignatti P, Morimoto T, Rifkin DB: Basic fibroblast growth factor, a protein devoid of secretory signal sequence, is released by cells via a pathway independent of the endoplasmic reticulum–Golgi complex. J Cell Physiol 151:81–93, 1992.

321. Rifkin DB, Moscatelli D, Bizik J, et al: Growth factor control of extracellular proteolysis. Cell Differ Dev 32:313–318, 1990.

322. Dionne CA, Crumley G, Bellot F, et al: Cloning and expression of two distinct high-affinity receptors cross-reacting with acidic and basic fibroblast growth factors. EMBO J 9:2685–2692, 1990.

323. Xu J, Nakahara M, Crabb JW, et al: Expression and immunochemical analysis of rat and human fibroblast growth factor receptor (flg) isoforms. J Biol Chem 267:17792–17803, 1992.

324. Bottaro DP, Rubin JS, Ron D, et al: Characterization of the receptor for ketatinocyte growth factor: Evidence for multiple fibroblast growth factor receptors. J Biol Chem 265:12767–12770, 1990.

325. Gospodarowicz D, Greene G, Moran J: Fibroblast growth factor can substitute for platelet factor to sustain the growth of BALB/c3T3 cells in the presence of plasma. Biochem Biophys Res Commun 65:779–787, 1975.

326. Gospodarowicz D, Mescher AL: Fibroblast growth factor and vertebrate regeneration. Adv Neurol 29:149–171, 1981.

327. Gospodarowicz D, Bialecki H: Effects of epidermal and fibroblast growth factors on replicative life span of cultured bovine granulosa cells. Endocrinology 103:854–865, 1978.

328. Gospodarowicz D, Vlodavsky I, Savion N: The role of fibroblast growth factor and the extracellular matrix in the control of proliferation and differentiation of corneal endothelial cells. Vision Res 21:87–103, 1981.

329. Folkman J: Tumor angiogenesis. Adv Cancer Res 43:175–203, 1985.

330. Shing Y, Folkman J, Haudenschild C, et al: Angiogenesis is stimulated by a tumor-derived endothelial cell growth factor. J Cell Biochem 29:275–287, 1985.

331. Broadley KN, Aquino AM, Woodward SC, et al: Monospecific antibodies implicate basic fibroblast growth factor in normal wound repair. Lab Invest 61:571–575, 1989.

332. Levi-Montalcini R, Hamburger V: Selective growth stimulating effects of mouse sarcoma on the sensory and sympathetic nervous system of the chick embryo. J Exp Zool 116:321–362, 1951.

333. Cohen S: Purification of a nerve growth promoting protein from the mouse salivary gland and its neurocytotoxic antiserum. Proc Natl Acad Sci USA 46:302–311, 1960.

334. Green LA, Shooter EM: The nerve growth factor: Biochemistry, synthesis, and mechanism of action. Annu Rev Neurosci 3:353–402, 1980.

335. Frazier WA, Angletti RH, Bradshaw RA: Nerve growth factor and insulin: Structural similarities indicate an evolutionary relationship reflected by physiological action. Science 175:482–488, 1972.

336. Thomas KA, Baglan NC, Bradshaw RA: The amino acid sequence of the gamma-subunit of mouse submaxillary gland 7S nerve growth factor. J Biol Chem 256:9156–9168, 1981.

337. Aloe L, Cozzari C, Calissano P, Levi-Montalcini R: Somatic and behavioural postnatal effects of fetal injections of nerve growth factor antibodies in the rat. Nature 291:412–415, 1981.

338. Hamburger V, Bruno-Bechtold JK, Yip JW: Neuronal death in the spinal ganglia of the chick embryo and its reduction by nerve growth factor. J Neurosci Res 1:60–71, 1981.

339. Gorin PD, Johnson EM Jr: Effects of long-term nerve growth factor deprivation on the nervous system of the adult rat: An experimental autoimmune approach. Brain Res 198:27–42, 1980.

340. Thoenen H, Barde Y-A: Physiology of nerve growth factor. Physiol Rev 60:1284–1335, 1980.

341. Korsching S, Thoenen H: Quantitative demonstration of the retrograde axonal transport of endogenous nerve growth factor. Neurosci Lett 39:1–4, 1983.

342. Heumann R, Korsching S, Scott J, Thoenen H: Relationship between levels of nerve growth factor (NGF) and its messenger RNA in sympathetic ganglia and peripheral target tissues. EMBO J 3:3183–3189, 1984.

343. Gee AP, Boyle MDP, Münger KL, et al: Nerve growth factor: Stimulation of polymorphonuclear leukocyte chemotaxis in vitro. Proc Natl Acad Sci USA 80:7215–7218, 1983.

344. Aloe L, Levi-Montalcini R: Mast cells increase in tissues of neonatal rats injected with the nerve growth factor. Brain Res 133:358–366, 1977.

345. Thorpe LW, Jerrells TR, Perez-Polo JR: Mechanisms of lymphocyte activation by nerve growth factor. Ann NY Acad Sci 594:78–84, 1990.

346. Thorpe LW, Perez-Polo JR: The influence of nerve growth factor on the in vitro proliferative response of rat spleen lymphocytes. J Neurosci Res 18:134–139, 1987.

347. Barde Y-A: The nerve growth factor family. Prog Growth Factor Res 2:237–248, 1990.

348. Acheson AL, Naujoks K, Thoenen H: Nerve growth factor–mediated enzyme induction in primary cultures of bovine adrenal chromaffin cells—specificity and level of regulation. J Neurosci Res 4:1771–1780, 1984.

349. Yamamoto H, Gurney ME: Human platelets contain brain-derived neurotrophic factor. J Neurosci Res 10:3469–3478, 1990.

350. Schubert D, Kimura H, LaCorbiere M, et al: Activin is a nerve cell survival molecule. Nature 344:868–870, 1990.

351. Hempstead BL, Chao MV: The nerve growth factor receptor: Biochemical and structural analysis. Recent Prog Horm Res 45:441–466, 1989.

352. Lamballe F, Klein R, Barbacid M: trkC, a new member of the trk family of tyrosine protein kinases, is a receptor for neurotrophin-3. Cell 66:967–979, 1991.

353. Klein R, Nanduri V, Jing SA, et al: The trkB tyrosine protein kinase is a receptor for brain-derived neurotrophic factor and neurotrophin-3. Cell 66:395–403, 1991.

354. Cordon Cardo C, Tapley P, Jing SQ, et al: The trk tyrosine protein kinase mediates the mitogenic properties of nerve growth factor and neurotrophin-3. Cell 66:173–183, 1991.

355. Walker PA, Weil ML, Weichsel ME Jr, Fisher DA: Effect of thyroxine on nerve growth factor concentration in neonatal mouse brain. Life Sci 28:1777–1787, 1981.

356. Walker P, Weichsel ME Jr, Eveleth D, Fisher DA: Ontogenesis of nerve growth factor and epidermal growth factor in submaxillary glands and nerve growth factor in brains of immature male mice: Correlation with ontogenesis of serum levels of thyroid hormones. Pediatr Res 16:520–524, 1982.

357. Fabricant RN, Todaro GJ: Increased serum levels of nerve growth factor in von Recklinghausen's disease. Arch Neurol 38:401–405, 1981.

358. Bigazzi M, Revoltella R, Casciano S, Vignetti E: High level of a nerve growth factor in the serum of a patient with medullary carcinoma of the thyroid gland. Clin Endocrinol 6:105–112, 1977.

358a. Lin L-FH, Mismer D, Lile JD, et al: Purification, cloning, and expression of ciliary neurotrophic factor (CNTF). Science 246:1023–1025, 1989.

358b. Giovannini AJ, Romo AJ, Evans GA: Chromosomal localization of the human ciliary neurotrophic factor gene (CNTF) to 11q12 by fluorescence in situ hybridization. Cytogenet Cell Genet 63:62–63, 1993.

358c. Clatterbuck RE, Price DL, Koliatsos VE: Ciliary neurotrophic factor prevents retrograde neuronal death in the adult central nervous system. Proc Natl Acad Sci USA 90:2222–2226, 1993.

358d. Apfel SC, Arezzo JC, Moran M, Kessler JA: Effects of administration of ciliary neurotrophic factor on normal motor and sensory peripheral nerves in vivo. Brain Res 604:1–6, 1993.

358e. Ip NY, Yancopoulos GD: Ciliary neurotrophic factor and its receptor complex. Prog Growth Fac Res 4:139–155, 1992.

358f. Bruce AG, Linsley PS, Rose TM: Oncostatin M. Prog Growth Fac Res 4:157–170, 1992.

358g. Stahl N, Yancopoulos GD: The alphas, betas, and kinases of cytokine receptor complexes. Cell 74:587–590, 1993.

358h. Kelly PA, Ali S, Rozakis M, et al: The growth hormone/prolactin receptor family. Rec Prog Horm Res 48:123–164, 1993.

358i. Lopez-Casillas F, Wrana JL, Massague J: Betaglycan presents ligand to the TGF-β signalling receptor. Cell 73:1435–1444, 1993.

358j. Kurzrock R, Estrov Z, Wetzler M, Gutterman U, Talpaz M: LIF: not just a leukemia inhibitory factor. Endocr Rev 12:208–217, 1991.

358k. Yamamori T, Sarai A: Coevolution of cytokine receptor families in the immune and nervous systems. Neurosci Res 15:151–161, 1992.

358l. Lo DC: A central role for ciliary neurotrophic factor? Proc Natl Acad Sci USA 90:2557–2558, 1993.

359. Bottenstein J, Hayashi I, Hutchings S, et al: The growth of cells in serum-free hormone-supplemented media. In Jakoby WB, Pastan IH (eds): Methods in Enzymology, vol 58. New York, Academic Press, 1978, pp 94–109.

360. Walsh JH, Wong HC, Dockray GJ: Bombesin-like peptides in mammals. Fed Proc 38:2315–2319, 1979.

361. Spindel ER, Giladi E, Segerson TP, Nagalla S: Bombesin-like peptides: Of ligands and receptors. Recent Prog Horm Res 48:365–391, 1993.

362. Spindel ER, Giladi E, Brehm P, et al: Cloning and functional characterization of a complementary DNA encoding the murine fibroblast bombesin/gastrin-releasing peptide. Mol Endocrinol 4:1956–1963, 1990.

363. Pekonen F, Suikkari AM, Mäkinen T, Rutanen EM: Different insulin-like growth factor binding species in human placenta and decidua. J Clin Endocrinol Metab 67:1250–1257, 1988.

364. Davenport ML, Clemmons DR, Miles MV, et al: Regulation of serum insulin-like growth factor-I (IGF-I) and IGF binding proteins during rat pregnancy. Endocrinology 127:1278–1286, 1990.

365. Pert A, Moody TW, Pert CB, et al: Bombesin: Receptor distribution in brain and effects on nociception and locomotor activity. Brain Res 193:209–220, 1980.

366. Ghatei MA, Sheppard MN, Henzen-Logman S, et al: Bombesin and vasoactive intestinal polypeptide in the developing lung: Marked changes in acute respiratory distress syndrome. J Clin Endocrinol Metab 57:1226–1232, 1983.

367. Viallet J, Minna JD: Gastrin-releasing peptide (GRP, mammalian bombesin) in the pathogenesis of lung cancer. Prog Growth Factor Res 1:89–97, 1989.

368. Cuttitta F, Carney DN, Mulshine J, et al: Autocrine growth factors in human small cell lung cancer. Cancer Surv 4:707–727, 1985.

369. Avis IL, Kovacs TO, Kasprzyk PG, et al: Preclinical evaluation of an anti-autocrine growth factor monoclonal antibody for treatment of patients with small-cell lung cancer. J Natl Cancer Inst 83:1470–1476, 1991.

370. Nakamura T, Kitazawa T, Ichihara A: Partial purification and characterization of masking protein for B-type transforming growth factor from rat platelets. Biochem Biophys Res Commun 141:176–184, 1986.

371. Michalopoulos G, Houck KA, Dolan ML, Luetteke C: Control of hepatocyte replication by two serum factors. Cancer Res 44:4414–4419, 1984.

372. Ghoda E, Tsubouchi H, Nakayama H, et al: Purification and partial characterization of hepatocyte growth factor from plasma of a patient with fulminant hepatic failure. J Clin Invest 81:414–419, 1988.

373. Weidner M, Arakaki N, Hartmann G, et al: Evidence for the identity of human scatter factor and human hepatocyte growth factor. Proc Natl Acad Sci USA 88:7001–7005, 1991.

374. Higashio K, Shima N, Goto M, et al: Identity of a tumor cytotoxic factor from human fibroblasts and hepatocyte growth factor. Biochem Biophys Res Commun 170:397–404, 1990.

375. Nakamura T, Nishizawa T, Hagiya M, et al: Molecular cloning and expression of human hepatocyte growth factor. Nature 342:440–443, 1989.

376. Bottaro DP, Rubin JS, Faletto DL, et al: Identification of the hepatocyte growth factor receptor as the c-met proto-oncogene product. Science 251:802–804, 1991.

377. Naldini L, Vigna E, Narsimhan RP, et al: Hepatocyte growth factor (HGF) stimulates the tyrosine kinase activity of the receptor encoded by the proto-oncogene c-met. Oncogene 6:501–504, 1991.

378. Kan M, Zhang G, Zarnegar R, et al: Hepatocyte growth factor/hepatopoietin A stimulates the growth of rat kidney proximal tubular epithelial cells (RPTE), rat nonparenchymal liver cells, human melanoma cells, mouse keratinocytes and stimulates anchorage independent growth of SV-40 transformed RPTE. Biochem Biophys Res Commun 174:331–337, 1991.

379. Zarnegar R, Muga S, Rahija R, Michalopoulos G: Tissue distribution of hepatopoietin-A: A heparin-binding polypeptide growth factor for hepatocytes. Proc Natl Acad Sci USA 87:1252–1256, 1990.

380. Kinoshita T, Tashiro K, Nakamura T: Marked increase of HGF mRNA in non-parenchymal liver cells of rats treated with hepatotoxins. Biochem Biophys Res Commun 165:1229–1234, 1989.

381. Schirmacher P, Geerts A, Pietrangelo A, et al: Hepatocyte growth factor/hepatopoietin A is expressed in fat-storing cells from rat liver but not myofibroblast-like cells derived from fat-storing cells. Hepatology 15:5–11, 1992.

382. Zarnegar R, Michalopoulos G: Purification and biological characterization of human hepatopoietin A, a polypeptide growth factor for hepatocytes. Cancer Res 49:3314–3320, 1989.

383. Lindroos PM, Zarnegar R, Michalopoulos GK: Hepatic growth factor (hepatopoietin A) rapidly increases in plasma before DNA synthesis and liver regeneration stimulated by partial hepatectomy and carbon tetrachloride administration. Hepatology 13:743–750, 1991.

384. Michalopoulos GK, Zarnegar R: Hepatocyte growth factor. Hepatology 15:149–155, 1992.

385. Zarnegar R, DeFrances MC, Kost DP, et al: Expression of hepatocyte growth factor mRNA in regenerating rat liver after partial hepatectomy. Biochem Biophys Res Commun 177:559–565, 1991.

386. Kinoshita T, Hirao S, Matsumoto K, Nakamura T: Possible endocrine control by hepatocyte growth factor of liver regeneration after partial hepatectomy. Biochem Biophys Res Commun 177:330–335, 1991.

387. Matsumoto K, Tajima H, Hamanque M, et al: Identification and characterization of "injurin," an inducer of expression of the gene for hepatocyte growth factor. Proc Natl Acad Sci USA 89:3800–3804, 1992.

388. Nagaike M, Hirao S, Tajima H, et al: Renotropic functions of hepatocyte growth factor in renal regeneration after unilateral nephrectomy. J Biol Chem 266:22781–22784, 1991.

389. Chiu IM: Growth factor genes as oncogenes. Mol Chem Neuropathol 10:37–48, 1989.

390. Mansukhani A, Moscatelli D, Talarico D, et al: A murine fibroblast growth factor (FGF) receptor expressed in CHO cells is activated by basic FGF and Kaposi FGF. Proc Natl Acad Sci USA 87:4378–4382, 1993.

391. Weinberger C, Thompson CC, Ong ES, et al: The c-erb-A gene encodes a thyroid hormone receptor. Nature 324:641–646, 1986.

392. Hunter T, Cooper JA: Protein-tyrosine kinase. Annu Rev Biochem 54:897–930, 1985.

393. Wahl MI, Olashaw NE, Nishibe S, et al: Platelet-derived growth factor induces rapid and sustained tyrosine phosphorylation of phospholipase C-gamma in quiescent BALBc/3T3 cells. Mol Cell Biol 9:2934–2943, 1989.

394. Van de Woude GF, Blair DG, McGeady ML, et al: Properties of the mouse MOS proto-oncogene locus. Haematologica 72 (Suppl 6):3–5, 1987.

395. Morrison DK, Kaplan DR, Rapp U, et al: Signal transduction from membrane to cytoplasm: Growth factors and membrane bound oncogene products increase Raf-1 phosphorylation and associated protein kinase activity. Proc Natl Acad Sci USA 85:8855–8859, 1988.

396. Konkel DA: What do ras oncogenes do? Mol Endocrinol 2:883–885, 1988.

397. Wigler MH: GAPs in understanding ras. Nature 346:696–697, 1990.

398. Sassone-Corsi P, Ransone LJ, Lamph WW, et al: Direct interaction between fos and jun nuclear oncoproteins: Role of the "leucine zipper" domain. Nature 336:692–695, 1988.

399. Rollins BJ, Stiles CD: Regulation of c-myc and c-fos proto-oncogene expression by animal cell growth factors. In Vitro Cell Dev Biol 24:81–84, 1988.

400. Van Wyk JJ: Remembrances of our founders: Will growth factors, oncogenes, cytokines, and gastrointestinal hormones return us to our beginnings? Endocrinology 130:3–5, 1992.

143

The Syndromes of Obesity: An Endocrine Approach

GEORGE A. BRAY

Obesity has been identified in numerous stone-age artifacts, some of which are more than 25,000 years old.[1] Of these, the Venus of Willendorf with abdominal obesity is the best known. In spite of this long prehistoric record of obesity and the long-known risks to health posed by obesity, which were identified in writings of Hippocrates 2000 years ago, we are only now beginning to understand the complexity that underlies this problem.

When confronted with a clinical observation such as obesity, one approach to providing a framework for its understanding is to isolate individual elements of the problem as a basis for beginning to comprehend the more complex interactions of the whole organism. This reductionist approach, necessarily eliminates important elements that arise in any integrated functional system. Studies of metabolism are largely reductionist and often ignore the impact of other organs and systems. Food intake as a behavioral phenomenon requires a more integrated approach because it cannot be measured in the absence of the animal. The study of obesity provides an excellent model problem because it requires integration of reductionist approaches into an understanding of the whole organism. This chapter is intended to provide this framework and to explore the implications for treatment.

DEFINITION AND MEASUREMENT OF BODY FAT AND FAT DISTRIBUTION

Overweight is defined as an increase in body weight above a standard related to height. Obesity, on the other hand, is defined as an abnormally high percentage of body fat. Overweight and fat distribution are useful predictors of excess mortality and the risks of heart disease, hypertension, diabetes mellitus, and gallbladder disease, among others. In order to determine whether an individual is obese or simply overweight due to increased muscle mass, one needs techniques for measuring body fat and standards against which to compare these numbers. Table 143–1 shows a list of the various methods that can be used for assessing body fat and its distribution. It also provides an assessment of the relative ease, reliability, accuracy, and expense of these various methods.[2]

Techniques for Measuring Body Fat

Techniques are available to measure total body fat, the pattern of subcutaneous fat distribution, and the amount of visceral fat.[3–8]

Anthropometric Methods

Measurements of height and weight and of circumferences of the chest, waist, hips, or extremities and skinfolds in the triceps, biceps, subscapula, abdomen, thigh, calf, and sometimes other regions are relatively inexpensive to perform and have been widely used in epidemiological studies to assess total body fat, fat distribution, or the degree of overweight. Of these techniques, height and weight can be measured with the greatest accuracy (coefficient of variation [CV] less than 1 per cent). Circumferences can also be measured accurately (CV = 2.5 per cent), but skinfolds have more variability in their measurement (CV = 11 per cent).[9] Interobserver variation and variability in precise site location for skinfolds limit their use to studies involving trained investigators. Because of the variability in skinfolds, they are of limited value in determining changes in body fat of individuals.

Quantitative Methods to Measure Body Compartments

TWO-COMPARTMENT MODELS. The data obtained from quantitative measurements of body composition can be used to partition the body into several compartments,[10]

some of which are summarized graphically in Figure 143–1.[3] Several methods provide two-compartment models, in which the first compartment is body fat and the second can be fat free mass, lean body mass, body potassium, or body water.

A third two-compartment model is obtained by estimating total body potassium.[11] The naturally occurring isotope of potassium, ^{40}K, can be estimated from its emission using a whole-body scintillation counter. Assuming that lean body mass has 60 mEq/kg of K in females and 66 mEq/kg of K in males, one can calculate lean body mass and by subtracting that from total body weight can calculate fat mass. In a study by Heymsfield and his colleagues[3] of a large group of men and women aged 52 to 58, the assumptions used in estimating total fat from total body water were shown to be highly reliable. Similarly, the density of fat free mass was also shown to be very close to the assumed values. However, the potassium concentrations were lower for both men and women than the values used in most equations, indicating that calculating body fat from ^{40}K could produce considerably larger errors.

Two other techniques for providing two-compartment models of body fat use electrical conductivity.[12] The first measures total body electrical conductivity using an expensive instrument called TOBEC (total body electrical conductivity). In contrast, determination of body electrical impedance, using either a fixed or a variable frequency electrical input at the wrist and ankle, can provide a relatively inexpensive method for calculating body fat, provided that the degree of hydration is satisfactory. Using appropriate equations that include height, impedance, age, and gender can provide good estimates for body fat in all but the most obese individuals.[13] Correlations between laboratories can provide interlaboratory co-efficients of between r = 0.95 and v = 0.99. Because this method measures water, variation in hydration may bias the interpretation.[14]

MULTICOMPARTMENT MODELS. The dual photon absorptiometer (DPA) and the dual energy x-ray absorptiometer (DEXA) were originally developed for determination of bone mass for studies of osteoporosis. This technique pro-

TABLE 143–1. METHODS OF ESTIMATING BODY FAT AND ITS DISTRIBUTION

METHOD	COST	EASE OF USE	ACCURACY	MEASURES REGIONAL FAT
Height and weight	$	Easy	High	No
Skin folds	$	Easy	Low	Yes
Circumferences	$	Easy	Moderate	Yes
Density				
Immersion	$$	Moderate	High	No
Plethysmograph	$$$	Difficult	High	No
Heavy water				
Tritiated	$$	Moderate	High	No
Deuterium oxide, or heavy oxygen	$$	Moderate	High	No
Potassium isotope (^{40}K)	$$$$	Difficult	High	No
Conductivity, total body electrical	$$$	Moderate	High	No
Bioelectric impedance	$$	Easy	High	No
Fat-soluble gas	$$	Difficult	High	No
Computed tomography	$$$$	Difficult	High	Yes
Magnetic resonance imaging	$$$$	Difficult	High	Yes
Ultrasonography	$$$	Moderate	Moderate	Yes
Dual energy x-ray or photon absorptiometry	$$$	Easy	High	±
Neutron activation	$$$$	Difficult	High	No

$, low cost; $$, moderate cost; $$$, high cost; $$$$, very high cost.

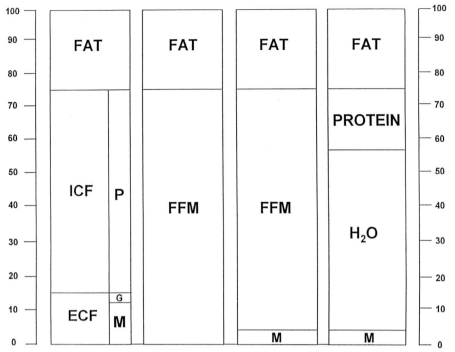

FIGURE 143–1. **Compartmental models of body composition.** Two-, three-, four-, and six-compartment models are shown. In each case, the fat is 25 per cent of total weight. Mineral is 4 per cent in the three-, four-, and six-compartment model. Protein is 22 per cent.

vides body mineral, body fat, and fat free mass (Fig. 143–1). Comparison of the estimated three-compartment model obtained with these instruments to that obtained with neutron activation ^{40}K and body water determinations shows a very high correlation.[15] Thus, the accuracy of fat mass estimated with DPA or DEXA is high, and it is probably the most appropriate gold standard for comparison of individuals who can be measured with this technique. Its current limitation is the mass of the individual who can be fitted on the table of these instruments—approximately 150 kg.

The most expensive procedure for determination of total body mass and its components is neutron activation. At present only the Brookhaven National Laboratory in New York is carrying out these highly expensive procedures.[3, 16] Coupling whole-body counting for potassium (^{40}K) and tritiated water dilution for body water with measurements from neutron activation can provide data on the amount of potassium, sodium, chloride, calcium, nitrogen, and carbon in the body as well as a number of minor elements. The limitation of the method is its radiation dose, which is on the order of 500 mrem. With knowledge about the proportion of calcium in the hydroxyapatite of bone crystal and the fact that nitrogen represents 16 per cent of protein mass, one can calculate a four- or six-compartment model based on neutron activation (see Fig. 143–1).

Fat Distribution

Subcutaneous fat distribution can be determined by several methods. The first is skinfold measurement on the trunk and on limbs.[17, 18] A second technique is the use of ultrasound, which measures subcutaneous fat thickness at defined trunk and limb sites. In addition to these two methods it is possible to use MR imaging and CT to assess the proportion of fat to muscle and bone in limbs or trunk.[4, 19] The limitation of multiple CT scans is again radiation exposure, a problem that does not occur with MR imaging.

Visceral fat is one of the most important fat depots but is the most difficult to measure. The only reliable methods for measuring visceral fat at present are CT or MR imaging. With either technique a cut through the L4–L5 region provides a good estimate of the visceral-to-subcutaneous fat ratio.

Summary

BODY COMPOSITION. DPA and DEXA appear to have replaced density, total body water, and ^{40}K as the gold standard for body composition. For regional fat distribution, the ratio of trunk to peripheral skinfolds or the ratio of waist circumference divided by hip circumference is the most widely used. Visceral fat can be adequately estimated at present only by MR imaging or CT scans.

COMPONENTS FOR MEASUREMENTS. Once measured, body fat can be divided into three main components. The first component is the total amount of body fat expressed as a per cent of body weight. The second component is the regional distribution of subcutaneous fat into male, android, or upper body patterns versus female, gynoid, or lower body patterns. This can best be done by determining the ratio of truncal skinfolds to limb skinfolds or with gender-specific measurements of waist circumference divided by hip circumference (waist-to-hip ratio). The third component of body fat is the amount of visceral fat located in the abdomen. This appears to be controlled differently from total fat or the regional distribution of subcutaneous fat and can be accurately estimated only with CT or MR imaging.

BODY WEIGHT FOR EPIDEMIOLOGICAL STUDIES. For epidemiological studies two methods of relating body weight to height have been most widely used. These are relative weight and body mass index. Relative weight compares actual weight to the appropriate weight table for a given height obtained from life insurance or other tables.

$$\text{Per cent overweight} = \frac{\text{Actual weight for height}}{\text{Table weight for height}} \times 100$$

One problem with this approach is that many tables divide weight into "frame" sizes, for which standards may be of dubious value.

The preferred method of relating height and weight is the body mass index, which was developed by Quetelet more than 100 years ago. This relationship is expressed below and is usually called the body mass index (BMI) but might be more appropriately called the *Quetelet index* (QI).

$$\text{BMI or QI} = \frac{\text{Weight (kg)}}{[\text{Ht(m)}]^2}$$

A nomogram for determining the body mass index is presented in Figure 143–2.

FAT DISTRIBUTION FOR EPIDEMIOLOGICAL STUDIES. Measurement of the ratio of the circumference of the abdomen at the minimal point between the ribs and iliac crest and the circumference of the gluteal region at the maximal gluteal protuberance—waist to hip circumference ratio, or WHR—is most widely used. A nomogram for WHR is shown in Figure 143–3. The ratio of trunk and peripheral skinfolds, including biceps, triceps, subscapula, abdomen, suprailiac area, lateral calf, and lateral thigh, can also be used. No satisfactory way exists to estimate visceral fat for epidemiological studies.

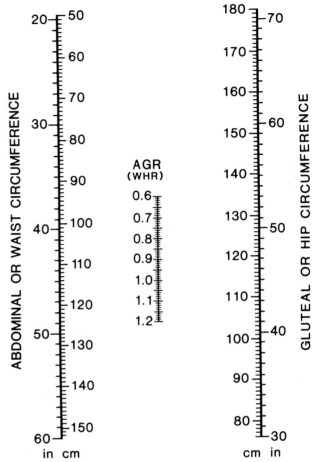

FIGURE 143–3. **Nomogram for determining waist-to-hips ratio.** Place a straight edge between the column for waist circumference and the column for hip circumference and read the ratio from the point where this straight edge crosses the AGR (WHR) line. The waist or abdominal circumference is the smallest circumference below the rib cage and above the umbilicus, and the hip or gluteal circumference is taken as the largest circumference at posterior extension of the buttocks. (Copyright 1987, George A. Bray.)

Criteria for Determining Overweight and Obesity

Setting weight standards can be done in three ways. First, the normal distribution of body weight in relation to height can be measured in a large sample of the population and then arbitrarily divided into overweight and severely overweight categories. This approach has been used by the National Center for Health Statistics. They define overweight as individuals above the 85th percentile of weight for height, using as reference the weights of 20- to 29-year-old American men and women. With this technique, overweight is defined as BMI greater than 27.8 kg/m² for men and 27.3 kg/m² for women. The top 5th percentile is considered severely overweight or obese—BMI values above 31.1 kg/m² for men and above 32.3 kg/m² for women. There are four problems with this approach. First, the standards change as the weight distribution of the population changes. Second, the decimal values of BMI at the 85th and 95th percentile make these numbers difficult to remember and use. Third, this approach defines 15 per cent of the adult population as overweight and 5 per cent as obese and by definition it is impossible

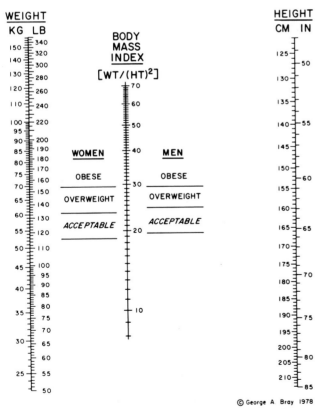

FIGURE 143–2. **Nomogram for determining body mass index (BMI).** To use this nomogram, place a ruler or other straight edge between the body weight in kilograms or pounds (without clothes) located on the left-hand line and the height in centimeters or inches (without shoes) located on the right-hand line. The BMI is read from the middle of the scale and is in metric units. (Copyright 1978, George A. Bray.)

to reduce these percentages. Finally, the most serious problem with this approach is the underlying assumption that an average weight is a healthy weight. Little evidence supports this idea.

A second approach to arriving at healthy weights is to use body weights associated with the lowest overall risk to health. The minimal death rate in several prospective studies is associated with a BMI between 22 and 25 kg/m². In an analysis of the data from the Build Study for 1979,[20] the population study from Norway,[21] and the American Cancer Society study,[22] Andres et al.[23] showed that the BMI associated with the lowest mortality for women increased with each decade of life. For men, on the other hand, the weight with the lowest mortality did not change with age in two of these three studies (Andres, personal communication). Based on these data, the Dietary Guidelines of the US Department of Agriculture and the US Department of Health and Human Services[24] have adopted BMI standards of 19 to 25 kg/m² for men and women aged 19 to 35 and a BMI of 21 to 27 kg/m² for men and women over 35 years of age. These data are similar to standards adopted in Canada and in Europe, although they differ in some details. Table 143–2 translates these numbers into weights and provides a middle target weight.

The third approach to arriving at weight standards is based on weights associated with the lowest morbidity rather than the lowest mortality. Two studies have used this method.[25, 26] Because body fat increases with age and is substantially higher for any given height/weight relationship in women than in men, assigning standards in terms of per cent body fat is more difficult and on less solid ground. Rough guidelines for defining obesity in relation to sex are provided in Table 143–3.

Criteria for Regional Fat Distribution

Several approaches have been used to estimate body fat distribution. The simplest is the circumference of the waist divided by the circumference of the hips (WHR). A nomogram for determining this is presented in Figure 143–3. The ratio of skinfolds on the trunk to the skinfolds on the extremities (T/E ratio) provides a second index of fat distribution. A third approach is the ratio of skinfold to circumference measurements on the upper arm and upper thigh, as originally proposed by Vague.[27] At present the only population-based criteria for the distribution of fat are the data from the Canadian National Survey in which waist and hip circumference were measured. These data are plotted in Figure 143–4 for both sexes.

Visceral Fat

Visceral fat can be estimated reliably with CT or MR imaging taken at the fourth to fifth lumbar vertebrae. Other estimates of visceral fat remain to be validated. Visceral fat increases with age and changes pari passu with changes in body fat or fat distribution. At this writing no standards are available.

TABLE 143–2. GOOD BODY WEIGHTS FOR ADULTS*

HEIGHT	19 to 34 Years		Over 35 Years	
	Target	Range	Target	Range
5'0"	112	97–128	123	108–138
5'1"	116	101–132	127	111–143
5'2"	120	104–137	131	115–148
5'3"	124	107–141	135	119–152
5'4"	128	111–146	140	122–157
5'5"	132	114–150	144	126–162
5'6"	136	118–155	148	130–167
5'7"	140	121–160	153	134–172
5'8"	144	125–164	158	138–178
5'9"	149	129–169	162	142–183
5'10"	153	132–174	167	146–188
5'11"	157	136–179	172	151–194
6'0"	162	140–184	177	155–199
6'1"	166	144–189	182	159–205
6'2"	171	148–195	187	164–210
6'3"	176	152–200	192	168–216
6'4"	180	156–205	197	173–222
6'5"	185	160–211	202	177–228
6'6"	190	164–216	208	182–234
BMI kg/m²	22	19–25	24	21–27

*Subject's height is measured without shoes; subject is weighed without clothes. Derived from National Research Council, 1989.

Stability of Body Weight in Childhood, Adolescence, and Adult Life

Several epidemiological studies have examined the relationship between weight at two or more ages in the same population. The mean upward shift in body weight during adult life may well camouflage considerable individual and year-to-year fluctuations. In 1302 women from Gothenburg, Sweden, the mean weight gain over a six-year period was 1.4 ± 5.1 kg (SD); 28 of the women lost more than 10 kg and 59 gained more than 10 kg.[28] In the normative aging study from Boston, 168 of 1396 men increased their weight more than 10 per cent, whereas 75 lost more than 10 per cent. The baseline weight for those gaining weight was higher (84.1 kg) than for those losing weight (77.3 Kg).[29] Williamson and colleagues[30] at the National Center for Health Statistics have also reported on 10-year changes in body weight. As expected, younger people gained more weight than older ones. In men the gain was less than in women before age 55. After 55 men tended to lose less than women. Fourteen to 16 per cent became overweight between age 35 and 44. The 10-year incidence of gaining more than 10 kg (≥ 5 kg/m²) peaks between ages 25 and 34 and is 3.9 per cent in men and 8.4 per cent in women. Thus women are more than twice as likely as men to gain weight in middle life.

TABLE 143–3. CRITERIA FOR OBESITY IN MEN AND WOMEN

CATEGORY	BODY FAT	
	MALES (%)	FEMALES (%)
Normal	12–20	20–30
Borderline	21–25	31–33
Obesity	>25	>33

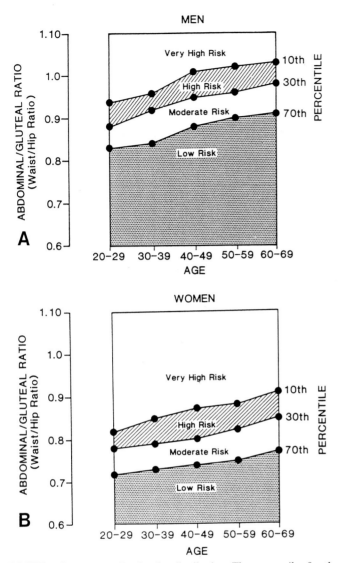

FIGURE 143-4. Percentiles for fat distribution. The percentiles for the ratio of abdominal circumference to gluteal circumference (ratio of waist to hips) are depicted for men *(A)* and women *(B)* by age groups. The relative risks for these percentiles are based on the available information. (Plotted from tabular data in the Canadian Standardized Test of Fitness (ed 3), 1986. Copyright 1987, George A. Bray.)

A number of studies have tracked childhood weight into adult life. An issue raised by this work is whether overweight adolescents remain overweight as adults. Although many studies have examined this question,[31–35] only a few of them[36–38] have calculated the relative risk of being in the top weight category as an adult based on the weight status in childhood or adolescence. According to these reports, it is between 1.6 and 2.5 times more likely for the heaviest youngster to be overweight than lightest youngster. In a 50-year follow-up of the Harvard Longitudinal Studies of Child Health and Development, the same group used by Must et al.,[38a] Casey et al.[39] found that the BMI of females in childhood had essentially no correlation with their BMI as adults. Adolescent BMI of females showed a better, but still low, correlation with BMI at age 50 (r = 0.25 to 0.35). The low correlation of adolescent weight with later adult weights in women may account for the failure of Must et al. to show an effect of overweight in adolescent girls on mortality of adult women. In men, on the other hand, the correlation of BMI in childhood or adolescence with BMI at age 50 was better (r = +0.44 to +0.55). Because the information on tracking of childhood and adolescent weight into adult life is of a low order, one must be careful in making public health recommendations to adolescents based on their adolescent weight status.[34] A prospective follow-up over 36 years points to the variability of body weight with age.[29] At age 36, 3322 people born in 1946 were divided into weight categories according to BMI. In this cohort, 5.3 per cent of the men and 8.4 per cent of the women had a BMI greater than 30 kg/m² and 38 per cent of the men and 24.2 per cent of the women were overweight with a BMI between 25 and 29.9 kg/m.² The correlation between BMI at age 26 and 36 was r = 0.64 for men and r = 0.66 for women. The authors draw the following important conclusions about weight stability. First, 25 per cent of the obese cohort, men as well as women, were obese both as children and adults. Second, the remaining 75 per cent of this cohort became obese when adults—an event that could not be predicted from weights before age 20. Those who became obese between ages 11 and 36 were often not the heaviest during childhood. Only 50 to 60 per cent of the men and women in the top decile at age 36 could be correctly predicted at age 26 using all socioeconomic, demographic, and other available weight data.

PREVALENCE

PREVALENCE OF OBESITY IN THE UNITED STATES. Several studies suggest a progressive increase in the weight for height ratio throughout the past century in the United States. For example, the weight of a man 68 inches tall inducted into military service rose from 67 kg in 1863 to 76 kg in 1962.[26] Life insurance data[22] and data from the National Center for Health Statistics also report a small increase in the average body weight for height and the percentage who are obese by similar criteria within this century. For example, Wong and Trowbridge[40] showed an increase in the percentage of both black and white women who were defined as obese between three surveys, one in 1960-62, a second in 1971-74, and a third in 1976-80. Black males showed a similar increase, but white males showed this increase only in the latter period of time.

During adult life BMI increases with age in both men and women. Proportional increases are greater in women than in men (Fig. 143–5). Black women have a higher percentage of obesity at all ages than do white women. In almost all populations, more women are obese and overweight than men.[41] Obesity appears to be more common among certain ethnic and racial groups than others. North American Indians, notably the Pimas and Papagos who live in the Southwest, have a very high prevalence of obesity.[42]

Socioeconomic status also plays an important role in the prevalence of obesity, particularly in women. For all women above age 25, the percentage in the overweight category was higher among individuals living below the poverty line, as assigned by the US government, than in the nonpoverty group. The differences among men were small and not statistically significant.

PREVALENCE OF OBESITY IN OTHER COUNTRIES. The prevalence of overweight, defined as the percentage of the population with a BMI between 25 and 29.9 and obesity as

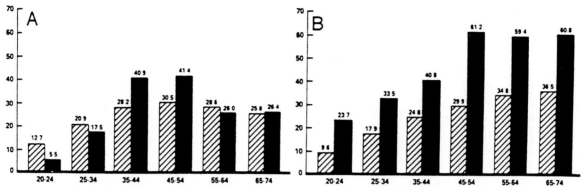

FIGURE 143–5. **Prevalence of obesity.** Data from the National Center for Health Statistics show the percentage of overweight men *(A)* and women *(B)* by age and socioeconomic status using the 85th percentile of weights for height of 20- to 24-year olds as the upper limits for weight.

a BMI above 30 kg/m², is summarized in Table 143–4. Two observations are clear. First, the percentage of men with a BMI between 25 and 29.9 kg/m² is higher than in women in all countries listed. Second, the prevalence of obesity, defined as a BMI greater than 30 kg/m², is similar in men and women.[43, 44]

PATHOGENESIS

Nutrient Balance Model for Obesity

One approach to integrating the data about the pathogenesis of obesity is through a feedback model, shown in Figure 143–6.[45, 46] A control system consisting of body fat and the circulating nutrients provides carbon and nitrogen for oxidation to produce ATP for production of heat and for physical work as well as repairing body tissues. Circulating hormones, primarily insulin, growth hormone, and cortisol, along with the autonomic and somatosensory nervous systems, modulate nutrient storage and metabolism and thus play a key integrating role. This control system generates afferent feedback signals that tell the controller about the state of the organism. The central controller receives these afferent signals and transduces them into efferent signals to the endocrine and autonomic nervous system as

well as the neuromuscular system involved with physical recognition, selection, and ingestion of food. We examine each of these components below.

Controlled System

In the normal adult, energy intake is between 1500 and 2500 kcal/d, divided among energy sources from protein, carbohydrate, and fat. For this model, I have partitioned daily energy intake into 20 per cent from protein, 40 per cent from fat, and 40 per cent from carbohydrate, which provides 2000 kcal/d. One requirement for maintenance of body weight and body fat stores is that the amount of fat and carbohydrate ingested in the diet be oxidized by the metabolic processes in the body. Failure to match the oxidation with intake of fat and carbohydrate eventually leads to obesity. In careful experimental studies on nutrient balance, Flatt[47, 48] has related the carbohydrate and fat balances from day to day with food intake. Carbohydrate intake has a highly significant inverse relationship with carbohydrate balance. That is, when carbohydrate balance is negative on one day, the following day there is an increase in carbohydrate, that is, food, intake. Conversely, when carbohydrate balance is positive on one day, the next

TABLE 143–4. PREVALENCE OF OBESITY IN SEVERAL COUNTRIES

	YEARS	AGE	OVERWEIGHT		OBESE		REFERENCES
			Men	Women	Men	Women	
United States	1976–80	35–44	46	21	12	16	Millar & Stephens, Am J Publ Health 77:38–41, 1987
Canada	1981	35–44	43	21	11	8	Millar & Stephens, Am J Publ Health 77:38–41, 1987
Britain	1980	35–44	38	24	8	8	Millar & Stephens, Am J Publ Health 77:38–41, 1987
Australia	1983–89	35–44	43	20	8	8	
Germany	1984–86	25–69	49	45[a]	16	16	Greiser et al, Int J Epidemiol 18(3 Suppl 1):S118–124, 1989
Sweden	1980–81	16–84	35	26	7	8	Kuskowska-Wolk & Rossner, J Intern Med 227:241–246, 1990
Netherlands	1981–88	35–49	38	21	5	6	Verweij, Maandbericht Gezondheidsstat 11:5–10, 1989

Overweight = BMI 25–<30 kg/m²
Obese = BMI ≥ 30 kg/m²
Adapted from Blokstra A, Kromhout D: Trends in obesity in young adults in the Netherlands from 1974 to 1986. Int J Obes 15(8):513–521, 1991.

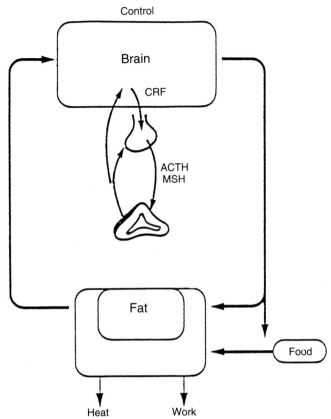

Control

Brain

CRF

ACTH
MSH

Fat

Food

Heat   Work

FIGURE 143–6. **Diagram of a controlled system.** The controller for food intake is located in the brain, which receives afferent signals from the periphery and integrates them into efferent controls that modulate food intake and the controlled system of nutrient intake storage and oxidation. The critical role of the adrenal steroids is indicated by the feedback between brain/pituitary and adrenal gland.

day is associated with a decrease in carbohydrate intake. In contrast, the day-to-day relationship between fat balance and fat intake is much less significant than the day-to-day relationship between carbohydrate balance and carbohydrate intake. The daily intakes of carbohydrate, fat, and protein are related to the body stores of protein, carbohydrate, and fat. The daily intake of carbohydrate approximates the daily stores. In contrast, the intake of fat is substantially less than 1 per cent of total stores. It is thus not unreasonable to anticipate that the regulation of carbohydrate stores would have a greater impact on carbohydrate intake than would small changes in body fat stores.

Several important clinical implications arise from the studies by Flatt[47, 48] indicating the strong relationship between carbohydrate intake and carbohydrate balance. First, to maintain body weight, fat oxidation on average must equal fat intake. Second, it is harder to become obese eating a high-carbohydrate diet because the feedback between carbohydrate stores and carbohydrate intake appears to be a strong and significant one. In contrast, it is easier to get fat eating a high-fat diet, a phenomenon well observed with the affluent western diet, which contains more than 30 per cent fat. Finally, physical activity, which increases muscle training, enhances fat oxidation and can serve as one buffer against storage of fat.

Adipose tissue provides the major site for storage of triglyceride. The normal 70-kg male has about 12 kg of body fat which stores about 110,000 kcal of energy, whereas the normal 55-kg female has about 14 kg of fat storing approximately 125,000 kcal of energy. On the other hand, only 24,000 kcal are stored as protein and only a few hundred kcal as carbohydrate. The triglycerides of the adipocyte contain predominately fatty acids of dietary origin. In individuals whose weight is stable, the dietary fat eaten is digested and then repackaged as chylomicrons. The chylomicrons enter the circulation through the lacteals and are cleared from the circulation through the action of lipoprotein lipase (LPL), which is made and secreted by adipocytes and then attaches to the endothelial surfaces (Fig. 143–7). LPL, when activated by apoCII, hydrolyzes the triglycerides with the production of intermediate and low density lipoproteins that remain in the circulation until cleared by other tissues. The fatty acids released by LPL move through the interstitial space to the adipocyte, where they are re-esterified with α-glycerophosphate and stored as triglycerides. The α-glycerophosphate is in turn formed from glucose taken up by the adipocyte. Although the human adipocyte can synthesize fatty acids, this appears to be of importance only during periods of positive caloric balance. In addition, adipocytes appear to be a major source of lactate during metabolism of glucose.

Fatty acids are the major metabolic fuel, and adipose tissue is their major repository. Control of fatty acid release from adipose tissue is under a variety of controls. First, blood flow provides binding sites on albumen to remove fatty acids. Second, as the blood flow through adipose tissue capillaries changes in rate, so does the relation of lipolysis to re-esterification in the adipocyte. The breakdown of triacylglycerol to free fatty acids (FFA) and glycerol is increased by catecholamines, which act on cell wall receptors as well as other hormones, which activate the hormone-sensitive lipase by a phosphorylation-dephosphorylation cascade with cAMP and protein kinase A as activators. Counteracting the effect of lipolytic hormones are insulin and adenosine, both of which are antilipolytic.[49] The net release of fatty acids is thus under the integrated effect of several control mechanisms.[50, 51]

The fat cell hypothesis for development of obesity[52] is based on the concept of critical periods in the cellular proliferation and development of adipose tissue.[53] Fat cells first appear at the beginning of the third trimester of gestation. They rapidly increase in size until birth, when fat represents more than 10 per cent of total birth weight. From the early postnatal period through adolescence there is an increase in the number and size of adipocytes.[54] It is now clear, however, that fat cells can be induced in adult life.[55] Preadipocytes can be induced to proliferate by a variety of growth factors as well as the nutritional state, both of which are limited and modulated by the genetic potential of the tissue. Once proliferation is initiated, fat cells can be induced to differentiate by nutritional and hormonal factors into mature adipocytes.[53]

Periods of fat cell enlargement are observed in the first year of life, during which the doubling of body fat occurs almost entirely by an increase in the size of individual adipocytes. In addition, numerous studies with acute overfeeding of adults have demonstrated hypertrophy of existing adipocytes with no evidence for a change in total number of fat cells. Conversely, acute weight loss appears to be accompanied by decreased size of individual adipocytes with little or no change in fat cell number. The number of

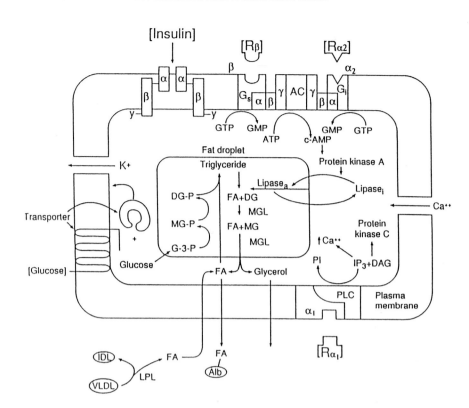

FIGURE 143–7. **Diagram of a fat cell.** The biochemical pathways for lipogenesis are shown on the left-hand side, and the pathways for lipolysis are shown on the right.

adipocytes may also be increased by chronic exposure to excess nutrients and/or an altered hormonal environment.

Afferent Signals

Afferent signals may be either positive (that is, they may stimulate feeding) or negative (they produce aversion or satiety). The good taste of food or pleasant social ambiance can enhance the amount of food eaten over what would occur in the absence of these signals. Negative feedback signals that produce satiety and the termination of eating may be generated by gastrointestinal distention, by the release of gastrointestinal hormones, or by the absorption and action of digested nutrients.

The afferent vagus nerve provides an important relay from the periphery to the CNS. The release of gastrointestinal hormones into the gut or circulation provides another source of afferent signals. Of these, cholecystokinin[56] and enterostatin[57] are the most interesting. Cholecystokinin (CCK) exists in several forms (CCK-8, CCK-33, and CCK-39), all of which decrease food intake when injected into the peritoneal cavity but not into the portal vein. Vagotomy blocks the inhibition of food intake by CCK-8, indicating that vagal afferents are involved in relaying information to the brain. The CCK-A receptors in the pyloric ring or in the liver produce afferent vagal signals to decrease food intake. Enterostatin is a pentapeptide, Val-Pro-Asp-Pro-Arg (VPDPR), released from the N-terminal end of pancreatic procolipase by tryptic digestion when this proenzyme is secreted into the intestine and activated by trypsin. This peptide is of particular interest because it specifically reduces fat intake and not protein or carbohydrate intake.[57]

Modulation of either glucose or fatty acid oxidation can influence feeding. 2-Deoxy-D-glucose stimulates food intake when injected peripherally or into the CNS. This effect of 2-deoxy-D-glucose, an analogue of glucose that blocks glucose oxidation, is not blocked by vagotomy, implying that this drug acts directly on the CNS, probably on the glucose receptors in the vagal complex of the hind brain. In animals and in human beings, a dip in the circulating glucose level of 10 to 12 per cent is a reliable signal for impending onset of a meal.[58] When the drop in glucose is first detected, an infusion of glucose to prevent a further drop delays or eliminates the next meal. A rise in insulin immediately precedes the fall in glucose, suggesting a coordinated neuroendocrine loop for control of meals. Blockade of fatty acid oxidation in the liver also increases food intake. Either mercaptoacetate or methyl palmoxirate, two drugs that inhibit fatty acid oxidation, stimulates food intake. This effect is blocked by vagotomy, indicating that hepatic vagal receptors are activated by fatty acid oxidation.[59, 60]

Central Controller

The messages from the periphery must be received, integrated, amplified, transduced, and relayed to appropriate sites to initiate or inhibit feeding and to modulate the control of metabolism. Figure 143–8 shows the anatomy of the human hypothalamus in relation to hyperphagia and anorexia. It has been known for many years that damage to the ventromedial hypothalamus in many species, including human beings, consistently produces obesity, whereas destruction of the lateral hypothalamus produces hyperphagia or anorexia.[61] Careful anatomical studies in experimental animals have shown that destruction of either the paraventricular (PVN) or the ventromedial (VMN) nucleus produces this syndrome of obesity.[46, 62] The mechanisms for these two types of obesity are quite different, however, and are presented schematically in Figure 143–9. The PVN lesion produces hyperphagia but little or no alteration in the function of the autonomic nervous system. In contrast,

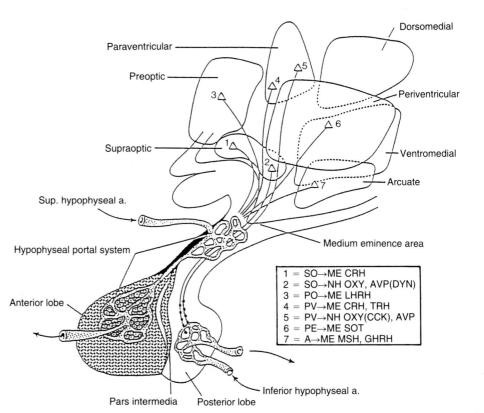

FIGURE 143–8. **The anatomical location of the hypothalamic nuclei.** Damage to the ventromedial or paraventricular nucleus produces obesity. Damage to the more lateral hypothalamus produces weight loss and anorexia.

1 = SO→ME CRH
2 = SO→NH OXY, AVP(DYN)
3 = PO→ME LHRH
4 = PV→ME CRH, TRH
5 = PV→NH OXY(CCK), AVP
6 = PE→ME SOT
7 = A→ME MSH, GHRH

damage to the VMN produces increased parasympathetic activity, decreased sympathetic activity, impaired growth hormone release with stunted growth, disturbed diurnal rhythms, and decreased physical activity. These two syndromes often occur together because most destructive hypothalamic lesions that damage the ventromedial nucleus also damage the paraventricular nucleus.

A variety of neurotransmitters are involved with modulation of food intake. These are summarized in Table 143–5. Norepinephrine, acting through α_2-adrenergic receptors in the PVN, as well as several peptides stimulate food intake, whereas serotonin, norepinephrine acting through β-adre-

nergic receptors, and a larger group of peptides decrease food intake. Several recent studies have shown that many of these peptides can stimulate or inhibit the intake of specific nutrients. For example, neuropeptide-Y, injected into the PVN, specifically increases carbohydrate intake. In contrast, galanin injected into the same area increases fat intake. On the other hand, our laboratory has shown that corticotropin-releasing hormone, enterostatin, and vasopressin specifically decrease fat intake. Glucagon has been reported to decrease protein intake, and angiotensin, injected peripherally or centrally, is known to increase sodium intake. Thus, a nutrient-specific hypothesis for peptide effects is consistent with a considerable amount of data.

A clinical phenomenon that can be explained by the nutrient-specific effect hypothesis of peptide action has been called *sensory-specific satiety*.[63] When a number of preferred foods are presented to a hungry subject, the prefer-

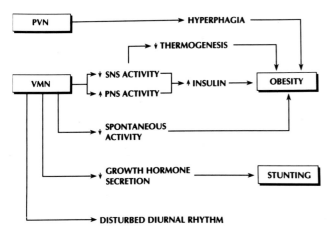

FIGURE 143–9. **Comparison of hypothalamic lesions in the ventromedial (VMN) and paraventricular nuclei (PVN).** Destruction of the PVN increases food intake but has no effect on the autonomic nervous system, the diurnal pattern of food intake, or the level of activity. In contrast, VMH lesions may not increase food intake, but they impair growth hormone secretion and alter the balance between the sympathetic and parasympathetic nervous system.

TABLE 143–5. PEPTIDES THAT STIMULATE OR SUPPRESS FEEDING

INCREASE FOOD INTAKE	DECREASE FOOD INTAKE
Dynorphin	Anorectin
β-Endorphin	Bombesin
Galanin	Calcitonin
Growth hormone–releasing hormone (low dose)	Cholecystokinin (CCK)
Neuropeptide Y (NPY)	Corticotropin-releasing hormone (CRH)
Somatostatin (low dose)	Cyclo-His-Pro
	Enterostatin
	Glucagon
	Insulin
	Neurotensin
	Oxytocin
	Thyrotropin-releasing hormone
	Vasopressin

ence rating is high for all of them. When one of these foods is then eaten and all of the foods are subsequently re-rated, the rating for the ingested food has fallen compared with the uneaten foods. If a second choice is now provided between the previously ingested food and other uneaten foods, individuals usually choose a new food rather than one of the previously eaten foods. Sensory-specific satiety describes the ability to eat desserts even though you no longer want "seconds" from other items on a menu. Such specificity for nutrient intake must have a neurochemical basis. The findings of specific alterations in nutrient preferences in association with specific peptides may provide the neurochemical basis for understanding the clinical phenomenon of sensory-specific satiety.[57]

In addition to the effect of peptides on specific nutrients, many peptides have a reciprocal relationship between their effects on the thermogenic part of the sympathetic nervous system and food intake. This is summarized in Table 143–6. It can be seen that hypothalamic lesions which increase food intake decrease sympathetic activity and vice versa, the PVN lesion being one exception. This relationship has been observed for several different peptides, two of which increase food intake and six or more of which decrease food intake. Each peptide has an opposing effect on the sympathetic nervous system and food intake. Three drugs—fenfluramine, 2-deoxyglucose, and muscimol—also show this relationship. The model shown in Figure 143–10 may help to understand this phenomenon. The generalized wiring of the hypothalamus is presented schematically at the left. The hypothalamus has three major functions: (1) control of the pituitary; (2) relay of fibers rostrally to the cortex from the reticular system in the hindbrain; and (3) descending control over the medial forebrain bundle. The addition of a feeding center in the hypothalamus with efferent connections to the reticular formation could provide the needed negative feedback

TABLE 143–6. RELATIONSHIP OF FOOD INTAKE AND SYMPATHETIC ACTIVITY

	FOOD INTAKE	SYMPATHETIC ACTIVITY
Lesion		
Ventromedial nucleus	↑	↓
Lateral hypothalamus	↓	↑
Peptides		
Neuropeptide Y	↑	↓
β-Endorphin	↑	↓
Anorectin	↓	↑
Cholecystokinin	↓	↑
Corticotropin-releasing hormone	↓	↑
Glucagon	↓	↑
Fibroblast growth factor-α	↓	↑
Interleukin-β	↓	↑
Neurotensin	↓	↑
Thyrotropin-releasing hormone	↓	↑
Vasopressin	↓	↑
Drugs and neurotransmitters		
Norepinephrine	↓	↓
Serotonin	↓	↑
Amphetamine	↓	↑
Fenfluramine	↓	↑
2-Deoxyglucose	↑	↓
4-Butene-1-olide	↓	↑

control (right hand panel). Such a model would provide a basis for explaining the inhibitory or stimulatory effects of various peptides on sympathetic activity and food intake.

Efferent Control Systems

A major element in the efferent control system is the regulation of feeding. It is well known that stimulation of the lateral hypothalamus activates feeding pathways, suggesting that this area has the wiring controls to make this possible. The lateral and ventromedial hypothalami also have major controls over the activity of the sympathetic and parasympathetic nervous system. The parasympathetic nervous system is involved with control of gastric emptying, because an increase in vagal activity increases gastric emptying. Vagal stimulation also increases insulin secretion. The sympathetic nervous system is involved with control of thermogenesis in smaller animals and with modulation of food intake, blood pressure control, and metabolic activity, modulated by both circulating epinephrine from the adrenal medulla and direct sympathetic innervation.

The model presented in Figure 143–8 can be redrawn to include the concept of nutrient partitioning, that is, the distribution of nutrient intake into body fat or protein. This is shown in Figure 143–11. Diet composition clearly affects a regulator, which must increase fat oxidation if the percentage of fat in the diet increases and fat storage is to be avoided. If the brain senses the altered nutrient composition of the diet, it has a variety of mechanisms by which it can adapt, as shown in the middle of the diagram under efferent systems. They include alterations of food intake, which can be depressed. Alternatively, the autonomic nervous system, both parasympathetic and sympathetic components, can be modulated to alter the metabolism of the incoming nutrient stream. A similar effect is observed with hormonal systems and finally with physical activity. Drugs that act on β_2/β_3-adrenergic receptors increase protein storage and decrease fat storage in cattle, sheep, and pigs.[64] Similarly, nutrient partitioning between lean and fat tissue is produced by growth hormone. In growing animals growth hormone increases lean tissue; in lactating cattle it increases milk production dramatically. Thus, both the autonomic nervous system and several hormonal systems have the potential for modulating nutrient partitioning between protein and fat stores and may be involved in the defect(s) in nutrient partitioning that represent obesity.

Clinical Aspects of Nutrient Balance

Natural History of Body Fat

At birth the human body contains about 12 per cent fat.[65] This is higher than any other mammal except the whale! During the first months of life, body fat rises rapidly to reach a peak of about 25 per cent at six months of age. It then declines to between 15 and 18 per cent in the prepubertal years for both males and females. At puberty there is a significant increase in the percentage of body fat in girls and a significant decrease in boys, particularly on the extremities. By age 18 males have approximately 12 to 18 per cent body fat and females 20 to 25 per cent body fat. Fat increases in both genders after puberty, and during adult life fat rises to between 25 and 35 per cent of body

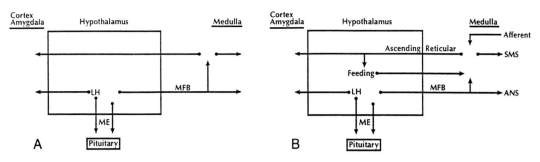

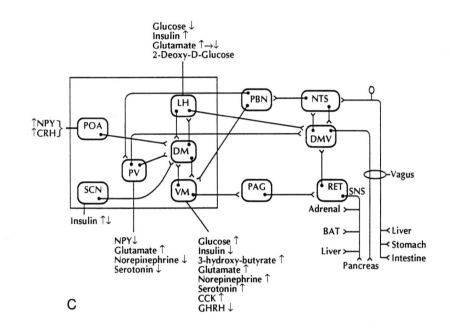

FIGURE 143–10. **Model for reciprocal control of food intake and sympathetic activity.** *A*, Elements of hypothalamus. *B*, Essential feedback circuit from medulla to hypothalamic feeding center and input from this feeding center to medulla. *C*, Sites at which various nutrients and peptides have been found to affect the sympathetic nervous system (SNS). LH, lateral hypothalamus; ME, medulla; MFB, medial forebrain bundle; SMS, somatomotor system; ANS, autonomic nervous system; POA, preoptic area; SCN, suprachiasmic nucleus; PV, paraventricular nucleus; DM, dorsomedial-hypothalamus; VM, ventromedial hypothalamus; PBN, parabrachial nucleus; PAG, periage rectal gray; NTS, nucleus tractus solitarii; DMV, dorsal motor nucleus of the vagus; RET, reticular formation; NPY, neuropeptide Y; CRH, corticotropinreleasing hormone; CCK, cholecystokinin; GHRH, growth hormone–releasing hormone; BAT, brown adipose tissue.

weight in women and between 15 and 25 per cent in men. Between the ages of 20 and 50 the fat content of men approximately doubles, and that of women increases by about 50 per cent. Because total body weight rises by only 10 to 15 per cent, this indicates a reduction in lean body mass with aging.

Energy Expenditure

A number of methods are available for assessing energy expenditure.[66] Both direct calorimeters, which measure heat loss, and indirect calorimeters, which measure oxygen consumption and carbon dioxide production, provide similar data. Thus most of the data on human energy expenditure has come from measurements using indirect calorimeters, either whole-body indirect calorimeters or ventilated hood indirect calorimeters, because they are technically simpler.

Doubly labeled water has provided a powerful new tool for the study of energy expenditure.[67] Administration of $^2H_2^{18}O$ provides a way of assessing oxygen and deuterium disposal from the body. Because deuterium can leave only as water, whereas ^{18}O can leave as water or carbon dioxide, it is possible to measure the separate rates of elimination for deuterium and ^{18}O in body fluids and obtain an estimate of carbon dioxide production over an interval of 7 to 14 days in free-living individuals. Estimation of energy expenditure requires either a measurement or estimate of respiratory quotient and the assumption that the natural supply of water during the study period maintains a stable ratio of $^2H_2^{18}O$ to $H_2^{16}O$. Because this method uses stable isotopes, it is appropriate for studies in children and pregnant women as well as other adults. Activity diaries, the measurement of heart rate, and the use of inertial movement counters have also been utilized, but the availability of doubly labeled water and a growing number of indirect calorimetry systems appear to provide the most useful information.

The components of energy expenditure are depicted in Figure 143–12.

RESTING METABOLIC RATE. Resting metabolism is defined as the total energy required by the body in the resting state. It is influenced by age, gender, body weight, body composition, drugs, climate, and genetics. Resting metabolic rate, or RMR, is approximately two thirds of total energy expenditure and is directly related to fat free mass or body surface area. This *Law of Surface Area* was discovered by Rubner[68] and applies to homeotherms. The surface area can be approximated by [body weight] $\times$ 0.75.[68, 69] The highest metabolic rates are observed in infants, with a gradual decline during childhood and a further slow de-

CONTROL

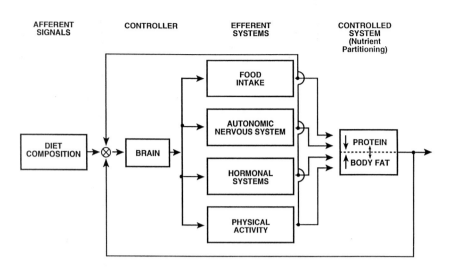

FIGURE 143–11. **Control model of nutrient partitioning.** Diet composition feeds into a "mixer" (indicated by the circled X) along with feedback signals from the controlled system *(lower line)* and each of the efferent systems *(upper lines).*

cline of approximately 2 per cent per decade in adult life. Much of this decline may represent a decrease in lean body mass with aging. A strong linear relationship exists between energy expenditure and fat free mass (Fig. 143–13), with approximately 80 per cent of the variance in energy expenditure being accounted for by variations in fat free mass.[70]

There is also a familial component to metabolic rate. In studies of the Pima Indians, a familial clustering was observed, with some families having lower metabolic rates than other families.[71] In prospective studies with the Pima Indians, three factors appear to relate to the likelihood of developing obesity. The first is resting metabolic rate. Ravussin and his colleagues[72] observed that over a four-year time interval, those individuals who initially had a low metabolic rate had a substantially higher risk for developing

obesity than individuals with a normal metabolic rate. Of interest was the observation that at the end of the period of weight gain, the metabolic rate per unit fat free mass was normal. A second predictor of fat storage was the respiratory quotient (RQ), defined as the ratio of the carbon dioxide produced to the oxygen taken up.[73] A higher RQ occurs when oxidizing more carbohydrates. Individuals with a high RQ are at higher risk to gain body fat. On any given diet, the higher the RQ, the more fat is stored, because it is not being oxidized. Thus, a higher RQ predicts future risk of gaining weight. The third predictive factor was insulin resistance. Individuals with lower insulin resistance had a greater likelihood of developing increased fat stores over the period of follow-up.[74]

THERMIC EFFECT OF FOOD. When food is eaten, the metabolic rate rises and then returns to baseline. This process requires several hours, and during this time the increase in energy expenditure can approximate 10 per cent or more of the total caloric value of the ingested food. One explanation for this thermogenic response to a meal is that it results from enhanced activity of the thermogenic part of the sympathetic nervous system.[75] When thermogenesis is

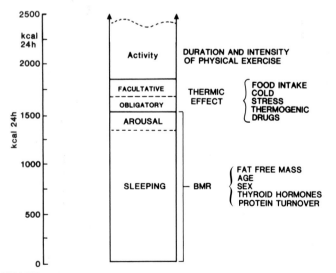

FIGURE 143–12. Daily energy expenditure can be divided into three major components: basal metabolic rate (sleeping metabolic rate [SMR] + energy cost of arousal), which represents 50 to 70 per cent of daily energy expenditure; the thermic effect of food, which represents about 10 per cent of daily energy expenditure; and the energy cost of physical activity (spontaneous physical activity [SPA] + unrestricted/voluntary physical activity), which represents 20 to 40 per cent of daily energy expenditure.

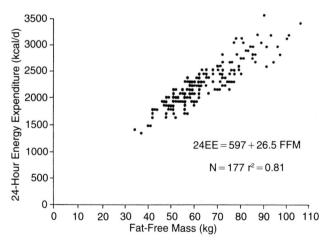

FIGURE 143–13. Relationship between 24-hour energy expenditure and free fat mass in 177 subjects. Twenty-eight observations are hidden.

stimulated by the infusion of glucose, approximately half of this effect can be blocked by propranolol, a beta-adrenergic blocking drug.[76] However, the thermogenic effects of oral administration of foods are not blocked by propranolol, suggesting that the primary mechanisms are other than the activation of the sympathetic nervous system.

The concept that a reduced thermic response to food may serve as a mechanism for the extra energy needed to develop obesity is both intriguing and controversial. Some studies have found a difference between obese and lean subjects in the energy produced following a meal, but others have not. This discrepancy may lie in the size of the meal used, the techniques of recording the palatability of the food, and the subjects selected. This problem has recently been addressed by Segal and her colleagues,[77] who have carefully compared three groups of individuals: (1) those with comparable body weight but different percentages of body fat; (2) those with comparable percentages of body fat but different body weights; and (3) those with the same percentage of body fat but differing in the degree of insulin resistance. They conclude that the impaired thermic response to a meal that occurs in obesity is related to the percentage of body fat and insulin resistance. Thus it now seems most likely that obesity, that is, an increased percentage of body fat, reduces the thermic effect of a meal.

PHYSICAL ACTIVITY. There are two approaches to studying the relationship of physical activity to obesity. One of them is in the laboratory and the other in naturalistic settings. Laboratory methods involve measuring energy expenditure when individuals are walking on a treadmill or riding a cycle ergometer. In both obese and lean individuals, the efficiency for coupling energy production to muscular exercise is approximately 30 per cent.[78] That is, the incremental work of turning a fly wheel on a bicycle ergometer accounted for 30 per cent of the extra energy expended during cycling. No evidence indicates an abnormality in the metabolic coupling of substrate oxidation to the contraction of muscular tissue in moderately or massively obese subjects compared with normal-weight subjects, whether in a condition of steady body weight or following acute weight gain.

A second approach to studying energy expenditure is with naturalistic observation. The obese are often observed to be less active than are normal-weight individuals. When given the choice of an escalator or stairs, for example, the obese are more likely to choose the escalator.[79] However, a lower level of spontaneous movement does not necessarily imply reduced energy expenditure because the overweight individual uses more energy for any given movement. When observing lean and obese boys on a playground, Waxman and Stunkard[80] noted that the obese boys expended more energy on the playground but similar amounts inside the home compared with their lean siblings. Thus, spending less time in physical activity does not necessarily result in a reduction in total energy expenditure, because of the extra mass associated with physical activity in the obese. Exercise has been reported to affect food intake in lean but not in obese subjects. In normal-weight individuals, graded increases in physical activity are associated with an increase in food intake to match the increment in energy expenditure. In obese subjects, on the other hand, changing the level of physical activity produces a much smaller increase in food intake.[81]

Energy Intake

Several techniques are available for determining energy intake and its composition. These can include epidemiological techniques measuring the frequency with which foods are eaten, a weighed dietary intake, and dietary recall using either one- or three-day dietary records. Alternatively, food intake can be determined in laboratory settings, where people eat either natural foods or formula diets over short or long periods of time. Food disappearance data can also be used to assess available energy.

Using the 24-hour food recall method, Beaton et al.[82] found that the mean daily energy intake was 2639 kcal/d for men and 1793 kcal/d for women. Data from the National Center for Health Statistics based on 24-hour recall showed reported intakes of 2359 kcal/d for men and 1639 kcal/d for women.[83] In several cross-sectional studies of overweight and normal-weight subjects that have been compared, the food intake of overweight subjects was comparable to that of lean subjects.[84] The validity of reported low energy intake in obese subjects has been questioned by data using doubly labeled water. Using this technique Bandini and her colleagues[85] and Prentice et al.[86] found significant underreporting of intake relative to energy expenditure measured by the use of doubly labeled water. This discrepancy was up to 41.3 per cent for obese subjects and 19.1 per cent for normal-weight subjects. Using carefully weighed dietary intakes, Mertz and his associates[87] have also reported a discrepancy between estimated food intake based on dietary records and recall and the actual amounts of nutrient intake required for weight maintenance. There is thus significant concern about the value that can be attached to measurements of food intake in epidemiological and field studies. This was highlighted by measurements in an individual who claimed to be a small eater but whose metabolic rate was much higher than the reported intake.[88]

In contrast to these problems with dietary recall, food intake can be quantitatively studied in metabolic wards and in some outpatient trials. Food intake is characterized by a parabolic curve with an initial rapid increase and a deceleration.[89] A variety of factors influence the quantity of food eaten in any one meal, including the interval since the last meal, perceptions about the characteristics of the food to be eaten, and a variety of environemental distractions and intrusions. Suffice it to say that both obese and lean subjects are significantly influenced by the emotional content of their eating experience.

Nutrient Partitioning and the Effects of Overfeeding

A number of laboratories have completed studies with voluntary overfeeding of normal or overweight men and women.[90–93] In these studies, an increase in body weight and body fat stores is related to the number of excess calories eaten. For any given level of calorie surplus, however, there is a large interindividual variation in the amount of weight and body fat that are gained. To identify the genetic and environmental components involved in this variability, Bouchard and his colleagues performed two overfeeding studies in identical twins, one lasting 22 days and the second 84 days.[92, 93] The daily increment was 1000 kcal for six days out of seven for each subject. The best correlations with the changes in body weight and body fat were found using the ratio of fat mass to fat free mass (FM/FFM), an index of nutrient partitioning. These observations are consistent with the discussion of nutrient partitioning presented earlier and suggest that important inter-individual differences exist in the mechanisms for nutrient partitioning and the fraction of excess calories converted to fat as opposed to other routes of metabolism.

RISKS TO HEALTH OF OBESITY AND ABDOMINAL FAT

It is a cliché to say that "overweight is risking fate." However, the data presented below argue that an excess quantity of fat is risky and also that increased abdominal fat distribution may be an even more important external guide to health risks.

Epidemiological data on the relationship between BMI and a given risk such as overall mortality, heart disease, diabetes, or gallbladder disease, are curvilinear and often described as J- or U-shaped. This effect on overall mortality is shown in Figure 143–14. Mortality or morbidity increases as BMI increases. There may also be an increase in excess mortality at weights below a BMI of 18 to 19 kg/m², but this may also be related largely to smoking.

Effects of Obesity and Fat Distribution on Overall Mortality

Both retrospective and prospective studies have contributed to our understanding of the relationship between overweight, fat distribution, and mortality. Overweight generally increases the risk of death, especially sudden death, although in many studies it may not be an independent variable. Three major problems plague the interpretation of studies in this area.[94] First, many studies fail to separate smokers from nonsmokers. Second, early mortality may bias the interpretation of weight status on life expectancy, because individuals who are losing weight at the time of initial survey may die early. Third, the failure to identify obesity as an independent risk factor has led many people to suggest that it is unimportant. This denies the important relationship that obesity has to diabetes, hypertension, and hyperlipidemia, through the effects of which the increase in body weight may cause ill health. Because obesity must modify some intermediate mechanism such as cardiac function or the metabolism of lipids or glucose to produce death or disease, overweight may serve as a useful identifier of risk factors.

The primary retrospective studies looking at the relationship of weight and obesity have come from the life insurance industry. Life insurance statistics have shown that excess weight is associated with higher mortality rates.[20] The minimal mortality for both men and women occurs among individuals 10 per cent below average weight. Deviations in body weight above or below this figure are associated with an increase in mortality. Based on the 1979 data, a body weight that is 10 per cent above average weight is accompanied by an 11 per cent increase in excess mortality for men and a 7 per cent increase for women. If body weight is 20 per cent above average weight, the excess mortality rises to 20 per cent for men and 10 per cent for women.

A second major retrospective study has examined the relationship between body weight and mortality in Norwegian men and women.[21] The same curvilinear relationship is observed in this study, with the minimum BMI observed between 23 and 27 kg/m². Individuals with lower body weights showed an increase, giving the U-shaped relationship described above.

PROSPECTIVE STUDIES OF OBESITY AND MORTALITY. A large number of prospective studies have now been published relating obesity and mortality. Interpretation of these data has varied because some studies found no relationship between weight and excess mortality, whereas others did. In a careful re-evaluation of these data, Sjostrom[95] plotted the relationship between the numbers of subjects studied, the duration of follow-up, and the mortality experience. He demonstrated that smaller studies of long duration or shorter studies with large numbers of subjects led to similar conclusions—that there was a relationship between initial body weight and subsequent excess risk of mortality.

EFFECTS OF CHANGE IN BODY WEIGHT ON MORTALITY. Weight gain in adults[29, 96–100] and children[101, 102] has been associated with an increase in blood pressure and blood lipids as well as glucose and uric acid and risk of heart disease. Losing and regaining weight, so-called *weight cycling*, may also be hazardous. Data from the Chicago Gas and Electric Company Study[103] showed that those who gained and lost weight had a significantly higher risk of death from cardiovascular disease than the group of individuals with no change in weight. More recently, Lissner et al,[104] using data from the Framingham Study, showed that significant changes in weight, whether in the obese or nonobese, were associated with higher likelihood of mortality. This is currently a controversial area.

Effects of Regional Fat Distribution

More than half a dozen studies are now published showing that central adiposity is positively correlated with increased mortality as well as the risk for developing cardiovascular disease, diabetes mellitus, breast cancer, and stroke. Most of these studies[6, 105–107] have provided information about men. Only the Gothenburg cohort has also provided data on women.[5] Among 14,462 women between age 38 and 60 years of age, the 12-year age-specific incidence rates for myocardial infarction and stroke and the overall death rate were related to central adiposity. Among the highest quintile for central body fat, the relative risk of myocardial infarction was 8.2 times higher than that for the lowest quintile. For stroke and overall death rate, the relative risk was 3.8 and 2.8 times higher for those in the highest quintile than for those in the lowest quintile. When women in the top 5 per cent for central adiposity, measured as the ratio of the circumference of the waist divided by the circumference of the hips (WHR), were compared with women in the lowest quintile, the risk for myocardial infarction was increased 14.8 times, the risk of having a stroke was increased 11.0 times, and the risk of death from all causes was increased 4.8 times. The Swedish data allow a comparison of men and women in the same town. Lars-

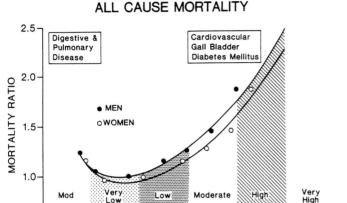

FIGURE 143–14. **Mortality ratio and body mass index (BMI).** Data from the American Cancer Society study have been plotted for men and women to show relationship of BMI to overall mortality. At a BMI below 20 kg/m² and above 25 kg/m², there is an increase in relative mortality. The major causes for this increased mortality are listed along with division of BMI groupings into various levels of risk. (Copyright 1987, George A. Bray.)

son et al.[108] have suggested that differences in fat distribution between men and women may account for most of the gender differences in rates of myocardial infarction.

Morbidity Related to Individual Systems

Cardiovascular Morbidity

Increased weight and central adiposity both produce a number of important changes in cardiovascular function.[109] Heart mass increases both on postmortem examination[110] and as assessed by echocardiographic measurements of posterior wall and interventricular septal thickness.[111] The increased cardiac mass is associated with increased blood volume and an increase in both intracellular and extracellular fluid volumes. Both cardiac output and cardiac stroke volume are elevated and positively correlated with body weight and with the degree of excess weight. Left and right ventricular end-diastolic pressures are also high, as are the pulmonary artery and pulmonary capillary wedge pressures. Studies using cardiac catheterization and echocardiography with pulsed Doppler techniques have revealed the presence of impaired left ventricular function in some obese patients,[111] and a cardiomyopathy of obesity has been clearly identified.[110] Abnormalities in both atrial and ventricular filling have been identified in 50 per cent of morbidly obese patients. Heart rate, however, does not increase in obesity. Thus the increased cardiac output occurs by increased stroke volume from an enlarged heart. Electrocardiographic alterations show a leftward shift in the mean QRS complex with increased fatness for both men and women. The PR interval, QRS duration, and QTc interval increase with increasing obesity. A prolonged QTc interval was present in 28.3 per cent of those tested.[109]

A number of lipoprotein abnormalities are associated with obesity.[112] First, high density lipoprotein cholesterol (HDL₂) decreases in obese males and females. Second,

serum total cholesterol is usually normal or only slightly elevated, although the transport of low density lipoproteins (LDL) cholesterol through the plasma compartment increases. This increased transport is consistent with the correlation between cholesterol production and obesity.[113, 114] As body fat accumulates, approximately 20 mg of additional cholesterol is synthesized for each extra kilogram of body fat. Third, the production of very low density lipoprotein triglyceride (VLDL) and the corresponding apoprotein B100 by liver tends to increase in relation to the degree of obesity in Caucasians and Pima Indians. The increased hepatic VLDL production in obesity is probably a reflection of the associated hyperinsulinemia. Fourth, the high rate of apoprotein-B synthesis in LDL is probably related to the high rate of synthesis apoprotein-B for incorporation into VLDL. Fifth, LPL, the enzyme that hydrolyzes acyltriglycerols in VLDL and chylomicrons, decreases in muscle and increases in adipose tissue in obese subjects. In contrast to most abnormalities in obesity, LPL in adipose tissue frequently rises with significant weight loss,[115, 116] whereas most other abnormalities return toward normal. Finally, free fatty acid concentrations frequently increase in obesity, reflecting their higher rate of turnover.

Hypertension

Increased blood pressure, like increased levels of insulin, is characteristic of obesity. Indeed, these two events may be related through the mechanism of insulin resistance.[117, 118] The use of sphygmomanometric methods for indirect determination of blood pressure requires an appropriately sized blood pressure cuff. When the blood pressure cuff is too short, greater differences are observed between systolic and diastolic pressures measured by direct intra-arterial methods than those obtained by indirect measurements.[109]

The cardiac response to hypertension can include both concentric hypertrophy and dilation.[119] Both central body fat distribution and an increase in total body fat appear to be related to the appearance of hypertension. During periods of severe caloric deprivation, such as occurred in World War I and World War II, hypertension was almost nonexistent. In clinical studies correlating changes in blood pressure with weight reduction, approximately 50 to 70 per cent of those who lose weight have a fall in blood pressure.[120, 121] Careful studies have shown that blood pressure falls even if sodium intake is preserved by giving salt supplements.[122, 123] Weight reduction is more effective in lowering systolic blood pressure than diastolic blood pressure.

Pulmonary Function

A number of abnormalities in pulmonary function have been observed in obese subjects. The first is the obesity-hypoventilation syndrome (OHS, pickwickian syndrome), characterized by somnolence, obesity, and alveolar hypoventilation. It is usually associated with obstructive sleep apnea and can represent a respiratory emergency.[124] Weight loss markedly reduces the detrimental effects of this syndrome, as does oxygenation of the patient's airway by using nocturnal compressed positive airway pressure (C-pap).[125]

Impairments in work capacity and pulmonary function are related to obesity per se.[126] Extensive alterations in pulmonary function are observed primarily in massively obese individuals or in obese individuals with some other underlying respiratory or cardiovascular problem. Thus, vital capacity, inspiratory capacity, residual volume, and diffusing capacity remain fairly constant over a wide range of body weights, except in subjects who are massively overweight, that is, those with a weight-to-height ratio greater than 1 kg/cm.

Diabetes Mellitus and Obesity

The US Diabetes Commission reported that the chance of becoming diabetic more than doubles for every 20 per cent of excess body weight. A curvilinear relationship between diabetes and obesity clearly exists. This has been demonstrated in the studies from Oslo, Norway,[127] in studies with the Pima Indians,[42] and in members of a weight-loss group in the United States ("TOPS").[128] The excess mortality for individuals with a BMI of 35 kg/m^2 increased by nearly eight-fold compared with those of normal weight.[21] The data suggest a threshold effect for overweight and the development of Type II diabetes, with a BMI of 20 kg/m^2 or less having essentially no risk for developing Type II diabetes.

Central fat deposition increases the risk of diabetes. This was first suggested by Vague[129] and has been demonstrated repeatedly since that time.[130, 131] There is a greater risk for developing diabetes as WHR increases (that is, with increased abdominal fat). For those in the lowest tertile for central fat distribution, increasing total fat had no significant effect on the risk of developing diabetes. Haffner and his colleagues[132] in the San Antonio Heart Study have demonstrated that the presence of central adiposity in Mexican-Americans was associated with high rates of Type II diabetes. In the women in this population, the BMI, a high WHR, and the ratio of subscapular to triceps skinfold measurements all made independent contributions to the risk of developing NIDDM.

Gallbladder Disease and Obesity

The association of obesity with gallbladder disease has been documented in several studies. In one study 88 per cent of the variation in frequency of gallbladder disease could be accounted for by weight, age, and parity, with weight being the most important variable.[133] Within each age group, however, the frequency of gallbladder disease increases at higher body weights. Women with a BMI greater than 30 kg/m^2 had a yearly incidence of gallstones of 1 per cent; those with a BMI greater than 45 kg/m^2 had an annual rate of approximately 2 per cent.[134] One mechanism for the increased risk of gallbladder disease is increased cholesterol production and secretion. As noted above, each kilogram of excess body fat increases cholesterol production by 20 mg/d.[113, 114] With weight loss, bile becomes more highly saturated with cholesterol and, if nidation factors are present, the risk of gallstone formation may increase sharply. Several recent studies have examined the formation of gallstones during the period of rapid weight loss. The incidence rates in these studies can be 15- to 25-fold higher than in the population of general obese subjects.[135] The stones that form appear to produce symptoms in approximately one third of the subjects and a

significant fraction—up to one half of them—may require surgery.

Cancer and Obesity

The American Cancer Society cohort study reported positive associations between excess weight and cancers of the gallbladder, biliary duct, endometrium, ovary, breast, and cervix among women and cancers of the colon and prostate among men.[21] An increase in the risk for endometrial cancer with increasing weight has been a consistent finding in the majority of case control studies, including those in northern Italy,[136] Denmark,[137] and the United States.[138] The relation of obesity to breast cancer has been observed primarily in postmenopausal women in studies in the Netherlands, Northern Italy, and Israel. Premenopausal women less frequently show an association of breast cancer and obesity. Indeed, Willett and his colleagues,[139] using data from the Nurses Health Trial, found an inverse relationship between BMI and age-adjusted relative risk for breast cancer in premenopausal women. However, this study does not consider fat distribution. Schapira et al.[140] have shown that central and probably visceral fatness carry increased risks of breast cancer.

Obesity and Joint Disease

Increasing body weight might be expected to add additional trauma to the weight-bearing joints and thus accelerate the development of osteoarthritis. The National Health and Nutrition Examination Survey (NHANES I) examined the prevalence of osteoarthritis in the hands and ankles in relation to weight status, race, and physical demands.[141] Within each age group, however, there was a clear increase in the prevalence of osteoarthritis in relation to body weight for all groups. The slope of increase with weight was sharpest below 90 kg, suggesting that body weight is only one factor.[142] Weight loss was associated with a significant reduction in risk for osteoarthritis of the knee.[143] In contrast with osteoarthritis, the risk of osteoporosis is reduced in the obese, possibly because of increased bone mass accrued during the early years of bone formation. Obesity is also associated with an increased risk of gout. In individuals whose weights were 115 per cent of desirable, the frequency of gout was 3.0 times that of individuals who were less than 110 per cent of desirable weight. There is also a significant correlation between uric acid levels and body weight.[144]

Obstetrics and the Overweight Patient

Body weight before pregnancy and weight gain during pregnancy both influence the course of labor and its outcome. Infants born to heavy women weigh more than those born to light women. There is also a direct relationship between placental weight and prepregnancy body weight. When these infants were compared with weight changes at age seven, 50 per cent of the incremental weight gain could be accounted for by the differences in placental weight at birth. The remaining 50 per cent of the difference was accounted for by the postnatal environment. Naeye[145] found that the fewest fetal and postnatal deaths occurred with mothers who were overweight at the beginning of pregnancy and who gained an average of 7.3 kg or less. The optimal weight gain during pregnancy was 9.1 kg for normal-weight women and 13.6 kg for those who were underweight.

Endocrine Function

Obesity produces a number of changes in endocrine function, but in almost all instances these appear to be secondary to the obesity rather than causative.[146]

GROWTH HORMONE (GH). The responses to most of the physiological and pharmacological stimuli that increase GH are diminished in obesity. Basal concentrations of GH are normal or slightly reduced. Although fasting increases basal GH levels in normal-weight subjects, this is not observed in obese individuals. The 24-hour secretory pattern, however, is impaired in both obese adults and children. This is manifested by reduced frequency of the secretory peaks, which nonetheless maintain a normal amplitude and duration when they do occur. Daily GH production, however, was reduced by 75 per cent in the obese, and there was an inverse correlation between the integrated GH release and the degree of obesity.[147]

Stimulation of somatomedin-C or insulin-like growth factor I (IGF-I) production by the liver is one of the major consequences of GH. Although one might thus expect reduced levels of IGF-I in obesity, levels have been reported to be normal or even elevated. IGF-I inhibits GH release at the hypothalamic or pituitary level. The differences between normal, elevated, and subnormal levels of IGF-I may reflect differences in the contribution of differing levels of the IGF-I–binding proteins. The maintenance of normal levels of IGF-I may also reflect, in part, the effects of hyperinsulinemia. This hypothesis deserves additional investigation.

Secretion of GH by the pituitary is under inhibitory and stimulatory control. Somatostatin, a 14-amino-acid peptide, is secreted from somatostatin-containing neurons in the hypothalamus and directly inhibits GH secretion. Conversely, GH-releasing factor (GRF), a 41-amino-acid peptide, is secreted from the ventromedial and arcuate hypothalamic nuclei directly into the hypothalamic portal circulation, with stimulation of GH release from the somatotropes in the pituitary. The stimulation of GH by insulin-induced hypoglycemia and by arginine appears to result from inhibition of somatostatin release from the hypothalamus. In obesity, the response to both insulin and arginine is reduced, suggesting a lowered activity of the somatostatin inhibitory system. Direct stimulation of the somatotroph by peripheral injections of GRF produces a significantly smaller release of GH in obese subjects than in normal-weight subjects or in obese subjects following weight loss. Williams et al.[148] have demonstrated an inverse correlation between GH secretion in response to GRF and the degree of overweight.

Table 143–7 summarizes the altered responses in obesity. Agents that act on the GRF system, such as the α_2-adrenergic receptor agonist clonidine and the enkephalin (opioid) analogue DAMME, result in GH release that is significantly less in obese subjects than in controls. Naloxone, which blocks opioid responses, suppresses GH secretion in normal-weight subjects but not in obese subjects.[149] Naloxone has also been reported to improve arginine-me-

TABLE 143–7. GROWTH HORMONE (GH) SECRETION IN OBESITY

Basal GH	N/↓
Nocturnal GH surge	↓
24-hour integrated GH output	↓
Insulin-like growth factor-I	↓/N/↑
GH response to	
Fasting	↓
Glucose	↓
Hypoglycemia	↓
Arginine	↓
GHRH	↓
Clonidine	↓
L-dopa	↓
Opioids	↓
Improvement of stimulated GH release by	
Naloxone (endogenous opioid system)	+/−
D,L-Fenfluramine (serotoninergic system)	+
Pyridostigmine (cholinergic system)	+
Weight reduction	+

N, Normal; ↑, increased; ↓, decreased; +, improvement; −, no improvement.

diated GH release in obese subjects but to be without effect following insulin-induced hypoglycemia or the injection of GRF. The appetite-suppressant drug fenfluramine has been shown to improve the GH response to arginine and to insulin-induced hypoglycemia, whereas basal GH levels are not affected. In summary, the state of overnutrition reflected in obesity is associated with reduced inhibitory and reduced stimulatory control of GH secretion.

PROLACTIN (PRL). PRL secretion is primarily under inhibitory dopaminergic control from hypothalamic neurons, but secretion can also be modified by thyrotropin-releasing hormone (TRH). In most studies, basal plasma PRL levels are normal in obese subjects, and there is no correlation with body weight or body fat distribution. The nocturnal rise in PRL, which normally occurs shortly after the onset of sleep, may be blunted or delayed in obese subjects, but 24-hour PRL production appears to be normal.

In contrast to the normal basal production of PRL, the secretion of PRL in response to pharmacological maneuvers is impaired in obese subjects. These effects are summarized in Table 143–8. L-Dopa is a precursor of dopamine which produces a normal suppression of pituitary PRL release in obesity. In contrast, chlorpromazine, a dopamine antagonist that normally stimulates PRL release by blocking dopamine-secreting neurons, produces a decreased response in obese subjects. The stimulation of PRL by TRH is frequently blunted in obese adults or children. However, no correlation exists between the degree of obe-

TABLE 143–8. PROLACTIN SECRETION IN OBESITY

Basal prolactin	N
Stimulation of prolactin release by	
Thyrotropin-releasing hormone	↓/N
Chlorpromazine	↓
Arginine	↓
Insulin-induced hypoglycemia	↓
Metoclopramide	↑/↓
Domperidone	↓/N
Suppression of prolactin release by	
L-Dopa	N

N, Normal; ↑, increased; ↓, decreased.

sity and the peak PRL response to TRH. Administration of the dopamine antagonist metoclopramide produced an increased response in obese subjects. Kopelman et al.[150] have observed differential responsiveness to metoclopramide and domperidone among obese subjects who responded with a release of PRL after insulin-induced hypoglycemia (the responders) versus those who exhibited no response to insulin-induced hypoglycemia. The response to metoclopramide was significantly impaired in subjects who failed to respond with a release of PRL after inducing hypoglycemia with insulin, whereas the release of PRL following domperidone was comparable whether or not subjects responded to insulin-induced hypoglycemia with a release of PRL. This suggested the possibility of a disturbance in the central pathways involving dopamine control of PRL secretion in obese subjects. Two groups of obese subjects can thus be separated based on the rise in PRL following insulin-induced hypoglycemia. The meaning of this difference in terms of etiology and therapy is currently unknown.

THYROTROPIN AND THE THYROID GLAND. Thyroxin concentrations are normal in obese subjects and are relatively uninfluenced by overfeeding or by weight loss. In contrast, plasma T_3 changes rapidly in response to nutrition. Both normal and elevated levels of plasma T_3 have been reported in obesity. This difference may reflect the differences in food intake in subjects because the T_3 concentration in plasma depends on total caloric intake as well as the composition of the diet. Decreasing the carbohydrate content in the diet and total fasting both acutely decrease serum T_3 levels and increase the concentrations of reverse T_3 (rT_3). Danforth and his colleagues[151] have reported that overfeeding of normal and obese subjects increases both the production rate of T_3 and its turnover in normal and obese Caucasian subjects, but less so in the obese Pima Indians.

Plasma thyrotropin levels are usually normal in obese subjects and in most studies are unaffected by fasting. In contrast, exaggerated, normal, or blunted responses of TSH to the administration of TRH have been reported in obesity. Fasting is associated with a decrease in TSH response to administered TRH. A summary of the effects of obesity, fasting, and overfeeding on thyroid parameters is presented in Table 143–9.

ENDORPHIN AND THE OPIOID SYSTEM. Met-enkephalin and leu-enkephalin are produced from pre-pro-prodynorphin A; dynorphin is produced from pre-pro-dynorphin B; and β-endorphin is produced from the precursor pre-pro-opiomelanocortin. These peptides are of interest because both dynorphin and β-endorphin stimulate food intake. Naloxone, a drug that inhibits the action of opioids, re-

TABLE 143–9. CHANGES IN THYROID FUNCTION TESTS IN OBESITY AND IN CONDITIONS OF FASTING AND OVERFEEDING

	OBESITY	FASTING	OVER-FEEDING
T_4	N	N (↑)	N
T_3	N/↑	↓	↑
rT_3	N	↑	↓
TSH basal	N	N (↓)	N
TSH after TRH	↓/N/↑	↓	↓/↑

N, Normal; ↑, increased; ↓, decreased; parentheses indicate limited number of studies.

TABLE 143–10. β-ENDORPHIN (βE) IN OBESITY

Basal βE	↑
βE circadian rhythm	absent
Basal βE after weight reduction	=/↓
Stimulation of βE by	
Insulin-induced hypoglycemia	↓
Corticotropin-releasing hormone	↓
Suppression of βE by	
Dexamethasone (1 mg)	↓

=, Unchanged; ↑, increased; ↓, decreased.

duces feeding in animals and in human beings.[152, 153] Clinical trials with naltrexone, a long-acting derivative of naloxone, have failed to show a significant effect on weight loss compared with the placebo-treated group.

β-Endorphin is produced in both the hypothalamus and the pituitary and is released in a pulsatile manner, mirroring the ACTH and cortisol rhythm. Both ACTH and β-endorphin secretion are stimulated by the peripheral administration of corticotropin-releasing hormone (CRH) and are inhibited by glucocorticoids. In obese adults and children the basal plasma level of β-endorphin is elevated. The secretion of β-endorphin from the pituitary may be abnormally controlled because in children administration of CRH did not result in the expected rise in β-endorphin. The administration of dexamethasone, however, adequately suppressed β-endorphin levels. Current information on β-endorphin in obesity is summarized in Table 143–10.

THE ADRENAL GLAND. In genetic, hypothalamic, and dietary forms of experimental obesity, adrenalectomy or blockade of glucocorticoid action reverses or prevents further development of obesity.[62] Only small quantities of glucocorticoid are required, however, for obesity to progress. Glucocorticoids can also modulate human obesity. A centripetal form of obesity is characteristic of Cushing's syndrome, and obesity may occasionally be its presenting feature. Addison's disease resulting from adrenal insufficiency is associated with a depletion of body fat.

ACTH, like β-endorphin, is produced from pro-opiomelanocortin (POMC). A normal diurnal rhythm for ACTH as well as cortisol has been shown in obesity. Moreover, basal plasma cortisol and its diurnal rhythm are normal in obesity. Although the excretion of urinary free cortisol is normal, the metabolic products of glucocorticoid metabolism, such as urinary 17-hydroxycorticosteroids, are increased, suggesting increased hepatic metabolism of cortisol. This is supported by data showing increased cortisol production rates. The enhanced cortisol metabolism may result from the oxidation of cortisol to cortisone in adipose tissue, because cortisone is a weaker suppressor of ACTH than cortisol and would require increased ACTH stimulation of the adrenal to provide adequate cortisol output. The stimulation of ACTH release from the pituitary of obese subjects by CRH is normal. However, in some studies, the cortisol response to CRH appears to be reduced, particularly in adults, in contrast to the normal stimulation of ACTH production.

A key criterion for the diagnosis of Cushing's disease is suppression of plasma ACTH and plasma cortisol levels following the administration of dexamethasone. Most studies in the obese have reported normal suppression, but in other studies between 10 and 16 per cent of obese patients fail to suppress cortisol adequately.[154-156] This failure of some individuals to suppress cortisol completely may reflect the larger distribution volume for dexamethasone in the obese and thus the lower plasma concentration that is achieved. This problem can be avoided by measuring plasma dexamethasone levels and showing that they reach appropriate levels. Table 143–11 summarizes the effects of obesity on the hypothalamic-pituitary-adrenocortical axis.

OBESITY AND GONADOTROPIN FUNCTION. In obese males the plasma concentration of testosterone is decreased.[157] This reduction in total testosterone is weight-related and results from a reduction in the level of sex hormone–binding globulin (SHBG). The level of free testosterone is normal in moderately obese men, but in massively obese men, there may be a decrease in free testosterone as well.[158] A weight-related rise in both estradiol and estrone also occurs, whereas the basal concentration of the pituitary gonadotropins, follicle-stimulating hormone (FSH), and luteinizing hormone (LH) are normal.[159] Similarly, the pituitary release of LH and FSH in response to an injection of gonadotropin-releasing hormone (GnRH) is normal, as is the concentration of these pituitary peptides during treatment with clomiphene, a drug that blocks the effects of estrogen. The testes in obese men are unaltered.

In girls, the onset of menarche may occur at a younger age than in normal-weight girls. One explanation for this phenomenon is the Frisch-Revelle hypothesis,[160] which is based on the observation that menstruation is initiated when body weight reaches a "critical mass." As the growth rate accelerates in late childhood, the percentage of fat rises and initiates the pubertal process. According to this hypothesis, the growth spurt begins at a body weight of approximately 31 kg. The maximum rate of weight gain occurs at 39 kg, and menstruation begins when body weight reaches 48 kg, or approximately 22 per cent body fat. Because obese girls grow faster and enter this critical weight range at a younger age than normal-weight girls, menstruation usually starts at an earlier age in overweight girls.

The obese patient often has irregular menstrual cycles as well as an increase in the frequency of menstrual abnormalities. The ovaries in obese women often show an increase in hyalinization as well as an increase in frequency of atretic follicles. As in obese men, the concentration of SHBG is reduced in obese women.

Women with hirsutism and anovulatory cycles were on average 14 kg heavier than women with no menstrual abnormalities.[161] There was also an increasing number of women with anovulatory cycles as the degree of excess weight increased. Only 2.6 per cent of women less than 20 per cent overweight had anovulatory cycles, compared with 8.4 per cent of women who are more than 74 per cent overweight. The longer the duration of obesity, the greater the amount of facial hair which was identified. Obesity occurring in the teenage years was associated with an increased number of married women who never became pregnant and with a higher likelihood of surgery for polycystic ovaries.

These findings indicate that alterations in body weight can influence both the onset of menstruation and the subsequent initiation of menstruation in women who have developed secondary amenorrhea. In a detailed endocrine analysis of the menstrual cycle in six obese women, two abnormalities were noted: first, the rise in FSH levels in the first half of the cycle was lower than normal; and second, progesterone failed to rise normally in the second half of the menstrual cycle. Although the mechanism for these disorders in obese women is unknown, attendant hormonal abnormalities in obese women are reversible with weight loss.

The function of the reproductive system in women is complicated by the metabolism of steroids in other organs, with the resulting production of biologically active steroidal products. Δ^4-Androstenedione, which is produced by the adrenal, can be converted to estrone by stromal elements of adipose tissue.[162] Muscle may also convert estrone to estradiol. Despite the enhanced rate of conversion of Δ^4-androstenedione to estrone in obesity, most studies in premenopausal obese women do not show an increase in the circulating concentration of estrogens. However, in obese postmenopausal women, the concentration of estrogens does appear to increase. When castrated obese and non-obese women are given implants of estradiol, the obese women had higher levels of Δ^4-androstenedione and free testosterone. Studies of estradiol metabolism showed that obese women had decreased hydroxylation at the C-2 position and increased oxidation at the 17-α position. Hydroxylation at the 16-α position was not significantly influenced by obesity, however. The final complicating factor is regional fat distribution. Women with upper body obesity had higher testosterone and estradiol but lower levels of SHBG.[163]

Just as the onset of menarche is earlier in obese women, so data suggest that the onset of ovarian failure and increased FSH production is four years earlier in obese than in normal weight women. This and other features of ovarian failure occurred at significantly younger age in the obese.

CLINICAL TYPES OF OBESITY

Classification of Obesities

The classification described below is adapted from a classification used for heart disease. It involves three components: (1) an anatomical classification, (2) an etiological classification, and (3) a functional classification (Table 143–12).

TABLE 143–11. HYPOTHALAMIC-PITUITARY-ADRENOCORTICAL-AXIS IN OBESITY

Basal cortisol	N
Basal ACTH	N
Diurnal rhythm cortisol/ACTH	N
Free cortisol urinary excretion	N (↑)
Cortisol metabolism	↑
Cortisol production rate	↑
ACTH stimulation of cortisol	N
CRH stimulation of ACTH	N
CRH stimulation of cortisol	N/↓
Insulin-induced hypoglycemia mediated stimulation of ACTH/cortisol	N/↓
Dexamethasone suppressibility of cortisol	N/↓

CRH, Corticotropin-releasing hormone; N, normal, ↑, increased; ↓, decreased; parentheses indicate limited number of studies.

TABLE 143–12. CLASSIFICATION OF OBESITY

I. Anatomical classification
   A. Microscopic
      1. Fat cell size
      2. Fat cell number
   B. Macroscopic
      1. Total body fat
      2. Subcutaneous fat distribution
      3. Visceral fat
      4. Abnormal or unusual fat deposits
II. Etiologic classification
   A. Hypothalamic
   B. Endocrine
   C. Dietary
   D. Physical inactivity
   E. Genetic
   F. Drug-induced
III. Functional classification
   A. Degree of risk estimated from body mass index
      1. Very low   (Class 1 or Grade 0)—BMI 20 <25 kg/m²
      2. Low   (Class 2 or Grade 1)—BMI 25–<30 kg/m²
      3. Moderate (Class 3 or Grade 2)—BMI 30–<35 kg/m²
      4. High   (Class 4 or Grade 2)—BMI 35–<40 kg/m²
      5. Very high (Class 5 or Grade 3)—BMI >40 kg/m²
   B. Associated risks
      1. High blood pressure
      2. Insulin resistance or diabetes
      3. Low HDL-C/LDL-C ratio
      4. LVH by ECG
      5. Sleep apnea or high $PaCO_2$
      6. Hirsutism or high LH/FSH ratio
      7. Smoking
      8. Restrained eaters
      9. Low physical activity

Anatomical Classification

The anatomical classification includes both the number of adipocytes and the distribution of body fat, but the major emphasis should be on distribution of body fat. In many of the obese whose problem begins in childhood, the number of adipocytes may be increased by two- to four-fold, with a normal number being 20 to 60 × 10⁹ fat cells. Individuals with increased numbers of fat cells have hyperplastic obesity, which is to be distinguished from the hypertrophic form of obesity, in which the total number of adipocytes is normal but the size of individual fat cells is increased.[52, 164] In general, all obesity is associated with an increase in the size of adipocytes, but only the markedly obese individual has an increase in the total number of fat cells. Individuals who are 75 per cent or more overweight almost always have an increase in the number of fat cells. The duration of weight loss that follows successful dietary treatment of obesity is shorter and the rate at which weight is regained is more rapid in individuals with hypercellular obesity than with hypertrophic obesity.[165]

The distribution of adipose tissue or body fat can be divided into four parts. The first is in the percentage of body fat. The second is the distribution of fat between upper segment, android or male-type obesity, in which fat is primarily on the trunk and shoulders, and lower body, gynoid or female-type obesity, in which the major fat deposits are located on the thighs or hips. Women with upper body fat distribution show impaired glucose tolerance and substantially increased insulin secretion following an oral glucose load compared with women with lower body fat distribution but similar total body fat levels.[166] Women with

upper segment obesity also show an increased circulating level of free testosterone, reduced levels of SHBG, increased insulin resistance, and reduced hepatic clearance of pancreatic insulin.[163, 167] Men with upper body obesity often have lower levels of testosterone, which has prompted studies using testosterone to reduce upper body fat in men.[168] The third part of this anatomical classification is the quantity of visceral fat. This intra-abdominal depot increases with age and carries the highest risk. The final part of the anatomical classification is unusual fat deposits. This includes the lipomas, which can be single or multiple and may have a genetic component. It also includes lipodystrophy, in which upper body, lower body, or total body fat is lost. Steatopygia also belongs in this group.

Age at Onset

Progressive childhood obesity is one syndrome of hypercellular obesity. These individuals develop obesity early in life and show a continuing weight gain and deviation from the upper limits of normal thereafter. However, progressive childhood obesity cannot be detected at birth. Birth weights of children who become obese are in general not different from those who maintain normal weight. However, individuals born to diabetic mothers are very fat at birth and develop more obesity in later life. So do children born to mothers who were starved during mid-pregnancy.

The crucial periods for the appearance of progressive childhood obesity are between ages 4 and 11. In a follow-up of 504 overweight children, 47 per cent were still obese as adults. Excessive overweight in puberty in this group was associated with increased morbidity and mortality in adult life.[32] Progressive childhood obesity can be identified by the progressive deviation of weight from the 95th percentile for children based on age and height. In our experience, young girls and boys who reach 100 kg by age 20 show a progressive weight gain thereafter, which may be as much as 5 kg/yr or 50 kg/decade. This form of progressive childhood obesity becomes a serious risk for mortality in middle adult life.

Most studies show that less than one third of the obese adults were obese in childhood. Thus, most obesity develops in adult life. For women, pregnancy is the central event associated with significant obesity. Almost all of the existing studies suggest that the woman who becomes pregnant will be several kilograms heavier two years after the pregnancy than a woman of the same age, weight, and occupation who was not pregnant. In addition, pregnancy may be a time of major weight gain, with reports of weight increasing by more than 50 kg. For fetal outcome the optimal weight gain for a normal weight woman is 10 to 12 kg. As body weight increases, the optimal weight gain to minimize fetal loss declines. For women who are more than 50 kg above desirable weight levels, a weight gain of 6 to 8 kg is optimal for minimal fetal loss. Weight loss during pregnancy is never desirable.

For men, the transition from the active life of adolescence to the more sedentary lifestyle associated with adult years in Western culture may be associated with weight gain. Clear evidence both from the Framingham study and from data on induction of men into the military service indicates that men have become progressively heavier for height during this century. This change has been particularly marked in the decades since 1970, but the reasons for this are unclear.

The middle years of life (age 30 to 60) are also important periods of weight gain for most adults. This is a time in which bone mass gradually declines, as do GH and testosterone levels in men. The decline in the levels of these anabolic agents may play an important role in the increasing deposition of visceral and abdominal fat in adults. For women, the continual monthly menstrual cycle with progestational preparation for pregnancy may play a role in the weight gain to which most women who do not restrain their eating are susceptible.

Etiological Classification

A number of causes of obesity are summarized in Table 143–12.

Neuroendocrine Obesity

HYPOTHALAMIC OBESITY. Hypothalamic obesity has been reported in human beings after a variety of injuries,[61, 169] including trauma, malignancy, and inflammatory diseases. Three groups of findings accompany the syndrome of hypothalamic obesity. The first is related to increased intracranial pressure and includes headaches and diminished vision due to papilledema or swelling of the optic nerve. The second group of symptoms are manifestations of endocrine alterations following disturbance of the hypothalamic-pituitary axis and include amenorrhea, impotence, diabetes insipidus, thyroid insufficiency, or adrenal insufficiency. The third group of symptoms are a variety of neurological and physiological derangements including convulsions, coma, somnolence, temperature disturbances, and disturbances of thirst. Treatment of the syndrome requires treating the underlying disease and giving appropriate endocrine and neurological support.

CUSHING'S DISEASE. Cushing's disease is described in considerable detail elsewhere in this volume (Ch. 100). Among clinical series of patients with Cushing's syndrome, obesity is a common finding and in some cases it can be the presenting symptom. One four-year-old boy was brought to our endocrine clinic by his mother because of weight gain. Evaluation revealed elevated plasma and urinary free cortisol and loss of the diurnal rhythm for cortisol. The most common cause of hyperadrenalism in children is an adrenal tumor, but this boy proved to be suffering from bilateral adrenal hyperplasia; appropriate treatment was given, and his obesity disappeared.

HYPOTHYROIDISM. Obesity may also occur with hypothyroidism, but this is usually not substantial. The primary increases in weight with the myxedematous state are in the increases of subcutaneous tissues, thickening of skin, and retention of fluid (see Ch. 45).

POLYCYSTIC OVARY SYNDROME. The syndrome of polycystic ovaries was originally described in 1844 as sclerocystic ovaries. It is characterized clinically by oligomenorrhea or amenorrhea, hirsutism, hyperandrogenism, an elevated LH/FSH ratio, and polycystic ovaries.[170, 171] Obesity is present in 16 to 49 per cent of the cases in various series.[170] When a group of very obese women with polycystic ovaries were compared with a group of women with a similar degree of obesity but without polycystic ovaries, the SHBG

concentration was reduced in both groups compared with that in control women. However, testosterone and albumin-bound testosterone levels were higher than normal, as were Δ⁴-androstenedione levels in those with polycystic ovaries. The level of dehydroepiandrosterone-sulfate (DHEA-S) was not increased. Estradiol and estrone were significantly higher in the women with polycystic ovaries than in the control women. An increased and pulsatile pattern of LH secretion was seen in both groups, but the value was higher in the less obese women.

Insulin resistance is also characteristic of the polycystic ovary syndrome. These changes are not due to alterations in the insulin receptors.[172] Insulin secretion during the 24 hours is higher in women with polycystic ovaries than in control-matched obese women. The levels of IGF-binding proteins (IGFBP) are altered in women with polycystic ovaries. The level of one of these binding proteins, IGFBP I, is low and may be associated with the high degree of insulin resistance observed in some of these patients. Obese women with the polycystic ovaries show a blunted secretion of GH and a low GH response to the injection of GRF. This contrasts with the normal levels of GH and normal response to GRF in normal-weight women with polycystic ovaries, suggesting an important role of obesity. In women with polycystic ovary syndrome, IGF-I, IGF-II, and GH are normal, but the level of IGFBP-I is decreased. One sequence relating these events may be the following: The increased insulin resistance associated with this syndrome leads to a decrease in IGFBP-I, which in turn leads to increase in bioavailability of IGF-I to its receptors. IGF-I can stimulate the ovary to increase androgen production, leading to the syndrome of polycystic ovaries.

PSEUDOHYPOPARATHYROIDISM. Pseudohypoparathyroidism is a genetic disease with impaired response to parathyroid hormone. These individuals may look obese, but their problem can be diagnosed by measuring serum calcium (see Ch. 67).

HYPOGONADISM. Hypogonadism is associated with reduced gonadal steroid hormone production and in both males and females with an increase in body fat. Appropriate replacement therapy restores the lean-to-fat ratios to normal (see Chs. 122 and 131).

GROWTH HORMONE DEFICIENCY. GH deficiency is likewise associated with increased subcutaneous adipose tissue deposition. Treatment with GH has been shown to reduce the level of subcutaneous adipose tissue (see Ch. 20).

INSULINOMA. Insulin has been reported to increase body fat. In patients with insulinomas, however, the degree of increase of body fat is very modest, suggesting that insulin levels alone are not often the major cause of obesity (see Ch. 92).

Iatrogenic Obesity

DRUG TREATMENT. A number of drugs can produce weight gain or weight loss. These are summarized in Table 143–13. The two largest and most important groups are the psychotropic drugs and the steroids. The involvement of norepinephrine, serotonin, histamine, and a variety of peptides in regulating food intake provides a basis for understanding the receptor systems through which drugs can modulate food intake and body weight when these drugs are used as treatment for depression and behavioral distur-

TABLE 143–13. DRUGS THAT INCREASE BODY WEIGHT

Phenothiazines (chlorpromazine > thioridazine ≥ trifluoperazine ≥ mesoridazine > promazine ≥ mepazine ≥ perphenazine ≥ prochlorperazine > haloperidol ≥ loxapine)
Antidepressants (amitriptyline > imipramine = doxepin = phenelzine > amoxapine = desipramine = trazodone = tranylcypromine)
Antiepileptics (valproate; carbamazepine)
Steroids (glucocorticoids; megestrol acetate)
Antihypertensives (terazosin)

bances. The phenothiazine drugs characteristically produce some weight gain, but the tricyclic antidepressant amitriptyline produces the most weight gain. Amitriptyline increases not only weight but the preference for carbohydrate.

HYPOTHALAMIC SURGERY. The syndrome of hypothalamic obesity has been described above. In approximately half of the patients with this problem, the obesity developed after neurosurgical intervention rather than as a presenting symptom. This is not surprising considering the difficulty of operating in this area. The surgically induced form of this syndrome might be called iatrogenic hypothalamic obesity.

HIGH FAT INTAKE. In experimental animals, one of the most robust techniques for producing obesity is to give animals a high-fat diet. The association of obesity with the high-fat Western type of diet is also suspected to be important in humans, but documenting this has been difficult. Support comes mainly from an epidemiological study from Brazil which shows the relationship between indices of obesity and the intake of fat.[173] Similar support for this concept comes from the increasing prevalence of obesity in Japan as the fat content of the Japanese diet has increased from below 15 per cent in the early years after World War II to values above 25 per cent at the present time. Several other reports also suggest this relationship.[174, 175]

PHYSICAL INACTIVITY. Individual patients frequently re-

port that their obesity began following surgery or other events that impede physical activity. Because physical activity is an important element in the energy balance equation, such an observation is not surprising. The epidemiological data of Kromhout[176] support a role for decreased activity in adult weight gain. In a 10-year interval between age 50 and 60, the energy intake of a cohort of Dutch men declined on average 500 kcal/d. Over this same interval of time body weight increased 3.5 kg, indicating that energy expenditure must have declined by slightly more than 500 kcal/d.

Genetic Factors in Obesity

Dysmorphic obesities are a group of rare diseases, with associated obesity and dysmorphic features, in which the evidence suggests that genetic factors are of major importance. Table 143–14 is a comparison of several such syndromes.

Genetic Predisposition

FAMILY, TWIN, AND ADOPTION STUDIES. Genetic and environmental factors interact in the development of obesity. Three sets of studies support this contention: the aggregation of obesity in families; obesity in adopted children; and studies of obesity in twins.

FAMILY STUDIES. Obesity in the parents of obese children has been noted in many studies. In well over 1000 patients, the frequency of obesity in one or both parents ranged from a low of 44 per cent to a high of 83 per cent. The mother was most frequently obese, with the father much less often so. This association between obesity in the parents and its presence in children, however, does not help us to separate environmental factors in the development of obesity, and more critical studies are needed.

The most recent examination of adopted children ap-

TABLE 143–14. A COMPARISON OF SYNDROMES OF OBESITY—HYPOGONADISM AND MENTAL RETARDATION

FEATURE	SYNDROME				
	Prader-Willi	**Bardet-Biedl**	**Ahlstrom**	**Cohen**	**Carpenter**
Inheritance	Sporadic; 2/3 have defect	Autosomal recessive	Autosomal recessive	Probably autosomal recessive	Autosomal recessive
Stature	Short	Normal; infrequently short	Normal; infrequently short	Short or tall	Normal
Obesity	Generalized moderate to severe; onset 1–3 yrs	Generalized; early onset, 1–2 yrs	Truncal; early onset, 2–5 yrs	Truncal; mid-childhood, age 5	Truncal Gluteal
Cranofacies	Narrow bifrontal diameter Almond-shaped eyes Strabismus V-shaped mouth High arched palate	Not distinctive	Not distinctive	High nasal bridge Arched palate Open mouth Short philtrum	Acrocephaly Flat nasal bridge High arched palate
Limbs	Small hands and feet Hypotonia	Polydactyly	No abnormalities	Hypotonia Narrow hands and feet	Polydactyly Syndactyly Genu valgum
Reproductive status	Primary hypogonadism	Primary hypogonadism	Hypogonadism in males but not in females	Normal gonadal function or hypogonadotropic hypogonadism	Secondary
Other features	Enamel hypoplasia Hyperphagia Temper tantrums Nasal speech			Dysplastic ears Delayed puberty	
Mental retardation	Mild to moderate		Normal IQ	Mild	Slight

pears to be both the most extensive and the most rigorous and concludes that genetic factors account for more than 30 per cent of the variance in BMI. Using the Danish registry, Stunkard and his colleagues[177] examined a sample of 800 adoptees aged 33 to 56, who were selected from a population of 3651 subjects. Four hundred men and 400 women were selected to represent thin, median, overweight, and obese, using BMI as the criterion. There was no relationship between BMI of the adoptive parents and their children. On the other hand, the BMI of the biological parents increased with increasing weight status of the children. This relationship was stronger for the mothers than for the fathers. This same conclusion was reached when the siblings of the adopted children were examined.[178] These data suggest that inheritance plays a role in the risk of developing obesity. Estimates suggest that about one third of the variations between BMI can be accounted for by genetic factors. Environment in the first year of life plays little role in the development of obesity because 55 per cent of the adoptees had been placed in the adoptive homes within the first months of life and 90 per cent within the first year of life. Of interest is the fact that the adoptive fathers of obese adopted children, male or female, tended to be leaner.

TWIN STUDIES. To approach the question of genetic versus environmental factors in obesity in still a more systematic way, several authors have examined the relationship between body weight in twins.[179–183] Because monozygotic twins presumably have identical genetic material, whereas dizygotic twins have the genetic diversity of brothers and/or sisters, evaluation of these two groups of twins should make it possible to separate nature from nurture most clearly. In one of the early studies, Verschuer[184] examined the per cent differences in weight between monozygotic and dizygotic twins. The 80 pairs of monozygotic twins had nearly half the mean differences in body weights that was observed in 38 pairs of dizygotic twins.

Bouchard and his colleagues[91] have utilized twins to provide an important dimension to the understanding of obesity. They have examined the relationships of skinfolds and total body fat in various groups of individuals with differing degrees of genetic relationship, as well as the effects of exercise training and overfeeding, in an attempt to identify some of the genetic and environmental interactions.[87, 89] In these studies, skinfold thickness at six sites was measured along with estimating of total body fat and calculating BMI. In adopted siblings, there was a very low order of correlation. Biological siblings, however, showed a somewhat higher correlation, and this correlation became highest, as might be expected, among the monozygotic twins. The fact that the biological siblings had a lower correlation for all of the variables than did the dizygotic twins, although they all had the same genetic variability, implies that an important environmental influence was operative in the dizygotic twins which was less important in the biological siblings.

The relative importance of biological and cultural inheritance can be estimated from various models using the data from families with different degrees of genetic variability—cousins, siblings, twins, and parents. Using a regression technique called path analysis,[19] it is possible to separate the transmissible variability into its genetic and environmental components. The amount of subcutaneous fat has about 40 per cent transmissibility, very little of which is inherited according to this model. For total body fat, on the other hand, the total transmissible variance is about 50 per cent, of which the genetic effect is about 20 per cent; that is, environment and genetics have nearly equal weight in determining total body fat. The highest transmissible effects are observed in the ratio of extremity to trunk fat, for which the transmissible variance is 60 per cent, again with nearly equal genetic and environmental components.

It is thus fair to conclude that both genetic and environmental factors are important in the development of obesity. The best estimates suggest that they are of approximately equal overall importance.

Functional Impairments

A number of associated events can enhance the degree of impairment associated with obesity per se. Pulmonary function in general remains normal until the weight in kilograms equals the height in centimeters (wt > 150 kg). Above this weight significant alterations begin to occur. Sleep apnea, the so-called pickwickian syndrome associated with the obesity-hypoventilation syndrome, carries substantial functional limitations and increases risk of congestive heart failure. Marked obesity enhances the risk of a cardiomyopathy and congestive heart failure. Hypertension is an obvious additional burden on the cardiovascular system and should be identified if present. Diabetes mellitus is likewise an additional problem for which obesity is a confound. The presence of hypertriglyceridemia and a low HDL cholesterol produces problems. The incidence of gallbladder disease is significantly increased, with a 1 per cent annual incidence for individuals with a BMI above 30 and approximately 2 per cent incidence for individuals with a BMI above 45 kg/m². Finally, many obese individuals have behavioral impairments. Nearly one third of the obese have been identified as binge eaters.[178] Many who are potentially obese are restrained eaters who occasionally lose control with unwanted consequences.

CLINICAL EVALUATION OF THE OBESE PATIENT

Because all treatments for obesity entail some risk, it is important to decide whether treatment is appropriate, and if so what that treatment should be. To do this requires an assessment of the risk associated with adiposity and its distribution in relation to the various treatments. Two variables can be used to make this assessment. The first is the BMI, and the second is the distribution of body fat.

The relationship between BMI and mortality is shown in Figure 143–14 (see above). Underweight individuals have increased risk for respiratory disease, tuberculosis, digestive disease, and some cancers. For overweight individuals the risks are cardiovascular disease, gallbladder disease, high blood pressure,[2] and diabetes. Body weights associated with a BMI of 20 to 25 kg/m² are good weights for most people. When BMI is below 18 kg/m² or above 27 kg/m², risk increases in a curvilinear fashion. Individuals with a BMI between 25 and 30 kg/m² in men of any age and between 25 and 30 kg/m² for women under 35 or 27 kg/m² in women over 35 may be described as having low risk. Those with a BMI between 30 and 35 kg/m² have moderate risk, those with a body mass index between 35 and 40 kg/m² are at high risk, and those with a BMI above 40 kg/m² are at very high risk from their obesity. The relative risk is shifted by a number of factors including insulin resistance, hypertension, elevated ratio of total or LDL cholesterol to HDL-cholesterol, and smoking.

From epidemiological data it is clear that increased abdominal and particularly visceral fat carries increased risks. The top tertile in abdominal fat distribution has a nearly two-fold increase in risk of mortality and morbidity from heart disease, diabetes, breast cancer, and hypertension. This extra risk is observed in men and women and rises sharply for the top 10th percentile of abdominal fat distribution. When the difference in fat distribution is corrected statistically, the excess mortality observed between men and women is largely, if not completely, eliminated.[185] The risk associated with excess central accumulation of fat probably reflects the increase in visceral fat. Abnormal glucose tolerance, hypertension, and hyperlipidemia are more closely associated with the amount of visceral fat than with WHR or total body fat. The sagittal diameter has been proposed as a way to estimate visceral fat, but at the present time the only reliable way to determine visceral fat is with a CT scan or MR imaging. The availability of newer, less expensive methods will be an important clinical advance.

The algorithm in Figure 143–15 provides a way of including both the degree of overweight, as estimated from the BMI, and the presence of other factors, including the distribution of body fat, hypertension, and lipids in making decisions about relative risk from obesity. At any given BMI, the risk to health is increased with higher WHR, blood pressure, smoking, fasting insulin, or lipid levels. Table 143–12 provides some guidelines for arriving at estimated risk that incorporates BMI and the risk associated with other factors including hyperlipidemia, hypertension, and central fat.

TREATMENT

Diet

Basic Considerations

Before considering specific diets, a number of important general points should be made about all diets. First, calories do count. During World War II, Keys and his colleagues[186] showed a clear-cut, predictable reduction in body weight and body fat stores when caloric intake of healthy young men was reduced to 1650 kcal/d. The rate of weight loss is largely independent of dietary composition despite wide variations in proteins, carbohydrate, and total fat intake.

Prediction of weight loss for an individual patient can prove difficult. In one study,[187] the variation in weight loss of women hospitalized for three weeks on a metabolic ward while eating an 800 kcal/d diet (3.4 MJ/d) varied from 1 kg to more than 10 kg. However, the rate of weight loss could be predicted from the metabolic expenditure of these women. Body weight in turn was the major predictor of metabolic expenditure. In general, the heavier the patient, the faster he or she loses weight. Moreover, no adult patient who has been studied in a metabolic chamber or with doubly labeled water has needed fewer than 1000 kcal/d for weight maintenance. As a rule of thumb, an obese individual requires about 10 kcal/lb (22 kcal/kg). Thus, an individual weighing 100 kg (220 lb) would require approximately 2200 kcal/d. Thus an individual who weighed 10 kg (22 lb) more than another would require approximately 220 kcal/d more to maintain that extra weight. If caloric intake is restricted to the same level as part of a treatment program, the individual with the higher body weight withdraws more energy from fat stores and loses weight more rapidly. Within any weight group, however, there is a variability of energy expenditure. The expected or calculated energy expenditure for a woman weighing 100 kg is 2650 kcal/d. The variability of ± 20 per cent could give energy needs as high as 3180 kcal/d and as low as 2120 kcal/d. The lower figure is more likely in older individuals and the higher one in younger individuals with more fat free body mass.

Energy requirements are modified by age and gender. On any given diet, males will lose greater amounts of weight than females of similar height and weight because they have more lean body mass and thus a higher energy expenditure. Older individuals of either gender at comparable weights have lower metabolic expenditures than younger ones because metabolic rate declines by approximately 2 per cent per decade as body fat increases and lean body mass decreases. In summary, calories do count. This means that the rate of weight loss is a function of the difference between energy intake and energy require-

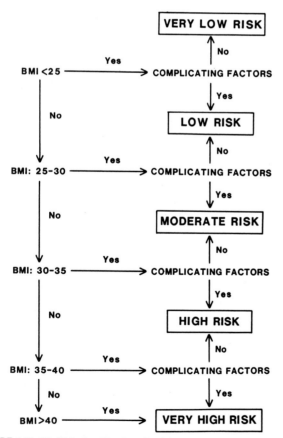

FIGURE 143–15. **Risk classification algorithm.** The patient is first placed into a category based on body mass index. The presence or absence of complicating factors include elevated abdominal-gluteal ratio (male 0.95, female 0.85), diabetes mellitus, hypertension, hyperlipidemia, male gender, and age less than 40 years. (Copyright 1987, George A. Bray.)

ments, which is primarily related to body weight and in turn fat free mass.

Second, the carbohydrate level in the diet is a determinant of the rate of short-term weight loss. Restriction of carbohydrate in the diet leads to glycogen mobilization, a sodium diuresis, and the loss of intracellular and extracellular fluids with resulting weight loss. Alternatively, adding carbohydrate to a carbohydrate-restricted diet leads to sodium retention and may be associated with transient weight gain. Dietary carbohydrate may also affect the activity of the sympathetic nervous system and the concentration of T_3. A very low carbohydrate diet reduces T_3 levels. Because this is the major calorigenic hormone, it may be that carbohydrate plays an important role in modulating metabolic rate.

The third element of any diet is the amount of nitrogen in relation to calories. When calorie levels are below those required to maintain body weight, a higher quantity of dietary nitrogen is required to minimize nitrogen loss in individuals eating a low-calorie diet. Factors that affect the rate of protein breakdown include the duration of the diet, the total energy of the diet, and the ratio of fat to carbohydrate in the diet. The nature of the diet consumed prior to initiating a new diet also influences nitrogen balance. If the nitrogen content of a weight-maintaining diet is low, less nitrogen is lost when the calorie intake is reduced than if the diet were high in nitrogen.

The work of Forbes and Drenick[188, 189] suggested that total body fat stores may also influence the rate of nitrogen loss. Markedly overweight individuals lose less nitrogen than normal-weight individuals when caloric intake is restricted. Finally, there are important differences between individuals in the amount of nitrogen lost. Hood et al[190] tested diets containing 3, 6, 12, 25, and 50 per cent of energy from carbohydrate in a total caloric intake of 1000 kcal (4.2 MJ). Nitrogen equilibrium was not obtained on any of these diets. However, nitrogen loss was smaller with diets having a high carbohydrate content than when ketosis develops with a low-carbohydrate diet. Thus ketosis does not have a protein-sparing effect. The longer an individual stays on a reducing diet, the smaller the rate of nitrogen loss.

A final consideration in the selection of a diet is the frequency with which food is eaten.[191] Eating less than two meals a day has been associated with increased skinfold thickness compared with eating more than two meals per day. Studies[23] have shown that eating one to two meals per day is associated with an increase in serum cholesterol compared with eating more frequently. Finally, Garrow[187] showed that the amount of nitrogen lost on a fixed caloric intake is lower with five meals than with one or three meals, whether the diet contains 10, 13, or 15 per cent protein. It thus seems desirable to eat five meals per day at whatever level of protein is selected.

Estimating Caloric Need

The rate of weight loss is directly related to the difference between nutrient or energy intake and an individual's energy requirements. An average deficit of 500 kcal/d (2.1 MJ/d) produces an expected weight loss of 0.45 kg/week (1 lb/week).

Although there are several methods of estimating caloric

expenditure, we suggest the following modification of formulas derived by Owen et al.[192, 193] (Table 143–15). This allows a direct estimate of resting metabolic rate and calculation of daily energy requirement. The low activity level includes individuals who lead a sedentary life. The high activity level applies to people in jobs requiring manual labor or people with regular daily physical exercise programs. Moderate activity is between low and high.

Fat stores provide the major source of fuel energy when caloric intake is below expenditure. During the adaptation to any calorically restricted diet, an initial disproportionate loss of protein and water occurs. As long as intake is below energy requirements, there will be a continuing loss of nitrogen from protein breakdown. This is not surprising when one considers the composition of tissue accumulated during periods of weight gain. When weight increases as a result of overeating,[92] approximately 75 per cent of the extra energy is fat, and the remaining 25 per cent is lean tissue. If the lean tissue contains 20 per cent protein, then 5 per cent of the extra weight gain would be protein. One would thus anticipate that 5 per cent of weight loss would be protein and 25 per cent lean tissue. During dieting, small continuing losses of protein are thus to be expected. Indeed, they are a necessary part of a calorie-reduced diet. A desirable feature of any reduced caloric intake, however, is that it provides the lowest possible loss of protein, recognizing that this cannot be less than 5 per cent of the weight loss.

Planning a diet requires a selection of caloric intake and then a selection of foods to meet that caloric level. Because it is desirable to ingest foods with adequate nutrients in addition to protein, carbohydrate, and essential fatty acids, diets should eliminate alcohol, sugar-containing beverages, and highly concentrated sweets because these rarely contain nutrients other than energy.

The long-term success of treatment programs utilizing nutritional advice alone is hard to quantify because most programs now use more than one therapeutic approach. In one study with a 14-year follow-up,[194] 27 of 32 patients were re-examined. Five of the 27 (18 per cent) were lighter than at the end of the original diet program, with an average loss of 13 kg. In a seven- to nine-year follow-up of 19 obese women, nine were lighter than initially.[55] The duration of success after treatment in this clinic could be predicted by fat cell morphology. Patients with hyperplastic obesity did less well than those with hypertrophic obesity.[165] In a five-year follow-up of 67 overweight individuals initially weighing 89.2 kg, Stamler et al.[195] reported that the mean weight loss of 6 per cent of initial body weight was achieved between one and two years and was maintained for five years. Thus with careful and thorough treatment, long-term, modest reductions in weight are possible for more than 20 per cent of individuals.

TABLE 143–15. ESTIMATING ENERGY NEEDS

RESTING METABOLIC RATE	DAILY ENERGY REQUIREMENT*	
	Activity Level	*Activity Factor*
Men = 900 ± 10 × (wt in kg)	Low	1.2
Women = 800 ± 7 × (wt in kg)	Moderate	1.4
	High	1.6

*Resting metabolic rate times the activity factor.

Very Low Calorie Diets

For practical purposes, diets with energy levels between 200 and 800 kcal/d are called "very low calorie diets" and those below 200 kcal/d "starvation diets." Because the energy withdrawn from body fat stores is a function of the energy deficit, the lower the calorie intake the more energy must be withdrawn from fat and the more rapid the weight loss. Hence the development of very low calorie diets. Starvation produces the most rapid weight loss, but hypotension and protein loss are major drawbacks. To prevent this, protein can be provided at levels of 30 to 50 g/d. Diets composed predominately of protein were introduced in the 1970's and contained 240 to 400 kcal/d.[196] Most diets of this type now contain more protein, with casein being the main source of protein.[196] Recent data have shown no difference in the rate of weight loss by patients using 400 or 800 kcal very low calorie diets.[197]

A second approach to developing a very low calorie diet is to determine the quantity of nutrients desirable for human nutrition, with an energy level as low as practical. The Recommended Dietary Allowances (RDA)[198] are one basis for these calculations. The RDA recommends 0.8 g/kg of protein per day. Using this figure, the minimum desirable protein intake would be 56 g/d for a 70-kg man. However with low caloric intake a higher nitrogen level may further reduce protein loss. For this reason we recommend 70 g/d for protein. Carbohydrate at 50 g/d minimizes ketosis and helps maintain circulating levels of T_3. With 10 g of essential fatty acids added to the diet, we arrived at a diet of no less than 570 kcal/d.[199] Some very low calorie diets use predominately fish and fowl to provide the protein foods for the diet. Other diet programs provide formulas with casein, soy protein, or egg albumin as the source of protein along with other added nutrients.

An early catastrophe with formula diets occurred when a formula containing collagen as the sole source of protein was sold widely to the American public. Data on 16 women and one man who died while consuming this diet were reported by the Center for Disease Control.[200] The 16 women had lost an average of 37.7 kg (83 lbs) at a rate of 2.1 kg/week (4.6 lb/week), which represented 34 per cent of their initial body weight. Six of these women died outside the hospital, and another six died after being admitted for syncopal events. The remaining four had cardiac arrest outside the hospital. Ventricular tachycardia and fibrillation were documented in 10 of these women. It became clear that long-term adherence to a diet with low-quality protein could be hazardous to the cardiovascular system of otherwise healthy individuals. In the past 10 years, formula diets containing high-quality protein (casein, egg albumin, or soy) as well as carbohydrate and adequate quantities of other nutrients, especially potassium, magnesium, vitamins, and minerals, have been used with no recurrence of these arrhythmias and deaths.[201]

Weight loss with very low calorie diets is more rapid than with conventional calorie diets because the caloric intake is lower and because adherence may be easier. In studies of up to 20 weeks in duration, the rate of weight loss appears to be related directly to the duration of treatment, and averages 1.5 kg/week or more.[202] As with all diets, the weight loss initially contains a larger quantity of protein than after adaptation, when protein breakdown slows. Patients adhering to very low calorie diets usually experience

a reduction in blood pressure, which drops most rapidly during the first week. Antihypertensive medications, especially those acting by ionic mechanisms such as calcium channel blockers and sodium-potassium exchange in the kidney, should be discontinued at the beginning of a very low calorie diet. Most Type II diabetics on very low calorie diets experience marked improvement in their diabetic control. Blood glucose drops within the first one to two weeks and remains low for as long as the diet is continued. Patients taking less than 50 units of insulin per day and those taking oral hypoglycemic drugs are usually able to discontinue these medications.

A number of side effects have been observed with very low calorie diets, including hair loss, thinning of the skin, and coldness.[196] Because marked caloric restriction is undesirable for lactating and pregnant women, these diets are contraindicated in that group, as well as in children who still require protein for linear growth. Finally, as with all diets, there is increased cholesterol mobilization from peripheral fat stores, enhancing the quantity of cholesterol moving through the biliary system and increasing the potential risk of cholesterol-containing gallstones.

Starvation

Starvation is the ultimate very low calorie diet and is defined as an intake of less than 200 kcal/d. During starvation the loss of protein and cellular components is the most rapid.[203] The rate of weight loss is also most rapid, but 50 per cent or more of this initial loss represents fluid and thus problems with hypotension are common. Likewise, an increase in serum uric acid enhances the risk of precipitating gout or uric acid kidney stones. Weight regain to initial level occurs over months to a few years in almost all patients treated by starvation. Because use of starvation diets should be conducted in a carefully supervised medical setting, its use has largely disappeared except under experimental settings.

Exercise

The addition of regular exercise to programs involving moderate to severe caloric restriction has produced variable effects on weight loss. Warwick and Garrow[204] compared three women who were observed for 12 weeks on a metabolic ward while eating a constant reducing diet containing 800 kcal/d (3.4 MJ/d). These authors were unable to find any increase in weight loss when subjects bicycled for two hours a day compared with when they did no additional exercise. They similarly found no effects of physical training on nitrogen balance and suggested that the failure to lose weight despite the greater energy deficit caused by exercise may have been due to glycogen deposition in trained muscles. This conclusion was supported by the work of Hill,[205] who compared five obese females who walked up to six km/d with three who had no exercise, during an inpatient study in which all subjects received an 800-kcal liquid diet each day. Both groups lost approximately eight kg. The only significant difference was that the group that exercised lost more fat and less lean body mass than the group that did not exercise. Effects on body composition were also observed by Pavlou et al.,[206] who randomized moderately obese policemen who were eating a variety of reduced-calorie diets to exercise and nonexercise groups. The officers who exercised for 20 to 45 minutes three times per week at 85 per cent of their maximal heart rates showed no greater weight loss (11.8 kg versus 9.2 kg) but lost significantly more fat and less lean body mass than did the nonexercising group. However, other studies have failed to demonstrate a sparing of lean body mass by exercise during caloric restriction. For example, Van Dale et al.[207] randomly assigned 6 of 12 obese females who were on a 12-week restricted diet of approximately 800 kcal/d (3.4 MJ/d) to exercise for one hour, four days per week at 50 to 60 per cent of their maximum aerobic capacity. Both groups lost 12 to 13 kg, and there was no difference between them in the loss of body weight, body fat, or lean body mass. Thus, it appears that exercise usually does not increase the rate of weight loss during a period of calorie restriction, although the reasons for this are not yet clear. However, exercise probably reduces the loss of lean body mass during dieting, although research is not consistent on this point. Such factors as gender, age, quality and type of diet, and frequency and intensity of exercise may explain some of the discrepancies.

Several studies with long-term follow-up have suggested that the inclusion of exercise in a weight control program leads to an improvement in long-term results. Harris and Hallbauer[208] studied 35 women and 11 men in a program that lasted for 12 weeks and used behavior modification and a contingency contract with or without daily exercise. Weight losses ranged from 2.0 to 3.2 kg (4.4 to 7.0 lb) and were not significantly different from those of a control group. However, when the subjects were examined six months later, the control subjects showed a net gain in weight of 0.82 kg (1.8 lb) whereas both of the other groups continued to lose weight after completing the program. The weight loss of 4.0 kg (8.7 lb) in the exercise group was significantly greater than the 2.9 kg (6.3 lb) loss of the nonexercise group. After one year of follow-up, Stalonas et al.[209] noted a nonsignificant trend and Wing et al.[210] a significant further weight loss in a behavior modification and exercise group compared with other subjects treated only with behavior modification. Finally, Dahlkoetter et al.[211] studied 44 women who were at least 6.8 kg above ideal weight. Those using behavior modification alone lost 3.2 kg, which was slightly more than the weight loss of those treated with exercise alone. The individuals who received a combination of exercise plus behavior modification lost 6.1 kg. At follow-up six months later, those in the exercise-only group were 2.5 kg lighter than initially, having regained only 0.3 kg. Those in the behavior modification group showed no change from the end of treatment, and those treated with exercise plus behavior modification lost an additional 1.1 kg, for a total of 7.3 kg. Thus, although the addition of exercise to a calorie-restricted diet often does not increase weight loss during treatment, exercise training as part of a treatment program for obesity appears to improve results over the long term and may reduce loss of lean tissue.

Drugs

Only a few drugs are currently approved for the treatment of obesity, and many of these are under the FDA dictum that they should be used only "for a few weeks." This section deals with the drugs that can be used to treat obesity, drugs that may be the newer avenues of research to find effective therapy for obesity, and the drugs that have been or should be abandoned for treatment of obesity.

Appetite-Suppressing Drugs

This is the largest group of drugs currently approved for use in treating obesity. They act by two different mechanisms and are discussed under those mechanisms.

DRUGS ACTING ON NORADRENERGIC NEUROTRANSMITTERS. Most appetite-suppressing drugs possess many of the pharmacological properties of norepinephrine, and all of the drugs listed in Table 143–16 can, to a variable degree, stimulate the CNS and increase locomotor activity. Their relative potencies, however, differ considerably.

Pharmacological Effects. Appetite suppressants have three types of pharmacological effects: First, most of these drugs can stimulate the CNS, but this is highly variable. Methamphetamine and amphetamine are the most stimulatory and should not be used for treatment of obesity. Diethylpropion, mazindol, and phentermine show much less stimulation. Second, appetite-suppressing drugs have cardiovascular effects including an increase in heart rate and blood pressure which has been observed with amphetamine and methamphetamine, but is also observed with ephedrine, phenmetrazine, and methylphenidate. The other drugs listed in Table 143–16 have few of these effects. Third, metabolic effects expressed as a rise in the concentration of free fatty acids and/or glycerol in plasma have been observed after administration of amphetamine, methamphetamine, and phenmetrazine. Methamphetamine has been found to antagonize the lipolytic effects of norepinephrine in vitro but has no direct lipolytic effect itself. Mazindol has been reported to increase the uptake of glucose following intra-arterial administration in humans.

The peak blood concentration for these drugs usually occurs shortly after oral administration, but the half-life of the drugs in the serum varies considerably. There are also important pharmacological differences among the stereoisomers of these compounds. The dextro isomer of amphetamine, for example, is four times more potent than the levo isomer. Urinary excretion of several drugs depends upon urine pH.

Clinical Use of Noradrenergic Appetite-Suppressing Drugs. In evaluating the clinical usefulness of appetite suppressants, two questions need to be answered: (1) Are they effective? (2) Are they safe?

The FDA has provided one of the largest reviews on the effectiveness of these drugs[212]—an analysis of 105 new drug applications containing data on 4543 placebo-treated and 3182 drug-treated patients. In studies comparing placebo and active drug, the drop-out rate after four weeks of therapy was 18.5 per cent for subjects on placebo and 24.3 per cent for those receiving active drug. At the end of the study periods, whether lasting three, four, eight, or more weeks, equal percentages of patients receiving placebo and active drugs remained in treatment (49 per cent for placebo versus 47.9 per cent for active drugs). Drug-treated patients lost an average 0.25 kg/week (0.56 lb/week) more than subjects receiving placebos. In clinically effective doses, there was no basis on which to choose between these drugs

TABLE 143–16. Appetite-Suppressing Drugs

GENERIC DRUG AND SOME PROPRIETARY NAMES	SUPPLIER	DOSAGE (mg)	ADMINISTRATION (mg)	PEAK BLOOD CONCENTRATION (HOURS AFTER ORAL DOSE)	HALF-LIFE IN BLOOD (HOURS)	EXCRETED UNCHANGED IN ACIDIC URINE (%)
Schedule II*						
(+) Amphetamine sulfate		5, 10, 15	5–10 before meals (tid)	1–2	5	55
Methamphetamine HC Desoxyn	Abbott	5, 10, 15	2.5 or 5 before meals (tid) 10 or 15 in morning	1–2	13	45
Phenmetrazine HC Preludin	Boehringer Ingelheim	25, 50, 75	25 bid or tid	—	—	19
Schedule III*						
Phendimetrazine tartrate Plegine	Ayerst	35	35 before meals	—	4	??
Benzphetamine HC Didrex	Upjohn	25, 50	25–50 before meals	1–2	—	??
Schedule IV*						
Diethylpropion HC Tenuate Tepanil	Merrell Dow Riker	25, 75	24 before meals (tid) 75 in morning	1–2	8–13	24
Fenfluramine HC Pondimin	Wyeth-Ayerst	20	20–40 before meals	1	20	20
Mazindol Sanorex Mazanor	Sandoz Wyeth	1, 2	1 before meals 2 in morning	2	13	22
Phentermine Fastin	Beecham	15,30	15 tid 30 in morning	—	Free 7–8	75
Ionamin (resin)	Pennwalt			1	20–24	

bid, twice a day; HC, hydrochloride; tid, three times a day.

*The Federal Controlled Substances Act of 1970 places the prescription anorexiants into five schedule categories going from high abuse potential (schedule I) to low abuse potential (schedule V).

in terms of their rates of weight loss or the duration over which that weight loss occurred.

Additional data are available from trials lasting from 6 to 190 weeks.[213] In one trial combining phentermine with fenfluramine, Weintraub et al.[214] showed that drug treatment was significantly more effective than placebo treatment (Fig. 143–16). More importantly, they showed that continuous drug treatment remained effective for nearly four years. Tolerance did not develop because increased amounts of drug were not required to maintain weight loss. Continuous therapy was more effective than intermittent therapy.

Safety of Appetite Suppressants. The safety of appetite-suppressant drugs has been the subject of considerable discussion. Griffiths et al.,[215] using baboons as subjects, have examined the reinforcing properties of intravenous preparations of several appetite-suppressing drugs and compared these effects with the potency of each drug to reduce food intake. The ratio of anorexiant dose to reinforcing dose was used as a measure of abuse potential. At one extreme were diethylpropion and amphetamine, at the other fenfluramine and phenylpropanolamine. Although the ratio of appetite-suppressant dose to reinforcing dose is of some utility in predicting abuse potential, it does not always correlate with clinical experience. For example, diethylpropion has been widely used as an appetite-suppressing drug, yet episodes of misuse are few. However, its appetite-suppressant to reinforcing ratio in baboons is greater than that of amphetamine or phenmetrazine, both of which are classified in Schedule II. There is no indication for use of

drugs in Schedule II (see Table 143–15) for the treatment of obesity. Drugs in Schedule IV are obviously preferred, but the two drugs in Schedule III also have a low abuse potential.

Drugs Acting on Serotonin Neurotransmitters. One of the general biobehavioral properties of serotonin

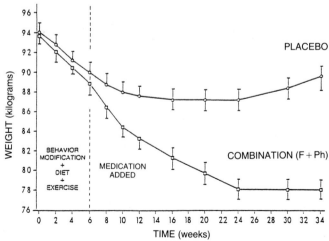

FIGURE 143–16. Participant body weight (kg) by study week. Open circles represent placebo group mean ± SEM (n=54). Open squares represent fenfluramine plus phentermine group mean ± SEM (n=58). (From Weintraub M, Fundaresan PR, Schuster B, et al: National Heart, Lung and Blood Institute long-term weight control study: I–VII. Clin Pharmacol Ther 51:581–585, 1992.)

is a reduction in the physiological level of activity, including food intake. Drugs modulating serotonin metabolism influence body weight. The administration of tryptophan or 5-hydroxytryptophan, two precursors which are converted to serotonin after entering the brain, reduces food intake. Similarly, drugs that release serotonin from nerve endings and/or block its reuptake decrease food intake and body weight.

d,f-Fenfluramine (racemic or rac-fenfluramine) was the first clinically useful appetite-suppressing drug of this type. In one trial,[216] rac-fenfluramine was administered continuously for one year, followed by a second year of placebo. A plateau of weight loss occurred by the eighth month, and weight remained 10 to 11 kg lower for the remainder of the year. When transferred to placebo, patients regained weight. Three clinical findings from this study argue against tolerance. First, subjects regained weight when fenfluramine was discontinued. Second, weight loss continued for six months until a new plateau was reached. Third, hunger did not increase during several months of treatment. One interpretation of this is that the drug had readjusted the weight-control mechanism to a lower level.

Fluoxetine, a serotonin-reuptake inhibitor, marketed as Prozac for the treatment of depression, has been shown to produce weight loss. Fluoxetine inhibits reuptake of serotonin and produces a dose-related decrease in body weight over eight weeks.[217] Longer trials show two differences from rac-fenfluramine.[218] First, the amount of weight lost appears to be less with fluoxetine than with fenfluramine. Second, after an interval of 12 to 20 weeks of treatment the average patient taking fluoxetine tends to regain weight while continuing to take the drug.[219] The reason for this weight regain is unknown, but the mechanism is of considerable interest.

Phenylpropanolamine. Phenylpropanolamine (PPA), a nasal decongestant, is also used as an over-the-counter drug for weight control.[220] It is thought to work on α_1 receptors in the hypothalamus. In a critical review of published and unpublished studies with this drug, Weintraub[221] concluded that PPA is effective in producing weight loss. In one group of five clinical trials with phenylpropanolamine, the drug-treated individuals lost an average of 0.24 kg/week more than the placebo-treated group. This is similar to the extra weight loss of 0.25 kg/week reported when prescription appetite-suppressing drugs and placebo are compared.[212]

BARRIERS TO THE TREATMENT OF OBESITY. The profile outlined above of relatively safe drugs with long-term effectiveness leads one to ask why they are not used more widely. The answer is that there are a number of barriers to the effective use of these drugs.[222] First, obesity is a stigmatized condition. That is, the public perceives obesity not as a "disease," as proposed by the 1985 NIH Consensus Conference,[223] but rather as the result of gluttony and a lack of willpower. Most people believe that willpower, the power to push oneself away from the table, is all that is needed to treat obesity. This simplistic public perception of obesity is reflected in attitudes of most professional health care workers.

The fact that obese patients regain weight after treatment is terminated is almost universally attributed to a "failure" of the drugs because health professionals expect that following drug treatment of obesity there should be no weight regain. That is, the drugs are expected to cure obesity. These professional attitudes have led to a demand for higher therapeutic standards for medications used in treating obesity than for medications used in treating other chronic conditions. In a recent review, Weintraub and Bray[213] described this unrealistic expectation as follows:

> We accept the fact that serum cholesterol values will rise following the cessation of therapy with hypocholesterolemic drugs. We also accept that peptic ulcers will also recur following cessation of the H_2-blocking medications. We understand that rising intraocular pressure when pilocarpine treatment is stopped means that glaucoma has been controlled, but not cured. Even in the absence of a cure, patients and physicians still view ocular hypotensive agents, cholesterol lowering medications, and H_2-blockers as valuable. All of these failures to cure a problem of malregulation in the human organism are acceptable. Yet, for obesity, this is unacceptable.

Barriers to the effective use of anorectic drugs are also provided by state licensing agencies. Many physicians have been questioned and disciplinary action brought for using appetite-suppressant drugs for "more than a few weeks." Yet the available data argue that they are effective for as long as they have been used.

Additional barriers in the regulatory rigidity in scheduling and labeling of anorexiant drugs are also barriers to effective use of appetite-suppressant drugs. The FDA has labeled these drugs for "the management of exogenous obesity as a short term (a few weeks) adjunct" to the treatment of obesity. There is no definition of "exogenous," a term of dubious and outmoded merit in describing obesity. The data do not support "a few weeks" unless this means 34 to 190 weeks. Clearly, regulations do not make truth, and current regulations appear to bear little relationship to the realities associated with these medications. Even worse, untruthful regulations can serve as the basis for criminal prosecutions without the perpetrators of the regulations being liable for the negligence that they have produced. Moreover, current regulations inhibit future developments because they indicate a closed and unresponsive legalistic mentality on the part of regulatory authorities.

Thermogenic Drugs

Thermogenic drugs that cause heat loss are a second category of agents that have been used to treat obesity. The agents in this group are either outmoded (thyroid and dinitrophenol), in need of additional evaluation (ephedrine), or new (β_3 agonists).

THYROID HORMONE. Thyroid hormone is the prototype of a thermogenic drug. It produces a dose-related increase in metabolic expenditure. Pharmacological doses of thyroid hormone are associated with increased breakdown of protein, increased calcium loss from bone, and an increased risk of cardiovascular dysfunction. There is thus no indication for using thyroid hormone for treatment of obesity except as replacement therapy for clinical and laboratory-documented hypothyroidism. In spite of these drawbacks, interest in T_3 as a treatment for obesity has been revived by two observations. First, during very low carbohydrate diets the concentration of T_3 falls.[151] Second, the administration of T_3 can prevent the decline in metabolic rate which occurs during treatment with very low calorie diets. However, as much as 75 per cent of the extra weight loss produced by T_3 can be accounted for by the loss of fat free mass. Moreover, the reduction in T_3 when dieting with very low calorie diets may facilitate the oxidation of visceral proteins. Thus, in obesity per se, thyroid hormones are not recommended.

EPHEDRINE. Ephedrine is a synthetic adrenergic drug that can increase energy expenditure when administered orally. Its potential for weight loss was first reported when asthmatic subjects being treated with a compound containing ephedrine, caffeine, and phenobarbital lost weight. In additional studies with ephedrine and caffeine compared with placebo and diethylpropion, the mean weight loss over 12 weeks was 4.1 kg in the placebo-treated group, compared with 8.4 kg in those treated with diethylpropion and 8.1 kg in those treated with the ephedrine.[224] The differences between active compounds and placebo were highly significant, but there was no significant difference between diethylpropion and ephedrine. The comparison of ephedrine alone or in combination with caffeine shows a significantly greater effect with the combination than with either drug alone.[225] Thus, the combination of ephedrine and caffeine may have a place in the treatment of obesity.

β AGONISTS. The observation that β-adrenergic drugs could enhance thermogenesis in experimental animals[226] has led to the development of compounds by several companies. Treatment of experimental animals with these drugs decreases body weight and body fat content without reducing food intake, suggesting that they work by increasing energy expenditure. In three clinical trials with the one β agonist (BRL 26830A), two have shown more weight loss than placebo,[227] but a third study was equivocal. Clinical trials with a second β agonist (Ro34-8714) showed a dose-response increase in both metabolic rate and heart rate.[228] The third drug has been reported only in animal studies.[229] Others are yet to reach the stage of publication.

Drugs and Fiber Affecting the Gastrointestinal Tract

Because the taste of food, its digestibility, and its metabolism are related to the control of food intake, it is not surprising that these approaches have been selected for development of therapeutic drugs to treat obesity. Several different drugs that modify the digestive or absorptive process in the gastrointestinal tract have been tested.

FIBER. Dietary fiber comprises the various cell-wall polysaccharides such as alginates, gums, hemicellulose, and lignin, which resist hydrolysis by human gut enzymes. Dietary fiber has been suggested as a therapeutic agent in obesity because it can cause gastrointestinal distention. In one trial, methylcellulose produced relatively little weight loss in patients with refractory obesity when compared with placebo or phenmetrazine.[230] In another trial mucilage was reported to be mildly effective. Twenty-eight patients were recruited and 16 completed a double-blind cross-over period of 30 days each. During the second 30-day period following the cross-over, the group receiving mucilage lost significantly more weight than those on diet alone. Fiber may enhance weight loss by restricting energy intake and aiding in compliance to a diet. When dietary fiber tablets were added to a reducing diet, the obese women treated with fiber lost 19 kg more than the placebo-treated patients.[231] Thus dietary fiber may have some limited value in treating obesity.

ENZYME INHIBITORS. Inhibition of fat digestion or absorption induces malabsorptions and thus reduces the available energy from fats in the diet. The antibiotic neomycin increases the fecal excretion of fat, but the changes in the intestinal mucosa while on this drug make it unacceptable for treatment of obesity.[27] Cholestyramine is a resin that binds bile salts and thus disturbs micelle formation and fat digestion. When given to obese patients in large doses, this drug does not increase fat loss sufficiently and it is thus ineffective in obesity.[27] Acarbose, a drug that inhibits disaccharidase in the intestine has also been tried as a treatment for obesity but has not been shown to increase weight loss over diet alone. Finally, a lipase inhibitor called orlistat (tetrahydrolipstatin) has recently been described. In animal studies this drug increases weight loss and in one reported clinical trial, drug-treated patients lost twice as much weight as placebo-treated patients (4.2 versus 2.1 kg in 12 weeks).[232]

SUCROSE POLYESTER. Sucrose polyester (Olestra) is an indigestible fat produced by esterifying sucrose with fatty acids of appropriate length to give it the characteristics of a normal cooking oil. Addition of this agent to the diet reduces the absorption of cholesterol, vitamin E, and vitamin A. In some clinical trials with Olestra, it was observed that overweight subjects lost weight.[233] A subsequent study,[234] however, failed to demonstrate any significant effect of substituting sucrose polyester for fat in the diet of five obese subjects. The reasons for the reduction in caloric intake in one study and the failure to detect a reduction in the second study remain unexplained. Recent studies in healthy volunteers show that after covert replacement of dietary fat with Olestra, caloric compensation occurs within 24 hours.[235]

Human Chorionic Gonadotropin

The treatment of obesity with diet and injections of human chorionic gonadotropin (hCG) has been used for more than 40 years. The rationale for this drug was the observation that in individuals with "pituitary" obesity, injections of hCG were associated with weight loss. Three double-blind, placebo-controlled studies[236] have compared injections of chorionic gonadotropin with placebo injections plus a low calorie diet. In no instance was there a statistically significant improvement in the rate of weight loss during treatment with chorionic gonadotropin compared with placebo. Thus, hCG is not effective in the treatment of obesity.

Regional Fat Mobilization

Lipolysis in human adipose tissue is stimulated by drugs that act on β-adrenergic receptors and is inhibited by drugs that act on α_2-adrenergic receptors. These clinical observations suggested that it might be possible to mobilize fat locally by β-adrenergic stimulation or inhibition of α_2-adrenergic receptors. This possibility has received support by finding that local injection of isoproterenol, a β-adrenergic agonist, into one thigh of women on a diet increased the rate of fat loss from the treated thigh. Local application of a cream containing aminophylline to increase β-adrenergic–like effects of yohimbine, an α_2-adrenergic blocking drug, also increased mobilization of fat from the treated thigh. The possibility of treating regional fat deposits by topical means has thus been proposed and awaits further testing.[237]

Invasive Surgical Treatments for Obesity

Gastric Bubble

Two different gastric bubbles have been developed. The rationale for this procedure is that placing a distensible object in the stomach causes smaller quantities of food to be eaten. The first bubble was developed in Europe and is known as the Ballobos bubble.[238] Clinical trials with this balloon are currently under way in a number of countries. The second bubble, the Garren-Edwards bubble, was invented in the United States and up to 20,000 were inserted during 1985 and 1986 at a cost of $2 to $4 million. In controlled trials comparing the gastric bubble with sham insertions, there was no evidence that the bubble was more effective than the diet with which it was associated.[239]

Jaw Wiring

Jaw wiring (mandibular fixation) has been used to reduce the intake of solid foods in overweight patients. Several clinical trials have demonstrated that individuals with jaws wired lose weight steadily while the jaws remain wired. In one study of 17 patients, two dropped out in less than one month, but in the remaining 15 the median weight loss at six months was 25.3 kg, which is comparable to that from the more drastic operative procedures described below. However, following removal of the wires two thirds of the patients regained some or all of their weight. Recently, Bjorvell et al.[239a] reported that two years following mandibular fixation, women maintained a 13.8-kg loss, compared with a maximum loss of 19 kg at the time wires were removed. To improve the long-term results, Garrow and Gardiner[240] have introduced an abdominal nylon cord that is attached around the abdomen at the end of the weight-loss period. According to their report, use of the nylon cord has improved the long-term maintenance of weight loss following mandibular fixation.

Vagotomy

The vagus nerve controls gastric emptying as well as a variety of other gastrointestinal and metabolic functions. Between 1977 and 1979, Gortz et al.[241] performed bilateral truncal vagotomy without gastric drainage procedure in 11 women and 2 men who were morbidly obese. The mean weight loss was 18.2 kg, with a range from 2 to 24 kg. A second small series was reported in 1981, but these patients experienced problems with gastric emptying due to vagotomy. The use of vagotomy in one patient with Prader-Willi syndrome and in one patient with hypothalamic obesity was of limited success. Recently Kral[242] has coupled vagotomy with gastroplasty and suggests that this may improve the effectiveness of the gastric operation as a treatment for morbid obesity.

Liposuction or Suction-Assisted Lipectomy

Local fat deposits can be altered cosmetically by liposuction, an operative procedure developed in the past 20 years.[243] It can be performed under local anesthesia, and the published pictures suggest that it is a promising technique for contouring or remodeling small to modest amounts of local fat. Both wet and dry suction lipectomy procedures have been developed. The difference is the quantity of fluid injected prior to aspiration of the fat. Successful operations have usually been performed on younger individuals with limited quantities of fat to be removed and in whom underlying elastic properties of the skin are sufficient to allow tightening over the aspirated areas. Difficulties such as dimpling or wavy contours have been observed, and seromas and infections and even death have also been reported.

Gastrointestinal Procedures

A variety of surgical methods have been used to decrease the quantity of food entering or its duration of time in the gastrointestinal tract. These include esophageal banding, gastric bypass with various kinds of diversion from the small upper pouch, gastroplasties including the vertically banded gastroplasty, and the jejunoileal bypass operations. There is little doubt that weight loss can be substantial with all of these procedures, but appropriate guidelines for patients should be used.[243]

GASTRIC OPERATIONS. The idea of reducing the size of the gastric pouch as an approach to obesity was introduced by Mason and Ito in 1967.[244] Since that time, a variety of different procedures have been developed, and these are shown in Figure 143–17. At one end of the spectrum are banding procedures, which have been used on both the esophagus and stomach. At the other end of the spectrum are the gastrointestinal anastomoses, in which the antrum and fundus of the stomach are anatomically or functionally separated and the fundal pouch is drained into the intestine through a loop enterostomy or a Roux-en-Y anastomosis. We refer to this group of operations as gastrointestinal bypass. The other group of operations narrow the connection between the fundus and antrum but leave them intact. These include wrapping procedures, transverse banding procedures, and vertical banding procedures. The number of operative procedures now available raises some concern about whether the most desirable procedure has yet been identified. This concern was expressed by Freeman and Burchett[245] as follows: "Despite 12 years of experience with gastric operations for morbid obesity in the surgical literature, the ideal technique remains unknown."

A reduction in food intake is the mechanism for weight loss with all of the gastric operations. The distribution of calories between carbohydrate, protein, and fat does not change, but the frequency of eating is increased.

Several good trials exist, comparing gastrointestinal bypass with gastroplasty. In general, patients with gastric (antral) bypass lose more weight than those with gastroplasty.

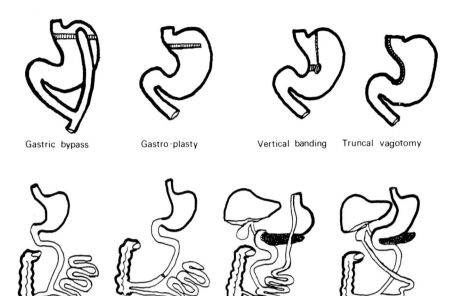

Gastric bypass   Gastro-plasty   Vertical banding   Truncal vagotomy

FIGURE 143-17. Operative treatments for obesity are shown schematically.

End-to-side   End-to-end   Biliopancreatic bypass   Biliointestinal bypass

Pories et al.[246] reported a prospective randomized trial comparing 42 patients who had gastric (antral) bypass with 45 patients who had a gastroplasty. In this group, patients with the gastric bypass lost 15 per cent more weight at 12 months and 24 per cent more weight at 18 months than those with gastroplasty. There were no technical failures in the gastric (antral) bypass group, but 28 of the 45 operations using gastroplasty were counted as failures. Sugerman et al.[247] recently provided one possible explanation for some of these failures. He divided patients into "non-sweets eaters" and "sweets eaters," who were defined as those who ate at least 300 kcal of sweets three times a week. The difference in rate of weight loss between patients with gastroplasty and those with gastric-antral bypass (Roux-en-Y) was among the "sweets-eaters." Among the "non-sweets eaters" there was no difference in the rate of weight loss between these two operations. This suggests that a dietary history of eating "sweets" frequently should lead the surgeon to select a gastric bypass.

Complications associated with gastric operations can be summarized in several categories. First are the operative problems. Operative mortality is usually less than 1 per cent. Problems with anastomotic connections can require reoperations. Other perioperative difficulties are also within reasonable bounds. Although weight loss with the gastroplasty procedures is substantial, failure rates as high as 50 per cent have been reported when all reversals, revisions, and patients lost to follow-up are considered. The complications in the third group are the result of metabolic changes and include anemia due to iron and vitamin B_{12} deficiency as well as thiamine deficiency and its associated neuropathy.

These operations also have advantages. The most obvious advantage is substantial weight loss. Another advantage of operative intervention is an improvement in the quality of life. In one series, 10 out of 44 patients had returned to school and another 10 had reported a change in their occupation. Self-concept improved after surgery, and there were fewer reports of feeling angry. Individuals tended to feel more attractive, more calm, and less depressed. Forty-one of these 44 patients were definitely glad that they had the surgery, and 43 per cent stated spontaneously that "surgery was the best thing that ever happened to me." In summary, although both gastric bypass and gastroplasty produce large losses of weight, long-term results appear to be more consistent with the gastric bypass operation.

JEJUNOILEAL BYPASS OPERATIONS. Four variants of the jejunoileal bypass have been performed (Fig. 143-17). In comparative trials with gastric and jejunoileal bypass operations, several groups of workers have reported similar rates of weight loss. However, there is a higher frequency of metabolic complications following the jejunoileal bypass. For these reasons almost all surgeons have now abandoned the jejunoileal bypass.

Two modifications of the intestinal bypass are currently still used. The first of these is a bilio-intestinal bypass,[248] in which the defunctionalized loop of ileum is attached to the gallbladder, allowing drainage of bile through the ileum. This provides a volume of flow through the defunctionalized bowel and allows bile salts to be reabsorbed in the ileum rather than lost in the colon. Bile acid–induced diarrhea and bacterial overgrowth are thus markedly reduced. An intact gallbladder is essential for this operation, and with the high frequency of cholelithiasis in obese patients the gallbladder is often absent.

The second operation, called the biliopancreatic bypass, was developed by Scopinaro et al.[249] and is depicted in Figure 143-17. In this operation, the gastrointestinal circuit at the stomach is divided into two conduits, one draining the fundal portion of the stomach into a long segment of intestine, which at a distal point is connected to the drainage from the gastric antrum, the pancreas, and bile ducts. This maintains adequate flow through the biliary tree and through the duodenojejunal segment. Anastomosis of these two intestinal segments can occur at a point determined by the surgeon. Weight losses with this operation have been very satisfactory. However, this operation is technically more difficult than the other procedures described earlier, and operative problems are more likely to occur.

SUMMARY AND CONCLUSION

RATE OF WEIGHT LOSS. The rate of weight loss varies substantially among treatments. Surgical treatment with gastroplasty or gastric bypass, starvation, and very low calorie diets produce the most rapid weight loss. Intermediate rates are seen with conventional diets, appetite-suppressing drugs, and behavior modification. The least rapid rate of weight loss is seen with exercise alone.

SAFETY. In general, safety is the inverse of the rate of weight loss. Surgery clearly has the highest risk. Renal stones, cholelithiasis, and death have also been reported during starvation and very low calorie diets. Conventional diets and behavior modification have the lowest risks, with exercise and appetite-suppressing drugs also carrying little risk.

COMPARATIVE EFFECTIVENESS OF TREATMENTS. Gastric bypass, gastroplasty, and biliopancreatic bypass have the best long-term outlook, but a substantial number of patients regain weight and many others require reoperation. Among the noninvasive treatments good long-term comparative studies are few in number. A five-year follow-up of patients treated with behavior modification or nutritional advice in a doctor's office[250] showed an initial result that favored behavior modification. After five years, however, the two treatments were essentially identical.

Several studies have compared pharmacological treatment and behavior modification in the short term, but only a few provide longer-term follow-up. In one of them fenfluramine was the active agent. At six months the drug-treated patients fared better.[251] However, over the next 12 months the regain by the drug-treated patients was greater, with a net preference for behavior modification.

Although rates of weight loss with very low calorie diets are among the most rapid, long-term maintenance of weight loss appears to be no better than with behavior modification.[252]

Finally, jaw wiring and behavior modification have been compared over a four-year period. The maximal weight loss was greatest in those with jaws wired. However, after four years with a high level of follow-up, the behavioral treatment group and formerly jaw-wired patients receiving behavioral modification treatment were still maintaining a reduction of 30 per cent of their initial overweight.[253]

MAINTENANCE. It seems clear that behavior modification is a key element of success for those individuals who achieve and maintain long-term weight loss. Epstein et al.[254] have shown a 10-year success using behavior modification in obese children. This may be because these patients are continuing to be treated, albeit often by themselves. As noted above, treatment for obesity has many similarities with treatment of other chronic diseases. Pharmacological agents can control hypertension in most patients, but few, if any, physicians would believe that hypertension will remain under control if drugs are discontinued. So it is with obesity. It is unrealistic and unreasonable to expect patients who lose weight to remain thinner when treatment is terminated. Thus behavior modification and a regular exercise program are essential continuing treatments that are necessary if people who lose weight are to remain thinner.

COSTS. The cost of individual treatments for obesity is highly variable, but the total expenditure is substantial. Those treatments, such as surgery, very low calorie diets, psychoanalysis, and physician-run programs are the most expensive. Those using behavioral modification, large groups, and work-site settings have the potential for being the most cost-effective.

REFERENCES

1. Bray GA: Obesity: Historical development of scientific and cultural ideas. Int J Obes 14:909–926, 1990.
2. Bray GA, Gray DS: Obesity: Part I—Pathogenesis. West J Med 149:429–441, 1988.
3. Heymsfield SB, Waki M, Kehayias J, et al: Chemical and elemental analysis of humans in vivo using improved body composition models. Am J Physiol 261(2 pt1):E190–E198, 1991.
4. Kvist H, Chowhury B, Grangard U, et al: Total and visceral adipose-tissue volumes derived from measurements with computed tomography in adult men and women: Predictive equations. Am J Clin Nutr 48:1351–1361, 1988.
5. Lapidus L, Bengtsson C, Larsson B, et al: Distribution of adipose tissue and risk of cardiovascular disease and death: A 12 year follow-up of participants in the population study of women in Gothenburg, Sweden. BMJ 289:1257–1261, 1984.
6. Larsson B, Svardsudd K, Welin L, et al: Abdominal adipose tissue distribution, obesity, and risk of cardiovascular disease and death: 13 year follow-up of participants in the study of men born in 1913. BMJ 288:1401–1404, 1984.
7. Sjostrom LV: A computer-tomography based multicompartment body-composition technique and anthropometric predictions of lean body-mass, total and subcutaneous adipose-tissue. Int J Obes 15(Suppl 2):19–30, 1991.
8. Tokunaga K, Matsuzawa Y, Ishikawa K, Tarui S: A novel technique for the determination of body fat by computed tomography. Int J Obes 7:437–445, 1983.
9. Bray GA, Greenway FL, Molitch ME, et al: Use of anthropometric measures to assess weight loss. Am J Clin Nutr 31:769–773, 1978.
10. Wang Z-M, Pierson RN, Heymsfield SB: The five-level model: A new approach to organizing body-composition. Am J Clin Nutr 56:19–28, 1992.
11. Forbes GB: Human Body Composition: Growth, Aging, Nutrition, and Activity. New York, Springer-Verlag, 1987.
12. Lukaski HC: Methods for the assessment of human body composition: Traditional and new. Am J Clin Nutr 46:537–556, 1987.
13. Segal KR, Van Loan M, Fitzgerald PI, et al: Lean body mass estimation by bioelectrical impedance analysis: A four-site cross-validation study. Am J Clin Nutr 47:7–14, 1988.
14. Forbes GB, Simon W, Amatruda JM: Is bioimpedance a good predictor of body-composition change? Am J Clin Nutr 56:4–6, 1992.
15. Heymsfield SB, Wang J, Heshka S, et al: Dual-photon absorptiometry: Comparison of bone mineral and soft tissue mass measurements in vivo with established methods. Am J Clin Nutr 49:1283–1289, 1989.
16. Cohn SH, Vaswani AN, Yasumura S, et al: Improved models for determination of body fat by in vivo neutron activation. Am J Clin Nutr 40:255–259, 1984.
17. Lohman TG: Skinfolds and body density and their relation to body fatness: A review. Hum Biol 53:181–225, 1981.
18. Bouchard C, Perusse L, Leblanc C, et al: Inheritance of the amount and distribution of human body fat. Int J Obes 12:205–215, 1988.
19. Seidell JC, Bakker CJ, van der Kroog K: Imaging techniques for measuring adipose-tissue distribution—a comparison between computed topography and 1.5-T magnetic resonance. Am J Clin Nutr 51:953–957, 1990.
20. Society of Actuaries and Association of Life Insurance Medical Directors of America: Society of Actuaries Build Study of 1979. Chicago, 1980.
21. Waaler HT: Height, weight and mortality: The Norwegian experience. Acta Med Scand 679:1–56, 1984.
22. Lew EA, Garfinkel L: Variations in mortality by weight among 750,000 men and women. J Chronic Dis 32:563–576, 1979.

23. Andres R, Elahi D, Tobin J, et al: Impact of age on weight goals. Ann Intern Med 10:1030–1033, 1985.
24. US Dept. of Agriculture: Nutrition and Your Health: Dietary Guidelines for Americans. Home and Garden Bulletin 232 (ed 3): 1990.
25. Fujioka S, Matsuzawa Y, Tokunaga K, Tarui S: Contribution of intraabdominal fat accumulation to the impairment of glucose and lipid metabolism in human obesity. Metabolism 36:54–59, 1987.
26. Garrison RJ, Kannel WB: A new approach to estimating healthy body weights. Int J Obes 17:417–423, 1993.
27. Bray GA: The Obese Patient. Major Problems in Internal Medicine. Philadelphia, WB Saunders, 1976.
28. Noppa H, Hallstrom T: Weight gain in adulthood in relation to socioeconomic factors, mental illness and personality traits: A prospective study of middle-aged women. J Psychosom Res 25:83–89, 1981.
29. Borkan GA, Sparrow D, Wisniewski C, Vokonas PS: Body weight and coronary disease risk: Patterns of risk factor change associated with long-term weight change. Am J Epidemiol 124:410–419, 1986.
30. Williamson DF, Kahn HS, Remington PL, et al: The 10-year incidence of overweight and major weight gain in US adults. Arch Intern Med 150:665, 1990.
31. Bradden FE, Rodgers B, Wadsworth ME, Davies JM: Onset of obesity in the 36-year birth cohort study. BMJ 293:299–303, 1986.
32. Charney E, Goodman HC, McBride M, et al: Childhood antecedents of adult obesity. N Engl J Med 295:6–9, 1976.
33. Khoury P, Morrison JA, Mellies MJ, Glueck CJ: Weight change since age 18 years in 30 to 55 year-old whites and blacks. JAMA 250:3179–3187, 1983.
34. Mossberg H-O: 40-Year follow-up on overweight children. Lancet 2:491–493, 1989.
35. Zack PM, Harlan WR, Leaverton PE, Cornoni-Huntley J: A longitudinal study of body fatness in childhood and adolescence. J Pediatr 95:126–130, 1979.
36. Garn SM, LaVelle M, Rosenberg KR, Hawthorne VM: Maturational timing as a factor in female fatness and obesity. Am J Clin Nutr 43:879–883, 1986.
37. Johnston FE, Mack RW: Obesity in urban black adolescents of high and low relative weight at 1 year of age. Am J Dis Child 123:862–864, 1978.
38. Melbin T, Vuille J-C: Weight gain in infancy and physical development between 7 and 10 1/2 years of age. Br J Prev Soc Med 30:233–238, 1976.
38a. Must A, Jacques PF, Dallel GE, et al: Long-term morbidity and mortality of overweight adolescents: A follow-up of the Harvard Growth Study of 1922 to 1935. N Engl J Med 327(19):1350–1355, 1993.
39. Casey VA, Dwyer JT, Coleman KA, Valadian I: Body mass index from childhood to middle age: A 50-year follow-up. Am J Clin Nutr 56:14–18, 1992.
40. Wong FL, Trowbridge FL: Nutrition surveys and surveillance: Their application to clinical practice. Clin Nutr 3:94–99, 1984.
41. Van Itallie TB, Lew EA: Assessment of morbidity and mortality risk in the overweight patient. In Wadden TA, Van Itallie TB (eds): Treatment of Seriously Obese Patient. New York, The Guilford Press, 1992, pp 3–32.
42. Knowler WC, Pettitt DJ, Savage PJ, Bennett PH: Diabetes incidence in PIMA Indians: Contributions of obesity and parental diabetes. Am J Epidemiol 113:144–156, 1981.
43. Seidel JC: Prevalence of obesity in Europe. Bibl Nutr Dieta 44:1–7, 1989.
44. Laurier D, Guiguet M, Chau NP, et al: Prevalence of obesity: A comparative survey in France, the United Kingdom and United States. Int J Obes 16:565–572, 1992.
45. Bray GA: Obesity—a disease of nutrient or energy balance? Nutr Rev 45:33–43, 1987.
46. Bray GA: Obesity, a disorder of nutrient partitioning: The MONA LISA hypothesis. J Nutr 121:1146–1162, 1991.
47. Flatt JP: Opposite effects of variations in food-intake on carbohydrate and fat oxidation in ad-libitum fed mice [technical note]. J Nutr Bioc 2:186–192, 1991.
48. Flatt JP: Assessment of daily and cumulative carbohydrate and fat balances in mice [technical note]. J Nutr Bioc 2:193–202, 1991.
49. Kather H, Scheurer A, Schlierf G: Antilipolytic action of insulin in abdominal adipocytes of obese subjects before and during energy restriction: Influence of adenosine deaminase. Int J Obes 11:191–200, 1987.
50. Arner P: Adrenergic receptor function in fat cells. Am J Clin Nutr 55:228S–236S, 1992.
51. Rebuffe-Scrive M, Bronnegard M, Nilsson A, et al: Steroid hormone receptors in human adipose tissues. J Clin Endocrinol Metab 71:1215–1219, 1990.
52. Hirsch J, Batchelor B: Adipose tissue cellularity in human obesity. J Clin Endocrinol Metab 5:299–311, 1976.
53. Ailhaud G, Grimaldi P, Negrel R: Cellular and molecular aspects of adipose tissue development. Annu Rev Nutr 12:207–233, 1992.
54. Knittle JL, Timmers K, Ginsberg-Fellner F, et al: The growth of adipose tissue in children and adolescents: Cross-sectional and longitudinal studies of adipose cell number and size. J Clin Invest 3:239–246, 1979.
55. Sjostrom LV, William-Olsson T: Prospective studies on adipose tissue development in man. Int J Obes 5:597–604, 1981.
56. Smith GP, Gibbs J: Are gut peptides a new class of anorectic agents? Am J Clin Nutr 55(Suppl 1):283S–285S, 1992.
57. Bray GA: Peptides affect the intake of specific nutrients and the sympathetic nervous system. Am J Clin Nutr 55:265S–271S, 1992.
58. Campfield LA, Brandon P, Smith FJ: On-line continuous measurement of blood glucose and meal pattern in free-feeding rats: The role of glucose in meal initiation. Brain Res Bull 14:605–616, 1985.
59. Friedman MI, Tordoff MG: Fatty acid oxidation and glucose utilization interact to control food intake in rats. Am J Physiol 251(5 pt2):R840–R845, 1986.
60. Ritter RC, Slusser PG, Stone S: Glucoreceptors controlling feeding and blood glucose: Location in the hindbrain. Science 213:451–452, 1981.
61. Bray GA: Syndromes of hypothalamic obesity in man. Ann Pediatr 13:525–536, 1984.
62. Bray GA, York DA, Fisler JS: Experimental obesity: A homeostatic failure due to defective nutrient stimulation of the sympathetic nervous system. Vitam Horm 45:1–125, 1989.
63. Rolls BJ: Sensory-specific satiety. Nutr Rev 44:93–101, 1986.
64. Reeds P, Fioroito ML, Davis TA: Nutrient partitioning: An overview. In Bray GA, Ryan DH (eds): The Science of Food Regulation. Food Intake, Taste, Nutrient Partitioning, and Energy Expenditure. Proceedings of the Pennington Center Nutrition Series. Baton Rouge, LA, Louisiana State University Press, 1992, pp 103–120.
65. Fomon SJ, Haschke F, Ziegler EE, Nelson SE: Body composition of reference children from birth to age 10 years. Am J Clin Nutr 35:1169, 1982.
66. Garrow J: Energy Balance and Obesity in Man. New York, Elsevier/North Holland, 1978.
67. Schoeller DA, Van Santen E, Peterson DW, Dietz W, et al: Total body water measurement in humans with O and H labeled water. Am J Clin Nutr 33:2686–2693, 1980.
68. Rubner M: The Laws of Energy Consumption in Nutrition. New York, Academic Press, 1982.
69. Kleiber M: The Fire of Life: An Introduction to Animal Energetics. New York, John Wiley & Sons, 1961.
70. Ravussin E, Lillioja S, Anderson TE, et al: Determinants of 24-hour energy expenditure in man: Methods and results using a respiratory chamber. J Clin Invest 78:1568–1578, 1986.
71. Bogardus C, Lillioja S, Ravussin E, et al: Familial dependence of the resting metabolic rate. N Engl J Med 315:96–100, 1986.
72. Ravussin E, Lillioja S, Knowler WC, et al: Reduced rate of energy expenditure as a risk factor for body-weight gain. N Engl J Med 318:467–472, 1988.
73. Zurlo F, Lillioja S, Esposito-Del Puente A, et al: Low ratio of fat to carbohydrate oxidation as predictor of weight gain: Study of 24-h RQ. Am J Physiol 259(5 pt1):E650–657, 1990.
74. Swinburn BA, Nyomba BL, Saad MF, et al: Insulin resistance associated with lower rates of weight gain in Pima Indians. J Clin Invest 88:168–173, 1991.
75. Glick Z, Teague RJ, Bray GA: Brown adipose tissue: Thermic response increased by a single low protein meal. Science 213:1125–1127, 1981.
76. Acheson K, Jequier E, Wahren J: Influence of beta-adrenergic blockade on glucose-induced thermogenesis in man. J Clin Invest 72:981–986, 1983.
77. Segal KR, Chun A, Coronel P, et al: Reliability of the measurement of postprandial thermogenesis in men of three levels of body fatness. Metabolism 41:754–762, 1992.
78. Whipp BJ, Bray GA, Koyal SN: Exercise energetics in normal man following acute weight gain. Am J Clin Nutr 26:1284–1286, 1973.
79. Brownell KD, Stunkard AJ, Albaum JM: Evaluation and modification of exercise patterns in the natural environment. Am J Psychiatry 137:1540–1545, 1980.
80. Waxman M, Stunkard AJ: Caloric intake and expenditure of obese boys. J Pediatr 96:187–193, 1980.

81. Woo R, Garrow JS, Pi-Sunyer FX: Effect of exercise on spontaneous calorie intake in obesity. Am J Clin Nutr 36:470–477, 1985.

82. Beaton GH, Milner J, Corey P, et al: Sources of variance in 24-hour dietary recall data: Implications for nutrition study design and interpretation. Am J Clin Nutr 32:2546–2559, 1979.

83. Braitman LE, Adlin EV, Stanton JL: Obesity and caloric intake: The National Health and Nutrition Examination Survey of 1971–1975 (NHANES I). J Chron Dis 38:727–732, 1985.

84. National Research Council: Diet and health, implications for reducing chronic disease risk. Washington, DC, National Academy Press, 1989.

85. Bandini LG, Schoelle DA, Dietz WH: Energy expenditure in obese and non-obese adolescents. Pediatr Res 27:198–203, 1990.

86. Prentice AM, Black AE, Coward WA, et al: High levels of energy expenditure in obese women. BMJ 292:983–987, 1986.

87. Mertz W, Tsui JC, Judd JT, et al: What are people really eating—the relation between energy-intake derived from estimated diet records and intake determined to maintain body-weight. Am J Clin Nutr 54:291–295, 1991.

88. Tremblay A, Seale J, Almeras N, et al: Energy requirements of a postobese man reporting a low-energy intake at weight maintenance. Am J Clin Nutr 54:506–508, 1991.

89. Kissileff HR, Thornton J, Becker E: A quadratic equation adequately describes the cumulative food intake curve in man. Appetite 3:255–272, 1982.

90. Sims EA, Danforth E, Horton ES, et al: Endocrine and metabolic effects of experimental obesity in man. Recent Prog Horm Res 29:457–487, 1973.

91. Bouchard C, Tremblay A, Després JP, et al: The response to long-term overfeeding in identical twins. N Engl J Med 322:1477–1482, 1990.

92. Forbes GB, Brown MR, Welle SL, Lipinski BA: Deliberate overfeeding in women and men: Energy cost and composition of the weight gain. Br J Nutr 56:1–9, 1986.

93. Poehlman ET, Tremblay A, Després JP, et al: Genotype-controlled changes in body composition and fat morphology following overfeeding in twins. Am J Clin Nutr 43:723–731, 1992.

94. Manson JE, Stampfer MJ, Hennekens CH, Willett WC: Body weight and longevity. A reassessment. JAMA 257:353–358, 1987.

95. Sjostrom LV: Morbidity of severely obese subjects. Am J Clin Nutr 55(Suppl 2):508S–515S, 1992.

96. Ashley FW, Kannel WB: Relation of weight change to changes in atherogenic traits: The Framingham Study. J Chron Dis 27:103–114, 1974.

97. Manson JE, Colditz GA, Stampfer MJ, et al: A prospective study of obesity and risk of coronary heart disease in women. N Engl J Med 322:882–889, 1990.

98. Noppa H: Body weight change in relation to incidence of ischemic heart disease and change in risk factors for ischemic heart disease. Am J Epidemiol 111:693–704, 1980.

99. Rissanen AM, Heliovaara M, Knekt P, et al: Determinants of weight-gain and overweight in adult Finns. Eur J Clin Nutr 45:419–430, 1991.

100. Rissanen A, Heliovaara M, Knekt P, et al: Risk of disability and mortality due to overweight in Finnish population. BMJ 301:835–837, 1990.

101. Abraham S, Collins G, Nordsieck M: Relationship of childhood weight status to morbidity in adults. HSMHA Health Report 86:273–284, 1971.

102. Clarke WR, Woolson RF, Lauer RM: Changes in ponderosity and blood pressure in children: The Muscatine Study. Am J Epidemiol 124:195–206, 1986.

103. Hamm P, Shekelle RB, Stamler J: Large fluctuations in body weight during young adulthood and twenty-five-year risk of coronary death in men. Am J Epidemiol 129:312–318, 1989.

104. Lissner L, Odell PM, D'Agostino RB, et al: Variability of body weight and health outcomes in the Framingham population. N Engl J Med 324:1839–1844, 1991.

105. Donahue RP, Abbott RD, Bloom E, et al: Central obesity and coronary heart disease in men. Lancet 1:821–824, 1987.

106. Ducimetiere P, Richard J, Cambien F: The pattern of subcutaneous fat distribution in middle-aged men and the risk of coronary heart disease: The Paris Prospective Study. Int J Obes 10:229–240, 1986.

107. Stokes J III, Garrison RJ, Kannel WB: The independent contributions of various indices of obesity to the 22-year incidence of coronary heart disease: The Framingham Heart Study. In Vague J, Bjorntorp P, Guy-Grand B, et al (eds): Metabolic Complications of Human Obesities. Amsterdam, Excerpta Medica, 1985, pp 49–57.

108. Larsson B, Bjorntorp P, Tibblin G: The health consequences of moderate obesity. Int J Obes 5:97–116, 1981.

109. Bray GA: Obesity and the heart. Mod Concepts Cardiovasc Dis 56:67–71, 1987.

110. Alexander JK: The cardiomyopathy of obesity. Prog Cardiovasc Dis 27:325–334, 1985.

111. Zarich SW, Kowalchuk GJ, McGuire MP, et al: Left ventricular filling abnormalities in asymptomatic morbid obesity. Am J Cardiol 68:377–381, 1991.

112. Grundy SM, Barnett JP: Metabolic and health complications of obesity [review]. Dis Mon 36:641–696, 1990.

113. Miettinen TA: Cholesterol production in obesity. Circulation 44:842–850, 1971.

114. Nestel PJ, Schreibman PH, Ahrens EH Jr: Cholesterol metabolism in human obesity. J Clin Invest 52:2389–2397, 1973.

115. Schwartz RS, Brunzell JD: Increase of adipose tissue lipoprotein lipase activity with weight loss. J Clin Invest 67:1425–1430, 1981.

116. Kern PA, Ong JM, Saffari B, Carty J: The effects of weight loss on the activity and expression of adipose tissue lipoprotein lipase in very obese humans. N Engl J Med 322:1053–1059, 1990.

117. DeFronzo RA, Ferranni E: Insulin resistance—a multifaceted syndrome responsible for NIDDM obesity, hypertension, dyslipidemia, and atherosclerotic cardiovascular disease [review]. Diabetes Care 14:173–194, 1991.

118. Reaven GM: Banting Lecture 1988: Role of insulin resistance in human disease. Diabetes 37:1596–1607, 1988.

119. Messerli FH: Cardiovascular effects of obesity and hypertension. Lancet 1:1165–1168, 1982.

120. Chiang BN, Perlman LV, Epstein FH: Overweight and hypertension: A review. Circulation 39:403–421, 1969.

121. MacMahon SW, Wilcken DE, MacDonald GJ: The effect of weight reduction on left ventricular mass. A randomized controlled trial in young, overweight hypertensive patients. N Engl J Med 314:334–339, 1986.

122. Reisin E, Abel R, Modan M, et al: Effect of weight loss without salt restriction on the reduction of blood pressure in overweight hypertensive patients. N Engl J Med 298:1–6, 1978.

123. Tuck ML, Sowers J, Dornfeld L, et al: The effect of weight reduction on blood pressure, plasma renin activity, and plasma aldosterone levels in obese patients. N Engl J Med 304:930–933, 1981.

124. Rochester DF, Enson Y: Current concepts in the pathogenesis of the obesity-hypoventilation syndrome: Mechanical and circulatory factors. Am J Med 57:402–420, 1974.

125. Sharp JT, Barrocas M, Chokroverty S: The cardiorespiratory effects of obesity. Clin Chest Med 1:103–118, 1980.

126. Ray CS, Sue DY, Bray GA, et al: Effects of obesity on respiratory function. Am Rev Respir Dis 128:501–506, 1983.

127. Westlund K, Nicolaysen JM: Ten-year mortality and morbidity related to serum cholesterol: A follow-up of 3,751 men aged 40–49. Scan J Clin Lab Invest 30(Suppl 127):3–24, 1972.

128. Rimm AA, Werner LH, Yserloo BV, Bernstein RA: Relationship of obesity and disease in 73,532 weight-conscious women. Public Health Rep 90:44–54, 1975.

129. Vague J: Degree of masculine differentiation of obesities: Factor determining predisposition to diabetes, atherosclerosis, gout, and uric calculous disease. Am J Clin Nutr 4:20–34, 1956.

130. Hartz AJ, Rupley CC, Rimm AA: The association of girth measurements with disease in 32,856 women. Am J Epidemiol 119:71–80, 1984.

131. Ohlson LO, Larsson B, Svardsudd K, et al: The influence of body fat distribution on the incidence of diabetes mellitus. 13.5 Years of follow-up of the participants in the study of men born in 1913. Diabetes 34:1055–1058, 1985.

132. Haffner SM, Stern MP, Hazuda HP, et al: Do upper body and centralized adiposity measure different aspects of regional body-fat distribution? Relationship to non–insulin-dependent diabetes mellitus, lipids, and lipoproteins. Diabetes 36:43–51, 1987.

133. Bernstein RA, Geifer EE, Vieira JJ, et al: Gallbladder disease: II. Utilization of the life table method in obtaining clinically useful information: A study of 62,739 weight-conscious women. J Chron Dis 30:529–541, 1977.

134. Stampfer MJ, Maclure KM, Colditz GA, et al: Risk of symptomatic gallstones in women with severe obesity. Am J Clin Nutr 55:652–658, 1992.

135. Weinsier R, Ullmann DO: Gallstone formation and weight loss: A review. Obesity Research 1:51–56, 1993.

136. La Vecchia C, DeCarli A, Fasoli M, Gentile A: Nutrition and diet in the etiology of endometrial cancer. Cancer 7:1248–1253, 1986.

137. Jensen H: Endometrial carcinoma: A retrospective, epidemiological study. Dan Med Bull 32:219–228, 1985.
138. Henderson BE, Casagrande JT, Pike MC, et al: The epidemiology of endometrial cancer in young women. Br J Cancer 47:749–756, 1983.
139. Willett WC, Browne ML, Bain C, et al: Relative weight and risk of breast cancer among premenopausal women. Am J Epidemiol 122:731–740, 1985.
140. Schapira DV, Kumar NB, Lyman GH: Obesity, body fat distribution, and sex hormones in breast cancer patients. Cancer 67:2215–2218, 1991.
141. Anderson JJ, Felson DT: Factors associated with osteoarthritis of the knee in the first National Health and Nutrition Examination Survey (HANES I): Evidence for an association with overweight, race and physical demands of work. Am J Epidemiol 128:179–189, 1988.
142. Davis MA, Ettinger WH, Neuhaus JM, Hauck WW: Sex differences in osteoarthritis of the knee: The role of obesity. Am J Epidemiol 127:1019–1030, 1988.
143. Felson DT, Zhang Y, Anthony JM, et al: Weight loss reduces the risk for symptomatic knee osteoarthritis in women. Ann Intern Med 116:535–539, 1992.
144. Kannel WB, Gordon T: Physiological and medical concomitants of obesity: The Framingham study. In Bray GA (ed): Obesity in America. Washington, DC, Department of Health, Education and Welfare, #79–249, 1979, pp 125–153.
145. Naeye RL: Weight gain and the outcome of pregnancy. Am J Obstet Gynecol 135:3–9, 1979.
146. Zelissen PMJ: Nerve endurance regulation in obesity. Thesis, University of Utrecht, 1991.
147. Veldhuis JD, Iranmane A, Ho KKY, et al: Dual defects in pulsatile growth-hormone secretion and clearance subserve the hyposomatotropism of obesity in man. J Clin Endocrinol 72:51–59, 1991.
148. Williams T, Berelowitz M, Joffe SN, et al: Impaired growth hormone responses to growth hormone–releasing factor in obesity: A pituitary defect reversed with weight reduction. N Engl J Med 311:1403–1407, 1984.
149. LaLa VR, Ray A, Jamias P, et al: Prolactin and thyroid status in prepubertal children with mild to moderate obesity. J Am Coll Nutr 7:361–366, 1988.
150. Kopelman PG, Pilkington TR, White N, Jeffcoate SL: Evidence for existence of two types of massive obesity. BMJ 280:82–83, 1980.
151. Danforth E Jr, Horton ES, O'Connel M, et al: Dietary-induced alterations in thyroid hormone metabolism during overnutrition. J Clin Invest 64:1336–1347, 1979.
152. Atkinson RL: Naloxone decreases food intake in obese humans. J Clin Endocrinol Metab 55:196–198, 1982.
153. Holtzman SG: Suppression of appetite behavior in the rat by naloxone: Lack of effect of prior morphine dependence. Life Sci 24:219–226, 1979.
154. Cohen MR, Picker D, Cohen RM, et al: Plasma cortisol and beta-endorphin immunoreactivity in human obesity. Psychosom Med 46:454–462, 1984.
155. Crapo L: Cushing's syndrome: A review of diagnostic tests. Metabolism 28:955–977, 1979.
156. Facchinetti F, Giovannini C, Petraglia F, et al: Plasma β-endorphin resistance to dexamethasone suppression in obese patients. J Endocrinol Invest 11:119–123, 1988.
157. Kley HK, Edelman P, Kruskemper HL: Relationships of plasma sex hormones to different parameters of obesity in male subjects. Metabolism 29:1041–1045, 1980.
158. Strain GW, Zumoff B, Miller LK, et al: Effect of massive weight loss on hypothalamic-pituitary-gonadal function in obese men. J Clin Endocrinol Metab 66:1019–1023, 1988.
159. Glass AR, Burman KD, Dahms WT, Boehm TM: Endocrine function in human obesity. Metabolism 30:89–104, 1981.
160. Frisch RE, McArthur JW: Menstrual cycles: Fatness as a determinant of minimum weight for height necessary for their maintenance or onset. Science 185:949–951, 1974.
161. Hartz AJ, Barboriak PN, Wong A, et al: The association of obesity with infertility and related menstrual abnormalities in women. Int J Obes 3:57–73, 1979.
162. Longcope C, Pratt JH, Schneider SH, Fineberg SE: Aromatization of androgens by muscle and adipose tissue in vivo. J Clin Endocrinol Metab 46:146–152, 1978.
163. Kirschner MA, Samojlik E, Drejka M, et al: Androgen-estrogen metabolism in women with upper body versus lower body obesity. J Clin Endocrinol Metab 70:473–479, 1990.
164. Bjorntorp P: Effects of age, sex, and clinical conditions on adipose tissue cellularity in man. Metabolism 11:1091–1102, 1974.
165. Krotkiewski M, Sjostrom L, Bjorntorp P, et al: Adipose tissue cellularity in relation to prognosis for weight reduction. Int J Obes 1:395–416, 1977.
166. Kissebah AH, Vydelingum N, Murray R, et al: Relation of body fat distribution to metabolic complications of obesity. J Clin Endocrinol Metab 54:254, 1982.
167. Evans DJ, Hoffmann RG, Kalkhoff RK, Kissebah AH: Relationship of androgenic activity to body fat topography, fat cell morphology, and metabolic aberrations in premenopausal women. J Clin Endocrinol Metab 57:304–310, 1983.
168. Rebuffe-Scrive M, Marin P, Bjorntorp P: Effect of testosterone on abdominal adipose tissue in men. Int J Obes 15:791–795, 1991.
169. Bray GA, Gallagher TF Jr: Manifestations of hypothalamic obesity in man: A comprehensive investigation of eight patients and a review of the literature. Medicine 54:301–330, 1975.
170. Franks S, Kiddy D, Sharp P, et al: Obesity and polycystic ovary syndrome. Ann NY Acad Sci 626:201–206, 1991.
171. Yen SCC: The polycystic ovary syndrome. Clin Endocrinol 12:177–207, 1980.
172. Ciaraldi TP, el-Roeiy A, Madar Z, et al: Cellular mechanisms of insulin resistance in polycystic ovarian syndrome. J Clin Endocrinol Metab 75:577–583, 1992.
173. World Health Organization: Diet, Nutrition, and Prevention of Chronic Diseases: Technical Report Series 797. Geneva, World Health Organization, 1990.
174. Lissner L, Levitsky DA, Strupp BJ, et al: Dietary fat and the regulation of energy intake in human subjects. Am J Clin Nutr 46:886–892, 1987.
175. Romieu I, Willett WC, Stampfer MJ, et al: Energy intake and other determinants of relative weight. Am J Clin Nutr 47:406–412, 1988.
176. Kromhout D: Changes in energy and macronutrients in 871 middle-aged men during 10 years of follow-up (the Zutphen Study). Am J Clin Nutr 37:287–294, 1983.
177. Stunkard AJ, Thorkild IA, Sorensen TIA, et al: An adoption study of human obesity. N Engl J Med 314:193–198, 1986.
178. Sorensen TIA, Price RA, Stunkard AJ, Schulsinger F: Genetics of obesity in adult adoptees and their biological siblings. BMJ 298:87–90, 1989.
179. Borjeson M: The aetiology of obesity in children: A study of 101 twin parts. Acta Paediatr Scand 65:279–287, 1976.
180. Brook CG, Huntley RM, Slack J: Influence of heredity and environment in determination of skinfold thickness in children. BMJ 2:719–721, 1975.
181. Newman HH, Freeman FN, Holzinger KJ: Twins: A Study of Heredity and Environment. Chicago, University of Chicago Press, 1937.
182. Stunkard AJ, Foch TT, Hrubec Z: A twin study of human obesity. JAMA 256:51–54, 1986.
183. Stunkard AJ: The body-mass of twins who have been reared apart. N Engl J Med 322:1483–1487, 1990.
184. Verschuer O: Die vererbungsbiologische Zwillingsforschung. Ergeb Inn Med Kinderheilkd 31:35–120, 1927.
185. Larsson B, Bengtsson C, Bjorntorp P, et al: Is abdominal body fat distribution a major explanation for the sex difference in the incidence of myocardial infarction? Am J Epidemiol 135:266–273, 1992.
186. Keys A, Brozek J, Henschel A, et al: The Biology of Human Starvation, vols 1 & 2. Minneapolis, University of Minnesota University Press, 1950.
187. Garrow JS: Treat Obesity Seriously. Philadelphia, WB Saunders, 1981.
188. Forbes GB: Lean body mass–body fat interrelationships in humans. Nutr Rev 45:225–231, 1987.
189. Forbes GB, Drenick EJ: Loss of body nitrogen on fasting. Am J Clin Nutr 32:1570–1574, 1979.
190. Hood CEA, Goodhart JM, Fletcher RF, et al: Observations on obese patients eating isocaloric reducing diets with varying proportions of carbohydrate. Br J Nutr 24:39–44, 1970.
191. Jenkins DJ, Wolever TM, Vuksan V, et al: Nibbling versus gorging: Metabolic advantages of increased meal frequency. N Engl J Med 321:929–934, 1989.
192. Owen OE, Kavle E, Owen RS, et al: A reappraisal of caloric requirements of healthy women. Am J Clin Nutr 44:1–19, 1986.
193. Owen OE, Holup JL, D'Alessio DA, et al: A reappraisal of the caloric requirements of men. Am J Clin Nutr 46:875–885, 1987.
194. Sohar E, Sneh E: Follow-up of obese patients: 14 years after a successful reducing diet. Am J Clin Nutr 26:845–848, 1973.
195. Stamler J, Farinaro E, Mojonnier LM, et al: Prevention and control of hypertension by nutritional-hygienic means: Long-term experience of the Chicago Coronary Prevention Evaluation Program. JAMA 243:1819–1823, 1980.

196. Atkinson RL, Pi-Sunyer FX (eds): Very low calorie diets. Am J Clin Nutr 56(Suppl 1):175S–305S, 1992.
197. Hoerr RA, Kohl HW, Nichaman MZ, et al: Differences in weight loss between two levels of energy intake during a 26 week very low calorie weight loss program: Institute for Aerobics Research. Dallas, TX, NAASO Abstracts, 1992.
198. National Research Council (US): Recommended Dietary Allowances/Subcommittee on the Tenth Edition of the RDAs, Food and Nutrition Board, Commission on Life Sciences, 10th rev. ed., 1989.
199. Bray GA: The Physician's Diet Plan. Unpublished manuscript, 1982.
200. Sours HE, Frattali VP, Brand CD, et al: Sudden death associated with very low calorie weight reduction regimens. Am J Clin Nutr 34:453–461, 1981.
201. Amatruda JM, Biddle TL, Patton ML, Lockwood DH: Vigorous supplementation of hypocaloric diet prevents cardiac arrhythmias and mineral depletion. Am J Med 74:1016–1022, 1983.
202. Wadden TA, Stunkard AJ, Brownell KD: Very low calorie diets: Their efficacy, safety, and future. Ann Intern Med 99:675–684, 1983.
203. Fisler JS, Drenick EJ: Starvation and semistarvation diets in the management of obesity. Ann Rev Nutr 7:465–484, 1987.
204. Warwick PM, Garrow JS: The effect of addition of exercise to a regime of dietary restriction on weight loss, nitrogen balance, resting metabolic rate and spontaneous physical activity in three obese women in a metabolic ward. Int J Obes 5:25–32, 1981.
205. Hill JO: Exercise, energy expenditure, and fat oxidation. In Bray GA, Ryan DH (eds): The Science of Food Regulation. Food Intake, Taste, Nutrient Partitioning, and Energy Expenditure. Baton Rouge, Louisiana State University Press, 1992, pp 103–120.
206. Pavlou KN, Steffee WP, Lerman RH, Burrows BA: Effects of dieting and exercise on lean body mass, oxygen uptake and strength. Med Sci Sport Med 17:466–471, 1985.
207. Van Dale D, Saris WHM, Tenhoor F: Weight maintenance and resting metabolic rate 18–40 months after a diet exercise treatment. Int J Obes 14:347–359, 1990.
208. Harris MB, Hallbauer ES: Self-directed weight control through eating and exercise. Behav Res Ther 11:523–529, 1973.
209. Stalonas PM, Perri MG, Kerzner AB: Do behavioral treatments of obesity last? A five-year follow-up investigation. Addict Behav 9:175–183, 1984.
210. Wing RR, Epstein LH, Paternostro-Bayles M, et al: Exercise in a behavioral weight control programme for obese patients with Type 2 (non–insulin-dependent) diabetes. Diabetologia 31:902–909, 1988.
211. Dahlkoetter J, Callahan EJ, Linton J: Obesity and the unbalanced energy equation: Exercise versus eating habit change. J Consult Clin Psychol 47:898–905, 1979.
212. Scoville BA: Review of amphetamine-like drugs by the Food and Drug Administration: Clinical data and value judgements. In Bray GA (ed): Obesity in Perspective. DHEW Publ No. (NIH) 75–708. Bethesda, MD, National Institutes of Health, 1975, pp 441–443.
213. Weintraub M, Bray GA: Drug treatment of obesity. Med Clin North Am 73:237–250, 1989.
214. Weintraub M, Fundaresan PR, Schuster B, et al: National heart, lung and blood institute long-term weight control study: I–VII. Clin Pharmacol Ther 51:581–585, 1992.
215. Griffiths M, Rivers PW, Hoinville EA: Obesity in boys: The distinction between fatness and heaviness. Human nutrition: Clinical Nutrition 39C:259–269, 1985.
216. Guy-Grand B, Apfelbaum M, Crepaldi G, et al: International trial of long term dexfenfluramine in obesity. Lancet 2:1142–1144, 1989.
217. Levine LR, Enas GG, Thompson WL, et al: Use of fluoxetine, a selective serotonin-uptake inhibitor, in the treatment of obesity—a dose response study. Int J Obes 13:635–645, 1989.
218. Gray DS, Fujioka K, Devine W, Bray GA: Fluoxetine treatment of the obese diabetic. Int J Obes 16:193–198, 1992.
219. Darga LL, Carroll-Michals L, Botsford SJ, Lucas CP: Fluoxetine's effect on weight loss in obese subjects. Am J Clin Nutr 54:321–325, 1991.
220. Lasagna L: Phenylpropanolamine—A Review. New York, John Wiley & Sons, 1988.
221. Weintraub M: Phenylpropanolamine as an anorexiant agent in weight control: A review of published and unpublished studies. In Morgan JP, Kagan DV, Brody JS (eds): Phenylpropanolamine. Risks, Benefits, and Controversies. New York, Praeger Scientific, 1985, pp 53–79.
222. Bray GA: Barriers to the treatment of obesity. Ann Intern Med 115:152–153, 1991.
223. National Institutes of Health: Health implications of obesity. Ann Intern Med 103:1073–1077, 1985.
224. Pasquali R, Casimirr F, Melchion N, et al: Effects of chronic administration of ephedrine during very-low-calorie diets on energy-expenditure, protein-metabolism and hormone levels in obese subjects. Clin Sci 82:85–92, 1992.
225. Astrup A, Breum L, Toubro S, et al: The effect and safety of an ephedrine/caffeine compound compared to ephedrine, caffeine and placebo in obese subjects on an energy restricted diet: A double blind trial. Int J Obes 16:269–277, 1992.
226. Arch JRS, Ainsworth AT, Cawthorne MA, et al: Atypical beta-adrenoceptor on brown adipocytes as target for anti-obesity drugs. Nature 309:163–165, 1984.
227. Connacher AA, Jung RT, Mitchell PE: Weight loss in obese subjects on a restricted diet given BRL 26830A, a new atypical beta adrenoceptor agonist. BMJ 296:1217–1220, 1988.
228. Henny CH, Buckert A, Schutz Y, et al: Comparison of thermogenic activity induced by the new sympathomimetic Ro 16–8714 between normal and obese subjects. Int J Obes 12:227–236, 1988.
229. Holloway BR, Howe R, Rao BS, et al: ICI-D7114 a novel selective beta-adrenoceptor agonist selectively stimulates brown fat and increases whole-body oxygen-consumption. Br J Pharm 104:97–104, 1991.
230. Enzi G, Inelmen EM, Crepaldi G: Effect of hydrophilic mucilage in the treatment of obese patients. Pharmatherapeutica 2:421, 1980.
231. Solum TT, Ryttig KR, Solum E, Larsen S: The influence of high-fibre diet on body weight, serum lipids and blood pressure in slightly overweight persons, a randomized, double-blind, placebo-controlled investigation with diet and fibre tables (dumo vital). Int J Obes 11(Suppl 1):67–71, 1987.
232. Hauptman JB, Jeunet FS, Hartmann D: Initial studies in humans with the novel gastrointestinal lipase inhibitor Ro 18–0647 (tetrahydrolipstatin)1,2. Am J Clin Nutr 55:309S–313S, 1992.
233. Glueck CJ, Hastings MM, Allen C, et al: Sucrose polyester and covert caloric dilution. Am J Clin Nutr 35:1352–1359, 1982.
234. Mellies MJ, Vitale C, Jandacek RJ, et al: The substitution of sucrose polyester for dietary fat in obese, hypercholesterolemic outpatients. Am J Clin Nutr 41:1–12, 1985.
235. Rolls BJ, Pirraglia PA, Jones MB, Peters JC: Effects of olestra, a noncaloric fat substitute, on daily energy and fat intakes in lean men. Am J Clin Nutr 56:84–92, 1992.
236. Bray GA, Gray DS: Treatment of obesity: An overview. Diabetes Metab Rev 4:653–679, 1988.
237. Greenway FL, Bray GA: Regional fat loss from the thigh in obese women after adrenergic modulation. Clin Ther 9:663–669, 1987.
238. Nieben OG, Harboe H: Intragastric balloon as bezoar for treatment of obesity. Lancet 1:198–199, 1982.
239. Lindor KD, Hughes RW Jr, Ilstrup DM, Jensen MD: Intragastric balloons in comparison with standard therapy for obesity—a randomized, double-blind trial. Mayo Clin Proc 62:992–996, 1987.
239a. Bjorvell H, Rossner S: Long term treatment of severe obesity: Four year follow up of results of combined behavioral modification programme. Br Med J 291:379–382, 1985.
240. Garrow JS, Gardiner GT: Maintenance of weight loss in obese patients after jaw-wiring. Br J Med 282:858–860, 1981.
241. Gortz L, Wallin G, Kral JG: Vertical banded gastroplasty with and without vagotomy. Clin Nutr 5(Suppl):79–81, 1986.
242. Kral JG: Overview of surgical techniques for treating obesity. Am J Clin Nutr 55(Suppl 2):552S–555S, 1992.
243. Teimourian B, Rogers WB: A national survey of complications associated with suction lipectomy: A comparative study. Plas Reconstr Surg 84:628–631, 1989.
244. Mason EE, Ito C: Gastric bypass. Ann Surg 170:329–339, 1970.
245. Freeman JB, Burchett H: Failure rate with gastric partitioning for morbid obesity. Am J Surg 145:113–117, 1983.
246. Pories WJ, Flickinger EG, Meelheim D, et al: The effectiveness of gastric bypass over gastric partition in morbid obesity. Ann Surg 196:389–399, 1982.
247. Sugerman HJ, Starkey JV, Birkenhauer R: A randomized prospective trial of gastric bypass versus vertical banded gastroplasty for morbid obesity and their effects on sweets versus non-sweets eaters. Ann Surg 205:613–624, 1987.
248. Hallberg D: A survey of surgical techniques for treatment of obesity and a remark on the bilio-intestinal bypass method. Am J Clin Nutr 33(Suppl 2):499–501, 1980.
249. Scopinaro N, Gianetta E, Civalleri D, et al: Partial and total biliopancreatic bypass in the surgical treatment of obesity. Int J Obes 5:421–429, 1981.
250. Stunkard AJ, Penick SB: Behavior modification in the treatment of obesity. Arch Gen Psychiatry 36:801–806, 1979.

251. Craighead LW, Stunkard AJ, O'Brien RM: Behavior therapy and pharmacotherapy for obesity. Arch Gen Psychiatry 38:763–768, 1981.
252. Stunkard AJ: Conservative treatments for obesity. Am J Clin Nutr 45:1142–1154, 1987.
253. Bjorvell H, Rossner S: Long term treatment of severe obesity: Four year follow up of results of combined behavioural modification programme. BMJ 291:379–382, 1985.
254. Epstein LH, Vvaloski A, Wing RR, McCurley J: Ten-year follow-up of behavioral, family-based treatment for obese children. JAMA 264:2519–2523, 1991.

Endocrine Responses to Starvation, Malnutrition, and Illness

DAVID HEBER

The interplay of the endocrine system and major metabolic pathways is illustrated in the adaptive response to uncomplicated starvation. This essential adaptation provides a fascinating, teleologically appropriate sequence of changes in which different endocrine glands work synergistically toward a critical metabolic response.[1] By understanding this normal response, the changes observed in malnourished children[2] and those occurring in malnourished adults with a variety of serious illnesses can be classified into a series of pathophysiological syndromes.[3] In many instances, recently discovered cytokines that are produced during the host immune response to illness and infection interfere with the normal adaptation to starvation.[4] The combination of altered hormonal responses and cytokine actions leads to a hypermetabolic state, which must be considered in the nutritional therapy of the critically ill hospitalized patient. Therapeutic protocols integrating knowledge of the normal and maladaptive responses to undernutrition have been integrated into the intensive care unit treatment of the critically ill patient.[5] In this critical-care setting, nutritional therapy has been shown to be essential to survival. Despite this realization in the critical-care setting, 50 to 60 per cent of patients hospitalized on general medical and surgical wards suffer from significant malnutrition. In the face of the multitude of procedures and tests conducted on hospitalized patients, house officers and many physicians fail to diagnose malnutrition. A better understanding of the endocrine response to illness, including the neuroendocrine, hormonal, and metabolic mediators involved, and earlier recognition of malnutrition in the ambulatory patient and patients on general medical and surgical wards can lead to improved outcomes. This chapter will attempt to provide an integrated view of the diagnosis and treatment of malnutrition based on an understanding of the endocrine response to starvation, malnutrition, and illness.

ADAPTATION TO UNCOMPLICATED STARVATION

Until the middle of the twentieth century, at which time fortified foods were made widely available in the industrialized nations of the world, humans survived throughout history in the face of scarcity or temporary absence of food by adapting to starvation. In well-nourished individuals, short-term adaptations occur each day between bedtime and breakfast to maintain normal blood sugar levels in the absence of food intake, with changes in hormones and metabolites similar to those seen in the earliest stages of the adaptation to starvation. If fasting is continued for up to 6 weeks, a series of adaptations occur to maintain the integrity of body protein stores which are essential to survival. Ironically, the bulk of the information available on the physiology of the adaptation to uncomplicated starvation has been developed in studies of massively obese subjects fasting voluntarily under metabolic ward conditions.[6–8]

Dietary Sources and Body Stores of Energy

The average distribution of dietary macronutrients consumed in the diet is roughly 20 to 40 per cent as fat, 40 to 60 per cent as carbohydrate, and 10 to 20 per cent as protein. There are variations in the dietary sources of these nutrients throughout the world and some variations in the proportions of these macronutrients. For example, in countries consuming a low-fat, high-fiber diet, complex carbohydrates are obtained from cereals, grains, fruits, and vegetables, while in industrialized countries consuming a high-fat, low-fiber diet, simple sugars from processed foods will comprise a large portion of the carbohydrate consumed. Despite wide variations in the dietary intake of macronutrients among various populations, the body stores these dietary macronutrients in a fairly uniform but different pattern from the ingested proportions. The distribution of stored calories is ideally adapted to the metabolic needs under conditions of stress and starvation.

In the average 70-kg man, the largest store of calories is in the form of fat in adipose tissue, with approximately 135,000 calories stored in 13.5 kg of adipose tissue. This storage compartment can be greatly expanded with long-term overnutrition in obese individuals. There are approximately 54,000 calories stored as protein both in muscle and viscera. Only half these calories can be mobilized for energy, since depletion below 50 per cent of total protein stores is incompatible with life.[9] In addition to being an energy source, protein plays a functional role in many organs, including the liver, and depletion is associated with impaired immunity to infection.[10] In fact, the most common cause of death in an epidemic of starvation is typically simple bacterial pneumonia. Conservation of protein is an adaptation tightly linked to survival during acute starvation.

There are only 1200 calories stored as carbohydrate in liver and muscle glycogen. There are clear adaptive advantages to storing calories as fat, since fat can provide more energy per gram than carbohydrate or protein. However, since carbohydrate stores are so small, they are depleted in 3 days of uncomplicated starvation or sooner under conditions of increased energy expenditure. This dependence on fat and protein stores in starvation requires metabolic adaptations to minimize the loss of protein stores and shift to metabolic pathways predominantly utilizing the large fat stores available (Fig. 144–1).

Metabolic Requirements of the Starved Host

The postabsorptive period is defined as 8 to 16 hours after eating and has been defined operationally as the timepoint after an overnight fast when a number of hormonal determinations can be made under standard conditions. It can be thought of as a period of very early adaptation to starvation. During this period, the primary metabolic priority is the provision of adequate glucose for essential functions of the brain, red blood cells, peripheral nerves, and renal medulla.

During this postabsorptive phase, insulin levels fall as blood glucose falls from a range of 4 to 5 mmol/L to 3 to 4 mmol/L.[7] Glucose is released from the liver into the circulation via glycogenolysis of stores accumulated after feeding under the influence of insulin. The fall in glucose level is associated with depletion of glycogen stores. Skeletal muscle does not release glucose from stored glycogen directly into the circulation because myocytes lack the enzyme glucose-6-phosphatase. However, muscle releases lactate and amino acids such as alanine which can enter the

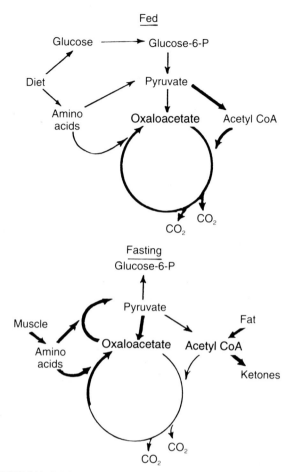

FIGURE 144–1. The flow of substrate during the fed and fasting states.

circulation and are converted to glucose in the liver via gluconeogenesis. Glucagon in the presence of lowered insulin concentrations promotes gluconeogenesis during the postabsorptive period.[11]

In addition, glucagon in the presence of lowered insulin levels promotes lipolysis. As the stored triglyceride in adipocytes is mobilized as free fatty acids, those tissues which do not require glucose as their primary fuel (e.g., skeletal muscle) begin to oxidize free fatty acids. These changes during the early postabsorptive period act to increase free fatty acid oxidation in order to spare protein breakdown. During the first few days of starvation, free fatty acid concentrations increase from a range of 0.5 to 0.8 mmol/L up to 1.2 to 1.6 mmol/L and plateau thereafter as starvation is prolonged.[7] These free fatty acids circulate bound to albumin and are oxidized in the liver to water-soluble ketone bodies, including acetoacetate and β-hydroxybutyrate. In obese subjects with more than adequate triglyceride stores, acetoacetate concentrations rise 25-fold and β-hydroxybutyrate concentrations rise 100-fold from the levels observed in the postabsorptive phase following 4 to 6 weeks of uncomplicated starvation (Fig. 144–2). These are the largest fluctuations seen in any circulating fuel with prolonged starvation.[12]

Protein synthesis and catabolism have been estimated to account for approximately 40 per cent of resting energy expenditure. In addition, the changes in protein metabolism are critical to maintaining the body cell mass during starvation, which directly affects survival.[13] Plasma amino

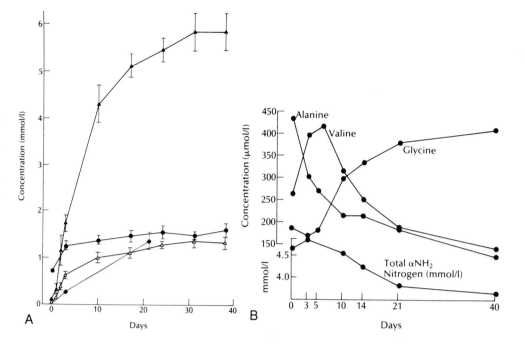

FIGURE 144–2. *A*, Blood 3-hydroxybutyrate (▲) and acetoacetate (△) and plasma acetone (◆) and free fatty acid (●) concentrations during starvation. *B*, Total alpha-amino nitrogen and three representative amino acids during prolonged starvation. (Reproduced with permission from Cahill GF: Starvation in man. N Engl J Med 282:668–675, 1970.)

acids measured in venous blood give nonspecific indications of the adaptations taking place in protein metabolism during the course of starvation. In addition, the excretion of protein from the body as urinary urea nitrogen expressed as nitrogen balance provides further insights into overall protein nutriture (Fig. 144–2).

The total alpha-amino nitrogen concentration, which reflects total amino acids, increases transiently from 4.6 to 4.8 mmol/L over the first few days of starvation and then decreases to 3.6 mmol/L.[14] These total amino acid changes obscure the changes in several different classes of amino acids. First, the branched-chain amino acids—leucine, isoleucine, and valine—increase transiently approximately twofold in the blood between 3 and 5 days after the onset of starvation. Alanine, which is the primary glucogenic amino acid in the liver during starvation, is released from muscle in amounts larger than the measurable alanine stores of muscle. This is explained by the formation of alanine in muscle through what is known as the *alanine cycle* (Fig. 144–3). Pyruvate from the liver as well as pyruvate derived by glycolysis of glucose from glycogen stores enters the muscle, where the branched amino acids donate

an amino group via the action of a specific branched-chain amino acid–targeted enzyme to produce alanine. This alanine is then released to the liver, where alanine accounts for a significant portion of glucose synthesis. During the period between 3 and 5 days after the onset of starvation, the branched-chain amino acids in the circulation support an increased rate of gluconeogenesis until the full adaptation to a fat-fuel economy has progressed significantly. Second, blood and muscle alanine concentrations decline rapidly over the first 10 days of starvation and then continue to decrease progressively to about 30 per cent of postabsorptive levels several weeks later. Third, blood and muscle glutamine concentrations also decrease progressively during starvation.

In the first few days of starvation, the gut plays an important role in regulating protein and amino acid metabolism. The intestinal synthesis of glutamine increases with a subsequent increase in alanine and ammonia formation. The alanine is used for hepatic gluconeogenesis, while the increased ammonia levels in the portal circulation trigger the liver to produce glutamine, which is utilized by the kidney for gluconeogenesis.[13] After 30 days of fasting, the kidney

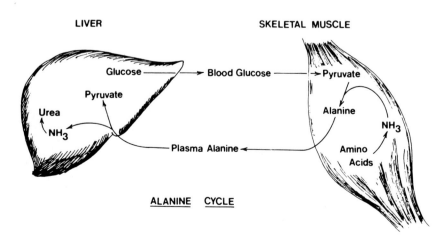

FIGURE 144–3. The alanine cycle allows carbon chains and ammonia to be shuttled from skeletal muscle to the liver, where they are used to synthesize glucose and urea, respectively.

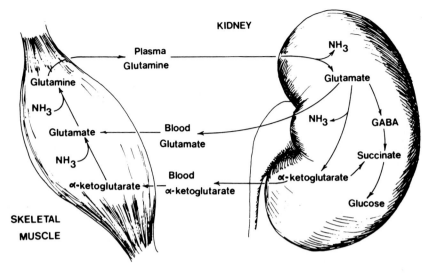

FIGURE 144–4. The glutamine cycle is a shuttle analogous to the alanine cycle which exists between skeletal muscle and the kidney. This cycle increases in importance as a fast extends beyond 30 days.

GLUTAMINE CYCLE

becomes an important gluconeogenic organ, contributing about half the body's glucose need. Most of this glucose is derived from the *glutamine cycle* (Fig. 144–4). Glutamine from the muscle and liver is converted to glutamate and ammonia in the kidney. Glutamate is then deaminated to α-ketoglutarate, which enters the gluconeogenic pathway.

The basic mechanisms underlying these adaptive changes in protein synthesis and degradation are still not completely understood. Proteolysis occurs in cellular lysosomes via autophagy. This process is stimulated by a shortage of critical regulatory amino acids, including phenylalanine, tryptophan, methionine, leucine, tyrosine, glutamic acid, proline, and histidine.[16] While not conclusively established, it appears that decreased concentrations of specific amino acyl transfer RNA's for these amino acids trigger proteolysis (Fig. 144–5). In terms of protein synthesis, there is a decrease in the amount and activity of RNA subunits involved in initiation, elongation, and termination of protein synthesis. Insulin is the primary hormone known to regulate protein metabolism.[17] Insulin deficiency leads to net protein breakdown, and hyperinsulinemia under euglycemic conditions inhibits proteolysis. There is also evidence that glucagon participates in this regulatory process by stimulating splanchnic proteolysis.[18] Plasma cortisol levels are increased for several hours and inhibit protein synthesis while increasing protein breakdown. Elevations in epinephrine, previously thought to increase protein breakdown, lead to decreases in the rate of whole-body protein breakdown. Growth hormone (GH) has been shown to increase protein synthesis but to oppose insulin's antiproteolytic effects. The role of insulin-like growth factor I (IGF-I) is still not established. Recent studies[19] have demonstrated that plasma amino acid levels and amino acid availability play an important role in modulating the rate of protein breakdown. The magnitude of these amino acid–mediated antiproteolytic effects was equivalent to that of insulin.

The impact of the adaptation to a fat-fuel economy is reflected in the rapid changes in urinary nitrogen excretion, showing net protein sparing through two processes. First, there is less protein breakdown. It has been estimated that protein synthesis decreases in the whole body by 40 per cent between the postprandial and postabsorptive phases,[13] with a further decrease over the first several days of starvation. Second, there is increased reutilization of nitrogen, evidenced by decreased urea formation in the

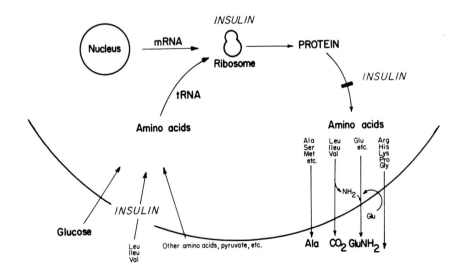

FIGURE 144–5. Effect of insulin in promoting glucose and amino acid uptake into muscle, activation of protein synthesis at the ribosome, and inhibition of proteolysis. Also shown is the predominant release of alanine (Ala) and glutamine (GluNH₂).

liver through the arginine-citrulline cycle. In obese subjects fasting for 7 days, protein breakdown and urinary urea nitrogen excretion decrease in parallel. Overall nitrogen is conserved so that nitrogen excretion decreases from 12 g/day in the postabsorptive state to 5 g/day 7 to 10 days later. This decrease translates into a decrease in muscle protein breakdown from 75 to 20 g/day. Based on theoretical calculations of the time necessary to reach the crucial 50 per cent of body cell mass, survival is extended through these adaptations from approximately 60 days to over 260 days, provided that adequate fluid and electrolytes are administered.[20]

Hormonal Mediators of Metabolic Adaptation

As discussed earlier, insulin is the primary hormone regulating fuel metabolism in the fed and fasted states. However, a number of other hormones participate in the adaptation to uncomplicated starvation. One group of hormones is called *counterregulatory* in recognition of their ability to antagonize the hypoglycemic action of administered insulin. Glucagon, for example, promotes glycogenolysis, gluconeogenesis, ketogenesis, proteolysis, and lipolysis. The levels of circulating catecholamines, norepinephrine, and epinephrine, which rise following insulin-induced hypoglycemia, also increase following acute starvation.[21]

Lipolysis is central to the adaptation to starvation and is regulated by catecholamines, glucagon, and GH. Catecholamines help to inhibit insulin secretion, which permits lipolysis. The lipolytic effects of epinephrine are more pronounced early in starvation,[22] and the rise in catecholamines promotes the metabolic utilization of fat. These hormones act through stimulatory and inhibitory G proteins and the cAMP cascade to modulate hormone-sensitive lipase. Beta$_1$-adrenergic stimulation increases glucagon secretion and inhibits muscle glucose metabolism.[23] Beta$_1$-adrenergic stimulation mediates the effects of glucagon, GH, cortisol, and vasopressin to increase lipolysis.[22] Thyroid hormones and glucocorticoids may act permissively on the processes stimulating lipolysis, while the actions of vasopressin, β-lipotropin, β-endorphin, and D-melanocyte–stimulating hormone have not been established.

Adipsin is a serine protease synthesized by adipocytes. Its exact physiological role is unknown, but its synthesis and secretion are inhibited by insulin or glucose and stimulated under catabolic conditions.[24] Its exact role in the adaptation to starvation, if any, remains to be determined.

Insulin-like growth factor I (IGF-I)/somatomedin-C stimulates amino acid uptake and protein synthesis while inhibiting lipolysis.[25] During growth and development, IGF-I secretion is dependent on GH. During starvation, this linkage is broken. In the presence of elevated GH levels, IGF-I levels remain low, and the concentration of IGF-I inhibitors in the circulation is increased.[26]

Within 7 to 10 days of starvation, there is a marked adaptive decrease in energy expenditure. Normally, resting energy expenditure is proportional to lean body mass. However, after 7 to 10 days of starvation, there is a 20 per cent decrease in resting energy expenditure, at a time when lean body mass has decreased by less than 5 per

cent.[27] Changes in the peripheral metabolism of thyroid hormones occur which may contribute significantly to the observed decrease in energy expenditure. Among these changes, there is less production of triiodothyronine (T$_3$), the most metabolically active thyroid hormone, via a decreased activity of 5'-monodeiodinase in the liver and other peripheral tissues.[28] There is a reciprocal rise in reverse T$_3$, an inactive metabolite, while thyroxine levels remain constant.[29] The overall decrease in energy expenditure with starvation is an adaptive change that results in a decreased rate of whole-body lipolysis, proteolysis, and gluconeogenesis (Fig. 144–6). Aerobic exercise in obese dieters does not reverse this adaptive change in energy regulation.[30]

There is a good correlation between the adaptive hormonal changes that occur during starvation (Table 144–1) and the decrease in whole-body protein breakdown that occurs as a result.[31]

Clinical Implications for the Endocrinologist

There are a number of clinical situations in which an understanding of the adaptive changes to uncomplicated starvation is useful. First, a number of patients with questions on the use of fad diets for weight loss will hope to find special ways of increasing their rate of weight loss on

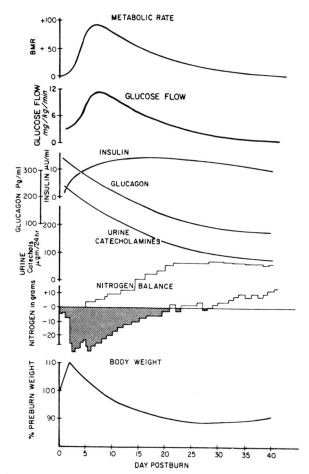

FIGURE 144–6. The hypermetabolism of injury during the flow phase is accompanied by increased glucagon and catecholamines relative to insulin. The hormonal mediators return to normal with recovery.

TABLE 144–1. CHANGES IN SERUM LEVELS OF HORMONES IN
NINE OBESE SUBJECTS AFTER 12 HOURS AND AFTER
7 DAYS OF FASTING

	12-H FAST	7-DAY FAST
T_3 (ng/dl)	130 ± 15	59 ± 5*
Free T_3 (pg/dl)	322 ± 32	159 ± 13*
rT_3 (ng/dl)	35 ± 3	57 ± 5*
T_4 (μg/dl)	9.1 ± 0.7	9.3 ± 0.8
Free T_4 (ng/dl)	4.7 ± 0.2	3.0 ± 0.3
Insulin	34 ± 6	15 ± 2*
Morning cortisol (mg/dl)	19.1 ± 2.1	26.4 ± 3.4*
Urinary free cortisol (μg/24 h)	27.1 ± 3.2	41.8 ± 6.3*

Data are expressed as the mean ± SEM for nine subjects
*$p < 0.05$.

a diet. However, some of the above adaptations to starvation can occur with decreased caloric intake.[32] Therefore, it is not uncommon to observe a 15 per cent decrease in resting energy expenditure with a subsequent slight decrease in the rate of weight loss on a hypocaloric regimen in normal obese women. On the other hand, most "clinical plateaus" in weight loss velocity that are encountered in practice are due to nonadherence to the diet regimen rather than metabolic adjustments to the diet.[33] Second, there are fluctuations in body weight during dieting which are the result of changes in water balance. The drop in insulin levels with dieting results in an acute sodium chloride diuresis in patients on a very low calorie diet (500 to 600 kcal/day). This diuresis is not due to ketonuria but can be accounted for by urinary sodium and chloride excretion.[34] The amount of weight lost during the first week on such a diet will be accelerated due to the loss of body water. Each quart accounts for 2 lb of weight loss. After the first 1 or 2 weeks when this diuresis is completed, the rate of weight loss decreases in most patients on a constant hypocaloric diet. If these patients suddenly increase their calorie intake due to dietary nonadherence, their weight will increase rapidly as water is reaccumulated. It is important to assure such patients that the increase in body weight is due to water, not fat. Third, there are a number of subjects who develop a syndrome of cyclic edema due to increased water intake (psychogenic polydipsia).[35] These patients are usually but not invariably women who combine dieting with excessive water intake. This combination of increased water intake together with diuresis can lead to a washing out of the renal medullary urea gradient. Loss of the urea gradient leads to an inability to excrete free water, resulting in the accumulation of edema. Serum albumin is usually normal, and the cause of the edema is not typically apparent, leading to the diagnosis of idiopathic cyclic edema. Despite the presence of edema, water restriction rather than diuresis is the indicated treatment of this condition. A daily regimen of recording body weight while monitoring fluid intake can be helpful in assessing adherence to a water-restriction regimen. Diuretics worsen the loss of renal medullary urea and can lead to hypokalemia and arrhythmias. Water restriction leads to a gradual reaccumulation of urea in the renal medulla with improvement in edema within 10 days. Through application of an understanding of the complex adaptation to starvation, the endocrinologist can establish management plans for each of these situations.

ADAPTATION TO PROTEIN-ENERGY MALNUTRITION

Observations of epidemics of starvation in third world countries led to the classification and definition of two different pathophysiological syndromes occurring in response to uncomplicated starvation as well as the undernutrition associated with illness. These concepts, while useful as classifications, are oversimplified, and the entire spectrum of protein and energy malnutrition has been observed in malnourished children throughout the world. Infants and children under 5 years of age have the highest energy requirements per unit body weight of any age group. Since their visceral organs account for a good portion of total body weight, energy expenditures between 50 and 100 kcal/kg/day are commonly measured compared with average energy expenditures of 20 to 30 kcal/kg/day in adults.[36] In fact, in epidemics of starvation, children will die first, men second, and women last, since women have the largest fat stores to allow protein sparing in the face of starvation.

Clinical Spectrum

Intrauterine undernutrition, prematurity, failure of lactation, and use of dilute formulas can lead to a wasting syndrome called *marasmus* that usually presents in the first 6 months of life.[37] The infant adapts to undernutrition by decreasing its linear growth rate and thereby decreasing energy requirements. If the condition persists, there is loss of muscle and fat tissue. There are no signs of edema or biochemical abnormalities, and immune function is maintained in this condition.

In many parts of Africa, custom dictates that after 1 year of breast feeding, children are weaned and sent to an adoptive aunt to be fed cassava fruit, a source of carbohydrates but not protein. The Swahili word for "separated from the breast" is *kwashiorkor*, and this name was given to the syndrome observed in children suffering from protein but not calorie deprivation. The condition occurs most frequently after weaning.[38] The major distinguishing features from marasmus are edema and hypoalbuminemia. In addition, a fatty liver, mucous membrane sores, and relative preservation of fat stores occurs. Since it often occurs in response to acute events, linear growth is not as severely retarded.

Growth retardation without any clinical features is the most common presentation of protein-energy malnutrition in children. The GH–IGF-I axis in children is the most sensitive in demonstrating changes due to malnutrition,[39] just as the reproductive hormonal axis is the most sensitive in adult women who develop amenorrhea in response to undernutrition.

Etiology and Pathophysiology

Marasmus is the childhood equivalent of semistarvation, and the hormonal and metabolic adaptations to acute starvation occur as expected. The changes in insulin, GH, and cortisol observed in obese normal individuals subjected to starvation can be seen in these children even before the development of obvious marasmus.[40]

On the other hand, it is not clear why some children develop kwashiorkor in the same nutritional environment while others develop marasmus. Kwashiorkor is more common in areas where protein intake is lower.[41] However, within a particular population it has not been possible to demonstrate that those children developing kwashiorkor indeed had the lowest protein intake.[42] One of the clearest causes of kwashiorkor due to decreased protein intake comes from North American infants fed coffee creamers containing only 1 per cent protein, 30 per cent carbohydrate, and 69 per cent fat calories in place of milk.[43] Rats fed a low protein-to-energy ratio will consume excess calories.[44] This leads to fatty liver and hypoalbuminemia. Lipolysis is thought to occur secondary to sympathetic stimulation combined with relative insulin resistance, while the fatty liver occurs due to the failure of apoprotein B synthesis to export triglycerides synthesized from the influx of fatty acids. Hepatic ketone production is also impaired. It is not uncommon for up to 40 per cent of the liver mass to be fat compared with the usual 5 per cent.

Higher plasma insulin and lower cortisol levels have been found in children with kwashiorkor than in children with marasmus.[40] It has been proposed that the higher insulin levels will direct amino acids toward muscle protein synthesis at the expense of liver protein synthesis. Overall protein synthesis is reduced in perfused rat liver systems when blood from protein-depleted rats is used.[45] Protein synthesis can be restored by adding branched-chain amino acids. While GH levels are usually elevated in kwashiorkor, these elevated levels are associated with reduced growth. In addition, administration of GH in these children will fail to stimulate growth.[46] These phenomena are accounted for by the decreased levels of IGF-I observed in both kwashiorkor and marasmus.

Since kwashiorkor also tends to occur acutely, there may be processes interfering with the adaptation to starvation, resulting in increased loss of muscle and visceral protein. In this way, kwashiorkor may be a model for the malnutrition seen in the adult with infection or traumatic injuries (see below).

ENDOCRINE RESPONSES TO ILLNESS AND UNDERNUTRITION

Illness and undernutrition are closely related in a number of chronic conditions. In fact, anorexia is one of the earliest symptoms of infectious, inflammatory, and neoplastic diseases. In a number of medical and surgical conditions, the hormonal changes associated with the adaptations to starvation described above do not occur. Nutritional assessment is focused on determining the severity of malnutrition, the underlying metabolic adaptations which pertain, and the form of therapy to be utilized. Following surgical or traumatic injury, there is a well-described series of events in which a specific sequence of hormonal changes occurs and must be considered in evaluating nutritional therapy. In the patient with critical illness, a hypermetabolic state caused by the endocrine and immune responses to illness results in a situation where nutritional therapy is recognized to be essential to the survival of the patient. Nutritional therapy can be used to support the malnourished patient, but special modifications are indicated in the metabolic support of patients with renal disease, pulmonary disease, cardiac disease, hepatic insufficiency, critical illness, and multiple organ system failure.

Etiology

Malnutrition in the hospitalized patient can result from decreased intake, increased losses, or increased requirements due to the metabolic effects of injury, sepsis, surgical trauma, or chronic disease. Reduced intake can result from decreased appetite or anorexia. Abnormal tastes, acquired food aversions, and decreased taste may occur in diabetes, renal failure, and cancer, especially following chemotherapy or radiation therapy.[47] Psychosocial disorders, including depression and isolation, can be associated with decreased food intake. When nausea or vomiting is induced as a side effect of any medication, reduced food intake can occur.

Both maldigestion and malabsorption can lead to losses of ingested nutrients.[48] Maldigestion in patients with exocrine pancreatic insufficiency can result from pancreatitis or pancreatic tumors. Malabsorption due to gastrointestinal dysfunction or absence can result from infarction of bowel segments, intestinal pseudo-obstruction due to defects in the neuromuscular functions mediating normal bowel motility, or diseases affecting the absorptive capacity of the gastrointestinal epithelium. Actual loss of nutrients from body stores can occur in so-called protein-losing enteropathies, which can occur in Ménétriere's disease, Crohn's disease, celiac sprue, and Whipple's disease.

Chronic diseases, surgical injury, trauma, and sepsis result in a redistribution of nutrients from reserves in muscle and fat tissue to the liver and bone marrow for host defense, visceral protein synthesis, and thermogenesis.[49–51] These responses interfere with the normal response to undernutrition and thereby make the patient more likely to develop malnutrition in a short period of time. Protein conservation, which is the hallmark of the adaptation to uncomplicated starvation, does not occur. Instead, protein turnover is increased, leading to increased loss of urinary nitrogen and an increase in resting energy expenditure. In fact, rates of hypermetabolism have been found to correlate with increased losses of urinary nitrogen in patients with major burns, sepsis, infection, or surgical trauma. For instance, in patients undergoing elective surgery, urinary nitrogen losses typically are between 7 and 9 g/day, while in patients with sepsis or skeletal trauma, nitrogen losses increase to between 11 and 14 g/day.[52]

Organ failure can result from a combination of factors in the critically ill patient, including regional hypoperfusion and hypoxia, toxic medications, immune responses, endocrine dysfunction, and acute starvation. Metabolic support can play a critical role in the survival of such patients.

Pathophysiology

The metabolic response associated with the stress of surgery or infection or the inflammation associated with the active phases of chronic illnesses, including cancer, differs markedly from the metabolic and hormonal adaptations occurring with uncomplicated starvation. This response can be considered to have evolved to help the previously well-nourished individual survive life-threatening injury or hemorrhage. In addition, the immune system is mobilized to counter any infection that might occur. The presence of an illness or chronic disease essentially provides a stimulus to this response system that is not quickly and easily eradicated. The resulting prolonged stress response can cause nutritional status to deteriorate and represents a particularly hazardous response for the previously malnourished individual with an illness.

The injury/stress response can be divided into two phases[53] (see Fig. 144–6). The ebb phase, which lasts for approximately 24 hours after an injury or insult, is dominated by the hemodynamic response to injury, which includes hypoperfusion, hypometabolism, and cardiac instability. There is a brisk release of hormones during this period, accompanied by a resistance to their action. Following successful resuscitation and restoration of perfusion, the flow phase begins and predominates between 48 and 72 hours after the initial stress. During this phase, metabolic responsiveness to circulating hormones returns, with resulting hypermetabolism, increased glucose production, increased protein breakdown, and lipolysis. In critical illnesses such as sepsis and multiple system organ failure, this phase is prolonged. During this phase, protein loss cannot be reversed despite the administration of apparently adequate nutritional support. During this phase, nutritional support can reduce the net loss of protein, and this is reflected in changes in urinary nitrogen excretion. Only correction of the underlying disease process will halt catabolism in this phase. Nonetheless, the temporizing influence of nutritional support can provide critical maintenance of pulmonary function[54] and gastrointestinal integrity[55] until the therapies directed at the primary disease process can have their intended effects.

The hormones mediating the metabolic changes noted in the ebb and flow phases of the stress response include insulin, glucagon, GH, cortisol, and catecholamines.[56] The secretion of both glucagon and insulin from the pancreas is critically influenced by the balance of alpha- and beta-adrenergic stimulation during the stress response. During the ebb phase, the alpha-adrenergic inhibition of insulin release predominates even in the face of hyperglycemia. Glucose production rises during this phase, resulting in the characteristic hyperglycemia of injury or sepsis. In the flow phase, beta-adrenergic stimulation predominates, with an increase in insulin to normal or higher levels. This phase is characterized by insulin resistance and results in abnormal glucose tolerance. The secretion of glucagon is not affected by alpha-adrenergic effects immediately after injury, but beta-adrenergic stimulation increases glucagon secretion. Therefore, glucagon levels are increased during both phases of the injury response.[57] Inhibition of glucagon but not catecholamines will result in a decrease in endogenous glucose production.[58] The decreased insulin-to-glucagon ratio is consistent with the changes seen in glucose metabolism, but these changes are associated with alterations in the secretion of other hormones as well.

The hypothalamic response to stress results in the release of ACTH, which stimulates adrenal glucocorticoid secretion. This response is stimulated directly by nerves originating in the area of injury or surgical trauma and does not occur with anesthesia of or experimental dener-

vation of the area before injury.[59] Cortisol stimulates hepatic gluconeogenesis and the release of amino acids from muscles via proteolysis. These effects result in a shunting of protein reserves from the periphery to the liver.

While cortisol is permissive of lipolysis, GH stimulates a rise in plasma free fatty acids and lipid oxidation.[60] Following an injury, GH is elevated even in the presence of hyperglycemia. Administration of GH can reverse some of the catabolic effects of glucocorticoids observed in malnourished patients receiving prednisone therapy.[61]

In addition to these hormonal changes, there is an increase in the synthesis of acute phase proteins such as fibrinogen, C-reactive protein, serum amyloid A protein, ceruloplasmin, haptoglobin, alpha$_2$-macroglobulin, alpha$_1$-acid glycoprotein, and certain complement components as well as procoagulants.[62] There is also a prominent leukocytosis with neutrophilia and a redistribution of plasma trace minerals evidenced by a decrease in zinc and iron and an increase in copper secondary to increased ceruloplasmin.[63]

The fever, negative nitrogen balance, increased protein metabolism, and other metabolic changes associated with the injury response are mediated in part through the action of cytokines released into the bloodstream as part of the immune response described. A complete review of all the actions of the cytokines and their interaction is beyond the scope of this chapter but is available in several excellent reviews[64-66] (see also Ch. 157). In brief summary, a number of studies have investigated the actions and interactions of tumor necrosis factor (TNF-α) and interleukin 1 (IL-1) on energy expenditure and intermediary metabolism during the injury/stress response. For instance, TNF-α infusion into animals can increase muscle proteolysis, increase net protein oxidation, increase energy expenditure, and increase hepatic anabolism of secreted and nonsecreted proteins.[67] IL-1β co-infused with TNF-α synergistically potentiates these metabolic shifts.[68] TNF-α has been shown to increase glucose uptake in peripheral tissues and to cause insulin resistance in rats. TNF-α also inhibits the development of lipogenic enzymes in 3T3L1 preadipocytes.[69] However, TNF has no direct effect on human adipocytes in vitro. Interleukins potentially act to affect both lipoprotein lipase and hormone-sensitive lipase. From the preceding work it is clear that cytokines may be involved in the injury/stress metabolic response.

Many components of the injury response have been shown to benefit the host in the presence of infection or inflammation.[70] For instance, fever, reduction of serum iron levels, and acute-phase proteins may help to fight certain infections. A prolonged injury response leading to malnutrition can impair the host immune response to pathogens. For instance, protein-malnourished patients fail to become febrile despite obvious sepsis. The ability of malnourished patients to synthesize leukocyte endogenous mediator (a combination of cytokines isolated from white cells) is impaired but can be restored following intravenous nutritional support. This improvement in immune responsiveness also has been associated with improved survival in these individuals.

The increasing recognition of the importance of cytokines, together with recombinant technology, is leading to advances in the treatment of shock and sepsis. Some approaches to counteracting the negative effects of the injury/stress response on anorexia and nutritional status may be possible through interference with the actions of certain cytokines. On the other hand, the administration of cytokines to malnourished patients with impaired immune responsiveness may improve outcome. As discussed below, there is a close interaction of nutritional therapy with immunity. Overfeeding and the use of certain lipids may impair immune response.[71] It is clear that this is an area where a great deal of additional research must be done to improve the nutritional therapy of the injured, septic, or chronically ill patient.

Clinical Spectrum

Malnutrition in the hospitalized patient and the patient with chronic illness is classified into two major types. First, a kwashiorkor-like malnutrition occurs when sufficient calories are provided but protein is not or when the acute response to stress interferes with the normal adaptation to starvation. These patients have hypoalbuminemia and edema but do not invariably have decreased body weight or wasting. This process can be relatively acute, accounting for the lack of a wasting response, and the replacement of lean tissue with water accounts for the lack of marked weight loss in many patients. Second, a marasmus-like malnutrition or protein-energy malnutrition can occur in which lean tissue and body weight are somewhat decreased, but immune function and albumin secretion are maintained due to the ketoadaptation and energy conservation characteristic of starvation physiology. The imposition of acute stress on preexisting nutrition of either type can lead to a severe form of malnutrition called *combined marasmus-kwashiorkor type malnutrition*.

While global clinical assessment of nutritional status has been shown to be as effective as formal nutritional assessment in discovering malnutrition,[72] the exercise of assessing the patient serves as a device enabling the diet technicians, house officers, and other physicians attending malnourished patients with complex problems to focus on the nutritional needs of patients under their care.

DIAGNOSTIC PROTOCOLS

Nutritional Assessment

A nutritionally oriented history should inquire as to the patient's preillness weight, height, rate of weight loss prior to presentation, nausea, vomiting, anorexia, and specific ingestive, metabolic, or absorptive problems that could impair nutritional status. Based on these assessments, the per cent ideal body weight from standard tables and the per cent usual weight at presentation can be calculated. Body weight changes may be misleading in patients with fluid overload, including those with congestive heart failure, liver disease, and renal failure. In uncomplicated starvation, there is an increase in extracellular fluid volume which tends to maintain weight despite loss of metabolically active tissues.

The sensitivity of nutritional evaluation is enhanced by including certain assessments of the functional indices of the body cell mass, including certain proteins synthesized in the liver[73] and the status of host immune function.[74]

Albumin is the major protein synthesized in the liver and carries out significant functions as a carrier protein and to provide oncotic pressure. Its half-life is approximately 20 days, and it does not reflect recent changes in nutritional status. Transferrin has a half-life of only 8.8 days and so can reflect more recent changes in nutritional status. However, transferrin levels are increased in iron deficiency, reducing the specificity of this measurement for nutritional status. Prealbumin has a half-life of 24 hours and can be used to reflect changes in nutritional status over the short term as patients receive nutritional support to assess response to therapy. Biochemical assessment should include, at a minimum, measurement of albumin. An albumin level of greater than 3.5 g/dl is normal. Albumin levels of 3.0 to 3.5 g/dl indicate significant hypoalbuminemia, while levels below 3.0 g/dl indicate severe albumin deficiency.

Immune function is impaired in malnutrition.[70] The quantitation of absolute lymphocyte counts derived from a complete blood cell count and differential and the assessment of delayed hypersensitivity using skin test antigens are techniques used to assess the impact of nutritional status on immune function. The routinely utilized skin test antigens include tuberculin (as purified protein derivative, or PPD), mumps, streptokinase-streptodornase (SKSD), *Candida albicans*, and *Trichophyton*. These tests were chosen on the basis that most normal individuals are exposed to them and would be expected to have a positive skin test reaction. In uncomplicated starvation or protein-energy malnutrition, skin test reactivity can be restored with renutrition. Anergy is not specific to malnutrition and can be a feature of certain diseases such as Hodgkin's disease, while decreased white blood cell counts can be depressed transiently in the postoperative period and following infection with human immunodeficiency virus. Therefore, these estimations of immunocompetence are not simply specific to malnutrition.

Given the variety of nutritional assessment techniques available, most clinicians will have to select a small group of routinely available tests to use on a regular basis. Most clinical centers will have available skin testing, albumin, and transferrin for routine use. These tests should make it possible to assess whether patients are mildly, moderately, or severely malnourished and whether marasmic, kwashiorkor-like, or combined severe malnutrition is present (Table 144-2).

The status of the lean body mass can be assessed by measuring urinary creatinine excretion over 24 hours. Creatinine production in most individuals is directly related to skeletal muscle mass, provided that no rapid catabolism of muscle is in progress as with severe sepsis or trauma and that large amounts of dietary creatinine found in animal skeletal muscle are not being ingested. A creatinine-height index is calculated based on the measured 24-hour excretion of creatinine and that expected in a normal adult of the same height as the patient. This index has limited sensitivity, with values between 60 and 80 per cent of ideal representing moderate skeletal muscle depletion and 40 to 50 per cent representing severe skeletal muscle depletion.[75] For purposes of estimation, the ideal creatinine excretion for adults is taken as 23 mg/kg/24 hours for males and 18 mg/kg/24 hours for females.[76]

TABLE 144–2. DIAGNOSTIC FEATURES OF ADULT MALNUTRITION

	MARASMUS	KWASHIORKOR
Clinical setting	Decreased caloric intake	Decreased protein intake plus stress
Time course to develop	Months to years	Weeks to months
Physical examination	Cachectic; fat depletion, muscle wasting	May look well nourished
Anthropometrics		
TSF	Depressed	Relatively preserved
AMC	Depressed	Relatively preserved
Weight for height	Depressed	Relatively preserved
Creatinine-height index	Depressed	Relatively preserved
Skin test responses	Normal or depressed	Relatively preserved
Visceral proteins		
Albumin	Relatively normal	Low
Transferrin	Relatively normal	Low
Lymphocyte cell	Relatively normal	Low

Assessment of Risk of Nutritional Depletion

Assessment of risk of nutritional depletion can be used to determine which patients require consideration for nutritional therapy, as described below. The presence of any of the following criteria should motivate the physician to conduct a complete nutritional assessment[77] with consideration of appropriate forms of nutritional therapy: (1) recent involuntary weight loss of greater than 5 per cent in 1 month or over 10 per cent in 6 months, especially when associated with anorexia, fatigue, or weakness, (2) history of recent significant physiological stresses such as organ dysfunction, major surgery, infection, or illness within the last 3 months, (3) absolute lymphocyte count less than 1200 cells/mm³, or (4) serum albumin less than 3.2 g/dl.

Determining Route and Dose of Nutritional Therapy

Nutritional therapy ranges from dietary counseling urging increased voluntary intake of foods and nutritional supplements to forced intake of nutrients via the gastrointestinal tract (enteral nutrition) or via the venous circulation (parenteral nutrition). The therapy of malnutrition is based on meeting the nutritional requirements of the patient for total energy, macronutrients, and micronutrients.

Total energy requirements can be measured using indirect calorimetry or estimated using approximate formulas. For well-nourished normal subjects, the estimated energy expenditure using the Harris-Benedict formula[78] is within 10 per cent of the measured energy expenditure in approximately 90 per cent of all individuals. However, in subjects with a variety of illnesses, hypermetabolism or hypometabolism may occur.[79] For these individuals, measurement of resting energy expenditure using indirect calorimetry is practical and more accurate than estimation methods (Fig. 144–7). In this method, data obtained from the rate of oxygen consumption and carbon dioxide production measured under controlled conditions together with information on urinary nitrogen excretion can be used to assess resting energy expenditure. The patient is placed under a ventilated plastic canopy at rest, and measurements are made for approximately 15 minutes. The equipment required for this measurement is available in most hospital pulmonary function laboratories, and newer portable models for bedside use are also available. Many of these newer pieces of equipment perform all necessary calculations internally to provide information on the energy requirements of patients. The ratio of the volume of carbon dioxide produced to oxygen consumed is defined as the respiratory quotient (RQ). Glucose has an RQ of 1.0, and the oxidation of glucose yields 5.0 kcal/L of oxygen consumed. Fat has an RQ of approximately 0.7, yielding significantly less energy per liter of oxygen consumed. The respiratory quotients and calorie equivalents of different mixtures of carbohydrate and fat per liter of oxygen consumed are shown in Table 144–2. These values are the nonprotein RQ values used to assess energy expenditure once an adjustment has been made for protein oxidation based on an estimate of the amounts of energy liberated (26.51 kcal/g of nitrogen), oxygen consumed (5.91 L/g of nitrogen), and carbon dioxide produced (4.76 L/g of nitrogen) by the metabolism of protein (Table 144–3). The daily excretion of urinary nitrogen is converted to the rate of nitrogen excretion per hour and is used to calculate resting energy expenditure, as shown in the example adapted from Cantarow and Trumper[80] in Table 144–4.

Once resting energy expenditure (REE) has been measured or basal energy expenditure (BEE) estimated using the Harris-Benedict equation, the total caloric require-

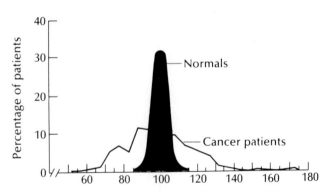

FIGURE 144–7. The distribution of measured resting energy expenditure in "normals" and in cancer patients. (From Knox L, Crosby L, Feurer I, et al: Energy expenditure in malnourished cancer patients. Ann Surg 197:152–162, 1983.)

TABLE 144–3. RESPIRATORY QUOTIENT FOR METABOLISM OF FUEL MIXTURES

RQ*	PERCENTAGE OF TOTAL O_2 CONSUMED BY:		PERCENTAGE OF HEAT PRODUCED BY:		CALORIES PER LITER O_2
	Carbohydrate	Fat	Carbohydrate	Fat	
0.707	0	100	0	100	4.686
0.75	14.7	85.3	15.6	84.4	4.739
0.80	31.7	68.3	33.4	66.6	4.801
0.82	38.6	61.4	40.3	59.7	4.825
0.85	48.8	51.2	50.7	49.3	4.862
0.90	65.8	34.2	67.5	32.5	4.924
0.95	82.9	17.1	84.0	16.0	4.985
1.00	100	0	100	0	5.047

*Nonprotein RQ

From Cantarow A, Trumper M: Clinical Biochemistry. Philadelphia, WB Saunders Co, 1955, p 367.

ments of subjects can be estimated. In general, these estimates range from 1.2 to 2.0 times the measured or estimated values based on observations of patients undergoing treatment for a variety of medical and surgical conditions. In moderately catabolic surgical patients, enteral nutrition has been found to lead to positive nitrogen balance at approximately 1.5 times the BEE, while in parenteral nutrition, 1.75 to 2.0 times the BEE is required.[81] Utilization of estimates of 1.75 times the BEE as a standard practice for all patients receiving parenteral nutritional therapy regardless of metabolic needs has led to overnutrition with resulting complications in certain disease states, as described below.[82]

Evaluation of Response to Nutritional Support

Since the goal of nutritional support is the attainment of an anabolic state or reduction of nitrogen losses, assess-

TABLE 144–4. ENERGY EXPENDITURE DETERMINATION BY INDIRECT CALORIMETRY AND ESTIMATION

EXAMPLE CALCULATION

The calculation of energy expenditure using indirect calorimetry is illustrated by the following example adapted from Cantarow and Trumper. These data were obtained from a patient under basal conditions: (1) urinary nitrogen, 0.18 g/h, (2) oxygen consumption, 12.2 L/h, and (3) carbon dioxide production, 9.2 L/h.

0.18 g of urinary N represents:
0.18 × 5.91 = 1.06 L oxygen
0.18 × 4.76 = 0.85 L carbon dioxide
0.18 × 26.51 = 4.77 kcal

Nonprotein oxygen consumption = 12.2 − 1.06 = 11.14 L
Nonprotein carbon dioxide production = 9.2 − 0.85 = 8.35 L
Nonprotein RQ = 0.75, representing the liberation of 4.739 kcal/L of oxygen
Nonprotein energy expenditure = 4.739 × 11.14 = 52.79 kcal/h
Total energy expenditure = 52.79 + 4.77 = 57.56 kcal/h
For men: RME (kcal/day) = 66.4730 + 13.7516(W) + 5.0033(H) − 6.7750(A)
For women: RME (kcal/day) = 655.095 + 9.563(W) + 1.8496(H) − 4.6756(A)
  where W = present weight in kilograms, H = height in centimeters, and A = age in years

ment of nitrogen balance is the most useful clinical assessment to determine whether nutritional therapy is effective. *Nitrogen balance* is defined as the difference between nitrogen intake and nitrogen excretion. Nitrogen intake is taken as the protein intake determined from dietary records divided by 6.25 g nitrogen per gram of "average" protein ingested. Nitrogen excretion is taken as the urinary nitrogen excreted per 24 hours plus a fixed estimate of 4.0 g/24 hours for unmeasured nitrogen losses from cellular sloughing into the feces (1 g), losses from the skin (0.2 g), and nonurea nitrogen losses in the urine (2 g).[83] Since nitrogen balance is most usefully applied in a serial fashion in the same patient, the particular constants used to estimate unmeasured excretion are only important for comparison of published results.

At any given level of nitrogen intake, nitrogen balance improves with increased administration of nonprotein calories to a maximum achieved at a ratio of 150:1 of nonprotein calories per gram of nitrogen.[84] Proteins vary in their biological value based on the mixture of essential and nonessential amino acids which they contain. Albumin has the ideal mixture of amino acids for optimal utilization of protein and is assigned a biological value of 100. Casein is close to albumin in its biological quality, followed by meat proteins such as those found in steak or tuna, which have a biological value of 80. Corn and beans, each with biological values of 40 or less, can be combined in a protein mixture with a biological value of 80 because the amino acid patterns of the two proteins are complementary. The protein requirement for normal individuals is 0.55 g/kg protein for a high-biological-value protein such as milk or albumin but 0.8 g/kg for the mixture of proteins found in the average United States diet.[85]

SPECIAL THERAPEUTIC PROBLEMS

Complications

Complications can occur following either enteral or parenteral nutrition. Complications of enteral nutrition are either mechanical or metabolic, while complications of parenteral nutrition can be mechanical, infectious, or metabolic.[86]

Mechanical problems of enteral feeding include aspiration, especially in semiconscious patients or patients with abnormalities of swallowing. This problem can be minimized by proper feeding tube placement and determination of the residual gastric contents eight hours after feeding to eliminate the possibility of gastric outlet obstruction or gastric atony. If these latter problems occur, the feeding tube can be placed into the jejunum. Proper placement should be ensured radiologically to avoid misplacement of the feeding tube. Irritation of the oropharynx and the gastric mucosa can occur, especially with the use of larger-bore and less flexible feeding tubes. This problem can be minimized by using inert silicone rubber and polyurethane tubes.

Diarrhea is the most common complication associated with tube feeding.[87] Carefully increasing the rate of administration will help avoid this problem. Most enteral formulations are lactose-free, so lactose intolerance is not likely to cause diarrhea. Nonetheless, prolonged starvation can lead to gastrointestinal epithelial atrophy and maldigestion, which, in turn, could result in diarrhea. Diarrhea also can be due to the effects of other medications, colonic infections (e.g., *Clostridium difficile*), or overly rapid administration of hypertonic enteral formulations. Dehydration with hypernatremia also can be a problem in infants and the elderly, in whom inadequate fluid intake can occur during the administration of a hypertonic enteral formula. Glucosuria can occur in patients without a prior history of diabetes when high-carbohydrate enteral formulas are used.

The complications of parenteral nutrition are in many cases more serious than those associated with enteral nutrition.[88] Pneumothorax and subclavian vein thrombosis are the most common catheter-related complications. Pneumothorax should occur in only about 1 to 2 per cent of catheter insertions, but this rate is higher when transthoracic puncture is used rather than open surgical placement of catheters or when less experienced individuals insert the catheters.[89] Radiological confirmation of proper placement and to exclude the presence of pneumothorax is essential. Pneumothorax usually will resolve spontaneously, but a chest tube may be required in some cases. Thrombosis of the catheter in the central veins has been reported in 5 to 10 per cent of patients receiving parenteral nutrition, especially when hypercoagulable states are present, as in sepsis, inflammatory bowel disease, pancreatitis, or cancer.[90] Heparin is given daily in prophylactic doses of 6000 units routinely, but when thrombosis occurs, the catheter must be removed. Peripheral venous nutrition is used while a full course of heparin or other treatment is undertaken to treat thrombosis. Infections most commonly occur from skin contaminants such as gram-positive organisms but can include fungi and unusual bacteria, especially if acquired during hospitalization. Infected catheters must be removed prior to the systemic treatment of catheter-related sepsis. In patients committed to lifelong parenteral nutrition, this decision is made carefully, since only eight external sites are available for central vein catheter placement.

There are a variety of metabolic complications that can occur during parenteral nutrition. The most common is overfeeding, which results in respiratory quotients of greater than 1.0. This results in excessive carbon dioxide production, which can complicate the care of patients with chronic lung disease.[91] Hyperglycemia can occur in many patients due to transient insulin resistance or relative insulin deficiency. Both subcutaneous insulin and insulin added to the parenteral solutions can be used to treat this complication.[92] Metabolic acidosis, which occurred commonly when potassium and sodium were administered only as chloride salts, is less frequently a problem since the use of acetate buffers in parenteral solutions. Abnormalities of phosphate, potassium, calcium, and magnesium can occur due to excessive or inadequate administration in the presence of underlying disorders such as renal failure or gastrointestinal fistulas that predispose to electrolyte abnormalities.[93, 94] Deficiencies of trace minerals such as zinc, copper, and chromium rarely occur, since these are now added routinely to parenteral solutions.[95] Azotemia can occur in renal failure patients or with excessive administration of amino acids relative to nonprotein calories given and is treated simply by reducing the amino acid load administered.[96] Essential fatty acid deficiency rarely occurs since the use of intravenous lipid emulsions has become so common.[97] In most cases, the metabolic complications associated with parenteral nutrition respond to fluid and electrolyte management with careful monitoring of input and output on a daily basis.

SPECIAL CLINICAL PRESENTATIONS/PROBLEMS

Multiple Organ Failure Syndrome

Multiple organ failure syndrome can develop in the critically ill patient secondary to a decline in cellular oxygen consumption, leakage of intracellular enzymes, and cell death.[98] A cascade of events leads to these terminal events, including at different times hypoperfusion/hypoxia, toxic mediator action, immunodysfunction, endocrine dysfunction, acute starvation, and metabolic derangement. Early organ failure usually appears from 5 to 7 days after the initial insult but can occur as late as 21 days after the initial injury.

The nutritional therapy provided to such patients has been called *metabolic support* to differentiate it from the nutritional support given to more stable patients with chronic anorexia and starvation. In nutritional support, the goals are simply to provide adequate calories and nutrients to restore nutritional deficiencies and to maintain protein synthesis, positive nitrogen balance, and lean body mass.[99] Metabolic support of the critically ill patient at risk of multiple organ failure syndrome is directed at partial caloric replacement, sustenance of important cellular and organ metabolism, and the avoidance of overfeeding and the metabolic costs of overfeeding, including lipogenesis, gluconeogenesis, and thermogenesis related to inefficient metabolism.

Excessive infusion rates and the choice of the wrong mixture of macronutrients can be harmful in the critically ill patient. One of the most common problems encountered in intravenous nutrition is hepatomegaly resulting from increased hepatic lipogenesis. This occurs when glucose is used as the sole energy source or is given at greater than the endogenous production rate of 3 g/kg/day. Cholestasis also can result from these changes. Replacement of glucose with long-chain triglycerides (LCT's) derived from soybean or safflower oil has been shown to reduce fatty infiltration of the liver. These LCT's are associated with problems related to poor clearance by the reticuloendothelial system leading to hypertriglyceridemia and possible adult respiratory distress syndrome and increased production of 2- and 4-series prostaglandins and leukotrienes which can enhance vasoconstriction, platelet aggregation, immunosuppression, inhibition of monokine responses, and free radical formation.[100]

The use of medium-chain triglycerides (MCT's) can avoid some of these problems, at least in experimental systems.[101] MCT oils do not require acylcarnitine transferase action for transport into mitochondria and are metabolized to ketone bodies readily. They contain no essential fatty acids and so should not be used alone. There are research efforts to combine the effects of LCT's and MCT's in structured lipids where the triglyceride contains both types of fatty acids. Additional structured lipids containing n-3 fatty acids or so-called fish oils are also being studied actively.[102]

A breakdown in the physical barrier and immunological defense function of the gastrointestinal tract can promote multiple organ failure syndrome. The gastrointestinal tract is particularly susceptible to ischemic and reperfusion injury. Glutamine, a preferred fuel in the gut epithelium, may promote gastrointestinal tract epithelial healing after an injury.[103] In animal studies, an enteral formula containing glutamine has been shown to improve gastrointestinal epithelial mucosal integrity and nitrogen balance.[104] Research is under way on the incorporation of these physiological properties of specific nutrients into therapeutic regimens to prevent multiple organ failure syndrome. However, the crucial difference between the multiple organ failure syndrome and chronic malnutrition is recognized in the need to avoid overfeeding by providing a hypocaloric protein-sparing nutritional regimen.

Specific Patient Groups

Patients with gastrointestinal fistulas often evidence fluid and electrolyte abnormalities, sepsis, and malnutrition. Retrospective analyses suggest that nutritional therapy is beneficial in promoting the closure of these fistulas.[105] It has been noted that 90 per cent of fistulas destined to close did so within 1 month of the control of sepsis. Prior to the advent of total parenteral nutrition, intensive enteral nutrition resulted in a favorable effect on mortality and a rate of closure comparable with that later observed following parenteral nutrition. While fistula output is more effectively managed with parenteral than enteral nutrition, enteral feedings may be as effective in very proximal or very distal fistulas. Moreover, with chronic low-output fistulas, even oral feeding may be tolerated. In any case, surgery is indicated for those fistulas not closing within 40 days after nutritional support is initiated. Crohn's disease, radiation enteritis, residual tumor, distal intestinal obstruction, epithelialization of a short fistulous tract (less than 2 cm from bowel to skin), and complete interruption of the gastrointestinal tract make it unlikely that healing will occur. In these instances, early surgical repair should be undertaken.

Short bowel syndrome results when greater than 75 per cent of the small intestine is absent secondary to extensive disease or massive resection.[106] This syndrome can occur secondary to trauma, infarction, severe Crohn's disease, radiation enteritis, and cancer. Loss of the ileum is more significant than loss of jejunum, since ileal loss leads to decreased enterohepatic circulation of bile salts. This results in entry of bile salts into the colon with resulting diarrhea and decreased absorption of vitamin B_{12}. Compensatory growth occurs in the small intestine following resection, with epithelial hyperplasia.[107] The intensity of epithelial hyperplasia is related directly to the length of intestine resected. The stimuli promoting this response are poorly understood but may include food, enteric secretions, and hormones. Immediately following the initial injury, diarrhea, fluid, and electrolyte disorders are controlled together with provision of parenteral nutrition. After several weeks, fecal output may fall to less than 2 L/day, at which point a trial of enteral feeding may be attempted using a predigested diet which is low in long-chain triglycerides (elemental diet). As the small bowel adapts, carbohydrates and protein are provided, with fat

limited to less than 30 g/day utilizing medium-chain triglycerides. After 6 months to 2 years, complete oral nutrition is possible in many patients. Dietary supplements of calcium and fat-soluble vitamins are prescribed for these patients even after gastrointestinal adaptation, since steatorrhea often persists with malabsorption of fat-soluble vitamins and precipitation of calcium in soaps.

Patients with chronic renal failure can be given nutrition during hemodialysis with improved nitrogen retention. During acute renal failure, electrolyte and fluid abnormalities as well as azotemia occur commonly and require appropriate alterations of the parenteral nutrition regimen.[108] Patients with cardiac disease often require fluid and sodium restriction and may benefit from diuretic administration so that protein and calorie requirements can be met.[109]

Diabetic patients developing hyperglycemia either can be given insulin as described or can be provided with an increased percentage of calories as fat to reduce insulin requirements.[110]

Patients with hepatic insufficiency have abnormal amino acid profiles with increased concentrations of aromatic amino acids and decreased levels of branched-chain amino acids.[111] Decreased plasma levels of branched-chain amino acids are thought to lead to increased central nervous system levels of aromatic amino acids, since these two classes of amino acids compete for uptake at the blood-brain barrier. Increased levels of aromatic amino acids interfere with catecholamine metabolism, resulting in shunting of tyrosine to produce octopamine, a false neurotransmitter. Excess serotonin is thought to develop from increased levels of tryptophan. The combination of decreased catecholamines, false neurotransmitters, and increased serotonin levels is proposed to lead to hepatic coma. Specialized formulas have been used to treat patients with hepatic encephalopathy. Some improvements in neurologic function with administration of specially formulated enteral supplements are noted in patients with chronic hepatic failure. However, in acute hepatic insufficiency, these formulas provided by the parenteral route have not proven beneficial when compared with ordinary parenteral formulations.

THERAPEUTIC PROTOCOLS

Enteral and Parenteral Nutrition

Once malnutrition has been diagnosed and classified as mild, moderate, or severe marasmic, kwashiorkor, or combined protein-energy malnutrition, the choice of the route of administration of nutritional therapy depends on the functional status of the gastrointestinal tract, the methods available for provision of nutritional support, and a working understanding of the various nutritional products and types of equipment used for parenteral and enteral nutritional support.

As a general rule, the enteral feeding route should be used whenever the gastrointestinal tract is functional.[88] Enteral feeding results in higher rates of visceral protein synthesis than similar nutrients provided parenterally. Enteral feeding results in a physiological release of gut peptides, including insulinotropic peptides which enhance anabolism. In addition, provision of nutrients in the gastrointestinal lumen has been shown in animal studies to maintain the barrier function of the gut to translocation of endotoxin and gram-negative bacteria.[112]

Prior to initiation of enteral feeding, every attempt should be made to utilize voluntary feeding techniques. Changes in meal frequency and size, use of flavorings, preparation of favorite foods in the patient's home, consideration of nutrition in the scheduling of diagnostic and therapeutic procedures, and the use of nutritional supplements between meals, should be considered.

Consideration should be given as to whether the patient's primary illness is best treated by putting the bowel to rest. For example, patients with gastrointestinal fistulas often require avoidance of enteral feeding.

The gastrointestinal tract must be truly functional. The stomach must be capable of delivering the nutritional mixture to the small intestine, and then digestion and absorption must proceed normally. If there is functional gastric obstruction due to a problem with gastric emptying, diabetic gastropathy, or prior surgery, then a tube can be placed directly into the jejunum.

When the gastrointestinal tract is not functional and there are clear therapeutic goals, parenteral nutrition should be used. There are a number of accepted indications for parenteral nutrition, including short bowel syndrome, when there is inadequate small bowel surface area for digestion and absorption of nutrients even after adaptation. The ability of this therapy to maintain life under these circumstances is established. The role of parenteral nutrition has been under careful scrutiny in view of the expense and potential side effects of this form of nutritional therapy.[113] While not therapeutic in terms of the conditions themselves, a useful role of parenteral nutrition has been defined in subgroups of patients with pancreatitis, gastrointestinal fistulas, and inflammatory bowel disease.

In some situations, transitional feeding is utilized in which parenteral and enteral nutrition are combined. For example, parenteral nutrition can be used in burn and head trauma patients when the gastrointestinal tract is functional but the total caloric requirement cannot be met by the enteral route.

Prognosis

While it is simple to demonstrate the impact of renutrition on the patient with uncomplicated starvation or an inability to absorb calories due to a loss of intestinal tissue, it is much more difficult to demonstrate the beneficial effects of nutrition in patients with a number of chronic illnesses, including common forms of cancer. Often the course of the underlying illness will mask the beneficial effects of nutritional therapy. In patients with mild disease or elective surgery, malnutrition is relatively well tolerated from a clinical point of view. In such cases, nutritional rehabilitation usually occurs without special efforts as the self-limited underlying medical or surgical condition runs its course. In patients with severe disease, the patient's nutrition is often relegated to the secondary list of problems as the progress of the primary illness dictates therapeutic decisions. In both these instances, nutritional therapy may play a beneficial role in either preventing or retarding malnutrition in individual patients. The benefits of nutritional support have been well-documented in selected reviews.[114] On the other hand, an extensive meta-analysis of 51 published studies of parenteral and enteral nutrition interventions[115] indicated that survival was improved in 6 studies, the same in 43 studies, and worse in 2 studies.

For a number of indications, the use of total parenteral nutrition (TPN) is controversial.[113] While many cancer and AIDS patients benefit from renutrition, the routine use of TPN in all cancer patients receiving chemotherapy or in all AIDS patients regardless of nutritional status is not appropriate. In some patients receiving chemotherapy or radiation therapy, mucosal inflammation, nausea, and vomiting impair normal intake. In such patients, TPN may be needed as an adjunct to restore the patient's functional status in order to continue therapy or undertake radiation therapy, chemotherapy, or surgical therapy.

The use of nutrition support in many instances is not supported by clinical trial data. However, a judgment must be made by the physician as to the severity of the effects of malnutrition and whether nutrition can reverse these effects to affect the overall prognosis of the patient. There are many instances where nutrition has become a routine part of patient care prior to a careful evaluation of its real benefit. It remains a challenge for nutrition researchers to define the benefits of nutrition support and to determine its best application in clinical practice.

REFERENCES

1. Cahill GF: Starvation in man. N Engl J Med 282:668–675, 1970.
2. Jelliffe DB: The Assessment of the Nutritional Status of the Community (Monograph Series 53). Geneva, World Health Organization, 1966.
3. Bistrian BR, Blackburn GL, Vitale J, et al: Prevalence of malnutrition in general medical patients. JAMA 235:1567–1570, 1976.
4. Wan JM, Han M, Blackburn GL: Nutrition, immune function, and inflammation: An overview. Proc Nutr Soc 48:315–335, 1989.
5. Blackburn GL, Wan JM, Teo TC, et al: Metabolic support of organ failure. In Bihari DJ, Cerra FB (eds): New Horizons: Multiple Organ Failure. Fullerton, CA, Society of Critical Care Medicine, 1989, pp 337–370.
6. Owen OE, Morgan AP, Kemp HG, et al: Brain metabolism during fasting. J Clin Invest 48:574–583, 1969.
7. Owen OE, Felig P, Morgan AP, et al: Liver and kidney metabolism during prolonged starvation. J Clin Invest 48:574–583, 1969.
8. Owen OE, Reichard GA: Human forearm metabolism during progressive starvation. J Clin Invest 50:1536–1545, 1971.
9. Bistrian BR, Blackburn GL, Hallowell E, Heddle R: Protein status of general surgical patients. JAMA 230:858–860, 1974.
10. Chandra RK: Nutrition, immunity, and infection: Present knowledge and future directions. Lancet 1:688–691, 1983.
11. Marliss EB, Aoki TT, Unger RH, et al: Glucagon levels and metabolic effects in fasting man. J Clin Invest 49:2256–2270, 1970.
12. Owen OE, Reichard GA, Kinney JM, et al: Metabolism during catabolic states of starvation, diabetes, and trauma in humans. In Bleicher SJ, Brodoff BN (eds): Diabetes Mellitus and Obesity. Baltimore, Williams & Wilkins, 1982, pp 172–184.
13. Waterlow JC: Protein turnover with special reference to man. Q J Exp Physiol 169:409–438, 1984.
14. Felig P, Owen OE, Wahren J, Cahill GF: Amino acid metabolism during prolonged starvation. J Clin Invest 48:584–594, 1969.
15. Cersosimo E, Williams PE, Radosevich PM, et al: Role of glutamine in adaptations in nitrogen metabolism during fasting. Am J Physiol 250:E622–628, 1986.
16. Mortimore GE, Poso AR: Lysosomal pathways in hepatic protein

degradation: Regulatory role of amino acids. Fed Proc 434:1289–1294, 1984.

17. Fukagawa NK, Minaker DL, Rowe JW, et al: Insulin-mediated reduction of whole body protein breakdown: Dose-response effects on leucine metabolism in postabsorptive men. J Clin Invest 76:2306–2311, 1985.

18. Nair KS, Halliday D, Matthews DE, Welle SL: Hyperglucagonemia during insulin deficiency accelerates protein catabolism. Diabetes 36(Suppl. II):74A, 1987.

19. Flakoll PJ, Brown LL, Frexes-Steed M, Abumrad NN: Use of amino acid clamps to investigate the role of insulin in regulating protein breakdown in vivo. J Parent Ent Nutr 15:81S–85S, 1991.

20. Young VR: Energy metabolism and requirements in the cancer patient. Cancer Res 37:2336–2347, 1977.

21. Arner P, Engfeldt P, Nowak J: In vivo observations on the lipolytic effect of noradrenaline during therapeutic fasting. J Clin Endocrinol Metab 53:1207–1212, 1981.

22. Jensen MD, Haymond MW, Gerich JE, et al: Lipolysis during fasting. J Clin Invest 79:207–213, 1987.

23. Unger RH: Insulin-glucagon relationship in the defense against hypoglycemia. Diabetes 32:575–583, 1983.

24. Flier JS, Cook KS, Usher P, Spiegelman BM: Severely impaired adipsin expression in genetic and acquired obesity. Science 237:405–408, 1987.

25. Froesch ER, Schmid C, Schwander J, Zapf J: Actions of insulin-like growth factor. Annu Rev Physiol 47:443–467, 1985.

26. Phillips LS: Nutrition, somatomedins, and the brain. Metabolism 35:78–87, 1986.

27. Bray GA: The Obese Patient. Philadelphia, WB Saunders Co, 1976, p 141.

28. Chopra IJ, Huang TS, Beredo A, et al: Evidence for an inhibitor of extrathyroidal conversion of thyroxine to 3,5,3'-triiodothyronine in sera of patients with non-thyroidal illnesses. J Clin Endocrinol Metab 60:666–672, 1985.

29. Spencer CA, Lum SM, Wilber JF, et al: Dynamics of serum thyrotropin and thyroid hormone changes in fasting. J Clin Endocrinol Metab 56:883–888, 1983.

30. Henson LC, Poole DC, Donahoe CP, Heber D: Effects of exercise training on resting energy expenditure during caloric restriction. Am J Clin Nutr 46:893–899, 1987.

31. Henson LC, Heber D: Whole body protein breakdown rates and hormonal adaptation during fasting in obese subjects. J Clin Endocrinol Metab 57:316–319, 1984.

32. Garrow JS: Energy Balance and Obesity in Man. Amsterdam, North Holland Publishing Co, 1974.

33. Brownell K, Marlatt GA, Lichtenstein E: Understanding and preventing relapse. Am Psychol 41:765–778, 1986.

34. Spark RF, Arky RA, Boulter PR, et al: Renin, aldosterone and glucagon in the natriuresis of fasting. N Engl J Med 292:1335–1340, 1975.

35. Streeten DHP, Luis LH, Conn JW: Secondary aldosteronism in idiopathic edema. Trans Assoc Am Physicians 73:227–239, 1960.

36. Golden BE, Golden MHN: Protein deficiency, energy deficiency, and the edema of malnutrition. Lancet 1:1261–1265, 1982.

37. Barltrop D, Sandhu BK: Marasmus, 1985. Postgrad Med J 61:915–923, 1985.

38. Frenk S: Protein-energy malnutrition. In Arneil GC, Metcoff J (eds): Pediatric Nutrition. London, Butterworth, 1985, pp 151–193.

39. Hintz RL, Suskind R, Amatayakul K, et al: Plasma somatomedin and growth hormone values in children with protein-energy malnutrition. J Pediatr 92:153–156, 1978.

40. Whitehead RG, Coward WA, Lunn PG, Rutishauser I: A comparison of the pathogenesis of protein-energy malnutrition in Uganda and Gambia. Trans R Soc Trop Med Hyg 71:189–195, 1977.

41. Truswell AS: Protein vs energy in protein energy malnutrition. S Afr Med J 59:753–756, 1981.

42. Gopalan C: Kwashiorkor and marasmus: Evolution and distinguishing features. In McCance RA, Widowson EM (eds): Calorie Deficiencies and Protein Deficiencies. London, Churchill Livingstone, 1968, pp 49–58.

43. Sinatra FR, Merritt RJ: Iatrogenic kwashiorkor in infants. Am J Dis Child 135:21–23, 1981.

44. Kirsch RE, Saunders SJ, Frith L, et al: Plasma amino acid concentration and the regulation of albumin synthesis. Am J Clin Nutr 22:1559–1562, 1969.

45. Lumn PG, Whitehead RG, Baker BA: The relative effects of a low-protein high-carbohydrate diet on free amino acid composition of liver and muscle. Br J Nutr 36:219–230, 1976.

46. Hadden DR, Rutishauer IHE: Effect of human growth hormone in kwashiorkor and marasmus. Arch Dis Child 42:29–33, 1967.

47. Schiffman SS: Taste and smell in disease. N Engl J Med 308:1275–1277, 1983.

48. Baron RB: Malnutrition in hospitalized patients: Diagnosis and treatment. West J Med 144:63–67, 1986.

49. Birkhan RH, Long CL, Fitkin D, et al: Effects of major skeletal trauma on whole body protein turnover in man measured by 14C-leucine. Surgery 88:294–299, 1980.

50. Long CL, Jeevanandam M, Kim BM, Kinney JM: Whole body protein synthesis and catabolism in septic man. Am J Clin Nutr 30:1340–1344, 1977.

51. Bistrian BR, Schwartz J, Istfan NW: Cytokines, muscle proteolysis, and the catabolic response to infection and inflammation. Proc Soc Exp Biol Med 200:220–223, 1992.

52. Blackburn GL, Bistrian BR, Maini BS: Nutritional and metabolic support of the hospitalized patient. J Parenter Enter Nutr 1:11, 1977.

53. Cuthbertson DP, Tilstone WJ: Metabolism during the post-injury period. Adv Clin Chem 12:1–4, 1969.

54. Bassili HR, Dietel M: Effects of nutritional support on weaning patients off of mechanical ventilators. J Parenter Enter Nutr 5:161–163, 1981.

55. Alverdy J, Chi HS, Sheldon G: The effect of parenteral nutrition on gastrointestinal immunity: The importance of enteral stimulation. Ann Surg 202:681–684, 1985.

56. Alberti KGMM, Batstone GF, Foster KJ, Johnston DG: Relative roles of various hormones on mediating the metabolic response to injury. J Parenter Enter Nutr 4:141–145, 1980.

57. Nair KS, Halliday D, Matthews DE, Welle SL: Hyperglucagonemia during insulin deficiency accelerates protein catabolism. Diabetes 36(Suppl 1):74A, 1987.

58. Matthews DE, Pesola G, Campbell RG: Effect of epinephrine on amino acid and energy metabolism in humans. Am J Physiol 258(Endo Metab 21):E948–E956, 1990.

59. Hjortso NC, Christensen NJ, Andersen T, Kehlet H: Effects of the extradural administration of local anesthetic agents and morphine on the urinary excretion of cortisol, catecholamines, and nitrogen following elective surgery. Br J Anesth 57:400–406, 1985.

60. Ziegler TR, Young LS, Manson JM, Wilmore DW: Metabolic effects of recombinant human growth hormone in patients receiving parenteral nutrition. Ann Surg 208:6–16, 1988.

61. Horber FF, Haymond MW: Human growth hormone prevents the protein catabolic side effects of prednisone in humans. J Clin Invest 86:265–272, 1990.

62. Dinarello CA: Interleukin 1 and the pathogenesis of the acute phase response. N Engl J Med 311:1413–1418, 1984.

63. Kushner I: The phenomenon of the acute phase response. Ann NY Acad Sci 389:39–48, 1982.

64. Old LJ: Polypeptide mediator network. Nature 326:330–331, 1987.

65. Nathan CF: Secretory products of macrophages. J Clin Invest 79:319–326, 1987.

66. Dinarello CA: Interleukin 1. Rev Infect Dis 6:51–95, 1984.

67. Flores EA, Bistrian BR, Pomposelli JJ, et al: Infusion of tumor necrosis factor/cachectin promotes muscle catabolism in the rat. J Clin Invest 83:1614–1622, 1989.

68. Tredgett EE, Yong MY, Zhong S: Role of interleukin 1 and tumor necrosis factor on energy metabolism in rabbits. Am J Physiol 255:E760–768, 1988.

69. Beutler B, Cerami A: Cachectin: More than a tumor necrosis factor. N Engl J Med 316:379–385, 1987.

70. Chandra RK: Nutrition, immunity and infection: Present knowledge and future directions. Lancet 1:688–691, 1983.

71. Hammaway KJ, Moldawer LL, Georgieff M: The effect of lipid emulsions on reticuloendothelial system function in the injured animal. J Parenter Enter Nutr 9:559–565, 1985.

72. Jeejeebhoy KN: Muscle function and malnutrition. Gut 27(Suppl. 1):25–39, 1986.

73. Shetty PS, Watrasiewicz KE, Jung RT, James WPT: Rapid-turnover proteins: An index of subclinical protein-energy malnutrition. Lancet 2:230–232, 1979.

74. Kahan BD: Nutrition and host defense mechanisms. Surg Clin North Am 61:557–570, 1981.

75. Bistrian BR, Blackburn GL, Hallowell E, Heddle R: Protein status of general surgical patients. JAMA 230:858–870, 1974.

76. Bistrian BR, Blackburn GL, Shermann M: Therapeutic index of nutritional depletion in hospitalized patients. Surg Gynecol Obstet 141:512–518, 1975.

77. Irving M: ABC of nutrition: Enteral and parenteral nutrition. Br Med J 291:1404–1408, 1985.

78. Harris JA, Benedict FG: Biometric Studies of Basal Metabolism in Man. Washington, Carnegie Institute Publication 279, 1919.

79. Knox L, Crosby L, Feurer I, et al: Energy expenditure in malnourished cancer patients. Ann Surg 197:152–162, 1983.

80. Cantarow A, Trumper M: Clinical Biochemistry. Philadelphia, WB Saunders Co, 1955, p 367.

81. Ang SD, Leskiw MJ, Stein TP: The effect of increasing total parenteral nutrition on protein metabolism. J Parenter Enter Nutr 7:525–529, 1983.

82. Askanazi J, Rosenbaum SH, Hyman AI: Respiratory changes induced by the large glucose loads of total parenteral nutrition. JAMA 243:1444–1447, 1980.

83. Sirba E: Effect of reduced protein intake on nitrogen loss from the human integument. Am J Clin Nutr 20:1158–1161, 1978.

84. Calloway D, Spector H: Nitrogen balance as related to caloric and protein intake in active young men. Am J Clin Nutr 2:405–412, 1954.

85. Recommended Dietary Allowances (ed 10). Washington, National Academy Press, 1989.

86. Bethel RA, Jansen RD, Heymsfield SB, et al: Nasogastric hyperalimentation through a polyethylene catheter: An alternative to central venous hyperalimentation. Am J Clin Nutr 32:1112–1120, 1979.

87. Voit KAJ, Echave V, Brown RA, Gund FN: Use of elemental diet during the adaptive stage of short gut syndrome. Gastroenterology 65:419–426, 1973.

88. Heymsfield SB, Bethel RA, Ansley JD, et al: Enteral hyperalimentation: An alternative to central venous hyperalimentation. Ann Intern Med 90:63–71, 1979.

89. Feliciano DV, Mattox KL, Graham JM: Major complications of percutaneous subclavian catheters. Am J Surg 138:869–874, 1979.

90. Ryan A, Abel M, Abbot WM: Catheter complications in total parenteral nutrition. N Engl J Med 290:757–761, 1974.

91. Covelli HD, Black JW, Olsen MS, Beekman JF: Respiratory failure precipitated by high carbohydrate loads. Ann Intern Med 95:579–581, 1981.

92. Ryan JA: Complications of total parenteral nutrition. In Fischer JE (ed): Total Parenteral Nutrition. Boston, Little, Brown, 1976, pp 55–100.

93. Ruberg R, Allen T, Goodman M: Hypophosphatemia with hypophosphaturia in hyperalimentation. Surg Forum 22:87–88, 1971.

94. Fleming CR, McGill DB, Hoffman HN, Nelson RA: Total parenteral nutrition. Mayo Clin Proc 51:187–189, 1976.

95. Fleming CR, Hodges RE, Hurley LS: A prospective study of serum copper and zinc levels in patients receiving total parenteral nutrition. Am J Clin Nutr 29:70–77, 1976.

96. Chen WJ, Ohashi E, Kasai M: Amino acid metabolism in parenteral nutrition: With special reference to the calorie/nitrogen ratio and the blood urea nitrogen level. Metabolism 23:1117–1123, 1974.

97. Goodgame JT, Lowry SF, Brennan MF: Essential fatty acid deficiency in total parenteral nutrition: Time course of development and suggestions for therapy. Surgery 84:271–277, 1978.

98. Blackburn GL, Wan JMF, Teo TC, et al: Metabolic support in organ failure. In Bihari DJ, Cerra FB (eds): New Horizons—Multiple Organ Failure, Fullerton, CA, Society of Critical Care Medicine, 1989, pp 337–370.

99. Cerra FB: Hypermetabolism, organ failure, and metabolic support. Surgery 101:1–14, 1987.

100. Kinsella JE, Lokesh B, Broughton S, Whelan J: Dietary polyunsaturated fatty acids and eicosanoids: Potential effects on modulation of inflammatory and immune cells: An overview. Nutrition 6:24–44, 1990.

101. Holman RT: Nutritional and metabolic interrelationships between fatty acids. Fed Proc 23:1062–1067, 1964.

102. DeMichele SJ, Karlstad MD, Bistrian BR, et al: Enteral nutrition with structured lipid: Effect on protein metabolism in thermal injury. Am J Clin Nutr 50:1295–1302, 1989.

103. Windmueller HG: Glutamine utilization by the small intestine. Adv Enzymol 53:210, 1982.

104. Fox AD, Kripke SA, DePaula JA: Glutamine supplemented diets prolong survival and decrease mortality in experimental enterocolitis. J Parenter Enter Nutr 12(Suppl. 1):8S, 1988.

105. Thomas RJS: The response of patients with fistulas of the gastrointestinal tract to parenteral nutrition. Surg Gynecol Obstet 153:77–80, 1981.

106. Weser E, Fletcher JT, Urban E: Short bowel syndrome. Gastroenterology 77:575–579, 1979.

107. Williamson RCN: Intestinal adaptation. N Engl J Med 298:1393–1402, 1444–1450, 1978.

108. Blumenkrantz MJ, Kopple JD, Koffler A: Total parenteral nutrition in the management of acute renal failure. Am J Clin Nutr 31:1830–1840, 1978.

109. Heymsfield SB, Bethel RA, Ansley JD: Cardiac abnormalities in cachectic patients before and during nutritional repletion. Am Heart J 95:584–594, 1978.

110. Fischer JE: Nutritional support in the seriously ill patient. Curr Prob Surg 17:466–532, 1980.

111. Fischer JE, Bower RH: Nutritional support in liver disease. Surg Clin North Am 61:653–660, 1981.

112. Peck MD, Alexander JW, Gonce SJ: Low-protein diets improve survival from peritonitis in guinea pigs. Ann Surg 209:448–454, 1989.

113. Pillar B, Perry S: Evaluating total parenteral nutrition: Final report and statement of the technology assessment and practice guidelines forum. Nutrition 6:313–317, 1990.

114. Meguid MM, Mughal MM, Meguid V, Terry JJ: Risk-benefit analysis of malnutrition and perioperative nutritional support: A review. Nutr Int 3:25–34, 1987.

115. Koretz RL: What supports nutritional support? Dig Dis Sci 29:577–588, 1984.

Anorexia Nervosa

MICHELLE P. WARREN

The syndrome of anorexia nervosa was first described in the nineteenth century by William Gull.[1] Presumably an old disease, it has received considerable attention in the scientific literature in recent years because the symptom complex that occurs with this syndrome combines medical, endocrine, and psychological manifestations, which appear to be reversible with weight gain. The combination of findings suggests a unique endocrine abnormality that is probably hypothalamic in origin and represents an adaptation to the starvation state.

INCIDENCE

Anorexia nervosa is a syndrome generally seen in young white women under age 25 and is particularly common in adolescence. The person with this condition presents with a classic triad: amenorrhea, weight loss, and behavioral changes. This group of symptoms usually occurs together, although any one group of symptoms may precede another.[2, 2a] The new criteria for the diagnosis of anorexia nervosa in the *Diagnostic and Statistical Manual of Mental Disorders* (DSM-IV) is shown in Table 145–1.[2b] This new definition contains bulimic subgroups. Although the overall incidence of anorexia nervosa is 0.24[3] to 1.6[4] per 100,000 people, the incidence differs greatly in different

TABLE 145–1. PROVISIONAL DIAGNOSTIC CRITERIA: ANOREXIA NERVOSA

A. Refusal to maintain body weight over a minimal normal weight for age and height, e.g., weight loss leading to maintenance of body weight 15 per cent below that expected; or failure to make expected weight gain during period of growth, leading to body weight 15 per cent below that expected.

B. Intense fear of gaining weight or becoming fat, even though underweight.

C. Disturbance in the way in which one's body weight, size, or shape is experienced. (The person claims to "feel fat" even when emaciated, believes that one area of the body is "too fat" even when obviously underweight.) *Denial of the seriousness of current low body weight or undue influence of body shape and weight on self-evaluation.*

D. In females, absence of at least three consecutive menstrual cycles when otherwise expected to occur (primary or secondary amenorrhea). (A woman is considered to have amenorrhea if her periods occur only following hormone, e.g., estrogen, administration.)

Bulimic subtype. During the episode of anorexia nervosa, the person engages in recurrent episodes of binge eating.

Nonbulimic subtype. During the episode of anorexia nervosa, the person does not engage in recurrent episodes of binge eating.

From Wilson GT, Walsh BT: Eating disorders in the DSM-IV. J Abnorm Psychol 100(3):362–365, 1991.

population groups.[5] Recent work reveals that an at-risk population appears to exist. This syndrome occurs in 1 of every 100 middle-class adolescent girls,[6] and professional ballet dancers have an incidence ranging from 1 in 20[7] to 1 in 5,[8] depending on the competitive level of the company from which the survey originated. The striking incidence of this disorder may relate to the rigid standards for thinness as well as the significantly greater number of hours of exercise,[8] particularly in the highly competitive ballet companies. These environmental factors may be fertile ground for the development of anorexia nervosa. Interestingly, animal studies suggest that increased levels of activity and restricted eating can induce self-starvation in rats, indicating an animal model for an activity-based anorexia.[9] Recent work also indicates that some ethnic groups have a much lower incidence of the syndrome of anorexia nervosa; for instance, it is very rare among blacks, including black ballet dancers, who are exposed to the same rigid standards of competition and weight restriction.[8] The low incidence of this problem among blacks may relate to different socio-cultural influences or, conceivably, this group may possess more efficient metabolic mechanisms for dealing with the high activity level and lowered caloric intake. Some recent reports are appearing on the disorder in blacks, but it is generally thought to be rare.[10] It is interesting in this regard that studies on monozygous twins have suggested a genetic factor in the emergence of the syndrome. The risk for female siblings is 6 per cent,[11] suggesting that inborn metabolic factors may be contributing to the syndrome. Anorexia is seen in association with Turner's syndrome,[12] diabetes mellitus,[13, 14] and Cushing's disease.[15] Although rare in men (female:male ratio is 9:1),[16] the syndrome has been reported in men who are training for competitive activity while restricting their weight.[17] Recent data indicate that the incidence of this syndrome is definitely increasing.[18]

Bulimia, although more common in slightly older age groups, is also generally a condition of young women and often related to previous anorectic behavior. In this syndrome, individuals gorge themselves and use artificial means to purge themselves of calories. The DSM-IIIR[18a] estimates that the rate of anorexia in girls between the ages of 12 and 18 ranges from 1 in every 800 to 1 in every 100 girls. Thus between 15,000 and 120,000 adolescent girls are expected to be anorectic at some time during adolescence. Four and a half per cent of girls and young women under age 20 will be bulimic, with other source[18b] estimating that at least 20 per cent of girls in this age range will exhibit bulimic behaviors. These include vomiting and laxative or diuretic abuse. Gorging episodes may alternate with periods of severe food restriction. This syndrome occurs in high school and college students (incidence varies from 2 per cent in community-based samples to 4 to 13 per cent in college-age groups)[19–21] and may be more common than anorexia nervosa in males. In addition, others have described a separate condition known as bulimia nervosa,[22, 23] in which the bulimic behavior evolves from the completely restricting anorexia nervosa–type pattern. Bulimics have a wide variety of medical problems that may be superimposed on the anorectic syndrome. These include severe tooth decay, parotid enlargement, stomach rupture, metabolic alkalosis, carpal pedal spasm, hypercarotenemia,[24–27] and pancreatitis.[24–28]

CLINICAL SYNDROME OF ANOREXIA NERVOSA

The syndrome of anorexia nervosa has fascinated reproductive endocrinologists because it represents a prototype of hypothalamic amenorrhea, and the reproductive abnormalities are potentially reversible with weight gain. The reproductive and physiological adjustments, which appear to be an adaptive phenomenon appropriate for the semistarved state, have been the subject of intense study by endocrinologists interested in the neuroendocrine signals that initiate and maintain normal reproductive cyclicity. The amenorrhea, weight loss, and psychiatric disturbance appear to occur together, and generally recovery parallels the weight gain. Unfortunately, there is no blood test or specific physical findings that enable one to make the diagnosis of anorexia nervosa. Thus the clinician makes the diagnosis based on a symptom complex[29] that includes severe weight loss (usually down to less than 80 per cent of ideal body weight), behavioral changes such as hyperactivity and preoccupation with food, and perceptual changes—in particular a distorted view of the body, generally with an unreasonable concern about being "too fat." The physical and metabolic adaptation to a self-induced semistarved state is thought to induce these diverse physical changes. Common signs and symptoms are listed in Table 145–1. The amenorrhea may occur at any time during the syndrome and may even precede it, but it often can be related to the onset of the food restriction, even if weight loss has been slight. If weight loss occurs prior to menarche, the patient may present with primary amenorrhea. The familiar syndrome, which ensues with the onset of the weight loss, is accompanied by findings shown in Table 145–2. In addition, hyperactivity is commonly seen, and the syndrome may begin in the guise of an athletic pursuit. There may be preoccupation with food, intense interest in low-calorie foods and diet sodas, large intakes of lettuce and other raw vegetables, and avoidance of fried foods and other products high in calories. Hypercarotenemia has been reported in anorexia nervosa, and elevated levels of carotenes in the blood give a yellow cast to the skin. This is only in part due to an increased intake of raw vegetables. Recent investigations have suggested that a metabolic deficit that occurs in the setting of dieting prevents the normal metabolism of carotene, a precursor of vitamin A.[30] This yellow substance is deposited in the subcutaneous layer of the skin and is seen in hypothalamic amenorrhea

TABLE 145–2. LABORATORY FINDINGS IN ANOREXIA NERVOSA

Chemical

Normal results on most laboratory tests early in process
Elevated BUN levels, secondary to dehydration
Hypercarotenemia
Elevated serum cholesterol levels (early; may decrease later)
Decreased transferrin (usually normal protein and albumin-globulin ratio); low complement, fibrinogen, and prealbumin
Elevated serum lactic dehydrogenase and alkaline phosphatase (possibly related to growth)
Depressed phosphorus level (a late and ominous sign); depressed magnesium and calcium levels (calcium may be elevated)
Possible depression of plasma zinc, urinary zinc, and urinary copper levels

Endocrine

Low luteinizing hormone (LH); low or pseudo-normal follicle-stimulating hormone (FSH); deficiency of gonadotropin-releasing hormone (GnRH); normal prolactin; low testosterone in men and low estradiol in women
Elevated circulating cortisol (normal production; does not suppress with dexamethasone)
Low normal fasting glucose (increased insulin binding by red blood cells and growth hormone deficiency reported)
Low normal thyroxine (T_4); reduced triiodothyronine (T_3); elevated reverse T_3; normal TSH
Possible elevation of parathyroid hormone (PTH) secondary to hypomagnesemia with resultant hypercalcemia
Elevated resting growth hormone levels

Hematologic

Leukopenia with relative lymphocytoses (bone marrow hypoplasia), absolute lymphopenia
Thrombocytopenia
Very low erythrocyte sedimentation rate, almost always
Anemia late (especially with rehydration)

From Comerci GD: Medical complications of anorexia nervosa and bulimia nervosa. Med Clin North Am 74(5):1293–1310, 1990.

related to dieting. The yellowish hue can be seen in the palms and soles, but the sclerae remain clear. One study suggests that limiting intake of foods high in vitamin A and thus lowering carotene levels may reverse the amenorrhea.[31]

Other clinical laboratory findings include a leukopenia with a relative lymphocytosis and electrocardiographic changes with an extreme bradycardia, low voltage, and low and inverted T waves. Interestingly, although pitting edema may occur, especially with refeeding, hypoalbuminemia is rare. Chemistry profiles may reflect dehydration, with elevated blood urea nitrogen (BUN) and a return to normal after rehydration. Common values are summarized in Table 145–2.

Numerous medical problems also have been reported in this syndrome, including salivary gland enlargement,[32] cardiac arrhythmias,[33] pericardial effusion,[34] pancreatitis,[35–37] pancreatic insufficiency,[38–40] liver dysfunction,[39] pneumomediastinum,[40, 41] kidney stones,[42] trace metal deficiencies, including hypoproteinemia and zinc deficiency,[43] thiamine deficiency,[44] coagulopathies,[32, 45] electrolyte imbalance,[46, 47] hypophosphatemia,[48] bilateral peroneal nerve palsies, and acrocyanosis.[49] Marked vasoconstriction of the extremities also may occur as a heat-conserving mechanism,[50] and if the weight loss occurs at or before the growth spurt, permanent growth deficiencies may occur.[51] Interestingly, although there is a marked leukopenia, increased risk of infection has not been documented, and cell-mediated immunity appears intact.[52–54] Ulcers may occur with anorexia,[55] as well as acute vascular compression of the duo-

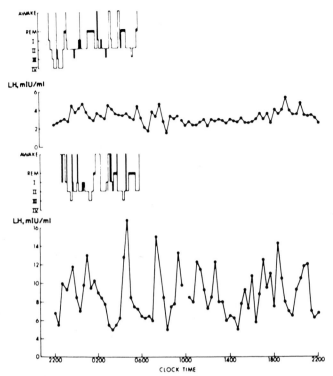

FIGURE 145–1. Plasma LH concentration every 20 min for 24 h during acute exacerbation of anorexia nervosa *(top)* and after clinical remission with a return of body weight to normal *(bottom)*. The latter represents a normal adult pattern. (Reprinted with permission from Boyar RN, Katz J, Finkelstein JW, et al: Anorexia nervosa: Immaturity of the 24-hour luteinizing hormone secretory pattern. N Engl J Med 291:861–865, 1974.)

denum and the superior mesenteric artery syndrome,[56–58] so that it is unwise to dismiss complaints of abdominal pain without detailed history and appropriate workup. Abnormal secretion of gastrointestinal peptides has been noted, including an increase in pancreatic polypeptide, decreased gastrin, and increased cholecystokinin. The latter is thought to be involved in a signal for satiety, and the earlier and greater risk of this peptide may perpetuate the

disorder.[59] Pancreatic function may be abnormal, and basal insulin levels are low. Insulin sensitivity has been reported.[60, 61] Hypoglycemia has been associated with coma and low or absent insulin and C-peptide levels, suggesting that this problem is due to malnutrition.[62] Osteoporosis and fractures are also being reported, problems that most likely have multiple causes and are the result of long-term poor nutritional intake as well as prolonged estrogen deficiency.[63–65] Altered adrenoceper activity may account for other physiological changes seen in anorexia, such as platelet hyperaggregatability.[66]

ENDOCRINOPATHY

The endocrine changes associated with anorexia nervosa have been studied in depth in the setting of anorexia nervosa, and only the endocrine profiles in particular provide strong evidence for hypothalamic dysfunction. Low levels of plasma luteinizing hormone (LH) and follicle-stimulating hormone (FSH) are accompanied by a profound estrogen deficiency.[2, 16] The hypogonadotropism can be accompanied by a low thyroxine (T_4) and a high plasma cortisol level, which differentiates anorexia nervosa from pituitary insufficiency.[2] In addition to the low levels of LH, there is a lack of the normal episodic variation of LH secretion and, in some cases, a reversion to a prepubertal low pattern of secretion over a 24-h period.[67] Nocturnal spurting of LH is also seen in adults, a pattern usually observed only in early puberty[67] (Fig. 145–1). A reversion to the normal adult-like pattern occurs with recovery (weight gain). Artificially, the pattern of gonadotropin secretion can be made to revert to a normal adult-like secretion by the pulsatile administration of gonadotropin-releasing hormone (GnRH). If this drug is given intravenously or subcutaneously every 2 h, a normal adult-like pattern of gonadotropin secretion results, and menstrual bleeding and ovulation can be induced[68] (Fig. 145–2). Recent research indicates that neurons containing GnRH are situated in the arcuate nucleus of the hypothalamus, and axons de-

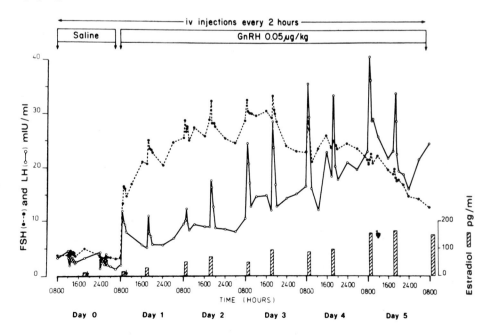

FIGURE 145–2. Plasma FSH (closed circles), LH (open circles), and estradiol responses to GnRH (0.05 μg/kg) every 2 hours in patient 1. The arrow indicates values below the sensitivity of the estradiol assay. (From Marshall JC, Kelch RP: Low dose pulsatile gonadotropin-releasing hormone in anorexia nervosa: A model of human pubertal development. J Clin Endocrinol Metab 49:712–718, copyright by the Endocrine Society, 1986.)

scend into the median eminence, where they terminate. From this vascular area a message is sent from the nerve terminals via the hypophyseal portal vein to pituitary gonadotrophs situated in the anterior pituitary.[69] These findings suggest that the amenorrhea seen in anorexia nervosa is probably due to faulty signals reaching the medial central hypothalamus from the arcuate nucleus, the center most likely responsible for the important episodic stimulation of GnRH.

Also of interest is the fact that the response of the pituitary to GnRH is reduced by a factor that is directly correlated with the weight loss.[69] In addition, the pattern of response to GnRH is immature, resembling that seen in prepubertal children; the FSH response is much greater than the LH response.[71] With weight gain, the normal ratios develop, with the LH response being much greater than that of FSH.[69] This adult-like response also can be induced artificially with the episodic administration of GnRH.[68] The return of normal levels and of normal LH/FSH ratios with repeated injections of GnRH suggests that the pituitary gonadotrophs have become sluggish owing to the lack of endogenous stimulation with LHRH and that the episodic stimulation may be important in determining the relative amounts of LH and FSH secreted. Recent evidence indicates that this is in fact the case.[72] Moreover, patients who are partially recovered from anorexia nervosa tend to have exaggerated responses to GnRH.[70, 73, 74] These changes have been seen in children in early puberty, suggesting that the hypothalamic signals of the central nervous system (CNS) revert to a prepubertal or pubertal state. Physiological experiments with opioid inhibitors such as naltrexone have shown variable effect on LH pulsatility, suggesting that the suppression of LH secretion seen with undernutrition is not consistently opioid-linked.[75–77] One study showed that naltrexone caused a further decrease in LH level.[77] Dopamine receptor blockade in the form of metoclopramide can increase LH pulsatility in hypothalamic amenorrhea but has not been specifically studied in anorexia.[78] The defect of neurotransmission which underlies the dysfunction of the GnRH pulse generator with the amenorrhea of anorexia nervosa is unclear.

It is well recognized that weight loss and food restriction can affect the normal menstrual cycle. Menstrual irregularities occur frequently in this setting, particularly if weight falls below 90 per cent of ideal, but appear to be generally reversible on return to a normal nutrition status. The fundamental physiological insult appears to be to the GnRH pulse generator; this is reflected in a decreased number and/or decreased amplitude of both LH and to some extent FSH pulses. Occasionally, signs of ovarian dysfunction are present prior to detectable changes in gonadotropin secretion.[2a, 79, 80]

Menstrual irregularities may involve a clinical spectrum ranging from a prolongation of the follicular phase or a shortening of the luteal phase to prolonged amenorrhea.[80, 81] Simple weight loss and diet-associated weight loss cause a menstrual dysfunction and amenorrhea which are qualitatively similar to the amenorrheic syndrome seen in anorexia nervosa but are less pronounced.[2a, 70, 82–85] Amenorrhea may be the presenting symptom, but a history of weight loss may not be volunteered. LH secretion is lowered, and there may be a reversal to a 24-hour pubertal secretory pattern, with sleep-entrained nocturnal spurting. The LH/FSH ratio is generally decreased, while pro-

lactin levels are normal.[70, 77, 80, 81] A history of a recent diet and amount of weight loss are important adjuncts to the history. Response to GnRH is extremely variable, but estrogen levels are generally low. Patients occasionally may become anovulatory with a positive response to a progesterone challenge, a good prognostic sign. Pituitary disease should be ruled out as part of the workup for this syndrome. The condition usually reverses with weight gain, but amenorrhea may persist for prolonged periods, even after gain of weight to near normal levels.[2a, 80, 81]

Dieting with weight loss can produce a variety of other changes in normal women, including a reduction in estradiol levels and anovulation and luteal phase defects in the face of apparently normal LH concentrations and LH pulse frequency[80, 81] (24-hour circadian studies, however, have not been reported). Changes in circulating LH also have been reported during the process of weight recovery in underweight infertile women.[86] These changes also have been seen with experimental starvation.[87]

Qualitative changes in the type of diet also may affect reproductive function. A vegetarian diet, for example, is associated with a higher than expected incidence of reproductive disorders and anovulation[88]; depressed LH and estrogen levels have been documented. A high-fiber vegetarian diet may affect estrogen levels by increasing fecal estrogen excretion in a bulky stool and preventing a normal enterohepatic circulation.[89] In general, however, these syndromes have not been well studied.

Minor menstrual irregularities with prolonged follicular phases, anovulation, and luteal phase deficiencies also may occur in women of normal weight but with high "restrained eating" scores. These women do not exhibit psychological features of women with eating disorders, but when tested with standardized scales, they exhibit high scores reflecting dieting behavior.[90]

Bulimia, although more common in slightly older age groups than anorexia nervosa, is also generally a condition seen in young women and often related to previous anorectic behavior. In fact, the new DSM-IV criteria for the diagnosis of anorexia recognize two subgroups: with and without bulimia.[2b] With bulimia, individuals gorge themselves and then use artificial means to purge calories; these include vomiting and laxative or diuretic abuse. Gorging episodes may alternate with periods of severe food restriction. The bulimic's weight may fluctuate but usually not to dangerously low levels. There is often a history of other impulsive behaviors, such as alcohol or drug use (some features of this disorder are not unlike those seen with drug addiction), stealing and shoplifting, as well as unrestrained promiscuity. This is unlike the restrictive anorectic, who remains generally asexual. A separate condition known as *bulimia nervosa* has been described in which the bulimic behavior evolves from the completely restricting anorexia nervosa type of pattern.

Bulimics often have medical problems and may or may not have menstrual irregularities.[2a] When present, menstrual irregularities often are accompanied by adequate estrogen secretion and anovulation.[2a] The menstrual disorder and amenorrhea may develop even when the weight remains normal. Bulimic behavior is often secretive, and patients will not admit to these patterns even when questioned directly. Thus the problem may be difficult to pinpoint. The behavior is often chronic, and increased anxiety, irritability, depression, and poor social functioning are common.[23, 91] Weight may remain within a reasonable range, but protein-calorie malnutrition must usually supervene and most likely contributes to the development of the reproductive disorder.

Bulimia may have an organic cause, and the association of neurological abnormalities and bulimia raises the intriguing possibility of underlying neuroendocrine dysfunction as a cause of both the nutritional and the menstrual disorder. Hypothalamic diseases may be associated with excess appetite and lack of satiety inhibition.[92, 93]

THE HYPOTHALAMIC SYNDROME

In addition to the reproductive changes, a number of other abnormalities in anorexia nervosa have been described that suggest hypothalamic dysfunction.[16, 74, 94, 95] These observations include the following: a deficiency in the handling of a water load, thought to result from a mild diabetes insipidus; abnormal thermoregulatory responses with exposure to temperature extremes; and lack of shivering. These abnormalities are all controlled by mechanisms that most likely involve hypothalamic pathways, as shown in Table 145–3. These alterations probably represent a syndrome too diffuse to be anything but "metabolic" and may be largely due to starvation. The lowered triiodothyronine (T_3) levels and, in some cases, the low T_4 levels that have been reported probably also represent a metabolic adaptation to starvation.[96]

Despite their marked cachexia, patients with anorexia nervosa have clinical and metabolic signs suggestive of hypothyroidism. These include constipation, cold intolerance, bradycardia, hypotension, dry skin, prolonged ankle reflexes, low basal metabolic rates, and hypercarotenemia.[16, 96, 97] The metabolism of certain steroids such as testosterone is analogous to that seen in hypothyroidism.[98] Some of these changes do suggest a compensatory hypometabolism, and studies on the circulatory system show that during maximal exercise, the attainable oxygen uptake and heart rate are low in children with anorexia nervosa. The $\dot{V}O_2$ max (maximal aerobic power) appears to be decreased out of proportion to the circulatory and body dimensions, indicating an adaptation to the low caloric intake.[99]

Serum levels of T_4 and T_3 in patients with anorexia nervosa are significantly lower than in normal individuals. In anorexia nervosa, as in starvation, the peripheral deiodi-

native conversion of T_4 is diverted from formation of the active T_3 to the production of reverse T_3, an inactive metabolite.[100] Evidence also indicates that fasting decreases hepatic uptake of T_4, with a proportionate decrease in T_3 production.[101] The low T_4 value is somewhat more difficult to explain. Low T_4 euthyroidism has been seen in seriously ill patients.[102, 103] Some studies indicate that in ill patients there is a unique dysfunctional state with abnormal T_4 binding with a normal free T_4 availability to peripheral tissue sites, but tissue hypothyroidism has not been excluded. Presumably, similar mechanisms may be operative in anorexia nervosa. Interestingly, the so-called low-triiodothyronine syndrome may mask hyperthyroidism, although this complication is rare.[104] Secretion of thyroid-stimulating hormone (TSH), however, appears to be normal, but the peak TSH response to thyroid-releasing hormone (TRH) stimulation is delayed from 30 to 60 to 120 minutes[105] and is also augmented.[106] This may reflect an altered setpoint for endogenous TRH regulation and is also characteristic of hypothalamic hypothyroidism. Another study shows subnormal response of T_4 and T_3 to TRH with a normal TSH response, suggesting chronic understimulation of thyroid, and also suggesting hypothalamic hypothyroidism.[107]

Mean levels of cortisol are elevated, and random sampling may suggest an absence or even a reversal in the normal circadian rhythm. The 24-h studies have shown that both the episodic and the circadian rhythms are normal but that the levels are considerably higher[113] (Fig. 145–3). This change, which also has been seen in malnutrition, is due to a prolonged half-life of the cortisol resulting from reduced metabolic clearance. As could be expected, the levels of the urinary steroids, including the 17-hydroxysteroids and the 17-ketosteroids, are usually low.[16] Other studies have suggested that the production rates may be elevated.[114] Recent studies indicate that suppression with dexamethasone is incomplete,[115] and the cortisol concentrations may exceed the binding capacity of cortisol-binding globulin (CBG). There appears also to be a decreased affinity of CBG for cortisol. Thus unbound cortisol may be

TABLE 145–3. ABNORMALITIES SUGGESTIVE OF HYPOTHALAMIC DYSFUNCTION IN ANOREXIA NERVOSA

ABNORMALITY	AREA OF DYSFUNCTION
Amenorrhea	
Gonadotropin release and control	Medial central
Thermoregulatory control	Anterior
	Posterior
Water conservation	Supraoptic
	Paraventricular
Behavioral	Ventromedial
Altered food intake	
Activity	

Reproduced with permission from Warren MP: Anorexia nervosa. *In* Speroff L (ed): Gynecology and Obstetrics, Reproductive Endocrinology, Infertility and Genetics, vol V. Hagerstown, MD, Harper & Row, 1981, pp 1–99.

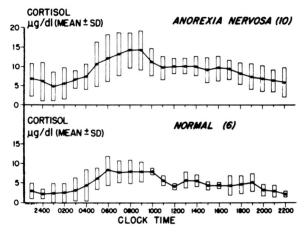

FIGURE 145–3. Hourly mean cortisol level (derived from average of the sample 20 minutes before, on, and after the hour) in 10 patients with anorexia nervosa, as compared with 6 normal controls matched for age and sex. Circadian rhythm remains intact in anorexia nervosa but at a higher level. (Reprinted with permission from Boyar RN, Hellman LD, Roffwarg H, et al: Cortisol secretion and metabolism in anorexia nervosa. N Engl J Med 296:190, 1977.)

significantly increased and more available to the tissues in patients with anorexia nervosa. One would expect the higher levels of cortisol measured in these patients to suppress ACTH. The observation of a retained circadian rhythm at higher cortisol levels suggests that a new setpoint has been determined by the hypothalamic-pituitary-adrenal axis. Recent work on the hypothalamic-pituitary-adrenal pathways suggests activation of this axis. Cortisol is elevated, and responses to CRH (corticotropin-releasing hormone) are abnormal. CRH is increased in the cerebrospinal fluid of patients with anorexia.[107–109, 113] CRH is known to suppress LH pulses in both humans and animals and may augment dopaminergic and opiodergic inhibition of GnRH.[110–112]

Other parameters of pituitary-hypothalamic function have been studied. Growth hormone levels are known to be elevated in starvation or any situation with restriction of food beyond the normal 12- to 15-hour "overnight" fast. In general, basal growth hormone levels are significantly higher than normal in anorexia nervosa but respond normally to provocative stimuli. Insulin-like growth factor is suppressed, and both these abnormalities resolve with nutritional therapy.[116] Nutritional deprivation may alter the GH-IGF axis by down-regulation of GH receptor or postreceptor.[117] Occasionally, low levels are seen, with blunted responses to insulin hypoglycemia.[16] The growth hormone levels associated with δ-wave sleep are normal.[94] The basal prolactin level is indistinguishable from normal. TRH-stimulated prolactin levels are also normal, although the time of the peak prolactin response is delayed.[94] With recovery (weight gain), the described endocrine abnormalities revert to normal.

Despite the return of normal gonadotropin secretory patterns,[72, 118] amenorrhea may persist in almost 30 per cent of patients with anorexia nervosa.[16, 119, 120] Thus other mechanisms, yet to be elucidated, are at fault. Of interest also are the low estradiol levels, which are partially due to lack of ovarian stimulation, but estrogen metabolism appears to be altered. With weight loss, the metabolism of estradiol via 16-α-hydroxylation is decreased in favor of 2-hydroxylation and the formation of catechol estrogen (2-hydroxyestrone).[121] This compound has features of an antiestrogen in that it has no intrinsic biological activity.[122] Thus the extraordinarily low estrogen levels seen in this syndrome are compounded by the presence of an endogenously produced antiestrogen, and in addition, the lack of fat tissue may deny the patient extraovarian sources of estrogen (fat being a site of estrone conversion from androstenedione).

The altered behavior patterns in this syndrome are also distinctive and include preoccupation with food and hyperactivity. Sometimes periods of gorging (bulimia) alternate with starvation and food avoidance. Altered food intake combined with change in activity has been seen in patients with hypothalamic tumors[123, 124] and other hypothalamic syndromes[125] and has been documented in rats with lesions of the ventromedial nucleus of the hypothalamus.[126] These lesions have led investigators to conclude that the ventromedial nucleus can inhibit food intake and promote activity, as seen in anorexia nervosa.

The unique combination of symptoms seen in anorexia nervosa is summarized in Table 145–4 and suggests a diffuse metabolic hypothalamic lesion. The hormonal and metabolic changes suggest a generalized adaptive state reflected in the hypothalamic changes. The hypometabolism

TABLE 145–4. PHYSICAL SYMPTOMS AND SIGNS IN ANOREXIA NERVOSA

Presenting Physical Symptoms
Weight loss
Amenorrhea, no cyclic symptoms or physical changes or menstruation (anovulatory)
Hyperactivity (mental and motor)
Aberrant behavior, irritability, isolation or withdrawal, sleep disturbances
Hyperacusis or optic hyperesthesia
Physical Signs
Cachexia, emaciation, debilitation or dehydration, possible signs of shock or impending shock
Covert infectious processes (pneumonia or sepsis; immunologic problems [late], anergy-negative skin tests)
Skin changes (dryness, yellowish palms and soles, desquamation, and "dirty" appearance to skin)
Scalp and pubic hair loss or lanugo hair or increased pigmented body hair
Hypothermia (rectal temperature below 96.6°F)
Bradypnea (respiratory compensation for alkalosis)
Bradycardia, "quiet" heart (decreased basal metabolic rate); pulse below 60 bpm usual
Hypotension often below 80/50 mm Hg
Heart murmur (infrequent)
Edema of lower extremities
Signs of estrogen deficiency (skin dryness; osteoporosis; small uterus and cervix; vaginal mucosa is pink, dry; and gross and microscopic evidence of deficient estrogen)
Signs of decreased androgen (no acne, no oily skin)

of anorexia nervosa has been studied recently and will reverse with refeeding. There is a decrease in resting energy expenditure and thermic response to food.[127, 128] This hypometabolism appears to be an appropriate mechanism to conserve energy.

The metabolic changes—including lowered metabolic rate, decrease in attainable oxygen uptake and maximal aerobic power ($\dot{V}O_2$ max), increase in cortisol (which stimulates gluconeogenesis and decreases peripheral glucose utilization), and decrease in gonadotropins (with a loss of fertility)—are all appropriate adaptations to starvation.[16, 129]

The association of psychological and neuroendocrine changes in patients with anorexia nervosa has led investigators to speculate that abnormalities of neurotransmission may be involved in the pathogenesis of the syndrome.[130] Excessive dopamine and norepinephrine in particular have well-documented effects on behavior and appetite,[131] and β-endorphin also has effects on feeding behavior.[132, 133] It is interesting in this regard that β-endorphin is thought to modulate secretion of GnRH from the hypothalamus.[134–136] It is most likely at this level that the episodic secretion of GnRH is altered in anorexia nervosa.

Osteoporosis

Amenorrhea in adolescence and young adulthood appears to have permanent effects on bone density, since a rapid increase in bone density occurs at puberty[137–148] and a delay related to retarded sexual development[149, 150] and further increase occur after age 20.[138–143, 147, 148, 151] This suggests that peak bone mass must be achieved before age 20 or a permanent deficiency may occur.

A leading complication of amenorrhea seen with anorexia and weight loss is the loss of bone mineral content and bone density[137, 218, 219, 221] present in spinal, radial, and femoral sites[152–156] and fractures.[152–155] Longitudinal studies on bone density show little[157, 158] or no[153] reversal with resolution of the amenorrhea. These observations are important because hypoestrogenism in young adulthood may predispose to premature osteoporosis in later life. Recent studies also suggest that increases in bone mass may occur in young individuals prior to return of normal menses but despite these increases still remain below normal controls, possibly due to prolonged hypoestrogenism in adolescence, and thus may have permanent effects on peak bone mass.[159] The effects of estrogen replacement on these changes need to be studied to determine if the trend toward lowered bone mass can be reversed by therapy.

Reduced bone mineral density associated with unusual and frequent fractures has been reported recently in women with anorexia nervosa.[152–155] Both cortical and trabecular bones are reduced in this syndrome, as reflected in studies of spinal, radial, and femoral bone density.[152–156] A number of factors appear to predict low bone mass, including the low caloric and calcium intake, low body weight, early onset and long duration of amenorrhea, reduced physical activity, and hypercortisolism. In general, physiological indices of bone activity, such as alkaline phosphatase and parathormone levels, are normal, although the former may rise with resumption of bone growth.[155] In general, 25-hydroxyvitamin D and 1,25-dihydroxyvitamin D and osteocalcin are normal, although osteocalcin may be depressed due to lower bone turnover.[153, 156] When reversal of osteoporosis occurs, it is more often seen with recovery from anorexia and is more tightly associated with weight gain that return of menses. Some studies suggest, however, that bone mass does not appear to recover even with weight gain, calcium supplementation, and exercise. Increased cortisol seen in anorexia has been suggested as a mechanism for the osteopenia.[160–162]

ANTECEDENTS OF ANOREXIA NERVOSA

At-Risk Groups

The striking incidence of anorexia nervosa in professional ballet dancers suggests that the chronic dieting behavior followed by members of this profession to achieve a thin body image may be important in the pathogenesis of anorexia nervosa. A number of investigators have been interested in the concept that anorexia nervosa occurs as a continuum of chronic dieting behavior. Weight loss–related amenorrhea and exercise-induced amenorrhea have similar endocrine profiles, suggesting that they have similar hypothalamic mechanisms.[163] Regression to prepubertal patterns of gonadotropin secretion and nocturnal LH spurts have been seen in weight loss–related amenorrhea similar to patterns seen in amenorrhea with anorexia nervosa.[164] Retrospective studies of the emergence of eating disorders suggest that anorexia nervosa often first occurs during the first half of adolescence, while bulimia nervosa has a later onset. Subclinical behaviors such as excessive dieting, weight concerns, and binging are pervasive across the adolescent years. Despite a burgeoning literature on eating disorders (over 800 articles published in the previous two years), little prospective work has been conducted to chart the onset of clinical or subclinical prob-

lems or the predictors of such problems.[165, 166] One study has shown that two-thirds of a sample of adolescent girls showed at least one symptom of disturbed eating behavior during adolescence prior to entering college and that early physical maturation presents a definite risk factor.[167] Bulimia has been reported to vary from 3 to 15 per cent in university students,[20, 21, 168] with a similar incidence of 15 per cent in high school students.[169] Other groups at risk include ballet dancers, models, gymnasts, endurance runners, figure skaters, and people in sports or professions in which low body weight is valued.[170–174] Recent studies on menstrual patterns in ballet dancers indicate that amenorrhea (or absence of menses for more than five months) is more significantly related to abnormal eating patterns and a history of anorexia nervosa than to exercise training.[175] In fact, in this group the incidence of anorexia nervosa was 20 per cent and was significantly higher in the more competitive companies.[8] The contribution of exercise training, weight loss, lowered body fat, dieting, and anorexia nervosa to the genesis of amenorrhea seen with exercise training remains unresolved. The fact that some of these activities are fertile breeding ground for the development of anorexia nervosa is becoming evident. The recognition of the syndrome in its early stages and a study of the syndrome to determine significant abnormalities have particular appeal. Early intervention has been shown to have a more favorable outcome.

Psychological Changes

A number of studies examine psychological changes in anorexia nervosa patients and at-risk groups. Patients with anorexia nervosa and secondary amenorrhea may share a need to achieve and a need for approval compared with control subjects.[176] The most outstanding differences were shown in "fear of failure" scales, in which anorectics scored highest. However, this study included as a comparison group all patients with secondary amenorrhea on a hypothalamic basis, not just those in the setting of weight loss. Another study on weight-preoccupied women (ballet dancers) suggested that some of this group displayed psychopathology similar to that in anorexia nervosa, whereas others only superficially resembled patients suffering serious eating disorders.[177, 178] The menstrual characteristics of the group with weight preoccupation were not examined, and numerous studies indicate that secondary amenorrhea may be an early marker for anorexia nervosa.[179] Another early marker for the illness may be the perceptual distortion that develops in patients with anorexia nervosa. These patients consider themselves to be too fat despite their low weight. Attempts have been made to measure this perceptual distortion, but different studies have shown that perceptual accuracy can be affected by age and that distortion can be caused by a high-carbohydrate diet.[180, 181] Patients with anorexia nervosa consistently overestimate body size and size of other objects, and this overestimation tends to disappear with weight gain. Thus the perceptual distortion would seem to reinforce dieting behavior and perpetuate the illness. Studies of high-risk groups such as ballet dancers and gymnasts reveal that overestimation depends on the protocol used.[182] Although methodology has much to do with results, most investigators feel that patients who have anorexia nervosa have severe body image disturbances that are present even in the early stages but difficult to measure.

Depression and obsessive-compulsive behavior often coexist with the eating disorder, particularly when bulimia is also present. Other comorbid problems include drug abuse and alcoholism.[183–192]

Studies also have been performed to evaluate the behavior disorder seen in anorexia as well as the perceptual abnormality. "Anorexic behavior scales" have been devised by a number of investigators and claim to differentiate individuals with anorexia nervosa from those who have secondary amenorrhea due to other causes. The scale may consist of a psychological profile, which is self-administered or administered by a doctor, a nurse, or a clinical psychologist. One study indicates that the anorectic behavior scale is very useful and accurate in distinguishing healthy females from those with anorectic behavior.[179] These scales may therefore be useful in the early diagnosis of anorexia nervosa, particularly in patients presenting with only secondary amenorrhea and little, if any, weight loss.[179]

In contrast to the perceptual disorder, the degree of anorectic behavior does not always correlate with the malnutrition.[179]

Along with the behavioral disorder, objective changes in the brain have been demonstrated by computed tomography. Enlargement of the cortical sulci and subarachnoid spaces, as well as cerebral atrophy, has been demonstrated in a small number of cases, with reversal of the atrophy with weight gain in one patient.[193–196]

Anorexia nervosa continues to be a perplexing syndrome, most likely psychogenic in nature. The large preponderance of girls at or near puberty from upper socioeconomic backgrounds would suggest the importance of environmental influences. The fact that the amenorrhea may precede the development of the full-blown syndrome has often been emphasized, although in most studies amenorrhea most often coincided with the onset of food restriction. Many of the signs and symptoms, including psychological changes, seen in anorexia nervosa have been reported in starvation, and it is difficult to tell when "anorexia" leaves off and starvation predominates.

On the other hand, the early development of amenorrhea and behavioral symptoms and the hypothalamic symptoms also suggest a primary hypothalamic syndrome. In addition, the association of psychological and neuroendocrine changes in patients with anorexia nervosa has led investigators to speculate that abnormalities of neurotransmission may be involved in the pathogenesis of the syndrome.[2a]

MANAGEMENT AND THERAPY

Mortality of anorexia nervosa ranges from 8 to 18 per cent, with a lower mortality in pediatric and adolescent groups. Morbidity persists with eating disorders with depression, obsessive-compulsive behavior, and poor sexual adjustment.[197, 198] Eating problems persist in more than half.[199–203] Death is due to starvation or its complications, including infections, renal or cardiac failure, arrhythmias, and complications of fluid imbalance.[199–203] Suicide also occurs with an incidence of 5 to 7 per cent.[203]

Management and therapy for this syndrome are still a subject of wide debate.[2, 204–206] Treatment of anorexia nervosa will depend on the amount of weight loss, the extent of the electrolyte abnormalities, the presence of other problems such as diuretic, laxative, or substance abuse, and the presence of immediately life-threatening medical complications.[200, 207] All therapeutic modalities are geared toward the reestablishment of normal weight. Treatment includes various combinations of psychotherapy, including family therapy, psychoanalysis, and, occasionally, drug therapy. Tricyclic antidepressants, cyproheptadine, L-dopa, fluoxetine, and metoclopramide have all been used and have met with variable success.[208, 209] Behavior modification is used with some success, although opinions on its efficacy vary.[210, 211] It is disconcerting that despite impressive studies on the cause and psychogenesis of anorexia nervosa, few specific or new therapeutic modalities are available. Emphasis has been placed on early diagnosis and recognition of anorectic behavior so that the patient may be treated before the full-blown syndrome sets in.[179] Since amenorrhea occurs as an early part of the disease process, it is usually the first symptom that causes the patient to seek help. Physicians, therefore, should be particularly attentive to a history of dieting and weight loss in their young patients. Generally, patients who are 75 per cent of ideal body weight or lower need immediate and aggressive intervention. Dietary therapy is important, since response to psychotherapy is improved with nutritional rehabilitation.[212, 213] This is usually best done in a hospital setting by a team consisting of psychiatrists or psychologists, internists or pediatricians, and, if possible, a nutritionist with special interest and expertise in anorexia nervosa and related eating disorders.[214]

The syndrome of anorexia nervosa and all associated symptoms appear to be reversible with weight gain. Although the majority of patients will have complete recovery, the insult to the reproductive system may be permanent in up to 30 per cent of patients with a history of prolonged illness (greater than a year). A poorer prognosis is also associated with bulimia.[209] The reproductive system remains particularly sensitive to fluctuations in weight, and this should be avoided. The resumption of normal cyclical menses is first dependent on resumption of normal weight. Patients who exercise heavily may need to weigh more to menstruate normally during periods when they are highly active.[163] Cyclical function may not return for almost a year after return of normal weight, although some estrogen secretion is detectable prior to the resumption of menses. Follow-up over a 10-year period shows that amenorrhea persists in 49 per cent of patients but in only 11 per cent (2 of 19) of those who have a normalization of weight.[215] LH response to GnRH may be a good predictor of outcome.[157]

In those who do not have a return of menstrual function, fertility may be restored by induction of ovulation. Agents such as clomiphene citrate or human menopausal gonadotropins can induce ovulation in almost all cases. The patient should have an evaluation to rule out other causes of amenorrhea, such as pituitary tumor or ovarian failure, prior to therapeutic induction of ovulation, and with these causes definitely eliminated, the patient can be reassured of future fertility. Recent research indicates that cyclical menstrual function can be restored in patients with weight-related hypothalamic amenorrhea, such as that in anorexia nervosa, with GnRH administered in a pulsatile fashion with the use of a pump by subcutaneous or intravenous routes.[216] These therapeutic modalities hold much promise for the future, as weight loss–related amenorrheas represent a group of disorders that respond particularly well to this form of therapy. These and other therapeutic modalities will soon be available to treat the deficiencies that remain after the illness is cured. Despite return of weight, some patients continue to have permanent problems. Preoccupation with food and persistent dieting behavior are not uncommon in weight-recovered patients.[7] For those patients with recovered anorexia nervosa who never menstruate again, estrogen replacement is definitely indicated. Estrogen replacement is needed to circumvent premature osteoporosis. Reports of osteoporosis-related problems in the patient with anorexia nervosa are appearing in the literature and should be of some concern.[65, 217] Recent evidence suggests that hypoestrogenism of a prolonged nature (greater than six months) in young women may predispose to osteopenia and premature osteoporosis.[218–223] Unfortunately, many patients who remain underweight will refuse estrogen therapy because of anxiety about gaining weight. The treatment of anorexia nervosa remains a major therapeutic challenge that has yet to be met.

ACKNOWLEGMENT: The author wishes to thank Ms. Farnaz Vossoughian for her efforts on revising the manuscript.

REFERENCES

1. Gull WW: Anorexia nervosa. Trans Clin Soc (Lond) 7:22–34, 1874.
2. Warren MP: Anorexia nervosa. In Sciarra JJ (ed): Gynecology and Obstetrics. Hagerstown, MD, Harper & Row, 1981, pp 1–9.
2a. Warren MP: The effects of undernutrition on reproductive function in the human. Endocr Rev 4:363–377, 1983.
2b. Wilson GT, Walsh BT: Eating disorders in the DSM-IV. J Abnorm Psychol 100(3):362–365, 1991.
3. Theander S: Anorexia nervosa. Acta Psychiatr Scand Suppl 214:1–194, 1970.
4. Kendell RE, Hall DJ, Harley A, Babigan HM: The epidemiology and anorexia nervosa. Psychol Med 2:200–203, 1973.
5. Kalucy RC, Crisp AH, Lacy JH, Harding B: Prevalence and prognosis in anorexia nervosa. Aust NZ J Psychiatry 11:251–257, 1977.
6. Crisp AH, Palmer RL, Kalucy RS: How common is anorexia nervosa? A prevalence study. Br J Psychiatry 128:549, 1976.
7. Garner DM, Garfinkel PE: Sociocultural factors in anorexia nervosa. Lancet 2:674, 1978.
8. Hamilton LH, Brooks-Gunn J, Warren MP: Sociocultural influences on eating disorders in professional female ballet dancers. Int J Eating Disorders 4(4):465–477, 1985.
9. Epling WF, Pierce WD, Stephan L: A theory of activity-based anorexia. Int J Eating Disorders 3:27–43, 1983.
10. Aumariega AJ, Edwards P, Mitchell CB: Anorexia nervosa in black adolescents. J Am Acad Child Psychiatry 1:111–114, 1984.
11. Askevold F, Heiberg A: Anorexia nervosa—Two cases in discordant MZ twins. Psychother Psychosom 32:223–228, 1979.
12. Darby PL, Garfinkel PE, Vale JM, et al: Anorexia nervosa and "Turner syndrome": Cause or coincidence? Psychol Med 11:141–145, 1981.
13. Brooks SA: Diabetes mellitus and anorexia nervosa: Another view. Br J Psychiatry 144:640–642, 1984.
14. Roland JM, Bhanji S: Anorexia nervosa occurring in patients with diabetes mellitus. Postgrad Med J 58:354–356, 1982.
15. Kontula K, Mustajoik P, Paetau A, Pelkonen R: Development of Cushing's disease in patient with anorexia nervosa. J Endocrinol Invest 7:35–40, 1984.
16. Warren MP, Vande Wiele RL: Clinical and metabolic features of anorexia nervosa. Am J Obstet Gynecol 117:435, 1973.

17. Smith NJ: Excessive weight loss and food aversion in athletes stimulating anorexia nervosa. Pediatrics 66:139–142, 1980.
18. Willi J, Grossmann S: Epidemiology of anorexia nervosa in a defined region of Switzerland. Am J Psychiatry 140:564–567, 1983.
18a. American Psychiatric Association: Diagnostic and Statistical Manual of Mental Disorders (3d ed rev) (DSM-IIIR). Washington, American Psychiatric Association, 1987.
18b. Schwartz DM, Thompson MG, Johnson CL: Anorexia nervosa and bulimia: The sociocultural context. In Emmett SW (ed): Theory and Treatment of Anorexia Nervosa and Bulimia. New York, Brunner/Mazel, 1985, pp 95–112.
19. Pyle RL, Mitchell JE, Eckert ED, et al: The incidence of bulimia in freshman college students. Int J Eating Disorders 2:75–85, 1983.
20. Stangler RS, Printz AM: DSM-III: Psychiatric diagnosis in a university population. Am J Psychiatry 137:937, 1980.
21. Halmi KA, Falk JR: Binge-eating and vomiting: A survey of a college population. Psychol Med 4:697, 1981.
22. Russell GFM: Bulimia nervosa: An ominous variant of anorexia nervosa. Psychol Med 9:429–448, 1979.
23. Fairburn CG, Cooper PJ: Self-induced vomiting and bulimia nervosa: An undetected problem. Br Med J 284:1153–1155, 1982.
24. Mitchell JE, Pyle RL: The bulimic syndrome in normal weight individuals: A review. Int J Eating Disorders 1:61–73, 1982.
25. Pyle RL, Mitchel JE: Bulimia: A report of 34 cases. J Clin Psychiatry 42:60–64, 1981.
26. Harris RT: Bulimarexia and related serious eating disorders with medical complications. Ann Intern Med 99:800–807, 1983.
27. Hasler JF: Parotid enlargement: A presenting sign in anorexia nervosa. Oral Surg 53:567–573, 1982.
28. Marano AR, Sangree MH: Acute pancreatitis associated with bulimia. J Clin Gastroenterol 6:245–248, 1984.
29. Feighner JP, Robins E, Guze SB, et al: Diagnostic criteria for use in psychiatric research. Arch Gen Psychiatry 26:57, 1972.
30. Frumar AM, Meldrum DR, Judd HL: Hypercarotenemia in hypothalamic amenorrhea. Fertil Steril 32:261–264, 1979.
31. Kemmann E, Pasquale SA, Skaf R: Amenorrhea associated with carotenemia. JAMA 249:926–929, 1983.
32. Walsh BT, Croft CB, Katz JL: Anorexia nervosa and salivary gland enlargement. Int J Psychiatry Med 11:255–261, 1981.
33. Brotman AW, Stern TA: Case report of cardiovascular abnormalities in anorexia nervosa. Am J Psychiatry 140:1227–1228, 1983.
34. Silverman JA, Krongrad E: Anorexia nervosa: A cause of pericardial effusion? Pediatr Cardiol 4:125–127, 1983.
35. Schoettle UC: Pancreatitis: A complication, a concomitant, or a cause of an anorexia nervosalike syndrome. J Am Acad Child Psychiatry 18:384–390, 1979.
36. Rampling D: Acute pancreatitis in anorexia nervosa. Med J Aust 2:194–195, 1982.
37. Cox KL, Cannon RA, Ament ME, et al: Biochemical and ultrasonic abnormalities of the pancreas in anorexia nervosa. Dig Dis Sci 28:225–229, 1983.
38. Nordgren L, von Schéele C: Hepatic and pancreatic dysfunction in anorexia nervosa: A report of two cases. Biol Psychiatry 12:681–686, 1977.
39. Lüthi M, Zurbrügg RP: A puzzling triad: Anorexia nervosa, high sweat electrolytes and indication to partial exocrine pancreatic insufficiency. Helv Paediatr Acta 38:149–158, 1983.
40. Al-Mufty NA, Bevan DH: A case of subcutaneous emphysema, pneumomediastinum and pneumoretroperitoneum associated with functional anorexia. Br J Clin Pract 31:160–161, 1977.
41. Brooks AP, Martyn C: Pneumomediastinum in anorexia nervosa (letter). Br Med J 1:125, 1979.
42. Silber TJ, Kass EJ: Anorexia nervosa and nephrolithiasis. J Adolesc Health Care 5:50–52, 1984.
43. Esca SA, Brenner W, Mach K, Gschnait F: Kwashiorkor-like zinc deficiency syndrome in anorexia nervosa. Acta Derm Venereol 59:361–364, 1979.
44. Smith DK, Ovesen L, Chu R, et al: Hypothermia in a patient with anorexia nervosa. Metabolism 32:1151–1154, 1983.
45. Niiya K, Kitagawa T, Fujishita M, et al: Bulimia nervosa complicated by deficiency of vitamin K–dependent coagulation factors. JAMA 250:792–793, 1983.
46. Warren SE, Steinberg SM: Acid-base and electrolyte disturbances in anorexia nervosa. Am J Psychiatry 136:415–418, 1979.
47. Lefebvre J: Treatment of undernutrition and electrolyte disturbances in anorexia nervosa. Acta Psychiatr Belg 80:551–556, 1980.
48. Sheridan PH, Collins M: Potentially life-threatening hypophosphatemia in anorexia nervosa. J Adolesc Health Care 491:44–46, 1983.

49. Schott GD: Anorexia nervosa presenting as foot drop. Postgrad Med J 55:58–60, 1979.

50. Freyschuss U, Fohlin L, Thorén C: Limb circulation in anorexia nervosa. Acta Paediatr Scand 67:225–228, 1978.

51. Rappaport R, Prevot C, Czernichow P: Somatomedin activity and growth hormone secretion. I. Changes related to body weight in anorexia nervosa. Acta Paediatr Scand 69:37–41, 1980.

52. Bowers TK, Eckert E: Leukopenia in anorexia nervosa. Lack of increased risk of infection. Arch Intern Med 138:1520–1523, 1978.

53. Golla JA, Larson LA, Anderson CF, et al: An immunological assessment of patients with anorexia nervosa. Am J Clin Nutr 34:2756–2762, 1981.

54. Pertschuk MJ, Crosby LD, Barot L, Mullen JL: Immunocompetency in anorexia nervosa. Am J Clin Nutr 35:968–972, 1982.

55. Kline CL: Anorexia nervosa: Death from complications of ruptured gastric ulcer. Can J Psychiatry 24:153–156, 1979.

56. Pentlow BD, Dent RG: Acute vascular compression of the duodenum in anorexia nervosa. Br J Surg 68:665–666, 1981.

57. Sours JA, Vorhaus LJ: Superior mesenteric artery syndrome in anorexia nervosa: A case report. Am J Psychiatry 138:519–520, 1981.

58. Froese AP, Szmuilowicz J, Bailey JD: The superior-mesenteric-artery syndrome: Cause or complication of anorexia nervosa? Can Psychiatr Assoc J 23:325–327, 1978.

59. Harty RF, Pearson PH, Solomon TE, McGuigan JE: Cholecystokinin, vasoactive intestinal peptide and peptide histidine methionine responses to feeding in anorexia nervosa. Regul Pept 36:141–150, 1991.

60. Uhe AM, Szmukler GI, Collier GR, et al: Potential regulators of feeding behavior in anorexia nervosa. Am J Clin Nutr 55:28–32, 1992.

61. Bassie HH: Anorexia/bulimia nervosa: The development of anorexia nervosa and of mental symptoms. Treatment and the outcome of the disease. Acta Psychiatr Scand Suppl 361:7–13, 1990.

62. Rich LM, Caine MR, Findling JW, Shaker JL: Hypoglycemic coma in anorexia nervosa: Case report and review of the literature. Arch Intern Med 150:894–895, 1990.

63. McAnarney ER, Greydanus DE, Campanella VA, Hoekelman RA: Rib fractures and anorexia nervosa. J Adolesc Health Care 4:40–43, 1983.

64. Ayers JW, Gidwani GP, Schmidt IM, Gross M: Osteopenia in hypoestrogenic young women with anorexia nervosa. Fertil Steril 41:224–228, 1984.

65. Rigotti NA, Nussbaum SR, Herzog DB, Neer RM: Osteoporosis in women with anorexia nervosa. N Engl J Med 311:1601–1606, 1984.

66. Gill J, DeSouza V, Wakeling A, et al: Differential changes in alpha- and beta-adrenoceptor–linked uptake in platelets from patients with anorexia nervosa. J Clin Endocrinol Metab 74:441–446, 1992.

67. Boyar RN, Katz J, Finkelstein JW, et al: Anorexia nervosa: Immaturity of the 24-hour luteinizing hormone secretory pattern. N Engl J Med 291:861–865, 1974.

68. Marshall JC, Kelch RP: Low dose pulsatile gonadotropin-releasing hormone in anorexia nervosa: A model of human pubertal development. J Clin Endocrinol Metab 49:712–718, 1979.

69. Fritz MA, Speroff L: Current concepts of the endocrine characteristics of normal menstrual function: The key to diagnosis and management of menstrual disorders. Clin Obstet Gynecol 26:647–689, 1983.

70. Warren MP, Jewelewicz R, Dyrenfurth I, et al: The significance of weight loss in the evaluation of pituitary response to LHRH in women with secondary amenorrhea. J Clin Endocrinol Metab 40:601–611, 1975.

71. Roth JC, Kelch RP, Kaplan SL, Grumbach MM: FSH and LH response to luteinizing hormone–releasing factor in prepubertal and pubertal children, adult males and patients with hypogonadotropic and hypergonadotropic hypogonadism. J Clin Endocrinol Metab 35:926–930, 1972.

72. Wildt L, Hausler A, Marshall G, et al: Frequency and amplitude of gonadotropin releasing hormone stimulation and gonadotropin secretion in the Rhesus monkey. Endocrinology 109:376, 1981.

73. Beaumont PJV, George GCW, Pimstone BL, Vinik AL: Body weight and pituitary response to hypothalamic releasing hormone in patients with anorexia nervosa. J Clin Endocrinol Metab 43:487, 1976.

74. Mecklenburg RS, Loriaux DL, Thompson RH, et al: Hypothalamic dysfunction in patients with anorexia nervosa. Medicine 53:147, 1974.

75. Giusti M, Delitala G, Mazzocchi G, et al: The role of opioid receptors on the secretion of LH, FSH and PRL in anorexia nervosa. In Endroczi E, Angelucci L, Scapagnini U, De Wied D (eds): Neuropeptides and Psychosomatic Processes. Budapest, Akademiai Kiado, 1983, p 701.

76. Grossman A, Moulte PJA, McIntyre H, et al: Opiate mediation of amenorrhea in hyper-prolactinemia and in weight loss–related amenorrhea. Clin Endocrinol (Oxf) 17:379–388, 1983.

77. Giusti M, Cavagnaro P, Torre R, et al: Endogeneous opioid blockade and gonadotropin secretion: Role of pulsatile luteinizing hormone–releasing hormone administration in anorexia nervosa and weight loss amenorrhea. Fertil Steril 49:797–801, 1988.

78. Berga SL, Loucks AB, Rossmanith WG, et al: Acceleration of luteinizing hormone pulse frequency in functional hypothalamic amenorrhea by dopaminergic blockade. J Clin Endocrinol Metab 72:151–156, 1991.

79. Warren MP: Anorexia nervosa and bulimia. In Sciarra JW (ed): Gynecology and Obstetrics. Hagerstown MD, Harper & Row, 1988, pp 1–14.

80. Schweiger U: Menstrual function and luteal-phase deficiency in relation to weight changes and dieting. Clin Obstet Gynecol 34:191–197, 1991.

81. Pirke KM, Schweiger U, Lemmel W, et al: The influence of dieting on the menstrual cycle of healthy young women. J Clin Endocrinol Metab 60:1174–1179, 1985.

82. Graham RL, Grimes DL, Gambrele RD Jr: Amenorrhea secondary to voluntary weight loss. South Med J 72:1259–1261, 1979.

83. Hall MGR, Murray MAF, Franks S, Jacobs HS: Endocrinopathy of weight recovered anorexia nervosa in women presenting with secondary amenorrhea. J Endocrinol 66:43–44, 1976.

84. Holmberg NG, Nylander I: Weight loss in secondary amenorrhea. Acta Obstet Gynecol Scand 50:241–246, 1971.

85. Knuth UA, Hull MGR, Jacobs HS: Amenorrhea and loss of weight. Br J Obstet Gynaecol 84:801–807, 1977.

86. Bates GW: Body weight control practice as a cause of infertility. Clin Obstet Gynecol 28:632–644, 1985.

87. Fichter MM, Pirke KM: Hypothalamic pituitary function in starving healthy subjects. In Pirke KM, Ploog D (eds): The Psychobiology of Anorexia Nervosa. Berlin, Springer-Verlag, 1984, pp 124–135.

88. Pirke KM, Schweiger U, Laessle R, et al: Dieting influences the menstrual cycle: Vegetarian versus nonvegetarian diet. Fertil Steril 46:1083–1088, 1986.

89. Goldin BR, Adlercreutz H, Gorbach SL, et al: Estrogen excretion patterns and plasma levels in vegetarian and omnivorous women. N Engl J Med 307:1542–1547, 1982.

90. Warren MP, Holderness CC, Lesobre V, et al: Hypothalamic amenorrhea and hidden nutritional insults. Am J Obstet Gynecol (in press).

91. Herzog DB, Copeland PM: Medical progress—Eating disorders. N Engl J Med 313:295–303, 1985.

92. Rau JH, Green RS: Compulsive eating: A neuropsychologic approach to certain eating disorders. Compr Psychiatry 16:223, 1975.

93. Rau JH, Green RS: Soft neurological correlates of compulsive eaters. J Nerv Ment Dis 166:435, 1978.

94. Vigersky RA, Loriaux DL: Anorexia nervosa as a model of hypothalamic dysfunction. In Vigersky R (ed): Anorexia Nervosa. New York, Raven Press, 1977, p 109.

95. Walsh BT: The endocrinology of anorexia nervosa. Psychiatr Clin North Am 3:299, 1980.

96. Moshang T Jr, Utiger RD: Low triiodothyronine euthyroidism in anorexia nervosa. In Vigersky R (ed): Anorexia Nervosa. New York, Raven Press, 1977, p 263.

97. Fowler PBS, Banim SO, Ikram H: Prolonged ankle reflex in anorexia nervosa. Lancet 2:307, 1972.

98. Boyar RM, Bradlow HL: Studies of testosterone metabolism in anorexia nervosa. In Vigersky R (ed): Anorexia Nervosa. New York, Raven Press, 1977, p 271.

99. Fohlin L: Exercise, performance, and body dimensions in anorexia nervosa before and after rehabilitation. Acta Med Scand 204:61, 1975.

100. Moshang T Jr, Parks JS, Baker L, et al: Low serum triiodothyronine in patients with anorexia nervosa. J Clin Endocrinol Metab 40:470, 1975.

101. Jennings AS, Ferguson DC, Utiger RD: Regulation of the conversion of thyroxine to triiodothyronine in the perfused rat liver. J Clin Invest 64:1614, 1979.

102. Cyrus J, Wood D, Samols E, Sudhakaran E: Low T4 and FT4I in Seriously Ill Patients. Presented at the 61st Annual Meeting of the Endocrine Society, Anaheim, CA, June 13–15, 1979, p 297.

103. Kaptein EM, Wheeler WS, Spencer CA, et al: Thyroid hormone economy in critical illness. Presented at the 61st Annual Meeting of the Endocrine Society, Anaheim, CA, June 13–15, 1979, p 240.

104. Byerley B, Black DW, Grosser BI: Anorexia nervosa with hyperthyroidism: Case report. J Clin Psychiatry 44:308–309, 1983.

105. Vigersky RA, Loriaux DL, Andersen AE, Lipsett MB: Anorexia nervosa: Behavioral and hypothalamic aspects. Clin Endocrinol Metab 5:517, 1976.
106. Leslie RD, Isaacs AJ, Gomez J, et al: Hypothalamo-pituitary-thyroid function in anorexia nervosa: Influence of weight gain. Br Med J 2:526–528, 1978.
107. Kiyohara K, Tamai H, Takaichi Y, et al: Decreased thyroidal triiodothyronine secretion in patients with anorexia nervosa: influence of weight recovery. Am J Clin Nutr 50:767–772, 1989.
108. Gold P, Gwirtsman H, Avgerinos P, et al: Abnormal hypothalamic-pituitary-adrenal function in anorexia nervosa. N Engl J Med 314:1335–1342, 1986.
109. Hotta I, Shebasoki K, Masuda A, et al: The responses of plasma adrenocorticotropin and corticotropin-releasing hormone (CRH) and cerebrospinal fluid immunoreactive CRH in anorexia nervosa patients. J Clin Endocrinol Metab 62:319–324, 1986.
110. Sapolsky RM, Krey LC: Stress-induced suppression of luteinizing hormone concentrations in wild baboons: Role of opiates. J Clin Endocrinol Metab 66:722–726, 1988.
111. Petraglia F, Vale W, Rivier C: Opioids act centrally to modulate stress-induced decrease in luteinizing hormone in the rat. Endocrinololgy 119:2445–2450, 1986.
112. Xiao E, Luckhaus J, Niemann W, Ferin M: Acute inhibition of gonadotropin secretion by CRH in the primate: Are the adrenal glands involved? Endocrinology 124:1632–1637, 1989.
113. Boyar RN, Hellman LD, Roffwarg H, et al: Cortisol secretion and metabolism in anorexia nervosa. N Engl J Med 296:190, 1977.
114. Casper RC, Chatterton RT, Davis JM: Alterations in serum cortisol and its binding characteristics in anorexia nervosa. J Clin Endocrinol Metab 49:406, 1979.
115. Walsh BT, Katz JL, Levin J, et al: Adrenal activity in anorexia nervosa. Psychosom Med 40:499–506, 1978.
116. Newman MM, Halmi KA: The endocrinology of anorexia nervosa and bulimia nervosa. Neurol Clin North Am 6:195–212, 1988.
117. Counts DR, Gwirtsman H, Carlsson LMS, et al: The effect of anorexia nervosa and refeeding on growth hormone-binding protein. The insulin-like growth factors (IGFs), and the IGF-binding proteins. J Clin Endocrinol Metab 75:762–767, 1992.
118. Sherman BM, Halmi KA, Zamudio R: LH and FSH response to gonadotropin-releasing hormone in anorexia nervosa: Effect of nutritional rehabilitation. J Clin Endocrinol Metab 41:135, 1975.
119. Starkey TA, Lee RA: Menstruation and fertility in anorexia nervosa. Am J Obstet Gynecol 105:374, 1969.
120. Eisenberg E: Toward an understanding of reproductive function in anorexia nervosa. Fertil Steril 36:543–550, 1981.
121. Fishman J, Boyar RM, Hellman L: Influence of body weight on estradiol metabolism in young women. J Clin Endocrinol Metab 41:989, 1975.
122. Gordon S, Cantrall EW, Leklenick WP, et al: Steroid and lipid metabolism: The hypocholesterolaemic effects of estrogen metabolites. Steroids 4:257, 1964.
123. Reeves AG, Plum F: Hyperphagia, rage and dementia accompanying a ventromedial hypothalamic neoplasm. Arch Neurol 20:616, 1969.
124. Haugh RM, Markesbery WR: Hypothalamic astrocytoma: Syndrome of hyperphagia, obesity, and disturbances of behavior and endocrine and autonomic function. Arch Neurol 40:560–563, 1983.
125. Stricker EM, Andersen AE: The lateral hypothalamic syndrome: Comparison with the syndrome of anorexia nervosa. Life Sci 26:1927–1934, 1980.
126. Kennedy GC, Mitra J: Hypothalamic control of energy balance and the reproductive cycle in the rat. J Physiol 166:395–407, 1963.
127. Vaisman N, Clarke R, Rossi M, et al: Protein turnover and resting energy expenditure in patients with undernutrition and chronic lung disease. Am J Clin Nutr 55:63–69, 1992.
128. Vaisman N, Rossi MF, Corey M, et al: Effect of refeeding on the energy metabolism of adolescent girls who have anorexia nervosa. Eur J Clin Nutr 45:527–537, 1991.
129. Hurd HP 2d, Palumbo PJ, Gharib H: Hypothalamic-endocrine dysfunction in anorexia nervosa. May Clin Proc 52:711–716, 1977.
130. Casper RC: Hypothalamic dysfunction and symptoms of anorexia nervosa. Psychiatr Clin North Am 7:201–213, 1984.
131. Barry VC, Klawans HL: On the role of dopamine in the pathophysiology of anorexia nervosa. J Neural Transm 38:107, 1976.
132. Lord JA, Waterfield AA, Hughes J, Kosterlitz HW: Endogenous opioid peptides: Multiple agonists and receptors. Nature 267:495, 1977.
133. Margules DL, Lewis MJ, Shibuya H, Pert CB: β-Endorphin is associated with overeating in genetically obese mice (ob/ob) and rats (fa/fa). Science 202:988, 1978.
134. Wardlaw SL, Thoron L, Frantz AG: Effects of sex steroids on beta-endorphin. Brain Res 245:327, 1982.
135. Wehrenberg WB, Wardlaw SL, Frantz AG, Ferin M: Beta-endorphin in hypophyseal portal blood: Variations throughout the menstrual cycle. Endocrinology 111:879, 1982.
136. Wardlaw SL, Wehrenberg WB, Ferin M, et al: Effect of sex steroids on beta-endorphin in hypophyseal portal blood. J Clin Endocrinol Metab 55:877, 1982.
137. Emans SJ, Grace E, Hoffer FA, et al: Estrogen deficiency in adolescents and young adults: Impact on bone mineral content and effects of estrogen replacement therapy. Obstet Gynecol 76:585–592, 1990.
138. Ponder SW, McCormick DP, Fawcett HD, et al: Spinal bone mineral density in children aged 5.00 through 11.99 years. Am J Dis Child 144:1346–1348, 1990.
139. Glastre C, Braillon P, David L, et al: Measurement of bone mineral content of the lumbar spine by dual energy x-ray absorptiometry in normal children: Correlations with growth parameters. J Clin Endocrinol Metab 70:1330–1333, 1990.
140. Gilsanz V, Gibbens DT, Carlson M, et al: Peak trabecular vertebral density: A comparison of adolescent and adult females. Calcif Tissue Int 43:260–262, 1988.
141. Gilsanz V, Gibbens DT, Roe TF, et al: Vertebral bone density in children: Effect of puberty. Radiology 166:847–850, 1988.
142. McCormick DP, Ponder SW, Fawcett HD, Palmer JL: Spinal bone mineral density in 335 normal and obese children and adolescents: Evidence for ethnic and sex differences. J Bone Miner Res 6:507–513, 1991.
143. Bonjour JPH, Theintz G, Buchs B, et al: Critical years and stages of puberty for spinal and femoral bone mass accumulation during adolescence. J Clin Endocrinol Metab 73:555–563, 1991.
144. Gilsanz V, Roe TF, Mora S, et al: Changes in vertebral bone density in black girls and white girls during childhood and puberty. N Engl J Med 325:1597–1600, 1991.
145. Lloyd T, Rollings N, Andon MB, et al: Determinants of bone density in young women: I. Relationships among pubertal development, total body bone mass, and total body bone density in premenarchal females. J Clin Endocrinol Metab 75:383–387, 1992.
146. Ott SM: Editorial: Attainment of peak bone mass. J Clin Endocrinol Metab 71:1082A–1082C, 1990.
147. Theintz G, Buchs B, Rizzoli R, et al: Longitudinal monitoring of bone mass accumulation in healthy adolescents: Evidence for a marked reduction after 16 years of age at the levels of lumbar spine and femoral neck in female subjects. J Clin Endocrinol Metab 75:1060–1065, 1992.
148. Mazess RB, Barden HS: Bone density in premenopausal women: Effects of age, dietary intake, physical activity, smoking, and birth-control pills. Am J Clin Nutr 53:132–142, 1991.
149. Dhuper S, Warren MP, Brooks-Gunn J, Fox RP: Effects of hormonal status on bone density in adolescent girls. J Clin Endocrinol Metab 71:1083–1088, 1990.
150. Finkelstein JS, Neer RM, Biller BMK, et al: Osteopenia in men with a history of delayed puberty. N Engl J Med 326:600–604, 1992.
151. Sowers MF, Kshirsagar A, Crutchfield M, Updike S: Body composition, age, and femoral bone mass of young adult women. Ann Epidemiol 1:245–254, 1991.
152. Bachrach LK, Guido D, Katzman D, et al: Decreased bone density in adolescent girls with anorexia nervosa. Pediatrics 86(3):440–447, 1990.
153. Rigotti NA, Neer RM, Skates SJ, et al: The clinical course of osteoporosis in anorexia nervosa: A longitudinal study of cortical bone mass. JAMA 265:1133–1138, 1991.
154. Warren MP, Shane E, Lee MJ, et al: Femoral head collapse associated with anorexia nervosa in a 20-year-old ballet dancer. Clin Orthop 251:171–176, 1990.
155. Salsbury JJ, Mitchell JE: Bone mineral density and anorexia nervosa in women. Am J Psychiaty 148:768–773, 1991.
156. Davies K, Pearson P, Huseman C, et al: Reduced bone mineral in patients with eating disorders. Bone 11:143, 1990.
157. van Binsbergen CJM, Coelingh Bennink HJT, Odink J, et al: A comparative and longitudinal study on endocrine changes related to ovarian function in patients with anorexia nervosa. J Clin Endocrinol Metab 71:705–711, 1990.
158. Bachrach LK, Katzman DK, Litt IF, et al: Recovery from osteopenia in adolescent girls with anorexia nervosa. J Clin Endocrinol Metab 72:602–606, 1991.
159. Jonnavithula S, Warren MP, Fox RP, Lazaro MI: Bone density compromised in amenorrheic women despite return of menses: A 2-year study. Obstet Gynecol 81:669–674, 1993.

160. Fonseca VA, D'Souza V, Houlder S, et al: Vitamin D deficiency and low osteocalcin concentrations in anorexia nervosa. J Clin Pathol 41:195–197, 1988.
161. Newman MM, Halmi KA: Relationship of bone density to estradiol and cortisol in anorexia nervosa and bulimia. Psychiatry Res 29:105–112, 1989.
162. Biller BMK, Saxe V, Herzog DB, et al: Mechanisms of osteoporosis in adult and adolescent women with anorexia nervosa. J Clin Endocrinol Metab 68:548–554, 1989.
163. Warren MP: The effects of exercise on pubertal progression and reproductive function in girls. J Clin Endocrinol Metab 51:1150–1157, 1980.
164. Kapen S, Sternthal E, Braverman L: Case report: A pubertal 24-hour luteinizing hormone (LH) secretory pattern following weight loss in the absence of anorexia nervosa. Psychosom Med 43:177, 1981.
165. Rodin J, Silberstein L, Striegel-Moore R: Women and weight: A normative discontent. In Sonderegger TB (ed): Nebraska Symposium on Motivation: Psychology and Gender. Lincoln, University of Nebraska Press, 1984, pp 267–307.
166. Attie I, Brooks-Gunn J, Petersen AC: A developmental perspective on eating disorders and eating problems. In Lewis M, Miller S (eds): Handbook of Developmental Psychopathology. New York, Plenum Press, 1990, pp 409–420.
167. Graber JA, Brooks-Gunn J, Paikoff RL, Warren MP: Prediction of eating problems and disorders: An eight-year study of adolescent girls. Submitted for publication.
168. Hawkins RC, Clement PF: Development and construct validation of a self-report measure of binge eating tendencies. Addict Behav 5:219, 1980.
169. Johnson C: The development of bulimia in high school and college women (abstract). Society for Research in Child Development Biennial Meeting, Detroit, Michigan, 1983.
170. Borgen JS, Corbin CB: Eating disorders among female athletes. Phys Sports Med 15:89–95, 1987.
171. Brooks-Gunn J, Burrow C, Warren MP: Attitudes toward eating and body weight in different groups of female adolescent athletes. Int J Eating Disord 7:749–757, 1988.
172. Brownell KD, Steen SN, Wilmore JH: Weight reduction practices in athletes: Analysis of metabolic and health effects. Med Sci Sports Exerc 19:546–556, 1986.
173. Grunewald KK: Weight control in young college women: Who are the dieters? J Am Dietetic Assoc 85:1445–1450, 1985.
174. Rosen LW, McKeag BD, Hough DO, et al: Pathogenic weight control behavior in female athletes, Phys Sports Med 14:79–86, 1986.
175. Brooks-Gunn J, Warren MP, Hamilton LH: The relationship of eating disorders to amenorrhea in ballet dancers. Med Sci Sport Exer 19(1):41–44, 1987.
176. Weeda-Mannak WL, Drop MJ, Smits F, et al: Toward an early recognition of anorexia nervosa. Int J Eating Disorders 2:27–37, 1983.
177. Garner DM, Olmsted MP, Polivy J, Garfinkel PE: Comparison between weight-preoccupied women and anorexia nervosa. Psychosom Med 46:255–266, 1984.
178. Garner DM, Olmsted MP, Garfinkel PE: Does anorexia nervosa occur on a continuum? Int J Eating Disorders 2:11–20, 1983.
179. Fries H: Studies on secondary amenorrhea, anorectic behavior and body image perception: Importance for the early recognition of anorexia nervosa. In Vigersky R (ed): Anorexia Nervosa. New York, Raven Press, 1977, p 163.
180. Slade RD, Russell GFM: Awareness of body dimensions in anorexia nervosa: Cross-sectional and longitudinal studies. Psychol Med 3:188, 1973.
181. Crisp AH, Kalucy RS: Aspects of the perceptual disorder in anorexia nervosa. Br J Med Psychol 47:349, 1974.
182. Meermann R: Experimental investigation of disturbances in body image estimation in anorexia nervosa patients, and ballet and gymnastics pupils. Int J Eating Disorders 2:91–100, 1983.
183. Gershon ES, Schreiber JL, Hamovit JR, et al: Clinical findings in patients with anorexia nervosa and affective illness in their relatives. Am J Psychiatry 141:1419–1422, 1984.
184. Rivinus TM, Biederman J, Herzog DB, et al: Anorexia nervosa and affective disorders: A controlled family history study. Am J Psychiatry 141:1414–1418, 1984.
185. Herzog DB: Are anorexia and bulimic patients depressed? Am J Psychiatry 141:1594–1597, 1984.
186. Holderness CC, Brooks-Gunn J, Warren MP: The co-morbidity of eating disorders and substance abuse: A review of the literature. Int J Eating Disorders (in press).
187. Simpson SG, Al-Mufti R, Andersen AE, DePaulo JR Jr: Bipolar II affective disorder in eating disorder inpatients. J Ment Nerv Dis 180:719–722, 1992.
188. Smith C, Steiner H: Psychopathology in anorexia nervosa and depression. J Am Acad Child Adolesc Psychiatry 5:841–843, 1992.
189. Holden NL: Is anorexia nervosa an obsessive-compulsive disorder? Br J Psychiatry 157:1–5, 1990.
190. Kerr JK, Skok RL, McLaughlin TF: Characteristics common to females who exhibit anorexic or bulimic behavior: A review of current literature. J Clin Psychol 47(6):846–853, 1991.
191. Rastam M: Anorexia nervosa in 51 Swedish adolescents: Premorbid problems and comorbidity. J Am Acad Child Adolesc Psychiatry 31(5):819–829, 1992.
192. Herzog DB, Keller MB, Sacks NR, et al: Psychiatric comorbidity in treatment-seeking anorexia and bulimics. J Am Acad Child Adolesc Psychiatry 31(5):810–818, 1992.
193. Enzmann DR, Lane B: Cranial computed tomography findings in anorexia nervosa. J Comput Assist Tomogr 4:410, 1977.
194. Heinz RE, Martinez J, Haenggeli A: Reversibility of cerebral atrophy in anorexia nervosa and Cushing's syndrome. J Comput Assist Tomogr 4:415, 1977.
195. Nussbaum M, Shenker IR, Marc J, Klein M: Cerebral atrophy in anorexia nervosa. J Pediatr 96:867–869, 1980.
196. Kohlmeyer K, Lehmkuhl G, Poutska F: Computed tomography of anorexia nervosa. AJNR 4:437–438, 1983.
197. Cooper PJ, Fairburn CG: The depressive symptoms of bulimia nervosa. Br J Psychiatry 148:268–274, 1986.
198. Swift WJ, Kalin NH, Wambolt FS, et al: Depression in bulimia at 2 to 5 years follow-up. Psychiatry Res 16:111–122, 1985.
199. Bryant-Waugh R, Knibbs J, Fosson A, et al: Long-term follow-up of patients with early onset anorexia nervosa. Arch Dis Child 63:5–9, 1988.
200. Comerci GD: Medical complications of anorexia nervosa and bulimia nervosa. Med Clin North Am 74(5):1293–1310, 1990.
201. Hsu LKG, Crisp AH, Callender JS: Psychiatric diagnoses in recovered and unrecovered anorectics 22 years after onset of illness: A pilot study. Compr Psychiatry 33(2):123–127, 1992.
202. Takei M, Nozoe S, Tanaka H, et al: Clinical features in anorexia nervosa lasting 10 years or more. Psychother Psychosom 52:140–145, 1989.
203. Crisp AH, Callender JS, Halek C, Hsu LKG: Long-term mortality in anorexia nervosa: A 20-year follow-up of the St. George's and Aberdeen cohorts. Br J Psychiatry 161:104–107, 1992.
204. Warren MP: Anorexia nervosa. In Kreiger DT, Bardin CW (eds): Current Therapy in Endocrinology. Toronto, BC Decker, 1985.
205. Halmi KA: Pragmatic information on the eating disorders. Psychiatr Clin North Am 5:371–377, 1982.
206. Anyan WR Jr, Schowalter JE: A comprehensive approach to anorexia nervosa. J Am Acad Child Psychiatry 2:122–127, 1983.
207. Warren MP: Anorexia, bulimia, and exercise-induced amenorrhea: Medical approach. In Bardin CW (eds): Current Therapy in Endocrinology and Metabolism (ed 4). Philadelphia, BC Decker, 1991, pp 12–16.
208. Rockwell WJ, Ellinwood EH Jr, Dougherty GG, Brodie HK: Anorexia nervosa: Review of current treatment practices. South Med J 75:1101–1107, 1982.
209. Johnson C, Stuckey M, Mitchell J: Psychopharmacological treatment of anorexia nervosa and bulimia. J Nerv Ment Dis 9:524–534, 1983.
210. Garner DM, Bemis KM: A cognitive-behavioral approach to anorexia nervosa. Cognitive Ther Res 2:123–151, 1982.
211. Halmi KA, Larson L: Behavior therapy in anorexia nervosa. In Feinstein SC, Giovacchini PL (eds): Adolescent Psychiatry, vol 5, New York, Jason Aronson, 1977, pp 323–351.
212. Walker J, Roberts SL, Halmi KA, Goldberg SC: Caloric requirements for weight gain in anorexia nervosa. Am J Clin Nutr 32:1396–1400, 1979.
213. Huse DA, Lucas AR: Dietary treatment of anorexia nervosa. J Am Diet Assoc 83:687–690, 1983.
214. Liebman R, Minuchin S, Baker L: An integrated treatment program for anorexia nervosa. Am J Psychiatry 4:431–436, 1974.
215. Kohmura H, Miyake A, Aono T, Tanizawa O: Recovery of reproductive function in patients with anorexia nervosa: a 10-year follow-up study. Eur J Obstet Gynecol Biol 22:293, 1986.
216. Hurley D, Brian R, Dutch K, et al: Induction of ovulation and fertility in amenorrheic women by pulsatile low-dose gonadotropin-releasing hormone. N Engl J Med 310:1069–1074, 1984.
217. Ayers JWT, Gidwant GP, Schmidt IMV, Gross M: Osteopenia in hypoestrogenic young women with anorexia nervosa. Fertil Steril 41:224–228, 1984.

218. Cann CE, Martin MC, Genant HK, Jaffe RB: Decreased spinal mineral content in amenorrheic women. JAMA 251:626–629, 1984.
219. Drinkwater BL, Nilson K, Chesnut CH, et al: Bone mineral content of amenorrheic and eumenorrheic athletes. N Engl J Med 311:277–281, 1984.
220. Linnell SK, Stager JM, Blue PW, et al: Bone mineral content and menstrual regularity in female runners. Med Sci Sports Exerc 16:343–348, 1984.
221. Lindberg JS, Fears WB, Hunt MM, et al: Exercise-induced amenorrhea and bone density. Ann Intern Med 101:647–648, 1984.
222. Marcus R, Cann C, Madvig P, et al: Menstrual function and bone mass in elite women distance runners: Endocrine and metabolic features. Ann Intern Med 102:158–163, 1985.
223. Athletic women, amenorrhea and skeletal integrity (editorial). Ann Intern Med 102:258–260, 1985.

146

Integrated Endocrine Responses and Exercise

HENRIK GALBO

REGULATION OF THE HORMONAL RESPONSE TO EXERCISE

The autonomic neuroendocrine system serves the coordination of the various functions of the body to allow coping with the physical challenges of life. In humans who perform severe exercise with big muscle groups, oxygen uptake may increase 14-fold due to increased metabolic rate in the working muscles. In these, arterioles and capillaries dilate and intra- and extracellular edema is formed. Cardiac output increases to about 20 L/min to meet the needs of the muscles. Some of the produced heat is accumulated in the body, and the core temperature may exceed 40°C. Most of the heat is removed by evaporation, however, and the sweat rate during exercise in hot and humid air may be 2 L/h. Potassium is released from contracting muscles, and the concentration in plasma may rise in response to maximum exercise to 8 mEq/L. It appears that in exercise there is a major need for substrate mobilization from energy stores, for cardiac stimulation and redistribution of fluid within the body, for diminution of renal fluid losses, and for counteracting electrolyte changes. Accordingly, the exercise-induced autonomic neuroendocrine changes are extensive and resemble those seen in hypoglycemia, early fasting, hyperthermia, and hemorrhage, i.e., including a decrease in plasma insulin as well as an increase in sympathetic nervous activity, insulin counterregulatory hormones, and hormones retaining sodium and water in the kidneys[1–4] (Table 146–1). Evidently, the various components of the hormonal response will react to different ex-

tents to the multiple perturbations in electrolyte and substrate levels, osmolality, temperature, distribution of blood flow, and intravascular pressures during exercise. Furthermore, these perturbations depend on the environment (e.g., ambient pressure and temperature) and the state of the organism prior to exercise (e.g., with regard to nutrition, physical fitness, age, disease, and menstrual cycle phase). Finally, the response to exercise of some hormones may have peculiar features regarding relationship to exercise intensity or time course during exercise of constant intensity. These facts have been carefully described previously[1–5] and will not be presented in detail here.

Here, emphasis will be on recent research that makes it possible to regard essential parts of the endocrine response to exercise as highly integrated. The research has pursued the unifying idea[1] that exercise offers a specific stimulus to the endocrine system consisting of nervous activity originating in motor centers and somatic afferent nerves from contracting muscle. This "feedforward" stimulus is determined by workload relative to the individual's maximum capacity rather than by absolute workload. It is, in contrast to traditional bloodborne feedback mechanisms, characteristic of exercise. In response to this "exercise factor" or specific exercise stress, changes in hormone secretion essential for homeostasis (e.g., controlling cardiovascular dynamics, fuel mobilization, and electrolyte transport) as well as changes merely reflecting that the system is stressed (e.g., increases in prolactin secretion) are elicited. Exercise-induced changes in hormone clearances are modest and only of major importance for the decrease in cortisol and gonadal hormone concentrations seen during mild exercise and for the increase in gonadal hormones seen during brief, heavy exercise.[1, 5–7]

The validity of the unifying hypothesis is so far not sufficiently evaluated for all components of the endocrine response to exercise. However, it is very attractive because it is based on the same fundamental regulatory principles that are thought to control circulatory, respiratory, and

TABLE 146–1. Important Changes in Plasma Hormone Concentrations During Prolonged Heavy Exercise

Decrease	Insulin
Increase	Norepinephrine, epinephrine, GH, ACTH, cortisol, glucagon, angiotensin, aldosterone, ADH

thermoregulatory responses in exercise.[8, 9] The fact that regulation of the major physiological systems during exercise can be fit into the same framework implies coherence in their responses to this condition.

Control by Feedforward Versus Traditional Feedback Mechanisms

Arguments Provided from Studies of Glucose Turnover in Exercise

It was long assumed that during exercise changes in plasma hormone concentrations and derived target cell functions were elicited entirely by feedback mechanisms. Feedback principles were well established in general endocrinology, and studies of glucose turnover in exercise seemed to indicate that these principles also were essential in exercise. Hepatic glucose production and muscular glucose uptake are well matched during exercise, and it was assumed that an increase in glucose metabolism was accompanied by a small decrease in plasma glucose concentration, which triggered an increase in glucose production.[2, 11]

The feedback theory was supported by some studies in which glucose was infused during exercise to mimic the increase in glucose production in control experiments. In humans[12] as well as in rats,[13] glucose infusion abolished the increase in endogenous glucose production during light exercise. Since the infusion was accompanied by an increase in plasma glucose of only a few milligrams per deciliter above levels seen without infusion and by no decrease in fat mobilization and muscle glycogenolysis, the experiments indicated that hepatic glucose production is very sensitive to feedback inhibition.

Also supporting the feedback theory for the exercise-induced increase in hepatic glucose production, some signals probably contributing to the stimulation of glucose production (e.g., epinephrine, glucagon, growth hormone, ACTH, cortisol) vary inversely with exogenous glucose administration and the plasma glucose concentration during exercise.[13–15] For example, after consuming a diet rich in fat, the exercise-induced decrease in glucose and increase in epinephrine and glucagon concentrations are more rapid than after consuming a diet rich in carbohydrate[15] (Fig. 146–1). Furthermore, when the plasma glucose concentrations are restored to preexercise levels by glucose infusion late during exercise in such conditions, concentrations of epinephrine and glucagon decrease markedly.[15]

Another approach to demonstrating the existence of feedback mechanisms has been to infuse phlorizin during exercise. Phlorizin causes a renal loss of glucose, resulting in an increased overall clearance of glucose. In experiments in which phlorizin was infused in rats in a dose lowering the plasma glucose level without causing hypoglycemia, a compensatory increase in glucose production and in plasma glucagon concentration in phlorizin compared to control experiments was found during light exercise.[16]

Interestingly, the metabolic feedback theory for the regulation of glucose production in exercise was analogous to the original theories concerning the regulation of cardiac output and ventilation in exercise. According to these theories, vasodilation and increased metabolism in muscle during exercise would result in a small decrease in blood

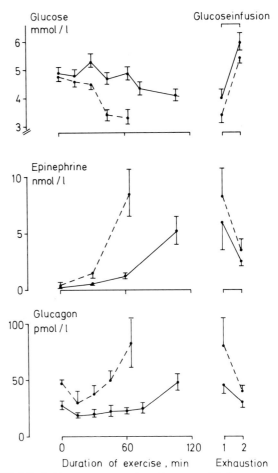

FIGURE 146–1. Plasma concentrations (mean ± SE) in seven subjects running at 70 per cent $\dot{V}O_{2,max}$ after having eaten a diet rich in carbohydrate (—) or fat (– –) for 4 days. At exhaustion, the subjects were encouraged to run for 10 min more while glucose was infused. (Modified with permission from H Galbo et al: The effect of different diets and of insulin on the hormonal response to prolonged exercise. Acta Physiol Scand 107:19–32, 1979.)

pressure and a small increase in arterial carbon dioxide tension, respectively, which, via arterial baro- and chemoreceptor feedback, would stimulate the heart and the respiratory muscles. However, the theory was not in accordance with the fact that during heavy exercise marked increases in cardiac output and ventilation are seen in the face of increased blood pressure and decreased arterial carbon dioxide tension. Now it is thought that exercise-specific feedforward stimulation from motor centers in the brain and stimulation by afferent nerve impulses directly from working muscles are the main determinants of heart rate and ventilation in exercise.[8, 9]

The metabolic feedback theory for the regulation of glucose production in exercise is also not in complete agreement with the behavior of the proposed error signal. Thus the plasma glucose concentration often does not tend to decrease during exercise. It may, in fact, increase, and this is more likely to happen at high-work-rate intensities, during which glucose production is also higher than during low-work-rate intensities.[17, 18] This indicates that increases in glucose production do not fall behind increases in glucose uptake. In accordance with this and using tracer methodology, it was found both in humans[19] and in rats[17] that in response to exercise a rapid increase in glucose production may precede a rise in glucose utilization, leading to an increase in plasma glucose concentration. Similarly, using catheterization techniques in dogs, a rapid and marked increase in net hepatic glucose production has been found early in exercise, long before arterial glucose concentration has decreased.[20]

It may be argued that rather than directly reflecting a decrease from the resting plasma glucose concentration, the metabolic error signal is intimately related to intramuscular glucose needs. Accordingly, even an increase in plasma glucose concentration could be hypothesized as necessary to allow a flux of glucose from muscle capillaries to sarcoplasma, which would meet the demand during exercise. It follows that intramuscular glucose deficiency should result in signals that enhance glucose production, and this might involve a resetting of glucoreceptors to respond at higher than basal glucose concentrations.[13]

Speaking against the possibility that intramuscular glycolytic deficiency triggers glucose production in exercise, glucose production increases from the onset of exercise, at which time intramuscular glycogen stores are plentiful. Furthermore, at high cycle-ergometer work rates, leg glucose uptake exceeds leg glucose utilization, and both glucose and glucose-6-phosphate and other glycolytic intermediates accumulate intramuscularly.[21]

Because the metabolic feedback theory did not sufficiently explain the regulation of glucose production in exercise, a theory including feedforward components was advanced, analogous to that accepted for regulation of cardiac output and ventilation in exercise.[1, 2] According to this hypothesis, from the onset of exercise, nervous impulses from motor centers in the brain as well as from the working muscles stimulate higher neuroendocrine centers to elicit a work-rate-dependent autonomic neuroendocrine signal that enhances glucose production. During continued exercise, feedback stimulation of glucose production may be added if the plasma glucose concentration declines. Since the proposed primary nervous mechanisms should be intimately coupled to exercise intensity rather than to a demand for the supply of extramuscular fuel, one would expect the exercise-induced increase in glucose production to be unaffected to some extent by exogenous glucose administration.

In agreement with this, at high work intensities in both the dog[22] and the rat,[13] overall glucose production is not diminished fully proportionally to the amount of glucose infused. Similarly, if rats exercising at a high intensity have glucose infused at a rate that is more than twice the rate of hepatic glycogenolysis in exercising control rats and which results in a dramatic increase in blood glucose, hepatic glycogen breakdown is only reduced by 40 per cent.[23] Further demonstrating the independence of metabolic feedback mechanisms, in rats exercising at more than a light intensity the increase in glucose production is identical whether plasma glucose (and accordingly the glucose supply to muscle) is lowered by phlorizin or not.[16]

According to the feedforward concept, the increase in glucose production in exercise is a primary event, and glucose is, so to speak, forced on the working muscles. The fact that during exercise in the fasting state (the condition most commonly studied) the plasma glucose concentration is often essentially unchanged from levels at rest must thus reflect that, in this nutritional state, the capacity to mobilize carbohydrate and accordingly the exercise-induced increase in glucose production, just by coincidence, matches the exercise-induced increase in glucose clearance. In agreement with this, in rats the increases in production and plasma concentration of glucose in response to exercise vary directly with the carbohydrate intake in the days prior to exercise.[24] Furthermore, supranormal hepatic glycogen levels achieved by a fasting/refeeding regimen are accompanied by exaggerated increases in the production and plasma concentration of glucose.[25]

When liver glycogen is low, gluconeogenesis contributes much more to the exercise-induced glucose production than when it is high.[24] Dietary experiments have underlined the role of muscle glycogen in the production of the major gluconeogenic substrate in exercise, lactate, and it has been pointed out that not only hepatic glycogen phosphorylase but also muscle glycogen phosphorylase is flux generating for glycolysis from glucose in muscle.[24] In this context, it is interesting to note that at a given rate of muscle contractions, muscle glycogen breakdown and lactate release vary directly with the preexercise glycogen concentration, glycogenolysis being subject to feedforward regulation and not accurately adjusted to fuel needs.[26] Furthermore, epinephrine enhances glycogen breakdown in working muscle by increasing glycogen phosphorylase a activity and decreasing glycogen synthase activity.[1, 17]

An increase in glucose uptake in muscle consequent to an increased glucose supply is only possible if the membrane transport of glucose is not overtaxed. This claim is fulfilled, since the Michaelis constant for glucose transport in exercised muscle is 5 to 17 mmol/L, depending on fiber type,[27] and because the $\dot{V}_{max}$ for glucose transport is increased by contractions.[27, 28] That glucose delivery is very important for glucose uptake in contracting muscle has been demonstrated most clearly in perfused preparations in which the composition of the perfusate is controlled.[29] This is in accord with the recent finding in humans that the addition of arm exercise increases both glucose delivery and glucose uptake in exercising legs.[30]

The view that glucose delivery is not accurately matched to glucose utilization by feedback mechanisms, but rather is forced on the working muscles, is supported by the finding that during maximal exercise, glucose delivery peaks, whereas glucose utilization in muscle (despite marked intracellular glucose accumulation) actually decreases compared with findings during submaximal exercise.[21] Furthermore, it has been shown that during exercise, the glucose produced in the liver may be subjected to futile cycling, becoming incorporated into glycogen in working muscle.[31]

Arguments Provided from Studies Interfering with the Putative "Exercise Stimulus"

The time course of hormonal changes during exercise and in the postexercise period, at the start of which activity in motor centers within the central nervous system and the flow of impulses from mechanoreceptors suddenly cease, indicates that the regulation of the autonomic neuroendocrine response to exercise has a fast nervous component.[32] In humans, the most direct evidence favoring an immediate activation of neuroendocrine centers from motor centers in the brain ("central command") comes from studies involving partial neuromuscular blockade with tubocurarine.[33, 34] Tubocurarine weakens the muscles and probably makes a higher motor center activity necessary to sustain a given absolute work rate. In agreement with this, subjects in experiments with blockade had a higher perceived exertion at the same absolute oxygen uptake than did those without blockade. Despite identical "metabolic needs," the augmented motor center activity during curarization was accompanied by exaggerated responses of catecholamines and of the pituitary hormones growth hormone (GH) and ACTH, indicating that motor center activity induces the neuroendocrine changes rather directly (Fig. 146–2). The exaggerated hormonal changes in tubocurarine compared with control experiments were accompanied by a more rapid increase in hepatic glucose production and enhanced lipolysis.[34] Arguments were given against a major role of emotional stress in these experiments, but psychological factors can never be excluded in conscious subjects. However, a direct neural interpretation of the findings is supported by the fact that in paralyzed, decorticated cats, electrical stimulation of subthalamic motor centers elicits a hormonal response similar to that seen during exercise (Fig. 146–3), with an accompanying increase in glucose production.[35]

In humans, experiments with tubocurarine also have lent support to the view that afferent nervous activity may enhance the hormonal response to exercise. During maximal effort, the activity of the relevant motor centers is probably maximal and, accordingly, is identical in experi-

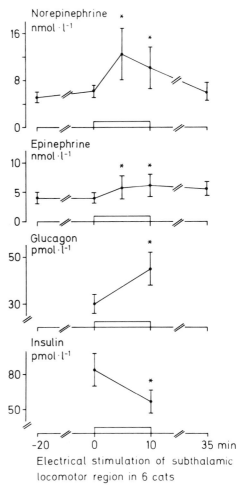

FIGURE 146–3. Plasma concentrations of four hormones (±SE) measured in decorticated cats paralyzed by neuromuscular blockade. (Modified with permission from Vissing J et al: Mobilization of glucoregulatory hormones and glucose by hypothalamic locomotor centers. Am J Physiol 257:E722–728, 1989.)

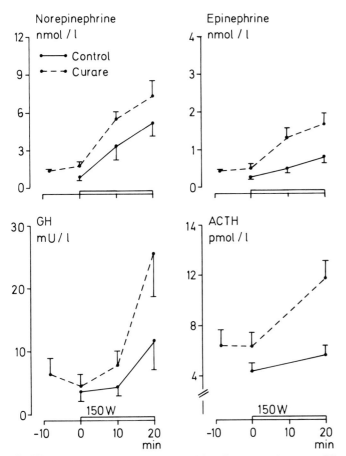

FIGURE 146–2. Plasma concentrations of four hormones (mean ± SE) during semisupine cycle exercise in seven subjects studied with or without partial neuromuscular blockade. (Modified with permission from M Kjaer et al: Role of motor center activity for hormonal changes and substrate mobilization in humans. Am J Physiol 253:R687–695, 1987.)

ments with and without partial neuromuscular blockade, but concentrations of catecholamines, GH, and β-endorphin in plasma are higher in the experiments without blockade (in which work rate, oxygen uptake, and probably afferent nervous activity are much larger than in experiments with motor blockade).[34] Furthermore, during the fading of neuromuscular blockade, maximal effort was accompanied by a gradually increasing work intensity and oxygen uptake, and in parallel with this, catecholamine levels increased.[33] Differences between these experiments could not be ascribed to the influence of blood-borne factors.

More direct evidence favoring an influence of afferent nervous feedback from working muscle on the hormonal response to exercise has come from studies using epidural anesthesia of the thin afferent nerve fibers from the lower body. Compared with control experiments, responses of ACTH and β-endorphin were diminished during submaximal cycle ergometer exercise (Fig. 146–4), and during static exercise, diminished catecholamine responses were seen.[36, 37] Since some reduction in muscle strength cannot be avoided during epidural anesthesia, a compensatory increase in motor center activity may have enhanced hormone secretion and blurred more extensive inhibitory ef-

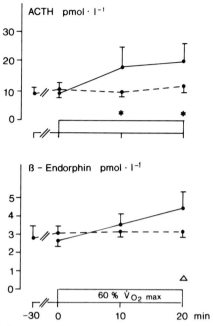

FIGURE 146–4. Plasma concentrations of ACTH and β-endorphin (mean ± SE) in six subjects during semisupine cycle exercise with (– –) or without (—) epidural blockade at the level of vertebrae L3–L4. (Modified with permission from M Kjaer et al: Hormonal and metabolic responses to exercise in humans: Effect of sensory nervous blockade. Am J Physiol 257:E95–101, 1989.)

the patients could not be explained by blood-borne feedback. However, although the exaggerated hormonal responses and substrate mobilization could be abolished by glucose infusion,[40] it is still possible that the difference in response to exercise between patients and controls was due directly to a difference in motor center activity or reflected a difference in afferent nerve activity in consequence of different fiber recruitment rather than of different substrate needs.

Endocrine Changes in Exercise

As is the case for glucoregulatory hormones, changes in ordinary feedback stimuli (i.e., osmolality and blood pressures) far from fully explain the exercise-induced changes in renin and antidiuretic hormone (ADH) secretion.[42, 43] Furthermore, renal sympathetic nerve activity stimulates renin release in exercise.[44] Accordingly, available evidence indicates that the hormonal response to exercise is regulated as follows:[1–3] At the onset of exercise, nervous impulses from motor centers in the brain and from working muscles elicit a work-rate–dependent increase in sympathoadrenal activity and in the release of some pituitary hormones (e.g., GH, ACTH, β-endorphin, prolactin,[2, 3] ADH, and possibly thyroid-stimulating hormone [TSH][2, 3]). These responses control the changes in secretion of subordinate endocrine cells: Sympathoadrenal activity depresses insulin secretion by alpha-receptor–mediated mechanisms,[41] and it also stimulates the renin-angiotensin-ADH system and the release of pancreatic polypeptide (PP) by beta-receptor mechanisms. Erythropoietin secretion also

fects on the exercise responses. Furthermore, one cannot be sure that a complete blockade of all relevant afferent nerve fibers was achieved. These difficulties were circumvented in recent studies of the impact of both central command and afferent muscle nerve activity (Kjaer and Galbo, unpublished material). Healthy subjects carried out bicycle exercise by functional electrical stimulation of their leg muscles during simultaneous lower body epidural anesthesia. The anesthesia was marked, as judged from the fact that voluntary leg raising was abolished. In contrast to voluntary exercise without anesthesia, insulin levels did not decrease during electrical stimulation, a fact indicating the importance of somatic nerve activity for splanchnic sympathetic activity.

In studies with epidural anesthesia, it is difficult to exclude effects of circulating anesthetic. However, in support of a role of neural feedback from working muscle, it has been demonstrated in rats that static muscle contraction, evoked by low-intensity electrical stimulation of the tibial nerve, elicits a reflex increase in adrenal sympathetic nerve activity.[38] Furthermore, electrical stimulation of muscle afferents in the femoral nerves of anesthetized and paralyzed cats increases glucose production and glucose, ACTH, β-endorphin, and metenkephalin concentrations and decreases insulin concentrations[39] (Fig. 146–5). These animal experiments are compatible with roles of afferent nerve activity from both mechano- and chemoreceptors in muscle.[38, 39] Pointing at neural feedback related to metabolism in working muscle, higher increases during exercise in concentrations of catecholamines, GH, ACTH, cortisol, glycerol, and free fatty acids and in glucose production and a greater decrease in plasma insulin are seen in McArdle patients with impaired muscle glycogenolysis compared with healthy subjects.[40] The higher hormonal response in

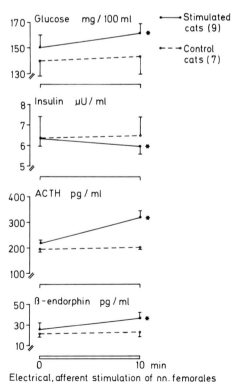

FIGURE 146–5. Plasma concentrations of three hormones and glucose (±SE) in anesthetized cats in which the central parts of the cut femoral nerves were stimulated to mimic the afferent activity anticipated during running. (From J Vissing, H Galbo, and JH Mitchell, unpublished data.)

may be stimulated by sympathoadrenal activity.[45, 46] ACTH stimulates the adrenal cortical secretion of cortisol.

The fast nervous mechanisms related to motor activity operate throughout exercise, but the hormonal responses may be gradually intensified due to a feedback from metabolic error signals (among which a decrease in glucose availability is the most important) (see Fig. 146–1), as well as from nonmetabolic error signals sensed by pressure, volume, osmolality, electrolyte, and temperature receptors.[1–3, 14, 47, 48] At high work rates, feedforward control from motor centers and working muscle, intimately related to contractile activity, dominates. At low exercise intensities, such as at rest, a feedback regulation secondary to changes in the internal milieu dominates the hormonal changes, and at least in humans, an increase in plasma glucagon concentration is always predominantly determined by a decrease in glucose availability.[1, 14, 48] The primary setting of the hormonal response to exercise depends on the state of the organism with respect to training, nutrition, hydration, phase of menstrual cycle, and state of health.[1–4, 47, 49–53] The hormonal response is more closely related to work rate expressed relative to actual work capacity ($\%\dot{V}_{O_{2,max}}$) than to absolute work rate.[1–3, 53]

Probably due to parallel changes in atrial filling pressure, the concentration of atrial natriuretic peptide (ANP) increases during exercise and may decrease afterward.[45, 49, 54] In humans, the secretion of gonadotropins is not influenced by acute exercise, and increases in the concentrations of gonadal hormones are due to decreases in plasma volume and hormone clearance.[3, 4] After long-term exercise, the plasma testosterone concentration may be lower than before exercise. This probably reflects a reduced secretion rate, the cause of which is unknown.[3, 4] During graded short-term exercise, the plasma calcium ion activity increases due to decreasing pH; this, in turn, may (as expected from known feedback relationships) stimulate the secretion of calcitonin and suppress the secretion of parathyroid hormone (PTH).[55] Similarly, during prolonged low-intensity exercise, a decrease in ionized calcium is accompanied by an increase in PTH.[56] Exercise also may elicit an increase in plasma concentrations of many putative hormones and neurotransmitters found in endocrine cells in the gastrointestinal tract and elsewhere in the body, including the central nervous system [e.g., vasoactive intestinal polypeptide (VIP), peptide histidine isoleucine amide (PHI), somatostatin (SRIF), secretin, substance P, and gastrin].[57] We know neither the exact origin of these substances nor the stimuli for their release in exercise or their role during physical activity.[1, 3, 4]

EFFECTS OF THE HORMONAL RESPONSE TO EXERCISE

Cardiovascular System, Water and Electrolyte Balance

The rapid onset of autonomic neuroendocrine changes in response to exercise implies that the needs for endocrine adjustments are, so to speak, anticipated. Sympathetic nervous activity is important to cardiovascular adaptation and thermoregulation in exercise.[1, 3, 8] Cardiac output is enhanced, and blood volume and flow are redistributed in favor of skin and working muscle. Sweat production is increased. Although studies involving experimental manipulations with the actual hormones are lacking, it is reasonable to assume that during exercise renal sodium and water excretion is restricted by angiotensin, aldosterone, and ADH as well as by direct effects of sympathetic activity in the kidneys.[1, 3] Furthermore, adrenergic activity and aldosterone secretion also counteract the tendency to hyperkalemia in exercise. During training, the increases in aldosterone and ADH induced by each exercise bout contribute to expansion of the extracellular volume, while increases in erythropoietin are responsible for increases in red blood cell mass.[1, 45, 46, 54]

Metabolism

Glucose Turnover

The overall hormonal response to exercise appears to be geared to stimulation of hepatic glucose production. However, which components are the more important, particularly in humans[45] is not clear. A decrease in plasma insulin concentration is always essential, glucose production during exercise varying inversely with modest artificial changes in insulin levels.[1, 45, 58] In rats[1, 17] and dogs,[45, 59] the exercise-induced increases in glucagon and epinephrine concentrations are major determinants of the increase in glucose production. Furthermore, the potency of the rise in glucagon has been shown to be enhanced by the accompanying fall in insulin.[60] On the other hand, both in these species and in humans, sympathetic liver nerves do not influence glucose production in exercise.[17, 45, 58] Strange to say, neither epinephrine[58] nor glucagon[1] seems to be major stimuli in humans. In humans, arterial glucagon does not increase above basal levels until after more than 1 hour of submaximal exercise, and it even decreases markedly during maximal exercise, when glucose production peaks.[1]

It may seem surprising that during exercise the glucose uptake in muscle varies inversely with the rate of secretion and the plasma concentration of insulin.[1] However, muscle contractions per se enhance muscle glucose uptake by mechanisms that are independent of insulin.[61] In isolated skeletal muscle, contractions are a more powerful stimulus to glucose transport than insulin, and the two stimuli are fully additive.[26, 27] This indicates that contractions and insulin enhance glucose transport at least partly by differing mechanisms. However, the protein mediating the membrane transport is believed to be the same for the two stimuli.[62]

During exercise, the decrease in plasma insulin curbs glucose uptake in muscle, and the same is true for the increase in plasma epinephrine.[1] The effect is due to the direct actions of hormonal changes on glucose transport as well as to the inhibition of hexokinase by glucose-6-phosphate accumulating secondary to an enhancement of both glycogen breakdown[1, 17, 26, 45] and intracellular availability of FFA.[1, 17, 26, 45]

Lipolysis

A decrease in the plasma insulin concentration and an increase in sympathoadrenal activity are probably the major determinants of lipolysis during exercise. Thus various indices of lipolysis vary directly with these neurohormonal changes, both under physiological conditions and during experiments in which the changes are artificially exaggerated or counteracted.[1, 45] Interestingly, fat and muscle cell lipolysis seem to be regulated by the same enzyme, the hormone-sensitive lipase, and to be enhanced by the same hormonal changes.[1, 45] During prolonged exercise, the responsiveness of the fat cells to catecholamines increases.[45] The relative importance of circulating catecholamines and sympathetic nervous activity for lipolysis in exercise has not been clarified. However, adrenergic activity is exerted by local beta-receptor mechanisms.[1, 45] Other hormones than those mentioned also may influence lipolysis, but they have not been studied thoroughly. However, neither changes in plasma glucagon nor in hormones from the pituitary or subordinate glands are indispensable for exercise-induced lipolysis.

Essential Features of the Hormonal Interference with Exercise Metabolism

The following characteristics are essential for an understanding of substrate metabolism in exercise:[1, 2, 45]

1. The hormonal response to exercise is essentially indiscriminate, promoting mobilization of both glycogen and triglyceride from extra- as well as intramuscular stores. Breakdown of the latter is further enhanced directly by contractions. The quantity of fuel mobilized from the different stores depends not only on the hormonal response and contractile activity but also on the size of the fuel depots, the state of hormone receptors, and the capacity of the enzymes involved in these depots. Normally, protein is not an important fuel during exercise.

2. The different intra- and extramuscular energy stores can substitute for each other. The uptake of blood-borne substrates depends in part on mass effects, extra- and intramuscular fuels being burned in competition with each other. Mobilization of intramuscular fuel is not called on simply when the delivery of exogenous fuel is insufficient. The final choice of fuel depends on the availability of substrates and on the capacity of the metabolizing, energy-yielding enzymatic pathways.

3. During exercise of a fixed intensity, the state of the organism before the studied moment of exercise influences the induced hormonal changes, the sensitivity of fuel depots to stimulation, and the capacity of the recruited muscle fibers to metabolize the different substrates.

4. While feedback mechanisms directly coupled to metabolic needs are characteristic at rest, during exercise the mobilization of both extra- and intramuscular fuel is regulated in part by feedforward mechanisms that are intimately related to contractile activity.

5. Mobilization of extra- and intramuscular fuel is neither accurately nor optimally matched to the energy demands of the contractile machinery. Exact regulation would hardly be compatible with the preceding four characteristics. Nor would it be compatible with the fact that, during exercise, changes in plasma levels of hormones influencing metabolism are not geared exclusively to metabolic needs but are also adjusted to control the circulation, the volume and osmolality of body fluids, and the body temperature. In fact, the mobilization of energy sources

during exercise may exceed energy expenditure, some of the mobilized fuel being accumulated extracellularly or stored in intra- or extramuscular depots. Nevertheless, fuel mobilization also may be suboptimal, limiting performance at a time when triglyceride stores are plentiful.

TRAINING-INDUCED ADAPTATIONS

Target Cell Responses

Endurance training enhances catecholamine-stimulated fat cell lipolysis.[45] This is not due to altered receptor binding but rather reflects an attenuated inhibition of adenylate cyclase as well as an enhanced responsiveness to cAMP.[45, 63] Conversely, the suppressant action of insulin on lipolysis is enhanced in trained subjects.[64, 65] Furthermore, the replenishment of fat cell triglyceride stores between exercise bouts is facilitated by an enhanced insulin-mediated glucose transport.[45] This reflects the fact that training increases the number of recruitable GLUT-4 glucose transporters in fat cells.[66] In trained subjects, both the sensitivity of hepatic glucose-producing mechanisms to stimulation by catecholamines[45] and insulin-mediated inhibition of glucose production[65] are enhanced. Insulin-mediated stimulation of whole-body glucose disposal is also higher in trained than in untrained subjects.[65] This is predominantly due to an increase in GLUT-4 protein in trained muscle.[67]

Endocrine Responses

Training diminishes the hormonal response at a given work rate[1-3, 53] (Fig. 146–6). This may reflect the fact that the signals influencing autonomic neuroendocrine activity

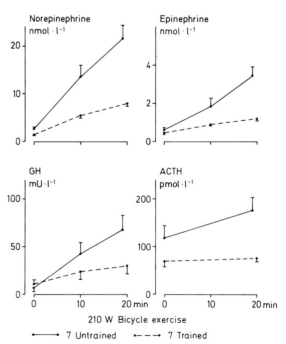

FIGURE 146–6. The response to exercise of plasma hormone concentrations ($\pm$SE) in trained and untrained men. (Modified with permission from M Kjaer et al: Hormonal response to exercise in humans: Influence of hypoxia and physical training. Am J Physiol 254:R197–203, 1988.)

are modified during training. However, training also may change the secretory capacity of the endocrine glands. An augmented adrenal medullary secretory capacity is found in elite athletes who have performed endurance training for several years.[68] In contrast, training diminishes the capacity to secrete insulin.[69, 70] This is justified by the smaller need for insulin to handle a given carbohydrate load in target tissues.[65] Interestingly, studies of bed rest have confirmed that pancreatic beta cell function is inversely and insulin effect directly related to the level of daily physical activity.[45] The training-induced adaptations within the beta cells and insulin target cells have been thought beneficial to health by reducing the strain on the beta cells as well as plasma glucose and insulin levels. However, these effects are to a large extent offset by the fact that training necessitates an increased food intake.[64, 72]

Aerobic training can cause all sorts of menstrual irregularities, including delayed menarche, oligomenorrhea, and primary and secondary amenorrhea.[1, 3, 5, 72, 73] Corresponding to the variation in menstrual function from normal to amenorrhea, in training women, plasma sex hormone levels may vary from normal to low levels reflecting hypothalamic hypogonadotropism (decreased levels of follicle-stimulating hormone, luteinizing hormone, estradiol, and progesterone).[3, 74] Even if athletes have regular menstrual cycles of normal length, detailed analysis may reveal an abnormality consisting in luteal phase shortening and reduced progesterone secretion.[72, 75] Essential for training-induced defects in gonad function is probably impairment of the hypothalamic gonadotropin-releasing hormone (GnRH) pulse generator resulting in reduced frequency and regularity in pulsatile luteinizing hormone release.[75] This phenomenon has been demonstrated in both female and male athletes.[76] Correspondingly, the finding of reduced testosterone levels and spermatogenesis in some intensely training males[5, 76] parallels the hypogonadism seen in female athletes.

Menstrual irregularities correlate positively with amount of training and are seen particularly in girls with late menarche and in girls who start training prior to menarche.[1, 3, 5, 73, 76] Putative pathophysiological mechanisms involved in exercise-induced reproductive dysfunction have been explored intensively. It may be concluded that inadequate fatness, psychological factors, hyperandrogenism, hyperprolactinemia, and increased secretion of β-endorphin are not of major significance.[1, 3, 5, 73, 75, 76] Hypothetically, repeated direct influence of nervous activity from motor centers and contracting muscle may cause hypothalamic adaptations. Alternatively, this "exercise factor" may act indirectly by increasing cortisol levels over the day or by causing a "low-energy state," at which energy balance is maintained at the lowest possible energy intake.[74-76] While the above-mentioned responses to training appear immediately meaningful, this is not the case for the adaptations within the reproductive system. The latter imply reduced fertility and, secondary to loss of bone, an increased risk of fractures.[73, 77] The hypogonadism is only appropriate in the sense that a very high daily physical activity level may not be compatible with pregnancy and maternal care. While exercise-induced menstrual irregularities are completely reversible upon reduction in amount of training,[1, 3, 72, 73] this may not be so for hypogonadotropic bone losses.[73]

EXERCISE IN DIABETES

Type I diabetics always balance between taking either too little insulin and developing hyperglycemia and ketosis or too much insulin and developing hypoglycemia. However, exercise aggravates the problem. The tendency toward hyperglycemia and ketosis is enhanced by the exercise-induced increase in counterregulatory hormones, and this increase, as well as its effects, is even exaggerated in insulin deficiency.[51] On the other hand, hypoglycemia is favored by the fact that insulin absorption from the subcutis may be enhanced.[51, 52] Furthermore, the effect of insulin on glucose uptake in muscle may be enhanced in exercise compared with rest because muscle blood flow and, in turn, glucose delivery are increased, and because the indirect effect via inhibition of fat cell lipolysis may be augmented because lipolysis is accelerated.[51, 52] Also, the depressing effect of insulin on glucose production will be more marked in exercise when glucose production is increased. Exercise is less likely to cause metabolic problems in Type II diabetics. Interestingly, however, in response to exercise, these patients also may experience an exaggerated counterregulatory hormonal response and ensuing increase in plasma glucose[78] as well as a marked decrease in glucose, which will be enhanced by drug-induced stimulation of insulin secretion.[52] In both Type I and Type II diabetics, the occurrence of long-term complications represents a further obstacle to exercise.[51, 52, 79] The benefits diabetics can obtain from exercise are physiological, medical, psychological, and social.[45, 52] However, Type I diabetics should not expect improved metabolic control during training, and Type II diabetics, only if they achieve a considerable weight loss by restricted calorie intake.[51, 52]

REFERENCES

1. Galbo H: Hormonal and Metabolic Adaptation to Exercise. New York, Thieme-Stratton, 1983.
2. Galbo H: The hormonal response to exercise. Proc Nutr Soc 44:257–266, 1985.
3. Galbo H: Autonomic neuroendocrine responses to exercise. Scand J Sports Sci 8:3–17, 1986.
4. Galbo H: The hormonal response to exercise. Diabetes Metab Rev 1:385–408, 1986.
5. Sutton JR, Farrell PA, Harber VJ: Hormonal adaptation to physical activity. In Bouchard C, Shephard RJ, Stephens T, et al (eds): Exercise, Fitness, and Health. Champaign, IL, Human Kinetics Books, 1990, pp 217–257.
6. Montagnani CF, Arena B, Maffulli N: Estradiol and progesterone during exercise in healthy untrained women. Med Sci Sports Exerc 24:764–768, 1992.
7. Kjær M, Christensen NJ, Sonne B, et al: Effect of exercise on epinephrine turnover in trained and untrained male subjects. J Appl Physiol 59:1061–1067, 1985.
8. Rowell LB: Human Circulation: Regulation during Physical Stress. New York, Oxford University Press, 1986.
9. Dempsey JA, Henke KG, Aaron EA: Pulmonary physiology: Feedback and feed-forward mechanisms. In Skinner JS, Corbin CB, Landers DM, et al (eds.) Future Directions in Exercise and Sports Science Research. Champaign, IL, Human Kinetics Books, 1989, pp 313–337.
10. Issekutz B: Energy mobilization in exercising dogs. Diabetes 28:39–44, 1979.
11. Vranic M, Berger M: Exercise and diabetes mellitus. Diabetes 28:147–163, 1979.
12. Jenkins AB, Chisholm DE, James DE, et al: Exercise-induced hepatic glucose output is precisely sensitive to the rate of systemic glucose supply. Metabolism 34:431–436, 1985.

13. Vissing J, Sonne B, Galbo H: Regulation of hepatic glucose production in running rats studied by glucose infusion. J Appl Physiol 65:2552–2557, 1988.

14. Tabata I, Atomi Y, Miyashita M: Blood glucose concentration dependent ACTH and cortisol responses to prolonged exercise. Clin Physiol 4:299–307, 1984.

15. Galbo H, Holst JJ, Christensen NJ: The effect of different diets and of insulin on the hormonal response to prolonged exercise. Acta Physiol Scand 107:19–32, 1979.

16. Vissing J, Sonne B, Galbo H: Role of metabolic feedback regulation in glucose production of running rats. Am J Physiol 255:R400–406, 1988.

17. Sonne B, Galbo H: Carbohydrate metabolism during and after exercise in rats: Studies with radioglucose. J Appl Physiol 59:1627–1639, 1985.

18. Wahren J, Felig P, Ahlborg G, Jorfeldt L: Glucose metabolism during leg exercise in man. J Clin Invest 50:2715–2725, 1971.

19. Kjær M, Farrell PA, Christensen NJ, Galbo H: Increased epinephrine response and inaccurate glucoregulation in exercising athletes. J Appl Physiol 61:1693–1700, 1986.

20. Wasserman DH, Lacy DB, Green DR, et al: Dynamics of hepatic lactate and glucose balances during prolonged exercise and recovery in the dog. J Appl Physiol 63:2411–2417, 1987.

21. Katz A, Broberg S, Sahlin K, Wahren J: Leg glucose uptake during maximal dynamic exercise in humans. Am J Physiol 251:E65–70, 1986.

22. Issekutz B: Effects of glucose infusion on hepatic and muscle glycogenolysis in exercising dogs. Am J Physiol 240:E451–457, 1981.

23. Winder WW, Arogyasami J, Yang HT, et al: Effects of glucose infusion in exercising rats. J Appl Physiol 64:2300–2305, 1988.

24. Sonne B, Mikines KJ, Galbo H: Glucose turnover in 48-hour-fasted running rats. Am J Physiol 252:R587–593, 1987.

25. Vissing J, Wallace JL, Galbo H: Effect of liver glycogen content on glucose production in running rats. J Appl Physiol 66:318–322, 1989.

26. Richter EA, Galbo H: High glycogen levels enhance glycogen breakdown in isolated contracting skeletal muscle. J Appl Physiol 61:827–831, 1986.

27. Ploug T, Galbo H, Vinten J, et al: Kinetics of glucose transport in rat muscle: Effects of insulin and contractions. Am J Physiol 253:E12–20, 1987.

28. Ploug T, Galbo H, Ohkuwa T, et al: Kinetics of glucose transport in rat skeletal muscle membrane vesicles: effects of insulin and contractions. Am J Physiol 262:E700–711, 1992.

29. Schultz TA, Lewis SB, Westbie DK, et al: Glucose delivery: A modulator of glucose uptake in contracting skeletal muscle. Am J Physiol 233:E514–518, 1977.

30. Kjær M, Kiens B, Hargreaves M, Richter EA: Influence of active muscle mass on glucose homeostasis during exercise in humans. J Appl Physiol 71:552–557, 1991.

31. Sonne B, Galbo H: Carbohydrate metabolism in fructose-fed and food-restricted running rats. J Appl Physiol 61:1457–1466, 1986.

32. Galbo H, Gollnick PD: Hormonal changes during and after exercise. In Jokl E, Hebbelinck M (eds): Medicine and Sport Science, vol 17. Basel, Karger, 1984, pp 97–110.

33. Galbo H, Kjær M, Secher NH: Cardiovascular, ventilatory and catecholamine responses to maximal dynamic exercise in partially curarized man. J Physiol 389:557–568, 1987.

34. Kjær M, Secher NH, Bach FW, Galbo H: Role of motor center activity for hormonal changes and substrate mobilization in humans. Am J Physiol 253:R687–695, 1987.

35. Vissing J, Iwamoto GA, Rybicki KJ, et al: Mobilization of glucoregulatory hormones and glucose by hypothalamic locomotor centers. Am J Physiol 257:E722–728, 1989.

36. Kjær M, Secher NH, Bach FW, et al: Hormonal and metabolic responses to exercise in humans: Effect of sensory nervous blockade. Am J Physiol 257:E95–101, 1989.

37. Kjær M, Secher NH, Bach FW, et al: Hormonal metabolic, and cardiovascular responses to static exercise in humans: Influence of epidural anesthesia. Am J Physiol 261:E214–220, 1991.

38. Vissing J, Wilson LB, Mitchell JH, Victor RG: Static muscle contraction reflexly increases adrenal sympathetic nerve activity in rats. Am J Physiol 261:R1307–1312, 1991.

39. Vissing J, Iwamoto GA, Fuchs IE, et al: Reflex control of glucoregulatory exercise responses by group III and IV muscle afferents. Am J Physiol, in press.

40. Vissing J, Lewis SF, Galbo H, Haller RG: Effect of deficient muscular glycogenolysis on extramuscular fuel production in exercise. J Appl Physiol 72:1773–1779, 1992.

41. Galbo H, Christensen NJ, Holst JJ: Catecholamines and pancreatic hormones during autonomic blockade in exercising man. Acta Physiol Scand 101:428–437, 1977.

42. Gleim GW, Zabetakis PM, De Pasquale EE, et al: Plasma osmolality, volume, and renin activity at the "anaerobic threshold." J Appl Physiol 56:57–63, 1984.

43. Wade CE: Response, regulation, and actions of vasopressin during exercise: A review. Med Sci Sports Exerc 16:506–511, 1984.

44. Zambraski EJ, Tucker MS, Lakas CS, et al: Mechanism of renin release in exercising dog. Am J Physiol 246:E71–76, 1984.

45. Galbo H: Exercise physiology: Humoral function. Sport Sci Rev 1:65–93, 1992.

46. Schwandt H-J, Heyduck B, Gunga H-C, Röcker L: Influence of prolonged physical exercise on the erythropoietin concentration in blood. Eur J Appl Physiol 63:463–466, 1991.

47. Brandenberger G, Candas V, Follenius M, Kahn JM: The influence of the initial state of hydration on endocrine responses to exercise in the heat. Eur J Appl Physiol 58:674–679, 1989.

48. Sotsky MJ, Shilo S, Shamoon H: Regulation of counterregulatory hormone secretion in man during exercise and hypoglycemia. J Clin Endocrinol Metab 68:9–16, 1989.

49. Richards AM, Tonolo G, Cleland JGF, et al: Plasma atrial natriuretic peptide concentrations during exercise in sodium replete and deplete normal man. Clin Sci 72:159–164, 1987.

50. Viinamäki O: The effect of hydration status on plasma vasopressin release during physical exercise in man. Acta Physiol Scand 139:133–137, 1990.

51. Galbo H: Exercise and diabetes. Scand J Sports Sci 10:89–95, 1988.

52. Galbo H, von Linstow M, Dela F, et al: Exercise and diabetes. Med Sport Sci 37:227–236, 1992.

53. Kjær M, Bangsbo J, Lortie G, Galbo H: Hormonal response to exercise in humans: Influence of hypoxia and physical training. Am J Physiol 254:R197–203, 1988.

54. Fellmann N, Bedu M, Giry J, et al: Hormonal, fluid, and electrolyte changes during a 72-h recovery from a 24-h endurance run. Int J Sports Med 10:406–412, 1989.

55. Aloia J, Rasulo P, Deftos J, et al: Exercise-induced hypercalcemia and the calciotropic hormones. J Lab Clin Med 106:229–232, 1985.

56. Ljunghall S, Joborn H, Roxin LE, et al: Prolonged low intensity exercise raises the serum parathyroid hormone levels. Clin Endocrinol 25:535–542, 1986.

57. Galbo H, Kjær M, Mikines KJ: Neurohormonal system. In Skinner JS, Corbin CB, Landers DM, et al (eds): Future Directions in Exercise and Sport Science Research. Champaign, IL, Human Kinetics Books, 1989, pp 329–345.

58. Kjær M, Engfred K, Fernandes A, et al: Regulation of hepatic glucose production during exercise in man: Role of sympathoadrenergic activity. Am J Physiol 265:E275–E283, 1993.

59. Moates JM, Lacy DB, Goldstein RE, et al: Metabolic role of the exercise-induced increment in epinephrine in the dog. Am J Physiol 255:E428–436, 1988.

60. Wasserman DH, Spalding JA, Lacy DB, et al: Glucagon is a primary controller of hepatic glycogenolysis and gluconeogenesis during muscular work. Am J Physiol 257:E108–117, 1989.

61. Ploug T, Stallknecht BM, Pedersen O, et al: Effect of endurance training on glucose transport capacity and glucose transporter expression in rat skeletal muscle. Am J Physiol 259:E778–786, 1990.

62. Henriksen EJ, Bourey RE, Rodnick KJ, et al: Glucose transporter protein content and glucose transport capacity in rat skeletal muscles. Am J Physiol 259:E593–598, 1990.

63. Izawa T, Kombabayashi T, Shinoda S, et al: Possible mechanism of regulating adenylate cyclase activity in adipocyte membranes from exercise-trained male rats. Biochem Biophys Res Commun 151:1262–1268, 1988.

64. Dela F, Mikines KJ, von Linstow M, Galbo H: Effect of training on response to a glucose load adjusted for daily carbohydrate intake. Am J Physiol 260:E14–20, 1991.

65. Mikines KJ, Sonne B, Farrell PA, et al: Effect of training on the dose-response relationship for insulin action in men. J Appl Physiol 66:695–703, 1989.

66. Stallknecht B, Andersen PH, Vinten J, et al: Effect of physical training on glucose transporter protein and mRNA levels in rat adipocytes. Am J Physiol 265:E128–E134, 1993.

67. Dela F, Handberg A, Mikines KJ, et al: GLUT-4 and insulin receptor binding and kinase activity in trained human muscle. J Physiol 469:615–624, 1993.

68. Kjær M, Mikines KJ, von Linstow M, et al: Effect of 5 weeks detraining on epinephrine response to insulin-induced hypoglycemia in athletes. J Appl Physiol 72:1201–1204, 1992.

69. Mikines KJ, Sonne B, Tronier B, Galbo H: Effects of training and detraining on dose-response relationship between glucose and insulin secretion. Am J Physiol 256:E588–596, 1989.

70. Dela F, Mikines KJ, Tronier B, Galbo H: Diminished arginine-stimulated insulin secretion in trained men. J Appl Physiol 69:261–267, 1990.

71. Dela F, Mikines KJ, von Linstow M, Galbo H: Twenty-four-hour profile of plasma glucose and glucoregulatory hormones during normal living conditions in trained and untrained men. J Clin Endocrinol Metab 73:982–989, 1991.

72. Prior JC: Reproduction: Exercise-related adaptations and the health of women and men. *In* Bouchard C, Shephard RJ, Stephens T, et al (eds): Exercise, Fitness, and Health. Champaign, IL, Human Kinetics Books, 1990, pp 661–675.

73. Drinkwater B: Training of female athletes. *In* Dirix A, Knuttgen HG, Tittel K (eds): Encyclopaedia of Sports Medicine, vol 1. Oxford, Blackwell Scientific Publications, 1988, pp 309–327.

74. Loucks AB, Vaitukaitis J, Cameron JL, et al: The reproductive system and exercise in women. Med Sci Sports Exerc 24:S288–293, 1992.

75. Loucks AB: Effects of exercise training on the menstrual cycle: Existence and mechanisms. Med Sci Sports Exerc 22:275–280, 1990.

76. Cumming DC: Discussion: Reproduction: Exercise-related adaptations and the health of women and men. *In* Bouchard C, Shephard RJ, Stephens T, et al (eds): Exercise, Fitness, and Health. Champaign, IL, Human Kinetics Books, 1990, pp 677–685.

77. Lloyd T, Myers C, Buchanan JR, Demers LM: Collegiate women athletes with irregular menses during adolescence have decreased bone density. Obstet Gynecol 72:639–642, 1988.

78. Kjær M, Hollenbeck CB, Frey-Hewitt B, et al: Glucoregulation and hormonal responses to maximal exercise in non-insulin-dependent diabetes. J Appl Physiol 68:2067–2074, 1990.

79. Hilsted J: Pathophysiology in diabetic autonomic neuropathy: Cardiovascular, hormonal and metabolic studies. Diabetes 31:730–737, 1982.

147

Endocrinology and Aging

MARC R. BLACKMAN
DARIUSH ELAHI
S. MITCHELL HARMAN

INTRODUCTION

Biological aging is a process of progressive loss of function with time that leads to a decreased capacity of the organism to maintain homeostasis, initially in the face of stress and subsequently under baseline conditions. Growing appreciation of the complexities and heterogeneity of the aging process has forced revision of the simplistic but once popular concept that aging is a consequence of one or more hormone deficiency states. It is now clear that aging results from multiple changes in the molecular, biochemical, and physiological functions of cells, tissues, and organisms.

A number of paradigms for understanding biological aging exist that, although not mutually exclusive, are not easily synthesized into a single coherent theory. The two major schools of thought can be summarized as genetic and environmental. The genetic paradigm assumes that aging is a continuation of the developmental process in which a program of successive gene activations and inactivations leads to differentiation and maturation from embryogenesis through puberty. From the evolutionary point of view, aging may be considered as adaptive (i.e., having some selective advantage for the species, if not for the individual) or nonadaptive (i.e., the result of a random accumulation of deleterious genes that, because expressed in old age, do not reduce reproductive potential and, hence, are not selected out).[1] The fact that rates of aging are variable among but characteristic for particular species suggests that the genetic model is at least partially valid. Evidence in favor of the genetic hypothesis also comes from experiments with cultured fibroblasts in which the number of population doublings achievable in vitro is less in cultures derived from species with shorter life spans and, within species, from individuals of greater ages.[2, 3] The lat-

ter results suggest the presence of some sort of genetic counter that limits cell replications.

The hypothesis that apoptosis, or genetically programmed cell death, contributes to the biological aging process as well as to age-related disease has gained increasing experimental support.[4, 5] Examples include the involvement of apoptosis in ovarian follicular atresia and reproductive senescence,[6] in cholinergically mediated neuronal cell death in Alzheimer's disease,[7] and in adrenalectomy-induced granule cell degeneration in the rat hippocampal dentate gyrus.[8]

The environmental paradigm assumes that aging results from the gradual accumulation of damage to cells and tissues caused by interactions with their milieu. Various mechanisms of damage have been implicated, but oxidation of cell components (i.e., lipid, protein, DNA) by free radicals generated by oxidative metabolism[9] and the nonenzymatic glycation of proteins,[10] or some combination of both processes,[11] are among the leading candidates. Cumulative damage hypotheses are insufficient to explain biological aging because they do not take into account the considerable autoreparative capacity of cells and tissues. Nonetheless, there is evidence of increased oxidative damage to proteins in older organisms.[12] In addition, experiments in which total life span of animals is lengthened and the appearance of markers of aging delayed by dietary caloric restriction have been interpreted as favoring the environmental hypothesis because this treatment is thought to reduce rates of both oxidation and glycation.[13]

An interaction of the genetic and environmental influences on chromosomal stability could provide a unifying concept between these two models. Thus various environmental influences (e.g., oxidation, glycation) could provide a constant source of chromosomal breaks and errors, and variation in a number of different alleles that influence chromosomal stability and modulate repair processes might account for both individual and characteristic species life spans.[14]

Whatever the underlying mechanisms, the aging process almost certainly leads to a state in which there are reductions in the number and/or functional reserve capacity of various types of differentiated cells and in the ability to repair or replace them by proliferation and/or differentiation of stem cells. This state of affairs may well apply to endocrine organs and their regulatory centers. In fact, many aspects of the aging phenotype bear marked similarities to various states of hormone deficiency or excess. Thus, for example, the increase in and more centripetal distribution of body fat, reduced glucose tolerance, loss of bone mineral and muscle mass, and fragility of vascular and connective tissues are suggestive of glucocorticoid excess. Similarly, the slowing of reflexes, drying of skin, and reduced bowel motility are consistent with hypothyroidism. Loss of virility and fertility and decreased sex drive and performance suggest loss of sex steroid hormones. Loss of lean body mass, increased percentage of body fat, and reduced rates of protein synthesis and tissue healing occur both in aging and in growth hormone (GH) and growth factor deficiency. Therefore, even though the primary mechanisms of the aging process are more complex than simple hormone deficiency (or excess), it is reasonable to ask how the aging process affects hormonal balance and, of obvious clinical significance, what role alterations in hormonal balance, which may themselves be secondary events, play in the cascade of multiple causes and effects leading ultimately to the aged phenotype.

To successfully pursue scientific inquiry into the effects of aging on hormonal balance, certain caveats must be observed. Advances in clinical and laboratory research in gerontological endocrinology have led to an increasing recognition of the need to discriminate between the effects on hormone physiology of aging per se and those of a variety of age-associated potentially confounding comorbid variables.[15–17] For example, biochemical perturbations of hormone physiology arise as a result of acute and chronic nonendocrine illnesses; use of various medications and drugs; alterations in diet, body composition, and weight; and variations in states of the sleep-wake cycle and in levels of physical and autonomic nervous system activity, all of which may occur coincidentally during the aging process. The practical results of factoring out such variables in carefully designed clinical studies have been to establish more precise normative data on the effects of aging on the endocrine system, to improve interpretation of diagnostic endocrine testing during illness in elderly people, and, perhaps most important, to identify some endocrine changes that may contribute to the normal aging process.

Until recently most clinically useful endocrine data in older people were derived from measurements (e.g., radioimmunoassay [RIA] or bioassay) of circulating hormone concentrations or urinary hormone excretion under baseline conditions and after various physiological stimulation (or suppression) tests. Blood hormone concentrations, however, represent the composite expression of numerous complex determinants. Moreover, plasma (or serum) hormone levels must ultimately be related to the responsivity of the target tissue or cell to that hormone.[15–20] Thus it is apparent that for each endocrine axis, genetic and/or environmental influences intrinsic to the aging process (and

as yet incompletely understood) may affect the mass and cellular composition of endocrine secretory tissue; hormone secretion rate and distribution space; circulating concentrations of certain specific and nonspecific carrier proteins that determine the free or metabolically active concentration of hormone; the rates and characteristics of hormone degradation and excretion; the amplitude and frequency of hormone-specific rhythmic secretory cycles; the ratios of biological activity to immunoreactivity (B/I ratios) of certain hormones (e.g., by way of alterations in the sialylation or glycosylation of glycoprotein hormones); sensitivity of hormone secretion to feedback regulation (e.g., by way of long, short, or ultrashort feedback loops); avidity of hormone receptor binding (usually number and less often affinity of receptors) for specific and nonspecific (e.g., receptor spillover) ligands; hormone receptor structure and function (e.g., by altering membrane fluidity by means of dietary changes); and, finally, hormone receptor–mediated cell-specific biological responses (e.g., by altering postreceptor signal transduction mediated by generation of cyclic nucleotides, various calcium-dependent subcellular processes, stimulation of phosphoinositol pathways, alterations in cellular cytoskeleton).

The sophisticated technology of basic endocrine research increasingly is being applied to in vivo and in vitro animal model systems (e.g., in the rodent) so as to investigate fundamental mechanisms of the biology of aging.[21] Although much data adduced from such studies provide important insights into the aging system being studied, one must exercise caution in extrapolating such findings to human biology.

HYPOTHALAMUS

Much experimental information supports the hypothesis that there are physiologically important endocrine-related alterations in the structure and function of the hypothalamus (and other areas of the CNS) in old versus mature rats.[21] Moreover, it has been postulated that aging results in part from a time-dependent dysregulation of the highly integrative neuroendocrine system, with a consequent cascade of effects at numerous target tissues.[22] Not unexpectedly, there are no reports in healthy aging people that directly assess basal and/or regulated content and turnover of hypothalamic releasing hormones or neurotransmitters known to affect pituitary hormone secretion. However, certain morphofunctional alterations in the hypothalami of normal older people or of those suffering from Alzheimer's disease have been described. For example, hypertrophy of a subpopulation of neurons that contains NKB, substance P, and estrogen receptor gene transcripts, in association with augmented tachykinin gene expression, has been observed in the infundibular or arcuate nuclei from postmenopausal women and has been proposed to contribute to age-related alterations in feedback regulation by estrogen and the pathogenesis of hot flashes.[23] In other studies aging has been associated with a reduced cell number in the suprachiasmatic nucleus,[24] with increased cell numbers in the supraoptic nucleus[25] and the parvicellular corticotropin-releasing hormone (CRH) neurons of the paraventricular nucleus,[24] and with an unchanged oxytocin cell number in the paraventricular nucleus.[26] In addition, hypothalamic α_2-adrenergic receptor density is decreased,[27] whereas hypothalamic activities of monoamine oxidase A and B are increased[28] with normal aging and, to an even greater extent, in patients with Alzheimer's disease. Much further research is needed to elucidate the functional significance of these age-related alterations.

Although caution must be exercised before assuming that the data and concepts generated from neuroendocrine studies of the aging rodent are applicable to humans, a number of reports suggest that some of the apparent differences in the neuroendocrine effects of aging between the two species are more quantitative than qualitative. For example, (1) old rats of both sexes may exhibit hyperprolactinemic hypogonadotropinemic hypogonadism,[29-33] a phenomenon that has been explained in part by the findings of age-related damage to hypothalamic dopaminergic neurons[34] and consequent decreased content and turnover of dopamine as well as by observations[32] that hypothalamic content and turnover of catecholamines are decreased, whereas those of serotonin are increased. In contrast, most old women and men exhibit hypergonadotropic hypogonadism,[35-38] with basal serum prolactin (PRL) levels that have been reported variously to be increased, decreased or unaltered (see Anterior pituitary, prolactin). Neither depletion of dopamine[39] nor reduction in the activity of tyrosine hydroxylase[40] has been observed in the hypothalami of aging humans. Nonetheless, studies reveal that basal and gonadotropin-releasing hormone (GnRH)-stimulated luteinizing hormone (LH) and follicle-stimulating hormone (FSH) levels are lower in older versus younger postmenopausal women[41] and decrease with advancing age in elderly men.[42-44] Moreover, repetitive administration of GnRH to old men improves gonadotropin production to that of younger men.[45, 46] (2) In old rats there are marked reductions in the amplitude but not the frequency of spontaneous GH secretory pulses.[47] There are as well age-related decreases in basal and growth hormone–releasing factor (GRF)-stimulated GH levels[48] and in contents of pituitary GH and hypothalamic somatostatin.[49] The finding that antisomatostatin antiserum evokes a greater increase in serum GH levels in older rats,[49] coupled with the observation that GRF mediates a lesser in vitro release of GH and adenylate cyclase by isolated pituitary cells from old rats,[48] suggests that aging in the rat is associated with both increases in somatostatin tone and intrinsic derangements in pituitary somatotropic function. By comparison, an age-related decrease in GRF-stimulated serum GH levels has been reported in women[50, 51] and in some[52-54] but not other[55-57] studies in men. Moreover, studies (see Growth Hormone) suggest that both augmented somatostatinergic tone and reduced endogenous GRF release contribute to the decline in GH secretion with age in humans. (3) Administration of CRH or exposure to various stressors evokes a lesser rise in circulating ACTH levels in older versus younger rats.[58] In addition, interleukin-1 (IL-1)-stimulated CRH release in vitro, hypothalamic and pituitary CRH receptor density, and basal and immobilization stress-induced levels of CRH messenger RNA in the paraventricular nucleus are all diminished in old rats.[58a, b] In contrast, spontaneous and CRH-stimulated ACTH release are similar in healthy young and old men both before and after dexamethasone administration.[59, 60]

As is evident from the discussion preceding, many inferences regarding the physiological integrity of hypothalamic neuroendocrine functions in humans have been derived, perforce, from clinical studies in which anterior pituitary responsivity to hypothalamic releasing hormones has been examined either indirectly (e.g., after administration of clomiphene or metyrapone or after insulin-induced hypoglycemia) or directly (e.g., after administration of GnRH, thyrotropin-releasing hormone [TRH], GRF, or CRH). Similarly, hypothalamic-neurohypophyseal function has been studied by measuring antidiuretic hormone (ADH) release after stimulation of osmoreceptor and baroreceptor pathways.

Hypothalamic sensitivity to feedback regulation by sex steroids, glucocorticoids, and thyroid hormones has been assessed in aging men, although the data are inconclusive. Of interest are conflicting reports that in healthy older men, administration of exogenous androgens leads to either increased[61] or decreased[62] suppression of serum gonadotropin levels, presumably by means of enhanced or reduced hypothalamic sensitivity.

Finally, ample evidence exists for age-related alterations in certain nonendocrine hypothalamic functions, such as thermoregulation, sensation of thirst, and blood pressure control. The interplay between each of the latter processes and the neuroendocrine functions of the hypothalamus in aging humans awaits clearer definition. Research suggests that altered metabolism of extrahypothalamic CRH may contribute to behavioral abnormalities in patients with Alzheimer's disease.[63] The interrelations among neuropeptides, behavior, and aging in healthy people are subjects for further scrutiny.[64, 65]

POSTERIOR PITUITARY

Hyponatremia is a common condition in both hospitalized and ambulatory elderly people. Although prevalence data for this phenomenon vary depending on the clinical setting, in one study 22.5 per cent of chronically institutionalized patients exhibited clinically significant hyponatremia, as evidenced by muscle cramps, hyporeflexia, lethargy, and seizures.[66] That significant neurological abnormalities can result from hyponatremia in the outpatient setting has also been reported.[67] Although elderly patients are more likely to harbor illnesses (e.g., congestive heart failure, renal failure, hypothyroidism), consume medications (e.g., diuretics, oral sulfonylureas), or be exposed to other agents (e.g., anesthesia) that promote hyponatremia, a disproportionate percentage (>60 to 75 per cent) of patients with idiopathic syndrome of inappropriate antidiuretic hormone are elderly.[66-68]

Numerous clinical studies have documented age-related decrements in both nephron mass and function.[69] Among the alterations in function are decreases in the ability to maximally concentrate or dilute urine after appropriate challenge by fluid restriction or water-loading tests. Studies in well-screened, healthy, ambulatory subjects exposed to 12 hours of dehydration have revealed that, independent of the associated age-related fall in glomerular filtration rate, the ability to maximally concentrate urine (Umax) falls less than previously believed, by perhaps 10 to 12 per cent after the eighth decade.[70] Possible causes for the physiological decline in Umax with age include a decreased hypothalamic-neurohypophyseal release of, or renal response to, ADH. The findings of augmented sensitivity of hypothalamic osmoreceptors for ADH release (see below) and of insignificant differences in urinary concentrating ability in older versus younger subjects after administration of submaximal doses of exogenous ADH[71] suggest that age-related alterations in Umax occur by means of ADH-independent mechanisms.

Abundant morphological and functional data indicate that aging in the rat is associated with a decline in hypothalamic-neurohypophyseal function.[72] In contrast, morphological studies in humans have revealed no evidence for significant age-related degenerative changes in the complex hypothalamic-neurohypophyseal pathways that control ADH synthesis and secretion.[72] In fact, in older people, cells in the hypothalamic paraventricular and supraoptic nuclei exhibit cytological changes characteristic of augmented hormone synthesis,[25] findings that correlate well with independent observations that hypothalamic ADH content and basal plasma ADH levels are normal to increased in older people.[72] Moreover, clinical studies have revealed that healthy older versus younger subjects matched for their basal plasma osmolalities exhibit a 2- to 2.5-fold greater rise in circulating ADH levels when similar increments in plasma osmolality are produced by infusion of hypertonic saline.[73] In addition, ethanol ingestion (a known inhibitor of ADH release) leads to a persistent suppression in plasma ADH levels in younger subjects but to only an evanescent decrease followed by a rise in ADH levels in older subjects.[73] Alterations in plasma volume also play an important role in the physiological regulation of ADH release, the effects being additive to but generally of lesser magnitude than those of changes in plasma osmolality. The rises in plasma levels of ADH but not of norepinephrine after an orthostatic challenge (overnight recumbency followed by eight minutes of standing still) are significantly reduced in older subjects.[74]

Taken together with prior reports that the volume of distribution and metabolic clearance rate (MCR) of ADH are age-invariate,[75] the morphological and functional data above support the hypothesis that there are age-related augmentations in basal and osmoreceptor-mediated ADH release. At the same time there appears to be an age-related defect in baroreceptor-mediated ADH release, with the defect seemingly located distal to the vasomotor center in the afferent limb of the baroreceptor arc.[74] Whether the age-related decreased sensitivity to the volume-pressure changes elicited by hypertonic saline infusion is responsible for the apparent enhancement in osmoreceptor sensitivity (i.e., increased ADH/Osm) of elderly people remains to be determined.

Although the ADH response to osmotic stimuli is enhanced in older people, the concomitant thirst response usually is reduced with age. It is possible that the hypothalamic osmoreceptor neurons that regulate ADH release and thirst may be discordantly affected by age, but it seems more likely that age-related hypodipsia results from other, ill-defined mechanisms. The observation that after overnight fluid deprivation and naloxone injection, older men exhibited a significantly lesser inhibition of fluid intake than did younger men suggests that there may be an age-related diminution in the opioid-mediated drinking drive.[76]

Release of ADH also occurs after stimulation of various other centers, such as those for nociception (by pain or

stress), emesis (by nausea, motion sickness, labyrinthitis, or drugs), and chemoreception (by hypercapnia). In addition, hypoglycemia, angiotensin II, atrial natriuretic hormone, and various drugs (e.g., nicotine, metoclopramide, chlorpropamide, clofibrate, cholinergic agents, β-adrenergic receptor agonists) can stimulate ADH release. There is little information as to whether these other stimuli of ADH release exert different effects in older versus younger people. In one study in healthy men age-related increases in ADH responses were observed after metoclopramide ingestion or cigarette smoking but not after insulin-induced hypoglycemia.[77]

ANTERIOR PITUITARY

Anatomical and histopathological studies have revealed the anterior pituitary gland in aging humans to be somewhat decreased in size, with increases in patchy fibrosis, focal necrosis, vascular alterations, iron deposition, and (micro)adenoma formation.[17] It is uncertain whether the increased numbers of adenomas are of the nonsecretory variety, or are associated with the hypersecretion of hormones (e.g., PRL) or other proteins (e.g., glycoprotein hormone subunits) of normal, altered, or absent biological activity. Earlier cytochemical investigations revealed no significant age-dependent changes in anterior pituitary content of PRL, GH, or thyrotropin (TSH) but increased contents of FSH and, to a lesser extent, LH.[17] Increased LH content has been reported in the anterior pituitary glands of older men and women. More recent immunocytochemical studies using antisera of greater specificity have demonstrated no age-related alterations in absolute or relative numbers of stainable GH or PRL cells.[78] The latter finding correlates well with the observation in several necropsy series that the prevalence of (micro)prolactinomas[79] and other pituitary tumors[80] is age-invariated.

Numerous caveats cloud the interpretation of the possible functional significance of the aforementioned findings. As already noted (see Introduction), age-related alterations might occur in the amount or biological activity of hypothalamic releasing hormones or other neurotransmitters impacting on, for example, the adenohypophysis, the binding of such hormones to specific pituitary cell surface receptors, and the mechanisms of signal transduction. More important from a physiological perspective are studies in which the basal and regulated secretion of various anterior pituitary hormones have been assessed.

Prolactin

An increasing number of studies of PRL secretory physiology in older people have been reported, with more recent investigations emphasizing the apparent interactive effects of aging and gender, diurnal rhythmicity, and/or dopaminergic tone. Baseline and TRH-stimulated serum concentrations of PRL (as well as pituitary PRL content) are 30 to 50 per cent greater in women than in men at all ages. Some[81, 82] but not other[83] studies have shown a decrease in basal serum PRL levels in women beginning in the mid-to-late fifth decade, in temporal association with the estrogen-deficient state of the menopause. In one study using a serial blood sampling technique, no age-related differences in the frequency or amplitude of spontaneous PRL secretion were observed in seven older (mean age 80 years) versus six younger (mean age 53 years) postmenopausal women.[84] In contrast, both unchanged and increased basal and 24-hour integrated serum PRL levels have been reported in older men.[81, 83, 85–87] Although circadian rhythmicity of PRL secretion was reported to be unchanged in one study,[85] several reports now clearly document a decreased amplitude but unchanged frequency of nocturnal PRL release in healthy older versus younger men.[88–90]

Aging in men has been variously reported to be accompanied by unchanged,[91] augmented and delayed,[92] and delayed[83] PRL responses to bolus intravenous injections of TRH. In one study of 85 healthy, ambulatory men aged 30 to 96 years, there were age-related increases in basal serum PRL levels; in addition, peak PRL responses to constant low-dose infusions of TRH were of greater magnitude and occurred earlier in the oldest men.[87] The observation that the administration of the dopamine antagonist metoclopramide elicits a greater increase in the amplitude of nocturnal PRL release in older versus younger men is compatible with the hypothesis that aging in humans, as in the rat, is associated with diminished hypothalamic dopaminergic tone.[90] By contrast, older and younger men exhibited no differences in the acute PRL secretory response to the guanyl derivative of an opioid analogue of met-enkephalin.[93] Finally, a qualitative, age-related alteration in the PRL molecule has been suggested by the observation of an absolute and relative decrease in the proportion of PRL biological activity to immunoreactivity in sera from postmenopausal versus premenopausal women.[82]

Growth Hormone

Growth hormone is a major anabolic hormone that exerts important stimulatory effects on protein synthesis (especially in the liver, spleen, kidneys, thymus, and red blood cells) and lipolysis.[94] Most of the peripheral tissue effects of GH are mediated by insulin-like growth factor I (IGF-I), also known as somatomedin C. IGF-I exerts its effects by way of endocrine, paracrine, and autocrine mechanisms (see Ch. 142). Most circulating IGF-I is generated in the liver by the action of GH,[95] and regulates GH secretion by negative feedback at the pituitary somatotropic level. The fact that aging in humans is accompanied by a generalized decrease in protein synthesis and a concomitant reduction in lean body mass suggests that GH secretion or action might decrease with advancing age.[94]

The effects of human aging on GH secretion have been evaluated by a number of researchers.[96] Early studies reported unchanged baseline plasma GH levels.[97] More recent studies of 24-hour secretion of GH, assessed by sampling every 20 minutes, have shown variable reductions (15 to 70 per cent) in most 24-hour GH secretory parameters in middle-aged (40 to 65 years)[98, 99] and older (over 60 years)[56, 100, 101] men and women. In a study performed in healthy nonobese men aged 21 to 71, deconvolution analysis has revealed that with each advancing decade, the GH production rate decreases by 14 per cent and the GH half-life falls by 6 per cent.[102] Reductions in the number and

amplitude of GH spontaneous pulses during sleep have been reported in adults over 50 years of age[103] and in two studies[104, 105] were found to be confined to the first three to four nighttime hours. Although nocturnal GH secretion is reduced with age in men, old men, like younger men, still have twofold to fourfold greater secretion at night than during the day.[56, 101]

Responses of GH to indirect stimuli have also been studied in older people. For example, the GH response to insulin-induced hypoglycemia has been reported to show no change[106] or a decrease[107] with age, a discrepancy that may be partly explained by the inclusion of subjects up to 50 years of age in the young control group in one of the studies.[106] The acute GH response to an intravenous arginine infusion has been found to be similar in young and old men,[52, 97, 108] whereas an arginine infusion potentiates GH responsivity to GRF in old men.[52] Administration of an oral arginine-lysine preparation (6 g of each amino acid per day) for two weeks did not increase spontaneous GH release (as assessed by overnight frequent sampling), plasma IGF-I levels, or GRF-stimulated GH secretion in old men.[109]

The acute GH response to exercise is reduced with age.[110, 111] In one study exercise training for 12 weeks improved the acute GH response after one hour of exercise in older men, although trained older men still had a lower GH response to exercise than did trained or even sedentary younger men.[110] In another study older men, unlike younger men, failed to demonstrate an increase in resting or one-hour postexercise plasma GH levels after 12 weeks of resistance strength training.[111]

The acute secretory response of GH to direct pituitary stimulation with GRF has been reported to be present but significantly reduced in healthy old women[50, 51] and in some[52–54] but not other[55–57] studies of old men. Variations in published findings in old men may have been caused in part by differences in race and/or life-style (e.g., exercise, diet), by the amount and/or regional distribution of body fat, or by other unidentified factors.

In one study of a large group of subjects aged 20 to 80 years, GH-binding protein (GH-BP) levels were observed to decrease after the fifth decade in healthy men but not in women.[112] In another investigation GH-BP levels were reduced in a group of healthy men and women beyond age 60.[113] This decrease with age could reflect either a loss of peripheral GH receptors (the putative source of GH-BP's) or the known decrease in GH secretion with aging (plasma GH-BP increases after each GH pulse).[114] The physiological significance of age-related changes in serum GH-BP's and in the extramembranous portion of the GH receptors from which they are derived remains to be established.

It has not been possible to accurately measure GRF or hypothalamic somatostatin in peripheral blood of humans. Because arginine is known to inhibit somatostatin secretion,[115] the observation that intravenous infusion of arginine potentiates GH responsivity to GRF in old men[52] suggests that in humans, as in the rat, somatostatin tone is increased with age. Conversely, the findings that repetitive administration of GRF to old men[53] and women[116] partly reverses their diminished GH responsiveness to GRF suggest that there may also be a reduction with age in GRF input to the pituitary. In addition, although only nonsignificant changes have been found in GH content of pituitary cells from old people,[117, 118] reductions with age in the number and size of somatotrophs have been reported in one immunocytochemical study.[78] Finally infusion of theophylline, a phosphodiesterase inhibitor that increases intracellular cAMP, improves GH responses to GRF in old but not young men,[119] suggesting that there may be an intrinsic alteration in GRF signal transduction in the aging somatotroph.

Levels of IGF-I in unextracted or acid-ethanol extracted serum or plasma decrease with age in both men and women,[96] so that in subjects in the seventh decade IGF-I values may fall to levels about 30 to 50 per cent of those in people in the third decade. The prevalence of low IGF-I serum concentrations increases progressively from 11 to 55 per cent from the fourth through the ninth decades.[96] The strong positive relation between baseline serum IGF-I levels and spontaneous 24-hour GH secretion in young adults has not been observed consistently in older subjects. Several studies have shown that circulating IGF-I levels increase similarly in young and old men after exogenous administration of either GH[120, 121] or GRF.[57]

Plasma IGF-I was inversely correlated with adiposity in one study,[104] whereas in another[122] there was an age-independent inverse correlation between body mass index (BMI) and IGF-I in men but not in women. There is also a significant inverse correlation of IGF-I levels with age that is independent of adiposity.[104, 122] Thus increased adiposity exerts an effect, independent of age, to decrease IGF-I levels. One possible mechanism for these effects is increased insulin action on hypothalamic and/or pituitary IGF-I receptors, resulting in enhanced feedback inhibition of GH, and hence IGF-I, secretion. Decreased physical activity may also contribute to the reduction in serum IGF-I levels with age. Maximum oxygen consumption and cardiorespiratory performance has been significantly correlated with IGF-I levels, independent of age, in healthy people.[123] This association is weaker in old versus young men.

Circulating levels of IGF-binding protein-3 (IGFBP-3), the major plasma IGF-I binding protein, decrease with advancing age in both women and men.[124] Prior reports have shown that changes in plasma IGF-I are positively correlated with IGFBP-3 binding activity, and a strong, age-independent positive correlation of IGFBP-3 with IGF-I levels has been described in men aged 22 to 79 years.[125] It seems likely that the decreases in GH and IGF-I release with aging are, at least in part, responsible for the reported reductions in IGFBP-3 levels.

Loss of cellular and tissue regenerative capacity and impairment of growth are concomitants of the aging process. Studies in cultured human fibroblasts from young, old, and progeric donors have revealed no age-related alterations in IGF-I binding or sensitivity to IGF-I action in either the absence or the presence of low (synergistic) concentrations of serum.[126] It has been demonstrated, however, that the synergism between IGF-I and dexamethasone in stimulating DNA synthesis and fibroblast multiplication is decreased in cells from old and progeric donors.[127] The possible physiological significance of the latter phenomenon to cellular aging remains to be elucidated.

The reported experience in administering GH to healthy or frail older patients has been reviewed.[96] In the longest duration study of GH administration to old people yet reported, 12 healthy men aged 61 to 81 years who had reduced basal plasma IGF-1 levels were treated with subcutaneous injections of recombinant human GH three times weekly, with the dose adjusted monthly based on IGF-I responses.[128] Administration of GH produced an 8.8 per cent increase in lean body mass, a 14.4 per cent decrease in adipose tissue mass, and a significant increase in skin thickness. A number of studies are assessing whether the GH-induced increase in lean body mass or decrease in fat mass elicits substantial improvements in muscle mass and strength, physical endurance or mobility, or the quality of life in older people.

Alternate-day intravenous injections of GRF for 12 days restore the acute GH responses to GRF of older men to levels comparable to those of young men.[53] Similar acute GH responses, accompanied by significant increases in IGF-I levels, also occur after administration of intravenous GRF for eight days to postmenopausal women.[116] Administration of GRF to healthy old men for 14 days was found to reverse age-related reductions in circulating levels of GH and IGF-I, with preservation of spontaneous diurnal GH secretory patterns, and without adverse effects on blood pressure, serum glucose, or urinary C-peptide.[55, 56] These observations suggest that administration of GRF or GRF analogues may represent an alternative and perhaps more physiological method of increasing subnormal GH and IGF-I levels in healthy old men and women.

Adrenocorticotropin

In early studies of the effects of age on pituitary corticotropic function, inferences regarding ACTH secretion were derived from measurements of plasma cortisol levels or urinary 17-hydroxycorticosteroid excretion under baseline conditions or after indirect stimulation of the pituitary by insulin-induced hypoglycemia or challenge with oral or intravenous metyrapone. Such investigations revealed no evidence in older people for age-related alterations in basal or stimulated levels of cortisol,[107, 129] although daily urinary 17-hydroxycorticosteroid excretion was found to be decreased.[130, 131]

Subsequent studies in which plasma ACTH levels were measured directly by RIA confirmed the lack of an age-related alteration in plasma levels of ACTH basally or after administration of intravenous metyrapone.[132] In a single report the diurnal rhythmicity of ACTH secretion was found to be altered in aged subjects.[133] In many of the aforementioned studies the exact health status of the elderly subjects was not specified. It is especially important to control for stress, depression, alcohol use, and states of obesity or malnutrition in studies of the hypothalamic-pituitary-adrenal axis.

Basal and stimulated levels of ACTH, cortisol, and dehydroepiandrosterone (DHEA) were measured after direct pituitary stimulation with ovine corticotropin-releasing hormone (oCRH) in a well-screened group of healthy aging men.[59] Older men exhibited slight but nonsignificant trends to higher plasma ACTH levels both before and after oCRH. There were no age-related alterations in the magnitude or timing of peak ACTH responses to oCRH. In addition, there was a modestly significant increase in basal plasma cortisol levels and a nonsignificant trend to higher oCRH-stimulated cortisol levels in older men. The findings in the latter study were compatible with a reduced hypothalamic-pituitary sensitivity to feedback inhibition by glucocorticoids. These same investigators subsequently found no age-related alterations in spontaneous or oCRH-stimulated ACTH or cortisol release before or after various doses of dexamethasone in a similar group of healthy young and old men.[60] In one study the ACTH responses to an oCRH stimulation test were found to be similar in old women and men, but basal, peak, and nadir cortisol levels were all higher only in old women.[134] The latter observations suggest that there may be gender differences in the effects of aging on pituitary-adrenocortical function.

Earlier investigations had suggested plasma cortisol levels to be disproportionately higher in older patients during perioperative stress[135] or depressive disease.[136] More recently, levels of cortisol but not of ACTH have been reported to be higher in old women after hip fracture than in their healthy age-matched counterparts.[137] An age-related reduction in hypothalamic-pituitary corticotropic sensitivity to feedback inhibition by glucocorticoids was postulated based on the findings of a lesser inhibition by dexamethasone of serum 11-hydroxysteroid levels in a small number of apparently healthy older people[138] and of plasma cortisol levels in older depressed patients.[136] Studies in both endurance athletes[139] and depressed patients[140] have revealed age-related increases in cortisol responses to oCRH after pretreatment with dexamethasone. Thus in humans it appears that glucocorticoid feedback regulation of pituitary-adrenocortical function is altered with age in the presence but not the absence of various exogenous or endogenous stressors.

Thyrotropin

Early studies in which relatively small numbers of subjects were examined revealed either no change or increased plasma (or serum) TSH levels with age.[17] Two subsequent reports in which larger numbers of apparently healthy community-dwelling subjects were investigated revealed age-related TSH elevations in as many as 3 per cent of men and 8 per cent of women.[141, 142] In one of the latter studies[142] subjects with TSH elevations also exhibited subnormal levels of peripheral thyroid hormones, suggesting that they had primary thyroid failure, presumably secondary to autoimmune thyroid disease. In some elderly people basal TSH elevations are unaccompanied by alterations in peripheral thyroid hormone levels, a condition that may represent incipient or compensated primary hypothyroidism. Moreover, in a study of healthy aging men, basal TSH levels were measured using a TSH RIA capable of detecting variations in TSH levels within (and below) the customary normal range.[143] In the latter study there were small but significant age-dependent increases in TSH levels and corresponding decreases in values for T_3 and free thyroxine index (FT_4I) (but not T_4) that fell within the respective normal ranges. Because the fractional turnover rate of TSH does not seem to vary with age (as measured in only a few subjects),[144] these data suggest that basal pituitary TSH secretion increases somewhat in older people.

Artefactual elevations in circulating TSH levels can be produced by the presence in the circulation of heterotypical antibodies (i.e., antibodies that cross-react with one or more of the polyclonal antibodies used in most TSH RIA's).[145] There have been no reports of the age-related prevalence of such heterotypical antibodies, although it seems possible that they would be more common in older people. Spurious increases or decreases in TSH measurements by RIA might also result from an age-dependent increase in the polymorphism of the TSH molecule. Prior gel chromatographic studies of serum TSH in old rats have revealed the TSH to be of larger apparent molecular size,[146] presumably because of an increase in sialylation or glycosylation of the TSH-α and/or TSH-β subunits. Analogous studies have yet to be reported in humans.

Screening studies using ultrasensitive TSH RIA's have revealed that low serum TSH levels commonly occur in older people and most often are unassociated with clinical or biochemical evidence of hyperthyroidism.[147] Moreover, TSH levels tend to be elevated to a lesser extent in older versus younger patients with primary hypothyroidism.[148] These findings suggest that aging is associated with an absolute or a relative reduction in spontaneous TSH secretion, a hypothesis that is further supported by the results of investigations of the effects of aging on the diurnal pattern of spontaneous TSH release. In one 24-hour study the amplitudes of daytime and nighttime TSH release were significantly lower in healthy older versus younger men, whereas older men exhibited a phase advance in peak hormone release and rapid-eye-movement sleep of 1 to 1.5 hours.[89] In another investigation older versus younger postmenopausal women were found to have significantly reduced T_3 levels but only a nonsignificant trend to greater TSH release.[84] These studies suggest that aging is associated with altered and presumably augmented feedback inhibition of TSH release by peripheral thyroid hormones. Lewis and colleagues detected subnormal free T_4 index values with nonelevated TSH levels in 2.5 per cent of a group of ambulatory older people and provided evidence for increased thyroid hormone feedback inhibition of TSH secretion with age, possibly because of enhanced intrapituitary T_4-to-T_3 conversion, increased T_4 uptake by pituitary thyrotropes, or other factors.[149]

The effects of age on TRH-stimulated TSH secretion have also been examined in several studies. Thus TSH responses to bolus intravenous injections of TRH have been reported to be decreased in men but not in women[150, 151]; decreased in women but not in men[152]; and increased in both men and women.[153] Demographic and other population differences and variable control for certain potentially confounding variables may explain some of the discrepancies. The responses of TSH to low-dose constant infusions of TRH have been reported in healthy aging men.[143] Older men demonstrated biphasic (i.e., early and late) TSH responses that were similar in frequency, magnitude, and timing to those in younger men. Because the older men exhibited slight but significant increases in basal levels of TSH and decreased levels of certain peripheral thyroid hormones, the failure to demonstrate augmented early or late TSH responses was interpreted as being consistent with a modest decrease in pituitary thyrotropic function in older men.

The effects of aging on dopaminergic and glucocorticoid regulation of TSH release have been described in several recent studies. In one study acute administration of L-dopa led to suppression of plasma TSH levels in healthy old but not young men.[154] These same investigators subsequently reported that the amplitude of nocturnal TSH release was blunted in older versus younger subjects and that after metoclopramide nighttime TSH release was augmented in older people, whereas daytime TSH release increased in younger subjects.[155] In another investigation impaired sensitivity to the inhibitory effects of dexamethasone on TRH-stimulated TSH release was evident in older versus younger men.[156]

THYROID

Typical age-related alterations in thyroid morphology include increased fibrosis, decreased follicular cellularity and size, and increased microscopic nodularity.[17] Although in early studies total size of the thyroid gland had been reported to decrease slightly with age,[157] in more recent investigations of apparently healthy people thyroid volume, as assessed by thyroid ultrasonography, has been shown to increase with age.[158–160] In one of these studies thyroid volume increased about 4.5 per cent per year and an age-related progression from simple nontoxic goiter to multinodular goiter with associated thyroid autonomy was evident.[159] In another report of 569 healthy persons beyond 60 years of age living in an iodine-deficient area, the prevalence of goiter was found to be 54 per cent in women and 22.5 per cent in men.[160] Single or multiple thyroid nodules occurred in 17.6 per cent and thyroid cysts in 7.6 per cent of the latter population. Not surprisingly the prevalence of clinically evident nodular goiters has also been reported to increase with age in most[159–161] but not all[141] studies.

The alterations in thyroid structure are relatively inconsequential, however, because baseline function and reserve capacity of the thyroid are sufficient to maintain a clinically euthyroid condition in most healthy elderly people.[17, 162, 163] Numerous investigators have reported various age-related alterations in the secretion, binding to circulating proteins, metabolic disposition, and (in rodents) target tissue actions of thyroid hormones. Some controversy remains as to the nature and magnitude of these various alterations because in many earlier studies the confounding effects of chronic illnesses, medication use, and abnormalities of nutrition or physical activity were not rigorously controlled. Thus with advancing age baseline plasma (or serum) levels of T_4 have been reported to be unchanged[142, 144, 150, 152, 153] or slightly decreased,[143, 164] the latter particularly in men. Serum levels of thyroxine-binding globulin (TBG) are unchanged[143] or slightly increased[164] with age, whereas levels of thyroid-binding prealbumin (TBPA), the in vitro T_3 resin uptake (T_3RU), and FT_4I ($FT_4I = T_4 \times T_3RU$) are unchanged[17] or slightly decreased.[143] The metabolic disposal of T_4 is reduced by as much as 50 per cent with age,[17] probably as a result of decreased peripheral conversion of T_4 to T_3. It has been speculated that the impaired cellular degradation of T_4 with aging may be partly caused by the concomitant age-related decline in physical activity,[17] although this hypothesis remains to be proved. Maintenance with aging of unaltered or slightly reduced serum levels of T_4 in the setting of a decreased MCR or T_4 implies that the thyroidal secretion rate of T_4 is also reduced. The latter has been confirmed directly by kinetic studies[165] and by inference from observations of decreased absolute thyroidal uptake of iodine in older people.[166] Because the thyroidal response to exogenous administration of large doses of bovine TSH remains normal in older people, as does the

capacity to greatly increase thyroidal T_4 turnover during stress (e.g., acute infections), the decreased thyroidal T_4 secretion rate with age has been considered to be a homeostatic adjustment to the reduced metabolic disposition of T_4.[17] A subtle reduction in thyroid cell responsiveness to TSH is suggested by the report that in vitro aging of each of two transfected human thyroid cell lines was associated with progressive increases in cell doubling time, decreases in binding of the high-affinity TSH receptor, and reductions of cAMP responsiveness to exogenous TSH.[167]

The effects of age on serum levels of T_3 have been extensively studied. In unscreened populations of elderly people (often nursing home residents or other chronically institutionalized people), basal serum levels of T_3 have been reported to be 40 to 50 per cent decreased.[150, 152, 164] In contrast, in several studies of apparently healthy populations, either modest (10 to 20 per cent) or no decreases in T_3 levels have been found.[142, 165, 168] In one study only 27 per cent of 190 elderly, hospitalized patients had normal values for all thyroid function studies. Low serum T_3 levels were present in 66 per cent of patients, and regression analysis revealed that severity of illness was a stronger predictor of the T_3 level than was age.[169] Alterations in free T_3 levels, or the free T_3 index, occur in parallel with those of total T_3. Whereas a reciprocal relation between plasma levels of T_3 and reverse T_3 (rT_3) has been described in many illnesses and with various medications,[170] most studies have shown rT_3 levels to be unaltered with advancing age.[143] In a single report derived from an inpatient population in a geriatric hospital, rT_3 levels were found to be increased.[171] The effects of age on the metabolic disposal of T_3 and rT_3 are unknown.

Studies of the effects of age on target organ responsiveness to thyroid hormones have been conducted primarily in rodents. Thyroid hormone–mediated effects have been variously reported to be unaltered, decreased and/or delayed, or increased, depending on the particular tissue and parameter being investigated.[17] The applicability of any of these findings to the physiology of aging in humans remains to be determined.

Hyperthyroidism

Although it is not commonly appreciated, the incidence of hyperthyroidism increases considerably in older patients.[145, 162, 163] In fact, in one study a sevenfold greater frequency of newly detected disease was evident in patients beyond the age of 60 years.[172] Clinical manifestations, laboratory results and therapeutic strategies frequently differ in older, as compared with younger, thyrotoxic patients (Table 147–1).[145, 162, 163] Older patients usually exhibit fewer systemic symptoms, such as decreased energy, increased fatigue, and heat intolerance. Symptoms and signs often are limited to a single system (especially cardiovascular or gastrointestinal) or are so nonspecific as to be attributable to coexistent nonendocrine illnesses. Toxic multinodular goiter is much more common in older patients, occurring as often as Graves' thyrotoxicosis. Interestingly, the absence of palpable thyromegaly is also encountered more often in older patients. Proptosis, especially the most severe variants, is uncommon in older patients presumably because of the decreased frequency of Graves' disease. The latter

TABLE 147–1. COMPARISON OF HYPERTHYROIDISM IN OLDER VERSUS YOUNGER PATIENTS

	OLDER PATIENTS	YOUNGER PATIENTS
Incidence Signs/Symptoms	7-fold more common (0.98/1000/yr)	0.14/1000/yr
Systemic		
Multisystem	Uncommon	Common
Single system	Common	Uncommon
Ophthalmological		
Stare, lid lag, etc.	Common	Common
Proptosis: Mild	Uncommon	Common
Severe	Rare	Uncommon
Thyromegaly		
Palpation	30% nonpalpable; of remainder, 50% (multi)nodular goiter, 50% diffusely enlarged	>90% palpable; most diffusely enlarged, smooth, firm nontender
Ultrasound	10–15%, no detectable enlargement	Most diffusely enlarged
Cardiac		
Palpitations	50%	75%
Tachycardia	50%	50%
Atrial fibrillation	Common	Rare
Congestive heart failure	>50%	Uncommon
New increased angina	Common	Uncommon
Gastrointestinal		
↓ Appetite	10%	Common
Anorexia	30%	Uncommon
Nausea, vomiting, diarrhea, abdominal pain	Occasional	Rare
Anorexia, constipation, weight loss	15%	Rare
Neuromuscular		
Anxious, irritable	<50%	Most
Tremor	50%	Common
Proximal muscle weakness	<5%	20%
Depression, withdrawal	Uncommon	Uncommon
Laboratory		
↑ RAI uptake	30–50%	70–90%
↑ T_4, ↑ free T_4 index	90%	90%
↑ T_3 RIA	60–70%	90–95%
T_3 toxicosis	5%	5%
Euthyroid hyperthyroxinemia	Common	Uncommon
Diagnosis		
Graves' thyrotoxicosis	50%	>90%
Toxic (multi)nodular goiter	50%	<10%
Treatment		
A. RAI[131]	1 or more ablative doses of 15–30 mCi	1 or more doses of 5–15 mCi to euthyroidism
B. β-Blockers	Common	Common
C. Thionamides (e.g., PTU, Tapazole) pre-RAI[131]	Uncommon	Common
post-RAI[131]	Common	Common
D. Inorganic iodides post-RAI[131]	Uncommon	Common
E. Surgery	Rare	Uncommon

Adapted from Gregerman RI: Thyroid diseases. *In* Andres R, Bierman EL, Hazzard WR (eds): Principles of Geriatric Medicine. New York, McGraw-Hill, 1985, pp 727–749.

phenomenon also accounts for the decreased frequency of diagnostic elevations of the radioactive iodine uptake (RAIU) in older patients. Serum T_4 and FT_4I values usually are elevated in older thyrotoxic patients, but levels of T_3 often are nonelevated, usually because of the concomitant presence of comorbid variables known to be associated with decreased peripheral conversion of T_4 to T_3. Nonetheless, the age-related increase in nodular thyrotoxicosis probably is primarily responsible for the increased frequency of isolated T_3 thyrotoxicosis in older people. A nonreduced basal TSH level in an ultrasensitive assay or a diagnostic rise in serum TSH levels after bolus injection of TRH usually excludes the diagnosis of hyperthyroidism. Conversely, a reduced basal TSH level or a blunted or absent TSH response does not prove the presence of thyrotoxicosis because some elderly euthyroid patients exhibit this finding, as do a significant number of patients with euthyroid multinodular goiters. Occasional diagnostic confusion arises in the elderly patient with euthyroid hyperthyroxinemia,[173] but follow-up with serial clinical and endocrine testing usually distinguishes this entity from true thyrotoxicosis.

Rapid thyroid ablation with relatively high doses (e.g., 15 to 30 mCi) of radioactive iodine (RAI[131]) followed by appropriate thyroid hormone repletion is the therapy of choice for most elderly thyrotoxic patients. Adjunctive pre- or post-RAI[131] use of inorganic iodides (e.g., SSKI) usually is inadvisable because of the increased risk of iodide-induced (or exacerbated) thyrotoxicosis, particularly in patients with multinodular goiters.[174] Post-RAI[131] institution of antithyroid drug therapy, using propylthiouracil or methimazole, often is of benefit in relieving symptoms while awaiting the beneficial effects of RAI[131]. Use of nonselective or selective β-adrenergic-blockers both pre- and post-RAI[131] may also be helpful, although contraindications to their use (e.g., bronchospasm, congestive heart failure, insulin-treated diabetes mellitus) are more common in older patients.

Hypothyroidism

Surveys of apparently healthy outpatient populations have revealed the prevalence of clinically and/or biochemically detectable hypothyroidism to be about 1 to 4 per cent, with the frequency as high as 17 per cent in patients beyond the age of 60 years.[145, 162, 163, 175] Because many of the signs and symptoms of hypothyroidism are nonspecific and often can be attributed to coexistent nonendocrine illness or medication use (the frequency of which increases with age), early manifestations of hypothyroidism are less often recognized and myxedema and myxedema coma are more common in elderly patients. Clinical manifestations of hypothyroidism often encountered in older patients include the following[145, 162, 163, 175]: dry, scaly, parchment-like skin; subcutaneous deposition of mucopolysaccharides; water bags (lymph-filled sacs) below the lower eyelids; a nonpalpable thyroid gland; hypertension; cardiomegaly; pleural and/or pericardial effusions; ischemic heart disease (especially in women with Hashimoto's disease) possibly related to secondary hyperlipidemia; severe obstipation (rarely, megacolon); severe myopathy-associated musculoskeletal symptoms; gait disturbances; and depression. Some older patients with ocular manifestations of undiagnosed hypothyroidism seek surgical consultation for aesthetic blepharoplasty.[176] Studies have shown no increase in the frequency of dementia or in the efficacy of thyroid hormone to ameliorate dementia symptoms in older hypothyroid patients.[177] In contrast, hyponatremia and SIADH (see Posterior pituitary), macrocytic anemia (with normal white blood cell count and platelet morphology), and hypercholesterolemia (increased total and low-density lipoprotein (LDL) cholesterol) are more common in elderly hypothyroid patients.[145, 162, 163, 175]

Diagnostic difficulty often arises in the acutely or chronically ill older patient with decreased T_4 and FT_4I and non-elevated basal and TRH-stimulated TSH levels. Most of these patients have the low-T_4 (euthyroid sick) syndrome (see Ch. 40). Evidence exists that derangements in both pituitary thyrotropic function[178] and peripheral thyroid hormone economy[179] are operative in certain of these patients. There is no convincing evidence to suggest that thyroid hormone therapy reduces morbidity or mortality in such patients.

Autoimmune chronic thyroiditis is especially prevalent in older women and is the most common cause of hypothyroidism in elderly people. Recognition that thyroid peroxidase is the antigen for the thyroid microsomal antibody has led to the development of RIA's to measure antithyroid peroxidase antibodies. In one geriatric study that analyzed data from 342 older subjects, antithyroid peroxidase antibody measurements were found to be more useful than measurements of antithyroid microsomal and antithyroglobulin antibodies in the diagnosis of autoimmune thyroid disease.[180] In another investigation the prevalence of diagnostic elevations in thyroid autoantibodies was found to be significantly greater in 40 subjects aged 70 to 85 years than in 436 persons less than 50 years of age or in 34 healthy centenarians. By contrast, cytofluorimetric analysis of peripheral blood lymphocytes revealed progressive and proportionate age-related decreases in total and CD5+ B cells.[181]

Therapy for hypothyroidism in elderly patients should be instituted early. The presence of stable ischemic or (tachy)dysrhythmic cardiac disease usually is not a contraindication to therapy, although an unstable cardiac condition should prompt more cautious decisions regarding the timing and dosage of hormone treatment. In view of the known age-related decrease in the thyroidal secretion rate of T_4, it is not surprising that elderly hypothyroid patients require lower doses of thyroid hormone to restore both the T_4 and the TSH to normal. In general, the goals of therapy should be to alleviate symptoms, if possible, and to normalize the T_4 and FT_4I. Use of sensitive TSH assays allows for convenient monitoring of the return of TSH to values within, rather than below, the normal range. These goals usually can be accomplished with doses of L-thyroxine (Synthroid) between 0.05 and 0.1 mg daily by mouth. By using lower maintenance doses of thyroid hormone, one presumably reduces the enhanced risk of adverse (cardiac, CNS) consequences of higher-dose suppressive therapy.

Goiter

The de novo occurrence of diffuse simple goiter is an uncommon event in elderly people.[145, 159] Newly detected diffuse goiters in older patients usually signal Graves' thyrotoxicosis, silent (lymphocytic) or subacute thyroiditis, or drug effect. Rarely, lymphoma or amyloid of the thyroid is responsible.

In contrast, the incidence of sporadic nontoxic multinodular goiter increases with age.[159, 161] As a result of the widespread use of iodized salt in the United States and the near elimination of iodine deficiency, most such goiters are of indeterminate cause. The thyroid glands typically exhibit both histopathological and radiographic evidence of numerous, variably sized nodules often with cystic and/or hemorrhagic degeneration. Although tracheal or esophageal deviation is common in patients with large goiters, the new onset of hoarseness, dysphagia, and other symptoms should prompt evaluation for malignant thyroid disease. Nearly 20 to 25 per cent of nontoxic nodular goiters fail to suppress with thyroid hormone, and attempts at such therapy are inadvisable in patients beyond 50 years of age.

Neoplasms

Data from the Framingham study reveal the prevalence of thyroid nodules to be about 3 per cent in people between 30 and 60 years of age, with an incidence of 1 case/1000 persons/year.[145] The peak incidence of new nodule detection occurs at about age 50; by age 80 new nodule formation is distinctly uncommon. The major considerations in evaluating an elderly patient with a newly detected apparently single thyroid nodule relate to determining whether the nodule is in fact both new and single, its functional status, and whether it harbors clinically significant malignant disease. The clinical, laboratory, and radiological evaluations required to accomplish these tasks have been detailed elsewhere (see Ch. 50). More than 90 per cent of nodules in the euthyroid patient with a new, single, cold, solid thyroid nodule of significant size (i.e., >2 cm) are benign lesions, and the incidence of malignant thyroid disease, like that of new nodule detection, declines gradually after age 50. Most of the 5 to 10 per cent of patients with papillary and/or follicular carcinomas of the thyroid have relatively benign clinical courses, although it has been shown that the worst prognoses in patients with these neoplasms occur in women and men beyond the ages of 50 and 40, respectively.[182]

Decisions related to adjunctive diagnostic use of thyroidal percutaneous fine-needle aspiration and cytology or cutting-needle biopsy should be tempered by the availability of pathologists skilled in evaluating such specimens. Most elderly patients with highly suspect or even cytologically or histologically confirmed malignant thyroid disease can be treated initially with appropriate doses of thyroid hormone suppression. If nodule size should increase during a 3-to-6-month observation period, surgical treatment usually is indicated. Details of combined therapy with surgery, RAI[131], and thyroid hormone suppression are reviewed elsewhere (see Ch. 50).

The presence of a rapidly expanding painful neck mass associated with symptoms of hoarseness and dysphagia in an elderly patient with a prior nodular goiter should prompt suspicion of anaplastic thyroid carcinoma. The prevalence of this highly malignant neoplasm increases progressively from midadulthood, accounting for nearly 10 per cent and 50 per cent respectively, of newly detected thyroid carcinomas in patients beyond the ages of 50 and 80.[145] Care must be taken by the pathologist to distinguish the small cell type of disease from the histopathologically similar but far more treatable thyroid lymphoma. In 20 to 30 per cent of patients with intracapsular or extracapsular thyroid disease but no other discernible metastases, early surgery may improve longevity. For the remainder no definite benefit has been shown using surgery, external radiation, and/or chemotherapy, and most patients succumb after a rapid clinical course.

ADRENAL CORTEX

Glucocorticoids

Although aging exerts striking effects on adrenal gland anatomy in several species, no major alterations occur in the human. Gross adrenal cortical weight decreases slightly, whereas microscopically, there are increases in cortical nodule formation, fibrosis, and pigment deposition.[15, 17] There are in addition decreases in epithelial cells and steroid-containing lipid, but there have been no correlative reports of age-related alterations in cell numbers in the zonae glomerulosa, fasciculata, and reticularis.

Basal plasma concentrations of glucocorticoids, whether measured as 17-hydroxycorticosteroids or as immunoreactive cortisol, tend not to change with age,[107, 129, 130] despite a corresponding decrease in the MCR of cortisol.[129, 130] This had been thought to result from a concomitant decrease in the production rate of cortisol, a finding supported by

observations that the 24-hour urinary excretion of major cortisol metabolites decreased by about 25 per cent later in life.[129, 130] In one study, however, cortisol production rates and 24-hour urinary free cortisol excretion were similar in healthy older and younger subjects, although the excretion of 6β-hydroxycortisol was reduced with age.[183] Neither corticosteroid-binding globulin (CBG) amount nor binding decreases significantly with age.[15, 17, 59] Diurnal rhythmicity of cortisol secretion has been reported to remain essentially intact with age,[133] although trends toward higher evening levels of cortisol[59, 184] and higher morning and evening levels of free cortisol[185] have been described. Three studies in men in which cortisol levels have been assessed after frequent blood sampling have led to somewhat differing results. In the first, men beyond the age of 40 were reported to have a three-hour phase advance in diurnal plasma cortisol levels, with peak, nadir, and acrophase all occurring earlier, but without significant age-related alterations in cortisol levels at comparable phases of the cycle.[186] In a second investigation older versus younger men exhibited a reduction in the mean amplitude of and a 1- to 1.5-hour phase advance in diurnal plasma cortisol levels.[89] In the third report no age-related alterations in the magnitude or pattern of spontaneous nocturnal cortisol release were evident.[60]

Direct stimulation of the adrenal glands with ACTH or indirect provocation with metyrapone or insulin-induced hypoglycemia results in normal or slightly prolonged cortisol secretory responses in older people.[107, 129, 130, 187] The maximal plasma cortisol responsivity to injections of increasing doses of ACTH was found to be reduced in old versus young men, whereas the slope of the dose-response curve was increased in old versus young women.[188] The cortisol response to endogenous ACTH incremented by administration of oCRH has been reported to be unchanged with age in men[59, 134] but greater in older women versus older men.[134]

Of particular interest are studies of the glucocorticoid secretory capacity of aged people in stress situations. Perioperative stress or femoral fracture results in higher and more prolonged elevations of plasma cortisol[135, 137, 189] as well as increased urinary excretion of cortisol metabolites[135] in older versus younger patients. Basal urinary cortisol excretion is greater[190] and plasma cortisol levels after a single-dose (2-mg) dexamethasone suppression[136] or combined administration of dexamethasone plus CRH[140] are higher in older, seriously depressed patients. As already discussed (see Adrenocorticotropin), these and other data are compatible with the hypothesis that there is an age-related diminution in feedback regulation of ACTH secretion by circulating glucocorticoids during stressful states and depression. By contrast, the observations that plasma cortisol levels were similarly decreased in old and young subjects after graded doses of dexamethasone[60] and after repetitive administration of a single dose of dexamethasone[191] suggest that normal aging, at least in men, is not associated with altered glucocorticoid feedback regulation of pituitary-adrenocortical function.

Adrenal Androgens

In contrast to the minimal effects of aging on adrenal secretion of cortisol, levels of DHEA and DHEA-sulfate

(DHEAS) diminish progressively from the third decade onward. As a result, elderly people have plasma levels of adrenal androgens only one fourth to one third those of young adults.[59, 192] Studies using frequent sampling techniques in older postmenopausal women versus younger, normally cycling women have revealed that the age-related reduction in DHEA results from a decrease in pulse amplitude and circadian amplitude, without changes in the timing or pulse frequency of DHEA secretion.[193] In addition, adrenal stimulation with exogenous[194, 195] or endogenous[59, 193] ACTH elicits markedly decreased DHEA responses in older subjects.

There are several possible explanations for the striking discordance between preserved glucocorticoid and decreased adrenal androgen secretory capacity in older people.[59] (1) Aging may be associated with decreased production of the presumptive adrenal androgen–stimulating hormone, the ACTH-independent pituitary factor thought to regulate adrenal androgen secretion. Because this substance has not been identified or characterized with certainty, no data exist regarding the effects of aging on its circulating levels or actions.[16] (2) Aging may lead to preferential utilization by the adrenal zonae fasciculata and reticularis of the common Δ^5-pregnenolone precursor for cortisol production. Although the effects of age on relative activities of the enzymes involved in adrenal steroid synthesis have yet to be reported, it has been observed that stimulation with exogenous CRH[193] or ACTH[194] elicits comparable responses of the Δ^4-steroids (i.e., progesterone, 17-hydroxyprogesterone, androstenedione, cortisol) but decreased Δ^5-steroid responses (pregnenolone, 17-hydroxypregnenolone, DHEA) in older versus younger men and women. Conceivably, adrenopause may be associated with decreased activity of the 17,20-desmolase, in contrast to adrenarche, in which the activity of this enzyme increases.[196] (3) Aging may be associated with a selective or disproportionate dropout of cells in the adrenal androgen–producing zona reticularis, in contrast to adrenarche, in which the corresponding cell mass increases.[197]

Epidemiological evidence suggests that there is an inverse relation between DHEAS levels and the incidence of coronary artery disease in men[198] but not in women.[199] In one study DHEA was administered to six healthy postmenopausal women for four weeks. There were no changes in body weight or percentage of body fat as measured by hydrodensitometry. The response of glucose to a three-hour oral glucose tolerance test was unaltered and that of insulin was increased. Levels of total and high-density lipoprotein cholesterol were significantly reduced, and there were nonsignificant trends toward lower LDL cholesterol and triglyceride values.[200]

Mineralocorticoids and Renin/Angiotensin

The effects of age on function of the renin-angiotensin-aldosterone axis have also been examined. Age-related decreases occur in the basal plasma concentrations, MCR, production rate, and 24-hour urinary excretion of aldosterone.[15–17, 201–203] In addition, the ability to augment plasma aldosterone levels in response to sodium restriction[17] or volume contraction[204] decreases in older subjects. Clinicians should be alert to the more frequent occurrence of

hyperkalemia and the syndrome of hyporeninemic hypoaldosteronism in elderly patients,[205] a phenomenon almost certainly related to the decrease in function of the renin-aldosterone system with age.

Concomitant with the changes in aldosterone, basal plasma renin activity (PRA) and PRA responses to sodium restriction or upright posture also decrease with age.[17, 203] In nearly one third of women beyond 70 years of age, the latter stimuli to renin release evoke no measurable rise in PRA.[17] In fact, it has been stated that there is a "close temporal and directional relationship between the age-related decrease in plasma renin activity and the age-related decrease in plasma aldosterone,"[201] suggesting that the low aldosterone levels are secondary to the reduction in PRA in older people.

Plasma concentrations of renin substrate, total renin, and inactive renin do not vary with age, but the corresponding plasma concentration of active renin does decrease in older subjects.[206] This raises the possibility that decreased conversion of inactive renin to active renin occurs with advancing age. These observations have important implications for categorizing hypertensive patients by means of their renin status and emphasize the need for improved normative data on basal and modulated plasma levels of renin, angiotensin, and aldosterone in elderly people.

The age-related decrease in PRA has been hypothesized to be caused by the known increase with age in plasma levels of atrial natriuretic peptide (ANP)[207] (see Atrial Natriuretic Peptide), which is a known inhibitor of renin secretion. This explanation is refuted by two findings; that (1) ANP infusion in doses sufficient to decrease PRA in young people resulted in no change in activity of the renin-angiotensin-aldosterone system in older men,[208] and (2) the circadian rhythms of PRA and ANP in elderly people show divergence from the reciprocal relation seen in younger people.[209] The latter results suggest a resistance to the inhibitory action of ANP on renin production in elderly people. Another possible explanation is related to the major decrease in baroreceptor sensitivity in older people.[210, 211] Despite the failure of older people to increase peripheral vascular resistance in response to acute lowering of central pressure, the increase in plasma renin activity was no different than that seen in younger subjects.[210] Thus the reduction with age in PRA remains unexplained.

ATRIAL NATRIURETIC PEPTIDE

Atrial natriuretic peptide, a 28-amino acid peptide hormone produced by cardiac myocytes, is stored inside myocyte granules and secreted into the circulation primarily in response to atrial stretch, usually induced by an expanded intravascular volume.[212] ANP has numerous actions, including natriuresis, diuresis, vasorelaxation, and interaction with other hormones, including suppression of vasopressin, aldosterone, and, possibly, renin.[212]

Basal ANP levels vary widely depending on the state of hydration and renal and cardiac function. Nearly all investigators report that ANP levels in nondiseased elderly people are up to threefold greater than those in healthy young people.[213–215] Although the reason for higher ANP levels in elderly people is not known, it seems unlikely that elevated levels result from clinically inapparent cardiac or renal disease because most of the studies involved carefully screened healthy subjects. In this regard a study of more than 300 frail elderly volunteers in a chronic-care facility demonstrated that ANP levels had significant predictive value for risk of congestive heart failure.[216]

ANP levels increase in healthy young subjects in response to volume expansion and catecholamine infusion.[212, 217, 218] In contrast, in older people the ANP response to norepinephrine infusion appears to be blunted[218] and the normal circadian rhythm of ANP is blunted or absent.[209] Moreover, the response of ANP levels in older subjects to volume expansion has been variously reported to be normal, supranormal, or blunted.[215, 218, 219] Differences among these results may be caused by inhomogeneity of the populations studied; nonetheless, there appears to be some age-related alteration in ANP release in response to certain stimuli. Blunted ANP secretion has been reported in response to volume expansion in hypertension-prone people.[220] Altered ANP secretion in response to volume expansion may be a predictor for hypertension in elderly people.

The actions of ANP appear to be similar independent of age. However, the relations between circulating ANP levels and end-organ responses are different between young and old. One study that examined the natriuretic response to infusion of ANP demonstrated a relative resistance to the natriuretic actions of ANP in young versus old subjects at levels within the physiological range.[217] In older men a resistance has also been observed to the plasma renin-inhibiting activity of an ANP infusion.[208] Although aging may be associated with production of a circulating form of ANP with reduced biological activity, no such molecular variants of ANP have yet been identified. In contrast, older people show greater degrees of peripheral capillary vasodilatation and decreases in mean arterial blood pressure in response to ANP infusions than do younger subjects.[217] This may be partially caused by a less vigorous sympathetic nervous system responsiveness in association with impaired baroreflexes in older people.[221]

ANP is a powerful inhibitor of aldosterone secretion.[222-224] It suppresses aldosterone secretion in humans despite upright posture, angiotensin II infusion, or potassium infusion.[222-224] Elevated ANP levels have been described in some patients with the syndrome of hyporeninemic hypoaldosteronism.[224] Elevated ANP levels in healthy elderly people may also be related to the relative hypoaldosteronism of normal aging.

CATECHOLAMINES

The sympathetic nervous system participates in the regulation of heart rate, respiratory rate, blood pressure, and body temperature and forms a crucial link in the physiological response to stress. Therefore, alterations in the function of this system with age could contribute importantly to an overall decline in homeostatic regulation. Alterations could take the form of increases or decreases in end-organ exposure to catecholamine signaling or changes in the sensitivity of the target organs themselves to catecholamine stimulation.

Plasma norepinephrine levels are significantly higher in older people compared with young controls.[225, 226] There is also a circadian variation in plasma norepinephrine in elderly people. Nocturnal levels have been reported to be 75 per cent higher than those of young controls and correlate with the decrease in stage IV sleep of older subjects.[227] Steady-state plasma levels are a result of the interaction of norepinephrine release, re-uptake, metabolism, distribution, and clearance. Endogenous norepinephrine is released into the extravascular compartment, and vascular concentrations do not accurately reflect sympathetic nervous system activity. Studies of norepinephrine kinetics by constant infusion to steady state have shown no difference in norepinephrine clearance and an increase in the rate of norepinephrine appearance with age.[228, 229] It is assumed that endogenous release is not affected by the infusion, despite the use of relatively large doses.

Estimation of turnover with radiolabeled norepinephrine, which allows a reduction of the concentration of the infusate by as much as 50-fold, has shown norepinephrine clearance to be decreased in older people[230-235]; however, the decrease was statistically significant in only half of the studies.[230, 231, 233] Using a two-compartment model, no difference between young and elderly people was observed.[236] Increased plasma norepinephrine levels in elderly people cannot be attributed to differences in neuronal uptake[237] but appear to result from an increased rate of appearance.[235-239] The mechanisms responsible for the increased turnover rate are not clear. Activity of the enzyme dopamine β-hydroxylase, which converts dopamine to norepinephrine, is enhanced with age.[240] In addition, hyperinsulinemia has been shown to be associated with a progressive increase in plasma norepinephrine levels in a dose-response manner.[241] This finding has not been confirmed in other older[242] or obese[243] people.

In contrast to norepinephrine, plasma levels of dopamine and epinephrine (including nocturnal levels) are not altered with age.[225, 244] The rate of appearance or clearance of epinephrine is not significantly different in older versus younger people.[233] These findings are consistent with an age-related increase in peripheral sympathetic nerve (mainly α-adrenergic) activity but no change in adrenal medullary (mainly β-adrenergic) activity.

Concomitant with the increased norepinephrine secretion with age, tissue responsiveness to α-adrenergic stimulation decreases, as evidenced by lesser chronotropic responses to stimuli such as hypoxia, hypercarbia, exercise, and handgrip.[245-247] However, α₂-adrenergic inhibition (as mediated by the α₂-adrenergic receptor agent clonidine) is functionally intact in older people and cannot account for the increased rate of appearance of norepinephrine in older people.[235] In fact, it is possible that the rise in plasma norepinephrine levels is compensatory for a primary reduction in tissue responsivity. Tissue responses to β-adrenergic stimulation also diminish with age, as shown by a decreased chronotropic response to isoproterenol and by lesser diminutions of heart rate and cardiac output after β-receptor blockade with propranolol.[248-250] The observations of an age-related decrease in the affinity but not number of β-adrenergic receptors on circulating lymphocytes[251] and of impaired postreceptor activation of lymphocyte adenylate cyclase[252] suggest that alterations in the structure and/or function of adrenergic receptors or in postreceptor signal transduction events may account for decreased catecholamine responsivity in certain cells and tissues from elderly people. Concepts related to the effects of aging on adrenergic receptor structure and function and associated post-receptor events have been reviewed.[253–256]

One clinical consequence of the decrease with age in responsivity of end-organs to catecholamine action might be orthostatic hypotension, observed with increased frequency in older people (see Ch. 156).[257] In addition, the relative decrease in β- versus α-adrenergic responsivity[258] may contribute to the increase with age in the prevalence of hypertension, to the reduced ability to maximize cardiac rate during exercise, to the diminished capacity to mobilize fatty acids from adipose tissue[259] (possibly related to the increased tendency to obesity), and to the increased risk of hypothermia.

PARATHYROID HORMONE

Until recently controversy existed regarding the effects of age on the secretion and peripheral action of parathyroid hormone (PTH). This situation arose mostly from the use of PTH RIA's using antisera of varying specificity, most of which cross-reacted with biologically inactive fragments of PTH. For example, using antisera directed against the biologically inactive COOH-terminal fragment, plasma levels of immunoassayable PTH were reported to be increased from twofold to ninefold in elderly people.[260–263] More recent studies using assays specific for the intact PTH molecule have also shown increased PTH levels with age,[264–269] but these increases were smaller (about 30 per cent) than those reported with older COOH-terminal assays. In one of these studies[264] there were also progressive age-related increases in nephrogenous cAMP and decreases in plasma levels of cAMP, total calcium, and albumin as well as in creatinine clearance, tubular reabsorption of phosphate, and the calciuric response to an oral calcium load. These findings suggest that biologically active PTH does increase with age. Because PTH remains normally suppressible by calcium infusion in older people,[268] it is likely that the rise with age in PTH is caused by a small decrease in ionized calcium rather than by increased autonomy of the parathyroid glands. In one study multivariate analysis revealed the age-related rise in PTH levels to be nonsignificant after correction for the concomitant fall in glomerular filtration rate.[264] In another larger study[265] creatinine clearance showed only a modest colinear relation with PTH and that only in men. Thus the major stimulus to PTH hypersecretion in elderly people is probably the known age-related decrease in gastrointestinal absorption of calcium (see Vitamin D) rather than a decrease in renal function. Invariably, the increase in PTH with age has been greater in women than in men, a finding attributed to the loss in postmenopausal women of the restraining effect of estrogens on PTH secretion.

Hypercalcemia

Serum levels of total calcium have been reported to both increase and decrease[16, 264, 268, 270] slightly with advancing age. Concurrent illness or the use of certain medications (e.g., thiazides, sex steroids) can alter levels of total serum calcium as well as serum calcium-binding proteins (principally albumin), with disproportionate changes in the levels of ionized calcium. Therefore, to ascertain the effects of age per se, these variables must be considered. In a large study of healthy men and women,[265] no change was found in either total or ionized calcium in women, whereas small (4 per cent) but significant ($p < .05$) decreases were observed in men.

Numerous studies indicate that primary hyperparathyroidism is the most common cause of hypercalcemia in outpatient populations, whereas cancer-associated hypercalcemia is more common in hospitalized patients. The peak annual incidence of primary hyperparathyroidism occurs in people 50 to 65 years of age, with 25 to 50 per cent of all cases reported in patients between 60 and 90 years of age.[271] In people beyond the age of 60, women are nearly twice as commonly affected as men (188 versus 92 cases/100,000).[272] As many as 50 per cent of patients, regardless of age, present with asymptomatic or minimally symptomatic disease. In elderly people neuropsychiatric and musculoskeletal symptoms as well as hypertension are particularly common nonspecific manifestations of primary hyperparathyroidism.[271]

The incidence and prevalence of most malignant diseases associated with hypercalcemia also increase with advancing age, so that cancer-associated hypercalcemia, with or without co-existent primary hyperparathyroidism, also occurs more commonly in older patients.

The general approach to the evaluation and management of hypercalcemia in older patients is similar to that in younger people (see Chs. 61 through 65). Diagnostically, many elderly patients have only mildly elevated serum levels of calcium and PTH, so that care must be taken to use age and sex-adjusted normative data in making the diagnosis of primary hyperparathyroidism. Although age per se is not a contraindication to parathyroid surgery, many older patients with clinically proved or highly suspect mild primary hyperparathyroidism can be managed without resort to parathyroidectomy.[271, 273] In patients with adequate renal function, oral phosphate or bisphosphonate therapy may be effective in decreasing the risk of renal stone formation. In some postmenopausal women with mild disease, estrogen replacement therapy alone can normalize the level of calcium and PTH. Hypercalcemic crisis is treated similarly in older and younger patients, save for the more judicious manipulation of fluid and electrolyte balance in the elderly person with cardiorespiratory disease.

Hypocalcemia

Hypocalcemia occurs most commonly in elderly patients as a result of metabolic bone disease (i.e., osteomalacia; see Ch. 72), renal failure, hypoalbuminemia secondary to acute or chronic nonendocrine illness or malnutrition, or the use of certain medications (e.g., sex hormones, anabolic steroids, aminoglycosides).[16] Hypoparathyroidism is uncommon, most often resulting from prior inadvertent removal of or damage to the parathyroid glands. Idiopathic hypoparathyroidism is rare in elderly patients but has been associated with seizures and/or incontinence.[274, 275]

CALCITONIN

In view of the osteoclastic inhibitory activity of calcitonin, it has been suggested that an age-related calcitonin deficiency may contribute to the pathogenesis of primary osteoporosis.[276] Calcitonin has been reported to decrease with age in some studies.[277, 278] Others have reported that although calcitonin levels are lower in women than in men before and after either calcium infusion or calcium clamp procedures, there are no significant age- or gender-related changes in basal calcitonin concentrations or calcitonin responses to calcium.[279, 280] Basal plasma levels of calcitonin in osteoporotic patients are similar to those in age-matched controls,[281] but the rise in calcitonin levels in response to calcium infusions may be blunted or absent in osteoporotic patients.[282] It is as yet uncertain whether the response to other calcitonin secretagogues (e.g., pentagastrin) is also diminished in osteoporotic patients. Treatment of postmenopausal women for one year with estrogen-progestin replacement produced a progressive increase of calcitonin secretory reserve, evaluated by calcium infusion test, suggesting augmentation of calcitonin secretion by estrogen.[283]

VITAMIN D

Decreased gastrointestinal absorption of calcium is a concomitant of normal aging and may result from deficiencies in calcium intake, $1,25(OH)_2D_3$ bioavailability, or $1,25(OH)_2D_3$ activity on the intestinal epithelium. It has been reported that the dermal production of 7-dehydrocholesterol, the precursor of previtamin D_3, decreases with age, leading to diminished production of vitamin D_3 and lower levels of serum $25(OH)D_3$.[284] Some studies corroborate a decrease in circulating $25(OH)D_3$ in older people,[267, 268] but in others no such change was observed.[265, 285–287] Similarly, healthy older men and women exhibit reduced plasma levels of $1,25(OH)_2D_3$ in some[268, 288] but not other[265, 266, 286, 287] investigations. In one study increased levels of serum $1,25(OH)_2D_3$ were found[269] and were thought to be caused by the increase with age in PTH. In contrast, when dietary calcium and phosphorus were normal and glomerular filtration rate was not reduced, the serum concentrations, MCR's, and production rates of $1,25(OH)_2D_3$ in old men and young men were found to be equivalent.[289]

The variability of the findings may reflect the relation of endogenous vitamin D production to exposure to sunlight, so that diminished vitamin D levels in elderly people occur seasonally (mainly in winter),[265, 290] are more prominent in higher latitudes,[267, 291] and are more severe in confined than in ambulatory people.[290] Even when serum $1,25(OH)_2D_3$ levels are unchanged, the amount detectable in bone may be reduced.[287] Finally, evidence exists for age-related reductions in intestinal vitamin D receptors and intestinal responsiveness to $1,25(OH)_2D_3$, requiring increases in PTH and, hence, $1,25(OH)_2D_3$ levels to maintain normal fractional absorption of calcium.[269] This concept is corroborated in another study[292] in which hourly fractional calcium absorption, corrected for levels of serum $1,25(OH)_2D_3$, was significantly lower in osteoporotic than in normal women, suggesting peripheral resistance to $1,25(OH)_2D_3$.

Administration of exogenous PTH produces similar increases in $1,25(OH)_2D_3$ levels in older and younger subjects, suggesting that if there is an age-related impairment in conversion of $25(OH)D_3$ to $1,25(OH)_2D_3$, factors other than a deficiency of renal 1α-hydroxylase response to PTH are responsible.[288] The serum levels of $24,25(OH)_2D_3$ and vitamin D–binding protein appear not to change with age.[285, 286]

Although the effects of aging on vitamin D activity remain somewhat controversial, it is of considerable interest to know whether supplementation of vitamin D might help to prevent the progressive loss of bone mineral and increased susceptibility to bone fractures characteristic of old age. Roentgenographic analyses of the spines of Dutch women living in Curacao did not show vertebral compression fractures commonly encountered in women living at higher latitudes.[267] In a study in Finland[293] annual fall injections of ergocalciferol given prospectively to old men and women for five years led to a 44 per cent reduction in fracture rate. This difference was significant only for women, in whom most of the fractures occurred. In a study of healthy older men with a high basal dietary calcium intake in Portland, Oregon, calcium and cholecalciferol supplementation did not affect the substantial bone loss at axial and appendicular sites.[294] These studies suggest that vitamin D supplementation may be most useful in sunlight-deprived populations and particularly in women. Gallagher[295] has suggested that up to 800 IU/day of vitamin D (four times the recommended daily allowance of 200 IU/day) may be required in elderly people for optimal calcium absorption, but further studies are needed to confirm this assertion.

MALE REPRODUCTIVE AND SEXUAL FUNCTION

Reproductive Function

In contrast to the clearly demarcated event of the menopause in women, aging of the reproductive system in men is a more gradual and highly variable process. Although controversy remains, it seems likely that a true male climacteric is a relatively uncommon event. Nonetheless, and despite the documentation of successful paternity in a 94-year-old man,[296] as healthy men age there usually are decreases in male fertility, as measured both by semen analysis (see below) and conception rate, as well as noticeable declines in sexual interest and activity and in erectile capacity. Equally important, there are decreases in lean body, bone, and muscle mass; a redistribution of body fat; and a reduction in sexual hair, with a consequent loss of strength and virile appearance. Whether and to what extent these changes are caused by decreases in the circulating levels or action of testosterone or other testicular androgens remain controversial questions.

Because both hypothalamic-pituitary-testicular physiology and sexual behavior are greatly influenced by various factors, including psychological stress, acute or chronic nonendocrine illnesses, malnutrition, obesity, and drug or medication use, it is important to discriminate between the effects of such confounding variables and the effects of aging per se in studies of male reproductive senescence.

Prior studies of testis morphology of aging men performed at necropsy or incidental surgery or on routine clinical examination have revealed a progressive decrease in testis size with advancing age.[36, 38] However, in a study of 1056 consequent necropsies in men between the ages of 18 and 96, paired testicular volumes and weights decreased slightly as a function of age only in men in the eighth decade and were independent of the effects of chronic illness, malnutrition, or alcohol use.[297] The latter findings correlate well with the observation that there was only a small decrease with age in testis size in vivo as measured by Prader orchidometer in highly selected healthy men aged 22 to 86.[298]

Age-related alterations in seminiferous tubular histology, demonstrable in most men beyond the age of 50, include thickening of the basement membrane, peritubular fibrosis, sclerotic narrowing or collapse of the tubular lumen, patchy impairment of spermatic maturation with accompanying immaturity or degeneration of germ cells, and increases in multinucleated Sertoli cells. Semen analyses in men beyond 50 years of age reveal a relative preservation of sperm numbers but declines in sperm motility and increased numbers of abnormal forms.[36, 38] The percentage of semen samples that contain mature spermatozoa decreases from 70 per cent at age 50 to 50 per cent at age 80. Basal levels of FSH measured by RIA[299–301] increase with age more consistently than do LH levels, suggesting tubular failure to be a more predictable effect of aging than Leydig cell dysfunction. This increase occasionally is monotropic and is most prominent in men with the most marked changes in seminiferous tubular morphology, suggesting that there may be an age-related decrease in the secretion or action of inhibin. In fact, decreases with age in basal serum inhibin levels[302] and in 24-hour integrated secretion of inhibin[303] have been reported.

Previous necropsy studies have revealed an age-related decrease in Leydig cell number with an increase in morphological abnormalities, associated in some studies with decreased serum levels of testosterone.[36, 38] In some of these investigations patients had died of a malignant disease or other protracted illness, thus confounding interpretation of the data. Early studies demonstrating a reduction in bioassayable urinary androgen excretion in men beyond the age of 40 probably reflected decreased adrenal, rather than testicular, androgen production. Subsequent studies of small numbers of older men showed decreased testicular vein testosterone levels[304] as well as reductions in both the metabolic clearance and the production rates of testosterone.[305] Several investigators then reported mean basal plasma levels of radioimmunoassayable testosterone to decrease progressively in men beyond 50 years of age[299, 306, 307]; however, the men studied were not drawn from a carefully screened, healthy population, so that the confounding effects of illness, medications, and so on could not be eliminated. The latter findings were called into question by a number of studies of highly screened, exceptionally healthy men in which no age-related difference in circulating testosterone levels was found.[298, 308] It is possible that altered circadian rhythmicity of testosterone secretion could have obscured an age-related decrease in serum testosterone in the latter studies. Two subsequent investigations demonstrated that peak levels of testosterone in the morning, but not nadir levels in the afternoon, were reduced in older men,[309, 310] whereas in another study 24-hour

mean integrated plasma testosterone levels were found to be decreased in healthy older men.[311] No significant alteration in circadian[312] or morning[313] levels of testosterone were observed in other investigations.

The issue of the effect of age on androgenicity is made more complex by the finding of age-related increases in sex hormone–binding globulin (SHBG) capacity, with consequent reductions in free testosterone disproportionate to those of total testosterone, in a number of studies.[300, 314] Because hepatic SHBG production is stimulated by estrogens, an increase in levels of total estradiol and/or estrone in older men, possibly as a result of the known increase in aromatization of androstenedione to estrone in peripheral (principally adipose) tissue,[315] could explain this change in SHBG. Increased total and free plasma levels of estradiol and estrone have been observed in older men in some studies[300, 306] but not in others.[298, 313] Moreover, in exceptionally healthy men there appears to be only a slight age-related increase in plasma testosterone binding to SHBG, which is insufficient to significantly alter the apparent free testosterone concentration.[298, 313]

Although there are no longitudinal studies of the effects of age on sex steroids of sufficient power to draw definite conclusions, two large, cross-sectional surveys (more than 1500 carefully studied men in each) have failed to demonstrate an age-related increase in the number of men with truly hypogonadal androgen levels, despite significant downward trends in free and total testosterone concentrations in one study[316] but not the other.[317] A meta-analysis of studies of androgens in aging men[318] revealed a highly significant inverse relation between total plasma testosterone and age but a near-zero slope when only studies excluding ill subjects are analyzed. This report underscores the fact that investigations including ill or institutionalized subjects showed lower levels of testosterone, a conclusion supported by a study comparing levels of total and free testosterone in healthy men with those in men with benign and malignant lung disease.[319]

Data on the effects of age on plasma levels of dihydrotestosterone (DHT) are conflicting. Reduced testicular vein DHT levels as well as reduced or unaltered plasma levels of total or free DHT have all been reported in older men.[298, 306, 320] In one study of elderly men with a high frequency of benign prostatic hyperplasia, increased plasma levels of DHT but subnormal levels of testosterone were observed, suggesting there to be increased peripheral (i.e., by excess prostatic tissue) reduction of testosterone, with subsequent release of DHT.[321] The significance of age-related alterations in plasma DHT levels as an indirect index of target tissue exposure to testicular androgens remains to be clarified.

The cause of decreased reproductive endocrine function with age appears to vary in an aging population. Mean basal plasma levels of LH measured by RIA[299–301] as well as urinary excretion of bioassayable gonadotropins[36, 38] increase progressively in men beyond the age of 50. Plasma gonadotropin levels in some men in their 80's and 90's may reach values encountered in postmenopausal women or castrated men. Furthermore, human chorionic gonadotropin stimulation tests have uniformly revealed absolute or relative diminutions in the testosterone secretory response in older men, consistent with an age-related decrease in Leydig cell number and/or reserve secretory capacity.[298, 300, 322] Thus the elevated basal LH levels presumably represent full or partial compensation for primary Leydig cell failure in older men, although decreases in sensitivity to feedback regulation by androgens (see above) or in the B/I ratio of circulating LH could also be responsible. In a single report a decreased B/I ratio of plasma LH was found in older men.[323]

Some reduction in baseline hypothalamic–pituitary gonadotropic function is likely, as shown by the finding of low or normal plasma levels of LH in a significant fraction of healthy older men with low testosterone levels.[319] The effects of age on pituitary gonadotropin reserve capacity have been assessed directly by stimulation with exogenous GnRH and indirectly using the antiestrogen clomiphene citrate. The results of GnRH testing have been variable but in general have revealed absolute or relative decreases in the magnitude of LH and/or FSH responses and delayed timing of peak LH responses in older men.[300, 301, 324] It is uncertain whether the latter finding results in part from age-related alterations in the MCR of LH and/or GnRH, although the MCR of LH is similar in postmenopausal and premenopausal women.[325] Clomiphene testing has uniformly revealed decreased gonadotropin responsivity in older men.[300, 326] The relative contributions of hypothalamic versus pituitary dysfunction to the reduced gonadotropic function of older men remain uncertain, but it has been shown that repeated pulsing of GnRH restores LH secretory responsiveness in healthy older men to that of young men,[45, 46] suggesting that the decrease in pituitary function is secondary to reduced hypothalamic GnRH stimulation. The observation of an attenuation of LH secretory burst amplitude in normal older men[42, 43] adds further evidence of a hypothalamic contribution to age-related reproductive failure.

Relatively little information exists in humans as to the effects of age on sensitivity of target tissues to circulating androgens. Binding of DHT to sex hormone–responsive skin is reduced in older men,[327] suggesting that responsivity to androgens may decrease with age, perhaps as a result of alterations in receptor and/or postreceptor actions of sex steroids. On the other hand, both decreased[62] and increased[61] sensitivity of pituitary gonadotropin secretion to feedback regulation by androgens has been reported in older men.

Certainly some of the discrepancies among investigations of reproductive hormone physiology in aging men are explainable by noncomparability among study groups with regard to potentially confounding variables. Nonetheless, even in exceptionally healthy men there are discernible age-related alterations in seminiferous tubular and Leydig cell structure and functions as well as subtle changes in the regulation of secretion of pituitary gonadotropins and, possibly, hypothalamic GnRH.

Sexual Activity

Many investigators have observed that sexual interest, activity, and performance in men decline progressively from late adolescence onward.[36, 38, 328] In healthy men between the fourth and eighth decades of life, the percentage of men expressing any interest in sex declines modestly with age, the reported interval after sexual release during which men feel comfortable without sex increases, and

actual sexual activity (as measured by the number of ejaculatory episodes/unit time) declines by 50 to 80 per cent.[329, 330] Nonetheless, as many as 15 per cent of healthy men may experience a period of heightened libido and sexual activity after the age of 60.[331] The most important predictors of sexual interest and activity in older men appear to be their characteristic sexual behavior in young adulthood, their general health, and those of the surviving spouse. Various age-related alterations in the patterns of male sexual response have also been described.[332]

Although it is clear from replacement studies in hypogonadal men that testosterone has an important influence on human male sexual behavior,[333] the absolute level of testosterone required for normal adult male sexuality and the interrelations among circulating androgen levels, libido, sexual activity, and sexual performance remain incompletely understood. In one study plasma levels of total testosterone were significantly correlated with frequency of sexual activity in older but not younger men.[334] Groups of old men with relatively high sexual activity also appear to have greater total[334] or bioavailable[330] testosterone levels than do age-matched men with lower activity, but whether these findings reflect a need for greater testosterone action to achieve the same CNS effect or whether heightened activity itself leads to increased testosterone secretion is unknown. Other studies have shown weak but significant inverse correlations of free or bioavailable testosterone levels with sexual thoughts, sexual activity, and morning erections in groups of aging men,[330, 335] but in one of these investigations statistical significance was lost when data were adjusted for the effects of age.[330] Moreover, in another study, after adjustment for age and BMI, there was no difference in bioavailable testosterone levels in potent versus impotent older men. The investigators concluded that hypogonadism and impotence were two common but independently distributed conditions in their study population.[336] Thus it appears that reduced serum testosterone levels contribute relatively little to the reported decrease in sexual activity in healthy older men, as compared with the contributions of age-related alterations in psychological, social, neurological, vascular, and other factors.[36, 38]

Most elderly men with decreased sexual function complain of impotence, with decreased libido, failure of ejaculation, or a combination of these abnormalities being somewhat less common. Although the frequency of impotence is probably underestimated, most studies reveal a striking increase with age from as little as 0.1 per cent at age 20 to as much as 50 to 75 per cent in men beyond age 75.[337] Because most men at some time experience transient symptoms of impotence, usually related to employment stress, fatigue, marital discord, or depression, only symptoms lasting more than two months should be investigated.[36, 38] The value of replacing testosterone to improve sexual function in older men, except those who are frankly hypogonadal, remains questionable and is the subject of research.

Other Effects of Gonadal Steroids

There is considerable interest in evaluating the interrelations between altered gonadal steroids in older men and age-related changes in body composition (i.e., decreases in muscle and bone, increases and redistribution of body fat) and associated metabolic variables, such as glucose and lipid homeostasis. Effects of altered androgen concentration or action on emotional and psychological function and quality of life are also possible and the subjects of contemporary research.

Male gender is associated with lower levels of HDL cholesterol and a greater risk of cardiovascular disease. A decrease in serum testosterone might a priori be expected to reduce the risk of atherosclerosis. In fact, a study[338] of 391 men aged 30 to 79 years found HDL cholesterol levels to be positively correlated with serum free testosterone, suggesting that endogenous testosterone might actually be protective against coronary heart disease. In a study by Marin and co-workers[339] testosterone treatment of middle-aged men led to decreases in visceral fat mass as measured by computed tomography and in insulin resistance as measured by euglycemic-hyperinsulinemic glucose clamp. Fasting blood glucose, diastolic blood pressure, and serum cholesterol also decreased. Finally, it is known that testosterone is important for maintaining bone mass and that it has positive effects on skeletal muscle mass and strength when supplied to hypogonadal men. Whether age-related decreases in testosterone (or other androgens) contribute to the 20 to 30 per cent loss of skeletal muscle mass or the reduction in bone mass that occurs between ages 40 and 80 is unknown.

One study[340] has shown a small but highly significant positive correlation between levels of free (but not total) testosterone and aggressive dominant behavior as measured psychometrically. The relationships, if any, between age-related changes in psychological and emotional function and changes in sex hormones remain to be elucidated.

FEMALE REPRODUCTIVE FUNCTION

Menopause is the dominant age-related alteration in reproductive tract physiology in healthy aging women. It is defined simply as the final episode of spontaneous menstrual bleeding, but this event actually is the culmination of a gradual irreversible loss of ovarian follicular development and responsivity to gonadotropins.[35, 37] The female climacteric, which temporally encompasses the menopause, refers to the period between the onset of reproductive senescence, typically between the ages of 35 and 40 years, and the early postmenopausal years. During the perimenopausal period there is a gradual shortening of the menstrual cycle because of a reduction in the length of the follicular phase, a decrease in the mean follicular phase estradiol levels, and an increase in the FSH levels.[341] The relative roles in these events of follicular depletion caused by atresia versus loss of gonadotropin responsiveness of the residual primary follicles are unknown, but the number of primary follicles in the human ovary approaches zero within one to two years after the menopause. The climacteric is accompanied by various endocrinological, physiological, and psychological changes, among which only vasomotor instability (e.g., hot flashes), urogenital atrophy, altered plasma lipid profile, and accelerated loss of bone mineral are clearly related to ovarian failure and estrogen deficiency.[35, 37, 342]

Although the age of onset of menarche in the United States has gradually become earlier, the median age of menopause has remained stable at about 50 years, seemingly unrelated to a host of sociodemographic, nutritional, or other factors. It has been suggested but not proved that women who smoke cigarettes experience earlier menopause.[343] Removal, destruction, or spontaneous cessation of ovarian function before age 40 is considered premature menopause.

Between the 1980's and the year 2000 nearly 40 million women in the United States will be beyond the age of 50 years. Given that the life expectancy for women is about 78 years, today's women will spend nearly one third of their lives in a postmenopausal state. Clearly, these facts mandate an ongoing public health need for continued improvement in our understanding and management of the perimenopausal and postmenopausal years. Considerable research effort is focused on the pathophysiology and treatment of vasomotor and psycho-behavioral symptoms, osteoporosis, and cardiovascular disease and on safer, more physiological modes of hormone replacement therapy with estrogens and/or progestogens. These topics are reviewed in detail in Chapters 73 and 122.

OBESITY

In healthy people body weight increases gradually from early adulthood until the fifth to sixth decade, after which weight tends to plateau. The prevalence of obesity also increases as a function of age. In addition, major changes in body composition occur, causing a redistribution of body fat mass and lean body mass even without a concomitant alteration in body weight. In one study comparing healthy younger versus older subjects of similar body weight, fat constituted 18.3 per cent versus 26.2 per cent of weight, respectively.[344] Obesity is accompanied by hyperinsulinemia and an increased prevalence of morbid conditions, including hypertension, dyslipoproteinemia, and diabetes mellitus.[345, 346]

Body mass index (wt/ht²), a measure of relative weight, does not distinguish fat from muscle in people with the same height and weight. In elderly people this is especially pertinent because total body weight may even decrease during an increase in the percentage of fat. Computation of BMI from the 1983 Metropolitan Tables of relative weight (Table 147–2) reveals that BMI decreases as height increases in both sexes (the 1959 Metropolitan tables held BMI constant). The average BMI's for people in the third and fourth decades of life are 20.4 and 22.1 kg/m², respectively, and increase by 1.6 kg/m², or about 10 lb, with each subsequent decade (Table 147–3). Andres and associates[347] examined mortality rates by gender as a function of body mass and age and demonstrated that the mortality ratio follows a J- or U-shaped distribution with high mortality at both the very low and the very high BMI's, with the lowest mortality at intermediate BMI values. The BMI associated with the lowest mortality increases with advancing age in both men and women.[348]

The pattern of body fat distribution appears to have important health implications beyond those of obesity per se. Research has shown that the distribution of fat plays a dominant role in determining the effects of obesity on various risk factors. The increased obesity of advancing age is thought to be causally related to age-related decreases in glucose tolerance only if fat is accumulated in the upper

TABLE 147–2. COMPARISON OF THE WEIGHT FOR HEIGHT TABLES FROM ACTUARIAL DATA (BUILD STUDY 1979); NON-AGE-CORRECTED METROPOLITAN LIFE INSURANCE COMPANY AND AGE-SPECIFIC GERONTOLOGY RESEARCH CENTER RECOMMENDATIONS

Height Feet Inches	METROPOLITAN 1983 WEIGHTS* Men 25–59 Yr	Women 25–59 Yr	GERONTOLOGY RESEARCH CENTER Age-Specific Weight Range* for Men and Women 20–29 Yr	30–39 Yr	40–49 Yr	50–59 Yr	60–69 Yr
4 10	100–131	84–111	92–119	99–127	107–135	115–142	
4 11	101–134	87–115	95–123	103–131	111–139	119–147	
5 0	103–137	90–119	98–127	106–135	114–143	123–152	
5 1	123–145	105–140	93–123	101–131	110–140	118–148	127–157
5 2	125–148	108–144	96–127	105–136	113–144	122–153	131–163
5 3	127–151	111–148	99–131	108–140	117–149	126–158	135–168
5 4	129–155	114–152	102–135	112–145	121–154	130–163	140–173
5 5	131–159	117–156	106–140	115–149	125–159	134–168	144–179
5 6	133–163	120–160	109–144	119–154	129–164	138–174	148–184
5 7	135–167	123–164	112–148	122–159	133–169	143–179	153–190
5 8	137–171	126–167	116–153	126–163	137–174	147–184	158–196
5 9	139–175	129–170	119–157	130–168	141–179	151–190	162–201
5 10	141–179	132–173	122–162	134–173	145–184	156–195	167–207
5 11	144–183	135–176	126–167	137–178	149–190	160–201	172–213
6 0	147–187	129–171	141–183	153–195	165–207	177–219	
6 1	150–192	133–176	145–188	157–200	169–213	182–225	
6 2	153–197	137–181	149–194	162–206	174–219	187–232	
6 3	157–201	141–186	152–199	166–212	179–225	192–238	
6 4	157–205	144–191	171–218	184–231	197–244		

*Values in this table are for height without shoes and weight without clothes.
From Andres R, Elahi D, Tobin JD, et al: Impact of age on weight goals. Ann Intern Med 103:1030–1033, 1985.

body (i.e., android obesity). In a recent report it has been shown that for women with upper body obesity aged 18 to 45 years, the risk of developing diabetes mellitus or cardiovascular disease is stronger in Caucasians than in African-Americans.[349] Intra-abdominal fat content as measured by computed tomography was significantly correlated with the two-hour serum glucose level after an oral glucose challenge in 41 men aged 41 to 76 years.[350] In healthy older men (47 to 73 years) the use of the euglycemic clamp has revealed that insulin sensitivity and glucose tolerance are affected primarily by regional fat distribution and not by age, physical fitness (assessed as maximal oxygen consumption), or obesity.[351, 352] Upper-body fat accumulation is associated with insulin resistance, hyperinsulinemia, diminished glucose tolerance, lower sensitivity to insulin in skeletal muscle, and a reduced rate of hepatic insulin extraction.[353–355] The distribution of adipose tissue is also a risk factor in the development of hypertension, gallbladder disease, non–insulin-dependent diabetes mellitus (NIDDM), cardiovascular disease, and some types of cancer.[346, 350, 356–360] Study of the influence of aging on body fat distribution in humans has relied historically on anthropometric measurements and hydrodensitometry, which do not quantify intra-abdominal fat accumulation as reliably as con-

temporary techniques such as magnetic resonance imaging and computed tomography.[361] People with increased fat in the hips, thighs, and buttocks (i.e., lower body or gynoid obesity) have been found to be metabolically more stable and not at greater risk for cardiovascular disease.

DIABETES MELLITUS

Glucose tolerance deteriorates with increasing age. Glucose homeostasis is regulated by the balance between glucose production (mainly by the liver) and utilization (mainly in muscle), which is in turn regulated by the plasma glucose level per se and by the effects of glucose on several hormones. It has been argued that the deterioration in glucose tolerance with age is not caused by aging per se but by such age-related confounding variables as medications, acute or chronic disease, diet, level of physical activity, stress, and obesity, all of which can interfere with glucose tolerance.[362] Increasing carbohydrate ingestion experimentally from 45 to 49 per cent to 85 per cent of total caloric intake improves insulin sensitivity and glucose tolerance in healthy old men but does not restore it to that of young men.[363, 364] The fact that community-dwelling people tend to increase their carbohydrate intake with age suggests that inadequate carbohydrate intake is an unlikely cause of glucose intolerance in aging.[365]

In one study of older men and women regular, prolonged exercise (longer than three months) improved glucose tolerance and insulin sensitivity[366] and was associated with changes in body weight and body composition,[367] which may have been responsible for the observed improvements. Shimokata and co-workers[368] measured glucose tolerance, obesity, fat distribution, and oxygen consumption during maximal treadmill exercise tolerance testing as well as overall physical activity level in a large

TABLE 147–3. RANGES OF NORMAL BODY MASS INDEX (WEIGHT IN KILOGRAM DIVIDED BY HEIGHT SQUARED IN CENTIMETERS)

AGE RANGE	LOWER LIMIT	AVERAGE	UPPER LIMIT
20–29	17.6	20.4	23.3
30–39	19.2	22.1	25.0
40–49	20.8	23.7	26.6
50–59	22.4	25.3	28.2
60–69	24.0	26.9	29.8

number of community-dwelling people aged 17 to 92 years. Using multivariate analysis, differences in glucose tolerance between young (17 to 39 years) and middle-aged (40 to 59 years) groups was fully attributable to activity level, fitness, and fat mass. In the elderly group (60 to 92 years) age remained a significant independent determinant of glucose tolerance.

Other important factors that significantly affect glucose tolerance are obesity and the pattern of fat distribution. Obesity has been shown to be the most powerful risk factor for the development of NIDDM, and this risk is increased severalfold with an increased accumulation of abdominal fat.[369-371] In aging a redistribution of fat toward the abdominal area occurs from early adult to middle-age years in men and postmenopausally in women.[372]

One mechanism for the age-related impairment of insulin action (see below) might be an alteration in the amount or action of the muscle glucose transporter GLUT-4. Results from human studies reveal no differences in muscle GLUT-4 levels in various glucose-intolerant states.[373] The effects of 12 weeks of exercise training were examined in 18 older, glucose-intolerant people.[374] Despite the absence of changes in body composition, peripheral insulin action improved and GLUT-4 concentration increased. There was, however, no direct relation between changes in GLUT-4 protein and the change in glucose disposal rate.

The major hormonal regulators of plasma glucose are insulin and insulinotropic hormones. Basal insulin levels do not change with increasing age in nonobese people.[375] Similarly, during euglycemic and hyperglycemic clamp studies no differences in either early-phase or late-phase insulin responses were observed among young, middle-aged, and older men.[376] An age-related decrease in the metabolic rate of insulin has been reported by some[377] but not all[378] investigators. Insulin is the most potent regulator of hepatic glucose production. Basal hepatic glucose production and hepatic sensitivity to physiological levels of insulin are normal[379, 380] or slightly decreased in elderly people.[381] The glucose intolerance of aging occurs primarily from decreased peripheral tissue sensitivity at physiological insulin levels; maximal responsivity remains unchanged.[379-382]

The important action of gut hormones to potentiate β-cell secretion is referred as to the incretin effect.[383] The most important insulinotropic gut hormones are gastric inhibitory polypeptide (GIP) and glucagon-like peptide-1 (GLP-1).[384] β-cell sensitivity to GIP is decreased with advancing age[385] and lost in NIDDM.[386, 387] β-cell sensitivity to GLP-1 has not been examined in older people but remains preserved in NIDDM patients.[387, 388]

Other potentially important modulators of glucose homeostasis include the IGF's, especially IGF-I, which decreases with aging (see Growth Hormone). Although IGF-I binds to and activates insulin receptors, the molar potency is lower than that of insulin[389]; in addition, IGF-I exerts a lesser hypoglycemic effect as glucose intolerance increases. Alterations in the other glucose regulatory hormones (glucagon, GH, cortisol, catecholamines) do not appear to contribute to the glucose intolerance of aging. For more detailed discussions of NIDDM in general and in older people, see Chapter 84 and recent reviews.[390, 391]

The decrease in glucose tolerance that accompanies normal aging confounds the diagnosis of diabetes mellitus in elderly people. In 1980 the National Institutes of Health

National Diabetes Data Group (NDDG) and the World Health Organization (WHO) established new criteria for the classification of diabetes mellitus,[392-394] but these criteria include no adjustment for changes with normal aging. The American Diabetes Association (ADA) has also made recommendations for screening and diagnostic testing, the aging implications of which have been reviewed.[395] In the long-term follow-up of men in the Baltimore Longitudinal Study of Aging, an exponentially increasing relation has been observed between the predictive value of the fasting glucose level and the subsequent development of clinically overt diabetes mellitus. This was a continuous relation so that even fasting glucose levels as low as 100 mg/dl had predictive value.[395]

The recommended diagnostic test for diabetes mellitus is the 75-g oral glucose tolerance test. The rationale for the use of a fixed dose is not clear because body size varies considerably in the overall population, and in elderly people there is a progressive loss of muscle mass with age. The ADA has recommended that the dose be adjusted for body size (40 g/m² body surface area). The fixed criteria for diagnosing diabetes mellitus and impaired glucose tolerance, as formulated by the NDDG and WHO panels (see Ch. 82), have resulted in a shift from the high prevalence of diabetes, especially in older people, to impaired glucose tolerance in both African-Americans and Caucasians (Table 147–4). Despite the reclassification from diabetic to impaired glucose tolerance, the latter group needs to be carefully monitored because impaired glucose tolerance is a strong risk factor for the development of diabetes.[396] For example, in a 10-year follow-up of 70-year-old men and women the conversion to frank diabetes mellitus was five-fold higher in the impaired glucose tolerance group versus the normal group.[397]

The announced results of the Diabetes Control and Complications Trial provide strong evidence that tight control of hyperglycemia (i.e., self-monitoring, diet, exercise, multiple daily injections of insulin) significantly reduces and delays the microangiopathic complications associated with insulin-dependent diabetes mellitus.[398] This trial suggests that tight control may also prevent or delay diabetic complications in aged patients with NIDDM. Most older patients with diabetes mellitus seldom test their own blood glucose. Overall, based on a questionnaire consisting of 116,929 persons from the 1989 National Center for Health Statistics, the probability of self-glucose testing decreased 18 per cent with each advancing decade in age.[399]

LIPIDS

Interest in plasma lipids, lipoproteins, and apolipoproteins derives primarily from their strong relations to the development of premature atherosclerosis of the coronary and peripheral vasculature.[400] Because these conditions often are associated with early demise, the prevalence and severity of most of the major dyslipoproteinemias (see Ch. 148), as assessed in cross-sectional studies, decrease with age.[401]

Table 147–5 lists plasma levels of the major lipids and lipoproteins in aged participants in the Lipid Research Clinics program. Detailed age-specific data for men and women beyond age 70 have yet to be reported, thus making diagnosis of dyslipoproteinemias in very old people more difficult.

TABLE 147–4. RATES OF DIABETES (SUM OF DIAGNOSED AND UNDIAGNOSED),* IMPAIRED GLUCOSE TOLERANCE (IGT), AND TOTAL GLUCOSE INTOLERANCE AMONG AFRICAN-AMERICANS AND CAUCASIANS IN THE US POPULATION AGED 20–74 YEARS

	AGE (YR)				
	20–44	*45–54*	*55–64*	*65–74*	*20–74*
African-American Males					
Diabetes	3.1	11.2	14.5	29.1	9.0
IGT	4.8	19.3	17.7	23.9	11.4
Total glucose intolerance	7.8	30.4	32.2	53.0	20.3
Caucasian Males					
Diabetes	1.1	7.5	9.0	18.4	5.5
IGT	4.6	12.7	17.1	22.5	10.2
Total glucose intolerance	5.6	20.3	26.1	40.9	15.7
African-American Females					
Diabetes	3.7	12.8	23.3	23.5	10.7
IGT	14.6	15.7	12.3	8.4	13.8
Total glucose intolerance	18.3	28.5	35.6	31.9	24.6
Caucasian Females					
Diabetes	2.2	8.4	14.8	16.9	7.2
IGT	6.5	14.6	13.6	23.0	11.1
Total glucose intolerance	8.7	23.0	28.5	40.0	18.3

*Percentage of population.
IGT, impaired glucose tolerance.

A longitudinal drop in total serum cholesterol across the adult life span, which can be explained in part by changes in diet, has been reported.[402] Cross-sectional studies conducted by health and nutrition examination surveys also report a progressive drop in cholesterol levels for cohorts examined in 1960–62, 1971–74, and 1976–80. Age, gender, level of physical activity and dietary habits were the most relevant factors responsible for variations in plasma lipoprotein levels. Concentrations of HDL cholesterol are higher in women than in men until women reach the menopause, after which the levels decrease to those found in men.[403] In men triglyceride concentrations increase until about 50 years of age, after which they decline. The triglyceride concentrations in women tend to increase progressively with age, with levels slightly higher in women taking estrogens.[404]

Many studies have found that the increased body weight associated with aging and, especially, the enhanced centripetal fat distribution contribute substantially to abnormal lipid concentrations in older people, thus increasing the risk for cardiovascular disease. Upper-body obesity is more strongly associated with diabetes, hypertension, altered lipid profiles, and gallbladder disease than is lower-body obesity.[345, 405] Upper-body fat excess and the associated insulin resistance and hyperinsulinemia lead to increased hepatic production of triglycerides and cholesterol-rich lipoproteins.[406]

Whether changes in lipoprotein levels that occur with age are caused by biological aging per se or are a consequence of age-related alterations in life-style factors (i.e., physical activity, diet) remains controversial. In the Bronx Aging Study 488 elderly subjects (75 to 85 years) were studied for 10 years to determine risk factors for coronary and cerebrovascular diseases.[407] In men low levels of HDL cholesterol were a coronary heart disease (CHD) risk factor, whereas in women elevated levels of LDL cholesterol were associated with myocardial infarction. In this study there was no control for factors such as medication use, nutrition, and exercise.

The Bronx Aging Study is one of the few studies to

TABLE 147–5. NORTH AMERICAN POPULATION PLASMA TOTAL AND LIPOPROTEIN CHOLESTEROL AND TRIGLYCERIDE VALUES IN OLDER, FREE-LIVING WHITE MEN AND WOMEN NOT TAKING HORMONES

SEX	AGE	TRIGLYCERIDE, mg/dL*	CHOLESTEROL, mg/dL*			
			Total	*HDL*	*LDL*	*VLDL*
Men	60–64	142 (58–291)	231 (159–276)	52 (30–74)	146 (83–210)	19 (3–44)
	65–69	137 (57–267)	213 (158–274)	51 (30–78)	150 (98–210)	20 (0–45)
	70+	130 (58–258)	207 (151–270)	51 (31–75)	143 (88–186)	17 (0–38)
Women	60–64	127 (56–239)	231 (172–297)	62 (36–91)	156 (100–234)	18 (1–45)
	65–69	131 (60–243)	233 (171–303)	61 (34–89)	162 (97–223)	18 (0–40)
	70+	132 (60–237)	228 (169–289)	60 (33–91)	149 (96–207)	16 (0–52)

*Means; 5th to 95th percentiles in parentheses below.
From Hazzard WR: Disorders of lipoprotein metabolism. *In* Andres R, Bierman EL, Hazzard WR (eds.): Principles of Geriatric Medicine. New York, McGraw-Hill, 1985, pp 764–775.

prospectively evaluate lipid and lipoprotein profiles in older people. Because people younger than age 75 were not studied, premature deaths from CHD were excluded. The results of the Bronx Aging Study suggest that treatment for lipid abnormalities, even at advanced ages, may improve the quality of life.

Other studies also support the hypothesis that abnormal lipid or lipoprotein profiles continue to be significant risk factors for CHD later in life. In this regard Sorkin and associates[408] have also demonstrated that cholesterol is a significant risk factor for CHD in people 75 to 97 years of age. In addition, in the Framingham Heart Study[409] serum cholesterol remained a risk factor for CHD in patients older than 65 years. After controlling for other risk factors such as obesity, the Framingham investigators observed a linear association of weight with CHD in men but not in women, perhaps because of a smaller sample size. The Framingham study report recommended that patients be educated on how to increase their HDL cholesterol levels through exercise and weight control.[410]

Despite the recognition that abnormal lipid and lipoprotein profiles remain as significant CHD risk factors in older people, the clinician must exercise caution in the management of elderly patients with dyslipidemias because dietary, exercise, and drug therapy[400, 401] may cause adverse consequences that are more frequent and serious in aged people.

REFERENCES

1. Kirkwood TBL, Rose MR: Evolution of senescence: Late survival sacrificed for reproduction. Philos Trans R Soc Lond (Biol) 332:15–24, 1991.
2. Hayflick L, Moorhead PS: The serial cultivation of human diploid cell strains. Exp Cell Res 25:586–621, 1961.
3. Martin GM, Sprague CA, Epstein CJ: Replicative lifespan of cultivated human cells. Effect of donor's age, tissue, and genotype. Lab Invest 23:86–92, 1970.
4. Monti D, Troiano L, Tropea F, et al: Apoptosis-programmed cell death; a role in the aging process? Am J Clin Nutr 55(6 Suppl): 1208S–1214S, 1992.
5. Koli K, Keski-Oja J: Cellular senescence. Ann Med 24:313–318, 1992.
6. Tilly JL, Kowalski KI, Johnson AL, Hsueh AJ: Involvement of apoptosis in ovarian follicular atresia and postovulatory regression. Endocrinology 129:2799–2801, 1991.
7. Branconnier RJ, Branconnier ME, Walshe TM, et al: Blocking the Ca$^{(2+)}$-activated cytotoxic mechanisms of cholinergic neuronal death: A novel treatment strategy for Alzheimer's disease. Psychopharmacol Bull 28:175–181, 1992.
8. Sloviter RS, Sollas AS, Dean E, Neubort S: Adrenalectomy-induced granule cell degeneration in the rat hippocampal dentate gyrus: Characterization of an in vivo model of controlled neuronal death. J Comp Neurol 330:324–336, 1993.
9. Sohal RS: The free radical hypothesis of aging: An appraisal of the current status. Aging Clin Exp Res 5:3–17, 1993.
10. Reiser KM: Nonenzymatic glycation of collagen in aging and diabetes. Proc Soc Exp Biol Med 196:17–29, 1991.
11. Kristal BS, Yu BP: An emerging hypothesis: Synergistic induction of aging by free radicals and Maillard reactions. J Gerontol 47:B107–114, 1992.
12. Stadtman ER, Oliver CN: Metal-catalyzed oxidation of proteins. J Biol Chem 266:2005–2008, 1991.
13. Masoro EJ: Retardation of aging processes by food restriction: An experimental tool. Am J Clin Nutr 55(6 Suppl):1250S–1252S, 1992.
14. Martin GM: Genetic and environmental modulations of chromosomal stability: Their roles in aging and oncogenesis. Ann NY Acad Sci 621:401–417, 1991.
15. Minaker KL, Meneilly GS, Rowe JW: Endocrine systems. In Finch CE, Schneider EL (eds): Handbook of the Biology of Aging (ed 2). New York, Van Nostrand Reinhold, 1985, pp 433–456.
16. Green MF: The endocrine system. In Pathy MSJ (ed): Principles and Practice of Geriatric Medicine. New York, John Wiley, 1985, pp 909–973.
17. Gregerman RI, Bierman EL: Aging and hormones. In Williams RH (ed): Textbook of Endocrinology (ed 5). Philadelphia, WB Saunders, 1981, pp 1192–1212.
18. Korenman SG: In Endocrine Aspects of Aging. New York, Elsevier Biomedical, 1982, p 1.
19. Eckel R, Hofeldt F: Endocrinology and metabolism in the elderly. In Schreir R (ed): Clinical Internal Medicine in the Aged. Philadelphia, WB Saunders, 1982, pp 222–225.
20. Goldstein S: Cellular senescence. In DeGroot L (ed): Endocrinology (ed 2). Philadelphia, WB Saunders, 1989, pp 2525–2549.
21. Finch CE, Schneider EL: Handbook of the Biology of Aging (ed 2). New York, Van Nostrand Reinholdt, 1985.
22. Meites J, Goya R, Takahashi S: Why the neuroendocrine system is important in aging processes. Exp Gerontol 22:1–15, 1987.
23. Rance NE: Hormonal influences on morphology and neuropeptide expression in the infundibular nucleus of postmenopausal women. Prog Brain Res 93:221–235, 1992.
24. Swaab DF, Hofman MA, Lucassen PJ, et al: Functional neuroanatomy and neuropathology of the human hypothalamus. Anat Embryol 187:317–330, 1993.
25. Hofman MA, Goudsmit E, Purba JS, Swaab DFJA: Morphometric analysis of the supraoptic nucleus in the human brain. J Anat 172:259–270, 1990.
26. Wierda M, Goudsmit E, Van der Woude PF, et al: Oxytocin cell number in the human paraventricular nucleus remains constant with aging and in Alzheimer's disease. Neurobiol Aging 12(5):511–516, 1991.
27. Meana JJ, Barturen F, Garro MA, et al: Decreased density of presynaptic alpha 2-adrenoceptors in postmortem brains of patients with Alzheimer's disease. J Neurochem 58(5):1896–1904, 1992.
28. Sparks DL, Woeltz VM, Markesbery WR: Alterations in brain monoamine oxidase activity in aging, Alzheimer's disease, and Pick's disease. Arch Neurol 48(7):718–721, 1991.
29. Haji M, Roth GS, Blackman MR: Excess in vitro prolactin secretion by pituitary cells from ovariectomized old rats. Am J Physiol 247 (Endocrinol Metab 10):E483–E488, 1984.
30. Takahashi S, Kawashima S, Wakabayashi K: Effects of gonadectomy and chlorpromazine treatment on prolactin, LH and FSH secretion in young and old rats of both sexes. Exp Gerontol 15:185–194, 1980.
31. Lu KH, Hopper BR, Vorgo TM, Yen SSC: Chronological changes in sex steroid, gonadotropin, and prolactin secretion in aging female rats displaying different reproductive states. Biol Reprod 21:193–203, 1979.
32. Simpkins JW, Mueller GP, Huang HH, Meites J: Evidence for depressed catecholamine and enhanced serotonin metabolism in aging male rats: Possible relation to gonadotropin secretion. Endocrinology 100:1672–1678, 1977.
33. Shaar CJ, Euker JS, Riegle GD, Meites J: Effects of castration and gonadal steroids on serum luteinizing hormone and prolactin in young and old rats. J Clin Endocrinol Metab 66:45–51, 1975.
34. Sarkar DK, Gottschall PE, Meites J: Damage to hypothalamic dopaminergic neurons is associated with development of prolactin-secreting pituitary tumors. Science 218:684–686, 1982.
35. Carr BR, MacDonald PC: The menopause and beyond. In Andres R, Bierman EL, Hazzard WR (eds): Principles of Geriatric Medicine. New York, McGraw-Hill, 1985, pp 325–336.
36. Harman SM: Alterations in reproductive and sexual function: Male. In Andres R, Bierman EL, Hazzard WR (eds): Principles of Geriatric Medicine. New York, Mc-Graw-Hill, 1985, pp 337–353.
37. Judd HL, Korenman SG: Effects of aging on reproductive function in women. In Korenman SC (ed): Endocrine Aspects of Aging. New York, Elsevier Biomedical, 1982, pp 163–197.
38. Swerdloff RS, Heber D: Effects of aging on male reproductive function. In Korenman SG (ed): Endocrine Aspects of Aging. New York, Elsevier Biomedical, 1982, pp 119–135.
39. Adolfsson R, Gottfries CG, Roos BE, Windblad B: Post-mortem distribution of dopamine and homovanillic acid in human brain, variations related to age, and a review of the literature. J Neurol Transm 45:81–105, 1979.
40. Robinson DS, Sourkes RL, Nies A, et al: Monoamine metabolism in human brain. Arch Gen Psychiatry 34:89–92, 1977.
41. Rossmanith WG, Scherbaum WA, Lauritzen C: Gonadotropin secretion during aging in postmenopausal women. Neuroendocrinology 54:211–218, 1991.
42. Vermeulen A, Deslypere JP, Kaufman JM: Influence of antiopioids

on luteinizing hormone pulsatility in aging men. J Clin Endocrinol Metab 68:68–72, 1989.

43. Veldhuis JD, Urban RJ, Lizarralde G, et al: Attenuation of luteinizing hormone secretory burst amplitude as a proximate basis for the hypoandrogenism of healthy aging in men. J Clin Endocrinol Metab 75:52–58, 1992.

44. Giusti M, Marini G, Traverso L, et al: Effect of pulsatile luteinizing hormone-releasing hormone administration on pituitary-gonadal function in elderly man. J Endocrinol Invest 13:127–32, 1990.

45. Pontiroli AE, Ruga S, Maffi P, et al: Pituitary reserve after repeated administrations of releasing hormones in young and in elderly men: Reproducibility on different days. J Endocrinol Invest 15:559–566, 1992.

46. Kaufman JM, Giri M, Deslypere JM, et al: Influence of age on the responsiveness of the gonadotrophs to luteinizing hormone–releasing hormone in males. J Clin Endocrinol Metab 72:1255–1260, 1991.

47. Sonntag WE, Steger RW, Forman LJ, Meites J: Decreased pulsatile release of growth hormone in old male rats. Endocrinology 107:1875–1879, 1980.

48. Ceda GP, Valenti G, Butturini U, Hoffman AR: Diminished pituitary responsiveness to growth hormone–releasing factor in aging male rats. Endocrinology 118:2109–2114, 1986.

49. Sonntag WE, Forman LJ, Miki N, et al: Effects of CNS active drugs and somatostatin antiserum on GH release in young and old male rats. Neuroendocrinology 33:73–78, 1981.

50. Lang I, Schernthaner G, Pietschmann P, et al: Effects of sex and age on growth hormone response to growth hormone releasing hormone in healthy individuals. J Clin Endocrinol Metab 65:535–540, 1987.

51. Bellantoni MF, Harman SM, Cho D, Blackman MR: Effects of progestin-opposed transdermal estrogen administration on GH and IGF-I in postmenopausal women of different ages. J Clin Endocrinol Metab 72:172–178, 1991.

52. Ghigo E, Goffi E, Nicolosi M, et al: Growth hormone (GH) responsiveness to combined administration of arginine and GH-releasing hormone does not vary with age in man. J Clin Endocrinol Metab 71:1481–1485, 1990.

53. Iovino M, Monteleone P, Steardo L: Repetitive growth hormone–releasing hormone administration restores the attenuated growth hormone (GH) response to GH releasing hormone testing in normal aging. J Clin Endocrinol Metab 69:910–913, 1989.

54. Shibasaki T, Shizume K, Nakahara M, et al: Age-related changes in plasma growth hormone response to growth hormone–releasing factor in man. J Clin Endocrinol Metab 58:212–214, 1984.

55. Corpas E, Harman SM, Piñeyro MA, et al: Continuous subcutaneous infusions of GHRH 1-44 for 14 days increase GH and IGF-I levels in old men. J Clin Endocrinol Metab 76:134–138, 1993.

56. Corpas E, Harman SM, Piñeyro MA, et al: GHRH 1-29 twice daily reverses the decreased GH and IGF-I levels in old men. J Clin Endocrinol Metab 75:530–535, 1992.

57. Pavlov EP, Harman SM, Merriam GR, et al: Responses of growth hormone (GH) and somatomedin-C to GH-releasing hormone in healthy aging men. J Clin Endocrinol Metab 62:595–600, 1986.

58. Hylka VW, Sonntag WE, Meites J: Reduced ability of old male rats to release ACTH and corticosterone in response to CRF administration. Proc Soc Exp Biol Med 175:1–4, 1984.

58a. Bernardini R, Mauceri G, Iwato MP, et al: Response of the hypothalamic-pituitary-adrenal axis to interleukin I in the aging rat. PNEI 5:166–171, 1992.

58b. Hevoux JA, Gigoviadis DE, DeSouza EB: Age-related decreases in corticotropin-releasing factor (CRF) receptors in rat brain and anterior pituitary gland. Brain Res 542:155–158, 1991.

59. Pavlov EP, Harman SM, Chrousos GP, et al: Responses of plasma adrenocorticotropin, cortisol and dehydroepiandrosterone to ovine corticotropin releasing factor in healthy aging men. J Clin Endocrinol Metab 62:767–772, 1986.

60. Waltman C, Blackman MR, Chrousos GP, et al: Spontaneous and glucocorticoid-inhibited adrenocorticotropic hormone and cortisol secretion are similar in healthy young and old men. J Clin Endocrinol Metab 73:495–502, 1991.

61. Winters SJ, Sherins RJ, Troen P: The gonadotropin-suppressive activity of androgen is increased in elderly men. Metabolism 33:1052–1059, 1984.

62. Muta K, Kato K, Akamine Y, Ibayashi H: Age-related changes in the feedback regulation of gonadotropin secretion by sex steroids in men. Acta Endocrinol (Copenh) 96:154–162, 1981.

63. DeSouza EB, Whitehouse PJ, Kuhar MJ, et al: Reciprocal changes in corticotropin-releasing factor (CRF)-like immunoreactivity and CRF receptors in cerebral cortex of Alzheimer's disease. Nature 319:593–595, 1986.

64. Van Ree JM: Memory and neuropeptides. In Morley JE, Korenman SG (eds): Endocrinology and Metabolism in the Elderly. Boston, Blackwell Scientific, 1992, pp 500–524.

65. Morley JE: Neuropeptides, behavior and aging. J Am Geriatr Soc 34:52–62, 1986.

66. Kleinfeld M, Casimir M, Borra S: Hyponatremia as observed in a chronic disease facility. J Am Geriatr Soc 27:156–161, 1979.

67. Ashraf N, Locksley R, Arieff AI: Thiazide-induced hyponatremia associated with death or neurologic damage in outpatients. Am J Med 70:1163–1168, 1981.

68. Goldstein CS, Braunstein S, Goldfarb S: Idiopathic syndrome of inappropriate antidiuretic hormone secretion possibly related to advanced age. Ann Intern Med 99:185–188, 1983.

69. Rowe JW: Alterations in renal function. In Andres R, Bierman EL, Hazzard WR (eds): Principles of Geriatric Medicine. New York, McGraw-Hill, 1985, pp 319–324.

70. Rowe JW, Shock NW, DeFronzo RA: The influence of age on the renal response to water deprivation in man. Nephron 17:270–278, 1976.

71. Lindeman RD, Lee TD Jr, Yiengst MJ, Shock NW: Influence of age, renal disease, hypertension, diuretics, and calcium on the antidiuretic responses to suboptimal infusions of vasopressin. J Lab Clin Med 68:206–223, 1966.

72. Helderman JH: The impact of normal aging on the hypothalamic-neurohypophyseal-renal axis. In Korenman SG (ed): Endocrine Aspects of Aging. New York, Elsevier Biomedical, 1982, pp 9–32.

73. Helderman JH, Vestal RE, Rowe JW, et al: The response of arginine vasopressin to intravenous ethanol and hypertonic saline in man: The impact of aging. J Gerontol 33:39–47, 1978.

74. Rowe JW, Minaker KL, Sparrow D, Robertson GL: Age-related failure of volume-pressure–mediated vasopressin release. J Clin Endocrinol Metab 54:661–664, 1982.

75. Engel PA, Rowe JW, Minaker KL, Robertson GL: Effect of exogenous vasopressin on vasopressin release. Am J Physiol 246 (Endocrinol Metab):E202–E207, 1984.

76. Silver AJ, Morley JE: Role of the opioid system in the hypodipsia associated with aging. J Am Geriatr Soc 40:556–560, 1992.

77. Chiodera P, Capretti L, Marchesi M, et al: Abnormal arginine vasopressin response to cigarette smoking and metoclopramide (but not to insulin-induced hypoglycemia) in elderly subjects. J Gerontol 46:M6–M10, 1991.

78. Sun Y-K, Xi Y-P, Fenoglio CM, et al: The effect of age on the number of pituitary cells immunoreactive to growth hormone and prolactin. Hum Pathol 15:169–180, 1984.

79. Burrows GN, Wortzman G, Rewcastle RB, et al: Microadenomas of the pituitary and abnormal sellar tomograms in an unselected autopsy series. N Engl J Med 304:156–158, 1981.

80. Annegers JF, Coulam CB, Laws ER: Pituitary tumors: Epidemiology. In Givens JR, Kitabchi AE, Robertson JT (eds): Hormone-Secreting Pituitary Tumors. Chicago, Year Book Medical Publishers, 1982.

81. Vekemans M, Robyn C: Influence of age on serum prolactin levels in women and men. BMJ 4:738–739, 1975.

82. Maddox PR, Jones DL, Mansel RE: Basal prolactin and total lactogenic hormone levels by microbioassay and immunoassay in normal human sera. Acta Endocrinol (Copenh) 125(6):621–627, 1991.

83. Yamaji T, Shimamoto K, Ishibashi M, et al: Effect of age and sex on circulating and pituitary prolactin levels in humans. Acta Endocrinol (Copenh) 83:711–718, 1976.

84. Rossmanith WG, Szilagyi A, Scherbaum WA: Episodic thyrotropin (TSH) and prolactin (PRL) secretion during aging in postmenopausal women. Horm Metab Res 24:185–190, 1992.

85. Touitou Y, Fevre M, Lagogouey M, et al: Age- and mental health-related circadian rhythms of melatonin, prolactin, luteinizing hormone and follicle-stimulating hormone in man. J Clin Endocrinol Metab 91:467–475, 1981.

86. Polleri A, Mastarzo P, Murialdo G, Agnoli A: Circadian rhythmicity of prolactin secretion in elderly subjects: Changes during bromocriptine treatment. J Endocrinol Invest 4:317–321, 1981.

87. Blackman MR, Kowatch MA, Wehmann RE, Harman SM: Basal serum prolactin levels and prolactin responses to constant infusions of thyrotropin releasing hormone in healthy aging men. J Gerontol 41:699–705, 1986.

88. Marrama P, Carani C, Baraghini GF, et al: Circadian rhythm of testosterone and prolactin in the aging. Maturitas 4:131–138, 1982.

89. van Coevorden A, Mockel J, Laurent E, et al: Neuroendocrine rhythms and sleep in aging men. Am J Physiol 260:E651–E661, 1991.

90. Greenspan SL, Klibanski A, Rowe JW, Elahi D: Age alters pulsatile

prolactin release: Influence of dopaminergic inhibition. Am J Physiol 258:E799–E804, 1990.

91. Wasada T: The changes in serum levels of FSH, LH, LH and β-subunit, and prolactin and their responses to synthetic LH-RH and TRH in normal subjects with aging. Fukuoka Acta Med 69:506–518, 1978.

92. Hossdorf T, Wagner H: Secretion of prolactin in healthy men and women of different ages. Aktuel Gerontol 10:119–126, 1980.

93. Giusti M, Delitala G, Marini G, et al: The effect of a met-enkephalin analogue on growth hormone, prolactin, gonadotropins, cortisol and thyroid stimulating hormone in healthy elderly men. Acta Endocrinol (Copenh) 127:205–209, 1992.

94. Rudman D: Growth hormone, body composition and aging. J Am Geriatr Soc 33:800–807, 1985.

95. Clemmons D, Van Wyk JJ: Somatomedin C in blood. J Clin Endocrinol Metab 13:113–143, 1984.

96. Corpas E, Harman SM, Blackman MR: Human growth hormone and human aging. Endocr Rev 14:20–39, 1993.

97. Dudl J, Ensinck J, Palmer E, Williams R: Effect of age on growth hormone secretion in man. J Clin Endocrinol Metab 37:11–16, 1973.

98. Zadik Z, Chalew SA, McCarter RJ, et al: The influence of age on the 24-hour integrated concentration of growth hormone in normal individuals. J Clin Endocrinol Metab 60:513–516, 1985.

99. Finkelstein J, Roffwarg H, Boyar P, et al: Age-related changes in the twenty-four-hour spontaneous secretion of growth hormone in normal individuals. J Clin Endocrinol Metab 35:665–670, 1972.

100. Ho KY, Evans WS, Blizzard RM, et al: Effects of sex and age on 24-hour profile of growth hormone secretion in men: Importance of endogenous estradiol concentrations. J Clin Endocrinol Metab 64:51–58, 1987.

101. Vermeulen A: Nyctohemoral growth hormone profiles in young and aged men: Correlations with somatomedin-C levels. J Clin Endocrinol Metab 64:884–888, 1987.

102. Iranmanesh A, Lizarralde G, Veldhuis JD: Age and relative adiposity are specific negative determinants of the frequency and amplitude of growth hormone (GH) secretory bursts and the half-life of endogenous GH in healthy men. J Clin Endocrinol Metab 73:1081–1088, 1991.

103. Carlson HE, Gillin JC, Gorden P, Snyder F: Absence of sleep-related growth hormone peaks in aged normal subjects and in acromegaly. J Clin Endocrinol Metab 34:1102–1105, 1972.

104. Rudman D, Vintner MH, Rogers CM, et al: Impaired growth hormone secretion in the adult population. Relation to age and adiposity. J Clin Invest 67:1361–1369, 1981.

105. Prinz PN, Weitzman ED, Cunningham GR, Karacan I: Plasma growth hormone during sleep in young and aged men. J Gerontol 38:519–524, 1983.

106. Kalk WJ, Vinik AI, Pimstone BL, Jackson WP: Growth hormone responses to insulin hypoglycemia in the elderly. J Gerontol 28:431–433, 1973.

107. Muggeo M, Fedele D, Tiengo A, et al: Human growth hormone and cortisol responses to insulin stimulation in aging. J Gerontol 30:546–551, 1975.

108. Blichert-Toft M: Stimulation of the release of corticotrophin and somatotrophin by metyrapone and arginine. Acta Endocrinol (Copenh) 195:65–85, 1975.

109. Corpas E, Blackman MR, Roberson R, et al: Oral arginine/lysine does not increase growth hormone and insulin-like growth factor-I secretion in old men. J Gerontol 48:M128–M133, 1993.

110. Hagberg JM, Seals DR, Yerg JE, et al: Metabolic responses to exercise in young and old athletes and sedentary men. J Appl Physiol 65:900–908, 1988.

111. Craig BW, Brown R, Everhart J: Effects of progressive resistance training on growth hormone and testosterone levels in young and elderly subjects. Mech Ageing Dev 49:159–169, 1989.

112. Hattori N, Kurahachi H, Ikekubo K, et al: Effects of sex and age on serum GH binding protein levels in normal adults. Clin Endocrinol (Oxf) 35:295–297, 1991.

113. Daughaday WH, Trivedi B, Andrews BAJ: The ontogeny of serum GH binding protein in man: A possible indicator of hepatic GH receptor development. J Clin Endocrinol Metab 65:1072–1074, 1987.

114. Hochberg Z, Amit T, Zadick Z: Twenty four hour profile of plasma growth hormone–binding protein. J Clin Endocrinol Metab 72:236–239, 1991.

115. Alba-Roth J, Muller OA, Schopohl J, Von Werder K: Arginine stimulates growth hormone secretion by suppressing endogenous somatostatin secretion. J Clin Endocrinol Metab 67:1186–1189, 1988.

116. Franchimont P, Urbain-Choffray D, Lambelin P, et al: Effects of repetitive administration of growth hormone–releasing hormone on growth hormone secretion, insulin-like growth factor I, and bone metabolism in postmenopausal women. Acta Endocrinol (Copenh) 120:121–128, 1989.

117. Pasteels JL, Gausset P, Danguy A, et al: Morphology of the lactotropes and somatotropes of man and rhesus monkeys. J Clin Endocrinol Metab 34:959–967, 1972.

118. Calderon L, Ryan N, Kovacs K: Human pituitary growth hormone cells in old age. J Gerontol 24:441–447, 1978.

119. Coiro V, Volpi R, Cavazzini U, et al: Restoration of normal growth hormone responsiveness to GHRH in normal aged men by infusion of low amounts of theophylline. J Gerontol 46:M155–M158, 1991.

120. Rudman D, Kutner MH, Rogers CM, et al: Impaired growth hormone secretion in the adult population: Relation to age and adiposity. J Clin Invest 67:1361–1369, 1981.

121. Johanson AJ, Blizzard RM: Low somatomedin-C levels in older men rise in response to growth hormone administration. Johns Hopkins Med J 149:115–117, 1981.

122. Copeland KC, Colletti RB, Devlin JD, McAuliffe TL: The relationship between insulin-like growth factor-1, adiposity and aging. Metabolism 39:584–587, 1990.

123. Poehlman ET, Copeland KC: Influence of physical activity on insulin-like growth factor in healthy younger and older men. J Clin Endocrinol Metab 71:1468–1473, 1990.

124. Baxter RC, Martin JL: Radioimmunoassay of growth hormone–dependent insulin-like growth factor binding protein in human plasma. J Clin Invest 78:1504–1512, 1986.

125. Corpas E, Harman SM, Blackman MR: Serum IGF-binding protein-3 is related to IGF-I, but not to spontaneous GH release, in healthy old men. Horm Metabol Res 24:543–545, 1992.

126. Conover CA, Dollar LA, Hintz RL, Rosenfeld RG: Somatomedin binding and action in fibroblasts from aged and progeric subjects. J Clin Endocrinol Metab 60:685–691, 1985.

127. Conover CA, Rosenfeld RG, Hintz RL: Aging alters somatomedin-C–dexamethasone synergism in the stimulation of deoxyribonucleic acid synthesis and replication of cultured human fibroblasts. J Clin Endocrinol Metab 61:423–428, 1985.

128. Rudman D, Feller AG, Nagraj HS, et al: Effect of human growth hormone in men over 60 years old. N Engl J Med 323:1–6, 1990.

129. Blichert-Toft M, Blichert-Toft B, Kaalund-Jensen H: Pituitary–adrenocortical stimulation in the aged as reflected in levels of plasma cortisol and compound S. Acta Chir Scand 136:665–670, 1970.

130. West CD, Brown H, Simons EL, et al: Adrenocorticol function and cortisol metabolism in old age. J Clin Endocrinol Metab 21:1197–1207, 1961.

131. Romanoff LP, Morris CW, Welch P, et al: The metabolism of cortisol-C14 in young and elderly men. I. Secretion rate of cortisol and daily excretion of tetrahydrocortisol allotetrahydrocortisol, tetrahydrocortisone and cortolone (20 alpha and 20 beta). J Clin Endocrinol Metab 21:1413–1425, 1961.

132. Jensen HK, Blichert-Toft M: Serum corticotrophin, plasma cortisol and urinary secretion of 17-ketogenic steroids in the elderly (age group 66–94 years). Acta Endocrinol (Copenh) 66:25–34, 1971.

133. Lakatua DJ, Nicolau GY, Bogdan C, et al: Circadian endocrine time structure in humans above 80 years of age. J Gerontol 39:648–654, 1984.

134. Greenspan SL, Rowe JW, Maitland LA, et al: The pituitary-adrenal glucocorticoid response is altered by gender and disease. J Gerontol 48:M72–M77, 1993.

135. Blichert-Toft M: Secretion of corticotrophin and somatotrophin by the senescent adenohypophysis in man. Acta Endocrinol (Copenh) 195 (Suppl):13–17, 1975.

136. Asnis GM, Sachar EJ, Halbreich U, et al: Cortisol secretion in relation to age in major depression. Psychosom Med 43:235–242, 1981.

137. Doncaster HD, Barton RN, Horan MA, Roberts NA: Factors influencing cortisol-adrenocorticotropin relationships in elderly women with upper femur fractures. J Trauma 34:49–55, 1993.

138. Dilman VM, Ostroumova MN, Tsyrlina EV: Hypothalamic mechanisms of ageing and of specific age pathology. II. On the sensitivity threshold of hypothalamo-pituitary complex to homeostatic stimuli in adaptive homeostasis. Exp Gerontol 14:175–181, 1979.

139. Heuser IJ, Wark HJ, Keul J, Holsboer F: Hypothalamic-pituitary-adrenal axis function in elderly endurance athletes. J Clin Endocrinol Metab 73(3):485–488, 1991.

140. von Bardeleben U, Holsboer F: Effect of age on the cortisol response to human corticotropin-releasing hormone in depressed patients pretreated with dexamethasone. Biol Psychol 29:1042–1050, 1991.

141. Turnbridge WMG, Evered DC, Hall R, et al: The spectrum of thyroid

disease in a community: The Wickham survey. Clin Endocrinol (Oxf) 7:481–493, 1977.

142. Sawin CT, Chopra D, Azizi F, et al: The aging thyroid: Increased prevalence of elevated serum thyrotropin levels in the elderly. JAMA 242:247–250, 1979.

143. Harman SM, Wehmann RE, Blackman MR: Pituitary-thyroid hormone economy in healthy aging men: Basal indices of thyroid function and thyrotropin responses to constant infusions of thyrotropin releasing hormone. J Clin Endocrinol Metab 58:320–326, 1984.

144. Cuttelod S, Lemarchand-Beraud T, Magnenat P, et al: Effect of age and role of kidneys and liver on thyrotropin turnover in man. Metabolism 23:101–113, 1974.

145. Gregerman RI: Thyroid diseases. *In* Andres R, Bierman EL, Hazzard WR (eds): Principles of Geriatric Medicine. New York, McGraw-Hill, 1985, pp 727–749.

146. Klug TL, Adelman RC: Evidence for a large thyrotropin and its accumulation during aging in rats. Biochem Biophys Res Commun 77:1431–1437, 1977.

147. Sawin CT, Geller A, Kaplan MM, et al: Low serum thyrotropin (thyroid-stimulating hormone) in older persons without hyperthyroidism. Arch Intern Med 151:165–168, 1991.

148. Wiener R, Utiger RD, Lew R, Emerson CH: Age, sex, and serum thyrotropin concentrations in primary hypothyroidism. Acta Endocrinol (Copenh) 124(4):364–369, 1991.

149. Lewis GF, Alessi CA, Imperial JG, Refetoff S: Low serum free thyroxine index in ambulating elderly is due to a resetting of the threshold of thyrotropin feedback suppression. J Clin Endocrinol Metab 73(4):843–849, 1991.

150. Snyder P, Utiger RD: Response to thyrotropin releasing hormone (TRH) in normal man. J Clin Endocrinol Metab 34:380–385, 1972.

151. Snyder PJ, Utiger RD: Thyrotropin response to thyrotropin releasing hormone in normal females over forty. J Clin Endocrinol Metab 34:1096–1098, 1972.

152. Wenzel KW, Meinhold H, Herpich M, et al: TRH-stimulations test mit alters-und geschlechtsabhangigem TSH anstieg bei normal person. Klin Wochenschr 52:722–727, 1974.

153. Ohara H, Kobayashi T, Shiraishi M, Wada T: Thyroid function of the aged as viewed from the pituitary thyroid system. Endocrinol Jpn 21:377–386, 1974.

154. Greenspan SL, Sparrow D, Rowe JW: Dopaminergic regulation of gonadotropin and thyrotropin hormone secretion is altered with age. Horm Res 36:41–46, 1991.

155. Greenspan SL, Klibanski A, Rowe JW, Elahi D: Age-related alterations in pulsatile secretion of TSH: Role of dopaminergic regulation. Am J Physiol 260:E486–E491, 1991.

156. Iovino M, Steardo L, Monteleone P: Impaired sensitivity of the hypothalamo-pituitary-thyroid axis to the suppressant effect of dexamethasone in elderly subjects. Psychopharmacology 105:481–484, 1991.

157. Frolkis VV, Verzhikovskaya NV, Valueva GV: The thyroid and age. Exp Gerontol 8:285–296, 1973.

158. Hegedus L, Perrild H, Poulsen LR, et al: The determination of thyroid volume by ultrasound and its relationship to bodyweight, age and sex in normal subjects. J Clin Endocrinol Metab 56:260–263, 1983.

159. Berghout A, Wiersinga WM, Smits NJ, Touber JL: Interrelationships between age, thyroid volume, thyroid nodularity, and thyroid function in patients with sporadic nontoxic goiter. Am J Med 89:602–608, 1990.

160. Hintze G, Windeler J, Baumert J, et al: Thyroid volume and goitre prevalence in the elderly as determined by ultrasound and their relationships to laboratory indices. Acta Endocrinol (Copenh) 124:12–18, 1991.

161. Studer H, Riek MM, Greer MA: Multinodular goiter. *In* DeGroot LJ (ed): Endocrinology. New York, Grune & Stratton, 1979, pp 489–499.

162. Levy EG: Thyroid disease in the elderly. Med Clin North Am 75:151–167, 1991.

163. Francis T, Wartofsky L: Common thyroid disorders in the elderly. Postgrad Med 92:225–230, 233–236, 1992.

164. Hesch RD, Gatz J, Juppner H, Stubbe P: TBG dependency of age-related variations of thyroxine and triiodothyromine. Horm Metab Res 9:141–146, 1977.

165. Wenzel KW, Horn WR: Triiodothyromine (T_3) and thyroxine (T_4) kinetics in aged men. *In* Robbins J, Utiger RD (eds): Thyroid Research. Amsterdam, Excerpta Medica, 1976, pp 270–273.

166. Hansen JM, Skovsted L, Siersbaeck-Nielsen K: Age dependent changes in iodine metabolism and thyroid function. Acta Endocrinol (Copenh) 79:60–65, 1975.

167. Page SR, Taylor AH, Whitley GS, et al: Effects of ageing on the growth and differentiated function of transfected human thyrocytes. Mol Cell Endocrinol 82:143–150, 1991.

168. Azizi F, Vagenakis AG, Portnay GI, et al: Pituitary-thyroid responsiveness to intramuscular thyrotropin releasing hormone based on analyses of serum thyroxine, triiodothyromine, and thyrotropin concentrations. N Engl J Med 292:273–277, 1975.

169. Simons RJ, Simon JM, Demers LM, Santen RJ: Thyroid dysfunction in elderly hospitalized patients. Effect of age and severity of illness. Arch Intern Med 150:1249–1253, 1990.

170. Chopra IJ, Chopra U, Smith SR, et al: Reciprocal changes in serum concentrations of 3,3′,5′ tri-iodothyroxine (reverse T_3) and 3,5,3′-triiodothyroxine (T_3) in systemic illnesses. J Clin Endocrinol Metab 41:1043–1049, 1975.

171. Nicod P, Burger A, Staeheli V, Vallotton ME: A radioimmunoassay for 3,3′,5′-triiodo-L-thyronine in unextracted serum. J Clin Endocrinol Metab 42:823–829, 1976.

172. Ronnøv V, Kirkegaard C: Hyperthyroidism—a disease of old age? BMJ 1:41–45, 1973.

173. Borst GC, Eil C, Burman K: Euthyroid hyperthyroxinemia. Ann Intern Med 98:366–378, 1983.

174. Fradkin JE, Wolff J: Iodide-induced thyrotoxicosis. Medicine 62:1–20, 1983.

175. Griffin JE: Hypothyroidism in the elderly. Am J Med Sci 299:334–345, 1990.

176. Klatsky SA, Manson PN, Surg AP: Thyroid disorders masquerading as aging changes. Ann Plast Surg 28:420–426, 1992.

177. Bahemuka M, Hodkinson HM: Screening for hypothyroidism in elderly inpatients. BMJ 2:601–603, 1975.

178. Wehmann RE, Gregerman RI, Burns WH, et al: Suppression of thyrotropin in the low-thyroxine state of severe nonthyroidal illness. N Engl J Med 312:546–552, 1985.

179. Wartofsky L, Burman KD: Alterations in thyroid function in patients with systemic illness: The "euthyroid sick syndrome." Endocr Rev 3:164–217, 1982.

180. Roti E, Gardini E, Minelli R, et al: Prevalence of anti-thyroid peroxidase antibodies in serum in the elderly: Comparison with other tests for anti-thyroid antibodies. Clin Chem 38:88–92, 1992.

181. Mariotti S, Sansoni P, Barbesino G, et al: Thyroid and other organ-specific autoantibodies in healthy centenarians. Lancet 339:1506–1508, 1992.

182. Samaan NA, Maheshwari YK, Nader S, et al: Impact of therapy for differentiated carcinoma of the thyroid: An analysis of 706 cases. J Clin Endocrinol Metab 56:1131–1138, 1983.

183. Barton RN, Horan MA, Weijers JWM, et al: Cortisol production rate and the urinary excretion of 17-hydroxycorticosteroids, free cortisol, and 6 beta-hydroxycortisol in healthy elderly men and women. J Gerontol 48:M213–M218, 1993.

184. Kaalund-Jensen H, Blichert-Toft M: Serum corticotrophin, plasma cortisol, and urinary excretion of 17-ketogenic steroids in the elderly (age group: 66–94 years). Acta Endocrinol Scand 66:25–34, 1971.

185. Touitou Y, Sulon J, Bogdan J, et al: Adrenal circadian system in young and elderly human subjects: A comparative study. J Clin Endocrinol Metab 93:201–210, 1982.

186. Sherman B, Wysham C, Pfohl B: Age-related changes in the circadian rhythm of plasma cortisol in man. J Clin Endocrinol Metab 61:439–443, 1985.

187. Oshashi M, Kato K, Nawata H, Ibayashi H: Adrenocortical responsiveness to graded ACTH infusions in normal young and elderly subjects. Gerontology 32:43–51, 1986.

188. Roberts NA, Barton RN, Horan MA: Ageing and the sensitivity of the adrenal gland to physiological doses of ACTH in man. J Endocrinol Invest 126:507–513, 1990.

189. Langer P, Balazova E, Vician M, et al: Acute development of low T_3 syndrome and changes in pituitary-adrenocortical function after elective cholecystectomy in women: Some differences between young and elderly patients. Scand J Clin Lab Invest 52:215–220, 1992.

190. Jacobs S, Mason J, Kosten T, et al: Urinary free cortisol excretion in relation to age in acutely stressed persons with depressive symptoms. Psychosom Med 46:213–221, 1984.

191. Friedman M, Green MF, Sharland DE: Assessment of hypothalamic-pituitary-adrenal function in the geriatric age groups. J Gerontol 24:292–297, 1969.

192. Orentreich N, Brind JL, Rizer RL, Vogelman JH: Age changes and sex differences in serum dehydroepiandrosterone sulfate concentrations from puberty through adulthood. J Clin Endocrinol Metab 59:551–555, 1984.

193. Liu CH, Laughlin GA, Fischer UG, Yen SS: Marked attenuation of ultradian and circadian rhythms of dehydroepiandrosterone in postmenopausal women: Evidence for a reduced 17,20-desmolase enzymatic activity. J Clin Endocrinol Metab 71:900–906, 1990.

194. Vermeulen A, Deslypere JP, Schelfhout W, et al: Adrenocortical function in old age: Response to acute adrenocorticotropin stimulation. J Clin Endocrinol Metab 54:187–191, 1982.
195. Yamaji T, Ibayashi H: Plasma dehydroepiandrosterone sulphate in normal and pathological conditions. J Clin Endocrinol Metab 29:273–278, 1969.
196. Shiebinger R, Albertson B, Cassorla F, et al: The developmental changes in plasma adrenal androgens during infancy and adrenarche are associated with changing activities of adrenal microsomal 17-hydroxylase and 17,20-desmolase. J Clin Invest 67:1177–1182, 1981.
197. Dohm G: The prepubertal and pubertal growth of the adrenal (adrenarche). Beitr Pathol 150:357–377, 1973.
198. Barrett-Connor E, Khaw KT, Yen SS: A prospective study of dehydroepiandrosterone sulfate, mortality, and cardiovascular disease. N Engl J Med 315:1519–1524, 1986.
199. Barrett-Connor E, Khaw KT: Absence of an inverse relation of dehydroepiandrosterone sulfate with cardiovascular mortality in postmenopausal women [letter]. N Engl J Med 317:711, 1987.
200. Mortola JF, Yen SS: The effects of oral dehydroepiandrosterone on endocrine-metabolic parameters in postmenopausal women. J Clin Endocrinol Metab 71:696–704, 1990.
201. Bauer JH: Age-related changes in the renin-aldosterone system. Physiological effects and clinical implications. Drugs Aging 3:238–245, 1993.
202. Hallengren B, Elmstahl S, Galvard H, et al: Eighty-year-old men have elevated plasma concentrations of catecholamines but decreased plasma renin activity and aldosterone as compared to young men. Aging (Milano) 4:341–345, 1992.
203. Tuck M, Sowers J: Hypertension and aging. In Korenman SG (ed): Endocrine Aspects of Aging. New York, Elsevier Biomedical, 1982, pp 81–117.
204. Luft FC, Fineberg NS, Weinberger MH: The influence of age on renal function and renin and aldosterone responses to sodium-volume expansion and contraction in normotensive and mildly hypertensive humans. Am J Hypertens 5:520–528, 1992.
205. Michelis MF: Hyperkalemia in the elderly. Am J Kidney Dis 16:296–269, 1990.
206. Tsunoda K, Abe K, Goto T, et al: Effect of age on the renin-angiotensin-aldosterone system in normal subjects: Simultaneous measurement of active and inactive renin, renin substrate, and aldosterone in plasma. J Clin Endocrinol Metab 62:384–389, 1986.
207. Phillips PA, Hodsman GP, Johnston CI: Neuroendocrine mechanisms and cardiovascular homeostasis in the elderly. Cardiovasc Drugs Ther 4(Suppl 6):1209–1213, 1991.
208. Or K, Richards AM, Espiner EA, et al: Effect of low dose infusions of ile-atrial natriuretic peptide in healthy elderly males: Evidence for a postreceptor defect. J Clin Endocrinol Metab 76:1271–1274, 1993.
209. Cugini P, Lucia P, Di Palma L, et al: Effect of aging on circadian rhythm of atrial natriuretic peptide, plasma renin activity, and plasma aldosterone. J Gerontol 47:B214–B219, 1992.
210. Kuwajima I, Suzuki Y, Hoshino S, et al: Effects of aging on the cardiopulmonary receptor reflex in hypertensive patients. Jpn Heart J 32:157–166, 1991.
211. Mancia G, Cleroux J, Daffonchio A, et al: Reflex control of circulation in the elderly. Cardiovasc Drugs Ther 4(Suppl 6):1223–1228, 1991.
212. Ballerman BJ, Brenner BM: Biologically active atrial peptides. J Clin Invest 76:2041–2048, 1985.
213. Clark BA, Elahi B, Epstein FH: Influence of gender and age on atrial natriuretic peptide levels in man. J Clin Endocrinol Metab 70:349–353, 1990.
214. Ohashi M, Fujio N, Nawata H, et al: High plasma concentrations of human atrial natriuretic polypeptide in aged men. J Clin Endocrinol Metab 64:81–85, 1987.
215. Haller BGD, Zust H, Shaw S, et al: Effects of posture and aging on circulating natriuretic peptide levels in men. J Hyperten 5:551–556, 1987.
216. Davis KM, Fish LC, Elahi D, et al: Atrial natriuretic peptide levels in the prediction of congestive heart failure risk in frail elderly. JAMA 267:2625–2629, 1992.
217. Clark BA, Elahi D, Shannon RP, et al: Influence of age and dose on the end-organ responses to atrial natriuretic peptide in humans. Am J Hyperten 4:500–507, 1991.
218. Morrow LA, Morganroth GS, Hill TJ, et al: Atrial natriuretic factor in the elderly: Diminished response to epinephrine. Am J Physiol 257:E866–E870, 1990.
219. Clark BA, Elahi D, Fish L, et al: Atrial natriuretic peptide suppresses osmostimulated vasopressin release in young and elderly humans. Am J Physiol 261:E252–E256, 1991.
220. Ferrari P, Weidman P, Ferrier C, et al: Dysregulation of atrial natriuretic factor in hypertension-prone man. J Clin Endocrinol Metab 71:944–951, 1990.
221. Shannon RP, Wei JY, Rosa RM, et al: The effect of age and sodium depletion on cardiovascular response to orthostasis. Hypertension 8:438–443, 1986.
222. Tuchelt H, Eschenhagen G, Bahr V, et al: Role of atrial natriuretic factor in changes in the responsiveness of aldosterone to angiotensin II secondary to sodium loading and depletion in man. Clin Sci 79:57–65, 1990.
223. Williams TDM, Walsh KP, Lightman SL, Sutton R: Atrial natriuretic peptide inhibits postural release of renin and vasopressin in humans. Am J Physiol 255:R368–R372, 1988.
224. Clark BA, Brown RS, Epstein FH: Effect of atrial natriuretic peptide on potassium-stimulated aldosterone secretion: Potential relevance to hypoaldosteronism in man. J Clin Endocrinol Metab 75:399–403, 1992.
225. Ziegler MB, Lake CR, Kopin IJ: Plasma noradrenaline increases with age. Nature 261:333–335, 1976.
226. Rowe JW, Troen BR: Sympathetic nervous system and aging in man. Endocr Rev 1:167–179, 1980.
227. Printz PN, Harter J, Benedetti C, Raskind M: Circadian variation of plasma catecholamines in young and old men—relation to rapid eye movements and slow wave sleep. J Clin Endocrinol Metab 49:300–304, 1979.
228. Young JB, Rowe JW, Pallotta J, et al: Enhanced plasma norepinephrine response to upright posture and oral glucose administration in elderly subjects. Metabolism 29:532–537, 1980.
229. Rubin X, Scott PJ, McLean K, Reid JL: Noradrenaline release and clearance in relation to age and blood pressure in man. Eur J Clin Invest 12:121–125, 1982.
230. Esler M, Skews H, Leonard P, et al: Age-dependence of noradrenaline kinetics in normal subjects. Clin Sci 60:217–219, 1981.
231. Featherstone JA, Veith RC, Flatness D, et al: Age and alpha-2 adrenergic regulation of plasma norepinephrine kinetics in humans. J Gerontol 42:271–276, 1987.
232. Hoeldtke RD, Cilmi KM: Effects of aging on cathecholamine metabolism. J Clin Endocrinol Metab 60:479–484, 1985.
233. Morrow LA, Linares OA, Hill TJ, et al: Age differences in the plasma clearance mechanisms for epinephrine and norepinephrine in humans. J Clin Endocrinol Metab 65:508–511, 1987.
234. Schwartz RS, Jaeger LF, Veith RC: The importance of body composition to the increase in plasma norepinephrine appearance rate in elderly men. J Gerontol 42:546–551, 1987.
235. Veith RC, Featherstone JA, Linares OA, Halter JB: Age differences in plasma norephinephrine kinetics in humans. J Gerontol 41:319–324, 1986.
236. Supiano MA, Linares OA, Smith MJ, Halter JB: Age-related differences in norepinephrine kinetics: Effect of posture and sodium-restricted diet. Am J Physiol 259:E422–E431, 1990.
237. Stromberg JS, Linares OA, Supiano MA, et al: Effect of desipramine on norepinephrine metabolism in humans: Interaction with aging. Am J Physiol 261:R1484–R1490, 1991.
238. Poehlman ET, McAuliffe T, Danforth EJ: Effects of age and level of physical activity on plasma norepinephrine kinetics. Am J Physiol 258:E256–E262, 1990.
239. MacGilchrist AJ, Hawksby C, Howes LG, Reid JL: Rise in plasma noradrenaline with age results from an increase in spillover rate. J Gerontol 35:7–13, 1989.
240. Freedman LS, Ohuchi T, Goldstein M, et al: Changes in human serum dopamine β-hydroxylase activity with age. Nature 236:310–311, 1972.
241. Rowe JW, Young JB, Minaker KL, et al: Effect of insulin and glucose infusions on sympathetic nervous system activity in normal man. Diabetes 30:219–225, 1981.
242. Minaker KL, Rowe JW, Young JB, et al: Effect of age on insulin stimulation of sympathetic nervous system activity in man. Metabolism 31:1181–1184, 1982.
243. O'Hare JA, Minaker KL, Meneilly GS, et al: Effect of insulin on plasma norepinephrine and 3,4-dihydroxyphenylalanine in obese men. Metabolism 38:322–329, 1989.
244. Franco-Morselli R, Elghozi JL, Joby E, et al: Increased plasma adrenalin in benign essential hypertension. BMJ 2:1251–1254, 1977.
245. Yin FC, Spurgeon HA, Greene HL, et al: Age-associated decrease in heart rate response to isoproterenol in dogs. Mech Ageing Dev 10:17–25, 1979.
246. Petrofsky JS, Lind AR: Isometric strength endurance and the blood pressure and heart rate responses during isometric exercise in

healthy men and women with special reference to age and body fat content. Pflugers Arch 360:49–61, 1975.

247. Kronenberg RS, Draze CJ: Attenuation of the ventilatory and heart rate responses to hypoxia and hypercapnia with aging in normal men. J Clin Invest 58:1812–1819, 1973.

248. Lakatta EG: Age-related alterations in the cardiovascular response to adrenergic mediated stress. Fed Proc 39:3173–3177, 1980.

249. Conway J, Whaler R, Sannersteldt R: Sympathetic nervous activity during exercise in relation to age. Cardiovasc Res 5:577–581, 1971.

250. Parker RJ, Berkowitz BA, Lee CH, Denckla WD: Vascular relaxation, aging and thyroid hormones. Mech Ageing Dev 8:397–405, 1978.

251. Feldman RD, Limbird LE, Nadeau J, et al: Alterations in leukocyte beta-receptor affinity with aging: A potential explanation for altered beta-adrenergic sensitivity in the elderly. N Engl J Med 310:815–819, 1984.

252. Krall JF, Connelly M, Weisbart R, Tuck ML: Age-related elevation of plasma catecholamine concentration and reduced responsiveness of lymphocyte adenylate cyclase. J Clin Endocrinol Metab 52:863–867, 1981.

253. Dax EM: Receptors and associated membrane events in aging. In Rothstein M (ed): Review of Biological Research in Aging (vol 2). New York, Alan R Liss, 1985, pp 315–336.

254. Dax EM: Age-related changes in membrane receptor interactions. Endocrinol Metab Clin North Am 16:947–963, 1987.

255. Heinsimer JA, Lefkowitz RJ: The impact of aging on adrenergic receptor function: Clinical and biochemical aspects. J Am Geriatr Soc 33:184–188, 1985.

256. Roth GS, Hess GD: Changes in the mechanisms of hormone and neurotransmitter action during aging: Current status of the role of receptor and post receptor alterations. A review. Mech Ageing Dev 20:175–194, 1982.

257. Mader SL: Aging and postural hypotension: An update. J Am Geriatr Soc 37:129–137, 1989.

258. Vestal RE, Wood AJ, Shand OG: Reduced beta-adrenoreceptor sensitivity in the elderly. Clin Pharmacol Ther 26:181–186, 1979.

259. Gregerman RI: Aging and hormone sensitive lipolysis: Reconciling the literature. J Gerontol (in press).

260. Chapuy MC, Ourr F, Chapuy P: Age-related changes in parathyroid hormone and 25-hydroxycholecalciferol levels. J Gerontol 38:19–22, 1983.

261. Insogna KL, Lewis AN, Lipinski BA, et al: Effect of age on serum immunoreactive parathyroid hormone and its biological effects. J Clin Endocrinol Metab 53:1072–1075, 1981.

262. Gallagher JC, Riggs LB, Jerpbak CM, Arnaud CD: The effect of age on serum immunoreactive parathyroid hormone in normal and osteoporotic women. J Lab Clin Med 95:373–385, 1980.

263. Wiiske PS, Epstein S, Bell NH, et al: Increases in immunoreactive parathyroid hormone with age. N Engl J Med 300:1419–1421, 1979.

264. Marcus R, Madvig P, Young G: Age-related changes in parathyroid hormone and parathyroid hormone action in normal humans. J Clin Endocrinol Metab 58:223–230, 1984.

265. Sherman SS, Hollis BW, Tobin JD: Vitamin D status and related parameters in a healthy population: The effects of age, sex, and season. J Clin Endocrinol Metab 71:405–413, 1990.

266. Eastell R, Yergey AL, Vieira NE, et al: Interrelationship among vitamin D metabolism, true calcium absorption, parathyroid function, and age in women: Evidence of an age-related intestinal resistance to 1,25-dihydroxyvitamin D action. J Bone Mineral Res 6:125–132, 1991.

267. Dubbelman R, Jonxis JH, Muskiet FA, Saleh AE: Age-dependent vitamin D status and vertebral condition of white women living in Curacao (The Netherlands Antilles) as compared with their counterparts in The Netherlands. Am J Clin Nutr 58:106–109, 1993.

268. Quesada JM, Coopmans W, Ruiz B, et al: Influence of vitamin D on parathyroid function in the elderly. J Clin Endocrinol Metab 75:494–501, 1992.

269. Ebeling PR, Sandgren ME, DiMagno EP, et al: Evidence of an age-related decrease in intestinal responsiveness to vitamin D: Relationship between serum 1,25-dihydroxyvitamin D_3 and intestinal vitamin D receptor concentrations in normal women. J Clin Endocrinol Metab 75:176–182, 1992.

270. Yendt ER, Cohanim M, Rosenberg GM: Reduced serum calcium and inorganic phosphate levels in normal elderly women. J Gerontol 41:325–330, 1986.

271. Eliel LP: Primary hyperparathyroidism. In Andres R, Bierman EL, Hazzard WR (eds): Principles of Geriatric Medicine. New York, McGraw-Hill, 1985, pp 776–780.

272. Heath H, Hodgson SF, Kennedy MA: Primary hyperparathyroidism. Incidence, morbidity, and potential economic impact in a community. N Engl J Med 302:189–193, 1980.

273. Block MA, Xavier A, Brush BE: Management of primary hyperparathyroidism in the elderly. J Am Geriatr Soc 23:385–389, 1975.

274. Baker S: Idiopathic hypoparathyroidism presenting as urinary and faecal incontinence. BMJ 2:963–964, 1982.

275. Graham K, Williams BO, Rowe MS: Idiopathic hypoparathyroidism: A cause of fits in the elderly. BMJ 1:1460–1461, 1979.

276. Chestnut C: Osteoporosis. In Andres R, Bierman EL, Hazzard WR (eds): Principles of Geriatric Medicine. New York, McGraw-Hill, 1985, pp 801–812.

277. Deftos LJ, Weisman MH, Williams GW, et al: Influence of age and sex on plasma calcitonin in human beings. N Engl J Med 302:1351–1353, 1980.

278. Pedrazzoni M, Mantovani M, Ciotti G, et al: Calcitonin levels in normal women of various ages evaluated with a new sensitive radioimmunoassay. Horm Metab Res 20:118–119, 1988.

279. Torring O, Bucht E, Sjoberg HE: Plasma calcitonin response to a calcium clamp. Influence of sex and age. Horm Metab Res 17:536–539, 1985.

280. Tiegs RD, Body JJ, Barta JM, Heath H III: Secretion and metabolism of monomeric human calcitonin: Effects of age, sex, and thyroid damage. J Bone Mineral Res 1:339–349, 1986.

281. Chestnut CH, Baylink DJ, Sison K, et al: Basal plasma immunoreactive calcitonin in postmenopausal osteoporosis. Metabolism 29:559–562, 1980.

282. Taggart HM, Chestnut CH, Ivey JL, et al: Deficient calcitonin response to calcium stimulation in postmenopausal osteoporosis. Lancet 1:475–478, 1982.

283. Gennari C, Agnusdei D: Calcitonin, estrogens and the bone. J Steroid Biochem Mol Biol 37:451–455, 1990.

284. MacLaughlin J, Holick MF: Aging decreases the capacity of human skin to produce vitamin D_3. J Clin Invest 76:1536–1538, 1985.

285. Fujisawa Y, Kida K, Matsuda H: Role of change in vitamin D metabolism with age in calcium and phosphorus metabolism in normal human subjects. J Clin Endocrinol Metab 59:719–726, 1984.

286. Hartwell D, Rodbro P, Jensen SB, et al: Vitamin D metabolites—relation to age, menopause and endometriosis. Scand J Clin Lab Invest 50:115–121, 1990.

287. Sagiv P, Lidor C, Hallel T, Edelstein S: Decrease in bone level of 1,25-dihydroxyvitamin D in women over 45 years old. Calcif Tissue Int 51:24–26, 1992.

288. Riggs L, Hamstra A, DeLuca HF: Assessment of 25-hydroxyvitamin D 1-hydroxylase reserve in postmenopausal osteoporosis by administration of parathyroid extract. J Clin Endocrinol Metab 53:833–835, 1981.

289. Halloran BP, Portale AA, Lonergan ET, Morris RCJ: Production and metabolic clearance of 1,25-dihydroxyvitamin D in men: Effect of advancing age. J Clin Endocrinol Metab 70:318–323, 1990.

290. Webb AR, Pilbeam C, Hanafin N, Holick MF: An evaluation of the relative contributions of exposure to sunlight and of diet to the circulating concentrations of 25-hydroxyvitamin D in an elderly nursing home population in Boston. Am J Clin Nutr 51:1075–1081, 1990.

291. McKenna MJ: Differences in vitamin D status between countries in young adults and the elderly. Am J Med 93:69–77, 1992.

292. Morris HA, Need AG, Horowitz M, et al: Calcium absorption in normal and osteoporotic postmenopausal women. Calcif Tissue Int 49:240–243, 1991.

293. Heikinheimo RJ, Inkovaara JA, Harju EJ, et al: Annual injection of vitamin D and fractures of aged bones. Calcif Tissue Int 51:105–110, 1992.

294. Orwoll ES, Oviatt SK, McClung MR, et al: The rate of bone mineral loss in normal men and the effects of calcium and cholecalciferol supplementation. Ann Intern Med 112:29–34, 1990.

295. Gallagher JC: Vitamin D metabolism and therapy in elderly subjects. South Med J 85:2S43–2S47, 1992.

296. Seymour FI, Duffy C, Koerner A: A case of authenticated fertility in a man of 94. JAMA 105:1423–1425, 1935.

297. Handelsman DJ, Staraj S: Testicular size: The effects of aging, malnutrition and illness. J Androl 6:144–151, 1985.

298. Harman SM, Tsitouras PD: Reproductive hormones in aging men. I. Measurement of sex steroids, basal LH, and Leydig cell response to hCG. J Clin Endocrinol Metab 51:35–40, 1980.

299. Stearns EL, MacDonald JA, Kauffman EJ, et al: Declining testis function with age: Hormonal and clinical correlates. Am J Med 57:761–766, 1974.

300. Rubens R, Dhont M, Vermeulen A: Further studies on Leydig cell function in old age. J Clin Endocrinol Metab 39:40–45, 1974.

301. Harman SM, Tsitouras PD, Costa PT, Blackman MR: Reproductive hormones in aging men. II. Basal pituitary gonadotropins and gonadotropin responses to luteinizing hormone-releasing hormone. J Clin Endocrinol Metab 54:547–551, 1982.

302. MacNaughton JA, Bangah ML, McCloud PI, Burger HG: Inhibin and age in men. Clin Endocrinol (Oxf) 35:341–346, 1991.
303. Tenover JS, Bremner WJ: Circadian rhythm of serum immunoreactive inhibin in young and elderly men. J Gerontol 46:M181–M184, 1991.
304. Hollander N, Hollander VP: The microdetermination of testosterone in human spermatic vein blood. J Clin Endocrinol Metab 38:966–971, 1958.
305. Kent JZ, Acone AB: Plasma androgens and aging. In Vermeulen A, Exley D (eds): Androgens in Normal and Pathological Conditions. Amsterdam, Excerpta Medica (ICS No. 101), 1966, pp 31–40.
306. Pirke KM, Doerr P: Age related changes in free plasma testosterone, dihydrotestosterone and oestradiol. Acta Endocrinol (Copenh) 80:171–178, 1975.
307. Vermeulen A, Rubens R, Verdonck L: Testosterone secretion and metabolism in male senescence. J Clin Endocrinol Metab 34:730–735, 1972.
308. Nieschlag E, Lammer U, Freischem CW, et al: Reproductive function in young fathers and grandfathers. J Clin Endocrinol Metab 51:675–681, 1982.
309. Bremner WJ, Prinz PN: A loss of circadian rhythmicity in blood testosterone levels with aging in normal men. J Clin Endocrinol Metab 56:1278–1281, 1983.
310. Marrama P, Carani C, Baraghini GF, et al: Circadian rhythm of testosterone and prolactin in the ageing. Maturitas 4:131–138, 1982.
311. Zumoff B, Strain GW, Kream J, et al: Age variation of the 24 hour mean plasma concentration of androgens, estrogens, and gonadotropins in normal adult men. J Clin Endocrinol Metab 54:534–538, 1982.
312. Murono EP, Nankin HR, Lin T, Osterman J: The aging Leydig cell. VI. Response of testosterone precursors to gonadotropin in men. Acta Endocrinol (Copenh) 100:455–461, 1982.
313. Sparrow D, Bosse R, Rowe JW: The influence of age, alcohol consumption, and body build on gonadal function in men. J Clin Endocrinol Metab 51:508–512, 1980.
314. Nahoul K, Roger M: Age related decline of plasma bioavailable testosterone in adult men. J Steroid Biochem Mol Biol 35:293–299, 1990.
315. Hemsell DL, Grodin JM, Brenner PF, et al: Plasma precursors of estrogen. II. Correlation of the extent of conversion of plasma androstenedione to estrone with age. J Clin Endocrinol Metab 38:476–479, 1974.
316. Gray A, Feldman HA, McKinlay JB, Longcope C: Age, disease, and changing sex hormone levels in middle-aged men: Results of the Massachusetts Male Aging Study. J Clin Endocrinol Metab 73:1016–1025, 1991.
317. Waldstreicher J, Gormley G, Cook T, et al: Absence of an age-associated decline in testosterone (T) and dihydrotestosterone (DHT) in men with benign prostatic hyperplasia (BPH) [Abstract]. Endocrine Society Program and Abstracts 380:145, 1993.
318. Gray A, Berlin JA, McKinlay JB, Longcope C: An examination of research design effects on the association of testosterone and male aging: Results of a meta-analysis. J Clin Epidemiol 44:671–684, 1991.
319. Blackman MR, Weintraub BD, Rosen SW, Harman SM: Comparison of the effects of lung cancer, benign lung disease and normal aging on pituitary-gonadal function in men. J Clin Endocrinol Metab 66:88–95, 1988.
320. Giusti G, Gonelli P, Borrelli D, et al: Age related secretion of androstenedione, testosterone, and dihydrotestosterone by the human testis. Exp Gerontol 10:241–245, 1975.
321. Horton R, Hsieh P, Barberia J, et al: Altered blood androgens in elderly men with prostate hyperplasia. J Clin Endocrinol Metab 41:793–796, 1975.
322. Nankin HR, Lin T, Murono ER, Osterman J: The aging Leydig cell. III. Gonadotropin stimulation in men. J Androl 2:181–189, 1981.
323. Marrama P, Montanini V, Celani MF, et al: Decrease in luteinizing hormone biological activity/immunoreactivity ratio in elderly men. Maturitas 5:223–231, 1984.
324. Winters SJ, Troen P: Episodic luteinizing hormone (LH) secretion and the response of LH and follicle-stimulating hormone to LH-releasing hormone in aged men: Evidence for coexistent primary testicular insufficiency and an impairment in gonadotropin secretion. J Clin Endocrinol Metab 55:560–565, 1982.
325. Kohler PO, Ross GT, Odell WD: Metabolic clearance and production rates of human luteinizing hormone in pre- and postmenopausal women. J Clin Invest 47:38–47, 1968.
326. Tenover JS, Bremner WJ: The effects of normal aging on the response of the pituitary-gonadal axis to chronic clomiphene administration in men. J Androl 12:258–263, 1991.
327. Desleypere JP, Vermeulen A: Aging and tissue androgens. J Clin Endocrinol Metab 53:430–434, 1981.
328. Schiavi RC, Schreiner-Engel P, Mandeli J, et al: Healthy aging and male sexual function. Am J Psychiatry 147:766–771, 1990.
329. Martin CE: Sexual activity in the aging male. In Money J, Musaph N (eds): Handbook of Sexology. New York, Elsevier-North Holland, 1977, p 813.
330. Schiavi RC, Schreiner-Engel P, White D, Mandeli J: The relationship between pituitary-gonadal function and sexual behavior in healthy aging men. Psychosom Med 53:363–374, 1991.
331. Butler RN, Lewis MI: Aging and Mental Health (vol 2). St Louis, Mosby, 1977, pp 112–117.
332. Masters WH, Johnson VE: Human sexual response. London, Churchill, 1966.
333. Davidson JM, Camargo CA, Smith ER: Effects of androgen on sexual behavior in hypogonadal men. J Clin Endocrinol Metab 48:955–958, 1979.
334. Tsitouras PD, Martin CE, Harman SM: Relationship of serum testosterone to sexual activity in healthy elderly men. J Gerontol 37:288–293, 1982.
335. Davidson JM, Chen JJ, Crapo L, et al: Hormonal changes and sexual function in aging men. J Clin Endocrinol Metab 57:71–77, 1983.
336. Korenman SG, Morley JE, Mooradian AD, et al: Secondary hypogonadism in older men: Its relation to impotence. J Clin Endocrinol Metab 71:963–969, 1990.
337. Burger H, Rose N: Sexual impotence. Med J Aust 2:24–26, 1979.
338. Khaw KT, Barrett-Connor E: Endogenous sex hormones, high density lipoprotein cholesterol, and other lipoprotein fractions in men. Arterioscler Thromb 11:489–494, 1991.
339. Marin P, Holmang S, Jonsson L, et al: The effects of testosterone treatment on body composition and metabolism in middle-aged obese men. Int J Obes 16:991–997, 1992.
340. Gray A, Jackson DN, McKinlay JB: The relation between dominance, anger, and hormones in normally aging men: Results from the Massachusetts Male Aging Study. Psychosom Med 53:375–385, 1991.
341. Sherman BM, Korenman SG: Hormonal characteristics of the human menstrual cycle throughout reproductive life. J Clin Invest 55:699–706, 1975.
342. Sacks FM: The effects of reproductive hormones on serum lipoproteins: Unresolved issues in biology and clinical practice. Ann NY Acad Sci 592:272–285, 1990.
343. Lindquist O, Bengtsson C: Menopausal age in relation to smoking. Acta Endocrinol Scand 205:73–79, 1979.
344. Lesser GT, Deutsch S, Markofsky J: Use of independent measurements of body fat to evaluate overweight and underweight. Metabolism 20:792–804, 1971.
345. Blackman MR: Obesity. In Barker LR, Burton JR, Zieve PD (eds): Principles of Ambulatory Medicine (ed 4). Baltimore, Williams & Wilkins (in press).
346. Stout RW: Insulin and atheroma. Diabetes Care 13:631–654, 1990.
347. Andres R, Muller DC, Sorkin JD: Long-term effects of change in body weight on all-cause mortality: A review. Ann Intern Med 119:737–743, 1993.
348. Andres R: Mortality and obesity: The rationale for age-specific height-weight tables. In Hazzard WR, Andres R, Bierman EL, Blass JP (eds): Principles of Geriatric Medicine and Gerontology (ed 2). New York, McGraw-Hill, 1990, pp 759–765.
349. Dowling HJ, Pi-Sunyer X: Race-dependent health risks of upper body obesity. Diabetes 42:537–543, 1993.
350. Sparrow D, Borkan GA, Gerzof SG, et al: Relationship of fat distribution to glucose tolerance. Results of computed tomography in male participants of the Normative Aging Study. Diabetes 35:411–415, 1986.
351. Coon PJ, Rogus EM, Drinkwater D, et al: Role of body fat distribution in the decline in insulin sensitivity and glucose tolerance with age. J Clin Exp Med 75:1125–1132, 1992.
352. Kohrt WM, Kirwan JP, Staten MA, et al: Insulin resistance in aging is related to abdominal obesity. Diabetes 42:273–281, 1993.
353. Peiris BN, Mueller RA, Smith GA, et al: Splanchnic insulin metabolism in obesity: Influence of body fat distribution. J Clin Invest 78:1648–1657, 1986.
354. Evans DJ, Hoffmann RG, Kalkhoff RK, Kissebah AH: Relationship of body fat topography to insulin sensitivity and metabolic profiles in premenopausal women. Metabolism 33:68–75, 1984.
355. Kissebah AH, Vyjdelingum N, Murray R, et al: Relation of body fat distribution to metabolic complications of obesity. J Clin Endocrinol Metab 54:254–260, 1982.
356. Kaplan NM: The deadly quartet: Upper body obesity, glucose intolerance, hypertriglyceridemia and hypertension. Arch Intern Med 149:14–20, 1989.
357. Larsson B, Svardsudd K, Welin L, et al: Abdominal adipose tissue distribution, obesity and risk of cardiovascular disease and death: 13

year follow up of participants in the study of men born in 1913. BMJ 288:1401–1404, 1984.

358. Ohlson LO, Larsson B, Svardsudd K: The influence of body fat distribution on the incidence of diabetes mellitus: 13.5 years of follow-up of the participants in the study of men born in 1913. Diabetes 34:1055–1058, 1985.

359. Selby JV, Freidman GD, Quesenberry CP: Precursors of essential hypertension. Am J Epidemiol 129:43–53, 1989.

360. Folsom AR, Keys SA, Prineas RJ, et al: Increased incidence of carcinoma of the breast associated with abdominal adiposity in postmenopausal women. Am J Epidemiol 131:794–803, 1990.

361. Borkan G, Hults DE, Gerzof SG, et al: Age changes in body composition revealed by computed tomography. J Gerontol 38:673–677, 1983.

362. Harris MIPC: Classification and diagnostic criteria for diabetes mellitus and other categories of glucose intolerance. Prim Care 15:205–225, 1993.

363. Chen M, Halter JB, Porte DJ: The role of dietary carbohydrate in the decreased glucose tolerance of the elderly. J Am Geriatr Soc 35:417–424, 1987.

364. Chen M, Bergman N, Porte DJ: Insulin resistance and B-cell dysfunction in aging: The importance of dietary carbohydrate. J Clin Endocrinol Metab 67:951–957, 1988.

365. Elahi VK, Elahi D, Andres R, et al: A longitudinal study of nutritional intake in man. J Gerontol 38:162–180, 1983.

366. Kirwan JP, Kohrt WM, Wojta DM, et al: Endurance exercise training reduces glucose-stimulated insulin levels in 60- to 70-year-old men. J Gerontol 48:M84–M90, 1993.

367. Kohrt WM, Obert KA, Holloszy JO: Exercise training improves fat distribution patterns in 60- to 70-year-old men and women. J Gerontol 47:M99–M105, 1992.

368. Shimokata H, Muller DC, Fleg JL, et al: Age as independent determinant of glucose tolerance. Diabetes 40:44–51, 1991.

369. Kissebah AH, Peiris AN: Biology of regional fat distribution: Relationship to non-insulin-dependent diabetes mellitus. Diabetes Metab Rev 5:83–109, 1989.

370. Pedersen O: The impact of obesity on the pathogenesis of non-insulin-dependent diabetes mellitus: A review of current hypotheses. Diabetes Metab Rev 5:495–509, 1989.

371. Bjorntorp P: Abdominal obesity and the development of non-insulin dependent diabetes mellitus. Diabetes Metab Rev 4:615–622, 1988.

372. Shimokata H, Tobin JD, Muller DC, et al: Studies in the distribution of body fat: Effect of age, sex and obesity. J Gerontol 44:M66–M73, 1989.

373. Davidson MB: Editorial: Role of glucose transport and GLUT4 transporter protein in type 2 diabetes mellitus. J Clin Endocrinol Metab 77:25–26, 1993.

374. Hughes VA, Fiatarone MA, Fielding RA: Exercise increases muscle GLUT-4 levels and insulin action in subjects with impaired glucose tolerance. Am J Physiol 264:E855–E862, 1993.

375. Elahi D, Muller D, Tzankoff S, Andres RJT: Effect of age and obesity on fasting levels of glucose, insulin, glucagon, and growth hormone in man. J Gerontol 37:385–391, 1982.

376. Elahi D, Muller DC, McAloon-Dyke M, et al: The effect of age on insulin response and glucose utilization during four hyperglycemic plateaus. J Exp Gerontol (in press).

377. Minaker KL, Rowe JW, Tonino R, Pallotta JA: Influence of age on clearance of insulin in man. Diabetes 31:851–855, 1982.

378. McGuire EA, Tobin JD, Berman M, Andres R: Kinetics of native insulin in diabetic, obese, and aged men. Diabetes 28:110–120, 1979.

379. DeFronzo RA: Glucose intolerance and aging: Evidence for tissue insensitivity to insulin. Diabetes 28:1095–1101, 1979.

380. Meneilly GS, Minaker KL, Elahi D, Rowe JW: Insulin action in aging man: Evidence for tissue-specific differences at low physiologic insulin levels. J Gerontol 42:196–201, 1987.

381. Fink RI, Kolterman OG, Griffin J, Olefsky JM: Mechanisms of insulin resistance in aging. J Clin Invest 71:1523–1535, 1983.

382. Rowe JW, Minaker KL, Pallotta J, Flier JS: Characterization of the insulin resistance of aging. J Clin Invest 71:1581–1587, 1983.

383. Creutzfeldt W, Nauck M: Gut hormones and diabetes mellitus. Diabetes Metab Rev 8:149–177, 1992.

384. Orskov C: Glucagon-like peptide-1, a new hormone of the entero-insular axis. Diabetologia 35:701–711, 1992.

385. Elahi D, Andersen DK, Muller DC, et al: The enteric enhancement of glucose-stimulated insulin release. The role of GIP in aging, obesity, and non-insulin-dependent diabetes mellitus. Diabetes 33:950–957, 1984.

386. Segal KR, Van Loan M, Fitzgerald PI, et al: Lean body mass estimation by bioelectrical impedance analysis: A four-site cross-validation study. Am J Clin Nutr 47:7–14, 1988.

387. McAloon-Dyke M, Fukagawa NK, Habener J, et al: The insulinotropic effect of GIP and GLP-1 in healthy and diabetic subjects. Regul Pept 40:205, 1992.

388. Nauck MA, Heimesaat MM, Orskov C, et al: Preserved incretin activity of glucagon-like peptide 1 [7-36] but not of synthetic human gastric inhibitory polypeptide in patients with type-2 diabetes mellitus. J Clin Invest 91:301–307, 1993.

389. Elahi D, McAloon-Dyke M, Fukagawa NK: The effects of recombinant human IGF-I on glucose and leucine kinetics in man. Am J Physiol 265:E831-E838, 1993.

390. DeFronzo RA, Bonadonna RC, Ferrannini E: Pathogenesis of NIDDM. Diabetes Care 15:318–368, 1992.

391. Jarrett RJ: Epidemiology and public health aspects of non-insulin-dependent diabetes mellitus. Epidemiol Rev 11:151–171, 1989.

392. National Diabetes Data Group: Classification and diagnosis of diabetes mellitus and other categories of glucose intolerance. Diabetes 28:1039–1057, 1979.

393. WHO Expert Committee on Diabetes Mellitus: Second report. WHO Technology Report Service 646:9–14, 1980.

394. World Health Organization: Diabetes mellitus—report of a WHO study group. Geneva, WHO Tech Rep Ser, 1985.

395. Andres R: Diabetes and aging. In Brocklehurst JC, Tallis RC, Fillit HM (eds): Textbook of Geriatric Medicine and Gerontology. London, Churchill Livingstone, 1992, pp 724–728.

396. Harris MI: Noninsulin-dependent diabetes mellitus in black and white Americans. Diabetes Metab Rev 6:71–90, 1990.

397. Agner E, Thorsteinsson B, Erikson M: Impaired glucose tolerance and diabetes mellitus in elderly subjects. Diabetes Care 5:600–604, 1982.

398. Dawson LY: DCCT and primary care: Prescription for change. Clin Diabetes 11:88–90, 1993.

399. Harris MI, Cowie CC, Howie LJ: Self-monitoring of blood glucose by adults with diabetes in the United States population. Diabetes Care 16:1116–1123, 1993.

400. Blackman MR, Busby-Whitehead J: Clinical implications of abnormal lipoprotein metabolism. In Barker LR, Burton JR, Zieve PD (eds): Principles of Ambulatory Medicine (ed 4). Baltimore, Williams & Wilkins (in press).

401. Hazzard WR: Disorders of lipoprotein metabolism. In Andres R, Bierman EL, Hazzard WR (eds): Principles of Geriatric Medicine. New York, McGraw-Hill, 1985, pp 764–775.

402. Hershcopf RJ, Elahi D, Andres R: Longitudinal changes in serum cholesterol in man: An epidemiological search for an etiology. J Chronic Dis 35:101–114, 1982.

403. Kirby B: Lipoproteins in the elderly. J Int Med Res 19:425–432, 1991.

404. Kreisberg RA, Kasim S: Cholesterol metabolism and aging. Am J Med 82(Suppl 1B):54–60, 1987.

405. Stern MP, Haffner SM: Body fat distribution and hyperinsulinemia as risk factors for diabetes and cardiovascular disease. Arteriosclerosis 6:123–130, 1986.

406. Bierman EL: Aging and atherosclerosis. In Hazzard WR, Andres R, Bierman EL, Blass JP (eds): Principles of Geriatric Medicine and Gerontology. New York, McGraw-Hill, 1990, pp 458–465.

407. Zimetbaum P, Frishman WH, Ooi WL: Plasma lipids and lipoproteins and the incidence of cardiovascular disease in the very elderly: The Bronx Aging Study. Arterioscler Thromb 12:416–423, 1992.

408. Sorkin JD, Andres R, Oller DC, et al: Cholesterol as a risk factor for coronary heart disease in elderly men. The Baltimore Longitudinal Study of Aging. Ann Epidemiol 2:59–67, 1992.

409. Castelli WP, Wilson PW, Levy D, Anderson K: Cardiovascular risk factors in the elderly. Am J Cardiol 63:12h–19h, 1989.

410. Wilson PF: High-density lipoprotein, low-density lipoprotein and coronary artery disease. Am J Cardiol 66:7A–10A, 1990.

Disorders of Lipoprotein Metabolism

H. BRYAN BREWER, Jr.
SALVIA SANTAMARINA-FOJO
JEFFREY M. HOEG

Plasma lipids are transported by lipoproteins composed of several classes of lipids (including cholesterol, triglycerides, and phospholipids) and proteins designated *apolipoproteins*. The roles of lipoprotein receptors, enzymes, apolipoproteins, and transfer proteins in lipoprotein metabolism have been elucidated, and this new information provides a conceptual framework for understanding lipid transport in normal subjects and in patients with genetic disorders of lipoprotein metabolism.

Human plasma lipoproteins may be classified based on their hydrated density or migration on electrophoresis. There are six major classes of human plasma lipoproteins. The five classes of lipoproteins separated by hydrated density include chylomicrons, very low density lipoproteins (VLDL), intermediate-density lipoproteins (IDL), low-density lipoproteins (LDL), and high-density lipoproteins (HDL).[1] Lp(a) has a hydrated density between LDL and HDL.[2] HDL can be further separated into HDL_2 and HDL_3. On electrophoresis, the lipoproteins which remain at the origin are equivalent to chylomicrons, the pre-β-lipoproteins to VLDLs, the β-lipoproteins to LDL, and the α-lipoproteins to HDL.[3] Lp(a) migrates in the pre-β position. Triglycerides are transported primarily by chylomicrons and VLDL. Plasma LDL and HDL transport approximately 70 and 20 per cent of plasma cholesterol, respectively.

PLASMA APOLIPOPROTEINS

Ten major human plasma apolipoproteins have been identified (Table 148–1) and their physiological role in lipoprotein metabolism established[4–9] (Table 148–2). Apo-lipoproteins A-I, B-100, B-48, C-II, E, and apo(a) are the most clinically relevant apolipoproteins because they are associated with specific genetic dyslipoproteinemias. The two principal apolipoproteins on HDL are apoA-I and apoA-II. In human plasma, apoB exists as two isoproteins, designated apolipoproteins B-100 and B-48, with molecular weights of 512 and 250 kDa, respectively.[10] ApoB-100 and apoB-48 are synthesized from a single apoB gene[11] by a unique RNA editing mechanism.[12–15] ApoB-100 has 4536 amino acids and is the translation product of the full-length apoB mRNA. ApoB-100 is synthesized by the liver and is the principal apolipoprotein on LDL. ApoB-48 contains 2152 amino acids and is synthesized from an apoB mRNA containing a premature in-frame translational stop codon introduced by RNA editing. ApoB-48 is synthesized by the intestine and is the major B apolipoprotein present on chylomicrons. The apoB isoproteins are the major structural apolipoproteins on chylomicrons, VLDL, IDL, and LDL.

Apo(a) is a unique apolipoprotein present only on Lp(a) and is used to quantitate the plasma levels of Lp(a).[16–18] ApoE is a 299 amino acid apolipoprotein that is primarily associated with VLDL and HDL.[19] ApoE is a genetically determined polymorphic apolipoprotein with three common codominantly inherited alleles, designated ε-2, ε-3, and ε-4.[7, 20–23] The E apolipoproteins coded for by these three alleles are apoE-2, apoE-3, and apoE-4. The relative frequencies of the three common alleles for the apoE gene locus are 0.073 (E-2), 0.783 (E-3), and 0.143 (E-4). In the general population there are three major classes of homozygous and three major classes of heterozygous genotypes, resulting in a total of six phenotypes. The structural differ-

TABLE 148–1. MAJOR HUMAN PLASMA APOLIPOPROTEINS

APOLIPOPROTEINS	APPROX. MW (kDa)	MAJOR SITE OF SYNTHESIS	MAJOR DENSITY CLASS
ApoA-I	28	Liver, intestine	HDL
ApoA-II	18	Liver	HDL
ApoA-IV	45	Intestine	Chylomicrons
ApoB-48	250	Intestine	Chylomicrons-VLDL-IDL
ApoB-100	500	Liver	Chylomicrons-VLDL-IDL-LDL
ApoC-I	7	Liver	Chylomicrons-VLDL-IDL
ApoC-II	10	Liver	Chylomicrons-VLDL-IDL
ApoC-III	10	Liver	Chylomicrons-VLDL-IDL
ApoE	34	Liver	VLDL-IDL-LDL
Apo(a)	500	Liver	LDL-HDL

ences between the common E-2, E-3, and E-4 isoproteins are due to the substitution of amino acids at residues 112 and 158. ApoE-2 contains two cysteines at positions 112 and 158, apoE-3 contains a cysteine and arginine, and apoE-4 has two arginines. The charge differences in the apoE isoproteins readily permit the determination of the six common apoE phenotypes by isoelectrofocusing gel electrophoresis.

In addition to serving as structural constituents of the lipoproteins, the functions of the apolipoproteins include participating as a cofactor or activator of enzymes involved in lipoprotein-lipid metabolism and interacting with a specific receptor site on cells, thereby directing lipoprotein catabolism. The well-established functions of the different apolipoproteins are summarized in Table 148–2.

LIPOPROTEIN METABOLISM

The metabolism of the human plasma lipoproteins can be separated conceptually into two separate pathways. One pathway is composed of the apoB-containing lipoproteins (chylomicrons, VLDL, IDL, and LDL), and the second pathway involves HDL. Schematic overviews of the two pathways for lipoprotein biosynthesis, transport, and catabolism are illustrated in Figures 148–1 and 148–2.

ApoB Metabolic Cascades

The pathway of metabolism of the lipoproteins containing apoB-48 and apoB-100 consists of two separate *apoB*

TABLE 148–2. FUNCTIONS OF THE PLASMA APOLIPOPROTEINS IN LIPOPROTEIN METABOLISM

FUNCTION	APOLIPOPROTEIN
I. Structural protein on lipoprotein particles	
Intestinal chylomicron	ApoB-48, ApoB-100
Hepatic VLDL	ApoB-100
HDL	ApoA-I
II. Ligand on lipoprotein particles for interaction with receptor sites on cells	
Remnant receptor	ApoE
LDL receptor	ApoB-100, ApoE
HDL receptor	ApoA-I, ApoA-II
III. Cofactor for enzymes	
Lipoprotein lipase	ApoC-II
Lecithin:cholesterol acyltransferase	ApoA-I

metabolic cascades (for general reviews, see refs. 7 and 24 to 26). This first apoB cascade involves the stepwise delipidation of triglyceride-rich chylomicron particles which transport dietary cholesterol and triglycerides from the intestine to peripheral tissues and the liver. Following secretion, chylomicrons acquire apoE and apoC-II present on HDL. As reviewed above, apoC-II activates lipoprotein lipase, which results in triglyceride hydrolysis and remodeling of the triglyceride-rich lipoprotein particles. Concomitant with the hydrolysis of triglyceride, apolipoproteins as well as lipid constituents are transferred from chylomicrons to HDL, resulting in the generation of small chylomicron remnants with a hydrated density of initially VLDL and then IDL.

The second apoB cascade involves triglyceride-rich VLDL containing apoB-100 secreted by the liver. ApoC-II and apoE dissociate from HDL and reassociate with the hepatogenous triglyceride-rich VLDL secreted from the liver. ApoC-II activates LDL as outlined above, and VLDL are serially converted to VLDL remnants, IDL, and finally LDL. Hepatic lipase, a second lipolytic enzyme, and apoE have been proposed to be necessary for the efficient conversion of IDL to LDL. Hepatic lipase functions in lipoprotein particle metabolism as both a phospholipase and a triglycerol hydrolase. During the metabolic conversion of VLDL to LDL, approximately 50 per cent of VLDL remnants and IDL are removed from the plasma by the liver.

Remnants of triglyceride-rich lipoproteins from the chylomicron and VLDL cascades have been proposed to be removed from the plasma primarily by the interaction of apoE on the remnant particles with the putative hepatic remnant and LDL receptors. The identification and characterization of the remnant receptor has been a challenge for the lipoprotein field. Initial studies revealed that apoE and chylomicron remnants were bound to hepatic membranes.[27] Hepatic membranes and intact hepatocytes isolated from normolipidemic subjects as well as from patients with homozygous familial hypercholesterolemia with a defect in the LDL receptor were able to bind[28] and internalize lipoproteins.[29] The best candidate for the putative remnant receptor is a glycosylated 600-kDa protein that has been designated the LDL receptor–related protein (LRP).[30] The major apolipoprotein ligand for the putative remnant receptor is apoE, and the clearance of triglyceride-rich chylomicron remnants has been proposed to involve an apoE–remnant lipoprotein particle pathway.

Recent studies have indicated that the importance of LRP may not be limited to lipoprotein metabolism, since

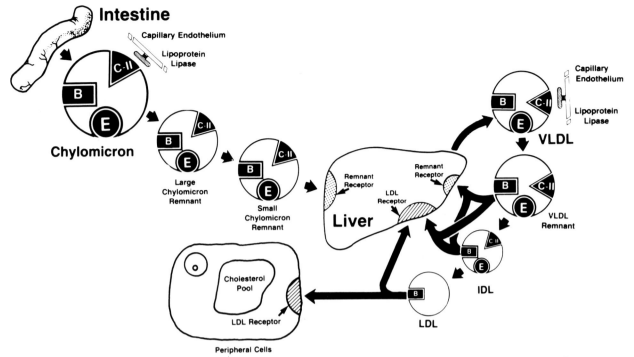

FIGURE 148–1. Overview of the metabolic pathways of the major apoB-containing lipoprotein particles, including chylomicrons, VLDL, IDL, and LDL. The intestinal apoB cascade involves the metabolic cascade of the intravascular metabolism of the triglyceride-rich chylomicrons secreted from the intestine. Chylomicron triglycerides undergo hydrolysis by lipoprotein lipase, and chylomicron remnant particles are formed which have an initial hydrated density of VLDL and finally IDL. The small chylomicron remnants are removed from the plasma and taken up by the liver via the putative remnant receptor. The hepatic apoB cascade involves the metabolic conversion of triglyceride-rich VLDL secreted by the liver. VLDL triglycerides are hydrolyzed by lipoprotein lipase, and remnants undergo stepwise delipidation with the formation of particles with a hydrated density of IDL and finally LDL. VLDL remnants are cleared from the plasma by interacting with the putative remnant and LDL receptors. Plasma LDL interacts with the LDL receptor, which initiates receptor-mediated endocytosis and LDL degradation. (See text for additional details.)

the LRP is identical to the α_2-macroglobulin receptor, which has been shown to bind several different ligands.[31] Thus LRP may play an important role in the clearance of several different plasma proteins as well as lipoproteins. Additional studies will be required to definitively understand the mechanisms that are involved in the metabolism and cellular uptake of the remnants of triglyceride-rich lipoproteins.

LDL, the final product of the VLDL cascade, contain

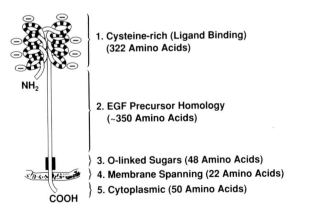

1. Cysteine-rich (Ligand Binding)
   (322 Amino Acids)

2. EGF Precursor Homology
   (~350 Amino Acids)

3. O-linked Sugars (48 Amino Acids)
4. Membrane Spanning (22 Amino Acids)
5. Cytoplasmic (50 Amino Acids)

FIGURE 148–2. Schematic model of the low-density lipoprotein (LDL) receptor. The 839-amino-acid receptor contains five separate functional domains.[35, 36] (See text for further details.)

virtually only apoB-100 and interact with the LDL receptors present on the plasma membranes of liver, adrenal, and peripheral cells, including fibroblasts and smooth-muscle cells.[32, 33] The interaction of LDL with the LDL receptor initiates receptor-mediated endocytosis and transport of LDL to intracellular lysosomes, where the protein moiety is degraded and cholesteryl esters are hydrolyzed to free cholesterol, which is then transferred to the intracellular cholesterol pool. Approximately 50 per cent of plasma LDL is catabolized by the liver and peripheral cells, respectively.

The LDL receptor also has been proposed to play an important role in the clearance of the remnants of triglyceride-rich lipoproteins. The two major apolipoproteins that serve as ligands for the LDL receptor are apoB-100 and apoE.[23, 32–34] Both apoB-100 and apoE are ligands involved in the uptake of apoB-containing lipoproteins in VLDL and IDL, whereas apoB-100 is the principal ligand for interaction with the LDL receptor pathway on LDL.

The LDL receptor is an 839-residue glycosylated protein containing five separate domains.[35, 36] These include a 322-residue amino-terminal cysteine-rich ligand-binding domain, a 350-amino acid domain which displays a high degree of homology to the epidermal growth factor precursor, a 48-amino acid domain containing O-linked carbohydrates, a 22-residue membrane-spanning domain, and a 50-amino-acid cytoplasmic domain (Fig. 148–3). The expression of the LDL receptor gene is under transcrip-

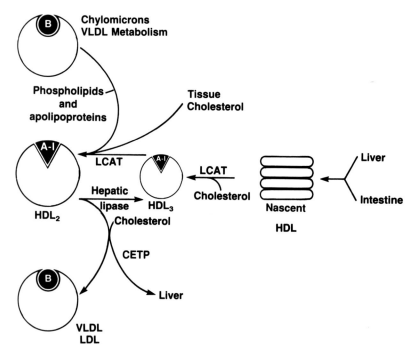

FIGURE 148–3. Pathways for the biosynthesis of plasma HDL. Disk-shaped nascent HDL are synthesized by both the liver and the intestine. Nascent HDL remove excess cellular cholesterol and are converted to spherical lipoprotein particles with a hydrated density of HDL_3. Addition of cholesterol, phospholipids, and apolipoproteins from the metabolism of triglyceride-rich lipoproteins and the uptake of cholesterol from peripheral tissues result in the conversion of lipoproteins in HDL_3 to particles with a hydrated density of HDL_2. Cholesterol in the lipoprotein particles is converted to cholesteryl esters by the enzyme lecithin:cholesterol acyltransferase (LCAT). Cholesteryl esters are transferred to VLDL-IDL-LDL by the cholesterol ester transfer protein (CETP). Lipoproteins in HDL_2 are converted back to HDL_3 by the enzyme hepatic lipase. (See text for additional information.)

tional regulation with *cis*-acting DNA sequences required for both basal and sterol-regulated control. A reduction in the concentration of intracellular cholesterol initiates a coordinate up-regulation of hydroxymethylglutaryl coenzyme A (HMG-CoA) reductase with increased synthesis of both intracellular cholesterol and the LDL receptor, resulting in an increased number of LDL receptors on the cell surface and enhanced binding as well as degradation of plasma LDL. This compensatory mechanism maintains the intracellular cholesterol concentration within the normal range. Drugs (e.g., lovastatin) which inhibit HMG-CoA reductase and reduce intracellular cholesterol levels result in an increased expression of the LDL receptor and a subsequent decrease in the plasma levels of LDLs.

HDL Metabolism

Lipoproteins within HDL are synthesized by four major pathways (Fig. 148–4; for reviews, see refs 4, 7, 37, and 38). Nascent HDL, composed primarily of apoA-I phospholipid disks, are secreted from both the human intestine and liver. Nascent HDL acquire excess cholesterol from tissues,

and the enzyme lecithin cholesterol acyltransferase (LCAT) catalyzes the esterification of lipoprotein cholesterol to cholesteryl esters. With the formation of cholesteryl esters, the nascent HDL are converted to spherical lipoproteins with a hydrated density of HDL_3. HDL_3 are converted to the larger HDL_2 by the acquisition of apolipoproteins and lipids released during the stepwise delipidation and remodeling of the triglyceride-rich chylomicrons and VLDL as well as by the esterification of the cholesterol removed from peripheral tissues. HDL_2 are converted back to HDL_3 by removal of phospholipids and triglycerides by hepatic lipase, by the transfer of cholesteryl esters to VLDL-IDL-LDL by the cholesterol ester transfer protein (CETP), and by the transfer of cholesterol to the liver and other tissues.[39] As lipoproteins within HDL are interconverted from HDL_3 to HDL_2 and back to HDL_3, cholesterol is picked up and transferred from peripheral tissues to the liver or to the apoB-containing lipoproteins. This hypothetical process, termed *reverse cholesterol transport*, is summarized schematically in Figure 148–4.[40, 41] VLDL are secreted from the liver and undergo stepwise delipidation to LDL as outlined above. LDL, the major cholesterol-transporting lipoproteins, bind to LDL receptors in the liver and periph-

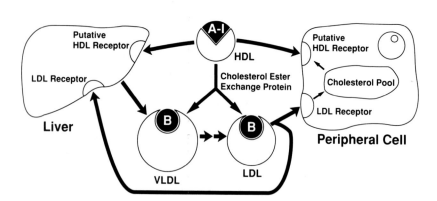

FIGURE 148–4. General overview of HDL and reverse cholesterol transport. VLDL are secreted by the liver and undergo intravascular remodeling with the formation of LDL. LDL are taken up by the liver and peripheral cells by interaction with the LDL receptor. Excess cellular cholesterol is removed by HDL following interaction with the putative HDL receptor. Cholesterol is converted to cholesteryl esters by LCAT, and the cholesteryl esters are transferred to either the liver or VLDL-IDL-LDL by CETP, the lipid transfer protein. (See text for additional details.)

eral cells, supplying cholesterol to the intracellular cholesterol pool. Excess cholesterol is removed from peripheral cells by HDL. In this proposed model, HDL interact with a putative HDL receptor that facilitates the transfer of cellular cholesterol to HDL (see Fig. 148–4). HDL transport this cholesterol in plasma and deliver it to the liver via the putative HDL receptor for removal from the body by direct secretion into bile or following conversion to bile acids. As outlined above, an additional major pathway for the transport of cholesterol from peripheral cells to the liver is mediated by CETP, which transfers cholesteryl esters from HDL to VLDL-IDL-LDL. Thus cholesterol may be transported back to the liver either directly by HDL or following exchange to VLDL-IDL-LDL. A variable portion of tissue cholesterol also has been proposed to be delivered to the liver by HDL particles containing apoE which may interact with both the hepatic remnant and LDL receptors.

The precise nature of the specific HDL receptor involved in the transport of cholesterol from peripheral cells back to the liver, where it can be excreted from the body, remains to be established. An HDL receptor has been postulated to be present on cellular membranes based on the results of saturable, specific binding of HDL to hepatic, endothelial, and adipose cells, as well as fibroblasts and steroidogenic tissues.[42–46] Ligand blot analyses have suggested that the HDL receptor has an apparent molecular weight of 80 to 110 kDa. Several different apolipoprotein ligands have been reported to bind to the putative 80- to 110-kDa HDL receptor in different tissues, including A-II and A-IV.[45]

It has been reported recently that the interaction of HDL with a specific cellular receptor in several cells initiates a second messenger pathway with protein kinase C activation.[47, 48] Activation of the protein kinase C pathway is associated with translocation of intracellular cholesterol to the cell membrane, where it can be removed by a variety of different plasma lipoproteins.

Over the last decade, several lines of evidence have indicated that HDL are heterogeneous. Thus HDL contain several separate lipoprotein particles which may have different functions in lipoprotein metabolism and reverse cholesterol transport.[4, 49, 50] The most effective current method available to classify lipoprotein particles in HDL is based on the apolipoprotein composition of the lipoprotein particle.[49] The two major lipoprotein particles within HDL classified by apolipoprotein composition are LpA-I and LpA-I,A-II. Several lines of evidence have suggested that LpA-I is more effective than LpA-I,A-II in facilitating the efflux of cellular cholesterol and protecting against premature heart disease. Further studies will be required to determine if LpA-I is the major antiatherogenic particle within HDL as well as the clinically important apoA-I–containing lipoprotein particles within HDL.

Lp(a)

An elevated plasma level of Lp(a), a cholesterol-rich lipoprotein that closely resembles LDL in lipid composition, is an independent risk factor for the development of premature cardiovascular disease.[16–18] Lp(a) has a hydrated density intermediate between LDL and HDL. The protein moiety of Lp(a) consists of apoB-100 and a unique apolipoprotein, designated apo(a).[51–53] Apo(a) is linked by a single disulfide bridge to apoB-100 on LDL to form Lp(a). Apo(a) is a large glycoprotein ranging in size from 400 to 700 kDa. The amino acid sequence of apo(a) is similar to the sequence of plasminogen and contains cysteine-rich domains of 80 to 114 amino acids in length termed *kringles* because of their structural similarity to a Danish pastry.[54, 55] Apo(a) contains a variable number of copies of kringle 4 and a single copy of kringle 5 followed by the protease domain of plasminogen. In contrast to plasminogen, apo(a) has no serine protease enzymic activity, and it cannot be converted to an active plasmin-like enzyme by tissue plasminogen activator, streptokinase, or urokinase. Of clinical importance is the observation that there is a correlation of the size of the apo(a) isoprotein and the plasma Lp(a) levels.[56] The Lp(a) isoproteins of higher and lower molecular weights are associated with lower and higher plasma concentrations, respectively. The different molecular weights of Lp(a) in human plasma are due to a variable number of copies of kringle 4 in the amino acid sequence of apo(a).[57, 58]

Current data suggest that Lp(a) is synthesized and secreted directly into plasma independent of the pathways of the apoB-containing lipoproteins. The physiological function(s) of Lp(a) in lipoprotein metabolism is as yet unknown.

MAJOR ATHEROGENIC AND ANTIATHEROGENIC PLASMA LIPOPROTEINS

Increased plasma levels of three classes of lipoproteins, LDL, β-VLDL, and Lp(a), and decreased levels of HDL have been associated with an increased risk of premature cardiovascular disease. A schematic representation of the interactions of the three major atherogenic lipoproteins and the antiatherogenic HDL in the development of the plaque is presented in Figure 148–5. An increased concentration of atherogenic lipoproteins accumulating in the vessel wall has been proposed to be associated with an increase in macrophage uptake of cholesterol-rich lipoproteins by the scavenger receptor, resulting in the formation of foam cells, which characterize the early atherosclerotic lesion. Smooth-muscle cells also may take up lipoproteins and undergo conversion to foam cells.

The scavenger receptor pathway in macrophages is a distinct system from the LDL receptor pathway[59] (Fig. 148–6). The scavenger receptor is a trimer of 77-kDa subunits containing six distinct domains:[59] the amino-terminal 110-amino acid cysteine-rich domain, a 72-residue collagen-like domain, a 163-amino acid α-helical coiled-coil domain, a 32-amino acid spacer, a 26-residue transmembrane-spanning domain, and a 50-amino acid cytoplasmic domain. The functional role of the scavenger receptor in lipoprotein metabolism has been postulated to be the clearance of chemically modified lipoproteins. This receptor has been proposed to play a central role in the macrophage uptake of modified lipoproteins and the development of foam cells in the atherosclerotic lesion.

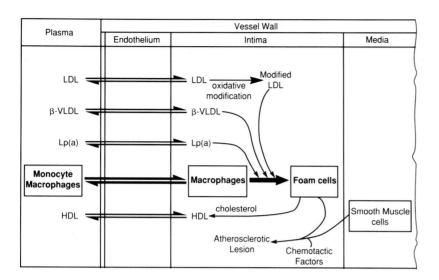

FIGURE 148–5. Schematic model of the interaction of the plasma lipoproteins with macrophages. Elevated levels of three major classes of plasma lipoproteins, LDL, β-VLDL, and Lp(a), have been associated with an increased risk of premature cardiovascular disease. Increased plasma levels of the atherogenic lipoproteins cause increased lipoprotein uptake by the macrophages, resulting in the formation of foam cells, the lesion characteristic of early atherosclerosis. LDL undergo oxidative modification with the generation of modified LDL, which are rapidly taken up by macrophages with the formation of foam cells. Elevated intimal levels of β-VLDL and Lp(a) are also associated with foam cell formation. Foam cell formation, macrophage activation, lipid oxidation, and endothelial cell injury all lead to the release of chemotactic agents, which contribute to the development of the atherosclerotic lesion. (See text for further details.)

LDL

The pathophysiological mechanisms involved in the development of the atherosclerosis associated with elevations of plasma LDL recently have been studied extensively (for reviews, see refs. 60 to 63). Native LDL is not readily taken up by the macrophage in vitro, and incubation with LDL does not result in the formation of foam cells. It is now know that oxidative modification of LDL in vitro results in markedly enhanced LDL uptake by the scavenger receptor

on macrophages, with foam cell formation. Oxidative modifications of LDL were observed following in vitro incubation with endothelial cells, smooth muscle cells, and macrophages or following modification with malondialdehyde. Malondialdehyde is a metabolic by-product of arachidonic acid metabolism in the biosynthesis of prostaglandins and is also formed during lipid peroxidation. Recent studies also have indicated that oxidized lipids within LDL may play an important role in the pathophysiology of the atherosclerotic lesion by stimulating the secretion of cytokinins and other factors which modulate endothelial cell function as well as facilitate the recruitment of plasma monocytes into the vessel wall. Based on an increasing body of data, it has been proposed that oxidative modification of LDL may be a prerequisite for the macrophage uptake of LDL and foam cell formation.

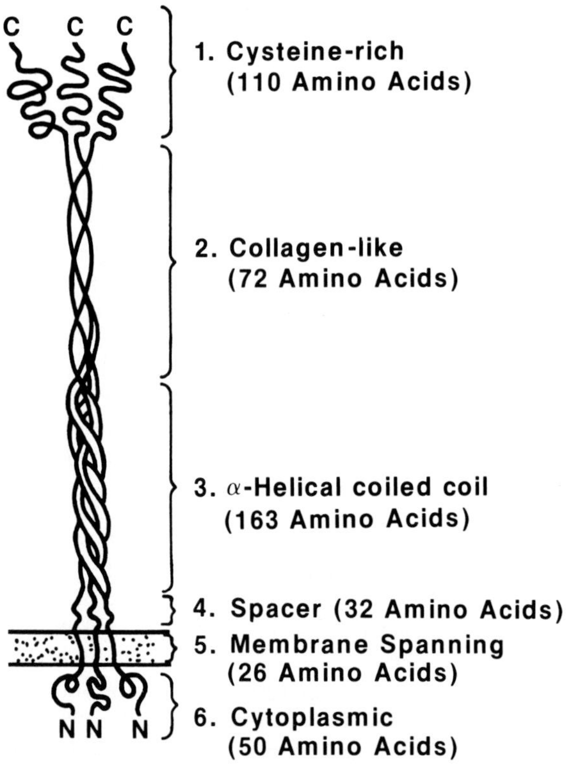

C C C

1. **Cysteine-rich (110 Amino Acids)**

2. **Collagen-like (72 Amino Acids)**

3. **α-Helical coiled coil (163 Amino Acids)**

4. **Spacer (32 Amino Acids)**
5. **Membrane Spanning (26 Amino Acids)**

N N N

6. **Cytoplasmic (50 Amino Acids)**

FIGURE 148–6. Schematic structural model of the type I macrophage scavenger receptor. The receptor is a triple-helix structure with each subunit containing seven separate domains. The cysteine-rich domains are similar in covalent structure to the LDL binding domain of the LDL receptor. (From Kodama T, Freeman M, Rohrer L, et al: Type I macrophage scavenger receptor contains alpha-helical and collagen-like coiled coils. Nature 343:531–535, 1990.)

β-VLDL

The metabolic remnants of triglyceride-rich chylomicrons and VLDL accumulate in type III hyperlipoproteinemia and in experimental animals fed diets high in cholesterol and saturated fat (for reviews, see refs. 64 to 67). Efficient clearance of the β-VLDL remnant chylomicrons and hepatic VLDL requires apoE. ApoE functions as a ligand for binding to both the putative remnant and LDL receptors, facilitating lipoprotein remnant clearance by the liver. In addition, apoE is required for the effective conversion of IDL to LDL. An absence or structural mutation in apoE results in defective removal of remnants of triglyceride-rich lipoproteins and the accumulation of plasma β-VLDL characteristic of type III hyperlipoproteinemia[22, 23, 64–67] (see below). The β-VLDL remnant lipoproteins have been proposed to be taken up by macrophages to form foam cells by either the LDL receptor or a specific macrophage β-VLDL receptor pathway.

Lp(a)

A considerable body of data has accumulated to establish that an elevated plasma level of Lp(a) is an important independent risk factor for the development of premature cardiovascular disease (as discussed above). Plasma Lp(a) levels range from less than 1 to more than 100 mg/dl. Approximately 20 per cent of the population have levels above 30 mg/dl, which are associated with a twofold increase in the relative risk of premature cardiovascular disease. The mechanism(s) by which elevated plasma levels of Lp(a) increase the risk of premature heart disease remains to be established. Lp(a) may be taken up by macrophages, resulting in cholesterol deposition and foam cell formation. Alternatively, its atherogenic properties may be related to its role in increasing thrombosis. Lp(a) has been reported to interact with fibrin peptides, inhibit thrombolysis, and be a competitive inhibitor of plasminogen for the plasminogen receptor present on endothelial cells.[68, 69]

HDL

As reviewed earlier, HDL has been regarded as the principal antiatherogenic lipoprotein in plasma.[70–73] The proposed mechanism for the protective effect of HDL is to facilitate the transport of excess cholesterol from peripheral cells back to the liver by a reverse cholesterol transport process.[40, 41] The higher the plasma levels of HDL, the more efficient is the transport of excess cholesterol from peripheral cells back to the liver. As previously indicated, the importance of the different lipoprotein particles within HDL in mediating the protective effect of HDL on premature cardiovascular disease remains to be established definitively.

GENETIC DYSLIPOPROTEINEMIAS

Hyperlipoproteinemia

Specific defects in lipoprotein metabolism usually involve either abnormal increases (hyperlipoproteinemias) or decreases (hypolipoproteinemias) in plasma levels of specific classes of plasma lipoproteins. Separation of the dyslipoproteinemias based on alterations in the plasma lipoproteins rather than changes in the plasma lipids assists in the classification of these disorders. For example, the hypolipoproteinemias can be further separated into those associated with decreased plasma levels of either HDL or the apoB-containing lipoproteins (i.e., chylomicrons, VLDL, IDL, and LDL). In some lipid disorders, characteristic abnormal plasma lipoproteins also accumulate in plasma.

Several of the genetic dyslipoproteinemias have distinct clinical syndromes. History, physical examination, and laboratory evaluation all contribute to establishing the diagnosis. As part of the initial differential diagnosis, it is important to separate the primary (genetic) lipoprotein disorders from dyslipoproteinemias secondary to other diseases in order to anticipate the clinical course and to select the most effective therapy.

During the last decade there have been major advances in our understanding of the molecular defects which lead to the well-characterized familial lipoprotein disorders. The major genetic dyslipoproteinemias will now be reviewed.

Chylomicronemia Syndrome

Severe chylomicronemia with or without eruptive xanthomas occurs in lipoprotein lipase deficiency and apoC-II deficiency (type I hyperlipoproteinemia) as well as in type V hyperlipoproteinemia (for reviews, see refs. 74 to 76).

CLINICAL SYNDROME. Plasma triglyceride concentrations are variable depending primarily on the temporal relationship between the time of sampling and that of fat intake. In general, fasting plasma concentrations over approximately 250 mg/dl are considered to be abnormal. Chylomicrons are normally seen in plasma only a few hours after a fatty meal has been consumed. At plasma concentrations of triglycerides exceeding 1500 mg/dl, there is usually a distinct accumulation of chylomicrons, which are visible as a creamy layer on the top of plasma left overnight in a refrigerator at 4°C. A cloudy infranatant indicates significant elevations of VLDL (or IDL) (Fig. 148–7). The clinical manifestations of the chylomicronemia syndrome often occur when triglyceride concentrations are greater than 1500 to 2000 mg/dl and may include creamy plasma, eruptive xanthomas, lipemia retinalis, and pancreatitis. Additional symptoms may include dry eyes and mouth, numbness or tingling in the extremities, abdominal pains of uncertain origin, depression, memory loss, and emotional lability. Most of these symptoms are ameliorated with the reduction in plasma triglycerides. A history of prior exploratory surgery because of abdominal pain is not unusual, and patients may ultimately develop chronic pancreatitis.

PHYSICAL EXAMINATION. The characteristic physical findings in patients with the chylomicronemia syndrome are lipemic plasma, lipemia retinalis, and eruptive xanthomas[74–76] (see Fig. 148–7). Lipemia retinalis can be detected in the fundus of the eye when triglyceride levels reach 3000 to 4000 mg/dl. The retinal arterioles and venules appear pale pink due to light scattering of the large chylomicron particles. Vision is not impaired, and there are no clinical sequelae of lipemia retinalis.

Eruptive xanthomas are usually asymptomatic, discrete papules 5 to 6 mm in size with a yellow center and red halo (see Fig. 148–7). During resolution, the inflammatory character of the lesions decreases and the papules become waxy yellow in appearance. These xanthomas result from the phagocytosis of triglyceride-rich lipoproteins by macrophages in the skin. Eruptive xanthomas may suddenly appear in showers and gradually disappear with a decrease in the acute transient elevations in plasma triglycerides. Occasionally, the xanthomas persist if the triglycerides remain elevated.

Hepatosplenomegaly associated with abdominal pain and tenderness is a frequent physical finding in the chylomicronemia syndrome. The hepatosplenomegaly is secondary to lipid accumulation in parenchymal and reticuloendothelial cells. Acute right and left upper quadrant pain may develop with rapid elevations in plasma triglycerides, often mimicking an acute abdominal emergency. With reduction in plasma triglycerides, the hepatosplenomegaly may decrease and the symptoms abate. Abdominal pain in patients with the chylomicronemia syndrome is frequently due to acute pancreatitis, which can have a fatal outcome. Chronic pancreatitis is an important sequela of the syndrome. The evaluation of abdominal pain in the patient

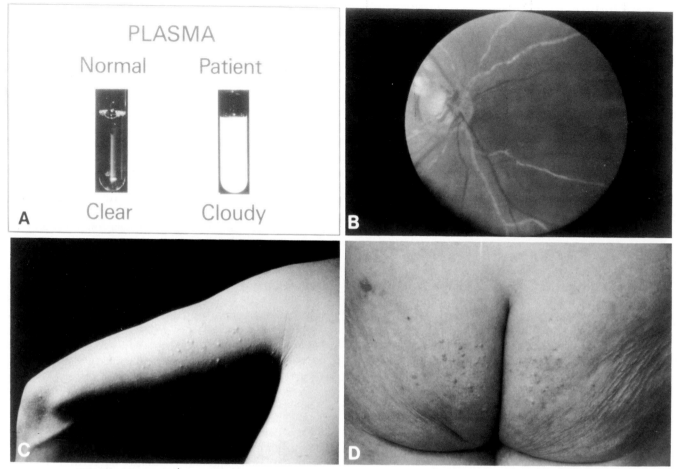

FIGURE 148–7. Clinical manifestations of the chylomicronemia syndrome include lipemic or "cream of tomato soup" plasma *(A)*, lipemia retinalis *(B)*, and eruptive xanthomas *(C,D)*.

with chylomicronemia is often a test of the clinical acumen of the physician.

Neuropsychiatric symptoms are frequently present in patients with severe elevations in plasma triglycerides. The symptoms are often bizarre, follow no neurological patterns, and include parasthesias, dysthesias, acute memory loss, personality changes, depression, and mild dementia. Physical findings are not consistent with any specific neurological deficit. The severity of the symptoms appears to be correlated generally with the elevation in the plasma triglycerides.

MOLECULAR DEFECT. Over the years, patients with severe chylomicronemia have been codified into two separate classes based on the time of onset of the clinical symptoms. Thus the age of onset of the chylomicronemia syndrome may suggest a specific genetic defect in patients with severe hypertriglyceridemia. In the first class, patients with signs and symptoms before puberty nearly always have genetic defects in triglyceride metabolism resulting from a deficiency of the lipoprotein lipase system. A genetic defect resulting in loss of lipoprotein lipase activity due to either a structural defect or absence of either lipoprotein lipase or the apoC-II cofactor results in defective lipolysis of chylomicrons and hepatogenous VLDL with accumulation of very large triglyceride-rich lipoprotein particles in plasma.[74–76] The clinical manifestations of apoC-II deficiency tend to be less severe than in familial lipoprotein lipase deficiency.

In the second class of defects, the patients develop severe hypertriglyceridemia in the fourth and fifth decades. There is no detectable abnormality in lipoprotein lipase or apoC-II, and the precise genetic defect(s) in these patients is as yet unknown. These patients have persistent elevations in the plasma levels of chylomicrons as well as VLDL and are classified as having type V hyperlipoproteinemia. The diagnosis must be pursued to separate primary or familial forms of type V hyperlipoproteinemia from secondary hypertriglyceridemia due to uncontrolled diabetes and other diseases. The differentiation of whether the hyperlipidemia is secondary to chronic pancreatitis or vice versa may sometimes be academic with respect to the clinical care of the patient.

A number of other patients have dyslipoproteinemias that are characterized by mild hypertriglyceridemia with plasma triglyceride levels of 250 to 500 mg/dl. These patients have a type IV lipoprotein pattern (elevations of plasma VLDL without chylomicrons). Two other heritable disorders, familial hypertriglyceridemia and familial combined hyperlipidemia (multiple lipoprotein phenotypes), have been identified as subgroups within this cadre of hypertriglyceridemic patients. The majority of patients with the type IV phenotype are asymptomatic and have few physical manifestations of hyperlipidemia. Patients with combined hyperlipidemia have an increased incidence of premature cardiovascular disease (see below). Occasionally, mildly affected patients with familial hypertriglyceridemia or combined hyperlipidemia may develop the chylomicronemia syndrome secondary to the additive effect of environmental factors (alcohol, obesity), separate diseases (hypothyroidism, diabetes), or medications (estrogens).

Genetic Hypercholesterolemia

The important clinical sequelae resulting from hypercholesterolemia associated with an increased level of plasma LDL is the development of premature coronary artery disease. The dyslipoproteinemia characterized by an increased plasma LDL level has been designated classically as type II hyperlipoproteinemia. This phenotype can be further subdivided into type IIa hyperlipoproteinemia, which is characterized by an isolated increase in LDL, and type IIb hyperlipoproteinemia, which is associated with an increase in both LDL and VLDL. Type II hyperlipoproteinemia represents a generic lipoprotein phenotypic classification system, and several underlying molecular defects that lead to the expression of a type II hyperlipoproteinemia phenotype have been elucidated. Three different genetically determined diseases which have been well characterized include familial hypercholesterolemia (FH), familial combined hyperlipidemia (FCH), and familial defective apobetalipoproteinemia. A fourth genetic disease, polygenic hypercholesterolemia, has not been definitively characterized and the molecular defect(s) are as yet unknown. Patients with these genetic disorders have variable clinical manifestations with respect to the degree of hypercholesterolemia and severity of premature cardiovascular disease.

FAMILIAL HYPERCHOLESTEROLEMIA

Clinical Syndrome. Familial hypercholesterolemia (FH) is a relatively common co-dominant disease with a gene frequency of approximately 1 in 500 in the general population (for reviews, see refs. 32 and 77 to 79). Patients with FH have elevated plasma cholesterol and LDL levels at birth. Heterozygotes for FH have plasma cholesterol levels in the 300 to 400 mg/dl range, and the most significant clinical sequela is the increased risk of the development of premature coronary artery disease. The onset of premature heart disease occurs in female heterozygotes approximately 10 years later than in male heterozygotes. One third of women and two thirds of men heterozygous for FH manifest coronary artery disease before age 60.

Homozygotes for FH have markedly elevated levels of cholesterol and LDL at birth, and during the first few years of life, plasma cholesterol values range from 700 to 1200 mg/dl. Of paramount clinical importance in homozygous patients is the very early development of severe coronary artery disease; myocardial infarction can occur in the first and second decades of life, and life expectancy rarely extends beyond the third decade.

Physical Examination. The hallmark of FH are tendon xanthomas located in the dorsum of the hand and Achilles tendons. Histologically, these xanthomas contain fibrous stroma packed with lipid-filled foam cells derived from macrophages. The cytoplasmic lipid droplets contain predominantly cholesteryl esters, which are birefringent and stain positively with the oil red O stain.

In FH heterozygotes, clinical manifestations typically do not develop until the third and fourth decades of life.

Xanthelasmas, xanthomas around eyes, are often present (Fig. 148–8). Arcus juvenilis, a grayish white ring in the cornea, resulting from the accumulation of lipid droplets is also characteristically present in FH. Tendon xanthomas are present in the tendons on the dorsum of the hands and Achilles tendons (see Fig. 148–8).

Homozygotes for FH develop tendon xanthomas and unique yellowish planar xanthomas (Fig. 148–9). During the first few years of life, the planar xanthomas are typically located in the interdigital webs of the hands and at pressure points or sites of trauma, particularly over the knees, elbows, and buttocks. Large xanthomas also may develop in Achilles tendons and over the elbows, ankles, and hands. Arcus in children is virtually always a sign of hypocholesterolemia. In older subjects its diagnostic value gradually diminishes with age.

Molecular Defect. In FH, a structural defect or an absence of the LDL receptor results in defective cellular uptake and degration of LDL, producing a marked increase in circulating plasma LDL.[78, 79] Patients with homozygous FH were initially categorized into receptor "negative" or "defective" depending on the residual binding activity of the LDL receptor. Mutations in the LDL receptor gene are currently characterized into four classes.[77–79] Class 1 mutations result in the failure of biosynthesis of the LDL receptor protein, while class 2 mutations lead to the synthesis of an LDL receptor that cannot be transported effectively from the endoplasmic reticulum to the cell surface. In class 3 mutations, the LDL receptor reaches the cell surface but is unable to bind LDL normally. Class 4 mutations lead to receptors that cannot be internalized normally by the cell. The degree of residual LDL receptor function is correlated with the clinical onset of symptoms, severity of disease, and response to treatment. Patients with the most severe deficiencies of LDL receptor function are symptomatic at an earlier age, develop more severe heart disease, and are more difficult to treat effectively. The spectrum of clinical disease in patients with heterozygous FH is broad, in keeping with the considerable polymorphism underlying the mutations in the LDL receptor gene.

FAMILIAL COMBINED HYPERLIPIDEMIA

Clinical Syndrome. Familial combined hyperlipidemia (FCH) is one of the most common monogenetic disorders in humans, with a gene frequency, assuming a single defect, as high as 1 in 300.[80–82] The clinical manifestations of FCH generally appear in the fourth and fifth decades. A characteristic feature of FCH is the variability in the elevations of plasma lipoproteins in the proband and affected relatives. The lipoproteins that are most frequently elevated are LDL, LDL + VLDL, and VLDL (lipoprotein phenotypes IIa, IIb, and IV). Patients with FCH have two changes in their plasma lipoproteins that are useful in establishing the diagnosis of FCH. The first is the presence of a plasma LDL containing an abnormal cholesterol-to-apoB ratio (normal < 1.3, FCH > 1.3) which is designated *dense LDL.* The second is an LDL apoB level greater than 130 mg/dl. In addition, HDL levels are frequently reduced, particularly in patients with hypertriglyceridemia. The most significant clinical manifestation of FCH is the development of premature cardiovascular disease, which is very similar in severity and clinical course to that observed in FH heterozygotes.

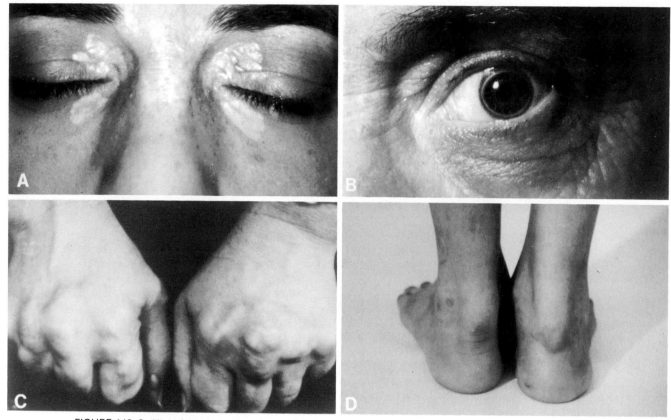

FIGURE 148–8. Clinical features of a patient with heterozygous familial hypercholesterolemia include xanthelasma (A), arcus juvenilis (B), and tendon xanthomas in the extensor tendons of the hand (C) and Achilles tendons (D).

A subset of patients with FCH with elevated levels of LDL apoB (>130 mg/dl) but normal LDL cholesterol levels have been identified. This syndrome, termed *hyperapobetalipoproteinemia*, is characterized by increased plasma levels of LDL apoB and the presence of dense LDL in the absence of hyperlipidemia.[81, 82] Kinetic studies of radiolabeled VLDL and LDL revealed an increase in VLDL apoB synthesis and a relatively normal rate of LDL catabolism.[83, 84] Of major clinical significance is the predisposition of patients with hyperapoabetalipoproteinemia to develop premature cardiovascular disease. It is also important to note that patients with premature heart disease and normal LDL cholesterol may have hyperapobetalipoproteinemia.

Physical Examination. The majority of patients with FCH have no tendon xanthomas, although arcus juvenilis and xanthelasma may be observed. The lack of tendon xanthomas is often a useful clinical feature to distinguish FH and FCH.

Molecular Defect. The molecular defect(s) in FCH remains to be established. The diagnosis of FCH is presumptive, being established only by the identification of a characteristic pattern of dyslipoproteinemia in the propositus and family members. The metabolic defect observed in FCH patients is an oversynthesis of VLDL and triglycerides and a mild increased catabolism of both VLDL and LDL.[83, 84] The conversion of VLDL to IDL and ultimately to LDL is relatively normal. No homozygotes for FCH have been definitively identified. Affected individuals in a number of kindreds with FCH may be genetic compounds,

containing two defective genes, one for FCH and a second one for another underlying genetic dyslipoproteinemia.

FAMILIAL DEFECTIVE APOB-100

Clinical Syndrome. Recently, a new genetic disease, familial defective ApoB-100 (FDB), which is characterized by elevated plasma levels of cholesterol and LDL, has been identified.[85, 86] These patients may have an increased risk of premature cardiovascular disease.

Physical Examination. Patients with FDB may have several of the clinical features of patients with familial hypercholesterolemia, including tendon xanthomas, arcus juvenilis, and xanthelasma.

Molecular Defect. The molecular defect in FDB involves a G to A mutation in apoB-100 which results in the substitution of a glutamine for arginine at amino acid 3500.[86] This amino acid substitution in apoB-100 results in decreased binding of the mutant LDL to the LDL receptor and delayed clearance of plasma LDL.[87] Thus LDL containing the arginine for glutamine mutation is a poor ligand for the LDL receptor, resulting in hypercholesterolemia and the potential for premature heart disease. The increased risk of premature cardiovascular disease in FDB with the apoB 3500 mutation is comparable with that observed in familial hypercholesterolemia, where the structural defect resides in the LDL receptor. Thus a defect has now been identified in both the ligand and the receptor in the LDL receptor pathway. A patient presenting with type II hyperlipopro-

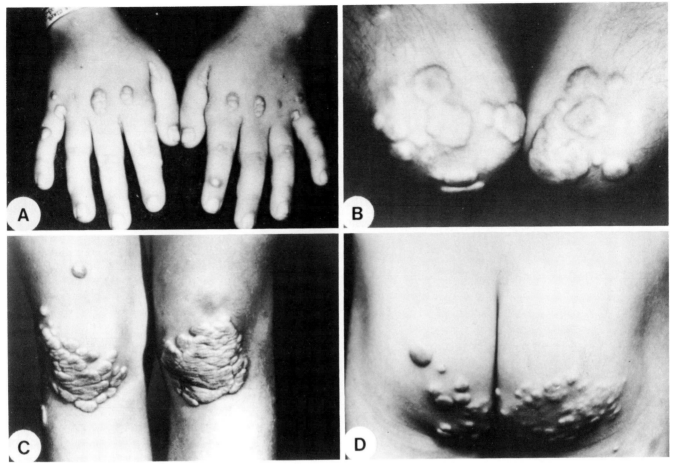

FIGURE 148-9. Tuberous and tendon xanthomas characteristic of a patient with homozygous familial hypercholesterolemia.

teinemia may have a defect in either the ligand, apoB-100, resulting in FDA or the LDL receptor, leading to FH.

Cerebrotendinous Xanthomatosis

CLINICAL SYNDROME. Cerebrotendinous xanthomatosis (CTX) is a rare autosomal recessive lipid storage disease characterized by the accumulation of cholestanol (5,6-dihydroxycholesterol) in plasma lipoproteins and tissues.[88–90] The cardinal manifestations of CTX include cataracts, xanthomas, severe neurological deficiences, mental retardation, dementia, and cardiovascular disease. The xanthomas may be widespread and most commonly occur in tendons as well as in the brain and lungs.

The onset of the clinical manifestations of CTX is frequently insidious, with variable presentation. The presenting symptoms, which may be related to xanthomas, neurological dysfunction with dementia, ataxia, or cataracts, are often not clearly manifested until the teenage years. Neurological symptoms, often devastating in the late stages of the disease, initially may be only a minor manifestation of the disease. Premature cardiovascular disease is an important clinical complication of patients with CTX. The diagnosis of CTX should be considered in a young person presenting with tendon xanthomas, cataracts, and normal plasma lipids. The diagnosis of CTX is established by the presence of an elevated cholestanol level in plasma or tissues. Bile contains a characteristic pattern with an increase in biliary cholestanol, decreased chenodeoxycholic acid, and a marked elevation in glucuronide-conjugated bile alcohols.

Plasma levels of VLDL and LDL are usually normal, and the plasma HDL level may be low. The HDL has an abnormal composition with increased triglycerides, reduced cholesteryl esters, increased ratio of protein to cholesteryl ester, and a relative increase in the ratio of the concentrations of apoA-I to apoA-II. The importance of the low plasma levels of HDL in the pathogenesis of the premature cardiovascular disease in CTX has not been established definitively. The cholestanol present in CTX appears to be derived almost exclusively from cholesterol. Cholestanol, like cholesterol, exists both in the free and the fatty acyl ester form, and cholestanol and cholestanol esters are transported in the plasma primarily by LDL.

The clinical features of CTX reflect the tissue accumulation of sterols, including cholestanol. In the final stages of the disease, the neurological deterioration may be severe. Death often occurs in the fourth or fifth decade due to either severe neurological deficiencies with pseudobulbar paralysis or acute myocardial infarction.

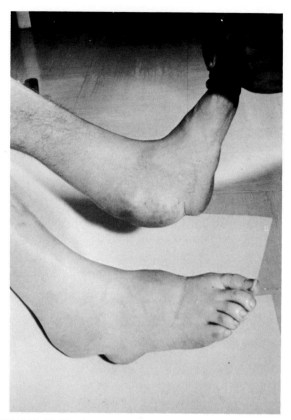

FIGURE 148–10. Tendon xanthomas observed in a patient with cerebrotendinous xanthomatosis. (Courtesy of Dr. Gerald Salens, Veterans Administration Hospital Center, East Orange, N.J.)

PHYSICAL EXAMINATION. The characteristic triad present in patients with CTX includes tendon xanthomas, cataracts, and neurological deficiencies. By the second and third decades, large tendon xanthomas are usually present in the Achilles tendons, extensor tendons of the hand, and tibial tuberosities (Fig. 148–10). The xanthomas in CTX are indistinguishable in appearance from the xanthomas present in other patients with hypercholesterolemia. Xanthomas also occur at unique sites, including the cerebellum, forebrain, lung, and bone, sites that are virtually never involved in familial hypercholesterolemia. The major lipids deposited are cholesteryl esters. The presence of a significant cholestanol content provides a definitive diagnosis of CTX.

Zonular cortical len cataracts are also a well-documented feature of CTX. The devastating neurological involvement may result in dementia, mental retardation, spasticity, ataxia, tremors, muscular atrophy, and pseudobulbar paralysis. The neurological symptoms are correlated anatomically with lipid accumulation and demyelination.

MOLECULAR DEFECT. The precise molecular defect(s) in CTX has not been established definitively. Several lines of evidence indicate that the genetic defect involves the hepatic enzymes involved in the biosynthesis of bile acids,[88-90] and in a recent report a mutation in sterol 27-hydroxylase has been identified in two unrelated kindreds.[91] The block in biosynthesis of bile acids results in a marked deficiency of biliary cholic and chenodeoxycholic acid and increased biliary secretion of cholestanol and glucuronide C27 bile alcohols. The accumulation of both cholesteryl and choles-

tanyl esters in tissues may be due to an increased hepatic synthesis of cholesterol and cholestanol resulting in a deficiency of bile acids in the enterohepatic circulation as well as the loss of normal feedback control of sterol biosynthesis. Treatment of patients with CTX with chenodeoxycholic acid alone or in combination with a HMG-CoA reductase inhibitor results in decreased plasma cholestanol levels and a reduction in the size of tendon xanthomas.[92]

Sitosterolemia

CLINICAL SYNDROME. Sitosterolemia is a rare autosomal recessive disease characterized by plasma and tissue accumulation of plant sterols, including sitosterol, campesterol, and stigmasterol. Increased plasma concentrations of plant sterols are frequently accompanied by an increase in cholesterol levels (for review, see refs. 88, 89, and 93). The clinical manifestations begin in childhood or the first and second decades of life. Although tendon xanthomas may develop, plasma cholesterol levels may be normal. The presence of a tendon xanthoma in a child without hypercholesterolemia may be a clue to the diagnosis of sitosterolemia. The disease also should be considered in young patients with tendon xanthomas and hypercholesterolemia. In these individuals, LDL receptor function is normal, and some of these patients have been codified as *pseudofamilial hypercholesterolemia*.

The diagnosis of sitosterolemia can be established definitively by finding increased plasma levels of plant sterols (upper limit of normal 0.5 per cent of total plasma sterols), which are transported primarily within LDL. The plant sterol content of xanthomas is greater than 10 per cent; however, the major sterol present in xanthomas is cholesterol. The fecal bile acid pattern is unusual, with increased levels of deoxycholic and lithocholic acids and fecal bile alcohols.

PHYSICAL EXAMINATION. The characteristic manifestations of sitosterolemia are tendon as well as subcutaneous xanthomas, xanthelasma, and premature cardiovascular disease (Fig. 148–11). Physical findings of cardiovascular disease, including arcus juvenilis and xanthomata, also may be present. Hemolytic anemia may occur in sitosterolemia; however, cataracts have not been reported.

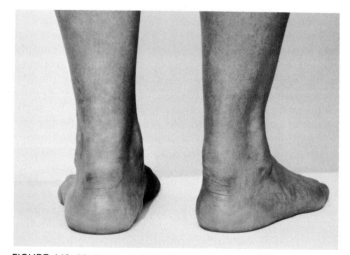

FIGURE 148–11. Tendon xanthomas characteristic of the clinical manifestations of sitosterolemia.

MOLECULAR DEFECT. The molecular defect in sitosterolemia is as yet unknown. Recent studies have established a very low rate of hepatic cholesterol synthesis due to a deficiency of HMG-CoA reductase activity, which is accompanied by an increased intestinal absorption of all sterols, including cholesterol and plant and shellfish sterols.[94, 95] In addition, a defect in the hepatic excretion of plant and shellfish sterols results in delayed hepatic clearance of the absorbed sterols; thus both cholesterol and plant sterols increase in plasma, resulting in tendon as well as subcutaneous tissues xanthomas. Premature cardiovascular disease is an important complication of sitosterolemia. Treatment of homozygous sitosterolemia patients with bile acid sequestrants results in substantial lowering of plasma sterols and regression of xanthomas, suggesting that treatment may be effective in reducing the risk of premature atherosclerosis.

Dysbetalipoproteinemia: Type III Hyperlipoproteinemia

CLINICAL SYNDROME. Individuals with this lipoprotein disorder are often classified as having dysbetalipoproteinemia when low or normal plasma lipid values are present and as type III hyperlipoproteinemia when hyperlipidemia has developed.[64–67, 96] Patients with dysbetalipoproteinemia often develop hyperlipidemia and clinical symptomatology in the fourth and fifth decades. This lipoprotein disorder is of particular importance because it is associated with an increased risk of both premature cardiac disease and peripheral vascular disease. The latter is particularly frequent in this dyslipoproteinemia.

Plasma concentrations of both triglycerides and cholesterol are elevated (frequently about equally), and the principal plasma lipoproteins which are increased are remnants of triglyceride-rich lipoproteins with a hydrated density of IDL. These lipoproteins are cholesterol-rich, migrate as an extra β band on high-resolution agarose gel electrophoresis of plasma, and are in the β position on lipoprotein electrophoresis following separation of the plasma lipoproteins by ultracentrifugation at a density of less than 1.006 g/ml. The β migrating lipoproteins present in a density of less than 1.006 g/ml have been designated *floating β-lipoproteins*. An additional important diagnostic feature of this dyslipoproteinemia is a VLDL cholesterol–to–plasma triglyceride ratio of greater than 0.3 (control subjects < 0.3).[64–67, 96]

PHYSICAL EXAMINATION. One of the fascinating features of type III hyperlipoproteinemia is the presence of palmar xanthomas (xanthoma striata palmaris), which are nearly pathognomonic of this dyslipoproteinemia (Fig. 148–12). Palmar xanthomas are frequently accompanied by tuberous lesions over the elbows, knees, and buttocks. Occasionally, patients may develop Achilles tendon xanthomas, characteristic of FH. The xanthomas in type III hyperlipoproteinemia, like those in FH, contain foam cells filled with cholesteryl esters.

MOLECULAR DEFECT. ApoE plays a key role in the metabolism and cellular uptake of triglyceride-rich lipoproteins. Population studies have indicated that apoE is controlled at a single genetic locus with an unusual degree of polymorphism. As outlined above, there are three common

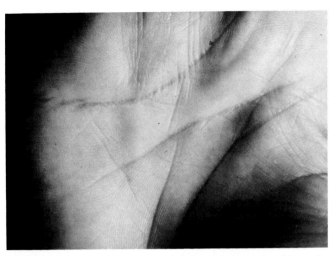

FIGURE 148–12. Palmar xanthomas (xanthoma striata palmaris), xanthomas in the creases of the palm, are virtually pathognomonic for type III hyperlipoproteinemia.

alleles in the general population which have been designated E-2, E-3, and E-4. The three E apolipoproteins encoded by these three alleles are separable by isoelectrofocusing and are codified as apoE-2, apoE-3, and apo-4. Six major apoE phenotypes are present in the population, including homozygotes for apolipoprotein E-2, E-3, and E-4 as well as heterozygotes for apolipoproteins E-2,3, E-2,4, and E-3,4. As reviewed above, differences in the apoE isoproteins have been shown to be due to one or two amino acid substitutions involving cysteine and arginine exchanges at amino acid residues 112 and 158.

Epidemiological studies have established the frequency of the E alleles and lipoprotein profiles in the general and hyperlipidemic populations. The predominant E isoprotein in the normolipidemic population is apoE-3, and it is considered the normal isoprotein. An increased frequency of the E-2 allele (apoE-2,2 phenotype) or E⁰ allele (apoE absence) has been observed in patients with type III hyperlipoproteinemia. As outlined above, subjects with the apoE-2,2 phenotype are frequently normocholesterolemic or hypocholesterolemic.[22, 23, 34] Subjects with the apoE-2,2 phenotype and no hyperlipidemia have been categorized as normolipidemic E-2 dysbetalipoproteinemic homozygotes. The development of the hyperlipidemia has been proposed to require the presence of an additional environmental or genetic abnormality such as obesity, hypothyroidism, or a second dyslipoproteinemia. Thus a second genetic defect may be necessary for the patient to become hyperlipidemic and develop type III hyperlipoproteinemia.

The majority of individuals with type III hyperlipoproteinemia have the autosomal recessive form of the disease. The most frequent apoE phenotype in these patients is the apoE-2,2 phenotype with the arginine 158 to cysteine substitution (Table 148–3). Patients with the dominant form of inheritance of type III hyperlipoproteinemia develop hyperlipidemia as heterozygotes. The apoE mutations associated with the dominant form of the dyslipoproteinemia include mutations at residue 142, residue 146, or a 7-amino-acid insertion at residue 121 of apoE[23, 97–100] (see Table 148–3).

The lipoproteins that accumulate in type III hyperlipo-

TABLE 148–3. CLASSIFICATION OF MODE OF INHERITANCE OF THE GENETIC DEFECTS IN ApoE ASSOCIATED WITH TYPE III HYPERLIPOPROTEINEMIA

MUTATION	ApoE PHENOTYPE
Dominant Inheritance	
ApoE-1$_{Harrisburg}$ (lys$_{146}$ → glu)	E-1
Lys$_{146}$ → gin	E-2
Arg$_{142}$ → cys	E-2
7 amino acid insertion at amino acid 121	E-3
Recessive Inheritance	
Arg$_{158}$ → cys	E-2

proteinemia contain both apoB-48 and apoB-100, indicating that there is defective metabolism of lipoproteins of both intestinal (chylomicron) and liver (VLDL) origin. The delay in catabolism of these lipoproteins is due to the absence of apoE or the presence of a mutation in apoE which results in defective binding to the hepatic remnant and LDL receptors.[34, 66] Remnants of the triglyceride-rich lipoproteins, therefore, persist in the circulation for an abnormally long period of time and are susceptible to uptake by macrophages, resulting in the formation of foam cells and the development of xanthomas. Elevated plasma remnants are also the basis for an increased incidence of coronary and peripheral arterial disease in patients with type III hyperlipoproteinemia.

Individuals with the apoE-4 variant have elevated plasma levels of total as well as LDL cholesterol when compared with subjects with the apoE-3,3 phenotype. Kinetic studies utilizing radiolabeled apoE isoproteins have established that apoE-4 is catabolized more rapidly than apo-3.[34, 101] Based on these results, it has been proposed that patients with the apo-4 phenotype have a more rapid clearance of plasma chylomicrons and VLDL remnants by the liver than apoE-3 subjects. The increased rate of hepatic clearance of the remnant particles leads to down-regulation of the LDL receptor, resulting in higher plasma concentrations of cholesterol, LDL, and remnant particles. An increased level of plasma LDL would be expected to increase the risk of premature cardiovascular disease in patients with the apoE-4 phenotype.

Hypolipoproteinemias

The dyslipoproteinemias, characterized by abnormally low concentrations of plasma lipoproteins, involve primarily HDL or all the apoB-containing lipoproteins (i.e., chylomicrons, VLDL, IDL, and LDL).

HDL Deficiency

TANGIER DISEASE

Clinical Syndrome. Tangier disease is a genetic dyslipoproteinemia characterized clinically by orange tonsils, cloudy corneas, hepatosplenomegaly, lymphadenopathy, and intermittent peripheral neuropathy.[102, 103] The diagnosis of Tangier disease should be suspected when the plasma cholesterol level is below 120 mg/dl and the triglycerides are

normal or slightly elevated. Marked decreases in the plasma levels of HDL, apoA-I, and apoA-II (less than 2 to 5 per cent of normal) are characteristic of Tangier disease.

The onset of the clinical manifestations of Tangier disease is insidious, reflecting the slow accumulation of cholesteryl esters in tissues. The most characteristic site of deposition, the pharyngeal tonsils, can provide the diagnosis of Tangier disease at a glance. However, the tonsils often have been removed prior to the physician examining the patient. Hepatosplenomegaly may be present and is due to lipid accumulation in the reticuloendothelial system. Hypersplenism is rare. The removal of the spleen, however, may lead to hyperplasia of the reticuloendothelial cells in the omentum and other areas of the body. Transient and recurrent peripheral neuropathy also appears to be due to an accumulation of lipid within the nerve sheaths. Neurological symptoms, including motor weakness, paresthesias, and dysesthesias, may occur but often wax and wane. The clinical course of patients with Tangier disease is extremely variable, and the diagnosis may not be made until the third or fourth decade. Despite the low plasma HDL levels, premature cardiovascular disease is not a prominent feature.

Physical Examination. The unique clinical feature of Tangier disease is the presence of lobulated, bright orange-yellow tonsils (Fig. 148–13). If the tonsils have been removed, pharyngeal tags of orange-yellow tissue may still be evident upon examination. The rectal mucosa has a similar appearance, and the identification of cholesteryl esters in foam cells in the rectal mucosa may be used to establish the diagnosis. Asymptomatic corneal opacities often require slit-lamp examination for identification. Mild hepatosplenomegaly and lymphadenopathy also may be present. The neuropathy in Tangier disease may be detected by decreased deep tendon reflexes and sensory motor abnormalities.

Molecular Defect. The molecular defect in Tangier disease has not been elucidated. Kinetic studies using radiolabeled HDL have established that the low plasma HDL levels in Tangier disease are due to markedly increased HDL catabolism.[104]

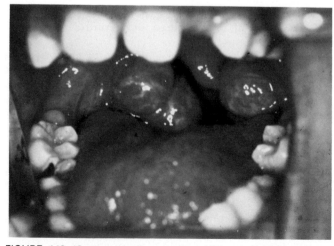

FIGURE 148–13. Orange-yellow tonsils, which are virtually pathognomonic for Tangier disease.

ApoA-I Gene Defects. ApoA-I, the major structural apolipoprotein of HDL, is of clinical interest because of the observed inverse association of both apoA-I and HDL cholesterol with the development of premature cardiovascular disease.[70-73] Most of the structural mutations identified in apoA-I do not affect HDL levels. However, identification of structural mutation in apoA-I which are associated with reduced HDL levels has important clinical implications for the diagnosis and treatment of patients with early heart disease. Two point mutations in apoA-I, the deletion of apoA-I lysine 107 and the substitution of apoA-I of proline 165 to arginine, are associated with reduced levels of HDL cholesterol.[105]

Mutations in the apoA-I gene complex which lead to the virtual absence of plasma apoA-I and HDL cholesterol are associated with severe premature heart disease. Three illustrative kindreds will be reviewed with premature cardiovascular disease, markedly reduced HDL levels, and a deficiency of apoA-I alone or in combination with apoC-III and apoA-IV. ApoA-I is in close proximity to the genes for apolipoproteins C-III and A-IV on chromosome 11.

ApoA-I Deficiency. The proband in the first kindred with apoA-I deficiency is a 5-year-old Turkish female with planar xanthomas and a markedly reduced level of plasma HDL.[106] Family history was positive for early heart disease. Clinical features included mild hepatomegaly but no splenomegaly, neuropathy, or orange tonsils. Plasma apoA-I was absent, apoA-II was reduced to 10 per cent of normal, and apoC-III as well as apoA-IV levels were similar to those of controls. The molecular defect in this kindred was shown to be a deletion of a base resulting in a frameshift introducing a premature stop codon at residue 27 in apoA-I.

ApoA-I + ApoC-III Deficiency. The affected individuals in the second kindred are two females identified at ages 31 and 32 years with mild corneal opacities and planar xanthomas on the trunk, neck, and eyelids and severe coronary artery disease.[107, 108] Plasma levels of VLDL were reduced, LDL was normal, and HDL was severely decreased. ApoA-I and apoC-III were absent, and apoA-II was reduced to less than 5 per cent of normal. The molecular defect in this kindred was an arrangement in the apoA-I and apoC-III genes resulting in the failure of synthesis of both apoA-I and apoC-III.[108]

ApoA-I + ApoC-III + ApoA-IV Deficiency. The proband in the third kindred was a 45-year-old female with mild corneal opacities and severe premature heart disease.[109] There were no xanthomas, organomegaly, or orange tonsils. Plasma triglycerides and VLDL were reduced, LDL and plasma apoB were normal, and HDL was markedly deficient. Plasma apolipoproteins A-I, C-III, and A-IV were not detectable, and apoA-II was decreased to less than 10 per cent of normal. The genetic defect in this kindred is a 7.5-kilobase deletion resulting in the failure of synthesis of all three apolipoproteins, A-I, C-III, and apoA-IV.[110]

These three kindreds illustrate two important points. First, the close proximity of the genes for apolipoproteins A-I, C-III, and A-IV on chromosome 11 permits loss of expression of up to three apolipoproteins by a single mutation, and second, the absence of plasma apoA-I alone or in combination with a deficiency of apoC-III or apoC-III + apoA-IV results in a virtual total absence of HDL and the development of severe premature heart disease.

FAMILIAL LECITHIN:CHOLESTEROL ACYLTRANSFERASE (LCAT) DEFICIENCY

Clinical Syndrome. LCAT deficiency is a rare autosomal recessive disease in which a deficiency of the plasma LCAT activity leads to a characteristic dyslipoproteinemia and lipid deposition in selected organs.[111] Plasma lipid changes include an increase in unesterified cholesterol as well as lecithin and a reduction in cholesteryl esters and lysolecithin. HDL levels are reduced to less than 15 mg/dl. Plasma triglyceride concentrations are frequently elevated, and total cholesterol is reduced. Plasma lipoproteins have an abnormal lipid composition, and vesicular lipoproteins are present in VLDL as well as in LDL. Moreover, discoidal particles containing predominantly apoE or apoA-I and apoA-II are present within HDL. The changes is the plasma lipoproteins are due to the failure of the normal esterification of free cholesterol and the transfer of the cholesteryl esters to the hydrophobic core of the plasma lipoproteins, including HDL as well as VLDL-IDL-LDL.

Two distinct clinical syndromes, classic LCAT deficiency[111] and fish eye disease,[112-114] have been recognized in patients with LCAT deficiency. In classic LCAT deficiency, the onset of clinical manifestations begins in childhood with the development of corneal opacities. During the next two decades, anemia may appear, and frequently, there is a gradual development of progressive renal failure with proteinuria. In fish eye disease, the only clinical manifestations are the dyslipoproteinemia and corneal opacifications, which may become so severe as to require corneal transplantation.

Physical Examination. Corneal opacities are the characteristic clinical feature of classic LCAT deficiency and fish eye disease (Fig. 148–14). The severity of the corneal opacities is variable, usually being more severe in patients with fish eye disease than in patients with classic LCAT deficiency. The corneal deposits are punctate stromal deposits resembling those present in Tangier disease. No characteristic xanthomas are present in patients with LCAT deficiency. Signs of renal failure and hemolytic anemia are frequently present in the latter stages of the disease in those patients with classic LCAT deficiency.

Molecular Defect. A deficiency or a structural mutation in the LCAT enzyme results in both classic LCAT deficiency[115-119] and fish eye disease.[116, 120-122] The variability in the clinical course of patients with classic LCAT deficiency and fish eye disease is due to the residual enzymic activity present in the mutant LCAT enzyme.[122] No residual LCAT enzymic activity is present in patients with classic LCAT deficiency, while a variable amount of residual LCAT enzymic activity is still present in fish eye disease patients. A relatively small amount of residual LCAT activity appears to be able to prevent the clinical features of hemolytic anemia and progressive renal disease.[122]

Deficiency of ApoB-Containing Lipoproteins

ABETALIPOPROTEINEMIA

Clinical Syndrome. Abetalipoproteinemia is a rare disease inherited as an autosomal recessive trait characterized in homozygotes by the absence of all lipoproteins containing apolipoproteins B-48 and B-100, including chylomicrons,

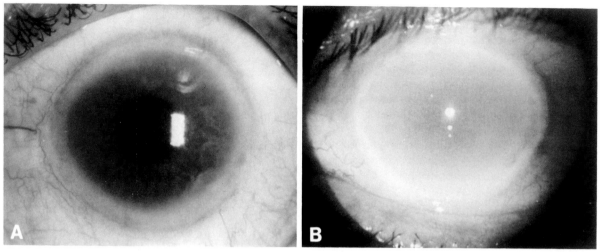

FIGURE 148–14. Clinical manifestations of patients with lecithin:cholesteryl acyltransferase deficiency observed in classic LCAT deficiency *(A)* and fish eye disease *(B)*.

VLDL, IDL, and LDL.[123, 124] Heterozygotes with abetalipoproteinemia have no detectable clinical or biochemical abnormalities. The clinical manifestations of abetalipoproteinemia include steatorrhea, retinitis pigmentosa, hemolytic anemia, and neurological dysfunction. The first symptoms to appear are often related to malabsorption of fat during the first years of life. Radiographic findings are not diagnostic, and biopsy of the small intestine reveals a snow-white mucosa with unblunted, well-formed villi containing lipid-laden mucosal cells. These mucosal findings are characteristic and distinguish abetalipoproteinemia from celiac disease. Of major clinical importance is the severe malabsorption of fat-soluble vitamins, particularly A and E. Visual symptoms often present as night blindness due to vitamin A deficiency. During the course of the disease, nystagmus develops, and progressive retinal degeneration may result in decreased visual acuity. Acanthocytes with altered cholesterol and phospholipid content are present, often leading to episodes of hemolysis and anemia. The most serious sequela of abetalipoproteinemia is the progressive neurological dysfunction, resulting in the loss of motor as well as sensory functions and ability to walk. The neurological defects have been proposed to be due to a profound deficiency of vitamin E. Death usually occurs in the fourth or fifth decade and may be related to cardiac arrhythmias.

The plasma concentrations of both triglycerides and cholesterol are extremely low (<50 mg/dl) and are a clue to the diagnosis. HDL are the only lipoproteins detected in plasma, and their composition is abnormal, with increased ratios of free to esterified cholesterol and sphingomyelin to phosphatidylcholine.

Physical Examination. The cardinal physical findings include nystagmus, retinitis pigmentosa, and decreased visual acuity (Fig. 148–15). In the latter stages of the disease, loss of deep tendon reflexes, decreased sensory discrimination, dysarthria, and severe ataxia may develop. Cardiac arrhythmias also may be present.

Molecular Defect. The characteristic feature of abetalipoproteinemia is the absence of plasma apoB-100 and apoB-48. However, intracellular apoB mRNA and protein are several-fold increased, and linkage studies have established

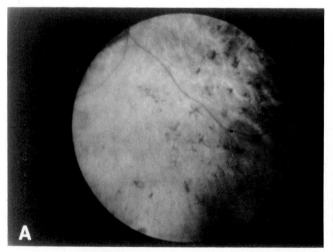
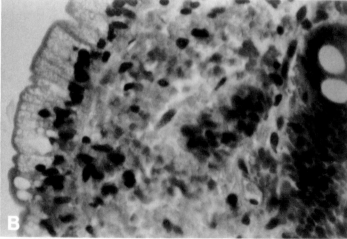

FIGURE 148–15. Abetalipoproteinemia is characterized clinically by atypical retinitis pigmentosa *(A)* and lipid-laden columnar epithelial cell in the intestinal tract *(B)*.

that the molecular defect in abetalipoproteinemia does not segregate with the apoB gene.[125] These results indicate that the defect in abetalipoproteinemia is most consistent with an abnormality in the assembly and/or secretion of apoB-containing lipoproteins. The microsomal triglyceride transfer protein has been proposed to be important in the assembly of the plasma lipoproteins.[126] Recently, a deficiency in the microsomal triglyceride transfer protein activity has been reported in intestinal biopsies of patients with abetalipoproteinemia, suggesting that a structural mutation in the triglyceride transfer protein may be the genetic basis of abetalipoproteinemia.[127] The inability to assemble and secrete chylomicrons by the intestine results in malabsorption and deficiency of fat-soluble vitamins, while the absence of hepatic production of VLDL severely diminishes the transport of endogenous triglycerides and abolishes the transport of cholesterol to peripheral cells via the LDL receptor pathway. Treatment of abetalipoproteinemia with high doses of vitamins A and E has ameliorated the progressive retinopathy and neuropathy observed in these patients.[128-130]

FAMILIAL HYPOBETALIPOPROTEINEMIA

Clinical Syndrome. Homozygous familial hypobetalipoproteinemia is a rare autosomal disease which, like classical abetalipoproteinemia, is characterized by the absence of apoB-48– and apoB-100–containing lipoproteins in plasma.[124] There are two major differences between these two clinical syndromes. First, the clinical manifestations of homozygous hypobetalipoproteinemia are milder than those of abetalipoproteinemia. Second, the heterozygous carrier state of familial hypobetalipoproteinemia is associated with reduced concentrations of plasma apoB and LDL. In homozygotes, malabsorption leads to a mild deficiency of fat-soluble vitamins. Intestinal biopsy reveals lipid-laden columnar epithelial cells similar to those observed in patients with abetalipoproteinemia. Circulating acanthocytes are present; however, the hemolytic anemia is milder than in abetalipoproteinemia. Ocular manifestations include night blindness and the development of progressive retinal degeneration. Of particular importance in the clinical course of patients with homozygous hypobetalipoproteinemia is the relative sparing of the neurological system. The majority of the patients have minimal ataxia, cerebellar signs, or motor-sensory dysfunction which is in marked contrast to the severe ataxia and neurological disease observed in abetalipoproteinemia.

Molecular Defect. The biochemical defect in familial hypobetalipoproteinemia, unlike that in abetalipoproteinemia, is due to a structural mutation in the apoB gene leading to decreased biosynthesis of apoB and the inability to secrete chylomicrons and hepatogenous VLDL effectively. Several different structural mutations in the apoB gene have been identified that lead to a defect in the biosynthesis of apoB.[131-134]

TREATMENT OF DYSLIPOPROTEINEMIAS

The treatment of patients with hyperlipoproteinemia has entered the mainstream of clinical medicine. The sequelae of dyslipoproteinemias, including pancreatitis, coronary ar-

tery disease, and peripheral vascular disease, can be prevented by the use of dietary and pharmacological strategies. Several angiographic trials have demonstrated the prevention of reinfarction and regression of atheromatous lesions with treatment of the dyslipoproteinemia. Using approaches designed to modulate critical steps in the synthesis, secretion, and catabolism of the lipoprotein particles, the vast majority of hyperlipidemic patients can now be treated successfully.

The first demonstration that modification of plasma lipoproteins could favorably prevent cardiovascular disease was reported in 1984 by the Lipid Research Clinics' Coronary Primary Prevention Trial.[135, 136] This study established that a 1 per cent reduction in the LDL cholesterol concentration in middle-aged men reduced their risk of developing symptomatic coronary artery disease by 2 per cent over 5 to 7 years of treatment. This observation led to the development of the National Cholesterol Education Program (NCEP), which was designed to parallel the efforts in public health which had facilitated the treatment of hypertension in the early 1970's. The first recommendations for the treatment of hypercholesterolemia were made by the Adult Treatment Panel (ATP-I) in 1988.[137] Subsequently, there has been an explosion of information relevant to the details of treating patients to prevent coronary artery disease. This new information has led to the second Adult Treatment Panel (ATP-II), which has provided a revision of the original guidelines for treating patients with hypercholesterolemia.

The vast majority of patients requiring treatment present with primary hyperlipoproteinemia. With routine screening for hypercholesterolemia, nearly 40 per cent of the population have total cholesterol concentrations above 200 mg/dl, which has been defined as "desirable." In routine clinical practice, particularly in the setting of an Internal Medicine or Endocrinology practice, however, many patients will manifest hyperlipoproteinemia that is secondary to other conditions such as hypothyroidism, diabetes mellitus, collagen-vascular disease, or renal failure. Most treatment guidelines, such as those of the National Cholesterol Education Program (NCEP), have been formulated based on primary and secondary intervention trials designed to test the efficacy of dietary and drug treatment of primary hyperlipoproteinemia. The applicability of these clinical trial strategies on the prevention of the cardiovascular sequelae present in secondary hyperlipoproteinemias is an active area of clinical investigation. Until the results of ongoing trials are evaluated, the clinician caring for patients with secondary hyperlipoproteinemias can selectively utilize therapeutic strategies that have proven successful in the treatment of primary hyperlipoproteinemias.

Prevention of Cardiovascular Disease

All individuals over age 20 should be screened for hypercholesterolemia by obtaining a random blood sample for total and HDL cholesterol concentrations. If desirable total cholesterol concentrations (<200 mg/dl) and HDL cholesterol concentrations (>35 mg/dl) are present, no specific treatment is recommended, and the patient should simply be reevaluated within 5 years. However, if the screening cholesterol concentration is greater than 200 mg/dl or if the HDL cholesterol concentration is less than 35 mg/dl, a fasting lipoprotein analysis should be performed. After a 9- to 12-hour fast, the triglycerides, cholesterol, and HDL cholesterol concentrations are determined, and the LDL cholesterol concentration is calculated using the formula [LDL cholesterol] = [total cholesterol] − ([triglyceride]/5) − [HDL cholesterol]. The calculated LDL cholesterol concentration is the basis for subsequent therapeutic decisions, which are also influenced by the absence (primary prevention strategy) or presence (secondary prevention) of coronary artery disease.

Primary Prevention

The threshold for treatment and the intensity of therapy for patients without symptoms of heart disease differ from those for patients who already manifest disease based on safety/benefit as well as cost-effectiveness considerations. If the LDL cholesterol concentration is less than 130 mg/dl, no further treatment is recommended for patients without clinically evident coronary artery disease. However, if the LDL cholesterol concentration is greater than 130 mg/dl, other "positive" and "negative" risk factors for cardiovascular disease affect treatment decisions. Patients with diabetes mellitus, HDL cholesterol concentrations less than 35 mg/dl, or hypertension and those who smoke cigarettes all are at increased risk for atherosclerotic disease by virtue of these "positive" risk factors. In addition, a positive family history for coronary heart disease, men older than 45 years, and women older than 55 years of age or who have undergone premature menopause and are not receiving estrogen replacement therapy are considered as having additional risk. In contrast, patients with HDL cholesterol concentrations of greater than 60 mg/dl are less prone to atherogenesis and are assigned a "negative" risk. For the patient with an LDL cholesterol concentration of 130 to 159 mg/dl but with fewer than two positive risk factors, the patient should be instructed on a step I diet and have the lipoproteins analyzed annually. For patients with LDL cholesterol concentrations of 130 to 150 mg/dl with two or more risk factors and for patients with an LDL cholesterol concentration of greater than 160 mg/dl, a repeated lipoprotein analysis should be performed to confirm the concentrations. If the first two LDL cholesterol determinations differ by more than 30 mg/dl, a third test should be obtained within 1 to 8 weeks, and the average value of the three tests should be used. If the average of two determinations falls within these same ranges, a full history, physical examination and laboratory testing to search for familial disorders and secondary causes for hyperlipidemia are indicated. The underlying disease should be treated in those patients with secondary hyperlipoproteinemias, and diet therapy should then be initiated for those with primary hyperlipoproteinemia.

Secondary Prevention

A more aggressive lipid-modifying approach is warranted in the patient who already manifests cardiovascular disease. Clinical trial data indicate substantial reduction in the atherogenic process angiographically with treatment of the hyperlipidemic patient. Aggressive drug treatment has been shown to reduce reinfarction, development of new symptoms, need for coronary artery bypass grafting, and even all-cause mortality.[138–145] The optimal LDL cholesterol concentration for the patient with symptomatic ischemic heart disease is less than 100 mg/dl. For those patients with LDL cholesterol concentrations greater than 100 mg/dl, a thorough history, physical examination, and laboratory evaluation to identify secondary hyperlipidemia and familial disorders should be undertaken.

Diet Therapy and Physical Activity

Since diet is the cornerstone for treatment, almost all patients* should be started on diet therapy. Dietary modification can prevent atherosclerotic lesion formation and reduce cardiovascular disease events.[144] Increasing physical activity augments the efforts directed toward diet. Dietary treatment is relatively inexpensive, safe, and can prevent many patients, particularly those with primary hyperlipoproteinemias, from advancing to drug treatment with its attendant risk, cost, and adverse effects. In addition, drug treatment is rendered more effective in patients who comply with a healthy diet. The three dietary factors that most affect the circulating LDL particles include high saturated fat intake, high intake of dietary cholesterol, and an imbalance between caloric intake and expenditure.

Modification of diet occurs in two steps. The first step is one that can be initiated from the routine office setting and is achievable by many patients making relatively minor adjustments to their food purchases and food preparation. Reducing the total fat intake to less than 30 per cent of total calories, the saturated fatty acid intake to less than 10 per cent of total calories, and total cholesterol intake to less than 300 mg/day can be achieved by eating leaner cuts of meat, smaller portion sizes, altered preparation methods, and substitutions of oils to those less saturated. Dietary studies in free-living populations have shown 3 to 14 per cent reduction in total cholesterol concentrations with the step I diet.

The step II diet is more stringent, with the saturated fat intake reduced to less than 7 per cent of calories and the cholesterol intake restricted to 200 mg/day. Advancing to step II is more difficult to achieve without the help of a registered dietitian. The more substantial changes required for long-term success necessitate customizing the diet to each patient. An additional 3 to 7 per cent reduction in the total cholesterol concentration compared with the step I diet can be expected. With proper dietary instruction, many patients can achieve their "goal" LDL cholesterol concentration and avoid further intervention.

Screening for Abnormalities in Triglyceride Concentrations

A great deal more is known about the benefits of cholesterol reduction in hypercholesterolemic patients than the lowering of triglyceride concentrations in hypertriglyceri-

---

*Excluding patients with familial hypercholesterolemia who manifest LDL cholesterol concentrations > 190 mg/dl, tendinous xanthomata, and an autosomal co-dominant inheritance pattern for premature (<60 years) cardiovascular disease.

demic individuals. Triglycerides are carried primarily in the VLDL and chylomicron particles, which are increased in concentration after a meal. Since elevated fasting triglyceride concentrations are also associated with disease, screening patients for hypertriglyceridemia may be of benefit. Fasting triglyceride concentrations greater than 200 mg/dl are elevated and concentrations greater than 1000 mg/dl are at risk for pancreatitis. Therefore, patients with recurrent pancreatitis should be screened for hypertriglyceridemia, since patients with increased concentrations of plasma chylomicrons (types I and V hyperlipoproteinemia) develop this complication. Since many patients with pancreatitis from other etiologies develop transient hypertriglyceridemia, the screening for hyperchylomicronemia should be performed after an acute pancreatitis episode. However, patients with pancreatitis rarely manifest the profoundly elevated total triglyceride concentrations that are seen with types I and V. These latter patients generally have triglyceride concentrations greater than 1000 mg/dl which are carried in the large chylomicron particles. These strikingly elevated levels can be observed by the inspection of the blood, which has a characteristic "cream of tomato soup" appearance and eruptive xanthomas (see Fig. 148–7). Once these patients have been identified, dietary/drug intervention can reduce their risk for subsequent episodes of pancreatitis.

Screening for hypertriglyceridemia also should be considered in patients who are started on treatment with either estrogen replacement therapy or with treatment with 13-cis-retinoic acid for the treatment of acne. If the fasting triglyceride concentrations are greater than 500 mg/dl, either avoiding these drugs or modifying the preparations may reduce the risk of developing profound hypertriglyceridemia (>1000 mg/dl) and pancreatitis.

Elevated concentrations of fasting plasma triglycerides also have been associated with cardiovascular disease, and this is particularly true in women. This association is generally not as strong as that for either LDL cholesterol or HDL cholesterol concentrations. Although the recent NIH Consensus Conference on High Triglyceride and Low HDL did not recommend universal screening for hypertriglyceridemia to assess cardiovascular disease risk, the determination of the fasting triglyceride concentration is important

for interpreting the plasma lipoproteins in hypercholesterolemic patients, as was outlined earlier in this chapter. In addition, the triglyceride concentrations are important in selecting the drugs that are used to treat hypercholesterolemia, since bile acid sequestrants can exacerbate hypertriglyceridemia (>250 mg/dl). Therefore, the use of triglyceride determinations for evaluating cardiovascular disease risk is principally related to the evaluation of hypercholesterolemia.

The treatment of profound hypertriglyceridemia (>1000 mg/dl) includes refraining from ethanol use, reducing the fat in the diet to less than 20 per cent of calories as fat, and avoiding estrogen therapy. Some patients with hyperchylomicronemia respond to niacin and fibric acid derivatives, and some investigators have advocated the use of these medications in patients with fasting triglyceride levels from 200 to 1000 mg/dl to reduce cardiovascular disease risk. Unfortunately, no studies have yet been reported which directly test the hypothesis that treatment of hypertriglyceridemia reduces cardiovascular disease risk.

Drug Treatment

Many patients who require treatment to reduce their cardiovascular disease risk by modifying their plasma lipoprotein concentrations respond to diet-only therapy. A 3- to 6-month trial of dietary intervention is warranted since habit and life-style modifications require a persistent effort over this period of time. The goals of therapy differ for primary and secondary interventions. Drug therapy should be considered in primary intervention if, after an adequate trial of diet therapy, the LDL cholesterol is greater than 190 mg/dl or greater than 160 mg/dl if the patient has two or more positive coronary heart disease risk factors. For secondary prevention, the target goal of therapy is an LDL cholesterol concentration of less than 100 mg/dl, and drug therapy should be considered if diet-only treatment does not achieve this level.

The principal classes of drugs for the treatment of hyperlipoproteinemia are shown in Table 148–4. All the listed drugs (except for fenofibrate) are currently available in the United States. Because of the long experience and favora-

TABLE 148–4. SUMMARY OF THE MAJOR CLASSES OF DRUGS FOR CONSIDERATION

DRUG CLASS	SPECIFIC DRUGS	REDUCE CHD RISK	LONG-TERM SAFETY	LDL CHOLESTEROL LOWERING	COMMENTS
Bile acid sequestrants	Cholestyramine Colestipol	Yes	Yes	15–30%	Avoid in patients with hypertriglyceridemia Can alter efficacy of other medications
Nicotinic acid	Crystalline Sustained release	Yes	Yes	15–30%	Can cause hepatitis; induces gout and diabetes mellitus
Statins	Lovastatin Pravastatin Simvastatin	Not proven	Preliminary data	25–45%	Monitor liver function
Fibrates	Gemfibrozil Fenofibrate*	Yes	Preliminary data	5–15%	May increase LDL levels
Antioxidants	Probucol	Not proven	Not established	10–15%	Prolongs QT interval and lowers HDL cholesterol concentration

*Not FDA approved for use as a cholesterol-lowering drug.

TABLE 148–5. DRUGS EFFECTIVE IN LOWERING LDL CHOLESTEROL

DRUG	STARTING DOSE	MAXIMUM DOSE	USUAL TIME AND FREQUENCY	MOST COMMON SIDE EFFECTS
Cholestyramine	4 g twice daily	24 g/day	Twice daily, within an hour of major meals	Constipation, bloating sensation
Colestipol	5 g twice daily	30 mg/day		
Crystalline nicotinic acid	100–250 mg as single dose	3 g/day (1.5 g/day tolerated by most patients)	Three times per day, with meals to avoid nausea and gastrointestinal upset	Skin flushing and itching, nausea, hepatitis symptoms
Sustained-release nicotinic acid	125–250 mg/dose	3 g/day (1.5 g/day tolerated by most patients)		Nausea, abdominal pain, and exacerbation of peptic ulcer disease symptoms
Lovastatin	20 mg once daily with evening meal	80 mg/day	Once in the evening or twice daily with meals	Occasional transaminase elevations or skin rash
Pravastatin	10–20 mg once daily with evening meal	40 mg/day		Occasional signs or symptoms of hepatitis or myopathy
Simvastatin	5–10 mg once daily with evening meal	40 mg/day		Occasional signs or symptoms of hepatitis or myopathy
Gemfibrozil	600 mg twice daily	1200 mg/day	600 mg twice daily 30 min before meals	Gastrointestinal symptoms
Fenofibrate	100 mg three times a day	300 mg/day	100 mg three times a day with meals	Gastrointestinal symptoms
Probucol	500 mg twice daily	1000 mg/day	500 mg twice daily with meals	Can prolong QT interval; cause GI side effects

ble clinical responses, the bile acid sequestrants and nicotinic acid have long been favored. Further experience and preliminary evidence indicates that the statins are also reasonable alternatives for the treatment of hypercholesterolemia. For these reasons, these three classes of drugs are preferred in treating hypercholesterolemia due to increased LDL cholesterol concentrations. The use of the fibrates and the antioxidants is more controversial, since clinical trial data supporting their use, especially in secondary prevention, are lacking.

However, the use of the fibrates is approved for the treatment of hypertriglyceridemia, since these drugs can induce profound reductions in the concentrations of plasma triglycerides. Nicotinic acid preparations are also effective in treating hypertriglyceridemia.

The important prescription details for these medications are outlined in Table 148–5. With encouragement and anticipation of adverse side effects, many patients can tolerate bile acid sequestrant and nicotinic acid preparations. The advantage to using these drugs is that they have a record of safety and efficacy not matched by other medications.

The advantage of the statins revolves around both efficacy and the lack of annoying side effects. The safety of these compounds appears to be excellent, and ongoing clinical trials will reveal the impact that these compounds have on preventing cardiovascular and total mortality in both primary and secondary trial settings.

The benefits of the fibric acid derivatives and probucol are more speculative.

SUMMARY

The insights provided by the analysis of lipoprotein and apolipoprotein metabolism have provided a framework that permits the effective diagnosis and classification of patients with disorders of lipid metabolism. Diet and drug treatment are now available which profoundly alter the metabolism of lipoprotein particles. Effective treatment of patients can prevent the morbidity and mortality associated with the genetic dyslipoproteinemias.

REFERENCES

1. Gofman JW, deLalla O, Glazier R, et al: The serum lipid transport system in health, metabolic disorders, atherosclerosis, and coronary artery disease. Plasma 2:413–484, 1954.
2. Berg K, Dahlen G, Frick MH: Lp(a) lipoprotein and pre-beta₁-lipoprotein in patients with coronary heart disease. Clin Genet 6:230–235, 1974.
3. Lee RS, Hatch RT: Sharper separation of lipoprotein species by paper electrophoresis in albumin containing buffer. J Lab Clin Med 61:518–528, 1963.
4. Osborne JC Jr, Brewer HB Jr: The plasma lipoproteins. Adv Protein Chem 31:253–337, 1977.
5. Scanu AM, Landsberger FR: Lipoprotein structure. Ann NY Acad Sci 384:1–436, 1980.
6. Brewer HB Jr: Current concepts of the molecular structure and metabolism of human apolipoproteins and lipoproteins. Klin Wochenschr 59:1023–1035, 1981.
7. Brewer HB Jr, Gregg RE, Hoeg JM, Fojo SS: Apolipoproteins and lipoproteins in human plasma: An overview. Clin Chem 34:4–8, 1988.
8. Breslow JL: Apolipoprotein genetic variation and human disease. Physiol Rev 68:85–132, 1988.
9. Li WH, Tanimura M, Luo CC, et al: The apolipoprotein multigene family: Biosynthesis, structure, structure-function relationships, and evoluation. J Lipid Res 29:245–271, 1988.
10. Kane JP: Apolipoprotein B: Structural and metabolic heterogeneity. Annu Rev Physiol 45:637–650, 1983.
11. Blackhart BD, Ludwig EM, Pierotti VR, et al: Structure of the human apolipoprotein B gene. J Biol Chem 261:15364–15367, 1986.
12. Hospattankar AV, Higuchi K, Law SW, et al: Identification of a novel in-frame translational stop codon in human intestine apoB mRNA. Biochem Biophys Res Commun 148:279–285, 1987.
13. Powell LM, Wallis SC, Pease RJ, et al: A novel form of tissue-specific

RNA processing produces apolipoprotein-B48 in intestine. Cell 50:831–840, 1987.

14. Chen SH, Habib G, Yang CY, et al: Apolipoprotein B-48 is the product of a messenger RNA with an organ-specific in-frame stop codon. Science 238:363–366, 1987.

15. Higuchi K, Hospattankar AV, Law SW, et al: Human apolipoprotein B (apoB) mRNA: Identification of two distinct apoB mRNAs, an mRNA with the apoB-100 sequence and an apoB mRNA containing a premature in-frame translational stop codon, in both liver and intestine. Proc Natl Acad Sci USA 85:1772–1776, 1988.

16. Kostner GM, Avagaro P, Zazzolato G, et al: Lipoprotein Lp(a) and the risk for myocardial infarction. Arteriosclerosis 38:51–61, 1981.

17. Armstrong VW, Cremer P, Eberle E, et al: The association between serum Lp(a) concentrations and angiographically assessed coronary atherosclerosis: Dependence on serum LDL levels. Atherosclerosis 62:249–257, 1986.

18. Utermann G: The mysteries of lipoprotein(a). Science 246:904–910, 1989.

19. Rall SC Jr, Weisgraber KH, Mahley RW: Human apolipoprotein E: The complete amino acid sequence. J Biol Chem 257:4171–4178, 1982.

20. Utermann G, Vogelberg KH, Steinmetz A, et al: Polymorphism of apolipoprotein E: II. Genetics of hyperlipoproteinemia type III. Clin Genet 15:37–62, 1979.

21. Zannis VI, Just PW, Breslow JL: Human apolipoprotein E isoprotein subclasses are genetically determined. Am J Hum Genet 33:11–24, 1981.

22. Mahley RW, Innerarity TL, Rall SC Jr, Weisgraber KH: Plasma lipoproteins: Apolipoprotein structure and function. J Lipid Res 25:1277–1294, 1984.

23. Davignon J, Gregg RE, Sing CF: Apolipoprotein E polymorphism and atherosclerosis. Arteriosclerosis 8:1–21, 1988.

24. Brewer HB Jr, Gregg RE, Hoeg JM: Apolipoproteins, lipoproteins, and atherosclerosis. In Braunwald E (ed): Heart Disease: A Textbook of Cardiovascular Medicine. New York, WB Saunders Co, 1989, pp 121–144.

25. Vega GL, Denke MA, Grundy SM: Metabolic basis of primary hypercholesterolemia. Circulation 84:118–128, 1991.

26. Schaefer EJ: Diagnosis and management of lipoprotein disorders. In Rifkind BM (ed): Drug Treatment of Hyperlipidemia. New York, Marcel Dekker, 1991, pp 17–52.

27. Mahley RW, Hui DY, Innerarity TL, Weisgraber KH: Two independent lipoprotein receptors on hepatic membranes of dog, swine, and man: Apo-B,E and apo-E receptors. J Clin Invest 68:1197–1206, 1981.

28. Hoeg JM, Edge SB, Demosky SJ Jr, et al: Metabolism of low-density lipoproteins by cultured hepatocytes from normal and homozygous familial hypercholesterolemic subjects. Biochim Biophys Acta 876:646–657, 1986.

29. Edge SB, Hoeg JM, Triche T, et al: Cultured human hepatocytes: Evidence for metabolism of low density lipoproteins by a pathway independent of the classical low density lipoprotein receptor. J Biol Chem 261:3800–3806, 1986.

30. Herz J, Hamann U, Rogne S, et al: Surface location and high affinity for a calcium of a 500-kDa liver membrane protein closely related to the LDL receptor suggest a physiological role as a lipoprotein receptor. EMBO J 7:4119–4127, 1988.

31. Strickland DK, Ashcom JD, Williams S, et al: Sequence identity between alpha$_2$-macroglobulin receptor and low-density-lipoprotein receptor–related protein suggests that this molecule is a multifunctional receptor. J Biol Chem 265:17401–17404, 1990.

32. Goldstein JL, Brown MS: The LDL receptor locus and the genetics of familial hypercholesterolemia. Annu Rev Genet 13:259–289, 1979.

33. Goldstein JL, Brown MS, Anderson RG, et al: Receptor-mediated endocytosis: Concepts emerging from the LDL receptor system. Annu Rev Cell Biol 1:1–39, 1985.

34. Gregg RE, Brewer HB Jr: The role of apolipoprotein E and lipoprotein receptors in modulating the in vivo metabolism of apolipoprotein B-containing lipoproteins in humans. Clin Chem 34:28–32, 1988.

35. Sudhof TC, Goldstein JL, Brown MS, Russell DW: The LDL receptor gene: A mosiac of exons shared with different proteins. Science 228:815, 1985.

36. Yamamoto T, Davis CG, Brown MS, et al: The human LDL receptor: A cysteine-rich protein with multiple Alu sequences in its mRNA. Cell 39:27–38, 1984.

37. Eisenberg S: High density lipoprotein metabolism. J Lipid Res 25:1017–1058, 1984.

38. Rader DJ, Ikewaki K, Schaefer JR, Brewer HB Jr: Metabolism of HDL particles LpA-1 and LpA-I,A-II in normal and hyperalphalipoproteinemic subjects. In Catapano AL, Bernini F, Corsini A (eds): High Density Lipoproteins: Physiopathology and Clinical Relevance. New York, Raven Press, 1993, pp 43–55.

39. Tall AR: Plasma lipid transfer proteins. J Lipid Res 27:361–367, 1986.

40. Glomset JA, Janssen ET, Kennedy R, Dobbins J: Role of plasma lecithin:cholesterol acyltransferase in the metabolism of high density lipoproteins. J Lipid Res 7:638–648, 1966.

41. Glomset JA: The plasma lecithins:cholesterol acyltransferase reaction. J Lipid Res 9:155–167, 1968.

42. Oram JF, Brinton EA, Bierman EL: Regulation of high density lipoprotein receptor activity in cultured human skin fibroblasts and human arterial smooth muscle cells. J Clin Invest 72:1611–1621, 1983.

43. Suzuki N, Fidge N, Nestel P, Yin J: Interaction of serum lipoproteins with the intestine: Evidence for specific high density lipoprotein-binding sites on isolated rat intestinal mucosal cells. J Lipid Res 24:253–264, 1983.

44. Schmitz G, Niemann R, Brennhausen B, et al: Regulation of high density lipoprotein receptors in cultured macrophages: Role of acyl-CoA:cholesterol acyltransferase. EMBO J 4:2773–2779, 1985.

45. Barbaras R, Puchois P, Grimaldi P, et al: Relationship in adipose cells between the presence of receptor sites for high density lipoproteins and the promotion of reverse cholesterol transport. Biochem Biophys Res Commun 149:545–554, 1987.

46. McKnight GL, Reasoner J, Gilbert T, et al: Cloning and expression of a cellular high density lipoprotein-binding protein that is up-regulated by cholesterol loading of cells. J Biol Chem 267:12131–12141, 1992.

47. Theret N, Delbart C, Aguie G, et al: Cholesterol efflux from adipose cells is coupled to diacylglycerol production and protein kinase C activation. Biochem Biophys Res Commun 173:1361–1368, 1990.

48. Mendez AJ, Oram JF, Bierman EL: Protein kinase C as a mediator of high density lipoprotein receptor-dependent efflux of intracellular cholesterol. J Biol Chem 266:10104–10111, 1991.

49. Alaupovic P: Conceptual development of the classification systems of plasma lipoproteins: Protides of the biological fluids. In Proceedings of the 19th Colloquium. 1972, pp 9–19.

50. Kostner G, Alaupovic P: Studies of the composition and structure of plasma lipoproteins: Separation and quantification of the lipoprotein families occurring in the high density lipoproteins of human plasma. Biochemistry 11:3419–3428, 1972.

51. Utermann G, Weber W: Protein composition of Lp(a) lipoprotein from human plasma. FEBS Lett 154:357–361, 1983.

52. Gaubatz JW, Heideman C, Gotto AM Jr, et al: Human plasma lipoprotein[a]: Structural properties. J Biol Chem 258:4582–4589, 1983.

53. Fless GM, Rolih CA, Scanu AM: Heterogeneity of human plasma lipoprotein(a): Isolation and characterization of the lipoprotein subspecies and their apoproteins. J Biol Chem 259:11470–11478, 1984.

54. Eaton DL, Fless GM, Kohr WJ, et al: Partial amino acid sequence of apolipoprotein(a) shows that it is homologous to plasminogen. Proc Natl Acad Sci USA 84:3224–3228, 1987.

55. McLean JW, Tomlinson JE, Kuang WJ, et al: cDNA sequence of human apolipoprotein(a) is homologous to plasminogen. Nature 330:132–137, 1987.

56. Utermann G, Menzel HJ, Kraft HG, et al: Lp(a) glycoprotein phenotypes: Inheritance and relation to Lp(a)-lipoprotein concentrations in plasma. J Clin Invest 80:458–465, 1987.

57. Koschinsky ML, Beisiegel U, Henne-Bruns D, et al: Apolipoprotein(a) size heterogeneity is related to variable number of repeat sequences in its mRNA. Biochemistry 29:640–644, 1990.

58. Azrolan N, Gavish D, Breslow JL: Lp(a) levels correlate inversely with apo(a) size and KIV copy number but not with apo(a) mRNA levels in a cynomolgus monkey model (abstract). Circulation 82:111-90, 1990.

59. Kodama T, Freeman M, Rohrer L, et al: Type I macrophage scavenger receptor contains alpha-helical and collagen-like coiled coils. Nature 343:531–535, 1990.

60. Steinberg D: Lipoproteins and atherosclerosis: A look back and a look ahead. Arteriosclerosis 3:283–301, 1983.

61. Steinberg D: Antioxidants and atherosclerosis: A current assessment. Circulation 84:1420–1425, 1991.

62. Van Lenten BJ, Fogelman AM: Processing of lipoproteins in human monocyte-macrophages. J Lipid Res 31:1455–1466, 1990.

63. Haberland ME, Fogelman AM: The role of altered lipoproteins in the pathogenesis of atherosclerosis. Am Heart J 113:573–577, 1987.

64. Brewer HB Jr, Zech LA, Gregg RE, et al: Type III hyperlipoprotein-

emia: Diagnosis, molecular defects, pathology, and treatment. Ann Intern Med 98:623–640, 1983.

65. Mahley RW: Dietary, fat, cholesterol, and accelerated atherosclerosis. Atherosclerosis Rev 5:1–34, 1979.

66. Gregg RE, Zech LA, Schaefer EJ, Brewer HB Jr: Type III hyperlipoproteinemia: Defective metabolism of an abnormal apolipoprotein E. Science 211:584–586, 1981.

67. Havel RJ: Familial dysbetalipoproteinemia: New aspects of pathogenesis and diagnosis. Med Clin North Am 66:441–454, 1982.

68. Loscalzo J: Lipoprotein(a): A unique risk factor for atherothrombotic disease. Arteriosclerosis 10:672–679, 1990.

69. Miles LA, Plow EF: Lp(a): An interloper in the fibrinolytic system. Thromb Haemost 63:331–335, 1990.

70. Miller GJ, Miller NE: Plasma high-density-lipoprotein concentration and development of ischaemic heart disease. Lancet 1:16–19, 1975.

71. Gordon T, Castelli WP, Hjortland MC, et al: High density lipoprotein as a protective factor against coronary heart disease: The Framingham study. Am J Med 63:707–714, 1977.

72. Miller NE, Thelle DS, Forde OH, Mjos OD: The Tromso heart study: High-density lipoproteins and coronary heart-disease: A prospective case-control study. Lancet 1:965–968, 1977.

73. Gordon DJ, Rifkind BM: High-density lipoprotein—The clinical implications of recent studies. N Engl J Med 321:1311–1316, 1989.

74. Brunzell JD: Familial lipoprotein lipase deficiency and other causes of the chylomicronemia syndrome. In Scriver CR, Beaudet AL, Sly WS, Valle D (eds): The Metabolic Basis of Inherited Disease. New York, McGraw-Hill, 1989, pp 1165–1180.

75. Fojo SS, Brewer HB Jr: Hypertriglyceridaemia due to genetic defects in lipoprotein lipase and apolipoprotein C-II. J Intern Med 231:669–677, 1992.

76. Santamarina-Fojo S: Genetic dyslipoproteinemias: Role of lipoprotein lipase and apoC-II. Curr Opin Lipidol 3:186–195, 1992.

77. Goldstein JL, Brown MS: Familial Hypercholesterolemia. In Scriver CR, Beaudet AL, Sly WS, Valle D (eds): The Metabolic Basis of Inherited Disease. New York, McGraw-Hill, 1989, pp 1215–1250.

78. Van der Westhuyzen DR, Fourie AM, Coetzee GA, Gevers W: The LDL receptor. Curr Opin Lipidol 1:128–135, 1990.

79. Russell DW, Esser V, Hobbs HH: Molecular basis of familial hypercholesterolemia. Arteriosclerosis 9(Suppl 1):1–8, 1989.

80. Goldstein JL, Schrott HG, Hazzard WR, et al: Hyperlipidemia in coronary heart disease: II. Genetic analysis of lipid levels in 176 families and delineation of a new inherited disorder, combined hyperlipidemia. J Clin Invest 52:1544–1568, 1973.

81. Sniderman A, Shapiro S, Marpole D, et al: Association of coronary atherosclerosis with hyperapobetalipoproteinemia [increased protein but normal cholesterol levels in human plasma low density (beta) lipoproteins]. Proc Natl Acad Sci USA 77:604–608, 1980.

82. Sniderman AD, Wolfson C, Teng B, et al: Association of hyperapobetalipoproteinemia with endogenous hypertriglyceridemia and atherosclerosis. Ann Intern Med 97:833–839, 1982.

83. Janus ED, Nicoll AM, Turner PR, et al: Kinetic bases of the primary hyperlipidaemias: Studies of apolipoprotein B turnover in genetically defined subjects. Eur J Clin Invest 10:161–172, 1980.

84. Thompson GR, Teng B, Sniderman AD: Kinetics of LDL subfractions. Am Heart J 113:514–557, 1987.

85. Innerarity TL, Weisgraber KH, Arnold KS, et al: Familial defective apolipoprotein B-100: Low density lipoproteins with abnormal receptor binding. Proc Natl Acad Sci USA 84:6919–6923, 1987.

86. Soria LF, Ludwig EH, Clarke HR, et al: Association between a specific apolipoprotein B mutation and familial defective apolipoprotein B-100. Proc Natl Acad Sci USA 86:587–591, 1989.

87. Vega GL, Grundy SM: In vivo evidence for reduced binding of low density lipoproteins to receptors as a cause of primary moderate hypercholesterolemia. J Clin Invest 78:1410–1414, 1986.

88. Bhattacharyya AK, Connor WE: Familial diseases with storage of sterols other than cholesterol (cerebrotendinous xanthomatosis and beta-sitosterolemia and xanthomatosis). In Stanbury JB, Wyngaarden JB, Fredrickson DS, et al (eds): Metabolic Basis of Inherited Disease. New York, McGraw-Hill, 1983, pp 656–669.

89. Salens G, Shafer S, Berginer VM: Familial disease with storage of sterol other than cholesterol: Cerebrotendinous xanthomatosis and sitosterolemia with xanthomatosis. In Stanbury JB, Wyngaarden JB, Fredrickson DS, et al (eds): Metabolic Basis of Inherited Disease. New York, McGraw-Hill, 1983, pp 713–730.

90. Kuriyama M, Fujiyama J, Yoshidome H, et al: Cerebrotendinous xanthomatosis: Clinical and biochemical evaluation of eight patients and review of the literature. J Neurol Sci 102:225–232, 1991.

91. Cali JJ, Hsieh CC, Francke U, Russell DW: Mutations in the bile acid biosynthetic enzyme sterol 27-hydroxylase underlie cerebrotendinous xanthomatosis. J Biol Chem 266:7779–7783, 1991.

92. Nakamura T, Matsuzawa Y, Takemura KK, et al: Combined treatment with chenodeoxycholic acid and provastatin improves plasma cholestanol levels associated with marked regression of tendon xanthomas in cerebriotendinous xanthomastosis. Metabolism 40:741–746, 1991.

93. Salens G, Shefer S, Nguyen L, et al: Sitosterolemia. J Lipid Res 33:945–955, 1992.

94. Bhattacharyya AK, Connor WE, Yin DS, et al: Sluggish sitosterol turnover and hepatic failure to excrete sitosterol into bile cause expansion of body of sitosterol in patients with sitosterolemia and xanthomatosis. Arteriosclerosis Thrombosis 11:1287–1294, 1991.

95. Salens G, Tint GS, Shefer S, et al: Increased sitosterol absorption is offset by rapid elimination to prevent accumulation in heterozygotes with sitosterolemia. Arteriosclerosis Thrombosis 12:563–568, 1992.

96. Lohse P, Mann WA, Stein EA, Brewer HB Jr: Apolipoprotein E-4$_{Philadelphia}$ (Glu^{13} → Lys,Arg^{145} → Cys): Homozygosity for two rare point mutations in the apolipoprotein E gene combined with severe type III hyperlipoproteinemia. J Biol Chem 266:10479–10484, 1991.

97. Mann WA, Gregg RE, Sprecher DL, Brewer HB Jr: Apolipoprotein E-1Harrisburg: A new variant of apolipoprotein E dominantly associated with type III hyperlipoproteinemia. Biochim Biophys Acta 1005:239–244, 1989.

98. Rall SC Jr, Newhouse YM, Clarke HR, et al: Type III hyperlipoproteinemia associated with apolipoprotein E phenotype E3/3: Structure and genetics of an apolipoprotein E3 variant. J Clin Invest 83:1095–1101, 1989.

99. Wardell MR, Weisgraber KH, Havekes LM, Rall SC Jr: Apolipoprotein E3-Leiden contains a seven-amino acid insertion that is a tandem repeat of residues 121–127. J Biol Chem 264:21205–21210, 1989.

100. Brewer HB Jr, Santamarina-Fojo S, Hoeg JM: Genetic defects in the human plasma apolipoproteins. Atherosclerosis Rev 23:51–61, 1991.

101. Gregg RE, Zech LA, Schaefer EJ, et al: Abnormal in vivo metabolism of apolipoprotein E4 in humans. J Clin Invest 78:815–821, 1986.

102. Assmann G, Schmitz G Brewer HB Jr: Familial high density lipoprotein deficiency: Tangier disease. In Scriver CR, Beaudet AL, Sly WS, Valle D (eds): The Metabolic Basis of Inherited Disease. New York, McGraw-Hill, 1989, pp 1267–1282.

103. Schaefer EJ, Zech LA, Schwartz DE, Brewer HB Jr: Coronary heart disease prevalence and other clinical features in familial high-density lipoprotein deficiency (Tangier disease). Ann Intern Med 93:261–266, 1980.

104. Schaefer EJ, Blum CB, Levy RI, et al: Metabolism of high-density lipoprotein apolipoproteins in Tangier disease. N Engl J Med 299:905–910, 1978.

105. von Eckardstein A, Funke H, Henke A, et al: Apolipoprotein A-I variants: Naturally occurring substitutions of proline residues affect plasma concentration of apolipoprotein A-I. J Clin Invest 84:1722–1730, 1989.

106. Schmitz G, Lackner K: High density lipoprotein deficiency with xanthomas: A defect in apoA-I synthesis. In Crepaldi G, Baggio G (eds): Atherosclerosis VIII. Rome, Tekno Press, 1989, pp 399–403.

107. Norum RA, Lakier JB, Goldstein S, et al: Familial deficiency of apolipoproteins A-I and C-III and precocious coronary artery disease. N Engl J Med 306:1513–1519, 1982.

108. Karathanasis SK, Zannis VI, Breslow JL: A DNA insertion in the apolipoprotein A-I gene of patients with premature atherosclerosis. Nature 305:823–825, 1983.

109. Schaefer EJ, Ordovas JM, Law SW, et al: Familial apolipoprotein A-I and C-III deficiency, variant II. J Lipid Res 26:1089–1101, 1985.

110. Ordovas JM, Cassidy DK, Civeira F, et al: Familial apolipoprotein A-I, C-III, and A-IV deficiency and premature atherosclerosis due to deletion of a gene complex on chromosome 11. J Biol Chem 264:16339–16342, 1989.

111. Norum KR, Gjone E, Glomset JA: Familial lecthin:cholesterol acyltransferase deficiency including fish eye disease. In Scriver CR, Beaudet AL, Sly WS, Valle D (eds): The Metabolic Basis of Inherited Disease. New York, McGraw-Hill, 1989, pp 1181–1194.

112. Carlson LA: Fish eye disease: A new familial condition with massive corneal opacities and dyslipoproteinaemia. Eur J Clin Invest 12:41–53, 1982.

113. Carlson LA, Holmquist L: Evidence for deficiency of high density lipoprotein lecithin:cholesterol acyltransferase activity (alpha-LCAT) in fish eye disease. Acta Med Scand 218:189–196, 1985.

114. Carlson LA, Holmquist L: Evidence for the presence in human

plasma of lecithin:cholesterol acyltransferase activity (beta-LCAT) specifically esterifying free cholesterol of combined pre-beta- and beta-lipoproteins: Studies of fish eye disease patients and control subjects. Acta Med Scand 218:197–205, 1985.

115. Taramelli R, Pontoglio M, Candiani G, et al: Lecithin:cholesterol acyltransferase deficiency: Molecular analysis of a mutated allele. Hum Genet 85:195–199, 1990.

116. Assmann G, von Eckardstein A, Funke H: Lecithin-cholesterol acyltransferase deficiency and fish-eye disease. Curr Opin Lipidol 2:110–117, 1991.

117. Bujo H, Kusunoki J, Ogasawara M, et al: Molecular defect in familial lecithin:cholesterol acyltransferase (LCAT) deficiency: A single nucleotide insertion in LCAT gene causes a complete deficient type of the disease. Biochem Biophys Res Commun 181:933–940, 1991.

118. Skretting G, Blomhoff JP, Solheim J, Prydz H: The genetic defect of the original Norwegian lecithin:cholesterol acyltransferase deficiency families. FEBS Lett 309:307–310, 1992.

119. Klein H-G, Lohse P, Duverger N, et al: Two different allelic mutations in the lecithin:cholesterol acyltransferase (LCAT) gene resulting in classic LCAT deficiency: LCAT (tyr83 → stop) and LCAT (tyr156 → asn). J Lipid Res 34:49–58, 1993.

120. Klein H-G, Lohse P, Pritchard PH, et al: Two different allelic mutations in the lecithin-cholesterol acyltransferase gene associated with the fish eye syndrome: Lecithin-cholesterol acyltransferase (Thr$_{123}$ → Ile) and lecithin-cholesterol acyltransferase (Thr$_{347}$ → Met). J Clin Invest 89:499–506, 1992.

121. Skretting G, Prydz H: An amino acid exchange in exon I of the human lecithin:cholesterol acyltransferase (LCAT) gene is associated with fish eye disease. Biochem Biophys Res Commun 182:583–587, 1992.

122. Klein H-G, Santamarina-Fojo S, Duverger N, et al: Fish eye syndrome: A molecular defect in the lecithin-cholesterol acyltransferase (LCAT) gene associated with normal alpha-LCAT specific activity. J Clin Invest (in press).

123. Illingworth DR, Connor WE, Miller RG: Abetalipoproteinemia: Report of two cases and review of therapy. Arch Neurol 37:659–662, 1980.

124. Herbert PN, Assmann G, Gotto AM Jr, Fredrickson DS: Familial lipoprotein deficiency: Abetalipoproteinemias, hypobetalipoproteinemias, and Tangier disease. In Stanbury JB, Wyngaarden JB, Fredrickson DS, et al (eds): Metabolic Basis of Inherited Disease. New York, McGraw-Hill, 1983, pp 589–621.

125. Lackner KJ, Monge JC, Gregg RE, et al: Analysis of the apolipoprotein B gene and messenger ribonucleic acid in abetalipoproteinemia. J Clin Invest 78:1707–1712, 1986.

126. Wetterau JR, Aggerbeck LP, Laplaud PM, McLean LR: Structural properties of the microsomal triglyceride-transfer protein complex. Biochemistry 30:4406–4412, 1991.

127. Wetterau JR, Aggerbeck LP, Bouma ME, et al: Absence of microsomal triglyceride transfer protein in individuals with abetalipoproteinemia. Science 258:999–1001, 1992.

128. Muller DPR: Effect of large oral doses of vitamin E on the neurological sequelae of patients with abetalipoproteinemia. In Lubin B Machlin LJ (eds): Vitamin E: Biochemical, Hematological, and Clinical Aspects. New York, New York Academy of Sciences, 1982, pp 133–144.

129. Bieri JG, Hoeg JM, Schaefer EJ, et al: Vitamin A and vitamin E replacement in abetalipoproteinemia. Ann Intern Med 100:238–239, 1984.

130. Hegele RA, Angel A: Arrest of neuropathy and myopathy in abetalipoproteinemia with high dose vitamin E therapy. Can Med Assoc J 12:41–44, 1985.

131. Cottrill C, Glueck CJ, Leuba V, et al: Familial homozygous hypobetalipoproteinemia. Metabolism 23:779–791, 1974.

132. Leppert M, Breslow JL, Wu L, et al: Inference of a molecular defect of apolipoprotein B in hypobetalipoproteinemia by linkage analysis in a large kindred. J Clin Invest 82:847–851, 1988.

133. Ross RS, Gregg RE, Law SW, et al: Homozygous hypobetalipoproteinemia: A disease distinct from abetalipoproteinemia at the molecular level. J Clin Invest 81:590–595, 1988.

134. Gabelli C: The lipoprotein metabolism of apolipoprotein B mutants. Curr Opin Lipidol 3:208–214, 1992.

135. Lipid Research Clinics Program: The Lipid Research Clinics coronary primary prevention trial results: I. Reduction in incidence of coronary heart disease. JAMA 251:351–364, 1984.

136. Lipids Research Clinics Program: The Lipid Research Clinics coronary primary prevention trial results: II. The relationship of reduction in incidence of coronary heart disease to cholesterol lowering. JAMA 251:365–374, 1984.

137. Report of the National Cholesterol Education Program Expert Panel on detection, evaluation, and treatment of high blood cholesterol in adults. Arch Intern Med 148:36–69, 1988.

138. Blankenhorn DH, Johnson RL, Mack WJ, et al: The influence of diet on the appearance of new lesions in human coronary arteries. JAMA 263:1646–1652, 1990.

139. Cashin-Hemphill L, Mack WJ, Pogoda JM, et al: Beneficial effects of colestipol-niacin on coronary atherosclerosis. JAMA 264:3013–3017, 1990.

140. Blankenhorn DH: Angiographic trials testing the efficacy of cholesterol lowering in reducing progression or inducing regression of coronary atherosclerosis. Coronary Artery Dis 2:875–879, 1991.

141. Brown G, Albers JJ, Fisher MD, et al: Regression of coronary artery disease as a result of intensive lipid-lowering therapy in men with high levels of apolipoprotein B. J Med 323:1289–1298, 1990.

142. Brown G, Albers W, Dodge HT, et al: Regression of coronary artery disease as a result of intensive lipid-lowering therapy in men with high levels of apolipoprotein B (abstract). N Engl J Med 323:1289–1298a, 1990.

143. Ornish D, Brown SE, Gould KL, et al: Can lifestyle changes reverse coronary heart disease? The lifestyle heart trial (abstract). Lancet 336:129–133, 1990.

144. Watts GF, Lewis B, Brunt JNH, et al: Effects on coronary artery disease of lipid-lowering diet, or diet plus cholestyramine, in the St Thomas' Atherosclerosis Regression Study (STARS). Lancet 339:563–569, 1992.

145. Canner PL, Berge KG, Wenger NK, et al: Fifteen year mortality in Coronary Drug Project patients: Long-term benefit with niacin. J Am Coll Cardiol 8:1245–1255, 1986.

149

Paraneoplastic Endocrine Disorders (Ectopic Hormone Syndromes)

LOUIS M. SHERWOOD

Systemic manifestations of malignant disease that are independent of the physical presence of tumor or its metastatic lesions have been of considerable interest to clinicians for years. With increasing recognition of malignant disorders and the shift in hospital populations to include more patients with cancer, there is even greater interest in early recognition of paraneoplastic manifestations. This subject has been the basis of a number of excellent reviews.[1] A number of synonymous terms refer to this fascinating group of disorders, including *ectopic hormone syndromes, endocrine phenocopies, paraendocrine tumors, paraneoplastic syndromes,* and *production of hormones by nonendocrine tumors.* Although this chapter will deal primarily with those protein hormones released by tumors that produce biochemical or clinical endocrine disorders, there are a number of paraneoplastic manifestations (not yet proved to be

due to a specific protein) that are of general importance and which also will be discussed.

Malignant tumors may be associated with a variety of clinical manifestations of a primary, secondary, or tertiary nature. The tumor itself, depending on the organ or site of origin, may lead to clinical suspicion because of presenting symptoms such as gastrointestinal bleeding, cough, dysphagia, or a lump in the breast. Second, it is not uncommon for tumors to present to the clinician as a metastatic lesion well before evidence of a primary tumor is even detected. Examples include hepatomegaly due to carcinoma of the colon, abnormal behavior or neurological disorders due to brain metastases from carcinoma of the lung or breast, a skeletal fracture due to a metastatic lesion, or cord compression from a metastatic tumor to the extradural space. Third, a malignant disorder may present one

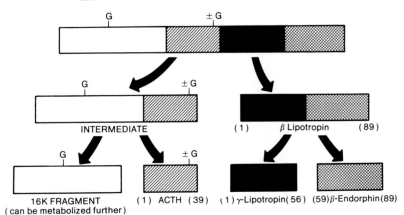

FIGURE 149–1. Conversion of proopiomelanocortin precursor to ACTH, lipotropins, and endorphin (G, glycosylation). Numbers refer to residues in hormone sequence. See text for further details.

of a variety of paraneoplastic manifestations which could be due to the production of polypeptide hormones, antibodies to tumor antigens, enzymes, or other substances. In some instances, the association is based on clinical or empirical observations, without documentation of production of a normal or abnormal substance by the tumor itself.

DEFINITION

Ectopic Versus Eutopic

The term *ectopic hormone secretion* refers to a release of a peptide hormone from a neoplasm arising in a site different from the endocrine gland normally synthesizing the hormone.[1] The production in endocrine tissue or a tumor of endocrine tissue that normally synthesizes the hormone is labeled, conversely, as *eutopic*. There is considerable confusion at the present time as to the precise definition of ectopic versus eutopic production. In order to determine that the production of a hormone is truly ectopic, it is necessary to know all the tissues in which the hormone is normally produced.[1] Extensive use of radioimmunoassays in recent years has suggested that hormone production is much more widespread than previously believed.[2] Polypeptide hormones have been identified by radioimmunoassay not only in many malignant tissues but also in many normal tissues.[3] Thus the precise definition of ectopic versus eutopic in individual tumors remains uncertain until all sites of normal hormone production are identified.

Endocrine, Paracrine, and Autocrine Factors

In order to facilitate our understanding of ectopic hormone syndromes, an altered definition of the term *hormone* might be considered. For example, classical concepts of endocrinology involve the production of hormone by an endocrine gland, its release into the bloodstream, and its action on distal target tissues as a chemical messenger. In recent years, it has become increasingly apparent that cells in various parts of the body produce peptide factors that operate locally on other cells without circulating in the blood (*paracrine* factors) and that some cells even produce polypeptides that feed back on the cell producing the peptide (*autocrine* factors). It has even been suggested that

hormones may have been derived from single-celled organisms, where they served as intracellular transmitters.[4] Tumors that synthesize ectopic peptides may release into the circulation factors that normally operate only in paracrine or autocrine fashion; thus clinical syndromes or biochemical abnormalities could be produced by factors not normally circulating (see discussion below of parathyroid hormone–related peptide).

Biochemical Concepts

Recent progress in molecular and cellular biology and in understanding the biosynthesis and processing of DNA, RNA, and proteins is helpful in evaluating ectopic hormone syndromes. Proteins that are released from cells (whether they be polypeptide hormones or other secreted proteins such as albumin or gamma globulin) are initially synthesized as a preprotein or prehormone containing a "leader" or "signal" sequence of 15 to 30 amino acid residues at the amino terminus that is hydrophobic in nature.[5] This hydrophobic sequence is needed to facilitate the transport of the newly synthesized hormone through the membrane of the endoplasmic reticulum into the subcellular transport system of the cell and on to the Golgi region for packaging and ultimate secretion. This complex process of the signal sequence being identified, bound, transported, and cleaved has been elucidated in much detail.[6] Prehormones or preproteins are not released from cells because the signal sequences are always cleaved within the cell. In the biosynthesis of some hormones such as ACTH, insulin, glucagon, gastrin, somatostatin, and parathyroid hormone, the prehormone is transformed to one or more prohormone precursors that are subsequently modified to produce mature hormones in other parts of the cell (Fig. 149–1). In some cases, prohormones can be released from stimulated normal (e.g., insulin) or tumor cells (e.g., ACTH). Specific enzymes generally present in the secretory granules and having trypsin-like activity carry out such conversion as part of posttranslational processing. A study of insulin secretory granule lysates showed normal processing of proopiomelanocortin (POMC).[7] Furthermore, carbohydrate residues are added to glycoprotein hormones as an essential feature of posttranslational processing to the mature hormone.

Ectopic hormones are always peptides, proteins, or glycoproteins. Steroid hormones, thyroid hormones, or catecholamines are not generally produced ectopically, since a cascade of enzymes would be necessary for their production.[1] On the other hand, tumors may metabolize such hormones and thus produce altered hormonal states [e.g., conversion of 25-(OH)D$_3$ to 1,25-(OH)$_2$D$_3$ by granuloma or lymphoma].

The process of hormone production by tumors is not a random one. There are specific histological associations between certain tumor types and the nature of the hormone produced[1] (Table 149–1). So-called ectopic tumors do not produce new hormones. They synthesize hormones that are normally made by endocrine tissues or other cells. Subcellular processing many be different, and thus tumors may release precursors or posttranslationally altered forms of the hormone, but they do not generally produce novel peptides. As DNA from ectopic tumors is increasingly subjected to sequence analysis, further insight into this important area will be documented. Recent studies of both neoplastic and normal tissues with a riboprobe for POMC-like mRNA suggest that mRNA molecules of 1200 or more bases were found in tumors or normal tissues that synthesize ACTH and were considerably shortened (<900 base pairs) in those that do not.[8]

PARANEOPLASTIC SYNDROMES NOT YET PROVEN TO BE DUE TO A SPECIFIC PROTEIN

Although the major emphasis of this chapter is on ectopic hormone syndromes, there are many paraneoplastic manifestations of importance that may be proven at a later date to have a humoral or immune basis. They are described briefly as follows.

Fever

Patients with malignant disease often have fever. Because of a debilitated physical condition and exposure to radiotherapy and potent cytotoxic chemotherapy, they are susceptible to infection or drug reaction, common and well-known causes of fever. In some cases, necrosis of tumor or hemorrhage into the tumor may cause fever. There are, nonetheless, instances in which fever associated with a tumor has not been due to infection or tumor necrosis and yet is related to the tumor itself. Atkins et al.[9] initially provided evidence for experimental production of fever from pyrogens. In an animal model, they described the production of endogenous leukocyte pyrogens by polymorphonuclear leukocytes, monocytes, and peritoneal and alveolar macrophages, as well as phagocytic cells of the reticuloendothelial system of the liver, spleen, and lymph nodes. At least one endogenous pyrogen is thought to be interleukin 1 (IL-1), a cytokine produced by monocyte-macrophages which acts on thermal-regulating centers in the hypothalamus as well as targets such as lymphocytes, myeloid cells, neutrophils, muscle, and brain.[10, 11] The action of IL-1 on the hypothalamus is known to be mediated through induction of the synthesis of prostaglandins, particularly PGE. Known as *exogenous pyrogens*, activators such as endotoxins of gram-negative bacteria, viruses, yeasts, drugs, particles that can be phagocytized, and hormonal pyrogenic steroids such as progesterone can provoke the release of endogenous pyrogen. Likewise, immune reactions also function as activators of the system, releasing IL-1, which also causes an enhanced immune response.[11] Other interleukins are also produced by tumors.

The situation in humans is not quite as clear, and circulating endogenous pyrogens have not been demonstrated often in human blood during febrile episodes. However, pyrogen was extracted from renal carcinoma tissue in two febrile patients and not from normal kidney by Rawlins et al.[12] Human leukocytes incubated in vitro do not release pyrogen spontaneously unless activated. Therefore, human tumor cells have been incubated in vitro and the supernatant fluid used to stimulate pyrogen release in animals. The generation of fever in the animal models does not always correlate, however, with the presence of fever in the patients. In some cases, it is believed that tumor antigens associated with antibody complexes might serve as activators of the release of IL-1. A recent report[13] on a patient with fever and pheochromocytoma suggested that IL-6 could cause the same syndrome. Although further studies of tumor-associated pyrogens need to be performed, it is clear that some tumors can produce proteins that cause pyrogenic reactions in experimental animals and humans, while in other cases, tumor-associated products (e.g., antigens) might stimulate inflammatory cells of the host to release cytokines. These experimental observations suggest an etiological basis for episodes of fever that occur frequently in patients with Hodgkin's disease, renal cell carcinoma, and other instances in which infection, tissue necrosis, abnormalities in liver function, or drug reaction cannot be implicated to explain the fever.

Weight Loss and Other Metabolic Abnormalities

Extreme weight loss and cachexia are frequent findings in patients with widespread malignancy. Anorexia, abnormalities in taste and smell, decreased food intake, gastrointestinal dysfunction, emotional depression, and combination chemotherapy are often described as factors directly related to weight loss and cachexia. Nevertheless, decreased food intake and anorexia cannot account completely for the progressive wasting of some patients, as evidenced by experimental studies in animals using forced feeding, paired feeding, and caloric restrictions.[14] Likewise, clinical observations suggest that hyperalimentation results in only transient improvement of nutritional status which cannot be maintained for long periods. Forced feeding in some cases actually has a detrimental effect.[15]

Since the normal mechanisms for controlling appetite and hunger are quite complex, it is difficult to determine how tumor factors might have an effect on these processes. Regulation of hunger involves a central control system in the brain, with specific areas in the hypothalamus controlling satiety and feeding. Some of the regulatory influences include reflexes generated from the gastrointestinal tract (e.g., gastric contractions); thermal factors related to the specific dynamic action of food substances; concentrations of hormones such as insulin, growth hormones, glucagon, and some of the gut hormones; glucose, lipid, and other metabolic products in blood; osmoregulatory factors; and a variety of environmental and emotional factors related to

TABLE 149–1. TUMOR TYPE AND SPECIFIC HORMONE PRODUCTION

HORMONE	TUMOR TYPE
ACTH and lipotropin (β-MSH, endorphin, and enkephalin)	Oat cell carcinoma of the lung
	Thymoma
	Islet cell tumor
	Bronchial carcinoid
	Also ovarian tumors, pheochromocytoma, gastrointestinal, prostate, neurogenic, and parotid tumors, and medullary thyroid carcinoma
	Inactive POMC precursor in a wide variety of tumors
Growth hormone–releasing hormone	Bronchial carcinoid, pancreatic carcinoid
Human placental lactogen	Undifferentiated carcinoma of the lung
	Hepatoma
	Lymphoma
	Pheochromocytoma
Prolactin (rare)	Renal cell carcinoma
	Undifferentiated carcinoma of the lung
	Breast carcinoma
Thyrotropin	Choriocarcinoma, hydatidiform mole
	Epidermoid carcinoma of the lung
	Mesothelioma
Gonadotropin	Choriocarcinoma of male and female; other testicular tumors; hydatidiform mole
	Hepatoblastoma, pancreatic, other gastrointestinal tumors
	Adenocarcinoma and other carcinomas of the lung
	Islet cell tumor (malignant)
	Breast carcinoma
	Melanoma
	Normal tissues (liver and colon)
hCG β subunit	Adenocarcinoma of the pancreas
	Islet cell tumor (malignant)
hCG α subunit	Carcinoid
	Islet cell tumor (malignant)
Vasopressin	Oat cell carcinoma of the lung
	Pancreatic adenocarcinoma
Calcium-mobilizing peptide hormones (parathyroid hormone–related peptide, or PTH-RP)	Epidermoid carcinoma of the lung
	Renal cell carcinoma and carcinoma of bladder
	Hepatoma, pancreatic, and gastrointestinal carcinoma
	Other epidermoid tumors
	Lymphoma
Prostaglandin E$_2$	Renal cell carcinoma
	Carcinoma of the lung
Osteoclast-activating factor	Multiple myeloma
	Burkitt's and other lymphomas
Calcitonin	Oat cell carcinoma of the lung
	Breast, pancreatic, and other carcinomas
Somatomedin (NSILA, IGF)	Mesodermal and mesenchymal tumors
	Adrenal carcinoma
Glucagon	Nonbeta islet cell tumors
	Undifferentiated lung cancer
Gastrin	Nonbeta islet cell tumor
	Duodenal wall carcinoma
	Ovarian carcinoma
Vasoactive intestinal peptide	Nonbeta islet cell tumor
	Carcinoma of the lung
	Pheochromocytoma and ganglioneuroblastoma
Erythropoietin	Renal cell carcinoma
	Cerebellar hemangioblastoma
	Pheochromocytoma
	Hepatoma
	Uterine fibroids
Renin	Juxtaglomerular tumor
	Wilms' tumor
	Renal cell carcinoma
Serotonin and 5-hydroxytryptophan	Nonbeta islet cell tumor
	Oat cell carcinoma of the lung
	Carcinoid (also growth hormone–releasing activity)
	Pancreatic adenocarcinoma

normal appetite mechanisms. The disruption of these mechanisms in patients with malignancy can be complex and multifactorial. Older studies suggested that there were peptides in the urine of fasted animals that were believed to have anorexic properties.[16] These substances also have been found in the urine of patients with malignant neoplasms,[17] and although it has been speculated that the tumor could produce such a peptide, there is as yet no confirmatory evidence. Likewise, there are humoral factors apparently generated during the fed state that can suppress food intake when infused into hungry animals.[18, 19] Theologides[20] proposed that tumors might produce anorexia or cachexia because of peptides or other substances that could modulate the activity of various enzymes (activating or inactivating them in host tissues). Alterations in metabolic patterns of the host could disrupt homeostatic mechanisms. If host metabolism were chaotic, nutritional substances normally used for body growth would be used principally to support growth of the tumor. A recently identified cytokine known as *tumor necrosis factor,* or *cachectin,* is produced by macrophages and has been associated with cachexia in experimental animals.[21] Whether it will be helpful in explaining such clinical syndromes in humans remains to be determined.

A number of metabolic abnormalities have been described in patients with neoplastic disorders. For example, it is well known that patients with malignancy have a high rate of anaerobic glycolysis.[22, 23] If anaerobic glycolysis were used as a principal means of energy production by tumors, oxidative phosphorylation and formation of adenosine triphosphate (ATP) would be much less than that associated with aerobic glycolysis. Anaerobic glycolysis is also a relatively inefficient pathway of energy production, since it produces large quantities of lactic acid. Although some lactic acid can be metabolized to water and carbon dioxide, most of it is regenerated to glucose via the Cori cycle (lactate is not excreted or oxidized in the Krebs cycle). Furthermore, there is an increased mobilization of protein to amino acids from steroids and other factors contributing to gluconeogenesis. Energy required for the regeneration of glucose from lactate leads to increasing demands on host energy resources. The tumor thus utilizes glucose for its own needs at the expense of loss of energy from the host, a theoretically efficient way of producing a thermodynamically cachexic state. One approach, therefore, is to provide more efficient energy utilization by using inhibitors of gluconeogenesis (such as inhibiting conversion of oxaloacetate to phosphoenolpyruvate or pyruvate to oxaloacetate).

Many of the adaptive mechanisms which are normally observed in an individual during starvation or semistarvation seemed impaired in the patient with uncontrolled malignant growth.[24] There is failure to reduce caloric expenditure, a continued utilization of amino acids and lactate for gluconeogenesis, and an inability to oxidize exogenous glucose normally. Nevertheless, the malignant tumor, which usually makes up less than 5 per cent of the total body mass, manages to maintain its rate of growth. There are many questions that remain to be answered about the cachexia of malignancy. A number of host and tumor factors are involved, but there is a possibility that specific proteins (such as cachectin) will be identified that lead to alterations in host metabolism.[21] This is a promising and important area for further investigation.

Abnormal Immunological Function and Connective-Tissue Disorders

Malignant disorders are associated with a wide variety of immunological syndromes (involving both excessive and impaired immune response) as well as connective-tissue disorders. These vary from disorders associated with a clone of immunoglobulin-producing cells (some of which may have antibody characteristics) to connective-tissue disorders such as dermatomyositis and neurological syndromes (see below) believed to be related to tumor antigens. It is beyond the scope of this chapter to discuss tumor immunology and current theories related to the development of tumors through blocking antibodies. On the other hand, it is pertinent to describe briefly a few of the immunological syndromes that may be associated with malignant disorders. Specific production of tumor proteins such as carcinoembryonic antigen and alpha-fetoprotein will be discussed later.

Some malignant disorders are associated with failure of cell-mediated and/or humoral immunity as well as macrophage dysfunction. These observations may be complicated by the use of radiotherapy and immunosuppressive and cytotoxic agents in the treatment of cancer and the presence of immunosuppressive viruses. As early as the first part of the century, Reed[25] noted cutaneous anergy (negative tuberculin reactions) in patients with advanced Hodgkin's disease. More recently, it has been appreciated that there is a generalized deficiency of cell-mediated immunity in Hodgkin's disease.[26] The lymphocytes of these patients respond poorly to in vitro stimulation by phytohemagglutinin,[27] and skin allografts are tolerated much better than in normal subjects.[28] Humoral immune responses also may be impaired in Hodgkin's disease, with hypogammaglobulinemia being a feature of advanced Hodgkin's disease.[29] In general, the degree of immunological impairment tends to correlate with the extent and histology of the disease.[30] Although some patients who have positive responses to skin tests and other tests of cellular immune function tend to have a better prognosis, this is a controversial area. Recent studies evaluating immune function in patients with lymphoid malignancies indicate many immunological disturbances similar to those noted earlier in Hodgkin's disease.[30] Such observations have led to the use of bacille Calmette-Guérin (BCG) and other agents to stimulate immune responses.

Of interest is the observation that patients with malignancy may have a factor in plasma that suppresses immunological activity. Glasgow et al.[31] examined 53 patients with malignant disease for hypersensitivity to skin antigen and 2,3-dinitrochlorobenzene. Of 41 patients with negative skin tests, 66 per cent had immunosuppressive factors in serum. Most of the activity was found in a peak of protein on gel filtration with a molecular weight less than 10,000. Other chemical studies suggested that the factor was peptide and that it suppressed human lymphocytes in vitro and the plaque-forming response to sheep erythrocytes. It primarily suppressed cellular immune mechanisms and was not antigen-specific.[31] This factor had no resemblance to blocking factors found in the serum of patients with malignancies by Sjögren and others.[32] It would be intriguing if the tumor were responsible for the production of this abnormal protein.

At the other extreme are hyperimmune phenomena which have been associated with malignancy. A number of connective tissue disorders, e.g., polymyositis, dermatomyositis, scleroderma, and hypertrophic osteoarthropathy, have been noted.[33] The pathogenesis of polymyositis and dermatomyositis is of considerable interest in relation to current theories of immune function. This disorder of skin and muscle that occurs in individuals with tumors appears to be similar to that in patients without tumors, but there is a higher incidence of malignancy in older individuals (over age 50) who have dermatomyositis. This occurs most frequently in patients with carcinoma of the breast, ovary, and lung, as well as lymphoma. On the other hand, children and young adults seem to have no increased association. There are a number of reports suggesting a regression of the connective disorder after resection of the tumor. This is particularly exciting in view of the considerable evidence that dermatomyositis is an autoimmune disorder.[34-38]

Polymyositis has been produced in guinea pigs by immunization with homogenized rabbit skeletal muscle in Freund's adjuvant,[34, 35] and it is believed that the animal model has some resemblance to human disease. Studies of human dermatomyositis show evidence of cytotoxic lymphocytes in vitro, specific transformation of lymphocytes in response to muscle antigens, cytotoxicity of lymphocytes for muscle cells in tissue culture, and specific release of lymphotoxin from lymphocytes on exposure to muscle antigen.[36-38] Relatively few studies of patients with both dermatomyositis and malignancy have been performed, but the immunological findings in those few cases seem similar. The obvious question is whether there is a cross-reacting antigen between muscle and the tumor so that the development of antibodies to a tumor antigen precipitates muscle destruction through the production of cytotoxic lymphocytes. An alternate theory is that tumor enzyme or other secretory products could modify muscle, perhaps during invasion, and stimulate production of antibodies against muscle.[36-38] There are patients with tumors who do not present the clinical manifestations of dermatomyositis or polymyositis but who have muscle antibodies in their serum or whose lymphocytes can be demonstrated to be cytotoxic for muscle tissues.

If a parallel is to be drawn between such immune phenomena and the humoral syndromes associated with cancer, it is that biochemical and immunological evidence will be present in many patients who do not necessarily manifest clinical syndromes. It is in these areas that the usefulness of humoral immune markers for malignancy might lead to earlier diagnosis. Other antibodies against tissues have been described in a wide variety of patients with malignant disease, particularly with the technique of immunofluorescence.[32] Antibodies to smooth muscle using an immunofluorescence technique were detected in nearly 70 per cent of patients with cancer. Such antibodies are not specific, however, since they also have been found in patients with liver disease and other disorders.[33]

Neurological Disorders

A large number of neurological and neuromuscular disorders have been described in association with malignancy.

These syndromes have been appreciated since the early part of the century and were popularized by the British neurologist Brain.[39] Patients with malignant disease often have neurological findings that cannot be attributed directly to metastatic lesions in the central or peripheral nervous system. These syndromes include peripheral neuropathy (both sensory and motor), radiculopathy, degeneration of the dorsal roots, myelopathic disorders, cerebellar degeneration, and a myasthenia gravis–like syndrome. It is important to recognize these disorders because they often cause disability far in excess of the neoplastic disease itself.[40] The abnormalities also may precede the more direct effects of the malignancy so that syndrome recognition can lead to early diagnosis of the malignancy. If they are recognized as complications of the neoplasm, unnecessary neurosurgery or other therapeutic maneuvers also can be avoided. Although the reports in the literature consider principally the peripheral neuropathy and myelopathy, central nervous system complications can be significant. In an extensive study of 250 males with bronchogenic carcinoma and 250 females with breast cancer, 16 per cent of the men and 4.4 per cent of the women had neurological or muscular signs.[41] Of these patients, only 7 had involvement of the central nervous system, while the rest had peripheral nerve and muscular dysfunction. The same authors subsequently expanded their series to over 1400 patients with various types of malignancy.[42] Of this group, 162 had some form of neuromyopathy, and 41 had manifestations in the central nervous system (11 motor neuron, 157 myelopathic, 15 cerebellar). One must be cautious, however, in ascribing these abnormalities to the malignancy, since other causes of neuropathy can occur in these patients. The types of disorders encountered clinically are described below.

Cerebral Disorders

Dementia is one of the most common manifestations and was noted by Brain[43] in 14 of 43 patients with neurological complications and by Posner[44] in a significant number of patients. The abnormalities involve a spectrum from confusion to severe organic brain syndrome with loss of memory and cerebral function; they may develop acutely or over a long period of time. Pathological abnormalities may or may not be found at postmortem examination, but these sometimes include degenerative changes in the hippocampus and amygdala.[45, 46]

Brain Stem Abnormalities

A variety of brain stem abnormalities including ophthalmoplegia, bulbar palsy, opsoclonus-myoclonus ("dancing eyes–dancing feet" syndrome), ataxia, vertigo, dysarthria, and nystagmus may be observed. Optic neuritis and photoreceptor degeneration are also occasionally found in association with extensive demyelination.[46]

Cerebellar Disorders

Degeneration of the cerebellum is said to be one of the more frequent central nervous system complications of malignancy.[46] The signs are usually bilateral and symmetrical and involve ataxia of the extremities, tremors of intention, and dysarthria, which may be severe; it is unusual to find vertigo or nystagmus. The course is usually severe, and the patient may become completely disabled. Pathologically, there may be degeneration of the Purkinje fibers with perivascular and leptomeningeal inflammation and accompanying degeneration of brain stem nuclei. Cord signs may be associated. An autoimmune basis has been strongly suggested by recent studies (see below).

Myelopathic Disorders

These may involve large tract and/or motor neuron degeneration, sometimes resembling amyotrophic lateral sclerosis and subacute necrosis. Norris[47] noted some form of malignancy in approximately 10 per cent of 130 patients with amyotrophic lateral sclerosis. Subacute necrosis of the cord occurs as a rapidly ascending motor and sensory paralysis to the thoracic cord level. At autopsy, there may be degeneration of both white and gray matter.[48]

Neuromuscular and Muscular Disorders

Myasthenia gravis–like syndromes have been reported in patients with carcinoma and are frequently given the eponym *Eaton-Lambert syndrome*.[49] The myasthenia may be mild or have a typical onset like myasthenia gravis. However, many of the patients have symptoms in the extremities before bulbar muscles are affected, making it somewhat different from classical myasthenia. Likewise, the responses to medication are much more variable than in the classical disease, and there is a marked sensitivity to curare-like medication. Weakness is often most marked in the pelvic and thigh muscles, although some of the patients have difficulty swallowing. In the cases described by Eaton and Lambert, there was strong male predominance. Definitive findings were noted by these authors on electromyographic testing (increase in amplitude on repetitive stimulation).

The defect seems to be due to decreased release of acetylcholine from motor neurons and is probably on an autoimmune basis.[50] Injection of mice with serum from patients reproduces the syndrome, including abnormalities in the release of presynaptic hormone from the myoneural junction. Most of the reported cases of the syndrome have been associated with pathology in the chest, particularly bronchogenic carcinoma of the small cell or oat cell type, although the association of myasthenia and thymoma is well known. The prognosis of the small cell carcinoma may be somewhat better than in patients without myasthenia. Myasthenia also has been associated with lymphosarcoma and lymphoma, as well as carcinoma of the pancreas, breast, prostate, ovary, thyroid, palate, cervix, kidney, and rectum.[40, 49] Although there is an overlap between classical myasthenia gravis and the Eaton-Lambert syndrome, the syndrome can be distinguished by the electromyographic features and by the fact that classical myasthenia usually presents with bulbar symptoms and is not usually associated with the depression of reflexes common in patients with carcinoma.[40] Guanidine hydrochloride, which increases acetylcholine release, may provide moderate improvement, and some benefit has been observed with immunosuppression and plasmapheresis.[51] Tumor removal also may be associated with improvement.

Peripheral Neuropathy

Peripheral neuropathy is probably the most frequent of the neurological syndromes associated with malignancy.[52] Peripheral neuropathy and polyneuropathy have been described in association with Hodgkin's disease (Guillain-Barré–like), Waldenström's macroglobulinemia, and osteosclerotic forms of multiple myeloma. The neuropathic disorders are sometimes associated with myelopathy and signs in the central nervous system. Many of the myopathic disorders are associated with considerable involvement of the peripheral nerves as well, and the patient may have an abnormal electromyogram, even if it is not expected clinically. Neuropathy may take the form of either a mild symmetrical sensory disease that occurs late in the course of a malignant disorder or an acute and severe sensory and motor myopathy that may occur early in the disease and progress to severe paralysis. The latter type may be noted before the presence of the neoplasm is even recognized, and it occasionally remits.[40, 52] Protein concentration in the cerebrospinal fluid may be elevated, suggesting pathology at the root (neuronopathy), and there is occasional pleocytosis. The peripheral nerves may show loss of both myelin and axon, although the myelin loss usually predominates, and degeneration of the dorsal root ganglia has been detected. Removal of the tumor usually causes no improvement in the peripheral neuropathy, and it is refractory to vitamins. It most commonly occurs in association with oat cell carcinoma of the lung and tumors of the breast, stomach, and thymus. An autoimmune etiology has been suggested.

Theories about the etiology of the neurogenic syndromes are multiple, and the actual relationship between underlying neoplasm and neurological disturbance is unclear. Theories include infectious, metabolic, toxic, and autoimmune etiologies as well as nutritional deficiencies.[40, 46] The multifocal leukoencephalopathy frequently associated with Hodgkin's disease and other tumors has been ascribed to a papovavirus (on the basis of electron microscopic and tissue culture evidence).[53] Likewise, in some of the dementias, there may be evidence for viral encephalitis. In disorders associated with metabolic derangements such as hypercalcemia or hypokalemia, a pathogenic basis for some of the neurological or muscular abnormalities is present. There is evidence for toxin production by some tumors, as well as evidence for autoimmune mechanisms.

A significant contribution to the pathogenesis of three neurological syndromes (visual, cerebellar, and sensory neuronopathy) associated with small cell carcinoma of the lung by autoimmune mechanisms has been well documented.[54] Immunoglobulins produced in response to tumor antigens cross-react with retinal, Purkinje, and peripheral neural proteins, causing clinical neurological abnormalities. At the same time, antibodies against tumor antigens may slow the growth of the neoplasm. Nutritional deprivation and cachexia also could be used to explain some of the neurological abnormalities, particularly if one postulates that metabolic disorders might affect the nervous system as well. These syndromes represent an interesting group of disorders that are frequently associated with malignancy. Our knowledge of pathogenesis is incomplete, but the importance of these syndromes in terms of patient morbidity and disability is considerable.

Vascular Disorders

A number of vascular disorders may be associated with malignancy, including migratory thrombophlebitis, hemorrhage and marantic (or nonbacterial) endocarditis.[55] Slichter and Harker[56] studied 77 patients with malignancy, some of whom were receiving antithrombotic therapy, including anticoagulants and/or platelet-function inhibitors. In general, they noted decreased survival of ^{51}Cr-labeled platelets and [^{125}I]fibrinogen. The hemostatic abnormalities were, in general, related to the extent of the malignant process and tended to regress with therapy. Requirement for transfusion was most often present when platelets were decreased. Possible causes for the low platelet count included decreased production, increased destruction, or a combination of factors. They tried to isolate these factors from chemotherapy and concluded that a failure of platelet production was the principal cause of thrombocytopenia in malignancy.

The same authors studied a number of patients having venous thromboembolism associated with solid tumors or Hodgkin's disease. These individuals had increased platelet and fibrinogen consumption up to four times normal.[56] The authors speculated that the circulating platelets were removed directly by reacting with tumor tissue surfaces (presumably because of inadequate or abnormal endothelialization of the blood-tumor interface) and that fibrinogen might be consumed as a result of platelet or surface initiation of fibrin formation. Fibrinogen levels, but not platelet survival, were improved with heparin therapy. Several patients treated with dipyridamole and/or aspirin showed improvement in platelet and fibrinogen survival. Although these inhibitors prevent tumor-induced consumption of platelet and fibrinogen, they probably would not provide helpful therapy for bleeding problems because they cause platelet dysfunction. Furthermore, platelet consumption is a less important cause of thrombocytopenia than impaired production or increased pooling. The patients with cancer-associated venous thromboembolism may be benefited by heparin or warfarin therapy but not by inhibitors of platelet function.

There is interesting evidence that mucin-producing tumors may be associated with increased intravascular coagulation.[55, 57] Entrance of mucus derived from the adenocarcinoma into the circulation is believed to act as a stimulus to coagulation, and there is a higher incidence of postoperative deep vein thrombosis in these patients. Crude tumor extracts contain partially purified mucin activated factor X and coagulation factors, while thromboplastic activity could be inactivated by the removal of sialic acid with neuraminidase.[57, 58] The actual incidence of deep vein thrombosis in association with carcinoma is not known. In general, the chances of finding a malignancy in a patient with clinical deep vein thrombosis are small, but some of the newer techniques used to diagnose deep vein thrombosis (such as radioactive fibrinogen scanning) turn up a much higher incidence of thrombosis than had been suspected previously. This is particularly true in patients with malignant disease who undergo surgery.

In patients with widespread neoplastic disease, microangiopathic hemolytic anemia may result from diffuse fibrin deposition. These patients may have several clotting defects, and this has been noted particularly in patients with promyelocytic leukemia and adenocarcinoma of the prostate.[58] The most likely cause of intravascular coagulation is contact of circulating blood with thromboplastic substances produced by the neoplastic cells. In some cases, heparin therapy may reverse some of the hemostatic problems.

The etiology of marantic endocarditis is a complete enigma, and there is little information available on its pathogenesis. Theoretically, tumors may produce substances that cause thrombosis or other changes on the endocardium or on heart valves.

Dermatological Disorders

There is a well-known association between neoplastic disorders and dermatological lesions. A number of abnormalities are related to genetic endocrine disorders (such as the mucosal neuromas of the lid in multiple endocrine neoplasia) (see Ch. 151), but others seem to be associated with malignant disease. In addition to disorders such as lymphoma, leukemias, and specific carcinomas where malignant cells are actually present in the skin, a number of paraneoplastic dermatological disorders exist. The association with dermatomyositis has already been described and may involve bluish-red discoloration around the face, neck, chest, and extremities, as well as heliotrope discoloration of the eyes.

Of considerable interest is the entity acanthosis nigricans, a velvety, verrucous, and hyperpigmented lesion that occurs frequently in body folds such as the axilla. It also may be associated with increased keratin production of the palms and soles. There is a significant association of acanthosis with visceral malignancy, usually adenocarcinoma. The two manifestations usually occur simultaneously, although the dermatological lesion may precede the cancer by a considerable period of time.[59] An unusual syndrome of marked resistance to insulin has been described in patients with acanthosis by Kahn et al.[60] (see Ch. 91). This group of patients does not have an associated malignancy, nor do those with acanthosis and other metabolic disorders such as lipoatrophic diabetes.

Additional dermatological abnormalities associated with malignant tumors include erythema gyratum repens (an unusual zebra-like abnormality noted most prominently on the back) and ichthyosis, which may be present in patients with lymphoma, usually Hodgkin's disease or carcinoma.[61] A number of bullous abnormalities also have been associated with tumors. These include dermatitis herpetiformis and bullous pemphigoid, a disorder in which antibodies to basal lamina in the skin can be demonstrated.[61] An association between glucagon-producing tumors and a necrolytic bullous skin disease also has been noted,[62] but the pathogenesis is unclear. A number of patients with lymphoma and other malignancies have herpes zoster, and the disseminated form has been noted in some patients on immunosuppressive therapy.[61] Hypertrichosis associated with lanugo-type hair has been described in adults with malignancy.

The dermatological manifestations associated with the carcinoid syndrome have been described elsewhere in this book (Ch. 150) and will not be reviewed here. Hyperpigmentation in ACTH-producing tumors, dermal melanosis associated with malignant melanoma, nodular fat necrosis associated with pancreatic tumors, Raynaud's syndrome related to myeloma, and porphyria cutanea tarda in patients with hepatocellular carcinoma have all been well documented. In addition, external manifestations in Gardner's syndrome and Peutz-Jegher's syndrome have been noted.

Evidence[59] supporting the association of dermatological lesions with visceral malignancy is as follows:

1. Specific action of a tumor product that causes the dermatological lesion (e.g., flushing associated with carcinoid)
2. A genetic relationship between the dermatological abnormality and the malignancy (Gardner's syndrome or Peutz-Jegher's syndrome)
3. Dermatological abnormalities caused by autoimmune disorders (dermatomyositis or bullous pemphigoid)
4. Simultaneous onset of the dermatological abnormality and the malignancy
5. Remission of the dermatological abnormality after removal or cure of the tumor.

In many cases the nature of the relationship is at present unknown (e.g., acanthosis nigricans)

Renal Disorders

There is an interesting association between malignancy and immune disease of the kidney. Bilateral renal vein thrombosis and amyloidosis can be complications of malignancy or myeloma-like syndromes. Lee et al.[63] reported an 11 per cent incidence of carcinoma in 101 patients presenting with the nephrotic syndrome. Eight of the patients showed evidence of membranous glomerulonephritis, one patient had lobular glomerulonephritis, and another had only minimal abnormalities. These included tumors of the bronchus, cervix, ovaries, kidneys, and oropharynx; breast, colon, and gastrointestinal tumors also have been reported. In addition, patients with lymphoma and leukemia have been reported to have nephrotic syndrome in association with these diseases without evidence of invasion of the renal parenchyma.[63–65] Not infrequently, treatment of lymphoma or Hodgkin's disease with immunosuppressive drugs or radiation results in remission of lymphoma as well as the nephrotic syndrome. Electron microscopy of renal biopsies in such patients usually shows minimal change disease. In carcinoma, on the other hand, there is strong evidence that the nephrotic syndrome frequently results from the deposition of antigen-antibody complexes on the basal lamina. It was postulated and then proven that renal biopsies from patients with carcinoma and the nephrotic syndrome would have deposition of IgG and IgM on the basal lamina by immunofluorescence.[65] An identical antigen was then obtained from a lung tumor extract and from elution of the involved glomerulus. This association proved a direct relationship between the synthesis of tumor antigens and associated circulating immune complexes which deposit in the kidney.

A wide variety of other renal problems may be seen in association with malignant tumors. These include problems related to mechanical compression or obstruction of the genitourinary tract, infection associated with obstruction, renal failure associated with hypercalcemia, hypoka-lemia, and hyperuricemia, renal tubular acidosis, and nephrogenic diabetes insipidus noted in hyperglobulinemic states.

Summary

The various tumor-related syndromes described in this section represent systemic and organ-specific manifestations associated with malignancy. In most instances, a definite association between production of a protein by the tumor and these manifestations has not yet been proven. Suggestive evidence has been provided in the case of pyrogen (IL-1) production, anorexigenic peptides (tumor necrosis factor), tumor antigens that produce autoimmune or immune-complex disease, and thromboplastic substances that lead to accelerated coagulation. Precise characterization of such tumor proteins is still in progress. In the ectopic hormone syndromes, on the other hand, more readily definable peptide hormones have been associated with tumors and have caused clinical syndromes or biochemical abnormalities that duplicate in many instances the abnormalities produced by endocrine hyperplasia or an endocrine tumor. In the section that follows, major emphasis will be placed on the endocrine and metabolic syndromes associated with ectopic hormone production. Prior to a detailed description of these syndromes, their importance as well as some of the theories concerning their pathogenesis will be reviewed.

GENERAL ASPECTS OF THE ECTOPIC HORMONE SYNDROMES

Significance and Incidence

The ectopic hormone syndromes are of considerable interest not only to the clinician and pathologist but also to the developmental biologist and molecular biologist.[1, 2] For the clinician, they represent a fascinating spectrum of endocrine and biochemical disorders associated with malignant disease. It is important to emphasize that they have been identified with increasing frequency as clinical problems; they are not medical curiosities! As the number of patients with malignant disease occupying hospital beds increases, greater recognition is being given to the elaboration by tumors of hormones, growth factors, cytokines, antigens, and other proteins. The concept of tumor markers and earlier potential diagnosis of malignant disease is important for current and future research in clinical medicine. These tumors are of considerable interest to the pathologist because of the association of the specific histologic types with discrete clinical syndromes and because of the identification of secretory granules in many of the tumors.[66] To the developmental biologist and molecular biologist, such tumors are extremely important because they may hold the key to a better understanding of normal embryological and ontogenetic development.

Of considerable interest to the clinician is the idea that elaboration of a humoral or protein substance may provide a clue to the presence of a neoplasm while it is still resectable and before metastases appear. Occasionally, this can be a frustrating search, as evidenced by the study of Rudnick and Odell[67] of a male patient with an elevated concentration of chorionic gonadotropin and no obvious testicular neoplasm. There was no evidence for a tumor in this patient until metastases suddenly appeared. At postmortem examination, a microscopic neoplasm was found in the testis which was producing the gonadotropic substance. Because there is increasing recognition of a variety of substances produced by tumors, one might theoretically predict a time when individuals above a certain age may be screened for a variety of hormonal and antigenic substances in pursuit of asymptomatic neoplasms. Moreover, evidence derived from experimental models and clinical sources indicates that dysplastic nonneoplastic cells may develop structural and functional alterations in their secretory apparatus, suggesting the possibility of diagnosing and monitoring preneoplastic changes through laboratory determinations of secretory products.[68, 69] Although such early diagnosis has been expected for years, it has unfortunately not become a reality. There are many problems with the sensitivity and specificity of hormones as "tumor markers" (see below), and many are more useful for tumor management than for early diagnosis.

At times, the metabolic and hormonal effects of the tumor hormone may be more devastating to the patient than the neoplasm itself. This may be particularly true for the marked hypokalemia and weakness associated with an ACTH-producing tumor, life-threatening hyponatremia in the inappropriate ADH syndrome, and symptomatic hypercalcemia of tumors associated with ectopic production of parathyroid hormone–related protein. Persistence or regression of the metabolic manifestations following surgery, radiotherapy, or chemotherapy is of considerable importance to the clinician.

In patients who present with tumors and associated endocrine manifestations, it is extremely important to determine whether the tumor itself is responsible or whether there is a concomitant endocrine disorder. Common endocrine or metabolic disorders may coexist with neoplastic disease and present a somewhat confusing picture (e.g., hyponatremia, hypercalcemia).

The incidence of ectopic hormone production depends on one's definition of the term (refer to earlier comments about ectopic versus eutopic production). It is probably true that hormone production by tumors is extremely widespread. Odell and others have argued on the basis of radioimmunoassay that the widespread appearance of peptides such as ACTH and related peptides, calcitonin, vasopressin, and chorionic gonadotropin suggests that ectopic hormone production may be more the rule than the exception.[2–4, 70, 71] On the other hand, actual clinical symptomatology, as opposed to biochemical or radioimmunoassay abnormalities, is much less common. The clinical findings are often subtle, but in some instances the metabolic abnormality may be a serious clinical problem for patient and physician.

There are a variety of factors that may obscure the frequency with which ectopic hormone production occurs.[1, 72] Such factors include lack of adequate clinical suspicion as well as follow-up of cancer patients, clinician or investigator bias, laboratory techniques available to establish the diagnosis, the short course of the illness, obscure clinical presentations, unidentified hormones, and release of precursors, subunits, or metabolic fragments with little or no biological activity.

Documentation and Criteria for Diagnosis

A number of indirect as well as direct methods have been utilized to document the presence of the ectopic hormone syndrome. In many cases, the observations are empirical and based on clinical phenomena, but recently, more direct immunological, biochemical, and even molecular data have been available to provide accurate documentation. Under each of the hormonal syndromes to be detailed, specific evidence for the methods of documentation will be provided, but basic principles covering all ectopic hormone syndromes are reviewed below. Documentation for the existence of an ectopic hormone syndrome[1] is generally provided by one or more of the following pieces of evidence:

1. Recognition of a known clinical endocrine syndrome in the presence of a malignant neoplasm. One must be careful to exclude a coexisting endocrine gland disorder such as primary hyperparathyroidism in a patient with hypercalcemia and malignancy.
2. Biochemical manifestations suggesting production of a hormone in the presence of a neoplasm (e.g., a high serum calcium or low serum sodium level in a patient with a lung tumor).
3. Disappearance or remission of the endocrine or metabolic abnormalities after surgery, radiotherapy, or chemotherapy.
4. Reappearance of the endocrine or biochemical abnormalities associated with recurrence of the tumor.
5. Measurement of increased levels of circulating hormones in the blood or urine of a patient with a malignancy.
6. Extraction of hormone from tumor tissue.
   a. Measurement of hormonal activity by bioassay.
   b. Measurement of hormonal activity by immunological, radioimmunoassay, or radioreceptor methods.
   c. Biochemical and physiological characterization of tumor peptides.
7. Evidence for synthesis of hormone by the tumor in vitro (e.g., continuous release of hormone in tissue culture or the incorporation of radioactive amino acids into labeled hormone).
8. Cell-free synthesis of ectopic hormone (using mRNA) or hybridization of labeled complementary DNA to mRNA in tumor extract or in situ hybridization studies of tumor sections.
9. Cloning and DNA sequencing of hormonal mRNA from a tumor.
10. An arteriovenous difference in hormone concentration across the tumor bed, with a higher concentration in the venous circulation.
11. Reproduction of the clinical or biochemical syndrome in the nude athymic mouse with a transplanted tumor.

Pathogenesis

Although considerable progress in recognizing the widespread synthesis of hormones by nonendocrine tumors has been made, the etiology of ectopic hormone production remains obscure.[1, 2] When the process is understood completely, we also will understand more fully the processes of normal cell proliferation, differentiation, maturation, and oncogenesis. Any single hypothesis that would adequately explain the process must take into account the following points:

1. The presence of polypeptide and protein hormones is extremely widespread in normal tissues as well as in malignancies.

2. Nonendocrine tumors synthesize protein hormones and not steroids, thyroid hormone derivatives, or catecholamines.

3. Tumors may release precursors of hormones, subunits of hormones, abnormally processed hormones, or metabolic fragments of hormones, but they generally do not release new proteins that have not been identified in normal physiology. (Sometimes, identification of the tumor product precedes its identification in normal tissues.)

4. There are distinct associations between histological tumor type and the specific hormone produced (see Table 149–1).

5. Ectopic hormone production is often unresponsive to negative- or positive-feedback control.

6. Multiple protein hormones may be produced by single tumors.

7. Ectopic synthesis of hormones by tumors is rarely caused by the expression or activation of abnormal genes but of known genes for recognized protein hormones and/or their precursors.

If the pathogenesis were well understood, there would not be as many hypotheses. Following is a description of the current pathogenetic mechanisms that have been suggested.

The APUD Concept and Its Implications and Limitations

Specific relationships of hormone production and neuroectodermal tissue have been suggested by a number of authors. The notion of a complex endocrine system comprising isolated cells scattered throughout the gastrointestinal tract and related viscera is not new. Feyrter[73] originally presumed them to be of endodermal derivation, but solid evidence pointing to the existence of a neuroectodermally derived endocrine system has accumulated.

The basic features shared by these cells are cytochemical and ultrastructural. Properties include high levels of amine precursors such as dihydroxyphenylalanine (DOPA) or 5-hydroxytryptophan (5-HT) and enzymes such as α-glycerophosphate dehydrogenase, esterase, and cholesterase.[74, 75] Additional properties were subsequently described, and the acronym *APUD* (*a*mine *p*recursor *u*ptake and *d*ecarboxylation) was introduced by Pearse and colleagues.[76, 77] The essential feature of these cells is their capability to take up substances such as DOPA and 5-HT, decarboxylate them, and subsequently produce biogenic amines that can be demonstrated in tissue sections by formalin-induced fluorescence.

On electron microscopy, APUD cells display a prominent rough endoplasmic reticulum and Golgi complex and are generally rich in free ribosomes. However, their most characteristic feature is the consistent presence of round secretory granules that display an inner core of variable electron density, a pale surrounding halo, and a single encompassing membrane (Figs. 149–2 and 149–3). The diameter of the granules varies considerably but falls mostly within the 100 to 250 nm range and is often fairly uniform within a given cell type. The electron density and configuration of the core also vary greatly, but they may be quite characteristic, as exemplified by the paracrystalline profiles seen in nonneoplastic pancreatic β cells and in some of the tumors as well (see Figs. 149–2 and 149–3).

The experimental methods used to show the migration of APUD cells from their origin in neural crest through the mesoderm to their final destination in the primitive intestine include the following:

1. Neural crest cell identification using tritiated thymidine incorporation

2. Grafting of neural crest elements between two related but morphologically distinct avian species

3. Formalin-induced fluorescence of biogenic amine–producing neural crest cells

These methods have been applied and embryos sacrificed

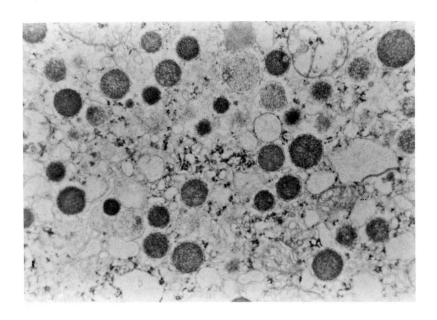

FIGURE 149–2. Electron micrograph showing secretory granules in islet cell adenoma of the pancreas. Paracrystalline profiles are shown in some granules (× 72,500).

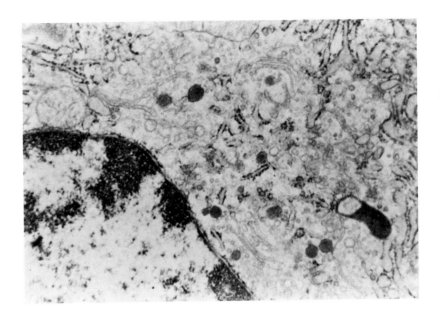

FIGURE 149–3. Electron micrograph of pulmonary oat cell carcinoma in patient with Cushing's syndrome, demonstrating secretory granules (× 22,500).

at sequential developmental phases, leading to the demonstration of neural crest derivation and APUD characteristics of numerous cells populating the gastrointestinal tract and related tissues.[78–80] The APUD system includes all peptide-producing cells of the stomach, duodenum, intestine, pancreatic islets, adrenal medulla, extra-adrenal paraganglia cells, adenohypophysis, parafollicular thyroid cells, and melanoblasts.[81] Additional cells with APUD characteristics have been found in the respiratory tree and in the gastrointestinal and urogenital tracts, although their secretory products and function remain unclear.[79, 81, 82] The parathyroid chief cells pose an important hurdle; although they produce a peptide hormone and display secretory granules, their cytochemical characteristics differ from those of the APUD-type cells.[81, 83] However, other investigators have strongly advocated the inclusion of the parathyroids within the APUD system,[84] and they have been shown to secrete a chromogranin A–like protein (parathyroid secretory protein or secretory protein I) which is generally found in neuroendocrine cells.[85]

The introduction of the APUD concept has resulted in considerable controversy, since its acceptance would imply revision of long-held notions of embryology, pathology, and so on. A taxonomic proliferation has already occurred, and generic terms to designate APUD-cell–derived neoplasms such as *APUDoma*,[85, 86] *neurolophoma*,[81] and *neuroendocrinoma*[87, 88] have been introduced. Neoplasms that might be included under such umbrella terms include islet-cell tumors, carcinoid, pheochromocytoma, ganglioneuroma, neuroblastoma, paraganglioma, medullary carcinoma of the thyroid, bronchial neuroendocrinoma (carcinoid), oat cell carcinoma of the lung, and some thymomas. Certain poorly understood, "undifferentiated" neoplasms of such areas as the gastrointestinal tract and mediastinum, which display typical neurosecretory granules under the electron microscope, also may be shown to contain considerable quantities of vanillylmandelic acid (VMA) and 5-hydroxyindoleacetic acid (5-HIAA). Clinically active and inactive tumors may display granules indistinguishable from each other and from those of normal endocrine cells.

Only some of the aforementioned neoplasms are associated with clinically obvious hormonal syndromes. This might be explained quantitatively or on the basis of aberrations in the secretory apparatus of the neoplastic cells. Some of these tumors may be able to complete the hormonal synthetic process to the prohormone level (e.g., proinsulin, proopiomelanocortin) but may lack the crucial enzyme-converting systems necessary to yield fully active biological hormones.[1, 66] However, even the presence of mature granules (and presumably active hormone) within tumor cells does not guarantee a clinically recognizable hormonal syndrome.

Both benign and malignant tumors can display chromosomal abnormalities that could result in alterations in appropriate gene expression. Therefore, structural and functional abnormal secretory activity on the part of tumors is hardly surprising. If one considers that most, if not all, above-mentioned tumors may actually derive from neuroectodermal cell lines, many of their puzzling features become clarified:

1. The cytochemical commonality of the APUD cells could explain the secretion of more than one hormone by a single tumor. Multiple secretory activity may be synchronous or asynchronous and may or may not be reflected in clinically detectable hormonal syndromes.[89]

2. The widespread distribution of APUD cells could indicate that a number of hormone-secreting tumors derived from them and generally believed to be "ectopic" (e.g., ACTH-producing oat cell carcinoma) may be so in terms of differentiated cell function but not so from the viewpoint of histogenesis.

3. Some neuroendocrine-type neoplasms (pheochromocytomas) may occur in association with important developmental anomalies of the neural crest such as von Recklinghausen's and Hirschsprung's diseases. This association has led to the term *neurocristopathy*.[90]

4. Finally, the APUD concept may be useful in explaining certain aspects of the multiple endocrine neoplasia syndrome.

The APUD system may have developed from primitive neural transmitter cells, these simple elements having migrated from their original location to populate other tissues as environmental requirements changed. While their basic cytochemical makeup and ability to synthesize biogenic amines remained unchanged, some components of the system acquired the capacity to produce more complex peptides.[81] Given this premise, neoplastic transformation of these cells may result in severe structural and functional changes in the secretory apparatus; as a result, neoplastic APUD cells may

1. Remain similar to the cells from which they were derived and synthesize and secrete active hormone(s).

2. Synthesize a hormone or a precursor but fail to release it.

3. Revert to the secretion of simpler amines.

4. Synthesize and release larger peptide hormone precursors not normally secreted by the cells from which they are derived.

5. Develop more than one secretory pattern.

The APUD concept has stimulated interest and research, offering a rational but highly speculative explanation for many obscure features of tumor-associated hormone production. However, many aspects of abnormal endocrine activity related to tumors remain unclear, and it seems unlikely that the APUD concept will explain them. Even if all current APUD-related ideas are accepted, many neoplasms associated with abnormal peptide material cannot be included, and it is likely that some cells may be excluded from the APUD system by further investigations. Moreover, some premises basic to the APUD concept have now been challenged. Experiments involving ablation of the ectoderm in rat embryos failed to prevent the appearance of pancreatic β cells, reopening the question of their embryogenesis; they might acquire neuroendocrine characteristics on their own.[91] Investigations involving heterologous grafts provided negative data regarding origin of some of the intestinal endocrine cells from neuroectoderm.[92] Alternatively, one might speculate that neuroectodermal cells migrated toward and populated the primitive gut far earlier than previously suspected. Possibly, APUD characteristics may not be the exclusive domain of neuroectodermal cells and could be generated by endodermal cells as well. As our knowledge of embryology and physiology increases, rigid notions attributing a specific function to cells of precise embryonal derivation have been shown to be mistaken (e.g., not only mesenchymal cells but also various epithelial cells are capable of collagen synthesis[93]).

Clinical Counterpart of the APUD Hypothesis

Weichert[84] presented arguments to support a common origin of the ectopic hormone syndromes and multiple endocrine neoplasia. Based on similarities in their development, histological and biochemical capabilities, the frequent production of ectopic hormone syndromes, and the development of multiple endocrine neoplasia, he suggested their origin from common neuroectodermal cell precursors. He cited evidence as follows: Common histochemical characteristics can be noted in tumors of all foregut derivatives, and argentaffin cells have been described along the entire alimentary tract. Islets of tissue have been described not only in their classical location in the foregut but also extending into the exocrine system, emphasizing the migration of these cells in the budding and branching of the primordial endodermal cell cords. Cells of the neu-

rogenic system that can give rise to carcinoid tumors are carried into the endodermal primordial pancreas during development and can be traced to the site of the islets. Occasional argentaffin cells are left behind in the ducts and acini and can be transformed into hormone-producing tumor tissue. The parathyroid, thymus, and ultimobranchial body developed similarly but have no remaining connection with the gastrointestinal tract. If hormone-secreting cells are argentaffin in nature, then functioning islet cell tumors could be expected wherever argentaffin cells are found. Islet cell tumors producing a variety of hormones such as insulin, gastrin, glucagon, and secretin have been reported from the lung, stomach, pancreas, duodenum, and biliary tree. Furthermore, carcinoid tumors associated with serotonin production also have been described in the same sites.

Carcinoid tumors may have their origins in the foregut, midgut, or hindgut and may be associated with a variety of syndromes [84] (Ch. 150). Foregut carcinoids (e.g., gastric) tend to produce an atypical carcinoid syndrome in which 5-HT rather than serotonin is produced, while midgut carcinoids frequently produce the typical carcinoid syndrome. Hindgut carcinoids are not generally active. There are many histological similarities among carcinoid, oat cell, and thymic tumors, and carcinoid has frequently been confused with the oat cell carcinoma histologically.

Levine and Metz[94] have taken a somewhat different approach to classifying ectopic hormone-producing tumors. They noted the association of hormone production with specific tumor cell types and focused on selective aspects of derepression rather than a random process. They classified almost all known ectopic hormone-producing tumors into one of two major groups and described the remainder as transitional. Tumors defined in group I have characteristics similar to APUD cells and appear to be biochemically related to cells having embryological origin in the neural crest.[79] All tumors in this group can synthesize and secrete all the other hormones characteristic of group I but not group II, with rare exception. They suggest that group I tumors are derived from neural crest cells which traveled through the primitive endoderm and in which migratory cells became incorporated into the bronchial tree, pancreatic anlagen, and various derivatives of the branchial arches. Although these cells earlier in their development lacked differentiated secretory capacity, they can be identified by histochemical techniques as precursors of secretory cells. The differences in cells of common ancestry might be due to different tissue environments in which they come to rest, origins in different parts of the neural crest, or varying periods of time in the neural crest prior to migration. The tumors in this group include the foregut carcinoid, oat cell carcinoma, pancreatic islet cell tumor, tumors of pancreatic and biliary ducts, thyroid medullary carcinoma, and malignant epithelial thymoma. The hormones produced by tumors of group I include corticotropin and growth hormone–releasing hormones, insulin, calcitonin, ACTH, lipotropin, vasopressin, gastrin, glucagon, secretin, and various biogenic amines and precursors, including serotonin, histamine, and the catecholamines.

The tumors they classified in group II include hepatoma, cholangioma, Wilms' tumor, renal cell carcinoma, adrenal cortical tumor, nongerminal gonadal tumor, vascular tumor, connective tissue and mesodermal tumor, reticuloendothelial tumor, squamous cell lung carcinoma, gastrointestinal tumors (excluding tumors of group I), and melanoma. Hormones of placental origin (particularly those associated with glycoprotein hormones) and fetal antigens such as α-fetoglobulin and placental-type enzymes are exclusively associated with group II tumors. The characteristic secretory granules noted in group I tumors are not generally noted in the group II tumors, but there may be heterogeneous cellular inclusion bodies suggesting secretory activity. The unifying characteristics of the group II tumors, despite their heterogeneity, are the hormones secreted, which include hypercalcemic peptide(s), erythropoietin, gonadotropins, human placental lactogen, prolactin, growth hormone, insulin-like growth factors, renin, and thyrotropin. In the third group were transitional tumors such as the pheochromocytoma, paraganglioma, neuroblastoma, and ganglioneuroma. While these tumors derive from neural crest, they proceed directly from the neural crest to ultimate locations in the adrenal medulla and sympathetic ganglia. These tumors have been characterized as transitional because of the hormones they secrete. They definitely produce some of the group I hormones, but secretion of group II hormones also has been shown. Levine and Metz[94] support their system by indicating the unusual crossovers that occur between the groups of tumors they have defined. A major problem the authors noted was the kind of information available in the literature. In many cases the descriptions of the ectopic syndrome have been based on clinical criteria, with only limited or speculative biochemical information.

Derepression or Dedifferentiation Hypothesis

A traditional mechanism suggested for the etiology of the ectopic hormone syndrome was dedifferentiation of cells in the course of the malignancy to explain the production of peptides by tumors, including hormones.[1] This is a theory that is nearly impossible to prove or disprove, but the nonrandom nature of the process and the association of specific histological types with specific hormones (see Table 149–1) make it unlikely. This theory would suggest that ectopic hormones are identical to normal ones, even if hormone precursors or subunits are produced. It is also consistent with the production of hormones and proteins of the placenta and other fetal tissues such as chorionic gonadotropin, placental lactogen, and α-fetoprotein. It does not explain the high and low incidence of the hormones of various types or why hormone production is not observed in every tumor. All somatic cells contain the same complement of DNA, but if this theory were valid, one might expect a totally random association between tumors and hormone production, and yet this is not true.

Recent advances in understanding of the biosynthesis of polypeptide hormones in normal cells and tumors have provided new perspectives on these issues, particularly the first intracellular product being a prehormone. Some tumors release precursor forms of the hormone rather than the hormone itself, and the difference between normal and malignant tissue may be in the ability of the tumor to process hormone precursors rather than in its ability to synthesize the precursor.

The suggestion that derepression or dedifferentiation of cells might be a plausible mechanism really comes from embryological studies. For example, Ellison et al.[68] showed that an undifferentiated rat renal cell carcinoma in organ co-culture with mouse embryo spinal cord produced differentiated renal tubules. The kind of embryonic induction that allowed transformation from anaplastic to normal tissue was thought to duplicate the differentiation process. Ectopic hormone production could theoretically occur through dedifferentiation of tumor cells and acquisition of previously competent functions, followed by misprogramming and abnormal activation of genes. Tumors arising from different embryological layers would therefore undergo differentiation to a varying degree. One group of tumors, for example, might acquire functions previously endowed in that germ layer, whereas other groups would undergo more extensive dedifferentiation and acquire characteristics of another germ layer (e.g., the acquisition of ectodermal properties by endodermal cells). Despite these embryological experiments, there is little or no credence given currently to the idea that ectopic hormone production occurs through derepression of DNA or dedifferentiation of tumor cells in an orderly reversal of normal cell development.

Dysdifferentiation Hypothesis

A model for the pathogenesis of ectopic production of hormones by tumors has been suggested by Baylin and Mendelsohn[95, 96] on the basis of observations they have made in medullary carcinoma of the thyroid, neuroblastoma, and small cell carcinoma. Their model suggests that a completely normal epithelial layer of cells such as the mucosa of the gastrointestinal tract or bronchial mucosa, which includes a modest number of cells with hormone-secreting characteristics, is derived from a single cell precursor. The development of tumor cells with multipotential capability would be analogous to the hemopoietic system, in which the primitive "stem cell" can differentiate along multiple pathways (e.g., developing into red cell precursors and erythrocytes, granulocytes, platelets, or histiocytes) and sometimes malignancy. Thus differentiation is a forward process from the primitive cell, influenced by local environmental factors, interactions between cells, and possibly autocrine, paracrine, or circulating factors. The primitive tumor cells thus have the capacity to express both fetal antigens or hormones and mature to phenotypic cells that look like epithelial cells or hormone-producing cells, depending on their state of proliferation and maturation. Hormones of the fetoplacental unit, such as human chorionic gonadotropin (hCG), placental lactogen, α-fetoprotein, and carcinoembryonic antigen, would be more likely expressed by cells in their "fetal" state of differentiation and less prominently in cells in their "adult" stage of differentiation. In the mature epithelial layer of the bronchus or intestine, these proteins would be minimally expressed. Certain other hormones or proteins such as L-dopa decarboxylase would be expressed prominently in the adult differentiated state in cells that have the capability to produce hormones and amines. The differentiated cells with fetal characteristics would have the capacity to either produce trophoblastic proteins such as hCG or placental lactogen or yolk sac epithelial proteins such as α-fetoprotein or carcinoembryonic antigen. Thus cells with APUD characteristics could be derived not only from the neural crest but also from epithelial cells that differentiate along these lines. Since production of various fetal proteins or placental hormones by tumors is not a random process, but highly specific and associated, some plausibility to this hypothesis is provided. However, even as Baylin and Mendelsohn[95] suggested, it is still a highly speculative model whose confirmation requires more data. While embryological models suggest that differentiation involves progressive specialization or irreversible suppression of DNA through development, the dysdifferentiation hypothesis supports a forward-moving model in which there are different lines of development for primitive tumor cells, with factors in the local environment affecting their development. Malignancy at any stage of differentiation could come from a clone of transformed tumor cells rather than being a "universal concomitant of neoplasia."[2] Production of tumor antigens and peptide hormones would be the result of progressive cell differentiation, and they would serve as tumor markers.[97]

The dysdifferentiation hypothesis could explain ectopic hormone production in tumors from epithelial cells that consist mostly of cells that do not have hormone-synthesizing capacity, tumors that are heterogeneous in morphology and hormone production, and metastatic lesions that differ in their hormone-synthesizing capacity. The heterogeneous population of cells is supported by immunochemical and immunoperoxidase studies of tumor tissues which show the presence of various tumor markers and hormones in different cells within the same tumor.[98, 99] The development of characteristics of APUD cells is only one of several directions that might be possible for immature and as yet uncommitted epithelial cells. The production of oncoplacental proteins and hormones by tumors is not a random process. Tumors of the gonad are most likely to produce such hormones, particularly when there are trophoblastic elements.[100, 101] Disturbances of endodermal epithelial surfaces such as the bronchus or intestine by either tumors or benign processes such as inflammation could affect the level of differentiation and result in production of specific hormones. Thus the appearance of distinct proteins and antigens implies a specific stage of differentiation, not necessarily dedifferentiation. Germ cell tumors are often heterogeneous, and the antigens or hormones expressed are determined by histological type. α-Fetoprotein and carcinoembryonic antigen would tend to be expressed by cells having the characteristics of the yolk sac, primitive liver, or gastrointestinal tract.

For example, different types of carcinoma of the lung could arise by similar origin. It has been known that epidermoid-type tumors tend to produce hypercalcemic factors, whereas small cell or oat cell tumors produce ACTH and related peptides as well as vasopressin. There may be heterogeneity of cells even in a small cell tumor.[102, 103] Small cell carcinoma is usually an advanced tumor when first diagnosed, and it is characterized by variability and heterogeneity. The content of calcitonin and histaminase is greater than in normal lung, and L-dopa decarboxylase is also usually high, but there may be much variability. These differences are quantitative, not qualitative. In medullary carcinoma, histaminase, L-dopa decarboxylase, and calcitonin are usually found, whereas in an earlier stage of C-cell hyperplasia, histaminase is not usually present.[98] Similarly, expression of hCG or its subunits in a pancreatic

tumor may suggest that it is malignant rather than benign.[104]

Oncogenes and Ectopic Hormone Production

Recent evidence indicates that one or more gene mutations (oncogenes) in normal cells may be related to the initiation and maintenance of the neoplastic state.[105–107] Such oncogenes are altered forms of normal proto-oncogenes that have important cellular functions; in some cases, a retrovirus may introduce the proto-oncogene into a normal cell. There is a high degree of sequence homology between oncogenes or proto-oncogenes and transforming genes of retroviruses.[108] Some retroviruses are associated with neoplastic disease in animals, while others are nontumorigenic. An example is the Rous sarcoma virus containing the src oncogene. Currently, there is considerable interest in the function of normal cellular oncogenes and their role in nonviral tumor formation. They are highly conserved in nature, suggesting that they have vital functions in normal cells and that oncogenic potential is acquired only after mutations or rearrangements of the so-called proto-oncogenes.[109] Well over 20 proto-oncogenes have been described in normal cells, and many of their nucleotide sequences have been determined.[105] The proteins encoded by oncogenes and their homologous cellular genes include tyrosine kinases, serine-threonine kinases, and a variety of transcription factors. The ras-encoded proteins and G proteins that couple receptors to enzymes on the inner membrane layer of the cell also can be converted to oncogenes.

Oncogenes are now recognized as an invariant concomitant in human cancer, although the specific oncogenes that are expressed in different tumors are still being defined.[110] Examples include the src oncogene in avian sarcomas, c-ras in human bladder carcinoma and neuroblastoma, erb B-2 in breast cancer, and c-myc in Burkitt's lymphoma. There is increasing evidence that neoplastic cells accumulate multiple oncogenes during the progression to malignancy, presumably acting on different aspects of cell function.

Until we have more information about the role of oncogenes in carcinogenesis, their relationship to ectopic hormone production will be unclear. On the other hand, products of some oncogenes resemble paracrine or autocrine growth factors or their receptors or subunits. For example, platelet-derived growth factor is associated with a proto-oncogene, c-sis,[111–114] and v-erb B generates a protein that resembles part of the epidermal growth factor receptor.[115] Production of these proteins thus mimics growth factor receptor activity, thereby stimulating or inhibiting paracrine or autocrine growth.[111] From analysis of cytogenic changes in human neoplasms, it is conceivable that genes at or near the sites of DNA rearrangements also play a role in the development of tumors.[116] For example, there are translocations between chromosomes 8 and 14 in Burkitt's lymphoma, with the c-myc gene (which is normally found on chromosome 8 in humans) being translocated to the heavy-chain locus of immunoglobulin on chromosome 14. In this case, the myc gene is brought under the regulatory control of the immunoglobulin gene enhancers and provides a model for ectopic hormone production. Rearrangement of the PTH gene to come under the control of an ovarian gene enhancer provides an analogous circumstance that leads to ectopic expression of PTH by the ovary.[117]

Gene amplification (or an increase in gene copy number per se) can occasionally be identified by the formation of double-minute chromosomes or homogeneous staining regions on regular chromosomes. Such regions contain multiple copies of genes. In some cases, gene amplification causes a high level of expression of oncogenes in human tumor cells. C-myc amplification has been identified in some gastric and other gastrointestinal neoplasms as well as in small cell carcinoma of the lung. Neuroblastomas have a high frequency of double-minute chromosomes, and there is amplification of the n-myc gene in neuroblastoma and in other neuroendocrine tumors. L-myc is amplified in small cell carcinoma and correlates with disease progression. Studies of some of the proteins that are encoded by oncogenes may provide further insight into the functions of these genes.

An additional class of oncogenes (known as recessive oncogenes or antioncogenes) has been identified initially in work on the retinoblastoma Rb gene.[118] Tumor-suppressor genes are inactivated either by mutation or by deletion (loss of heterozygosity). The number of different tumor suppressor genes is probably equal to that of activating oncogenes. Many tumors contain a combination of mutated oncogenes such as ras and inactivated suppressor genes such as P-53. The suppressor gene P-53 has been shown to be inactivated by mutations in colon cancer, brain neoplasms, and sarcomas.[118] These are growth-limiting or tumor-suppressor genes, whose inactivation leads to tumor formation in such disorders as lung cancer, bladder cancer, and bilateral acoustic neurofibromatosis.

The exact relationship of genetic control mechanisms to expression of hormones by tumors is probably important, and future studies should help to clarify precisely how tumor cells are altered at various control sites of polypeptide synthesis and processing. Cell hybridization has been suggested as a potential mechanism for the acquisition of new competence by tumor cells.[119] While experiments using hybridization techniques in vitro have noted the development of new characteristics or cells that have been hybridized, there is no definitive evidence that this is the case for neoplastic cells making hormones. Brown[120] reviewed mechanisms that may be operative in eukaryotic organism gene expression. Such mechanisms involve those in which the genes themselves are altered by amplification, diminution, rearrangement, or modification and those in which there is a change or modulation in gene expression through altered control mechanisms affecting transcription, posttranscription, or translation. It is likely that oncogenes act in this manner and ultimately induce ectopic hormone gene expression by effects on cell differentiation and cellular signaling pathways.

Experimental evidence strongly supports the fact that hormones made by ectopic tumors are the same as those made by the related endocrine organ.[1, 121] Some data are already available from DNA sequencing.[122] The most sophisticated techniques of molecular biology are thus being applied to the study of the biosynthesis of polypeptide hormones and an understanding of endocrine and tumor cell biology. It is important that ectopic hormones be purified and characterized biochemically, although it is easier to clone and sequence DNA. The presence of DNA or mRNA for the peptide may be associated with variable levels of transcription or translation, respectively. Detailed studies have clarified the precursor forms of hormones and allowed us to understand how precursors rather than the mature hormone may be synthesized and possibly released.

An interesting finding has been the widespread appearance of polypeptide hormones in tumors, much more than previously recognized.[97, 123] Such has been noted for ACTH, vasopressin, calcitonin, and hCG and its subunits. In addition, proteins such as hCG have been identified in normal testis,[124, 125] liver, and colon.[126] Ectopic hormone synthesis may thus be characteristic of malignant cells (even if clinical syndromes are unusual), and thus quantitative expression of hormones might be a form of "tumor marker." A basal level of hormone could be synthesized by cells in normal nonendocrine tissues. When such cells became malignant, the capacity to produce the proteins in question might be enhanced, as suggested by the work of Baylin et al.[95] This brings us back to the definition of ectopic and eutopic hormones, which is still controversial but serves as a basis for future research.[2] Understanding of the ectopic syndromes will be furthered by progress in developmental biology and molecular biology that provides new evidence concerning the nature of epigenetic mechanisms, phase-active genomes, oncogenes, and cell differentiation. The remainder of this chapter discusses specific hormonal syndromes reported in the literature.

ECTOPIC ACTH SYNDROME

Historical Aspects

In 1928, Brown, a London pathologist, described the first ectopic hormone syndrome, although he was not aware of the nature of the disorder.[127] Brown described an obese, pigmented, and plethoric 45-year-old woman with polydipsia, anorexia, weakness, blurred vision, baldness, hirsutism, and purpura. Laboratory studies showed polycythemia, hyperglycemia, and a normal sella turcica on skull x-ray. At autopsy, the patient had a 1-cm oat cell carcinoma of the lung and enlarged adrenal glands. This patient was reported several years before the description of Cushing's syndrome, and the association of the tumor with adrenal hyperplasia was not yet recognized. Since that time, several hundred patients with adrenal hyperplasia in association with tumors have been reported,[128] and many more have been diagnosed by criteria that are now standard.

The term ectopic ACTH syndrome was first defined by Meador et al.,[129] who demonstrated the presence of ACTH-like activity in extracts of nonendocrine tumors associated with Cushing's syndrome. Further studies by Liddle et al.[130] showed similarities between ACTH extracted from tumors and the hormones from pituitary glands in tests of biological activity, chromatographic behavior, and physical and chemical properties.

Tumor Types

The ectopic ACTH syndrome has been associated principally with tumors of the lung, thymus, and pancreas which tend to be similar histologically and also may produce related hormones. The following tumors[128] account for the majority of cases:

1. Oat cell carcinoma of lung, 60 per cent
2. Thymic tumors, 15 per cent
3. Pancreatic carcinoma (usually islet cell), 10 per cent
4. Bronchial adenoma (carcinoid type), 4 per cent
5. The remaining 11 per cent includes pheochromocytoma, medullary carcinoma of the thyroid, various neurogenic tumors, and tumors of the parotid, ovary, prostate, and kidney. Carcinoma of the breast, esophagus, colon, gallbladder, testis, or uterus are rare causes.

Biochemical and Physiological Characteristics of Ectopic ACTH and Related Peptides

Knowledge about the pathogenesis of this disorder has grown, in part through the progress made in understanding the molecular biology and biochemistry of ACTH and related peptides. ACTH is synthesized through a higher-molecular-weight precursor known as *proopiomelanocortin* (POMC), which is glycosylated and contains the sequences of ACTH and β- and γ-lipotropin (1–58), β-endorphin (61–91), and the enkephalins (see Ch. 22).

The data supporting the structure of the ACTH and lipotropin gene and precursor come from two major sources. One approach used radioactive amino acid incorporation to show that animal and human pituitary cells in tissue culture synthesized higher-molecular-weight forms of ACTH.[131, 132] Several forms of ACTH-related peptides were detected within cells and culture medium by immunoprecipitation, and other studies showed that higher-molecular-weight forms could be converted to ACTH by endopeptidases. A precursor-product relationship could not be demonstrated on the basis of size and structural data alone, and it was therefore necessary to show through radioactive pulse-chase experiments that the higher-molecular-weight precursor was converted to the smaller forms. The incorporation studies in cells were supported by work with ACTH mRNA in cell-free systems which demonstrated the existence of a 29-kDa precursor.[133] The polypeptide precursor is glycosylated posttranslationally and can reach molecular weights as high as 34 kDa. A second major approach by Nakanishi et al.[134] involved determination of the structure of cloned cDNA for bovine ACTH-lipotropin that included the coding sequences for the preceding peptides (see Fig. 149–1). In addition to the sequences of ACTH and lipotropin in POMC, there was a 16-kDa peptide amino-terminal to the ACTH sequence whose function has not yet been determined. The 16-kDa fragment is cleaved to a smaller NH₂-terminal 76-amino acid glycopeptide whose function is unknown but could be a growth factor for the adrenal cortex.[135] The 16-kDa region is preceded by the "signal" sequence for the pre-POMC molecule. These studies have pointed definitively to the existence of a common precursor for the pituitary peptides of the ACTH family. These findings are of considerable importance in understanding both normal physiological function of the pituitary and the pathogenesis of the ectopic ACTH syndrome.

In addition to data supporting a common precursor, there is also evidence that the metabolism of the precursor may vary in different tissues.[136, 137] For example, it appears that the normal anterior pituitary gland can process POMC to make ACTH, β-lipotropin, and β-endorphin.[132] This is supported by the fact that levels of ACTH, lipotropin, and endorphin are all elevated in patients with Addison's disease and Nelson's syndrome. In the pars intermedia of animal pituitary glands, human fetuses, and pregnant women, on the other hand, a different type of cleavage takes place in which α-MSH [or acetyl-ACTH (1–13)], a potent pigmentary peptide, γ-MSH (a weak ACTH-like and pigmentary peptide), and corticotropin-like intermediate peptide (CLIP) [ACTH (18–39)] are produced. Various permutations of posttranslational processing are possible, depending on the tissue in which the precursor is present and presumably the presence of different enzymes, sites of processing, or secretory granules in which processing can take place, leading to different sized proteins, varying degrees of glycosylation, and the like. The precursor protein in various tissues could theoretically vary, and evidence for expression of the POMC gene from an alternate promoter has been obtained.[138] There has been no evidence for activation of abnormal genes or the production of peptides not known to be synthesized in normal tissues. More likely is variable processing and metabolism in different tissues and tumors.

Amino-terminal glycopeptides have been identified in patients with both Cushing's syndrome and ectopic ACTH production.[139] Furthermore, a number of peptides ranging in molecular weight between the size of the amino-terminal glycopeptide of 76 amino acids and γ-MSH have been identified in a number of such tumors.[140] The production of γ-MSH occurs from cleavage of amino-terminal glycopeptide. It is less potent than ACTH in its adrenotropic activity,[141, 142] but it has been suggested that it might be a stimulator of aldosterone production.[143] Tumors also may produce CLIP, which has no ACTH-like activity but may stimulate insulin release.[144, 145]

Earlier studies by Gewirtz and Yalow[146] and subsequently by Odell et al.[147] indicated that ACTH was present by radioimmunoassay in many tumors of patients who did not have clinical Cushing's syndrome or in whom it was not even suspected. The presence of ACTH-like activity was unrelated to the histological type of tumor. Furthermore, these studies suggested that the form of ACTH that might be synthesized and released was higher in molecular weight than 39-amino acid ACTH and could be converted to ACTH by trypsin. The peptide(s) had little or no biological activity and were presumably an ACTH precursor. Wolfsen and Odell[148] examined both plasma and extracts of lung cancer for the presence of pro-ACTH by column chromatography and radioimmunoassay. In 100 patients who were admitted with abnormal chest x-rays, 53 of 74 with lung cancer had increased plasma ACTH. In evaluating 101 patients with chronic obstructive lung disease, 5 of 20 with increased ACTH and only 2 of 81 with normal ACTH developed lung cancer within 2 years. The mean level of ACTH in the patients with cancer was 131.8 pg/ml, compared with 52.5 pg/ml in normal subjects. Of the 74 per cent of patients with cancer who exceeded the normal level, all had mean values about 107 pg/ml. The patients with benign lung disease had a mean level of 55 pg/ml. Immunoreactive ACTH was increased in the serum of patients with lung cancer and tumors of other organs, including the colon, breast, kidney, and pancreas, although concentrations by radioreceptor assay were within the normal range. This immunoreactive ACTH was believed to be a precursor form of ACTH, since it eluted in the void volume on gel filtration and did not react in the receptor assay. In normal subjects, plasma values for ACTH by radioimmunoassay and radioreceptor assay were equivalent. Radiation therapy and chemotherapy lowered plasma ACTH in patients with lung cancer (values falling from a mean of 131.8 to 87.0 pg/ml in treated patients).

When tumor extracts were assayed, 38 lung cancer specimens each contained more than 1 ng/g of ACTH-like immunoreactivity, with most containing more than 5 ng. Normal lung at postmortem from patients who died without cancer contained less than 2 ng. Chromatography of tissue extracts showed that more than 50 per cent of the ACTH immunoreactivity was in the void volume, with little or no immunoreactivity in the area of elution of ACTH (1–39). The weight of the pro-ACTH in these studies was 20-kDa or greater.[26]

Both pituitary cells and tumors that produce ACTH have been shown to contain higher-molecular-weight forms. Orth and Nicholson[149] showed that higher-molecular-weight forms of human ACTH also were glycoproteins. In their studies, normal pituitary ACTH and ACTH from ectopic tumors and patients with Nelson's syndrome were separated according to molecular weight on Sephadex G-50. A total of 29 to 61 per cent of "big" ACTH from tumors bound to Con A–agarose and could be eluted with α-methyl-D-mannopyranoside, while "little" ACTH in most cases did not bind the lectin. This group established a human oat cell carcinoma in continuous culture and provided strong evidence for production therein of a higher-molecular-weight precursor.[150–152] By means of three radioimmunoassays with antibodies directed against ACTH (1–39), β-MSH, and β-endorphin, respectively, five immunoreactive components were identified on gel filtration. There was a void volume peak that was recognized by antibodies against the three peptides, a second peak co-eluting with β-endorphin that was recognized by antibodies against MSH and endorphin, and smaller peaks co-eluting with γ-lipotropin, β-endorphin, and ACTH. These studies provided very strong evidence for a common precursor both in normal pituitary cells and in the ectopic tumors. As indicated earlier, crucial factors in the generation of clinical ectopic hormone syndromes may be the presence or

absence of enzymes that convert larger- to smaller-molecular-weight forms.[153]

Although Upton and Amatruda[154] described the presence of peptides with corticotropin-releasing factor or hormone (CRF or CRH)–like activity in the tumors of patients with ectopic ACTH syndrome, a variety of indirect observations had suggested that such peptides might be found. Christy[155] described two patients with ectopic ACTH syndrome who responded to the adrenal inhibitor metyrapone, suggesting that such tumors enhanced pituitary ACTH secretion by "unknown means." Landon et al.[156] noted stimulation of steroid production by vasopressin and hypoglycemia in a patient with the ectopic ACTH syndrome and suggested that CRH peptides might be released. The response of some patients with the ectopic syndrome to metyrapone has suggested that the tumors produce factors that cause secretion of ACTH from the normal pituitary[157, 158] (Fig. 149–4). Imura et al.[159] studied six tumors from patients with the ACTH syndrome and found CRH-like activity in all of them. These studies were performed in vitro. Hirata et al.[160] performed extensive studies in vitro on tumor tissues from four patients with ectopic ACTH syndrome. All but one of the patients lacked classical features of Cushing's syndrome and showed, instead, muscle weakness, edema, hypertension, hypokalemia, and glycosuria. Variable responses in the physiological activity of these tumors were noted during incubations in vitro. In one tumor, biogenic amines, norepinephrine, and serotonin caused increased production of tissue cAMP without increasing the release of ACTH. These findings led to speculation on the possible dissociation of adenyl cyclase and hormone release or altered tumor receptors, as suggested by Shorr et al.[161] Incorporation of radioactive amino acids into two tumors showed that the labeled hormone was predominantly or exclusively ACTH precursor.[159] Whether there are abnormalities in the glucocorticoid regulatory element in POMC or ACTH genes in tumors is unknown.

The variable responses of the tumors to regulators of adenylate cyclase production and hormone release suggest that some of our concepts of tumor autonomy in the ectopic ACTH syndrome may have to be revised. Production of CRH by ectopic tumors suggests that normal hypothalamic and pituitary functions can be modulated by the tumor, whereas the findings in the in vitro studies suggest

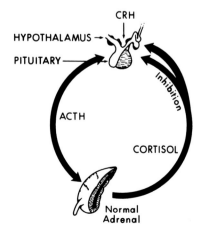
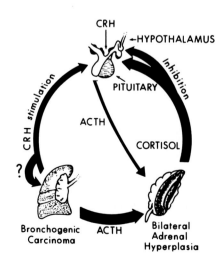

FIGURE 149–4. Comparison of the normal pituitary-adrenal feedback relationships (left) with those of an ACTH-producing tumor (right).

regulation by the tumor itself. The response to dexamethasone or metyrapone by tumors may be more common than suggested. Because of the relatively infrequent application of the radioimmunoassay for ACTH to serum measurements in such patients in response to stimulators or suppressors of ACTH secretion, further investigation is needed. While identification of both ACTH and CRH in tumor extracts is common, identification of circulating CRH is quite rare.[162] A nice experimental model for chronic overproduction of CRH in transkaryotic rats was recently reported.[163]

Clinical Characteristics

Most patients with the ectopic ACTH syndrome do not have the classical clinical features of Cushing's syndrome.[130] Even though they may have very high levels of ACTH and cortisol in the blood, the signs and symptoms may be subtle. It has been argued that the excess cortisol must be present for several years in order to produce the classical physical abnormalities of Cushing's syndrome. Furthermore, the catabolic effects of malignant tumors (see above) also may be responsible for aspects of the clinical presentation. The acute consequences of marked cortisol excess in terms of both glucocorticoid and mineralocorticoid actions and the effects of ACTH excess tend to predominate. A recent comparison of medical outcomes in patients with small cell carcinoma with and without Cushing's syndrome has shown that patients with the syndrome fared much more poorly, i.e., showing clinical deterioration and death from opportunistic infection shortly after starting chemotherapy.[164]

Common among the major physical abnormalities in patients with this disorder are the following:

1. Weight loss, in contrast to classical Cushing's syndrome, in which weight gain, centripetal obesity, and livid striae are common.

2. Generalized muscle weakness, related to hypokalemic alkalosis, steroid myopathy, and carcinomatous neuropathy and/or myopathy.

3. Hyperpigmentation, related to high levels of ACTH as well as tumor production of lipotropin and other melanotropic peptides.

4. More frequent appearance in men, in contrast to pituitary Cushing's disease, which is more common in women. There is a growing incidence in women because of relative increase in cigarette use.

5. Peripheral edema, related to the mineralocorticoid effects of cortisol.

6. Hypertension.

7. Polyuria, polydipsia, and other manifestations of glucose intolerance.

8. Hirsutism and acne in some cases.

9. Pulmonary congestion.

10. Lymphadenopathy or evidence of obstruction of the superior vena cava.

11. Signs and symptoms of lung or other tumors, including metastatic disease.

Laboratory Diagnosis

Routine laboratory tests included the following:

1. Unexplained hypokalemic alkalosis, particularly when observed in the absence of diuretics, is more common than in patients with pituitary Cushing's disease and suggests ectopic Cushing's syndrome or primary aldosteronism.

2. Elevated levels of urinary 17-hydroxysteroids, 17-ketosteroids, and urinary free cortisol. Extraordinarily high levels of both 17-hydroxysteroids and 17-ketosteroids are noted due to the high levels of ACTH. The selective increases of 17-ketosteroids, which tend to be found in adrenal carcinoma, are not generally present in this syndrome.

3. Hyperresponsiveness to ACTH administration.

4. Response to metyrapone is not usually present, but because of CRH production by tumors, it may occur (see above).

5. Dexamethasone suppression (both low-dose and high-dose) is usually absent. Because of CRH production, partial suppression might theoretically occur in some. This has been noted particularly with thymomas and bronchial carcinoids.[155–157]

6. Elevated plasma ACTH without diurnal variation. Elevated immunoreactive ACTH is the hallmark of the diagnosis. Simple elevation of ACTH, however, does not differentiate absolutely between ectopic and Cushing's disease due to pituitary hormone excess or tumors that release biologically inactive precursors. The levels of ACTH in the ectopic syndrome are, in general, higher than those in pituitary diseases. Elevation of immunoreactive ACTH both in the blood and in the tumor tissue, particularly of the POMC variety, is a much more frequent finding than previously suspected. Increases may be noted even in patients without clinical or biochemical evidence of Cushing's syndrome.

7. Increased secretion of 5-hydroxyindoleacetic acid. Oat cell carcinoma may be extremely difficult to distinguish from carcinoid tumors. A number of tumors have been reported in which production of serotonin as well as ectopic ACTH has been described.[165] This has been particularly true for the bronchial carcinoid and medullary carcinoma of the thyroid.

8. Occasionally, the presence of the syndrome is detected clinically or biochemically even before the tumor becomes apparent in the patient. Since the most likely cause is an oat cell carcinoma of the lung, such a tumor may appear at a later date than the clinical syndrome. Careful examination of chest radiographs and tomograms looking for mediastinal widening, atelectasis, and abnormal densities should be performed. In some cases where the disease was initially thought to be pituitary in origin, bilateral adrenalectomy was done, with the malignant tumor appearing at a much later date.[166]

9. Electron microscopy of ACTH-producing tumors shows neurosecretory-type granules and similarities to carcinoid.[167–170]

Gomi et al.[171] described two patients who had a combination of ectopic ACTH and amylase production. The latter was reflected in zymogen granules present in the tumor. These cases raised interesting questions about possible relationships between neurosecretory-type granules and zymogen granules, not previously known to be associated. Chin[172] described a patient with a lateral neck mass and Cushing's syndrome who had ectopic ACTH production. The mRNA extracted directly from the tumor directed the translation of a precursor of calcitonin in a cell-free system, leading to the ultimate diagnosis of medullary carcinoma of the thyroid. Although the authors were looking for the translation of an ACTH precursor from the tumor tissue, they found a dominant protein of 15 kDa that was immunoprecipitated by antibodies to human calcitonin and a small amount of higher-molecular-weight precursor to ACTH. Pierce et al.[173] reported the simultaneous production of ACTH and arginine vasopressin from a small cell carcinoma associated with both syndromes.

Several patients with ACTH secretion from pheochromocytoma also have been described.[174] In one case, episodes of secretion of ACTH and catecholamines followed each other. Review of the outcome of patients with ACTH production by pheochromocytoma[175–177] revealed a mortality of over 50 per cent. It is suggested that all patients with ectopic ACTH or with Cushing's syndrome be screened for catecholamine production. Molecular studies suggest that gene expression of POMC may occur in all pheochromocytomas, but only when a 1300 or larger base pair mRNA is transcribed does Cushing's syndrome result.[177] ACTH secretion also has been described from carcinoma of the breast[178] and prostate,[179] from carcinoid in a child with multiple endocrine neoplasia,[180] and from pulmonary tumorlets (small peripheral nodules in the lung field that bear an uncertain relationship to the bronchial carcinoid).[181] In a patient with medullary carcinoma of the thyroid and ectopic ACTH production described by Rosenberg et al.,[182] osteoporosis was the presenting manifestation, and the course was more chronic and indolent than in most other reports. Drasin et al.[183] described a patient with mediastinal lipomatosis masquerading as a mediastinal tumor in a patient with ectopic ACTH production due to bronchial carcinoid. Although the latter has been well described in Cushing's syndrome, it had not been reported previously in the ectopic ACTH syndrome.

Differential Diagnosis

With the laboratory diagnoses outlined, documentation of the ectopic ACTH syndrome is usually straightforward, although differential diagnosis can occasionally be confusing. The marked excess of urinary 17-ketosteroids compared with 17-hydroxysteroids found in patients with carcinoma of the adrenal gland is not present in the ectopic syndrome, and the ratio is usually between 2 and 3 to 1, as in normal individuals or those with Cushing's syndrome. Patients with adrenal adenoma tend to synthesize predominantly glucocorticoids. There is generally hyperresponsiveness to ACTH in the ectopic ACTH syndrome, but only about 50 per cent of adrenal adenomas respond to ACTH, and adrenal carcinomas rarely respond.[184] Following the use of an inhibitor of cortisol synthesis such as metyrapone, there is no increase (and usually a decrease) in patients with adrenal tumors, but they are unchanged or increased in patients with the ectopic ACTH syndrome and with pituitary Cushing's disease. The presence of CRH, as already indicated, in ectopic tumors can make the test occasionally confusing. Plasma ACTH is usually over 100 pg/ml in patients with ectopic ACTH production, less than that in pituitary Cushing's disease, and below 10 pg/ml in patients with adrenal tumors, but the differentiation between ectopic and pituitary ACTH is not definitive. On the other hand, selective venous sampling for ACTH radioimmuno-

assay from petrosal sinuses, the internal jugular vein, or mediastinal or other veins compared with the periphery can resolve the differential diagnosis.[185] After CRH administration, 203 patients with Cushing's syndrome had a peak inferior petrosal plasma ratio of 3 or more (with no false positives), and patients with ectopic ACTH were lower or failed to respond.[185] Although it has been recommended that CRH stimulation can differentiate patients with ectopic ACTH production (who do not respond) from patients with pituitary Cushing's syndrome (who do), like other tests, it may not be absolutely definitive.[186] Patients with severe stress and terminal illness may not regulate ACTH or cortisol secretion normally and may be difficult to differentiate from patients with the ectopic ACTH syndrome.

New methods of anatomical localization, including computed axial tomography and nuclear magnetic resonance imaging, may be useful in documenting both adrenal and pituitary tumors and ectopic tumors that may produce ACTH. Occasionally, an ectopic tumor that is not yet visible by radiologic or other means may be associated with ACTH excess.[187] Furthermore, some tumors may produce hormones in cycles, so-called *periodic hormonogenesis*.[188] Studies by Garroway et al.[189] of a human ACTH-producing melanoma that was unresponsive to steroid suppression showed that the cortisol receptor was lacking from the cell line, indicating a possible mechanism for the failure of steroid responsiveness. A report by Himsworth et al.[190] described a patient with a hepatoma associated with ectopic ACTH production which also produced melanotropin and calcitonin. A geometric increase in ACTH release was noted throughout the course, particularly following adrenalectomy, and the tumor was not appreciated. Although immunoreactive ACTH increased markedly with time, biological potency was not present, and release of a precursor was indicated. Spontaneous remission[191] and intermittent disease[192] can make differential diagnosis confusing.

A review of the diagnostic tests in Cushing's syndrome has suggested that the overnight dexamethasone suppression test was the best screening technique. The importance of urinary free cortisol determinations and late-evening plasma cortisol with a 2-mg daily test dose of dexamethasone is also emphasized. The high-dose suppression test has remained the principal test for differentiating various causes of the syndrome.[193] Findling et al.[194] emphasized the use of selective venous sampling for ACTH in differentiating Cushing's disease from the ectopic ACTH syndrome. Ratios obtained at the level of the jugulobulbar vein were not diagnostic, and blood from the inferior petrosal sinus was believed to be much more reliable. An arteriovenous gradient of 6.8 across the pulmonary circulation was found in a patient with a bronchial carcinoid tumor.

Therapy

Therapy for patients with the ectopic ACTH syndrome is complex and depends principally on the underlying tumor.[195] Since the most common cause of the syndrome is oat cell carcinoma, the prognosis is usually extremely poor. There have been significant advances in the chemotherapy of this disorder with combination chemotherapy, but the prognosis nonetheless remains grim. A similar outlook exists for patients with islet cell carcinomas or malignant thymomas, although occasional surgical cures have been described. The prognosis is usually better for patients with pheochromocytoma, paraganglioma, thymoma, or bronchial carcinoid.

In some cases, the major clinical manifestations of the tumor are due to hypercorticism and its effects such as hypokalemia, muscle weakness, and diabetes. Administration of oral or intravenous potassium, sodium restriction, and the administration of spironolactone may be helpful. One might consider bilateral total adrenalectomy in patients in whom a more favorable prognosis warrants the procedure. Under exceptional circumstances, a primary malignant neoplasm producing ACTH might be removed successfully by surgery.[196] This would definitely be true for the benign tumors associated with the disorder. Normally, however, some form of medical management of adrenal steroid production is necessary and can be performed with one or more inhibitors of adrenal steroid biosynthesis or cytolytic therapy. The agents include metyrapone (which blocks the 11β-hydroxylase enzyme converting 11-deoxycortisol to cortisol), aminoglutethimide (which blocks the conversion of cholesterol to pregnenolone), and o,p'-DDD (which is an adrenal cytolytic agent). Successful use of metyrapone in the management of ectopic ACTH has been described.[197–199] Double blockade with aminoglutethimide[195, 200, 201] in combination with metyrapone may be even more effective, and there is no compensatory increase in ACTH. The simultaneous use of o,p'-DDD and the other two agents will result in cytolytic activity while steroid hormone production is being inhibited and will allow lower doses with fewer side effects. Cooper and Schucart[202] have emphasized the value of o,p'-DDD in treatment of the ectopic ACTH syndrome, particularly in combination with aminoglutethimide and metyrapone. Ketoconazole also has been used with some success.[203] More recently, the long-acting analogue of somatostatin octreotide has been used with some success to control ectopic ACTH secretion.[204, 205] Octreotide has found even greater usage in pituitary as well as gastroenteropancreatic tumors,[205] a clinical observation that is supported by the presence of somatostatin receptors in many tumors.[206]

Ectopic Production of Lipotropins and Opioid-Like Peptides

Hyperpigmentation is a common clinical manifestation in patients with chronic and debilitating illness, especially in gastrointestinal disorders such as sprue, adenocarcinoma, and Whipple's disease. Increased pigmentation in these disorders has not been associated clearly with ectopic production of peptides that increase melanocyte activity. On the other hand, the hyperpigmentation frequently associated with the ectopic ACTH syndrome has been partially associated with the production of melanotropic peptides.[130, 205] It is now known that most of the melanotropic activity is actually contained in lipotropin. Hyperpigmentation also can be produced by large quantities of ACTH because of homologies in structure between the amino-terminal end of the ACTH molecule and MSH. The same cell that produces ACTH in the normal pituitary is also responsible for producing β-lipotropin. Shimizu et

al.[207] demonstrated that tumors contain more melanotropic activity than can be accounted for by their content of ACTH alone and that tumor lipotropin can be separated from ACTH.[208] Extensive studies of tumors were performed by Abe et al.,[209, 210] who noted that less than 5 per cent of the biological MSH-like activity of human pituitary glands was due to α-MSH and that the tumors also contained a minority of their MSH as α-MSH. They[210, 211] showed that over 95 per cent of the biologically active MSH in human pituitary glands and serum was due to β-MSH or a related peptide. It is apparent that ectopic tumors may produce not only ACTH and β-lipotropin but also fragments. Whether the fragments are produced spontaneously or are due to degradation by enzymes will require further studies involving protein synthesis. Isolated production of lipotropin by tumors has not been reported, and the hyperpigmentation associated with chronic nonmalignant disease is not due to lipotropin.[209, 210] Some of the β-MSH activity being measured in the pituitary and plasma may be material of higher molecular weight than the native hormone.[212, 213] The normal pituitary gland synthesizes the molecule β-lipotropin (β-LPH), which has 89 amino acids,[214] and γ-lipotropin (γ-LPH), which is identical to the first 56 amino acids of β-LPH. Since β-MSH corresponds to a sequence in the lipotropin molecule, and since all three peptides have melanotropic properties, antibodies directed against MSH would measure other peptides as well. Studies by Gilkes et al.[215] suggest strongly that most of what has been measured heretofore as β-MSH is actually lipotropin activity.

Odell et al.[147] found evidence of increased lipotropin in tumor extracts and in the serum of the same patients whose tumors produced ACTH. The frequency of its occurrence was not as great as that of ACTH[148] but was significant nonetheless. Comparative statistics are as follows: In lung cancer, 72 per cent of patients had increased plasma proACTH and 36 per cent had increased lipotropin; in colon cancer, comparable values were 27 and 10 per cent, respectively; in pancreatic cancer, 92 and 25 per cent; in gastric or esophageal cancer, 54 and 14 per cent; and in breast cancer, 41 and 0 per cent. Of 79 acetic acid extracts of carcinoma of the lung, colon, stomach, esophagus, and breast, lipotropin concentrations greater than those in blood were found in 61. Lipotropin also was present in larger amounts than in control tissues from patients without cancer. Thus lipotropin was frequently increased in the blood and tumor tissue of patients with various types of carcinoma and served as a useful marker of ectopic production.

Jeffcoate et al.[216] developed a specific radioimmunoassay for human β-lipotropin isolated from human pituitary glands, and the plasma assays were done after extraction with ground glass. Normal levels in the morning were 25 pg/ml. In normal subjects, there was a rise in secretion following the administration of metyrapone and a fall after dexamethasone; insulin-induced hypoglycemia increased values to 200 pg/ml. In patients with Cushing's disease, Nelson's syndrome, and the ectopic ACTH syndrome, there was an excellent correlation between ACTH and β-lipotropin, supporting the concept that they are co-secreted. Measurements of the 30-amino acid joining peptide separating N-terminal peptide and ACTH show excellent correlations in plasma with ACTH and lipotropin.[217] The function of lipotropin has not yet been determined, although it has been suggested that β-lipotropin is the precursor of β-endorphin. The potential role of β-lipotropin in the control and awareness of pain, appetite, release of other hormones, and etiology of mental disorders has not yet been defined. There is great interest in the potential importance of the enkephalin-endorphin peptides in these areas.

Guillemin et al.[218] showed that ACTH and β-endorphin in the rat were co-secreted by the pituitary. Tanaka et al.[219] also suggested that the enkephalin-endorphin peptides and ACTH were secreted in parallel during both physiological and pathological conditions. Studies by Deftos et al.[220] suggested that immunoreactive CT might be present within the anterior lobe of the rat pituitary gland and could be part of the 31-kDa precursor molecule for ACTH and β-lipotropin, but this has not been confirmed. Mendelsohn et al.[217] were unable to demonstrate CT in normal human pituitary glands using conditions that demonstrated it in medullary carcinoma; they also were unable to find any evidence of immunoreactive β-lipotropin in medullary carcinoma of the thyroid. Xavier et al.[221] reported a small cell carcinoma of the lung that made both calcitonin and ACTH, but there was evidence for separate biosynthetic precursors.

Ueda et al.[222] used antibodies against β-MSH and α-endorphin to evaluate extracts of human pituitaries and ectopic tumors producing ACTH. On gel filtration, β-lipotropin was identified by antibodies developed against both β-MSH and α-endorphin, while γ-lipotropin was identified only by antibodies to β-MSH. Gel filtration studies of extracts of five normal human pituitary glands showed both β- and γ-lipotropin peaks, but a clear β-lipotropin peak was observed in only three tumor extracts. β-MSH comprised 3 to 55 per cent of total immunoreactive β-lipotropin. Whether these studies show that β-MSH was actually present in some of the tumors has not yet been determined. Differing enzyme characteristics of tumors compared with normal tissues may have accounted for these findings. Whether these are physiological effects or nonspecific effects due to protease activity remains to be determined.

It appears that β-lipotropin is a major opioid-like peptide in human pituitary glands and in the plasma of normal human subjects.[223, 224] High concentrations of β-endorphin are present in the plasma of patients with endocrine disorders associated with increased ACTH and β-lipotropin, but the latter is not completely converted to β-endorphin in vivo in normal subjects. Studies of pituitary adenomas in patients with Cushing's syndrome showed that the conversion of β-lipotropin to β-endorphin was enhanced in ACTH/β-lipotropin–producing adenomas.[225] β-Endorphin in the normal pituitary gland is more likely to exist in the β-lipotropin form. Wiedermann et al.[226] developed a specific radioimmunoassay for human β-endorphin in unextracted plasma in which there was minimal cross-reactivity with β-lipotropin. In normal fasting subjects, morning levels ranged from 5 to 45 pg/ml, and β-endorphin was elevated in patients with untreated Cushing's disease, Nelson's syndrome, and bronchogenic carcinoma. In normal subjects with an intact pituitary-adrenal axis, endorphin was undetectable following dexamethasone administration and increased after metyrapone and insulin-induced hypoglycemia. It thus appears to respond to the same stimuli as ACTH and β-lipotropin. Patients in remission from pituitary-adrenal disease had normal levels. Pullan et al.[227] looked for met-enkephalin and β-endorphin in tissue extracts of nonendocrine tumors. High concentrations of the two peptides that were undetectable in control lung tissue were identified in three carcinoid tumors from patients with the ectopic ACTH syndrome. In one patient, the met-enkephalin concentration in veins draining the tumor was twice that in a peripheral vein. The presence of increased quantities of neural peptides in the tumors and blood of patients with malignancy suggests that some of the confusing and diverse paraneoplastic syndromes (particularly neurological) associated with malignancy could be related to such peptides. In patients with renal failure, levels of both γ- and β-lipotropin may be significantly elevated, and they must be considered possible factors in causing some of the clinical phenomena.[228]

Pullan et al.[229] studied extracts from seven tumors. Four tumors contained the complete family of peptides, including ACTH, lipotropin, α-MSH, CLIP, β-endorphin, and met-enkephalin, although the proportions varied in different tumors. In addition, high-molecular-weight forms of ACTH and met-enkephalin were observed. None of these peptides was detectable in normal lung tissue. These data suggest that the common precursor is synthesized by all tumors but that the subsequent pattern of metabolism depends on the particular enzyme activity present in the particular tumor. There was a high-molecular-weight, enkephalin-like peptide that reacted in the met-enkephalin assay but not in the β-endorphin assay, supporting the concept that the precursor for met-enkephalin might be distinct from that for ACTH and lipotropin.[230] The presence of enkephalin, as well as precursors for the ACTH-lipotropin genes for these polypeptides, might have resulted either from gene duplication or from genes closely related to each other in structure. Whether these non-ACTH peptides have physiological effects in cancer patients remains to be determined, but they could have important actions, including stimulation of insulin secretion (by CLIP), production of analgesia (by β-endorphin and met-enkephalin), as well as behavioral effects. The multiple effects of β-lipotropin and the endorphins in a wide variety of physiological systems, such as hormone release,[231, 232] stress-induced eating,[233, 234] blood pressure control,[235] exercise,[236] and behavior,[237] suggest that in the future these peptides will likely be shown to be responsible for important clinical phenomena. Their effects could potentially explain a number of poorly understood clinical phenomena in cancer patients.

ECTOPIC PITUITARY, HYPOTHALMIC, AND PLACENTAL HORMONES

Growth Hormone and Growth Hormone–Releasing Hormone

Ectopic production of human growth hormone (hGH) is one of the least frequently documented hormonal syndromes. Since major fluctuations in plasma hGH in response to exercise, dietary intake, and sleep are observed, it may be difficult to differentiate clinically between hGH production from tumors and increases in secretion related to normal physiological events.[238] Steiner et al.[239] first showed elevated circulating levels of hGH in a patient with a lung tumor. Following surgical resection of the adenocarcinoma, immunoreactive hGH in plasma fell from 38 to 3 ng/ml. The patient's symptoms rapidly disappeared, but the tumor was not analyzed for growth hormone. Cameron et al.[240] reported a similar patient in whom hGH was not elevated, but it failed to suppress normally. The physiological abnormality was still present after partial resection of an undifferentiated adenocarcinoma of the lung, but the osteoarthropathy was improved. With immunofluorescent antibodies, the tissue showed reactivity for both hGH and human placental lactogen (hPL). Only one of three patients with hypertrophic osteoarthropathy described by DuPont et al.[241] had elevated levels of hGH. Increased GH concentrations in 7 of 18 bronchogenic and 5 of 8 gastric adenocarcinomas have been reported by Beck and Burger.[242]

More convincing documentation was suggested by the work of Greenberg et al.,[243] who showed that GH could be synthesized and secreted from a poorly differentiated large cell lung tumor in tissue culture and that there was disappearance of an elevated plasma level of hGH and hypertrophic osteoarthropathy after surgical resection. Cells were maintained in continuous culture for 4 months, and synthesis of hGH in vitro was documented by incorporation of radioactive amino acids into a protein that had chromatographic and molecular weight characteristics similar to hGH. Release of hormone from the cultured cells was stimulated by activators of the adenylate cyclase system.[243] Whether hypertrophic osteoarthropathy is related directly to hGH or might be associated with some other peptide or substance produced by the tumor is not clear. Since the clinical and radiological manifestations of hypertrophic osteoarthropathy are different from those of the pure GH excess noted in acromegaly, the relationship has not yet been documented.[244] The tumor concentration of hGH was 190 ng/g compared with adjacent nontumorous lung of 60 ng/g.

An interesting pancreatic islet tumor associated with acromegaly included a lack of growth hormone–releasing hormone (GRH) in plasma, high levels of hGH, and an arteriovenous gradient in hGH across the pancreas. There were normal responses to GRH and glucose following surgery and a fall in serum hGH to normal within hours of excision. The tumor showed incorporation in vitro of [³H]leucine into GH, some of it being larger than the native molecule. In plasma, tumor, and culture medium, there was a molecule the size of GH. A recent report[246] from a pancreatic tumor extract using molecular hybridization with a cDNA probe showed an mRNA transcript compatible with that of GH. These well-documented cases emphasize what is a very unusual syndrome.

A number of reports document the association of acromegaly with nonpituitary tumors that produce GRH and stimulate the normal pituitary gland to release GH, causing acromegaly. Saeed et al.[247] described a patient with a bronchial carcinoid and acromegaly, pituitary enlargement, and elevated GH. Symptoms of active acromegaly and elevated GH persisted for 11 years after hypophysectomy, and resection of the pulmonary tumor reduced GH to normal levels. No GH was present in the carcinoid tumor, but when extracts of it were added to isolated pituitary cells in culture, GRH activity was noted. Frohman et al.[248] reported studies on a number of additional tumors containing GRH activity. They studied extracts of a pancreatic islet tumor that contained a large amount of activity, as did extracts of a small-cell carcinoma of the lung and carcinoid. Each of the tumors also contained somatostatin-like immunoreactivity, but the levels did not correlate with the biological activity of the tumor. The material with GRH activity had a molecular weight greater than 6000, was adsorbed on DEAE-cellulose at low ionic strength, and was removed at higher ionic strength. When purified further by HPLC, the preparation increased GH release by pituitary monolayer cultures up to five times baseline. The activity was resistant to exopeptidase digestion but could be destroyed by trypsin and chymotrypsin. It was suggested that this finding could explain the possible presence of pituitary tumors in some patients with multiple endocrine neoplasia type 1. The stimulatory effects of the GRH factor were inhibited by somatostatin. It had not been clear whether the releasing hormone was the same peptide produced by the median eminence of the hypothalamus; there were differences between them in size and chromatographic behavior, although the tumor material might be a precursor. Purification and chemical characterization of the peptides suggest that they are identical.[249] A number of both biologically active and inactive forms may be found in plasma, tumor extracts, and some normal tissues.[250]

It has been suggested that the possibility of an extrapituitary tumor be considered in every patient with acromegaly. The presence of pituitary tumors suggests that prolonged stimulation of GH release by GRH can cause tumor formation, supporting the possibility that pituitary acromegaly might be primarily a hypothalamic disease. The radioimmunoassay for somatomedin C has been used as a highly reliable means for confirming the diagnosis of acromegaly and assessing clinical disease activity, since it correlates extremely well with GH concentrations.[251] The mean fasting levels were 6.8 U/ml in acromegalic patients and 0.67 U/ml in normal subjects. Following therapy, somatomedin C measurements were extremely useful as an index of improvement.

Before irradiation or transsphenoidal surgery of the pituitary gland, ectopic GRH secretion should be ruled out, but the latter is a relatively rare cause of acromegaly.[252] The results of specific testing may be unusual in ectopic GRH secretion, as they are in the standard variety of acromegaly.[253, 254] Most of the tumors associated with this syndrome have been carcinoid or pancreatic islet cell tumors, but a hypothalamic gangliocytoma also can be present in patients with acromegaly.[255]

The initial identification and isolation of GRH (the hypothalamic factor) was from a patient with an islet cell tumor who had acromegaly. The protein and DNA sequences were identical to those of hypothalamic GRH when determined from an extract of this tumor.[256] The peptide also has been identified by immunohistochemical means in small cell carcinoma, even in the absence of the clinical syndrome.[257] Somatostatin as well as long-acting somatostatin analogues have now been shown to be useful in treating acromegaly as well as ectopic tumors secreting GRH.[258, 259]

Human Placental Lactogen

Human placental lactogen (hPL) (or human chorionic somatomammotropin, hCS) is a protein hormone produced by the trophoblastic layer of the placenta which is closely related to hGH in its biological and immunological properties as well as its amino acid sequence.[260] It is representative of the structural homologies that are present between placental and pituitary hormones—pituitary ACTH with human chorionic corticotropin, luteinizing hormone with human chorionic gonadotropin, pituitary growth hormone and prolactin with human placental lactogen. Grumbach et al.[261] reported increased concentrations of hPL (normally only a female hormone during pregnancy) in the serum of a male with gynecomastia and an anaplastic large cell carcinoma of the lung. The patient's tumor previously had been reported to contain gonadotropin by bioassay. Weintraub and Rosen[262] noted that 11 of 128 patients with nontrophoblastic tumors had elevated levels of hPL. Seven of 64 patients with lung tumors had increased hPL in sera; 5 of these patients had gynecomastia and increased secretion of estradiol (4 of the 5 also had evidence for increased production of chorionic gonadotropin). In 89 nonneoplastic sera studied by Weintraub and Rosen[262] and in other sera studied by Payne and Ruan,[263] no hPL was noted. Thus the presence of this protein in nonpregnant sera was truly indicative of a hormone-producing tumor. In some cases, Weintraub and Rosen[262] were only able to detect hPL in the sera after concentration by affinity chromatography. In their normal subjects, even affinity chromatography provided no evidence for the peptide hormone, indicating concentrations of less than 0.002 ng/ml. Of the patients with nontrophoblastic tumors, hPL was detected in seven with lung tumors (four undifferentiated, one oat cell, one adenocarcinoma, and one epidermoid tumor) and one each with lymphoma, pheochromocytoma, hepatoma, and hepatoblastoma. The series was biased in terms of patients who had gynecomastia; the only other individuals having elevated values of hPL in blood consisted of both male and female patients with trophoblastic tumors. In patients with nontrophoblastic tumors, hPL concentration varied from 0.007 to 14 ng/ml; in patients with trophoblastic tumors, from 3 to 180 ng/ml; and in normal third-trimester subjects, from 2 to 7 µ/ml. There was a reasonable correlation between the level of hPL in patients with trophoblastic tumors and effective therapy. The hormone in tissue extracts and plasma behaved identically in the radioimmunoassay to native hPL, but the level was well below that required for lactogenic or somatotropic assay activity in most bioassay systems.

The presence of ectopic hPL has been shown to be associated with the production of other placental proteins, such as chorionic gonadotropin (hCG) and placental alkaline phosphatase.[264, 265] The concordance of these three markers in indicating the presence of cancer was suggested by Sussman et al.,[264] who studied sera from eight patients with nontrophoblastic malignancy. Three sera contained all three marker proteins, three sera contained two of the three markers (alkaline phosphatase and hCG or hCG and hPL), and two sera contained only one marker (alkaline phosphatase or hPL). Concordance of biochemical markers and clinical responses was noted, however, when this was studied in detail.[264, 265]

There has been considerable interest in the identification of placental hormones as tumor markers. In two reports,[266, 267] hPL was identified as a marker of breast cancer. Horne et al.[266] studied 50 carcinomas of the breast by an enzyme-bridge immunoperoxidase technique to deter-

mine the presence of a pregnancy-specific β_1-glycoprotein, hPL, and hCG. In their studies, β_1-glycoprotein was present in 76 per cent, hPL in 82 per cent, and hCG in 60 per cent. In 60 per cent of the tumors, all three proteins were present. Appropriate controls were used to rule out nonspecific findings, although the results were qualitative rather than quantitative. Of interest was the observation that an improved prognosis was associated with the absence rather than the presence of the β_1-glycoprotein and hPL. Sheth et al.[267] found that 10 of 72 women with carcinoma of the breast had detectable hPL in sera; 12 had detectable hCG-β subunits. Control studies of patients with cystic mastitis, fibroadenoma, and breast inflammation and of normal men and women did not show detectable hormones. The concentration of hPL varied from 3 to 5 ng/ml and of hCG-β from 3 to 25 ng/ml. There was no correlation between circulating concentrations of hPL and size of the tumor. More premenopausal than postmenopausal women had detectable hPL, while the reverse was true of hCG-β. None of the tumors secreted both hCG and hPL simultaneously, unlike the findings in trophoblastic tumors. Although the levels of hPL were significant, they were considerably below those found in the third trimester of normal pregnancy (mean of 4.3 µg/ml).

Evidence has accumulated that there is a "big" form of hPL in placental tissue and in the blood of pregnant women[268, 269] that is closely related to "big" forms of hGH and prolactin. Further studies have shown this larger material to be a disulfide dimer of the native molecule.[270] This does not appear to be a precursor hormone, but its significance needs to be determined. Further studies of ectopic tumors that produce hPL will have to be examined carefully for the presence of larger forms of the molecule in tumor tissue extracts and in blood.

Prolactin

Pituitary prolactin has significant chemical homologies with both pituitary growth hormone and placental lactogen.[271] Turkington[272] demonstrated elevated concentrations of prolactin in the serum of a man with undifferentiated carcinoma of the lung and a woman with galactorrhea who had renal-cell carcinoma. Following therapy with radiation and nephrectomy, serum concentrations of prolactin by radioimmunoassay decreased. The renal-cell carcinoma was shown to produce prolactin in tissue culture, which was verified by bioassay and neutralized by prolactin antibodies. Measurements of prolactin in the sera of 20 additional patients with carcinoma of the lung failed to show any increase. Rees et al.[273] also have identified immunoreactive prolactin in a bronchogenic tumor.

Immunocytochemistry has been used to show prolactin in both normal breast and prostate tissue as well as in carcinoma of the prostate and infiltrating breast carcinoma.[274] Since breast and prostate cancers may have receptors for prolactin as well, this could represent an autocrine-type function. Ectopic prolactin synthesis remains a relatively rare event.

Glycoprotein Hormones: Gonadotropins

The clinical association between tumors of the lung and gynecomastia was first described[275] in 1915, and ectopic production of gonadotropin has been associated with abnormalities of the breast. Furthermore, a number of boys with precocious puberty secondary to production of a luteinizing hormone (LH)–like substance have been described by McArthur et al.[276] These patients also had other associated abnormalities such as spina bifida occulta and hemihypertrophy of the tongue and extremities. Hepatomegaly in these subjects was associated with accelerated growth and virilization, and increased LH activity was demonstrated. At autopsy, the liver revealed a tumor or hepatoblastoma, and the testes showed proliferation of Leydig cells. Ectopic hormone production in these patients could not be suppressed with estrogen therapy.

Gynecomastia is frequently found in adults with malignant disease, especially when they have liver disease or are receiving drugs such as chlorpromazine, digitalis, reserpine, or spironolactone.[276] Gynecomastia has been associated with carcinoma of the lung and sometimes with hypertrophic pulmonary osteoarthropathy. Increased estrogen production has been reported in patients with carcinoma of the lung, and this may be related to the production of gonadotropin by lung tumors or metabolism of estrogen precursors.[261] The presence of increased gonadotropin and gynecomastia may even antedate the appearance of the lung tumor.[277, 278] In some patients, gynecomastia was felt to be due to gonadotropin production with secondary increases in estrogen production. A low content of gonadotropin was measured in the pituitary at autopsy, supporting the concept that gonadotropin production occurred from the tumor.

Faiman et al.[279] reported a step-up in the arteriovenous concentrations for follicle-stimulating hormone (FSH) across an adenocarcinoma of the lung, providing direct evidence for production of this hormone by the tumor. Although precocious puberty in boys and gynecomastia in men have been the principal syndromes associated with ectopic gonadotropin secretion, levels of hCG in excess of levels found in the first trimester of pregnancy also have been documented in patients without any clinical manifestations.[280] In addition to carcinoma of the lung and hepatoblastoma, tumors of the testis, ovary, pineal gland, mediastinum, adrenal, breast, bladder, pancreatic islet, stomach, kidney, and melanoma may be associated with ectopic gonadotropin production.[1, 281, 282] Two types of gonadotropins are produced by the normal pituitary, FSH and LH. These glycoprotein hormones have been shown to consist of both α and β subunits. The α subunit is identical in the gonadotropins and thyroid-stimulating hormone. Immunologically, the α subunits are indistinguishable; the β subunit, on the other hand, is different and accounts for hormonal specificity.[283] Assays are available not only for the intact hormone but also for the α and β subunits, and they have been used in screening as tumor markers. Production of ectopic FSH by tumors is uncommon but has been suggested by Rosen et al.[278] To date, despite these very suggestive reports, unequivocal ectopic production of FSH and LH by tumors has not been demonstrated.[283]

Estrogen production in men with gonadotropin-producing neoplasms has been studied by Kirschner et al.[284] Urinary estradiol production rates were elevated in six men with gonadotropin-producing tumors (four with choriocarcinoma and two with tumors of stomach and lung) and were correlated with gonadotropin level and tumor mass.

The origin of the elevated estradiol was determined by administering dehydroepiandrosterone sulfate (DHEAS) intravenously and determining conversion to estradiol; radioactive DHEAS also was incubated with tumor tissue. Gonadotropin-producing tumors could convert DHEAS directly to estradiol, indicating that they behave like normal trophoblastic tissue. These findings provide an additional indication that the tumor behaves like placental tissue in that it can carry out the same biochemical function.

In recent years, there has been great interest in the production of gonadotropins, particularly hCG, by both nontrophoblastic tumors and normal cells.[125] hCG is a primary secretory product of the trophoblast and is known to be elevated early in pregnancy. In the past, its measurement was used principally for documentation of pregnancy and for the diagnosis, evaluation, and follow-up of patients with gestational neoplasms, particularly hydatidiform mole and choriocarcinoma. It is also elevated in males with histologically related tumors of the testis. Recent progress in this field has depended on the development of radioimmunoassays that are specific for the β subunit of hCG and that differentiate the placental marker protein from its closely related structural homologue pituitary LH. This permits measurement of concentrations of hCG as low as 1 ng in the presence of physiological quantities of LH.

Braunstein et al.[124] first called attention to an hCG-like substance in extracts of normal human testicular tissue. This protein was parallel with hCG standards in the radioimmunoassay, co-chromatographed with hCG on gel filtration, and was adsorbed to Con A. In subsequent studies by several workers, hCG-like substances were identified in a number of other tissues. Yoshimoto et al.[126] identified β-hCG by radioimmunoassay and radioreceptor assay in extracts of normal colon and liver, although they found that the material did not bind Con A well and suggested that it might have less carbohydrate by exoglycosidase digestion. There is heterogeneity in ectopic hCG, but in general, it is glycosylated similar to placental hCG.[285, 286] Using an antibody against the unique C-terminal portion of hCG, Chen et al.[287] found evidence in normal subjects of a protein that had physical-chemical, immunological, and biological similarities to hCG. Borkowski and Muquardt[288] extracted hCG from human plasma in normal nonpregnant subjects and found a level of 18 pg/ml in the plasma of 13 normal men. Braunstein et al.[125, 289] identified an hCG-like protein in numerous normal human tissues, including the ovary, pituitary, lung, liver, kidney, spleen, stomach, placenta, and small intestine. The techniques used involve both highly specific radioimmunoassays and radioreceptor assays. The concentrations were 1 to 11 ng/g in normal tissues, over 5000 ng/g in the placenta, and over 20,000 ng/g in the pituitary. The pituitary material was felt to be distinct from LH.

During Con A–binding studies, the extracts of various tissues varied widely in the degree of adsorption of the immunoreactive substance to the lectin. More of the material present in testes, ovaries, placenta, or small intestine adsorbed to Con A than was the case with the material in lung, liver, or kidney. These findings were similar to those of Yoshimoto et al.,[126] who identified hCG-like material in all extracts of normal human tissues studied (colon, liver, and lung) at concentrations varying from 1.2 to 7 ng/g.

Given that hCG production may be common to a variety of normal tissues, there has been extensive interest in examining the production of this protein by tumors. Prior to the development of specific assays for hCG, there were relatively few reports of ectopic hCG production. Braunstein et al.[290] studied sera from 906 patients with nontrophoblastic neoplasms and found that 11.4 per cent had detectable hCG. A number of other investigators examined multiple human sera, and the highest frequency of positives was found in patients with gynecological, breast, lung, and gastrointestinal tract tumors, as well as melanoma, with an average of approximately 19 per cent. The actual production of hCG by these tumors may be more frequent than that. Yoshimoto et al.[126] found that 7 of 30 tumors studied contained hCG-like material in amounts greater than those in normal tissue; the rest contained it in amounts similar to those in normal tissue. The values in cancer patients varied from 1 to greater than 100 ng/g. In their studies, Con A bound 92.5 per cent of hCG from the placenta, 31 per cent of cancer tissue hCG, and only 6 per cent of hCG from normal tissues. The discrepancy between the frequency of positive assays for hCG in sera and in tumor tissues may be related to defective glycosylation or the short half-life of desialated hCG in the circulation.

The levels of hCG in the circulation of cancer patients are low, usually in the range of 1 to 5 ng/ml (at the lower limit of detection of the hCG-β assay). The presence of hCG in serum is not absolutely specific for cancer, since 2.6 per cent of control subjects were found to have detectable hCG.[291] Further close follow-up of these positive controls may show some to harbor an occult neoplasm, but this needs to be determined. Braunstein et al.[290] examined serum samples from 1150 patients for the presence of the β subunit and found it to be present in 11.6 per cent of 876 patients with nontrophoblastic tumors and 1.5 per cent of 1074 patients with benign disorders. There were no significant differences in age, race, or histological type of tumor between patients with neoplasms who had hCG present and those who did not. More of the patients with metastatic disease who were positive were women. Patients over 50 years of age with benign disorders were more likely to have false-positive tests. The majority of patients had values between 1 and 5 ng/ml, while no patient with a benign disorder had levels greater than 10, and 13 per cent of patients with tumor production of hormone had levels above this. Thus serum hCG measurements were of limited usefulness in screening for nontrophoblastic malignancies.

Hattori et al.[292] found hCG in 10 of 100 plasma samples from patients with malignancy and in none of 56 control subjects. In tumor tissues, hCG was identified in 42 per cent, and it was suggested that APUD tumors might contain smaller amounts of hCG than non-APUD tumors. Papapetrou et al.[293] studied hCG in both the sera and urine of patients with malignant disease. They found 17.1 per cent of patients positive in sera and 44.3 per cent in urine; 20 patients were positive only in urine. The hCG-like immunoreactive material in the urine was mostly a species smaller than hCG and hCG-β, although its nature was not further known. Weymann and Nisula[294] studied the renal clearance rates of subunits of hCG in humans and found that excretion of unaltered subunit accounts for a very small fraction of the total metabolic removal of hCG. Twelve hours after injection of the hCG-β subunit, 90 per cent of the immunoreactivity in the urine was in a fragment that contained carbohydrate and had a molecular weight

about 25 per cent that of the injected peptide. Within the first 4 hours after injection, most of the material was intact.

Goldenberg et al.[295] used antibodies to hCG coupled to ^{125}I in an attempt to localize tumor tissue. In several patients this showed promise, and excision of one of the metastatic tumors located by this method indicated a tumor/nontumor radioactive ratio of 39. There are many technical problems, including sensitivity, that have to be resolved, but the use of this advanced technology may be promising in locating tumor tissue. On the other hand, the status of hormone production by the tumors may or may not be related to the amount of tumor tissue present. A similar approach has been used for tumors producing carcinoembryonic antigen.[296]

Production of hormones also may vary at different times in the life cycle of the tumor. In a patient who had large cell carcinoma of the lung and gynecomastia reported by Metz et al.,[297] preoperative levels of hCG were 109 ng/ml, with the α and β subunit concentrations being 3.2 and 21 ng/ml, respectively; after complete tumor resection and resolution of gynecomastia, hCG titers remained elevated at 3.3 ng/ml, indicating tumor recurrence. During this time, administration of luteinizing hormone–releasing hormone (LHRH) produced a markedly delayed increase in pituitary gonadotropins. Subsequent chemotherapy, helped by the use of hCG measurements, reduced it to undetectable levels, and the response to LHRH was then normal.

Considerable work in recent years has defined mechanisms for the biosynthesis of the subunits of hCG and other glycoprotein hormones.[298, 301] These studies have established the separate synthesis of the two subunits and identified posttranslational processing that involves carbohydrate addition. A variety of different-sized products may be produced, and in some cases, the released α subunit may be larger than the one in the cells due to carbohydrate addition.[302–305] These findings may have ultimate implications for the kinds of subunits and intact molecules produced by tumors. There are two reports of abnormal β subunits produced by ectopic tumor.[306, 307]

A major problem at present is the fact that normal tissues can produce hCG, and in a small percentage of normal subjects, there will be detectable hCG in blood. Although hCG measurements may be useful as a screening agent, they certainly do not prove cancer, but the patient with a positive assay needs to be followed up carefully. Further information on these points is necessary in order to improve the care of patients with hCG-producing tumors.

Considerable work has been performed with hCG and its subunits and with cells in tissue culture that produce them. This is a most promising area of research and may help to clarify some of the molecular mechanisms involved. The following specific observations have been made:

1. Desialation results in marked loss of biological potency in vivo but not in vitro for the gonadotropins. Immunological activity is also dependent on the peptide and is preserved in desialated molecules.[308]

2. Cross-reactivity of the glycoprotein hormones within a species resides primarily in the α subunit, while that between species is primarily in the β subunit.[308]

3. Large quantities of free hCG-α subunits have been identified in placental tissue from all trimesters of preg-

nancy, the tissue concentration of hCG-α being at least 10 times greater than that of hCG itself in the last two trimesters, although the concentration of the complete hormone in the blood exceeds that of the free subunit. The subunits have a shorter half-life in plasma, and no free hCG-β subunits are found in placental tissue or peripheral blood during pregnancy.[308]

4. Normal human pituitary extracts contain free α subunits.[309, 310] An increase in α subunits in sera of patients with hypothyroidism following TRH administration or following LHRH administration in postmenopausal women has been noted.

5. Elevated hCG concentrations are more likely to be present in carcinoma of the gastrointestinal tract (18 per cent), breast (21 per cent), or lung (10 per cent). Specificity for malignancy is not present in the gastrointestinal tract, since inflammatory bowel disease, cirrhosis, and peptic ulcer also can result in detectable hCG.[308] HeLa cell cultures have been shown to produce hCG and subunits in tissue culture. Ghosh and Cox[311] reported the production by HeLa cells of hCG-β, as measured by specific RIA. Sodium butyrate markedly increased the production rate of hCG-β, increasing both the intracellular and extracellular concentrations. Lieblich et al.[312] reported production of α subunits by HeLa cells in culture. Three different cell lines secreted a substance that was immunologically indistinguishable from hCG-α, the secretion rates varying by as much as 50-fold. No hCG-β was detected in these cultures, and hCG-α appeared to have a slightly higher molecular weight than the normal subunit. It is probably similar to the hCG-α produced by a gastric carcinoma in vivo and a bronchogenic carcinoma in vitro.[313] The α subunit could be a precursor of the normal subunit.

6. Lieblich et al.[314] compared the rate of release of hCG and subunits from a bronchogenic carcinoma in tissue culture with that from a choriocarcinoma under identical conditions. The choriocarcinoma secreted only hCG and the bronchogenic carcinoma only α subunits under identical conditions. Production of ectopic α subunits actually exceeded the ectopic production of hCG, although increased degradation was not ruled out. The choriocarcinoma had a relatively small intracellular pool of α subunits, in contrast to the large pool in normal placental tissue. Marked variation in the production of hCG and subunits by various tumors is quite likely and will be determined by further studies.

7. Weintraub et al.[315] studied in detail the α subunits produced by a gastric carcinoid and bronchogenic carcinoma. These subunits were slightly larger than the normal subunit but were co-chromatographed on ion-exchange chromatography. One α subunit showed decreased ability to combine with hCG-β, and the other had no detectable combining activity when incubated with hCG-β. The results were interpreted as reflecting either abnormalities of the protein synthesized by the tumors with respect to its polypeptide backbone or carbohydrate content or possibly the production of an hCG-α precursor.

8. Using the unique carboxyl-terminal peptide of hCG as an antigen, Chen et al.[287] developed a radioimmunoassay specific for hCG in contrast to LH. Studies with this assay provided clear evidence that there is hCG activity in postmenopausal urinary extracts and in normal human pituitary glands.

9. Weintraub et al.[315] looked exhaustively at the combi-

nation of α and β subunits in vitro, using both RIA and RRA to detect recombination. Caution must be observed, since alterations resulting from purification of the hormone or dissociation during purification of subunits is possible. Abnormalities in the combination of ectopic α subunits with β subunits were noted.

10. Cell-free translation of RNA from tumors produced α subunits of larger than normal size,[316] presumably the precursor.

The production of hCG by tumors leads to no symptoms, except for gynecomastia in some males. In these instances, it is not always clear whether increased estrogen is due to the gonad's response to gonadotropins or to the tumor's ability to produce estradiol or to convert dehydroepiandrosterone sulfate to estradiol.[284] The widespread identification of hCG and its subunits in both normal and abnormal tissues is of great interest but needs further clarification. Quantitative differences between patients may be as important as qualitative ones.

Glycoprotein Hormones: Thyrotropin

Hyperthyroidism has been described principally in patients with trophoblastic tumors, although a similar syndrome has been described with epidermoid carcinoma of the lung and mesothelioma.[1] The hyperthyroidism found in these patients is usually mild, although severe hyperthyroidism has been described, particularly in association with choriocarcinoma.[317, 318] The hyperthyroid state is more common in hydatidiform mole, however. Miyai et al.[319] studied 12 patients with trophoblastic disease, including 4 with hydatidiform mole, 3 with invasive mole, and 5 with choriocarcinoma. In 6 of the 12 patients, thyroid-stimulating activity was detectable by the McKenzie bioassay. In this group, pituitary thyroid-stimulating hormone (TSH) was usually undetectable and did not respond to thyrotropin-releasing hormone (TRH). In the group without detectable thyroid-stimulating activity, basal TSH was detectable in half the patients and responded to TRH in all. Serum concentrations of total thyroxin (T_4) were 18.7 versus 9.2 μg/100 ml; free T_4, 4.9 versus 2.0 ng/100 ml; and total T_3, 352 versus 156 ng/100 ml in the two groups, respectively. Following treatment of the patients with hyperthyroidism, thyroid-stimulating activity became detectable, and the serum TSH response to TRH was positive. These findings suggested strongly that the trophoblastic thyroid stimulator increased thyroid hormone secretion, which in turn suppressed pituitary TSH and its response to TRH. Of the patients with hyperthyroidism, 3 had hydatidiform mole, 1 had invasive mole, and 2 had choriocarcinoma.

There is fairly convincing evidence that the thyrotropic stimulator associated with trophoblastic disease is in fact hCG. Cave and Dunn[317] reported a 15-year-old girl with severe hyperthyroidism and metastatic choriocarcinoma whose serum contained high levels of hCG and thyroid-stimulating activity different from pituitary TSH or long-acting thyroid stimulator. Gradient ultracentrifugation, gel filtration, and gel electrophoresis showed that the tumor protein was similar to hCG. Morely et al.[318] described three patients with choriocarcinoma and hyperthyroidism in whom correction of thyrotoxicosis was parallel to the fall in hCG. In two of the three, the ratio of TSH biological activity to immunoassayable hCG was in the range of 0.37 to 0.59 (compared with a native hCG ratio of 0.42), while in the third it was 1.41, suggesting the possibility of an ectopic thyrotropin separate from hCG. Although there was evidence for chorionic thyrotropin in earlier studies, no definitive evidence for its existence or pathogenetic role in hyperthyroidism during abnormal pregnancy has been documented.

Since hCG has been postulated to be the thyrotropic factor in trophoblastic and nontrophoblastic neoplasms associated with hyperthyroidism, further studies have been performed on the thyroid-stimulating capabilities of hCG. Amir et al.[319] studied the interaction of both crude and purified hCG with receptors in human thyroid membranes by examining the binding of iodinated TSH and adenylate cyclase activation. These studies showed that crude preparations of hCG contained a factor that inhibited the binding of iodinated bovine TSH to human thyroid. There also was a factor in the crude preparations that inhibited the stimulation of adenylate cyclase by bovine TSH. Purified hCG did not stimulate adenylate cyclase directly or inhibit its response to bovine TSH. Pekonen and Weintraub[320, 321] conducted similar studies and found that the cross-reactivity in a TSH radioreceptor assay using bovine TSH and thyroid membranes was very great with crude hCG but very limited with the purified preparation. However, when "physiological" conditions were used, the crude and purified preparations behaved similarly, and the effect of the other protein inhibitors was abolished. Based on these studies, the authors concluded that the thyrotropic activity of 1 IU of hCG was equivalent to 0.5 to 0.8 µIU of bovine TSH. With the very high levels of hCG present in choriocarcinoma or hydatidiform mole, there would be sufficient thyrotropic activity to account for the hyperthyroid response.

The association of mild hyperthyroidism with trophoblastic neoplasms has been known for 25 years. Higgins and Herschman[322] studied 20 patients with hydatidiform mole and found that 12 were euthyroid, while 6 were severely and 2 mildly hyperthyroid. The 6 patients with more severe disease had clinical signs and symptoms, and all had a palpable goiter. Two patients developed supraventricular tachycardia and pulmonary edema, while a number of the other patients had significant symptoms. In the past, most studies showed that the patients were clinically euthyroid even though their circulating levels of free thyroid hormone were increased. Molar pregnancy is much more common in the Far East, being 10 times as frequent as in the West. The current data still point to hCG as the pathogenic factor in the disease. hCG increases adenylate cyclase activity in human thyroid membranes, although its effects are very slight. Harada and Herschman[323] extracted human term placentas and failed to obtain significant evidence for a separate human chorionic thyrotropin.

An interesting variant of TSH has been found in plasma by Kourides et al.[324] and Spitz et al.[325]; it is of higher molecular weight than the normal protein. In the three patients in whom a large form of TSH was described, the higher molecular weight of TSH could be related to posttranslational processing and probably does not represent a precursor. The patients studied by Spitz et al.[325] were euthyroid with an elevated TSH level. The material showed normal binding to TSH receptor but decreased stimulation of adenylate cyclase.

Vasopressin (Antidiuretic Hormone) and Related Peptides (Propressophysin, Neurophysin)

The association of malignant disease and inappropriate secretion of antidiuretic hormone (ADH) is now recognized frequently. A possible connection between the tumor and production of ADH was described by Winkler and Cranshaw[326] when they noted increased excretion of sodium in some cases of lung cancer, but no definite suggestion of a hormonal link was made. In 1957, Schwartz and colleagues[327] reported two patients with bronchogenic tumors who had concentrated urine containing large quantities of sodium despite the fact that they had severe hyponatremia. The authors suggested correctly that the water and electrolyte disorder was due to inappropriate secretion of ADH, but they suggested that the tumor stimulated secretion of ADH by the posterior pituitary. Additional data concerning the relationship to the tumor were provided by Thorn and Transbol,[328] who showed the presence of large quantities of antidiuretic hormone in the urine of such a patient. Definitive evidence was provided by Amatruda et al.,[329] who showed evidence for ADH-like material in extracts of an oat cell carcinoma. Subsequently, a number of workers have reported ADH in extracts of tumor, with values ranging from 4 to 750 µU/mg dry tumor.[330–333] In 1967, Bartter and Schwartz[334] reported an additional 12 patients with the hyponatremic syndrome and indicated that an ADH-like substance in tumor extract behaved in the immunoassay like vasopressin. Most of the reports are from carcinoma of the lung (particularly oat cell carcinoma but also adenocarcinoma and large cell carcinoma), but the syndrome also has been described in duodenal and pancreatic carcinoma.[1, 130] Twenty-eight of 38 reported cases have been oat cell carcinoma of the lung, 7 being due to anaplastic carcinoma. Other cases have been mucin-secreting adenocarcinomas of the lung and pancreas,[130] as well as carcinoma of the ureter, bladder, and prostate, and lymphoma.[335, 336] It has been described in 7 or more per cent of patients with small cell carcinoma.[337]

Comis et al.[338] evaluated 41 patients with small cell carcinoma of the lung for water abnormalities using a standard water loading test; 68 per cent had abnormalities. They found these abnormalities in 47 per cent of patients with carcinoma in one hemithorax and in 86 per cent with more extensive disease. Forty-six per cent had the syndrome of inappropriate ADH secretion (SIADH). Zerbe et al.[339] reviewed the various types of vasopressin release in patients with SIADH and discussed the multiple possible mechanisms in patients with cancer, other than ectopic hormone production. These included hypovolemia, obstruction of the vena cava, invasion of the vagus nerve, metastases to the hypothalamus, drug administration, carcinomatous neuropathy, as well as ectopic production of a vasopressin-releasing factor.

Robertson[340] described a number of patients with elevated plasma levels of tumor vasopressin in the absence of the clinical syndrome. Because of the close physiological tie between serum osmolality and vasopressin, the magnitude of vasopressin secretion must be assessed in relation to serum osmolality. Normal physiological regulation involves a flat response of vasopressin secretion until the critical threshold of osmolality is reached, following which a large increase in secretion is observed. In patients with carcinoma, inappropriate levels of vasopressin are seen at lower than normal levels of serum osmolality.

Studies by Padfield et al.[341, 342] showed that the patterns of vasopressin secretion in patients with ectopic ADH production may be quite variable. In some cases, the physiological response to changes in osmolality is normal, but the osmostat appears to be set at an abnormal level. In the patient with malignant disease, a number of factors may cause SIADH, and it is important to differentiate potential tumor production of ADH from the multiple other causes. Perks et al.[343] described a patient with malignant mesothelioma and SIADH who had increased serum and urine concentrations of arginine vasopressin but no vasopressin in the tumor. It appears more likely that nonosmotic stimuli related to the patient's extensive chest diseases may have been factors in stimulating ADH, working through pulmonary baroreceptors or the vagus nerve.

Although Skrabanek and Powell[344] reviewed the evidence for ectopic ADH production and suggested that it was still incomplete, recent studies suggest that the documentation is more complete.[345] Pettingill et al.[346] reported a cell line from an oat cell carcinoma that synthesized small amounts of immunoreactive arginine vasopressin in vitro. Kondo et al.[347] obtained tumor tissue at autopsy from a 58-year-old man with bronchogenic oat cell carcinoma and SIADH. The tumor tissue was transplanted serially in nude mice, with 20 passages over more than 4 years, and the plasma levels of vasopressin in the mice were 24 to 50 pg/ml and in the tumor tissue 1.3 ng/g. Furthermore, neurophysin was detected in both plasma and tumor tissues (7.5 ng/ml and 2.8 μg/g, respectively). The nude mice had water retention with high sodium concentrations in the urine, and when they were hydrated, they had decreased water clearance. They did not become hyponatremic because they drank less, but when loaded with water, they developed a marked decrease in plasma sodium concentration. This tumor obviously produced ADH and induced SIADH in the nude mice. It is a useful experimental model and provides further convincing evidence for ectopic ADH production by human tumors.

Padfield et al.[342] studied 17 patients with SIADH associated with bronchogenic carcinoma and found that plasma arginine vasopressin (AVP) levels were elevated in most. In 14 patients with tumors but without overt SIADH, levels also were significantly higher than normal. This finding, together with the lower than normal osmolality, suggested that ADH excess might be more common than believed. The usual positive correlation between osmolality and plasma AVP is reversed in SIADH associated with ectopic tumors. Kelly and Morton[348] examined tumor tissues from 32 patients with carcinoma of the bronchus and found immunological activity in only three, all of whom had small cell tumors and two had hyponatremia. AVP levels varied between 28 and 164 pg/mg wet weight. These findings argue against the conclusion that ectopic secretion is the cause of raised ADH in patients with carcinoma of the bronchus and a normal serum sodium level. However, the study was not conclusive, since plasma levels were not known, and there could have been tissue destruction. In another study, Morton et al.[341, 348] found immunological activity only in small cell tumors. Perks et al.[344] studied 29 patients with histologically proven mesotheliomas and found 62 per cent with hyponatremia. The authors believed that the hyponatremia was not only caused by ectopic production of ADH but also could be due to reflex effects through the vagus nerve. Compression of pulmonary baroreceptors or infiltration of the vagus nerve by the mesothelioma could lead to reflex secretion of ADH.

The concentrations of ectopic ADH have been too small to permit purification and structural characterization, but the hormone behaves immunologically like arginine vasopressin, and indirect evidence suggests that it is very similar to the human hormone.[333] Certain properties of ectopic ADH make it similar to pituitary ADH,[130] as follows:

1. Inactivation by thioglycolate, which disrupts the disulfide bond
2. Persistence of biological activity similar to arginine vasopressin after the purification procedure
3. Similar behavior chromatographically on ion-exchange chromatography
4. Affinity for neurophysin
5. Susceptibility to inactivation by oxytocinase
6. Immunological similarities to arginine vasopressin
7. Inactivation by vasopressin antibodies
8. Synthesis of vasopressin by bronchogenic carcinoma in vitro[349]
9. Generation by limited trypsin digestion of labeled propressophysin precursor[350]
10. Release of ADH by tumor tissue in culture[351]
11. Cell-free translation of mRNA for vasopressin and neurophysin and reproduction of the syndrome in the nude mouse[347]
12. The mRNA for atrial natriuretic peptide (ANP) also has been found in some tumor extracts from patients with hyponatremia.[352] A recent report described ANP and ADH in both the plasma and tumor of a patient with small cell carcinoma and hyponatremia.

Since extraction of ADH from the tumors has been obtained and the hormone synthesized in vitro in tumor tissue by at least several investigators, it is clear that tumor production of hormone is at least one mechanism that accounts for the inappropriate ADH syndrome. However, a number of other causes exist, as follows:

1. Metastases to the hypothalamus stimulating production of ADH
2. A mediastinal or thoracic tumor affecting volume receptors and stimulating ADH secretion
3. Renal tubular defects in association with tumors, leading to natriuresis
4. Central nervous system infections such as tuberculosis, basilar meningitis, or complicating tumors
5. Cerebrovascular disease
6. Subdural hematoma
7. Systemic illnesses such as polyneuritis, systemic lupus erythematosus, and pulmonary infection
8. Administration of certain drugs such as chlorpropamide, tolbutamide, vincristine, morphine, and estrogen
9. Excessive use of cigarettes (bronchial epithelial dysplasia)
10. Pain, trauma, and emotional stress
11. Production of an ADH-like factor which is not ADH by tumors[354]

These and other factors must all be considered in the patient with malignancy who is noted to have inappropriate ADH secretion.[355] The hallmarks of the syndrome are hyponatremia, persistently concentrated urine in the face of hyponatremia, a low blood urea nitrogen (BUN), and the absence of peripheral edema. Although the syndrome is characterized by excessive secretion of ADH, it will not be clinically apparent unless there is intake of sufficient water parenterally or orally. In a patient who has excessive secretion of hormone, the syndrome is not demonstrable clinically when fluid intake is restricted.

The clinical findings in the severe syndrome include symptoms of water intoxication and complications such as anorexia, nausea, vomiting, headache, fatigue, confusion, pseudobulbar palsy, and ultimately coma if the serum sodium level is low enough.[334] Although treatment by fluid restriction is usually successful, hypertonic saline may occasionally be helpful in severely hyponatremic states. Hantman et al.[356] suggested that intravenous furosemide with hypertonic saline may produce negative water balance while conserving sodium and potassium. Other approaches to the treatment of inappropriate ADH syndrome include the use of lithium[357] and demethylchlortetracycline.[358] Administration of diphenylhydantoin (500 mg intravenously in 5 min) has been shown to correct the inappropriate antidiuresis of many disorders, but it has no effect when it is due to a neoplasm. Therapy for the inappropriate ADH syndrome is usually accomplished by fluid restriction below 1 L per day (for more severe cases below 500 ml/day). Fluid restriction does not remove the source of the ADH, but it controls the clinical manifestations. The actual quantity of fluid retained in these patients is approximately 3 to 4 L.

Decaux et al.[359] have described treatment with exogenous urea, the latter lowering urinary sodium excretion and increasing plasma sodium as long as the value was less than 130 mEq/L. Urea also induced a persistent osmotic diuresis, allowing a normal daily intake of water. Up to 30 g urea per day was administered over a number of weeks, and this was suggested as an alternative to other therapy. The potential risk of this therapy is dehydration if the patient does not drink enough. Demeclocycline is not well tolerated by some patients because of potential nephrotoxicity, although it is believed to be superior to lithium. Short-term treatment with urea[359] and chronic administration of oral furosemide together with adequate salt intake[360] also have been used in the syndrome.

Propressophysin, a 20-kDa polypeptide, has now been identified as the biosynthetic precursor for both vasopressin and neurophysin.[361] Hamilton et al.[362] reported that neurophysin may be produced by some tumors in patients with the syndrome. Neurophysin is a normal protein component of the posterior hypothalamus that is responsible for binding oxytocin and vasopressin, and its release is elevated by stimuli that cause the release of the two hormones.[363, 364]

North et al.[365] used the radioimmunoassay for two human neurophysins to study 61 patients with small cell carcinoma of the lung. They found that plasma levels of one or both of these proteins were elevated to more than three times normal in 62 per cent of patients before the beginning of therapy. Presumably, these elevations were the result of production and release by the tumor. Eighteen patients who had elevated values prior to therapy were followed, and there was an excellent correlation between decreases in neurophysin concentrations and the clinical

response of the patient. Partial or complete response in 12 patients was associated with a marked reduction in circulating concentrations and with a rise during progression. Relapse was associated with an increase over earlier values. Thus the radioimmunoassay of neurophysins may be an extremely useful guide to the management of patients with small cell carcinoma of the lung.

Placental Enzymes

Tumor proteins may not lead to any clinical or biochemical abnormality in the patient but may be useful as a marker for disease. This is characteristic of proteins such as enzymes or antigens produced by tumor tissue which give a clue to the presence of a neoplasm but do not cause any clinical manifestations. The alkaline phosphatase enzyme of the placenta not normally found in adult men or nonpregnant women has been well described in a number of tumors by Stolbach et al.[366] The tumors producing ectopic alkaline phosphatase were primarily from the lung,[366] but other tumors also have been reported. The alkaline phosphatase produced by the ectopic tumor tends to be the placental-type enzyme, which is heat-stable and can be distinguished as a separate enzyme. In 50 nonneoplastic sera, no evidence of placental alkaline phosphatase was identified by Sussman et al.[264] The crucial issues for tumor markers are specificity and sensitivity.

ECTOPIC PRODUCTION OF HYPOGLYCEMIC SUBSTANCES

Although the association of tumors with hypoglycemia is well documented, the pathogenesis of hypoglycemia in these patients is still not clear. There are two major causes of fasting hypoglycemia associated with tumors: (1) insulin production by islet cell tumors and (2) production of hypoglycemia from extrapancreatic tumors by other mechanisms (Table 149–2). Although they may be clinically indistinguishable, separation often can be achieved by various laboratory studies and measurements. Other disorders associated with fasting hypoglycemia include severe liver disease, hypopituitarism, hypothyroidism, hypoadrenalism, and decreased glucagon reserve. Islet cell tumors are discussed in Chapter 92 and will not be reviewed here.

TABLE 149–2. POSSIBLE CAUSES OF HYPOGLYCEMIA IN PATIENTS WITH NON–ISLET CELL TUMORS

1. Production of insulin by the tumor (rare)
2. Production of NSILA-s or insulin-like growth factor (particularly IGF-II) by the tumor
3. Production of an insulin-secreting substance by the tumor
4. Production of insulin receptors by the tumor
5. Excessive glucose consumption by the tumor because of size
6. Production of cytokines (e.g., tumor necrosis factor) which enhance general tissue glucose uptake
7. Suppression of counterregulatory hormones or mechanisms (e.g., growth hormone, epinephrine)
8. Production of metabolites which interfere with gluconeogenesis (e.g., tryptophan)
9. Acquired glycogen storage disease (e.g., hepatocellular carcinoma)
10. Malnutrition
11. Chemotherapy

The extrapancreatic tumors associated with hypoglycemia can be separated into several groups defined below. To date, several hundred such patients have been reported.[1, 367]

1. Large mesenchymal or mesodermal tumors in the abdomen and thorax (42 per cent). These tumors may be retroperitoneal, intraperitoneal, or intrathoracic. They are frequently large and include fibrosarcomas, mesotheliomas, neurofibromas, neurofibrosarcomas, spindle-cell sarcomas, rhabdomyosarcomas, and leiomyosarcomas. They range in weight from 800 to 10,000 g, are frequency benign, and the symptoms are alleviated by their removal.

2. Hepatocellular carcinoma or hepatoma (22 per cent).

3. Adrenal cortical cell carcinoma (9 per cent).

4. Pancreatic, bile duct, and other gastrointestinal tumors (10 per cent).

5. Miscellaneous tumors, including lung, cervix, ovary, kidney, neuroblastoma, pheochromocytoma, hemangiopericytoma, Wilms' tumor, and lymphoma (17 per cent).

Few of these patients have had increases in serum insulin described, although there are occasional reports.[368–375] In the patient reported by Unger et al.,[369] immunoreactive insulin and glucagon were demonstrated at autopsy in the tumor, but there was no evidence confirming hypoglycemia during life. The report by Saeed et al.[370] suggested the presence of insulin or insulin-like activity on immunofluorescent staining of the tumors. Shames et al.[371] showed evidence of a bronchial carcinoid histologically very similar to an islet cell tumor of the pancreas which may have been histologically related. The report of Lyall et al.[372] showed no evidence of immunoreactive insulin in extracts of the tumors and no β-type secretory granules, but the patient had a clear increase of insulin in the basal state. Following removal of the tumor, glucose returned to normal, and the authors suggested the possibility that the tumor might be stimulating insulin release and possibly suppressing glucagon secretion. Shetty et al.[374] described tumors having secretory granules, but ultrastructural studies of several retroperitoneal sarcomas associated with hypoglycemia failed to reveal secretory granules. Thus there is no definite evidence that the hypoglycemia associated with extrapancreatic tumors is due to insulin production. Furthermore, it is claimed that insulin is widely present in normal tissues.[376]

On the other hand, these tumors can clearly produce insulin-like growth factors, which can be demonstrated by stimulation of glucose uptake in vitro in bioassays using rat diaphragm or adipose tissue.[367] Insulin activity in serum normally consists of both immunoreactive insulin (which can be neutralized by specific antibodies) and nonsuppressible insulin-like activity (NSILA-s), which is capable of accomplishing in vitro insulin-like biological effects and cannot be neutralized by insulin antibodies. The latter substance is immunologically distinct from insulin and represents different peptides.[377] NSILA-s is related to one or more of the somatomedin-like peptides that are produced in the liver of animals in response to GH administration. The possibility that NSILA-s was related to somatomedins was suggested when it was noted that somatomedin could be extracted from plasma by an acid ethanol extraction method similar to that used for purification of NSILA-s.[378] NSILA-s consists primarily of peptides with a structure similar to proinsulin and includes insulin-like growth factor I (IGF-I) or somatomedin C and IGF-II or multiplication-stimulating activity.[379, 380]

IGF-I has a molecular weight of 7500 Da, resembles proinsulin chemically, and is bound to a circulating protein. IGF-I has specific receptors, but it also binds weakly to insulin receptors and is believed to mediate some of the effects of growth hormone.[381] IGF-I is produced by cells from many tissues and is thought to be a paracrine-type factor stimulated by growth hormone.[382, 383] IGF-II is similar in size to IGF-I, binds a separate receptor, and also promotes tissue growth, but its dependency on GH is less well documented.[384]

NSILA-s has been suggested as the pathogenic factor causing hypoglycemia in some patients with non–islet cell tumors, but more specific assays have not always confirmed this. The variety of assays used for NSILA-s may account for some of the findings of different investigators. Megyesi et al.[385] used a radioreceptor assay that detects predominantly IGF-II and identified increased NSILA-s in some patients. Gorden et al.[386] reviewed the variety of tumor types associated with non–islet cell tumor hypoglycemia using an assay for multiplication-stimulating activity. Nineteen of 52 samples had IGF-II–like levels greater than 150 per cent of controls. Elevations were found in patients with hemangiopericytoma (six of seven), hepatoma (two of four), adrenocortical carcinoma (one of three), and pheochromocytoma (two of two). Patients with lymphoma and hypoglycemia had distinctly low values. This material was thought to be similar to IGF-II. Daughaday et al.,[384] using a radioreceptor assay for IGF-II with rat placental membranes, showed increased circulating levels in 10 of 14 sera from patients with tumor-related hypoglycemia. IGF-I, on the other hand, was low or unmeasurable. Another study showed slight increases in IGF-II and marked decreases in IGF-I in patients with malignancy and hypoglycemia.[379] Daughaday[381] recently reported a large fibrosarcoma which contained IGF largely as 10- to 15-kDa molecules rather than 7.5 kDa, the molecular weight of IGF-II, with a similar protein being found in plasma. He suggested that the higher-molecular-weight form was due to incomplete processing and was predominant in the syndrome.[111, 387] In addition, he has suggested a deficiency in IGF-binding proteins which may account for failure to find increased levels of IGF-II in the plasma of many patients with the syndrome.[388] The mechanism of hypoglycemia in this syndrome is unclear, but a variety of insulin-like growth factors, including IGF-I (somatomedin C), somatomedin A, and IGF-II (multiplication-stimulating activity) are able to lower blood glucose.[111] A recent report[389] of a hepatocellular carcinoma provided good documentation of increased IGF-II in plasma and tumor associated with decreased IGF-I. Ron et al.[390] also described mRNA for IGF-II in tumor extract.

NSILA-p also has been reported to cause hypoglycemia.[391] This is a 90-kDa serum glycoprotein that exhibits insulin-like activity and has been characterized only partially. It apparently accounts for the major portion of serum insulin–like activity in bioassays. NSILA-p is not considered a member of the somatomedin family, since it has limited or no sulfation factor activity. NSILA-p levels increase moderately in pregnancy, and elevations have been found in patients with various types of cancer.[391]

Additional studies concerning the nature of the peptide

or peptides produced by these tumors clearly need to be done. It also has been suggested that oncogenes may stimulate tumor glucose metabolism and that tumor necrosis factor and other cytokines could increase glucose uptake by tissues more broadly.[392]

It is likely that no single mechanism accounts for the hypoglycemia tumor syndrome. Various mechanisms may be responsible in patients with different tumors. Table 149–2 lists the possible causes of hypoglycemia in these patients.[393]

There is evidence for a high rate of glycolysis by tumors, and the large size of such tumors could possibly contribute to excessive glucose utilization. August and Hiatt,[392] found an arteriovenous difference of 41 mg/100 ml across the tumor bed, but a glucose infusion was running at the time of measurement. Critical review of the literature suggests that glucose utilization by the tumor itself in the absence of deficient counterregulatory mechanisms is probably not sufficient to account for hypoglycemia, particularly since the compensatory response by the normal liver is capable, at least temporarily, of a fivefold increase in glucose production. McFadzean and Yeung[395] made observations on the etiology of hypoglycemia with hepatocellular carcinoma. They divided their patients with hypoglycemia and hepatocellular carcinoma into two groups, one of which seemed to have abnormally stable glycogen in liver tissue. They suggested from their histological and other observations that an acquired form of glycogen storage disease due to mechanical and other factors in the liver might be part of the hypoglycemic syndrome, but this has not been confirmed.

The differential diagnosis between islet cell tumors and non–islet cell tumors is not difficult. The hallmark of the islet cell tumor is the presence of a low blood sugar and elevated or high-normal plasma insulin (and sometimes proinsulin and/or C-peptide). Plasma free fatty acids and lactate tend to be elevated in patients with extrapancreatic tumors, while they are correspondingly low in patients with islet cell tumors. The prognosis in these patients is generally related to the tumor type. The large retroperitoneal mesenchymal tumors, although huge, are often slow-growing and tend to be of a relatively low grade of malignancy.

Amelioration of the hypoglycemia may result from partial or complete resection. Fortunately, many of these tumors are benign. Agents such as diazoxide, glucocorticoids, and glucagon, which may be extremely useful in treating islet cell tumors, are of limited use in the nonpancreatic tumors. Sometimes these patients require, during the hypoglycemic attacks, continuous intravenous and oral glucose. The symptoms they manifest are related to the acuteness and severity of the hypoglycemia. Occasionally, high doses of glucocorticoids to stimulate gluconeogenesis, long-acting glucagon, and streptozotocin may be helpful.

ECTOPIC PRODUCTION OF HYPERCALCEMIC (CALCIUM-MOBILIZING) SUBSTANCES

The association of malignant disease with hypercalcemia is well recognized, frequent, and often of clinical importance[396] (see Ch. 62). A number of potential mechanisms are responsible for this metabolic abnormality:

1. Direct invasion of bone by tumor. This is particularly true of tumors that metastasize commonly to bone such as carcinoma of the lung, breast, or kidney. Prostate cancer, which frequently metastasizes to bone, usually causes osteoblastic metastases which are not associated with hypercalcemia. Even where tumor cells are actually present in bone, it is probable that bone lysis is mediated by one or more known factors responsible for local bone destruction such as prostaglandin E_2 (PGE_2),[397] osteoclast-activating factor,[398, 399] epidermal growth factor,[400] or direct lysis of bone by tumor cells,[401] monocytes,[402] or macrophages.[403]

2. Production of parathyroid hormone (PTH) or PTH-like substance by tumor (renal cAMP-stimulating factors).[404]

3. Production of other bone-mobilizing substances such as prostaglandins, osteoclast-activating factor, or transforming growth factors.

4. Coexistence of tumor with primary hyperparathyroidism, a disorder with a prevalence rate of almost 1 per 1000.[405, 406]

5. Coexistence with another cause of hypercalcemia, such as vitamin D intoxication, sarcoidosis, hyperthyroidism, immobilization, and adrenal insufficiency.

6. Administration of estrogen or androgen to a patient with carcinoma of breast metastatic to bone.

The differential diagnosis of hypercalcemia of unknown etiology usually can be accomplished on clinical grounds. The principal difficulty at times is in differentiating between primary hyperparathyroidism and a latent malignancy, but this usually can be resolved with the immunoradiometric assay for PTH. Osteolytic lesions must be greater than 1 cm in size to be observed radiographically.[407] The accuracy of diagnosis is improved markedly with isotopic bone scans, and core bone marrow biopsy may be a significant aid in diagnosing metastatic disease to bone. Compounding this difficulty in differential diagnosis at times is the frequency of hyperparathyroidism, which may coexist with other causes of hypercalcemia.

The association of malignancy and PTH production by tumors was first suggested in a discussion by Albright in a clinicopathological conference at the Massachusetts General Hospital.[408] The patient was a 51-year-old man with renal-cell carcinoma associated with hypercalcemia and hypophosphatemia. Neck exploration revealed three normal parathyroid glands, and a large osteolytic lesion in the ileum was irradiated, with improvement in the serum calcium and phosphorus. Although bioassay tests at that time were negative, it was suggested by Albright that the tumor might be exerting its metabolic effects by producing a PTH-like substance.[408] Plimpton and Gellhorn[409] popularized the association when they reported 10 additional patients with tumors and hypercalcemia. Four patients had renal cell carcinoma, and, in three, resection of the tumors was associated with return of the serum calcium to normal. Connor et al.[410] described two patients with lung cancer and hypercalcemia, one of whom developed hypercalcemia associated with tumor recurrence.

In those patients without metastases to bone (and even in some of those with), it has been suggested that a humoral factor produced by the tumor itself and released into the circulation might mediate the hypercalcemia, causing increased bone resorption, calcium mobilization into the circulation, and the resultant clinical disorder.[409]

There has been considerable controversy concerning the factor(s) responsible for such calcium mobilization.[396] The first candidate to be studied intensively was PTH, since the well-recognized disorder of primary hyperparathyroidism is associated with similar biochemical abnormalities. There has been intensive study of the production of PTH or PTH-like substances of tumors.

The first evidence for ectopic production of a PTH-like substance was suggested by Goldberg et al.,[411] who reported a positive assay for PTH in a renal carcinoma and its metastases using the indirect technique of complement fixation inhibition.[412, 413] More definitive evidence using a radioimmunoassay for PTH was provided by Sherwood et al.,[414] who quantitated the presence of an immunoreactive PTH-like substance in carcinoma of the lung, an undifferentiated parotid tumor, an adrenal carcinoma, and a histiocytic lymphoma (reticulum cell sarcoma). PTH in these tumors varied from 0.75 to 8.93 ng bovine equivalent per gram dry weight, and the molecular weight of the tumor hormone by sucrose density gradient analysis was similar to that of bovine PTH. In a report by Knill-Jones et al.,[415] an arteriovenous gradient of PTH across the tumor bed of a carcinoma of the bile ducts was demonstrated. The elevated concentrations of hormone in blood fell to normal after partial hepatectomy. The increased concentration in hepatic veins confirmed the production of hormone by the tumor. Additional confirmation that ectopic tumors produce PTH was provided by the in vitro studies of Tashjian,[416] who showed that a tumor associated with ectopic PTH production released the hormone for months in tissue culture. Hamilton et al.[417] showed that a squamous cell carcinoma synthesized a peptide similar to but not necessarily identical with human PTH.

Confusing evidence has been provided in recent years by the extensive application of radioimmunoassays for PTH (both N- and C-terminal and midmolecule) to the sera of many patients with cancer and hypercalcemia. While most of these studies have shown detectable levels of PTH in the circulation, the levels have, in general, been relatively low or normal.[404] When elevated hormone levels occur, as they do occasionally, they might suggest PTH production by the tumor or, much more commonly, coexisting primary hyperparathyroidism. These observations are confounded by the complex metabolism of PTH and the persistence of biologically inert but immunoreactive C-terminal fragments with a relatively long half-life in the circulation. Nevertheless, if PTH itself were the usual mediator of tumor hypercalcemia, consistent elevation of PTH peptides in the circulation should be found. One cannot account for the lack of elevation of PTH in these patients by renal dysfunction or by abnormal metabolism of PTH by the tumors. From the well-understood biosynthesis of PTH, it is highly unlikely that precursors or other factors could explain the phenomenon, since pro-PTH is not known to enter the circulation and is also relatively inert biologically. A search for prepro-PTH mRNA in tumor extracts also was negative.[418] Yoshimoto et al.[419] recently provided excellent documentation of PTH production in a patient with small cell carcinoma and hypercalcemia by demonstrating increased PTH in plasma by three different radioimmunoassays, PTH in a liver metastasis, normal parathyroid glands at autopsy, and PTH mRNA on Northern blot analysis of tumor extract. Nussbaum et al.[117] reported ectopic PTH production by an ovarian carcinoma. In this case, a rearrangement of

the PTH gene brought it under the control of regulatory DNA elements that are active in the ovary. Because of the paucity of evidence supporting more than the occasional ectopic production of PTH in these clinical syndromes, there has been an intensive search for other possible factors.

Powell et al.[420] described 11 patients with tumors associated with hypercalcemia, low serum phosphorus, and the absence of demonstrable bony metastases. In these patients, therapy with surgery, radiation, or chemotherapy reversed the hypercalcemia. Bone resorption was subsequently demonstrated in tumor extracts from three patients using an in vitro mouse calvarium bioassay. Despite the evidence of a bone-mobilizing substance in tumor tissue, all radioimmunoassays for PTH or related substances were negative in extracts of the tumor and in the peripheral blood.

The nature of bone-mobilizing substances is now becoming more clear, and there has been active pursuit of the hypothesis that prostaglandins could be responsible for some cases of the syndrome. This was based on an experimental model in a mouse sarcoma in which Tashjian and colleagues[416] provided evidence to support this concept. Prostaglandins were first shown to cause local bone resorption in an in vitro system by Klein and Raisz[421] in 1970. Their studies showed that the PGE compounds were the most potent in mobilizing calcium and that they caused osteoclastic bone resorption. In the mediation of bone resorption by PG, it also was shown that there was increased collagenase activity and cAMP production. Subsequent studies by Tashjian and colleagues[422] suggested in two animal models, fibrosarcoma in the mouse and VX_2 carcinoma in the rabbit, that PG production accounted for the hypercalcemic state. These studies showed that tumor production of PG resulted in systemic hypercalcemia, that there was an arteriovenous difference in PG concentration across the tumor bed, and that the PG could be synthesized by the tumor in vitro as well. Similarly, inhibitors of PG synthesis ameliorated the hypercalcemia and decreased the circulating levels. Increased osteoclastic bone resorption was noted at sites distant from the tumor. They also provided evidence that PGE_2 infusion into rats produced a hypercalcemic state.[423]

Human studies have been much less clear, but there is some evidence that PG may account for hypercalcemia in patients with malignancy.[424–426] Robertson et al.[425] reported a patient with renal cell carcinoma and hypercalcemia who had low PTH and elevations of both plasma PGE and tissue PGE. Indomethacin-responsive hypercalcemia in patients with tumors also was described by others.[404] Seyberth[426] described 14 patients with hypercalcemia and malignancy who had increased PG metabolites in the urine (PGE-M), while patients with primary hyperparathyroidism and hypercalcemia had normal levels of urinary metabolites. In later studies, Robertson et al.[427] found increased levels of plasma PGE in a number of patients with hypercalcemia, and Cummings and Robertson[428] showed that renal cell carcinoma in monolayer tissue culture synthesized PGE. Furthermore, Atkins et al.[429] reported that hypernephroma in co-culture with mouse calvarium caused indomethacin-reversible bone resorption. In a review by Metz et al.,[397] 10 of 33 hypercalcemic patients with cancer had elevated levels of PGE and PGE metabolites in venous blood, although levels were not as high as those reported in the animal studies. In a review of the three largest series of human subjects studied, a total of 63 patients with this syndrome have been described.[397] There was considerable variability in the methods used to detect the PG in these studies, and the prevalence of elevated levels varied considerably. Problems to be resolved in this kind of work include the possible role of PG and metabolites other than PGE, the source of the PG, the importance of location of the tumor (because of the metabolism of PGE on first pass through the liver and lung), and the potential site of PG production that causes bone resorption. It is not known whether the problem is due to release of PG itself from the tumor or, as Minkin et al.[430] have suggested, to local production of PG in bone in response to a circulating humoral hypercalcemic factor.[431]

In addition to PTH and PG, Mundy and Raisz[399] have suggested that osteoclast-activating factor might be involved in the development of hypercalcemia in patients with certain types of malignancy, such as multiple myeloma and some lymphomas. Osteoclast-activating factor was first identified in human lymphocytes by Luben et al.[398] This substance is a soluble mediator of resorption which has been identified in supernatant fluid from peripheral human leukocytes grown in tissue culture in the presence of antigen or phytomitogen. In an organ culture bioassay system, it stimulated active osteoclastic resorption from fetal rat bones. Activity also has been found in supernatant fluid from cultured lymphoid cell lines in patients with multiple myeloma, Burkitt's lymphoma, and malignant lymphoma, but not from normal subjects or patients with other neoplasms.[431] The activity could be distinguished from prostaglandins, PTH, and vitamin D–like compounds and was sensitive to inhibition by glucocorticoids. Thus it appears that hypercalcemia in patients with multiple myeloma and certain lymphomas might be explainable on this basis rather than a PTH-like factor or other substance. Studies by Garrett et al.[432] suggest the possibility that osteoclast-stimulating activity of myeloma may be lymphotoxin, a cytokine present in the supernatant of activated leukocyte cultures.

Considering the prevalence of tumor-related hypercalcemia,[404] the etiological factors described above have not been adequate to account for the frequency of the phenomenon. In recent studies,[404, 433, 435] it has become apparent that immunoreactive PTH in the circulation is often normal or low in patients with cancer and hypercalcemia, despite the fact that urinary cAMP or nephrogenous cAMP is often increased. An elevated cAMP level in the urine had been considered to be the hallmark of hyperparathyroidism, and thus the studies seem paradoxical. Stewart et al.[435] investigated such patients in detail. On evaluating 50 consecutive individuals with cancer and hypercalcemia, they found that nephrogenous cAMP excretion was elevated in 41 and suppressed in 9 (5.85 versus 0.51 nmol/100 ml glomerular filtrate). They compared the group of patients with elevated nephrogenous cAMP with a group of 15 patients with primary hyperparathyroidism and found the following: The group with hypercalcemia, cancer, and increased nephrogenous cAMP had reduced tubular reabsorption of phosphorus (like patients with primary hyperparathyroidism), but unlike the latter, they had increased fasting calcium excretion (0.66 versus 0.25 mg/100 ml glomerular filtrate), substantial reduction in circulating levels of 1,25-dihydroxyvitamin D_3 (20 versus 83 pg/ml),

and low levels of immunoreactive PTH in four different radioimmunoassays (which measured both N- and C-terminal portions of the molecule). Thus the patients appeared to behave as if they had increased PTH, but the low levels of 1,25-dihydroxyvitamin D_3 and the increased fractional calcium excretion, as well as diminished or absent PTH, suggested that some factor other than PTH itself was responsible for increased urinary cAMP. Other workers[436] have found normal $1,25(OH)_2D_3$ values in patients with renal carcinoma and hypercalcemia.

There also was increased cytobiochemical activity in the peripheral plasma of 10 of 16 of these patients with hormonal hypercalcemia of malignancy.[437] This is a highly sensitive bioassay that depends on the activation of glucose-6-phosphate dehydrogenase in renal tubular cells (which is known to be stimulated by PTH and cAMP). The patients with hypercalcemia and cancer, like patients with primary hyperparathyroidism, had increased activity in their serum of a protein that mimics PTH. When this activity was fractionated by gel filtration, however, it appeared to elute from the column at a molecular weight higher than that of PTH. Furthermore, antiserum to PTH only partially neutralized the biological activity in the serum, whereas it neutralized completely the activity in patients with primary hyperparathyroidism. In similar studies by Rude et al.,[434] plasma and urinary cAMP levels were determined in 91 patients with hypercalcemia and malignancy. Plasma cAMP was elevated in cancer patients with both hypercalcemia and normocalcemia, but not in patients with primary hyperparathyroidism. The mean urinary cAMP level was increased at least two-fold in all patient groups. They found increased nephrogenous cAMP in 46 per cent of the patients with hypercalcemia and malignancy who had bone metastases and 60 per cent of the patients with normocalcemia and malignancy. Increased urinary cAMP was most likely to be found in patients with squamous cell carcinoma of the lung, upper gastrointestinal tumors, and renal-cell carcinomas, although it was not completely specific for these tumors. Only 4 of 91 patients had detectable IPTH, 3 of these having coexisting primary hyperparathyroidism. In further studies, Minkin et al.[430] utilized extracts of tumors from patients with this syndrome to examine bone resorption in vitro from labeled mouse calvaria. Extracts of three of five tumors caused a significant increase in ^{45}Ca release, and bone resorption was blocked by indomethacin. Further studies by Stewart et al.[438] evaluated bone histomorphometry in these subjects. Compared with patients with primary hyperparathyroidism, those with humoral hypercalcemia of malignancy (HHM) showed a threefold increase in bone resorption coupled with a reduction in bone formation, decreased bone volume, and the appearance of uncoupling of osteoclast and osteoblast activity. Over 10.5 per cent of the bone surface was covered with osteoclasts, compared with 2.7 per cent in primary hyperparathyroidism and 0.5 per cent in controls.

It has been possible to establish the humoral hypercalcemia syndrome in the nude mouse using cells from a human renal cell carcinoma line that stimulated renal adenylate cyclase in vitro.[439, 440] The tumor-bearing mice were hypercalcemic, hypophosphatemic, and had an increased concentration of $1,25(OH)_2D_3$. The hypercalcemia was reversed by removing the tumor, and the action of the PTH-like factor was inhibited in vitro by a synthetic analogue of PTH which inhibits PTH action.[439, 440] These studies have provided additional evidence that the PTH-like factor interacts with the PTH receptor in the kidney. In other animal models,[441] including a human squamous tumor model in the nude mouse, urinary cAMP has been increased. Studies using the Leydig C cell tumor in parathyroidectomized rats have shown that the tumor factor increases tubular reabsorption of calcium, decreases tubular reabsorption of phosphorus, and increases cAMP excretion, exactly like PTH.[442] Stewart et al.[443] reviewed the frequency with which adenylate cylase–stimulating activity was associated with tumors and HHM. In their studies, 18 of 20 HHM tumor extracts displayed cyclase-stimulating activity, compared with only 4 (all squamous cell tumors) of 37 controls. One tumor containing adenylate cyclase–stimulating activity was partially purified, and it also had potent bone-resorbing activity.

While it has been strongly suggested that the hypercalcemic factor is the adenylate cyclase–stimulating factor,[443] Mundy and colleagues[444] have argued for the role of tumor-derived transforming growth factors (TGF). It is possible that both theories have validity, but the cAMP-stimulating factors appear to be the dominant cause. The evidence in support of a PTH receptor agonist includes the increase in nephrogenous cAMP excretion in patients with hypercalcemia, the presence of adenylate cyclase–stimulating activity in human and animal tumors, extracts, and cultured cells, the inhibition of biological activity with a synthetic PTH analogue, failure of antisera to PTH to inhibit the factor, and the absence of prepro-PTH messenger RNA in tumor extracts. The tumors containing cyclase-stimulating activity are predominantly of squamous cell origin. Alternatively, Mundy and colleagues[445] have suggested that HHM tumors may contain more than one factor, and they have provided evidence for both cyclase-stimulating activity and transforming growth factor in tumor extracts. Transforming growth factors do not contain cyclase-stimulating activity.[445] TGF-α, which binds to epidermal growth factor receptor, may be responsible for bone resorption in some models of HHM, and other possible mediators are TGF-β and platelet-derived growth factor. TGF-α and -β have been shown to enhance bone resorption by stimulating local production of PGE_2 in bone cultures.[446] Mundy[444] suggests that the growth factors and cyclase-stimulating factors may work in concert to cause hypercalcemia and might be encoded, for example, on related genes or a single gene with variable splicing. The growth factors may predominantly resorb bone, while the cyclase-stimulating factor may cause calcium reabsorption by the kidney.

Dramatic progress has been made in the search for the factor(s) responsible for the hypercalcemia syndrome. It has been apparent that the proteins behaving like PTH in various tumor extracts have been, in general, higher in molecular weight than PTH in the range of 20 kDa or more.[447] Broadus et al.[448] injected Xenopus oocytes with polyA RNA from human and animal tumors associated with HHM. The mRNA from these tumors directed the synthesis in the oocyte of a factor which had positive cytochemical activity for PTH and was inhibited by a PTH analogue. Moseley et al.[449] purified from a human lung cancer cell line an 18-kDa protein with biological activity six times that of amino-terminal PTH in stimulating adenylate cyclase activity in osteoblast-like cells. This protein was purified, and partial amino acid sequence showed that 8 of the first 13 amino acid residues were homologous with those in human PTH. The factor has been called PTH-related protein or PTHrP (see Ch. 57). Antibodies against a synthetic peptide from the amino-terminal end reacted weakly with (1–34) PTH, but the peptide reacted weakly with antibodies to PTH. These workers then reported the cloning and expression of the protein and its complete amino acid sequence.[450] It consists of 141 amino acids and is homologous with PTH only in the amino-terminal region. There is also a prepro-peptide of 36 amino acids preceding the hormone sequence. A similar factor was purified by Stewart et al.[451] and Strewler et al.[452] PTHrP has been localized to the short arm of chromosome 12. The PTH gene on chromosome 11 is clearly related in evolution, and the two genes have similar intron and exon structures. Although this may not be the only factor responsible for HHM, it represents dramatic progress toward solving a vexing problem.[453]

Of considerable interest is the normal physiological role for the PTHrP. Merendino et al.[454] suggested that this protein may be produced normally in human keratinocytes. Conditioned medium from cultures of keratinocytes stimulated cAMP production in osteosarcoma cells, and the effects were inhibited by the PTH analogue. Since substances produced by keratinocytes probably do not circulate normally, it might normally be a paracrine factor, exerting its effects locally. This could explain why the factor does not usually play a role in calcium homeostasis, unless it reaches the plasma (i.e., from a tumor). PTHrP also has been identified in the sheep fetus and in mammalian milk, suggesting that it also could play some role in maternal-fetal calcium hemostasis.[454]

In a study of patients with breast cancer, PTHrP was identified by immunohistochemistry in 53 per cent of tumors from patients without hypercalcemia who had bone metastases and in 88 per cent of tumors from patients with metastases who ultimately developed hypercalcemia.[455] All tumors from patients with hypercalcemia were positive, and there was close correlation of PTHrP in plasma with the presence of hypercalcemia. Thus a circulating humoral factor may be more important in breast cancer hypercalcemia than previously believed and also has been reported in mammary hyperplasia associated with hypercalcemia.[456] The recent availability of a radioimmunoassay for PTHrP has clearly identified the hormone in the plasma of many patients with HHM and has facilitated differential diagnosis as well as monitoring of cancer therapy.[256, 257]

A new mechanism of tumor hypercalcemia has been suggested in some patients with hematological and related malignancies. It has been demonstrated that cells of the monocyte-macrophage type have the ability to convert 25-hydroxyvitamin D_3 to $1,25(OH)_2D_3$.[458] Reports of patients with T-cell lymphomas (associated with the HTLV-I virus) have suggested an incidence of hypercalcemia as high as 25 per cent.[459] Increased levels of $1,25(OH)_2D_3$ have been described in patients with both non-Hodgkin's lymphoma[460] and Hodgkin's lymphoma,[461] as well as with plasma cell granuloma.[462] It also has been described in small cell carcinoma of the lung and melanoma.

On clinical grounds alone, it may be extremely difficult among patients with malignancy and hypercalcemia to determine whether they are producing PTH-like substances, prostaglandin, osteoclast-activating factor, transforming growth factors, or even other substances. Definitive responses of hypercalcemia to indomethacin or aspirin therapy may point to prostaglandin production. Bringhurst et al.[463] recently described a transitional-cell carcinoma that releases a unique factor that stimulates prostaglandin release and stimulates bone resorption but does not increase cAMP and does not exhibit transforming growth factor activity. This may be another unique syndrome.

The following tumors[1] have been associated with ectopic production of PTH-like substances:

1. Lung: squamous cell carcinoma
2. Genitourinary: renal cell, bladder, testis, penis, adrenal, ovary, uterus, including cervix, vulva
3. Gastrointestinal: colon, esophagus, pancreas, liver, and biliary
4. Parotid
5. Melanoma and other epidermoid
6. Breast
7. Lymphoma

Mundy et al.[464] compared the efficacy of oral phosphate, mithramycin, glucocorticoids, indomethacin, and bisphosphonates in the management of hypercalcemia of malignancy (see Ch. 64). They found that mithramycin and oral phosphates were the most effective, although no agent was effective in all and there were disadvantages of each. The newer bisphosphonates,[465] such as amino hydroxypropylidene biphosphonate (APD), have proven to be effective in recent trials.[465–468] More recent aminobisphosphonates show even greater promise.[469] Calcitonin also has been used with variable results. It is more effective when given with steroids[464, 470] and also has been used effectively in suppository form.[470]

ECTOPIC PRODUCTION OF CALCITONIN

There have been numerous reports of the ectopic production of calcitonin (CT) by tumors other than medullary carcinoma of the thyroid.[471–474] As in patients with medullary carcinoma,[475] those with ectopic CT usually have no clinical effects from the production of the hormone, except possibly diarrhea in patients with medullary carcinoma. Serum calcium tends to be normal in both. It is the association of the disorder with the production of other proteins or substances by medullary carcinoma or by the ectopic tumor that leads to clinical consequences or symptoms, if they are present at all. Schwartz et al.[474] performed a prospective study to determine the value of CT as a tumor marker. In their studies, elevated concentrations of plasma CT were found in a number of common cancers such as those of the lung (38 per cent), colon (24 per cent), breast (38 per cent), pancreas (42 per cent), and stomach (30 per cent). In patients with small cell carcinoma of the lung, 58 per cent had elevated CT, and immunological activity was detected in 14 per cent of tumor extracts but not in normal tissue outside the thyroid. There was no clinical correlation of abnormal serum calcium with increased CT secretion, and control studies with [^{125}I]hCT suggested that the measurements were not an artifact of label degradation. That CT is not an absolute marker for neoplastic disease, however, was shown by elevations in some patients with renal failure, gastrointestinal bleeding, and chronic obstructive lung disease. It is known that CT secretion responds physiologically to calcium, gastrin, glu-

cagon, and catecholamines. Silva et al.[476] did a similar prospective study in 61 patients with bronchogenic cancer. Fifty-two per cent of these patients exhibited increased plasma CT without any correlation with particular histological type, and 78 per cent of those with increased CT remained normocalcemic, there being no correlation between CT concentrations and the presence of bony metastases. Release of CT from tumors was either ectopic or due to thyroidal release, the ectopic type being more closely correlated with small cell tumors.[476] With appropriate therapy, circulating concentrations decreased. A similar study of immunoreactive CT in lung cancer by Roos et al.[473] examined these issues in more detail; they not only measured plasma CT by radioimmunoassay but also validated it by immunoextraction and gel filtration. In their studies, plasma CT appeared to be elevated in 18 per cent of basal samples from patients with epidermoid or anaplastic cancer, although unequivocal increases in CT were not found in any. However, in patients with small cell or adenocarcinoma, unequivocal increases were found in 27 per cent, and the form of CT recovered in the latter patients was larger than the CT monomer.

In in vitro studies, Bertagna et al.[137] studied a line of human small cell carcinoma in culture which produced ACTH, lipotropin, endorphin, and CT. After gel exclusion chromatography, two forms of CT were found at 7000 and 14,000 Da. These appeared to be high-molecular-weight forms of CT that did not cross-react with ACTH antibodies; they supported the release of high-molecular-weight forms of CT from small cell carcinoma but not the existence of a common precursor for ACTH and CT. Immunoperoxidase staining also has been useful in documenting the presence of CT in lung cancer. Baylin and Mendelsohn[95] found increased quantities of L-dopa-decarboxylase in small cell and adenocarcinoma of the lung but not in other types of lung cancer.

In a study by Hansen et al.,[471] both basal and pentagastrin-stimulated levels of CT and serum histaminase were examined in a group of 79 patients with small cell carcinoma of the lung. Serum CT was increased in 68 per cent (54 of 79 patients), with 20 patients having a level as high as that usually found in medullary carcinoma of the thyroid gland. Levels of histamines were no different from control. In 3 of 19 patients who had pentagastrin testing, CT was significantly increased.

Hansen et al.[471] studied ACTH, ADH, and CT as markers of small cell carcinoma of the lung. No significant or consistent changes in these three hormones were found following lysis of tumor cells by cytotoxic agents. After the tumor had responded to treatment, plasma ACTH, ADH, and CT became normal in most patients, but recurrent or progressive disease was not always followed by increases in plasma ACTH or ADH. In 12 patients with disease progression, however, CT increased in 10 and plasma ADH in 11, although the changes were only moderate. Furthermore, in some patients, CT concentrations were found to be increased after tumor regression. Therefore, decisions concerning patient treatment cannot be based exclusively on the concentrations of these hormones, since the amounts may vary greatly at different times in the life cycle of the tumor. They also examined the pattern of metabolites in small cell tumors in relation to stage and subtype. Approximately one-third had the ectopic ADH syndrome. Twenty-nine per cent had elevated plasma ACTH, and 64 per cent had elevated serum calcitonin. Gastrin concentrations were increased in 20 per cent but only marginally. There was no elevation of glucagon, insulin, secretin, VIP, GH, hCG, hPL, or VMA. The concentrations of ACTH, CT, and ADH were found not to be correlated with the stage of the disease, and no correlation with histological subtypes of small cell carcinoma was identified.

Small cell carcinoma of the lung has been examined for both CT and somatostatin-like immunoreactivity.[473, 477] In 15 control subjects, Roos et al.[473] found the upper limit of normal of plasma somatostatin to be 37 pg/mg. In 26 patients with small cell lung cancer, 4 had significant elevations in the range of 136 to 6150 pg/mg, while none of 19 patients with epidermoid lung cancer had an increase. Immunoadsorbent chromatography confirmed that the plasma measurements were due to true measurement of somatostatin-like activity, although there was evidence on gel filtration for at least three species in the range of 13,000, 4000, and 1600 Da. It also was detectable in extracts of 5 of 9 small cell lung cancers in the range of 14 to 441 pg/mg compared with concentrations of 60 to 9200 pg/mg in medullary carcinoma of the thyroid and was not detectable in normal lungs or in epidermoid lung cancer. The presence of higher-molecular-weight forms may represent biosynthetic precursors. Baylin and Mendelsohn[95] also examined the content of histaminase, L-dopa-decarboxylase, and CT in small cell carcinoma of the lung. These three markers have regularly been used for medullary carcinoma of the thyroid. There was evidence that histaminase was increased in 6 lung tumors (to 3 to 14,000 times control), L-dopa-decarboxylase in 4 of 6 (to 6 to 30 times control), and CT in one of one. In some metastatic lesions, low or absent levels of these markers were found despite high values in the primary tumor lesions. Since the concentration of tumor markers varied between primary tumors and metastases, circulating levels may not correlate well with the tumor burden. Samaan et al.[478] studied patients with bronchogenic and breast cancer both before and after pentagastrin stimulation and compared the patients with those with medullary carcinoma of the thyroid. They found a number of patients with either bronchogenic tumors or breast cancer with increased CT. In some patients with normal basal CT, the level was abnormally high after pentagastrin stimulation. The degree of response was significantly less than that seen in patients with medullary carcinoma of the thyroid, however. CT also has been shown to be elevated in several patients with VIPomas[1] and in prostate cancer.[479]

The evidence for CT and related peptides in ectopic tumors, particularly small cell carcinoma, is interesting when viewed in relation to developments in the area of CT physiology and medullary carcinoma of the thyroid.[480] For over 20 years, research on CT has focused on the issue of its physiological role. Despite a great deal of investigation, this is very unclear, even though CT is a useful agent in the management of Paget's disease and hypercalcemia, and measurement of CT is useful in the diagnosis of medullary carcinoma of the thyroid.

CT, like other polypeptide hormones of similar molecular weight, is derived through synthesis of a higher-molecular-weight precursor.[481] Some variability of the assay of CT in normal plasma is related to the difference between serum samples and plasma; hemolysis, and other variations also account for differing values seen in various laboratories. Some of these factors affect the values obtained in plasma of patients with various tumors (see above). Furthermore, there is heterogeneity of plasma CT on gel filtration, and immunoassay reveals several peaks of CT-like immunoreactivity. Whether these multiple forms are the result of peripheral metabolism or of the synthesis of different peptides (including precursors) has not yet been resolved. Although monomeric CT equivalents are being measured, the value may actually represent the aggregate of multiple forms of CT. Thus the values for CT from any one laboratory must be interpreted in relation to the normal values from the same laboratory. Some ectopic tumors cannot process calcitonin, as is the case for ACTH.[484] The variability in expression of calcitonin, its multiple forms, and its lack of specificity make its use as a tumor marker (other than in medullary carcinoma) problematic.[483, 484]

METABOLIC BONE DISEASE ASSOCIATED WITH TUMORS (ONCOGENIC OSTEOMALACIA)

The association of osteomalacia with tumors has been well documented. The patients reported in the literature have primarily had mesenchymal tumors (usually benign) that included sclerosing hemangiomas, giant cell tumors of bone, fibromas and fibroangiomas, ossifying mesenchymomas, hemangiopericytomas, neuromas, neurofibromas, and a mesenchymal tumor of the pharynx.[485, 486] The soft-tissue mesenchymal tumors typically have prominent vessels, osteoclast-like giant cells, focal microcystic changes, osseous metaplasia, dystrophic calcifications, and/or cartilage-like areas.[486] More than 70 patients have now been described.[487] In these patients there is a common syndrome consisting of hyperphosphaturia and marked hypophosphatemia, normocalcemia, elevated serum alkaline phosphatase, and osteomalacia associated with bone pain, muscle weakness, and pseudofractures on x-ray.[1, 488] Most of the cases appeared in childhood, and some were familial. The tumor may be small and only identified several years after the bone disturbance. Glycosuria and aminoaciduria also may be present. In 1977, Drezner and Feinglos[489] described a 42-year-old woman with a giant cell tumor of the iliac bone who had osteomalacia and aminoaciduria. This patient had low levels of $1\alpha,25$-dihydroxyvitamin D_3, and it was suggested by these authors that a defect in the conversion of 25-hydroxyvitamin D_3 to the dihydroxy derivative might be an important part of the picture. Deficiency of the metabolite is known to contribute to renal phosphate loss, but the degree of hypophosphatemia and phosphaturia in this patient was inappropriately high. Daniels and Weisenfeld[486] reported a middle-aged man with sclerosing hemangiomas of bone who showed marked improvement following the administration of oral phosphate (1.5 g phosphorus) and 100,000 U/day of vitamin D. Fukumoto et al.[488] described a patient with a benign osteoblastoma associated not only with osteomalacia but also with marked proximal renal tubular dysfunction that included generalized aminoaciduria and glucosuria. The level of 1,25-dihydroxyvitamin D_3 was less than 4 pg/ml in this patient, and the level of 25-hydroxyvitamin D_3 was normal. The patient was treated with 1α-hydroxyvitamin D_3, and despite levels of 1,25 that were in the high-normal range, hypophosphatemia and phosphaturia persisted (suggesting that 1,25 deficiency was not the sole pathogenic defect). Correction of the abnormal tubular reabsorption of phosphorus and hypophosphatemia followed very quickly removal of the tumor. It is possible that a proximal renal tubular defect may explain both the phosphaturia and the vitamin D metabolite deficiency, since conversion to 1,25-dihydroxyvitamin D_3 occurs in the proximal tubule.

Lyles et al.[490] emphasized that hypophosphatemic osteomalacia may be associated not only with mesenchymal tumors but also with prostatic carcinoma and endodermal malignancy. They described two patients with hypophosphatemia associated with metastatic prostatic carcinoma who had significant osteomalacia; this abnormality had not been described previously in prostatic cancer. They were unable to remove the metastatic tumor and effect cure of the clinical problem. On bone biopsy, there was unequivocal osteomalacia demonstrated by excessive osteoid covering trabecular bone surfaces and inadequate mineralization. The level of 1,25-dihydroxyvitamin D_3 was 15 pg/ml, and there was significant renal phosphate wasting. This association is worth pursuing further because of the frequency of prostatic carcinoma and the possibility that osteomalacia might be contributing to the bone pain in this disease. There is one report of the syndrome in oat cell carcinoma[491] and another in hepatocellular carcinoma.[492] Miyauchi et al.[493] transplanted a hemangiopericytoma into nude mice and found hypophosphatemia, increased alkaline phosphatase, and increased urinary phosphate in the animals. Tumor extracts added to cultures of renal tubular cells did not change cAMP levels, but 1α-hydroxylase activity decreased markedly. Nitzan et al.[494] found no effect on phosphate transport in a tubule cell line, although tumor extracts caused hypophosphatemia and phosphaturia in nude mice. The pathogenesis of oncogenic osteomalacia remains an enigma, but there is presumably a factor(s) produced by the tumor which results in phosphaturia and a low serum $1,25(OH)_2D_3$.

Atkinson et al.[495] presented an interesting patient with stage IVB Hodgkin's disease (nodular sclerosis) who had hypertrophic pulmonary osteoarthropathy that was completely reversed by chemotherapy, including evidence of periosteal new bone formation on the tibia. They reviewed 13 additional cases of Hodgkin's disease associated with similar findings. The majority were patients with advanced disease (stage IIIB or IV), and mediastinal involvement was present in all. The mechanism remains obscure.

ECTOPIC PRODUCTION OF ERYTHROPOIETIN

The kidney is known to be the principal source of erythropoietin, the hormone that stimulates red blood cell production (Ch. 157). A number of benign as well as malignant disorders of the kidney may be associated with increased production of erythropoietin; these include hypernephroma and benign conditions such as renal cysts and hydronephrosis. Elevated erythropoietin associated with nonneoplastic renal disease such as benign renal cysts also suggests that dysplastic cells may be capable of hormone production. Strictly speaking, production of erythropoietin by a renal tumor is not an ectopic syndrome but rather a manifestation of the normal function of the organ.

In other situations, ectopic production of this hormone may be associated with lesions such as cerebellar hemangioblastoma (21 per cent), uterine fibroma (6 per cent), adrenal cortical tumors (3 per cent), ovarian neoplasms (3 per cent), hepatomas (2 per cent), and pheochromocytoma (1 per cent).[1, 496, 497] More than half the patients with excess erythropoietin production have malignant renal tumors or benign renal conditions.[1] Polycythemia occurs in 2 to 5 per cent of patients with renal neoplasms and 9 to 20 per cent of patients with cerebellar hemangioblastomas. Studies involving the synthesis and release of erythropoietin in vitro by renal tumors have confirmed the production of the hormone by renal tumors.[498] The production of hormone by the tumor does not necessarily correlate with polycythemia in the patient because the presence of a malignancy may interfere with the polycythemic response. Detection of elevated levels of erythropoietin has depended in the past principally on somewhat cumbersome bioassay techniques.

The development of a highly sensitive radioimmunoassay for the hormone in human blood has allowed its application to patients with a variety of neoplastic and other disorders.[499, 500] The production of recombinant erythropoietin has made it available not only for clinical trials but also as a reagent for radioimmunoassay.[501, 502] Erythropoietin is a 39-kDA glycoprotein which may be synthesized in the kidney as well as the liver.[503] Production of erythropoietin by renal tumors is not thought to be ectopic in nature, but whether hormone production in other organs such as the liver (which may be a source of normal hormone production) or cerebellum is ectopic is not certain. A number of recent reports have documented with more modern techniques the presence of erythropoietin in tumors.[503–506] DaSilva et al.[507] demonstrated a strong signal for erythropoietin in Northern blot analysis of tumor extracts with no evidence of gene alterations. In situ hybridization showed that the mRNA was in tumor cells. The syndrome has been reproduced in nude mice[508] and the messenger RNA translated in the *Xenopus* system.[506] More recently, the erythropoietin receptor itself has been cloned, and some patients with polycythemia may have a mutation in the receptor, leading to increased hormone levels.[509]

Like other ectopic syndromes, detection of a biochemical marker may or may not be associated with physiologic effects in the patient.[510, 511] In addition to secretion of erythropoietin by tumors, it is also possible that some tumors produce thrombopoietin[512] and also possibly leukopoietin or colony-stimulating factor.[55]

MISCELLANEOUS SYNDROMES ASSOCIATED WITH ECTOPIC HORMONE PRODUCTION

Renin-Secreting Tumors

A number of patients have been reported who have had hypertension associated with production of renin by tumors. These have principally been tumors of the kidney, particularly tumors of the juxtaglomerular apparatus (hemangiopericytoma), Wilms' tumor, and renal cell carcinoma.[513–515] It also has been described in oat cell carcinoma of the lung,[516] adenocarcinoma of the lung[517] and pancreas,[518] ovarian carcinoma,[519] and hepatocellular carcinoma.[520] Since the juxtaglomerular cell is normally the site of origin of renin, this could not be considered a truly ectopic syndrome. When produced from clear cell carcinoma, hepatic tumors, or other tumors outside the kidney, the designation *ectopic syndrome* seems more justified. Although some of these patients had severe hypertension, hypokalemia, increased peripheral vein renin activity, and secondary aldosteronism, this is by no means consistent; in some patients, only mild hypertension has been noted. Intravenous pyelography has not always shown the tumors because of their small size, and selective arteriography as well as renal vein renin assays to show the step-up in production of renin in the kidneys may be necessary. The differential diagnosis for the patient with hypertension requires excluding malignant hypertension or renal vascular hypertension, which also would be associated with excessive amounts of renin. Increased production of renin has been shown by the tumors in vitro in tissue culture.

Recent studies of renin in normal and tumor tissues has shown the presence of a higher-molecular-weight form of renin that has minimal biological activity and which is present in some human plasmas, tumor extracts, and amniotic fluid.[520-524] It is believed that some tumors may release large amounts of an inactive precursor form of renin.[520, 522] In other patients, excessive production of renin substrate (angiotensinogen) by hepatic tumors may be pathogenic.[520] Production of endothelin by a malignant hemangioendothelioma as a cause of hypertension also has been described.[525]

Prostaglandin Production

In the section on hypercalcemia and tumors, production of prostaglandin E by animal and human tumors was described. In another report, production of prostaglandin A from an anaplastic renal tumor was associated with antihypertensive activity.[526] This patient developed severe hypertension after removal of the tumor and developed hemiparesis 1 year after operation. Preoperatively, elevated levels of PGA (8.05 ng/ml) were found in the plasma, which were markedly reduced postoperatively to the normal range. It is likely that this and other instances of prostaglandin production by tumors may be associated with ectopic syndromes. With increased availability of the radioimmunoassays for prostaglandins A, E, and F, further syndromes are likely to be reported. Since prostaglandins are ubiquitous, however, it may be difficult to implicate them in the pathogenesis of ectopic hormone syndromes, and they may be more contributory than primary in pathogenesis.

Oncofetal Proteins and Tumor Markers

Production of proteins normally found in fetal life has been associated with certain neoplasms.[527] The two principal antigens have been α-fetoprotein associated with liver tumors and carcinoembryonic antigen associated with carcinoma of the bowel. Neither antigen has proven to be completely specific for the tumors and may even be pro-

duced in normal subjects. A discussion of their significance is beyond the scope of this chapter.

Nerve Growth Factor and Epidermal Growth Factor

Nerve growth factor, which has prominent effects on sympathetic and sensory ganglia, is produced by the normal mouse. Neuroblastoma cells in the mouse also have been shown to produce nerve growth factor, and it is likely that certain human tumors might do the same.[111, 528] The same is true of epidermal growth factor and transforming growth factors (see above).

Golde et al.[529] reviewed data concerning a variety of growth factors related to various cellular phenomena. In the section of this chapter concerning hypoglycemia, the potential importance of somatomedins or insulin-like growth factors was emphasized. Two very important growth factors that were originally identified in male mouse submaxillary glands may be important in humans. One is nerve growth factor, which consists of three distinct subunits, the β subunit of which is biologically active and consists of a dimer of two identical polypeptides of 118 amino acids.[530] Human nerve growth factor has now been purified from human placental tissue,[531] and it has a distinct structural homology with insulin. Although it cannot substitute for insulin action, it appears to have important effects on the growth of nerve cells in vitro and in vivo and also may have important effects on tyrosine hydroxylase. Both nerve growth factor and its receptors have been found on human melanoma cells, but no definite relationship has been identified as yet between overproduction or deficiency of nerve growth factor and a human disease. Subsequent studies by radioimmunoassay may change this perspective.

A second important growth factor also originally identified in mouse submaxillary tissue is a protein that causes early eyelid opening and incisor tooth eruption in animals that were used for the bioassay for nerve growth factor. This peptide (epidermal growth factor) was subsequently purified and shown to consist of 53 amino acids; its amino acid sequence has been determined.[532] Epidermal growth factor has been identified in human urine, and receptors have been identified in a number of target tissues, including human cornea, fibroblasts, glial cells, and granulosa cells.[533] It has been an important agent in the study of down-regulation of peptides using radiolabeled peptide. Its possible relationship to human disease, including cancer, remains to be explored.

Ectopic Hormone Receptors

In addition to producing abnormal protein substances, a tumor might develop abnormal protein receptors in the course of its growth and development. This situation has been identified in an adrenal tumor of the rat which developed receptors to inappropriate hormones.[161] In addition to responding to ACTH, the adenylate cyclase enzyme of the rat adrenal tumor was stimulated by thyrotropin, LH, FSH, and β-adrenergic agonists. Another report described ectopic β-adrenergic receptors in human adrenocortical carcinoma.[534]

Multiple Hormone Production

Many of the patients described in the literature have had production of more than one ectopic hormone by a single tumor. These have been outlined in some detail in the sections dealing with specific neoplasms. In addition to ACTH, some tumors, for example, may produce lipotropin, gastrin, glucagon, parathyroid hormone–related protein, antidiuretic hormone, serotonin, and/or epinephrine. Moreover, the production of multiple hormones may be asynchronous, and individual hormone production may be periodic. A recent report of elevated ACTH and ADH in the plasma and tumor of a patient with both syndromes is unique.[535] Production of multiple hormones may be very common.

Ectopic Production of Other Proteins

As already described and in the studies of Rosen et al.[536] of human tumor cell lines, widespread production of polypeptide hormones by tumors has been well documented. A number of immune disorders have been associated with the production of tumor antigens and appropriate immune responses.[1] The first description of the glucagonoma syndrome (skin rash, diabetes, weight loss, and anemia) from a nonpancreatic tumor was published.[537] It is highly likely that future studies will produce even more data suggesting that specific clinical or biochemical syndromes associated with cancer are due to proteins produced by the tumors themselves. More problematic is the cause(s) of this phenomenon, but the tremendous advances in molecular biology coupled with an intense interest in tumor cells in vitro should assist in resolving the remaining mysteries.

ACKNOWLEDGEMENTS: The author wishes to express his gratitude and appreciation to Ms. Barbara Brooks for her excellent assistance in the preparation of the manuscript.

REFERENCES

1a. Hall TC (ed): Paraneoplastic syndromes. Ann NY Acad Sci 230:1, 1974.
1b. Blackman MR, Rosen SW, Weintraub BD: Ectopic hormones. Adv Intern Med 23:85, 1978.
1c. Odell SD, Wolfsen AR: Humoral syndromes associated with cancer: Ectopic hormone production. Prog Clin Cancer 8:57, 1982.
1d. Sherwood LM: Ectopic hormone syndromes. In Ingbar SH (ed): Contemporary Endocrinology. New York, Plenum Press, 1985.
1e. Orth DN: Ectopic hormone production. In Felig, P, Baxter JD, Broadus AEK, Frohman LA (eds): Endocrinology and Metabolism. New York, McGraw-Hill, 1987, pp 1692–1735.
1f. Endocrine manifestations of systemic disease. Endocrinol Metab Clin North Am 20:483, 1991.
2. Odell WD: Paraendocrine syndromes of cancer. Adv Intern Med 34:325, 1989.
3. Saito E, Odell WD: Corticotropin/lipotropin common precursor-like material in normal rat extrapituitary tissues. Proc Natl Acad Sci USA 80:3792, 1983.
4. Roth J, LeRoith D, Shiloach J, et al: The evolutionary origins of hormones, neurotransmitters and other extracellular chemical messengers: Implications for mammalian biology. N Engl J Med 306:523, 1982.
5. Blobel G, Dobberstein B: Transfer of proteins across membranes, parts I and II. J Cell Biol 67:835, 1975.
6. Gilmore R, Blobel G, Walter P: Protein translocation across the endoplasmic reticulum: I. Detection in the microsomal membrane of a receptor for the signal recognition particle. J Cell Biol 95:463, 1982.
7. Rhodes CJ, Thorne BA, Lincoln B, et al: Processing of proopiomelanocortin by insulin secretory granule proinsulin processing endopeptidases. J Biol Chem 268:4267, 1993.
8. DeBold CR, Menefee JK, Nicholson WE, et al: Proopiomelanocortin gene is expressed in many normal human tissues and in tumors not associated with ectopic adrenocorticotropin syndrome. Mol Endocrinol 2:862, 1988.
9. Atkins E, Feldman JD, Francis L, Hursh E: Studies on the mechanism of fever accompanying delayed hypersensitivity: The role of the sensitized lymphocyte. J Exp Med 135:1113, 1972.
10. Farrar WL, Kilian PL, Ruff MR, et al: Visualization and characterization of interleukin 1 receptors in brain. J Immunol 139:459, 1987.
11. Dinarello CA: Interleukin 1 and the pathogenesis of the acute-phase response. N Engl J Med 311:1413, 1984.
12. Rawlins MD, Luff RH, Cranston WI: Pyrexia in renal carcinoma. Lancet 1:1371, 1970.
13. Fukumoto S, Matsumoto T, Harada S, et al: Pheochromocytoma with pyrexia and marked inflammatory signs. J Clin Endocrinol Metab 73:877, 1991.
14. Richardson GE, Johnson BE: Paraneoplastic syndromes in lung cancer. Curr Opin Oncol 4:323, 1992.
15. Terepka AR, Waterhouse C: Metabolic observations during the forced feeding of patients with cancer. Am J Med 20:225, 1956.
16. Stevenson JAF, Box BM, Szalvko AJ: A fat mobilizing and anorectic substance in the urine of fasting rats. Proc Soc Exp Biol Med 116:424, 1964.
17. Rudman D, Del Rio AE, Garcia LA, et al: Isolation of two lipolytic pituitary peptides. Biochemistry 9:99, 1970.
18. Davis JG: Food intake following broad mixing of hungry and satiated rats. Psychol Sci 3:177, 1965.
19. Davis JD, Gallagher RJ, Ladore RS, Turansky AJ: Inhibition of food intake by humoral factor. J Comp Physiol Psychol 67:407, 1969.
20. Theologides A: Pathogenesis of cachexia in cancer: A review and a hypothesis. Cancer 29:484, 1972.
21. Vassalli P: The pathophysiology of tumor necrosis factors. Annu Rev Immunol 10:411, 1992.
22. Gold J: Metabolic profiles in human solid tumors. Cancer Res 26:695, 1966.
23. Argiles JM, Garcia-Martinez C, Llovera M, Lopez-Soriano FJ: The role of cytokines in muscle wasting: Its reaction with cancer cachexia. Med Res Rev 12:637, 1992.
24. Heber D, Tchekmedyian NS: Pathophysiology of cancer: Hormonal and metabolic abnormalities. Oncology 49(Suppl 2):28, 1992.
25. Reed DM: On the pathological changes in Hodgkin's disease with special reference to its relation to tuberculosis. Johns Hopkins Rep 10:133, 1902.
26. Aisenberg AC: Studies on delayed hypersensitivity in Hodgkin's disease. J Clin Invest 41:1964, 1972.
27. Hersh EM, Oppenheim JJ: Impaired in vitro lymphocyte transformation in Hodgkin's disease. N Engl J Med 273:1006, 1965.
28. Keller WD, Lamb DL, Varco RL: Investigation of Hodgkin's disease with respect to the problems of homotransplantation. Ann NY Acad Sci 87:187, 1960.
29. Ultmann JE, Cunningham JK, Gellhorn A: The clinical picture of Hodgkin's disease. Cancer Res 26:1047, 1966.
30. Harris J, Copeland D: Impaired immunoresponsiveness in tumor patients. Ann NY Acad Sci 230:56, 1974.
31. Glasgow AH, Nimberg RB, Menzoian JO, et al: Association of anergy with an immunosuppressive peptide fraction in the serum of patients with cancer. N Engl J Med 291:1263, 1974.
32. Sjögren HO, Hellström I, Bansal SC, Hellström KE: Suggestive evidence that the "blocking antibodies" of tumor-bearing individuals may be antigen-antibody complexes. Proc Natl Acad Sci USA 68:1372, 1971.
33. Friou GJ: Current knowledge and concepts of the relationship of malignancy, autoimmunity, and immunologic disease. Ann NY Acad Sci 230:23, 1974.
34. Dawkins RL, Eghtedari A, Holborow EJ: Antibodies to skeletal muscle demonstrated by immunofluorescence in experimental autoallergic myositis. Clin Exp Immunol 9:329, 1971.

35. Morgan G, Peter JB, Newbould BB: Experimental allergic myositis in rats. Arthritis Rheum 14:599, 1971.

36. Currie S, Saunders M, Knowles M, Brown AE: Immunological aspects of polymyositis: The in vitro activity of lymphocytes on incubation with muscle antigen and with muscle cultures. Q J Med 157:63, 1971.

37. Dawkins RL, Mastaglia FL: Cell-mediated cytotoxicity to muscle in polymyositis: Effect of immunosuppression. N Engl J Med 288:434, 1973.

38. Johnson RL, Fink CW, Ziff M: Lymphotoxin formation by lymphocytes and muscle in polymyositis. J Clin Invest 51:2435, 1972.

39. Brain WR, Norris F Jr: Remote Effects of Cancer on the Nervous System. New York, Grune & Stratton, 1965.

40. Tyler HR: Paraneoplastic syndromes of nerve, muscle and neuromuscular junction. Ann NY Acad Sci 230:348, 1974.

41. Croft PB, Wilkinson M: Carcinomatous neuromyopathy: Incidence in patients with carcinoma of the lung and breast. Lancet 1:184, 1963.

42. Croft PB, Wilkinson M: The incidence of carcinomatous neuromyopathy in patients with various types of carcinoma. Brain 88:427, 1965.

43. Brain WR: The neurological complications of neoplasms. Lancet 1:179, 1963.

44. Posner JB: Neurological complications of systemic cancer. Med Clin North Am 55:625, 1971.

45. Wilner EC, Brody JA: An evaluation of the remote effects of cancer on the nervous system. Neurology 18:1120, 1968.

46. Joynt RJ: Neurogenic paraneoplastic syndromes: The brain's uneasy peace with tumors. Ann NY Acad Sci 230:342, 1974.

47. Norris FH Jr: Prognosis in amyotrophic lateral sclerosis. Trans Am Neurol Assoc 96:290, 1971.

48. Mancall EL, Rosales RK: Necrotizing myelopathy associated with visceral carcinoma. Brain 87:639, 1964.

49. Eaton LM, Lambert EH: Electromyography and electric stimulation of nerves in diseases of motor unit. JAMA 163:1117, 1957.

50. Lang B, Newsom-Davis J, Wray D, Vincent A: Autoimmune aetiology for myasthenia (Eaton-Lambert) syndrome. Lancet 2:224, 1981.

51. Engel AG: Myasthenia gravis and myasthenic syndromes. Ann Neurol 16:519, 1984.

52. Croft AB, Urich H, Wilkinson M: Peripheral neuropathy of sensorimotor type associated with malignant disease. Brain 90:31, 1967.

53. Richardson EP Jr: Our evolving understanding of progressive multifocal leukoencephalopathy. Ann NY Acad Sci 230:358, 1974.

54. Kornguth, SE: Neuronal proteins and paraneoplastic syndromes. N Engl J Med 321:1607, 1989.

55. Johnson RA, Roodman GD: Hematologic manifestations of malignancy. Dis Month 11:721, 1989.

56. Slichter SJ, Harker LA: Hemostasis in malignancy. Ann NY Acad Sci 230:252, 1974.

57. Pineo GF, Brain MC, Gallus AS, et al: Tumors, mucus production, and hypercoagulability. Ann NY Acad Sci 230:262, 1974.

58. Goodnight SH Jr: Bleeding and intravascular clotting in malignancy: A review. Ann NY Acad Sci 230:271, 1974.

59. Curth HO: Cutaneous manifestations associated with malignant internal disease. In Fitzpatrick CB, Arndt KA, Claude WH Jr, et al (eds): Dermatology in General Medicine. New York, McGraw-Hill, 1971.

60. Kahn CR, Flier JS, Archer JA, et al: The syndromes of insulin resistance and acanthosis nigricans: Insulin-receptor disorders in man. N Engl J Med 294:739, 1976.

61. Boyd AS, Neldner KH, Menter A: Erythema gyratum repens: A paraneoplastic eruption. J Am Acad Dermatol 26:757, 1992.

62. Mallison CN, Bloom SR, Warin AP, et al: A glucagonoma syndrome. Lancet 2:1, 1974.

63. Lee JC, Yamaguchi H, Hopper J Jr: The association of cancer and the nephrotic syndrome. Ann Intern Med 64:41, 1966.

64. Plager J, Stutzman L: Acute nephrotic syndrome as a manifestation of active Hodgkin's disease: Report of four cases and review of the literature. Am J Med 50:56, 1971.

65. Loughridge LW, Lewis MG: Nephrotic syndrome in malignant disease of non-renal origin. Lancet 1:256, 1971.

66. Gould VE, Benditt EP: Ultrastructural and functional relationships of some human endocrine tumors. Pathol Ann 8:205, 1973.

67. Rudnick P, Odell WD: In search of a cancer. N Engl J Med 284:405, 1971.

68. Ellison ML, Ambrose EJ, Easty GC: Differentiation in a transplantable rat tumor maintained in organ culture. Exp Cell Res 55:198, 1969.

69. Sherbert GV: Epigenetic processes and their relevance to the study of neoplasia. Adv Cancer Res 13:97, 1970.

70. Yoshimoto Y, Wolfsen AR, Odell WD: Human chorionic gonadotropin-like substance in nonendocrine tissues of normal subjects. Science 197:575, 1977.

71. Braunstein GD, Vaitukaitis JL, Carbone PP, Ross LT: Ectopic production of human chorionic gonadotrophin by neoplasms. Ann Intern Med 78:39, 1973.

72. Rees LH: Concepts in ectopic hormone production. Clin Endocrinol (Oxf) 5:363, 1976.

73. Feyrter T: Die peripheren endoKrinen (paraKrinen) Drusen. In Kaufmann-Staemler F, DeGuyter G (eds): Lehrbuch der speziellen pathologischen Anatome. Berlin, Springer-Verlag, 1969, p 12.

74. Pearse AG: Common cytochemical properties of cells producing polypeptide hormones with particular reference to calcitonin and the thyroid C cells. Vet Rec 79:587, 1966.

75. Pearse AG: 5-Hydroxytryptophan uptake by dog thyroid "C" cells, and its possible significance in polypeptide hormone production. Nature 211:598, 1966.

76. Pearse AG: Common cytochemical and ultrastructural characteristics of cells producing polypeptide hormones (the APUD series) and their relevance to thyroid and ultimobranchial cells and calcitonin. Proc R Soc Lond [Biol] 170:71, 1968.

77. Pearse AG: The cytochemistry and ultrastructure of polypeptide hormone-producing cells of the APUD series and the embryologic, physiologic and pathologic implications of the concept. J Histochem Cytochem 17:303, 1969.

78. LeDourain N, LeLievre C: Demonstration de l'origine neural des cellules a calcitonine du corps ultimobranchial chez l'embryon du poulet. CR Acad Sci Paris [D] 270:2857, 1970.

79. Pearse AG, Polak JM: Neural crest origin of the endocrine polypeptide (APUD) cells of the gastrointestinal tract and pancreas. Gut 12:783, 1971.

80. Pearse AG, Polak JM, Rust FW, et al: Demonstration of the neural crest origin of type I (APUD) cells in the avian carotid body, using a cytochemical marker system. Histochemie 34:191, 1973.

81. Pearse AG: The APUD cell concept and its implications in pathology. Pathol Ann 9:27, 1974.

82. Pearse AG, Polak JM: Cytochemical evidence for the neural crest origin of mammalian ultimobranchial C cells. Histochemie 27:96, 1971.

83. Pearse AG: The APUD concept and its implications in pathology (addendum). In Sommers SC (ed): Endocrine Pathology Decennial. New York, Appleton-Century-Crofts, 1975, p 162.

84. Weichert RF III: The neural ectodermal origin of the peptide secreting endocrine glands. Am J Med 49:232, 1970.

85. Friesen SR, Hermreck AS, Mantz FA Jr: Glucagon, gastrin, and carcinoid tumors of the duodenum, pancreas and stomach: Polypeptide apudomas of the foregut. Am J Surg 127:90, 1974.

86. Szijj I, Csapo Z, Laszlo FA, Kovacs K: Medullary cancer of the thyroid gland associated with hypercorticism. Cancer 24:167, 1969.

87. Gould VE, Benditt EP: Ultrastructural and functional relationships of some human endocrine tumors (addendum). In Sommers SC (ed): Endocrine Pathology Decennial. New York, Appleton-Century-Crofts, 1975, p 190.

88. Gould E: Neuroendocrinomas: APUD cell system neoplasms and their aberrant secretory activities. Pathol Ann 12, 1977.

89. Hammar S, Sale G: Multiple hormone producing islet cell carcinomas of the pancreas: A morphologic and biochemical investigation. Hum Pathol 6:349, 1975.

90. Bolande RP: The neurocristopathies: A unifying concept of diseases arising in neural crest maldevelopment. Hum Pathol 5:409, 1974.

91. Pictet RL, Rall LB, Phelps P, Rutter WJ: The neural crest and the origin of the insulin-producing and other gastrointestinal hormone-producing cells. Science 191:191, 1976.

92. Le Dourain NM, Teillet MA: The migration of neural crest cells to the wall of the digestive tract in avian embryo. J Embryol Exp Morphol 30:31, 1973.

93. Gould VE, Battifora H: Origin and significance of the basal lamina and some interstitial fibrillar components in epithelial neoplasms. Pathol Ann 11:353, 1976.

94. Levine RJ, Metz SA: A classification of ectopic hormone-producing tumors. Ann NY Acad Sci 230:533, 1974.

95. Baylin SB, Mendelsohn G: Ectopic (inappropriate) hormone production by tumors: Mechanisms involved and the biological and clinical implications. Endocr Rev 1:45, 1980.

96. Nelkin BD, de Bustros AC, Mabry M, Baylin SB. The molecular biology of medullary thyroid carcinoma: A model for cancer development and progression. JAMA 261:3130, 1989.

97. Hansen M, Pedersen AG: Tumor markers in patients with lung cancer. Chest 89:219S, 1986.

98. Baylin SB, Mendelsohn G, Weisburger WR, et al: Levels of histaminase and L-DOPA decarboxylase activity in the transition from C-cell hyperplasia to familial medullary thyroid carcinoma. Cancer 44:1315, 1979.

99. Abeloff MD, Eggleston JC, Mendelsohn G, et al: Changes in morphologic and biochemical characteristics of small cell carcinoma of the lung: A clinicopathologic study. Am J Med 66:757, 1979.

100. Abelev GI: Alpha-fetoprotein as a marker of embryo-specific differentiations in normal and tumor tissues. Transplant Rev 20:3, 1974.

101. Kurman RJ, Scardino PT, McIntire KR, et al: Cellular localization of alpha-fetoprotein and human chorionic gonadotropin in germ cell tumors of the testis using an indirect immunoperoxidase technique. Cancer 40:2136, 1977.

102. Bonikos DS, Benson KG: Endocrine cells of bronchial and bronchiolar epithelium. Am J Med 63:765, 1977.

103. Berger CL, Goodwin G, Mendelsohn G, et al: Endocrine-related biochemistry in the spectrum of human lung carcinoma. J Clin Endocrinol Metab 53:422, 1981.

104. Kahn CR, Rosen SW, Weintraub BD, et al: Ectopic production of chorionic gonadotropin and its subunits by islet-cell tumors. N Engl J Med 297:565, 1977.

105. Hunter T: The proteins of oncogenes. Sci Am 251:88–97, 1985.

106. Land H, Parada LF, Weinberg RA: Cellular oncogenes and multistep carcinogenesis. Science 222:771, 1983.

107. Bishop JM: The molecular genetics of cancer. Science 235:305, 1987.

108. Bishop JM, Varmus H: Functions and origins of retroviral transforming genes. In Wasset R, et al (eds): Molecular Biology of Tumor Viruses (ed 2). New York, Cold Spring Harbor Laboratory, 1982, p 999.

109. Cooper GM, Lane MA: Cellular transforming genes and oncogenesis. Biochim Biophys Acta 738:9, 1984.

110. Slamon DJ, deKernion JB, Verma IM, Cline MJ: Expression of cellular oncogenes in human malignancies. Science 224:256, 1984.

111. Daughaday WH, Deuel TF: Tumor secretion of growth factors. Endocrinol Metab Clin North Am 20:539, 1991.

112. Chiu IM, Reddy EP, Givol D, et al: Nucleotide sequence analysis identifies the human c-sis proto-oncogene as a structural gene for platelet-derived growth factor. Cell 37:123, 1984.

113. Josephs SF, Ratner L, Clarke MF, et al: Transforming potential of human c-sis nucleotide sequences encoding platelet-derived growth factor. Science 225:636, 1984.

114. Betsholtz C, Johnsson A, Heldin CH, et al: cDNA sequence and chromosomal localization of human platelet-derived growth factor A-chain and its expression in tumour cell lines. Nature 320:695, 1986.

115. Downward J, Yarden Y, Mayes E, et al: Close similarity of epidermal growth factor receptor and v-erb B oncogene protein sequences. Nature 307:521, 1984.

116. Leder P, Battey J, Lenoir G, et al: Translocations among antibody genes in human cancer. Science 222:765, 1983.

117. Nussbaum SR, Gaz RD, Arnold A: Hypercalcemia and ectopic secretion of parathyroid hormone by an ovarian carcinoma with rearrangement of the gene for parathyroid hormone. N Engl J Med 323:1324, 1990.

118. Friend SH, Dryja TP, Weinberg RA: Oncogenes and tumor-suppressing genes. N Engl J Med 318:618, 1988.

119. Warner TF: Cell hybridisation in the genesis of ectopic hormone-secreting tumours. Lancet 1:1259, 1974.

120. Brown DD: Gene expression in eukaryotes. Science 211:667, 1981.

121. Bunnett NW, Reeve JR Jr, Dimaline R, et al: The isolation and sequence analysis of vasoactive intestinal peptide from a ganglioneuroblastoma. J Clin Endocrinol Metab 59:1133, 1984.

122. Schworer ME, DeBold CR, Orth DN: Sequence of mRNA encoding ectopic proopiomelanocortin from a human small cell lung carcinoma maintained in tissue culture. Endocrinology 116:163, 1985.

123. Odell WD, Wolfsen AR: Hormones from tumors: Are they ubiquitous? Am J Med 68:317, 1980.

124. Braunstein GD, Rasor J, Wade ME: Presence in normal human testes of a chorionic-gonadotropin-like substance distinct from human luteinizing hormone. N Engl J Med 293:1339, 1975.

125. Braunstein GD, Kamdar V, Rasor J, et al: Widespread distribution of a chorionic gonadotropin-like substance in normal human tissues. J Clin Endocrinol Metab 49:917, 1979.

126. Yoshimoto Y, Wolfsen AR, Odell WD: Glycosylation, a variable in the production of hCG by cancers. Am J Med 67:414, 1979.

127. Brown WH: A case of pluriglandular syndrome: Diabetes in bearded women. Lancet 2:1022, 1928.

128. Amatruda TT Jr, Upton GV: Paraneoplastic syndromes: Hyperadrenocorticism and ACTH-releasing factor. Ann NY Acad Sci 230:168, 1974.

129. Meador CK, Liddle GW, Island DP, et al: Cause of Cushing's syndrome in patients with tumors arising from "non-endocrine" tissue. J Clin Endocrinol 22:693, 1962.

130. Liddle GW, Nicholson WE, Island DP, et al: Clinical and laboratory studies of ectopic humoral syndromes. Recent Prog Horm Res 25:283, 1969.

131. Mains RE, Eipper BA: Biosynthesis of adrenocorticotropic hormone in mouse pituitary tumor cells. J Biol Chem 251:4115, 1976.

132. Eipper BA, Mains RE: Structure and biosynthesis of pro-adrenocorticotropin endorphin and related peptides. Endocr Rev 1:1, 1980.

133. Roberts JL, Herbert E: Characterization of a common precursor to corticotropin and beta-lipotropin: Identification of beta-lipotropin peptides and their arrangement relative to corticotropin in the precursor synthesized in a cell-free system. Proc Natl Acad Sci USA 74:5300, 1977.

134. Nakanishi S, Inoue A, Kita T, et al: Nucleotide sequence of cloned cDNA for bovine corticotropin beta-lipotropin precursor. Nature 278:423, 1979.

135. Lowry PJ, Silas L, McLean C, et al: Pro-γ-melanocyte-stimulating hormone cleavage in adrenal gland undergoing compensatory growth. Nature 306:70, 1983.

136. Krieger DT, Martin JB: Brain peptides. N Engl J Med 304:876–885, 1981.

137. Bertagna XY, Nicholson WE, Sorenson GD, et al: Corticotropin, lipotropin, and beta-endorphin production by a human nonpituitary tumor in culture: Evidence for a common precursor. Proc Natl Acad Sci USA 75:5160, 1978.

138. deKeyzer Y, Bertagna X, Luton JP, Kahn A: Variable modes of proopiomelanocortin gene transcription in human tumors. Mol Endocrinol 3:215, 1989.

139. Hale AC, Ratter SJ, Tomlin SJ, et al: Measurement of immunoreactive γ-MSH in human plasma. Clin Endocrinol (Oxf) 21:139, 1984.

140. deKeyzer Y, Bertagna X, Lenne F, et al: Altered proopiomelanocortin gene expression in adrenocorticotropin-producing nonpituitary tumors. J Clin Invest 76:1892, 1985.

141. Tanaka K, Nicholson WE, Orth DN: The nature of the immunoreactive lipotropins in human plasma and tissue extracts. J Clin Invest 62:94, 1978.

142. Tanaka I, Nakai Y, Nakao K, et al: γ₁-Melanotropin-like immunoreactivity in bovine and human adrenocorticotropin-producing tissues. J Clin Endocrinol Metab 56:1080, 1983.

143. Pederson RC, Brownie AC, Ling N: Pro-adrenocorticotropin/endorphin–derived peptides: Coordinate action on adrenal steroidogenesis. Science 208:1044, 1980.

144. Ratcliffe JG, Scott AP, Bennett HP, et al: Production of a corticotrophin-like intermediate lobe peptide and of corticotrophin by a bronchial carcinoid tumour. Clin Endocrinol (Oxf) 2:51, 1973.

145. Ratcliffe JG, Podmore J, Stack BHR, et al: Circulating ACTH and related peptides in lung cancer. Br J Cancer 45:230, 1982.

146. Gewirtz G, Yalow RS: Ectopic ACTH production in carcinoma of the lung. J Clin Invest 53:1022, 1974.

147. Odell WD, Wolfsen AR, Bachelot I, Hirose FM: Ectopic production of lipotropin by cancer. Am J Med 66:631, 1979.

148. Wolfsen AR, Odell WD: ProACTH: Use for early detection of lung cancer. Am J Med 66:765, 1979.

149. Orth DN, Nicholson WE: High molecular weight forms of human ACTH are glycoproteins. J Clin Endocrinol Metab 44:214, 1977.

150. Orth DN, Nicholson WE: Different molecular forms of ACTH. Ann NY Acad Sci 297:27, 1977.

151. Orth DN, Guillemin R, Ling N, Nicholson WE: Immunoreactive endorphins, lipotropins and corticotropins in a human nonpituitary tumor: Evidence for a common precursor. J Clin Endocrinol Metab 46:849, 1978.

152. Bertagna XY, Nicholson WE, Sorenson GD, et al: Corticotropin, lipotropin, and β-endorphin production by a human nonpituitary tumor in culture: Evidence for a common precursor. Proc Natl Acad Sci USA 75:5160, 1978.

153. Schteingart DE: Ectopic secretion of peptides of the proopiomelanocortin family. Endocrinol Metab Clin North Am 20:453, 1991.

154. Upton GV, Amatruda TT Jr: Evidence for the presence of tumor peptides with corticotropin-releasing factor–like activity in the ectopic ACTH syndrome. N Engl J Med 285:419, 1971.

155. Christy NP: Adrenal corticotropic activity in the plasma of patients with Cushing's syndrome associated with pulmonary neoplasm. Lancet 1:85, 1961.

156. Landon J, James VH, Peart WS: Cushing's syndrome associated with "corticotrophin"-producing bronchial neoplasm. Acta Endocrinol (Copenh) 56:321, 1967.

157. Belsky JL, Cuello B, Swanson LW, et al: Cushing's syndrome due to ectopic production of corticotropin-releasing factor. J Clin Endocrinol Metab 60:496, 1985.

158. Carey RM, Varma SK, Drake CR Jr, et al: Ectopic secretion of corticotropin-releasing factor as a cause of Cushing's syndrome: A clinical, morphologic, and biochemical study. N Engl J Med 311:13, 1984.

159. Imura H, Matsukura S, Yamamoto H, et al: Studies on ectopic ACTH-producing tumors: II. Clinical and biochemical features of 30 cases. Cancer 35:1430, 1975.

160. Hirata Y, Yamamoto H, Matsukura S, Imura H: In vitro release and biosynthesis of tumor ACTH in ectopic ACTH producing tumors. J Clin Endocrinol Metab 41:106, 1975.

161. Schorr I, Hinshaw HT, Cooper MA, et al: Adenyl cyclase hormone responses of certain human endocrine tumors. J Clin Endocrinol Metab 34:447, 1972.

162. Muller OA, von Werder K: Ectopic production of ACTH and CRH. J Steroid Biochem Mol Biol 43:403, 1992.

163. Hammer GD, Mueller G, Liu B, et al: Ectopic corticotropin-releasing hormone produced by a transfected cell line chronically activates the pituitary adrenal axis in transkaryotic rats. Endocrinology 130:1975, 1992.

164. Dimopoulos MA, Fernandez JF, Samaan NA, et al: Paraneoplastic Cushing's syndrome as an adverse prognostic factor in patients who die early with small cell lung cancer. Cancer 69:66, 1992.

165. Horai R, Nishihara H, Tateishi R, et al: Oat-cell carcinoma of the lung simultaneously producing ACTH and serotonin. J Clin Endocrinol Metab 37:212, 1973.

166. Pimstone BL, Uys CJ, Vogelpoel L: Studies in a case of Cushing's syndrome due to ACTH-producing thymic tumor. Am J Med 53:521, 1972.

167. Hattori S, Matsuda M, Tateishi R, et al: Oat-cell carcinoma of the lung. Clinical and morphological studies in relation to its histogenesis. Cancer 30:1014, 1972.

168. Corrin B, McMillan M: Fine structure of an oat-cell carcinoma of the lung associated with ectopic ACTH syndrome. Br J Cancer 24:755, 1970.

169. Bensch KG, Corrin B, Pariente R, Spencer H: Oat-cell carcinoma of the lung: Its origin and relationship to bronchial carcinoid. Cancer 22:1163, 1968.

170. Mason AM, Ratcliffe JG, Buckle RM, Mason AS: ACTH secretion by bronchial carcinoid tumours. Clin Endocrinol (Oxf) 1:3, 1972.

171. Gomi K, Kameya T, Tsumuraya M, et al: Ultrastructural, histochemical, and biochemical studies of two cases with amylase, ACTH, and beta-MSH producing tumor. Cancer 38:1645, 1976.

172. Chin WW, Goodman RH, Jacobs JW, et al: Medullary thyroid carcinoma identified by cell-free translation of tumor messenger ribonucleic acid in a patient with a neck mass and the syndrome of ectopic adrenocorticotropin. J Clin Endocrinol Metab 52:572, 1981.

173. Pierce ST, Metcalfe M, Banks ER, et al: Small-cell carcinoma with two paraendocrine syndromes. Cancer 69:2258, 1992.

174. Forman BH: ACTH-secreting pheochromocytoma (letter). N Engl J Med 301:1399, 1979.

175. Forman BH, Marban E, Kayne RD, et al: Ectopic ACTH syndrome due to pheochromocytoma: Case report and review of the literature. Yale J Biol Med 52:181, 1979.

176. Spark RF, Connolly PB, Gluckin DS, et al: ACTH secretion from a functioning pheochromocytoma. N Engl J Med 301:416, 1979.

177. deKeyzer Y, Rousseau-Merck MF, Luton JP, et al: Pro-opiomelanocortin gene expression in human phaeochromocytomas. J Mol Biol 2:175, 1989.

178. Cohle SD, Tschen JA, Smith FE, et al: ACTH-secreting carcinoma of the breast. Cancer 43:2370–2376, 1979.

179. Molland EA: Prostatic adenocarcinoma with ectopic ACTH production. Br J Urol 50:358, 1978.

180. Amano S, Hazama F, Haebara H, et al: Ectopic ACTH-MSH producing carcinoid tumor with multiple endocrine hyperplasia in a child. Acta Pathol Jpn 28:721, 1978.

181. Rodgers-Sullivan RF, Weiland LH, Palumbo PJ, Hepper NG: Pulmonary tumorlets associated with Cushing's syndrome. Am Rev Respir Dis 117:799, 1978.

182. Rosenberg EM, Hahn TJ, Orth DN, et al: ACTH-secreting medullary carcinoma of the thyroid presenting as severe idiopathic osteoporosis and senile purpura. J Clin Endocrinol Metab 47:255, 1978.

183. Drasin GF, Lynch T, Temes GP: Ectopic ACTH production and mediastinal lipomatosis. Radiology 127:610, 1978.

184. Bertagna C, Orth DN: Clinical and laboratory findings and results of therapy in 58 patients with adrenocortical tumors admitted to a single medical center. Am J Med 71:855, 1981.

185. Oldfield EH, Doppman JL, Nieman LK, et al: Petrosal sinus sampling with and without CRH for the differential diagnosis of Cushing's syndrome. N Engl J Med 325:897, 1991 (Erratum N Engl J Med 326:1172, 1992).

186. Orth DN: Differential diagnosis of Cushing's syndrome. N Engl J Med 325:957, 1991.

187. Findling JW, Tyrrell JB: Occult ectopic secretion of corticotropin. Arch Intern Med 146:929, 1986.

188. Chajek T, Romanoff H: Cushing syndrome with cyclical edema and periodic secretion of corticosteroids. Arch Intern Med 136:441, 1976.

189. Garroway NW, Orth DN, Harrison RW: Binding of cytosol receptor–glucocorticoid complexes by isolated nuclei of glucocorticoid-responsive and nonresponsive cultured cells. Endocrinology 98:1092, 1976.

190. Himsworth RL, Bloomfield GA, Coombes RC, et al: "Big ACTH" and calcitonin in ectopic hormone secreting tumour of the liver. Clin Endocrinol (Oxf) 7:45, 1977.

191. Kammer H, Barter M: Spontaneous remission of Cushing's disease: A case report and review of the literature. Am J Med 67:519, 1979.

192. Bochner F, Burke CJ, Lloyd HM, Nurnberg BI: Intermittent Cushing's disease. Am J Med 67:507, 1979.

193. Trainer PJ, Grossman A: The diagnosis and differential diagnosis of Cushing's syndrome. Clin Endocrinol (Oxf) 34:317, 1991.

194. Findling JW, Aron DC, Tyrrell JB, et al: Selective venous sampling for ACTH in Cushing's syndrome. Ann Intern Med 94:647, 1981.

195. Schteingart DE: Ectopic secretion of peptides of the proopiomelanocortin family. Endocrinol Metab Clin North Am 20:453, 1991.

196. Sachs BA, Becker N, Bloomberg AE, Grunwald RP: "Cure" of ectopic ACTH syndrome secondary to adenocarcinoma of the lung. J Clin Endocrinol Metab 30:590, 1970.

197. Orth DN, Liddle GW: Results of treatment in 108 patients with Cushing's syndrome. N Engl J Med 285:243, 1971.

198. Coll R, Horner I, Kraiem Z, Gafni J: Successful metyrapone therapy of the ectopic ACTH syndrome. Arch Intern Med 121:549, 1968.

199. Carey RM, Orth DN, Hartmann WH: Malignant melanoma with ectopic production of adrenocorticotropic hormone: Palliative treatment with inhibitors of adrenal steroid biosynthesis. J Clin Endocrinol Metab 36:482, 1973.

200. Gorden P, Becker CE, Levey GS, Roth J: Efficacy of amino-glutethimide in the ectopic ACTH syndrome. J Clin Endocrinol Metab 28:921, 1968.

201. McMillan M, Maisey MN: Effects of aminoglutethimide in a case of ectopic ACTH syndrome. Acta Endocrinol (Copenh) 64:676, 1970.

202. Cooper PR, Shucart WA: Treatment of Cushing's disease with o,p'-DD (letter). N Engl J Med 301:48, 1979.

203. Farwell AP, Devlin JT, Stewart JA: Total suppression of cortisol excretion by ketoconazole in the therapy of the ectopic adrenocorticotropic hormone syndrome. Am J Med 84:1063, 1988.

204. Bertagna X, Favrod-Coune C, Escourolle H, et al: Suppression of ectopic adrenocorticotropin secretion by the long-acting somatostatin analogue octreotiols. J Clin Endocrinol Metab 68:988, 1989.

205. Ginsburg J: Looking ahead. Metabolism 41:121, 1992.

206. Reubi JC, Krenning E, Lamberts SW, Kvols L: In vitro detection of somatostatin receptors in human tumors. Metabolism 41:104, 1992.

207. Shimizu N, Ogata E, Nicholson WE, et al: Studies on the melanotrophic activity of human plasma and tissues. J Clin Endocrinol Metab 25:984, 1965.

208. Island DP, Shimizu N, Nicholson WE, et al: Methods for separating small quantities of MSH and ACTH with good recovery of each. J Clin Endocrinol 25:957, 1965.

209. Abe K, Nicholson WE, Liddle GW, et al: Normal and abnormal regulation of beta-MSH in man. J Clin Invest 48:1580, 1969.

210. Abe K, Nicholson WE, Liddle GW, et al: Radioimmunoassay of beta-MSH in human plasma and tissues. J Clin Invest 46:1609, 1967.

211. Shapiro M, Nicholson WE, Orth DN, et al: Differences between ectopic MSH and pituitary MSH. J Clin Endocrinol Metab 33:377, 1971.

212. Scott AP, Lowry PJ: Adrenocorticotrophic and melanocyte-stimulating peptides in the human pituitary. Biochem J 139:593, 1974.

213. Bloomfield GA, Scott AP, Lowry PJ, et al: A reappraisal of human beta-MSH. Nature 252:492, 1974.

214. Li CH, Barnafi L, Chretien M, Chung D: Isolation and amino-acid sequence of beta-LPH from sheep pituitary glands. Nature 208:1093, 1965.

215. Gilkes JJ, Bloomfield GA, Scott AP, et al: Development and validation of a radioimmunoassay for peptides related to beta-melanocyte-stimulating hormone in human plasma: The lipotropins. J Clin Endocrinol Metab 40:450, 1975.

216. Jeffcoate WJ, Rees LH, Lowry PJ, Besser GM: A specific radioimmunoassay for human β-lipotropin. J Clin Endocrinol Metab 47:160, 1978.

217. Philipponeau M, Lenne F, Proeschel MF, et al: Plasma immunoreactive joining peptide in man. J Clin Endocrinol Metab 76:325, 1993.

218. Guillemin R, Vargo M, Rossi J, et al: Beta-endorphin and adrenocorticotropin are secreted concomitantly by the pituitary gland. Science 197:1367, 1977.

219. Tanaka K, Nicholson WE, Orth DN: The nature of the immunoreactive lipotropins in human plasma and tissue extracts. J Clin Invest 62:94, 1978.

220. Deftos LJ, Burton D, Catherwood BD, et al: Demonstration by immunoperoxidase histochemistry of calcitonin in the anterior lobe of the rat pituitary. J Clin Endocrinol Metab 47:457, 1978.

221. Bertagna XY, Nicholson WE, Pettengill OS, et al: Ectopic production of high molecular weight calcitonin and corticotropin by human small cell carcinoma cells in tissue culture: Evidence for separate precursors. J Clin Endocrinol Metab 47:1390, 1978.

222. Ueda M, Takeuchi T, Abe K, et al: Beta-melanocyte-stimulating hormone immunoreactivity in human pituitaries and ectopic adrenocorticotropin-producing tumors. J Clin Endocrinol Metab 50:550, 1980.

223. Liotta AS, Suda T, Krieger DT: Beta-lipotropin is the major opioid-like peptide of human pituitary and rat pars distalis: Lack of significant beta-endorphin. Proc Natl Acad Sci USA 75:2950, 1978.

224. Suda T, Liotta AS, Krieger DT: Beta-endorphin is not detectable in plasma from normal human subjects. Science 202:221, 1978.

225. Suda T, Abe Y, Demura H, et al: ACTH, beta-LPH and beta-endorphin in pituitary adenomas of the patients with Cushing's disease: Activation of beta-LPH conversion to beta-endorphin. J Clin Endocrinol Metab 49:475, 1979.

226. Wiedemann E, Saito T, Linfoot JA, Li CH: Specific radioimmunoassay of human beta-endorphin in unextracted plasma. J Clin Endocrinol Metab 49:478, 1979.

227. Pullan PT, Clement-Jones V, Corder R, et al: Ectopic production of methionine enkephalin and beta-endorphin. Br Med J 280:758, 1980.

228. Bertagna XY, Stone WJ, Nicholson WE, et al: Simultaneous assay of immunoreactive β-lipotropin, α-lipotropin, and β-endorphin in plasma of normal human subjects, patients with ACTH/lipotropin hypersecretory syndromes, and patients undergoing chronic hemodialysis. J Clin Invest 67:124, 1981.

229. Pullan PT, Clement-Jones V, Corder R, et al: ACTH LPH and related peptides in the ectopic ACTH syndrome. Clin Endocrinol (Oxf) 13:437, 1980.

230. Clement-Jones V, Corder R, Lowry PJ: Isolation of human met-enkephalin and two groups of putative precursors (2K-pro-met-enkephalin) from an adrenal medullary tumor. Biochem Biophys Res Commun 95:665, 1980.

231. Grossman A, Besser GM, Milles JJ, Baylis PH: Inhibition of vasopressin release in man by an opiate peptide. Lancet 2:1108, 1980.

232. Matsuoka H, Mulrow PJ, Li CH: β-Lipotropin: A new aldosterone-stimulating factor. Science 209:307, 1980.

233. McCloy J, McCloy RF: Enkephalins, hunger, and obesity (letter). Lancet 2:156, 1979.

234. Margules DL, Moisset B, Lewis MJ, et al: Beta-endorphin is associated with overeating in genetically obese mice (ob/ob) and rats (fa/fa). Science 202:988, 1978.

235. Holaday JW, O'Hara M, Faden AI: Hypophysectomy alters cardiorespiratory variables: Central effects of pituitary endorphins in shock. Am J Physiol 241:H479, 1981.

236. Carr DB, Bullen BA, Skrinar GS, et al: Physical conditioning facilitates the exercise-induced secretion of beta-endorphin and beta-lipotropin in women. N Engl J Med 305:560, 1981.

237. Davis GC, Buchsbaum MS, Bunney WE Jr: Opiates, opioid peptides and psychiatry. Ann NY Acad Sci 362:67, 1981.

238. Krieger DT, Glick SM: Sleep EEG stages and plasma growth hormone concentration in states of endogenous and exogenous hypercortisolemia or ACTH elevation. J Clin Endocrinol Metab 39:986, 1974.

239. Steiner H, Dahlback O, Waldenström J: Ectopic growth-hormone production and osteoarthropathy in carcinoma of the bronchus. Lancet 1:783, 1968.

240. Cameron DP, Burger HG, DeKretzer DM, et al: On the presence of immunoreactive growth hormone in a bronchogenic carcinoma. Australas Ann Med 18:143, 1969.

241. Dupont B, Hoyer I, Borgeskov S, Nerup J: Plasma growth hormone and hypertrophic osteoarthropathy in carcinoma of the bronchus. Acta Med Scand 1–2:25, 1970.

242. Beck C, Burger HG: Evidence for the presence of immunoreactive growth hormone in cancers of the lung and stomach. Cancer 30:75, 1972.

243. Greenberg PB, Martin TJ, Beck C, Burger HG: Synthesis and release of human growth hormone from lung carcinoma in cell culture. Lancet 1:350, 1972.

244. Hammarsten JF, O'Leary J: The features and significance of hypertrophic osteoarthropathy. Arch Intern Med 99:431, 1957.

245. Melmed S, Ezrin C, Kovacs K, et al: Acromegaly due to secretion of growth hormone by an ectopic pancreatic islet-cell tumor. N Engl J Med 312:9, 1985.

246. Ezzat S, Ezrin C, Yamashita S, Melmed S: Recurrent acromegaly resulting from ectopic growth hormone gene expression by a metastatic pancreatic tumor. Cancer 71:66, 1993.

247. Saeed UZ Zafar M, Mellinger RC, et al: Acromegaly associated with a bronchial carcinoid tumor: Evidence for ectopic production of growth hormone releasing activity. J Clin Endocrinol Metab 48:66, 1979.

248. Frohman LA, Szabo M, Berelowitz M, Stachura ME: Partial purification and characterization of a peptide with growth hormone-releasing activity from extrapituitary tumors in patients with acromegaly. J Clin Invest 65:43, 1980.

249. Mayo KE, Cerelli GM, Lebo RV, et al: Gene encoding human growth hormone-releasing factor precursor: Structure, sequence, and chromosomal assignment. Proc Natl Acad Sci USA 82:63, 1985.

250. Melmed S, Ziel FH, Braunstein GD, et al: Medical management of acromegaly due to ectopic production of growth hormone–releasing hormone by a carcinoid tumor. J Endocrinol Metab 67:395, 1988.

251. Melmed S, Braunstein GD, Horvath E, et al: Pathophysiology of acromegaly. Endocr Rev 4:271, 1983.

252. Thorner MO, Frohman LA, Leong DA, et al: Extrahypothalamic growth-hormone–releasing factor (GRF) secretion is a rare cause of acromegaly: Plasma GRF levels in 177 acromegalic patients. J Clin Endocrinol Metab 59:846, 1984.

253. Glikson M, Gil-Ad I, Galun E, et al: Acromegaly due to ectopic growth hormone–releasing hormone secretion by a bronchial carcinoid tumor: Dynamic hormonal responses to various stimuli. Acta Endocrinol (Copenh) 125:366, 1991.

254. Melmed S. Extrapituitary acromegaly. Endocrinol Metab Clin North Am 20:507, 1991.

255. Bevan JS, Asa SL, Rossi ML, Esrimm EA: Intrasellar gangliocytoma containing gastrin and growth hormone-releasing hormone associated with a growth hormone-secreting pituitary adenoma. Clin Endocrinol (Oxf) 30:213, 1989.

256. Rivier J, Speiss J, Thorner M, Vale W: Characterization of a growth hormone–releasing factor from a human pancreatic islet tumour. Nature 300:276, 1982.

257. Asa SL, Kovacs K, Thorner MO, et al: Immunohistological localization of growth hormone–releasing hormone in human tumors. J Clin Endocrinol Metab 60:423, 1985.

258. Frohman LA: Therapeutic options in acromegaly. J Clin Endocrinol Metab 72:1175, 1991.

259. Gorden P, Comi RJ, Maton PN, Go VL: Somatostatin and somatostatin analogues (SMS 201-995) in treatment of hormone-secreting tumors of the pituitary and gastrointestinal tract and nonneoplastic diseases of the gut. Ann Intern Med 110:35, 1989.

260. Sherwood LM, Handwerger S, McLaurin WD, Lanner M: Amino-acid sequence of human placental lactogen. Nature 233:59, 1971.

261. Grumbach MM, Kaplan SL, Sciarra JJ, Burr IM: Chorionic growth hormone–prolactin (CGP): Secretion, disposition, biologic activity in man, and postulated function as the "growth hormone" of the second half of pregnancy. Ann NY Acad Sci 148:501, 1968.

262. Weintraub BD, Rosen SW: Ectopic production of human chorionic somatotropin by nontrophoblastic cancers. J Clin Endocrinol Metab 32:94, 1971.

263. Payne RA, Ryan RJ: Human placental lactogen in the male subject. J Urol 107:99, 1972.

264. Sussman HH, Weintraub BD, Rosen SW: Relationship of ectopic placental alkaline phosphatase to ectopic chorionic gonadotropin and placental lactogen. Cancer 33:820, 1974.

265. Muggia FM, Rosen SW, Weintraub BD, Hansen HH: Ectopic placental proteins in nontrophoblastic tumors. Cancer 36:1327, 1975.

266. Horne CH, Reid IN, Milne GD: Prognostic significance of inappropriate production of pregnancy proteins by breast cancers. Lancet 2:279, 1976.

267. Sheth NA, Suraiya JN, Sheth AR, et al: Ectopic production of human placental lactogen by human breast tumors. Cancer 39:1693, 1977.

268. Schneider AB, Kowalski K, Sherwood LM: "Big" human placental

lactogen: Disulfide-linked peptide chains. Biochem Biophys Res Commun 64:717, 1975.
269. Schneider AB, Kowalski K, Sherwood LM: Identification of "big" human placental lactogen in placenta and serum. Endocrinology 97:1364, 1975.
270. Schneider AB, Kowalski K, Russell J, Sherwood LM: Identification of the interchain disulfide bonds of dimeric human placental lactogen. J Biol Chem 254:3782, 1979.
271. Sherwood LM: Human prolactin. N Engl J Med 284:774, 1971.
272. Turkington RW: Ectopic production of prolactin. N Engl J Med 285:1455, 1971.
273. Rees LH, Bloomfield GA, Rees GM, et al: Multiple hormones in a bronchial tumor. J Clin Endocrinol Metab 38:1090, 1974.
274. Purnell DM, Hillman EA, Heatfield BM, Trump BF: Immunoreactive prolactin in epithelial cells of normal and cancerous human breast and prostate detected by the unlabeled antibody peroxidase-antiperoxidase method. Cancer Res 42:2317, 1982.
275. Locke EA: Secondary hypertrophic osteoarthropathy and its relationship to clubbed fingers. Arch Intern Med 15:659, 1915.
276. McArthur JW, Toll GD, Russfield AB, et al: Sexual precocity attributable to ectopic gonadotropin secretion by hepatoblastoma. Am J Med 54:390, 1973.
277. Treves N: Gynecomastia: The origins of mammary swelling in the male. An analysis of 406 patients with breast hypertrophy, 525 with testicular tumors and 13 with adrenal neoplasms. Cancer 11:1083, 1958.
278. Rosen SW, Becker CE, Schlaff S, et al: Ectopic gonadotropin production before clinical recognition of bronchogenic carcinoma. N Engl J Med 279:640, 1968.
279. Faiman C, Colwell JA, Ryan RJ, et al: Gonadotropin secretion from a bronchogenic carcinoma: Demonstration by radioimmunoassay. N Engl J Med 277:1395, 1967.
280. Vaitukaitis JL: Immunologic and physical characterization of human chorionic gonadotropin (HCG) secreted by tumors. J Clin Endocrinol Metab 37:505, 1973.
281. Castleman B, Scully RE, McNeely BU: Case records of the Massachusetts General Hospital. N Engl J Med 286:594, 1972.
282. Castleman B, Scully RE, McNeely BU: Case records of the Massachusetts General Hospital. N Engl J Med 286:713, 1972.
283. Herman-Bonert VS, Braunstein GD: Gonadotropin secretory abnormalities. Endocrinol Metab Clin North Am 20:519, 1991.
284. Kirschner MA, Cohen FB, Jespersen D: Estrogen production and its origin in men with gonadotropin-producing neoplasms. J Clin Endocrinol Metab 39:112, 1974.
285. Fein HG, Rosen SW, Weintraub BD: Increased glycosylation of serum human chorionic gonadotropin and subunits from eutopic and ectopic sources: comparison with placental and urinary forms. J Clin Endocrinol Metab 50:1111, 1980.
286. Cole LA, Hussa RO: Use of glycosidase digested human chorionic gonadotropin beta subunit to explain the partial binding of ectopic glycoprotein hormones to Con A. Endocrinology 109:2276, 1981.
287. Chen HC, Hodgen GD, Matsukura S, et al: Evidence for gonadotropin from nonpregnant subjects that has physical, immunological, and biological similarities to human chorionic gonadotropin. Proc Natl Acad Sci USA 73:2885, 1976.
288. Borkowski A, Muquardt C: Human chorionic gonadotropin in the plasma of normal, nonpregnant subjects. N Engl J Med 301:298, 1979.
289. Braunstein GD: Human chorionic gonadotropin in nontrophoblastic tumors and tissues. In Talwar GP (ed): Recent Advances in Reproduction and Regulation of Fertility. Amsterdam, Elsevier, 1979; p 389.
290. Braunstein G, Rasor J, Thompson R, et al: Prospective evaluation of serum chorionic gonadotrophin measurements for the immunodiagnosis of cancer. Clin Res 29:90, 1981.
291. Braunstein GD, Rasor J, Wade ME: Presence of an hCG-like substance in non-pregnant humans. In Segal SL (ed): Chorionic Gonadotropin. New York, Plenum Press, 1980, p 303.
292. Hattori M, Fukase M, Yoshimi H, et al: Ectopic production of human chorionic gonadotropin in malignant tumors. Cancer 42:2328, 1978.
293. Papapetrou PD, Sakarelou NP, Braouzi H, Fessas PH: Ectopic production of human chorionic gonadotropin (hCG) by neoplasms. Cancer 45:2583, 1980.
294. Weymann RE, Nisula BC: Renal clearance rates of the subunits of human chorionic gonadotropin in man. J Clin Endocrinol Metab 49:674, 1979.
295. Goldenberg DM, Kim EE, DeLand FH, et al: Clinical radioimmunodetection of cancer with radioactive antibodies to human chorionic gonadotropin. Science 208:1284, 1980.
296. Goldenberg DM, DeLand F, Kim E, et al: Use of radiolabeled antibodies to carcinoembryonic antigen for the detection and localization of diverse cancers by external photoscanning. N Engl J Med 298:1384, 1978.
297. Metz SA, Weintraub B, Rosen SW, et al: Ectopic secretion of chorionic gonadotropin by a lung carcinoma. Am J Med 65:325, 1978.
298. Bielinska M, Boime I: mRNA-dependent synthesis of a glycosylated subunit of hCG in cell-free extracts derived from ascites tumor cells. Proc Natl Acad Sci USA 75:1768, 1978.
299. Birken S, Canfield RE: Structural and immunochemical properties of human choriogonadotropin. In McKerns KW (ed): Structure and Function of the Gonadotropins. New York, Plenum Press, 1978, p 47.
300. Boime I, Landefeld T, McQueen S, McWilliams D: The biosynthesis of chorionic gonadotropin and placental lactogen in first- and third-trimester human placenta. In McKerns KW (ed): Structure and Function of the Gondaotropins. New York, Plenum Press, 1978, p 235.
301. Chin WW, Gharib SD: Organization and expression of gonadotropin genes. Adv Exp Biol Med 205:245, 1986.
302. Benveniste R, Conway MC, Puett D, Rabinowitz D: Heterogeneity of the human chorionic gonadotropin alpha-subunit secreted by cultured choriocarcinoma (JEG) cells. J Clin Endocrinol Metab 48:85, 1979.
303. Benveniste R, Lindner J, Puett D, Rabin D: Human chorionic gonadotropin alpha-subunit from cultured choriocarcinoma (JEG) cells: Comparison of the subunit secreted free with that prepared from secreted human chorionic gonadotropin. Endocrinology 105:581, 1979.
304. Dean DJ, Weintraub BD, Rosen SW: De novo synthesis and secretion of heterogeneous forms of human chorionic gonadotropin and its free alpha-subunit in the human choriocarcinoma clonal cell line JEG-3. Endocrinology 106:849, 1980.
305. Quigley MM, Tyrey L, Hammond CB: Alpha-subunit in sera of choriocarcinoma patients in remission. J Clin Endocrinol Metab 50:98, 1980.
306. Hussa RO, Fein HG, Pattillo RA, et al: A distinctive form of human chorionic gonadotropin β-subunit–like material produced by cervical carcinoma cells. Cancer Res 46:1948, 1986.
307. Nagelberg SB, Cole LA, Rosen SW: A novel form of ectopic human chorionic gonadotropin β-subunit in the serum of a woman with epidermoid cancer. J Endocrinol 107:403, 1985.
308. Vaitukaitis JL, Ross GT, Braunstein DG, Rayford PL: Gonadotropins and their subunits: Basic and clinical studies. Recent Prog Horm Res 32:289, 1976.
309. Kourides IA, Weintraub BD, Ridgway EC, Maloof F: Pituitary secretion of free alpha and beta subunit of human thyrotropin in patients with thyroid disorders. J Clin Endocrinol Metab 40:872, 1975.
310. Prentice LG, Ryan RJ: LH and its subunits in human pituitary, serum and urine. J Clin Endocrinol Metab 40:303, 1975.
311. Ghosh NK, Cox RP: Production of human chorionic gonadotropins in HeLa cell cultures. Nature 259:416, 1976.
312. Lieblich JM, Weintraub BD, Rosen SW, et al: HeLa cells secrete α subunit of glycoprotein tropic hormones. Nature 260:530, 1976.
313. Weintraub BD, Krauth G, Rosen SW, Rabson AS: Differences between purified ectopic and normal alpha subunits of human glycoprotein hormones. J Clin Invest 56:1043, 1975.
314. Lieblich JM, Weintraub BD, Krauth GH, et al: Ectopic and eutopic secretion of chorionic gonadotropin and its subunits in vitro: Comparison of clonal strains from carcinomas of the lung and placenta. J Natl Cancer Inst 56:911, 1976.
315. Weintraub BD, Stannard BS, Rosen SW: Combination of ectopic and standard human glycoprotein hormone alpha with beta subunits: Discordance of immunologic and receptor-binding activity. Endocrinology 101:225, 1977.
316. Landefeld T, Boguslawski S, Corash L, Boime I: The cell-free synthesis of the alpha subunit of human chorionic gonadotropin. Endocrinology 98:1220, 1976.
317. Braunstein GD: Placental proteins as tumor markers. Immunol Ser 53:673, 1990.
318. Cave WT Jr, Dunn JT: Choriocarcinoma with hyperthyroidism: Probable identity of the thyrotropin with human chorionic gonadotropin. Ann Intern Med 85:60, 1976.
319. Amir SM, Sullivan RC, Ingbar SH: In vitro response to crude and purified hCG in human thyroid membranes. J Clin Endocrinol Metab 51:51, 1980.
320. Pekonen F, Weintraub BD: Thyrotropin binding to cultured lymphocytes and thyroid cells. Endocrinology 103:1668, 1978.
321. Pekonen F, Weintraub BD: Interaction of crude and pure chorionic gonadotropin with the thyrotropin receptor. J Clin Endocrinol Metab 50:280, 1980.

322. Higgins HP, Hershman JM: The hyperthyroidism due to trophoblastic hormone. Clin Endocrinol Metab 7:167, 1978.
323. Harada A, Hershman JM: Extraction of human chorionic thyrotropin from term placentas: Failure to recover thyrotropic activity. J Clin Endocrinol Metab 47:681, 1978.
324. Kourides IA, Weintraub BD, Maloof F: Large molecular weight TSH-β: The sole immunoreactive form of TSH-β in certain human sera. J Clin Endocrinol Metab 47:24, 1978.
325. Spitz IM, LeRoith D, Hirsch H, et al: Increased high-molecular-weight thyrotropin with impaired biologic activity in a euthyroid man. N Engl J Med 304:278, 1981.
326. Winkler AW, Cranshaw OS: Chloride depletion conditions other than Addison's disease. J Clin Invest 17:1, 1938.
327. Schwartz WB, Bennett W, Curelop ES, Bartter FC: A syndrome of renal sodium loss and hyponatremia probably resulting from inappropriate secretion of antidiuretic hormone. Am J Med 23:529, 1957.
328. Thorn NE, Transbol I: Hyponatremia and bronchogenic carcinoma associated with renal excretion of large amounts of antidiuretic material. Am J Med 35:257, 1963.
329. Amatruda TT Jr, Mulrow PJ, Gallagher JC, Sawyer WH: Carcinoma of the lung with inappropriate antidiuresis: Demonstration of antidiuretic hormone-like activity in tumor extract. N Engl J Med 269:544, 1963.
330. Bower BF, Mason DM, Forsham PH: Bronchogenic carcinoma with inappropriate antidiuretic activity in plasma and tumor. N Engl J Med 271:934, 1964.
331. Vorherr H, Massry S, Utiger RD, Kleeman CR: Antidiuretic principle in malignant tumor extracts from patients with inappropriate ADH syndrome. J Clin Endocrinol Metab 28:162, 1968.
332. Utiger RD: Inappropriate antidiuresis and carcinoma of the lung: Detection of vasopressin in tumor extracts by immunoassay. J Clin Endocrinol Metab 26:970, 1966.
333. Sawyer WH: Pharmacological characteristics of the antidiuretic principle in a bronchogenic carcinoma for a patient with hyponatremia. J Clin Endocrinol Metab 27:1497, 1967.
334. Bartter FC, Schwartz WB: The syndrome of inappropriate secretion of antidiuretic hormone. Am J Med 42:790, 1967.
335. Kaye SB, Ross EJ: Inappropriate antidiuretic hormone (ADH) secretion in association with carcinoma of the bladder. Postgrad Med J 53:274, 1977.
336. Cassileth PA, Trotman BW: Inappropriate antidiuretic hormone in Hodgkin's disease. Am J Med Sci 265:233, 1973.
337. Hainsworth JD, Workman R, Greco FA: Management of the syndrome of inappropriate antidiuretic hormone secretion in small cell lung cancer. Cancer 51:161, 1983.
338. Comis RL, Miller M, Ginsberg SJ: Abnormalities in water homeostasis in small cell anaplastic lung cancer. Cancer 45:2414, 1980.
339. Zerbe R, Stropes L, Robertson G: Vasopressin function in the syndrome of inappropriate antidiuresis. Annu Rev Med 31:315, 1980.
340. Robertson GL: The regulation of vasopressin in function in health and disease. Recent Prog Horm Res 33:333, 1976.
341. Morton JJ, Kelly P, Padfield PL: Antidiuretic hormone in bronchogenic carcinoma. Clin Endocrinol (Oxf) 9:357, 1978.
342. Padfield PL, Morton JJ, Brown JJ, et al: Plasma arginine vasopressin in the syndrome of antidiuretic hormone excess associated with bronchogenic carcinoma. Am J Med 61:825, 1976.
343. Perks WH, Stanhope R, Green M: Hyponatraemia and mesothelioma. Br J Dis Chest 73:89, 1979.
344. Skrabanek P, Powell D: Is the evidence for ectopic antidiuretic hormone watertight? Med Hypotheses 6:193, 1980.
345. Moses AM, Scheinman SJ: Ectopic secretion of neurohypophyseal peptides in patients with malignancy. Endocrinol Metab Clin North Am 20:489, 1991.
346. Pettengill OS, Faulkner CS, Wurster-Hill DH, et al: Isolation and characterization of a hormone-producing cell line of human small-cell anaplastic carcinoma of the lung. J Natl Cancer Inst 58:511, 1977.
347. Kondo Y, Mizumoto Y, Katayama S, et al: Inappropriate secretion of antidiuretic hormone in nude mice bearing a human bronchogenic oat-cell carcinoma. Cancer Res 41:1545, 1981.
348. Kelly P, Morton JJ: Antidiuretic hormone immunoactivity in tumour tissue from patients with bronchogenic carcinoma: with and without hypernatraemia. Clin Endocrinol (Oxf) 12:99, 1980.
349. George JM, Capen CC, Phillips AS: Biosynthesis of vasopressin in vitro and ultrastructure of a bronchogenic carcinoma. J Clin Invest 51:141, 1972.
350. Yamaji T, Ishibashi M, Hori T: Propressophysin in human blood: A possible marker of ectopic vasopressin production. J Clin Endocrinol Metab 59:505, 1984.
351. Martin TJ, Greenberg PB, Beck C, Johnston CI: Synthesis of peptide hormones by human tumors in cell cultures. In Endocrinology Proceedings of the IV International Congress. Amsterdam, Excerpta Medica, 1973, pp 1198–1204.
352. Bliss DP, Battey JF, Linnoila RI, Birrer MJ, et al. Expression of the atrial natriuretic factor gene in small cell lung cancer tumors and tumor cell lines. J Natl Cancer Inst 82:305, 1990.
353. Shimizu K, Nakano S, Nakano Y, Ando M, et al: Ectopic atrial natriuretic peptide production in small cell lung cancer with the syndrome of inappropriate ADH secretion. Cancer 68:2284, 1991.
354. Kern PA, Robbins RJ, Bichet D, et al: Syndrome of inappropriate antidiuresis in the absence of arginine vasopressin. J Clin Endocrinol Metab 62:148, 1986.
355. Fichman MP, Bethune JE: The role of adrenocorticoids in the inappropriate antidiuretic hormone syndrome. Ann Intern Med 68:806, 1968.
356. Hantman D, Rossier B, Zohlman R, Schrier R: Rapid correction of hyponatremia in the syndrome of inappropriate secretion of antidiuretic hormone. Ann Intern Med 78:870, 1973.
357. White MG, Fetner CD: Treatment of the syndrome of inappropriate secretion of antidiuretic hormone with lithium carbonate. N Engl J Med 292:390, 1975.
358. Cherrill DA, Stote RM, Birge JR, Singer I: Demeclocycline treatment in the syndrome of inappropriate antidiuretic hormone secretion. Ann Intern Med 83:654, 1975.
359. Decaulx G, Brimioulle S, Genette F, Mockel J: Treatment of the syndrome of inappropriate secretion of antidiuretic hormone by urea. Am J Med 69:99, 1980.
360. Decaulx G, Waterlot Y, Genette F, Mockel J: Treatment of the syndrome of inappropriate secretion of antidiuretic hormone with furosemide. N Engl J Med 304:329, 1981.
361. Land H, Shutz G, Schmale H, Richter D: Nucleotide sequence of cloned cDNA encoding bovine arginine vasopressin-neurophysin II precursor. Nature 295:299, 1982.
362. Hamilton BP, Upton GV, Amatruda TT Jr: Evidence for the presence of neurophysin in tumors producing the syndrome of inappropriate antidiuresis. J Clin Endocrinol Metab 35:764, 1972.
363. Robinson AG, Zimmerman EA, Frantz AG: Physiologic investigation of posterior pituitary binding proteins neurophysin I and neurophysin II. Metabolism 20:1148, 1971.
364. Hamilton BP: Presence of neurophysin proteins in tumors associated with the syndrome of inappropriate ADH secretion. Ann NY Acad Sci 248:153, 1975.
365. North WG, Ware J, Maurer LH, et al: Neurophysins as tumor markers for small cell carcinoma of the lung. Cancer 62:1343, 1988.
366. Stolbac LL, Krant MJ, Fishman WH: Ectopic production of an alkaline phosphatase isoenzyme in patients with cancer. N Engl J Med 281:757, 1969.
367. Marks LJ, Steinke J, Podolsky S, Egdahl RH: Hypoglycemia associated with neoplasia. Ann NY Acad Sci 230:147, 1974.
368. Olefsky S, Bailey I, Samols E, Bilkus D: A fibrosarcoma with hypoglycemia in a high serum insulin level. Lancet 2:378, 1962.
369. Unger RH, Lochner J, Eisentraut AM: Identification of insulin and glucagon in bronchogenic metastasis. J Clin Endocrinol Metab 24:823, 1964.
370. Saeed SM, Fine G, Horn RC Jr: Hypoglycemia associated with extra-pancreatic tumors: An immunofluorescent study. Cancer 24:158, 1969.
371. Shames JM, Dhurandhar NR, Blackard WG: Insulin-secreting bronchial carcinoid tumor with widespread metastases. Am J Med 44:632, 1968.
372. Lyall SS, Marieb NJ, Wise JK, et al: Hyperinsulinemic hypoglycemia associated with a neurofibrosarcoma. Arch Intern Med 135:865, 1975.
373. Honicky RE, dePapp EW: Mediastinal teratoma with endocrine function. Am J Dis Child 126:650, 1973.
374. Shetty MR, Boghossian HM, Duffell D, et al: Tumor-induced hypoglycemia: A result of ectopic insulin production. Cancer 49:1920, 1982.
375. Smith NL, Janelli DE, Madariaga J, Mishriki Y: Hypoglycemia and Hodgkin's disease with hyperinsulinemia. J Surg Oncol 19:27, 1982.
376. Rosenzweig JL, Havrankova J, Lesniak MA, et al: Insulin is ubiquitous in extrapancreatic tissues of rats and humans. Proc Natl Acad Sci USA 77:572, 1980.
377. Jakob A, Hauri C, Froesch ER: Nonsuppressible insulin-like activity in human serum: III. Differentiation of two distinct molecules with non-suppressible ILA. J Clin Invest 47:2678, 1968.
378. Hall K, Uthne K: Some biological properties of purified sulfation factor (SF) from human plasma. Acta Med Scand 190:137, 1971.

379. Froesch ER, Zapf J, Widmer U: Hypoglycemia associated with non-islet-cell tumor and insulin-like growth factors (letter). N Engl J Med 306:1178, 1982.

380. Froesch ER, Schmid C, Schwander J, Zapf J: Actions of insulin-like growth factors. Ann Rev Physiol 47:443, 1985.

381. Sussenbach JS: The gene structure of the insulin-like growth factor family. Prog Growth Factor Res 1:33, 1989.

382. Russell SM, Spencer EM: Local injections of human or rat growth hormone or of purified human somatomedin-C stimulate unilateral tibial epiphyseal growth in hypophysectomized rats. Endocrinology 116:2563, 1985.

383. LeRoith D, Clemmons D, Nissley P, Rechler MM: NIH conference: Insulin-like growth factors in health and disease. Ann Intern Med 116:854, 1992.

384. Daughaday WH, Trivedi B, Kapadia M: Measurement of insulin-like growth factor II by a specific radioreceptor assay in serum of normal individuals, patients with abnormal growth hormone secretion, and patients with tumor-associated hypoglycemia. J Clin Endocrinol Metab 53:289, 1981.

385. Megyesi K, Kahn CR, Roth J, Gorden P: Hypoglycemia in association with extrapancreatic tumors: Demonstration of elevated plasma NSILA-s by a new radioreceptor assay. J Clin Endocrinol Metab 38:931, 1974.

386. Gorden P, Hendricks CM, Kahn CR, et al: Hypoglycemia associated with non-islet-cell tumors and insulin-like growth factors. N Engl J Med 305:1452, 1981.

387. Daughaday WH, Emanuele MA, Brooks MH, et al: Synthesis and secretion of insulin-like growth factor II by a leiomyosarcoma with associated hypoglycemia. N Engl J Med 319:1434, 1988.

388. Daughaday WH, Kapadia M: Significance of abnormal serum binding of insulin-like growth factor II in the development of hypoglycemia in patients with non-islet-cell tumors. Proc Natl Acad Sci USA 86:6778, 1989.

389. Yonei Y, Tanaka M, Ozawa Y, et al: Primary hepatocellular carcinoma with severe hypoglycemia. Liver 12:90, 1992.

390. Ron D, Powers AC, Pandian M, et al: Increased insulin-line growth factor II production and consequent suppression of growth hormone secretion: A dual mechanism for tumor-induced hypoglycemia. J Clin Endocrinol Metab 68:701, 1989.

391. Plovnick H, Ruderman NB, Aoki T, et al: Non-B-cell tumor hypoglycemia associated with increased nonsuppressible insulin-like protein (NSILP). Am J Med 66:154, 1979.

392. Daughaday WH: Hypoglycemia in patients with non-islet cell tumors. Endocrinol Metab Clin North Am 18:91, 1989.

393. Alexrod L, Ron D: Insulin-like growth factor II and the riddle of tumor-induced hypoglycemia. N Engl J Med 319:1477, 1988.

394. August JT, Hiatt HH: Severe hypoglycemia secondary to non-pancreatic fibrosarcoma with insulin activity. Ann Intern Med 2258:17, 1958.

395. McFadzean AJ, Yeung RT: Further observations on hypoglycemia and hepatocellular carcinoma. Am J Med 47:220, 1969.

396. Rodman JS, Sherwood LM: Disorders of mineral metabolism in malignancy. In Avioli LV, Krane S (eds): Metabolic Bone Disease. New York, Academic Press, 1978.

397. Metz SA, McRae JR, Robertson RP: Prostaglandins as mediators of paraneoplastic syndromes: Review and update. Metabolism 30:299, 1981.

398. Luben RA, Mohler MA, Nedwin GE: Production of hybridomas secreting monoclonal antibodies against the lymphokine osteoclast-activating factor. J Clin Invest 64:337, 1979.

399. Mundy GR, Raisz LG, Shapiro JL, et al: Big and little forms of osteoclast-activating factor. J Clin Invest 60:122, 1977.

400. Raisz LG, Simmons HA, Sandberg AL, Canalis E: Direct stimulation of bone resorption by epidermal growth factor. Endocrinology 107:270, 1980.

401. Eilon G, Mundy GR: Direct resorption of bone by human breast cancer cells in vitro. Nature 276:726, 1978.

402. Mundy GR, Altman AJ, Gondek MD, Bandelin JG: Direct resorption of bone by human monocytes. Science 196:1109, 1977.

403. Minkin C, Posek R, Newbrey J: Mononuclear phagocytes and bone resorption: Identification and preliminary characterization of a bone-derived macrophage chemotactic factor. Metab Bone Dis Relat Res 2:363, 1981.

404. Sherwood LM: The multiple causes of hypercalcemia in malignant disease (editorial). N Engl J Med 303:1412, 1980.

405. Mundy GR, Cove DH, Fisken R: Primary hyperparathyroidism. Lancet 1:1317, 1980.

406. Heath H III, Hodgson SF, Kennedy MA: Primary hyperparathyroidism: Incidence, morbidity, and potential economic impact in a community. N Engl J Med 302:189, 1980.

407. Bachman AL, Sproul EE: Correlation of radiographic and autopsy findings in suspected metastasis in the spine. Bull NY Acad Sci 31:146, 1955.

408. Albright FA: Case records of the Massachusetts General Hospital #27, 461. N Engl J Med 225:79, 1941.

409. Plimpton CH, Gellhorn A: Hypercalcemia in malignant disease without evidence of bone destruction. Am J Med 21:750, 1956.

410. Connor TB, Thomas WC Jr, Howard JE: Etiology of hypercalcemia associated with lung carcinoma. J Clin Invest 35:697, 1956.

411. Goldberg MR, Tashjian AH Jr, Order SE, Dammin GJ: Renal adenocarcinoma containing a parathyroid hormone–like substance and associated with marked hypercalcemia. Am J Med 36:805, 1964.

412. Tashjian AH Jr, Levine L, Munson TL: Immunochemical identification of parathyroid hormone in nonparathyroid neoplasms associated with hypercalcemia. J Exp Med 119:467, 1964.

413. Munson TL, Tashjian AH Jr, Levine L: Evidence of parathyroid hormone in non-parathyroid tumors associated with hypercalcemia. Cancer Res 25:1062, 1965.

414. Sherwood LM, O'Riordan JL, Aurbach GD, Potts JT Jr: Production of parathyroid hormone by nonparathyroid tumors. J Clin Endocrinol Metab 27:140, 1967.

415. Knill-Jones RP, Buckle RM, Parsons V, et al: Hypercalcemia and increased parathyroid-hormone activity in a primary hepatoma: Studies before and after hepatic transplantation. N Engl J Med 282:704, 1970.

416. Tashjian AH Jr: Tumor humors and the hypercalcemias of cancer (editorial). N Engl J Med 290:905, 1974.

417. Hamilton JW, Hartman CR, McGregor DH, Cohn DV: Synthesis of parathyroid hormone–like peptides by a human squamous cell carcinoma. J Clin Endocrinol Metab 45:1023, 1977.

418. Simpson EL, Mundy GR, D'Souza SM, et al: Absence of parathyroid hormone messenger RNA in nonparathyroid tumors associated with hypercalcemia. N Engl J Med 309:325, 1983.

419. Yoshimoto K, Yamasaki R, Sakai H, et al: Ectopic production of parathyroid hormone by small cell lung cancer in a patient with hypercalcemia. J Clin Endocrinol Metab 68:976, 1989.

420. Powell D, Singer FR, Murray TM, et al: Nonparathyroid humoral hypercalcemia in patients with neoplastic diseases. N Engl J Med 289:176, 1973.

421. Klein DC, Raisz LG: Prostaglandins: Stimulation of bone resorption in tissue culture. Endocrinology 86:1436, 1970.

422. Tashjian AH Jr: Role of prostaglandins in the production of hypercalcemia by tumors. Cancer Res 38:4138, 1978.

423. Franklin RB, Tashjian AH Jr: Intravenous infusion of prostaglandin E_2 raises plasma calcium concentration in the rat. Endocrinology 97:240, 1975.

424. Demers LM, Allegra JC, Harvey HA, et al: Plasma prostaglandins in hypercalcemic patients with neoplastic disease. Cancer 39:1559, 1977.

425. Robertson RP, Baylink DJ, Marini BJ, Adkison HW: Elevated prostaglandins and suppressed parathyroid hormone associated with hypercalcemia and renal cell carcinoma. J Clin Endocrinol Metab 41:164, 1975.

426. Seyberth HW: Prostaglandin-mediated hypercalcemia: A paraneoplastic syndrome. Klin Wochenschr 56:373, 1978.

427. Robertson RP, Baylink DJ, Metz SA, Cummings KB: Plasma prostaglandin E in patients with cancer with and without hypercalcemia. J Clin Endocrinol Metab 43:1330, 1976.

428. Cummings KB, Robertson RP: Prostaglandin: Increased production by renal cell carcinoma. J Urol 118:720, 1977.

429. Atkins D, Ibbotson KJ, Hillier K, et al: Secretion of prostaglandins and bone-resorbing agents by renal cortical carcinoma in culture. Br J Cancer 36:601, 1977.

430. Minkin C, Fredericks RS, Pokress S, et al: Bone resorption and humoral hypercalcemia of malignancy: Stimulation of bone resorption in vitro by tumor extracts is inhibited by prostaglandin synthesis inhibitors. J Clin Endocrinol Metab 53:941, 1981.

431. Luben RA, Mundy GR, Trummel CL, Raisz LG: Partial purification of osteoclast-activating factor from phytohemagglutinin-stimulated human leukocytes. J Clin Invest 53:1473, 1974.

432. Garrett IR, Durie BG, Nedwin GE, et al: Production of lymphotoxin, a bone-resorbing cytokine, by cultured human myeloma cells. N Engl J Med 317:526, 1987.

433. Kukreja SC, Shemerdiak WP, Lad TE, Johnson PA: Elevated nephrogenous cyclic AMP with normal serum parathyroid hormone levels in patients with lung cancer. J Clin Endocrinol Metab 51:167, 1980.

434. Rude RK, Sharp CF Jr, Fredericks RS, et al: Urinary and nephrogenous cyclic AMP in the hypercalcemia of malignancy. J Clin Endocrinol Metab 52:765, 1981.

435. Stewart AF, Horst R, Deftos LJ, et al: Biochemical evaluation of patients with cancer-associated hypercalcemia. N Engl J Med 303:1377, 1980.

436. Yamamoto I, Kitamura N, Aoki J, et al: Circulating 1,25-dihydroxyvitamin D concentrations in patients with renal cell carcinoma–associated hypercalcemia are rarely suppressed. J Clin Endocrinol Metab 64:175, 1987.

437. Goltzman D, Stewart AF, Broadus AE: Malignancy-associated hypercalcemia: Evaluation with a cytochemical bioassay for parathyroid hormone. J Clin Endocrinol Metab 53:899, 1981.

438. Stewart AF, Vignery A, Silverglate A, et al: Quantitative bone histomorphometry in humoral hypercalcemia of malignancy: Uncoupling of bone cell activity. J Clin Endocrinol Metab 55:219, 1982.

439. Strewler GJ, Williams RD, Nissenson RA: Human renal carcinoma cells produce hypercalcemia in the nude mouse and a novel protein recognized by parathyroid hormone receptors. J Clin Invest 71:769, 1983.

440. Strewler GJ, Wronski TJ, Halloran BP, et al: Pathogenesis of hypercalcemia in nude mice bearing a human renal carcinoma. Endocrinology 119:303, 1986.

441. Abramson EC, Kukla LJ, Shevrin DH, et al: A model for malignancy-associated humoral hypercalcemia. Calcif Tissue Int 36:563, 1984.

442. Rizzoli R, Caverzasio J, Fleisch H, Bonjour JP: Parathyroid hormone-like changes in renal calcium and phosphate reabsorption induced by Leydig cell tumor in thyroparathyroidectomized rats. Endocrinology 119:1004, 1986.

443. Stewart AF, Insogna KL, Burtis WJ, et al: Frequency and partial characterization of adenylate cyclase-stimulating activity in tumors associated with humoral hypercalcemia of malignancy. J Bone Miner Res 1:267, 1986.

444. Mundy GR, Ibbotson KJ, D'Souza SM: Tumor products and the hypercalcemia of malignancy. J Clin Invest 76:391, 1985.

445. Mundy GR, Ibbotson KJ, D'Souza SM, et al: The hypercalcemia of cancer. N Engl J Med 310:1718, 1984.

446. Tashjian AH Jr, Voelkel EF, Lazzaro M, et al: Alpha and beta human transforming growth factors stimulate prostaglandin production and bone resorption in cultured mouse calvaria. Proc Natl Acad Sci USA 82:4535, 1985.

447. Rabbani SA, Mitchell J, Roy DR, et al: Purification of peptides with parathyroid hormone–like bioactivity from human and rat malignancies associated with hypercalcemia. Endocrinology 118:1200, 1986.

448. Broadus AE, Goltzman D, Webb AC, Kronenberg HM: Messenger ribonucleic acid from tumors associated with humoral hypercalcemia of malignancy directs the synthesis of a secretory parathyroid hormone–like peptide. Endocrinology 117:1661, 1985.

449. Moseley JM, Kubota M, Diefenbach-Jagger H, et al: Parathyroid hormone-related protein purified from a human lung cancer cell line. Proc Natl Acad Sci USA 84:5048, 1987.

450. Suva LJ, Winslow GA, Wettenhall RE, et al: A parathyroid hormone-related protein implicated in malignant hypercalcemia: Cloning and expression. Science 237:893, 1987.

451. Stewart AF, Wu T, Goumas D, Burtis WJ: Amino-terminal sequence of a human HHM-associated adenylate cyclase-stimulating protein contains PTH-like and PTH-unlike domains. J Bone Miner Res 2(Suppl 1):392, 1987.

452. Nissensen R, Leung S, Diep D, et al: Purification of a low molecular weight form of the tumor-derived parathyroid hormone–like protein. J Bone Miner Res 2(Suppl 1):388, 1987.

453. Martin TJ, Ebeling PR: A novel parathyroid hormone-related protein: Role in pathology and physiology. Prog Clin Biol Res 332:1, 1990.

454. Merendino JJ Jr, Insogna KL, Milstone LM, et al. A parathyroid hormone–like protein from cultured human keratinocytes. Science 231:388, 1986.

455. Bundred NJ, Ratcliffe WA, Walker RA, et al: Parathyroid hormone-related protein and hypercalcemia in breast cancer. Br Med J 303:1506, 1991.

456. Burtis WJ, Brady TG, Orloff JJ, et al: Immunochemical characterization of circulating PTH-related protein in patients with humoral hypercalcemia of cancer. N Engl J Med 322:1106, 1990.

457. Grill V, Ho P, Body JJ, et al: Parathyroid hormone–related protein: Elevated levels in both humoral hypercalcemia of malignancy and hypercalcemia complicating metastatic breast cancer. J Clin Endocrinol Metab 73:1309, 1991.

458. Adams JS, Singer FR, Gacad MA, et al: Metabolism of 25-hydroxy D₃

459. by cultured pulmonary alveolar macrophages in sarcoidosis. J Clin Endocrinol Metab 60:960, 1985.

459. Bunn PA Jr, Schechter GP, Jaffe E, et al: Clinical course of retrovirus-associated adult T-cell lymphoma in the United States. N Engl J Med 309:257, 1983.

460. Breslau NA, McGuire JL, Zerwekh JE, et al: Hypercalcemia associated with increased serum calcitriol levels in three patients with lymphoma. Ann Intern Med 100:1, 1984.

461. Rieke JW, Donaldson SS, Horning SJ: Hypercalcemia and vitamin D metabolism in Hodgkin's disease. Cancer 63:1700, 1989.

462. Helikson MA, Havey AD, Zerwekh JE, et al: Plasma-cell granuloma producing calcitriol and hypercalcemia. Ann Intern Med 105:379, 1986.

463. Bringhurst FR, Bierer BE, Godeau F, et al: Humoral hypercalcemia of malignancy: Release of a prostaglandin-stimulating bone-resorbing factor in vitro by human transitional-cell carcinoma cells. J Clin Invest 77:456, 1986.

464. Mundy GR, Wilkinson R, Heath DA: Comparative study of available medical therapy for hypercalcemia of malignancy. Am J Med 74:421, 1983.

465. Stewart AF: Therapy of malignancy-associated hypercalcemia. Am J Med 74:475, 1983.

466. Kinirons MT: Newer agents for the treatment of malignant hypercalcemia. Am J Med Sci 305:403, 1993.

467. Ostenstad B, Andersen OK: Disodium pamidronate versus mithramycin in the management of tumour-associated hypercalcemia. Acta Oncol 31:861, 1992.

468. Dodwell DJ, Howell A, Morton AR, et al: Infusion rate and pharmacokinetics of intravenous pamidronate in the treatment of tumour-induced hypercalcemia. Postgrad Med J 68:434, 1992.

469. Zysset E, Ammann P, Jenzer A, et al: Comparison of a rapid (2-h) versus a slow (24-h) infusion of alendronate in the treatment of hypercalcemia of malignancy. Bone Miner 18:237, 1992.

470. Mundy GR: Ectopic production of calciotropic peptides. Endocrinol Metab Clin North Am 20:473, 1991.

471. Hansen M, Hansen HH, Tryding N: Small cell carcinoma of the lung: Serum calcitonin and serum histaminase (diamine oxidase) at basal levels and stimulated by pentagastrin. Acta Med Scand 204:257, 1978.

472. Mulder H: Ectopic secretion of calcitonin as a tumor marker (review). Anticancer Res 3:247, 1983.

473. Roos BA, Lindall AW, Baylin SB, et al: Plasma immunoreactive calcitonin in lung cancer. J Clin Endocrinol Metab 50:659, 1980.

474. Schwartz KE, Wolfsen AR, Forster B, Odell WD: Calcitonin in nonthyroidal cancer. J Clin Endocrinol Metab 49:438, 1979.

475. Lairmore TC, Wells SA Jr: Medullary carcinoma of the thyroid: Current diagnosis and management. Semin Surg Oncol 7:92, 1991.

476. Silva OL, Broder LE, Duppman JL, et al: Calcitonin as a marker for bronchogenic cancer. Cancer 44:680, 1979.

477. Sano T, Saito H, Yamasaki R, et al: Immunoreactive somatostatin and calcitonin in pulmonary neuroendocrine tumor. Cancer 57:64, 1986.

478. Samaan NA, Castillo S, Schultz PN, et al: Serum calcitonin after pentagastrin stimulation in patients with bronchogenic and breast cancer compared to that in patients with medullary thyroid carcinoma. J Clin Endocrinol Metab 51:237, 1980.

479. DiSantagnese PA: Neuroendocrine differentiation in carcinoma of the prostate. Cancer 70:254, 1992.

480. Austin LA, Heath H III: Calcitonin: Physiology and pathophysiology. N Engl J Med 304:269, 1981.

481. Goodman RH, Jacobs JW, Habener JF: Cell-free translation of messenger RNA coding for a precursor of human calcitonin. Biochem Biophys Res Commun 91:932, 1979.

482. Zajac JD, Martin TJ, Hudson P, et al: Biosynthesis of calcitonin by human lung cancer cells. Endocrinology 116:749, 1985.

483. Beastall GH, Cook B, Rustin GJ, Jennings J: A review of the role of established tumor markers. Ann Clin Biochem 28:5, 1991.

484. Jacobs EL, Haskell CN: Clinical use of tumor markers in oncology. Curr Probl Cancer 15:299, 1991.

485. Ryan EA, Reiss E: Oncogenous osteomalacia: Review of the world literature of 42 cases and report of two new cases. Am J Med 77:501, 1984.

486. Weidner N: Review and update: Oncogenic osteomalacia-rickets. Ultrastruct Pathol 15:317, 1991.

487. Nuovo MA, Dorfman HD, Sun CC, Chalew SA. Tumor-induced osteomalacia and rickets. Am J Surg Pathol 13:588, 1989.

488. Fukumoto Y, Tarui S, Tsukiyama K, et al: Tumor-induced vitamin D-resistant hypophosphatemic osteomalacia associated with proximal renal tubular dysfunction and 1,25-dihydroxyvitamin D deficiency. J Clin Endocrinol Metab 49:873, 1979.

489. Drezner MK and Feinglos MN: Osteomalacia due to 1 alpha, 25-dihydroxycholecalciferol deficiency: Association with a giant cell tumor of bone. J Clin Invest 60:1046, 1977.

490. Lyles KW, Berry WR, Haussler M, et al: Hypophosphatemic osteomalacia: Association with prostatic carcinoma. Ann Intern Med 93:275, 1980.

491. Taylor HC, Fallon MD, Velasco ME: Oncogenic osteomalacia and inappropriate antidiuretic hormone secretion due to oat-cell carcinoma. Ann Intern Med 101:786, 1984.

492. Mizuno Y, Masaki N, Hashimoto H, et al: Marked hypophosphatemia with decreased serum $1,25(OH)_2D_3$ in a patient with hepatocellular carcinoma complicating liver cirrhosis. Jpn J Med 30:81, 1991.

493. Miyauchi A, Fukase M, Tsutsumi M, Fujita T: Hemangiopericytoma-induced osteomalacia: Tumor transplantation in nude mice causes hypophosphatemia and tumor extracts inhibit renal 25-hydroxyvitamin D_1-hydroxylase activity. J Clin Endocrinol Metab 67:46, 1988.

494. Nitzan DW, Horowitz AT, Darmon D, et al: Oncogenous osteomalacia: A case study. Bone Miner 6:191, 1989.

495. Atkinson MD, McElwain TJ, Peckham MJ, Thomas PP: Hypertropic pulmonary osteoarthropathy in Hodgkin's disease. Cancer 38:1729, 1976.

496. Montag TW, Murphy RE, Belinson JL: Virilizing malignant lipid cell tumor producing erythropoietin. Gynecol Oncol 19:98, 1984.

497. Ghio R, Haupt E, Ratti M, Boccaccio P: Erythrocytosis associated with a dermoid cyst of the ovary and erythropoietic activity of the tumour fluid. Scand J Haematol 27:70, 1981.

498. Sherwood JB, Goldwasser E: Erythropoietin production by human renal carcinoma cells in monolayer culture. Endocrinology 99:504, 1976.

499. Sherwood JB, Goldwasser E: Radioimmunoassay for erythropoietin. Blood 54:885, 1979.

500. Sue JM, Sytkowski AJ: Site-specific antibodies to human erythropoietin directed toward the NH_2-terminal region. Proc Natl Acad Sci USA 80:3651, 1983.

501. Erslev A: Erythropoietin coming of age (editorial). N Engl J Med 316:101, 1987.

502. Eschbach JW, Egrie JC, Downing MR, et al: Correction of the anemia of end-stage renal disease with recombinant human erythropoietin: Results of a combined phase I and II clinical trial. N Engl J Med 316:73, 1987.

503. Jacobs K, Shoemaker C, Rudersdorf R, et al: Isolation and characterization of genomic and cDNA clones of human erythropoietin. Nature 313:806, 1985.

504. Sytkowski AJ, Bicknell KA, Smith GM, Garcia JF: Secretion of erythropoietin-like activity by clones of human renal carcinoma cell line GKA. Cancer Res 44:51, 1984.

505. Okabe T, Urabe A, Kato T, et al: Production of erythropoietin-like activity by human renal and hepatic carcinomas in cell culture. Cancer 55:1918, 1985.

506. Saito T, Saito K, Trent DJ, et al: Translation of messenger RNA from a renal tumor into a product with the biologic properties of erythropoietin. Exp Hematol 13:23, 1985.

507. DaSilva JL, Lacombe C, Bruneval P, et al: Tumor cells are the site of erythropoietin synthesis in human renal cancers associated with polycythemia. Blood 75:577, 1990.

508. Hagiwara M, Chin IL, McGonigle R, et al: Erythropoietin production in a primary culture of human renal carcinoma cells maintained in nude mice. Blood 63:828, 1984.

509. Winkelmann JC: The human erythropoietin receptor. Int J Cell Cloning 10:254, 1992.

510. Johnson RA, Roodman GD: Hematologic manifestations of malignancy. Dis Mon 35:721, 1989.

511. Rowe JM, Rapoport AP. Hemopoietic growth factors: A review. J Clin Pharmacol 32:486, 1992.

512. Levin J, Conley CL: Thrombocytosis associated with malignant disease. Arch Intern Med 114:497, 1964.

513. Robertson PW, Klidjian A, Harding LK, et al: Hypertension due to a renin-secreting renal tumor. Am J Med 43:963, 1967.

514. Eddy RL, Sanchez SA: Renin-secreting renal neoplasm and hypertension with hypokalemia. Ann Intern Med 75:725, 1971.

515. Hollifield JW, Page DL, Smith C, et al: Renin-secreting clear cell carcinoma of the kidney. Arch Intern Med 135:859, 1975.

516. Hauger-Klevene JH: High plasma renin activity in an oat cell carcinoma: A renin-secreting carcinoma? Cancer 26:1112, 1970.

517. Genest J, Rojo-Ortega JM, Kuchel O, et al: Malignant hypertension with hypokalemia in a patient with renin-producing pulmonary carcinoma. Trans Assoc Am Physicians 88:192, 1975.

518. Ruddy MC, Atlas SA, Salerno FG: Hypertension associated with a renin-secreting adenocarcinoma of the pancreas. N Engl J Med 307:993, 1982.

519. Atlas SA, Hesson TE, Sealey JE, et al: Characterization of inactive renin ("prorenin") from renin-secreting tumors of nonrenal origin. J Clin Invest 73:437, 1984.

520. Kew MC, Leckie BJ, Greef MC: Arterial hypertension as a paraneoplastic phenomenon in hepatocellular carcinoma. Arch Intern Med 149:2111, 1989.

521. Slater EE, Haber E: Inactive renin: "Through a glass darkly" (editorial). N Engl J Med 301:429, 1979.

522. Soubrier F, Devaux C, Galen F, et al: Biochemical and immunological characterization of ectopic tumoral renin. J Clin Endocrinol Metab 54:139, 1982.

523. Sealey JE, Atlas SA, Laragh JH: Prorenin and other large molecular weight forms of renin. Endocr Rev 1:365–391, 1980.

524. Poulsen K, Vuust J, Lykkegaard S, et al: Renin is synthesized as a 50,000-dalton single-chain polypeptide-free in cell translation systems. FEBS Lett 98:135, 1979.

525. Yokokawa K, Tahara H, Kohno M, et al: Hypertension associated with endothelin-secreting malignant hemangioendothelioma. Ann Intern Med 114:213, 1991.

526. Zusman RM, Snider JJ, Cline A, et al: Antihypertensive function of renal-cell carcinoma. N Engl J Med 290:843, 1974.

527. Seleznick MJ: Tumor markers. Prim Care 19:715, 1992.

528. Murphy RA, Pantazis NJ, Arnason BG, Young M: Secretion of a nerve growth factor by mouse neuroblastoma cells in culture. Proc Natl Acad Sci USA 72:1895, 1975.

529. Herschman HR, Lusis AJ, Groopman JE: Growth factors. Ann Intern Med 92:650, 1980.

530. Frazier WA, Angeletti RH, Bradshaw RA: Nerve growth factor and insulin: Structural similarity is indicated in evolutionary relationship reflected by physiologic action. Science 176:482, 1972.

531. Goldstein LD, Reynolds CP, Perez-Polo JR: Isolation of human nerve growth factor from placental tissue. Neurochem Res 3:175, 1978.

532. Carpenter G, Cohen S: Peptide growth factors. Trends Biochem Sci 9:169, 1984.

533. Ahronov A, Pruss RM, Herschman HR: Epidermal growth factor: Relationship between receptor regulation and mitogenesis in 3T3 cells. J Biol Chem 253:3970, 1978.

534. Katz MS, Kelly TM, Dax EM, et al: Ectopic beta-adrenergic receptors coupled to adenylate cyclase in human adrenocortical carcinomas. J Clin Endocrinol Metab 60:900, 1985.

535. Pierce ST, Metcalfe M, Banks ER, et al: Small cell carcinoma with two paraendocrine syndromes. Cancer 69:2258, 1992.

536. Rosen SW, Weintraub BD, Aaronson SA: Nonrandom ectopic protein production by malignant cells: Direct evidence in vitro. J Clin Endocrinol Metab 50:834, 1980.

537. Hunstein W, Trumper LH, Dummer R, Schwechheimer K: Glucagonoma syndrome and bronchial carcinoma. Ann Intern Med 109:920, 1988.

Neuroendocrine Tumors of Carcinoid Variety

AARON I. VINIK
IVANA PAVLIC RENAR

The term *carcinoid (Karzinoide)* was first used in 1907[1] and applied to an unusual ileal tumor, reported earlier,[2] which showed little mitotic activity. Histologically, the tumor consists of innocuous-appearing cells, uniform in their shape with rare mitotic figures. A symptom complex, *carcinoid syndrome*, accompanying these tumors, delineated in 1954,[3] occurs in less than 10 per cent of patients with these tumors.[4]

Classically, carcinoids derive from enterochromaffin and argentaffin cells of the digestive tract, but the term *carcinoid tumor* can be expanded to cover "gut" tumors of paracrine and endocrine-like cells of unknown function.[5] These tumors are neuroendocrine and derive from a primitive stem cell that may differentiate into any of a variety of adult endocrine-secreting cells, producing a variety of biogenic amines and peptides, hormones, and neurotransmitters, thus causing a wide array of symptoms and endocrine syndromes. Moreover, the secretory activity may change with time, and metastases can exhibit different hormonal activity than the parent tumor. A large fraction of carcinoid tumors may or may not produce peptides but show no clinical symptoms. In these "nonfunctioning" tumors, measurements of peptide levels may serve as tumor markers and help to monitor the rate of tumor growth and response to treatment. Finally, a number of carcinoids do not store, synthesize, or secrete peptides or amines and present because of a tumor mass and local effects but do not cause carcinoid syndrome.

The annual incidence of these tumors is estimated to be approximately 1.5 per 100,000 general population, i.e., 2500 new cases per year in the United States.[6] These tumors account for 56 per cent of all neuroendocrine tumors of gastroenteropancreatic axis, 13 to 34 per cent of all tumors of the small bowel, and 17 to 46 per cent of all malignant tumors in that location.[7]

HISTOPATHOLOGY

Because they are highly differentiated, carcinoids, like other neuroendocrine tumors, are often rather easily identified in routinely stained sections. These tumors occur in three sites: the foregut, comprising the lungs, stomach, and first part of the duodenum; the midgut, comprising the gut from the second part of the duodenum to the right colon; and the hindgut, which includes the transverse colon through the rectum. Midgut carcinoids have the most typical picture of insular-like formations of tumor cells surrounded by relatively pronounced fibrotic stroma. Foregut carcinoids usually show a mixed growth pattern, whereas hindgut carcinoids are mostly trabecular or solid.[8]

However, there are times when it may be difficult to distinguish carcinoids from other highly differentiated tumors of any origin, especially when staining for secretory granules or when appropriate immunohistochemical stains are not used. At the other extreme, although infrequent, they may be poorly differentiated and difficult to discriminate from poorly differentiated or undifferentiated carcinomas.[9-11] The occasional presence of a subpopulation of tumor cells in adenocarcinomas with neuroendocrine differentiation makes this issue even more complicated.[12-15] Generally this is of no diagnostic significance unless the tumor presents as the rare mixed type, such as goblet cell carcinoid of the appendix.

Carcinoids of the lung present a problem in classification. These tumors resemble small cell lung carcinoma, the opposite side of a spectrum whose other side consists of highly differentiated neuroendocrine tumors.[16] This cellular mimicry has great significance in terms of therapeutic options and prognosis. The advent of new tumor markers and immunohistochemistry has drawn attention to an apparent change in the "incidence" of tumors. For example, in the 20 years from 1960 to 1980, the lung accounted for less than 10 per cent of carcinoids, and in the decade after introduction of histochemistry, these tumors comprised 30 per cent of carcinoids. It is thus of critical importance to verify the neuroendocrine origin of a tumor using a variety of markers. Basically, two types of markers are used—nonspecific and specific.

Nonspecific Markers

The oldest nonspecific marker of normal or tumorous neuroendocrine cells is heavy metal salt staining[17]—thus the name *argentaffin* if ammoniacal silver nitrate is employed and *enterochromaffin* if potassium dichromate is used. Silver (or other metal) is precipitated in secretory granules. The granules are then visible by light microscopy; otherwise, they are only identifiable by electron microscopy. Precipitation of silver in the absence of a reducing agent is called an *argentaffin reaction*, whereas some secretory granules precipitate silver only in the presence of an external reducing agent; they are then called *argyrophylic*.[18] It is important to note, however, that a negative silver reaction does not absolutely rule out the possibility of a neuroendocrine tumor. Also, in poorly differentiated tumors which have low levels of cytoplasmic peptides, silver staining may be weak or absent. There is, again, a distinction within carcinoids according to their primary site: Almost all the tumors of foregut and midgut origin show the argyrophil reaction in the majority of cells, whereas hindgut carcinoids are often unreactive or weakly positive.[19-21] A variety of neuropeptide markers help to narrow the uncertainty.

Chromogranin A, a 431-amino-acid peptide encoded on chromosome 14, was originally identified in the adrenal medulla.[22] It was later shown, however, to be present in the majority of neuroendocrine cells.[23] It is found generally in the same distribution as the positive argyrophil reaction. However, it is more specific, since some intracellular components other than neurosecretory granules may react with silver.

Neuron-specific enolase (NSE), a glycolytic enzyme present in central neurons,[24-26] has been identified in the peripheral neuroendocrine cell system.[27, 28] It is not a component of secretory granules. It is very useful to identify argyrophil-negative neuroendocrine tissues, which do not react with chromogranin antibodies, and poorly differentiated tumors with low granular content, such as small cell carcinoma of the lung and adrenal neuroblastoma. Some nonneuroendocrine carcinomas can contain NSE, detectable both immunohistochemically and by analyses of tumor extracts. However, the amounts of NSE in such tumors are definitely lower than those found in neuroendocrine tumors.

In recent years synaptophysin, a vesicular membrane protein specifically expressed in neuroendocrine tissues, has emerged as a reliable marker for neuroendocrine tumors, including carcinoids.[29, 30] This is generally not available in most laboratories, but no doubt it will find a role because of its specificity.

Finally, the nonspecific argyrophil staining of Sevier-Munger[18] is almost completely discriminatory for enterochromaffin-like cells in the fundus and body of the stomach,[31] distinguishing these tumors from adenocarcinomas.

The surge of interest in these tumors arises from their association with atrophic gastritis and pernicious anemia, possibly nurtured by the trophic action of the reflex rise in gastrin. Critically important, however, is the need to identify the sporadic variety without these other elements, since these are potentially malignant, whereas those associated with pernicious anemia and multiple endocrine neoplasia (MEN) syndrome tend to be benign.

Specific Markers

Specific markers are used to detect tumor peptide products. Several methods are used for serotonin determination: formalin-induced fluorescence,[32] Masson's argentaffin reaction,[33] and poly- or monoclonal antibodies to serotonin.[34] Foregut carcinoids do not in general secrete serotonin but instead its precursor 5-hydroxytryptamine. Screening should therefore seek this product (Fig. 150–1). To further characterize the tumor with regard to its peptide content, a widening range of poly- and monoclonal antibodies to peptide hormones is available. Several peptides and amines are found in neuroendocrine tumors. These include substance P and neurokinin A, among others (Table 150–1).

CLASSIFICATION

A carcinoid can derive from virtually every endoderm-derived tissue. There are reports of anecdotal cases of primary carcinoids in almost every location in the human body. However, 95 per cent of all carcinoids are found in three sites: appendix, rectum, and small intestine. In 1 in every 200 to 300 appendectomies, a small tumor is found.

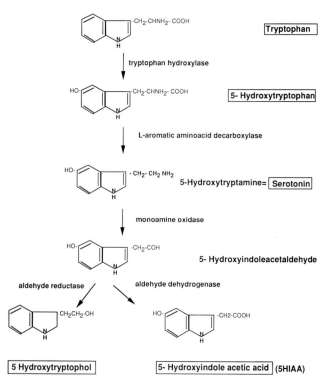

FIGURE 150–1. Serotonin metabolism, simplified.

TABLE 150–1. CLASSIFICATION OF CARCINOIDS ACCORDING TO THE SITE OF PRIMARY TUMOR

SITE	HISTOLOGY	ARGENTAFFIN REACTION	BIOCHEMISTRY*	CLINICAL PICTURE	METASTASES
Foregut Bronchi, stomach, first part of duodenum	Mixed growth pattern	Negative	5–HTP Often ACTH, GH, gastrin, GRH, or other hormones	Protracted, purplish or violaceous flush, telangiectasias and skin folds (leontine facies), manifestation of ectopic hormone secretion	Liver, bone
Midgut Second part of duodenum, jejunum, ileum, right colon	Insular-like formation of tumor cells	Positive	5-HT Kinins, neuropeptides, prostaglandins	Pink-red flush, cyanotic teleangiectasias, rare endocrine syndromes, tendency to multiple lesions	Liver
Hindgut Transverse, left, sigmoid colon and rectum	Trabecular or solid	Negative	None	Silent, only local symptoms	Liver, bone

*5–HT = 5-hydroxytryptamine, serotonin; 5–HTP = 5-hydroxytryptophan; GH = growth hormone; GRH = gastrin releasing hormone.

Its incidence declines with age. In a large series of 108 such patients followed for greater than 5 years (83 of them for 10 to 35 years), Moertel et al.[35] found no recurrence or metastases of tumor. It appears that simple appendectomy is adequate treatment for such patients, with the exception of rare tumors larger than 2 cm in diameter that metastasize.

A carcinoid nodule is expected in 1 in every 2500 middle-aged adults who undergoes a proctoscopy. Ninety-nine per cent of such rectal carcinoids are on the anterior and lateral rectal wall in a small zone 4 to 13 cm above the dentate line. They are usually inactive and argentaffin- and serotonin-negative. Much the same as tumors located in the appendix, the tendency to metastasis is related to size: Those less than 1 cm probably never metastasize, whereas those greater than 2 cm nearly always do. The "gray zone" is 1 to 2 cm. The treatment and follow-up of those patients have to be carefully evaluated.[36] The reported distribution of carcinoids (in 6965 cases) showed 2.8 per cent in stomach, 2.9 per cent in duodenum, 25.5 per cent in jejunoileum, 36.2 per cent in appendix, 6.0 per cent in colon, and 16.4 per cent in rectum. Of extragastrointestinal sites, the most common is bronchial carcinoid (9.9 per cent) and ovarian (0.5 per cent), whereas 0.2 per cent had miscellaneous primary sites and in 3.3 per cent the primary site remained unknown.[37]

It is notable that there is a major difference in prevalence of carcinoid tumors found in the jejunoileum at autopsy versus the clinical series (Table 150–2), indicating that these tumors are frequently silent.[38]

From the clinical point of view, the most useful classification seems to be one according to the site of the primary tumor (see Table 150–1). This classification provides guidelines for diagnosis, and if taken together with the rule that the larger the primary, the greater the likelihood of metastasis, this also provides prognostic implications.

NATURAL HISTORY

Carcinoid tumors grow slowly and may be present for years without overt symptoms. In the early stages, vague abdominal pain goes undiagnosed and is invariably as-cribed to "irritable bowel" or "spastic colon." One-third of patients present with years of intermittent abdominal pain. The spectrum of symptoms is extremely broad due to the potential of these tumors to produce a variety of hormones and bioactive amines. Moreover, carcinoid can be associated with MEN showing a sex distinction: In more than 75 per cent of female patients, the tumor is in the lungs, whereas in more than two thirds of male patients, it is in the thymus.[37]

Small, multiple gastric carcinoids are rare, less than 1 to 2.3 per cent of all carcinoids,[39] but are much more prevalent among patients with pernicious anemia and atrophic gastritis.[40, 41] They may represent the outcome of a loss of the inhibitory influence of gastric acid on the gastrin cell and enterochromaffin-like (ECL) cells with consequent hypergastrinemia.[42, 43] Gastrin is a trophic stimulus to ECL cells, and tumors have only been found in patients with gastrin levels greater than 1000 pg/ml.[44] This concept is becoming a topic of growing concern in the present age of widespread long-term use of powerful gastric acid inhibitors.[31] These tumors may show spontaneous regression[45] or be stable for years.[46]

The carcinoid syndrome only occurs in about 10 per cent of patients with tumors and occurs rarely, if ever, in hindgut tumors.[36] By the time the diagnosis is arrived at,

TABLE 150–2. ANATOMIC DISTRIBUTION OF CARCINOID TUMORS (PERCENTAGES)

TUMOR SITE	SURGICAL/CLINICAL (6965 CASES)	AUTOPSY (201 CASES)
Stomach	2.8	2.5
Duodenum	2.9	0.0
Jejunoileum	25.5	75.6
Appendix	36.2	3.5
Colon	6.0	6.5
Rectum	16.4	1.5
Bronchus	9.9	9.0
Ovary	0.5	0.0
Miscellaneous	0.2	0.0
Unknown primary	0.3	1.0

From Vinik AI, Moattari AR: Neuroendocrine tumors, secretory diarrhea, and responses to somatostatin. *In* Lebenthal E, Duffey M (eds.): Textbook of Secretory Diarrhea. New York, Raven Press, 1990, p 309.

there generally has been a history of symptoms which can be attributed to a carcinoid tumor for an average duration of 9 years[37] in our experience, although others report 2 years.[36] The principal features of carcinoid syndrome include flushing, sweating, wheezing, diarrhea, abdominal pain, and cardiac fibrosis with development of valvular disease, predominantly on the right (more often pulmonary stenosis and tricuspid incompetence than tricuspid incompetence and/or pulmonary regurgitation alone). The right-sided heart lesions lead to the development of right-sided heart failure.[46] However, features of heart disease are becoming less frequent with active intervention and concerted efforts to reduce serotonin production by controlling the tumor burden. Pellagra-like dermatosis due to niacin deficiency is found with extensive disease, since tryptophan is overutilized in serotonin metabolism. Some patients develop a proximal myopathy which can antedate the rest of the syndrome and resemble that found with Cushing's syndrome, certain carcinomas, and hyperthyroidism. Others even develop an arthropathy misdiagnosed as rheumatism but responding surprisingly well to somatostatin analogue treatment. Flushing is found in 84 per cent of patients, gastrointestinal hypermotility and diarrhea in 70 per cent, dyspnea in 37 per cent, abdominal pain in about 33 per cent, myopathy in 7 per cent, and bronchospasm in 6 per cent (Table 150–3). It is not clear which substance(s) mediate the various features of carcinoid syndrome. Serotonin,[47, 48] prostaglandins,[49] 5-hydroxytryptophan,[50, 51] dopamine,[52] kallikrein,[53] histamine,[51] and neurokinin A,[54] are thought to be involved in the clinical manifestations.

An additional problem is multihormone production, which may occur in foregut carcinoids. Hormones which may be produced are insulin, calcitonin, ACTH, vasopressin, glucagon, secretin, gastrin, and various biogenic amines and their precursors. Carcinoid is a cause of 4 per cent of ectopic ACTH syndromes.[55] The most commonly reported source of ectopic ACTH is a small cell carcinoma of the lung, but for the reasons discussed earlier, these tumors may have been neuroendocrine in nature. Ectopic ACTH syndrome accompanying carcinoid can present only a biochemical entity, without clinical manifestations of Cushing syndrome. The ACTH-like immunoreactivity may represent different, biologically inactive forms of ACTH or related peptides derived from pro-opiomelanocorticotropin (lipotropins, enkephalins, and β-endorphin) for which no clinical syndrome has been identified. The co-secretion of ACTH, as well as of gastrin, by a carcinoid tumor is generally a sign of a poor prognosis.

DIAGNOSIS

Only when there is a reasonable clinical suspicion should biochemical testing be done, and localization studies must be reserved for those cases *proven* biochemically. Presenting symptoms of unexplained chronic intermittent abdominal pain and a history of "irritable" or "spastic" colon probably deserve a screening evaluation, since almost all cases of carcinoid have at some stage of their development been labeled as "psychogenic" or "irritable bowel syndrome." However, a number of tumors on different sites only cause local symptoms without the characteristic features of carcinoid syndrome.

Diarrhea accompanying carcinoid tumor is usually secretory in nature. It persists with fasting and fails to disappear with prolonged intravenous nutrition. Relief of diarrhea with H_2-receptor antagonists is strongly suggestive of gastrinoma syndrome and not carcinoid. The diarrhea seldom causes hypokalemia, steatorrhea, or severe electrolyte disturbance unless the tumor co-secretes vasoactive intestinal peptide (VIP) or other secretory peptides. Hypercalcemia is found in 50 per cent of VIP-secreting tumors, and metabolic acidosis with bicarbonate wasting and hypokalemia is usually only a characteristic of tumors secreting VIP. Hypokalemia with steatorrhea suggests gastrinoma syndrome not carcinoid. Theoretically, the differential diagnosis of secretory diarrhea includes villous adenoma of the rectum; however, this is extremely rare. A much more frequent possibility that is extremely important (but difficult to differentiate) is laxative abuse. KOH preparation to detect a laxative is mandatory. Measurement of stool electrolytes and osmolarity should show that 2(Na + K) is equal to osmolarity. A large gap suggests the presence of non-ionic osmolytes likely to be laxatives. In difficult cases, measurement of intestinal secretions by passing a multilumen tube and quantitating electrolytes and water transport with concomitant stool electrolyte measurement helps distinguish secretory from nonsecretory diarrhea, thus establishing the diagnosis.

Two types of flushing are seen with carcinoid syndrome (see Table 150–2). The foregut variety is more intense, lasting sometimes for hours, purplish in hue, and frequently followed by telangiectasia and facial disfiguration. It involves the upper trunk and limbs, which may become acrocyanotic. The skin on the face often thickens, while the nose frequently resembles that of rhinophyma. In contrast, midgut flushing ("classic") is faint pink or red, usually ephemeral, and does not leave permanent discoloration. Initially, flushing is provoked by alcohol and tyramine-containing foods (blue cheese, chocolate, red sausage, red wine), but with time it may appear without provocation. It involves the face and upper trunk down to

TABLE 150–3. CLINICAL FEATURES OF CARCINOID SYNDROME

SYMPTOM	FREQUENCY (%)	CHARACTERISTICS
Flushing	84	Protracted, purplish foregut ephemeral, pink-red midgut
Diarrhea, gastrointestinal hypermotility	70	Secretory
Dyspnea	37	Due to right-sided heart disease
Abdominal pain	33	An unusually long history
Proximal myopathy	7	Resembles that of carcinoma, thyrotoxicosis, and Cushing's
Bronchospasm	6	Expiratory wheezing
Dermatosis	5	Hyperpigmentation, pellagra-like
Arthropathy	Rare	

Modified from Vinik AI, McLeod MK, Shapiro B, Lloyd RV: Clinical features, diagnosis, and localization of carcinoid tumors and their management. Gastrointest Clin North Am 18:865–896, 1989.

the nipple line. Why it is limited to this distribution is not known. Conditions to consider in the differential diagnosis include carcinoid, medullary carcinoma of thyroid, VIPoma, pheochromocytoma, diabetic autonomic neuropathy, chlorpropamide-alcohol flushing, menopause flushing, autonomic epilepsy, mastocytosis, drug or alcohol withdrawal, panic syndrome, and idiopathic flushing. Most can be excluded by careful history but may require measurement of calcitonin and histamine and an electroencephalogram.

Biochemical Markers

The rate-limiting step in synthesis of serotonin is the conversion of tryptophan into 5-hydroxytrypophan (5-HTP) by tryptophan hydroxylase (Fig. 150–1). In midgut tumors, 5-HTP is rapidly converted to 5-hydroxytryptamine (5-HT, serotonin) by amino acid decarboxylase (dopa-decarboxylase). Serotonin is either stored in neurosecretory granules or secreted into the vascular compartment. Most of the secreted serotonin is taken up by platelets and stored in their secondary granules. The rest is free in the plasma and converted into the urinary metabolite 5-hydroxyindoleacetic acid (5-HIAA) by monoamine oxidase (MAO) and aldehyde dehydrogenase. These enzymes are abundant in the kidney. In patients with foregut carcinoids, the urine contains relatively little 5-HIAA but large amounts of 5-HTP. It is presumed that these foregut tumors are deficient in dopa-decarboxylase; hence 5-HTP is not decarboxylated to serotonin. Measurement of serotonin and its metabolites permits the detection of 84 per cent of patients with neuroendocrine tumors. The reference method today is high-pressure liquid chromatography with electrochemical detection,[56, 57] significantly more specific than previously used colorimetric and fluorometric methods. Single measurement of 5-HIAA in the urine seems to be the best for screening, although no one single test is sufficient to identify all cases. Patients should be warned to avoid serotonin precursor–containing foods (such as avocados, bananas, eggplant, pineapples, pecans, walnuts, tomatoes) 3 days before testing. Although the levels of serotonin in tumor patients usually far exceed those found after food ingestion, this precaution helps to exclude carcinoid in people with borderline-high 5-HIAA levels.

Recent studies of serum chromogranin (CG) A and B levels[58, 59] show elevation in all carcinoid patients studied. Moreover, changes in serum levels seem to correlate well with other markers and tumor response to intervention. The co-secretion of chromogranin A with the primary tumor peptide can be expected, since it is a secretory peptide. It is sensitive but clearly not specific. Thus there have been further attempts to identify other tumor-specific peptides in the diagnostic evaluation.

The significance of elevated plasma concentrations of various peptides is still being investigated. High levels of neuropeptides that can be further elevated by the pentagastrin stimulation test have been reported.[60] However, neuropeptide abnormalities seem to occur in noncarcinoid flushing and might be of significance in the mechanism of this phenomenon.[61]

Several provocative tests are being used for carcinoid syndrome. Ahlman et al.[62] reported the results of pentagastrin stimulation in 16 patients with midgut carcinoids and hepatic metastases who had elevated urinary 5-HIAA levels. The stimulation uniformly induced flushing and gastrointestinal symptoms which did not happen in any of the healthy control subjects. Administration of a serotonin receptor antagonist aborted gastrointestinal symptoms.[62] Flushing was associated with a rise in circulating substance P in 80 per cent of patients with gastric carcinoid.[63] We, however, found that basal substance P levels were raised in 80 per cent of patients with carcinoid but that pentagastrin stimulation did not enhance the sensitivity of the measurement and that there was dissociation between the clinical and biochemical responses.[63] Norheim et al.[64] reported a twofold or greater increase in other tachykinins such as neurokinin A in 12 of 16 and substance P in 3 of 16 patients with metastatic carcinoid. In another recent series reported by Conlon et al.,[65] 5 patients who flushed after pentagastrin stimulation had undetectable values of neurokinin A and substance P, suggesting that elevation of this class of tachykinins is not a constant feature of carcinoid patients but undoubtedly contributes to the symptom complex in certain patients. In our previous experience, elevated (>50 pg/ml) basal levels of substance P identified tumors with a sensitivity of 71.4 per cent and specificity of 100 per cent.[63] Recently, we found similar results with neurokinin A (unpublished data). The role of neuropeptides and serotonin metabolites in the mechanism of flushing is still unclear. The traditional attribution of the symptom complex to serotonin and to its metabolites does not hold, since not all flushing patients have elevated serotonin levels, nor is serotonin elevation uniformly related to spontaneous or pentagastrin-provoked flushing.

In conclusion, it should be emphasized that blood levels of serotonin and urine levels of its metabolites remain the key to the biochemical diagnosis of carcinoid. The 14 per cent of undiagnosed cases dictate a need to pursue the search for as yet unidentified markers. An important biochemical secretory marker is serum chromogranin A. A variety of peptide hormones may cause symptoms, e.g., VIP and diarrhea; since these tumors have the ability to produce them, they should be included in the evaluation. However, the peptides produced may be structurally altered and inactive.[66] The role of neuropeptides in the symptom complex is still under investigation, but elevated kinins such as substance P[63] and neurokinin A are strongly suggestive of a carcinoid or other neuroendocrine tumor.

Localization

Primary carcinoids in several sites are relatively easy to detect, e.g., bronchial carcinoid by chest x-ray or computed tomography (CT) and carcinoids of the cecum, right colon, and rectum by barium enema and endoscopy. The greatest problems emerge in localizing common small bowel carcinoids and the uncommon ones in extraintestinal sites. Upper gastrointestinal radiographic studies are usually not helpful. Endoscopy can help, but only in detection of tumors in the stomach and duodenum. Barium examinations may demonstrate fixation, separation, thickening, and angulation of the bowel loops but are rarely diagnostic.

Primary tumors of the small intestine are usually below

the resolution capacity of CT or ultrasonography. However, CT is helpful in tumor staging and assessment of the extent of tumor spread to the mesentery and bowel wall as well as metastases to the lymph nodes and liver, where focal hypodense lesions appear.[67]

Scintigraphic imaging of carcinoid tissue is possible by the use of ^{125}I-labeled analogue of guanethidine (meta-iodobenzylguanidine, MIBG). MIBG is concentrated in chromaffin tissue by uptake into norepinephrine storage sites. Imaging is performed 24, 48, and 72 h after the administration of MIBG. This method is highly specific for pheochromocytoma. It is not that specific for other neuroendocrine tumors, but in combination with CT it seems to be the most useful test for the localization of metastatic carcinoids.[68]

Magnetic resonance imaging (MRI), although very sensitive for the detection of liver metastases, needs further evaluation before its use for the diagnosis and staging of carcinoid tumors can be recommended.[69]

The role of angiography has decreased with time with the development of noninvasive methods of investigation. However, it is still employed when the results of noninvasive techniques are equivocal and surgery is being considered. Liver metastases are usually vascular, with abundant neovascularity, which makes them appropriate for angiographic imaging. If angiography is done both with and without administration of somatostatin analogue, the effects on the vasculature of the liver metastases seems to predict the response to treatment.[70]

Finally, in unclear cases in which the tumor has been identified by none of the mentioned techniques, total-body venous sampling may be considered if there is production of a known and measurable peptide substance. Measurements of gradients of serotonin[71] and substance P[72] have been reported to be useful for localization of occult tumors.

A novel imaging technique still regarded as experimental is the use of radioactive iodine (^{123}I)–labeled somatostatin analogue.[73] Somatostatin receptors have been detected in a variety of tumors, especially of the neuroendocrine variety.[74] Autoradiography of endocrine pancreatic tumors and carcinoids has revealed a high density of binding sites[75] in tumors which are responsive to treatment. Thus these tracer studies not only may help to localize the tumors but also may predict those which would respond to octreotide.

TREATMENT

Several approaches to treatment have been applied to carcinoids. None with the exception of surgery for small, localized, nonmetastatic tumors is really curative. However, there are several defined end points in the treatment related to symptom relief, reduction of tumor mass, and normalization of biochemical tests. Bearing in mind that carcinoids are extremely slow-growing and that recurrence may occur decades after the initial diagnosis,[36] it is important to follow patients longitudinally (with the exception of noninvasive, resectable tumors less than 1 cm). The goals of treatment are:

1. Relief of symptoms—at least to a bearable level.

2. Reduction of tumor mass to less than 50 per cent, as assessed by serial CT scans or other localization studies.

3. Reduction of the blood or urine levels of biochemical markers(s) to less than 50 per cent or to normal. It is important to note, however, that no direct correlation between tumor mass and levels of any marker is uniformly present. There is often a discrepancy between the biochemical and radiologic assessments of tumor growth. For these reasons, it remains essential to monitor the symptoms, biochemistry, and tumor mass.

Surgery

Surgery is the primary treatment of certain small, localized carcinoid tumors but may be required in other situations. Surgery is especially important in emergency situations with gastrointestinal obstruction, hemorrhage, or intestinal perforation. Surgical debulking of tumors of any size, even those which are metastatic, may afford a relief of symptoms by reducing the tumor mass and render further treatment with octreotide or chemotherapy more effective. Different centers have different approaches to timing and extent of surgery in metastatic carcinoids. An aggressive surgical approach was adopted by Ahlman et al.[76] in 41 patients and seemed to give encouraging results. However, it is difficult to compare these effects of treatment in such a variable disease without data on comparable surgical treatment and tumor staging.

Antrectomy with resection of multicentric argyrophil gastric carcinoids seems the logical treatment,[77] although gastrin antagonists and somatostatin analogue have been explored with some success. However, a number of those tumors recur and metastasize,[44, 78] especially the sporadic tumors not associated with pernicious anemia or MEN syndrome. Treatment should be performed early in the course of disease, while there are still only hyperplastic changes without an invasive tumor.[78]

Medical Treatment

Mediators of Biological Response

SOMATOSTATIN. Somatostatin, an inhibitor of secretion of a variety of peptides, and its long-acting analogue octreotide have been shown to suppress symptoms in carcinoid syndrome.[79–81] There are even reports of arrest or reversal of the growth of tumors in up to two thirds of patients and of shrinkage of liver metastases.[81, 82] There can be little doubt that somatostatin is a useful agent for treatment of the symptom complex.

Flushing, the presenting symptom in 64 per cent of our patients, decreased in frequency in all patients on 1 to 2 mg/kg/day of octreotide.[83] Certain patients, however, experienced no significant change in the severity or duration of episodes. Other authors reported a 50 per cent reduction in flushing in 19 of 24 patients[82] and improvement in 6 of 8 patients.[83] In contrast to other studies,[84] we did not experience a relapse of flushing with continued treatment.[85] Carcinoid crisis can be regarded as an extreme example of flushing. With its profound fall in blood pressure, it is a life-threatening complication of carcinoid syndrome. The onset can be provoked by any stressful manipulation, such as induction of anesthesia. Kvols et al.[80] presented data of such a crisis in a patient who was unresponsive to intravenous fluids, calcium, and epinephrine but recovered within a minute after 100 mg IV octreotide. Octreotide is clearly a significant addition to the therapeutic armamentarium for carcinoid syndrome.

Octreotide may be useful for the diarrhea syndrome and has been shown to normalize water and electrolyte transport across the proximal intestine acutely.[86] However, long-term effects are not consistent with this observation. In 58 per cent of our patients, the diarrhea disappeared with the use of octreotide,[81] which is significantly less frequent than the response rate reported by Kvols et al.[82] The difference might be due to a complex etiology of carcinoid diarrhea. Besides increased motility and a secretory component to the diarrhea, there is also an effect of partial luminal obstruction, bacterial overgrowth, and short bowel syndrome due to gut resection. An additional variable is the steatorrhea that can emerge during octreotide treatment. As to etiology, the drug is known to suppress exocrine pancreatic function. However, supplementation of pancreatic enzymes does not uniformly improve the condition.[83] Steatorrhea has a complex pathogenesis, partly attributable to alterations in bile flow, but it also includes a direct effect of octreotide on nutrient absorption and intestinal motility.[84]

Improvement of pulmonary function, documented by spirometry, has been observed in three of our patients.[85] Octreotide treatment also has been shown to reverse proximal myopathy,[86] a rare feature of carcinoid syndrome,[87–89] as well as to relieve the pain of the arthropathy that occasionally accompanies carcinoid.

Reports of biochemical responses to octreotide are somewhat controversial. Richter et al.[83] reported a drop in 5-HTP without a change in urinary 5-HIAA and unchanged serotonin levels with prolonged treatment.[90] Others have reported a drop in urinary 5-HIAA.[43] We observed normalization of urinary 5-HIAA in one third of our patients, but the overall values of blood serotonin after treatment were not significanty different from those before treatment. Of particular note is the lack of correlation between changes in serotonin and its metabolites and the clinical response to treatment.

There are reports of shrinkage of liver metastases with octreotide treatment in patients with carcinoid[81, 82] and other neuroendocrine tumors.[91] There has been no clear relationship between the effects on tumor growth and peptide production.[64, 92] In our experience, in up to one third of patients, escalating doses of octreotide seems to stop or reverse growth. Kvols,[93] on the other hand, has shown a three-fold increase in life expectancy after octreotide and has found an even greater effect by increasing the dose to 1500 μg/day.[93] Anthony et al.[94, 95] have used very high doses (6000 μg/day). This group claims even more satisfactory results with continuous infusion of octreotide as well as with high doses of a new synthetic analogue, somatuline. Somatostatin treatment, however, is not universally favorable, and alternate therapies must be considered.

INTERFERON. Interferon is known to suppress growth of different types of tumors.[96] Öberg et al.[97, 98] reported the first studies on the use of human leukocyte interferon to treat carcinoids. The same Swedish group showed much better response to this treatment than to a streptozotocin and 5-fluorouracil combination.[86] In a recent report using recombinant 2β interferon, Rönnblom et al.[99] describe a total response in 36 per cent of 135 patients, partial response in 52 per cent, and no response in only 12 per cent. Similar results have been reported by others.[100] In another prospective trial,[104] a response was achieved in 9 of 23 patients (39 per cent) for a median of 4 weeks and 4 of 20 (20 per cent) for 7 weeks. However, in this study, patients received higher doses to achieve the effect and experienced severe side effects (extreme fatigue, flulike syndrome), for which the dose had to be decreased. It is not clear whether the difference is due to the different forms of recombinant interferon used (2α versus 2β) or choice of patients. The development of neutralizing antibodies was shown,[98] which might be the cause for secondary failure. Another serious side effect is the development of autoimmune disease.[101, 102] At the present time, it seems that this treatment should be reserved for failed octreotide treatment.

Chemotherapeutic Agents

Treatment of carcinoid tumors with chemotherapeutic agents has proven frustrating until recently. Different agents have been used with variable success, but eventual relapse and increasing resistance to drugs are encountered.[103, 104] The single most studied agent is 5-fluorouracil, which has had response rates of 26 and 18 per cent.[104, 105] In attempts to enhance efficacy, the drug was administered intra-arterially or via the portal venous system, and a high complication rate and little benefit were reported.[106] A few responses were observed with doxorubicin[36, 104, 107] and streptozotocin.[7, 101] The results with dacarbasine and dactinomycin[108] are also not encouraging, although there have been anecdotal reports of a response.[107, 109] Cisplatin[110] and etoposide[114] gave similarly disappointing results.

Early nonrandomized studies of combinations of cyclophosphamide and methotrexate, streptozotocin and 5-fluorouracil, or streptozotocin and doxorubicin reported responses sometimes exceeding 50 per cent. However, rigid criteria for measurement of response were not always employed, nor was a complete response ever seen.[7, 104, 105, 111, 112] Based on these observations, the Eastern Cooperative Oncology Group conducted multicentric randomized trials of combinations containing streptozotocin. The outcome of two such studies of 170 patients showed response rates of 23 to 33 per cent.[104, 105, 113] A suggestion of a beneficial effect of streptozotocin alone or in combination with cyclophosphamide on foregut carcinoid was reported,[114] contrasting with the negative results of the Eastern Oncology Group. However, this observation remains unsubstantiated. A prospective trial done by the Southwest Oncology Group reported response rates similar to those observed by the Eastern Oncology Group after use of a combination of 5-fluorouracil, cyclophosphamide, and streptozotocin with or without doxorubicin.[115] Another prospective study showed only a 10 per cent response after streptozotocin and 5-fluorouracil.[86] A more recent study showed effectiveness of combined etoposide and cisplatin in anaplastic variants of neuroendocrine carcinomas with an overall regression in 12 of 18 patients with these tumors in contrast with only 2 of 27 patients with well-differentiated carcinoids or

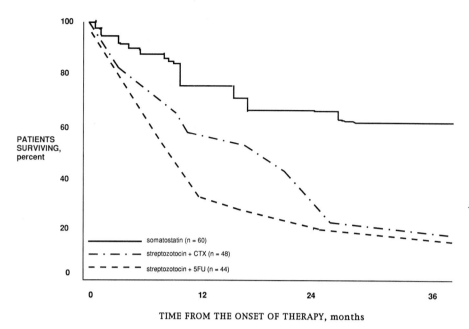

FIGURE 150–2. Malignant carcinoid syndrome survival: somatostatin analogue versus chemotherapy. (Reprinted by permission from Kvols LK, Martin JK, Marsh HM, Moertel CG: Rapid reversal of carcinoid crisis with a somatostatin analogue (letter). N Engl J Med 313:1229–1230, 1985.)

TIME FROM THE ONSET OF THERAPY, months

islet cell carcinomas.[116] It is thus apparent that except in the nonsecretory undifferentiated tumor, where combined cisplatinum and etoposide may be of value, results in the remaining cases have been singularly unimpressive, dictating a need for a continued search for improved therapy.

Hepatic Artery Embolization

Hepatic artery embolization[117-119] is a relatively safe procedure for palliation of hepatic metastases. The rationale for this form of treatment is to reduce the tumor mass. There is little or no evidence that it is curative. Gelfoam powder or Ivalon particles are usually used. Complications of the procedure include abscess formation, gas formation without infection at the site of embolization, severe pain in virtually all patients, and pyrexia in half. Renal failure may be prevented by vigorous hydration and allopurinol administration. There is always a risk of carcinoid crisis, although it seems to develop rarely. However, a large dose of octreotide before the procedure seems to be the proper prophylaxis.

Radiotherapy

There are no data available to support the use of external radiation treatment in these patients. The only indication for this type of therapy is spinal cord compression or painful bone metastases.

Internal radiotherapy using radiolabeled MIBG is still only experimental. Possible guidelines for its use, based on experience with pheochromocytoma and other neuroendocrine tumors,[120] would include its use for lesions not treatable by other modalities in patients with a sufficient life expectancy.[121] Future prospects of use of tracer octreotide[122] in treatment must still be evaluated.

Symptomatic Treatment

Symptomatic treatment with parachlorophenylalanine, cyproheptadine, methoprazine, and phenoxybenzamine helps to relieve the symptoms in some patients. There are some anectotal reports of effect of some of these agents on tumor regression (such as cyproheptadine[123]); however, this has not been confirmed.[36]

PROGNOSIS

For a malignant disease, the overall prognosis is rather good. Based on 2837 cases in the literature, the median 5-year overall survival is 82 per cent; for a localized tumor, it is 94 per cent; 64 per cent with lymph node involvement and 18 per cent with distant metastases.[39] The mean survival is 36 months after the first flushing episode, with 25 per cent 6-year survival.[4] With regional lymph node involvement, the median survival is 14 months, and it is only 11 months with 5-HIAA in excess of 150 µg/24 h for inoperable tumors.[36] The curve for metastatic tumors, however, has been altered drastically with the advent of octreotide (Fig. 150–2), with a three-fold increase in median survival time.

RESEARCH IN PROGRESS AND FUTURE DIRECTIONS

There are several fields of research interest in carcinoids: biological proprieties of tumors, their treatment, and mechanisms of the symptom complex. There are, however, problems that can only be studied in animal models.

Unfortunately, there are only a few established permanent carcinoid cell lines.[124] There is a growing interest in factors responsible for initiation of growth, increase in cell number and size, differentiation into endocrine cells, growth cessation, and maintenance of the viability of neuroendocrine cells. The finding that a loss of alleles on chromosome 11, on which the insulin gene is located,[125] is associated with multiple endocrine neoplasia type 1[126] and evidence that patients with MEN-1 might secrete parathyroid[127] and islet cell[128] mitogenic activity suggest a role for genetically determined circulating growth factors in at least the initiation of growth in neuroendocrine tumors. A role of tumor-produced growth factors as paracrine or autocrine moderators of growth was suggested 12 years ago[129] and recently was supported by observations of an effect of insulin-like growth factor I (IGF-I) on carcinoid cells in cultures expressing IGF-I receptors.[130] Oncoproteins have been demonstrated immunohistochemically in tumor tissues[131] and in carcinoid cell cultures.[132] Their role in tumor development, however, remains unclear. It thus seems that there may indeed be a cell line sensitive to growth promotion which is destined to become a carcinoid tumor. Studies of autocrine growth factors raise the possibility of future development of antagonists that act via inhibition of their autocrine secretion.[133]

One of the obstacles in developing a rational medical treatment of carcinoid is the lack of an appropriate experimental model. Recently reported tumors in nude mice resulting from inoculation of cultured carcinoid cells represent such an attempt.[134] These tumors responded to combined treatment with interferon, octreotide, and difluoromethylornithine.[134] The use of labeled octreotide analogues as tumor markers opens new experimental possibilities of localization of tumor tissue and even the possibility of delivery of concentrated radiotherapy for somatostatin receptor–positive tumors.[123]

Although recognized long ago, the mechanism of the symptom complex accompanying carcinoid tumors is not clear. Different vasoactive substances, in particular, products of pre-protachykinin and calcitonin–calcitonin gene–related peptide genes, are of major interest as potent mediators of the symptom complex and as tumor markers in a subset of patients with carcinoid tumors.[44, 50–62, 135]

CONCLUSION

Carcinoid tumors continue to fascinate clinicians and researchers with their meandering pace of growth; the diversity of hormones, amines, and prostanoids produced; differences in tumor biology based on site as well as endocrine nature; and the more recent success with endocrine therapy of an endocrine tumor. Treatment of patients with the symptom complex suggesting carcinoid is summarized on Figure 150–3. The first step in carcinoid diagnosis is heightened awareness of the complex constellation of symptoms and signs that are often mistakenly ascribed to some other condition. Once biochemical confirmation has been established unequivocally, only then does one embark on a search for the tumor. If and when the tumor can be localized, the next step in treatment of the carcinoid is surgery. In cases of small (up to 1 cm), localized tumors, this is the only treatment required. In patients with large and metastatic tumors, surgical debulking may still be beneficial to reduce tumor bulk prior to medical treatment. Patients with painful bony metastases may benefit from external irradiation.

Medical treatment consists of two lines of medication:

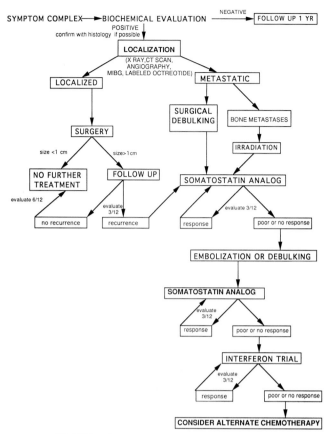

FIGURE 150–3. Carcinoid treatment flowchart.

octreotide and interferon. Because of the more serious side effects of interferon and beneficial effects of octreotide treatment of various features of carcinoid syndrome, we are inclined to advise it as a first step in medical treatment. Nevertheless octreotide has been shown to reverse the carcinoid crisis, so it is advisable to use it for prevention (before stressful procedures) and have it in the "emergency set" for urgent interventions such as may occur with angiography or anesthesia. Prolonged medical treatment, with, if necessary, surgical debulking of metastases or secondary tumors or dearterialization of liver metastases by embolization, can substantially improve expectancy and quality of life.

"Classic" antineoplastic agents have been shown to be ineffective. Experimental data on new combinations of treatment are expected in the next few years.

REFERENCES

1. Oberndorfer S: Karzenoide tumoren des dundarms. Frankfurt Z Pathol 1:426, 1907.
2. Lubarsch O: Uber der primaren krebs des ileum nebst bemerkingen uber das gleichzeitige norkommen von krebs und tuberculose. Virchows Arch [Pathol Anat] 3:280, 1988.
3. Thomson Å, Biörck C, Byörkman G, Waldenström J: Malignant carcinoid of the small intestine with metastases to the liver, valvular disease of the right side of the heart (pulmonary stenosis and tricuspid regurgitation without septal defects), peripheral vasomotor symptoms, bronchoconstriction, and an unusual type of cyanosis: A clinical and pathological syndrome. Am Heart J 47:795–817, 1954.
4. Davis Z, Moertel CG, McIlrath DC: The malignant carcinoid syndrome. Surg Gynecol Obstet 137:637–644, 1973.

5. Solcia E, Capella C, Buffa R, et al: Morphological and functional classification of endocrine cells and related growths in the gastrointestinal tract. *In* Glass GBJ (ed): Gastrointestinal Hormones. New York, Raven Press, 1980, p. 1.

6. Vinik AI, Thompson NV, Averbuch AD: Neoplasms of the gastroenteropancreatic endocrine system. *In* Holland JF (ed.): Cancer Medicine. Philadelphia, Lea & Febiger, 1992.

7. Buchanan KD, Johnston CF, O'Hare MM, et al: Neuroendocrine tumors: A European view. Am J Med 81:14–22, 1986.

8. Soja J: Carcinoids: Their changing concepts and a new histologic classification. *In* Fujita T (ed.): Gastro-entero-pancreatic endocrine system: A cell-biological approach. Baltimore, Williams & Wilkins, 1974, pp 101–119.

9. Rogers LW, Murphy RC: Gastric carcinoid and gastric carcinoma: Morphologic correlates of survival. Am J Surg Pathol 3:195–202, 1979.

10. Wilander E, El-Salhy M, Lundquist M: Atypical gastric carcinoids. Histopathology 8:183–193, 1984.

11. Wilander E: Diagnostic pathology of gastrointestinal and pancreatic neuroendocrine tumours. Acta Oncol 28:363–369, 1989.

12. Azzopardi JG, Pollock DJ: Argentaffin and argyrophil cells in gastric carcinoma. J Pathol Bacteriol 86:443–451, 1963.

13. Brodner OG, Grube D, Helmstaedter V, et al: [Endocrine cells in testicular teratomas (author's transl)]. Verh Dtsch Ges Pathol 61:148–151, 1977.

14. Eusebi V, Capella C, Bondi A, et al: Endocrine-paracrine cells in pancreatic exocrine carcinomas. Histopathology 5:599–613, 1981.

15. Partanen S, Syrjanen K: Argyrophilic cells in carcinoma of the female breast. Virchows Arch [Pathol Anat] 391:45–51, 1981.

16. Yousem SA: Pulmonary carcinoid tumors and well-differentiated neuroendocrine carcinomas. Is there room for an atypical carcinoid? (editorial). Am J Clin Pathol 95:763–764, 1991.

17. Grimelius L: A silver nitrate stain for alpha-2 cells in human pancreatic islets. Acta Soc Med Uppsala 73:243–270, 1968.

18. Servier AC, Munger BL: A silver method for paraffin sections of neural tissue. J Neuropathol Exp Neurol 24:130–135, 1965.

19. Wilander E, Portela-Gomes G, Grimelius L, Westermark P: Argentaffin and argyrophil reactions of human gastrointestinal carcinoids. Gastroenterology 73:733–736, 1977.

20. Grimelius L, Wilander E: Silver stains in the study of endocrine cells of the gut and pancreas. Invest Cell Pathol 3:3–12, 1980.

21. Wilander E, El-Salhy M, Pitkanen P: Histopathology of gastric carcinoids: a survey of 42 cases. Histopathology 8:183–193, 1984.

22. Smith AD, Winkler H: Purification and properties of an acidic protein from chromaffin granules of bovine adrenal medulla. Biochem J 103:483–492, 1967.

23. Fischer-Colbrie R, Lassmann H, Hagn C, Winkler H: Immunological studies on the distribution of chromogranin A and B in endocrine and nervous tissues. Neuroscience 16:547–555, 1985.

24. Moore BW, McGregor D: Chromatographic and electrophoretic fractionation of soluble protein in brain and liver. J Biol Chem 240:1647–1653, 1965.

25. Pickel VM, Reis DJ, Marangos PJ, Zomzely-Neurath C: Immunocytochemical localization of nervous system specific protein (NSP-R) in rat brain. Brain Res 105:184–187, 1976.

26. Schmechel D, Marangos PJ, Zis AP, et al: Brain endolases as specific markers of neuronal and glial cells. Science 199:313–315, 1978.

27. Tapia FJ, Polak JM, Barbosa AJ, et al: Neuron-specific enolase is produced by neuroendocrine tumours. Lancet 1:808–811, 1981.

28. Simpson S, Vinik AI, Marangos PJ, Lloyd RV: Immunohistochemical localization of neuron-specific enolase in gastroenteropancreatic neuroendocrine tumors: Correlation with tissue and serum levels of neuron-specific enolase. Cancer 54:1364–1369, 1984.

29. Wiedenmann B, Franke WW, Kuhn C, et al: Synaptophysin: A marker protein for neuroendocrine tumors and neoplasms. Proc Natl Acad Sci USA 83:3500–3504, 1986.

30. Wiedenmann B: Synaptophysin: A widespread constituent of small neuroendocrine vesicles and a new tool in tumor diagnosis. Acta Oncol 30:435–440, 1991.

31. Modlin IM, Esterline W, Kim H, Goldenring JR: Enterochromaffin-like cells and gastric argyrophil carcinoidosis. Acta Oncol 30:493–498, 1991.

32. Falck B, Hilrap NÅ, Thieme G, Torp A: Fluorescence of catecholamine and related compounds condensed with formaldehyde. J Histochem Cytochem 10:348–354, 1962.

33. Singh I: A modification of the Masson-Hamperl method for staining the argentaffin cells. Anat Anz 115:81–82, 1962.

34. Consolazione A, Milstein C, Wright B, Cuello AC: Immunocytochem-ical detection of serotonin with monoclonal antibodies. J Histochem Cytochem 29:1425–1430, 1981.

35. Moertel CG, Dockerty MB, Judd ES: Carcinoid tumors of the vermiform appendix. Cancer 21:270–278, 1968.

36. Moertel CG: Karnofsky memorial lecture: An odyssey in the land of small tumors. J Clin Oncol 5:1502–1522, 1987.

37. Vinik AI, McLeod MK, Fig LM, et al: Clinical features, diagnosis, and localization of carcinoid tumors and their management. Gastroenterol Clin North Am 18:865–896, 1989.

38. Vinik AI, Moattari AR: Neuroendocrine tumors, secretory diarrhea, and responses to somatostatin. In Lebenthal E, Duffey M (ed.): Textbook of secretory diarrhea. New York, Raven Press, 1990, pp 309–324.

39. Godwin JD: Carcinoid tumors: An analysis of 2837 cases. Cancer 36:560–569, 1975.

40. Lattes R, Grossi C: Carcinoid tumors of the stomach. Cancer 9:698–711, 1956.

41. Borch K, Renvall H, Liedberg G: Gastric endocrine cell hyperplasia and carcinoid tumors in pernicious anemia. Gastroenterology 88:638–648, 1985.

42. Borch K, Renvall H, Liedberg G: Endocrine cell proliferation and carcinoid development: A review of new aspects of hypergastrinaemic atrophic gastritis. Digestion 35(Suppl 1):106–115, 1986.

43. Wynick D, Williams SJ, Bloom SR: Symptomatic secondary hormone syndromes in patients with established malignant pancreatic endocrine tumors. N Engl J Med 319:605–607, 1988.

44. Eckhauser FE, Lloyd RV, Thompson NW, et al: Antrectomy for multicentric, argyrophil gastric carcinoids: A preliminary report. Surgery 104:1046–1053, 1988.

45. Harvey RF: Spontaneous resolution of multifocal gastric enterochromaffin-like cell carcinoid tumours (letter). Lancet 1:821, 1988.

46. Lundin L: Carcinoid heart disease: A cardiologist's viewpoint. Acta Oncol 30:499–502, 1991.

47. Feldman JM: Urinary serotonin in the diagnosis of carcinoid tumors. Clin Chem 32:840–844, 1986.

48. Melmon KL, Sjoerdsma A, Oates JA, Laster L: Treatment of malabsorbtion and diarrhea of carcinoid syndrome with methysergide. Gastroenterology 48:18–24, 1965.

49. Sandler M, Karim SM, Williams ED: Prostaglandins in amine-peptide-secreting tumours. Lancet 2:1053–1054, 1968.

50. Alumets J, Hakanson R, Ingemansson S, Sundler F: Substance P and 5-HT in granules isolated from an intestinal argentaffin carcinoid. Histochemistry 52:217–222, 1977.

51. Pernow B, Waldenström J: Determination of 5-hydroxytryptamine, 5-hydroxyindole acetic acid and histamine in 33 cases of carcinoid tumor (argentaffinoma). Am J Med 23:16–25, 1957.

52. Feldman JM: Increased dopamine production in patients with carcinoid tumors. Metabolism 34:255–260, 1985.

53. Lucas KJ, Feldman JM: Flushing in the carcinoid syndrome and plasma kallikrein. Cancer 58:2290–2293, 1986.

54. Theodorsson-Norheim E, Norheim I, Öberg K, et al: Neuropeptide K: A major tachykinin in plasma and tumor tissues from carcinoid patients. Biochem Biophys Res Commun 131:77–83, 1985.

55. Amatruda TT Jr, Upton GV: Paraneoplastic syndromes: Hyperadrenocorticism and ACTH-releasing factor. Ann NY Acad Sci 230:168–180, 1974.

56. Koch DD, Kissinger PT: Determination of tryptophan and several of its metabolites in physiological samples by reversed-phase liquid chromatography with electrochemical detection. J Chromatogr 164:444–455, 1979.

57. Flachaire E, Beney C, Berthier A, et al: Determination of reference values for serotonin concentration in platelets of healthy newborns, children, adults, and elderly subjects by HPLC with electrochemical detection. Clin Chem 36:2117–2120, 1990.

58. O'Connor DT, Deftos LJ: Secretion of chromogranin A by peptide-producing endocrine neoplasms. N Engl J Med 314:1145–1151, 1986.

59. Eriksson B, Arnberg H, Öberg K, et al: A polyclonal antiserum against chromogranin A and B—A new sensitive marker for neuroendocrine tumours. Acta Endocrinol (Copenh) 122:145–155, 1990.

60. Feldman JM, O'Dorisio TM: Role of neuropeptides and serotonin in the diagnosis of carcinoid tumors. Am J Med 81:41–48, 1986.

61. Aldrich LB, Moattari AR, Vinik AI: Distinguishing features of idiopathic flushing and carcinoid syndrome. Arch Intern Med 148:2614–2618, 1988.

62. Ahlman H, Dahlstrom A, Gronstad K, et al: The pentagastrin test in the diagnosis of the carcinoid syndrome: Blockade of gastrointestinal symptoms by ketanserin. Ann Surg 201:81–86, 1985.

63. Vinik AI, Gonin J, England BG, et al: Plasma substance-P in neuroendocrine tumors and idiopathic flushing: The value of pentagastrin stimulation tests and the effects of somatostatin analog. J Clin Endocrinol Metab 70:1702–1709, 1990.
64. Norheim I, Theodorsson-Norheim E, Brodin E, Öberg K: Tachykinins in carcinoid tumors: Their use as a tumor marker and possible role in the carcinoid flush. J Clin Endocrinol Metab 63:605–612, 1986.
65. Conlon JM, Deacon CF, Richter G, et al: Circulating tachykinins (substance P, neurokinin A, neuropeptide K) and the carcinoid flush. Scand J Gastroenterol 22:97–105, 1987.
66. Vinik AI, Thompson N, Eckhauser F, Moattari AR: Clinical features of carcinoid syndrome and the use of somatostatin analogue in its management. Acta Oncol 28:389–402, 1989.
67. Gould M, Johnson RJ: Computed tomography of abdominal carcinoid tumour. Br J Radiol 59:881–885, 1986.
68. Adolph JM, Kimmig BN, Georgi P, zum Winkel K: Carcinoid tumors: CT and I-131 meta-iodobenzylguanidine scintigraphy. Radiology 164:199–203, 1987.
69. Kressel HY: Strategies for magnetic resonance imaging of focal liver disease. Radiol Clin North Am 26:607–615, 1988.
70. Cho KJ, Vinik AI: Effect of somatostatin analogue (octreotide) on blood flow to endocrine tumors metastatic to the liver: angiographic evaluation. Radiology 177:549–553, 1990.
71. Åhlund L, Kindblom LG, Nilsson O, et al: Clinical and experimental studies on a midgut carcinoid tumor. J Surg Oncol 41:86–92, 1989.
72. Strodel WE, Vinik AI, Jaffe BM, et al: Substance P in the localization of a carcinoid tumor. J Surg Oncol 27:106–111, 1984.
73. Krenning EP, Bakker WH, Breeman WA, et al: Localisation of endocrine-related tumours with radioiodinated analogue of somatostatin. Lancet 1:242–244, 1989.
74. Reubi JC, Maurer R, von Werder K, et al: Somatostatin receptors in human endocrine tumors. Cancer Res 47:551–558, 1987.
75. Reubi JC, Hacki WH, Lamberts SW: Hormone-producing gastrointestinal tumors contain a high density of somatostatin receptors. J Clin Endocrinol Metab 65:1127–1134, 1987.
76. Ahlman H, Wängberg B, Jansson S, et al: Management of disseminated midgut carcinoid tumours. Digestion 49:78–96, 1991.
77. Borch K, Renvall H, Kullman E, Wilander E: Gastric carcinoid associated with the syndrome of hypergastrinemic atrophic gastritis: A prospective analysis of 11 cases. Am J Surg Pathol 11:435–444, 1987.
78. Wängberg B, Grimelius L, Granerus G, et al: The role of gastric resection in the management of multicentric argyrophil gastric carcinoids. Surgery 108:851–857, 1990.
79. Gyr NE, Kayasseh L, Keller U: Somatostatin as a therapeutic agent. In Bloom SR, Polak JM (ed.): Gut hormones. New York, Churchill Livingston, 1981, pp. 581–585.
80. Kvols LK, Martin JK, Marsh HM, Moertel CG: Rapid reversal of carcinoid crisis with a somatostatin analogue (letter). N Engl J Med 313:1229–1230, 1985.
81. Vinik AI, Tsai ST, Moattari AR, et al: Somatostatin analogue (SMS 201–995) in the management of gastroenteropancreatic tumors and diarrhea syndromes. Am J Med 81:23–40, 1986.
82. Kvols LK, Moertel CG, O'Connell MJ, et al: Treatment of the malignant carcinoid syndrome: Evaluation of a long-acting somatostatin analogue. N Engl J Med 315:663–666, 1986.
83. Richter G, Stöckmann F, Lembcke B, et al: Short-term administration of somatostatin analogue SMS 201–995 in patients with carcinoid tumors. Scand J Gastroenterol Suppl 21(Suppl 119):193–198, 1986.
84. Hengl G, Prager J, Pointner H: The influence of somatostatin on the absorption of triglycerides in partially gastrectomized subjects. Acta Hepatogastroenterol (Stuttg) 26:392–395, 1979.
85. Vinik AI, Moattari RA: Use of somatostatin analogue in the management of carcinoid syndrome. Dig Dis Sci 34(Suppl):14s–27s, 1989.
86. Öberg K, Eriksson B: Medical treatment of neuroendocrine gut and pancreatic tumors. Acta Oncol 28:425–431, 1989.
87. Berry EM, Maunder C, Wilson M: Carcinoid myopathy and treatment with cyproheptadine (Periactin). Gut 15:34–38, 1974.
88. Green D, Joynt RJ, van Allen MW: Neuromyopathy associated with a malignant carcinoid tumor—a case report. Arch Intern Med 114:494–496, 1964.
89. Wroe SJ, Ardron M, Bowden AN: Myasthenia gravis associated with a hormone producing malignant carcinoid tumour (letter). J Neurol Neurosurg Psychiatry 48:719–720, 1985.
90. Stöckmann F, Richter G, Lembcke B, et al: Long-term treatment of patients with endocrine gastrointestinal tumors with the somatostatin analogue SMS 201–995. Scand J Gastroenterol Suppl 21(Suppl 119):230–237, 1986.
91. Kraenzlin ME, Ch'ng JL, Wood SM, et al: Long-term treatment of a VIPoma with somatostatin analogue resulting in remission of symptoms and possible shrinkage of metastases. Gastroenterology 88:185–187, 1985.
92. Anderson JV, Bloom SR: Neuroendocrine tumours of the gut: Long-term therapy with the somatostatin analogue SMS 201–995. Scand J Gastroenterol Suppl 119:115–128, 1986.
93. Kvols LK: Personal communication, 1992.
94. Anthony LB, Winn S, Johnson DH, et al: Continuous Subcutaneous Octreotride Infusion for Carcinoid Tumor Syndrome. Presented at the ASCO Meeting, San Diego, CA, 1992.
95. Anthony LB, Krozely MG, Johnson DH, et al: Somatuline's Antitumor Efficacy and Phase I Clinical Trial in Neuroendocrine Tumors. Presented at the ASCO Meeting, San Diego, CA, 1992.
96. Strander H: Interferon treatment of human neoplasm. In Klein G, Weinhouse S (ed.): Advances in Cancer Research. London, Academic Press, 1986.
97. Öberg K, Funa K, Alm G: Effects of leukocyte interferon on clinical symptoms and hormone levels in patients with midgut carcinoid tumors and carcinoid syndrome. N Engl J Med 309:129–133, 1983.
98. Öberg K, Alm G, Magnusson A, et al: Treatment of malignant carcinoid tumors with recombinant interferon alfa-2β: Development of neutralizing interferon antibodies and possible loss of antitumor activity. J Natl Cancer Inst 81:531–535, 1989.
99. Rönnblom LE, Alm GV, Öberg KE: Autoimmunity after alpha-interferon therapy for malignant carcinoid tumors. Ann Intern Med 115:178–183, 1991.
100. Hanssen LE, Schrumpf E, Kolbenstvedt AN, et al: Treatment of malignant metastatic midgut carcinoid tumors with recombinant α-2β interferon with or without hepatic artery embolization. Scand J Gastroenterol 24:787–795, 1989.
101. Moertel CG, Rubin J, Kvols LK: Therapy of metastatic carcinoid tumor and the malignant carcinoid syndrome with recombinant leukocyte A interferon. J Clin Oncol 7:865–868, 1989.
102. Conlon KC, Urba WJ, Smith JW, et al: Exacerbation of symptoms of autoimmune disease in patients receiving alpha-interferon therapy. Cancer 65:2237–2242, 1990.
103. Kvols LK: Metastatic carcinoid tumors and the carcinoid syndrome: A selective review of chemotherapy and hormonal therapy. Am J Med 81:49–55, 1986.
104. Moertel CG: Treatment of the carcinoid tumor and the malignant carcinoid syndrome. J Clin Oncol 1:727–740, 1983.
105. Moertel CG, Hanley JA: Combination chemotherapy trials in metastatic carcinoid tumor and the malignant carcinoid syndrome. Cancer Clin Trials 2:327–334, 1979.
106. Melia WM, Nunnerley HB, Johnson PJ, Williams R: Use of arterial devascularization and cytotoxic drugs in 30 patients with the carcinoid syndrome. Br J Cancer 46:331–339, 1982.
107. Kvols LK, Buck M: Chemotherapy of endocrine malignancies: A review. Semin Oncol 14:343–353, 1987.
108. van Hazel GA, Rubin J, Moertel CG: Treatment of metastatic carcinoid tumor with dactinomycin or dacarbazine. Cancer Treat Rep 67:583–585, 1983.
109. Kessinger A, Foley JF, Lemon HM: Therapy of malignant APUD cell tumors: Effectiveness of DTIC. Cancer 51:790–794, 1983.
110. Moertel CG, Rubin J, O'Connell MJ: Phase II study of cisplatin therapy in patients with metastatic carcinoid tumor and the malignant carcinoid syndrome. Cancer Treat Rep 70:1459–1460, 1986.
111. Kelsen D, Fiore J, Heelan R, et al: Phase II trial of etoposide in APUD tumors. Cancer Treat Rep 71:305–307, 1987.
112. Mengel CE, Shaffer RD: The carcinoid syndrome. In Holland JF, Frei E (eds.): Cancer Medicine. Philadelphia, Lea & Febiger, 1973, pp 1584–1594.
113. Engstrom PF, Lavin PT, Moertel CG, et al: Streptozocin plus fluorouracil versus doxorubicin therapy for metastatic carcinoid tumor. J Clin Oncol 2:1255–1259, 1984.
114. Feldman JM: Carcinoid tumors and the carcinoid syndrome. Curr Probl Surg 26:835–885, 1989.
115. Bukowski RM, Johnson KG, Peterson RF, et al: A phase II trial of combination chemotherapy in patients with metastatic carcinoid tumors: A Southwest Oncology Group Study. Cancer 60:2891–2895, 1987.
116. Moertel CG, Kvols LK, O'Connell MJ, Rubin J: Treatment of neuroendocrine carcinomas with combined etoposide and cisplatin: Evidence of major therapeutic activity in the anaplastic variants of these neoplasms. Cancer 68:227–232, 1991.
117. Allison DJ, Jordan H, Hennessy O: Therapeutic embolisation of the hepatic artery: A review of 75 procedures. Lancet 1:595–599, 1985.

118. Carrasco CH, Charnsangavej C, Ajani J, et al: The carcinoid syndrome: Palliation by hepatic artery embolization. AJR 147:149–154, 1986.
119. Marlink RG, Lokich JJ, Robins JR, Clouse ME: Hepatic arterial embolization for metastatic hormone-secreting tumors: Technique, effectiveness, and complications. Cancer 65:2227–2232, 1990.
120. Sisson JC, Shapiro B, Beierwaltes WH, et al: Radiopharmaceutical treatment of malignant pheochromocytoma. J Nucl Med 25:197–206, 1984.
121. Sisson J, Hutchinson R, Johnson J, et al: Acute toxicity of therapeutic I-131-MIBG relates more to whole body than blood dosimetry (abstract). J Nucl Med 28:618, 1987.
122. Lamberts SW, Bakker WH, Reubi JC, Krenning EP: Treatment with Sandostatin and in vivo localization of tumors with radiolabeled somatostatin analogs. Metabolism 39:152–155, 1990.
123. Harris AL, Smith IE: Regression of carcinoid tumour with cyproheptadine. Br Med J (Clin Res Ed) 285:475, 1982.
124. Lundqvist M, Öberg K: In vitro culture of neuroendocrine tumors of the pancreas and gut. Acta Oncol 28:335–339, 1989.
125. Owerbach D, Bell GI, Rutter WJ, et al: The insulin gene is located on the short arm of chromosome 11 in humans. Diabetes 30:267–270, 1981.
126. Larsson C, Skogseid B, Oberg K, et al: Multiple endocrine neoplasia type 1 gene maps to chromosome 11 and is lost in insulinoma. Nature 332:85–87, 1988.
127. Marx SJ, Sakaguchi K, Green J, et al: Mitogenic activity on parathyroid cells in plasma from members of a large kindred with multiple endocrine neoplasia type 1. J Clin Endocrinol Metab 67:149–153, 1988.
128. McLeod MK, Tutera AM, Thompson NW, Vinik AI: Evidence for a Pancreatic Islet-Cell Mitogenic Factor in Patients with MEN-1. Association for Academic Surgery, Louisville, KY, 1989.
129. Sporn MB, Todaro GJ: Autocrine secretion and malignant transformation of cells. N Engl J Med 303:878–880, 1980.
130. Nilsson O, Wangberg B, Theodorsson E, et al: Presence of IGF-I in human midgut carcinoid tumours—An autocrine regulator of carcinoid tumour growth? Int J Cancer 51:195–203, 1992.
131. Roncalli M, Springall DR, Varndell IM, et al: Oncoprotein immunoreactivity in human endocrine tumours. J Pathol 163:117–127, 1991.
132. Nilsson O, Ahlman H, Wangberg B: The expression of oncogene products in midgut carcinoid tumor cells in tissue culture. Int J Cancer (in press).
133. Wigander A, Lundmark K, McRae A, et al: Production of transferable neuronotrophic factor(s) by human midgut carcinoid tumour cells; studies using cultures of rat fetal cholinergic neurons. Acta Physiol Scand 141:107–117, 1991.
134. Evers BM, Hurlbut SC, Tyring SK, et al: Novel therapy for the treatment of human carcinoid. Ann Surg 213:411–416, 1991.
135. Eriksson B, Öberg K: Peptide hormones as tumor markers in neuroendocrine gastrointestinal tumors. Acta Oncol 30:477–483, 1991.

Multiple Endocrine Neoplasia

MULTIPLE ENDOCRINE NEOPLASIA TYPE 1

RAJESH V. THAKKER

Multiple endocrine neoplasia[1] is characterized by the occurrence of tumors involving two or more endocrine glands within a single patient. The disorder has been referred to previously as multiple endocrine adenopathy[2] (MEA) or the pluriglandular syndrome.[3] However, glandular hyperplasia and malignancy also may occur in some patients and the term *multiple endocrine neoplasia* (MEN) is now preferred.[4, 5] There are two major forms of multiple endocrine neoplasia, referred to as type 1 and type 2, and each form is characterized by the development of tumors within specific endocrine glands (Table 151–1). Thus the combined occurrence of tumors of the parathyroid glands, the pancreatic islet cells, and the anterior pituitary is characteristic of multiple endocrine neoplasia type 1 (MEN 1), which is also referred to as *Wermer's syndrome.*[6] In addition to these tumors, adrenal cortical, carcinoid, and lipomatous tumors also have been described in patients with MEN 1. However, in multiple endocrine neoplasia type 2 (MEN 2), which is also called *Sipple's syndrome,*[7] medullary thyroid carcinoma (MTC) occurs in association with pheochromocytoma, and three clinical variants referred to as MEN 2A, MEN 2B, and MTC-only are recognized.[8, 9] In MEN 2A, which is the most common variant, the development of MTC is associated with pheochromocytoma and parathyroid tumors. However, in MEN 2B, parathyroid involvement is rare, and the occurrence of MTC and pheochromocytoma is found in association with a marfanoid habitus, mucosal neuromas, medullated corneal fibers, and intestinal autonomic ganglion dysfunction leading to a megacolon. In the variant MTC-only, medullary thyroid carci-

noma appears to be the sole manifestation of the syndrome. Although MEN 1 and MEN 2 usually occur as distinct and separate syndromes, some patients occasionally may develop tumors which are associated with both MEN 1 and MEN 2. For example, patients suffering from islet cell tumors of the pancreas and pheochromocytomas[10, 11, 12] or from acromegaly and pheochromocytoma[13, 14] have been described, and MEN in these patients may represent an "overlap" syndrome.[9, 10] All these forms of MEN may either be inherited as autosomal dominant syndromes[15] or may occur sporadically, i.e., without a family history.[1] However, this distinction between sporadic and familial cases may sometimes be difficult, since in some sporadic cases the family history may be absent because the parent with the disease may have died before developing symptoms.

The detailed clinical and biochemical features of each of these individual hormone syndromes together with their respective treatments have been reviewed in other chapters. This part of the chapter will discuss these individual hormone syndromes in the context of MEN 1 and will particularly review the recent progress in the molecular genetics of MEN 1.

HISTORICAL ASPECTS

Patients with MEN 1 are characterized by the combined occurrence of tumors of the parathyroid glands, the pancreatic islet cells, and the anterior pituitary gland. The first

TABLE 151–1. THE MULTIPLE ENDOCRINE NEOPLASIA (MEN) SYNDROMES AND THEIR CHARACTERISTIC TUMORS

TYPE	TUMORS
MEN 1	Parathyroids
	Pancreatic islets
	Gastrinoma
	Insulinoma
	Glucagonoma
	VIPoma
	PPoma
	Pituitary (anterior)
	Prolactinoma
	GH-secreting
	ACTH-secreting
	Nonfunctioning
	Associated tumors
	Adrenal cortical
	Carcinoid
	Lipoma
MEN 2A	Medullary thyroid carcinoma
	Pheochromocytoma
	Parathyroids
MEN 2B	Medullary thyroid carcinoma
	Pheochromocytoma
	Associated abnormalities
	Mucosal neuroma
	Marfanoid habitus
	Medullated corneal nerve fibers
	Megacolon

occurrence of such multiple endocrine tumors was described in a patient with acromegaly whose autopsy revealed the presence of an anterior pituitary tumor and enlarged parathyroid glands.[16] Pancreatic islet cell tumors were subsequently observed in association with parathyroid and pituitary tumors,[17, 18] and a familial occurrence was suggested by the finding of these tumors in two sisters.[19] Further case reports revealing the triad of parathyroid, pancreatic islet cell, and anterior pituitary tumors in individual patients led to the recognition of a unifying disorder,[2] and a familial basis was demonstrated by documenting its occurrence in a father and daughter of one family[20, 21] and in a father and four daughters of another family.[6] An autosomal dominant mode of inheritance was proposed[6] and established by further family studies which demonstrated inheritance of the syndrome in five generations with equal frequency in males and females.[22]

It was proposed that these tumors, which occurred in several different endocrine glands, had a common neuroectodermal origin[23, 24] within cells that were capable of amine precursor uptake and decarboxylation (APUD). However, the parathyroids, which are involved in the majority of MEN 1 patients, were found to have cytochemical characteristics which differed from APUD cells.[25] In addition, a consideration of the embryological development of the three major endocrine glands which are involved in MEN 1 revealed that they do not derive from the neuroectoderm. Thus the parathyroids are thought not to be of neuroectodermal origin but to derive from the pharyngeal pouch endoderm, and the origin of the pancreatic islet cells from neuroectoderm remains controversial.[26, 27] The anterior pituitary, unlike the posterior pituitary, is not of neuroectodermal origin but is from Rathke's pouch, which is not derived from the endoderm of the foregut but from the ectoderm anterior to the stomal plate.[28] Thus a neu-

roectodermal origin and a role for the APUD system in the etiology of MEN 1 tumors appears unlikely.[25] More recent studies utilizing the methods of molecular biology have further elucidated the genetic etiology of these tumors.[29]

CLINICAL FINDINGS AND TREATMENT

The incidence of MEN 1 has been estimated from randomly chosen postmortem studies to be 0.25 per cent[3, 8] and to be 18 per cent among patients with primary hyperparathyroidism.[30, 31] The disorder affects all age groups, with a reported age range of 5 to 81 years, and 80 per cent of patients have developed clinical manifestations of the disorder by the fifth decade.[22, 32–38] The clinical manifestations of MEN 1 are related to the sites of tumors and to their products of secretion. In addition to the triad of parathyroid, pancreatic, and pituitary tumors, which constitute the major components of MEN 1, adrenal cortical, carcinoid, and lipomatous tumors also have been described. The combinations of these affected glands and their pathological features—for example, hyperplasia or single or multiple adenomas of the parathyroid glands—have been reported to differ in members of the same family.[35–38] In the absence of treatment, these tumors have been observed to be associated with an earlier mortality in patients with MEN 1.[38a]

Parathyroid Tumors

Primary hyperparathyroidism is the most common feature of MEN 1 and occurs in more than 95 per cent of all MEN 1 patients.[22, 33, 35, 36, 39–41] Patients may present with asymptomatic hypercalcemia, nephrolithiasis, osteitis fibrosa cystica, or vague symptoms associated with hypercalcemia (e.g., polyuria, polydipsia, constipation, or malaise), or occasionally with peptic ulcers. Biochemical investigations reveal hypercalcemia usually in association with raised circulating parathyroid hormone (PTH) concentrations. No effective medical treatment for primary hyperparathyroidism is generally available, and surgical removal of the abnormally overactive parathyroids is the definitive treatment. However, all four parathyroid glands are usually affected with multiple adenomas or hyperplasia,[35, 42, 43, 43a] although this histological distinction may be difficult,[44] and parathyroidectomy for primary hyperparathyroidism in patients with MEN 1 has been associated with a high failure rate.[45, 46] Subtotal parathyroidectomy has resulted in persistent or recurrent hypercalcemia in 50 per cent of patients and in hypocalcemia, which required long-term therapy with vitamin D or its active metabolite calcitriol, in 10 per cent of patients with MEN 1.[45] These rates are markedly higher than those observed for parathyroidectomies in patients who do not have MEN 1, in whom recurrent hypercalcemia occurs in 4 to 16 per cent and hypocalcemia in 1 to 8 per cent of patients. In order to avoid neck reexploration, which is difficult, and to improve the treatment of primary hyperparathyroidism in patients with MEN 1, total parathyroidectomy with autotransplantation of parathyroid tissue in the forearm has been performed.[46–49] Both fresh and cryopreserved parathyroid tissue has been used for autotransplantation. The use of cryopreserved parathyroid tissue allows the confirmation of hypoparathyroidism in the patient prior to autotransplantation, but unfortunately, only 50 per cent of parathyroid grafts survive cryopreservation. The use of fresh parathyroid tissue for autotransplantation in the forearm results in viable grafts which secrete parathyroid hormone. However, the presence of functioning autotransplanted parathyroid tissue leads to recurrent hypercalcemia in more than 50 per cent of patients with MEN 1, and surgical removal of transplanted grafts has been required. Thus the management of primary hyperparathyroidism in patients with MEN 1 is difficult; parathyroid surgery in these patients is associated with a higher prevalence of persistent or recurrent hypercalcemia. Total parathyroidectomy, which would prevent this, has therefore been proposed as the definitive treatment for primary hyperparathyroidism in MEN 1, with the resultant lifelong hypocalcemia being treated with oral calcitriol (1,25-dihydroxyvitamin D).[45] It is recommended that such total parathyroidectomy should be reserved for the symptomatic hypercalcemic patient with MEN 1 and that the asymptomatic hypercalcemic MEN 1 patient should not have parathyroid surgery but have regular assessments for the onset of symptoms and complications, at which time total parathyroidectomy should be undertaken.

Pancreatic Tumors

The incidence of pancreatic islet cell tumors in MEN 1 patients varies from 30 to 80 per cent in different series.[22, 33, 35–42, 49a] The majority of these tumors produce excessive amounts of hormone, e.g., gastrin, insulin, glucagon, or vasoactive intestinal polypeptide (VIP), and are associated with distinct clinical syndromes.

Gastrinoma

Zollinger and Ellison initially described two patients in whom nonbeta islet cell tumors of the pancreas were associated with recurrent peptic ulceration and marked gastric acid production,[50] and gastrin was subsequently extracted from such tumors.[51, 52] These gastrin-secreting tumors (gastrinomas) represent over 50 per cent[33, 35, 37, 40] of all pancreatic islet cell tumors in MEN 1 and are the major cause of morbidity and mortality in MEN 1 patients. This is due to the recurrent severe multiple peptic ulcers which may perforate. This association of recurrent peptic ulceration, marked gastric acid production, and nonbeta islet cell tumors of the pancreas is referred to as the *Zollinger-Ellison syndrome*. Additional prominent clinical features of this syndrome include diarrhea and steatorrhea. The diagnosis is established by demonstration of a raised fasting serum gastrin concentration in association with an increased basal gastric acid secretion.[53] Occasionally, intravenous provocative tests with either secretin (2 units/kg) or calcium infusion (4 mg Ca^{2+} per kilogram per hour for 3 h) are required to distinguish patients with Zollinger-Ellison syndrome from other patients with hypergastrinemia, such as, for example, in antral G cell hyperplasia. However, in patients with MEN 1, the Zollinger-Ellison syndrome does not appear to occur in the absence of primary hyperparathyroidism,[36, 54] and hypergastrinemia also has been reported to be associated with hypercalcemia.[55] Thus

the diagnosis of Zollinger-Ellison syndrome may be difficult in some MEN 1 patients.

Medical treatment of MEN 1 patients with the Zollinger-Ellison syndrome is directed toward reducing basal acid output to less than 10 mmol/L, and this may be achieved by large doses of the histamine H_2-receptor antagonists cimetidine and ranitidine[56, 57] or by the parietal cell H^+, K^+-ATPase inhibitor omeprazole, which has proved efficacious and has become the drug of choice for gastrinomas.[58] Surgical treatment with total gastrectomy is recommended only for persistently noncompliant patients.[53] The ideal treatment for a nonmetastatic gastrinoma situated in the pancreas is surgical excision of the gastrinoma. In addition, duodenal gastrinomas, which occur more frequently in patients with MEN 1, have been treated successfully by surgery.[59] However, in the majority of patients with MEN 1, gastrinomas are frequently multiple or extrapancreatic, and with the exception of duodenal gastrinomas, surgery has often not been successful.[49a, 60, 61, 61a] The use of transhepatic selective venous gastrin sampling to localize the gastrinomas preoperatively in MEN 1 patients has been reported to improve the surgical outcome in one study.[62] Venous sampling in this study revealed that the MEN 1 patients with Zollinger-Ellison syndrome had either diffuse gastrin secretion from multiple pancreatic sites or localized gastrin secretion from a single region. The patients in whom gastrin secretion was localized benefited from resection of the gastrinoma by a partial pancreatectomy and required no drug therapy postoperatively. Other tumor localization studies using ultrasonography, computed tomography (CT), nuclear magnetic resonance imaging, selective abdominal angiography, or venous sampling have demonstrated that these techniques are often not useful and do not improve the surgical success rate.[63] The treatment of disseminated gastrinomas is difficult, and chemotherapy with streptozotocin and 5-fluorouracil,[49a, 64] hormonal therapy with octreotide, which is a human somatostatin analogue (SMS201–995),[65] hepatic artery embolization,[66] administration of human leukocyte interferon,[49a, 67] and removal of all resectable tumor[68] have all been successful occasionally.

Insulinoma

These beta islet cell tumors that secrete insulin represent one third of all pancreatic tumors in MEN 1 patients.[33, 37, 42, 49a] Insulinomas also occur in association with gastrinomas in 10 per cent[37, 69, 70] of MEN 1 patients, and the two tumors may arise at different times. Patients with an insulinoma present with hypoglycemic symptoms which develop after a fast or exertion and improve after glucose intake. Biochemical investigations reveal raised plasma insulin concentrations in association with hypoglycemia. Circulating concentrations of C-peptide and proinsulin, which are also raised, may be useful in establishing the diagnosis. Medical treatment, which consists of frequent carbohydrate feeds and diazoxide or octreotide, is not always successful, and surgery may be required. Most insulinomas are multiple and small, and preoperative localization with CT scanning, celiac axis angiography, and preoperative and perioperative percutaneous transhepatic portal venous sampling is difficult and success rates have varied.[49a, 71, 71a] Surgical treatment, which ranges from enucleation of a single tumor to a distal pancreatectomy or partial pancreatectomy, has been curative in some patients.[49a, 71a] Intraoperative direct pancreatic ultrasonography is proving very useful for localization. Chemotherapy, which consists of streptozotocin or somatostatin, is used for metastatic disease.[72]

Glucagonoma

These alpha islet cell, glucagon-secreting, pancreatic tumors have been reported in only five MEN 1 patients.[68, 73–76] The characteristic clinical manifestations of a skin rash (necrolytic migratory erythema), weight loss, anemia, and stomatitis may be absent, and the presence of the tumor may be indicated only by glucose intolerance and hyperglucagonemia. The tail of the pancreas is the most frequent site for glucagonomas, and surgical removal is the treatment of choice. However, treatment may be difficult, since approximately half the patients have metastases at the time of diagnosis.[76] Medical treatment with octreotide, streptozotocin, or dimethyltriazenoimidazole carboxamide (DTC) has been successful in some patients.[77, 78]

VIPoma

Patients with VIPomas, which are vasoactive intestinal peptide (VIP)–secreting pancreatic tumors, develop watery diarrhea, hypokalemia, and achlorhydria. This clinical syndrome has been referred to as the *Verner-Morrison syndrome*,[79] the *WDHA syndrome*,[80] or the *VIPoma syndrome*.[81] VIPomas have been reported in only a few MEN 1 patients,[36, 79, 82–84] and the diagnosis is established by excluding laxative and diuretic abuse, by confirming a stool volume in excess of 0.5 to 1.0 L/day during a fast, and by documenting a markedly raised plasma VIP concentration. Surgical management of VIPomas, which are mostly located in the tail of the pancreas, has been curative. However, in patients with unresectable tumor, treatment with streptozotocin,[85] a long-acting somatostatin analogue[84] (e.g., octreotide), corticosteroids,[86] indomethacin,[87] metoclopramide,[88] and lithium carbonate[89] has proved beneficial.

PPoma

These tumors, which secrete pancreatic polypeptide (PP), are found in a large number of patients with MEN 1.[32, 90] No pathological sequelae of excessive PP secretion are apparent, and the clinical significance of PP is unknown, although the use of serum PP measurements has been suggested for the detection of pancreatic tumors in MEN 1 patients.[91, 92]

Somatostatinoma

Somatostatin, which inhibits growth hormone (GH) secretion, has been demonstrated to be present in the gastrointestinal tract, particularly in the pancreatic islets.[93–95] Pancreatic tumors secreting somatostatin are associated with the somatostatinoma syndrome, which is characterized by diabetes mellitus, gallstones, low acid output, steatorrhea, and weight loss.[96] The somatostatinoma syndrome does not appear to have been reported in a MEN 1 patient, and this may possibly reflect the inhibitory action of somatostatin on endocrine cell proliferation and secretion.

Pituitary Tumors

The incidence of pituitary tumors in MEN 1 patients varies from 15 to 90 per cent in different series.[22, 33, 35–42] Approximately 60 per cent of MEN 1–associated pituitary tumors secrete prolactin, 25 per cent secrete GH, 3 per cent secrete ACTH, and the remainder appear to be nonfunctioning.[33, 40, 97–99] The clinical manifestations of these tumors in MEN 1 patients are similar to those in non-MEN 1 patients and depend on the hormone secreted and the size of the pituitary tumor. Thus patients may present with the symptoms of hyperprolactinemia, e.g., amenorrhea, infertility, and galactorrhea in women and impotence in men, or with acromegaly or Cushing's disease. In addition, enlarging pituitary tumors may compress adjacent structures such as the optic chiasm or normal pituitary tissue and cause bitemporal hemianopia or hypopituitarism, respectively. Treatment of pituitary tumors in MEN 1 patients is similar to that in non-MEN 1 patients and consists of medical therapy or selective hypophysectomy by the transsphenoidal approach if feasible, with radiotherapy being reserved for residual unresectable tumor.

Associated Tumors

Patients with MEN 1 may have tumors involving glands other than the parathyroids, pancreas, and pituitary. Thus carcinoid, adrenal cortical, thyroid, and lipomatous tumors have been described in association with MEN 1.

Carcinoid Tumors

Carcinoid tumors, which occur more frequently in patients with MEN 1, may be inherited as an autosomal dominant trait in association with MEN 1.[98, 100] The carcinoid tumor may be located in the bronchi,[101] the gastrointestinal tract,[102–104, 104a] the pancreas,[105] or the thymus.[98] Most patients are asymptomatic and do not suffer from the flushing attacks and dyspnea associated with the carcinoid syndrome, which usually develops after the tumor has metastasized to the liver.

Adrenocortical Tumors

The incidence of asymptomatic adrenocortical tumors in MEN 1 patients has been reported to be as high as 40 per cent.[22, 42, 106] The majority of these tumors, which may include cortical adenomas, hyperplasia, multiple adenomas, or nodular hyperplasia, are nonfunctioning.[106] However, functioning adrenocortical tumors in MEN 1 patients have been documented to cause hypercortisolemia and Cushing's syndrome,[99–107] as well as primary hyperaldosteronism, as in Conn's syndrome.[73, 108, 109]

Lipomas

Subcutaneous lipomas may occur in 2 per cent of patients with MEN 1,[22, 103] and frequently, they are multiple. In addition, pleural or retroperitoneal lipomas also may occur in patients with MEN 1.

Thyroid Tumors

Thyroid tumors consisting of adenomas, colloid goiters, and carcinomas have been reported to occur in over 25 per cent of MEN 1 patients.[22, 42] However, the prevalence of thyroid disorders in the general population is high, and it has been suggested that the association of thyroid abnormalities in MEN 1 patients may be incidental and not significant.

MOLECULAR GENETICS

In recent years, important advances in endocrinology have resulted from the application of the methods of molecular biology. Thus the molecular basis for mammalian sex development[110–112] and for Kallmann's syndrome[113, 114] has been elucidated. In addition, some of the susceptible genes involved in the development of hypertension,[115] insulin-dependent diabetes mellitus,[116, 117] and non–insulin-dependent diabetes mellitus[118, 119] have been identified. In these studies, the first important step toward elucidating the genetic abnormality and in subsequently characterizing the gene product (i.e., protein) was represented by the localization of the disease gene locus. This approach has been referred to as *reverse genetics*[120] or *positional cloning*.[121] The chromosomal localization of genes, which is also referred to as *gene mapping*, may be accomplished either by the cytogenetic detection of chromosomal abnormalities in affected individuals or by segregation studies in affected families using recombinant DNA genetic markers.[122, 123] Application of these techniques has made it possible to localize mutant genes that cause abnormal growth and activity of endocrine glands,[1, 29] such as, for example, in the clinical syndrome of MEN 1.

Genetic Models of Tumor Development

The development of tumors may be associated with mutations or inappropriate expression of specific normal cellular genes, which are referred to as *oncogenes*. Two types of oncogenes, referred to as *dominant* and *recessive*, have been described.[124–126] An activation of dominant oncogenes leads to malignant transformation of the cells containing them, and the genetic changes that cause this activation have been elucidated recently. For example, chromosomal translocations affecting such dominant oncogenes are associated with the occurrence of chronic myeloid leukemia and Burkitt's lymphoma.[127–130] In these conditions, the mutations that lead to activation of the oncogene are dominant at the cellular level; therefore, only one copy of the mutated gene is required for the phenotypic effect. Such dominantly acting oncogenes may be assayed in cell culture by first transferring them into recipient cells and then scoring the numbers of transformed colonies; this is referred to as the *transfection assay*. However, in some inherited neoplasms which also may arise sporadically, such as retinoblastoma,[131] tumor development is associated with two recessive mutations which inactivate oncogenes, and these are referred to as *recessive oncogenes*. In the inherited tumors, the first of the two recessive mutations is inherited via the germ cell line and is present in all the cells. This recessive mutation is not expressed until a second mutation, within a somatic cell, causes loss of the normal dominant allele (Fig. 151–1). The mutations causing the inherited and sporadic tumors are similar, but the cell types in which they occur are different. In the inherited tumors, the first mutation occurs in the germ cell, whereas in the sporadic tumors, both mutations occur in the somatic cell. Thus the risk of tumor development in an individual who has not inherited the first germ line mutation is much smaller, since both mutational events must coincide in the same somatic cell. In addition, the apparent paradox that the inherited cancer syndromes are due to recessive mutations but dominantly inherited at the level of the family is explained because in individuals who have inherited the first recessive mutation, a loss of a single remaining wild-type allele is almost certain to occur in at least one of the large number of cells in the target tissue. This cell will be detected because it forms a tumor, and almost all individ-

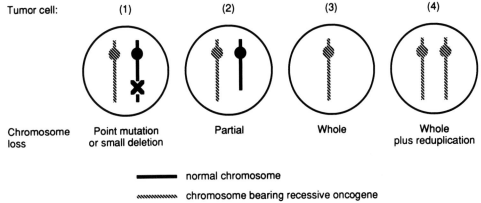

FIGURE 151–1. Chromosomal mechanisms involved in the "second hit" of Knudson's hypothesis. A pair of chromosomes—one normal and the other bearing the recessive oncogene—is represented schematically in each of four tumor cells (1 to 4). Four main forms of the "second hit" involving the normal chromosome, i.e., the normal dominant allele, are shown. In tumor cell 1, there has been a point mutation or a small deletion, whereas in tumor cells 2 and 3, partial and complete losses of the normal chromosomes have occurred, respectively. A complete loss of a chromosome, resulting in autosomal monosomy, may be disadvantageous to cell growth, and reduplication of the chromosome bearing the recessive oncogene may occur, as shown in tumor cell 4. These second hits involving the normal dominant allele would lead to an unmasking of the recessive oncogenic mutation and thereby result in tumor development. (Reproduced with permission from Thakker RV: The molecular genetics of the multiple endocrine neoplasia syndromes. Clin Endocrinol 38:1–14, 1993.)

uals who have inherited the germ line mutation will express the disease, even though they inherited a single copy of the recessive gene. This model involving two (or more) mutations in the development of tumors is known as the *"two-hit" hypothesis*.[132, 133] The normal function of these recessive oncogenes appears to be in regulating cell growth and differentiation, and these genes also have been referred to as *antioncogenes* or *tumor suppressor genes*.[125] An important feature which has facilitated the investigation of these genetic abnormalities associated with tumor development is that the loss of the remaining allele, which occurs in the somatic cell and gives rise to the tumor, often involves a large-scale loss of chromosomal material (Fig. 151–1). This represents a much larger target than the inherited mutation, which may be a small deletion or point mutation, in the search for the genetic loci involved in the development of different inherited tumors.[131, 134, 135]

The investigation of the genetic abnormalities involved in tumor development and the search for these inherited cancer genes have become possible as a result of advances in molecular biology[1, 29] that have provided cloned human DNA sequences to detect these mutations (Fig. 151–2). These cloned DNA probes identify restriction fragment length polymorphisms (RFLP's), which are the result of variations in the primary DNA sequence of individuals and may be due to either single base changes or deletions,

additions, or translocations.[136, 137] These changes in DNA sequence occur frequently (approximately once every 250 base pairs) in the noncoding regions, do not usually affect gene function, and are often at a distance away from the disease gene.[138] These polymorphisms may, however, lead to the presence or absence of a cleavage site for a restriction enzyme, which cleaves DNA in a sequence-specific manner. Two complementary approaches have been used to identify the mutations involved in the development of tumors in MEN 1. In one approach, RFLP's obtained from a patient's leukocyte DNA were compared with those obtained from tumor DNA, and differences were sought. In the second approach, RFLP's were used as genetic markers in linkage studies of affected families in order to localize the gene causing the MEN 1 syndrome.

Tumor Analysis

A comparison of the RFLP's obtained from leukocyte DNA and tumor DNA can facilitate detection of the chromosomal abnormalities associated with the "second hit" in tumor DNA, and this is illustrated in Figure 151–2. A restriction enzyme is used to cleave leukocyte and tumor DNA, and the resulting DNA fragments are separated according to size by agarose gel electrophoresis and transferred by Southern blotting[139] to a nylon membrane, which is hybridized with a single-stranded radiolabeled DNA probe. The labeled DNA probe will anneal to any fragments which have a complementary sequence, and these restricted fragments of varying lengths (RFLP's) are revealed by autoradiography. The exact number and size of RFLP's will vary in relation to the number of recognition sites for the restriction enzyme, as shown in Figure 151–2. In this example, the two chromosomes from the leukocytes differ in the number of restriction enzyme cleavage sites; one chromosome has three cleavage sites, and the other has two cleavage sites. Following digestion and hybridization, two fragments will be revealed at autoradiography. The chromosome bearing the recessive oncogenic mutation has three cleavage sites, and although two fragments of 4 and 1 kb will result from the enzymatic cleavage, only the 4-kb fragment will be visualized at autoradiography because it contains the complementary sequence to the radiolabeled DNA probe. However, the normal chromosome (i.e., the one not containing the recessive oncogenic mutation) has a loss of one restriction enzyme cleavage site due to a change in the DNA sequence, and following digestion, only restriction fragments of 5 kb in size will result. A single 5-kb RFLP is observed at autoradiography. Alleles can be designated to these RFLP's; for example, the larger, 5-kb RFLP is designated allele **1** and the smaller, 4-kb RFLP is designated allele **2**. Thus the leukocytes in this example are heterozygous (alleles **1,2**) and the chromosome bearing the recessive oncogenic mutation has allele **2**, while the normal chromosome with the dominant allele has allele **1**. A partial loss of the normal chromosome, i.e., the "second hit" (Fig. 151–1), associated with the development of the tumor would be detected by the loss of the 5-kb RFLP (allele **1**). Thus the tumor cells would be hemizygous (allele-**2**), as illustrated in Figure 151–2, or they may be homozygous (allele **2,2**) if a reduplication of the chromosome bearing the recessive oncogenic mutation had oc-

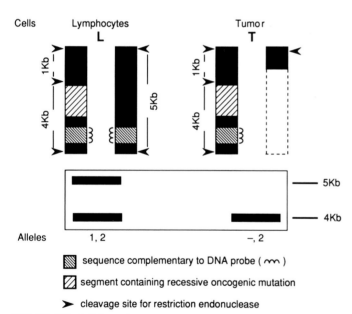

FIGURE 151–2. Schematic representation of the use of restriction fragment length polymorphisms (RFLP's) to investigate the chromosomal mechanisms involved in the "second hit." The example illustrated is that of a partial loss of the normal chromosome in the tumor, i.e., tumor cell 2 in Figure 151–1. RFLP's obtained from the leukocyte (L) and tumor (T) DNA of a patient are compared to detect deletions in the tumor tissue. The leukocytes are heterozygous (alleles **1,2**), and one of the pair of chromosomes in the leukocytes contains the segment with the recessive oncogenic mutation, whereas the other chromosome contains the normal dominant allele. In the example illustrated, there has been a partial loss of the normal chromosome in the tumor, i.e., tumor cell 2 in Figure 151–1, and this is detected by a loss of one of the RFLP's, which have been designated alleles. An example of such losses in a parathyroid tumor from a MEN 1 patient is illustrated in Figure 151–3. This abnormality in the tumor cells has been referred to as either loss of heterozygosity or loss of alleles (allelic deletions). (Reproduced with permission from Thakker RV: The molecular genetics of the multiple endocrine neoplasia syndromes. Clin Endocrinol 38:1–14, 1993.)

curred (Fig. 151–1). This type of analysis, involving paired leukocyte and tumor DNA, which has been referred to as the detection of a loss of alleles, allelic deletions, or a loss of heterozygosity in tumors, has been very useful in localizing tumor suppressor genes, e.g., those associated with retinoblastoma,[134, 135, 140] colorectal carcinomas,[141, 142] Wilms' tumor,[143, 144] MEN 1,[38, 145, 146] and MEN 2.[147–149]

Linkage Analysis

The investigation of the tumor suppressor gene involved in the MEN 1 syndrome has been facilitated by the use of RFLP's as genetic markers in studies of affected families. RFLP's are inherited in a mendelian manner, and their inheritance can be followed together with a disease in an affected family.[29, 120, 150] The consistent inheritance of an RFLP allele with the disease indicates that the two genetic loci are close together, i.e., *linked*. Genes that are far apart do not consistently co-segregate but show recombination because of the crossing over during meiosis. By studying recombination events in family studies, the distance between two genes and the probability that they are linked can be ascertained.[151, 152] The distance between two genes is expressed as the *recombination fraction* θ, which is equal to the number of recombinants divided by the total number of offspring resulting from informative meioses within a family. The value of the recombination fraction can range from zero to 0.5. A value of zero indicates that the genes are very closely linked, while a value of 0.5 indicates that the genes are far apart and not linked. The probability that the two loci are linked at these distances is expressed as a *LOD score*, which is $\log_{10}$ of the odds ratio favoring linkage. The odds ratio favoring linkage is defined as the likelihood that two loci are linked at a specified recombination versus the likelihood that the two loci are not linked. A LOD score of +3, which indicates a probability in favor of linkage of 1000:1, establishes linkage between two loci, and a LOD score of −2, indicating a probability against linkage of 100:1, is taken to exclude linkage between two loci. LOD scores are usually evaluated over a range of recombination fractions, thereby enabling the genetic distance and the maximum (or peak) probability favoring linkage between two loci to be ascertained. A fuller review of linkage in families with inherited metabolic and endocrine disorders has been described previously.[1, 122, 123]

Localization of the MEN 1 Gene

Linkage studies using classical genetic markers, e.g., the human leukocyte antigens (HLA), red cell antigens, serum proteins, and enzymes, were unable to localize the gene causing MEN 1.[153, 154] In addition, cytogenetic studies which indicated a segmental deletion of the short arm of chromosome 20 in MEN 1[155] remained unconfirmed. Combined tumor deletion mapping and family linkage studies utilizing RFLP's as genetic markers have successfully localized the MEN 1 gene to chromosome 11q13.[38, 145, 156]

Tumor Deletion Mapping Studies

A two-stage genetic mutational model has been proposed for the development of tumors in MEN 1,[133] and this is

analogous to that reported for retinoblastoma.[131] Studies of parathyroid tumors,[38, 146] insulinomas,[145] and anterior pituitary tumors[157, 158, 158a] from patients with MEN 1 have revealed that allelic deletions on chromosome 11 are involved in the monoclonal development of these tumors. An example is shown in Figure 151–3, in which a loss of alleles involving the whole of chromosome 11 is demonstrated in the parathyroid tumor of a patient with familial MEN 1.[159] This loss of alleles in the tumor results from the loss of chromosomal regions containing the marker loci; the complete absence of RFLP's suggests that this abnormality has occurred within all the tumor cells studied and indicates a monoclonal origin of the tumor. In addition, combined pedigree and tumor studies[38] demonstrated that these tumor-related allelic deletions of chromosome 11 occurred on the chromosome inherited from the normal parent and not the one from the affected parent (Fig. 151–

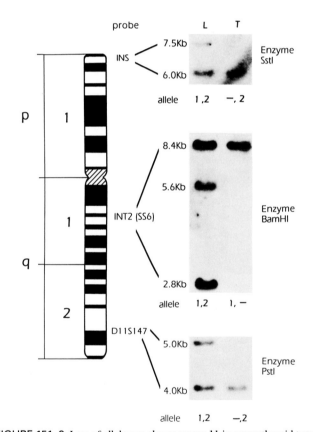

FIGURE 151–3. Loss of alleles on chromosome 11 in a parathyroid tumor from patient III.1 in Figure 151–4 with familial MEN 1. The RFLP's obtained from the patient's leukocyte (L) and parathyroid tumor (T) DNA using the probes *INS* (insulin), *INT2(SS6)*, and *D11S147* are shown. These probes are cloned human DNA sequences from chromosome 11 and are shown juxtaposed to their region of origin on the short (p) and long (q) arms of chromosome 11. The RFLP's are assigned alleles (Fig. 151–2). For example, two *PstI*-derived RFLP's were revealed by *D11S147*: the 5.0-kb fragment is assigned allele 1 and the 4.0-kb fragment is assigned allele 2. The leukocytes are heterozygous (alleles **1,2**), but the tumor cells have lost the 5.0-kb fragments (allele **1**) and are hemizygous (allele **2**). Similar losses of alleles are detected by the use of the DNA probes *INS* and *INT2(SS6)*, and an extensive loss of alleles involving the whole of chromosome 11 is observed in the parathyroid tumor of this patient with MEN 1. In addition, the complete absence of bands suggests that this abnormality has occurred within all the tumor cells studied and indicates a monoclonal origin for this MEN 1 parathyroid tumor. (Reproduced with permission from Thakker RV et al: *In* Cohn DV et al (eds): Calcium Regulation and Bone Metabolism, vol 10. London, Elsevier Science Publishers, 1990, pp 118–124.)

4). Thus this indicated that the second mutation involved the normal dominant allele and thereby provided additional evidence for the proposed two-stage recessive mutation model for the development of tumors in MEN 1. An examination of more tumors has revealed allele loss within tumors involving smaller regions of chromosome 11, and these studies have mapped the MEN 1 locus to the region within chromosome band 11q13.[146, 157] The results from one parathyroid tumor indicated that the MEN 1 gene is telomeric to the *PYGM* locus, which encodes human muscle glycogen phosphorylase. These studies also have demonstrated that such allelic deletions of chromosome 11 are involved in the development of sporadic non-MEN 1 parathyroid tumors, gastrinomas, prolactinomas, and somatotrophinomas.[157, 158, 158a, 160-162] Thus the region 11q13 appears to be involved in the development of non-MEN 1 and MEN 1 endocrine tumors.

Family Linkage Studies

In order to localize the gene causing MEN 1, family linkage studies were used as a parallel and complementary approach to deletion mapping studies. The segregation of

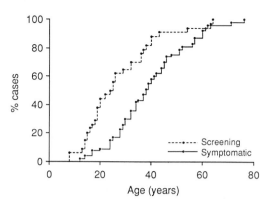

FIGURE 151–5. Age-related onset of familial MEN 1. The ages for diagnosis in 87 patients with familial MEN 1 were found to range from 8 to 76 years. The patients were subdivided, depending on the method used to detect MEN 1, into two groups. The symptomatic group consisted of 53 patients, and the age-related onset for MEN 1 in these patients at 20, 35, and 50 years of age was 9, 43, and 75 per cent, respectively. In another 34 asymptomatic patients, MEN 1 had been detected by biochemical screening, and the respective age-related onset for MEN 1 in these patients increased to 44, 74, and 91 per cent. Thus biochemical screening detected an earlier onset of MEN 1 in all age groups. (Calculated from refs. 37 and 159, and reproduced with permission from Thakker RV: The molecular genetics of the multiple endocrine neoplasia syndromes. Clin Endocrinol 38:1–14, 1993.)

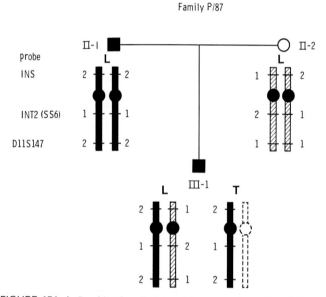

FIGURE 151–4. Combined pedigree and tumor analysis. The alleles obtained with probes from the short arm *(INS)* and the long arm [*INT2(SS6)* and *D11S147*] of chromosome 11 in patient III.1 and his parents (II.1 and II.2) are shown. These alleles were obtained by RFLP analysis of leukocytes (L) and parathyroid tumor (T) DNA, as illustrated in Figure 151–3. The father (II.1) was affected, and his leukocyte genotypes, which were homozygous at these three loci, are represented on the chromosomes as dark areas; the mother (II.2) was unaffected, and her leukocyte genotypes, which were heterozygous at the *INS* and *INT2(SS6)* loci and homozygous at *D11S147*, are represented on the chromosomes as hatched areas. The centromere is shown as a solid circle. The leukocyte genotypes of the affected son, III.1 (Fig. 151–3), which were heterozygous at all three loci, are represented on the chromosomes inherited from the father and the mother. An examination of the parathyroid tumor genotypes indicated hemizygosity with a loss of the maternal chromosome *(dotted lines)*. Thus a loss of the chromosome carrying the normal MEN 1 allele from the mother occurred in the tumor cells of this patient, and this is consistent with the "two hit" recessive oncogene model described (Fig. 151–1, cell 3) for the development of MEN 1 tumors. (Reproduced with permission from Thakker RV et al: Association of parathyroid tumors in multiple endocrine neoplasia type 1 with loss of alleles on chromosome 11. N Engl J Med 321:218–224, 1989.)

the disease and chromosome 11 RFLP's was investigated, and the MEN 1 gene was mapped to the region 11q13 by establishing linkage between MEN 1 and the genetic markers *PYGM* and *INT2(SS6)*.[38, 147, 156] This segregation analysis relies on an accurate assignment of the MEN 1 phenotype (i.e., affected or unaffected), and this depends on the methods used to detect MEN 1 and the age of the individual (Fig. 151–5). The age-related onset, which helps in the estimation of the penetrance of MEN 1 and is detailed below in screening studies, was used in the phenotypic assessment of individuals in MEN 1 families, and linkage was established (i.e., LOD score > 3) between MEN 1 and the 11q13 loci *PYGM* and *INT2(SS6)*.[38, 145, 156, 159] Recombinants between *INT2(SS6)* and MEN 1 have been observed, and this indicates that the oncogene *INT2(SS6)* is not the MEN 1 gene itself.[156, 163] No recombinants between MEN 1 and *PYGM* have been observed in affected individuals from two large studies of 6[164] and 27[165] families with MEN 1. The genetic map of this region (11q13) has been defined with polymorphic markers to be 11pter-D11S288-D11S149-11cen-PGA-PYGM-D11S97-D11S146-INT2-11qter,[165, 166, 166a] and the MEN 1 gene has been located by family linkage studies to a region distal to *PGA* and proximal to D11S97 and in the vicinity of *PYGM*.[164, 165, 166a] The region containing the MEN 1 gene has been identified by genetic and physical mapping studies using pulsed-field gel electrophoresis to be approximately 2 to 3 cM in size, which is equivalent to 2 to 3 million base pairs.[29, 167] The genetic markers defining this small region around the MEN 1 locus are proving useful in further studies of cloning the gene and in identifying individuals within a family who are at risk of developing the disorder.

The investigation and identification of such disease gene carriers in a family may be limited because many of the currently available DNA probes used to detect either RFLP's or variable numbers of tandem repetitive (VNTR's) sequences by Southern blotting are often not highly polymorphic. Thus information from the marker loci in the region of the MEN 1 gene may not be obtained from family studies. In order to gain maximal genetic information from these segregation studies, highly polymorphic genetic markers are required, and the polymerase chain reaction (PCR) is utilized to directly detect DNA sequence polymorphisms in one of two ways. First, PCR may be used to detect length variations in microsatellite tandem repeats,[168] e.g., $(CA)_n$, where $n = 10$ to 60. In addition to tandem repeats in the sequence (CA), microsatellite tandem repeats consisting of $(AT)_n$, $(GA)_n$, $(ATT)_n$, $(ATTT)_n$, and the hexanucleotide $[T(Pu)T(Pu)T(Pu)]_n$ also have been reported.[169–171] These tandem repeats, which are highly polymorphic and are inherited in a mendelian manner, are estimated to occur once in every 50 to 100 kilobase pairs. Thus they are a valuable technique in obtaining a detailed genetic map around a disease locus, e.g., MEN 1.[172] In this technique oligonucleotide primers are synthesized on either side of the repeat, and PCR is used to amplify the repeat sequence (Fig. 151–6). The smaller and larger fragment length polymorphisms in these repetitive sequences are detected by separation on a polyacrylamide sequencing gel or an agarose gel. In the second method PCR is used to detect either base-pair changes or length variations associated with the *Alu* sequence family.[173] These *Alu* sequence polymorphisms, which are ubiquitous in the human genome and appear to occur once every 6 kp are detected in a manner similar to that for the microsatellite tandem repeats. The use of one such polymorphic marker due to a $(CA)_{14}$ $(GA)_{25}$ repeat at the *PYGM* locus[174] in a family with MEN 1 is illustrated in Figure 151–7. The combined use of RFLP's and microsatellite polymorphisms enables the maximal yield of genetic information to be obtained from the study of polymorphisms in a single family. This has facilitated the construction of a precise genetic map around the MEN 1 gene, and the use of markers flanking the MEN 1 locus has made it possible to identify disease gene carriers with a predictive accuracy of 99.5 per cent.[164, 165, 166a] The cloning and characterization of the DNA sequence for the MEN 1 gene will further help in the identification of individuals at risk for this disorder by direct mutational analysis.

Screening for MEN 1

Detection by biochemical screening for the development of MEN 1 tumors in asymptomatic members of families with MEN 1 is important because earlier diagnosis and treatment of these tumors reduce morbidity and mortality. The attempts to screen for the development of MEN 1 tumors in the asymptomatic relatives of an affected individual have depended largely on measuring the serum concentrations of calcium, gastrointestinal hormones, and prolactin.[35–37, 176] Parathyroid overactivity causing hypercalcemia is invariably the first manifestation of the disorder, and this has become a useful and easy screening investigation.[35–37] Pancreatic involvement in asymptomatic individuals has been detected previously by estimating the fasting plasma concentrations of gastrin and PP. However, one recent study has reported that a stimulatory meal test is a better method for detecting pancreatic disease in individuals who have no demonstrable pancreatic tumors by CT.[92]

An exaggerated increase in serum gastrin and/or PP proved to be a reliable early indicator for the development of pancreatic tumors in these individuals. Some asymptomatic pituitary tumors may be detected by demonstration of hyperprolactinemia.

Screening in MEN 1 is difficult because the clinical and biochemical manifestations in members of any one family are not uniformly similar[35–38] and because the age-related penetrance (i.e., the proportion of gene carriers manifesting symptoms or signs of the disease by a given age) has not been established. The proportion of affected individuals who have been detected at a certain age by clinical symptoms or biochemical screening in different series[34, 35, 36, 176, 177, 177a] has ranged from 11 to 47 per cent at 20 years of age, 52 to 94 per cent at 35 years, and 83 to 100 per cent at 50 years; biochemical screening, which detects asymptomatic patients, increased the proportion of affected individuals at all ages. Thus the likelihood of wrongly attributing an "unaffected" status to an individual with no manifestations of the disease at age 35 may be as high as 1

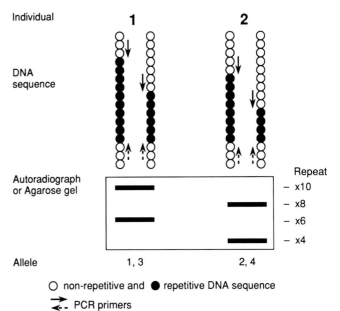

○ non-repetitive and ● repetitive DNA sequence

⇌· PCR primers

FIGURE 151–6. Schematic representation of polymorphisms in microsatellite tandem repetitive DNA sequences, which may consist, for example, of the dinucleotide CA, or the trinucleotide ATT, or the tetranucleotide ATTT, or the hexanucleotide TATATG. Oligonucleotide primers (⇌) corresponding to the nonrepetitive sequences (○) on either side of the repetitive DNA sequence (●) are synthesized, and the polymerase chain reaction (PCR) is utilized to amplify the repeat in genomic DNA obtained from different individuals. The resulting PCR products are separated either by polyacrylamide gel or agarose gel electrophoresis, and the polymorphisms are revealed by autoradiography or by viewing of an ethidium bromide–stained agarose gel under ultraviolet light. Thus, of the pair of chromosomes from individual 1, one has 10 repeats and the other has 6 repeats, whereas of the pair of chromosomes from individual 2, one has 8 repeats and the other has 4 repeats. Following PCR amplification and separation by gel electrophoresis, these variations in the length of the repeats will be revealed by the differences in the size of the bands, which have been designated alleles; for example, the larger band consisting of 10 repeats is designated allele 1, and those consisting of 8, 6, and 4 repeats are designated alleles **2, 3,** and **4,** respectively. These microsatellite tandem repetitive sequences, which are highly polymorphic, show mendelian inheritance (Fig. 151–7) and can be used as genetic markers in MEN 1 families. (Reproduced with permission from Thakker RV: The molecular genetics of the multiple endocrine neoplasia syndromes. Clin Endocrinol 38:1–14, 1993.)

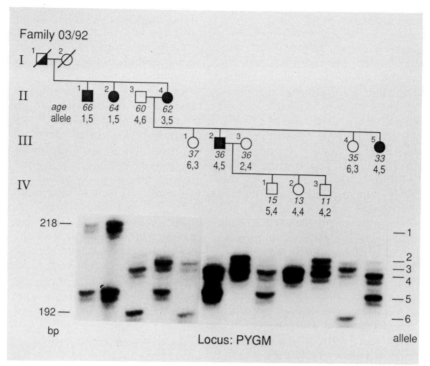

FIGURE 151–7. Segregation of *PYGM* and MEN 1 in family 03/92. Genomic DNA from the family members *(upper panel)* was used with [γ^{32}P]adenosine triphosphate (ATP) for PCR amplification of the polymorphic repetitive element $(CA)_{14}$ $(GA)_{25}$ at this locus.[174] The PCR amplification products were detected by autoradiography on a polyacrylamide gel and are shown in the lower panel. PCR products were detected from the DNA of each individual, and these ranged in size from 192 to 218 base pairs. Alleles were designated for each PCR product and are indicated on the right. For example, individuals II.1 and II.2 reveal two pairs of bands on autoradiography. The upper pair of bands is designated allele **1** and the lower pair of bands is designated allele **5**, and these two individuals are therefore heterozygous (alleles **1,5**). A pair of bands for each allele is frequently observed in the PCR detection of microsatellite repeats, and the upper band in the pair is the "true" allele and the lower band in the pair is its associated "shadow," which results from slipped-strand mispairing during the PCR.[175] The segregation of these bands and their respective alleles together with the disease can be studied in the family members whose alleles and ages are shown. In some individuals, the inheritance of paternal and maternal alleles can be ascertained, and in these the paternal allele is shown on the left. Individuals are represented as unaffected male (□), affected male (■), unaffected female (○), and affected female (●). Individual II.4 is affected and heterozygous (alleles **3,5**), and an examination of her affected children (III.2 and III.5) and her siblings (II.1 and II.2) reveals inheritance of allele **5** with the disease. In addition, her 15-year-old grandson, IV.1, has also inherited allele **5**, and this individual therefore is at a high risk of developing the disease and would require regular biochemical screening. However, the grandchildren IV.2 and IV.3 have not inherited allele **5** and would thus be at a low risk of developing the disease, as detailed in Figure 151–8.

in 2, or approaching 1 in 20, and depends on whether clinical symptoms alone or biochemical screening methods are used to detect the disease. In order to improve this situation, further biochemical screening and systematic family studies have been undertaken.[33, 35, 37, 159, 176] Results from two studies,[37, 159] in which 87 patients with familial MEN 1 were investigated, are shown in Figure 151–5. This reveals that the age-related onset for MEN 1 detected by clinical manifestations (symptomatic group) at 20, 35, and 50 years of age is 9, 43, and 75 per cent, respectively. The respective age-related onset for MEN 1 detected by biochemical screening is markedly improved to 44, 74, and 91 per cent. However, the identification of individuals at risk in an affected family can still be difficult (Fig. 151–8), and the recent availability of DNA markers for MEN 1 has helped to reduce these problems. These DNA markers enable carriers of the mutant MEN 1 gene to be detected within a family and thereby identify those individuals who need to undergo repeated screening tests for the development of tumors. This is illustrated in Figure 151–7 for a family suffering from MEN 1. The alleles of each individual at the *PYGM* locus, which reveals a less than 1 per cent

recombination rate with MEN 1,[164, 165, 166a] are shown. Individual II.4 is an affected female who is heterozygous (allele **3,5**) and is the mother of four children; her affected children, III.2 and III.5, and siblings, II.1 and II.2, indicate segregation of allele **5** and the disease. Her daughters, III.1 and III.4, who are 37 and 35 years old, respectively, are biochemically normal, and this indicates that they have a low probability (5 and 13 per cent, respectively) of being gene carriers (Fig. 151–8). In addition, the results of genetic marker analysis reveal that III.1 and III.4 have inherited allele **3**, which is not associated with the disease in this family, and this indicates a low probability (<1 per cent) for these being gene carriers. The combined use of flanking DNA markers and biochemical screening in this age group helps to reduce the risk for these individuals of being carriers to less than 0.05 per cent. The three children (IV.1, IV.2, and IV.3) of the affected male, III.2, who is heterozygous (alleles **4,5**), are in a younger age group (10 to 15 years) and have not developed the disease. The finding of normal serum biochemistry in these individuals still indicates a residual 40 per cent risk of their being gene carriers. However, individuals IV.2 and IV.3 have inherited

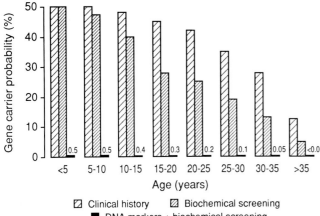

FIGURE 151–8. Probabilities for gene carriers of MEN 1. The probabilities (shown as per cents) for a child of an affected MEN 1 parent being a gene carrier following negative screening results using clinical history, biochemical screening (i.e., serum calcium, prolactin, and gastrointestinal hormone concentrations), and/or DNA marker studies (Fig. 151–7) are shown for eight age groups. The risk, assessed clinically at birth, of having inherited this autosomal dominant disorder is 50 per cent, and biochemical estimations are not useful in reducing this risk further. In contrast, DNA marker studies using flanking DNA probes can markedly reduce the risk of being a carrier to 0.5 per cent. With increasing age, the clinically assessed risk for the unaffected child of an affected parent declines gradually from 50 per cent to only 28 per cent at age 35. However, the risk as assessed by biochemical tests declines more rapidly from 50 per cent at birth to 25 per cent by age 25 and to 12.5 per cent by age 35. These risks can be further decreased by the combined use of flanking DNA markers, and the significantly lower 0.5 per cent risk of being a gene carrier at birth is reduced to 0.05 per cent at age 35. Thus the use of DNA markers can help considerably in reassuring those individuals who are not gene carriers for MEN 1 and in identifying those individuals who are MEN 1 gene carriers and who therefore require regular screening. (Calculated from Thakker RV: The molecular genetics of the multiple endocrine neoplasia syndromes. Clin Endocrinol 38:1–14, 1993.)

allele **4** from their affected father, III.2, and this indicates a low probability (<1 per cent) of their being gene carriers. The combined use of flanking DNA markers and biochemical screening in these individuals, who are 11 and 13 years old, reduces this risk to 0.4 per cent. In contrast, individual IV.1 has inherited allele **5** from his affected father and is at high risk of developing the disease, since the probability of being a gene carrier exceeds 99 per cent. This individual should undergo regular biochemical screening.

Thus the application of DNA markers has helped to determine the carrier risk status of many individuals, and this has substantially altered the screening strategy (Fig. 151–8) and clinical management of these patients. It is suggested that DNA analysis should now be introduced in the screening program of MEN 1 families.[164] The advantages of DNA analysis are that it requires a single blood sample and does not need to be repeated, unlike the biochemical screening tests. This is so because the analysis is independent of the age of the individual and provides an objective result. The limitations of DNA analysis are that blood samples for DNA analysis must be available from two or more affected family members to conclude which allele of the marker is inherited with the MEN 1 gene. In addition, DNA analysis may be subject to a small but significant error rate because of recombination between the marker and the gene. This error rate can be minimized by the use

of flanking DNA markers. The ultimate cloning of the gene itself will help to identify mutations directly and thereby remove this limited uncertainty. As of this writing an integrated program of both DNA screening, to identify gene carriers, and biochemical screening, to detect the development of tumors, is recommended.[29, 164, 165] Thus a DNA test identifying an individual as a mutant gene carrier is likely to lead not to immediate medical or surgical treatment but to earlier and more frequent biochemical screening, whereas a DNA result that leaves an individual with a residual carrier risk of less than 1 per cent will lead to a decision for either infrequent or no screening.

It is suggested that individuals at high risk of developing MEN 1 should be screened once per annum.[8, 37] Because the disease has developed in some individuals by the age of 5 years, screening should commence in early childhood and should continue for life, since some individuals have not developed the disease until the eighth decade.[33, 37, 38] Screening history and physical examination should be directed toward eliciting the symptoms and signs of hypercalcemia, nephrolithiasis, peptic ulcer disease, neuroglycopenia, hypopituitarism, galactorrhea and amenorrhea in women, acromegaly, Cushing's disease, visual field loss, and the presence of subcutaneous lipomata. Biochemical screening should include serum calcium and prolactin estimations in all individuals, and measurement of gastrointestinal hormones and more specific endocrine function tests should be reserved for individuals who have symptoms or signs suggestive of a clinical syndrome. Thus the recent advances in molecular biology, which have enabled the localization of the gene causing MEN 1, have helped in the clinical management of patients and their families with this disorder.

Dominant Oncogenes in Endocrine Tumors

Studies of parathyroid tumors and somatotrophinomas, which are GH-secreting tumors, have revealed roles for dominantly acting oncogenes in these tumors. The dominant oncogene associated with parathyroid tumors has been referred to as *PRAD1* (parathyroid adenomatosis type 1), and the dominant oncogene associated with somatotrophinomas involves mutation of the gene encoding the alpha chain of the guanine nucleotide (GTP) binding subunit of the stimulatory regulator of adenylyl cyclase, referred to as the $G_s\alpha$ *protein*.

PRAD1 Gene

The molecular basis of non-MEN 1 parathyroid tumors has been investigated, and a structural defect within the parathyroid hormone (PTH) gene itself identified. The human PTH gene has been localized to the short arm of chromosome 11 by using rodent-human hybrid cell lines[178] and its nucleotide sequence determined.[179] Further analysis of the organization of the pre-pro PTH gene revealed that it has two intervening sequences which separate the gene into three functional domains. The intervening sequences are called *introns*, and the gene sequences which encode the mature messenger RNA (mRNA) are called *exons*. The first exon, at the 5' end, encodes an untranslated regulatory domain; the second exon encodes the signal peptide and part of the "prohormone" sequence; and the third exon encodes the remainder of the "prohormone" sequence, together with the PTH peptide and the 3' untranslated region.[180] Structural abnormalities within the organization of the PTH gene have been identified in two non-MEN 1 parathyroid adenomas.[181] These abnormalities involved a separation of the first exon from the fragment containing the second and third exons together with a rearrangement in which the PTH regulatory elements became juxtaposed with "new" non-PTH DNA,[182] which was referred to as *D11S287*. Investigation of *D11S287* localized it to the long arm of chromosome 11, band 11q13, a region which contains the MEN 1 gene. Detailed analysis revealed that *D11S287* contained a sequence that was highly conserved in different species and that was expressed in normal parathyroids and in parathyroid adenomas. This expressed sequence from *D11S287* was designated *PRADI*, and its relationship to the MEN 1 gene was investigated. The *PRADI* gene is not the MEN 1 gene, since the two genes are separated by several million base pairs.[183] Thus the *PRADI* gene is located within 160 kilobase pairs proximal to *INT2*,[183] whereas the MEN 1 gene is located more than 4 million base pairs proximal to the INT2 locus.[164, 165, 166a, 167] The *PRADI* gene is therefore not the gene causing MEN 1, although it is overexpressed in some parathyroid adenomas.[184] The combination of the clonal rearrangement of one copy of the *PRADI* gene and the altered gene expression indicated that *PRADI* is a dominant oncogene whose activation is associated with the development of parathyroid tumors. Similar activation of cellular oncogenes through analogous rearrangements has been implicated in the pathogenesis of several tumors, e.g., Burkitt's lymphoma and chronic myeloid leukemia.[127–130] The *PRADI* complementary DNA (cDNA) was isolated from a human placental cDNA library, and an analysis revealed that this cDNA encoded a protein of 295 amino acids which had similarities to the cyclin family of proteins.[185] Cyclins were first identified in the dividing cells of clams and sea urchins,[186] in which they were associated with a cell cycle–regulated proteolysis in the immediate period preceding the onset of anaphase. Cyclins also have been identified in humans, in whom they also have an important role in regulating progress through the cell cycle. Thus *PRADI*, which appears to encode a novel cyclin, also may be a regulator of the cell cycle, and an overexpression of *PRADI* may be an important event in the development of parathyroid tumors. In addition, studies of lymphomas have revealed that *PRADI* is likely to be the B cell lymphoma type 1 *(BCL1)* oncogene.[187] A further characterization of the role of the *PRADI* gene in regulating the cell cycle and in mitosis will help to elucidate the etiology of these and parathyroid tumors.

$G_s\alpha$ Mutations

The G proteins are a family of guanine nucleotide (GTP)–binding proteins that mediate signal transduction across cell membranes.[188] These proteins couple cell surface receptors to their second-messenger signal-generation systems and thereby regulate the activity of intracellular effector enzymes and ion channels. The G proteins share a heterotrimeric structure composed of α, β, and γ subunits. The β and γ subunits are tightly associated with each other

as a $\beta\gamma$ complex and appear to be functionally interchangeable among some of the G proteins. The α subunits are the most diverse and are unique to each G protein. The α subunit which contains the guanine nucleotide–binding site and has intrinsic guanine triphosphatase (GTPase) activity is thought to confer specificity on each G protein and thereby allow it to discriminate among multiple receptors and effectors. For example, the hormone-sensitive adenylate cyclase system is regulated by at least two G proteins, one of which stimulates ($G_s\alpha$) and another which inhibits ($G_i\alpha$) the activity of the membrane-bound enzyme that catalyzes the formation of the intracellular second-messenger cAMP. The role of these G proteins in the development of GH-secreting tumors has been studied.[189, 190] GH-releasing hormone (GHRH) acts via cAMP to stimulate GH secretion and proliferation of somatotrophs,[191] and a subset of somatotrophinomas are associated with an elevation in basal adenylyl cyclase activity which is unresponsive to further stimulation by GHRH and GTP analogues.[192] This alteration in the hormone-sensitive adenylyl cyclase system has been further investigated, and a constitutive activation of $G_s\alpha$ which was associated with an inhibition of GTPase activity was demonstrated in these somatotrophinomas.[192] An analysis of the gene encoding $G_s\alpha$, which is located on chromosome 20,[193] has revealed four mutations at two codons in 40 per cent of somatotrophinomas.[189, 190, 194] These tumor-specific missense mutations of $G_s\alpha$ occurred either in codon 201, which is in exon 8, or in codon 227, which is in exon 9.[195] At codon 201, the mutation led to a replacement of arginine (wild-type codon CGT) with either cysteine (mutant codon TGT) or histidine (mutant codon CAT), and at codon 227, the mutation led to a replacement of glutamine (wild-type codon CAG) with either arginine (mutant codon CGG) or leucine (mutant codon CTG).[189, 190, 194] The mutation in the G_s protein α chain, which is referred to as a *gsp* mutation, occurred in only one copy of the gene and thus appeared to act as a dominant oncogene.[189] The roles of these dominantly acting *gsp* mutations together with the recessively acting gene located in chromosome 11q13 are being investigated.

Somatotrophinomas have been investigated further.[158a] These studies revealed that chromosome 11q13 allelic deletions and *gsp* mutations were specifically associated with the monoclonal development of somatotrophinomas, and a genetic model involving both these recessive and dominant oncogenes has been proposed for the multistep etiology and progression of these pituitary tumors.[158a]

CIRCULATING GROWTH FACTOR

Tumor development in MEN 1 may be associated with a circulating growth factor which is mitogenic for parathyroid cells[196] and which has similarities to basic fibroblast growth factor (bFGF).[197] This observation is of interest because initial genetic mapping studies of MEN 1 revealed linkage between MEN 1 and the oncogene *INT2*,[38, 156] which encodes a fibroblast growth factor. Although subsequent genetic mapping studies which revealed recombination between MEN 1 and *INT2* excluded *INT2* as the gene causing MEN 1,[163–165] the finding of this circulating mitogenic growth factor in the plasma of patients with MEN 1 remains of importance in elucidating the etiology of these tumors. The circulating growth factor which was identified in the plasma of MEN 1 patients by in vitro studies was detected by the use of bovine parathyroid cells maintained in a long-term culture system.[196] Plasma from MEN 1 patients stimulated these bovine parathyroid cells to rapidly incorporate [³H]thymidine and to proliferate. This plasma mitogenic activity was markedly reduced by heat, acid, and dithiothreitol treatment, indicating that the stimulatory properties may be due to protein-containing disulfide bonds. Gel-filtration analysis demonstrated the mitogenic activity to be within a single peak in a region between bovine serum albumin and ovalbumin, thereby indicating that the protein has a molecular weight in the range of 50,000 to 55,000. This mitogenic factor was demonstrated to be a distinct factor from other growth factors, such as epidermal growth factor (EGF), platelet-derived growth factor (PDGF), nerve growth factor (NGF), fibroblast growth factor (FGF), insulin-like growth factor I (IGF-I), and tumor growth factor β (TGF-β), and was shown not to be an autocrine product from the parathyroid glands themselves. Additional studies revealed that the parathyroid mitogenic factor had similarities to basic fibroblast growth factor (bFGF), in contrast to its acidic counterpart, and that the mitogenic factor appeared to act as a tumor angiogenic factor by stimulating endothelial cells.[197] The parathyroid mitogenic factor appeared to be specific for parathyroid cells and did not stimulate activity in anterior pituitary or pancreatic islet cells.[196, 198] In addition, plasma from some patients with familial hypocalciuric hypercalcemia, who do not suffer from MEN 1, also demonstrated this mitogenic activity.[196] More recent studies, using a novel sensitive specific two-site immunoradiometric assay for plasma bFGF, have revealed that plasma bFGF-like immunoreactivity decreases after surgery for pituitary tumor and after initiation of bromocryptine therapy, thereby indicating that this plasma mitogenic factor may originate from the pituitary.[198a] These findings require further study in order to elucidate the specific role for this circulating growth factor in the development of MEN 1 tumors.[198]

ANIMAL MODELS

An animal model for MEN 1 would greatly facilitate studies into the pathogenesis, gene expression, and pharmacological therapies for this disorder. Two animal models with multiple endocrine tumors which have some similarities to human MEN 1 disorder have been described. The first animal model resulted from the transplantation of functioning endocrine tumors in rats, and the second model resulted from the introduction of cloned recombinant DNA sequences into the germ cells of mice.

The transplantation of GH- and prolactin-secreting rat pituitary tumor tissue into syngeneic rats resulted in hypercalcemia and raised serum concentrations of parathyroid hormone, 1,25(OH)$_2$-vitamin D, GH, and prolactin.[199] Parathyroidectomy in these rats led to hypocalcemia, thereby revealing the parathyroid dependence of the hypercalcemia. The pathophysiological basis for these endocrine abnormalities remains unknown, and it has been suggested that prolactin or GH may directly stimulate parathyroid hormone secretion[199] and increase renal 1α-hydroxylase enzyme activity.[200, 201]

Transgenic Mouse

The introduction of cloned genes into the germ cells of mammals is one of the major recent technological advances in biology.[202, 203] The inserted cloned gene is stably transmitted from generation to generation and is referred to as a *transgene*. These advances have enabled animal models to be produced for human genetic diseases and thereby have permitted further study of these disorders. For example, the introduction of a recombinant oncogene containing the insulin gene promoter into fertilized mouse eggs resulted in an inherited form of insulinoma in transgenic mice.[204] Transgenic mice with pituitary and pancreatic tumors have been reported, and these may provide a model for the human disorder of MEN 1.[205] These transgenic mice developed from fertilized one-cell mouse eggs which had a hybrid oncogene introduced into them by microinjection. The hybrid oncogene consisted of the promoter region of the bovine arginine vasopressin (AVP) gene fused to the DNA sequence coding for the large-T antigen of simian virus 40 (SV40). The eggs surviving this procedure were returned by oviduct transfer to pseudopregnant recipient female mice, and the transgenic offspring in the litter were identified and bred for further studies. Tumors of the pancreatic islet cells and anterior pituitary developed in these transgenic mice. The pancreatic tumors consisted of insulin-producing cells, but those of the pituitary appeared to be nonfunctioning. Hypercalcemia and parathyroid tumors were not detected in preliminary studies. This intriguing transgenic mouse model may prove useful in investigating the pathogenesis of MEN 1 in humans.

CONCLUSIONS

Clinical, genetic, and epidemiological studies have improved our understanding of the manifestations of the MEN 1 syndrome. Thus the presentation, age at onset, diagnosis, and patterns of occurrence within families have been elucidated. This information has already helped in the biochemical screening for this disorder in family members. In addition, molecular genetic studies have localized the gene causing MEN 1 to 11q13, and the establishment of genetic markers flanking the disease locus has helped in the identification of those family members who are at a high risk of developing the disease. Molecular genetic studies also have helped to increase our understanding of the pathogenesis of endocrine tumors. The future cloning and characterization of the gene causing MEN 1 and the correlations of mutations within this gene with the clinical phenotype will further help to elucidate the basis for tumor development in multiple endocrine neoplasia type 1 (MEN 1).

ACKNOWLEDGMENTS: I am grateful to the Medical Research Council (U.K.) for support, to Ms. Joanna Pang (MRC Ph.D. student) for help in the preparation of some of the figures, and to Ms. Lesley Sargeant for typing the manuscript.

REFERENCES

1. Thakker RV, Ponder BAJ: Multiple endocrine neoplasia. *In* Sheppard MC (ed): Clinical Endocrinology and Metabolism, vol 2, no 4: Molec-

ular Biology and Endocrinology. London, Bailliere Tindall, 1988, pp 1031–1067.

2. Underdahl LO, Wootner LB, Black BM: Multiple endocrine adenomas: Report of 8 cases in which parathyroids, pituitary and pancreatic islets were involved. J Clin Endocrinol Metabol 13:20–47, 1953.

3. Berdjis CC: Pluriglandular syndrome: II. Multiple endocrine adenomas in man. A report of five cases and a review of the literature. Oncologia 15:288–311, 1962.

4. Steiner AL, Goodman AD, Powers SR: Study of a kindred with pheochromocytoma, medullary thyroid carcinoma, hyperparathyroidism and Cushing's disease: Multiple endocrine neoplasia, type 2. Medicine 47:371–409, 1968.

5. Wermer P: Multiple endocrine adenomatosis: Multiple hormone-producing tumors, a familial syndrome. Clin Gastroenterol 3:671–684, 1974.

6. Wermer P: Genetic aspects of adenomatosis of endocrine glands. Am J Med 16:363–371, 1954.

7. Sipple JH: The association of pheochromocytoma with carcinoma of the thyroid gland. Am J Med 31:163–166, 1961.

8. Lips CJM, Vaseu HFA, Lamers CBHW: Multiple endocrine neoplasia syndromes. CRC Crit Rev Oncol Hematol 2:117–184, 1984.

9. Schimke RN: Multiple endocrine neoplasia: How many syndromes? Am J Med Genet 37:375–383, 1990.

10. Tateishi R, Wada A, Ishiguro S, et al: Coexistence of bilateral pheochromocytoma and pancreatic islet cell tumor: Report of a case and review of the literature. Cancer 42:2928–2934, 1978.

11. Carney JA, Go VLW, Gordin H, et al: Familial pheochromocytoma and islet cell tumor of the pancreas. Am J Med 68:515–521, 1980.

12. Zeller JR, Kauffman HM, Komorowski RA, Itskovitz HD: Bilateral pheochromocytoma and islet cell adenoma of the pancreas. Arch Surg 117:827–830, 1982.

13. Kahn MR, Mullen DA: Pheochromocytoma without hypertension: Report of a case with acromegaly. JAMA 188:74–75, 1964.

14. Miller GL, Wynn J: Acromegaly, pheochromocytoma, toxic goiter, diabetes mellitus, and endometriosis. Arch Intern Med 127:299–303, 1971.

15. McKusick VA: Mendelian Inheritance in Man. Baltimore, Johns Hopkins University Press, 1988.

16. Erdheim J: Zur normalen und pathologischen histologie der glandular thyreoidea, parathyreoidea und hypophysis. Beitr Pathol Anat Allergy Pathol 33:158–236, 1903.

17. Cushing H, Davidoff LM: The pathological findings in four autopsied cases of acromegaly with a discussion of their significance. Rockefeller Institute of Medicine Research Monograph 22, 1927.

18. Lloyd PC: A case of hypophyseal tumor with associated tumor-like enlargement of the parathyroids and islands of Langerhans. Bull Johns Hopkins Hosp 45:1, 1929.

19. Rossier PH, Dressler M: Familiare erkrankung innersekretorischer Drusen kombiniert mit ulkuskrankheit. Schweiz Med Wochenschr 69:43, 1939.

20. Moldawer MP: Case records of the Massachusetts General Hospital, case 39501. N Engl J Med 249:990–993, 1953.

21. Moldawer MP, Nardi GL, Raker JW: Concomitance of multiple adenomas of the parathyroids and pancreatic islet cells with tumor of the pituitary: A syndrome with familial incidence. Am J Med Sci 228:190–206, 1954.

22. Ballard HS, Frame B, Hartstock C: Familial multiple endocrine adenoma–peptic ulcer complex. Medicine 43:481–515, 1964.

23. Pearse AGE: Common cytochemical and ultra structural characteristics of cells producing polypeptide hormones (the APUD series) and their relevance to thyroid and ultimobranchial C cells and calcitonin. Proc R Soc Lond [Biol] 170:71–80, 1968.

24. Pearse AGE: The cytochemistry and ultra structure of polypeptide hormone-producing cells of the APUD series and the embryologic, physiologic and pathologic implications of the concept. J Histochem Cytochem 17:303–313, 1969.

25. Le Douarin NM: Developmental relationship between the neural crest and the polypeptide-hormone-secreting cells. In The Neural Crest. London, Cambridge University Press, 1982, pp 91–107.

26. Pictet RL, Rall LB, Phelp P, Rutter W: The neural crest cells to the origin of the insulin-producing and other gastrointestinal hormone-producing cells. Science 191:191–192, 1976.

27. Le Douarin NM, Teillet MA: The migration of neural crest and the wall of the digestive tract in amnion embryo. J Embryol Exp Morphol 30:31–48, 1973.

28. Weichert RK III: The neural ectodermal origin of the peptide secreting endocrine glands. Am J Med 49:232–241, 1970.

29. Thakker RV: The molecular genetics of the multiple endocrine neoplasia syndromes. Clin Endocrinol 38:1–14, 1993.

30. Jackson CE, Boonstra CE: The relationship of hereditary hyperparathyroidism to endocrine adenomatosis. Am J Med 43:727–734, 1967.

31. Christensson T: Familial hyperparathyroidism. Ann Intern Med 85:614–615, 1976.

32. Gelston AL, Delisle MB, Patel YC: Multiple endocrine adenomatosis type I occurrence in an octogenarian with high levels of circulating pancreatic polypeptide. JAMA 247:665–666, 1981.

33. Trump D, Farren B, Wooding C, et al: Clinical and biochemical studies of multiple endocrine neoplasia type 1 in 44 families. J Endocrinol 132(S):123, 1992.

34. Shepherd JJ: Latent familial multiple endocrine neoplasia in Tasmania. Med J Aust 142:393–397, 1985.

35. Marx SJ, Vinik AI, Sauten RJ, et al: Multiple endocrine neoplasia type 1: Assessment of laboratory tests to screen for the gene in a large kindred. Medicine 65:226–241, 1986.

36. Benson L, Ljunghall S, Akerstrom G, Oberg K: Hyperparathyroidism presenting as the first lesion in multiple endocrine neoplasia type 1. Am J Med 82:731–737, 1987.

37. Vasen HFA, Lamers CBHW, Lips CJM: Screening for the multiple endocrine neoplasia syndrome type I. Arch Intern Med 149:2717–2722, 1989.

38. Thakker RV, Bouloux P, Wooding C, et al: Association of parathyroid tumors in multiple endocrine neoplasia type 1 with loss of alleles on chromosome 11. N Engl J Med 321:218–224, 1989.

38a. Wilkinson S, Teh BT, Davey KR, et al: Cause of death in multiple endocrine neoplasia type 1. Arch Surg 128:683–690, 1993.

39. Majewski JT, Wilson SD: The MEA-I syndrome: An all or none phenomenon. Surgery 86:474–484, 1979.

40. Eberle F, Grun R: Multiple endocrine neoplasia type I (MEN-I). Ergbeg Inn Med Kinderheilkd 46:76–149, 1981.

41. Marx SJ, Spiegel AM, Levine MA, et al: Familial hypocalciuric hypercalcemia: The relation to primary parathyroid hyperplasia. N Engl J Med 307:416–426, 1982.

42. Croisier JC, Azerod E, Lubetzki J: L'adenomatose polyendocrinienne (syndrome de Wermer). A propos d'une observation personnelle et revue de la literature. Semin Hop Paris 47:494–525, 1971.

43. Lamers CBHW, Froeling PGAM: Clinical significance of hyperparathyroidism in familial multiple endocrine adenomatosis type I (MEAI). Am J Med 66:422–424, 1979.

43a. Kraimps JL, Duh QY, Demeure M, Clark OH: Hyperparathyroidism in multiple endocrine neoplasia syndrome. Surgery 112:1080–1088, 1992.

44. Black WC, Utley JR: The differential diagnosis of parathyroid adenoma and chief cell hyperplasia. Am J Clin Pathol 49:761–765, 1968.

45. Rizzoli R, Green J, Marx SJ: Primary hyperparathyroidism in familial multiple endocrine neoplasia type 1: Long-term follow-up of serum calcium levels after parathyroidectomy. Am J Med 78:467–474, 1985.

46. Wells SA Jr, Farndon JR, Dale JK, et al: Long-term evaluation of patients with primary parathyroid hyperplasia managed by total parathyroidectomy and heterotopic autotransplantation. Ann Surg 192:451–458, 1980.

47. Wells SA Jr, Ellis GJ, Gunnells JC: Parathyroid auto transplantation in primary parathyroid hyperplasia. N Engl J Med 295:57–62, 1976.

48. Saxe AW, Brennan MF: Reoperative parathyroid surgery for primary hyperparathyroidism caused by multiple-gland disease: Total parathyroidectomy and auto transplantation with cryopreserved tissue. Surgery 91:616–621, 1982.

49. Mallette LE, Blevins T, Jordan PH, Noon GP: Autogenous parathyroid grafts for generalised primary hyperplasia: Contrasting outcomes in sporadic versus multiple endocrine neoplasia type I. Surgery 101:738–745, 1987.

49a. Grama D, Skogseid B, Wilander E, et al: Pancreatic tumours in multiple endocrine neoplasia type 1: Clinical presentation and surgical treatment. World J Surg 16:611–619, 1992.

50. Zollinger RM, Ellison EH: Primary peptic ulcerations of the jejunum associated with islet cell tumors of the pancreas. Ann Surg 142:709–728, 1955.

51. Gregory RA, Tracy H, French JM, Sircus W: Extraction of a gastrin-like substance from a pancreatic tumour in a case of Zollinger-Ellison syndrome. Lancet 1:1045–1048, 1960.

52. Gregory RA, Grossman MI, Tracy HJ, Bentley PH: Nature of gastric secretagogue in Zollinger-Ellison tumours. Lancet 2:543–544, 1967.

53. Wolfe MM, Jensen RT: Zollinger-Ellison syndrome: Current concepts in diagnosis and management. N Engl J Med 317:1200–1209, 1987.

54. Betts JB, O'Malley BP, Rosenthal FD: Hyperparathyroidism: A prerequisite for Zollinger-Ellison syndrome in multiple endocrine ade-

nomatosis type 1: A report of a further family and a review of the literature. Q J Med 49:69–76, 1980.

55. Thompson MH, Sanders DJ, Grund ER: The relationship of the serum gastrin and calcium concentrations in patients with multiple endocrine neoplasia type 1. Br J Surg 63:779–783, 1976.

56. Deveney CW, Stein S, Way LW: Cimetidine in the treatment of Zollinger-Ellison syndrome. Am J Surg 146:116–123, 1983.

57. Jensen RT, Collen MJ, McArthur KE: Comparison of the effectiveness of ranitidine and cimetidine in inhibiting acid secretion in patients with gastric hypersecretory states. Am J Med 77:90–105, 1984.

58. McArthur KE, Collen MJ, Maton PN: Omeprazole: Effective convenient therapy for Zollinger-Ellison syndrome. Gastroenterology 88:939–944, 1985.

59. Pipeleers-Marichal M, Somers G, Willems G, et al: Gastrinomas in the duodenums of patients with multiple endocrine neoplasia type 1 and the Zollinger-Ellison syndrome. N Engl J Med 322:723–727, 1990.

60. Delcore R, Hermreck AS, Friesen SR: Selective surgical management of correctable hypergastrinemia. Surgery 106:1094–1102, 1989.

61. Sheppard BC, Norton JA, Dopmann JL, et al: Management of islet cell tumors in patients with multiple endocrine neoplasia: A prospective study. Surgery 106:1108–1118, 1989.

61a. Ruszniewski P, Podevin P, Cadiot G, et al: Clinical, anatomical, and evolutive features of patients with the Zollinger-Ellison syndrome combined with type I multiple endocrine neoplasia. Pancreas 8:295–304, 1993.

62. Thompson NW, Bondeson AG, Bondeson L, Vinik A: The surgical treatment of gastrinoma in MEN 1 syndrome patients. Surgery 106:1081–1086, 1989.

63. Wise SR, Johnson J, Sparks J, et al: Gastrinoma: The predictive value of preoperative localization. Surgery 106:1087–1093, 1989.

64. Moertel CG, Hanley JA, Johnson LA: Streptozocin alone compared with streptozocin plus fluorouracil in the treatment of advanced islet cell carcinoma. N Engl J Med 303:1189–1194, 1980.

65. Kvols LIC, Buck M, Moertel CG: Treatment of metastatic islet cell carcinoma with somatostatin analogue (SMS 201–995). Ann Intern Med 107:162–168, 1987.

66. Carrasco CH, Chuang VP, Wallace S: Apudoma metastatic to the liver: Treatment of hepatic artery embolization. Radiology 149:79–83, 1983.

67. Erickson B, Oberg K, Alun G: Treatment of malignant endocrine pancreatic tumours with human leucocyte interferon. Lancet 2:1307–1309, 1986.

68. Norton JA, Collen MJ, Gardner JD: Prospective study of gastrinoma localization and resection in patients with Zollinger-Ellison syndrome. Ann Surg 204:468–479, 1986.

69. Croisier JC, Lehy T, Zeitoun P: A₂ cell pancreatic microadenomas in a case of multiple endocrine adenomatosis. Cancer 28:707–713, 1971.

70. Peurifoy JT, Gomez LG, Thompson JC: Separate pancreatic gastrin cell and beta-cell adenomas: Report of a patient with multiple endocrine adenomatosis type 1. Arch Surg 114:956–958, 1979.

71. Daggett PR, Goodburn EA, Kurtz AB, et al: Is pre-operative localisation of insulinomas necessary? Lancet 1:483–486, 1981.

71a. Demeure MJ, Klonoff DC, Karam JH, et al: Insulinomas associated with multiple endocrine neoplasia type I: The need for a different surgical approach. Surgery 110:998–1005, 1991.

72. Broder LE, Carter SK: Chemotherapy of malignant insulinomas with streptozotocin. In Proceedings of the 8th International Congress on Diabetes, Excerpta Medica International Congress Series 314. Amsterdam, Excerpta Medica, 1974, pp 714–727.

73. Croughs RJM, Hulsmans HAM, Israel DE, et al: Glucagonoma as part of the polyglandular adenoma syndrome. Am J Med 52:690–698, 1972.

74. Tiengo A, Fedek D, Marchiori E, et al: Suppression and stimulation mechanism controlling glucagon secretion in a case of islet cell tumor producing glucagon, insulin and gastrin. Diabetes 25:408–412, 1976.

75. Leclerc J, Vican F, Laurent J, et al: Tumeur insulaire avec diarrhee et diabete (glucagonoma) associee a un hyperparathyroidism-resultat eloingne du traitement par l. streptozotocine loco-regionale. Ann Endocrinol (Paris) 38:153–154, 1977.

76. Stacpoole PW, Jaspan J, Kasselberg AG, et al: A familial glucagonoma syndrome: Genetic, clinical and biochemical features. Am J Med 70:1017–1026, 1981.

77. Strauss GM, Weitzman SA, Aoki THT: Dimethyltriazenoimidazole carboxamide therapy of malignant glucagonoma. Ann Intern Med 90:57–58, 1979.

78. Marynick SP, Fagadan WR, Duncan LA: Malignant glucagonoma syndrome: Response to chemotherapy. Ann Intern Med 93:453–454, 1980.

79. Verner JV, Morrison AB: Islet cell tumor and a syndrome of refractory water diarrhea and hypokalemia. Am J Med 25:374–380, 1958.

80. Marks IN, Bank S, Louw JH: Islet cell tumor of the pancreas with reversible watery diarrhea and achlorhydria. Gastroenterology 52:695–708, 1967.

81. Bloom SR, Polak JM, Pearse AGE: Vasoactive intestinal peptide and watery diarrhea syndrome. Lancet 2:14–16, 1973.

82. Brown CH, Crile G Jr: Pancreatic adenoma with intractable diarrhea, hypokalemia and hypercalcemia. JAMA 190:30–34, 1964.

83. Burkhardt A: Das Verner-Morrison Zyndrome. Klin Pathol Anat. Klin Wochenschr 54:1–11, 1976.

84. Long RG, Bryant MG, Mitchell SJ, et al: Clinicopathological study of pancreatic and ganglioneuroblastoma tumour secreting vasoactive intestinal polypeptide (VIPoma). Lancet 2:764–767, 1979.

85. Kahn CR, Levy AG, Gardner JD, et al: Pancreatic cholera: Beneficial effects of treatment with streptozotocin. N Engl J Med 292:941–945, 1975.

86. Kingham JGC, Dick R, Bloom SR, Frankel RJ: VIPoma: Localization of percutaneous transhepatic portal venous sampling. Br Med J 2:1682–1683, 1978.

87. Jaffe BM, Kopen DF, de Schrijver-Kecskcemeti K, et al: Indomethacin-responsive pancreatic cholera. N Engl J Med 297:817–821, 1977.

88. Long RG, Bryant MG, Yuille PM, et al: Mixed pancreatic APUDoma with symptoms of excess vasoactive intestinal polypeptide and insulin: improvement of diarrhea with metoclopramide. Gut 22:505–511, 1981.

89. Pandol SJ, Korman LY, McCarthy DM, Gardiner JD: Beneficial effect of oral lithium carbonate in the treatment of pancreatic cholera syndrome. N Engl J Med 302:1403–1404, 1980.

90. Friesen SR, Kimmel JR, Tomita T: Pancreatic polypeptide as screening marker for pancreatic polypeptide apudomas in multiple endocrinopathies. Am J Surg 139:61–72, 1980.

91. Lamers CBHW, Diemel CM: Basal and postatropine serum pancreatic polypeptide concentrations in familial multiple endocrine neoplasia type I. J Clin Endocrinol Metab 5:774–778, 1982.

92. Skogseid B, Oberg K, Benson L, et al: A standardized meal stimulation test of the endocrine pancreas for early detection of pancreatic endocrine tumors in multiple endocrine neoplasia type 1 syndrome: Five years experience. J Clin Endocrinol Metab 64:1233–1240, 1987.

93. Bloom SR, Polak JM, West AM: Somatostatin content of pancreatic endocrine tumors. Metabolism 27:1235–1238, 1978.

94. Guillemin R: Some thoughts on current research with somatostatin. Metabolism 27:1453–1461, 1978.

95. Lundbeck K: Somatostatin: Clinical importance and outlook. Metabolism 27:1463–1469, 1978.

96. Krejs GJ, Orci L, Conlon JM, et al: Somatostatinoma syndrome. N Engl J Med 301:285–292, 1979.

97. Prosser PR, Karom JH, Townsend JJ, Forsham PH: Prolactin-secreting pituitary adenomas in multiple endocrine adenomatosis type 1. Ann Intern Med 91:41–44, 1979.

98. Farid NR, Buchler S, Russell NA, et al: Prolactinomas in familial multiple endocrine neoplasia syndrome type I: Relationship to HLA and carcinoid tumors. Am J Med 69:874–880, 1980.

99. Maton PN, Gardner JD, Jensen RT: Cushing's syndrome in patients with the Zollinger-Ellison syndrome. N Engl J Med 325:1–5, 1986.

100. Duh QY, Hybarger CD, Geist R, et al: Carcinoids associated with multiple endocrine neoplasia syndromes. Am J Surg 154:142–148, 1987.

101. Williams ED, Celestin LR: The association of bronchial carcinoid and pluriglandular adenomatosis. Thorax 17:120–127, 1962.

102. Fisher ER, Hicks J: Further pathologic observations on the syndrome of peptic ulcer and multiple endocrine tumors. Gastroenterology 38:458–466, 1960.

103. Snyder N III, Murphy TS, Deiss WP: Five families with multiple endocrine adenomatosis. Ann Intern Med 76:53–58, 1972.

104. Rode J, Dhillon AP, Cotton PB, et al: Carcinoid tumor of stomach and primary hyperparathyroidism: A new association. J Clin Pathol 40:546–551, 1987.

104a. Cadiot G, Laurent-Puig P, Thuille B, et al: Is the multiple endocrine neoplasia type I gene a suppressor for fundic argyrophil tumors in the Zollinger-Ellison syndrome? Gastroenterology 105:579–582, 1993.

105. Lee CH, Ching KN, Lui WY, et al: Carcinoid tumor of the pancreas causing the diarrheogenic syndrome: Report of a case combined with multiple endocrine neoplasia type 1. Surgery 99:123–129, 1980.

106. Skogseid B, Larsson C, Lindgren P-G, et al: Clinical and genetic features of adrenocortical lesions in multiple endocrine neoplasia type 1. J Clin Endocrinol Metab 75:76–81, 1992.

107. Raker JW, Henneman PH, Graf WS: Co-existing primary hyperparathyroidism and Cushing's syndrome. J Clin Endocrinol Metab 22:273–280, 1962.

108. Dluhy RG, Williams GH: Primary aldosteronism in a hypertensive acromegalic patient. J Clin Endocrinol 29:1319–1324, 1969.

109. Fertig A, Welsley M, Lynn JA: Primary hyperparathyroidism in a patient with Conn's syndrome. Postgrad Med J 56:45–47, 1980.

110. Sinclair AH, Berta P, Palmer MS, et al: A gene from the human sex-determining region encodes a protein with homology to a conserved DNA-binding motif. Nature 346:240–244, 1990.

111. Gubbay J, Collignon J, Koopman P, et al: A gene mapping to the sex-determining region of the mouse Y chromosome is a member of a novel family of embryonically expressed genes. Nature 346:245–250, 1990.

112. Koopman P, Gubbay J, Vivian N, et al: Male development of chromosomally female mice transgenic for Sry. Nature 351:117–121, 1991.

113. Franco B, Guioli S, Pragliola A, et al: A gene deleted in Kallmann's syndrome shares homology with neural cell adhesion and axonal path-finding molecules. Nature 353:529–536, 1991.

114. Legouis R, Hardelin JP, Levilliers J, et al: The candidate gene for the X-linked Kallman syndrome encodes a protein related to adhesion molecules. Cell 67:423–435, 1991.

115. Hilbert P, Lindpainter K, Beckmann JS, et al: Chromosomal mapping of two genetic loci associated with blood-pressure regulation in hereditary hypertensive rats. Nature 353:521–529, 1991.

116. Todd JA, Aitman TJ, Cornall RJ, et al: Genetic analysis of autoimmune type 1 diabetes mellitus in mice. Nature 351:542–547, 1991.

117. Cornall RJ, Prins J-B, Todd JA, et al: Type 1 diabetes in mice is linked to the interleukin-1 receptor and Lsh/Ity/Bcg genes on chromosome 1. Nature 353:262–265, 1991.

118. Julier C, Hyer RN, Davies J, et al: Insulin-IGF2 region on chromosome 11p encodes a gene implicated in HLA-DR4–dependent diabetes susceptibility. Nature 354:155–159, 1991.

119. Froguel Ph, Vaxillaire M, Sun F, et al: Close linkage of glucokinase locus on chromosome 7p to early-onset non-insulin-dependent diabetes mellitus. Nature 356:162–164, 1992.

120. Ruddle FH: The William Allan Memorial Award Address: Reverse genetics and beyond. Am J Hum Genet 36:944–953, 1984.

121. Collins FS: Positional cloning: Let's not call it reverse any more. Nature Genet 1:3–6, 1992.

122. Thakker RV, O'Riordan JLH: Inherited forms of rickets and osteomalacia. In Martin TJ (ed): Clinical Endocrinology and Metabolism, vol 2, no 1: Metabolic Bone Disease. London, Bailliere Tindall, 1988, pp 157–191.

123. Thakker RV, Davies KE, Whyte MP, et al: Mapping the gene causing X-linked recessive idiopathic hypoparathyroidism to Xq26-Xq27 by linkage studies. J Clin Invest 86:40–45, 1990.

124. Varmus HE: The molecular genetics of cellular oncogenes. Annu Rev Genet 18:533–612, 1984.

125. Friend SH, Dryja TP, Weinberg RA: Oncogenes and tumor-suppressor genes. N Engl J Med 318:618–622, 1988.

126. Ponder B: Gene losses in human tumours. Nature 335:400–402, 1988.

127. de Klein A, van Kessel AG, Grosveld G: A cellular oncogene is translocated to the Philadelphia chromosome in chronic myelocytic leukemia. Nature 300:765–767, 1982.

128. Dalla-Favera R, Bregni M, Erikson J, et al: Human c-myc oncogene is located on the region of chromosome 8 that is translocated in Burkitt lymphoma cells. Proc Natl Acad Sci USA 79:7824–7827, 1982.

129. Kurzrock R, Gutterman JN, Talpaz M: The molecular genetics of Philadelphia chromosome–positive leukemias. N Engl J Med 319:990–998, 1988.

130. Taub R, Kirsch I, Morton C: Translocation of the c-myc gene into the immunoglobulin heavy chain locus in human Burkitt lymphoma and murine plasmacytoma cells. Proc Natl Acad Sci USA 79:7837–7841, 1982.

131. Hansen MF, Cavanee WK: Retinoblastoma and the progression of tumor genetics. Trend Genet 4:125–128, 1988.

132. Knudson AG: Mutation and cancer: Statistical study of retinoblastoma. Proc Natl Acad Sci USA 68:820–823, 1971.

133. Knudson AG, Strong LC, Anderson DE: Heredity and cancer in man. Prog Med Genet 9:113–158, 1973.

134. Cavenee WK, Murphree AL, Shull MM: Prediction of familial predisposition to retinoblastoma. N Engl J Med 314:1201–1207, 1986.

135. Friend SH, Bernards R, Rogelj S, et al: A human DNA segment with properties of the gene that predisposes to retinoblastoma and osteosarcoma. Nature 323:643–646, 1986.

136. Little PFR, Annison G, Darling S, et al: Model for antenatal diagnosis of B thalassemia and other monogenic disorders by molecular analysis of linked DNA polymorphisms. Nature 285:144–147, 1980.

137. Orkin SH: The use of cloned DNA fragments to study human disease. Genet Eng 3:189–206, 1981.

138. Cooper DN, Schmidtke J: DNA restriction fragment length polymorphisms and heterozygosity in the human genome. Hum Genet 66:1–16, 1984.

139. Southern EM: Detection of specific sequences among DNA fragments separated by gel electrophoresis. J Mol Biol 98:503–517, 1975.

140. Dryja TP, Rapaport JM, Joyce JM, Petersen RA: Molecular detection of deletions involving band q14 of chromosome 13 in retinoblastomas. Proc Natl Acad Sci USA 83:7391–7394, 1986.

141. Solomon E, Voss R, Hall V: Chromosome 5 allele loss in human colorectal carcinomas. Nature 328:616–619, 1987.

142. Stanbridge EJ: Identifying tumor suppressor genes in human colorectal cancer. Science 247:12–13, 1990.

143. Fearon ER, Vogelstein B, Feinberg A: Somatic deletion and duplication of genes on chromosome 11 in Wilms' tumor. Nature 309:176–178, 1984.

144. Koufos A, Hansen MF, Lampkin BC, et al: Loss of alleles at loci on human chromosome 11 during genesis of Wilms' tumor. Nature 309:170–172, 1984.

145. Larsson C, Skogseid B, Oberg K, et al: Multiple endocrine neoplasia type I gene maps to chromosome 11 and is lost in insulinoma. Nature 332:85–87, 1988.

146. Friedman E, Sakaguchi K, Bale AE, et al: Clonality of parathyroid tumors in familial multiple endocrine neoplasia type 1. N Engl J Med 321:213–218, 1989.

147. Mathew CGP, Smith BA, Thorpe K, et al: Deletion of genes on chromosome 1 in endocrine neoplasia. Nature 328:524–526, 1987.

148. Mathew CGP, Chin KS, Easton DF, et al: A linked genetic marker for multiple endocrine neoplasia type 2A on chromosome 10. Nature 328:527–528, 1987.

149. Simpson NE, Kidd KK, Goodfellow PJ: Assignment of multiple endocrine neoplasia type 2a on chromosome 10 by linkage. Nature 328:528–530, 1987.

150. White R, Leppert M, Bishop DT, et al: Construction of linkage maps with DNA markers for human chromosomes. Nature 313:101–105, 1985.

151. Morton NE: Sequential tests for the detection of linkage. Am J Hum Genet 7:277–318, 1955.

152. Ott J: Estimation of the recombination fraction in human pedigrees: Efficient computation of the likelihood for human linkage studies. Am J Hum Genet 26:588–597, 1974.

153. Bear JC, Briones-Urbina R, Fahey JF, Farrid NR: Variant multiple endocrine neoplasia (MEN I Burin): Further studies and non-linkage of HLA. Hum Hered 351:15–20, 1985.

154. Bale SJ, Marx SJ, Langfield D, et al: Multiple endocrine neoplasia type 1 (MEN I): Genetic linkage studies. Cytogenet Cell Genet 46:575, 1987.

155. Jackson CE, van Dyke DL, Babu VR, Wurzel JM: Relationship between multiple endocrine neoplasia type 1 and type 2: Cytogenetic findings (abstract). In Program of the 68th Annual Meeting of the Endocrine Society, 1986, p 252.

156. Bale SJ, Bale AE, Stewart K, et al: Linkage analysis of multiple endocrine neoplasia type 1 with INT2 and other markers on chromosome 11. Genomics 4:320–322, 1989.

157. Bystrom C, Larsson C, Blomberg C, et al: Localization of the MEN 1 gene to a small region within chromosome 11q13 by deletion mapping in tumors. Proc Natl Acad Sci USA 87:1968–1972, 1990.

158. Thakker RV, Wooding C, Boscaro M, et al: Chromosome 11 abnormalities in somatotrophinomas from patients with acromegaly. Human gene mapping 11. Cytogenet Cell Genet 58:1971, 1991.

158a. Thakker RV, Pook MA, Wooding C, et al: Association of somatotrophinomas with loss of alleles on chromosome 11 and with gsp mutations. J Clin Invest 91:2815–2821, 1993.

159. Thakker RV, Bouloux P, Wooding C, et al: The molecular basis of parathyroid tumours in multiple endocrine neoplasia type 1. In Cohn DV, Glorieux FH, Martin TJ (eds): Calcium Regulation and Bone Metabolism, vol 10. London, Elsevier Science Publishers, 1990, pp 118–124.

160. Friedman E, Bale AE, Marx SJ, et al: Genetic abnormalities in sporadic parathyroid adenomas. J Clin Endocrinol Metab 71:293–297, 1990.

161. Bale AE, Norton JA, Wong EL, et al: Allelic loss on chromosome 11 in hereditary and sporadic tumors related to familial multiple endocrine neoplasia type 1. Cancer Res 51:1154–1157, 1991.
162. Sawicki MP, Wan Y-JY, Johnson CL, et al: Loss of heterozygosity on chromosome 11 in sporadic gastrinomas. Hum Genet 89:445–449, 1992.
163. Nakamura Y, Larsson C, Julier C, et al: Localization of the genetic defect in multiple endocrine neoplasia type 1 within a small region of chromosome 11. Am J Hum Genet 44:751–755, 1989.
164. Larsson C, Shepherd J, Nakamura Y, et al: Predictive testing for multiple endocrine neoplasia type 1 using DNA polymorphisms. J Clin Invest 89:1344–1349, 1992.
165. Thakker RV, Wooding C, Pang J, et al: Linkage analysis in 27 families with multiple endocrine neoplasia type 1 (MEN 1). Ann Hum Genet 57:17–25, 1993.
166. Julier C, Nakamura Y, Lathrop M, et al: A detailed genetic map of the long arm of chromosome 11. Genomics 7:335–345, 1990.
166a. Pang JT, Wooding C, Leigh SEA, et al: Molecular genetic mapping of 13 markers from chromosome 11q13 in 33 families with multiple endocrine neoplasia type I. J Bone Miner Res 8:5136, 1993.
167. Janson M, Larsson C, Werelius B, et al: Detailed physical map of human chromosomal region 11q12–13 shows high meiotic recombination rate around the MEN 1 locus. Proc Natl Acad Sci USA 88:10609–10613, 1991.
168. Weber JL, May PE: Abundant class of human DNA polymorphisms which can be typed using the polymerase chain reaction. Am J Hum Genet 44:388–396, 1989.
169. Litt M, Luty JA: A hypervariable microsatellite revealed by in vitro amplification of a dinucleotide repeat within the cardiac muscle actin gene. Am J Hum Genet 44:397–401, 1989.
170. Parkinson DB, Shaw NJ, Himsworth RL, Thakker RV: Parathyroid hormone gene analysis in autosomal hypoparathyroidism using an intragenic tetranucleotide $(AAAT)_n$ polymorphism. Hum Genet 91:281–284, 1993.
171. Eubanks JH, Selleri L, Hart R, et al: Isolation, localization and physical mapping of a highly polymorphic locus on human chromosome 11q13. Genomics 11:720–729, 1991.
172. Pang JT, Pook MA, Eubanks JH, et al: Molecular genetic mapping of the multiple endocrine neoplasia type 1 (MEN 1) locus. Henry Ford Hosp Med J 40:162–166, 1992.
173. Economou EP, Bergan AW, Warren AC, Antonarakis SE: The polydeoxyadenylate tract of Alu repetitive elements is polymorphic in the human genome. Proc Natl Acad Sci USA 87:2951–2954, 1990.
174. Iwasaki H, Stewart PW, Dilley WG, et al: A minisatellite and a microsatellite polymorphism within 1.5 kb at the human muscle glycogen phosphorylase (PYGM) locus can be amplified by PCR and have combined informativeness of PIC 0.95. Genomics 13:7–15, 1992.
175. Litt, M. PCR of TG microsatellites. In McPherson MJ, Quirke P, Taylor GR (eds): PCR: A Practical Approach. Oxford, IRL Press, 1991, pp 85–99.
176. Skogseid B, Eriksson B, Lundqvist G, et al: Multiple endocrine neoplasia type 1: A 10-year prospective screening study in four kindreds. J Clin Endocrinol Metab 73:281–287, 1991.
177. Anderson DE: Genetic varieties of neoplasia. In Genetic Concepts and Neoplasia. Baltimore, Williams & Wilkins, 1970, pp 85–109.
177a. Trump D, Farren B, Wooding C, Thakker RV, et al: Clinical and biochemical studies of multiple endocrine neoplasia type I in 220 patients. J Endocrinol 137(S): OC12, 1993.
178. Naylor SL, Sakaguchi AY, Szoka P, et al: Human parathyroid hormone gene (PTH) is on the short arm of chromosome 11. Somat Cell Genet 9:609–616, 1983.
179. Vasicek TJ, McDeviff BE, Freeman MW, et al: Nucleotide sequences of the human parathyroid hormone gene. Proc Natl Acad Sci USA 80:2127–2131, 1983.
180. Parkinson DB, Thakker RV: A donor slice site mutation in the parathyroid hormone gene is associated with autosomal recessive hypoparathyroidism. Nature Genet 1:149–152, 1992.
181. Arnold A, Staunton CE, Kim HG, et al: Monoclonality and abnormal parathyroid hormone genes in parathyroid adenomas. N Engl J Med 318:658–662, 1988.
182. Arnold A, Kim HG, Gaz RD, et al: Molecular cloning and chromosomal mapping of DNA rearranged with the parathyroid hormone gene in a parathyroid adenoma. J Clin Invest 83:2034–2040, 1989.
183. Bale AE, Wong E, Arnold A: The parathyroid breakpoint locus on 11q13 maps close to BCL1 and is not a candidate gene for MEN 1. Am J Hum Genet 47:A3, 1990.
184. Rosenberg CL, Kim HG, Shows TB, et al: Rearrangement and overexpression of D11S287E, a candidate oncogene on chromosome 11q13 in benign parathyroid tumors. Oncogene 6:449–453, 1991.
185. Motokura T, Bloom T, Kim HG, et al: A novel cyclin encoded by a bcl1-linked candidate oncogene. Nature 350:512–515, 1991.
186. Hunt T: Cell cycle gets more cyclins. Nature 350:462–463, 1991.
187. Rosenberg CL, Wong E, Petty EM, et al: PRAD1, a candidate BCL1 oncogene: Mapping and expression in centrocytic lymphoma. Proc Natl Acad Sci USA 88:9638–9642, 1991.
188. Simon MI, Strathmann MP, Gautam N: Diversity of G proteins in signal transduction. Science 252:802–808, 1991.
189. Landis CA, Masters SB, Spada A, et al: GTPase inhibiting mutations activate the chain of Gs and stimulate adenyl cyclase in human pituitary tumours. Nature 340:692–696, 1989.
190. Lyons J, Landis CA, Harsh G, et al: Two G protein oncogenes in human endocrine tumors. Science 249:655–659, 1990.
191. Billestrup N, Swanson LW, Vale W: Growth hormone–releasing factor stimulates proliferation of somatotrophs in vitro. Proc Natl Acad Sci USA 83:6854–6857, 1986.
192. Vallar L, Spada A, Giannattasio G: Altered GS and adenylate cyclase activity in human GH-secreting pituitary adenomas. Nature 330:566–568, 1987.
193. Blatt C, Eversole-Cire P, Cohn VH, et al: Chromosomal localization of genes encoding guanine nucleotide-binding protein subunits in mouse and human. Proc Natl Acad Sci USA 85:7642–7646, 1988.
194. Clementi E, Malgaretti N, Meldolesi J, Taramelli R: A new constitutively activating mutation of the Gs protein α subunit-gsp oncogene is found in human pituitary tumors. Oncogene 5:1059–1061, 1990.
195. Kozasa T, Ito H, Tsukamoto T, Kaziro Y: Isolation and characterization of the human $G_s\alpha$ gene. Proc Natl Acad Sci USA 85:2081–2085, 1988.
196. Brandi ML, Aurbach GD, Fitzpatrick LA: Parathyroid mitogenic activity in plasma from patients with familial multiple endocrine neoplasia type I. N Engl J Med 314:1287–1293, 1986.
197. Zimering MB, Brandi ML, DeGrange DA, et al: Circulating fibroblast growth factor-like substance in familial multiple endocrine neoplasia type 1. J Clin Endocrinol Metab 70:149–154, 1990.
198. Marx SJ, Sakaguchi K, Green J III, et al: Mitogenic activity on parathyroid cells in plasma from members of a large kindred with multiple endocrine neoplasia type 1. J Clin Endocrinol Metab 67:149–153, 1988.
198a. Zimering MB, Katsumata N, Sato Y, et al: Increased basic fibroblast growth factor in plasma from multiple endocrine neoplasia type I: Relation to pituitary tumor. J Clin Endocrinol Metab 76:1182–1187, 1993.
199. Carlson HE, Lamberts SWJ, Brickman AS, et al: Hypercalcemia in rats bearing growth hormone and prolactin secreting transplantable pituitary tumors. Endocrinology 117:1602–1607, 1985.
200. Spanos E, Colston KW, Evans IMS, et al: Effect of prolactin on vitamin D metabolism. Mol Cell Endocrinol 5:163–167, 1976.
201. Spanos E, Barrett D, MacIntyre I, et al: Effect of growth hormone on vitamin D metabolism. Nature 273:246–247, 1978.
202. Jaenisch R, Mintz B: Simian virus 40 DNA sequences in DNA of healthy adult mice derived from preimplantation blastocysts injected with viral DNA. Proc Natl Acad Sci USA 71:1250–1254, 1974.
203. Jaenisch R: Transgenic animals. Science 240:1468–1474, 1988.
204. Hanahan D: Heritable formation of pancreatic B cell tumors in transgenic mice expressing recombinant insulin/simian virus 40 oncogenes. Nature 315:115–122, 1985.
205. Murphy D, Bishop A, Rindi G, et al: Mice transgenic for a vasopressin-SV40 hybrid oncogene develop tumors of the endocrine pancreas and the anterior pituitary. Am J Pathol 129:552–566, 1987.

MULTIPLE ENDOCRINE NEOPLASIA TYPE 2

ROBERT F. GAGEL

DEFINITIONS

Multiple endocrine neoplasia type 2A (MEN 2A) is an autosomal dominant genetic syndrome which includes medullary thyroid carcinoma (MTC), pheochromocytoma, and hyperparathyroidism. *Multiple endocrine neoplasia type 2B* (MEN 2B) is an autosomal dominant genetic syndrome which includes medullary thyroid carcinoma, pheochromocytoma, multiple mucosal neuromas, and a marfanoid habitus. *Familial medullary thyroid carcinoma only syndrome* (FMTC) refers to a variant of MEN 2A in which MTC is the only clinical manifestation. The *MEN 2 locus* refers to the genetic locus on chromosome 10 for the predisposing gene(s).

HISTORICAL PERSPECTIVE

It was a chance autopsy observation by John Sipple in 1961 that led to the association of thyroid carcinoma and pheochromocytoma.[1] It was left to others to define the nature of the thyroid tumor (medullary thyroid carcinoma, or MTC),[2, 3] its derivation from the parafollicular C cell,[4, 5] and the nature of the hereditary syndrome and to separate this polyglandular syndrome from the other major hereditary tumor syndrome, multiple endocrine neoplasia type 1[6] (see earlier part of this chapter). During this *descriptive phase,* the clinical features of bilateral and multicentric medullary thyroid carcinoma, bilateral pheochromocytomas, and hyperparathyroidism (MEN 2A) were first delineated.[7–9] It was also during this period that the association of MTC, pheochromocytoma, and multiple mucosal neuromas (multiple endocrine neoplasia type 2B, or MEN 2B) was first delineated and differentiated from MEN 2A.[10, 11]

The isolation and characterization of the hypocalcemic peptide calcitonin and the realization that it was produced in large quantities by MTC introduced a second period in our understanding of this clinical syndrome, the *prospective screening phase.* The realization that provocative tests for calcitonin release and measurement of serum or urine catecholamines could be utilized to identify gene carriers early in the course of the clinical syndrome laid the groundwork for identification of hyperplasia of C cells or adrenal medulla as precursor lesions[12–14] and the prevention of death from metastatic MTC or pheochromocytoma.

The resurrection of genetic linkage techniques in the early 1980's and their application to MEN 2 led to mapping of a MEN 2 locus on chromosome 10 in 1987[15, 16] and the beginning of the current *genetic phase.* Over the past 5 years, all four variants of MEN 2 have been mapped to this locus, and a series of tightly linked polymorphic sequences has been identified. The use of these DNA sequences for genetic diagnosis of MEN 2 has quietly transformed the management of kindreds with this disorder. Efforts continue to identify and clone the MEN 2 predisposition gene.[17] The recent identification of point mutations of the RET protooncogene in MEN 2A and 2B will further affect diagnosis and management of this disorder.

INCIDENCE AND DISTRIBUTION

The MEN 2–related syndromes are uncommon. There are probably fewer than 10,000 affected individuals worldwide. Multiple affected families have been reported in North and South America, Australia, Europe, and South Africa, most thought to be transmitted by colonists from European countries. There are few reports of MEN 2 in Asia, except for Japan, where many families exist.[18] There is little information about the incidence in native Africans, although there are affected black families in the United States. The earliest deduced case of this disease occurred in approximately 1730.[19] The importance of these syndromes lies in their fascinating clinical presentations and their potential for unraveling molecular events leading to endocrine neoplasia.

PATHOPHYSIOLOGY

The parafollicular or calcitonin-producing cells (C cells) are dispersed within the parenchyma of the thyroid gland. This neuroendocrine cell migrates from the neural crest in early embryonic life to a position adjacent to the thyroid follicle. There is a characteristic distribution of C cells within the thyroid gland, with the greatest concentration of C cells located at the juncture of the upper one-third and lower two-thirds of each lobe of the thyroid gland along a hypothetical superior to inferior central axis (Fig. 151–9). This seemingly minor point may be of importance in the histological identification of early foci of abnormal C cells, which may be missed unless the gland is carefully sectioned and particular attention focused on this region. The histological definition of a normal C cell population has been difficult, in part because of the variation in the C cell population within the thyroid gland and the belief that there may be several genetic or pathophysiological determinants of C cell number. For example, increased numbers of C cells have been identified in such diverse conditions as autoimmune thyroiditis[20, 21] and hyperparathyroidism.[22]

The adrenal chromaffin cell is thought to migrate from the neural crest tissue,[23] although this point has not been established so clearly as for the C cell. These cells express the enzyme norepinephrine N-methyltransferase and are capable of converting norepinephrine to epinephrine, a point of some importance for diagnosis of pheochromocytoma in MEN 2. Differentiation of chromaffin cells is thought to be directed by several growth factors, including nerve growth factor.[24] The exact molecular defect leading to diffuse expansion of the adrenal medulla in MEN 2 is unknown.

The primary event in the development of neoplasia is a clonal expansion of the C, adrenal medullary, and parathyroid cell populations. The exact molecular events leading to hyperplasia are not known, but point mutations of the RET protooncogene are thought to be causative. One hypothesis is that mutation of this gene results in C cell hyperplasia and that other mutational events are required for transformation and tumor progression.

The normal C cell synthesizes and secretes calcitonin, a peptide hormone which is important for regulation of osteoclast function (see Ch. 58). Hyperplasia of the C cells is associated with an increased production and release of calcitonin and a change in the pattern of differential RNA processing, resulting in production of the alternative product, calcitonin gene–related peptide[25] (reviewed in Ch. 58). It is not known whether the increased calcitonin production results exclusively from the increased cell number or is related to an increased expression of the cell-specific transcription factor, a member of the helix-loop-helix family of transcription factors.[26, 27] Measurement of the serum calcitonin basally and after a provocative test has been used to detect C cell hyperplasia. Carcinoembryonic antigen (CEA) is normally produced by the C cell[28] and by medullary thyroid carcinoma[29]; the serum concentration of CEA correlates roughly with tumor mass and provides an independent method for monitoring the mass of MTC. Chromogranin A[30] and somatostatin[31, 32] are two other peptides produced frequently by the normal C cell and by MTC. Neither is specific for MTC, and therefore these two peptides have not been used extensively to diagnose or follow patients with MTC.

THE CLINICAL SYNDROMES

Multiple Endocrine Neoplasia Type 2A

Multiple endocrine neoplasia type 2A is the association of medullary thyroid carcinoma, pheochromocytoma, and hyperparathyroidism inherited as an autosomal dominant trait. The presenting features in the fully developed form of this syndrome include the presence of bilateral thyroid masses, clinical manifestations of pheochromocytoma, and less commonly, hyperparathyroidism. Other clinical features which occur include diarrhea, renal stones, and sudden death related to elevated levels of catecholamines.

Medullary Thyroid Carcinoma

Medullary thyroid carcinoma (MTC) is generally bilateral and multicentric and is set on a background of generalized hyperplasia of the C cells. Most commonly the tumor appears as a chalky-white lesion within the upper portion of each lobe of the thyroid gland (Fig. 151–9). The tumors are frequently multifocal, a finding which is thought to represent expansion of individual clones of cells rather than intrathyroidal metastasis[33] (Fig. 151–10).

The onset of prospective screening with provocative calcium or pentagastrin tests in the early 1970's led to the identification of C cell hyperplasia as a precursor lesion for MTC.[34] The progression from normal through hyperplasia, nodular hyperplasia, and microscopic and macroscopic carcinoma appears to occur over a number of years. Little is known about the age of initiation of clonal expansion, although C cell hyperplasia has been observed in gene

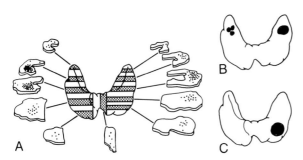

FIGURE 151–9. Distribution of C cells in the thyroid gland. *A*, A reconstruction of the distribution of C cells in the thyroid gland. (Adapted from Wolfe HJ, Voelkel EF, Tashjian AH Jr: Distribution of calcitonin containing cells in the normal adult human thyroid gland: A correlation of morphology with peptide content. J Clin Endocrinol Metab 38:688–694, 1974.) The greatest concentration of C cells occurs at the junction of the upper one-half and lower two-thirds of the gland. This distribution explains the characteristic location of hereditary medullary thyroid carcinoma. *B*, Hereditary medullary thyroid carcinoma is almost always bilateral, although the extent of involvement may not be equal. *C*, Sporadic medullary thyroid carcinoma is most commonly a unilateral process that may develop at any location within the thyroid gland. (*B* and *C* reprinted with permission from Grauer A, Raue F, Gagel RF: Changing concepts in the management of hereditary and sporadic medullary thyroid carcinoma. Endocrinol Metab Clin North Am 19:613–635, 1990.)

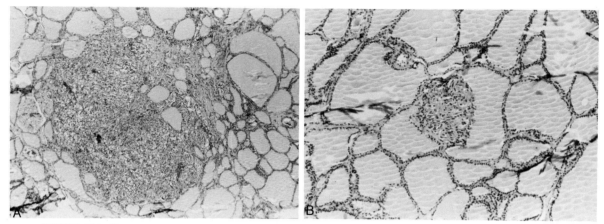

FIGURE 151–10. Histological features of hereditary medullary thyroid carcinoma. *A*, Nodular C cell hyperplasia which displaces an entire thyroid follicle. *B*, Microscopic medullary thyroid carcinoma.

carriers as young as 3 years of age. Metastasis has been described with microscopic MTC.[35]

The biological behavior of MTC in MEN 2A is variable. Metastasis to local lymph nodes occurs frequently with tumors greater than 1 cm in size. Despite the fact that metastasis may be present, the tumor pursues a relatively indolent course in 80 per cent of affected individuals. In about 5 to 10 per cent of patients, the tumor pursues a more aggressive course, which can include early metastasis and death.[36, 37] In some kindreds there is a familial pattern of aggressiveness; in others one or two members will display an aggressive pattern of behavior on a general background of benignity. This characteristic has allowed MEN 2A to remain undetected in some families over several generations, resulting in newly discovered kindreds even in the past decade.[38] Characteristics of aggressive behavior include early bone or liver metastasis, a loss of expression of the calcitonin gene, or a switch to production of calcitonin gene–related peptide, the alternatively produced product of the calcitonin gene. Distant metastasis occurs most commonly to liver, lung, and bone. Death is most commonly attributable to metastatic disease causing local airway obstruction or to liver and lung metastases. The presence of metastatic disease in the liver may or may not be a poor prognostic feature; a number of patients with hepatic metastasis have survived several decades.[37, 39]

Diarrhea may be the presenting complaint in medullary thyroid carcinoma. Initially the diarrhea may be a minor complaint, but with an increasing tumor burden the patient may have 10 to 20 stools per day. Unlike diarrhea associated with islet cell tumors, the stools are usually not voluminous.[40] The etiology of the diarrhea is unclear, although it is believed to be caused by a humoral factor produced by the tumor. Flushing has been observed in patients with MTC.

Another clinical finding associated with MTC is ectopic ACTH syndrome (see Chs. 22 and 100). The clinical syndrome is most frequently seen in patients with a large primary tumor or with metastatic MTC.[41] A detailed analysis of MTCs suggests that most express the pro-opiomelanocortin gene,[42] but the peptide precursor is processed to produce ACTH in only a few tumors. The clinical features of hypercorticism may be subtle (muscle weakness, edema, and mild centripetal obesity). The clinician should be aware of this clinical syndrome because patients with medullary thyroid carcinoma and ectopic ACTH may do well for long periods of time if the hypercorticism is controlled (see Ch. 100).

Pheochromocytoma

Approximately 50 per cent of known gene carriers will develop clinically detectable pheochromocytomas, although autopsy studies suggest a larger percentage of gene carriers are likely to have abnormalities of the adrenal medullae.[12, 43] There is the general belief that the adrenal medullary cell, like the C cell, passes through a hyperplastic stage before the development of multicentric pheochromocytomas. It seems likely that the histological abnormalities in the adrenal medulla occur in parallel with those observed in the C cell, although clinically apparent pheochromocytomas are only rarely detected prior to the diagnosis of C cell abnormalities.

UNIQUE FEATURES OF PHEOCHROMOCYTOMAS ASSOCIATED WITH MEN 2A. Pheochromocytoma in MEN 2A is generally limited to the adrenal gland. The occasional exception may be explained by the presence of ectopic adrenal rest tissue.[44] The pheochromocytomas are usually multicentric and set on a background of diffuse adrenal medullary hyperplasia.[12, 43] Although malignant pheochromocytoma in MEN 2A is rare,[45] capsular invasion is observed frequently. There appears to be no correlation between capsular invasion and recurrence of the tumor.

Pheochromocytoma associated with MEN 2A can be differentiated from sporadic pheochromocytoma by several unique features. The first is the relative overproduction of epinephrine by the tumor. The earliest biochemical abnormality is an increase in plasma or urine epinephrine[39, 46–48] (Fig. 151–11). A clinical observation, which may be attributable to this biochemical finding, is the relative lack of hypertension in patients with early pheochromocytomas and the predominance of beta-adrenergic–like symptoms such as palpitations, tachycardia, and nervousness. Rarely, adrenal medullary hyperplasia may be associated with symptoms suggestive of a pheochromocytoma with few or no detectable abnormalities of catecholamines. In larger pheochromocytomas there is also overproduction of norepinephrine, although the ratio of epinephrine to norepi-

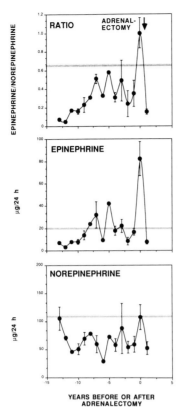

FIGURE 151–11. The mean 24-hour urinary norepinephrine and epinephrine excretion and the ratio of epinephrine/norepinephrine excretion in 11 prospectively screened patients subsequently proven to have pheochromocytoma. Each value shows the mean of values in 11 prospectively screened patients prior to adrenalectomy. The dashed line shows the upper limit of normal. To convert epinephrine values to nanomoles, multiply by 5.458; to convert norepinephrine values to nanomoles, multiply by 5.911. (Data from Gagel RF, Tashjian AH Jr, Cummings T, et al: The clinical outcome of prospective screening for multiple endocrine neoplasia type 2A: An 18-year experience. N Engl J Med 318:478–484, 1988.)

nephrine remains increased.[39] Hypertension may be a clinical problem in patients with larger tumors. Sudden death related to pheochromocytoma occurred with some frequency in kindreds prior to routine prospective screening.

Hyperparathyroidism

Hyperparathyroidism occurs in 15 to 20 per cent of patients with the fully developed form of MEN 2A. Parathyroid hyperplasia is the most common histological abnormality; when parathyroid adenomas are found, they are generally set on a background of hyperplasia.[7, 8] The clinical features of hyperparathyroidism do not differ from those associated with sporadic hyperparathyroidism (see Ch. 61). Unlike MEN 1, where hyperparathyroidism is generally the first manifestation of the syndrome, hyperparathyroidism in MEN 2 rarely occurs during the early phases of the syndrome. In addition, prospective screening of MEN 2A families has led to the observation that children who are thyroidectomized for C cell hyperplasia or early MTC have not developed hyperparathyroidism during a 10- to 15-year follow-up period.[39] Whether the failure of thyroidectomized children to develop hyperparathyroidism is related to partial removal of parathyroid tissue at the time of thyroid surgery and reflects an inadequate follow-up

period or is related to removal of a growth stimulus by total thyroidectomy is unclear. There are, however, families in which hyperparathyroidism occurs early and is a prominent part of the syndrome.[49] Whether this reflects a fundamental genetic difference is not clear.

The MEN 2A/Cutaneous Lichen Amyloidosis Variant

At least 12 kindreds have been identified in which MEN 2A is associated with the development of a pruritic skin lesion over the upper back.[38, 50] The first manifestation of the skin lesion is intermittent intense pruritus. The onset of pruritus generally precedes the development of a visible skin lesion by several years. The fully developed skin lesion has a lichenoid-papular appearance and may be unilateral or bilateral (Fig. 151–12A). Amyloid deposition analogous to that found in cutaneous lichen amyloidosis is found in more advanced lesions (Fig. 151–12B). Whether this variant represents a specific genetic mutation is not clear, but it is of interest that the skin lesion is found in a minority of kindreds and has not been observed in MEN 2B. Although the skin lesion is a minor component of MEN 2, its importance may lie in the identification of a genetic locus for cutaneous lichen amyloidosis, a common skin disorder in Asiatic populations.[51, 52]

Familial Medullary Thyroid Carcinoma

Familial medullary thyroid carcinoma (FMTC) is another variant of MEN 2A without other manifestations of MEN 2A.[67, 68] The clinical characteristics of medullary thyroid carcinoma in FMTC do not differ substantially from those of MEN 2A, although the observation has been made that the FMTC variant is less aggressive. One viewpoint is that the FMTC-only syndrome is MEN 2A but with a later onset of neoplasia, making it less likely that pheochromocytoma will develop during a normal lifetime.

Multiple Endocrine Neoplasia Type 2B

The association of medullary thyroid carcinoma, pheochromocytoma, mucosal neuromas, a marfanoid body habitus, and the absence of hyperparathyroidism has been classified as multiple endocrine neoplasia type 2B (MEN 2B). Although there are earlier descriptions, it was Williams and his colleagues who compiled the several components as a distinct clinical syndrome.[11] Most cases of this clinical syndrome are thought to represent new mutations because of a failure to find evidence of disease in parents, although germ line transmission of the disease with an autosomal dominant pattern of inheritance has been described in several kindreds.[53, 54]

Medullary Thyroid Carcinoma and Pheochromocytoma

Development of medullary thyroid carcinoma in MEN 2B is thought to follow a similar pattern of progression as described for MEN 2A but with a few differences. C cell hyperplasia and microscopic carcinoma, in general, develop much earlier in MEN 2B. Children have been de-

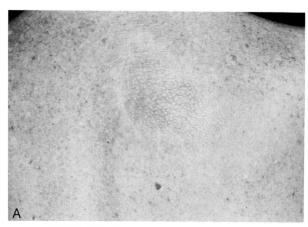
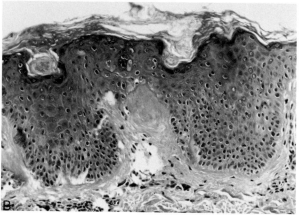

FIGURE 151–12. *A*, Characteristic cutaneous feature of lesion of cutaneous lichen amyloidosis. Patients with this lesion complain of intermittent pruritus and burning in the area of the skin lesion. *B*, Characteristic histological features of cutaneous lichen amyloidosis showing deposition of amyloid at the interface between the dermis and epidermis. (Reprinted with permission from Gagel RF, Levy ML, Donovan DT, et al: Multiple endocrine neoplasia type 2a associated with cutaneous lichen amyloidosis. Ann Intern Med 111:802–806, 1989.)

scribed with metastatic MTC shortly after birth.[55, 56] Death related to complications of metastatic MTC may occur before the onset of the third decade, although a larger experience which includes several multigenerational families suggests that the prognosis in an individual patient may be better than previously considered.[57, 58] Pheochromocytomas in MEN 2B occur in more than 50 per cent of affected individuals and also may develop at an early age. The clinical presentation of pheochromocytoma does not differ substantially from that observed in MEN 2A.

Mucosal Neuromas and Other Clinical Features

The most striking phenotypic feature of MEN 2B is the presence of multiple mucosal neuromas. The presence of multiple neuromas located on the tongue tip, within the lips, and on the eyelids makes for a characteristic facies identifiable even in childhood[59] (Fig. 151–13). Mucosal neuromas exist throughout the gastrointestinal tract. Gastrointestinal symptomatology is the second most common reason for recognition of this syndrome.[60] Children and

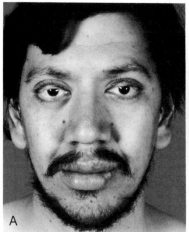
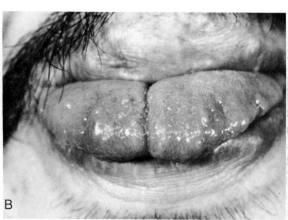
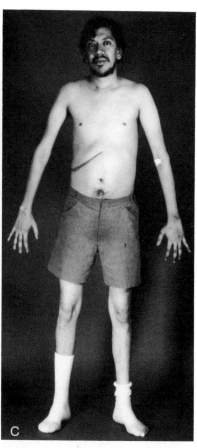

FIGURE 151–13. Characteristic facies with thickened lips and eyelids in a patient with MEN 2B. Note that this patient had extensive reconstructive surgery on the left side of his lower lip *(A)* and the tip of his tongue *(B)* during childhood in an attempt to excise the neuromas. *C*, The marfanoid features of MEN 2B, including the long arms, thin fingers, and altered body ratio. The abdominal scar resulted from removal of a unilateral pheochromocytoma.

adults will frequently present with complaints of increased gas, abdominal pain, and occasionally, obstruction caused by neuromatous tissue. Obstructive symptoms combined with diarrhea caused by MTC can produce a puzzling clinical syndrome characterized by alternating obstructive symptoms and diarrhea. It is important to exclude an anatomical cause of obstruction and, where possible, to debulk the mass of medullary thyroid carcinoma to reduce diarrhea. Abdominal exploration is generally indicated only in patients with proven obstruction. Gastrointestinal neuromas associated with MEN 2B can be confused with Hirschsprung's disease, a condition that has been associated with MEN 2A in a few kindreds.[64] Inactivating point mutations of the RET protooncogene have also been identified in familial Hirschsprung's disease.[61]

Hyperparathyroidism is rare in MEN 2B.[62] Other clinical features frequently found in this syndrome include a marfanoid habitus with long, thin arms, an altered upper/lower body ratio, long fingers, hyperextensible joints, and slipped femoral epiphyses.[63]

MEN 2A and 2B have been viewed as two separate syndromes, but some evidence of overlap exists. The identification of a mother with MEN 2B and two children with MTC, one with the characteristic MEN 2B phenotype and the second with no phenotypical features of MEN 2B, suggests that the mucosal neuroma phenotype may not be 100 per cent penetrant.[65] Recent reports of corneal nerve thickening, a finding associated with MEN 2B, in kindreds with MEN 2A provides additional evidence for overlap.[66] Recent studies have identified a germ-line point mutation of the RET protooncogene affecting exon 16 in MEN 2B.[66a]

SCREENING FOR MEN 2A

The primary goal of screening for MEN 2 is to identify and treat the several manifestations of MEN 2 before they become life-threatening. A secondary goal is to provide genetic counseling to family members about the potential for transmission to the next generation. These goals become closely intertwined because family decisions regarding the next generation are largely based on experience in the current generation. The two life-threatening manifestations of MEN 2 are metastasis from MTC and sudden death caused by pheochromocytoma. In selected kindreds, renal nephrolithiasis may be a cause of morbidity and renal failure. A 20-year experience now makes it reasonable to believe that death or serious morbidity caused by these manifestations can be prevented.

Medullary Thyroid Carcinoma

Measurement of the serum calcitonin basally and after a provocative test remains the preferred method for diagnosis of MTC associated with MEN 2. The sensitivity and specificity of the test are enhanced by the use of a provocative stimulus of calcitonin release such as calcium,[69] pentagastrin,[70] or a combination of the two.[71] The provocative stimulus results in a rapid (within 2 to 10 minutes) increase of the serum calcitonin concentration.

Experience with the pentagastrin (or combined cal-

cium/pentagastrin) testing over the past two decades indicates that it is a reliable predictor of C cell abnormalities, especially when combined with current sensitive assays. The test is performed by the injection of pentagastrin (Peptavlon), 0.5 μg/kg intravenously, over 5 to 10 seconds, generally in the fasting state. The serum calcitonin level is measured basally and 2, 5, 10, and 15 minutes after the injection, although measurement of basal, 2- and 5-minute samples will reduce the cost of the test without affecting sensitivity. The normal range is defined for each specific calcitonin assay, although pentagastrin-stimulated values greater than 50 pg/ml for women and 125 pg/ml for men are considered abnormal in most assays.[72] The major objections to use of the test are several unpleasant side effects, including nausea, substernal tightness, flushing, tingling of extremities, and the urge to void; these symptoms usually subside within 2 to 3 minutes of injection and are of variable severity. The patient should be warned of these side effects prior to the pentagastrin injection and provided with reassurance of their transient nature. In the author's experience, there have been no serious side effects when pentagastrin has been used for prospective screening in children. There have been anecdotal reports of hypotension and flushing in patients with a significant tumor mass; pentagastrin testing in patients with a sizable tumor mass generally provides no additional information, although its use in specific circumstances such as venous catheterization for localization of tumor may be appropriate.

Several facts have emerged from prospective annual screening studies during the 1970's and 1980's. First, it is possible to identify children with early C cell abnormalities by use of annual pentagastrin tests. Approximately 50 per cent of the children who developed abnormal tests had hyperplasia of the C cells, and 50 per cent had microscopic MTC without evidence of metastasis.[39, 73, 74] It is believed that total thyroidectomy in these children is likely to be curative, although some have low but detectable levels of calcitonin 10 to 15 years after thyroidectomy.[73, 75] Second, measurement of the basal calcitonin level alone is inadequate for screening purposes. Basal calcitonin measurements, even with the greater sensitivity of current assays, are normal in a significant percentage of children with early C cell disease.[75] Measurement of basal calcitonin alone may result in a delay of diagnosis for a period of 3 to 5 years (Fig. 151–14). Finally, utilization of the most sensitive and specific calcitonin assay available will result in earlier diagnosis of C cell abnormalities (Fig. 151–14).

There are several problems in the interpretation of test results during screening for hereditary MTC which occur with some regularity. The first is a test result in which the child has an elevated basal serum calcitonin level but no further increase after a provocative test result. This pattern of test result is most commonly associated with an artifactual elevation of the serum calcitonin concentration. Demonstration that the result is normal in another radioassay, either a standard radioimmunoassay, a concentration-type radioimmunoassay,[72] or a two-site immunoradiometric assay,[76] will provide reassurance that the abnormal value reflects an artifact. A second problem is the minimally abnormal result. In the past this problem has been dealt with by repetitive testing at 6-month intervals, with the expectation that there would be a persistence or progression of the abnormal result in gene carriers. The addition of genetic

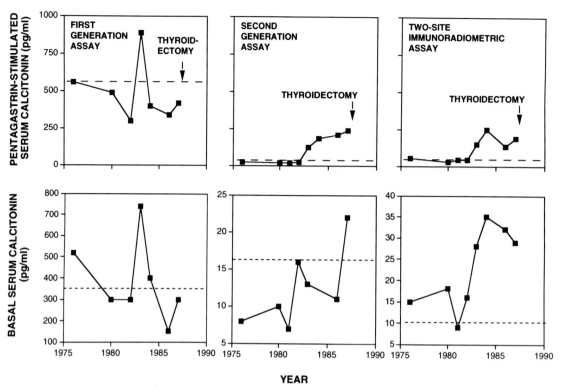

FIGURE 151–14. Retrospective comparison of serum calcitonin values measured in three calcitonin assays in a single MEN 2A gene carrier. This figure shows basal *(lower panels)* or pentagastrin-stimulated *(upper panels)* calcitonin values measured by a first, second, or two-site immunoradiometric (IRMA) assay in a single patient who was found to have several foci of microscopic MTC without metastasis at thyroidectomy 3 months after the last test shown. Measurements in the first-generation assay were made within a few weeks of the date shown; second-generation and two-site IRMA assays were performed on banked frozen samples in 1987–1988. Note that the ordinate scales for the lower portion of the figure differ for each panel. The dotted line shows the upper limit of normal for each measurement. This figure makes several points: First, the first-generation assays were relatively insensitive. At a point in time when the pentagastrin-stimulated values on banked samples were clearly abnormal in the second-generation assay and the two-site IRMA, the results in the first-generation assay were equivocal or normal. Second, basal measurements of calcitonin were never consistently abnormal in the first- and second-generation assays, whereas in this patient a basal measurement by IRMA might have predicted disease 3 to 4 years prior to the performance of the thyroidectomy. A larger experience in this same kindred, unfortunately, did not prove the basal calcitonin measurement by IRMA to be consistently predictive of disease status, leading to the conclusion that the measurement of the serum calcitonin value after a provocative test in either a second-generation or two-site IRMA remains the diagnostic test of choice for detecting early C cell disease. (The data shown in this figure were described in part in ref. 75; the data were kindly provided by Dr. Kaplan.)

testing (discussed below) provides an independent method for assessing the relevance of a single abnormal test result.

New mutations causing MEN 2A appear to be rare. Careful examination of isolated cases usually has led to a connection with a known kindred. The rarity of a new mutation causing MEN 2A suggests that the family of a newly identified case should be apprised of the genetic risks and offered screening.*

It is likely that provocative testing for calcitonin release will become less important for diagnosis of gene carrier

status as genetic testing is phased in over the next several years. Current recommendations are for a combined approach utilizing both genetic and selective pentagastrin testing to identify children likely to develop MTC.

Pheochromocytoma

The goal of screening for pheochromocytoma is to identify and treat excess catecholamine production prior to the development of life-threatening manifestations. Experience over the past 2 decades indicates that this can be accomplished by simple screening techniques repeated at regular intervals. A careful history is important and may provide the earliest clue to the presence of an adrenal abnormality. Each suspected gene carrier should be queried annually about the presence of palpitations, nervousness or attacks of jitteriness, headaches, or other unusual vascular symptoms. Screening for excessive catecholamine production can be accomplished by annual measurement of fractionated catecholamines (epinephrine and norepi-

---

*Families of affected individuals may or may not respond positively to the suggestion for family screening. It is important, however, to apprise the family of the genetic risks. To aid in this process, the author has developed a pamphlet which describes the major features of this syndrome in simple terms. The affected individual is encouraged to distribute this pamphlet to other first-degree relatives. This information source for family members is frequently more effective in soliciting enthusiasm for screening than is an attempt by a physician to contact family members directly. A family meeting frequently will provide a nonthreatening forum for hesitant family members to gain information about the disease and screening protocols. A copy of this pamphlet is available by writing the author.

nephrine) in a 12- to 24-hour urine collection or by annual measurement of plasma catecholamines. The earliest indication of increased adrenal medullary mass is an increase of the 12- to 24-hour excretion of epinephrine and an increase in the ratio of epinephrine/norepinephrine in this collection (see Fig. 151–11) or an elevated basal plasma epinephrine measurement.[77] The author has adopted an 8- to 12-hour urine collection for fractionated catecholamines as a compromise measure which most patients find acceptable. Measurement of vanillylmandelic acid is not useful for detection of pheochromocytoma, and there is little information available to permit comparison of urine metanephrines with fractionated catecholamines in the diagnosis of early adrenal medullary abnormalities in this syndrome.

Screening for pheochromocytoma should begin by age 6. Adrenal medullary hyperplasia or pheochromocytoma has been described in the 10- to 12-year age range,[39] and a 13-year-old child has presented with hypertensive encephalopathy caused by a large pheochromocytoma.[78] Parents should be instructed to be alert to symptoms of headaches or jitteriness in children. Screening should be intensified during the childbearing years, which are also the peak years for diagnosis of pheochromocytoma in this syndrome.

There are several radiographic studies which have been utilized for the diagnosis of pheochromocytoma in MEN 2. Preoperative evaluation by either computed tomography (CT) or magnetic resonance imaging (MRI) is important to define surgical anatomy and determine bilaterality. Considerable controversy has developed over the use of [^{131}I]metaiodobenzylguanidine for diagnosis of pheochromocytoma in MEN 2. Although most investigators agree that this radioisotope is a very sensitive indicator of adrenal medullary hyperfunction, it may be too sensitive, thereby resulting in detection of adrenal medullary hyperplasia (which is likely to be present in the majority of gene carriers over the age of 20 years) before there is a significant increase in production of catecholamines.[79] This technique may be used for preoperative localization of adrenal tissue to exclude the possibility of a pheochromocytoma in an adrenal rest[80] and in recurrent pheochromocytoma to exclude the rare extra-adrenal tumor. Arteriography is rarely indicated in the management of pheochromocytoma associated with MEN 2 and should be performed only after administration of adrenergic receptor antagonists (see Ch. 106).

Hyperparathyroidism

Screening for hyperparathyroidism in MEN 2 is straightforward. Measurement of the serum calcium concentration every other year after age 10 is adequate for early diagnosis.[39, 49, 81] The finding of an elevated serum calcium level should prompt measurement of a serum intact parathyroid hormone concentration. Pheochromocytoma is a rare cause of hypercalcemia in MEN 2 and should be excluded prior to parathyroid gland exploration.[39] Other, more common causes of hypercalcemia should be excluded by careful history and physical examination and additional laboratory tests where appropriate (see Ch. 63).

Unique Screening Issues

A question asked frequently is whether the family of a patient with apparent sporadic MTC should be screened for hereditary MTC, especially when a careful history fails to turn up any evidence of familial MTC. The key point to be considered in responding to this question is, How good is a family history in excluding hereditary disease? Some insight has been provided by a study of English and North American kindreds in which it was determined that only 60 per cent of predicted gene carriers were identified by methods other than calcitonin testing[82, 83]; screening by provocative calcitonin testing in these same families resulted in identification of over 90 per cent of predicted gene carriers. These results suggest that family history is likely to be a poor predictor of familial disease.

Based on this type of information, it is the author's belief that *first-degree* relatives of an individual with apparent sporadic MTC should be offered pentagastrin testing, especially if there is coexistent C cell hyperplasia present in the thyroid gland outside the area of the tumor. Even though C cell hyperplasia may be found in apparently sporadic MTC,[84] its presence should be considered suspicious for hereditary disease.[85] Unfortunately, this ideal screening goal is rarely met in clinical practice for a variety of reasons. It seems likely that a major impact of the identification of specific MEN 2 gene mutations will be the ability to determine directly whether a germ line mutation of the MEN 2 gene exists in an individual patient.

Unique Screening Features for MEN 2B

There is evidence that most patients with MEN 2B will develop medullary thyroid carcinoma at an early age. Metastatic carcinoma has been described in children with MEN 2B as young as 3 months of age. Because of this early expression of MTC, there is a consensus that thyroidectomy should be performed at the earliest possible age in children with phenotypic features of MEN 2B. It is also possible that the mucosal neuroma phenotype may not be 100 per cent penetrant, making it mandatory to screen (by pentagastrin or genetic analysis, where feasible) all children born to an MEN 2B parent.[65]

MOLECULAR GENETICS

Identification of RET Protooncogene Mutations in MEN 2A and 2B

The application of linkage analysis using restriction fragment length polymorphism to the many large and well-defined MEN 2 kindreds led to the linkage of MEN 2A to a centromeric chromosome 10 locus (Fig. 151–15) in 1987.[15, 16] Subsequent studies by several groups (reviewed in ref. 17) have led to the identification of flanking DNA sequences (*FNRB* and *H4JRBP* or *pMCK2*) for this locus. More recent studies have demonstrated that the predisposing gene(s) for all four variants of MEN 2 maps to the same genetic locus. Progress toward identification of the predisposing gene(s) was slowed by the low recombination rate (the normal exchange of parenteral DNA dur-

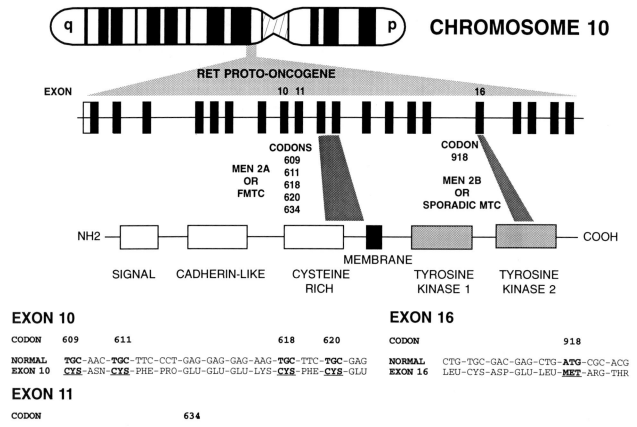

EXON 10

CODON	609	611					618	620	
NORMAL	**TGC**-AAC-**TGC**-TTC-CCT-GAG-GAG-GAG-AAG-**TGC**-TTC-**TGC**-GAG
EXON 10	**CYS**-ASN-**CYS**-PHE-PRO-GLU-GLU-GLU-LYS-**CYS**-PHE-**CYS**-GLU

EXON 16

CODON					918		
NORMAL	CTG-TGC-GAC-GAG-CTG-**ATG**-CGC-ACG
EXON 16	LEU-CYS-ASP-GLU-LEU-**MET**-ARG-THR

EXON 11

CODON		634
NORMAL	CTG-TGC-GAC-GAG-CTG-**TGC**-CGC-ACG
EXON 11	LEU-CYS-ASP-GLU-LEU-**CYS**-ARG-THR

FIGURE 151–15. Molecular abnormalities in MEN 2A and 2B. The causative gene was mapped to the proximal long arm of chromosome 10. Point mutations of the RET protooncogene have been identified in both MEN 2A and 2B. The germ-line point mutations in MEN 2A convert a highly conserved cysteine at one of 5 codons (609, 611, 618, 620, or 634) in exon 10 or 11 to another amino acid. These mutations fall in a highly conserved cysteine-rich region in the extracellular portion of this tyrosine kinase receptor. MEN 2B has been associated with germ-line mutations of codon 918 (methionine to threonine) in the intracellular tyrosine kinase region. This figure shows the specific mutations associated with MEN 2A (exon 10 or 11) and MEN 2B (exon 16). Polymerase chain reaction–based technology has been developed for rapid identification of these mutations.

ing meiosis) in the centromeric region of chromosome 10, making it difficult to utilize linkage approaches to further narrow the region containing the disease gene. Specific mutations of the RET protooncogene have recently been identified in MEN 2A (Fig. 151–15).

Genetic Screening for MEN 2

The low recombination rate around the MEN 2 locus, however, has made it possible to use closely linked polymorphic DNA sequences for genetic diagnosis.[91–97] Several DNA sequences have been described for which no recombination between the MEN 2 locus and the DNA sequence has been described (Fig. 151–15). The important point is that utilization of several closely linked or flanking DNA sequences permits prediction of gene carrier status with a high degree of certainty. The predictive usefulness of a particular DNA sequence is dependent on several factors, including closeness to the MEN 2 locus and its informativeness (the ability to separate the two parenteral alleles) in a particular family. If closely linked flanking markers are informative, the ability to correctly predict gene carrier status may be as high as 99 per cent. Informativeness of only a single DNA sequence will lower predictive ability. In interpreting results, the clinician also must consider the possibility of nonpaternity, which could lead to an incorrect assignation of gene carrier status. Blood samples for restriction fragment polymorphism analysis must be obtained not only from affected individuals but also from their spouses and other family members who are not gene carriers to establish on which allele the disease gene is located. Despite these caveats, the information obtained will in most cases have a major impact on management of this disease.[92] Identification of RET mutations make it possible to predict gene carrier status with certainty in MEN 2 families with identifiable mutations (Fig. 151–15).

Molecular and Cytogenetic Abnormalities Found in MEN 2 Tumors

There is currently no evidence that the MEN 2 gene functions as a tumor suppressor–type gene like that found in MEN 1[98] or retinoblastoma. Studies of many MTC's and pheochromocytomas from hereditary and sporadic cases have only rarely demonstrated findings consistent with this type of mechanism. Identification of point mutations of the RET photooncogene provides conclusive evidence against this type of mechanism. There is, however, evidence to suggest loss or abnormality of a tumor suppressor gene on chromosome 1p or 22[99, 100] and cytogenetic evidence to suggest abnormalities of chromosomes 3p and 9.[101] Current evidence suggests that the mutation represents the primary event involved in transformation; it seems likely that other molecular events on chromosomes 1p, 22, 3p, or 9 may be involved in progression of transformation.[102]

Integration of Genetic and Standard Screening Techniques in the Management of MEN 2A

Neither pentagastrin testing nor genetic testing applied individually provides 100 per cent certainty of diagnosis. There are several reported examples of false-positive pentagastrin tests leading to thyroidectomy in individuals who were not gene carriers[39, 103] and unreported examples in which the pentagastrin test has been normal on one annual test and very abnormal on a subsequent test with the finding of macroscopic carcinoma, suggesting either a false-negative test result or a sample mixup at the time of first test. Similarly, inherent in the approaches used for genetic testing is the small possibility of a polymerase chain reaction artifact leading to either a false-positive or false-negative test result. A combination of the two types of information, because they are based on different types of data, makes an incorrect diagnosis unlikely.[92]

There are distinct advantages to genetic testing as well. Figure 151–16 shows information obtained from earlier prospective studies during which the age of conversion from a negative to a positive pentagastrin test was determined in a large number of affected families. A priori, each family member has a 50 per cent probability of subsequently developing medullary thyroid carcinoma. By 20 years of age, an individual with a negative pentagastrin test has less than a 10 per cent probability of subsequent development of MTC.[104] The application of genetic screening in this same individual makes it possible to determine with 90 to 99 per cent certainty at birth whether he or she is or is not a gene carrier (the degree of certainty is dependent on the proximity of informative DNA sequences to the MEN 2

locus). Plotting this type of information on Figure 151–16 demonstrates that the probability of gene carrier status at birth goes from 50 per cent to as high as 90 to 99 per cent or as low as 1 to 10 per cent.

Clinicians who manage kindreds with MEN 2A or 2B are moving toward clinical decision making based solely on specific RET mutational analysis. There are, however, issues that need to be addressed regarding accuracy of testing protocols, incidence of false-positive or -negative genetic test results, and availability of these testing procedures. Most of these issues will probably be resolved within the next year or two, so that decisions can be made solely on the basis of the presence or absence of a RET mutation.

Another use of genetic information is in the interpretation of borderline pentagastrin test results. Differentiation of the minimally abnormal pentagastrin test result in the early stages of MTC from the occasionally positive test result in a child who is not a gene carrier is difficult.[105] The independent determination of gene carrier status by RET analysis permits the clinician to interpret abnormal test results with greater confidence. For example, it would not be reasonable to proceed with total thyroidectomy on the basis of a minimally abnormal test result in a child with a negative genetic test, whereas it would be reasonable in a child with a positive genetic test.

Identification of the RET protooncogene mutation suggests that these recommendations will shortly be changed.[88, 89] In most cases it will be possible to predict gene carrier status with 100 per cent certainty by means of a single blood sample utilizing polymerase chain reaction techniques to amplify and analyze the MEN 2 gene from DNA derived from the child at risk. It is likely that a recommendation will be made for total thyroidectomy at the earliest reasonable age in those children who are found to be gene carriers because of the overwhelming likelihood of development of medullary thyroid carcinoma. It also will be possible to exclude family members with negative genetic tests from screening. It is also possible that some family members will opt for some form of genetic selection at the time of conception to eliminate this gene from the germ line. The use of genetic testing is not likely to have an impact on screening for hyperparathyroidism or pheochromocytoma except to exclude the 50 per cent of family members with a normal copy of the MEN 2 gene from screening.

Clinical Management of Kindreds with MEN 2A or MEN 2B

MEDULLARY THYROID CARCINOMA. Total thyroidectomy is mandatory for treatment of hereditary medullary thyroid carcinoma because of the bilateral and multicentric nature of the disease. Metastatic disease to lymph nodes of the central compartment of the neck is seen in a high percentage of patients with a palpable or easily visualized mass, making central lymph node dissection at the time of primary operation mandatory in this group of patients.[49, 106] Although extensive lymph node dissection without proof of metastasis at the time of primary surgery may seem overly aggressive, there is abundant experience which indicates that surgical cure is possible even in individuals with local nodal metastasis.[107] The decision to extend the surgical procedure to include the mediastinum at the time of primary surgery should be based on operative findings, although it should be pointed out that the natural drain-

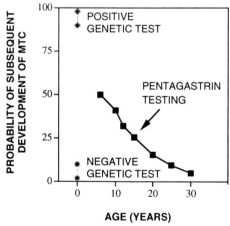

FIGURE 151–16. The impact of genetic screening on the management of MEN 2. Using data collected from many kindreds during the 1970's, it was possible to determine the age of conversion from a negative to a positive pentagastrin test.[104] This information can be used to predict the subsequent probability of conversion for an individual with a negative pentagastrin test. A priori, probability for a family member at birth was 50 per cent; each subsequent negative pentagastrin test result reduced the probability of subsequent conversion. By age 35 there was less than a 5 per cent probability of subsequent conversion. Superimposed on the same figure is the risk assessment utilizing genetic testing techniques for a child with either a positive or a negative genetic test at birth. It should be emphasized that current techniques for assessing genetic risk fall short of 100 per cent predictability because of the small possibility of a recombination between currently available DNA markers and the MEN 2 gene. The values shown for genetic prediction overstate the potential error for most families to make this point.

age patterns for the central lymph nodes of the neck make the upper mediastinum one of the logical places to search for metastatic MTC.

In children detected by prospective screening, a total thyroidectomy with sampling of lymph nodes in the central portion of the neck should be performed.[39, 73, 108, 109] In most centers, some form of central node dissection is also performed. Even with this type of treatment there are occasional patients who have detectable calcitonin values in the postoperative period.[73, 75] Whether the calcitonin in these few patients derives from an incomplete thyroidectomy, from metastatic disease, or from calcitonin-producing cells outside the neck is not clear. Fifteen-year follow-up studies suggest that there is no further increase of calcitonin values over time in the majority of these children.[39, 75]

In individuals who present with MTC and no history to suggest hereditary disease (apparently sporadic MTC), it is important to perform a total thyroidectomy and central lymph node dissection for several reasons. First, even sporadic MTC may be multifocal, and intrathyroidal metastasis is not uncommon. Second, the finding of characteristic C cell hyperplasia in the lobe contralateral to the tumor may provide evidence for a familial form of the disease. Finally, removal of the entire thyroid gland and performance of a central node dissection will simplify subsequent localization procedures if there is a postoperative calcitonin elevation.[110]

Perhaps the most controversial subject in the management of MTC is whether reoperation has therapeutic value in patients with a persistent elevation of the serum calcitonin concentration after an adequate primary operation. At present, data are scarce, but the most optimistic results suggest that 20 to 25 per cent of patients who have no detectable disease when assessed by radiographic techniques can be rendered calcitonin-negative by meticulous neck and, if necessary, mediastinal node dissection.[111] Before consideration of such extensive surgery, it is important to thoroughly exclude metastatic disease in lung, liver, and bone by appropriate radiologic techniques. Selective venous catheterization may provide a focus for surgical efforts and, importantly, may identify distant metastasis, making extensive neck or mediastinal dissection unwarranted.[112–114] Use of several scanning techniques, including [^{131}I]metaiodobenzylguanidine,[114, 115] thallium, dimercaptosuccinic acid,[116, 117] and somatostatin receptor imaging,[118] has met with variable success in finding macroscopic tumor, and the utility of these scanning approaches for finding microscopic tumor is unclear.

Finally, before consideration of thyroid surgery, individuals suspected of hereditary disease should have measurements of urine catecholamines or other appropriate studies to exclude pheochromocytoma. If a pheochromocytoma is found, surgical removal should be performed prior to thyroid surgery.

PHEOCHROMOCYTOMA. The goal of prospective screening for pheochromocytoma is to identify pheochromocytomas or adrenal medullary hyperplasia at a point prior to the development of significant neurological or cardiovascular manifestations. A patient with a proven pheochromocytoma should be started on combined alpha- and beta-adrenergic antagonists (see Ch. 106) for 2 to 4 weeks before surgery. Although intraoperative episodes of hypertension and tachycardia may occur at the time of removal of a small tumor, the profound clinical manifestations

which can occur with a large pheochromocytoma are less likely in patients with small tumors.

An anterior abdominal approach should be utilized to permit inspection of the liver (to exclude or localize metastatic MTC), to identify the rare extra-adrenal pheochromocytoma, and to examine the contralateral adrenal gland. Bilateral adrenalectomy should be performed if there is a family history of malignant pheochromocytoma,[45] if there are bilateral pheochromocytomas, or if there is a unilateral pheochromocytoma and a suspiciously enlarged contralateral adrenal gland.[119, 120] The majority of physicians who care for MEN 2 kindreds do not perform bilateral adrenalectomy at the primary operation unless one of these conditions exists. Although it is likely that a second operation will be required to remove an apparently unaffected adrenal gland, a period of 8 to 10 years may pass before a second operation is required.[39, 49, 119, 121] The issues to be balanced in the decision to perform unilateral or bilateral adrenalectomy at the primary operation include the risks of glucocorticoid deficiency (the author is aware of one death related to adrenal insufficiency in a MEN 2 patient) and the long-term risks of residual adrenal medullary tissue which may subsequently develop into a pheochromocytoma. Factors which may modify the decision-making process include cooperation of the individual with past screening efforts and access to emergency care for adrenal insufficiency.

Screening for pheochromocytoma should be conducted prior to pregnancy or, if this is not possible, early in pregnancy. Deaths during childbirth have occurred in MEN 2, and family histories include occasional mention of maternal death associated with childbirth.[122, 123] After careful consideration of the risks to fetus and mother, including the size of the tumor and its likely capacity for causing arrhythmia and sudden death, the physician will, in most cases, opt for removal of a pheochromocytoma at a suitable time during pregnancy.

HYPERPARATHYROIDISM. Development of hyperparathyroidism is uncommon in kindreds who are prospectively screened and affected children treated by thyroidectomy. In the unusual kindred in whom primary hyperparathyroidism is a prominent manifestation of the clinical syndrome, consideration should be given to total removal of parathyroid tissue with implantation into the nondominant forearm, an approach frequently used in MEN 1 patients.[49, 124, 125] Such an approach eliminates the necessity for repetitive neck exploration. Identification of candidates for this type of procedure can only be accomplished by a careful review of the clinical course of hyperparathyroidism in other family members.

REFERENCES

1. Sipple JH: The association of pheochromocytoma with carcinoma of the thyroid gland. Am J Med 31:163–166, 1961.
2. Hazard JB: The C-cells (parafollicular cells) of the thyroid gland and medullary thyroid carcinoma: A review. Am J Pathol 88:214, 1977.
3. Hazard JB, Hawk WA, Crile G Jr: Medullary (solid) carcinoma of the thyroid: A clinicopathologic entity. J Clin Endocrinol Metab 19:152–161, 1959.
4. Williams ED, Brown CL, Doniach I: Pathological and clinical findings in a series of 67 cases of medullary carcinoma of the thyroid. J Clin Pathol 19:103–113, 1966.
5. Williams ED: Histogenesis of medullary carcinoma of the thyroid. J Clin Pathol 19:114–118, 1966.

6. Steiner AL, Goodman AD, Powers SR: Study of a kindred with pheochromocytoma, medullary carcinoma, hyperparathyroidism and Cushing's disease: Multiple endocrine neoplasia, type 2. Medicine 47:371–409, 1968.
7. Melvin KEW, Tashjian AH Jr, Miller HH: Studies in familial (medullary) thyroid carcinoma. Recent Prog Horm Res 28:399–470, 1972.
8. Keiser HR, Beaven MA, Doppman J, et al: Sipple's syndrome: Medullary thyroid carcinoma, pheochromocytoma, and parathyroid disease. Ann Intern Med 78:561–579, 1973.
9. Jackson CE, Frame B: Relationship of hyperparathyroidism to multiple endocrine adenomatosis. Birth Defects 7:66–68, 1971.
10. Williams ED: A review of 17 cases of carcinoma of the thyroid and phaeochromocytoma. J Clin Pathol 18:288–292, 1965.
11. Williams ED, Pollock DJ: Multiple mucosal neuromata with endocrine tumours: A syndrome allied to Von Recklinghausen's disease. J Pathol Bacteriol 91:71–80, 1966.
12. DeLellis RA, Wolfe HJ, Gagel RF, et al: Adrenal medullary hyperplasia: A morphometric analysis in patients with familial medullary thyroid carcinoma. Am J Pathol 83:177–196, 1976.
13. Carney JA, Sizemore GW, Tyce GM: Bilateral adrenal medullary hyperplasia in multiple endocrine neoplasia, type 2: The precursor of bilateral pheochromocytoma. Mayo Clin Proc 50:3–10, 1975.
14. Wolfe HJ, Melvin KEW, Cervi-Skinner SJ, et al: C-cell hyperplasia preceding medullary thyroid carcinoma. N Engl J Med 289:437–441, 1973.
15. Simpson NE, Kidd KK, Goodfellow PJ, et al: Assignment of multiple endocrine neoplasia type 2A to chromosome 10 by linkage. Nature 328:528–530, 1987.
16. Mathew CG, Chin KS, Easton DF, et al: A linked genetic marker for multiple endocrine neoplasia type 2A on chromosome 10. Nature 328:527–528, 1987.
17. Simpson NE: The exploration of the locus or loci for the syndromes associated with medullary thyroid cancer (MTC) on chromosome 10. In Brandi ML and White R (eds): Hereditary Tumors. New York, Raven Press, 1991, pp 55–67.
18. Yamamoto M, Takai S, Miki T, et al: Close linkage of MEN2A with RBP3 locus in Japanese kindreds. Hum Genet 82:287–288, 1989.
19. Telenius-Berg M, Berg B, Hamberger B, et al: Impact of screening on prognosis in the multiple endocrine neoplasia type 2 syndromes: Natural history and treatment results in 105 patients. Henry Ford Hosp Med J 32:225–231, 1984.
20. Barbot N, Guyyetant S, Beldent V, et al: Thyroïdite chronique autoimmune et hyperplasie des cellules C etude de la sécrétion de calcitone chez 24 patients. Ann Endocrinol (Paris) 52:109–112, 1991.
21. Biddinger PW, Brennan MF, Rosen PP: Symptomatic C-cell hyperplasia associated with chronic lymphocytic thyroiditis. Am J Surg Pathol 15:599–604, 1991.
22. Livolsi VA, Feind CR: Incidental medullary thyroid carcinoma in sporadic hyperparathyroidism. Am J Clin Pathol 71:595–599, 1979.
23. Lallier TE: Cell lineage and cell migration in the neural crest. Ann NY Acad Sci 615:158–171, 1991.
24. Coupland RE: The natural history of the chromaffin cell—Twenty-five years on the beginning. Arch Histol Cytol 52S:331–341, 1989.
25. Rosenfeld MG, Amara SG, Roos BA, et al: Altered expression of the calcitonin gene associated with RNA polymorphism. Nature 290:63–65, 1981.
26. Peleg S, Abruzzese RV, Cote GJ, Gagel RF: Transcription of the human calcitonin gene is mediated by a C cell–specific enhancer containing E-box-like elements. Mol Endocrinol 4:1750–1757, 1990.
27. de Bustros A, Lee RY, Compton D, et al: Differential utilization of calcitonin gene regulatory DNA sequences in cultured lines of medullary thyroid carcinoma and small-cell lung carcinoma. Mol Cell Biol 10:1773–1778, 1990.
28. Kodama T: Identification of carcinoembryonic antigen in the C-cell of the normal thyroid. Cancer 45:98, 1980.
29. DeLellis RA, Rule AH, Spiler I, et al: Calcitonin and carcinoembryonic antigen as tumor markers in medullary thyroid carcinoma. Am J Clin Pathol 70:587–594, 1978.
30. Deftos LJ, Woloszczuk W, Krisch I, et al: Medullary thyroid carcinomas express chromogranin A and a novel neuroendocrine protein recognized by monoclonal antibody HISL-19. Am J Med 85:780–784, 1988.
31. Gagel RF, Palmer WN, Leonhart K, et al: Somatostatin production by a human medullary thyroid carcinoma cell line. Endocrinology 118:1643–1651, 1986.
32. Modigliani E, Alamowitch C, Cohen R, et al: The intratumoral immunoassayable somatostatin concentration is frequently elevated in medullary thyroid carcinoma: Results in 34 cases. Cancer 65:224–228, 1990.
33. Baylin SB, Gann DS, Hsu SH: Clonal origin of inherited medullary thyroid carcinoma and pheochromocytoma. Science 193:321–323, 1976.
34. Wolfe HJ, DeLellis RA: Familial medullary thyroid carcinoma and C-cell hyperplasia. Clin Endocrinol Metab 10:351–365, 1981.
35. Graham SM, Genel M, Touloukian RJ, et al: Provocative testing for occult medullary carcinoma of the thyroid: Findings in seven children with multiple endocrine neoplasia type IIa. J Pediatr Surg 22:501–503, 1987.
36. Kakudo K, Carney JA, Sizemore GW: Medullary carcinoma of thyroid: Biologic behavior of the sporadic and familial neoplasm. Cancer 55:2818–2821, 1985.
37. Samaan NA, Schultz PN, Hickey RC: Medullary thyroid carcinoma: Prognosis of familial versus sporadic disease and the role of radiotherapy. J Clin Endocrinol Metab 67:801–805, 1988.
38. Gagel RF, Levy ML, Donovan DT, et al: Multiple endocrine neoplasia type 2a associated with cutaneous lichen amyloidosis. Ann Intern Med 111:802–806, 1989.
39. Gagel RF, Tashjian AH Jr, Cummings T, et al: The clinical outcome of prospective screening for multiple endocrine neoplasia type 2a: An 18-year experience. N Engl J Med 318:478–484, 1988.
40. Isaacs P, Whittaker SM, Turnberg LA: Diarrhea associated with medullary carcinoma of the thyroid. Gastroenterology 67:521–526, 1974.
41. Deftos LJ, Murray SS, Burton DW, et al: A cloned chromogranin A (CgA) cDNA detects a 2.3 Kb mRNA in diverse neuroendocrine tissues. Biochem Biophys Res Commun 137:418–423, 1986.
42. Hoppener JW, Steenbergh PH, Moonen PJ, et al: Detection of mRNA encoding calcitonin, calcitonin gene related peptide and pro-opiomelanocortin in human tumors. Mol Cell Endocrinol 47:125–130, 1986.
43. Webb TA, Sheps SG, Carney JA: Differences between sporadic pheochromocytoma and pheochromocytoma in multiple endocrine neoplasia, type 2. Am J Surg Pathol 4:121–126, 1980.
44. Lips CJ, Minder WH, Leo JR, et al: Evidence of multicentric origin of the multiple endocrine neoplasia syndrome type 2a (Sipple's syndrome) in a large family in the Netherlands: Diagnostic and therapeutic implications. Am J Med 64:569–578, 1978.
45. Sisson JC, Shapiro B, Beierwaltes WH: Scintigraphy with I-131 MIBG as an aid to the treatment of pheochromocytomas in patients with the multiple endocrine neoplasia type 2 syndromes. Henry Ford Hosp Med J 32:254–261, 1984.
46. Miyauchi A, Masuo K, Ogihara T, et al: Urinary epinephrine and norepinephrine excretion in patients with medullary thyroid carcinoma and their relatives. Nippon Naibunpi Gakkai Zasshi 58:1505–1516, 1982.
47. Hamilton BP, Landsberg L, Levine RJ: Measurement of urinary epinephrine in screening for pheochromocytoma in multiple endocrine neoplasia type II. Am J Med 65:1027–1032, 1978.
48. Gagel RF, Melvin KE, Tashjian AH Jr, et al: Natural history of the familial medullary thyroid carcinoma–pheochromocytoma syndrome and the identification of preneoplastic stages by screening studies: A five-year report. Trans Assoc Am Physicians 88:177–191, 1975.
49. Cance WG, Wells SA Jr: Multiple endocrine neoplasia type IIa. Curr Probl Surg 22:1–56, 1985.
50. Nunziata V, Giannattasio R, di Giovanni G, et al: Hereditary localized pruritus in affected members of a kindred with multiple endocrine neoplasia type 2A (Sipple's syndrome). Clin Endocrinol 30:57–63, 1989.
51. Robinson MF, Furst EJ, Nunziata V, et al: The multiple endocrine neoplasia type 2/cutaneous lichen amyloidosis syndrome: Clinical features of a new variant. Calcium Reg Bone Metab (in press).
52. Robinson MF, Furst EJ, Nunziata V, et al: Characterization of the clinical features of five families with hereditary primary cutaneous lichen amyloidosis and multiple endocrine neoplasia type 2. Henry Ford Hosp Med J 40:249–252, 1992.
53. Lairmore TC, Howe JR, Korte JA, et al: Familial medullary thyroid carcinoma and multiple endocrine neoplasia type 2B map to the same region of chromosome 10 as multiple endocrine neoplasia type 2A. Genomics 9:181–192, 1991.
54. Norum RA, Lafreniere RG, O'Neal LW, et al: Linkage of the multiple endocrine neoplasia type 2B gene (MEN2B) to chromosome 10 markers linked to MEN2A. Genomics 8:313–317, 1990.
55. Moyes CD, Alexander FW: Mucosal neuroma syndrome presenting in a neonate. Dev Med Child Neurol 19:518–534, 1977.
56. Samaan NA, Draznin MB, Halpin RE, et al: Multiple endocrine syndrome type IIb in early childhood. Cancer 68:1832–1834, 1991.
57. Vasen HFA, van der Feltz M, Raue F, et al: The natural course of multiple endocrine neoplasia type IIb: A study of 18 cases. Arch Intern Med 152:1250–1252, 1992.

58. Sizemore GW, Carney JA, Gharib H, Capen CC: Multiple endocrine neoplasia type 2B: Eighteen-year followup of a four generation family. Henry Ford Hosp Med J 40:236–244, 1992.

59. Rashid M, Khairi MR, Dexter RN, et al: Mucosal neuroma, pheochromocytoma and medullary thyroid carcinoma: Multiple endocrine neoplasia type 3. Medicine 54:89–112, 1975.

60. Carney JA, Go VL, Sizemore GW, Hayles AB: Alimentary-tract ganglioneuromatosis: A major component of the syndrome of multiple endocrine neoplasia, type 2b. N Engl J Med 295:1287–1291, 1976.

61. Seri M, Ceccherini I, Pasin B, et al: Point mutations affecting the tyrosine kinase domain of the RET protooncogene in Hirschsprung's disease. Nature 367:377–378, 1994.

62. Carney JA, Roth SI, Heath H III, et al: The parathyroid glands in multiple endocrine neoplasia type 2b. Am J Pathol 99:387–398, 1980.

63. Carney JA, Bianco AJ Jr, Sizemore GW, Hayles AB: Multiple endocrine neoplasia with skeletal manifestations. J Bone Joint Surg 63A:405–410, 1981.

64. Verdy M, Weber AM, Roy CC, et al: Hirschsprung's disease in a family with multiple endocrine neoplasia type 2. J Pediatr Gastroenterol Nutr 1:603–607, 1982.

65. Sciubba JJ, D'Amico E, Attie JN: The occurrence of multiple endocrine neoplasia type IIb in two children of an affected mother. J Oral Pathol 16:310–316, 1987.

66. Kinoshita S, Tanaka F, Ohashi Y, et al: Incidence of prominent corneal nerves in multiple endocrine neoplasia type 2A. Am J Ophthalmol 111:307–311, 1991.

66a. Hofstra RMW, Landsvater RM, Ceccherini I, et al: A mutation in the RET protooncogene associated with MEN 2B and sporadic medullary thyroid carcinoma. Nature 367:376, 1994.

67. Houdent C, Avronsart B, Dubuisson M, et al: Familial medullary thyroid cancer: Contribution of genealogy and genetics to the study of two families. Presse Med 19:549–552, 1990.

68. Farndon JR, Leight GS, Dilley WG, et al: Familial medullary thyroid carcinoma without associated endocrinopathies: A distinct clinical entity. Br J Surg 73:278–281, 1986.

69. Parthemore JG, Bronzert D, Roberts G, Deftos LJ: A short calcium infusion in the diagnosis of medullary thyroid carcinoma. J Clin Endocrinol Metab 39:108–111, 1974.

70. Hennessey JF, Wells SA, Ontjes DA, Cooper CW: A comparison of pentagastrin injections and calcium infusion as provocative agents for the detection of medullary carcinoma of the thyroid. J Clin Endocrinol Metab 39:487, 1974.

71. Wells SA Jr, Baylin SB, Linehan WM, et al: Provocative agents and the diagnosis of medullary carcinoma of the thyroid gland. Ann Surg 188:139–141, 1978.

72. Gharib H, Kao PC, Heath H III: Determination of silica-purified plasma calcitonin for the detection and management of medullary thyroid carcinoma: Comparison of two provocative tests. Mayo Clin Proc 62:373–378, 1987.

73. Telander RL, Zimmerman D, van Heerden JA, Sizemore GW: Results of early thyroidectomy for medullary thyroid carcinoma in children with multiple endocrine neoplasia type 2. J Pediatr Surg 21:1190–1194, 1986.

74. Wells SA, Dilley WG, Farndon JA, et al: Early diagnosis and treatment of medullary thyroid carcinoma. Arch Intern Med 145:1248–1252, 1985.

75. Kaplan MM, Stall GM, Cummings T, et al: High-sensitivity serum calcitonin assays applied to screening for thyroid C-cell disease in multiple endocrine neoplasia type 2A. Henry Ford Hosp Med J 40:227–231, 1992.

76. Motte P, Vauzelle P, Gardet P, et al: Construction and clinical validation of a sensitive and specific assay for serum mature calcitonin using monoclonal anti-peptide antibodies. Clin Chim Acta 174:35–54, 1988.

77. Vistelle R, Grulet H, Gibold C, et al: High permanent plasma adrenaline levels: A marker of adrenal medullary disease in medullary thyroid carcinoma. Clin Endocrinol 34:133–138, 1991.

78. Jadoul M, Leo JR, Berends MJ, et al: Pheochromocytoma-induced hypertensive encephalopathy revealing MEN-IIa syndrome in a 13-year-old boy: Implications for screening procedures and surgery. Horm Metab Res Suppl 21:46–49, 1989.

79. Yobbagy JJ, Levatter R, Sisson JC, et al: Scintigraphic portrayal of the syndrome of multiple endocrine neoplasia type-2B. Clin Nucl Med 13:433–437, 1988.

80. Miyauchi A, Matsuzaka F, Kuma K, et al: Diagnosis of adrenal medullary diseases in patients with sporadic or hereditary medullary thyroid carcinoma: A report of 37 cases with 8-year follow-up study. Nippon Geka Gakkai Zasshi 88:1423–1429, 1987.

81. Heath H III, Sizemore GW, Carney JA: Preoperative diagnosis of occult parathyroid hyperplasia by calcium infusion in patients with multiple endocrine neoplasia, type 2a. J Clin Endocrinol Metab 43:428–435, 1976.

82. Ponder BA, Ponder MA, Coffey R, et al: Risk estimation and screening in families of patients with medullary thyroid carcinoma. Lancet 1:397–401, 1988.

83. Easton DF, Ponder MA, Cummings T, et al: The clinical and screening age-at-onset distribution for the MEN-2 syndrome. Am J Hum Genet 44:208–215, 1989.

84. Ekblom M, Valimaki M, Pelkonen R, et al: Familial and sporadic medullary thyroid carcinoma: Clinical and immunohistological findings. Q J Med 65:899–910, 1987.

85. Block MA, Jackson CE, Greenawald KA, et al: Clinical characteristics distinguishing hereditary from sporadic medullary thyroid carcinoma. Arch Surg 115:142–148, 1980.

86. Mulligan LM, Kwok JBJ, Healey CS, et al: Germline mutations of the RET protooncogene in MEN 2A. Nature 363:458–460, 1993.

87. Donis-Keller H, Shenshen D, Chi D, et al: Mutations in the RET protooncogene are associated with MEN 2A and FMTC. Hum Molec Genet 2:851–856, 1993.

88. Mulligan LM, Eng C, Healey CS, et al: Specific mutations of the RET protooncogene are related to disease phenotype in MEN 2A and FMTC. Nature Genet 6:70–74, 1994.

89. Gagel RF, Cote GJ: Decision making in multiple endocrine neoplasia type 2. Adv Endocrinol Metab, In press.

90. Thomas PM, Gagel RF: Advances in genetic screening for multiple endocrine neoplasia type 2 and implications for the management of children at risk. Endocrinologist 4:140–147, 1994.

91. Howe JR, Lairmore TC, Mishra SK, et al: Improved predictive test for MEN 2 using flanking dinucleotide repeats and RFLPs. Am J Hum Genet (in press).

92. Gagel RF, Robinson ML, Alford BR, Donovan DT: Medullary thyroid carcinoma: Clinical review. J Clin Endocrinol Metab (in press).

93. Brooks-Wilson AR, Smailus DE, Weier HU, Goodfellow PJ: Human repeat element-mediated PCR: Cloning and mapping of chromosome 10 DNA markers. Genomics 13:409–414, 1992.

94. Shimotake T, Iwai N, Yanagihara J, et al: Prediction of affected MEN2A gene carriers by DNA linkage analysis for early total thyroidectomy: A progress in clinical screening program for children with hereditary cancer syndrome. J Pediatr Surg 27:444–446, 1992.

95. Sobol H, Narod SA, Nakamura Y, et al: Screening for multiple endocrine neoplasia type 2a with DNA-polymorphism analysis. N Engl J Med 321:996–1001, 1989.

96. Mathew CG, Easton DF, Nakamura Y, Ponder BA: Presymptomatic screening for multiple endocrine neoplasia type 2A with linked DNA markers: The MEN 2A International Collaborative Group. Lancet 337:7–11, 1991.

97. Gagel RF: The impact of gene mapping techniques on the diagnosis of multiple endocrine neoplasia type 2. Trends Endocrinol Metab 2:19–25, 1991.

98. Larsson C, Skogseid B, Oberg K, et al: Multiple endocrine neoplasia type 1 gene maps to chromosome 11 and is lost in insulinoma. Nature 332:85–87, 1988.

99. Takai S, Tateishi H, Nishisho I, et al: Loss of genes on chromosome 22 in medullary thyroid carcinoma and pheochromocytoma. Jpn J Cancer Res 78:894–898, 1987.

100. Mathew CG, Smith BA, Thorpe K, et al: Deletion of genes on chromosome 1 in endocrine neoplasia. Nature 328:524–526, 1987.

101. Taylor LD, Elder FB, Knuth A, Gagel RF: Cytogenetic characterization of two human and three rat medullary thyroid carcinoma cell lines (abstract). Henry Ford Hosp Med J 37:207, 1989.

102. Nelkin BD, de Bustros AC, Mabry M, Baylin SB: The molecular biology of medullary thyroid carcinoma: A model for cancer development and progression. JAMA 261:3130–3135, 1989.

103. Lichter JB, Wu JS, Genel M, et al: Presymptomatic testing using DNA markers for individuals at risk for familial multiple endocrine neoplasia type 2A. J Clin Endocrinol Metab 74:368–373, 1992.

104. Gagel RF, Jackson CE, Block MA, et al: Age-related probability of development of hereditary medullary thyroid carcinoma. J Pediatr 101:941–946, 1982.

105. Body JJ, Heath HI: Nonspecific increases in plasma immunoreactive calcitonin in healthy individuals: Discrimination from medullary thyroid carcinoma by a new extraction technique. Clin Chem 30:511–514, 1984.

106. Miller HH, Melvin KEW, Gibson JM, Tashjian AH Jr: Surgical ap-

proach to early familial medullary carcinoma of the thyroid gland. Am J Surg 123:438–443, 1972.

107. Donovan DT, Gagel RF: Medullary thyroid carcinoma and the multiple endocrine neoplasia syndromes. *In* Falk (ed): Thyroid Disease: Endocrinology, Surgery, Nuclear Medicine, and Radiotherapy. New York, Raven Press, 1990, pp 501–525.

108. Leape LL, Miller HH, Graze K, et al: Total thyroidectomy for occult familial medullary carcinoma of the thyroid in children. J Pediatr Surg 11:831–837, 1976.

109. Graze K, Spiler IJ, Tashjian AH Jr et al: Natural history of familial medullary thyroid carcinoma: Effect of a program for early diagnosis. N Engl J Med 299:980–985, 1978.

110. Raue F, Winter J, Frank RK, et al: Diagnostic procedure before reoperation in patients with medullary thyroid carcinoma. Horm Metab Res Suppl 21:31–34, 1989.

111. Tisell L, Hansson G, Jansson S, Salander H: Reoperation in the treatment of asymptomatic metastasizing medullary thyroid carcinoma. Surgery 99:60–66, 1986.

112. Wells SA Jr, Baylin SB, Johnsrude IS, et al: Thyroid venous catheterization in the early diagnosis of familial medullary thyroid carcinoma. Ann Surg 196:505–511, 1982.

113. Mrad MDB, Gardet P, Roche A, et al: Value of venous catheterization and calcitonin studies in the treatment and management of clinically inapparent medullary thyroid carcinoma. Cancer 63:133–138, 1989.

114. Lupoli G, Lombardi G, Panza N, et al: (^{131}I)Metaiodobenzylguanidine scintigraphy and selective venous catheterization after thyroidectomy for medullary thyroid carcinoma. Med Oncol Tumor Pharmacother 8:7–13, 1991.

115. Itoh H, Sugie K, Toyooka S, et al: Detection of metastatic medullary thyroid cancer with ^{131}I-MIBG scans in Sipple's syndrome. Eur J Nucl Med 11:502–504, 1986.

116. Becker W, Borner W, Reiners C: Tc-99m-(V)-DMSA: The new sensitive and specific radiopharmaceutical for imaging metastases of medullary thyroid carcinomas? Horm Metab Res Suppl 21:38–42, 1989.

117. Clarke S, Lazarus C, Maisey M: Experience in imaging medullary thyroid carcinoma using [99m]Tc (V) dimercaptosuccinic acid (DMSA). Henry Ford Hosp Med J 37:167–168, 1989.

118. Lamberts SW, Bakker WH, Reubi JC, Krenning EP: Somatostatin-receptor imaging in the localization of endocrine tumors. N Engl J Med 323:1246–1249, 1990.

119. Tibblin S, Dymling JF, Ingemansson S, Telenius-Berg M: Unilateral versus bilateral adrenalectomy in multiple endocrine neoplasia IIA. World J Surg 7:201–208, 1983.

120. van Heerden JA, Sizemore GW, Carney JA, et al: Surgical management of the adrenal glands in the multiple endocrine neoplasia type II syndrome. World J Surg 8:612–621, 1984.

121. Jansson S, Tisell LE, Fjalling M, et al: Early diagnosis of and surgical strategy for adrenal medullary disease in MEN II gene carriers. Surgery 103:11–18, 1988.

122. Moraca Kvapilova L, Op de Coul AA, Merkus JM: Cerebral haemorrhage in a pregnant woman with a multiple endocrine neoplasia syndrome (type 2A or Sipple's syndrome). Eur J Obstet Gynecol Reprod Biol 20:257–263, 1985.

123. Chodankar CM, Abhyankar SC, Deodhar KP, Shanbhag AM: Sipple's syndrome (multiple endocrine neoplasia) in pregnancy: Case report. Aust NZ J Obstet Gynaecol 22:243–244, 1982.

124. Mallette LE, Blevins T, Jordan PH, Noon GP: Autogenous parathyroid grafts for generalized primary parathyroid hyperplasia: Contrasting outcome in sporadic hyperplasia versus multiple endocrine neoplasia type I. Surgery 101:738–745, 1987.

125. Wells SA Jr, Ellis GJ, Gunnells JC, et al: Parathyroid autotransplantation in primary parathyroid hyperplasia. N Engl J Med 195:57–62, 1976.

152

Endocrine Management of Malignant Disease

MARC E. LIPPMAN
EDWARD P. GELMANN

It is highly appropriate to include a chapter on the endocrine management of malignant disease in a textbook of endocrinology. Endocrinologists have long been closely involved in some of the most exciting developments in the therapy of human cancer. Many malignant counterparts of normal tissues provide extremely useful model systems for the study of hormone action. It is difficult to imagine that our understanding of the mechanisms of action of estrogens, androgens, and glucocorticoids would be nearly so far advanced without both in vivo and in vitro model systems for breast cancer, prostatic cancer, and leukemia and lymphoma. With the increasingly complex nature of cancer therapy and the constant search for less toxic treatments, it is reasonable for the oncologist and the endocrinologist to combine forces in attempting to both increase survival and improve the quality of life of patients with cancer.

While the general idea that some human neoplasms may be responsive to a variety of endocrine manipulations has been recognized for nearly a century, the precise role of hormones in the carcinogenic process and in the promotion of cancer growth is incompletely understood. It is widely appreciated that certain tissues of the body are under rigorous endocrine control. These obviously include breast, endometrium, and prostate, which are also sites of cancer that are of enormous public health importance. It is also known that malignancies arising from these tissues retain, to varying extents, the growth-regulatory responses of the normal tissues to endocrine manipulations, which provides an obvious basis for many successful endocrine therapies. This is, however, a substantial oversimplification of the role of hormones in human malignancy.

Responses are seen to a variety of endocrine therapies for which no obvious physiological equivalent is now known. Frequently, these responses are induced at concentrations of hormones which vastly exceed normal circulating levels and which induce effects opposite to those seen when replacement doses are provided. High concentrations of estrogens and progestins can induce worthwhile regressions of some human breast cancers. The mechanisms of these paradoxical responses to high concentrations of steroids remain mysterious. While it is common to consider the list of tumors that are hormone-responsive to be restricted to leukemia, lymphoma, and those of breast, endometrium, and prostate, this too is a very substantial oversimplification. Virtually all normal and malignant cell lines in culture can be shown to have complex hormonal requirements for their growth. A large number of specific growth factors—including insulin, insulin-like growth factors, epidermal growth factor, fibroblast growth factor, glucocorticoids, platelet-derived growth factor, and others—have all been shown to alter substantially the growth rate of many different cell lines in culture. Receptors for these hormones have been found to be equally widespread among many different varieties of cancer. While discussion of specific tumor-related growth factors such as the transforming growth factors will not be included in this chapter, it is well worth bearing in mind that most human cancers retain some degree of hormonal responsiveness, at least as evidenced by factor dependency in vitro, and may yet become candidates for therapies that attempt to alter the growth-promoting properties of their milieu in vivo.

The precise role of hormones in the evolution of a clinical cancer is complicated and probably different for different tumors. One can identify at least three sites of action of hormones that are likely to be important in the eventual development of gross malignancy. First, there is direct evidence that steroidal and nonsteroidal estrogens may function as true carcinogens. That is, they are capable of forming covalent adducts to DNA and, by this primary modification of the DNA structure as well as the resultant repair process set in motion, can induce mutations that may eventually lead to heritable expression of a malignant phenotype. Second, hormones clearly can function as promoters of some previously occurring carcinogenic event.

There are many examples both in animal models and from epidemiological studies which suggest that a tumor will not appear if hormonal stimulation is withdrawn following exposure to a carcinogen. Third, it is likely that hormones may play a permissive role in allowing carcinogenic events to occur. In this scenario, unless the target tissue is under hormonal stimulation, the carcinogen is ineffective. This may conceivably result from alterations in chromatin structure following hormonal stimulation which render those growth-regulatory genes under hormonal control accessible to carcinogenic action. A straightforward illustration of these processes is provided by carcinogen-induced breast cancers in rats. In this setting, the carcinogen dimethylbenzanthracene is ineffective if given to sexually immature animals. Similarly, it is ineffective if castration is performed following its administration to sexually mature animals. Tumors are seen only when sexually mature animals are treated with a carcinogen followed by continuous physiological exposure to sex steroids. Thus separate carcinogenic, promoter, and permissive actions of sex steroids can be identified in the evolution of cancer.

In this chapter we will consider four major endocrine-responsive tumors: breast cancer, endometrial cancer, carcinoma of the prostate, and leukemia and lymphoma. Thyroid cancer is excluded from this discussion because of its detailed consideration in Chapter 50. Although the number of hormone-regulated tumors is likely to be greater than these four groups of tumors, the most information available is about them, and for this reason, they provide useful paradigms for further work with other malignancies. Finally, endocrine therapy will be considered only in the context of management of these tumors. Glucocorticoids will not be discussed as nonspecific mood-elevating drugs or as drugs to avoid toxicity in prevention of either emesis from chemotherapy or cerebral edema following irradiation. Neither will androgens be considered as general anabolic agents or for simulation of hematopoiesis. These highly specific indications are more within the province of specialized cancer care and do not contribute much to the general principles of endocrine therapy of malignancy to be discussed here.

BREAST CANCER

In 1992, breast cancer was the second leading cause of cancer death in women (barely second to lung cancer). In 1992, there were approximately 180,000 newly diagnosed cases in the United States; approximately 40,000 will eventually prove fatal. The median age for developing breast cancer is the mid-50's, and it is therefore certain that even more women will eventually die of metastatic disease if they survive long enough. Unlike colon or lung cancer, in which 5-year survival without recurrence is essentially equivalent to cure, breast cancer continues to recur up to 25 years following primary diagnosis. Enormous attention has been focused on the crucial role of endocrine factors in the etiology of this disease. Given the current limitations on successful control of both localized and systemic breast cancer, rational endocrine approaches to disease prevention are of great interest. For this reason, we will briefly summarize some of the epidemiological data with respect to breast cancer risk, particularly as they pertain to endo-

crine factors. This will next lead to identification of those factors which suggest that clinically apparent breast cancer remains responsive to endocrine manipulations. Finally, a discussion of endocrine therapies of proven value for the management and prevention of breast cancer will be provided.

Epidemiology

The epidemiology of breast cancer in women has been studied extensively, and while many controversies yet remain to be resolved, a variety of important risk factors are widely agreed on.[1-3] Among the most important predictors of risk are sex, age, height, weight, age at menarche and menopause, age at birth of first child, country of origin, dietary factors, and a family history of breast cancer. In addition, certain exogenous factors such as hormone exposure are clearly of great importance. Many of these risk factors are interdependent, and it appears likely that the majority are related through endocrine factors. An understanding of the mechanisms by which these various risk factors increase breast cancer incidence is of extraordinary importance, since prophylactic endocrine measures of real significance may result. Unfortunately, although the impact of these risk factors is great, no risk factor, taken either by itself or in combination with others, is sufficiently discriminatory at the present time to identify women in whom special therapy aimed at intervention is warranted. This is particularly true given that therapeutic intervention at the present time is limited to prophylactic mastectomy in one of its various forms. The only exception to this is the very high risk to kindreds or women with first-degree relatives (mothers or sisters) with bilateral premenopausal breast cancer, for whom the risk of breast cancer may be as high as 65 per cent. Recent studies have identified several putative genes involved in familial breast cancer. Studies by Friend and colleagues have shown that the Li-Fraumeni syndrome, which includes breast cancer, is caused by an inherited mutation in one allele of the *p53* gene, which is a tumor suppressor gene. Somatic loss of function or mutation of the other allele leads to malignancy. King and co-workers have described a dominantly acting gene on 17q.[4] The precise sequence of this gene will be an invaluable aid in counseling relatives of patients with breast cancer. Furthermore, the absence of any known risk factors is not sufficient to rule out the possibility of breast cancer in a woman with a suspicious lump. Therefore, at the present time, the diagnostic approach to patients should be almost entirely without regard to a history of risk factors.

A detailed consideration of these risk factors is beyond the scope of this chapter, but brief information will be provided concerning four general groupings of risk factors in which endocrine influences almost certainly play a substantial role. These are reproductive history, international variation, familial clustering, and the endocrine environment.

Reproductive and menstrual history has been examined in numerous studies. Age at menarche is an important determinant of breast cancer risk. Women who begin menstruating at an earlier age have a higher risk of breast cancer. Thus, if onset of menses at age 13 or older is assigned a relative risk of 1, then women who begin menstruating before age 12 have nearly a two-fold increase in relative risk.[5] In addition, the interval from menarche to the establishment of regular cycles is also important. Women who take longer to establish regular menses have a decreased risk of breast cancer compared with women who develop regular cycles earlier.[6] Similarly, age of menopause is also an important factor for breast cancer risk. It has been estimated by Trichopolous and colleagues[7] that women whose natural menopause occurs before age 45 have only one half the risk of breast cancer of those whose menopause occurs after age 55. Surgical menopause is protective against breast cancer in proportion to the reduction in years of menstrual life.

Parity is also of crucial importance in estimating breast cancer risk. If one arbitrarily assigns a relative risk of 1 to nulliparous women, then there is nearly a threefold variation in risk of breast cancer varying from 0.5 for women who have their first child before age 15 to their first child after age 37.[8] It is interesting that this protective effect of early pregnancy and delivery is maintained throughout life, even among women age 70 and older. Pike and colleagues[5] recently have made the disturbing observation that a first-trimester abortion, whether spontaneous or induced, which occurs prior to a full-term pregnancy is associated with a substantial increase in breast cancer risk, whereas abortions after the first full-term pregnancy do not alter the risk of breast cancer. While the effects of parity, menarche, and menopause have been widely recognized, the enormous contribution that they might make to breast cancer risk when considered collectively had probably not been sufficiently appreciated until Pike and colleagues proposed a very thought-provoking means of explaining international variation with respect to breast cancer on these bases. In their proposal, early menarche and the length of menstrual life prior to first pregnancy are particularly important risk factors.[9] Since dietary practices are also likely to influence height and weight and thereby the onset and regularity of menses, this is a convenient way to incorporate multiple risk factors into a single hypothesis.

DeWaard and colleagues[10] demonstrated the important impact of height and weight on breast cancer risk. Of great interest is their observation that while an increased body weight (>70 kg versus <60 kg) can approximately double the breast cancer risk, this increase is limited exclusively to postmenopausal women, and the risk increases with age.[3, 11] These data are consistent with the general view that the etiology of pre- and postmenopausal breast cancers may be somewhat different, with the latter having the greater dependence on external endocrine factors.

International variation of breast cancer risk around the world[3, 11] is an enormously important epidemiological finding. For example, the incidence of breast cancer for women who are 50 years old is about six times higher in the United States than in Japan or Taiwan. For postmenopausal women, the difference increases to nearly 20-fold. While this might initially be interpreted as evidence for a genetic basis for breast cancer risk, this hypothesis has largely been discarded. This is based on numerous studies of the descendants of Chinese or Japanese people living in Western communities. In these observations, second-generation Japanese or Chinese have a breast cancer risk equivalent to that of the Caucasian individuals living in their surrounding communities.[12] It is of interest that the incidence of breast cancer in Japan is increasing rapidly.

This fits the hypothesis of Pike and colleagues[9] that altered dietary habits clearly lead to increased height and weight and early onset of menstruation and could result in increased breast cancer risk. These kinds of data lead one to the inescapable conclusion that environmental factors, most probably diet in the broadest sense, are responsible for nearly 90 per cent of all the breast cancer cases seen in the United States.

Studies of international variation also emphasize the potential difference between pre- and postmenopausal breast cancer. In those countries in which a high incidence of breast cancer has been observed, risk increases with age such that by age 50, the breast cancer risk in the United States is approximately 80 per 100,000 women but by age 70 rises to 350 per 100,000.

In low-risk countries, the rate of development of breast cancer decreases after menopause. This is further evidence in support of deWaard's observation that pre- and postmenopausal breast cancer may have different etiologies and that the chronic effects of some endocrine factor mediated through diet, height and weight, and menstrual history may alter the incidence of postmenopausal breast cancer.[10]

Family history is a major contributor to breast cancer risk.[13] Many patients and physicians overinterpret these data and presume that any relative with a history of breast cancer has an important impact on the eventual likelihood of developing breast cancer, which is not true. Breast cancer risk is primarily determined by a history in first-degree relatives. While the increase in risk is approximately two- to threefold for women with a single postmenopausal first-degree relative with breast cancer, it may rise to ninefold (approximately 65 per cent) in cases in which the first-degree relative is premenopausal and has bilateral breast cancer. It is not clear how much of this increase in familial risk may be attributed to shared environmental factors and how much to genetic predisposition. Unfortunately, studies of these patients from an endocrine point of view with respect to differences in prolactin and gonadotropins, estrogens, etc. have been almost completely negative. While older data were most consistent with an autosomal dominant mode of inheritance,[14] as mentioned earlier in this chapter, at least one specific gene responsible for familial breast cancer has been identified by segregation analysis.[4, 15]

If endocrine factors are important in the etiology of breast cancer, one would expect that either important endogenous differences in hormone levels would exist or that exogenous hormone administration would be an important risk factor between patients developing breast cancer and normal controls.

Since a promotional relationship between breast cancer and estrogen seems likely, the measurement of urinary estrogens was undertaken by several groups. There were, however, no consistent or reproducible differences between women with breast cancer and those in the normal population. These studies suffer from the shortcoming that estrogens should have been measured at the time of carcinogenesis rather than at some stage of clinical disease. Further, the large fluctuations in estrogen levels during the menstrual cycle and the alterations in route of metabolism with disease or with drugs make interpretation difficult. A recent review of this area generally concludes that hormonal patterns of presumptively high-risk groups of women did not differ from those of the normal population.[16]

As a result of some previous work suggesting that estriol is an estrogen antagonist, considerable attention was given to data showing a decreased risk for breast cancer in women with a high urinary excretion of estriol.[17] In support of this hypothesis was the finding that Japanese women (a low-risk group) had higher urinary estriol excretion than did Australian women.[18] However, this hypothesis should be abandoned for the following reasons: First, estriol is an estrogen whose receptor-binding characteristics make it act as an antagonist only when it is given intermittently with simultaneous administration of more potent estrogens.[19] When given continuously, it is a potent estrogen and will act as a promoter of mammary gland carcinogenesis in experimental systems. Second, continuous exposure to estriol can be shown to directly stimulate hormone-responsive human breast cancer.[20] Third, urinary estriol has no relationship to plasma estriol concentrations or production rates.[21] Further, the ratio of estriol to estrone plus estradiol is not related to differences between estrogen blood levels and production rates in normal women or in women with breast cancer. Henderson and colleagues[22] have found recently that teenage daughters of patients with breast cancer had significantly elevated estradiol and estrone concentrations compared with age-matched controls. Differences were quantitatively small, but the impact of such differences added over decades is difficult to assess.

Other work supports the idea that abnormalities in estrogen contribute to the development of breast cancer. Korenman and colleagues[23] suggest that unopposed estrogen action is a major risk factor. Their "estrogen window" hypothesis is based on five premises:

1. Human breast cancer is induced by carcinogens in a susceptible (i.e., a hormone-primed) mammary gland.

2. Unopposed estrogenic stimulation favors tumor induction.

3. There is a long latency between tumor induction and clinical disease.

4. The duration of the estrogen window is proportional to breast cancer risk.

5. Inducibility declines with establishment of normal ovulatory menses and becomes very low during pregnancy.

This hypothesis does not fit well with the epidemiological data of Pike and colleagues,[5] who found irregular (and presumably anovulatory) menses to be associated with a decreased breast cancer risk. Brown[24] reviewed daily endocrine profiles in young women entering puberty, during normal menstrual life, and at menopause. These studies document multiple anovulatory cycles at either extreme of menstrual life and provide a biological basis for Korenman's hypothesis.

Finally, Siiteri and colleagues re-examined the question of serum estrogen concentrations in breast cancer.[25, 26] They found that while total serum estrogen concentrations may be normal in women with breast cancer, abnormally high free estrogen concentrations occur owing to decreased plasma binding. The latter results both from a decrease in sex hormone–binding globulin (SHBG) or possibly in some cases because of an abnormal SHBG. More recently, it has been suggested that these differences

are due to sample storage. Further developments in this area should be followed closely.

The exact role of prolactin in the etiology of breast cancer in women remains controversial. Some investigators have found abnormalities in prolactin in patients with breast cancer,[5, 27] as well as in their daughters.[28] Others failed to detect significant abnormalities.[29] One excellent review of the subject[30] concluded that prolactin abnormalities are probably associated with breast cancer risk, but whether causally or not remains to be determined.

As will be discussed later, however, there is virtually no evidence that a significant subset of established breast cancers is dependent on prolactin as a trophic hormone.

Abnormalities of thyroid function, usually goiter or hypothyroidism, have been reported to be increased in patients with breast cancer. However, at least two critical reviews of this area[3, 31] failed to support these contentions. At present, little evidence links any thyroid abnormality to an altered breast cancer risk.

Studies of exogenous hormone administration are also confusing. Multiple retrospective case-control studies failed to reveal a significant overall increase in risk of developing breast cancer among oral contraceptive users.[32, 33] However, several observations prevent a totally sanguine view of this conclusion. In general, the time required for tumor promotion in humans is long, and there may not be sufficient experience as yet for firm conclusions. Two studies of younger women showed a relative risk ratio of 1.7 for users of oral contraceptives for more than 8 and 5 years, respectively,[34, 35] although this increase was not statistically significant. Two other studies failed to show an increase in risk with passage of time.[36, 37] However, in one of these studies,[37] oral contraceptives increased the risk of breast cancer in three subsets of patients—nulliparous women, women using the pill prior to the birth of their first child, and women with a history of benign breast disease.

Three major exceptions may exist. Women with previous benign breast disease may have striking increases in breast cancer risk following oral contraceptive use.[5, 38] Pike and colleagues[12] and others[39, 40] have shown that oral contraceptive use at either the beginning or the end of menstrual life may dramatically increase breast cancer risk. Thus the relative risk for women using oral contraceptives between the ages of 46 and 50 was 2.4 and 4 in the two studies cited. For women using oral contraceptives for more than 8 years prior to their first full-term pregnancy, the relative risk was 3.5. These data are badly in need of confirmation. They appear to be in direct conflict with the estrogen window hypothesis and imply an important promotional role for progestins. This fits the data of Fergusson and Anderson,[41] who found that cell division in the human breast is higher during the luteal phase. This area should be watched closely.

There have been many retrospective analyses of women using estrogens after the menopause, and few show a significant association between use and breast cancer risk.[33–35, 42] In one large retrospective study,[43] a relative risk ratio of 1.3 (of borderline statistical significance) was found for estrogen users. More alarmingly, risk was related to duration of administration, with a doubling of this risk ratio after 12 years of use. No follow-up of oral contraceptive users of this duration is available. A recent National Institutes of Health (NIH) study revealed a significant dose-dependent increase in breast cancer among users of menopausal estrogens.[44] The risk was greatest in women who took the highest-strength preparation, although it was not related to duration of use. Several recent well-done studies suggest small but significant (1.3 to 2) relative risk increases in long-term and high-dose users.[45–48] A recent meta-analysis of this subject clearly demonstrates a time- and dose-response relationship between postmenopausal estrogen replacement and breast cancer. While estrogen replacement therapy increases breast cancer incidence, this increase must be weighed carefully against the symptomatic benefits enjoyed by patients with significant menopausal symptoms and the objective benefits of reduction in cardiovascular and osteopenic events.[49] Many have advocated discontinuation of therapy, cyclical therapy with or without intermittent progestins, or low-dose therapy. None of these additional recommendations has been proven to either increase or decrease risk, nor is it possible to assess alternative repercussions of such therapeutic interventions on such conditions as osteoporosis or cardiovascular disease, for which postmenopausal hormone replacement therapy can be of real benefit. Particularly alarming is one report in which the addition of progestin to estrogen replacement therapy was associated with a substantial increase in breast cancer.[50] It remains to be confirmed whether a maneuver which clearly prevents estrogen replacement therapy–induced endometrial cancer results in an increase in breast cancer. To some extent, these issues may require individual considerations because of differences in risk for various diseases associated with estrogens.

Hormone Receptors and Endocrine Therapy of Breast Cancer

Human breast cancers have been known to respond to endocrine manipulations since Beatson[51] induced tumor regressions in patients following bilateral oophorectomy. Patients who respond to endocrine therapy not only have disease palliation but also a substantially longer survival rate than nonresponders. Unfortunately, only about one third of unselected patients show objective tumor regressions following hormonal therapy. With the advent of effective chemotherapy regimens, a more precise selection of different treatment modalities is necessary, since acceptable alternatives exist.

Several empirically derived clinical guidelines (long disease-free intervals, nonvisceral sites of involvement, good performance status), as well as a few biochemical tests (excretion of androgen metabolites, steroid sulfation), have been suggested as being of value in selecting patients with hormone-responsive tumors. None of these approaches is sufficiently reliable for treatment decision making. Developments in the field of hormone action have brought more accurate means of patient selection.

The first step in steroid hormone action in general, and estrogen action in particular, is the binding of the hormone to a specific receptor protein. Functional receptor molecules are a necessary, albeit insufficient, requirement for steroid hormone action.[52] In animal systems, regression of mammary cancer in response to hormonal therapy requires the presence of estrogen receptors.[53, 54] Subsequently, human breast cancer samples were shown to take up and specifically retain estrogen.[55, 56] Later, Jensen and colleagues[57] found specific estrogen-binding activity in human breast cancers and showed direct correlations between the presence of estrogen receptor and the likelihood of response to endocrine therapy.

Because of the clinical importance of these assays, they have been the focus of intense investigation. Comprehensive reviews of this field are available.[58–60] About two thirds of primary breast cancers contain significant concentrations of estrogen receptor, while a somewhat smaller proportion of metastatic samples are positive for estrogen receptor. Premenopausal patients have tumors that are less frequently estrogen receptor–positive and generally contain lower concentrations of receptor. These observations are only partially explained by the larger amounts of endogenous estrogen in plasma of premenopausal women which may mask the binding sites. Overall, there is a highly significant association between the presence of estrogen receptor and the likelihood of response to endocrine therapy. Predictive accuracy for the test is about 75 per cent. Thus about 60 per cent of the 60 per cent of patients with estrogen receptor–positive tumors respond to endocrine therapy, while 95 per cent of the 40 per cent of patients with estrogen receptor–negative tumors fail to respond. The greater the estrogen receptor content of the tumor, the higher is the response rate to endocrine therapy. Although the accuracy of estrogen receptor assays in selecting therapy for patients with advanced disease is substantial, a potentially more valuable use of these tests may be in selecting appropriate adjuvant regimens for patients with breast cancer. In this setting, correct therapy selection is particularly important for two reasons. First, there is no objective evidence on which to base conclusions concerning response to treatment, since the first indication of inadequate therapy is recurrence. Second, since adjuvant therapy has been shown to have survival benefit in some patient subgroups, others may be disadvantaged by adjuvant endocrine therapy, and all are at risk for toxicity,[61, 62] accurate assays are mandatory. Recently, substantially more attention has been paid to uniformity of assay and to quality control.[63]

While the response rate of tumors apparently lacking estrogen receptors is low, it is not zero. Therefore, a single negative assay should be considered as only one component in the selection of appropriate therapy. There are several explanations for the observation of an endocrine response in women with purportedly estrogen receptor–negative tumors. First, steroid receptors are thermolabile proteins; many methodological pitfalls may prevent detection of receptor activity. Particularly common problems include incorrect handling and storage of samples. Second, a pathological diagnosis of metastatic breast cancer may be based on a few tumor cells infiltrating nonmalignant tissue. A negative assay may result from an insufficient sampling of malignant cells or even inadvertent biopsy of neighboring nonmalignant tissue. Third, a variety of additive and ablative therapies employed in patients with breast cancer may act by mechanisms mediated by other receptors. Thus, even in the absence of estrogen receptor, a response to some endocrine manipulations may be observed. Fourth, breast tumors are heterogeneous with respect to receptor status; thus a biopsied site that is estrogen receptor–negative may not be representative of other tumor deposits. Fifth, it is possible that some assays are falsely negative, since most estrogen receptor analyses are performed on cytoplasmic extracts using conditions that do not permit detection of nuclear receptor sites occupied by endogenous hormone. Histochemical assays, while theoretically overcoming these disadvantages, are not as reliable. This can occur during the luteal phase of the menstrual cycle, during pregnancy, or while on exogenous hormone replacement. Sixth, it has been shown that even in the absence of endogenous hormone, receptor sites may be localized to the nucleus[64] and therefore may be missed by standard methodologies. It is thus somewhat surprising how rarely (about 5 per cent) so-called estrogen receptor–negative tumors respond to endocrine therapy. Recently, Fuqua and colleagues[65] have described a series of receptor mutants that have interesting properties. Some are hormone-binding mutants but still capable of activating transcription, while others retain ligand-binding sites but cannot activate transcription. The quantitative contribution of these mutants to altered hormone responsivity is unknown.

More commonly, tumors that contain estrogen receptor fail to respond to endocrine therapy. The most commonly invoked explanation for this observation is tumor cell heterogeneity. That is, a sufficient number of cells within the tumor sample contain receptor to give a positive assay result, although the majority are receptor-negative. This is supported by the quantitative relationship between the concentration of estrogen receptor and the likelihood of observing an endocrine response.[66] Direct observation of tumor samples using monoclonal antibodies directed against the estrogen receptor is also consistent with tumor heterogeneity.[67, 68] Second, the presence of estrogen receptor is generally correlated with a variety of endocrine therapies. If, for example, androgen administration induces tumor regression by a process involving interaction with androgen receptor, then some estrogen receptor–positive, androgen receptor–negative tumors might fail to respond to the endocrine therapy. Third, the presence of receptor may indicate hormone-dependent breast cancer, but the endocrine therapy may not sufficiently alter the hormonal milieu. For example, pituitary ablation may be incomplete. Additionally, it is well known that about 5 to 10 per cent of patients with metastatic breast cancer who fail to respond to oophorectomy will respond to a subsequent adrenalectomy. Presumably these patients can be assumed to have had hormone-dependent tumors at the time of their oophorectomy, and thus their tumors would have been estrogen receptor–positive pseudo-hormone–independent. Fourth, any step distal to the initial binding of hormone to receptor may be deranged. Binding of hormone to receptor is only the first step in hormone action.[52] Prediction of hormone dependence could be achieved more certainly if a tumor were assessed for a hormone-inducible function; this obviously presupposes the presence of receptor.

Overwhelmingly, the most useful test of estrogen receptor function is determination of the progesterone receptor.[58, 59] In both normal uterus and malignantly transformed uterine and mammary tissues, progesterone receptor synthesis is regulated by estrogen action through the estrogen receptor. Tumors lacking estrogen receptor are virtually never progesterone receptor–positive, whereas about two thirds of estrogen receptor–positive tumors are progesterone receptor–positive. Estrogen receptor–positive tumors lacking progesterone receptor respond to endocrine therapy about one third of the time (the same overall response rate seen in a cohort of unselected patients). The response rate to endocrine therapy in patients whose tumors contain both estrogen and progesterone receptors exceeds 75 per cent. Some of the responses seen in women whose tumors were categorized as being estrogen receptor–positive and progesterone receptor–negative can be explained on two bases. First, in premenopausal women during the later phase of their menstrual cycle or while pregnant, circulating progesterone concentrations may occupy receptor, translocate it to the nucleus, and obscure its detection.[69] Second, in some postmenopausal women with hormone-dependent tumors, circulating estrogen levels may be insufficient to induce progesterone receptor levels.[70] Measurement of other estrogen-inducible proteins such as *p52* also has been proposed to discriminate between hormone-responsive and hormone-unresponsive tumors.

Despite the many possible explanations for false-positive and false-negative results, steroid receptor studies in breast cancer are extremely valuable; for the majority of patients, response to endocrine therapy can be predicted with accuracy.

In addition, receptor determinations may be of value as a prognostic aid. Patients with estrogen receptor–positive primary breast cancer have a substantially prolonged disease-free interval independent of other known prognostic variables, including menopausal status, tumor size, histological grade, and axillary lymph node status.[71–75]

The development of specific monoclonal antibodies to the estrogen receptor protein allows detection of the receptor, independent of the binding of labeled hormone by the receptor.[67, 68] This assay, as well as others using immunoperoxidase or immunofluorescence methods, may provide a basis for simple, efficient detection and localization of estrogen receptor in clinical samples.

Management of Breast Cancer

Patterns of cancer management are often surprisingly idiosyncratic. For example, thyroid cancer is commonly managed by endocrinologists, while breast cancer is not. The data discussed here are presented in the hope of fostering closer interactions between these disciplines. Many aspects of the management of breast cancer fall outside the province of the endocrinologist; therefore, in order to place endocrine manipulations in a proper context, it is worthwhile to mention briefly certain aspects of the oncologist's approach to the patient with breast cancer. A reasonably comprehensive review of the subject has just been published.[76]

It is appropriate to divide the management of breast cancer into two phases: the approach to the patient with early-stage disease and the approach to the patient with advanced (metastatic) disease.

Early Breast Cancer

Nearly 90 per cent of women who develop breast cancer in the United States will initially present with apparently localized stage I or II disease. That is, clinical disease is confined to the breast and possibly to the ipsilateral axillary nodes. Many decisions concerning a variety of surgical and radiotherapeutic options need to be considered, and these should be separated in time from an initial diagnostic biopsy. Patients should be encouraged to seek out additional opinions concerning the therapy options available to them rather than being rushed into the first treatment plan suggested to them. Adequate staging is mandatory. All women with early breast cancer should have an estrogen receptor assay, if at all possible, on material obtained at biopsy or mastectomy. The assay has prognostic significance, as already mentioned. Adjuvant endocrine therapy decisions are also influenced by estrogen receptor status. Other data suggest that the estrogen receptor status of the primary cancer is likely to be maintained in the metastases. Thus knowledge of the receptor status of the primary tumor permits assignment to the appropriate treatment category when metastases develop, even if there is no readily accessible tissue for biopsy at that time.

Patients require therapy directed at the primary tumor which not only is sufficient for local control of disease but, at the same time, is as attentive as possible to cosmetic outcome. This is an area of active investigation, and therapy is becoming more individualized. Recently completed studies indicate that less than total mastectomy is equivalent to mastectomy for most patients.[77] Most (but not all) women who are adequately informed of their options will choose a breast-conservative procedure. Shockingly—although there are substantial regional differences—only about one third of United States women avoid mastectomy. Patients require adequate staging, including assessment of axillary lymph node involvement with tumor. On the basis of this evaluation, adjuvant therapy regimens are often indicated, although their exact role in individual subsets of patients remains to be completely defined. The current status of adjuvant endocrine therapy will be discussed. Close attention to a rapidly changing literature is important.[78, 79]

Metastatic Breast Cancer

Many patients with primary breast cancer will remain free of disease following local therapy (with or without the addition of systemic adjuvant therapy). Unfortunately, the disease recurs in more than 40,000 patients each year. At this time endocrine therapy is one of several possible options. Only about one third of unselected patients can be expected to achieve a partial response or better. The emphasis is on the word *unselected,* because with appropriate consideration of steroid receptor status and other prognostic variables, substantial improvement in response rates can be achieved. Following appropriate assessment of receptor status, patients may be assigned to differing treatment regimens. Obviously, other factors must be weighed in such decision making, including prognostic variables, such as performance status and sites of involvement, and issues involving individual patients, such as the relative impact of various treatment modalities on lifestyle. Furthermore, there is substantial latitude of choice for endocrine therapies, with emphasis on the use of antiestrogens and inhibitors of endogenous steroidogenesis and aromatization, since these provide the least toxicity without sacrificing efficacy.

Endocrine Therapy of Breast Cancer

Ablative Therapies

OOPHORECTOMY. Removal of the ovaries of premenopausal patients was first shown to be effective treatment for some women with inoperable breast cancer 80 years ago.[51] Using strict criteria, the regression rate is 25 to 30 per cent,[80, 81] and the median duration of remission is 9 months. Interpretation of absolute response rate and comparisons between different studies are extremely difficult. An enormous number of selection biases may strongly influence the apparent success of an endocrine therapy in breast cancer. Aside from the presence of estrogen and progesterone receptors in a tumor sample, good performance status, lack of visceral metastases, a long interval from local therapy to first recurrence, and response to previous endocrine therapy all tend to be correlated with response to endocrine therapy. Surgical ablation is the method of choice, since radiation may require several weeks to be effective and incomplete destruction of the follicles has been reported.

It is important to be able to accurately evaluate ovarian status. A high plasma follicle-stimulating hormone (FSH) level or a low plasma estradiol (<20 pg/ml) level is characteristic of cessation of ovarian function. In perimenopausal and postmenopausal patients, the regression rate from oophorectomy is well below that of women with ovarian function.[82] The use of oophorectomy by itself as an adjuvant to locoregional management of breast cancer is undergoing a re-evaluation. Although a drastic approach, recent meta-analysis has suggested that not only is the disease-free interval prolonged, but there is a significant improvement in survival following prophylactic castration. Early information from the Southwest Oncology Group's randomized comparison of five-drug chemotherapy with or without oophorectomy for estrogen receptor–positive premenopausal patients with axillary lymph node involvement also suggests a significant survival benefit for women receiving drugs plus oophorectomy.

In one trial of unique importance,[83] the addition of low daily doses of prednisone to oophorectomy led to a statistically significant improvement in survival in premenopausal women as compared with women treated with oophorectomy alone. The mechanism for this improved result versus oophorectomy alone is not clear but probably represents the additional benefit of some degree of adrenal suppression.

Currently, a reassessment of the role of oophorectomy as first-line endocrine therapy in premenopausal patients is underway. Further information will be found in the section on antiestrogens.

ADRENALECTOMY AND HYPOPHYSECTOMY. Estrogens persist in blood and urine after oophorectomy. The adrenal cortex secretes a small amount of estrone,[84] but the main source of estrone after castration is the transformation of androstenedione, secreted by the adrenal cortex, to estrone in peripheral tissues, including breast.[85] These low concentrations of estradiol and estrone characteristic of menopause are sufficient to support the growth of endocrine-sensitive tumors. Human breast cancer cells in culture respond to as little as 2 to 3×10^{-11} M estradiol.[86]

The absence of an estrogen receptor in tumor tissue, predicting that adrenalectomy will fail to be beneficial, is additional evidence for this concept.

While the mechanism of response to adrenalectomy appears to be removal of an additional source of estrogens, the mechanism of response to hypophysectomy is more obscure. Many patients respond because of the removal of ACTH, as demonstrated by the fact that the response to adrenalectomy is quite low after hypophysectomy. Lowering prolactin is probably not the means of response, since equivalent response rates are seen with pituitary stalk section, which actually raises plasma prolactin levels. Administration of prolactin-lowering agents such as L-dopa or bromocriptine is unsuccessful in treating breast cancer. Other incompletely characterized hypothalamic and pituitary peptides may well play important roles in regulation of tumor growth.[87] A re-evaluation of the role of growth hormone is warranted. Most breast cancers have insulin-like growth factor I (IGF-I) receptors and, at least in vitro, respond to IGF-IB. Further, as discussed later, there are responses to somatostatin administration.

The criteria for selecting patients for adrenalectomy or hypophysectomy are several. First, if an estrogen receptor can be identified in the metastatic tissue, then the chance of response is about 60 per cent. Whether these two criteria identify the same patients is not known, but it is likely. As with other endocrine therapies, a long disease-free interval, nonvisceral metastases, and good performance status increase response rate. Adrenalectomy can now be achieved by medical means (as discussed below). Direct comparison of medical and surgical adrenalectomy suggests that response rates and duration are approximately equivalent.

The rate of response to adrenalectomy or hypophysectomy has been variously estimated as equal to or somewhat in favor of hypophysectomy. The mean duration of remission in one study was longer after hypophysectomy (15 versus 8 months).[88] Although these data suggest that hypophysectomy may offer some advantages, the choice of operation usually must be made on the basis of more pragmatic considerations, such as the surgical skills available, the sites of metastases, and the age of the patient. The management of adrenal or pituitary insufficiency following ablative surgery should be carefully attended to. It is necessary only to state that the patient can be treated adequately in either case and, when a remission occurs, can often resume full activity. Rare spontaneous regressions of breast cancer have been shown to result from malignant destruction of ovaries or adrenal glands. For reasons more pertaining to adverse complications, surgical ablative procedures have been performed far less frequently in recent years.

Additive Therapies

ANDROGEN THERAPY. Lacassagne was the first to show that the growth of murine mammary tumors could be inhibited by testosterone propionate.[89] Androgen therapy of women with metastatic cancer was initiated 30 years ago. The mechanism by which androgens induce responses in women with breast cancer is unknown. An excellent review has weighed various possibilities.[90] Some tumors have androgen receptors,[91, 92] but their role in mediating the response of the tumor to androgens is not established. The overall response rate of 521 patients treated with testosterone propionate was 21 per cent.[93] The response rate was higher in postmenopausal women. Within a year of the menopause, the remission rate was less than 10 per cent, and it was highest 5 years after the menopause. Soft-tissue metastases responded most favorably, visceral metastases the least. The median period of remission was 8 months. Any androgen given in large amounts produces about the same rate of regression.

Testosterone may produce virilization that is severe and often distressing. A synthetic steroid, testolactone, has little or no androgenic activity and inhibits steroid aromatase activity. It has been reported to produce regression of disease.[94] Although the incidence of remissions was low, their occurrence is evidence that antitumor effect can be independent of androgenicity. Danazol also has been shown to be effective in breast cancer and has fewer virilizing effects.[95–97] One recent trial has shown that combined therapy employing an antiestrogen plus danazol and aminoglutethimide improves the response rate seen with the antiestrogen alone.[98] Despite the improvement in response rate, there was absolutely no improvement in overall survival when the combination was compared with sequential treatments. In fact, survival was somewhat better when these therapies were used sequentially.

ESTROGENS. For reasons that remain obscure, pharmacological concentrations of estrogens may induce remission in 30 to 37 per cent of patients when estrogen is used as the initial therapy.[99, 100] Possible explanations have included down-regulation of estrogen receptors and induction of growth-inhibiting peptides such as mammastatin. The duration of response to estrogen therapy has been longer than that to androgen therapy in most series. The response rate to pharmacological estrogen therapy increases with years after menopause. As with androgen therapy and the ablative procedures, the longer the disease-free interval, the higher is the probability of a therapeutic response to estrogen.

When estrogens are used in patients who have relapsed from other endocrine therapies, remission rates are low—the chances of response being less than 10 per cent. Also, estrogen is generally ineffective following hypophysectomy or adrenalectomy.

The toxicity from estrogens, even at high doses, is moderate. Endometrial hyperplasia and breakthrough bleeding are not uncommon and can usually be managed by giving a progestogen, followed by a short period of cessation of hormone therapy to permit sloughing to the endometrium. Salt and water retention, particularly in the elderly, may occur with any estrogen. Of greatest consequence, however, is hypercalcemia. This can occur abruptly in any patient but is rare in patients 10 or more years postmenopausal. Hypercalcemia almost certainly results from direct tumor stimulation; it is managed by withdrawal of estrogen and by saline diuresis. Mithramycin is not usually needed. Often, on gradual reinstitution of therapy, a regression will be obtained without recurrence of hypercalcemia. Patients developing hypercalcemia eventually have a higher response rate to endocrine therapy than patients who do not.

The phenomenon of a response following withdrawal of estrogen or of androgen has been recorded.[101] Withdrawal responses are more common after an initial response to the additive therapy has occurred; however, they can be seen even in the absence of a primary response. Thus, new attempts at therapy should generally not be started until six weeks after steroids have been stopped, unless clinical deterioration mandates immediate therapy. The mechanism of withdrawal responses is unknown.

PROGESTOGENS. Many progestogens have been used in patients with breast cancer. Their exact mechanism of action is unknown, although possibilities include blockade of progestin receptor, interference with estrogen receptor synthesis, androgen-like effects, and effects on other areas such as the immune system.[90] Remission rates have averaged about 20 per cent.[102] Responses to progestogens may be seen after successful or unsuccessful trials of castration, estrogen, androgen, or antiestrogens. In general, these agents are without important side effects except edema and weight gain. Regression appears to be more common with soft-tissue metastases and unusual with bone metastases. Interest in progestins has been rekindled by investigations using extremely large doses.[103, 104] Response rates of 30 to 40 per cent have been reported without significant toxicity. Randomized comparisons suggest approximately equivalent response rates to antiestrogen therapy, although time to progression and survival may favor tamoxifen therapy.[105] Failure to respond to the primary therapy generally has predicted minimal activity for the second regimen.

GLUCOCORTICOIDS. Large doses of any glucocorticoid (equivalent to 200 to 300 mg of cortisol daily) can induce regression of metastatic breast cancer in 10 to 15 per cent of patients.[106] Remissions are short-lived, but the rapid onset of effect of glucocorticoids makes them useful in rapidly advancing disease. A response to glucocorticoids is not predictive of response to other endocrine modalities. When combined with oophorectomy for early (stage I to II) breast cancer, glucocorticoids are associated with a substantial improvement in survival.[83] Glucocorticoids also have been shown to improve response rate and survival when combined with certain cytotoxic chemotherapy programs.[106] Glucocorticoids are also of value in managing such acute complications as hypercalcemia and intracranial metastases.

Antiestrogen Therapy

Any substance that antagonizes the action of estrogens may be termed an *antiestrogen*. Many compounds fit this definition, including a variety of nonspecific inhibitors of protein and RNA synthesis. However, with the possible exception of certain weak, short-acting agonists, such as estriol, all such compounds of clinical relevance developed thus far are derivatives of triphenylethylene. These include nafoxidine, clomiphene, tamoxifen, and toremifene (a chlorinated triphenylethylene derivative). Several "pure" steroidal antiestrogens devoid of partial agonistic activity are also about to enter clinical trial. These compounds compete with estradiol for binding to specific estrogen receptor sites. However, their biological activity cannot be explained in terms of this effect alone. Detailed information on this subject is available.[107, 108] It is likely that after binding to estrogen receptors, antiestrogenic compounds activate receptors and facilitate high-affinity binding of receptor to nuclear sites. Partially conflicting results make it impossible to establish with certainty whether these nuclear sites are identical to nuclear sites occupied by estrogen receptor complexes. In addition, subtle differences in es-

trogen response element (ERE) sequences and the protein components that interact with receptors binding to ERE sites add complexity to the picture.

In addition to interactions with the classic high-affinity estrogen receptor sites, several researchers have recently characterized distinct antiestrogen binding sites.[109–112] These sites have limited affinity for classic estrogens. They do not translocate from cytoplasm to nucleus. Their binding affinities for various antiestrogens are not perfectly correlated with antiestrogenic activity. While their definitive role in antihormone action remains unknown at present, it is not likely to be important.

Antiestrogens have proved extremely useful in the management of postmenopausal breast cancer.[113–116] Their role in premenopausal patients is complex, since they may continue to have apparently normal menstrual cycles while exhibiting objective tumor regressions.[117] Antiestrogens have many effects that must be termed *estrogenic*. In mice, tamoxifen is a complete agonist. The majority of postmenopausal women usually show an estrogenic effect during treatment. In addition, some women appear to show a brief "flare" of tumor following the institution of antiestrogen therapy.[118]

Antiestrogens are of value in both male and female breast cancer.[113–116] About one third of patients will benefit from antiestrogen therapy, given the aforementioned conditions concerning patient selection. Thus these drugs are at least as efficacious as other forms of endocrine manipulation. A particular advantage of the antiestrogens is their almost complete lack of significant toxicity. Tamoxifen administration is not associated with significant myelosuppression or with renal, hepatic, or central nervous system toxicity. Most commonly reported are hot flashes, uterine bleeding, and nausea. As mentioned before, tumor stimulation is occasionally seen with associated hypercalcemia.

Patterson and colleagues[119] collected 2889 patients treated with antiestrogens from 45 separate studies. The overall response rate was 971 of 2889, or 34 per cent, with somewhat less than 7 per cent of the total achieving a complete remission. The range of response rates reported varied from 14 to 57 per cent. Prior endocrine therapy strongly influenced response rate. Without prior systemic therapy, 176 of 407, or 43 per cent, had an objective response to tamoxifen. Prior chemotherapy did not have a significant effect on response to tamoxifen (96 of 233, or 41 per cent). Patients who had responded to prior endocrine therapy responded 109 of 201 times, or 59 per cent, whereas nonresponders to prior endocrine therapy responded far less frequently to subsequent endocrine therapy (34 of 165, or 21 per cent). In our own experience with a heavily pretreated cohort of women with advanced breast cancer,[120] only 17 per cent achieved an objective partial or better response using strict evaluation criteria. Although it is commonly stated that the response rate to endocrine therapy is about one in three patients, an extraordinary number of selection biases and prognostic variables can cause huge variations in expected response rates. Much lower response rates to endocrine therapy are found with visceral metastases, multiple sites of involvement, estrogen receptor negativity, perimenopausality, poor performance status, failure to respond to prior endocrine or chemotherapy, and age under 35.

For a variety of reasons one might imagine that age

would be an important prognostic variable in response rate. The effects of tamoxifen on circulating hormone levels have been well reviewed by Manni and colleagues.[121] In postmenopausal patients, tamoxifen had little effect on circulating gonadotropins or on plasma concentrations of estrone, estradiol, or estriol. In premenopausal patients, tamoxifen induced a profound increase in plasma estradiol and, at higher doses, increases in gonadotropins as well. On this basis one might anticipate a substantially lower response rate in premenopausal patients.

In the experience summarized by Patterson and associates,[119] the response rate in women under age 50 who achieved an objective response was 56 of 180, or 31 per cent. This was no different from the results in women aged 51 to 60 (76 of 255, or 30 per cent) and 61 to 70 (87 of 245, or 36 per cent). Of note, 46 per cent of 142 women over age 70 responded to tamoxifen.

Two studies[122, 123] comparing antiestrogen therapy with ovarian ablation concluded that the two therapies appeared equivalent. However, numbers are very small, and it is difficult to accept tamoxifen as the endocrine therapy of choice in younger women in light of its failure in the adjuvant setting. Several studies failed to define any dose-response relationship for tamoxifen. A rationale for this observation springs from information concerning the pharmacology and metabolism of the drug.[124, 125] Two critical facts have emerged. First, tamoxifen has a greatly prolonged terminal elimination half-life in plasma, in the range of 7 to 10 days. For example, 10- to 20-fold increases in tamoxifen concentration in plasma occur after a month of therapy as compared with peak plasma values after a single dose. Thus plasma values around 300 ng/ml are reported after a month of tamoxifen administered at a dose of 20 mg bid.[126] This is equivalent to approximately 10^{-6} M and may exceed by a thousand times or more premenopausal concentrations of estradiol. Second, tamoxifen is extensively metabolized to at least two other compounds: N-desmethyl tamoxifen and 4-OH-tamoxifen. While the former is only weakly antiestrogenic, the latter compound is at least 10 times more potent than tamoxifen. Since the relative binding affinities of 4-OH-tamoxifen and estradiol are roughly equivalent, it is likely even in premenopausal women that under many circumstances there is sufficient tamoxifen and/or active metabolites to antagonize the effects of circulating estrogens. Recently Osborne and colleagues have suggested that an alternative pathway for tamoxifen may exist, leading to its transformation to a more potent agonist. This may explain why some patients have withdrawal responses to tamoxifen and occasionally even respond to readministration of the drug after a prolonged period of withdrawal. Obviously, if resistance to tamoxifen is due to an abnormality of drug metabolism, patients may respond to other endocrine therapies.

New antiestrogens such as toremifine are in clinical trial, but it remains to be seen whether or not they have any advantage over tamoxifen. The data concerning antiestrogen therapy in early-stage breast cancer is encouraging and rapidly developing.

Because the only antiestrogen used in adjuvant clinical trials is tamoxifen and the doses are generally either 20 or 40 mg/day, meta-analyses of outcome provide very useful information of efficacy.[127] There is totally convincing evidence that administration of tamoxifen to either stage I or II patients following local therapy results in a substantial

(approximately 25 per cent) improvement in survival in women over age 50 and an even greater increase in relapse-free survival. While an improvement in disease-free survival has been seen in women under age 50, no consistent effect on overall survival has yet been seen. Improvements in overall and disease-free survival are associated with 2 years of use as compared with 1 year of administration; evidence that 5 years of therapy is superior to 2 years is less convincing. Improvement in overall and disease-free survival is associated with the presence of estrogen receptors. Relative improvement in overall and disease-free survival is unaffected by degree of axillary lymph node involvement.

Women who develop breast cancer are at increased risk of developing a second cancer in the opposite breast. Data from several of the larger adjuvant studies had suggested a reduction in these second primaries. Because of tamoxifen's favorable toxicity profile, and because tamoxifen has weak estrogen-like effects on bone mineralization and blood lipids, it has been proposed that tamoxifen be considered as a chemopreventative agent for women not yet diagnosed as having breast cancer. A nationwide study which will eventually enroll 16,000 women is under way, and results of this study may significantly affect the management of breast cancer.

Numerous other trials have asked whether or not tamoxifen added to a chemotherapy regimen is superior to chemotherapy alone. These studies by major cooperative oncology groups have been uniformly negative with respect to survival, although disease-free survival is generally improved. In most of these studies, tamoxifen was discontinued after 1 or 2 years, and longer use may be more successful. Routine tamoxifen use either alone or in combination in older women probably does no harm but does not help many women; it is of no benefit in young women. This is also an area of very rapid progress and should be followed closely.

Pharmacological Interference with Endogenous Steroidogenesis

Although major ablative endocrine therapies are effective for some patients, their morbidity and mortality have prompted efforts to achieve similar results pharmacologically. In 1973, Griffiths and colleagues[128] proposed the use of aminoglutethimide combined with dexamethasone to suppress adrenal function. Aminoglutethimide had been shown previously to be a potent inhibitor of the conversion of cholesterol to pregnenolone.[129] While this regimen was effective in some women, subsequent studies by Santen and colleagues[130] demonstrated that aminoglutethimide substantially shortened the plasma half-life of dexamethasone, and as a result, pituitary ACTH secretion resumed and overrode the adrenal blockade imposed by aminoglutethimide. By substituting hydrocortisone (whose metabolism was not altered by aminoglutethimide), it was possible to derive a fixed-dose regimen that gave adequate adrenal suppression in most patients.[131] Careful measurement of adrenal steroid concentrations in some of these patients suggested that although dehydroepiandrosterone levels declined, there was an initial rise in Δ^4-androstenedione, the immediate precursor of estrone. The rapidly falling levels of estrone suggested that an important additional activity of aminoglutethimide might be a blockade of peripheral aromatization. This has been substantiated by in vitro measurements in which aminoglutethimide has been shown to inhibit aromatization by human placenta.

The entire area of inhibitors of steroidogenesis has been extensively reviewed.[132] Aminoglutethimide in combination with hydrocortisone appears capable of inducing falls in plasma estrone and estradiol levels equivalent to those seen following surgical adrenalectomy. Most recent work has attempted to define the exact role of aminoglutethimide in comparison with other means of endocrine therapy. In a randomized comparison, response rate and duration were equivalent between surgical adrenalectomy and treatment with aminoglutethimide.[133] Recently, another potent inhibitor of aromatase (4-OH-androstenedione) has been introduced into clinical trials.[134] Early results are promising, and toxicity appears less than with aminoglutethimide.[135] Sedative and allergic responses are less common. Since 4-hydroxyandrostenedione, as well as another agent, CGS16949A,[136] are more specific for aromatase, glucocorticoid replacement is not required.

Antiprogestins

Recent data have suggested that antiprogestins may provide another modality of endocrine therapy. The best known is mifepristone (RU 486), initially developed as an inducer of medical termination of pregnancy. More recently, onapristine has been shown to have a higher degree of potency with significant activity in a variety of rodent mammary cancers.[137, 138] Clinical trials are planned.

Luteinizing Hormone–Releasing Hormone Analogues

For several decades it has been appreciated that hypophysectomy can induce antitumor effects in breast and prostate cancer. It is far from clear as to which pituitary peptides are contributory to disease stimulation. As one means of analyzing this problem and providing safer medical therapies, a variety of LHRH analogues have been explored in clinical trials. The rationale is simple. The chronic exposure of pituitary cells to these analogues with longer half-lives and higher potency induce down-regulation of LHRH receptors and desensitize the pituitary to LHRH, leading to a fall in gonatrophins which results in plasma estrogen and testosterone levels equivalent to surgical castration.

The three agents currently available are Buserelin (Hoechst), Leuprolide (Abbott), and Zoladex (ICI). While Buserelin, Zoladex, and Leuprolide have shown significant activity in breast cancer (partial response rates in excess of 40 per cent),[139–141] these data must be interpreted with extreme caution, since extensive patient selection in early phase II studies will undoubtedly bias results. A randomized trial comparing Zoladex with surgical oophorectomy is underway.[142]

Somatostatin Analogues

Recently, a somatostatin analogue (octreotide acetate, Sandoz) has been brought into clinical trial. This compound induces profound falls in IGF-I levels. In addition, somatostatin receptors have been demonstrated directly on the surfaces of breast cancer cells.[143] Somatostatin can directly inhibit the growth of some breast cancer cell lines.[144] Clinical trials with somatostatin analogues are underway, and data concerning efficacy should be available soon.

Combinations of Endocrine Therapy and Chemotherapy

A detailed review of systemic therapy of breast cancer is beyond the scope of this chapter. While one might imagine that endocrine therapy and chemotherapy combined might improve survival, such is not the case. There are at present no convincing data that such routine combinations add to survival, although initial response rates are often slightly higher than with chemotherapy alone.[145] Recently, attention has been paid to alternative means of using endocrine therapy to synchronize or recruit hormone-dependent cells and render them nonresponsive to chemotherapy.[146–148] These data are encouraging and also appear applicable to both prostate and endometrial cancer.

Male Breast Cancer

Male breast cancer is exceedingly rare (approximately 1 per cent of female incidence). It is commonly a hormone-dependent neoplasm and provides many interesting contrasts with female breast cancer. Several complete reviews are available.[148–151] Most of the known risk factors—exogenous estrogen exposure, atypical endogenous steroid metabolism and excretion, Klinefelter's syndrome, radiation, family history, gynecomastia, and orchitis—have underlying known or suspected endocrine components. A convincing argument for a role of exogenous estrogen was provided in a report of two 30-year-old transsexuals who developed male breast cancer after castration and continuous estrogen use.[152] The tumors usually contain estrogen receptor and are frequently positive for progestin, glucocorticoid, and androgen receptors as well.[153] Although male and female breast cancers have nearly identical stage-by-stage survival rates, a far greater proportion of men present with disease at an advanced stage. Approximately two thirds of cases cited in the literature will respond to orchiectomy; this is approximately twice the response rate of female breast cancer to endocrine therapy.[151] Adrenalectomy and hypophysectomy are frequently successful even in patients who failed to respond to primary endocrine manipulations. Patterson and colleagues[154] collected 31 patients with advanced male breast cancer who were treated with tamoxifen. Fifteen, or 48 per cent, achieved a complete or partial response with minimal toxicity. Antiestrogens may thus be the initial treatment of choice for patients with male breast cancer.

ENDOMETRIAL CANCER

Epidemiology

The endometrium has been studied as a target tissue for sex steroid hormone action in innumerable species. Its growth and morphology change cyclically in response to estradiol and progesterone. The identification of a specific uterine receptor for estradiol in 1960[155] began the modern era of steroid hormone action. Just as in the case of breast cancer, carcinogenic, permissive, and promotional activities are probably attributable to estrogens. The promotional activity of estrogens in leading to expression of endometrial cancer is the most important clinically.

Clinical, biological, and epidemiological data all show that prolonged or unopposed estrogenic stimulation increases the risk of endometrial carcinoma. The longer the endometrium is stimulated, the greater is the cancer risk, as shown by the association of endometrial carcinoma with the duration of use of exogenous estrogens after the menopause[156] and with late menopause. The increase in endometrial cancer among women with estrogen-secreting tumors and with the polycystic ovary syndrome[157] emphasizes the role of progesterone-induced endometrial sloughing as a protective mechanism. A higher incidence of endometrial cancer is also seen with several other ovarian abnormalities, such as cortical stromal hyperplasia and persistent stromal thecal cells. In these cases, estrogen secretion may not be excessive; it is, however, continuous, since there are no ovulatory cycles with their accompanying progesterone secretory periods and the subsequent endometrial sloughing. Endometrial cancer can occur in women with estrogens alone. The causal role of continued, unopposed estrogenic stimulus is further supported by the high incidence of irregular menses in women with endometrial cancer.[157] The resumption of cyclic ovarian function in response to ovarian wedge resection in the Stein-Leventhal syndrome results in regression of endometrial hyperplasia, and progesterone also has been shown to reverse estrogen-induced endometrial hyperplasia.[158]

Another risk factor for endometrial carcinoma (as with breast cancer) is obesity. In the premenopausal woman, the association of obesity with anovulatory cycles and amenorrhea may be the explanation. In the postmenopausal woman, the predominant blood estrogen is estrone, derived almost entirely from the conversion in peripheral tissues of androstenedione secreted by the adrenal cortex. The rate of this conversion increases with age[159] and with weight,[160] and plasma estrogen concentrations increase with increasing weight.[161] Fat has the capacity to aromatize androgens and quantitatively provides the greatest source of estrogens in postmenopausal women. This is a reasonable explanation of the association between weight and endometrial cancer risk. Plasma estrone production rates and concentrations are the same in women with endometrial cancer as in weight- and age-matched controls, but the higher incidence of obesity in the women with cancer means that, as a group, there is greater exposure to estrogen. The relationship between estrogen use by postmenopausal women and increased risk of endometrial cancer is impressive.[162] Relative risk ratios for the development of endometrial cancer vary from 4:1 to 9:1, the risk increasing with the duration of use. Increased risk with increasing duration of exposure is characteristic of tumor promoters in the classic two-step carcinogen-promoter model for cancer induction. Some workers have claimed that these estimates of excess risk are spurious because of detection bias owing to the vaginal bleeding that may accompany estrogen therapy.[162] This has been refuted by additional data and theoretical considerations,[156] and it is established that the use of estrogen after menopause is an important risk factor for endometrial cancer. It should be noted that in all studies of the use of estrogen in postmenopausal women, greater than physiological doses of estrogen have been used, and progestin-induced withdrawal bleeding has not generally been part of the regimens. Attention to both these factors would be expected to reduce the risk appreciably. It is also gratifying that after an expected lag period, the incidence of endometrial cancer has declined sharply following substantial reduction in the use of exogenous estrogens for menopausal symptomatology. Many arguments exist for continued use of postmenopausal estrogens, most notably protection against osteoporosis, hip fracture, and cardiovascular disease. Some have encouraged either cyclic use of estrogens, lower dosage, or the use of intermittent progestins. While all these (particularly the latter) may reduce endometrial cancer, they should not be adopted as useful therapy without appreciating the potential hazards involved in increasing breast cancer risk. In the absence of definitive studies, risk/benefit ratios of estrogen therapy in postmenopausal patients should be assessed on an individual basis with a well-informed patient.

Endocrinology and Receptors

The uterus is probably the best-studied example of an estrogen-responsive tissue, and a considerable amount of what is known concerning the molecular mechanism of action of sex steroids has been learned from studies on uteri from various animal sources. The estrogen receptor content of the endometrium is highest in the proliferative phase and is decreased in the luteal phase[163, 164] or by administration of progestins.[165] Progesterone receptor capacity is highest at the time of the estradiol peak[163] and can be induced by estrogens. Estrogen receptor persists in most endometrial carcinomas, and the receptor content is inversely correlated with the degree of differentiation,[163] whereas cytosol progesterone receptor capacity[163, 166] and nuclear progesterone receptors[167] are highest in well-differentiated cancer. The enzyme, 17β-hydroxysteroid dehydrogenase, which catalyzes the conversion of estradiol to estrone, is induced by progesterone[168] and can serve as an index of progestational effect. The recent development of a nude mouse model system for the study of hormone-dependent and -independent human endometrial cancer should provide an important means of better studying the mechanisms of hormone regulation of endometrial cancer.[169, 170]

The mechanism of action of progestins is still speculative. In the normal estrogen-primed uterus, progesterone causes specific maturational changes, followed by atrophy when a progestogen is continued for long periods. Following administration of progestogens to women with endometrial cancer, mitotic activity ceases, there is increased glandular differentiation, and an increase in cytoplasm/nucleus ratio is seen. Atrophy is also noted. These changes duplicate those of the normal endometrium during progesterone therapy. The finding that endometrial cancers contain progesterone receptors provides an explanation for the therapeutic effect. Thus progesterone decreases estrogen receptors and increases the capacity of the endometrium to metabolize estradiol (see above). As with breast cancer, these tumors may be heterogeneous with respect to cell content of progesterone receptors, thereby accounting for the variability of response. Nevertheless, progesterone receptor determinations are of only modest value. This is so because at present there is no effective alternative means of controlling systemic spread on endometrial cancer aside from endocrine treatment.

Therapy

Kelley and Baker reported that progestogens could cause regression in about one third of patients with metastatic endometrial cancer.[171] This has been confirmed in cooperative studies of patients at many centers.[172] A variety of progestins, including medroxyprogesterone acetate (Provera), megesterol acetate (Megace), and hydroxyprogesterone caproate (Delalutin), have been explored with differing dose schedules. None appears superior to another.[173–176] The response to therapy did not depend on age of patient, site of metastasis, or previous or concurrent therapy. However, women with slowly growing or more differentiated tumors responded better than those with aggressive cancers. Duration of life after initiation of therapy was 27 months in those who responded and only 7 months in those who did not. Thus far, there is no evidence that any progestin is superior to another with respect to response or survival.[177, 178] Efforts to use antiestrogens in the management of endometrial cancer have not been very encouraging.[179–182] Response rates have generally been low, although toxicity was, as expected, mild.

Given the lack of substantial activity of systemic cytotoxic chemotherapy, it is generally reasonable to attempt a trial of progestins in any patient with metastatic disease. It is claimed that the response of pulmonary metastases is better than that of bone metastases, but responses have been noted in all groups. The remissions seen with progestogens are particularly beneficial because they are accomplished with essentially no toxicity. Recently, several studies have reported improved results from chemotherapy in endometrial cancer.[183, 184] If confirmed in larger series, not only will receptor determinations become more important, but combined-modality approaches will need to be explored.

PROSTATE CANCER

Hormone therapy plays a more important role in prostate cancer than in any other human malignancy. Nearly all patients with metastatic prostate cancer will respond favorably to androgen ablation. Moreover, the past decade has seen the development of new therapeutic agents for androgen ablation that have reduced morbidity and improved survival in advanced prostate cancer. This section will provide an overview of our current understanding of prostate cancer and its treatment and will describe the new therapeutic agents that are now applied to this disease.

Epidemiology

Prostate cancer is a very common malignancy among males in Western countries. It has received increasing attention during the last 5 years. Estimates for 1991 indicate that prostate cancer will be the most common malignancy among males in the United States.[185] This is due to increased screening efforts, an increased proportion of older men in the population, and leveling off in the incidence of lung cancer. In 1991, there were approximately 122,000 new cases of prostate cancer and 32,000 deaths due to prostate cancer in the United States. Few specific risk factors for prostate cancer have been identified; however, the profound international variation in incidence of prostate cancer emphasizes the importance of environmental factors. Dietary fat intake may play a role in prostate cancer.[186–188] There is a family history of prostate cancer in 18 per cent of cases. Individuals in whom there is a strong family history appear to have a twofold increased risk for developing prostate cancer.[189] Since prostate epithelium depends on the presence of androgen for growth and development, it seemed logical to try to correlate serum androgen levels with the incidence of prostate cancer. Such studies have yielded mixed results.[190–193] There is no clear association between levels of serum testosterone and prostate cancer risk.

Prostate cancer incidence has a wide geographic variation. The disease is more common in North America and northwestern Europe.[194] Prostate cancer incidence is substantially lower in Japan and in African countries. In Africa, the incidence may be less than one tenth the incidence in the United States. Geographic differences in prostate cancer incidence suggest that environmental factors play a role in prostate carcinogenesis. This is further underscored by studies of latent or subclinical prostate cancer in different countries. Microscopic foci of prostate cancer develop in most men and increase in frequency with age; however, these foci represent subclinical cancer that is not associated with disease.[195, 196] The incidence of subclinical microscopic prostate cancer is similar in all countries regardless of the incidence of clinical prostate cancer.[197–199] For example, the incidence of latent prostate cancer is identical in the United States and Japan,[197, 198] but the incidence of clinical prostate cancer differs tenfold at least. Prostate cancer incidence increases with age at the same rate in both the United States and Japan, but the incidence curve is shifted by approximately 10 years for Japanese men. This suggests that the exogenous factors that change microscopic to clinical prostate cancer have an earlier impact in the United States than in Japan. Japanese men who move to Hawaii have an intermediate incidence of prostate cancer.[200, 201] Therefore, it appears that environmental or dietary factors play a major role in the development of clinical prostate cancer.

One of the most striking aspects of prostate cancer epidemiology is the incidence among blacks in the United States. Black Americans have the highest incidence of prostate cancer of any group in the world, nearly 100 new cases annually per 100,000 population.[202] Their incidence of prostate cancer is over twice that found in white Americans. Moreover, this appears to be due to environmental factors, since blacks in Africa have an extremely low incidence of prostate cancer.[203] Whereas prostate cancer is the number three cancer killer among white males in the United States, it is the number two cancer killer among black males.[185] Although this may be attributable to differences in stage at diagnosis and delays in diagnosis,[204] there appear to be suggestions that prostate cancer among black Americans is a more virulent disease. In a nationwide randomized trial of prostate cancer therapy, a group of black patients did significantly worse than a comparably matched group of white patients.[205]

Staging

Thorough staging of prostate cancer is critical both for an accurate assessment of prognosis and for planning appropriate therapy. Stage A describes cancers discovered during cystoscopic transurethral resection of the prostate (TURP) to treat urinary obstruction. Stage A_1 disease refers to those cases in which fewer than 5 per cent of the resected prostate chips contain histological evidence of malignancy. Except in young patients, stage A_1 patients are treated with watchful waiting after the diagnosis and stage have been confirmed. This treatment decision is based on the observation that between 5 and 10 years after the diagnosis of stage A_1 prostate cancer, approximately 8 per cent of patients develop metastases and only 2 per cent of patients suffer mortality from prostate cancer.[206–208] Stage A_2 disease designates those patients in whom greater than 5 per cent of the chips resected during TURP contain cancer. Patients with A_2 disease require additional local therapy, either definitive radiation therapy or a radical prostatectomy. Stage B disease includes those patients whose prostate cancer is detected by physical examination but whose cancer has not spread beyond the confines of the prostate gland capsule. Patients with a single subcapsular nodule on one side of the gland are staged as B_1, and patients in whom a tumor crosses the midline of the gland are staged as B_2. Patients with B_1 disease are thought to be curable, either by surgery or by radiation therapy. Patients with B_2 disease are often operated on, but their curability is more controversial. Even though stage B_2 prostate cancer may eventually recur, the best surgical series does report a 50 to 60 per cent 15-year survival with radical surgery for locally advanced prostate cancer.[209] These results surpass any published radiation therapy series. Thus for a 55-year-old man with stage B_2 prostate cancer, surgery may prove the best choice for therapy. However, for a 70-year-old man, radiation therapy may provide equivalent expectations for survival due to risks associated with surgery and the shorter life expectancy at age 70 compared with age 55.

When prostate cancer extends beyond the capsule of the gland and perhaps to adjacent structures such as the seminal vesicles, it is considered stage C. Although it may be prudent to treat stage C disease with local measures such as surgery or radiation therapy, stage C disease is generally not curable. Stage D describes those patients whose cancer has spread to distant sites. Stage D_1 disease refers to those individuals with involved pelvic lymph nodes and stage D_2 disease to those with involvement of more distant sites, most commonly bone metastases.

Prognostic Factors

In addition to staging, there are other indicators of prognosis when a patient is diagnosed with prostate cancer. The degree of differentiation of the individual cancer cells and the degree of disorder among the neoplastic ducts both have been used to grade prostate cancer. Grading systems are expected to correlate with disease recurrence and survival rates. One commonly used grading system was designed by Gleason[210] and depends on the glandular differentiation of the tumor as viewed microscopically under low magnification. Gleason observed that many prostate specimens had more than one pattern present. Therefore, he assigned a grade for the predominant pattern and a secondary grade for the minor pattern. Grades were assigned a number from 1 to 5, and the sum of the two grades gave a Gleason score from 2 to 10. The Gleason score has been shown to correlate with prognosis, presence of lymph node metastases, and other clinical parameters.[211, 212] Other histological grading systems have relied on cellular atypia (the system of Mostofi[213]) or both acinar structure and cellular differentiation, as in the Mayo Clinic system.[214] Many grading systems are valid predictors of survival.

Tumor cell DNA content, as determined by flow cytometry analysis of tumor tissue, has been shown to have substantial prognostic significance in prostate cancer. About 15 per cent of all prostate cancer cases contain populations of aneuploid cells. These cases have a substantially poorer prognosis.[215–217] Unlike other epithelial cancers, such as breast cancer, the search for molecular markers that have prognostic significance has, to date, failed to identify a single oncogene or other cellular component (other than prostate-specific antigen) whose altered structure, gene amplification, or altered expression have prognostic or etiological importance in prostate cancer.

Our ideas about staging and approaches to the treatment of localized prostate cancer are rapidly evolving due to an accumulation of information about the tumor marker prostate-specific antigen (PSA). PSA is a serine protease with a molecular weight of 34,000 that is synthesized only by prostate cells.[218] It is not found in women[219] and has not been reported to be synthesized by other cancers. In patients who have had total prostatectomies, PSA is a marker for the detection of recurrent disease.[220] It also is a useful indicator of residual disease after definitive surgery.[221] PSA also has been studied as a screening test.[222] Its utility for cancer screening is not well defined but is rapidly expanding. PSA levels are the best single test available to screen asymptomatic men for prostate cancer.[223] When combined with digital rectal examination, the combination of the two suspicious tests predicts a 33 per cent rate of positive biopsies for cancer.[223] PSA also may have some applicability as a staging tool. For example, studies have shown that initial PSA determinations that exceed certain levels have an extremely high likelihood of indicating the presence of metastatic disease.[224–226] All these measurements must be reviewed with some degree of caution. A high level of PSA can result from benign prostatic hypertrophy.[227] PSA levels should never be used per se to establish a cancer diagnosis, since this diagnosis can only be established by histological examination of a prostate biopsy. However, when an abnormal PSA is detected during a routine screening, the patient should be referred for transrectal ultrasound and directed biopsy of any abnormal areas.

Treatment of Localized Prostate Cancer

Most cases of stages A_1, A_2, and B_1 prostate cancers are curable by local treatments, either surgery or radiation therapy.[228] Except in men under 60 years of age, treatment of stage A₁ disease would involve watchful waiting after the pathological findings of the TURP. Therapy of more extensive localized disease (stages B₂ and C) can achieve good local control and provide an extended disease-free interval. Until the early 1980's, proponents of surgical treatment of early-stage prostate cancer alleged the superiority of treatment outcome as measured by disease-free survival. However, surgery used to result in almost certain loss of sexual potency. The pioneering work done by Walsh and co-workers at Johns Hopkins University is responsible for decreasing the rate of impotence after radical prostatectomy for localized prostate cancer.[229, 230] Walsh observed that preserving neurovascular bundles adjacent to the prostate decreased the rate of postoperative impotence from 100 per cent to approximately 30 per cent.

Localized radiation therapy also can be a definitive form of local treatment for prostate cancer.[231, 232] Overall, radiation therapy treatment of localized prostate cancer gives somewhat inferior results to surgical therapy. This is due partly to the fact that surgical candidates are generally younger and in better overall health. Many major surgical centers restrict their surgical candidates to patients who are under 70 years of age. Many older men or men who are felt to have localized but inoperable prostate cancer are referred for definitive radiation therapy. Therefore, radiation therapists treat patients who have more advanced disease and poorer performance status, both adverse prognostic indicators. There is only a single randomized trial comparing radical prostatectomy with radiation therapy for the treatment of localized prostate cancer.[233, 234] This single trial showed that radical prostatectomy was superior in overall survival to radiation therapy. The trial has been criticized for technical aspects and uniformity of the radiation therapy but remains the only randomized comparison between the two modalities.

Although no subsequent trials have compared directly the safety and efficacy of radical prostatectomy and definitive radiation therapy, both approaches have benefited over the last two decades from technical improvements. Currently, both surgery and radiation therapy have comparable morbidity rates with regard to maintenance of potency, incontinence, and bowel problems. A 1987 NIH Consensus Development Conference on the management of clinically localized prostate cancer concluded that both radical prostatectomy and radiation therapy were effective for the treatment of localized prostate cancer and had comparable 10-year survival rates.[235]

The treatment of advanced localized prostate cancer, stage B₂ or stage C, should emphasize local control and limited morbidity. Advanced localized prostate cancer should be viewed as incurable cancer in its early stages. Radiation therapy is most often employed for local control. Some surgeons prefer to operate on selected cases of stage B₂ prostate cancer. However, decisions regarding local therapy for locally advanced prostate cancer are guided by clinical judgment. The use of systemic hormonal therapy as an adjuvant to local treatment of stage B₂ or stage C disease can be considered. However, there are no data that suggest that survival is improved by the use of androgen ablation prior to the finding of metastatic prostate cancer.

Treatment of Disseminated Prostate Cancer

Once prostate cancer has spread beyond the gland itself, it is incurable. Even with current attempts to improve early diagnosis of prostate cancer by more widespread screening efforts and the emerging use of routine serum PSA determinations, more than half of prostate cancer patients present to the physician with disseminated disease. Although several therapeutic agents and approaches to treat disseminated prostate cancer have been in vogue during the past 50 years, treatment of stage D disease has been based on a single principle of endocrinology established by Huggins and Hodges in 1941 when they observed a beneficial effect of castration in patients with metastatic prostate cancer.[236, 237] To this day, the principal goal of therapy for stage D prostate cancer is the maximal reduction of systemic androgens. Between 85 and 90 per cent of patients with disseminated prostate cancer will manifest an objective tumor response to some therapeutic maneuver designed to lower serum testosterone to castrate levels.

Development of the fetal prostate is under control of androgens, which regulate development of the urogenital sinus.[238, 239] Aberrant responsiveness to androgen, associated with inborn errors of the androgen receptor gene or 5α-reductase deficiency, can result in a hypoplastic or underdeveloped prostate gland (see ref. 240 for a review). In the developing rat prostate gland, androgen receptors are expressed in stromal but not in epithelial cells.[241, 242] Since the development of prostate epithelium is androgen-dependent, it appears that androgen stimulation of stromal cells induces the expression of paracrine factors that influence epithelial cell development and replication. In the adult human prostate, androgen receptors are expressed both in the epithelial and stromal cells.[243–245] Androgen is essential for maintenance of the normal prostate gland. Castration of an adult male rat results in prostate epithelial involution within seven days.[246] Stromal elements remain intact, suggesting that androgen is necessary for the maintenance of the epithelial cells through stimulation of the stromal cells, but the stroma itself can survive without androgens. Androgen withdrawal from a normal prostate results in epithelial cell apoptosis or programmed cell death. In the prostate gland this has been shown to be an energy-requiring process characterized by the expression of specific genes that results in cellular involution.[247]

Malignant prostate epithelial cells express androgen receptor and respond directly to androgen stimulation. Androgen receptor expression has been demonstrated immunohistochemically in malignant prostate epithelial cells.[244] Two human prostate cancer cell lines, LNCaP[248, 249] and PC-82,[250] express androgen receptor and are dependent on androgens for their growth. In prostate cancer patients, metastatic deposits of prostate cancer respond to therapeutic androgen ablation even though the prostate cancer cells in the metastatic deposits are remote from the prostate stroma. Lastly, some prostate cancer tumor specimens have been found to contain point mutations in the androgen receptor gene.[251] Presumably these mutations were detected in the clonally expanded population of cancer cells. Had these mutations occurred sporadically in normal stroma surrounding the cancer cells, they would not have been detected by the molecular techniques used. The LNCaP cell line contains a mutation in the hormone-binding region of the androgen receptor that is responsible for aberrant responsiveness of these cells to antiandrogen treatment in vitro.[252, 253] The finding of androgen receptor mutations in prostate cancer and the antiandrogen resistance of LNCaP cells suggest that androgen receptor mutations may be a mechanism of clinical antiandrogen resistance. The evidence does suggest strongly that, unlike normal prostate epithelium, malignant prostate cells acquire androgen receptor expression and, in some cases, express mutant receptor molecules.

Dihydrotestosterone (DHT) is the predominant active androgen in the prostate gland. DHT is formed by action of 5α-reductase on circulating testosterone. Approximately 500 μg DHT is formed per day, most of it by 5α-reductase in the prostate gland. Each day 7 mg testosterone is produced in an adult male. Ninety percent of testosterone production occurs in the testes; the remaining 10 per cent is formed by the adrenal glands. For the first 40 years after Huggins and Hodges' paper, therapeutic approaches focused on testicular production of androgens. Orchiectomy has always been the definitive, relatively safe, and inexpensive approach to androgen ablation. This operation continues to be an important therapeutic option in treating prostate cancer, but because of the other options available today, it is chosen only about 20 per cent of the time by eligible patients.

Pharmacological doses of estrogens, particularly diethylstilbestrol (DES), have been used to suppress pituitary secretion of luteinizing hormone (LH) and thereby reduce testicular androgen secretion. DES was effective in reducing circulating testosterone to castrate levels. However, a series of randomized trials conducted by the Veterans Administration Cooperative Urological Research Group (VACURG) showed that DES, when used at the standard dose of 5 mg/day, had unexpected and substantial cardiovascular toxicity, mostly thromboembolic events from increased platelet aggregation caused by DES.[254] Subsequent studies demonstrated equal efficacy of 1 and 5 mg in controlling prostate cancer, but the lower doses obviated the cardiovascular complications. Since it has been shown that 1 mg DES suppresses testosterone to castrate levels in only 70 per cent of patients, 2.5 to 3 mg daily is currently recommended.[255] Although DES is an effective and inexpensive drug for the control of metastatic prostate cancer, other morbidities such as gynecomastia, gastrointestinal distress, and edema may influence decreased compliance and increased cost. Many patients required prophylactic breast radiation therapy to prevent painful gynecomastia.

Testosterone and LH secretion also can be affected at the level of the hypothalamus. In 1971, LHRH was isolated and subsequently modified, initially for the treatment of infertility. LHRH is a decapeptide that can be substituted at the sixth, ninth, and tenth positions to increase receptor affinity more than 100-fold. Substitution of glycine at position six with a D-amino acid stabilizes the peptide. LHRH is secreted episodically to stimulate LH secretion by the pituitary. When administered as single doses, LHRH agonists simulate this effect and cause transient increases in serum LH and testosterone (see ref. 256 for a review). However, when administered continuously, LHRH agonists induce suppression of gonadotropins, reducing testosterone secretion to castrate levels about 2 weeks after the initial burst of LH secretion that results from the first dose.[256]

Three LHRH agonists have been used clinically in the treatment of disseminated prostate cancer. Leuprolide and goserelin, administered by subcutaneous injection, are approved for use in the United States. Buserelin, another LHRH analogue, can be administered by subcutaneous injection or intranasally. Its use has not been approved in the United States. LHRH analogues, when administered chronically, reduce circulating testosterone to castrate levels and achieve therapeutic benefit in prostate cancer comparable with DES.[257] The benefits of LHRH agonists are in the reduced toxicity profile compared with DES. The major morbidities of LHRH agonists are hot flashes and loss of libido.[256]

Tumor flares have been reported to accompany the initiation of LHRH agonist therapy.[257, 258] These are due to transient increases in testosterone levels that occur during the first days of LHRH agonist administration. Tumor flares can be prevented by administration of antiandrogens such as flutamide or cyproterone acetate.[260] Although clinically important tumor flares are rare, they can cause significant morbidity, such as spinal cord compression caused by sudden growth stimulation of a vertebral metastasis. It is prudent to precede initiation of LHRH agonist therapy by 1 to 3 days of antiandrogen therapy, whether or not combined androgen blockade will be used for maintenance therapy.

Labrie and coworkers[261] popularized the notion that adrenal androgens were important stimulants of prostate cancer. They argued that blockade of the action of adrenal androgens would contribute to the efficacy of hormonal treatment for metastatic prostate cancer. This approach was termed *total androgen blockade* and was accomplished by simultaneous administration of leuprolide and the antiandrogen, flutamide, given as 125 or 250 mg orally three times a day. Flutamide is metabolized to 2-hydroxyflutamide after one transit through the liver. 2-Hydroxyflutamide competes for androgen binding to the androgen receptor.[262] Based on optimistic reports of substantially prolonged disease-free survival in selected patients treated with total androgen blockade by Labrie, several multicenter randomized trials were undertaken to assess the actual benefit of the combined therapy compared with an LHRH agonist alone.

The National Cancer Institute Intergroup 0036 trial has provided convincing data for the slight advantage of total androgen blockade over monotherapy with an LHRH agonist.[263] Six hundred and three patients were randomized to receive either daily injections of 1 mg leuprolide plus oral placebo three times per day or 250 mg leuprolide plus flutamide orally three times per day. Patients were stratified for extent of disease and performance status. After more than 5 years, there is a significant, but small survival advantage for the group that received the combined therapy. Median time to progression was 13.8 months for leuprolide plus placebo and 16.9 months for combined therapy. Median survival from initiation of therapy was 35.1 months for the combined-therapy group and 29.3 months for the leuprolide-alone group. Patients with minimal disease and excellent performance status benefited the most from combined therapy. Although this subgroup was relatively small compared with the entire trial population, results with the minimal disease group have focused further interest on additional trials and earlier use of total androgen blockade in disseminated prostate cancer.[264]

Other trials also have examined the issue of monotherapy with LHRH agonists and combined treatment. For example a Danish trial compared goserelin plus flutamide versus orchiectomy alone.[265] The trial was open to patients with stage C and D prostate cancer and accrued 262 patients. No significant differences in outcome have been observed between the two groups. The European Organization for the Research and Treatment of Cancer also conducted a trial of goserelin plus flutamide versus orchiectomy.[266] At early follow-up interval there was a trend in favor of the combination therapy. A third trial in France asked the same therapeutic question and compared goserelin with combination therapy of goserelin plus flutamide.[267] Since these European studies have each accrued between 200 and 300 patients, they may not possess the statistical power to show the same response and survival differences demonstrated by the NCI Intergroup 0036 study. In the future, a meta-analysis may have to be conducted to determine if a common conclusion can be made regarding the numerous clinical trials on total androgen blockade.

Hormonal therapy has been proposed as a means of downstaging locally advanced prostate cancer to reduce the size of local disease, thus potentially rendering a large inoperable cancer operable. Although large deposits of local prostate cancer can be shrunk by androgen ablation, there is no evidence that patients who achieve such a response have an improved survival if they are then subject to prostatectomy.

Treatment of metastatic prostate cancer with flutamide alone has been investigated in small trials. Flutamide monotherapy has the potential to preserve potency and libido, although it is unclear that antiandrogen monotherapy will have a sufficient inhibitory effect on prostate cancer to be used as the treatment of choice. In a randomized trial comparing flutamide, 250 mg three times a day, with DES, 1 mg three times a day, initial responses to therapy were similar, but median survival among the DES patients was 43.2 months compared with 26.2 months for the flutamide group ($p = 0.007$).[269]

Numerous other hormonal manipulations have been used previously as first-line therapy for metastatic prostate cancer and may be employed as second-line therapy for disease that has progressed after total androgen blockade. Although short-lived minor tumor responses or stabilization of disease can be achieved with second-line hormonal therapy, the administration of hormonal therapy after failure of total androgen blockade should not be viewed as anything more than palliative treatment that has no impact on survival. Second-line hormonal therapies may include glucocorticoids such as hydrocortisone or prednisone, inhibitors of adrenal androgenesis such as ketoconazole or newer analogues currently in clinical trials such as liriazole, inhibitors of adrenal steroidogenesis such as aminoglutethimide, and progestational agents such as megestrol acetate.

5α-Reductase Inhibition: Finasteride

The conversion of testosterone to DHT by 5α-reductase is largely carried out in the prostate gland. DHT appears to have selective importance for the prostate. Inherited deficiency of 5α-reductase produces prepubertal males with ambiguous genitalia. These individuals virilize normally at puberty but have hypoplastic prostate glands, little facial hair, no temporal hair loss, and no acne. This suggests that inhibition of 5α-reductase in the adult may be relatively specific for the prostate gland.[268] Finasteride was designed to be a specific inhibitor of 5α-reductase. Finasteride has been shown to inhibit DHT synthesis and cause up to twofold reflex increases in serum testosterone.[268] In a published pilot trial of finasteride versus placebo for treatment of benign prostatic hypertrophy (BPH), finasteride caused reduction in prostate size of about 25 per cent on average.[270] Symptomatic improvement of urinary flow was not statistically different from the placebo group in this relatively small study of 104 patients. Other antiandrogens have been used for the treatment of BPH; however, finasteride has the advantage of virtually no effect on potency or libido.[270] Although finasteride has not been shown to have any efficacy or role in the treatment of prostate cancer, it has a potential role as a preventative agent for prostate cancer. DHT is the major hormonal growth stimulus for the prostate and, therefore, is the physiological tumor promoter for prostate cancer. Consideration is being given to a trial of the administration of finasteride to men at high risk for prostate cancer to see if a protective effect can be demonstrated. Both organ specificity and relative safety suggest that finasteride may have a role as a chemopreventive agent for prostate cancer.

In the future, refinements in the hormonal treatment of prostate cancer will continue to be made. One of the remaining questions focuses on the role of androgen receptor mutations in prostate cancer and how these mutations may affect the response of cancer cells to antiandrogens. Other advances will come in the form of longer-acting antiandrogens with less gastrointestinal and hepatic toxicity than the agents currently used. New roles for hormonal therapy are in chemoprevention of prostate cancer by specific blockade of androgen, the primary tumor promoter of prostate cancer. Lastly, continued testing of chemotherapeutic agents may one day identify cytotoxic drugs that have efficacy against prostate cancer. To date, no cytotoxic agents have ever been shown to influence disease-free status or overall survival of prostate cancer patients.

LEUKEMIA AND LYMPHOMA

Glucocorticoids are hormones with wide-ranging effects on the growth, differentiation, and function of virtually every tissue and organ system of the body.[271] Inhibitory actions on lymphoid tissue have long been appreciated.[272, 273] Glucocorticoids produce marked lymphocytopenia and thymic atrophy in humans and in experimental animals. A major discovery was that glucocorticoids also kill some leukemic lymphoblasts in humans.[274] Despite this important observation, several difficulties prevent their most effective use. Variable response rates are observed in patients with differing histological types of acute and chronic leukemia and lymphoma.[275] Thus clinical data do not predict accurately which subset of patients is likely to benefit from glucocorticoid therapy. In addition, many patients who respond to glucocorticoid therapy eventually relapse, and inevitably these patients become unresponsive to further glucocorticoid therapy.[276] Thus, while initial response rates in pediatric acute lymphoblastic leukemia range between 45 and 65 per cent, after primary relapse, the rate of subsequent remission induction with glucocorticoids alone falls to 25 per cent.

Furthermore, glucocorticoid administration is associated with many complications. These include immunosuppression with concomitant nosocomial infections, Cushing's syndrome, diabetes mellitus, poor wound healing, psychosis, and other problems.[271, 277] Since most patients with leukemia and lymphoma die of infectious complications rather than of the cancer per se, it is likely that in some cases glucocorticoids may be a significant detriment to therapy. This particular difficulty is amplified by the fact that most patients with leukemia and lymphoma are currently managed by combinations of agents that include glucocorticoids along with cytotoxins. Thus possibly harmful components in the drug combination, such as the glucocorticoid, may be continued long after they cease to be of benefit.

It would therefore be of value to be able to predict in advance when glucocorticoid therapy is indicated. One obvious approach is to measure glucocorticoid sensitivity in vitro using some type of cytotoxic or inhibitory end point. Unfortunately, such methods have not proved useful.[278–280] It is difficult to reliably culture leukemic cell populations, and furthermore, in vitro effects of hormones may not be as easily demonstrated as in vivo responses. In fact, sometimes the response seen is that of hormonal stimulation rather than inhibition; thus the presence of receptor may not even correlate with the direction of in vitro response.

Studies performed in breast cancer and other malignant disease support the notion that quantification of specific steroid receptors for estrogen is useful in predicting response to endocrine therapy.[281] On the basis of this observation, plus a clearer understanding of the mechanism of action of glucocorticoids, several groups sought and found specific glucocorticoid receptors in various populations of human leukemic and lymphoid cells.[281–283]

Glucocorticoid receptors are readily demonstrable in normal peripheral blood lymphocytes as well as in partially purified subpopulations of lymphocytes and monocytes.[284–287] These receptor proteins are similar to the glucocorticoid receptor more extensively characterized in rat thymocytes.[288] Agents that induce blastic transformation of human lymphoid cells such as phytohemagglutinin or concanavalin A lead to several-fold increases in intracellular glucocorticoid receptor content similar to that of human leukemic lymphoblasts.

Early studies in human acute lymphoblastic leukemia suggested that quantitative glucocorticoid receptor analyses would be clinically relevant.[289–292] Glucocorticoid receptors are readily detectable by assay of either cytoplasmic extracts or intact whole cells in most previously untreated patients with acute lymphoblastic leukemia. Many more receptor sites are detectable by whole-cell assay, and they are more widely used. There is good agreement between concentrations of glucocorticoids that bind to receptor sites and concentrations that inhibit cellular processes. Early data in acute lymphoblastic leukemia suggest that a reasonable correlation may exist between loss of glucocorticoid receptor activity and in vitro resistance to glucocorticoids.[290] These early studies correlated lack of response

with absence of receptor, not with quantity of receptor. Other researchers have attempted correlations with brief trials of glucocorticoid therapy.[279, 293, 294] Each group has a high- and a low-receptor group. Overall, 18 of 19 patients with high glucocorticoid receptor content responded to glucocorticoids, whereas 4 of 16 with low values (generally less than 5000 sites per cell) responded. Wells and colleagues[295] have reported that glucocorticoid receptor levels ranged from 0 to 41,000 sites per cell (mean 17,000) in 6 patients resistant to chemotherapy, compared with 17,000 to 151,000 (mean 51,000) in 12 untreated patients. Furthermore, recent investigations suggest that there are substantial differences in receptor content of the various types of acute lymphoblastic leukemia of childhood—so-called T cell leukemias—having substantially fewer receptor sites than null cell leukemia.[291] The quantity of receptor in acute lymphoblastic leukemia has recently been shown to correlate with the duration of initial complete remission.[292] This correlation is independent of known prognostic factors such as cell type, initial white blood cell count, and sex. In 133 patients with common or undifferentiated acute lymphoblastic leukemia, low levels were noted in patients presenting with central nervous system disease.[296] After high-risk features were excluded, low receptor levels still correlated with a poor prognosis. These workers found that at 33 months, 29 per cent of patients with greater than 16,000 glucocorticoid receptors had relapsed, whereas 83 per cent had initial treatment failure if their initial receptor content was less than 16,000. Thus, at least in acute lymphoblastic leukemia, a role for analyses of glucocorticoid receptors appears established.

Glucocorticoid receptors also have been identified in other leukopathic states, including acute myelogenous leukemia,[297, 298] chronic myelogenous leukemia in blast crisis,[298] chronic lymphocytic leukemia,[299–301] and the Sézary syndrome. In none of these illnesses have significant correlations between receptor content and either clinical parameters or prognosis been reliably documented. Bloomfield and colleagues[302] have recently shown that quantitative glucocorticoid receptor determinations can accurately identify which patients with non-Hodgkin's lymphoma will respond to single-agent glucocorticoid therapy. Overall, receptor content did not correlate with any histological formulation. However, 39 patients with newly diagnosed lymphoma and 8 in relapse received single-agent glucocorticoid therapy for a minimum of 5 days, and response was correlated with receptor content. Mean glucocorticoid receptor content was 4031 sites per cell for responders and 2049 sites per cell for nonresponders ($p = 0.0006$). Clearly, "receptorology" as it pertains to glucocorticoid-responsive neoplasia is in an early stage of development and, with the possible exception of acute lymphoblastic leukemia, should be regarded as experimental. Nonetheless, these data are promising and deserve further study.

REFERENCES

1. MacMahon B, Cole P, Brown J: Etiology of human breast cancer: A review. J Natl Cancer Inst 50:21, 1973.
2. Miller AB: An overview of hormone-associated cancer. Cancer Res 38:3985, 1973.

3. Kelsey JL: A review of the epidemiology of human breast cancer. Epidemiol Rev 1:74, 1979.

4. Hall JM, Lee MK, Newman B, et al: Linkage of early-onset familial breast cancer to chromosome 17q21. Science 250:1684, 1990.

5. Pike MC, Henderson BE, Casagrande JT, et al: Oral contraceptive use and early abortion risk factors for breast cancer in young women. Br J Cancer 43:72, 1981.

6. Henderson BE, Pike MC, Casagrande JT: Breast cancer and the oestrogen window hypothesis. Lancet 2:363, 1981.

7. Trichopolous D, MacMahon B, Cole P: The menopause and breast cancer risk. J Natl Cancer Inst 48:605, 1972.

8. MacMahon B, Cole P, Lin TM, et al: Age at first birth and breast cancer risk. Bull WHO 43:209, 1970.

9. Pike MC, Henderson BE, Casagrande JT: The epidemiology of breast cancer as it relates to menarche, pregnancy and menopause. In Pike MC, Siiteri PK, Welsch CW (eds): Hormones and Breast Cancer. New York, CSH Publishing, 1981, pp 3–20.

10. deWaard F, Cornelis JP, Aoki K, et al: Breast cancer incidence according to weight and height in two cites of the Netherlands and in Aichi Prefecture. Jpn Cancer 40:1269, 1977.

11. Waterhouse J, Muir C, Correa P, et al: Cancer incidence in five continents. IARC (International Agency of Research in Cancer) Science Publication, vol 3, no 15, 1976.

12. Henderson BE, Pike MC, Ross RM: Epidemiology and risk factors. In Breast Cancer: Diagnosis and Management, vol 1. New York, John Wiley & Sons, 1984, pp 15–33.

13. Anderson DE: Breast cancer in families. Cancer 40:1855, 1977.

14. King MC, Go RCP, Elston RC, et al: Allele increasing susceptibility to human breast cancer may be linked to the glutamatepyruvate transaminase locus. Science 208:405, 1980.

15. Benedict WF, Hong-Ji X, Shi-Xue H, Takahashi R: Role of the retinoblastoma gene in the initiation and progression of human cancer. J Clin Invest 85:988, 1990.

16. Zumoff B: Abnormal plasma hormone levels in women with breast cancer. In Pike MC, Siiteri PK, Welsch CW (eds): Hormones and Breast Cancer. New York, CSH Publishing, 1981, pp 143–168.

17. Lemon HM, Wotiz HH, Parsons L, Mozden PJ: Reduced estriol excretion in patients with breast cancer prior to endocrine therapy. JAMA 196:1128, 1966.

18. MacMahon B, Cole P, Brown J, et al: Oestrogen profiles of Asian and North American women. Lancet 2:900, 1971.

19. Anderson JN: Estrogen-induced uterine responses and growth: Relationship to receptor estrogen binding by uterine nuclei. Endocrinology 96:160, 1975.

20. Lippman ME, Monaco ME, Bolan G: Effects of estrone, estradiol and estriol on hormone-responsive human breast cancer in long-term tissue culture. Cancer Res 37:1901, 1977.

21. Longcope C, Pratt JH: Relationship between urine and plasma estrogen ratios. Cancer Res 38:4025, 1978.

22. Henderson BE, Gerkins V, Rosario I, et al: Elevated serum levels of estrogen and prolactin in daughters of patients with breast cancer. N Engl J Med 293:790, 1975.

23. Korenman SG: Reproductive endocrinology and breast cancer in women. In Pike MC, Siiteri PK, Welsch CW (eds): Hormones and Breast Cancer. New York, CSH Publishing, 1981, pp 71–82.

24. Brown JB: Hormone profiles in young women at risk of breast cancer: A study of ovarian function during thelarche, menarche and menopause and after childbirth. In Pike MC, Siiteri PK, Welsch CW (eds): Hormones and Breast Cancer. New York, CSH Publishing, 1981, pp 33–54.

25. Siiteri PK, Hammond GL, Nisker JA: Increased availability of serum estrogens in breast cancer: A new hypothesis. In Pike MC, Siiteri PK, Welsch CW (eds): Hormones and Breast Cancer. New York, CSH Publishing, 1981, pp 87–101.

26. Moore JM, Clark CMG, Bulbrook RD, et al: Serum concentrations of total and non-protein-bound estradiol in patients with breast cancer and in normal controls. Int J Cancer 29:17, 1981.

27. Hill P, Wynder EL, Kumar J, et al: Prolactin levels in populations at risk for breast cancer. Cancer Res 36:4102, 1976.

28. Levin PA, Malarkey WB: Daughters of women with breast cancer have elevated mean 24-hour prolactin (PRL) levels and a partial resistance of PRL to dopamine suppression. J Clin Endocrinol Metab 53:179, 1981.

29. Fishman J, Fukushima D, O'Connor J, et al: Plasma hormone profiles of young women at risk for familial breast cancer. Cancer Res 38:4006, 1978.

30. Henderson BC, Pike MC: Prolactin—An important hormone in breast neoplasia? In Pike MC, Siiteri PK, Welsch CW (eds): Hormones and Breast Cancer. New York, CSH Publishing, 1981, pp 115–127.

31. Bulbrook RD, Thomas BS, Fantl VE, Hayward JL: A prospective study of the relation between thyroid function and subsequent breast cancer. In Pike MC, Siiteri PK, Welsch CW (eds): Hormones and Breast Cancer. New York, CSH Publishing, 1981, pp 131–140.

32. Kelsey JL, Holford TR, White C, et al: Oral contraceptives and breast disease. Am J Epidemiol 107:236, 1978.

33. Sartwell PE, Arthes FG, Tonascia JA: Exogenous hormones, reproductive history and breast cancer. J Natl Cancer Inst 59:1589, 1977.

34. Casagrande J, Gerkins V, Henderson BE, et al: Brief communication: Exogenous estrogens and breast cancer in women with natural menopause. J Natl Cancer Inst 56:839, 1976.

35. Craig TJ, Comstock GW, Geiser PB: Epidemiologic comparison of breast cancer patients with early and late onset of malignancy and general population controls. J Natl Cancer Inst 53:1577, 1974.

36. Paffenbarger RS, Fasal E, Simmons ME, Kampert JB: Cancer risk as related to the use of oral contraceptives during fertile years. Cancer 39:1887, 1977.

37. Boston Collaborative Drug Surveillance Programme: Oral contraceptives and venous thromboembolic disease, surgically confirmed, gallbladder disease, and breast tumours. Lancet 1:1399, 1973.

38. Brinton L, Williams R, Hoover R, et al: Breast cancer risk factors among screening program participants. J Natl Cancer Inst 63:37, 1979.

39. Jick H, Walker AM, Watkins RN, et al: Oral contraceptives and breast cancer. Am J Epidemiol 112:577, 1980.

40. Lippman ME, Huff K, Bolan G, Neifeld JP: Interactions of R5020 with progesterone and glucocorticoid receptors in human breast cancer and peripheral blood lymphocytes in vitro. In McGuire WL, et al (eds): Progesterone Receptors in Normal and Neoplastic Tissues. New York, Raven Press, 1977, pp 193–210.

41. Fergusson DJP, Anderson TJ: Morphological evaluation of cell turnover in relation to menstrual cycle in the "resting" human breast. Br J Cancer 44:177, 1981.

42. Boston Collaborative Drug Surveillance Programme: Lancet 1:1399, 1973.

43. Hoover R, Gray LA, Cole P, MacMahon B: Menopausal estrogens and breast cancer. N Engl J Med 295:410, 1976.

44. Brinton LA, Hoover RN, Szkio M, Fraumeni JF: Menopausal estrogen use and risk of breast cancer. Cancer 47:2517, 1981.

45. Hoover R, Gray L, Cole P, et al: Menopausal estrogens and breast cancer. N Engl J Med 295:401, 1976.

46. Hoover R, Glass A, Finkle WD, et al: Conjugated estrogens and breast cancer risk in women. J Natl Cancer Inst 67:815, 1981.

47. Jick H, Walker AM, Watkins RN, et al: Oral contraceptives and breast cancer. Am J Epidemiol 112:586, 1980.

48. Ross RK, Hill AP, Gerkins VR, et al: A case-control study of menopausal estrogen therapy and breast cancer. JAMA 243:1635, 1980.

49. Hunt H, Vessey M, McPherson K, Coleman M: Long term surveillance of mortality and cancer incidence in women receiving hormone replacement therapy. Br J Obstet Gynecol 94:620, 1987.

50. Bergkuist L, Adami H-O, Persson I, et al: The risk of breast cancer after estrogen and estrogen-progestin replacement. N Engl J Med 321:293, 1989.

51. Beatson GT: On the treatment of inoperable cases of carcinoma of the mamma: Suggestions for a new method of treatment of inoperable cases of carcinoma of the mamma. Lancet 2:162, 1896.

52. Grody WW, Schrader WT, O'Malley BW: Activation transformation and subunit structure of steroid hormone receptors. Endocr Rev 3:141, 1982.

53. McGuire WL, Julian JA, Chamness GC: A dissociation between ovarian-dependent growth and estrogen sensitivity in mammary carcinoma. Endocrinology 89:969, 1971.

54. Terenius L: Parallelism between oestrogen binding capacity and hormone responsiveness of mammary tumours in GR/A mice. Eur J Cancer 8:55, 1972.

55. Folca PJ, Glascock RF, Irvine WT: Studies with tritium labelled hexoestrol in advanced breast cancer. Lancet 2:796, 1966.

56. Korenman SG, Dukes BA: Specific estrogen binding by the cytoplasm of human breast carcinoma. J Clin Endocrinol 30:639, 1970.

57. Jensen EV, DeSombre ER, Jungblut PP: Estrogen receptors in hormone responsive tissues and tumors. In Wissler RV, Dao TL, Wood S (eds): Endogenous Factors Influencing Host Tumor Balance. Chicago, University of Chicago Press, 1967, pp 15–30.

58. Seibert K, Lippman ME: Hormone receptors in breast cancer. Clin Oncol 1:735, 1982.

59. Clark GM, McGuire WL: Progesterone receptors and human breast cancer. Breast Cancer Res Treat 3:157, 1983.

60. McGuire WL: Prognostic factors for recurrence and survival in human breast cancer. Breast Cancer Res Treat 10:5, 1987.

61. Fisher B, Redmond C, Brown A, et al: The influence of tumor estrogen and progesterone receptor levels on the response to tamoxifen and chemotherapy in primary breast cancer. J Clin Oncol 1:227, 1983.

62. Hill SM, Fuqua SAW, Chamness GC, et al: Estrogen receptor in human breast cancer associated with an estrogen receptor gene restriction fragment length polymorphism. Cancer Res 49:145, 1989.

63. Wittliff JL, Fisher B, Durant JR: Establishment of uniformity in steroid receptor analysis used in cooperative trials of breast cancer treatment. In Henningsen B, Linden F, Steichele C (eds): Recent Results in Cancer Research: Endocrine Treatment of Breast Cancer. New York, Springer-Verlag, 1980, p 198.

64. Panko WB, MacLeod RM: Uncharged nuclear receptors for estrogen in breast cancer. Cancer Res 38:1948, 1978.

65. Fuqua SAW, Krieg SL, Allred DC: Gel retardation assays help assess functional estrogen receptors in human breast tumors (abstract). Breast Cancer Res Treat 16:149, 1990.

66. McGuire WL: Steroid receptors in human breast cancer. Cancer Res 38:4289, 1978.

67. Greene GL, Nolan C, Engler JP, Jensen EV: Monoclonal antibodies to human estrogen receptor. Proc Natl Acad Sci USA 77:5115, 1981.

68. Greene GL, Closs LE, Fleming H: Antibodies to estrogen receptor: Immunochemical similarity of estrophilin from various mammalian species. Proc Natl Acad Sci USA 74:3681, 1977.

69. Saez S, Martin PM, Chouvet DC: Estradiol and progesterone receptor levels in relation to plasma estrogen and progesterone levels. Cancer Res 38:3468, 1978.

70. Degenshein GA, Bloom N, Ceccarelli F: Estrogen and progesterone receptor site studies as guides to the management of advanced breast cancer. Breast Dis Breast 3:23, 1977.

71. Knight WA, Livingston RB, Gregory EJ, McGuire WL: Estrogen receptor as an independent prognostic factor for early recurrence in breast cancer. Cancer Res 37:4669, 1977.

72. Maynard PV, Blamey RW, Elston CW, et al: Estrogen receptor assay in primary breast cancer and early recurrence of the disease. Cancer Res 38:4292, 1978.

73. Allegra JC, Lippman ME, Simon R, et al: Association between steroid hormone receptor status and disease-free interval in breast cancer. Cancer Treat Rep 1271, 1979.

74. Kinne DW, Ashikari R, Butler A: Estrogen receptor protein in breast cancer as a prediction of recurrence. Cancer 47:2364, 1981.

75. Leake RE, Laing L, McArdle C, Smith DC: Soluble and nuclear oestrogen receptor status in human breast cancer in relation to prognosis. Br J Cancer 43:59, 1981.

76. Harris JR, Lippman ME, Veronesi U, Willett W: Medical progress: Breast cancer. N Engl J Med 327:319–328, 1992.

77. Harris JR, Hellman S, Silen W (eds): Conservative Management of Breast Cancer. Philadelphia, JB Lippincott Co, 1983.

78. Lippman ME: Adjuvant systemic therapy of breast cancer therapy. In DeVita VT, Hellman S, Rosenberg S (eds): Current Topics in Oncology. Philadelphia, JB Lippincott Co, 1984.

79. Glauber JG, Kiang DT: The changing role of hormonal therapy in advanced breast cancer. Semin Oncol 19:308, 1992.

80. Hall TC, Dederick MM, NeVinney HB, Muench H: Prognostic value of response of patients with breast cancer to therapeutic castration. Cancer Chemother Rep 31:47, 1963.

81. Lewison EF: Castration in the treatment of advanced breast cancer. Cancer 18:1558, 1965.

82. Fracchia AA, Farrow JH, Miller TR, et al: Hypophysectomy as compared with adrenalectomy in the treatment of advanced carcinoma of the breast. Surg Gynecol Obstet 128:1226, 1969.

83. Meakin JW: Is there a place for adjuvant endocrine therapy of breast cancer? In Henningsen B, Linder F, Steichele C (eds): Recent Results in Cancer Research: Endocrine Treatment of Breast Cancer. New York, Springer-Verlag, 1980, p 178.

84. Longcope C: Metabolic clearance and blood production rates of estrogens in postmenopausal women. Am J Obstet Gynecol 111:778, 1971.

85. Grodin JM, Siiteri PK, MacDonald PC: Source of estrogen production in postmenopausal women. J Clin Endocrinol 36:207, 1973.

86. Aitken SC, Lippman ME: Steroid receptors in breast cancer. Arch Intern Med 142:363, 1982.

87. Schally AV, Reddin TW: Inhibition of cell growth by a hypothalamic peptide. Proc Natl Acad Sci USA 79:7014, 1982.

88. Henderson IC, Canellos GP: Cancer of the breast: The past decade. N Engl J Med 302:17, 1980.

89. Lacassagne MA: Apparition de cancers de la mamelle chez la souris male, soumise a des injections de folliculine. C R Acad Sci [III] 195:630, 1932.

90. Davies P, Nicholson RI: How do androgens and progestins cause regression of breast cancer? Rev Endocr Relat Cancer 10:19, 1981.

91. Allegra JC, Lippman ME, Thompson EB, et al: The distribution, frequency and quantitative analysis of estrogen, progesterone, androgen and glucocorticoid receptors in human breast cancer. Cancer Res 39:1447, 1979.

92. Allegra JC, Lippman ME, Thompson EB, et al: Relationship between the progesterone, androgen and glucocorticoid receptor and response rate to endocrine therapy in metastatic breast cancer. Cancer Res 39:1973, 1979.

93. Cooperative Breast Cancer Group: Testosterone propionate therapy in breast therapy. JAMA 188:1069, 1964.

94. Goldenberg IS: Clinical trial of delta-1-testolactone (NSC 23759), medroxyprogesterone acetate (NSC 26386), and oxylone acetate (NSC 47438) in advanced female mammary cancer. Cancer 23:109, 1969.

95. Mansel RE, Wisbey JR, Hughes LE: The use of danazol in the treatment of painful benign breast disease: Preliminary results. Postgrad Med J 55:61, 1979.

96. Madanos AE, Farber M: Danazol. Ann Intern Med 96:625, 1982.

97. Coombes RC, Dearnaley D, Humphreys J, et al: Danazol treatment of advanced breast cancer. Cancer Treat Rep 64:1073, 1980.

98. Powles TJ, Gordon C, Coombes RC: Clinical trial of multiple endocrine therapy for metastatic and locally advanced breast cancer with tamoxifen-aminoglutethemide-danazol compared to tamoxifen used alone. Cancer Res 42:3458, 1982.

99. Kennedy BJ: Hormone therapy in inoperable breast cancer. Cancer 24:1345, 1969.

100. Kennedy BJ: Diethylstilbestrol versus testosterone propionate therapy in advanced breast cancer. Surg Gynecol Obstet 120:1246, 1965.

101. Kaufman RJ, Escher GC: Rebound regression in advanced mammary carcinoma. Surg Gynecol Obstet 113:635, 1961.

102. Stoll BA: Progestin therapy of breast cancer: Comparison of agents. Br Med J 3:338, 1967.

103. Pannuti F, Martoni A, DiMarco AR, et al: Prospective, randomized clinical trial of two different high dosages of medroxyprogesterone acetate (MAP) in the treatment of metastatic breast cancer. Eur J Cancer 15:593, 1979.

104. Beretta G, Tabiadon D, Tedeschi L, Luporini G: Hormonotherapy of advanced breast carcinoma: Comparative evaluation of tamoxifen citrate versus medroxyprogesterone acetate. In Iacobelli S, Lippman ME, Della Cona GR (eds): The Role of Tamoxifen in Breast Cancer. New York, Raven Press, 1983, pp 113–120.

105. Muss HB, Well HB, Pasehold EH, et al: Mesestrol acetate versus tamoxifen in advanced breast care: 5-year analysis. J Clin Oncol 8:1797–1805, 1990.

106. Geiner NF, Donegan WL: Role and mechanism of corticosteroid therapy in breast cancer. Rev Endocr Relat Cancer 6:5, 1980.

107. Sutherland RL, Jordan VC: Non-steroidal anti-estrogen molecular pharmacology and antitumor activity. In Sutherland RL, Jordan VC (eds): Non-Steroidal Antioestrogens. Sydney, Academic Press, 1981.

108. Butta A, MacLennan K, Flanders KC, et al: Induction of transforming growth factor beta 1 in human breast cancer in vivo following tamoxifen treatment. Cancer Res 52:4261–4264, 1992.

109. Sutherland RL, Murphy LC, Foo MS, et al: High-affinity anti-estrogen binding site distinct from the oestrogen receptor. Nature 288:273, 1980.

110. Osborne CK, Coronado E, Wiebe V, et al: Acquired tamoxifen resistance in breast cancer correlates with reduced tumor accumulation of tamoxifen and trans-4-hydroxytamoxifen (Abstract). Proc Am Soc Clin Oncol 10:46, 1991.

111. Murphy LC, Sutherland RL: Modifications in the aminoether side chain of clomiphene influence affinity for a specific anti-estrogen binding site in MCF-7 cytosol. Biochem Biophys Res Commun 100:1353, 1981.

112. Eckert RL, Katzenellenbogen BS: Physical properties of estrogen receptor complexes in MCF-7 human breast cancer cells. J Biol Chem 257:8840, 1982.

113. Legha S, Muggia FM: Antiestrogens in the treatment of cancer. Ann Intern Med 84:751, 1976.

114. Mouridsen H, Palshof T, Patterson J: Tamoxifen in advanced breast cancer. Cancer Treat Rep 5:131, 1978.

115. Heel RC, Brogden RN, Speight TM: Tamoxifen—A review of its pharmacologic properties and therapeutic use in the treatment of breast cancer. Drugs 16:1, 1978.

116. Pearson OH, Manni A, Arafah BM: Antiestrogen treatment of breast cancer: An overview. Cancer Res 42:3424, 1982.

117. Manni A, Trujillo J, Marshall JS, Pearson OH: Antiestrogen-induced remissions in stage IV breast cancer. Cancer Treat Rep 60:1445, 1976.

118. McIntosh IH, Thynne GS: Tumour stimulation by anti-oestrogens. Br J Surg 64:900, 1977.

119. Patterson JS, Battersby LA, Edwards DG: Review of the clinical pharmacology and international experience with tamoxifen in advanced breast cancer: Rev Endocr Relat Cancer Suppl 9:563, 1982.

120. Tormey DC, Lippman ME, Edwards BK, Cassidy J: Evaluation of tamoxifen doses with and without fluoxymesterone in advanced breast cancer. Ann Intern Med 98:139, 1983.

121. Manni A, Arafah B, Pearson OH: Changes in endocrine status following antioestrogen administration to premenopausal and postmenopausal women. In Sutherland RL, Jordan VC (eds): Non-Steroidal Antioestrogens. Sydney, Academic Press, 1981, pp 435–452.

122. Pritchard KI, Thomson DB, Myers RE: Tamoxifen therapy in premenopausal patients with metastatic breast cancer. Cancer Treat Rep 64:787, 1980.

123. Manni A, Pearson OH: Antiestrogen-induced remissions in premenopausal women with stage IV breast cancer: Effects of ovarian function. Cancer Treat Rep 64:779, 1980.

124. Adam HK, Patterson JS, Kemp JV: Studies on the metabolism and pharmacokinetics of tamoxifen in normal volunteers. Cancer Treat Rep 64:761, 1980.

125. Fabian C, Sternson L, Barnett M: Clinical pharmacology of tamoxifen in patients with breast cancer: Comparison of traditional and loading dose schedules. Cancer Treat Rep 64:775, 1980.

126. Patterson JS, Settatree RS, Adam HK: Clinical use of antiestrogens. In Mouridsen H, Palshof T (eds): Breast Cancer: Experimental and Clinical Aspects. London, Pergamon Press, 1980, pp 89–92.

127. Valcuaara R, Tuominen J, Johansson R: Predictive value of tumor estrogen and progesterone receptor levels in postmenopausal women with advanced breast cancer treated with toremifene. Cancer 66:2264, 1990.

128. Griffiths CT, Hall TC, Saba Z, et al: Preliminary trial of aminoglutethimide in breast cancer. Cancer 32:31, 1973.

129. Fishman LM, Liddle GW, Island DP, et al: Effects of aminoglutethimide on adrenal function in man. J Clin Endocrinol Metab 27:481, 1967.

130. Santen RJ, Lipton A, Kendall J: Successful medical adrenalectomy with amino-glutethimide: Role of altered drug metabolism. JAMA 230:1661, 1974.

131. Santen RJ, Samojlik E, Lipton A, et al: Kinetic, hormonal and clinical studies with aminoglutethimide in breast cancer. Cancer 39:2948, 1977.

132. Harvey HA, Lipton A, Sonfert RJ: Aromatase: New perspectives for breast cancer. Cancer Res 42:3267, 1982.

133. Wells SA, Worsol TJ, Samojlik E, et al: Comparison of surgical adrenalectomy to medical adrenalectomy in patients with metastatic carcinoma of the breast. Cancer Res 42:3454, 1982.

134. Coombes RC, Dowsett M, Goss P, et al: 4-hydroxyandrostenedione in treatment of postmenopausal patients with advanced breast cancer. Lancet 1:1237, 1984.

135. Goss PE, Powles TJ, Dowsett M, et al: Treatment of advanced postmenopausal breast cancer with an aromatase inhibitor, 4-hydroxyandrostenedione: Phase II report. Cancer Res 46:4823–4826, 1986.

136. Kangas L, Mieminen AL, Blanco G, et al: A new triphenylethylene compound, Fc-1157a: II. Antitumor effects. Cancer Chemother Pharmacol 17:109–113, 1986.

137. Michna H, Schneider M, Nishino Y, et al: The antitumor activity of the antiprogestins ZK 98.299 and RU 38.486 in hormone-dependent rat and mouse mammary tumors: Mechanistic studies. Breast Cancer Res Treat 14:275–288, 1989.

138. Michna H, Schneider MR, Nishino Y, et al: The antitumor mechanism of progesterone antagonists is a receptor mediated antiproliferative effect by induction of terminal cell death. J Steroid Biochem 34:447–453, 1989.

139. Kaufman M, Jonat W, Kleeberg U, et al: Goserelin, a depot gonadotrophin-releasing hormone agonist in the treatment of premenopausal patients with metastatic breast cancer. J Clin Oncol 7:1113–1119, 1989.

140. Harvey HA, Lipton A, Max DT, et al: Medical castration produced by the GnRH analogue leuprolide to treat metastatic breast cancer. J Clin Oncol 3:1068–1072, 1985.

141. Hoffken K, Oesterdickhoff C, Becher R, et al: LHRH agonist treatment with Buserelin in premenopausal patients with advanced breast cancer: A phase II study. Cancer Ther Controv 1:13–20, 1989.

142. Robert NJ, Dalton WS, Osborne CK, et al: Therapy in premenopausal women with advanced, oestrogen positive or/and progesterone positive breast cancer: surgical oophorectomy versus the LHRH analogue, Zoladex. Horm Res 32(suppl 1):221–222, 1989.

143. Reubi JC, Torhorst J: The relationship between somatostatin, epidermal growth factor and steroid hormone receptors in breast cancer. Cancer 64:1254–1260, 1989.

144. Setyono-Han B, Henkelman MS, Foekens JA, et al: Direct inhibitory effects of somatostatin (analogues) on the growth of human breast cancer cells. Cancer Res 47:551–558, 1987.

145. Lippman ME: Efforts to combine endocrine and chemotherapy in the management of breast cancer: Do two and two equal three? Breast Cancer Res Treat 3:117, 1983.

146. Lippman ME, Cassidy J, Wesley M, Young RC: A randomized attempt to increase the efficacy of cytotoxic chemotherapy in metastatic breast cancer by hormonal synchronization. J Clin Oncol 2:28, 1984.

147. Suarez AJ, Lamm DL, Radwin HM, et al: Androgen priming and cytotoxic chemotherapy in advanced prostatic cancer. Cancer Chemother Pharmacol 8:261, 1982.

148. Allegra JC: Methotrexate and 5-fluorouracil following tamoxifen and premarin in advanced breast cancer. Semin Oncol 10:23, 1983.

149. Crichlow RW: Carcinoma of the male breast. Surg Gynecol Obstet 134:1011, 1972.

150. Meyskens FL, Tormey EC, Neifeld JP: Male breast cancer: A review. Cancer Treat Rep 3:83, 1976.

151. Everson RB, Lippman ME: Male breast cancer. In McGuire WL (ed): Breast Cancer Advances in Research and Treatment, vol 3. New York, Plenum Press, 1979, pp 239–267.

152. Symners WSC: Carcinoma of breast in transsexual individuals after surgical interference with the primary and secondary sex characteristics. Br Med J 2:83, 1968.

153. Everson RB, Lippman ME, Thompson EB, et al: Clinical correlations of steroid receptors and male breast cancer. Cancer Res 40:991, 1980.

154. Patterson JS, Battershy LA, Bach BK: Use of tamoxifen in advanced male breast cancer. Cancer Treat Rep 64:801, 1980.

155. Jensen EV, Jacobsen HI: Basic guides to the mechanism of estrogen action. Recent Prog Horm Res 18:387, 1962.

156. Antunes CMF, Sooley PD, Rosenshein NB, et al: Endometrial cancer and estrogen use (report of a large case-control study). N Engl J Med 300:9, 1979.

157. Nisker JA, Ramzy I, Collins JA: Adenocarcinoma of the endometrium and abnormal ovarian function in young women. Am J Obstet Gynecol 130:546, 1978.

158. Whitehead MI, Campbell SC, King RJ, McQueen J: Oestrogen treatment and endometrial carcinoma. Br Med J 2:453, 1977.

159. Hensell DL, Grodin JM, Brenner PF, et al: Plasma precursors of estrogen: II. Correlation of the extent of conversion of plasma androstenedione to estrone with age. J Clin Endocrinol Metab 38:476, 1974.

160. MacDonald PC, Edman CD, Hemsell DL, et al: Effect of obesity on conversion of plasma androstenedione to estrone in postmenopausal women with and without endometrial cancer. Am J Obstet Gynecol 130:448, 1978.

161. Judd HL, Lucas WE, Yen SC: Serum 17β-estradiol and estrone levels in postmenopausal women with and without endometrial cancer. J Clin Endocrinol Metab 43:272, 1976.

162. Feinstein AR, Horowitz RI: A critique of the statistical evidence associating estrogens with endometrial cancer. Cancer Res 38:4001, 1978.

163. Pollow K, Lubbert H, Boquoi E, et al: Characterization and comparison of receptors for 17β-estradiol and progesterone in human proliferative endometrium and endometrial carcinoma. Endocrinology 96:319, 1975.

164. Bayard F, Damilamo S, Robel P, Baulieu E: Cytoplasmic and nuclear estradiol and progesterone receptors in human endometrium. J Clin Endocrinol Metab 46:635, 1978.

165. King RJB, Dyer G, Collins WP, Whitehead MI: Intracellular estradiol, estrone and estrogen receptor levels in endometrial specimens from postmenopausal women receiving estrogens and progestins. J Steroid Biochem 13:377, 1980.

166. Young PCM, Ehrlick CE, Cleary RE: Progesterone binding in human endometrial carcinomas. Am J Obstet Gynecol 125:353, 1976.

167. Feil PD, Mann WJ, Mortel R, Bardin CW: Nuclear progestin receptors in normal and malignant human endometrium. J Clin Endocrinol Metab 48:327, 1979.

168. Gurpide E, Gusberg SB, Tseng L: Estradiol binding metabolism in human endometrial hyperplasia and adenocarcinoma. J Steroid Biochem 7:891, 1976.

169. Satyaswaroop PG, Zaino R, Murtel R: Human endometrial adenocarcinoma transplanted into nude mice: Growth regulation by estradiol. Science 219:58, 1983.

170. Satyaswaroop PG, Zaino R, Murtel R: Estrogen-like effects of tamoxifen on human endometrial carcinoma transplanted into nude mice. Cancer Res 44:4006, 1984.

171. Kelley RM, Baker WH: Progestational agents in the treatment of carcinoma of the endometrium. N Engl J Med 264:216, 1961.

172. Reifenstein EC Jr: Hydroxyprogesterone caproate therapy in advanced endometrial cancer. Cancer 27:485, 1971.

173. Reifenstein EC Jr: The treatment of advanced endometrial cancer with hydroxyprogesterone caproate (review). Gynecol Oncol 2:377, 1974.

174. Piver MS, Barlow JJ, Lurain JR, Blumenson LE: Medroxyprogesterone acetate (Depo-Provera) versus hydroxyprogesterone caproate O (Delalutin) in women with metastatic endometrial adenocarcinoma. Cancer 45:268, 1980.

175. Quinn MA, Cauchi M, Fortune D: Endometrial carcinoma: Steroid receptors and response to medroxyprogesterone acetate. Gynecol Oncol 21:314, 1985.

176. Podratz KC, O'Brien PC, Malkasian GD Jr, et al: Effects of progestational agents in treatment of endometrial carcinoma. Obstet Gynecol 66:106, 1985.

177. Malkasian GD Jr, Decker D, Mussey E, Johnson CE: Progesterone treatment of recurrent endometrial carcinoma. Am J Obstet Gynecol 110:15, 1971.

178. Park RC, Grigsby PW, Muss HB, Norris HJ: Corpus: Epithelial tumors. In Hoskins WJ, Perez CA, Young RC (eds): Principles and Practice of Gynecologic Oncology. Philadelphia, JB Lippincott Co, 1992, pp 663–693.

179. Swenerton KD: Treatment of advanced endometrial adenocarcinoma with tamoxifen. Cancer Treat Rep 64:805, 1980.

180. Bonte J, Ide P, Billiet G, Wynants P: Tamoxifen as a possible chemotherapeutic agent in endometrial adenocarcinoma. Gynecol Oncol 11:140, 1981.

181. Slavik M, Petty WM, Blessing JA, et al: Phase II clinical study of tamoxifen in advanced endometrial adenocarcinoma: A Gynecologic Oncology Group study. Cancer Treat Rep 68:809, 1984.

182. Edmonson J, Krook JE, Hilton JF, et al: Ineffectiveness of tamoxifen in advanced endometrial carcinoma after failure of progestin treatment. Cancer Treat Rep 70:1019, 1986.

183. Seski JC, Edwards CL, Gershman DM: Doxorubicin and cyclophosphamide chemotherapy for disseminated endometrial cancer. Obstet Gynecol 53:88, 1981.

184. Bruckner HW, Cohen CJ, Deppe G: Chemotherapy of gynecological tumors with platinum. J Clin Hematol Oncol 7:619, 1977.

185. Gloeckler Ries LA, Hankey BF, Miller BA: Cancer Statistics Review 1973–88. Bethesda, MD: US Department of Health and Human Services, 1991.

186. Rotkin ID: Studies on the epidemiology of prostate cancer: Expanded sampling. Cancer Treat Rep 61:173–180, 1977.

187. Graham S, Haughey B, Marshall J, et al: Diet in the epidemiology of carcinoma of the prostate gland. J Nat Cancer Inst 70:687–692, 1983.

188. Hirayama T: Epidemiology of prostate cancer with special reference to the role of diet. NCI Monogr 53:149–155, 1979.

189. Steinberg GD, Carter BS, Beaty TH, et al: Family history and the risk of prostate cancer. Prostate 17:337–347, 1990.

190. Ghanadian R, Puah CM, O'Donoghue EPN: Serum testosterone and dihydrotestosterone in carcinoma of the prostate. Br J Cancer 39:696–699, 1979.

191. Ahluwalia B, Jackson MA, Jones GW, et al: Blood hormone profiles in prostate cancer patients in high risk and low risk populations. Cancer 48:2267–2273, 1981.

192. Drafta D, Proca E, Zamfir V, et al: Plasma steroids in benign prostatic hypertrophy and carcinoma of the prostate. J Steroid Biochem 17:689–693, 1982.

193. Zumoff B, Levin J, Strain GW, et al: Abnormal levels of plasma hormones in men with prostate cancer: evidence toward a "two-disease" theory. Prostate 3:579–588, 1985.

194. Zaridze DG, Boyle P: Cancer of the prostate: Epidemiology and etiology. Br J Urol 59:493–502, 1987.

195. Frank LM: Latent carcinoma of the prostate. J Pathol Bacteriol 68:603–614, 1954.

196. Sheldon CA, Williams RD, Fraley EE: Incidental carcinoma of the prostate: A review of the literature and critical reappraisal of classification. J Urol 124:626–631, 1980.

197. Breslow N, Char CE, Dhom G, et al: Latent carcinoma of the prostate at autopsy in seven areas. Int J Cancer 20:680–688, 1977.

198. Yatani R, Chigusa K, Stemmerman GN: Geographic pathology of latent prostatic carcinoma. Int J Cancer 33:223–230, 1982.

199. Jackson MA, Ahluwalia BS, Herson J: Characterization of prostatic carcinoma among blacks: A continuation report. Cancer Treat Rep 61:167–172, 1977.

200. Akazaki K, Stemmerman GN: Comparative study of latent carcinoma of the prostate among Japanese in Japan and Hawaii. J Nat Cancer Inst 50:1137–1144, 1973.

201. Hanenszel W, Kurihari M: Studies of Japanese migrants: Mortality from cancer and other diseases among Japanese in the United States. J Nat Cancer Inst 40:43–68, 1968.

202. Ross RK, Paganini-Hill A, Henderson BE: Epidemiology of prostatic cancer. In Skinner DG, Lieskovsky G (eds): Diagnosis and Management of Genitourinary Cancer. Philadelphia, WB Saunders Co, 1988, pp 40–45.

203. Kovi J, Heshmat MY: Incidence of cancer in negroes in Washington, DC, and other selected American cities. Am J Epidemiol 96:401, 1972.

204. Levine RL, Wilchinsky M: Adenocarcinoma of the prostate: A comparison of the disease in blacks versus whites. J Urol 121:761–762, 1979.

205. Crawford ED, Nabors W: Hormone therapy of advanced prostate cancer: Where we stand today. Oncology 5:21–28, 1991.

206. Correa RJ, Anderson RG, Gibbons RP, Mason JT: Latent carcinoma of the prostate: Why the controversy? J Urol 111:644–646, 1974.

207. Haney JA, Chang HC, Daly JJ, Prout G: Prognosis of clinically undiagnosed prostate carcinoma and influence of endocrine therapy. J Urol 118:282–287, 1977.

208. Cantrell BB, DeKlerk DP, Eggleston JC, et al: Pathologic factors that influence prognosis in stage A prostatic cancer: The influence of extent versus grade. J Urol 125:516–520, 1981.

209. Olsson CA, Babyan R, deVere White R: Surgical management of stage B or C prostate carcinoma: Radical surgery versus radiotherapy. Urology Suppl 25:30–35, 1985.

210. Gleason DF: Classification of prostatic carcinomas. Cancer Chemother Rep 50:125–128, 1966.

211. Gleason DF, Mellinger GT: The Veterans Administration Cooperative Urologic Research Group: Prediction of prognosis for prostatic adenocarcinoma by combined histologic grading and clinical staging. J Urol 10:235–236, 1974.

212. Murphy GP, Whitmore WF Jr: A report of the workshops on the current status of the histologic grading of prostate cancer. Cancer 44:1490–1494, 1977.

213. Mostofi FK: Problems of grading carcinoma of the prostate. Semin Oncol 3:161–169, 1976.

214. Utz DC, Farrow GM: Pathologic differentiation and prognosis of prostatic carcinoma. JAMA 209:1701–1703, 1969.

215. Bandalament RA, O'Toole RV, Young DC, Drago JR: DNA ploidy and prostate-specific antigen as prognostic factors in clinically resectable prostate cancer. Cancer 67:3014–3023, 1991.

216. Montgomery BT, Nativ O, Blute ML, et al: Stage B prostate adenocarcinoma flow cytometric nuclear DNA ploidy analysis. Arch Surg 125:327–331, 1990.

217. Forsslund G, Esposti P-L, Nilsson B, Zetterberg A: The prognostic significance of nuclear DNA content in prostatic carcinoma. Cancer 69:1432–1439, 1992.

218. Wang MD, Valenzuela LA, Murphy GP, Chu TM: Purification of a human prostate specific antigen. Invest Urol 17:159, 1979.

219. Seamonds B, Yang N, Anderson K, et al: Evaluation of prostate-specific antigen and prostatic acid phosphatase as prostate cancer markers. Urology 28:472–479, 1986.

220. Stamey T, Yang N, Hay AR, et al: Prostate-specific antigen as a serum marker for adenocarcinoma of the prostate. N Engl J Med 317:900–916, 1987.

221. Oesterling JE, Chan DW, Epstein JI, et al: Prostate-specific antigen in the preoperative and postoperative evaluation of localized prostatic cancer treated with radical prostatectomy. J Urol 139:766–772, 1988.

222. Powell CS, Fielding AM, Rosser K, et al: Prostate-specific antigen: A screening test for prostatic cancer? Br J Urol 64:504–506, 1989.

223. Catalona WJ, Smith DS, Ratliff TL, et al: Measurement of prostate-specific antigen in serum as a screening test for prostate cancer. N Engl J Med 324:1156–1161, 1991.

224. Chan DW, Bruzek DJ, Oesterling JE, et al: Prostate-specific antigen as a marker for prostatic cancer: A monoclonal and polyclonal immunoassay compared. Clin Chem 33:1916–1920, 1987.

225. Hudson MA, Bahnson RR, Catalona WJ: Clinical use of prostate specific antigen in patients with prostate cancer. J Urol 142:1011–1017, 1989.

226. Stamey TA, Kabalin JN: Prostate-specific antigen in the diagnosis and treatment of adenocarcinoma of the prostate: I. Untreated patients. J Urol 141:1070–1075, 1989.

227. Stamey TA, Yang N, Hay AR, et al: Prostate-specific antigen as a serum marker for adenocarcinoma of the prostate. N Engl J Med 317:909–916, 1987.

228. Lange PH: Controversies in management of apparently localized cancer of the prostate. Urology 34(suppl 4):13–80, 1989.

229. Walsh PC, Donker PJ: Impotence following radical prostatectomy: Insight into etiology and prevention. J Urol 128:492–497, 1982.

230. Quinlan DM, Epstein JI, Carter BS, Walsh PC: Sexual function following radical prostatectomy: Influence of preservation of neurovascular bundles. J Urol 145:998–1002, 1991.

231. Bagshaw MA, Kaplan HS, Sagerman RH: Linear accelerator supervoltage radiotherapy: VII. Carcinoma of the prostate. Radiology 85:121–129, 1965.

232. Hanks GE: External-beam radiation therapy for clinically localized prostate cancer: Patterns of care studies in the United States. NCI Monogr 7:75–84, 1988.

233. Paulson DF: Randomized series of treatment with surgery versus radiation for prostate adenocarcinoma. NCI Monogr 7:127–131, 1988.

234. Paulson DF, Lin GH, Hinshaw W, et al: Radical surgery versus radiotherapy for adenocarcinoma of the prostate. J Urol 128:502–504, 1982.

235. NIH Consensus Development Conference: Management of clinically localized prostate cancer. Oncology 1:46–49, 1987.

236. Huggins C, Stevens RE, Hodges CL: Studies on prostatic cancer: II. The effect of castration on clinical patients with carcinoma of the prostate. Arch Surg 43:209, 1941.

237. Huggins C, Hodges CL: Studies on prostatic cancer: Effect of castration, of estrogen and of androgen injection on serum phosphatases in metastatic carcinoma of the prostate. Cancer Res 1:293–297, 1941.

238. Wilson JD, Siiteri PK: Developmental pattern of testosterone synthesis in the fetal gonad of the rabbit. Endocrinology 92:1182–1191, 1973.

239. Siiteri PK, Wilson JD: Testosterone formation and metabolism during male sexual differentiation in the human embryo. J Clin Endocrinol Metabol 38:113–125, 1974.

240. Griffin J: Androgen resistance: The clinical and molecular spectrum. N Engl J Med 326:611–618, 1992.

241. Shannon JM, Cunha GR, Vanderslice KD: Autoradiographic localization of androgen receptors in the developing urogenital tract and mammary gland. Anat Rec 199:232, 1981.

242. Shannon JM, Cunha GR: Autoradiographic localization of androgen binding in the developing mouse prostate. Prostate 4:367–373, 1983.

243. Takeda H, Miguno T, Lasnitzki I: Autoradiographic studies of androgen-binding sites in the rat urogenital sinus and postnatal prostate. J Endocrinol 104:87–92, 1985.

244. Lubahn DB, Joseph DR, Sar M, et al: The human androgen receptor: Complementary deoxyribonucleic acid cloning, sequence analysis, and gene expression in prostate. Mol Endocrinol 2:1265, 1988.

245. Chodak GW, Kranc DM, Puy LA, et al: Nuclear localization of androgen receptor in heterogeneous samples of normal, hyperplastic, and neoplastic human prostate. J Urol 147:798–803, 1992.

246. Kyprianou N, Isaacs JT: Activation of programmed cell death in the rat ventral prostate after castration. Endocrinology 122:552–562, 1988.

247. Buttyan R, Zaker Z, Lochshin R, Wolgemuth D: Cascade induction of c-fos, c-myc, and heat shock 70K transcripts during regression of the rat ventral prostate gland. Mol Endocrinol 2:650–657, 1988.

248. Horoszewicz JS, Leong SS, Chu TM, et al: The LNCaP line: A new model for studies on human prostatic carcinoma. In Murphy GP (ed): Progress in Clinical Biologic Research. New York, Alan R Liss, 1980, pp 115–132.

249. Horoszewicz JS, Leong SS, Kawinski E, et al: LNCaP model of human prostatic carcinoma. Cancer Res 43:1809–1818, 1983.

250. van Steenbrugge GJ, van Dongen JJW, Reuvers PJ, et al: Transplantable human prostatic carcinoma (PC-82) in athymic nude mice: I. Hormone-dependence and the concentration of androgens in plasma and tumor tissue. Prostate 11:195–210, 1987.

251. Newmark JR, Hardy DO, Tonb DC, et al: Androgen receptor gene mutations in human prostate cancer. Proc Natl Acad Sci USA 89:6319–6323, 1992.

252. Wilding G, Chen M, Gelmann EP: Aberrant response in vitro of hormone-responsive prostate cancer cells to antiandrogens. Prostate 14:103–115, 1989.

253. Veldscholte J, Ris-Stalpers C, Kuiper GGJ, et al: A mutation in the ligand binding domain of the androgen receptor of human LNCaP cells affects steroid binding characteristics and response to anti-androgens. Biochem Biophys Res Commun 173:534–540, 1990.

254. Byar DP: The Veterans Administration Cooperative Urological Research Group's studies of cancer of the prostate. Cancer 32:1126–1130, 1973.

255. Prout GR: Endocrine changes after diethylstilbestrol therapy: Effect on prostatic neoplasm and pituitary gonadal axis. Urology 7:148, 1976.

256. Schally AV, Coy DH, Arimura A: LH-RH agonist and antagonists. Int J Gynaecol Obstet 18:318–324, 1980.

257. The Leuprolide Study Group: Leuprolide versus diethylstilbestrol for metastatic prostate cancer. N Engl J Med 311:1281–1286, 1984.

258. Labrie F, Dupong A, Belanger A, et al: New approach in the treatment of prostate cancer: Complete instead of partial withdrawal of androgens. Prostate 4:579–594, 1983.

259. Waxman JH, Wass JAH, Hendry WF, et al: Treatment with gonadotrophin-releasing hormone analogue in advanced prostatic cancer. Br J Med 286:1309–1312, 1983.

260. Kuhn J-M, Billebaud MD, Navratil H, et al: Prevention of the transient adverse effects of a gonadotropin-releasing hormone analogue (Buserelin) in metastatic prostatic carcinoma by administration of an antiandrogen (Nilutamide). N Engl J Med 321:413–418, 1989.

261. Labrie F, Dupong A, Belanger A, et al: New approach in the treatment of prostate cancer: Complete instead of partial withdrawal of androgens. Prostate 4:579–594, 1983.

262. Sufrin G, Coffey DS: Flutamide: Mechanisms of action of a new nonsteroidal antiandrogen. Invest Urol 13:429–434, 1976.

263. Crawford ED, Eisenberger M, McCleod DG, et al: A controlled trial of leuprolide with and without flutamide in prostatic carcinoma. N Engl J Med 321:419–424, 1989.

264. Eisenberger M, Crawford D, McCleod D, et al: A comparison of leuprolide and flutamide versus leuprolide alone in newly diagnosed stage D2 prostate cancer: Prognostic and therapeutic importance of minimal disease subset. Proc Am Soc Clin Oncol 11:A619, 1992.

265. Iversen P, Christensen MG, Friis E, et al: A phase III trial of Zoladex and flutamide versus orchiectomy in the treatment of patients with advanced carcinoma of the prostate. Cancer Suppl 66:1058–1066, 1990.

266. Newling D, Pavone Macaluse M, Smith P, et al: Update of EORTC clinical trials in prostate cancer: The EORTC Genito-Urinary Group. Semin Urol 10:65–71, 1992.

267. Fourcade RO, Cariou G, Coloby P, et al: Total androgen blockade with Zoladex plus flutamide vs Zoladex alone in advanced prostate carcinoma: Interim report of a multicenter, double-blind, placebo-controlled study. Eur Urol Suppl 18:45–47, 1990.

268. McConnell JD, Wilson JD, George FW, et al: Finasteride, an inhibitor of 5 alpha-reductase, suppresses prostatic dihydrotestosterone in men with benign prostatic hyperplasia. J Clin Endocrinol Metab 74:505–508, 1992.

269. Chang A, Yeap B, Blum R, et al: A double-blind randomized study of primary treatment for stage D₂ prostate cancer: Diethylstilbestrol (DES) versus flutamide. Proc Am Soc Clin Oncol 11:A621, 1992.

270. Stoner E: The clinical effects of a 5 alpha-reductase inhibitor, finasteride, on benign prostatic hyperplasia: The Finasteride Study Group. J Urol 147:1298–1302, 1992.

271. Thompson EB, Lippman ME: Mechanism of action of glucocorticoids. Metabolism 23:159, 1974.

272. Baxter JD, Forsham PH: Tissue effects of glucocorticoids. Am J Med 53:573, 1972.

273. Selye H: Studies on adaptation. Endocrinology 21:169, 1937.

274. Claman HN: Corticoids and lymphoid cells. N Engl J Med 287:388, 1972.

275. Livingston RB, Carter SK (eds): Single Agents in Cancer Chemotherapy. New York, Plenum Press, 1970.

276. Vietti TJ, Sullivan MP, Berry DH, et al: The response of acute childhood leukemia to an initial and second course of prednisone. J Pediatr 66:18, 165.

277. Kjellstraad CM: Side effects of steroids and their treatment. Transplant Proc 7:123, 1975.

278. Cline MJ, Rosenbaum E: Prediction of in vivo cytotoxicity of chemotherapeutic agents by their in vitro effect on leukocytes from patients with acute leukemia. Cancer Res 28:2516, 1968.

279. Ho AD, Hunstein W, Ganeshaguru K, et al: Therapeutic and prognostic implications of glucocorticoid receptors and terminal deoxynucleotidyl transferase in acute leukemia. Leuk Res 6:1, 1982.

280. Costlow ME, Pui CH, Dahl GV: Glucocorticoid receptors in childhood acute lymphocytic leukemia. Cancer Res 42:4801, 1982.

281. Schmidt TJ, Thompson EB: Glucocorticoid receptors in human leukemia. *In* Sharma RK, Criss WE (eds): Endocrine Control in Neoplasia. New York, Raven Press, 1975, p 263.
282. Lippman ME, Konior-Yarbro G, Leventhal BG: Clinical implications of glucocorticoid receptors in human leukemia. Cancer Res 38:4251, 1978.
283. Crabtree GR, Smith KA, Munck A: Glucocorticoid receptors and sensitivity of isolated human leukemia and lymphoma cells. Cancer Res 38:4268, 1978.
284. Neifeld JP, Lippman ME, Tormey DC: Steroid hormone receptors in normal human lymphocytes: Induction of glucocorticoid receptor activity by phytohemagglutinin stimulation. J Biol Chem 254:2972, 1977.
285. Lippman ME, Barr R: Glucocorticoid receptors n purified subpopulations of human peripheral blood lymphocytes. J Immunol 118:1977, 1977.
286. Nanni P, Nicoletti G, Prodi G, et al: Glucocorticoid receptor and in vitro sensitivity to steroid hormones in human lymphoproliferative disease and myeloid leukemia. Cancer 49:623, 1982.
287. Ho AD, Hunstein W, Schmid W: Glucocorticoid receptors and sensitivity in leukemias. Blut 42:183, 1981.
288. Munck A, Wira C: Glucocorticoid receptors and action in rat thymocytes. *In* Raspe G (ed): Advances in the Biosciences: Schering Workshop on Steroid Hormone Receptors, vol 7. Oxford, Pergamon Press, 1971, p 301.
289. Lippman ME, Halterman R, Perry S, et al: Glucocorticoid binding proteins in human leukaemic lymphoblasts. Nature 242:157, 1973.
290. Lippman ME, Halterman R, Leventhal GF, et al: Glucocorticoid binding proteins in acute lymphoblastic leukemic blast cells. J Clin Invest 52:1715, 1973.
291. Yarbro GS, Lippman ME, Johnson GE, Leventhal BG: Glucocorticoid receptors in subpopulations of childhood acute lymphocytic leukemia. Cancer Res 37:2688, 1977.
292. Lippman ME, Konior-Yarbro G, Leventhal BG: Clinical implications of glucocorticoid receptors in human leukemia. Cancer Res 38:4251, 1978.
293. Mastrangelo R, Malandrino R, Riccardi R, et al: Clinical implications of glucocorticoid receptor studies in childhood acute lymphoblastic leukemia. Blood 56:1036, 1980.
294. Bloomfield CD, Smith KA, Peterson BA, Munch A: Glucocorticoid receptors in adult acute lymphoblastic leukemia. Cancer Res 41:4857, 1981.
295. Wells RJ, Mascaro K, Young PCM, et al: Glucocorticoid receptor in the lymphoblasts of patients with glucocorticoid-resistant childhood acute lymphocytic leukemia. Am J Pediatr Hematol Oncol 3:259, 1981.
296. McGuire WL (ed): Estrogen Receptors in Human Breast Cancer. New York, Raven Press, 1975.
297. Lippman ME, Perry S, Thompson EB: Glucocorticoid binding proteins in myeloblast of acute myelogenous leukemia. Am J Med 59:224, 1975.
298. Crabtree GR, Smith KA, Munck A: Glucocorticoid receptors and sensitivity of isolated human leukemia and lymphoma cells. Cancer Res 38:4268, 1978.
299. Gailiani S, Minowada J, Silvernail P, et al: Specific glucocorticoid binding in human hematopoietic cell lines and neoplastic tissue. Cancer Res 33:2653, 1978.
300. Homo F, Duval D, Meyer P, et al: Chronic lymphatic leukaemia: Cellular effects of glucocorticoid in vitro. Br J Haematol 38:491, 1978.
301. Terenius L, Simonsson B, Nilsson K: Glucocorticoid receptors, DNA synthesis, membrane antigens and their relation to disease activity in chronic lymphatic leukemia. J Steroid Biochem 7:905, 1976.
302. Bloomfield CD, Holbrook NJ, Munck AU, et al: Glucocorticoid receptors. *In* Bresciani F, King RJB, Lippman ME, et al (eds): Progress in Cancer Research and Therapy, vol 3: Hormones and Cancer 2. New York, Raven Press, 1984.

153

Hormones of the Gastrointestinal Tract

JOHN P. H. WILDING
MOHAMMAD A. GHATEI
STEPHEN R. BLOOM

In 1901 Bayliss and Starling performed a classic endocrine experiment: They denervated a segment of jejunum by careful dissection of its nerve supply and were able to show the release of pancreatic juice when hydrochloric acid was introduced to this isolated segment.[1] Furthermore, they demonstrated the release of pancreatic juice from the denervated pancreas following the injection of small intestinal extracts.[2] The existence of a novel means of communication between different tissues was postulated, mediated by a blood-borne signal released from the jejunum acting on the pancreas, which they named *secretin*, the first hormone to be described. This was followed in 1905 by the demonstration that gastric acid secretion was stimulated by another putative hormone, gastrin.[3] Thus hormones in the gastrointestinal tract hold a special place in the history of endocrinology.

The last 20 years have seen rapid expansion in our understanding of the variety and complexity of the gut endocrine system. This has been made possible by the wide range of techniques now available to study hormonal systems. These include classic techniques utilizing antibodies such as radioimmunoassay and immunocytochemistry, along with electron microscopy to localize and measure the cellular content of peptides. These methods are now complemented by molecular biological techniques using specific oligonucleotide probes to identify sites of synthesis. The effects of infusion of peptides into the blood or gut lumen have provided the first clues to the physiological role of the peptide, but this can be finally elucidated only as and when specific antagonists become available. The molecular characterization and cloning of hormone receptors provide further information on hormone action, for example, by demonstrating the existence of several distinct subtypes with different effects.

At the anatomical level the gut contains a diffuse population of endocrine cells, some of which communicate with, and are sensitive to, changes in the chemical environment of the gut lumen (e.g., to pH, amino acids); others lie within the gut wall and may perform other functions (paracrine, sensitive to stretch, tropic). Finally there is a wide variety of peptide-producing neuronal cells that form the rich myenteric plexus of the gut (Fig. 153–1).

These hormones and neurotransmitters, also found in the CNS ("brain-gut peptides"), are single-chain polypeptides, many of which bear structural similarities to each other (e.g., gastrin/CCK, VIP/secretin) although having somewhat different actions. Different peptides may also result from the same precursor molecule, which may pro-

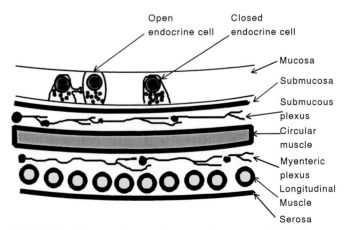

FIGURE 153–1. Section through the gut wall to show localization of the peptide-producing cells in the mucosa, which may be open to the gut lumen and may connect via cytoplasmic processes. The anatomical position of the submucous and myenteric nerve plexuses is also shown.

duce a different peptide subserving a completely different function elsewhere in the body (e.g., glucagon/entero-glucagon), or from differential splicing of the same gene (e.g., CGRP/calcitonin). These peptides frequently show marked evolutionary conservation, perhaps further support for their importance. It is of interest that the peptide-producing and secreting cells share many features, including the handling of biogenic amines, and many structural and histochemical properties. They have been classified as APUD (amine precursor, uptake and decarboxylation) cells for this reason[4] and have been claimed to derive from a common precursor cell that then differentiated to produce each endocrine or neuroendocrine cell line.

The functional role of this complex system is four-fold: (1) There is the regulation of the *mechanical* processes of digestion, gut motility; (2) there is regulation of the *chemical* and enzymatic processes involved in digestion, secretion; (3) there is control of the *postabsorbtive* processes involved in the assimilation of digested food and CNS feedback regulating intake; and (4) the diffuse endocrine system appears to have important *tropic* effects on the growth and development of the gastrointestinal tract.

Not all these gut "hormones" act in a strictly hormonal manner. Some functions are likely to be mediated by direct cell to cell communication (paracrine), or cells may act to regulate their own secretion (autocrine). Many gut regulatory peptides are neurotransmitters.

This chapter aims first to describe the normal physiology of the regulatory peptides found in the gastrointestinal tract. We have divided these into those that subserve predominantly hormonal or paracrine actions and those that act mainly as neurotransmitters. Peptides with structural similarities have been grouped together where possible. This classification is by necessity predominantly structural, as to adopt a purely functional approach would be confusing given the still limited knowledge available on the true functional role of this system. The final section deals with clinical aspects of gut regulatory peptides, both as abnormalities resulting in disease (mainly due to tumors) and secondary changes due to other conditions affecting the gastrointestinal tract.

PHYSIOLOGY

Hormones

Gastrin

Gastrin was one of the first gastrointestinal peptides to be isolated,[3] and its functions are now well understood. The main sites of gastrin synthesis are in the upper small intestine and in the G cells in the gastric antrum.[5, 6] The gastrin gene has been cloned and sequenced.[7] Gastrin is cleaved from its 101-amino acid prohormone in such a way as to produce several molecular forms. These all share a carboxy-terminal sequence of four amino acids that confer biological activity and amidation of the carboxy-terminal phenylalanine.[8] Three major forms of gastrin are found in the circulation, with variable length amino terminals; these are known as G_{34} (big gastrin), G_{17}, and G_{14} (minigastrin).[9–11] Larger molecular forms have been described, but these have yet to be fully characterized and may in fact be artefacts detected only with some antisera.[12, 13] G_{17}, the first

form of gastrin to be described, exists with sulfation of the tyrosine residue at position 11 (gastrin II) and without sulfation (gastrin I)[9]; sulfation does not appear to affect biological activity. G_{34} is the predominant form of gastrin found in the circulation, and G_{17} and G_{34} are biologically active, although the half-life is much longer for G_{34} (40 minutes), compared to G_{17} (5 minutes).[14] Tissue extracts from the gastric antrum and duodenum contain predominantly G_{17}.[15]

The biosynthesis of gastrin and its release into the circulation are under control of humoral and local factors and of the autonomic nervous system (Table 153–1). Studies of the role of these systems has been helped by the development of specific antagonists and monoclonal antibodies directed against putative regulatory factors. The predominant regulatory system is the presence of amino acids and proteins in the lumen of the stomach, which along with gastric distention, stimulate acid secretion.[16, 17] The vagus not only stimulates gastrin secretion but also has a direct effect on acid secretion; thus, vagotomy results in increased plasma gastrin and decreased acid secretion by the stomach.[18] Under some circumstances β-adrenergic stimulation affects gastrin release.[19] Gastrin secretion is itself inhibited when the pH of the lumen falls below pH 3.[20] A further important factor in this control system is the probable important paracrine control by neighboring somatostatin-producing cells in the gastric antrum. These cells extend cytoplasmic processes to the G cells,[21] and somatostatin inhibits gastrin release.[22] Immunoneutralization with the FAB fragment of a somatostatin monoclonal antibody has been shown to increase gastrin release,[23] and the two hormones are oppositely regulated by physiological stimuli, such as fasting and refeeding.[24] The effect of somatostatin may be to both decrease transcription of the gastrin gene and increase the rate of mRNA turnover.[25, 26] It has recently been suggested that calcitonin gene related peptide (CGRP) in gastric afferent neurons inhibits acid secretion by stimulation of somatostatin synthesis.[27]

The predominant action of gastrin is stimulation of acid release from the parietal cells of the fundus and body of the stomach. Clarification of the physiological importance of this effect has come with the development of a specific gastrin/cholecystokinin (CCK)-B receptor antagonist, L365,260.[28] The direct component of this effect, mediated by specific receptors on the parietal cell, occurs via an increase in cytosolic calcium.[29, 30] Indirect effects on acid release, via stimulation of histamine release from the enterchromaffin-like (ECL) cell, are also likely to be important.[31] Gastrin stimulates the release of pepsin and intrinsic

TABLE 153–1. CONTROL OF GASTRIN SECRETION

MECHANISM	STIMULATORY INFLUENCES	INHIBITORY INFLUENCES
Hormonal	Bombesin	Secretin
	Pancreastatin	GLP-1
		GIP
		VIP
Paracrine		Somatostatin
Neural	Acetylcholine	CGRP
	Norepinephrine	PYY
	(β-adrenergic)	Galanin
Local (metabolites, etc.)	Amino acids, gastric distention	pH <3

factor from the stomach.[32] Gastrin has important trophic effects on the growth of gastric mucosa and mucosa in the small and large intestine.[33, 34] Of particular interest is the observation that rats treated with the proton pump inhibitor, omeprazole, which renders them achlorhydric and causes very high levels of circulating gastrin, develop tumors of the ECL cell in the gastric fundus (gastric carcinoids) because of direct gastric stimulation of these histamine-producing cells.[35] Other actions of gastrin include stimulation of blood flow to the stomach and small intestine, contraction of the lower esophageal sphincter, stomach, and gallbladder, and relaxation of the pylorus and sphinctor of Oddi.[36, 37]

Cholecystokinin

Cholecystokinin (CCK) is produced in several molecular forms from a 114-amino-acid precursor.[38] In the gut, synthesis occurs in the open type of endocrine cells (I cells) in the upper small intestine, predominantly in the duodenum and upper jejunum.[39] CCK is a major neurotransmitter and is widely distributed throughout the central nervous system, particularly the hypothalamus, cerebral cortex, and neurohypophysis.[40, 41] It is also found in peripheral nerves, notably in the myenteric plexus and in the submucosal plexus of the large intestine. CCK shares the first five C-terminus amino acids with gastrin, but biological specificity is determined by the next three residues, of which the seventh (tyrosine) residue is sulfated. CCK-8 is the predominant form of CCK in the nervous system, but larger forms (CCK-33, 38, and 59) are the main ones found circulating and in the intestine[42, 43] (Fig. 153–2).

The predominant stimulus to CCK release is the presence of breakdown products of food in the upper small intestine, specifically fatty acids of 10–18 carbon atoms and L-amino acids such as phenylalanine and tryptophan.[44] In the case of fatty acids, the response is greater for unsaturated than saturated fats.[45] This release appears to occur independently of vagal innervation, as vagotomy does not inhibit CCK release in response to a meal.[46] It has been suggested that trypsin, one of the main pancreatic enzymes produced in response to CCK, may inhibit its release, possibly via a putative CCK-releasing peptide.[47] Bile salts also may act in a physiological manner to inhibit CCK release.[48] Other peptide hormones that may influence CCK release include somatostatin, which may act in a paracrine manner to inhibit release,[49] and bombesin, which stimulates release.[50]

The actions of CCK are mediated through two different classes of receptors; the CCK-A receptor is the predominant receptor found in the periphery, for example, in the pancreas and gallbladder, whereas the CCK-B receptor is found predominantly in the central nervous system. All the peripheral physiological effects of gastrin are also mediated by way of this latter type of receptor (CCK-B), which has recently been cloned.[51] CCK does not, however, affect gastric acid secretion, as there are CCK-A–type receptors on the parietal cell that are inhibitory, thus antagonizing the potential stimulatory effect of CCK on the CCK-B/gastrin receptor.

A number of additional actions have been proposed for CCK since its description as a blood-borne agent stimulating gallbladder contraction[52] and the recognition that CCK and pancreozymin (the proposed hormone that controlled pancreatic exocrine secretion) were the same hormone.[53] These include trophic effects on the growth of the pancreas, stimulation of endocrine pancreatic secretion including pancreatic polypeptide, somatostatin, glucagon, and insulin release (the latter as part of the incretin effect), inhibition of gastric emptying, effects on intestinal blood flow and motility, and the signaling of satiety.[54, 55] CCK has also been found to have a central action in the modulation of pain sensation, perhaps via antagonism of opioid receptors, although this effect appears to be weak.[56] The recent development of potent and selective antagonists to both peripheral- and central-type CCK receptors has enabled the study of the physiological relevance of these effects (Fig. 153–3).

The evidence that gallbladder emptying is primarily controlled by CCK is quite strong, as inhibition of CCK-A receptors completely inhibits gallbladder contraction in response to a meal,[57] and trials of CCK-A antagonists are under way for the treatment of biliary colic. In contrast, the effects on pancreatic enzyme secretion are less clear, and while some authors have demonstrated reductions in meal-stimulated responses with CCK antagonists,[58, 59] others have found little or no effect and suggest that pancreatic enzyme secretion may be primarily mediated via neural and other influences.[57, 60] The observation that infusions of physiological-concentrations of CCK influence intestinal motility has also been called into question by studies using antagonists.[60] Administration of CCK antagonists may inhibit duodenal and pancreatic DNA synthesis following refeeding, suggesting a trophic role for CCK, at least in the rat.[33] The effects of CCK on plasma insulin and pancreatic polypeptide responses to a mixed meal have been studied using the CCK-A antagonist loxiglumide: CCK appears to be important in the pancreatic polypeptide response, but not the insulin response, suggesting that it is not a major incretin hormone in man.[61] One of the most controversial

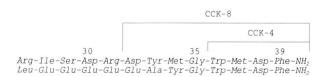

```
            1              5              10
CCK      Tyr-Ile-Gln-Gln-Ala-Arg-Lys-Ala-Pro-Ser-Gly-Arg-Val-
Gastrin                     pGlu-Leu-Gly-Pro-Gln-Gly-His-Pro-


            15             20             25
         Ser-Met-Ile-Lys-Asn-Leu-Gln-Ser-Leu-Asp-Pro-Ser-His-
         Ser-Leu-Val-Ala-Asp-Pro-Ser-Lys-Lys-Gln-Gly-Pro-Trp-

                        CCK-8

                                   CCK-4

            30             35             39
         Arg-Ile-Ser-Asp-Arg-Asp-Tyr-Met-Gly-Trp-Met-Asp-Phe-NH2
         Leu-Glu-Glu-Glu-Glu-Glu-Ala-Tyr-Gly-Trp-Met-Asp-Phe-NH2
```

FIGURE 153–2. Amino-acid sequences of CCK and gastrin, illustrating the various fragments.

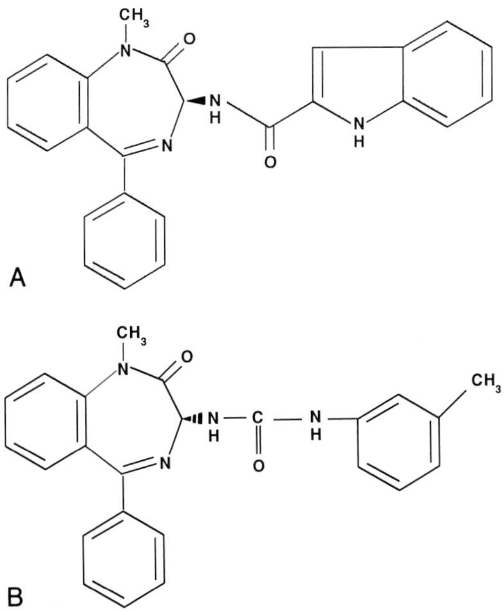

FIGURE 153–3. Structure of *A*, CCK-A receptor antagonist devazepide and *B*, CCK-B receptor antagonist L-365260.

areas has been the role of peripheral and central CCK in the development of postprandial satiety. It is well recognized that exogenous CCK decreases meal size in animals and humans.[62] However, the physiological role of endogenous CCK and the relative importance of peripheral (CCK-A) and central (CCK-B) receptors are uncertain and have been investigated by a number of workers using specific antagonists. It seems fairly clear that appetite is increased by the administration of CCK-A antagonists, suggesting that CCK, acting by way of a peripheral-type receptor, may constitute part of the meal termination signal.[63] It is of interest that blockade of central (CCK-B) type receptors also potently increases food intake after an oral preload in rats,[64] although this has been disputed.[65]

Secretin

Secretin is a 27 amino-acid linear peptide, with a helical configuration, secreted by the S cells of the duodenum, where it is colocalized with serotonin and chromogranin A.[66] Secretin-like immunoreactivity and secretin mRNA have also been found in the central nervous system, but the functional significance of this is not known.[67, 68] The genomic sequence of the secretin precursor gene is now known, and this along with peptide sequence data obtained from the preprohormone in the duodenum has enabled some interesting new insights into the biosynthesis of secretin.[67, 69–71] The coding region is divided into four sections coding for the different components of preprosecretin (secretin, the carboxy- and amino-terminal peptides, and the signal peptide), with three short introns separating these exons. This organization is similar to that of glucagon and VIP/PHI precursors, providing further support for the view gained from sequence homology that these peptides share a common evolutionary ancestry. It is of interest that similarities between rat and porcine secretin genes are confined to the exon coding for the biologically active peptide (only one amino acid change), with very poor conservation

of the C-terminal peptide (39 per cent homology), suggesting strong evolutionary pressure for conservation of the active peptide, but not of the C-terminal sequence.[70] Isolation of the secretin precursor from porcine intestine has suggested some differences from the deduced sequence from the cDNA, and it is therefore possible that differential splicing may occur during processing to mRNA.[71]

Secretin is released from the duodenum when the pH of the duodenal contents falls below 4.5. Other possible stimuli to secretin release include fat in the duodenum[72] and bile salts.[73] Recently a potential new antiulcer drug, geranyl-geranyl acetone, was found to stimulate pancreatic bicarbonate secretion indirectly by stimulating secretin release from the duodenum.[72] Secretin release is inhibited by the somatostatin analogue octreotide.[74]

The main physiological action of secretin is the stimulation of bicarbonate secretin by the pancreas in response to acid in the duodenum,[75] as identified by Bayliss and Starling. This effect is not confined to the pancreas, and secretion of bicarbonate by the liver into bile and by Brunner's glands in the duodenum also occurs in response to secretin and is likely to be of physiological importance.[76] The secretin receptor belongs to the family of G protein–coupled receptors with seven transmembrane domains, which includes the calcitonin, parathyroid hormone, and recently cloned VIP and GLP-1 receptors.[77] A number of other actions have been ascribed to secretin, including potentiation of vagally induced pancreatic enzyme secretion, inhibition of gastrin and gastric acid release, and synergy with CCK in stimulating gallbladder contraction.[78] Other observed actions, such as effects on the esophageal sphincter and stimulation of insulin release, occur only at high concentrations and may be considered pharmacological. One possible further role for secretin is in growth and development of the gastrointestinal tract, particularly in the early postnatal period, when secretin levels are high and gut growth is particularly rapid.[79]

GASTRIC INHIBITORY POLYPEPTIDE. Gastric inhibitory polypeptide (GIP) was isolated in 1970 and is a member of the secretin family of gastrointestinal regulatory peptides, sharing 15 of its 42 amino acids with glucagon and 9 with secretin.[80, 81] It is found in the K cells of the intestinal mucosa, predominantly in the duodenum and jejunum, but also in the ileum and colon in much lower concentrations.[82] GIP is released into the circulation following a mixed meal and also following ingestion of glucose, fat, or amino acids. The peak concentrations are achieved after 30 to 60 minutes, although this is delayed up to two hours following ingestion of fat.[83]

Two main actions have been attributed to GIP. The first is an enterogastrone, that is a substance released by the proximal small intestine in response to intraluminal nutrients that inhibits gastric acid secretion and gastric motility.[84] Infusions of GIP certainly produce this effect, but whether it is of physiological significance remains in doubt as the concentrations required in man are four times higher than those seen following a meal, although infusions of antibodies to GIP in dogs support a physiological role.[85, 86]

The second action is the stimulation of glucose-induced insulin release from the pancreas, and GIP is thought to be one component of the incretin effect—that is, the potentiation of insulin release seen after oral as opposed to intravenous glucose.[87] This has given rise to a second name for GIP, namely, glucose-dependent insulinotropic poly-peptide. The levels of GIP found after a meal are similar to those required to stimulate insulin secretion in the presence of glucose,[87, 88] and GIP has been found to promote insulin release from isolated perfused rat islets.[89, 90] The other main component of the incretin effect is glucagon-like peptide GLP-1 (7–36) amide (see below), which may act synergistically with GIP to account for the incretin effect.[91]

Peptide Products of Glucagon Gene

Glucagon, a 29-amino acid residue peptide synthesized and released by the α cells of the pancreatic islets, plays an important role in glycogenolysis, glucogenesis, and keto-genesis, opposing the action of insulin and turning the liver from an organ of glucose storage to an organ of glucose production.[92] With the development of the first radioimmunoassays for glucagon it became apparent that glucagon was synthesized as part of a larger precursor molecule "proglucagon" in the mammalian pancreas and gas-trointestinal tract.[93–96] Mammalian glucagon and its related peptides are encoded by a single preproglucagon mRNA that is expressed in the pancreas, intestine, and brain and gives rise to a 180-amino-acid proglucagon precursor.[97–101] However, the post-translational processing of this transcript differs markedly from tissue to tissue (Fig. 153–4). In the α cell of the pancreas, the main processing products of the proglucagon precursor are proglucagon 1–30 (glicentin-related pancreatic peptide: GRPP), glucagon (proglucagon 33–61), and a carboxy-terminal fragment containing the sequence of GLP-1 and GLP-2. In the mucosal L cell of intestine, proglucagon is chiefly processed to glicentin or enteroglucagon (proglucagon 1–69) and two smaller pep-tides, GLP-1 and GLP-2. Both glicentin (proglucagon 1–69) and GLP-1 (proglucagon 72–108) undergo further enzymatic cleavage to produce proglucagon 33–69 (oxyn-tomodulin) and proglucagon (78–107 amide) or GLP-1

7–36 NH₂, respectively.[102–105] In the hypothalamus, proglu-cagon appears to be processed as in the intestine,[106, 107] although glucagon is also present.[108] By this remarkable tissue-specific processing, glucagon is produced by the α cells, enteroglucagon, and GLP-1 by intestinal mucosa and a mixture of all these peptides by the hypothalamus. How-ever, the factors responsible in the generation of the diverse products of the glucagon gene remain to be eluci-dated.

GLUCAGON-LIKE PEPTIDE-1. The observation that GLP's are produced in the intestinal mucosa has led to intense investigations into their precise structure and functions. Although structural similarities between these two peptides and glucagon are moderate, the amino acid sequences of the GLP's themselves have been strongly conserved during evolution. Indeed, the sequence of GLP-1 is identical in rat, hamster, guinea pig, pig, and human and has only a few amino acid changes in fish, implying it has been nec-essary for survival across millions of years of vertebrate evolution.[109–111] Early investigations into the biological activ-ity of GLP's used GLP-1 (1,37), GLP-1 (1–36 NH₂), and GLP-2. Subsequently they were unable to show any signifi-cant biological effects of these peptides upon insulin re-lease.[112–114] Further sequence analysis of GLP-1 by Drucker et al. demonstrated that when GLP-1 was aligned with other members of glucagon family, greatest homology was observed when the histidyl residue at position 7 was aligned with position 1 of the others. Following this observation they demonstrated for the first time that the truncated form of GLP-1 (GLP-1 7–37 or GLP-1 7–36 NH₂) but not GLP-1 (1–37 or 1–36 NH₂) potently increases cAMP pro-duction, insulin release, and insulin gene expression from a rat insulinoma cell line.[115]

GLP-1 appears to be an important incretin in man. It is released from the intestine after a glucose load,[116] and GLP-1 infusion together with glucose greatly potentiates the effect of glucose on insulin secretion.[117] In addition, glucagon secretion is inhibited and somatostatin secretion potentiated.[118] Infusion of GLP-1 greatly reduces insulin

Preproglucagon

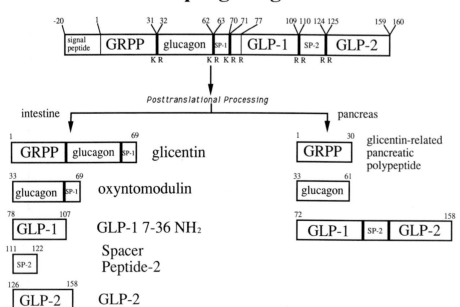

FIGURE 153–4. Post-translational processing of proglucagon in mammalian pancreatic α-cell and small-intestinal L-cell. In the α-cell, the main products are glucagon-related pancreatic peptide (GRPP), glucagon, and a carboxy-ter-minal fragment containing the sequence of gluca-gon-like peptide-1 (GLP-1) and glucagon-like peptide-2 (GLP-2). In the L-cell the main prod-ucts are glicentin, oxyntomodulin, GLP-1 (7–36) amide, spacer peptide-2 (SP-2), and GLP-2.

requirements following a meal in Type I and Type II diabetic patients, raising the possibility that analogues may prove to be a new form of treatment for diabetes mellitus.[119]

ENTEROGLUCAGON. Immunoreactive GLP's were detected as cross-reacting material in mammalian intestinal extracts in early pancreatic glucagon assays. It was later found that C-terminally directed antisera to pancreatic glucagon did not detect the intestinal material, which also had a higher molecular weight. To differentiate verbally between the two types of glucagon immunoreactivity, several alternative terms were suggested for the intestinal material, the most commonly used being glucagon-like immunoreactivity (GLI), gut glucagon, enteroglucagon, and glicentin. Early studies indicated that enteroglucagon is localized to intestinal mucosal L cells and released into circulation in several molecular forms.[120] The principal form is a 69-amino-acid single-chain peptide that contains the entire sequence of pancreatic glucagon (residue 33–61).

As only a small amount of enteroglucagon has been purified, there is almost no information on its pharmacology apart from its effect on inhibition of gastric acid secretion in the rat.[121] However, when pancreatic glucagon is administered in very large quantities a number of effects on the gastrointestinal tract have been observed, which might conceivably be due to stimulation of the enteroglucagon receptor. In humans, enteroglucagon is released after oral administration of long-chain fatty acids and carbohydrate and by ingestion of a normal mixed meal. Intrajejunal and intracolonic instillation of glucose and triglycerides stimulates the secretion of enteroglucagon directly. Intravenous bombesin or GRP infusion also stimulates considerable release of enteroglucagon.[122]

A number of lines of evidence favor enteroglucagon as a mediator of adaptive hyperplasia, but unfortunately this has all been circumstantial. The hypothesis was initiated with the observation that an enteroglucagon-secreting tumor was associated with villus hypertrophy and greatly increased intestinal transit time.[123] After removal of the tumor, the abnormalities disappeared and the circulating plasma enteroglucagon returned to normal. High concentrations of enteroglucagon have been found in circumstances in which there is loss of small-intestinal mucosal absorption surface due to mucosal damage such as celiac disease, tropical sprue, cystic fibrosis, and severe acute diarrhea, and after surgery (for review see ref. 124). Plasma enteroglucagon levels and crypt cell production rate are both elevated after intestinal resection[125] and in the lactating rat[126]; both are lowered after starvation and increased with refeeding.[127] Also, enteroglucagon correlated with crypt cell production when a variety of diets were given.[128] The location of the bulk of enteroglucagon (L) cells in the distal region of the gastrointestinal tract[129] suggests that they are in an ideal position to monitor the efficiency of the digestive process and signal if intestinal transit needs to be delayed or cell proliferation increased. Despite all of this evidence it has been difficult to demonstrate an enterotrophic role for enteroglucagon. Indeed, one study demonstrated that immunoneutralization of enteroglucagon by infusion of enteroglucagon-specific antibodies failed to inhibit the adaptive response to proximal small intestinal resection[130]; however, it has yet to be shown that these antibodies block enteroglucagon binding to its receptor. Relatively recently it has been shown that while enteroglu-

cagon concentrations increase moderately after epidermal growth factor administration, they do not increase in proportion to the proliferative response,[131] which could be interpreted as supporting the enteroglucagon hypothesis by showing that elevated plasma levels of enteroglucagon are not inevitable consequences of increased intestinal cell proliferation. Nevertheless, it has also been shown that enteroglucagon levels are very significantly elevated in germ-free animals to a level above those seen after intestinal resection,[132] without any concomitant changes in crypt cell production rates.[133]

Enteroglucagon is also elevated in the dumping syndrome after gastric surgery,[134] presumably because fast food transit to the terminal ileum stimulates a great number of enteroglucagon cells. The elevation in dumping has led to the postulate that enteroglucagon may also have an inhibitory role on gastrointestinal motor activity and gastric acid secretion. Enteroglucagon concentrations rise markedly after birth when neonates switch from in utero placental nutrition to their first oral feeding and thus require a fully functioning gut for the first time. Interestingly, if babies are fed intravenously after birth, no such enteroglucagon rise occurs.[135]

OXYNTOMODULIN. Oxyntomodulin, a peptide corresponding to the 33–69 sequence of mammalian glucagon, has been identified in extracts from porcine small-intestinal mucosa and circulation.[136] This peptide consists of the whole glucagon sequence extended at its C-terminal end by a basic octapeptide.[137] Oxyntomodulin is a potent inhibitor of pentagastrin-stimulated gastric acid secretion in both rat[138, 139] and man.[140] The peptide and its C-terminal octapeptide also inhibit liquid meal-stimulated acid secretion.[141] This activity seems to be mediated by high-affinity receptors present in the acid-secreting oxyntic gland,[142] resulting in stimulation of cAMP production and gastric somatostatin release.[143, 144] In addition, oxyntomodulin competes with glucagon for binding to cell membrane with molar potency of 20 per cent compared with glucagon[145] and promotes glucose production from hepatocytes.

Motilin

Motilin is a 22-amino-acid peptide, also found as a C-terminal extended form, first isolated from small intestine as a substance that stimulated gastric motor activity.[146, 147] The biological activity is thought to reside in the nine amino acids at the N terminus.[148] Although it shows limited amino acid homology with gastrin and secretin, motilin is dissimilar in structure to any other known gastrointestinal regulatory peptide. The genomic DNA sequence is interesting in that the exons encoding the motilin moiety are split by an intron.[149] Motilin immunoreactivity is found in the M cells, which are endocrine cells present in the epithelium throughout the small intestine, but with their population density decreasing from duodenum to ileum.[150] Motilin is also found throughout the large intestine, with the exception of the cecum, and in the gallbladder and biliary tract.

Plasma motilin concentrations are highest during phase III of the interdigestive migrating motor complex. Motilin release is stimulated by a lipid-rich meal or by intravenous lipid infusion, but inhibited by amino acids or glucose.[151] Gastric distention from a water load and duodenal acidification also promote motilin secretion.[152, 153] Electrical vagal stimulation increases motilin release, but basal motilin levels are not affected by vagotomy.[154] Other regulatory peptides may influence motilin release; these include bombesin, which is stimulatory, and somatostatin and pancreatic polypeptide, which are inhibitory.[155–157]

The main function ascribed to motilin is the regulation of intestinal motility, in particular that of the "activity front" or phase III of the interdigestive migrating motor complex (MMC); regulation of this wave of intestinal contraction is multifactorial and involves the integration of several nutritional, hormonal, and neural signals. Increases in plasma motilin concentrations occur immediately prior to the contractile events. Administration of exogenous motilin results in initiation of the activity front, and in dogs motilin antiserum inhibits the generation of the MMC.[158] The suppression of these complexes with food is consistent with the observation that certain nutrients inhibit motilin release. The neural regulation of the activity front and the relationship with motilin is more complex and depends on the region of the gut examined. In the small intestine vagotomy does not influence the response to exogenous motilin, whereas the esophagus and stomach do not then respond. Atropine suppresses the increase in plasma motilin usually observed with the MMC.[154] Spontaneous and motilin-induced phase III contractions can be inhibited by 5-HT_3 antagonists in the dog but not in a denervated gastric pouch, suggesting that serotoninergic mechanisms may also be important in regulating the cholinergic stimulation of the MMC.[159] Dopamine has also been shown to stimulate the MMC and motilin release.[160] The actions of motilin may also occur via modulation of opioid and VIP release from nerves in the myenteric plexus.[161] In addition to these effects on the contractility of the stomach and small bowel, motilin also causes smooth muscle contraction in the large intestine and influences jejunal salt and water absorption. Motilin may also act to inhibit pancreatic insulin secretion.[162]

The prokinetic effect of macrolide antibiotics such as erythromycin is mediated via the motilin receptor, and development of analogues to these antibiotics, which are potent agonists at the motilin receptor, may lead to a new class of prokinetic agents of potential use in a wide range of conditions in which intestinal motility is reduced, for example, in patients with diabetic gastroparesis.[163]

Somatostatin

Somatostatin (SS) was initially isolated from ovine hypothalamus as a factor that inhibited secretion of growth hormone from the pituitary; it exists in two main molecular forms—SS 14 and an N-terminally extended form, SS 28.[164, 165] Structurally it is a cyclic peptide with a disulfide bridge linking two cysteine residues at positions 3 and 14 (Fig. 153–5). The cDNA encoding SS has been isolated and cloned from a wide variety of species, including rat, pig, humans, and several teleost fish. The peptide itself is invariant in all mammalian species examined, and there are only minor variations in the sequence of the prohormone. In humans the SS gene consists of two exons encoding for the signal peptide and the mature hormone, respectively, split by a single intron.[166] Considerable effort has been applied to the understanding of the structure-function relationships of SS; first it should be noted that

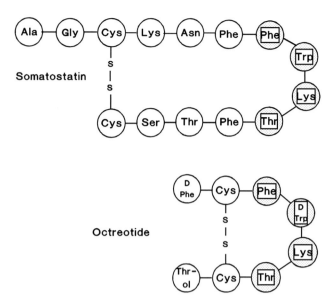

FIGURE 153–5. Amino-acid sequence and structure of somatostatin-14 and the synthetic somatostatin analogue octreotide.

the 14 amino acids at the N terminal of SS 28 have no intrinsic biological activity, although they may confer different specificity on the molecule. The essential structure resides in the beta-turn formed by the four amino acids Phe-Trp-Lys-Thr (residues 7–11).[167] Modifications in this region eventually led to the development of the long-acting SS analogue, octreotide, which has a number of therapeutic uses, particularly for the chronic suppression of hormone release in acromegaly and gut endocrine tumors.[168, 169]

SS is widely distributed in both the central and peripheral nervous system, where it acts as a neurotransmitter, and in endocrine cells in the gut and D cells of the pancreas, where it certainly has paracrine functions, whereas its role as a true circulating hormone remains uncertain. It is also found in the thyroid, genitourinary system, heart, thymus, and eye. Extensive discussion of the role of SS outside the gastrointestinal tract is, however, outside the scope of this chapter. SS is present in endocrine cells throughout the length of the intestine, particularly in the gastric fundus and antrum and in the colon.[170] In the fundus, SS-immunoreactive cells are closely associated with parietal cells, whereas in the antrum they are close to and extend cytoplasmic processes to the gastrin-producing G cells, thus providing anatomical evidence for a paracrine role.[171] These cells also communicate with the gut lumen, which may provide a means of sensing intragastric pH. SS is also found extensively in the enteric nervous system, where the predominant form is SS 14, as opposed to SS 28 in the endocrine cells.[172]

Release of SS into the circulation occurs after the ingestion of a mixed meal; this is probably due to a combination of nutritional, hormonal, and neural stimuli, the relative importance of which is unclear. The main component of the postprandial rise is somatostatin 28.[173] SS secretion can be stimulated by fat and protein, lowered gastric pH, GIP, CCK, secretin, and cholinergic and adrenergic stimulation and inhibited by opioids. However, the latter (neural) modulatory effects are not universal and vary according to the species studied and the conditions of the experiment, for example, cholinergic activation is stimulatory in humans and dogs but inhibitory in rats and pigs, whereas adrenergic stimulation promotes SS release in dogs but not in humans.[174] The opioid receptor antagonist naloxone can be shown to inhibit the meal-related increase in SS, but this depends on the carbohydrate content of the test meal.[175]

SS has extensive inhibitory actions on gut hormone release, intestinal secretion, and motility. It may even inhibit its own release via an autocrine mechanism.[176] One of the best studied roles of SS in the gut is its probable paracrine role as an inhibitor of gastrin release in the control of gastric acid secretion. The ability of SS to inhibit acid secretion was recognized early,[177] and a paracrine mechanism was initially postulated on the basis of anatomical studies.[171] This was confirmed by experiments in isolated luminally perfused stomach, in which direct perfusion of acid enhanced somatostatin secretion in the presence of tetrodotoxin, suggesting a direct effect of acid on the SS cell, and augmentation of basal and pentagastrin and histamine stimulated acid output with SS antiserum, suggesting a direct inhibitory effect of SS on the parietal cell.[178, 179] Inhibition of gastrin release from the antral G cells may occur through a similar paracrine mechanism. Pancreatic and biliary secretion are inhibited by SS. The effects on gut motility include delayed gastric emptying and reduced small bowel transit time, which may partly be due to inhibition of the secretion of other hormones and also due to a direct effect of somatostatin. Whether SS acts as a true circulating hormone remains uncertain, but the physiological increase in SS 28 seen after a meal is certainly sufficient to produce some of the known actions of SS.[180] It is therefore reasonable to suggest that the combination of local somatostatin release from nerves and endocrine cells and systemic release of SS acts to damp down the secretory and motor activity stimulated by the ingestion of a meal.

SS exerts these multiple effects via specific receptors, which are known to be coupled to G proteins and involve the activation of adenylyl cyclase, although G-protein independent mechanisms involving inositol phospholipid/protein kinase C have also been implicated.[181] Two human and mouse clones of SS receptors have recently been identified; these appear to have seven transmembrane domains and therefore are likely to belong to the superfamily of G protein–coupled receptors. The presence of multiple binding sites of probes directed against these receptors in DNA digests suggests that these may be the first of a larger family of SS receptors.[182]

Neurotensin and Neuromedin N

Neurotensin and neuromedin N are two structurally related peptides encoded in tandem on the same precursor gene.[183] Neurotensin is a 13-amino acid peptide, whereas neuromedin N is a hexapeptide. The carboxy-terminus is necessary for biological activity. Neurotensin is present in neurons throughout the central nervous system and in nerves and endocrine cells in the gut (N cells). These cells are present mainly in the ileum and to a lesser extent in the jejunum.[184] The role of neuromedin N is at present little understood.

Neurotensin is released into the circulation following a mixed meal, with fat ingestion being the most potent stim-

ulus, causing up to a four-fold rise in plasma immunoreactive neurotensin concentrations.[185] This meal-stimulated release of neurotensin appears to be dependent on intact cholinergic innervation, as the effect may be blocked by atropine. Intravenous bombesin has also been shown to stimulate neurotensin release in man.[186] This effect is not blocked by atropine.

Neurotensin was named from its ability to cause vasodilation, hypotension, and cyanosis.[187] A wide range of effects on the gut has been demonstrated following infusion of neurotensin. Many of these effects have been noted only at supraphysiological concentrations of the peptide, and it remains unclear whether they are truly hormonal or are mediated by paracrine or neural transmission. The main effects demonstrated at close to physiological doses are inhibition of gastric motility and secretion and stimulation of pancreatic exocrine secretion.[188, 189] Some of these effects may be indirectly mediated via release of dopamine.[190] Plasma pancreatic polypeptide and glucagon release are stimulated, whereas insulin release is inhibited. Other possible functions include stimulation of colonic contractile activity, stimulation of growth of the intestinal mucosa, and increases in intestinal blood flow.[191, 192] The actions of neurotensin are mediated via a specific receptor, which has now been cloned and characterized, and involve activation of a G protein–linked second messenger system.[193]

Peptide YY

Peptide tyrosine tyrosine (PYY) was isolated from procine intestine by Tatemoto in 1982.[194] It is a member of the family of peptides including pancreatic polypeptide and neuropeptide Y (all named because of the presence of a C-terminal tyrosine). It seems likely that these three peptides are products of one ancestral gene that has become duplicated, as their precursor peptides and genomic DNA sequences show remarkable structural similarity[195] (Fig. 153–6).

PYY is found predominantly in endocrine cells in the ileum, colon, and rectum, where it has been shown to be co-localized with enteroglucagon.[196] In contrast, in the fetus the main site of expression appears to be the pancreas.[195]

The main physiological stimulus to PYY release is the ingestion of a meal, particularly in response to fat.[197] This may be mediated via a direct effect on the open-type PYY-producing cells, but predominantly indirectly by neural and endocrine signals (both bombesin and CCK stimulate PYY release).[198] The response to a meal is prompt, long lasting, and proportional to meal size.[196]

PYY has been found to inhibit gastric acid secretion, gastric emptying, small intestinal motility, and pancreatic enzyme secretion. In contrast to other enterogastrone-like

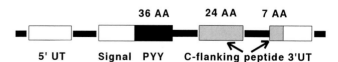

FIGURE 153–6. Structure of the PYY gene. The structural organization of the PP and NPY genes is similar, with four exons, separated by three introns, coding for a 5′ untranslated region, a signal peptide, and a C-terminal peptide, as well as for the final cleaved product.

peptides the inhibitory effect of PYY on gastric acid secretion does not appear to be mediated via stimulation of somatostatin[199] and may be due to inhibition of the vagal innervation. This also seems to be the case for the effects on gastric emptying and intestinal motility, as the effects are lost when denervated preparations are studied or following atropine administration. PYY inhibits the release of acetylcholine via a pertussus toxin–sensitive mechanism, suggesting that this action may occur via an inhibitory G protein.[200] At physiological concentrations PYY has few cardiovascular effects or effects on intestinal secretion unless these are first stimulated (e.g., by vasoactive intestinal peptide [VIP]).[201] PYY may therefore be an important hormone that acts to inhibit intestinal motility and secretion after a meal to allow sufficient time for absorption.

Pancreatic Polypeptide

Pancreatic polypeptide (PP) is a 36-amino-acid peptide closely related to neuropeptide Y (NPY) and PYY in structure. It is found in the PP cells at the periphery of the pancreatic islets, predominantly in the head of the pancreas, and in endocrine cells scattered throughout the exocrine pancreas.[202]

PP is released in a biphasic manner following a meal. The initial phase of secretion (cephalic phase) is vagally mediated and may be blocked by atropine.[203] The second phase is longer lasting and is due to stimulation by ingested nutrients, particularly amino acids, although even this phase has important neural and hormonal regulation, involving cholinergic and β-adrenergic stimulation and inhibition by dopaminergic or α-adrenergic pathways, perhaps via an enteropancreatic reflex.[204, 205] Several gut hormones have been shown to modulate PP release, including bombesin and motilin, which are stimulatory, and somatostatin, which inhibits its release.[206, 207] PP is also released in response to hypoglycemia and as such is a useful marker of parasympathetic stimulation of the islets.[208]

PP has been shown to inhibit gallbladder contraction, pancreatic exocrine secretion, and gastric acid secretion.[209] The physiological importance of these effects is not known, and there are no obvious effects of a deficiency or an excess of this hormone. However, it seems logical to suggest that PP is involved in damping down the pancreatic exocrine secretion following a meal, as these effects have been demonstrated at plasma concentrations in the physiological range. Finally, it has been observed that in the fasting state the concentrations of PP fluctuate with the interdigestive migrating motor complex in a way similar to motilin, suggesting a possible role in regulating gut motility.[210]

Chromogranins and Secretogranins

The chromogranins and secretrogranins are a family of acidic secretory proteins that are found in the large "dense-cored" vesicles of the secretory granules of endocrine cells and neurons, being stored together with many different peptide hormones and neuropeptides. The chromogranin family members are the most widespread marker for secretory granules of endocrine and neuronal cells currently available (for review see refs. 211 and 212).

The first three members of the family, chromogranin A (CgA), chromogranin B (CgB), and secretogranin II (SgII), share certain biochemical properties as well as widespread distribution in secretory granules of endocrine and neuronal cells. Such a distribution is also characteristic of three other acidic secretory proteins, 7B2, HISL-19 antigen, and the 1B1075 gene product, which may be related to CgA, CgB, and SgII.[213, 214]

Comparison of the primary structure of the chromogranins, obtained by cDNA cloning, has revealed that CgA and CgB are more closely related to each other than either protein is to the other members of the chromogranin family.[214] Two particular structural and biochemical properties of the chromogranins will be mentioned here, as these are probably related to their function(s). First, the presence of multiple proteolytic processing sites in the gene suggests that such proteins are precursors of biologically active peptides. This is further supported by the discovery of pancreastatin and chromostatin in the case of CgA[215, 216] and peptide GAWK in the case of CgB.[217, 218] Pancreastatin has been demonstrated to suppress insulin secretion and to alter pancreatic exocrine secretion.[219] Second, the chromogranins exhibit Ca^{2+} binding activity, suggesting a role in regulation of internal pH of the granule, a factor of importance in the activation of processing enzymes.[220]

Chromogranins are often oversecreted in certain neuroendocrine tumors, and measurements of circulating levels are extremely useful as nonspecific markers of such tumors.[221–223]

Neurotransmitters

VIP and Related Peptides

Vasoactive intestinal polypeptide (VIP) was first isolated by Said and Mutt in 1970,[224] as an intestinal peptide that produces systemic vasodilation. It is a straight-chain 28-amino-acid peptide and has close sequence homology with the 27-amino-acid peptide histidine isoleucine (PHI).[225, 226] The elucidation of the cDNA sequence encoding human prepro-VIP revealed that these peptides are synthesized from the same prohormone, although the human form of PHI differs by one amino acid (the isoleucine is substituted with methionine) and is known as peptide histidine methionine or PHM.[227] PHM is also found in a larger, C-terminal extended form (PHV). A recent addition to this group of peptides is pituitary adenylate cyclase-activating peptide (PACAP), which exists in two molecular forms (PACAP 27 and PACAP 38) and shows 68 per cent homology with VIP[228, 229]; although PACAP is encoded for by a different gene, they may have evolved from a single evolutionary precursor. These peptides also show some sequence homology with secretin, GIP, and pancreatic glucagon and can be considered part of this peptide family. VIP, PHI/PHM, and PACAP are found in nerves in a wide range of tissues both within and outside the gastrointestinal tract, as well as the central nervous system and autonomic ganglia, where they act as neurotransmitters or neuromodulators. In the gastrointestinal tract, VIP is found in the submucous and myenteric plexus; it is not found in endocrine cells. Likewise, PACAP is also found in nerves in the gastrointestinal tract.[230]

Plasma VIP concentrations are readily detectable by radioimmunoassay and have been found to increase following a number of stimuli, including duodenal acidification and gastric distention, as well as following a meal.[231, 232] This is thought to represent spillover into the circulation from VIP released from local nerve terminals. The half-life of circulating VIP is very short (less than one minute), as it is rapidly degraded in the liver. Tissue concentrations of VIP are low in conditions in which there is denervation such as Hirschprung's and Chagas' disease.[233] Although PHM is also detectable in plasma, this is unlikely to signify physiological significance as a circulating hormone.

The main actions of VIP in the gastrointestinal tract are modulation of gut motility and stimulation of secretion—specifically, contraction of the longitudinal muscle and relaxation of the circular muscle of the small intestine and relaxation of the lower esophageal and pyloric sphincters and of the gallbladder.[234, 235] VIP is a potent stimulus to intestinal secretion, both in the intestine, where it inhibits sodium reabsorption and stimulates chloride secretion, and in the pancreas and liver where it promotes secretion of bicarbonate.[236, 237] VIP inhibits gastric acid secretion, possibly mediated by stimulation of somatostatin release from neighboring D cells.[238] VIP-ergic nerves innervate the islets of Langerhans, and VIP and PHI stimulate insulin and glucagon release.[239] VIP is also a vasodilator and may be partly responsible for the hyperemia seen in the small intestine after a meal.[224] PACAP has also been found to have effects similar to VIP on intestinal secretion and motility[240, 241] and may be acting at the VIP receptor in this regard.[242]

VIP causes accumulation of intracellular cAMP, and the VIP receptor is thought to be coupled to the adenylate cyclase stimulating G protein, in common with other members of this peptide family, including secretin, PACAP, and PHI, which compete with VIP for receptor binding. A cDNA clone encoding a receptor for VIP has been identified that has seven transmembrane domains and significant homology with the secretin receptor[243]; however, receptor purification studies suggest the existence of more than one receptor, although these have yet to be identified.

Bombesin-like Family of Peptides

The bombesin-like peptides represent a large family of structurally related peptides, initially isolated from amphibian skin. The bombesin family includes bombesin, alytesin, ranatensins, and litorin (for review see ref. 244). The first and most extensively characterized of the group is bombesin, a 14-amino-acid residue that was isolated from the skin of the European frog, *Bombina-bombina*.[245] Pharmacological screening of bombesin and its analogues led, unexpectedly, to the finding that bombesin is a potent gastric acid secretagogue, mediated by its unique action to increase the release of plasma immunoreactive gastrin.[246] The mammalian counterparts of bombesin were appropriately named *gastrin-releasing peptide* (GRP) and isolated from porcine gastric and intestinal extracts.[247] Amino acid analysis verified that this peptide had remarkable sequence homology to bombesin, especially in its carboxy-terminal decapeptide. GRP, which is present in many mammalian tissues including lung, brain, and the nerve fibers of the gastrointestinal tract, has since been isolated from rat, human, dog, bird, and guinea pig. The smaller molecular form of bombesin is the carboxy-terminal decapeptide

(GRP 18–27), which appears to be present in all species that also produce the larger form. As GRP shares all of bombesin's biological actions, GRP and GRP 18–27 have been considered the mammalian equivalent of amphibian bombesin. The human bombesin gene is localized on chromosome 18[248] and when transcribed codes for three mRNAs encoding pro-GRP consisting of a signal sequence at the N terminus, GRP itself, and a C-terminal flanking peptide. The second and third messages differ from the first in having a 21 and 19 base deletion, respectively, in the region encoding the C-terminal flanking peptide.[249, 250] Thus all three mRNA's produce peptide sequences that are identical except at the C terminus of the C-flanking peptide. As of this writing little is known about the expression and biological activity of GRP gene-related peptides in mammalian tissues.

In vitro experiments with bombesin or GRP caused smooth muscle contractions in almost all kinds of peripheral tissue preparations. In vivo studies extend the in vitro data and revealed that GRP produces a wide spectrum of potent pharmacological actions in mammalian gastrointestinal tract and pancreas. In humans the action of GRP on gastric acid, pancreatic and biliary secretory responses, gallbladder contraction, and plasma hormone release has been shown to be equipotent to that of synthetic bombesin. Similar comparisons have been made in animals using bombesin and GRP, which provided comparable results.[251]

Compelling evidence implicates bombesin or GRP as a growth factor in normal development of mammalian gastrointestinal tract, pancreas, and respiratory tract, as well as in neoplasia of neuroendocrine cells (for review see ref. 244). In fact, bombesin appears to provide a novel and unique model for the elucidation of the signal transducing system leading to cell proliferation.[252] Ontogenetically GRP immunoreactivity and its mRNA's are present as early as nine weeks of gestation in human lung and increase during fetal development, reaching a peak at birth.[253, 254] In the lung the bombesin concentration, but not its mRNA, remains almost unchanged during early childhood but decreases to one tenth in the adult. The demonstration that bombesin or GRP stimulates the proliferation of cultured bronchial epithelial cells and its depletion in children with acute respiratory distress syndrome[253] suggests an important role for such peptides in lung development. GRP is synthesized by a large number of neuroendocrine tumors of the lung (small cell carcinoma and carcinoid) and thyroid and also by other neuroendocrine cells.[255, 256] Indeed a rapidly evolving research field for bombesin is based on the implication that it is an autocrine growth factor in both normal and neoplastic lung.

Neuromedin B

Neuromedin B is a bombesin-like peptide that shares sequence homology with ranatensin and was isolated from porcine spinal cord on the basis of its ability to contract uterine smooth muscle.[257] Neuromedin B is a 10-amino acid peptide that is also found as amino-terminally extended 27- and 32-amino acid forms.[258] The cDNA encoding neuromedin B has been cloned from both rat and human brain, and the two regions of the two precursor mRNA's that encode the N-terminally extended peptides display a high degree of structural homology.[259, 260] In the rat the pattern of expression of the neuromedin B mRNA precursor is different from that of bombesin,[259] while in humans neuromedin B mRNA has been found only in the pituitary, brain, and in some clonal cell lines derived from small cell carcinoma of the lung.[260–262]

Neuromedin B-like immunoreactivity has been found in many mammalian species, including humans, pig, cat, and rodent, where it is widely distributed throughout the central nervous system and various peripheral tissues.[263–265] In mammals neuromedin B is found in the pituitary gland and various brain regions where it has been shown to be present in the synaptosomes.[266] In peripheral tissue neuromedin B is present in the adrenal glands, pancreas, and gastrointestinal tract with the esophagus and rectum possessing the highest concentrations.[265]

Neuromedin B exerts effects on a variety of physiological systems that are similar to, although less potent than, those of bombesin.[267, 268] Taken with the widespread distribution of neuromedin B in mammalian tissues, this suggests that it is a physiologically important peptide.

In the anterior pituitary, where the concentrations of neuromedin B are highest, its synthesis was found to be altered following changes in hormonal status, and immunocytochemical staining revealed that neuromedin B is present in thyrotrophs.[269, 270] Further evidence of an involvement with thyrotroph function has come from the demonstration that neuromedin B exerts potent inhibitory effects on the release of TSH from the anterior pituitary cells both in vivo and in vitro.[271] It is known that locally acting autocrine/paracrine systems are regulators within endocrine tissue, including the anterior pituitary. These observations suggest that neuromedin B may function as a locally acting regulator of anterior pituitary function.

The receptor for neuromedin B has been isolated from a rat esophagus cDNA library, and the distribution of its mRNA has been mapped and found to be different from that of the bombesin receptor which has also been cloned.[272, 273] In the brain the receptor for neuromedin B was found to be expressed mainly in the olfactory and central thalamic regions, while the bombesin receptor was found mainly in the hypothalamus.[272]

Neuromedin U

Neuromedin U 8 and U 25 are two novel peptides, originally isolated from porcine spinal cord, that cause contraction of rat uterus and elevate blood pressure.[274] Structural analysis revealed that both peptides are C-terminally amidated and that the amino acid sequence of the octapeptide was contained at the carboxy-terminus of the larger form, with no structural similarity with any other known regulatory peptides.

In addition, neuromedin U (NmU) has also been isolated and sequenced from rat, rabbit, frog, guinea pig, and chicken.[275–279] Relatively recently the cDNA of a precursor molecule encoding NmU has been isolated from rat ileum,[280] showing the sequence coding NmU to be at the C-terminal end. This sequence is flanked on the N-terminal side by a similar-sized peptide bound by double basic amino acids suggesting that it is separately cleaved and secreted. High concentrations of NmU-like immunoreactivity have been found in the gastrointestinal tract, brain regions, spinal cord, and urogenital tract.[281] In the gastrointestinal tract the highest concentration of NmU is found in the ileum. Immunocytochemical studies demonstrate NmU exclusively within the nerves, particularly in the submucous plexus.[282]

Apart from its potent uterine contracting and hypertensive effects, NmU also reduces superior mesenteric artery and portal vein blood flow[283] and modifies electrogenic ion transport in the porcine distal jejunum.[284] NmU has been shown to have motor activity along the GI tract, although its site of action is species specific.

Calcitonin Gene–Related Peptide

Calcitonin gene–related peptide (α-CGRP) is the first neuropeptide to be discovered solely by a molecular approach, without the biological basis for chemical characterization that was used for many other biological active peptides. The expression of this 37–amino acid polypeptide results from the alternative splicing of RNA transcribed from the calcitonin gene. While in the thyroid C cells, the primary RNA transcripts are processed to mRNA for calcitonin; mRNA for CGRP is formed predominantly in neural tissues.[285] Thus, alternative processing of the calcitonin gene transcripts determines in a tissue-specific manner which of the two biologically active peptides encoded by the gene is expressed. CGRP is widely distributed throughout the central nervous system and peripheral tissues and has been shown to possess a number of biological actions, including potent effects on gastric acid secretion and food intake, pancreatic function, and on the cardiovascular systems (for review see refs. 286–288). Subsequently a second CGRP-encoding gene with no associated calcitonin-like sequence was discovered. This peptide, which has one amino-acid residue different from α-CGRP, is known as β-CGRP and has been demonstrated to occur in vivo.[289] β-CGRP possesses a very similar spectrum of biological actions to α-CGRP.[290] However, the peptides exhibit differential tissue distribution, which probably reflects the preferential actions of the two forms, such that α-CGRP is the predominant form in central nervous tissue and sensory innervation, while β-CGRP forms the main component of the gut and pancreatic intrinsic innervation.[290, 291]

Opioid Peptides

Endogenous opioid peptides, enkephalins and endorphins, are widespread in the nerves of the gastrointestinal tract, in both myenteric and submucous neurons. The main representatives of these two groups of opioid peptides found in the gut are leu- and met-enkephalin from preproenkephalin A and dynorphin from preproenkephalin B.

The circumstances affecting the release of endogenous opioids in the enteric nervous system is not clear, although they are likely to play an important role in the normal function of intestinal motility and secretion.

Opioid agonists, in the form of morphine and its derivatives, have long been used in the treatment of increased intestinal secretion and motility associated with diarrhea. Three main subtypes of opioid receptor have now been identified μ, δ, and κ. Leu-enkephalin is μ specific and met-enkephalin prefers the δ-receptor. Dynorphin appears to be the endogenous ligand for the κ-receptor subtype.

Actions of endogenous opioids in the gut are thought to include inhibition of intestinal secretion and increased smooth muscle contractility, with inhibition of intestinal transit.[292] In general, effects on transit may be mediated predominantly via μ-receptors, with agonists inhibiting and antagonists increasing intestinal transit. Kappa agonists tend to increase and μ-agonists decrease gastric acid secretion.[293] Opioids may also be involved in mucosal integrity of the stomach (perhaps via effects on prostaglandins), as morphine inhibits the mucosal damage associated with alcohol in rats.[294]

Substance P and the Tachykinins

Substance P was known for a considerable period prior to its isolation and purification. It was discovered by virtue of its ability to induce smooth muscle contraction and vasodilation in the 1930's, but it was not until 1971 that substance P was finally characterized (for detailed review see refs. 295–297). Substance P shares homology with a number of nonmammalian and mammalian peptides, collectively forming a family named tachykinins because of their characteristic rapid action on tissue preparations. All tachykinins share the common C-terminal sequence Phe-X-Gly-Met-Leu NH_2 where X is an aromatic or branched aliphatic amino acid. Substance P is an 11-amino acid peptide and is the most characterized mammalian tachykinin and perhaps the best-documented peptide as a neurotransmitter and/or neuromodulator. The other mammalian tachykinins are neurokinin α (substance K or neuromedin L) and neurokinin β (neuromedin K); the confusion in terminology is due to their independent discovery, isolation, and classification by different groups. There are also a number of amphibian tachykinins, including physalamin, eledoisin, and kassinin. In mammals, tachykinins are synthesized by two distinct but similar genes, preprotachykinin (PPT) genes A and B.[298, 299] PPT-A encodes both substance P and neurokinin α while PPT-B encodes neurokinin β. Alternative splicing of PPT-A mRNA can generate three different mRNA's, α-, β-, and δ-preprotachykinin, the first form encoding only substance P and the latter two both substance P and neurokinin α. Processing of the PPT polypeptide occurs at pairs of basic residues, with C-terminal glycine serving as a donor for C-terminal amidation. It is possible that the processing of PPT generates different peptides, which may have biological activity. One such candidate, neuropeptide K, has a tachykinin sequence at its C-terminal end and may therefore have a physiological role.[300]

Tachykinins are found throughout the peripheral and central nervous systems, including sensory organs, respiratory tract, skin, and urogenital tract. Within the brain and spinal cord their expression is very localized and concentrated, particularly in those regions thought to be involved in pain perception that also contain high levels of enkephalins.[301] PPT mRNA's are expressed in neurons of the myenteric plexus in both the esophagus and stomach, although they are more numerous in the latter tissue. The ganglion cells distributed in both the myenteric and submucosal plexus of the intestine also contain PPT mRNA, the distribution of which is parallel to that of the peptide,[302] suggesting that specific mRNA's and posttranslationally processed peptides are localized in the same structure. All three tachykinins excite neurons, act as potent vasodilators, and contract almost all smooth muscles. They are, however, distinguished by quantitative differences in the relative potencies of their pharmacological actions. There are at least three distinct G protein–coupled tachykinin receptors in mammals. These receptors interact differentially with the tachykinin peptides and are uniquely distributed throughout the nervous system.[303, 304] The neurokinin-1 receptor preferentially interacts with substance P, the neurokinin-2 receptor prefers neurokinin α, neuropeptide K, and neuropeptide δ, and the neurokinin-3 receptor interacts best with neurokinin β.

Our understanding of the molecular nature of multiple tachykinin-binding sites has recently been advanced by molecular cloning of these receptors.[305] The development of new chemical probes specific for different receptor subtypes has led to an explosion of information in the field of tachykinin research. Future investigations will undoubtedly reveal new and important functions of this neuropeptide family.

Neuropeptide Y

Neuropeptide Y (NPY) is a 36-amino acid peptide first isolated in 1982.[306] It is widespread in both the central and peripheral nervous system, where it is often co-localized with norepinephrine, as well as other peptide neurotransmitters.[307, 308] It is a member of the PYY and PP family of peptides, with which it shares close structural homology.[306] In the gastrointestinal tract, NPY is predominantly localized to intrinsic neurons in the submucous and myenteric nerve plexuses, innervating the mucosa, submucosa, and smooth muscle.[309] NPY neurons are also found in the pancreas.[308, 310]

Any release of NPY into the circulation is likely to involve neuronal spillover, and little is known about factors that regulate NPY release in the gut. However, NPY is often co-released with epinephrine and norepinephrine, and it may act as a sympathetic neuromodulatory transmitter.[311] Immunoreactive NPY has been reported to increase in peripheral blood after a meal.[312]

NPY is a powerful vasoconstrictor and has also been found to have potent antisecretory effects on the mucosa in the upper intestine.[313] In the pancreas it is an inhibitor of insulin release but is less potent than norepinephrine in this respect and may be important in regulating local blood flow.[314] Effects have also been reported on colonic motility. On the basis of studies using different fragments of NPY, there are likely to be at least two main subtypes of NPY receptor. The Y_1 or postsynaptic receptor binds the {Leu^{31} Pro^{34}} NPY analogue, whereas NPY 13–36 and other C-terminal fragments are inactive in this respect. In contrast, the Y_2-receptor subtype is predominantly presynaptic and can be stimulated by C-terminal fragments. Further receptor subtypes have also been postulated. While it is clear that many of the actions of NPY are mediated via a pertussis toxin–sensitive G protein linked to the receptor, there is considerable evidence that other second messenger systems, involving alterations in intracellular calcium, are also activated.[315] Recent isolation of a number of NPY receptor clones should help clarify this.[316]

Galanin

Galanin is a 29-amino acid peptide isolated from porcine intestine in 1983.[317] Following the identification of the cDNA-encoding porcine preprogalanin,[318] the sequences of rat and human preprogalanin have been identified.[319, 320] Human galanin differs from porcine galanin by six amino acids; notably it has a serine substituted for glycine at position 30 and is therefore likely to be 30 amino acids in length and not likely to be amidated. Galanin-like immunoreactivity and galanin mRNA have been found in the peripheral nervous system, notably in nerves supplying the pancreas, liver, and myenteric, mucous, and submucous plexuses of the gut as well as in the lung and urogenital tract.[318, 321] Galanin is also widespread in the CNS.[322] Galanin immunoreactivity in the gut has been found to be co-localized with many other neurotransmitters, most notably VIP.[321, 323]

Galanin has been found to be released into the circulation following sympathetic activation (presumably as a spill-over from neuronal release). This appears to originate both from nerves supplying the endocrine pancreas and from other areas of the gastrointestinal tract, notably the liver and gut.[324, 325] Whether there is local release of galanin in the gut following more physiological stimuli, for example, following a meal, is not known.

Galanin has several effects on the gastrointestinal tract, particularly on gut motility and pancreatic endocrine secretion. Galanin infusion inhibits gastric emptying and cecum-to-colon transit times and reduces the release of many gastrointestinal peptides, including insulin, PYY, neurotensin, enteroglucagon, SS, and pancreatic polypeptide.[326] The effects on smooth muscle in the gut are largely inhibitory and appear to occur both directly and by neuromodulatory effects interfering with the release of excitatory transmitters such as acetylcholine and substance P.[327] Direct stimulatory effects have also been described, and it is possible that different receptors may be involved in these actions, as inhibitory actions appear to require the intact galanin molecule, whereas some stimulatory effects require only the presence of the N-terminal 10-amino acids.[328] Galanin inhibits basal and pentagastrin-stimulated gastric acid secretion, but it is not known if this effect is direct or mediated via modulation of other gastric acid secretagogues.[329] Galanin potently inhibits glucose-induced insulin secretion from the pancreatic beta cell and may also have effects on pancreatic exocrine secretion.[328] The recent description of a synthetic chimeric peptide, galantide, consisting of galanin 1–13 and substance P(5–11) amide, which is a potent antagonist at the galanin receptor, is likely to clarify the physiological role of galanin in the enteric nervous system.[330]

Galanin exerts its actions by both calcium-independent mechanisms linked to a pertussis toxin–sensitive inhibitory G protein and by calcium-dependent mechanisms involving opening of potassium channels and the prevention of opening of calcium channels, for example, in the pancreatic beta cell and in inhibitory effects on excitatory myenteric neurons.[331]

Endothelin

Endothelin-1 was originally isolated from the conditioned medium of cultured porcine aortic endothelial cells (see Chapter 154).[332] It is one of the most potent vasoconstrictor peptides yet known. Endothelin-1 is produced not only by vascular endothelial cells, but also by a variety of other cell types such as neurons[333, 334] and epithelial cells.[335] High densities of endothelin-binding sites have been found on vascular smooth muscle cells,[336] nervous tissues,[337] lung,[338] and so on. Therefore, endothelin-1 is thought to be a ubiquitous peptide.

It is now known that there are three endothelin genes (endothelin-1, -2, and -3) in the human, porcine, and rat genome.[339, 340] There are two amino acid differences between endothelin-1 and -2, and six amino acid differences between endothelin-1 and -3. In addition, a vasoactive intestinal contractor peptide (VIC) with structural similarity to the endothelins has been cloned and sequenced from the mouse genome.[341] All these endothelins have two identically positioned disulfide bonds.

Endothelins have structural and functional similarities to a group of peptide toxins, sarafotoxins, that were purified and sequenced from the venom of the Israeli burrowing asp *Atractaspis engaddensis*.[342, 343] The presence of immunoreactive endothelin, its mRNA and high-affinity binding sites for endothelin have been reported in both rat[344] and human[345, 346] gastrointestinal tract. Endothelin appears to be produced by a variety of cells in the gastrointestinal tract, including mucosal epithelial cells[347] and plexus nerves. Its release and influence may form a hitherto unknown physiological regulatory system in the gastrointestinal tract. All the information so far supports the idea that endothelin is a locally produced regulator acting in the gastrointestinal tract. The possible implications of this, including a primary contribution to and/or secondary role in the etiology of gastric ulcers, are unclear,[348] and its formation by tumors remains to be investigated.

GUT HORMONES IN DISEASE

This section describes patterns of alteration of gut hormone secretion in a number of conditions affecting the gastrointestinal tract and the pathophysiology and treatment of the various clinical syndromes associated with dysfunction of many of the hormones already described. Syndromes may result from either overproduction of a particular hormone or neurotransmitter, usually from a tumor, or its deficiency.

Gastric Pathology

Achlorhydria

Achlorhydria may result from autoimmune destruction of the acid-producing cells in the stomach (pernicious anemia), from surgical vagotomy or medical treatment for peptic ulceration with H_2 receptor antagonists or proton pump inhibitors such as omeprazole. In these situations there are usually very high levels of gastrin secretion, stimulated predominantly by the rise in gastric pH,[349] although indirect effects may also be important, for example, the increase in gastric bacterial colonization.[350] Despite the large number of effects reported for gastrin on cells other than the parietal cell, no clinical sequelae of these high gastrin levels have been reported, although the possibility of the development of gastric carcinoid tumors should not be forgotten[35] (see Gastrin).

Peptic Ulcer Disease

While there is no doubt that elevated gastrin concentrations, as seen in the Zollinger-Ellison syndrome, can be a potent cause of peptic ulceration, it is far from clear whether gastrin is implicated in the more common form of the disease. Basal gastrin levels may be normal in duodenal ulcer, although there is often an exaggerated response to a meal. These subjects may also be more sensitive to the effects of gastrin on acid secretion.[351] The mucosal protective barrier may also be defective, resulting in increased likelihood of damage by acid. Recent attention has focused on the role of infection with the organism *Helicobacter pylori* (previously *Campylobacter pylori*).[352, 353] This organism is present in the mucous layer of the stomach of most patients with duodenal ulceration and appears to damage the protective layer and cause gastritis. It may also influence acid and gastrin secretion, although the relative importance of these factors is not known.[354] Eradication of *Helicobacter pylori* does cause a decrease in gastrin but not acid secretion.[355] Management of peptic ulcer is with H_2 antagonists, with the more effective but more expensive proton pump inhibitors reserved for resistant cases. Antibiotics in combination with colloidal bismuth are useful in eradicating *Helicobacter pylori* infection. Antibiotics administered on a background of complete gastric acid inhibition, using high-dose proton pump inhibitors, may be even more effective. Surgical treatment with vagotomy tends to be reserved for patients in whom bleeding or ulcer perforation has occurred and may become an operation of the past.

Gastric Surgery

Following partial or total gastrectomy and sometimes truncal vagotomy, patients may develop the dumping syndrome, related to rapid gastric emptying. This produces a constellation of symptoms, including tachycardia, hypotension, and abdominal bloating; it may sometimes also be associated with hypoglycemia. The postprandial increase of a number of gut hormones is grossly exaggerated in this condition, including VIP, PYY, enteroglucagon and neurotensin, with a decrease in motilin.[356] It has been suggested that these symptoms may be in part due to this hormone release and that the hypoglycemia is related to an exaggerated incretin effect; however, these associations remain unproven at present. Blockade of hormonal secretion with the somatostatin analogue, octreotide, has been used with some success in treating this condition.[357]

Other Gastrointestinal Conditions

Intestinal Surgery

A number of changes in gastrointestinal hormones can be demonstrated following ileal or colonic resection. These changes are largely compensatory and serve to increase growth and decrease transit to maximize the area of mucosa and time available for absorption of nutrients. Thus, after ileal resection, gastrin, enteroglucagon, PP, motilin, and PYY levels are all elevated, whereas only gastrin and PP are increased following colonic resection.[358] The operation of jejunoileal bypass, performed for morbid obesity, is associated with complete loss of the postprandial rise in GIP;

however, increases in many hormones, particularly enteroglucagon, that result in compensatory hypertrophy have a tendency to reduce the effectiveness of this operation.[359]

Malabsorption

The changes in many of the gut hormones observed with several malabsorption syndromes can often be understood given knowledge of the sites of synthesis and actions of these hormones.

CELIAC DISEASE. Celiac disease (gluten enteropathy) is a result of immune-mediated destruction of the upper intestinal mucosa, triggered by the presence of gluten in the diet. These patients develop villous atrophy and often severe malabsorption, which has been found to be partly due to reduced exocrine pancreatic secretion. The production of many mucosal hormones with effects on pancreatic hormone secretion, such as CCK, secretin, and GIP, is dramatically reduced in this condition, whereas PYY (which inhibits secretion) is increased, and together this may explain the reduced pancreatic and biliary secretion.[360, 361] In contrast, secretion of tropic hormones such as neurotensin and enteroglucagon from distal mucosa is increased and may partly explain the increased turnover of cells in the upper intestine seen in this condition, presumably as a futile attempt to increase growth.[360] These changes, and the villous atrophy, are completely reversed by a gluten-free diet.

TROPICAL SPRUE. Tropical sprue, or postinfective malabsorption, occurs predominantly in travelers to Asia, Central and South America, and the Southern Mediterranean, where it is sometimes also seen in the indigenous population. It is rarely seen in travelers to Africa. It is characterized by persistent diarrhea (arbitrarily defined as being of greater than two months' duration) and is often associated with bacterial overgrowth, although viral infection has also been implicated. These subjects tend to have high circulating concentrations of enteroglucagon, motilin, and PYY, which may be an attempt to enhance absorption by reducing intestinal transit rate and growth.[362, 363] Treatment is with tetracycline and folic acid.

PANCREATIC MALABSORPTION. Pancreatic malabsorption, whether produced by chronic pancreatitis or cystic fibrosis, is associated with reduced release of PP following a meal, presumably because of involvement of endocrine cells. Again there is increased release of PYY and enteroglucagon from the colon.[363, 364]

Neural Abnormalities

CHAGAS' DISEASE. This condition is due to chronic infection with *Trypanosoma cruzi*. It is endemic in Central and South America. The features of Chagas' disease are chronic inflammation of heart muscle and the smooth muscle of the gut—the latter results in denervation and loss of motility, resulting in functional obstruction and megaesophagus, megaduodenum, and megacolon. Not surprisingly the concentrations of peptidergic neurotransmitters such as VIP, enteroglucagon, substance P, and somatostatin in the gut wall are much reduced.[233]

SHY-DRAGER SYNDROME. In contrast to Chagas' disease, patients with chronic autonomic failure, who lose extrinsic nerves, have normal concentrations of the peptide neurotransmitters in rectal biopsy specimens. This is probably because these peptides are largely present in the intrinsic innervation of the gut.[233]

HIRSCHSPRUNG'S DISEASE. This congenital condition is due to the presence of an aganglionic segment of large bowel; this segment shows reduced concentrations of VIP and substance P.[365]

HUMAN IMMUNODEFICIENCY VIRUS (HIV) INFECTION. HIV infection is associated with the presence of diarrhea and malabsorption, and specific secondary infection may not always be present. HIV has been found to infect gastrointestinal epithelia and cause abnormalities in the nerves. One study has suggested reduced substance P, VIP, and somatostatin immunostaining in the bowel of patients with HIV infection; furthermore, this was correlated with reduced CD4+ lymphocyte count.[366] These interesting findings, suggesting a specific HIV-related gut neuropathy, are yet to be confirmed, however.

Inflammatory Diarrhea

INFECTION. Acute infective diarrhea, whether bacterial or viral, is associated with large increases in plasma enteroglucagon, PYY, and motilin, which return to normal after recovery. It seems likely that these changes are in response to the infection and may be responsible for the characteristic changes in motility seen in infection and in the stimulation of growth of new mucosa.[367]

INFLAMMATORY BOWEL DISEASE. Ulcerative colitis is associated with reduced gastric acid secretion, and these patients have a compensatory increase in fasting and stimulated gastrin secretion. Other peptides such as GIP, motilin, and PP are also moderately increased. Crohn's disease is characterized by histological abnormalities of VIP-ergic nerves, which appear dilated and tortuous.[368] PP, motilin, GIP, and enteroglucagon are also increased. These changes may be related to alterations in both motility and growth of the intestine.[369]

Carcinoma of the Colon

Both normal colonic mucosa and adenocarcinomas are known to contain gastrin receptors, and plasma gastrin is elevated in patients with colonic carcinoma. Given the known trophic effects of gastrin, gastrin antagonists have been tried with some success at inhibiting growth of colonic cell lines.[370] The clinical relevance of these findings in the etiology and treatment of colonic cancer remains unknown.

Irritable Bowel Syndrome

Although this condition is associated with functional abnormalities of gut motility, gut hormone responses appear to be normal. Recent work has suggested that abnormalities in sensitivity to the motor effects of CCK in the gallbladder, small bowel, and colon may be relevant to its etiology, as CCK infusion produces greater effects and mimics some symptoms in subjects with irritable bowel syndrome.[371] However, treatment with the CCK antagonist loxiglumide did not affect the colonic response to a meal in normal subjects or in patients with irritable bowel syndrome,[372] so these effects may be pharmacological.

Neuroendocrine Tumors

The pluripotential nature of the endocrine cells of the gastrointestinal tract means that tumors of this system may produce a wide range of hormones, which may or may not result in clinical syndromes. This is further complicated by the fact that an individual tumor may produce more than one hormone in the course of its natural history.[373] Some tumors do not produce a recognizable hormone and are classified as nonfunctioning tumors, which have been reported to account for up to 50 per cent of all tumors.[374] Gastrointestinal endocrine tumors are rare tumors, with an incidence of one per million population per year for the most common tumor, gastrinoma, to one per 10 million per year or less for the other tumors.[375] The majority of tumors arise in the pancreas, although some, notably gastrinomas, may occur in extrapancreatic sites. Approximately 25 per cent of tumors occur in association with parathyroid tumors and pituitary adenomas as a feature of multiple endocrine neoplasia type 1 (MEN 1), notably gastrinomas and nonfunctioning tumors.[376] Approximately 70 per cent of spontaneous tumors and 45 per cent of those associated with MEN 1 are malignant, with metastases to regional lymph nodes and the liver being most common. Gut hormone tumors, even when malignant, are relatively slow growing, and prolonged survival is often possible.

Gastrinoma (Zollinger-Ellison Syndrome)

Gastrinomas represent 20 to 25 per cent of pancreatic endocrine tumors and are most common between 30 and 50 years of age, although they may occur at any age.[377] Gastrinoma is associated with MEN 1 in 25 to 30 per cent of cases, and a family history and the possibility of hyperparathyroidism or pituitary tumor should be actively sought at the time of diagnosis. Sixty per cent of gastrinomas are malignant. Although the majority arise in the pancreas, extrapancreatic tumors do occur, predominantly in the duodenum (20 per cent of cases) but also in the stomach, spleen, ovary, and peripancreatic lymph nodes.[378] Histologically, these tumors have the typical appearance of endocrine tumors, with uniform cells and few mitoses, arranged in ribbons or in a glandular structure.

The clinical syndrome produced by gastrinomas was first recognized by Zollinger and Ellison in 1955[379] and is characterized by recurrent and severe peptic ulcer disease, associated with the presence of a pancreatic tumor. The diagnosis is made on the basis of an elevated fasting plasma gastrin level in the presence of peptic ulcer disease, assuming that other causes of a raised gastrin level are excluded (Table 153–2). Other features of the syndrome include diarrhea (30 per cent of patients) and steatorrhea, probably related to the low pH found in the duodenum and jejunum, which damages the mucosa and interferes with the activity of digestive enzymes. Gastrin also directly decreases intestinal salt and water absorption.[380] Abdominal pain is usually the result of peptic ulcer disease. When plasma gastrin is unequivocally elevated (>40 pmol/L) the diagnosis is usually straightforward. If there is doubt, basal and pentagastrin-stimulated acid output may also be measured, with basal levels above 15 mmol/h being diagnostic of gastrinoma, and a ratio of basal to stimulated greater than 0.6.[378] If there is still uncertainty, then a secretin test

TABLE 153–2. CAUSES OF INCREASES OF SOME COMMONLY MEASURED GUT HORMONES

HORMONE	CAUSES OF RAISED PLASMA CONCENTRATION
General	Postabsorptive
	Renal failure
	Hepatic failure
	Stress
Gastrin	Drugs: H₂ antagonists
	Omeprazole
	Pernicious anemia
	Intestinal resection
	Gastrinoma
	Inflammatory bowel disease
Glucagon	Drugs: oral contraceptives, danazol
	Diabetes mellitus
	Hypoglycemia
	Familial hyperglucagonemia
	Glucagonoma
Pancreatic polypeptide	Inflammatory bowel disease
	Other neuroendocrine tumors
	PPoma
Somatostatin	Somatostatinoma
VIP	VIPoma

can be considered. This exploits the exaggerated rise in plasma gastrin seen in patients with gastrinoma following intravenous secretin (2 U/kg given as a bolus over 30 to 60 sec) which should rise to over 40 pmol/L or 50 per cent above basal in patients with gastrinoma.[381] The secretin test has also been used in conjunction with selective arterial catheterization and may improve diagnostic accuracy. Imaging with CT, MRI, or selective angiography can then be used to localize the tumor, and if there are no metastases then the patient may be considered for surgery. Patients with biochemical evidence of hypergastrinemia, suggestive of gastrinoma, but in whom no tumor is found, may be considered for exploratory surgery as many of these patients will be found to have small pancreatic or duodenal gastrinomas at the time of surgery; however, this course of action is not without its risks, and patients may have multiple lesions that are not necessarily the cause of the increased gastrin.[382]

Increased acid secretion and peptic ulceration in Zollinger-Ellison syndrome can be effectively controlled with H₂ antagonists or with the proton pump inhibitor omeprazole, and many patients have now been treated, often for long periods, without problems, although there is the theoretical risk of gastric carcinoids with prolonged therapy[35] and the treatment of choice is surgical excision. Patients with metastatic disease have been treated with combination chemotherapy, using streptozocin and 5-fluorouracil, with varying degrees of success. Another treatment for metastatic disease is interferon-α.[383] Success of treatment can be assessed by serial measurement of plasma gastrin, along with other endocrine tumor markers, as a second syndrome may develop.

VIPoma

The VIPoma syndrome was originally described by Priest and Alexander in 1957 and Verner and Morrison in 1955[384, 385] as a syndrome associated with watery diarrhea, hypokalemia, and achlorhydria and with the presence of an islet cell tumor. The association with increased plasma VIP concentrations was observed in 1973,[386] and the syndrome was renamed the VIPoma syndrome. VIPomas account for approximately 2 per cent of gut hormone tumors.[387] The majority of tumors are found in the pancreas, but other tumors have been found to secrete VIP, including ganglioneuroblastomas (predominantly in children), pheochromocytomas, neuroblastomas, and bronchogenic carcinomas.[388]

The clinical features of the VIPoma syndrome can be predicted from the known actions of VIP on the enterocyte and on blood vessels, although these tumors have subsequently been shown to co-secrete peptide-histidine-methionine (PHM), which is a less potent stimulus to intestinal secretion than VIP, although it may act at the same receptor.[389] The diarrhea associated with the syndrome is severe, and patients frequently produce up to 3 L of watery stool daily, with up to 20 L having been reported. Loss of potassium and bicarbonate in the stool leads to a hypokalemic alkalosis, which may be life threatening. Hypomagnesemia is also recognized. Symptoms may initially be intermittent, and patients may be symptomatic for 3 years or more before diagnosis. Achlorhydria is a frequent feature, and glucose intolerance is seen in 20 to 50 per cent of cases, probably due to a glucagon-like action of VIP. Hypercalcemia may be due to production of parathyroid hormone-related protein (PTHrp) or hyperparathyroidism associated with MEN 1. Flushing and hypotension also occur, related to the direct effects of VIP to cause vasodilation.[390]

The diagnosis is based on clinical suspicion, and measurement of plasma VIP levels by radioimmunoassay. This can be supplemented by measurement of PHM, as concentrations of this peptide are much higher, because of a longer half-life.[389] Fifty per cent of tumors have metastasized at the time of diagnosis. Tumors may be localized by ultrasound and CT, supplemented by angiography when necessary. Transhepatic venous sampling has been used with some success.[391] A novel approach to tumor localization is the use of radiolabeled somatostatin analogues; although these have been used with some success, in our experience most of these tumors would be detected by other means. Exploratory laparotomy may be justified if these localizing procedures are unsuccessful, as removal of a small, benign tumor may be lifesaving.

Surgical resection is the treatment of choice for solitary lesions, and distal pancreatectomy or debulking procedures may be helpful in more extensive disease.[392] Medical treatment has been much improved with the use of the somatostatin analogue octreotide, which is effective in controlling diarrhea in many patients. Chemotherapy with streptozocin and 5-fluorouracil is particularly effective palliation for VIPomas. Interferon has also been used with mixed success.[383]

Glucagonoma Syndrome

The most dramatic feature of pancreatic tumors producing glucagon is the rash, necrolytic migratory erythema, which starts in the groin and then spreads to cover the perineum, buttocks, and limbs. The initial erythema may blister and become encrusted, and secondary infection may occur. As it heals, it leaves behind a pigmented area. The mechanism may relate either to zinc or amino-acid deficiency, the latter being due to the expected effect of glucagon to stimulate gluconeogenesis. However, zinc levels are usually normal, and correction of reduced plasma amino acids may not affect the rash.[393] It has been suggested that glucagon may directly affect the skin, but octreotide may cure the rash without affecting plasma glucagon levels. Other features such as weight loss and anemia may be related to the decreased availability of amino acids, perhaps exacerbated by the effects of tumor bulk.[394] Other clinical features include mild diabetes mellitus, venous thrombosis, and depression.[395, 396] The majority (75 per cent) of glucagonomas are malignant, and 50 per cent of patients have metastases at the time of diagnosis.[397] The diagnosis is usually straightforward, but other causes of increased glucagon, including renal impairment, diabetes mellitus, and hypoglycemia, should be considered, particularly if the elevation is only moderate. Treatment with danazol has been reported to result in very high glucagon concentrations.[398]

Management of glucagonoma is along the general principles already described, with surgical resection as the treatment of choice if this is practical and palliative treatment with chemotherapy, octreotide, and hepatic embolization all having a role.[383] Liver transplantation may be considered following tumor resection for metastatic disease.[399] The rash frequently responds to lowering of the plasma glucagon level, for example, with octreotide.[400] Diabetes is usually mild and can be managed on conventional lines. Prophylaxis against thromboembolic disease is important, and aspirin or dipyridamole should be considered.

PPoma

Pancreatic polypeptide levels are raised in 22 to 77 per cent of all patients with islet tumors; however, although pure PPomas have been described, there is no well-defined clinical syndrome.[401] A patient with an erythematous, scaly, papular rash that resolved after chemotherapy to reduce tumor bulk has been described, but this may not have been due to PP, but instead to another, unrecognized factor.[402] PPomas tend to be large, vascular tumors, and have usually metastasized at the time of presentation. Other causes of raised PP levels include diabetes mellitus and chronic renal failure. The finding of a raised PP level may be important supporting evidence for the presence of an islet cell tumor, but is not sufficiently sensitive or specific to act as a diagnostic test.[403]

Somatostatinoma

Somatostatinomas are rare tumors, with an incidence of about one in 40 million. It is important to distinguish between pancreatic somatostatinomas, which are large tumors and frequently associated with the features of SS excess, and duodenal tumors, which are often small and well localized and thus amenable to surgical resection. Duodenal somatostatinomas are frequently associated with neurofibromatosis type I (von Recklinghausen's neurofibromatosis).[404] Duodenal carcinoids associated with this syndrome are often also found to contain SS, although this rarely causes clinical problems.

Specific clinical features of the somatostatinoma syndrome include diabetes, which is present in up to 90 per

cent of patients with pancreatic tumors. The diabetic condition is often mild and may be present for many years before diagnosis, although ketoacidosis has been reported. Hypoglycemia may also occur, although this is rare. Nonspecific features such as abdominal bloating, diarrhea, weight loss, anemia, and cholelithiasis predominate, so the diagnosis is frequently not made until late in the course of the disease. Patients with duodenal tumors present earlier because of local symptoms such as cholestatic jaundice due to tumor obstructing the ampulla of Vater.[405–407] The diagnosis is confirmed by finding a raised plasma somatostatin concentration, and tumors are usually easily localized by ultrasound or CT. Duodenal tumors may be found at endoscopy. SS is released in a variety of forms, larger molecular forms possibly being precursor molecules. Differential rates of release of S 14 and S 28 may account for part of the heterogeneity of the clinical syndrome, with high levels of S 28 tending to inhibit glucagon release and result in hypoglycemia.[408] Treatment is mainly surgical, although palliation with chemotherapy or hepatic embolization can be helpful.

Other Hormones and Malignancy

PARATHYROID HORMONE-RELATED PROTEIN (PTHrp). This peptide is the usual mediator of humoral hypercalcemia of malignancy and is expressed in normal pancreatic islets.[409] It is the likely mediator of hypercalcemia observed with other tumors when hyperparathyroidism is not present. Several cases of malignant islet cell tumors producing only PTHrp have now been described. If surgical cure is not possible, the hypercalcemia may be controlled with octreotide and bisphosphonates.[410, 411]

ACTH AND CORTICOTROPIN-RELEASING FACTOR (CRF). Pancreatic tumors producing both CRF and ACTH are recognized, but only ACTH-secreting tumors are associated with Cushing's syndrome. If surgical treatment is not curative, effective palliation may be achieved with chemotherapy or hepatic artery embolization. Octreotide has been reported to normalize ACTH levels in four out of five patients in one small series, but adrenalectomy may be necessary in resistant cases.

GROWTH HORMONE–RELEASING HORMONE. A few patients have been identified with pancreatic tumors that produce growth hormone–releasing hormone (GHRH). These have resulted in acromegaly or gigantism due to somatotroph hyperplasia or adenoma in the pituitary gland. When surgical resection is not feasible, octreotide is effective treatment at both the pituitary and pancreatic level.[412]

ENTEROGLUCAGONOMA. A single renal enteroglucagon-producing tumor has been described. The patient had elongation of intestinal villi and markedly increased gastrointestinal transit time.[123]

Numerous other peptides have been found either in plasma or in tissue from endocrine tumors of the gastrointestinal tract, including NPY, neurotensin, neuromedin B, CGRP, bombesin, and motilin, but these have not been associated with specific clinical syndromes.

REFERENCES

1. Bayliss WM, Starling EH: The mechanism of pancreatic secretion. J Physiol 28:325–335, 1902.

2. Bayliss WM, Starling EH: On the causation of the so-called "peripheral reflex secretion" of the pancreas. Proc R Soc Lond 69:352–360, 1902.

3. Edkins JS: On the chemical mechanism of gastric secretion. Proc R Soc Lond 76:376, 1905.

4. Pearse AGE, Polak JM: Endocrine tumours of neural crest origin: Neurolophomas. APUDomas and the APUD concept. Med Biol 52:3–18, 1974.

5. McGuigan JE: Gastric mucosal intracellular localization of gastrin by immunofluorescence. Gastroenterology 55:315–327, 1968.

6. Buchan AMJ, Polak JM, Solcia E, Pearce AGE: Localisation of intestinal gastrin to a distinct endocrine cell type. Nature 277:138–140, 1979.

7. Wiborg O, Berglund L, Boel E: Structure of a human gastrin gene. Proc Natl Acad Sci USA 81:1067–1069, 1984.

8. Morley JS, Tracy HJ, Gregory RA: Structure-function relationships in the active C-terminal tetrapeptide sequence of gastrin. Nature 207:1356–1359, 1965.

9. Gregory RA, Tracy HJ: The constitution and properties of two gastrins isolated from hog antral mucosa. Gut 5:103, 1964.

10. Yalow RS, Berson SA: Size and charge distinctions between endogenous human plasma gastrin in peripheral blood and heptadecapeptide gastrins. Gastroenterology 58:609–615, 1970.

11. Gregory RA, Tracy HJ, Harris JI: Minigastrin: Corrected structure and synthesis. Hoppe Seyler's Z Physiol Chem 360:73–80, 1979.

12. Rehfeld JF, Stadil F, Vikelsoe J: Immunoreactive gastrin components in human serum. Gut 15:102–111, 1974.

13. Yalow RS, Berson SA: And now, "big, big" gastrin. Biochem Biophys Res Commun 48:391–395, 1972.

14. Walsh JH, Debas HT, Grossman MI: Pure human big gastrin: Immunochemical properties, disappearance half-time and stimulating action in dogs. J Clin Invest 54:477–485, 1974.

15. Rehfeld JF, Stadil F, Malmstrom J, et al: Gastrin heterogeneity in serum and tissue. A progress report. In Thompson JC (ed): Gastrointestinal Hormones. Austin, University of Texas Press, 1975, p 43.

16. Taylor IL, Byrne WJ, Christie DL, et al: Effect of individual L-amino acids on gastric acid secretion and serum gastrin and pancreatic polypeptide release in humans. Gastroenterology 83:273–278, 1982.

17. Ganguli PC: The effect of protein, carbohydrate, or fat on plasma gastrin concentration in human subjects. Gut 11:1061, 1970.

18. Kronborg O, Stadil F, Rehfeld J, Christiansen PM: Relationship between serum gastrin concentrations and gastric acid secretion in duodenal ulcer patients before and after selective and highly selective vagotomy. Scand J Gastroenterol 8:491–496, 1973.

19. Peters MN, Walsh JH, Ferrari J, Feldman M: Adrenergic regulation of distention-induced gastrin release in humans. Gastroenterology 82:659–668, 1982.

20. Woodward ER, Dragstedt LR: Role of the pyloric antrum in regulation of gastric secretion. Physiol Rev 40:490, 1960.

21. Solcia E, Capella C, Buffa R, et al: Endocrine cells of the digestive system. In Johnson LR (ed): Physiology of the Gastrointestinal Tract. New York, Raven Press, 1981, p 39.

22. Raptis S, Dollinger HC, von Berger L, et al: Effects of somatostatin on gastric secretion and gastrin release in man. Digestion 13:15–26, 1975.

23. McIntosh CH, Tang CL, Malcolm AJ, et al: Effect of a purified somatostatin monoclonal antibody and its Fab fragments on gastrin release. Am J Physiol 260:G489–G498, 1991.

24. Wu V, Sumii K, Tari A, et al: Regulation of rat antral gastrin and somatostatin gene expression during starvation and after refeeding. Gastroenterology 101:1552–1558, 1991.

25. Karnik PS, Wolfe MM: Somatostatin stimulates gastrin mRNA turnover in dog antral mucosa. J Biol Chem 265:2550–2555, 1990.

26. Karnik PS, Monahan SJ, Wolfe MM: Inhibition of gastrin gene expression by somatostatin. J Clin Invest 83:367–372, 1989.

27. Dimalane R, Forster ER, Evans D, Dockray GJ: Action of calcitonin gene–related peptide (CGRP) on gastric somatostatin mRNA abundance in the rat. Regul Pept 39:276, 1992.

28. Lott VJ, Chang RSL: A new potent and selective non-peptide gastrin antagonist and brain cholecystokinin receptor (CCK-B) ligand. Eur J Pharmacol 162:273–280, 1989.

29. Soll AH, Amirian DA, Thomas LP, et al: Gastrin receptors on isolated canine parietal cells. J Clin Invest 73:1434, 1984.

30. Delvalle J, Tsunoda Y, Williams JA, Yamada T: Regulation by secretogogue stimulation of canine gastric parietal cells. Am J Physiol 262:G420–G426, 1992.

31. Sandvik AK, Waldum HL: CCK-B (gastrin) receptor regulates gastric histamine release and acid secretion. Am J Physiol 260:G925–G928, 1991.

32. Eysselein V, Maxwell V, Reedy T, et al: Similar acid stimulatory potencies of synthetic human big and little gastrins in man. J Clin Invest 73:1284, 1984.

33. Dembinski A, Warzecha Z, Konturek SJ, et al: The effect of antagonist of receptors for gastrin, cholecystokinin and bombesin on growth of gastroduodenal mucosa and pancreas. J Physiol Pharmacol 42:263–277, 1991.

34. Johnson LR: New aspects of the trophic action of gastrointestinal hormones. Gastroenterology 72:788–792, 1977.

35. Polak JM, Bloom SR: Review: The enterochromaffin-like cell, intragastric acidity and the trophic effect of plasma gastrin. Aliment Pharmacol Ther 2:291–296, 1988.

36. Lin TM, Spry GF: Effect of pentagastrin, cholecystokinin, caerulin and glucagon on the choledochal resistance and bile flow of the conscious dog. Gastroenterology 56:1178, 1969.

37. Castell DO, Harris LD: Hormonal control of gastrooesophageal sphincter strength. N Engl J Med 282:886–890, 1970.

38. Gubler U, Chua AO, Hoffman BJ, et al: Cloned cDNA to cholecystokinin mRNA predicts an identical preprocholecystokinin in pig brain and gut. Proc Natl Acad Sci USA 81:4307, 1984.

39. Polak JM, Pearse AGE, Bloom SR, et al: Identification of cholecystokinin-secreting cells. Lancet 2:1016–1018, 1975.

40. Vanderhaegen JJ, Signeau JC, Gepts W: New peptide in the vertebrate CNS reacting with antigastrin antibodies. Nature 257:604–605, 1975.

41. Muller JE, Straus E, Yalow RS: Cholecystokinin and its COOH-terminal octapeptide in the pig brain. Proc Natl Acad Sci USA 74:3035–3037, 1977.

42. Mutt V, Jorpes JE: Structure of porcine cholecystokinin-pancreozymin. I. Cleavage with thrombin and with trypsin. Eur J Biochem 6:156–162, 1968.

43. Dockray GJ: Immunoreactive component resembling cholecystokinin octapeptide in intestine. Nature 270:359–361, 1977.

44. Welch IM, Saunders K, Read NW: Effect of ileal and intravenous infusions of fat emulsions on feeding and satiety in human volunteers. Gastroenterology 89:1293–1297, 1985.

45. Beardshall K, Frost G, Morarji Y, et al: Saturation of fat and cholecystokinin release: Implications for pancreatic carcinogenesis. Lancet 2:1008–1010, 1989.

46. Hopman WPM, Jansen JBMJ, Lamers CBHW: Plasma cholecystokinin response to a liquid fat meal in vagotomized patients. Ann Surg 200:693–697, 1984.

47. Lu L, Louie D, Owyang C: A cholecystokinin releasing peptide mediates feedback regulation of pancreatic secretion. Am J Physiol 256:G430–G435, 1989.

48. Miyasaka K, Funakoshi A, Shikado F, Kitani K: Stimulatory and inhibitory effects of bile salts on rat pancreatic secretion. Gastroenterology 102:598–604, 1992.

49. Abucham J, Reichlin S: Cysteamine induces cholecystokinin release from the duodenum. Evidence for somatostatin as an inhibitory paracrine regulator of cholecystokinin secretion in the rat. Gastroenterology 99:1633–1640, 1990.

50. Cuber JC, Vilas F, Charles N, et al: Bombesin and nutrients stimulate release of CCK through distinct pathways in the rat. Am J Physiol 256:G989–G996, 1989.

51. Kopin AS, Lee YM, McBride EW, et al: Expression cloning and characterisation of the canine parietal gastrin receptor. Proceedings of The Second International Conference on Gastrin, Dana Point, CA, 1992.

52. Ivy AC, Oldberg E: A hormone mechanism for gall bladder contraction and evacuation. Am J Physiol 86:599–613, 1928.

53. Jorpes JE, Mutt V: Cholecystokinin and pancreozymin, one single hormone? Acta Physiol Scand 66:196–202, 1966.

54. Cooper SJ, Dourish CT, Clifton PG: CCK antagonists and CCK monoamine interactions in the control of satiety. Am J Clin Nutr 55 (Suppl):291S–295S, 1992.

55. Fried M, Erlacher U, Schwiezer W, et al: Role of cholecystokinin in the regulation of gastric emptying and pancreatic enzyme secretion in humans. Studies with the cholecystokinin receptor antagonist loxiglumide. Gastroenterology 101:503–511, 1991.

56. Baber NS, Dourish CT, Hill DR: The role of CCK caerulin, and CCK antagonists in nociception. Pain 39:307–328, 1989.

57. Schmidt WE, Creutzfeldt W, Hocker M, et al: Cholecystokinin receptor antagonist loxiglumide: Influence on bilio-pancreatic secretion and gastrointestinal hormones in man. Digestion 46 (Suppl 2):232–239, 1990.

58. Fried M, Erlacher U, Schwizer W, et al: Role of cholecystokinin in the regulation of gastric emptying and pancreatic enzyme secretion

in humans. Studies with the cholecystokinin-receptor antagonist loxiglumide. Gastroenterology 101:503–511, 1991.

59. Schmidt WE, Creutzfeldt W, Schleser A, et al: Role of CCK in regulation of pancreaticobiliary functions and GI motility in humans: Effects of loxiglumide. Am J Physiol 260:G197–G206, 1991.

60. Cantor P, Motensen PE, Myhre J, et al: The effect of the cholecystokinin receptor antagonist MK-329 on meal stimulated pancreatobiliary output in humans. Gastroenterology 102:1742–1751, 1992.

61. Hildebrand P, Ensinck JW, Ketterer S, et al: Effect of a cholecystokinin antagonist on meal-stimulated insulin and pancreatic polypeptide release in humans. J Clin Endocrinol Metab 72:1123–1129, 1991.

62. Morley JE: Neuropeptide regulation of appetite and weight. Endocr Rev 8:256–287, 1987.

63. Miesner J, Smith GP, Gibbs J, Tyrka A: Intravenous infusion of CCKA-receptor antagonist increases food intake in rats. Am J Physiol 262:R216–R219, 1992.

64. Dourish CT, Rycroft W, Iversen SD: Postponement of satiety by blockade of brain cholecystokinin (CCK-B) receptors. Science 245:1509–1511, 1989.

65. Corwin RL, Gibbs J, Smith GP: Increased food intake after type A but not type B cholecystokinin receptor blockade. Physiol Behav 50:255–258, 1991.

66. Usellini L, Finzi G, Riva C, et al: Ultrastructural identification of human secretin cells by the immunogold technique. Their costorage of chromogranin A and serotonin. Histochemistry 94:113–120, 1990.

67. Kopin AS, Wheeler MB, Leiter AB: Secretin: Structure of the precursor and tissue distribution of the mRNA. Proc Natl Acad Sci USA 87:2299–2303, 1990.

68. O'Donohue TL, Charlton CG, Miller RL: Identification, characterization and distribution of secretin immunoreactivity in rat and pig brain. Proc Natl Acad Sci USA 78:5221–5224, 1981.

69. Itoh N, Furuya T, Ozaki K, et al: The secretin precursor gene. Structure of the coding region and expression in the brain. J Biol Chem 266:12595–12598, 1991.

70. Kopin AS, Wheeler MB, Nishitani J, et al: The secretin gene: Evolutionary history, alternative splicing, and developmental regulation. Proc Natl Acad Sci USA 88:5335–5339, 1991.

71. Gafvelin G, Jornvall H, Mutt V: Processing of prosecretin: Isolation of a secretin precursor from porcine intestine. Proc Natl Acad Sci USA 87:6781–6785, 1990.

72. Guan D, Spannagel A, Ohta H, et al: Role of secretin in basal and fat-stimulated pancreatic secretion in conscious rats. Endocrinology 128:979–982, 1991.

73. Hanssen LE: Pure synthetic bile salts release immunoreactive secretin in man. Scand J Gastroenterol 15:461–463, 1980.

74. Shiratori K, Watanabe S, Takeuchi T: Somatostatin analog, SMS 201-995, inhibits pancreatic exocrine secretion and release of secretin and cholecystokinin in rats. Pancreas 6:23–30, 1991.

75. Schaffalitzky de Muckadell OB, Fahrenkrug J: Secretion pattern of secretin in man: Regulation by gastric acid. Gut 19:812–818, 1978.

76. Ainsworth MA, Ladegaard L, Svendsen P, et al: Pancreatic, hepatic, and duodenal mucosal bicarbonate secretion during infusion of secretin and cholecystokinin. Evidence of the importance of hepatic bicarbonate in the neutralization of acid in the duodenum of anaesthetized pigs. Scand J Gastroenterol 26:1035–1041, 1991.

77. Ishihara T, Nakamura S, Kaziro Y, et al: Molecular cloning and expression of a cDNA encoding the secretin receptor. EMBO J 10:1635–1641, 1991.

78. Mate L, Sakemoto T, Greeley GH, Thompson JC: Regulation of gastric acid secretion by secretin and serotonin. Am J Surg 149:40–45, 1985.

79. Pollack PF, Wood JG, Solomon T: Effect of secretin on growth of stomach, small intestine, and pancreas of developing rats. Dig Dis Sci 35:749–758, 1990.

80. Brown JC, Pederson RA: A multiparameter study on the actions of preparations containing cholecystokinin-pancreozymin. Scand J Gastroenterol 5:537–541, 1970.

81. Brown JC, Dryburgh JR: A gastric inhibitory polypeptide II. The complete amino acid sequence. Can J Biochem 49:867–872, 1970.

82. Polak JM, Bloom SR, Kuzio M, et al: Cellular localization of gastric inhibitory polypeptide in the duodenum and jejunum. Gut 14:284–288, 1973.

83. Cleator IGM, Gourlay RH: Release of immunoreactive gastric inhibitory polypeptide (IRGIP) by oral ingestion of food substance. Am J Surg 130:128–135, 1975.

84. Pederson RA, Brown JC: Inhibition of histamine-pentagastrin and insulin stimulated gastric secretion by pure gastric inhibitory polypeptide. Gastroenterology 62:393–400, 1972.

85. Soon-Shiong P, Debas HT, Brown JC: The evaluation of gastric inhibitory polypeptide as the enterogastrone. J Surg Res 26:1681–1686, 1979.

86. Wolfe MM, Hocking MP, Maico DG, McGuigan ME: Effects of antibodies to gastric inhibitory polypeptide on gastric acid secretion and gastrin release in the dog. Gastroenterology 84:941–948, 1983.

87. Dupre J, Ross SA, Watson D, Brown JC: Stimulation of insulin secretion by gastric inhibitory polypeptide in man. J Clin Endocrinol Metab 37:826–828, 1973.

88. Ebert R, Illmer K, Creutzfeld W: Release of gastric inhibitory polypeptide (GIP) by intraduodenal acidification in rats and humans and abolishment of the incretin effect of acid by GIP antiserum in rats. Gastroenterology 76:515–523, 1979.

89. Tze WT: Gastric inhibitory polypeptide (GIP): A potent stimulator of insulin release. Gastroenterology 68:621–622, 1975.

90. Siegel EG, Creutzfeld W: Stimulation of insulin release in isolated rat islets by GIP in physiological concentrations; its relation to islet cyclic AMP content. Diabetologia 28:857–861, 1985.

91. Fehmann HC, Goke B, Goke R, et al: Synergistic stimulatory effect of glucagon-like peptide-1 (7–36) amide and glucose-dependent insulin-releasing polypeptide on the endocrine pancreas. FEBS Lett 252:109–112, 1989.

92. Unger RH, Orci L: Glucagon and the A cell: Physiology and pathophysiology. N Engl J Med 325:1518–1575, 1981.

93. Unger RH, Eisentraut AM, McCall MS, Madison LL: Glucagon antibodies and an immunoassay for glucagon. J Clin Invest 40:1280–1285, 1961.

94. Unger RH, Ketterer H, Eisentraut AM: Distribution of immunoassayable glucagon in gastrointestinal tissues. Metabolism 15:865, 1966.

95. Heding LG: Radioimmunological determination of pancreatic and gut glucagon in plasma. Diabetologia 7:10, 1971.

96. Holst JJ: Extraction, gel filtration pattern and receptor binding of porcine gastrointestinal glucagon-like immunoreactivity. Diabetologia 13:159, 1977.

97. Lopez LC, Frazier ML, Su CJ, et al: Mammalian pancreatic preproglucagon contains three glucagon related peptides. Proc Natl Acad Sci USA 80:5485, 1983.

98. Bell GI, Santerre RF, Mullenbach GT: Hamster preproglucagon contains the sequence of glucagon and two related peptides. Nature 302:716, 1983.

99. Bell GI, Sanchez-Pescador R, Lay-Bourn PJ, et al: Exon duplication and divergence in the human preproglucagon gene. Nature 304:368, 1983.

100. Heinrich G, Gros P, Lund PK, et al: Pre-pro glucagon messenger RNA: Nucleotide sequence and encoded amino acid sequence of the rat pancreatic cDNA. Endocrinology 115:2176, 1984.

101. Drucker DJ, Asa SL: Glucagon gene expression in vertebrate brain. J Biol Chem 263:13475, 1988.

102. Mojsov S, Heinrich G, Willson IB, et al: Preproglucagon gene expression in pancreas and intestine diversifies at the level of post-translational processing. J Biol Chem 261:11880, 1987.

103. Orskov C, Holst H, Knutsen S, et al: Glucagon-like peptides GLP-1 and GLP-2, predicted products of the glucagon gene are secreted separately from pig small intestine but not pancreas. Endocrinology 119:1467, 1986.

104. George SK, Uttenthal LO, Ghiglione M, et al: Molecular forms of glucagon-like peptides in man. FEBS Lett 192:275, 1985.

105. Patzett C, Schiltz E: Conversion of proglucagon in pancreatic alpha cells—the major end products are glucagon and a single peptide, the major proglucagon fragment, that contains two glucagon-like sequences. Proc Natl Acad Sci USA 81:5007, 1984.

106. Lui EY, Asa SL, Drucker DJ, et al: Glucagon and related peptides in the foetal rat hypothalamus in vivo and in vitro. Endocrinology 126:110, 1990.

107. Kreymann B, Ghatei MA, Burnet P, et al: Characterization of glucagon-like peptide-1 7-36 NH2 in the hypothalamus. Brain Res 502:325, 1989.

108. Ghatei MA, Bloom SR, Langevin H, et al: Regional distribution of bombesin and seven other regulatory peptides in the human brain. Brain Res 293:101, 1984.

109. Orskov C, Bersani M, Johnsen AH, et al: Complete sequence of glucagon-like peptide-1 from human and pig small intestine. J Biol Chem 264:1286, 1989.

110. Kreymann B, Yiangou Y, Kanse S, et al: Isolation and characterization of GLP-1 7-36NH2 from rat intestine. Elevated levels in diabetic rats. FEBS Lett 242:167, 1988.

111. Lund PK, Goodman RH, Dee PC, Habener JF: Pancreatic proglucagon cDNA contains two glucagon-related coding sequences arranged in tandem. Proc Natl Acad Sci USA 79:3345–3349, 1982.

112. Ghiglione M, Uttenthal LO, George SK, Bloom SR: How glucagon-like is glucagon-like peptide-1? Diabetologia 27:599–600, 1984.

113. Ghiglione M, Blazquez E, Uttenthal LO, et al: Glucagon-like peptide-1 does not have a role in hepatic carbohydrate metabolism. Diabetologia 28:920–921, 1985.

114. Schmidt W, Siegel EG, Creutzfeldt W: Glucagon-like peptide-1 but not glucagon-like peptide-2 stimulates insulin release from isolated rat islets. Diabetologia 28:704–707, 1985.

115. Drucker DJ, Philippe H, Mojsov S, et al: Glucagon-like peptide-1 stimulates insulin gene expression and increases cyclic AMP levels in a rat islet cell line. Proc Natl Acad Sci USA 84:3434–3438, 1987.

116. Orskov C, Jeppesen J, Madsbad S, Holst JJ: Proglucagon products in plasma in non-insulin dependent diabetics and non-diabetic controls in the fasting state and following oral glucose and intravenous arginine. J Clin Invest 87:415–423, 1990.

117. Kreymann B, Ghatei MA, Williams G, Bloom SR: Glucagon-like peptide 7-36: A physiological incretin in man. Lancet 2:1300–1303, 1987.

118. Orskov C, Holst JJ, Nielsen OV: Effect of truncated glucagon-like peptide 1 (proglucagon-(78–107) amide) on endocrine secretion from pig pancreas, antrum and non-antral stomach. Endocrinology 123:2009–2013, 1988.

119. Gutniak M, Orskov C, Holst JJ, et al: Antidiabetogenic effect of glucagon-like peptide-1 (7–36) amide in normal subjects and patients with diabetes mellitus. N Engl J Med 326:1316–1322, 1992.

120. Valverde I, Rigopoulou D, Marlo J, et al: Characterization of glucagon-like immunoreactivity (GLI). Diabetes 19:614–623, 1970.

121. Kiakegged P, Moody AJ, Holst JJ, et al: Glicentin inhibits gastric acid secretion in the rat. Nature 297:156, 1970.

122. McDonald TJ, Ghatei MA, Bloom SR, et al: A quantitative comparison of canine plasma gastroenteropancreatic hormone responses to bombesin and porcine gastric releasing peptide (GRP). Regul Pept 2:293, 1981.

123. Bloom SR: An enteroglucagon tumour. Gut 13:520–523, 1972.

124. Bloom SR: Gut hormones in adaptation. Gut 28 (Suppl 1):31–35, 1987.

125. Sagor GR, Ghatei MA, Al-Muktitar MYT, et al: Evidence for a humoral mechanism after intestinal resection exclusion of gastrin but not enteroglucagon. Gastroenterology 84:902–906, 1983.

126. Jacobs LR, Bloom SR, Dowling RH: Response of plasma and tissue levels of enteroglucagon immunoreactivity to tissue resection, lactation and hyperphagia. Life Sci 29:2003–2007, 1981.

127. Goodlad RA, Al-Mukhtar MYT, Ghatei MA, et al: Cell proliferation, plasma enteroglucagon and plasma gastrin in starved and refed rats. Virchows Arch 43:55–62, 1983.

128. Goodlad RA, Wilson TG, Lenton W, et al: Urogastrone-epidermal growth factor is trophic to the intestinal epithelium of parenterally fed rats. Experientia 41:1161–1163, 1985.

129. Bloom SR, Polak JM: The hormonal pattern of intestinal adaptation. A major role for enteroglucagon. Scand J Gastroenterol 17 (Suppl 74):93–104, 1982.

130. Gregor M, Menge H, Reicken EO: Effect of monoclonal antibodies to enteroglucagon on ileal adaptation after proximal small bowel resection. Gut 281 (Suppl 1):9–14, 1987.

131. Goodlad RA, Ghatei MA, Gregory H, et al: The effects of urogastrone-EGF on plasma hormone levels, a role for PYY. Experientia 45:168–169, 1989.

132. Goodlad RA, Ratcliffe BR, Fordham JP, et al: Plasma enteroglucagon, gastrin and peptide YY in conventional and germ free rats refed with fibre-free or fibre-supplemented diet. Q J Exp Physiol 74:437–442, 1989.

133. Goodlad RA, Ratcliffe BR, Fordham JP, Wright NA: Does dietary fibre stimulate intestinal epithelial cell proliferation in germ-free rats? Gut 30:820–825, 1989.

134. Sagor GR, Ghatei MA, McGregor SP, et al: The influence of an intact pylorus on post-prandial enteroglucagon and neurotensin release after upper gastric surgery. Br J Surg 68:190–192, 1981.

135. Aynsley-Green A, Lucas A, Lawson GR, Bloom SR: Gut hormones and regulatory peptides in relation to enteral feeding, gastroenteritis and necrotizing colitis in infancy. J Pediatr 117:24–32, 1990.

136. Bataille D, Tatemoto K, Gespach C, et al: Isolation of glucagon-37 (bioactive enteroglucagon/oxyntomodulin) from porcine jejunum-ileum. Characterisation of the peptide. FEBS Lett 146:79–86, 1982.

137. Holst JJ: Evidence that enteroglucagon (II) is identical with the C-terminal sequence (residue 33–69) of glicentin. Biochem J 207:381–388, 1982.

138. Dubrasquet JM, Bataille D, Gespach C: Oxyntomodulin (glucagon-37 or bioactive enteroglucagon): A potent inhibitor of pentagastrin-stimulated gastric secretion in the rat. Biosci Rep 2:391–395, 1982.

139. Jarrasse C, Audosset-Puech MP, Dubrasquet M, et al: Oxyntomodulin (glucagon-37) and its C-terminal octapeptide inhibit gastric secretion. FEBS Lett 188:81–84, 1985.

140. Schjoldger BTG, Baldissera FGA, Mortensen PE, et al: Oxyntomodulin: A potent hormone from the distal gut. Pharmacokinetics and effects on gastric acid and insulin secretion in man. Eur J Clin Invest 18:499–503, 1988.

141. Jarrouse C, Niel H, Audosset-Puech MP, et al: Oxyntomodulin and its C-terminal octapeptide inhibit liquid meal stimulated acid secretion. Peptides 7 (Suppl 1):253–256, 1986.

142. Bataille D, Jarrouse C, Keruran A, et al: The biological significance of "enteroglucagon": Present status. Peptides 7 (Suppl 1):37–42, 1986.

143. Gespach C, Emani S, Chastree E: Membrane receptors in the gastrointestinal tract. Biosci Rep 8:199–231, 1988.

144. Bado A, Bataille D, Accarg JP, et al: Luminal gastric somotostatin-like immunoreactivity in response to oxyntomodulin and derivatives in the cat. Biomed Res 53:195–199, 1988.

145. Baldissera FGA, Holst JJ, Knuhtsen S, et al: Oxyntomodulin (glicentin 33–69): Pharmacokinetics, binding to liver cell membranes, effects on isolated perfused pig pancreas, and secretin from isolated perfused lower small intestine of pigs. Regul Pept 21:151–156, 1988.

146. Brown JC, Cook MA, Dryburgh JR: Motilin, a gastric motor activity stimulating polypeptide: Further purification, amino acid composition, and C-terminal residues. Gastroenterology 62:401–404, 1972.

147. Brown JC, Cook MA, Dryburgh JR: Motilin, a gastric motor activity-stimulating polypeptide: The complete amino acid sequence. Can J Biochem 51:533–537, 1973.

148. Poitras P, Gagnon D, St Pierre S: N-terminal portion of motilin determines its biological activity. Biochem Biophys Res Commun 183:36–40, 1992.

149. Daikh DI, Douglass JO, Adelman JP: Structure and expression of the human motilin gene. DNA 8:615–621, 1989.

150. Pearse AGE, Polak JM, Bloom SR, et al: Enterochromaffin cells of the mammalian small intestine as the source of motilin. Virchows Arch 16:111–120, 1974.

151. Christofides ND, Bloom SR, Besterman HS, et al: Release of motilin by oral and intravenous nutrients in man. Gut 20:102–106, 1979.

152. Christofides ND, Sarson DL, Albuquerque RH, et al: Release of gastrointestinal hormones following an oral water load. Experientia 35:1521–1523, 1979.

153. Mitznegg P, Bloom SR, Domschke W, et al: Release of motilin after duodenal acidification. Lancet 1:888–889, 1976.

154. Hall KE, Greenburg GR, El-Sharkawy TY, Diamant NE: Relationship between porcine motilin-induced migrating motor complex activity, vagal integrity, and endogenous motilin release in dogs. Gastroenterology 87:76–85, 1984.

155. Adrian TE, Greenburg GR, Barnes AJ, et al: Effects of pancreatic polypeptide on motilin and circulating metabolites in man. Eur J Clin Invest 10:235–240, 1980.

156. Mori K, Seino Y, Itoh Z, et al: Motilin release by intravenous infusion of nutrients and somatostatin in conscious dogs. Regul Pept 1:265–270, 1981.

157. Poitras P, Tasse D, Laprise P: Stimulation of motilin release by bombesin in dogs. Am J Physiol 245:G249–G256, 1983.

158. Lee KY, Chang TM, Chey WY: Effect of rabbit antimotilin serum on myoelectric activity and plasma motilin concentration in the fasting dog. Am J Physiol 245:G547–G553, 1983.

159. Itoh Z, Mizumoto A, Iwanaga Y, et al: Involvement of 5-hydroxytryptamine$_3$ receptors in regulation of interdigestive gastric contractions by motilin in the dog. Gastroenterology 100:901–908, 1991.

160. Marzio L, Neri M, Pieramico O, et al: Dopamine interrupts gastrointestinal fed motility pattern in humans. Effect on motilin and somatostatin blood levels. Dig Dis Sci 35:327–332, 1990.

161. Fox Threlkeld JE, Manaka H, Manaka Y, et al: Mechanism of noncholinergic excitation of canine ileal circular muscle by motilin. Peptides 12:1047–1050, 1991.

162. Ebert R, Bornmann V, Bertsch A, Creutzfeldt W: Plasma motilin regulates insulin secretion in man. Diabetologia 34 (Suppl 2):A14 (abstract 55), 1991.

163. Catnach SM, Fairclough PD: Erythromycin and the gut. Gut 33:397–401, 1992.

164. Brazeau P, Vale W, Burgus R, et al: Hypothalamic polypeptide that inhibits the secretion of immunoreactive pituitary growth hormone. Science 179:77–79, 1973.

165. Pradayrol L, Jornvall H, Mutt V, Ribet A: N-terminally extended somatostatin: The primary structure of somatostatin 28. FEBS Lett 109:55–58, 1980.

166. Andrews PC, Dixon JE: Biosynthesis and processing of the somatostatin family of hormones. Scand J Gastroenterol 21 (Suppl 119):22–28, 1986.

167. Veber D, Freidinger R, Schwenk D, et al: A potent cyclic hexapeptide of somatostatin. Nature 292:55–58, 1981.

168. Wynick D, Bloom SR: Clinical review 23: The use of the long-acting somatostatin analogue octreotide in the treatment of gut endocrine tumours. J Clin Endocrinol Metab 73:1–3, 1991.

169. Brown NJ: Octreotide: A long-acting somatostatin analogue. Am J Med Sci 300:267–273, 1990.

170. Penman E, Wass JA, Butler MG, et al: Distribution and characterization of immunoreactive somatostatin in human gastrointestinal tract. Regul Pept 7:53–65, 1983.

171. Larsson LI, Goltermann N, DeMagistis L, et al: Somatostatin cell processes as pathways for paracrine secretion. Science 205:1393–1394, 1979.

172. Patel YC, Wheatley T, Ning C: Multiple forms of immunoreactive somatostatin: Comparison of distribution in neural and non-neural tissues and portal plasma of the rat. Endocrinology 109:1943–1949, 1981.

173. Ensinck JW, Vogel RE, Laschansky EC, Francis BH: Effect of ingested carbohydrate, fat and protein on the release of somatostatin-28 in humans. Gastroenterology 98:633–638, 1990.

174. Schusdziarra V, Schmid R: Physiological and pathophysiological aspects of somatostatin. Scand J Gastroenterol 21 (Suppl 119):29–41, 1986.

175. Schusdziarra V, Rewes B, Lenz L, et al: Evidence for a role of endogenous opiates in postprandial somatostatin release. Regul Pept 6:355–361, 1983.

176. Park J, Chiba T, Yokotani K, et al: Somatostatin receptors on canine fundic D-cells: Evidence for autocrine regulation of gastric somatostatin. Am J Physiol 257 (2 pt 1):G235–G241, 1989.

177. Bloom SR, Mortimer CH, Thorner MD, et al: Inhibition of gastrin and gastric acid secretion by growth hormone release inhibiting hormone. Lancet 2:1106–1109, 1974.

178. Schubert ML, Edwards NF, Makhlouf GM: Regulation of gastric somatostatin secretion in the mouse by luminal acidity: A local feedback mechanism. Gastroenterology 94:317–322, 1988.

179. Short GM, Doyle JW, Wolfe MM: Effect of antibodies to somatostatin on acid secretion and gastrin release by the isolated perfused rat stomach. Gastroenterology 88:984–988, 1985.

180. Hildebrand P, Ensinck JW, Gyr K, et al: Evidence for hormonal inhibition of exocrine pancreatic function by somatostatin 28 in humans. Gastroenterology 103:240–247, 1992.

181. Delvalle J, Park J, Chiba T, Yamada T: Cellular mechanisms of somatostatin action in the gut. Metabolism 39 (9 Suppl 2):134–137, 1990.

182. Yamada Y, Post SR, Wang K, et al: Cloning and functional characterisation of a family of human and mouse somatostatin receptors expressed in brain, gastrointestinal tract, and kidney. Proc Natl Acad Sci USA 89:251–255, 1992.

183. Kislauskis E, Bullock B, McNeil S, Dobner PR: The rat gene encoding neurotensin and neuromedin N: Structure, tissue specific expression and evolution of exon sequences. J Biol Chem 263:4963–4968, 1988.

184. Polak JM, Sullivan SN, Bloom SR, et al: Specific localisation of neurotensin to the N cell in human intestine by radioimmunoassay and immunocytochemistry. Nature 270:183–184, 1977.

185. Rosell S, Rokaeus A: The effect of ingestion of amino acids, glucose and fat on circulating neurotensin-like immunoreactivity (NTLI) in man. Acta Physiol Scand 107:263, 1979.

186. Lezoche E, Ghatei MA, Carlei F, et al: Gut hormone responses to bombesin in man. Gastroenterology 76:1185, 1979.

187. Carraway R, Leeman SE: The isolation of a new vasoactive peptide, neurotensin, from bovine hypothalami. J Biol Chem 248:6854–6861, 1973.

188. Blackburn AM, Fletcher DR, Bloom SR: Effect of neurotensin on gastric function in man. Lancet 1:987–989, 1980.

189. Fletcher DR, Blackburn AM, Adrian TE, et al: Effect of neurotensin on pancreatic function in man. Life Sci 29:2157–2161, 1981.

190. Iwatsuki K, Horiuchi A, Ren LM, Chiba S: Direct and indirect stimulation of pancreatic exocrine secretion by neurotensin in anaesthetized dogs. Clin Exp Pharmacol Physiol 18:475–481, 1991.

191. Evers BM, Izukura M, Chung DH, et al: Neurotensin stimulates growth of colonic mucosa in young and aged rats. Gastroenterology 103:86–91, 1992.

192. Thor K, Rosell S: Neurotensin increases colonic motility. Gastroenterology 90:27–31, 1986.

193. Tanaka K, Masu M, Nakanishi S: Structure and functional expression of the cloned rat neurotensin receptor. Neuron 4:847–854, 1990.

194. Tatemoto K: Isolation and characterisation of peptide YY (PYY), a candidate gut hormone that inhibits pancreatic exocrine secretion. Proc Natl Acad Sci USA 79:2514–2518, 1982.

195. Krasinski SD, Wheeler MB, Leiter AB: Isolation, characterisation and developmental expression of the rat peptide-YY gene. Mol Endocrinol 5:433–440, 1991.

196. Adrian TE, Ferri GL, Bacarese-Hamilton AJ, et al: Human distribution and release of a putative new gut hormone, peptide YY. Gastroenterology 89:1070–1077, 1985.

197. Aponte GW, Fink AS, Meyer JM, et al: Regional distribution and release of peptide YY with fatty acids of different chain length. Am J Physiol 249:G745–G750, 1985.

198. Greeley GH, Yeng YJ, Gomez G, et al: Evidence for regulation of peptide YY release by proximal gut. Endocrinology 124:1438–1443, 1989.

199. Greeley GH, Guo YS, Gomez G, et al: Inhibition of gastric acid secretion by peptide YY is independent of gastric somatostatin release in the rat. Proc Soc Exp Biol Med 189:325–328, 1988.

200. Wiley JW, Lu Y, Owyang C: Mechanism of action of peptide YY to inhibit gastric motility. Gastroenterology 100:865–872, 1991.

201. Playford RJ, Benito-Orfila MA, Nihoyannopoulous P, et al: Effects of peptide YY on the human cardiovascular system: Reversal of responses to vasoactive intestinal peptide. Am J Physiol 263:E740–E747, 1992.

202. Adrian TE, Bloom SR, Bryant MG, et al: Distribution and release of pancreatic polypeptide. Gut 17:940–944, 1976.

203. Floyd JC, Fajans SS, Pek S: Regulation in healthy subjects of the secretion of human pancreatic polypeptide, a newly recognised pancreatic islet polypeptide. Trans Assoc Am Physicians 89:146–158, 1976.

204. Wilson RM, Boden G, Owen OE: Pancreatic polypeptide responses to a meal and to intraduodenal amino acids and sodium oleate. Endocrinology 102:859, 1978.

205. Singer MV, Solomon TE, Wood J, Grossman MI: Latency of pancreatic enzyme response to duodenal stimulants. Am J Physiol 238:G23–G29, 1980.

206. Lezoche E, Carlei F, Vagni V, et al: Inhibition of food-stimulated pancreatic-polypeptide (PP) by bombesin in man. Gastroenterology 76:1185, 1979.

207. Marco J, Hedo JA, Villanueva ML: Inhibitory effect of somatostatin on human pancreatic polypeptide secretion. Life Sci 21:1729, 1977.

208. Bloom SR, Edwards AV, Hardy RN: The role of the autonomic nervous system in the control of glucagon, insulin and pancreatic polypeptide release from the pancreas. J Physiol 280:9–23, 1978.

209. Greenburg GR, McCloy RF, Adrian TE, et al: Inhibition of pancreatic and gall bladder functions by pancreatic polypeptide in man. Lancet 1:14–17, 1979.

210. Adrian TE, Bloom SR, Bryant MG, et al: Distribution and release of human pancreatic polypeptide. Gut 17:755–758, 1976.

211. Fischer-Colbrie H, Hagun C, Schober M: Chromogranins A, B, C: Widespread constituents of secretory vesicles. Ann NY Acad Sci 493:120–134, 1987.

212. Lloyd D, Cano M, Rosa P, et al: Distribution of chromogranin A and secretogranin I (chromogranin B) in neuroendocrine cells and tumours. Am J Pathol 130:296–304, 1988.

213. Eiden LE, Huttner WB, Mallet J, et al: A nomenclature proposal for the chromogranin/secretogranin proteins. Neuroscience 21:1019–1021, 1987.

214. Huttner WB, Gerdes HH, Rosa P: The granin (chromogranin/secretogranin) family. TIBS 16:27–30, 1991.

215. Tatemoto K, Efendie S, Mutt V, et al: Pancreastatin—A novel pancreatic peptide that inhibits insulin secretion. Nature 324:476–478, 1986.

216. Galindo E, Rill A, Bade MF, et al: Chromostatin, a 20-amino acid peptide derived from chromogranin A, inhibits chromaffin cell secretion. Proc Natl Acad Sci USA 88:1426–1430, 1991.

217. Benjannet S, Leduc R, Adrouche N, et al: Chromogranin B (secretogranin 1), a putative precursor of two novel pituitary peptides through processing at paired basic residues. FEBS Lett 224:142–148, 1987.

218. Salahuddin MJ, Sekiya K, Ghatei MA, et al: Regional distribution of chromogranin B 420–493-like immunoreactivity in the pituitary gland and central nervous system of man, guinea pig and rat. Neuroscience 30:231–240, 1989.

219. Schmidt WE, Creutzfeld W: Pancreastatin—A novel regulatory peptide? Acta Oncol 3:441–449, 1991.

220. Reiffen FU, Graztl M: Chromogranins widespread in endocrine and nervous tissue, bind Ca + +. FEBS Lett 195:327–330, 1986.

221. Deftos LJ: Chromogranin A: Its role in endocrine function and as an endocrine and neuroendocrine marker. Endocr Rev 12:181–186, 1991.
222. Sekiya K, Ghatei MA, Salahuddin MJ, et al: Production of GAWK (chromogranin B 420–493)-like immunoreactivity by endocrine tumours and its possible diagnostic value. J Clin Invest 83:1834–1842, 1988.
223. Weidemann B, Huttner WB: Synaptophysin and chromogranins/secretogranins—widespread constituents of distinct types of neuroendocrine vesicles and new tools in tumour diagnosis. Virchows Arch 58:95–121, 1989.
224. Said SI, Mutt V: Peptide with broad biological activity: Isolation from small intestine. Science 169:1217–1218, 1970.
225. Mutt V, Said SI: Structure of the porcine vasoactive intestinal octacosopeptide. The amino acid sequence. Use of kallikrein in its determination. Eur J Biochem 42:581–589, 1974.
226. Tatemoto K, Mutt V: Isolation and characterization of the intestinal peptide porcine PHI (PHI-27), a new member of the glucagon-secretin family. Proc Natl Acad Sci USA 78:6603–6607, 1981.
227. Itoh N, Obata K, Yanaihara N, Okamoto H: Human prepor-vasoactive intestinal polypeptide contains a novel PHI-27 peptide, PHM-27. Nature 304:547–549, 1983.
228. Miyata A, Arimura A, Dahl RR, et al: Isolation of a novel 38 residue-hypothalamic polypeptide which stimulates adenylate cyclase in pituitary cells. Biochem Biophys Res Commun 164:567–574, 1989.
229. Miyata A, Jiang RR, Dhal RR, et al: Isolation of a neuropeptide corresponding to the N-terminal 27 residues of the pituitary adenylate cyclase activating polypeptide with 38-residues (PACAP-38). Biochem Biophys Res Commun 170:643–648, 1990.
230. Koves K, Arimura A: Immunohistochemical demonstration of pituitary adenylate cyclase activating peptide in ovine gut. Clin Res 38:969A, 1990.
231. Burhol PC, Waldum HL, Jorde R, et al: The effect of a test meal on plasma vasoactive intestinal polypeptide (VIP), gastric inhibitory polypeptide (GIP) and secretin in man. Scand J Gastroenterol 14:939–943, 1979.
232. Schaffalitzky de Muckadell OB, Fahrenkrug J, Holst JJ, Lauritsen KB: Release of vasoactive intestinal polypeptide (VIP) by intraduodenal stimuli. Scand J Gastroenterol 12:793–799, 1977.
233. Long RG, Bishop AE, Barnes AJ, et al: Neural and hormonal peptides in rectal biopsy specimens from patients with Chagas' disease and chronic autonomic failure. Lancet 1:559–562, 1980.
234. Domschke W, Lux G, Domschke S, et al: Effects of vasoactive intestinal peptide on resting and pentagastrin stimulated lower oesophageal sphincter pressure. Gastroenterology 75:9–12, 1978.
235. Bennett A, Bloom SR, Ch'ng J, et al: Is vasoactive intestinal peptide an inhibitory transmitter in the circular but not the longitudinal muscle of guinea pig colon? J Pharm Pharmacol 36:787, 1984.
236. Krejs GJ, Fordtran JS, Bloom SR: Effect of VIP infusion on water and ion transport in the human jejunum. Gastroenterology 78:722–727, 1980.
237. Algazi M, Chen HS, Koss MA, et al: Effect of VIP antagonist on VIP-, PGE2- and acid stimulated bicarbonate secretion. Am J Physiol 256:G833–G836, 1989.
238. Schubert MI: The effect of vasoactive intestinal peptide on gastric acid secretion is predominantly mediated by somatostatin. Gastroenterology 100:1195–1200, 1991.
239. Holst JJ, Fahrenkrug J, Knuhtsen S, et al: VIP and PHI in the pig pancreas: Co-existence, co-release, and co-operative effects. Am J Physiol 252 (2 pt 1):G182–G189, 1987.
240. Mungan Z, Ozmen V, Ertan A, Arimura A: Pituitary adenylate cyclase activating polypeptide-27 (PACAP-27) inhibits pentagastrin-stimulated gastric acid secretion in conscious rats. Regul Pept 38:199–206, 1992.
241. Mungan Z, Ertan A, Hammer RA, Arimura A: Effect of pituitary adenylate cyclase activating polypeptide on rat pancreatic exocrine secretion. Peptides 12:559–562, 1991.
242. Suda K, Smith DM, Ghatei MA, Bloom SR: Investigation of the interaction of VIP binding sites with VIP and PACAP in human brain. Neurosci Lett 137:19–23, 1992.
243. Ishihara T, Shigemoto R, Mori K, et al: Functional expression and tissue distribution of a novel receptor for vasoactive intestinal polypeptide. Neuron 8:811–819, 1992.
244. Tache Y, Melchiorri P, Negri L: Bombesin-like peptides in health and disease. Ann NY Acad Sci 547:183–193, 1988.
245. Anastasi A, Erspamer V, Bucci H: Isolation and structure of bombesin and alytesin, two analogous active peptides from the strain of European amphibians bombina and alytes. Experientia 27:166–167, 1971.
246. Bertacinni G, Erspamer V, Melchiorri P, Sopranzi N: Gastrin release by bombesin in the dog. Br J Pharmacol 52:219–225, 1974.
247. McDonald TJ, Jornvall H, Nilsson G, et al: Classification of gastrin releasing peptide from porcine non-antral tissue. Biochem Biophys Res Commun 90:227–233, 1979.
248. Naylor SL, Sakaguchi AY, Spindel ER, Chin WW: Human gastrin releasing peptide gene is located on chromosome 18. Somatic Cell Mol Genet 13:87–91, 1987.
249. Sausville E, Lehacq-Verhey AM, Spindel ER, et al: Expression of the gastrin-releasing peptide gene in human small cell lung cancer. J Biol Chem 261:2451–2457, 1986.
250. Spindel ER, Zilberberg MD, Chin WW: Analysis of the gene and multiple mRNAs encoding human gastrin releasing peptide (GRP): Alternate RNA splicing occurs in neural and endocrine tissue. Mol Endocrinol 1:224–232, 1987.
251. McDonald TJ, Ghatei MA, Bloom SR, et al: Dose-response comparisons of canine plasma gastropancreatic hormone response to bombesin and the porcine gastrin-releasing peptide (GRP). Regul Pept 5:127–137, 1983.
252. Zachary I, Gil J, Lehmann W, et al: Bombesin, vasopressin and endothelin rapidly stimulate tyrosine phosphorylation in intact Swiss 3T3 cells. Proc Natl Acad Sci USA 88:4577–4581, 1991.
253. Ghatei MA, Sheppard MN, Henzen-Logman S, et al: Bombesin and vasoactive intestinal polypeptide in the developing lung: Marked changes in acute respiratory distress syndrome. J Clin Endocrinol 57:1226–1232, 1983.
254. Bhatnagar M, Springall DR, Ghatei MA, et al: Localisation of mRNA and co-expression and molecular forms of GRP gene products in endocrine cells of human foetal lung. Histochemistry 90:299–307, 1988.
255. Ghatei MA, Springall DR, Nicholl CG, et al: Gastrin-releasing peptide-like immunoreactivity in medullary thyroid carcinoma. Am J Clin Pathol 84:581–586, 1985.
256. Al-Saffar N, White A, Moore M, Hasleton PS: Immunoreactivity of various peptides in typical and atypical bronchopulmonary carcinoid tumours. Br J Cancer 58:762–766, 1988.
257. Minamino N, Kangawa K, Matsuo H: Neuromedin B: A novel bombesin-like peptide identified in porcine spinal cord. Biochem Biophys Res Commun 114:514–548, 1983.
258. Minamino N, Sudoh T, Kangawa K, Matsuo H: Neuromedin B-32 and B-30: Two "big" neuromedin Bs identified in porcine brain and spinal cord. Biochem Biophys Res Commun 130:685–691, 1985.
259. Wada E, Way J, Lebacq-Verhaden AM, Batley JF: Neuromedin B and gastrin-releasing peptide mRNAs differentially distributed in the rat nervous system. Neurosci 19:2917–2930, 1990.
260. Krane IM, Naylor SL, Helin-Davis D, et al: Molecular cloning of cDNAs encoding the human bombesin-like peptide neuromedin B. J Biol Chem 263:13317–13323, 1988.
261. Hearn SC, Jones PM, Ghatei MA, et al: The presence, characterization and synthesis of neuromedin B in the human pituitary gland. Neuroendocrinology 56:729–734, 1992.
262. Giaccone G, Batley J, Gazdar AF, et al: Neuromedin B is present in lung cancer cell lines. Cancer Res 52:2732S–2736S, 1992.
263. Namba M, Ghatei MA, Anand P, Bloom SR: Distribution and chromatographic characterisation of neuromedin B-like IR in human spinal cord. Brain Res 342:183–186, 1985.
264. Namba M, Ghatei MA, Gibson SJ, et al: Distribution and localisation of neuromedin B-like immunoreactivity in pig, cat and rat spinal cord. Neuroscience 15:1217–1226, 1985.
265. Namba M, Ghatei MA, Bishop AE, et al: Presence of neuromedin B-like immunoreactivity in the brain and gut of rat and guinea-pig. Peptides 6 (Suppl):257–263, 1985.
266. Minamino N, Kangawa K, Matsuo H: Neuromedin B is a major bombesin-like peptide in rat brain: Regional distribution of neuromedin B and C in rat brain, pituitary and spinal cord. Biochem Biophys Res Commun 124:925–932, 1984.
267. Namba M, Ghatei MA, Adrian TE, et al: Effect of neuromedin B on gut hormone secretion in the rat. Biomed Res 5:229–234, 1984.
268. Otsuki M, Fujii M, Nakamura T, et al: Effects of neuromedin B and neuromedin C on exocrine and endocrine pancreas. Am J Physiol 252:G491–G498, 1987.
269. Steel JH, Van-Noorden S, Ballesta J, et al: Localisation of 7B2, neuromedin B, and neuromedin U in specific cell types of rat, mouse, and human pituitary, and in 30 human pituitary and extrapituitary tumours. Endocrinology 122:270–282, 1988.
270. Jones PM, Withers D, Ghatei MA, Bloom SR: Neuromedin B synthesis in the rat anterior pituitary and its regulation by endocrine status. Endocrinology 130:1829–1836, 1992.

271. Rettori V, Milenkovic L, Fahim A, et al: Role of neuromedin B in the control of the release of thyrotrophin in the rat. Proc Natl Acad Sci USA 86:4789–4792, 1989.
272. Wada E, Way J, Shapira H, et al: cDNA cloning, characterisation, and brain region specific expression of a neuromedin preferring bombesin receptor. Neuron 6:421–430, 1991.
273. Batley JF, Way J, Corjoy MH, et al: Molecular cloning of the bombesin/GRP receptor from Swiss 3T3 cells. Proc Natl Acad Sci USA 88:395–399, 1991.
274. Minamino N, Kangawa K, Matsuo H: Neuromedin U 8 and U 25: Novel uterus stimulating and hypertensive peptides identified in porcine spinal cord. Biochem Biophys Res Commun 130:1078–1085, 1985.
275. Conlon JM, Domin JM, Thim L, et al: Primary structure of neuromedin U from the rat. J Neurochem 51:988–991, 1988.
276. O'Harte F, Bockman CS, Abel PW, Conlon JM: Isolation, structural characterization and pharmacological activity of dog neuromedin U. Peptides 12:11–15, 1991.
277. Domin J, Yiangou YG, Spokes RA, et al: The distribution, purification, and pharmacological action of an amphibian neuromedin U. J Biol Chem 264:20881–20885, 1989.
278. Murphy R, Turner CA, Furness JB, et al: Isolation and microsequence analysis of a novel form of neuromedin U from guinea pig small intestine. Peptides 11:613–617, 1990.
279. O'Harte F, Bockman CS, Zeng W, et al: Primary structure of a nonapeptide related to neuromedin U isolated from chicken intestine. Peptides 12:809–812, 1991.
280. Lo G, Legon S, Austin C, et al: Characterisation of complementary DNA encoding the rat neuromedin U precursor. J Mol Endocrinol 6:1538–1544, 1993.
281. Domin J, Ghatei MA, Chohan P, Bloom SR: Neuromedin U—a study of its distribution in the rat. Peptides 8:779–784, 1987.
282. Ballesta J, Carlei F, Bishop AE, et al: Occurrence and developmental pattern of neuromedin U-immunoreactive nerves in the gastrointestinal tract and brain of the rat. Neuroscience 25:797–816, 1988.
283. Gardiner SM, Compton AM, Bennett T, et al: Regional hemodynamic effects of neuromedin U in conscious rats. Am J Physiol 258:R32–R38, 1990.
284. Brown DR, Quito FL: Neuromedin U octapeptide alters ion transport in porcine jejunum. Eur J Pharmacol 155:159–162, 1988.
285. Rosenfeld MG, Mermond JJ, Amara SG, et al: Production of a novel neuropeptide encoded by the calcitonin gene via tissue specific RNA processing. Nature 304:129–135, 1983.
286. Tache Y, Holzer P, Rosenfeld MG: Calcitonin gene related peptide: First decade of a novel pleiotropic neuropeptide. Ann NY Acad Sci 657:1992.
287. Goodman EC, Iversen LL: Calcitonin gene-related peptide: Novel neuropeptide. Life Sci 38:2169–2178, 1986.
288. Zaidi M, Breimer H, MacIntyre I: Biology of peptides from the calcitonin genes. Q J Exp Physiol 72:371–408, 1987.
289. Amara SG, Arriza JA, Leff SE, et al: Expression in brain of a messenger RNA encoding a novel neuropeptide homologous to calcitonin gene-related peptide. Science 229:1094–1097, 1985.
290. Mulderry PK, Ghatei MA, Spokes RA, et al: Differential expression of α-CGRP and β-CGRP by primary sensory neurons and enteric autonomic neurons of the rat. Neuroscience 25:195–205, 1988.
291. Jamal H, Jones PM, Byrne J, et al: Peptide content of neuropeptide Y, vasoactive intestinal polypeptide, and β-calcitonin gene-related peptide and their messenger ribonucleic acids after dexamethasone treatment in the isolated rat islets of Langerhans. Endocrinology 129:3372–3380, 1991.
292. Olson GA, Olson RD, Kastin AJ: Endogenous opiates: 1988. Peptides 10:1253–1280, 1989.
293. Burks TF, Fox TA, Hirning LD, et al: Regulation of gastrointestinal function by multiple opioid receptors. Life Sci 43:2177–2181, 1988.
294. Gyires K: Morphine inhibits the ethanol-induced gastric damage in rats. Arch Int Pharmacodyn Ther 306:170–181, 1990.
295. Helke CJ, Krause JE, Mantyh PW, et al: Diversity in mammalian tachykinin peptidergic neurons: Multiple peptides, receptors and regulatory mechanisms. FASEB J 4:1606–1615, 1990.
296. Maggio JE: Tachykinins. Annu Rev Neurosci 11:13–88, 1988.
297. Arunin, Difiglia M, Leeman SE: Substance P. In Krieger DT, Brownstein MJ, Martin JB (eds): Brain Peptides. New York, Wiley, 1983, p 783.
298. Nawa H, Kotani H, Nakanishi: Tissue specific generation of two preprotachykinin mRNAs from one gene by alternative RNA splicing. Nature 312:729–734, 1984.
299. Krause JE, Chirgwin JM, Carter MS, et al: Three rat preprotachykinin

300. Tatemoto K, Lunberg JM, Jornvall H, et al: Neuropeptide K: Isolation, structure and biological activities of a novel brain tachykinin. Biochem Biophys Res Commun 128:947–953, 1985.
301. Weihe E, Nohre D, Muller S, et al: The tachykinin neuroimmune connection in inflammatory pain. Ann NY Acad Sci 632:283–295, 1991.
302. Sternini C: Tachykinin and calcitonin gene–related peptide in the mammalian enteric nervous system and sensory ganglia. Adv Exp Med Biol 298:39–51, 1991.
303. Nakanishi S: Mammalian tachykinin receptors. Annu Rev Neurosci 14:123–136, 1991.
304. Frossard N, Advenier C: Tachykinin receptors and the assays. Life Sci 49:1941–1953, 1991.
305. Ohkubo H, Nakanishi S: Molecular characterization of three tachykinin receptors. Ann NY Acad Sci 632:53–62, 1992.
306. Tatemoto K, Carlquist M, Mutt V: Neuropeptide Y—A novel brain peptide with structural similarities to peptide YY and pancreatic polypeptide. Nature 296:659–660, 1982.
307. Adrian TE, Allen JM, Bloom SR, et al: Neuropeptide Y distribution in human brain. Nature 308:584–586, 1983.
308. Pettersson M, Ahren B, Lundquist I, et al: Neuropeptide Y: Intrapancreatic neuronal localisation and effects on insulin secretion in the mouse. Cell Tissue Res 248:43–48, 1987.
309. Ekblad E, Winther C, Ekman R, et al: Projection of neuropeptide containing peptides in rat small intestine. Neuroscience 20:169–188, 1987.
310. Carlei F, Allen JM, Bishop AE, et al: Occurrence, distribution and nature of neuropeptide Y in the rat pancreas. Experientia 41:1554–1557, 1985.
311. Sheikh SP, Holst JJ, Shak-Nielsen T, et al: Release of NPY in pig pancreas: Dual sympathetic and parasympathetic regulation. Am J Physiol 255:G46–G54, 1988.
312. Balasubramaniam A, McFadden D, Rudnicki M, et al: Radioimmunoassay to determine postprandial changes in plasma neuropeptide Y levels in awake dogs. Neuropeptides 14:209–212, 1989.
313. Cox HM, Cuthbert AW, Hakanson R, Wahlestedt C: The effect of neuropeptide Y and peptide YY on electrogenic ion transport in rat intestinal epithelia. J Physiol 398:65–80, 1988.
314. Skoglund G, Gross RA, Bertrand GR, et al: Comparison of effects of neuropeptide Y and nor-epinephrine on insulin secretion and vascular resistance in perfused rat pancreas. Diabetes 40:660–665, 1991.
315. Dumont Y, Martel JC, Fournier A, et al: Neuropeptide Y and neuropeptide Y receptor subtypes in brain and peripheral tissues. Prog Neurobiol 38:125–167, 1992.
316. Eva C, Kienanen K, Monyer H, et al: Molecular cloning of a novel G protein-coupled receptor that may belong to the neuropeptide receptor family. FEBS Lett 271:81–84, 1990.
317. Tatemoto K, Rokaeus A, Jornvall A, et al: Galanin—A novel biologically active peptide from porcine intestine. FEBS Lett 164:124–128, 1983.
318. Rokaeus A: Galanin: A newly isolated biologically active neuropeptide. TINS 10:158–164, 1987.
319. Miralles P, Peiero E, Degano P, et al: Inhibition of insulin and somatostatin secretion and stimulation of glucagon secretion by homologous galanin in perfused rat pancreas. Diabetes 39:996–1001, 1990.
320. McKnight GL, Karlsen AE, Kowalyk S, et al: Sequence of human galanin and its inhibition of glucose stimulated insulin secretion from RIN cells. Diabetes 41:82–87, 1992.
321. Bishop AE, Polak JM, Bauer FE, et al: Occurrence and distribution of a newly discovered peptide, galanin, in the mammalian enteric nervous system. Gut 27:849–857, 1986.
322. Ch'ng JLC, Christofides ND, Anand P, et al: Distribution of galanin immunoreactivity in the central nervous system and the response of galanin-containing neural pathways to injury. Neuroscience 16:343–354, 1985.
323. Shimosegawa S, Moriizumi S, Koizumi M, et al: Immunohistochemical demonstration of galaninlike immunoreactive nerves in human pancreas. Gastroenterology 102:263–271, 1992.
324. Dunning BE, Havel PJ, Veith RC, Taborsky GJ: Pancreatic and extrapancreatic galanin release during sympathetic neural activation. Am J Physiol 258:E436–E444, 1990.
325. Kowalyk S, Veith R, Boyle M, Taborsky GJ: Liver releases galanin during sympathetic activation. Am J Physiol 262:E671–E678, 1992.
326. Bauer FE, Zintel A, Kenny MJ, et al: Inhibitory effect of galanin on postprandial gastrointestinal motility and gut hormone release in humans. Gastroenterology 97:260–264, 1989.

mRNAs encode the neuropeptides substance P and neurokinins A. Proc Natl Acad Sci USA 84:881–885, 1987.

327. Ekblad E, Hakanson R, Sundler F, Wahlestedt C: Galanin: Neuro-modulatory and direct contractile effects on smooth muscle preparations. Br J Pharmacol 86:241–246, 1985.
328. Dunning BE, Ahren B, Veith RC, et al: Galanin: A novel pancreatic neuropeptide. Am J Physiol 251:E127–E133, 1986.
329. Yagci RV, Alpetkin N, Rossowski WJ, et al: Inhibitory effect of galanin on basal and pentagastrin-stimulated gastric acid secretion in rats. Scand J Gastroenterol 25:853–858, 1990.
330. Bartfai T, Bedecs K, Land T, et al: High-affinity chimeric peptide that blocks the neuronal actions of galanin in the hippocampus, locus coeruleus, and spinal cord. Proc Natl Acad Sci USA 88:10961–10965, 1992.
331. Weile de J, Schmith-Antomarchi H, Fosset M, Lazdunski M: ATP-sensitive K⁺ channels that are blocked by hypoglycaemia-inducing sulphonylureas in insulin-secreting cells are activated by galanin, a hyperglycaemia-inducing hormone. Proc Natl Acad Sci USA 85:1312–1316, 1988.
332. Yanagisawa M, Kirihara H, Kimura S, et al: A novel potent vasoconstrictor peptide produced by vascular endothelial cells. Nature 332:411–415, 1988.
333. Giaid A, Gibson SJ, Ibrahim NBN, et al: Endothelin-1, an endothelium derived peptide, is expressed in neurons of the human spinal cord and dorsal root ganglia. Proc Natl Acad Sci USA 86:7634–7638, 1989.
334. Takahashi K, Ghatei MA, Jones PM, et al: Endothelin in human brain and pituitary gland: Presence of immunoreactive endothelin, endothelin messenger ribonucleic acid and endothelin receptors. J Clin Endocrinol Metab 72:693–699, 1991.
335. Black PN, Ghatei MA, Takahashi K, et al: Formation of endothelin by cultured airway epithelial cells. FEBS Lett 255:129–132, 1989.
336. Hirata Y, Yoshima H, Takata S, et al: Cellular mechanisms of action by a novel vasoconstrictor peptide in cultured rat vascular smooth muscle cells. Biochem Biophys Res Commun 154:868–875, 1988.
337. Koseki C, Imai M, Hirata Y, et al: Autoradiographic distribution in rat tissues of binding sites for endothelin: A neuropeptide? Am J Physiol 256:R858–R866, 1989.
338. Kanse SM, Ghatei MA, Bloom SR: Endothelin binding sites in porcine aortic and rat lung membrane. Eur J Biochem 182:175–179, 1989.
339. Yanagisawa M, Inoue A, Ishikawa T, et al: Primary structure, synthesis and biological activity of rat endothelin and endothelium derived vasoconstrictor peptide. Proc Natl Acad Sci USA 85:6864–6867, 1988.
340. Inoue A, Yanagisawa M, Kimura S, et al: The human endothelin family: Three structurally and pharmacologically distinct isopeptides predicted by three separate genes. Proc Natl Acad Sci USA 86:2863–2867, 1989.
341. Saidi K, Mitsui Y, Ishida N: A novel peptide, vasoactive intestinal contractor, of a new (endothelin) peptide family. Molecular cloning, expression and biological activity. J Biol Chem 264:14613–14616, 1989.
342. Takasaki K, Tamiya N, Bdolah A, et al: Sarafotoxins S6: Several isotoxins from Atractapsis engaddensis (borrowing asp) venom that attack the heart. Toxicol 26:543–548, 1988.
343. Lee CY, Chiapinelli VA, Takahashi C, et al: Similarity of endothelin to snake venom toxin. Nature 355:303, 1988.
344. Takahashi K, Jones PM, Kanse SM, et al: Endothelin in the gastrointestinal tract: Presence of endothelin-like immunoreactivity, endothelin-1 messenger RNA, endothelin receptors and pharmacological effect. Gastroenterology 99:1660–1667, 1990.
345. Inagaki H, Bishop AE, Escrig C, et al: Localization of endothelin-like immunoreactivity and endothelin binding sites in human colon. Gastroenterology 101:47–54, 1991.
346. Escrig C, Bishop AE, Inagaki H, et al: Localisation of endothelin-like immunoreactivity in adult and developing human gut. Gut 33(2):212–217, 1993.
347. Ghatei MA, Kirkland SC, Perera TPS, et al: Formation of endothelin by human colorectal adenocarcinoma cell lines. Digestion 46 (Suppl 1):35, 1990.
348. Whittle BJR, Esplugues JV: Induction of rat gastric damage by the endothelium derived peptide, endothelin. Br J Pharmacol 95:1011–1013, 1988.
349. Ganguli PC, Cullen DR, Irvine WJ: Radioimmunoassay of plasma gastrin in pernicious anaemia, achlorhydria, with gut pernicious anaemia, hypochlorhydria and controls. Lancet 1(691):155–158, 1993.
350. Calam J, Goodlad RA, Lee CY, et al: Achlorhydria-induced hypergastrinaemia; the role of bacteria. Clin Sci 80:281–284, 1991.
351. McGuigan JE, Trudeau WL: Differences in rates of gastrin release in normal persons and patients with duodenal ulcer disease. N Engl J Med 288:64–66, 1973.
352. Warren JR, Marshall B: Unidentified curved bacilli on gastric epithelium in active chronic gastritis. Lancet 1:1273–1275, 1983.
353. Marshall BJ, Warren JR: Unidentified curved bacilli in the stomach of patients with gastritis and peptide ulceration. Lancet 1:1311–1315, 1984.
354. Chittajallu S, Dorrian GA, Neithercut WD, et al: Is Helicobacter pylori associated hypergastrinaemia due to the bacterium's urease activity or the antral gastritis? Gut 32:1286–1290, 1991.
355. Prewett EJ, Smith JT, Nwokolo CU, et al: Eradication of Helicobacter pylori abolishes 24-hour hypergastrinaemia: A prospective study in healthy subjects. Aliment Pharmacol Ther 5:283–290, 1991.
356. Adrian TE, Long RG, Fuessl HS, Bloom SR: Plasma peptide YY (PYY) in dumping syndrome. Dig Dis Sci 30:1145–1148, 1985.
357. Mackie CR, Jenkins SA, Hartley MN: Treatment of severe postvagotomy/postgastrectomy syndromes with the somatostatin analogue octreotide. Br J Surg 78:1338–1343, 1991.
358. Besterman HS, Adrian TE, Mallinson CN, et al: Gut hormone release after intestinal resection. Gut 23:854–861, 1982.
359. Sarson DL, Scopinaro N, Bloom SR: Effect of partial ileal bypass on the gut hormone responses to food in man. Digestion 28:191–196, 1983.
360. Besterman HS, Bloom SR, Sarson DL, et al: Gut-hormone profile in coeliac disease. Lancet 1:785–788, 1978.
361. Maton PN, Selden AC, Fitzpatrick ML, Chadwick VS: Defective gallbladder emptying and cholecystokinin release in celiac disease: Reversal with a gluten free diet. Gastroenterology 88:391–396, 1985.
362. Besterman HS, Cook GC, Sarson DL, et al: Gut hormones in tropical malabsorbtion. Br Med J 1:1252–1255, 1979.
363. Adrian TE, Savage AP, Bacarese-Hamilton AJ, et al: Peptide YY abnormalities in gastrointestinal diseases. Gastroenterology 90:379–384, 1986.
364. Besterman HS, Adrian TE, Bloom SR, et al: Pancreatic and gastrointestinal hormones in chronic pancreatitis. Digestion 24:195–208, 1982.
365. Taguchi T, Tanaka K, Ikeda K, et al: Peptidergic innervation irregularities in Hirschsprung's disease. Virchows Arch 401:223–235, 1983.
366. Sharkey KA, Sutherland LR, Davison JS, et al: Peptides in the gastrointestinal tract in human immunodeficiency virus infection. Gastroenterology 103:18–28, 1992.
367. Besterman HS, Christofides ND, Welsby PD, et al: Gut hormones in acute diarrhoea. Gut 24:665–671, 1983.
368. Bishop AG, Polak JM, Bryant MG, et al: Abnormalities of vasoactive polypeptide containing nerves in Crohn's disease. Gastroenterology 79:853–860, 1980.
369. Besterman HS, Mallinson CN, Modigliani R, et al: Gut hormones in inflammatory bowel disease. Scand J Gastroenterol 18:845–852, 1983.
370. Hoosein NM, Kiener PA, Curry RC, et al: Antiproliferative effects of gastrin receptor antagonists and antibodies to gastrin on human colon carcinoma cell lines. Cancer Res 48:7179–7183, 1988.
371. Kellow JE, Phillips SF, Miller LJ, Zinsmeister AR: Dysmotility of the small intestine in irritable bowel syndrome. Gut 29:1236–1243, 1988.
372. Niederau C, Faber S, Karaus M: Cholecystokinin's role in regulation of colonic motility in health and in irritable bowel syndrome. Gastroenterology 102:1889–1898, 1992.
373. Chiang HC, O'Dorisio TM, Huang HC, et al: Multiple hormone elevations in Zollinger-Ellison syndrome. Prospective study of clinical significance and of the development of a second pancreatic endocrine tumour syndrome. Gastroenterology 99:1565–1575, 1990.
374. Thompson GB, van-Heerden JA, Grant CS, et al: Islet cell carcinoma of the pancreas: A twenty year experience. Surgery 104:1018–1023, 1988.
375. Krejs GJ: Gastrointestinal endocrine tumors. Am J Med 82(Suppl 5B):1–3, 1988.
376. Eriksson B, Oberg K, Skogseid B: Neuroendocrine pancreatic tumours. Clinical findings in a prospective study of 84 patients. Acta Oncol 28:373–377, 1989.
377. Ellison EH, Wilson SD: The Zollinger-Ellison syndrome: Reappraisal and evaluation of 260 registered cases. Ann Surg 160:512, 1964.
378. McGuigan JE: The Zollinger-Ellison syndrome. In Sleisinger MH, Fordtran JS (eds): Gastrointestinal Disease: Pathophysiology, Diagnosis and Management. Philadelphia, Saunders, 1989, pp 909–925.
379. Zollinger RM, Ellison EH: Primary peptide ulcerations of the jejunum associated with islet cell tumors of the pancreas. Ann Surg 142:709–723, 1955.
380. Mansbach CM, Wilkins RM, Dobbins WO, Taylor MP: Intestinal mucosal function and structure in the steatorrhea of Zollinger-Ellison syndrome. Arch Intern Med 212:487, 1968.

381. McGuigan JE, Wolfe MM: Secretin injection test in the diagnosis of gastrinoma. Gastroenterology 79:1324–1331, 1980.
382. Akerstrom G: Surgical treatment of carcinoids and endocrine pancreatic tumours. Acta Oncol 28:409–414, 1989.
383. Oberg K, Eriksson B: Medical treatment of neuroendocrine gut and pancreatic tumor. Acta Oncol 28:425–431, 1989.
384. Priest WM, Alexander MK: Islet cell tumour of the pancreas with peptic ulceration, diarrhoea and hypokalemia. Lancet 2:1145–1147, 1957.
385. Verner JV, Morrison AB: Islet cell tumor and a syndrome of refractory, watery diarrhoea and hypokalemia. Am J Med 25:374–380, 1955.
386. Bloom SR, Polak JM, Pearse AGE: Vasoactive intestinal polypeptide and watery diarrhoea syndrome. Lancet 2:14–16, 1973.
387. Buchanan KD, Johnston CF, O'Hare M, et al: Neuroendocrine tumors: A European view. Am J Med 81:14–27, 1986.
388. Rescorla FJ, Vane DW, Fitzgerald JF, et al: Vasoactive intestinal polypeptide secreting ganglioneuromatosis affecting the entire colon and rectum. J Pediatr Surg 23:635–637, 1988.
389. Yiangou Y, Williams SJ, Bishop AE, et al: Peptide-histidine-methionine immunoreactivity in plasma and tissue in patients with vasoactive intestinal peptide-secreting tumours and watery diarrhea syndrome. J Clin Endocrinol Metab 64:131–139, 1987.
390. Bloom SR, Polak JM: VIPomas. In Said SI (ed): Vasoactive Intestinal Peptides. New York, Raven Press, 1982, p 457.
391. Kingham JC, Dick R, Bloom SR, Frankel RJ: Vipoma: Localisation by percutaneous transhepatic portal venous sampling. Br Med J 2:1682–1683, 1978.
392. Fraker DL, Norton JA: The role of surgery in the management of islet cell tumors. Gastroenterol Clin North Am 18:805–829, 1989.
393. Abraira C, DeBartolo M, Katzen R, Lawrence AM: Disappearance of glucagonoma rash after surgical resection, but not during dietary normalization of amino acids. J Clin Nutr 39:351–355, 1984.
394. Almdal TP, Heindorff H, Bardram L, Vilstrup H: Increased amino acid clearance and urea synthesis in a patient with glucagonoma. Gut 31:946–948, 1990.
395. Mallinson DL, Bloom SR, Warin AP, et al: A glucagonoma syndrome. Lancet 2:1–3, 1974.
396. McGavran M, Unger RH, Recant L, et al: A glucagon secreting α-cell carcinoma of the pancreas. N Engl J Med 274:1408–1413, 1966.
397. Bloom SR, Polak JM: Glucagonoma syndrome. Am J Med 82:25–36, 1987.
398. Williams G, Lofts F, Fuessl H, Bloom SR: Treatment with danazol and plasma glucagon concentration. Br Med J 291:1155–1156, 1985.
399. Arnold J, O'Grady J, Bird G, et al: Liver transplantation for primary and secondary hepatic APUDomas. Br J Surg 76:248–249, 1989.
400. Santangelo WC, Unger RH, Orci L, et al: Somatostatin analogue-induced remission of necrolytic migratory erythema without changes in plasma glucagon concentration. Pancreas 1:464–469, 1986.
401. Tomita T, Friesen R, Kimmel JR, et al: Pancreatic polypeptide secreting islet cell tumors: A study of three cases. Am J Pathol 113:134–142, 1983.
402. Choksi U, Sellin RV, Hickey RC, Samaan NA: An unusual skin rash associated with a pancreatic polypeptide-producing tumor of the pancreas. Ann Intern Med 108:64–65, 1988.
403. Langstein HN, Norton JA, Chiang V, et al: The utility of circulating levels of pancreatic polypeptide as a marker for islet cell tumors. Surgery 108:1109–1115, 1990.
404. Ohtsuki Y, Sonobe H, Mizobuchi T, et al: Duodenal carcinoid (somatostatinoma) combined with von Recklinghausen's disease. A case report and review of the literature. Acta Pathol Jpn 39:141–146, 1989.
405. Krejs GJ, Orci L, Conlon JM, et al: Somatostatinoma syndrome. Biochemical, morphological and clinical features. N Engl J Med 301:285–292, 1979.
406. Harris GJ, Tio F, Cruz AB: Somatostatinoma: A case report and review of the literature. J Surg Oncol 36:8–16, 1987.
407. Jackson JA, Raju BU, Fachnie JD, et al: Malignant somatostatinoma presenting with diabetic ketoacidosis. Clin Endocrinol 26:609–621, 1987.
408. Penman E, Lowry PJ, Wass JAH, et al: Molecular forms of somatostatin in normal subjects and patients with pancreatic somatostatinoma. Clin Endocrinol 12:611, 1980.
409. Drucker J, Asa SL, Henderson J, Goltzman D: The parathyroid hormone-like peptide gene is expressed in the normal and neoplastic human pancreas. Mol Endocrinol 3:1589–1595, 1989.
410. Wynick D, Ratcliffe WA, Heath DA, et al: Treatment of a malignant pancreatic endocrine tumour secreting parathyroid hormone related protein. Br Med J 300:1314–1315, 1990.
411. Rizzoli R, Sappino AP, Bonjour JP: Parathyroid hormone related protein and hypercalcemia in pancreatic neuro-endocrine tumours. Int J Cancer 46:394–398, 1990.
412. Maton PN, Gardner JD, Jensen RT: Use of long-acting somatostatin analogue, SMS201-995 in patients with pancreatic islet cell tumours. Dig Dis Sci 34(Suppl):S28–S39, 1989.

CARDIAC NATRIURETIC PEPTIDES

Hormones of the Cardiovascular System

ERIC A. ESPINER

Body fluid volume and blood pressure regulation, crucial to maintaining organ perfusion and function, are maintained in health by the integrated actions of the autonomic nervous system (maintaining cardiac output and peripheral vascular resistance), renal modulation of sodium excretion,[1] and a complex series of interlocking neurohumoral (endocrine) responses. Traditionally the endocrine regulation of body fluid volume has focused on the renal-adrenal axis (renin-angiotensin-aldosterone system), nonosmotic release of vasopressin from the neurohypophysis, and changes in local (and possibly circulatory) levels of norepinephrine under the influence of the sympathetic nervous system. However, discoveries in the last decade have made it clear that cardiac and vascular tissues have the ability to synthesize hormones and local peptides and autocoids with important actions affecting body fluid volume and distribution. While some of these newly identified factors may act locally rather than circulate as hormones in the traditional sense, de Bold's discovery,[2] leading to the isolation and identity of a series of natriuretic peptides of cardiac origin, has uncovered an entirely novel hormonal system affecting renal, vascular, and neuroendocrine tissues concerned with sodium and blood pressure homeostasis.

This chapter is largely confined to circulating hormones synthesized by the heart (atrial natriuretic peptide [ANP], brain natriuretic peptide [BNP]), and peripheral vascular tissues (endothelins). A large number of other peptides with potent hemodynamic effects have also been identified. Many are neuropeptides whose principal function is more likely to be concerned with regulating transmission within key neural tissues (e.g., hypothalamic and medullary centers) concerned with cardiovascular function. In other instances, vasoactive peptides (e.g., neuropeptide Y, vasoactive intestinal peptide, calcitonin gene related peptide, kinins, opioid peptides) may be secreted by nerves supplying the vascular wall and affect vascular smooth muscle tone directly. Some (e.g., calcitonin gene related peptide[3] and neuropeptide Y[4]) may circulate in plasma, but their physiological role and possible hormone status are still unclear. Similarly a variety of peptides (other than cardiac natriuretic peptides) are localized within the heart muscle or associated with conducting tissue or coronary vessels. Readers are referred to recent texts[5] for more detailed discussion on the activity and possible role[6] of these factors in fluid and blood pressure regulation.

CARDIAC NATRIURETIC PEPTIDES

General Considerations and Classification of Natriuretic Peptides

The possibility that low pressure areas of the heart may be able to sense the fullness of the circulation and signal appropriately to the kidney has long intrigued the physiologist. Such a humoral link between atria and renal sodium excretion first received direct support in 1981 from de Bold's discovery that atrial muscle extracts contain peptides that when injected into rats had potent natriuretic, diuretic, and vasodepressor activities.[2, 7] In fact, 25 years earlier, Kisch[8] had noted membrane-bound granules in atrial but not ventricular myocytes of guinea pigs. This finding was confirmed in other species by Jamieson and Palade,[9] who likened the granules to those found in other endocrine tissues. De Bold's novel findings of natriuretic activity in atrial extracts spawned an enormous research effort culminating in the isolation, sequence identity, and synthesis[10] of a 28-amino acid residue peptide, α-human atrial natriuretic peptide (αhANP). Within 2 years of its discovery, sufficient pure material was available for experimental studies in vivo. These studies, together with the development of specific antisera allowing the hormone's detection in plasma, established the potential importance of ANP as a circulating hormone with diverse renal, hemodynamic, and endocrine actions affecting blood pressure and sodium homeostasis. The speed of these developments bears testimony to the efficacy of recombinant molecular biology tools in endocrine research. Perhaps for the first time, and in striking contrast to previous methods that had used laborious extraction procedures coupled with chemical assays and bioassays, endocrinologists were presented with an entirely novel and virtually "pure" hormone and asked to determine its role in cardiovascular health and disease.

Before this question could be fully settled, two distinct but clearly related peptides were isolated and identified from extracts of brain tissue. The first of these, BNP, was identified in porcine brain on the basis of muscle relaxant activity.[11] Although first identified in mammalian brain tissue, the peptide was subsequently found to be more abundant in cardiac atria than in the central nervous system.[12] In humans, brain natriuretic peptide is secreted by the heart, circulates in plasma, and has similar biological actions and potency to ANP and can therefore be classified as a true cardiac hormone. The most recently identified peptide, so-called *C-type natriuretic peptide* (CNP), was isolated from brain[13] on the basis of muscle relaxant and natriuretic activity (which were approximately 1 per cent of those of ANP). As shown in Figure 154–1, the structure and close amino acid sequence homology within the ring of the three peptides characterize a "family" of natriuretic peptides that for historical reasons[13] can be reclassified as A-type natriuretic peptide, B-type natriuretic peptide, and C-type natriuretic peptide (CNP). All contain a 17-member ring (required for biological activity) formed by a disulfide bridge between two cysteine residues. Despite this similarity, each of the three peptides is the product of a unique gene transcript, which in the case of CNP is the most highly conserved of the three (greater than 90 per cent homology among mammalian species of nucleic acids coding for the 126-amino-acid residue prohormone so far examined).[14] In human brain, the content of immunoreactive CNP is some 30-fold greater than that of ANP and 70-fold that of BNP.[15] Although all these three members of the natriuretic peptide family are synthesized within brain tissue, CNP differs in that the gene is expressed (if at all) at low levels in cardiac tissues.[15a] Further, there is controversy[15] on the presence of CNP in peripheral plasma.[15b] According to Tawaragi and colleagues[14] and Minamino and co-workers,[15] these findings suggest that unlike BNP and ANP, CNP may be a unique brain peptide without a systemic (circulating) hormonal role. Whereas this view appeared to be supported by studies of receptors unique to CNP[16] that are largely confined to tissues of neural crest origin, the detection of these same receptors within vascular and other non-neural tissues (see later) has reopened the question of CNP's systemic role. The interrelationships between neural and other tissue natriuretic peptide systems on the one hand and the circulating (hormonal) effects of ANP and BNP on the other are clearly complex and currently ill defined.

It should be noted that cardiac natriuretic peptides are chemically distinct (and unrelated functionally) from de Wardener's natriuretic factor[17] and other putative Na^+, K^+, ATPase inhibitors.[18] Similarly the term *third factor* (previously used to designate factor(s) additional to GFR and aldosterone-regulating sodium excretion) is now an anachronism in view of the multiple factors involved in the renal excretion of sodium.

Atrial Natriuretic Peptide

Structure and Synthesis

ANP 99–126*—the major bioactive and circulating form of the hormone in all mammalian species so far studied (also known as atrial natriuretic factor [ANF], atriopeptin, cardionatrin, and more recently A-type natriuretic peptide)—is cleaved during the process of secretion from the carboxy-terminus of a large parent peptide (pro-ANP, 1–126, also known as γ ANP) which is the main storage form and the chief constituent of atrial granules. The amino acid sequence of ANP has been determined in many species and is identical in all except for variation at residue 110, where isoleucine replaces methionine in the rat, mouse, and rabbit. Shortened forms of the hormone (e.g., ANP 101–126, and other C- and N-terminal–deleted forms), originally isolated from rat atrial tissue, are almost certainly extraction artefacts.[19] Homology among precursor forms has been elucidated by molecular studies identifying and characterizing the ANP gene and the encoded messenger RNA (mRNA).[20] Overall, amino-acid homology among pro-ANP forms derived from human, rat, mouse, dog, and rabbit is 74 per cent. The transcription of the ANP gene (which in humans resides on chromosome 1, band p36) yields an mRNA species encoding a 151-amino-acid precursor, prepro-ANP. Prepro-ANP contains a 25-amino acid hy-

*In this review ANP signifies hANP (99–126).

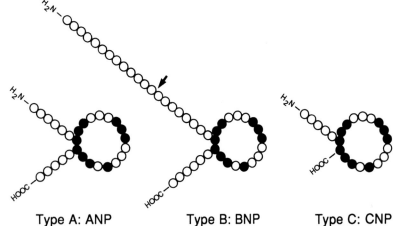

FIGURE 154–1. **Members of the natriuretic peptide family.** The structural homology between A-, B-, and C-type hormones is schematically shown. Amino acids within the 17-member ring that are identical in all natriuretic peptides are shown (*filled circles*). The *arrow* identifies the cleavage site that yields human BNP (32 amino acids). In humans and pigs, the brain also contains an amino-terminal extended form of CNP (CNP-53) in addition to CNP-22. (From Rosenzweig A, Seidman CE: Atrial natriuretic factor and related peptide hormones. Annu Rev Biochem 60:229–255, 1991. Reproduced, with permission, from the Annual Review of Biochemistry, Vol. 60, © 1991 by Annual Reviews Inc.)

Type A: ANP   Type B: BNP   Type C: CNP

drophobic leader sequence that is presumably cleaved in the rough endoplasmic reticulum prior to storage (as pro-ANP) in the atrial granule. The major site of ANP gene expression is the cardiac atrium where mRNA ANP constitutes 1 to 3 per cent of the total mRNA.[20] The normal mature ventricle, particularly the endocardium, also expresses the gene, but at a level 100-fold lower than the atrium.[21] However, with the development of left ventricular failure (and associated left ventricular strain and/or hypertrophy), ANP gene expression within the ventricle is much increased[20] so that the ventricle becomes an important source of circulating ANP (see later). This enhanced expression of the ANP gene appears to be related to activation of protein kinase C (possibly induced by the local action of α_1-adrenergic agonists, endothelin, or angiotensin II) which may be one of the mediators of both hypertrophy and ANP gene expression.[22] In contrast to the atrial cell, the ventricle does not appear to store the hormone (the ventricle contains few if any granules even in heart failure or hypertrophy), and secretion (like BNP, see later) is presumably constitutive rather than regulated as in atrial tissue. A number of factors (e.g., glucocorticoids, thyroxine, endothelin, $PGF_{2\alpha}$) can regulate ANP gene transcription, including volume-related "stretch," which is discussed further below. Outside the heart, evidence of ANP gene expression has been found in lung, aortic arch, kidney, pituitary, adrenal medulla,[20, 23] and the central nervous system, particularly specific nuclei within the hypothalamus.[21] While the mRNA abundance in all these extracardiac sites is much lower than either atrial or ventricular tissue, the ANP transcripts are identical. However, processing may be different—for instance, within the central nervous system smaller molecular weight forms (ANP 102–126 and 103–126) are synthesized.[24] Similarly, pro-ANP synthesized by renal cells[25] may be the source of urodilatin (ANP 95–126), a biologically active peptide identified in human urine[26] and which may play a paracrine role to promote natriuresis.[27] Although production of ANP transcripts by extracardiac tissues is likely to have important local actions, particularly within the central nervous system where ANP-related peptides are concentrated in neurons subserving cardiovascular regulatory function,[28] the precise role and regulation of the extracardiac peptides in organ function is unknown. Using the analogy of the tissue renin-angiotensin system, it is conceivable that local production of ANP within vascular tissue may inhibit growth of vascular smooth muscle cells and/or oppose angiotensin-induced vascular smooth muscle cell hypertrophy.[29]

Secretion and Regulation

Before or during secretion, cleavage of pro-ANP at Arg 98-Ser 99 occurs to yield the circulating peptide (ANP 99–126) and an N-terminal peptide (ANP 1–98), which are secreted in approximately equimolar amounts into coronary sinus blood. The latter fragment circulates in plasma at higher levels than ANP, presumably because of its reduced rate of metabolic clearance.[30] Its function, if any, is unknown, but evidence exists for a natriuretic and diuretic action of some of these N-terminal peptides.[30a] The enzyme(s) involved in the processing of pro-ANP to ANP have not yet been convincingly identified. Noncardiac contributions to circulating plasma ANP levels are probably insig-

nificant, although there is evidence in vivo that the lung and the hypothalamus[31] can secrete the hormone.

The most important stimulus to the secretion of ANP is increase in atrial wall tension as evidenced by the effects of acute[32] and chronic[33] volume expansion, congestive heart failure (CHF), and other conditions associated with increased intra-atrial pressure. The immediate stimulus is likely to be increased atrial transmural pressure (rather than increasing volume or intra-atrial pressure per se), since experimental and clinical studies of cardiac tamponade (a state in which atrial pressure is high but transmural pressure often unchanged) show that ANP secretion is relatively unaffected. Both atria probably contribute equally to secretion. In humans it has been calculated that for each 1-mmHg rise in atrial pressure there is an associated rise of approximately 10 to 14 pmol/L in plasma (venous) ANP concentration.[34] As expected, acute reduction of atrial pressure reduces ANP secretion.[35] Whereas ANP secretion appears to be unaffected by cardiac denervation,[36] an influence of the central nervous system on the heart's ANP response to acute volume expansion is suggested in other studies. For instance, the ANP response to volume loading is abolished in the pithed rat and can be restored by vasopressin. Sinoaortic (afferent) denervation in rats also inhibits the plasma ANP response to hypertonic saline.[37] Furthermore, lesions of specific hypothalamic areas (AV3V),[38] central injections of ANP immune serum intracerebroventricularly (icv),[39] and hypophysectomy all reduce the cardiac secretion of ANP in response to volume expansion. Conversely, centrally (icv) administered angiotensin II augments the ANP response to volume expansion via a central vasopressin-dependent pathway.[40] While some of these effects may be mediated by vagal or sympathetic pathways, the mechanism by which cardiac secretion is affected by brain (neural) events remains largely unexplained. Despite the generally strong relationship between atrial pressure (wall tension) and ANP secretion in vivo, discrepancies occur.

For example, plasma ANP levels remain elevated well beyond any increase in right atrial pressure associated with volume loading. Again, in both experimental and clinical heart failure the expected increase in ANP secretion in response to volume expansion is attenuated. Surprisingly, chronic volume expansion in normal humans reduced the expected plasma ANP response to an acute saline load administered intravenously.[41] Such discrepant findings could be due to changes in atrial wall compliance, feedback inhibition by plasma ANP, or, in the instance of heart failure, a change in signal/response coupling that accompanies myocardial fiber lengthening. "Exhaustion" of ANP from excessive and prolonged stimulation, for instance, in chronic severe heart failure, appears to be unlikely.[42]

In addition to atrial stretch, other mechanical factors, particularly heart rate, may affect ANP secretion. Supraventricular (atrial) tachyarrhythmias are important stimuli to hormone secretion, which in these circumstances may initiate a polyuric syndrome if secretion is sustained for long enough and cardiac output and renal blood flow are not compromised. Although rise in atrial pressure accompanying atrial tachycardia complicates interpretation, recent studies in both dogs and humans support a direct effect of heart rate on ANP synthesis and release independent of change in atrial pressure. In vitro studies using isolated perfused heart preparations or atrial muscle fragments have confirmed the independent roles of tension and heart rate in ANP release, although the intracellular signals transducing stretch (or rate) into hormone release have not yet been established. Such studies also indicate that several chemical stimuli—including adrenergic agonists, acetylcholine, glucocorticoids, endothelin, calcium ionophores, $PGF_{2\alpha}$, vasopressin, calcitonin gene related peptide, and angiotensin II—may directly stimulate ANP release. Some of these factors may have a paracrine role. With the possible exception of angiotensin II,[43] the relevance of these findings to pathophysiology is unclear. There is increasing evidence that the action of many ANP secretagogues is mediated by the phosphotidyl inositol system, but the precise mechanisms coupling signals to secretion (as already noted above in relationship to mechanical stimuli) remain in doubt.

Receptors and Intracellular Actions

The diverse biological effects of ANP, including natriuresis, vasorelaxation, and inhibition of renin-aldosterone, are mediated by binding of the hormone to specific membrane-associated receptors that have been identified in all of the hormone's known target tissues.[23] Initial studies using ^{125}I ANP binding to plasma membrane preparations or cultured cells identified only one high-affinity receptor (equilibrium dissociation constant, Kd, approximately 10^{-10} M). However, subsequent studies, using cross-linking or photo affinity methods to purify the labeled receptor, identified two distinct cell surface-binding proteins—one of 130,000 D coupled to guanylate cyclase (GC) and considered to mediate the biological actions of ANP, and a second smaller (65,000 D) homodimer receptor without GC activity and unassociated with any known intracellular (second messenger) system.[44] Both receptors displayed high affinity for ANP, but the smaller (non-GC containing) receptor was much less demanding in terms of specificity and bound many biologically inactive analogues of ANP. Because of its wide distribution and abundance in tissues and apparent lack of coupling to intracellular biological mediators, a "clearance" function for this receptor (so-called C receptor) has been proposed.[45] Recently the identity of at least three distinct ANP receptors has been clarified using recombinant DNA technology, which has enabled cloning, sequence, and expression of each receptor gene.[16] The structure and homology of these human

ANP receptors together with their putative physiological ligands of the natriuretic peptide family are shown in Figure 154–2. Two distinct types of GC (so-called B or R1) ANP receptors have now been identified in human tissue, each containing an extracellular ligand binding domain and an intracellular GC catalytic domain. Each molecule (which is a linear transmembrane polypeptide of 1030 amino acids) contains a cytoplasmic domain structurally homologous to protein kinase and which appears to function as a regulatory element. The first to be identified (hence, hANP receptor A, also known as GC-A receptor) is activated most efficiently (as judged by cGMP production) by ANP and to a lesser extent (10 per cent of ANP potency) by BNP. The second G-C receptor (ANP receptor B or GC-B) was originally considered to be a specific BNP receptor but has recently been identified as a specific receptor for C-type NP (CNP). Guanylate cyclase of the ANP-B receptor is selectively activated (in contrast to the action of ANP and BNP) by CNP at physiologically relevant (0.5 nM) concentrations.[16] The third ANP receptor (non-GC, or C receptor, also known as R2) contains an extracellular domain (440 amino acids), homologous with those of ANP-A and ANP-B receptors, but only a short (37 amino acid) cytoplasmic domain. The C receptor recognizes and binds a wide range of natriuretic peptides and analogues, though affinity for hBNP is appreciably less than for ANP or CNP.[16, 46] It is to be noted that a specific BNP receptor has not yet been identified.

The distribution of the three ANP receptors among various tissues determines, at least in part, physiological actions of natriuretic peptides. The C receptor is widely distributed and represents 60 to 95 per cent of ANP binding—and may be as high as 99 per cent in vascular smooth muscle cells.[47] Inactive ANP analogues, which bind to the C receptor but not to the more specific GC receptors, may reduce clearance of physiologically secreted hormone so that plasma levels and hence biological activity (acting via GC receptors) are promoted.[45] The abundance, location within the vascular system, and lack of obvious biological effector all fit with the concept of a clearance function. However, there is increasing evidence that the C receptor may not be biologically "silent."[20] For instance, C-receptor stimulation may inhibit adenyl cyclase[48] in several tissues (including vascular smooth muscle cells) and stimulate phosphoinositide hydrolysis,[49] though the physiological consequence of these actions is unclear. A recent

Hormones   Human Receptors

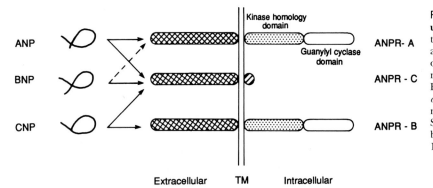

FIGURE 154–2. **Hormone specificity for the human natriuretic peptide receptors.** A schematic representation of the ability of the human natriuretic peptides to specifically activate the guanylyl cyclase of human ANPR-A or ANPR-B or bind to human ANPR-C. The *solid lines* connect the receptors with their preferred ligand. The ambiguity of BNP's role in activation of ANPR-A is represented by a *dashed line,* as described in the text. *TM,* transmembrane region. (From Koller JK, Lowe DG, Bennett GL, et al: Selective activation of the B natriuretic peptide receptor by C-type natriuretic peptide (CNP). Science 252:120–123, 1991. Copyright 1990 by the AAAS.)

report points to an inhibitory role of the C receptor (independent of change in cell nucleotides) in mitogenesis and proliferation of rat aortic smooth muscle cells.[50] Clearly more work is required before an "inert clearance" role for this receptor is proven.[50a]

In keeping with the known biological effects of ANP, regional tissue distribution of the ANP-A receptor (as indicated by expression of the gene receptor in primate tissues) shows high concentrations in the kidney glomerulus, adrenal zona glomerulosa, brain, and cardiac atria.[51] In contrast, the ANP-B receptor appears to be largely confined to tissues of neural origin,[51] findings consistent with the view that CNP acts chiefly within the CNS. However, more recent work indicates the presence of ANP-B receptors in peripheral tissues including blood vessels.[51a] There appear to be major variations in receptor type among different species—for instance, vascular smooth muscle cells from rat aorta and mesangial cells from human kidney both express the ANP-B receptor.[46]

The immediate effect of ANP-A (and/or -B) receptor stimulation is activation of the plasma membrane-associated guanylate cyclase in a concentration-dependent manner to increase the intracellular level of cGMP. The membrane ("particulate") form of guanylate cyclase is distinct from the cytoplasmic (soluble) form that is stimulated in vascular smooth muscle by nitric oxide and endothelium-derived relaxant factor (EDRF) and not affected by ANP. The magnitude of the cellular cGMP rise induced by ANP varies from five-fold in some tissues to greater than a thousand-fold in vascular endothelial cells and may be affected by other intracellular messenger systems, as well as by changes in ionic calcium and a specific cGMP phosphodiesterase. For example, ANP-induced cGMP accumulation is inhibited by angiotensin II, AVP, and an increase in cytosolic ionic calcium.[52] Regulation of ANP receptor number (as in the process of "down-regulation") may also af-

fect the long-term actions of the hormone. Apparently ANP-A receptors are desensitized by prolonged exposure to ANP[53]—a phenomenon that may also induce down regulation of the C receptor in vascular smooth muscle cells, implying cooperative interaction (and close association on the membrane) between the two receptors. In endothelial cells, C receptor numbers are increased and the activity of guanylate cyclase (presumably "A") receptors reduced by glucocorticoids.[54] The physiological relevance of the above findings is unclear, particularly since numerous clinical and physiological studies (both short- and long-term) have usually shown a good correlation of plasma cGMP levels (or increment) with plasma ANP concentrations.[55-57]

A number of observations strongly suggest that intracellular cGMP is the second messenger of ANP hormone action. For example, many of the actions of ANP, including enhanced glomerular filtration, inhibition of Na transport, and vasorelaxation, can be reproduced by exogenous cGMP analogues. Not all actions of ANP, however, can be attributed to cGMP-mediated mechanisms; in particular, inhibition of aldosterone by ANP has been difficult to relate to intracellular changes in this nucleotide. The precise intracellular mechanism of action of cGMP is complex and varies in different tissues but is likely to involve protein kinase activation, phosphorylation of intracellular proteins, and associated changes in cytosolic (ionic) calcium.[23]

Plasma ANP and Metabolism in Humans

A variety of radioimmunoassays have been used to measure ANP in human plasma. Most antisera are directed to the carboxy-terminus rather than the ring structure where bioactivity resides, so values obtained may not necessarily reflect biological activity. However, analysis of plasma extracts using high-pressure liquid chromatography (HPLC) and gas chromatography have in general shown a single immunoreactive peak corresponding to αhANP.[58, 59] Larger forms, including the prohormone (γhANP) and an unusual antiparallel dimer (βhANP) have been found in the plasma of patients with severe congestive heart failure.[60]

Analysis of coronary sinus plasma extracts, in addition to confirming the identity of hANP 99–126 as the main circulating hormone in humans, shows an isoform of the hormone in which the Cys Phe bond at 105/106 has been hydrolyzed to yield an open ring (biologically inactive) metabolite—"cleaved ANP."[61] As discussed below, the same metabolite can be generated in human plasma in vitro and is presumably the product of a specific tissue endopeptidase, EC 24.11. Cleaved ANP may represent up to 30 per cent of immunoreactive ANP in coronary sinus plasma extracts of heart failure subjects, but levels in peripheral venous plasma drawn from normal subjects are below the limit of assay detection. Mean plasma venous immunoreactive ANP in resting (sitting) young, adult subjects consuming a normal sodium intake ranges from approximately 5 to 20 pmol/L (15 to 60 pg/ml). Plasma levels of ANP (but not plasma cGMP) are higher in the elderly and are increased by supine posture, increasing sodium content of the diet, and sodium-retaining drugs[62] (Fig. 154–3). In supine subjects studied under controlled conditions, there is little evidence of pulsatile secretion or convincing evidence of diurnal rhythmicity. Plasma ANP levels are unaffected by acute stress such as insulin-induced

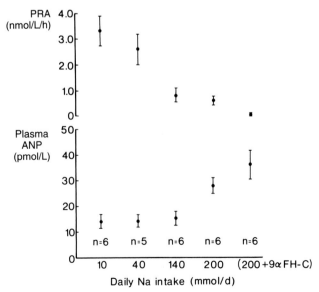

FIGURE 154–3. **Plasma renin activity (PRA) and ANP** in normal subjects receiving a range of different dietary sodium intakes. Blood samples (0800 h ambulant) were drawn after at least four days on each diet. Subjects receiving 200 mmol sodium daily were further treated with 0.4 mg 9α-fluorohydrocortisone (9αFH-C) daily for four days. (From Espiner EA, Nicholls MG: Human atrial natriuretic peptide. Clin Endocrinol 26:637–650, 1987.)

hypoglycemia. Evidence for tissue uptake of ANP is provided by the finding of higher levels in arterial plasma compared to matching venous samples. Thus the arteriovenous ratio across the lower limb, kidney, and liver is approximately 2:1.[63] These results are consistent with rapid uptake of the hormone by C receptors in the vascular beds and/or rapid degradation by tissue endopeptidase.

Consistent with these findings are the rapid disappearance rate (first phase half-life [t½] approximately 3 min) and large volume of distribution (VD approximately 10 to 12 L at plasma ANP concentrations of 300 pmol/L) after bolus injection or constant infusion of ANP.[64] Studies employing constant infusions of hormone (0.75 to 15 pmol/kg/min) indicate that the metabolic clearance rate is relatively high (2.4 to 8 L/min) and dose dependent, both VD and MCR being greater at lower infusion rates. Neither MCR nor disappearance rate of ANP appears to be affected by sodium intake or the presence of cardiac failure. As well as specific uptake by ANP receptors, it is likely that the hormone is subject to cleavage by EC 24.11 and subsequently rapid proteolysis by other enzymes such as kallikrein. EC 24.11 (also known as enkephalinase) is present in many epithelial tissues, particularly the luminal proximal tubular membrane of the nephron, and is also detectable in human plasma. Addition of endopeptidase inhibitors delays the degradation of ANP, delays the clearance of exogenous ANP,[65] and raises endogenous ANP levels in healthy normal subjects[66] as well as in patients with hypertension or heart failure.[67] These findings support the view that tissue endopeptidase plays a role in ANP metabolism. Since the enzyme itself may be subject to regulation it is possible that the membrane-bound ANP is regulated by tissue variation in the expression of the endopeptidase gene.

Small amounts of immunoreactive ANP are excreted in urine, although proof of the hormone's chemical identity (by amino acid sequencing) is still lacking. There is evidence that much of the filtered ANP is degraded in proximal tubules by endopeptidase; inhibition of the renal enzyme promotes both ANP and cGMP excretion and increases natriuresis, possibly by allowing ANP access to amiloride-sensitive sodium channels in the apical membrane of the inner medullary collecting duct. Urodilatin (ANP 95–126), a naturally occurring form of ANP produced intrarenally and excreted in human urine,[26] is less subject to endopeptidase action[67a] and could also act (in a paracrine sense) to regulate sodium excretion. Clearly, more studies are required to determine the physiological significance of ANP metabolites, endopeptidase activity, and the paracrine role of these factors in cardiovascular disease.

Plasma ANP in Pathological States

As already detailed, hypervolemic states such as congestive heart failure (CHF), chronic renal failure, and mineralocorticoid hypertension are associated with high levels of plasma ANP. Plasma levels in CHF may be raised 20- to 30-fold above normal values and are generally related to the magnitude of increase in right or left atrial pressure and to functional class (New York Heart Association classes I to IV). The percentage of immunoreactive ANP attributable to β-ANP is increased in severe heart failure[67b] and falls with effective treatment.[60] Many other disorders of cardiac muscle or valvular function are associated with elevated levels of ANP; in all of these situations (except cardiac tamponade), arterial and venous ANP levels are significantly correlated with indices of left or right atrial pressure and inversely correlated with cardiac output. Plasma cGMP similarly reflects the long-term increase in hormone level.[55] In chronic disorders of ventricular function (e.g., dilated cardiomyopathy) there is evidence that the overloaded left ventricle contributes to circulating ANP levels[68]—findings consistent with increased ventricular levels of ANP gene expression in states of experimental and human heart failure. Plasma ANP also tends to be raised after acute myocardial infarction and in patients with chronic obstructive pulmonary disease, in whom acute hypoxia is likely to be an additional stimulus to ANP secretion. Interestingly, a recent study of a large number of patients observed after myocardial infarction shows that plasma ANP is a good marker of mild ventricular impairment[69] and a useful prognostic marker of left ventricular dysfunction. ANP levels in other noncardiac edematous states such as nephrosis and cirrhosis are more variable, but elevated levels are reported in several studies. In many of these studies interpretation is difficult, since details of cardiac and other hemodynamic measurements are not provided, and often conditions of posture, sodium intake, fluid intake, and the like are uncontrolled. A number of other "noncardiac" disorders, for instance, syndrome of inappropriate antidiuretic hormone (SIADH), Cushing's syndrome, Bartter's syndrome, and orthostatic hypotension, are reported to be associated with raised plasma ANP. In most instances the mechanism for increase in ANP is unclear.

There is now a large body of evidence to support the original reports[70] of raised plasma ANP levels in subjects with hypertension. In a recent meta-analysis by Atlas and Laragh[71] significant elevation of ANP (above those of matched normotensive subjects) was reported in 6 of 10 studies reviewed. The increase is modest, amounting to an increase of 20 to 100 per cent, and could not be accounted for by age or renal dysfunction. Overall, ANP levels in hypertension are correlated with severity of blood pressure and the presence of left ventricular hypertrophy, raising the possibility that altered chamber compliance or geometry could be responsible for increased synthesis and secretion from either atrium or ventricle. Increased central blood volume and circulating secretagogues (such as angiotensin II or catecholamines) may also be involved. Interestingly, in this context basal plasma ANP levels are increased in patients with low-renin hypertension[72] when compared with age- and blood pressure-matched normoreninemic subjects. It has been argued that ANP levels should be supranormal in hypertensive subjects and that a "normal" level may indicate inadequate hormone secretion in the setting of hypertension—and point to a causal role in the development of the elevated pressure. Two studies—one in spontaneous hypertensive rats[73] and one in hypertension-prone men[74]—postulate that deficient ANP production during sodium loading predicates the subsequent development of systemic hypertension. These findings raise the possibility that ANP secretion may be impaired in the early (developmental) phase of the disorder. It is to be noted that with this one possible exception, a primary disorder of either excess or deficiency of ANP secretion has yet to be proved in humans. By analogy with transgenic models carrying an extra ANP gene,[75] and in which plasma ANP levels are chronically elevated, such a primary syndrome of excessive ANP secretion would be expected to show features of hypovolemia and hypotension. Claims that Bartter's syndrome may be such a primary disorder[76] are controversial and await confirmation by more detailed studies. In one report of possible ectopic ANP production from a small cell tumor of the lung,[77] evidence that there was inappropriate secretion of ANP by the tumor was not obtained, and the specific contribution of raised plasma ANP to the clinical syndrome was difficult to assess, since arginine vasopressin was also much increased.

Biological Actions

A vast amount of evidence on ANP's bioactivity in humans and experimental animals has been obtained since the hormone's discovery in 1981. Much of it is difficult to interpret, since early studies used suprapathophysiological doses that often elicited counterregulatory neurohormonal responses. The interdependence of renal hemodynamic and endocrine action was also slow to be appreciated. For example, a sustained natriuretic effect of ANP is critically dependent on the maintenance of renal perfusion pressure. Similarly, interpretation of neurohumoral responses to ANP (renin-angiotensin, aldosterone, sympathetic nervous activity, and arginine vasopressin) requires knowledge of the prevailing hemodynamic and renal effects of the hormone. Equally important is the time frame of experimental studies chosen, their duration, and the degree of ANP stimulation employed. Nonetheless, while doubt may still exist concerning the importance of the hormone in sodium and blood pressure homeostasis, it is clear that small increments in plasma ANP within the physiological range are natriuretic, inhibit renin-aldosterone, and exert vasodepression in humans and experimental animals.

RENAL ACTIONS. Constant short-term infusions or bolus injections of ANP in normovolemic states induce prompt natriuresis, diuresis, and smaller increases in divalent ions without significantly increasing potassium excretion.[78] Large doses of ANP increase GFR, but at more physiological levels this effect is difficult to demonstrate unless basal renovascular tone is high.[79] Apart from a dramatic increase in urine cGMP (and nephrogenous cGMP excretion), the most striking renal effect of ANP is to increase the fractional excretion of sodium (i.e., the fraction of the total sodium filtered at the glomerulus that is excreted in the urine). In most studies the filtration fraction (i.e., the fraction of the total blood flow that is filtered at the glomerulus) is also increased. Thus a hemodynamic contribution from ANP, probably due to increased glomerular efferent arteriolar resistance along with afferent arteriolar dilatation,[80] may explain some of the natriuretic effect.

Tubular sites of ANP action are necessary to explain the increased fractional sodium excretion, but the precise site and mechanisms of action are still debated.[23] A direct effect of ANP on proximal tubular epithelial cation transport has been difficult to show, and no ANP receptors (abundant in glomerulus, inner medullary collecting duct, and papilla) have been found in this segment of the nephron. Whereas direct (receptor-mediated) actions of ANP in the glomerulus and the collecting duct[30a] are generally agreed upon,

many of the proposed actions of ANP appear to be mediated by inhibition of the action of angiotensin II.

A characteristic effect of large and prolonged ANP infusions (which lower arterial pressure) is the lack of sustained natriuresis. Numerous studies have now shown that the natriuretic effect is unusually dependent on the maintenance of renal perfusion pressure[81] or closely related intrarenal event. Even low sustained infusion rates—barely raising plasma ANP levels—induce only transient natriuresis, which wanes as vasodepression ensues.[56, 82] In contrast, prolonged intrarenal ANP infusions in dogs, insufficient to affect systemic pressure or neurohumoral factors, induce sustained natriuresis.[83] On the other hand, increased renal perfusion pressure (as may occur in plasma volume–expanded states) augments the natriuretic effect of ANP. There is increasing evidence that intrarenal factors, particularly angiotensin II and renal sympathetic nervous activity, underlie these variations in the renal response to ANP.

As further discussed in the setting of prolonged (vasodepressor) ANP infusions, any transient natriuresis is followed by a return to basal excretion rates, i.e., sodium balance is again achieved but at a lower level of arterial perfusion pressure. In other words, the familiar pressure-natriuresis relationship is shifted to the left, and the kidney can continue to excrete sodium normally at a lower level of blood pressure.[84] These findings explain, at least in part, the hypotensive effect of chronic increases in ANP in the absence of conspicuous natriuresis.[84, 85] Further, the findings allow the possibility of important subtle natriuretic effects of elevated ANP even in "refractory" states such as congestive heart failure in which systemic and renal perfusion pressure is often much reduced. The natriuretic effect of exogenous ANP is clearly reduced in both human[86, 87] and experimental[88] heart failure but can be restored in one model of rat heart failure by inhibition of angiotensin using converting enzyme (ACE) inhibitors.[89] Similarly the natriuretic effect of neutral endopeptidase inhibitors (a means of increasing endogenous ANP levels) is potentiated by angiotensin II inhibition in dogs with congestive heart failure[90]—an effect that is abolished by intrarenal angiotensin II infusion. In sodium-replete normal humans, angiotensin inhibition has no effect on the natriuretic response to infused ANP.[91]

Taken together these studies further confirm the importance of increased angiotensin II in attenuating the renal response to ANP in congestive heart failure. Thus hemodynamic factors, local angiotensin II production, and increased sympathetic nervous activity are more likely to be responsible for the renal hyporesponsiveness to ANP than "down regulation" of ANP receptors, particularly since plasma cGMP levels are usually commensurate with elevated levels of ANP in congestive heart failure.[55] Reports of reduced renal production of cGMP (nephrogenous cGMP) in response to exogenous ANP in CHF[92] may be due to high levels of intrarenal angiotensin II, which has the potential to inhibit the cGMP response to ANP.[52]

In contrast to CHF and other hypoperfusion states, the renal response (especially natriuresis) in hypertension is enhanced,[93, 94] and more so in some volume expanded hypertensive models.[95] Whether this increased responsiveness is simply a reflection of increased renal perfusion pressure, relatively depressed SNA, and/or low local renin-angiotensin II is still unclear.

HEMODYNAMIC EFFECTS. The hemodynamic effects of ANP are multiple and complex in keeping with the abundance and diverse distribution of ANP receptors within the vascular system. Early in vitro studies using isolated precontracted blood vessels emphasize the direct (vasorelaxant) and cGMP-dependent action of ANP, which is not dependent on the presence of the endothelium. This effect was especially prominent in the setting of angiotensin II vasoconstriction[23] and appeared to be confirmed by the hypotensive effects of large bolus doses of the hormone in vivo. Subsequent in vivo studies, producing variable vasodepression after a large single-bolus dose or infusion, showed that vascular resistance increased in most regional beds.[96] These effects were presumably mediated by counterregulatory responses to initial and abrupt falls in blood pressure, as decreased peripheral vascular resistance occurred if the sympathetic nervous system was inhibited.[97] There is now general agreement that one of the main vasodepressor effects of ANP in normal health is mediated by reductions in cardiac filling pressure and consequently fall in cardiac output. Some of this effect of ANP is due to reduction in plasma volume and caused by a shift of plasma from vascular to the extravascular space[98] mediated by enhanced capillary hydraulic conductivity.[99] Additional venodilator[100] actions of ANP may also contribute to the reduction in preload. Cardiac muscle contractility is largely unaffected by ANP, and despite earlier concerns, coronary blood flow is likely to be unchanged or increased.[101] A direct effect of ANP on atrial (and ventricular) myocytes, reducing their tension or excitability, has also been proposed and may be a means whereby the hormone modulates (inhibits) its own secretion. A further important hemodynamic action of ANP is affected by changes in vagal and baroreceptor regulation.[102] ANP appears to sensitize vagal afferents (leading to reflex bradycardia), and in humans large doses dampen arterial baroreflex responses, an effect prevented by angiotensin II converting enzyme inhibition.[103] Similar effects are seen in rats given doses of ANP that do not lower blood pressure or affect heart rate.[104] Taken together these findings suggest that the vasodepressor action of ANP may involve capillaries, resistance vessels, veins, and neural elements—the proportionate effect depending upon resting or basal tone.

The hemodynamic effects of infused ANP in normotensive states vary according to dose, species, and duration of infusion.[23] In normotensive humans, large single doses cause a small and sustained fall in mean arterial pressure and a small rise in heart rate.[105] Whereas sudden (vasovagal-like) hypotension can occur during short-term infusions, a consistent hypotensive effect of ANP has been difficult to show, even when reduction in cardiac filling pressure is observed.[86, 106] More consistent are increases in hematocrit[106] (unrelated to diuresis), suggesting that fall in plasma volume is a sensitive feature of ANP's action at physiological levels.[107] However, longer-term infusions of low-dose ANP, in which there is less effect on counterregulatory reflexes, appear to reduce arterial pressure in dogs[84] and sheep.[108] Twenty-four-hour constant infusions in sheep induce significant falls in systolic arterial pressure, central venous pressure, and plasma volume (without activation of heart rate, sympathetic nervous activity, or renin-angiotensin-aldosterone) in response to small ANP increments of approximately 22 pmol/L.[56] Even smaller doses (0.8 pmol/kg/min) prolonged for 48 hours, and which

did not significantly raise venous plasma ANP concentration, lower systolic arterial pressure and peripheral vascular resistance.[109] After 48 hours of infusion, no change in baroreceptor function was found, but the pressor response to exogenous angiotensin II was reduced. Since no change occurred in cardiac output, plasma volume, sympathetic nervous activity, or renin-angiotensin levels, these results suggest that chronic subtle changes in ANP primarily affect blood pressure by reducing peripheral vascular resistance. Similar observations were made in sheep given more prolonged (5-day) infusions.[108]

The hemodynamic and blood pressure-lowering effects of ANP in hypertensive states have been studied extensively. In general the findings follow those observed in normotensive states. However, long-term low-dose ANP infusions in some rat models of hypertension (particularly renin dependent), impressively reduce blood pressure.[110] In humans, 5-day infusions of ANP (doubling basal plasma ANP levels) induced a prolonged hypotensive effect, first evident at 24 hours without change in plasma renin-angiotensin, but associated with significant fall in plasma volume.[82] These findings are similar to those reported in studies of normotensives (see above) and raise the possibility that prolonged small increases in ANP have important vasodepressor actions.

In contrast to the inconsistencies and debates surrounding the hemodynamic effects of ANP administration in normal and hypertensive states, there is more unanimity concerning the effects of ANP infusion in heart failure. Large infusions consistently lowered preload, mean arterial pressure, and peripheral vascular resistance and increased cardiac output without changing heart rate or sympathetic nervous activity in most studies.[86, 87, 111] These beneficial effects are presumably due to peripheral vasodilatation, which in heart failure may fail to evoke a normal neurohumoral response. As already noted, some of this fall in peripheral vascular resistance is likely to be due to inhibition of angiotensin II-induced vasoconstriction, since circulating levels of renin-angiotension II generally remain unaffected. The effects of prolonged administration of lower (and more physiological) doses of ANP in heart failure, including the use of ANP-promoting drugs such as neutral endopeptidase inhibitors, remain to be examined.

OTHER VASCULAR ACTIONS. The vascular endothelium contains both GC (A) and C receptors. The possibility that ANP may act to regulate vascular permeability is supported by studies showing inhibition by ANP of endothelial cell permeability to macromolecule egress induced by thrombin.[112] This action of ANP is mimicked by cGMP.[113] Thus, ANP may be importantly involved in maintaining the integrity of the endothelial barrier—for instance, in lung tissue—and thereby protect against the development of pulmonary edema. This action on the endothelium (to reduce permeability to large molecules) should be distinguished from the action of ANP on systemic capillary hydraulic pressure (reducing plasma volume), an action that is presumably mediated by the balance of vascular smooth-muscle afferent and efferent tone.

Other vascular effects of ANP include inhibition of endothelin-1 secretion stimulated by angiotensin II.[114] Again this action of ANP is mimicked by cGMP. Such endothelial actions of ANP may further contribute to the vasorelaxant effects of the hormone, as detailed above.

ENDOCRINE ACTIONS. One of the remarkable aspects of

ANP action is the near-universal inhibition of the action of angiotensin II (an exception appears to be the constrictor action of both hormones on the glomerular efferent arteriole). Many of these interactions have already been discussed in the context of the renal and hemodynamic actions of ANP. The antagonism extends to many of the endocrine actions, for instance, inhibition of angiotensin II-induced aldosterone secretion, angiotensin II-induced vasopressin secretion, and other central effects mediated by the brain-renin-angiotensin system.

As shown in Figure 154–4, short-term low-dose infusions of ANP, increasing plasma levels (by approximately 8 pmol/L) into the upper quartile of the normal range, significantly inhibit plasma renin activity (PRA) as well as plasma aldosterone in normal and hypertensive humans.[115] Although stimulated by massive doses of ANP eliciting abrupt hypotension and increased SNA,[116] inhibition of renin secretion appears to be a consistent and prompt effect of ANP in situations in which resting renin-angiotensin activity is near normal. Further, the expected renin response to the stimulation by erect posture, diuretic, or isoproteronol is inhibited by ANP. Similar results are obtained in experimental animals. Longer-term low-dose ANP infusions (up to 13 days in rats with "renal clip hyperten-

sion"[117]) appears to maintain renin suppression,[118] but the effect appears to be less or negligible in severe heart failure. The mechanism by which ANP inhibits renin secretion is still debated. A direct inhibitory effect on renin release is supported by some studies, but there is also strong support for an inhibitory effect mediated by increased sodium delivery (induced by ANP) to the macula densa.[119] The failure of even high doses of ANP to inhibit renin-angiotensin in patients with severe CHF, who are generally refractory to the natriuretic action of the ANP, is also consistent with this hypothesis.

Early in vitro studies established that ANP at physiological levels (10^{-11} M) has a selective inhibitory effect on the zona glomerulosa and aldosterone production—an effect that can be partially overcome by increasing the concentration of secretagogues such as angiotensin and/or ACTH.[120] Subsequent studies have shown that ANP inhibits steroidogenesis in glomerulosa cells, at a step just before mitochondrial cholesterol uptake, whereas steroidogenesis in fasciculata cells is largely unaffected by ANP. The aldosterone-stimulating effects of ACTH, angiotensin, and potassium (and metoclopramide in vivo) are all reduced by ANP, although once again it is the action of angiotensin that is most affected.[121] Although ANP-A receptors are present in glomerulosa cells, the evidence at present does not favor mediation by intracellular cGMP. Although the precise mechanism of ANP's potent adrenal action remains to be clarified, it almost certainly involves inhibition of intracellular pathways subsequent to angiotensin II–stimulated Ca^{2+} influx.[120, 122] In most clinical situations, infusions of ANP that inhibit aldosterone also cause proportionate falls in renin-angiotensin II, and similar observations have been made in experimental animals receiving prolonged low-dose infusion.[118] However, the responses of renin and aldosterone can be dissociated—for instance, in congestive heart failure (in which aldosterone is more inhibited than renin in some studies)[87, 123] and in experimental animals with renal ischemia.[124] Most of the studies of ANP's action on the adrenal cortex have been limited in duration so that the effect of chronic ANP elevation is largely unknown.

It is to be noted that ANP can also antagonize the action of aldosterone on the distal tubule and collecting duct,[125] actions that presumably also contribute to the hormone's natriuretic effect.

The inhibitory effect of ANP on thirst, vasopressin, and in some circumstances ACTH secretion may be further examples of the hormone's suppression of angiotensin II's action, including those within the brain renin-angiotensin system.[6] Whereas the central (icv) administration of ANP can suppress basal as well as dehydration-, hemorrhage-, or angiotensin II-stimulated release of vasopressin,[126] the inhibitory effects of *systemic* administration of ANP on vasopressin release are more controversial, especially at levels of ANP likely to be attained in health. Recent studies in humans suggest that physiological increments of ANP do not inhibit osmotically stimulated vasopressin but do blunt thirst perception,[127] supporting the view that the systemic elevations of plasma ANP have the potential to affect hypothalamic function. Despite numerous studies supporting an inhibitory effect of ANP on corticotropin-releasing hormone or ACTH secretion in vitro[128, 129] or less often in vivo,[130, 131] the acute effects of small increments of ANP in

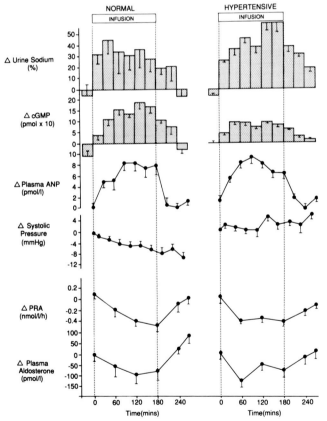

FIGURE 154–4. **Response to intravenous ANP** (2.25 ng/kg/min for 180 min) in six normotensive subjects and six hypertensive subjects equilibrated on a daily sodium intake of 150 mmol. Values are plotted as change (Δ) from time-matched levels on control day. Change in urine sodium excretion is expressed as % change from baseline (mean of first three collection periods before infusions = 100%). Change in systolic blood pressure is shown relative to values integrated for 30 min immediately before infusions. (Adapted from Espiner EA, Richards AM: Atrial natriuretic peptide; an important factor in sodium and blood pressure regulation. Lancet 1:707–710, 1989.)

humans do not appear to affect hypothalamic-pituitary-adrenal function.[132]

NEUROENDOCRINE AND NEUROTRANSMITTER ACTIONS. Readers are referred to recent reviews[133] for a detailed discussion of the central effects of ANP. The actions and role of ANP synthesis within brain tissue have been difficult to unravel. However, central administration of ANP shows potent effects, for instance, fentomole concentrations can inhibit the spontaneous firing rate of hypothalamic neurons in vivo.[134] The cardiovascular and renal effects of centrally administered ANP are also controversial.[135] Large doses given icv tend to be vasodepressor[136] and attenuate the pressor action of central angiotensin II.[137] Microinjections into known cardioinhibitory sites of the ambiguus nucleus (a major relay center for ANP immunoreactive neuronal projections from paraventricular and other hypothalamic nuclei) induce bradycardia and can be abolished by bilateral vagotomy or atropine.[138] Taken together these findings suggest that ANP has a role in the central processing of baroreceptor inputs. Other neuroendocrine actions of ANP, including inhibition of prolactin and LH secretion and inhibition of central dopamine neurons, have been proposed but await further confirmation. However, there seems little doubt that ANP has important central actions, particularly in the hypothalamus and circumventricular organs, in the brain's control of cardiovascular function.

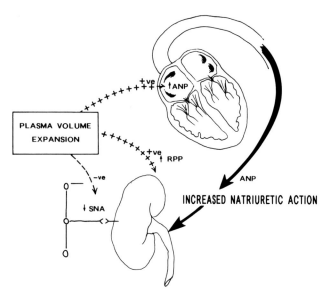

FIGURE 154–5. **Effect of plasma volume expansion on the renal response to ANP.** Increases in extracellular fluid (plasma) volume, in the setting of a competent cardiovascular system, will increase renal perfusion pressure (RPP), reduce renal sympathetic nervous activity (SNA), and thereby augment the natriuretic response to the evoked ANP release. Reduced intrarenal angiotensin II formation may also contribute to the enhanced natriuretic effect of ANP. Exactly opposite events accompany *decreases* in extracellular fluid (plasma) volume.

Integrated Actions and Role of ANP in Pathophysiology

The striking range of actions, including reductions in cardiac filling pressure, arterial vasodilation, promotion of sodium excretion, inhibition of renin-angiotensin-aldosterone, and reduced baroreflex sensitivity, strongly implicate ANP as a major hormone involved in the defense against hypervolemia. Parallels with the renin-angiotensin II system—the major hormone system concerned with maintaining homeostasis during volume contraction—are obvious and highlighted by the remarkable antagonism between ANP and angiotensin expressed at numerous physiological and intracellular levels. Nevertheless, the importance and significance of ANP in the regulation of volume has been questioned, chiefly because of the lack of consistent relationship between plasma hormone levels and natriuresis.[139] For example, the apparent dominance of angiotensin II actions (vasoconstriction and sodium retention) in severe heart failure in the face of very high plasma ANP levels has seriously questioned the potency, and role, of the cardiac hormone system.[140] However, the lack of consistent relationship between plasma ANP and natriuresis is not surprising when the integrated hemodynamic and renal effects of the hormones are considered.

As already discussed, the renal effects of ANP are augmented when plasma volume (or more specifically effective arterial blood volume)[141] is expanded (Fig. 154–5). Under normal conditions of health, increasing ANP secretion in response to small increases in atrial pressure will induce an appropriate brisk renal response. Exactly the opposite occurs when volume is reduced; ANP secretion lessens and the renal response to the hormone is attenuated so that sodium is conserved. This relationship tends to break down in heart failure, particularly when it is severe, since in this

setting plasma volume expansion (i.e., atrial hypertension) is associated eventually with reduced cardiac output, reduced renal perfusion pressure, and therefore reduced renal responsiveness to ANP, even though plasma levels may be greatly increased. However, other cardiovascular and renal effects of ANP may continue to play an important role even in established heart failure. For example, comparative studies of two types of experimental heart failure in dogs, one that increases plasma ANP (right ventricular pacing) and one that does not (thoracic inferior vena cava constriction), show much greater sodium retention and renin-aldosterone activation in the latter model despite comparable depression of cardiac output and arterial pressure. Similarly, total removal of the heart in calves and its replacement by an artificial pump markedly reduced plasma ANP. This fall in ANP is associated with salt retention, edema, renin-aldosterone and vasopressin stimulation, whereas calves with artificial ventricles of comparable function (but with intact atria and normal ANP production) fail to exhibit the severe heart failure syndrome.[142] Although these constitute complex models, these and other studies[143] indicate that ANP has an important role in counterbalancing the neurohumoral response (increased sympathetic nervous activity, increased renin-angiotensin II and vasopressin secretion) to diminishing cardiac output. The fact that ANP's actions are finally overwhelmed in severe congestive heart failure is entirely consistent with in vitro studies of ANP-angiotensin II interaction and presumably reflects the primacy of the body's defense of arterial pressure.

While the definitive role and importance of ANP must await the development of specific ANP inhibitors/antagonist, there is already substantial evidence that ANP does indeed participate in sodium and blood pressure homeostasis in several situations outside those of severe cardiac disease. Not only do volume loading maneuvers or dietary sodium changes[62] evoke corresponding and temporally associated changes in plasma ANP and urine sodium excretion, but, equally important, small sustained increments in plasma ANP (achieved during infusions of the hormone and mimicking those induced by increasing dietary sodium) are natriuretic and may account for more than half of the net increase in the rate of sodium excretion.[115, 144]

Surprisingly, some studies in experimental animals suggest that renin-aldosterone inhibition, as well as the natriuresis associated with acute saline loading are both ANP-dependent events, since they are almost completely blocked by injections of ANP antiserum.[145] In yet other studies the role of hormonal changes (including ANP) in the natriuresis associated with acute saline loading is reported to be insignificant.[146] Possibly the effects of ANP are more evident in the setting of chronic changes in sodium homeostasis. Recent studies on transgenic mice, in which prolonged increase in plasma ANP is achieved by constitutive secretion from a hepatic gene transcript, further confirm the potent effects of sustained ANP levels.[85] These mice are hypotensive, excrete sodium normally, and have an augmented natriuretic response to saline loading when compared to litter-mate controls. Such "whole-animal" studies are likely to significantly illuminate our understanding of the long-term effects on organ physiology of raising ANP levels.

Brain Natriuretic Peptide

As already discussed, BNP was first isolated from porcine brain extracts (hence its name), but is now recognized as a circulating hormone primarily of cardiac origin and analogous in many respects to ANP. However, a distinct gene and different pattern of secretion, regulation, and metabolism distinguish the hormone from ANP and warrant the reclassification[13] as B-type natriuretic peptide. It should be noted, however, that whereas BNP binds to ANP-A receptors, stimulates guanylate cyclase, and has many of the bioactions of ANP, a specific BNP receptor has not yet been identified.[16, 46]

In a series of reports by Sudoh and colleagues[11, 147] and Kojima and co-workers,[148] genomic clones from atrial tissue, and circulating forms of BNP, have been identified in pigs, humans, and rats. In all, the molecular construction of the prepro form is strikingly similar to those of ANP (and C-type natriuretic peptide, CNP). Thus, gene transcription yields a precursor form (prepro-BNP) containing a short (N terminal) hydrophobic leader segment that is cleaved at the C terminus to produce the prohormone (pro-BNP) containing the mature form of the hormone. However, in contrast to both CNP and ANP precursors, sequence homology among species is low and confined largely to the signal (leader) sequence and the C-terminal mature form of BNP.[148] Even here, in contrast to other members of the natriuretic peptide family, BNP mature forms are species specific with only short segments retaining sequence homology among species. Further, final processing to mature forms differs appreciably; rat BNP is a 45-amino acid peptide derived from a 95-amino acid prohormone; porcine BNP circulates as a 26- or 32-amino acid peptide (derived from a 106-amino acid pro form);

and human BNP is a 32-amino acid hormone (BNP 77–108) derived from a 108-amino acid prohormone. The same form (hBNP32) is present in human brain tissue. These variations in size and amino-acid sequence no doubt contribute to the species specificity of the hormone's receptor selectivity[46] and biological action[149] and account for the absence of or poor cross-reactivity of BNP antisera in different species. For these reasons, early studies involving cross-species experiments need to be interpreted with caution.

Although first isolated in porcine brain (where levels are some 10-fold higher than those of ANP[150]), the highest concentration of BNP is found in atrial tissue. In comparison, the BNP concentration in ventricular tissue is low (< 1 per cent of atrial concentration). Whereas the ventricular concentrations of ANP and BNP are similar, the concentration of BNP in atrial tissue is only 1 per cent (or less) of ANP. The form of stored hormone also differs. Unlike ANP, which is stored in atrial granules as the prohormone, immunoreactive forms of BNP extracted from cardiac tissue vary from predominantly pro-BNP in the pig[151] to mostly low-molecular weight (mature form) in humans[152] and rats. More instructive is the quantitation of gene expression by measurement of mRNA BNP in cardiac tissue. Several studies indicate that the ventricular mRNA level, compared to the concentration of immunoreactive BNP, is proportionately higher, and similar to that of atrial tissue. Thus when allowance is made for organ weight, the total amount of mRNA BNP in the ventricle is approximately 70 per cent of that of the whole heart.[153, 154] In the rat heart, the mRNA BNP content of the left ventricle is some 10-fold higher than that of the right.[153] Direct studies of BNP secretion from isolated perfused heart[153] and from in vivo studies in humans[152] further confirm that some 60 to 80 per cent of the cardiac secretion of BNP arises from the ventricle. These findings are in striking contrast to the pattern of mRNA distribution (and secretion) of ANP, which in health is predominantly synthesized and secreted from the atrium. Taken together, the findings also strongly suggest that BNP is secreted promptly from ventricular myocytes—presumably via constitutive pathways rather than released from preformed stores within myocytes, as occurs in the instance of atrial ANP. Not surprisingly, both ventricular gene expression and BNP secretion are increased in states of chronic left ventricular strain or overload. For example, the ventricular BNP mRNA content and BNP secretion rate are increased two-fold in spontaneously hypertensive stroke-prone rats[153] when compared with normal control rats. Similar observations have been made in the human heart of subjects with dilated cardiomyopathy.[152, 154] Thus the failing or hypertrophied ventricle has the ability to augment BNP production, whereas atrial mRNA BNP and secretion of BNP from the atria remain relatively unchanged in these circumstances. There is some evidence that the regulation of BNP secretion from atrial tissue may differ from that in the ventricle,[155] but further studies on the precise source, dynamics of the response (including rate of change in response to stimulation), and its importance in the heart's response to overloading are clearly required.

NONCARDIAC BNP. As shown previously for ANP, BNP has been isolated from brain tissue in several species. Immunoreactive BNP levels in porcine brain are 10-fold higher than those of ANP but similar to ANP content in human brain. The BNP gene does not appear to be expressed in rat brain. The distribution of BNP differs from that of ANP; highest concentrations of immunoreactive BNP in porcine brain occur in the medulla-pons, striatum, and hypothalamus.[156] The possibility that noncardiac sources (e.g., the brain) could contribute to circulating BNP levels seems unlikely. The role of BNP and interrelationships with ANP and CNP within the central nervous system are largely unknown.

Regulation and Secretion

As already discussed, increased ventricular immunoreactive BNP, mRNA BNP, and secretion of the mature hormone occur in hypervolemic states such as cardiac failure and hypertension. Deoxycorticosterone (DOC) administration and salt loading in rats also increase ventricular hormone concentration, whereas the atrial level is reduced.[157] In rats given salt and DOC there is significant positive correlation of both plasma BNP and ANP with increase in blood pressure; however, the relative increase in plasma immunoreactive BNP (compared to the control group) exceeded that of ANP.[155] Similar findings have been reported in human hypertension.[158] These findings together with the evidence of increased mRNA BNP in the left ventricle suggest that ventricular wall tension is an important stimulus to the hormone's synthesis and secretion.[158a] In this context it should be noted that increased production of ANP by the failing ventricle (up to 30-fold) is even more impressive (when expressed as a percentage of the normal ANP production from the ventricle) than the increase in BNP (approximately two-fold). Although the ventricular production of both hormones is commonly assumed to be constitutive in type (and therefore less responsive to exogenous stimuli), ventricular myocytes, at least in respect to ANP secretion, are responsive to endothelin[159] and phorbol esters.

Clearly, more studies are required to clarify the regulation of BNP and ANP within ventricular tissue. Other studies have found a clear relation of atrial tissue ANP and BNP content with hormone levels in blood or perfusate derived from atrial tissue. Such evidence is consistent with co-secretion of the two hormones, possibly from the same

atrial secretory granules[160] in some circumstances. Whether ANP secretogogues also stimulate atrial BNP synthesis and release is still unknown.

Plasma BNP and Metabolism in Humans

The development of species-specific antisera has enabled studies of circulating hormone levels in humans. Preliminary reports indicate that immunoreactive hBNP levels in venous plasma of normal adults, while correlating with plasma ANP levels and increasing with age, are significantly lower than plasma venous ANP levels determined at the same time.[152, 161] Much-increased levels[152, 161] (exceeding those of ANP in some cases) are found in subjects with heart failure, the rise being related in some studies to severity[152] (New York Heart Association functional class). This marked increase in plasma level is due at least in part to augmented ventricular secretion of the hormone. However, the molecular form of immunoreactive BNP in plasma of heart failure subjects may differ from that of normal subjects in containing a large proportion of high-molecular-weight immunoreactive material, closely similar to pro-BNP.[161, 162] This change in pattern of immunoreactive forms in heart failure is also shown (but to a lesser extent) by ANP and presumably reflects increasing constitutive secretion with incomplete processing of the prohormone to the mature form. As shown in Figure 154–6, venous levels of immunoreactive BNP are also raised soon after uncomplicated acute myocardial infarction (in which the acute rise in plasma BNP may exceed ANP levels[163]) and in subjects with chronic renal failure. The acute rise in BNP observed after myocardial infarction is not necessarily associated with clinical evidence of left ventricular dysfunction. Small elevations in plasma immunoreactive BNP are also reported in subjects with hypertension[158] and in normal subjects consuming high-sodium diets for 5 days.[164] More work is required to clarify the relative contributions of low- (hBNP32) and high-molecular-weight forms to these changes in circulating immunoreactive BNP levels.

The above findings are consistent with the view that augmented ventricular BNP production and secretion occur in response to hypervolemic states, particularly when ventricular dysfunction supervenes. In humans plasma BNP is

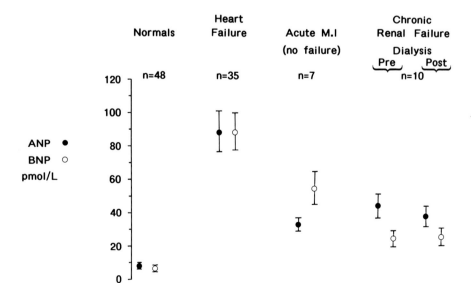

FIGURE 154–6. Venous plasma ANP (*filled circles*) and concurrent plasma BNP (*open circles*) levels in normal subjects and patients with circulatory disorders. Values are mean ± SEM. *n*, number of subjects in each group. Heart failure was of recent onset, New York Heart Association functional class II-IV. Blood was drawn within 24 h of admission in patients with acute (uncomplicated) myocardial infarction (M.I.). In patients with chronic renal failure, venous blood was drawn immediately pre and post routine hemodialysis. (From Yandle TG, Richards AM, Gilbert A, et al: Assay of brain natriuretic peptide (BNP) in human plasma: Evidence for high molecular weight BNP as a major plasma component in heart failure. J Clin Endocrinol Metab 76:832–838, © by the Endocrine Society, 1993.)

a good marker of left ventricular dysfunction and correlates better with measures of left ventricular ejection fraction than does plasma ANP.[164a] However, unlike ANP, the BNP hormonal system appears to be less responsive to abrupt changes in cardiac filling pressure, as may be observed for instance with changes in posture.[161] Similarly, brief exercise—increasing plasma ANP levels some two-fold to three-fold within 10 minutes—causes only a small (20 per cent) increase in hBNP in normal subjects.[164b] The findings suggest that at least in the uncompromised heart the response in BNP to acute stimulation[164c] is much less than that of ANP. Presumably this different pattern of secretion reflects the relative content of the two hormones in atrial granules.

Relatively little is known concerning the metabolism of hBNP. Consistent with a lower affinity of hBNP for the C receptor,[16, 46] the arteriovenous difference across the lower limb and the renal extraction of hBNP are significantly less than ANP. Further, the disappearance rate (first phase) of hBNP is considerably slower than that of ANP (22 and 3.2 min respectively). Prolonged half-life may therefore contribute to the greater rise of hBNP (compared to ANP) observed in congestive heart failure. The importance of endopeptidase 24.11 in BNP degradation is not yet clear, but hBNP appears to be relatively resistant to hydrolysis by the enzyme.[67a] Whereas human BNP is degraded by neutral endopeptidase in vitro,[165] the preferred site of cleavage is not the Cys/Phe bond which is the rate-limiting step in ANP degradation. The degradation of labeled BNP in human plasma is slower than ANP and less affected by endopeptidase 24.11 and other enzyme inhibitors.[161] A preliminary report suggests that endopeptidase 24.11 inhibitors further increase plasma immunoreactive BNP in subjects with heart failure,[166] but the clinical consequences of such increments remain to be determined.

Biological Actions

In vitro and in vivo studies indicate that BNP, like ANP, binds to A-type ANP receptors,[16, 46] stimulates guanylate cyclase,[167] and has natriuretic[11] and renin-aldosterone inhibitory actions.[168] However, compared to ANP, species homology among mature (circulating) forms of the hormone is much less striking and the biological actions of administered hormone in cross-species studies are more variable and difficult to predict.[149] For these reasons it is essential that the actions of the hormone are studied in the species of origin.

Whereas both ANP and hBNP (to a lesser extent) activate the guanylate cyclase A receptor, the affinity of the C receptor for hBNP is much less than ANP. The ANP-B receptor, originally proposed as a specific BNP receptor, is, in fact, selectively activated by CNP, and a specific BNP receptor has not yet been identified. Low infusion rates of hBNP in normal humans, sufficient to raise plasma levels seven-fold and into the range observed in mild heart failure or after an acute myocardial infarction, induce a two-fold rise in sodium excretion, increase plasma and urine cyclic GMP, and promptly inhibit renin-aldosterone.[169] Similar findings were observed in subjects with essential hypertension.

Although comparative studies of ANP and hBNP have not yet been undertaken in the same subjects, nor is there information over a wide range of doses, it appears that the biological effects of these two circulating hormones are similar, at least as judged by the results of short-term infusions. In humans, porcine BNP has similar potency and actions to human ANP.[168] The effects of short-term (30 min) hBNP infusions have also been studied in subjects with congestive heart failure.[170] High infusion rates achieving plasma levels approximating 2220 pmol/L (20-fold above baseline) were diuretic and natriuretic and lowered both atrial pressure and systemic vascular resistance. Since heart rate also increased, there was a significant increase in stroke volume index. These beneficial hemodynamic effects on left ventricular function in heart failure are similar to those described using ANP infusions,[86, 87] but the acute natriuretic effect of hBNP appeared to be greater. Surprisingly, despite falls in cardiac preload and afterload, plasma ANP levels increased by approximately 15 per cent. This effect was attributed to competition of high concentrations of BNP for ANP degradation sites (e.g., C receptors). Whether the observed natriuretic effect follows from the summated effects of the two natriuretic peptides or is due to some unique action of hBNP in heart failure remains to be clarified. Inhibition of aldosterone (but not necessarily renin secretion) appears to be a consistent effect of hBNP in both normal subjects and in those with heart failure.[169, 170]

Significance of BNP

Much more work is required to determine the role of BNP and its interrelationships with ANP in sodium and blood pressure regulation. For example, the biological effects of prolonged increases in BNP (to simulate the events of heart failure or hypertension) in the presence and absence of ANP are unknown. Untangling the individual roles of the two hormones will require specific antagonists and/or use of transgenic models. However, it is already apparent that there are striking differences in the source, secretion, regulation, and metabolism of the two hormones (Table 154–1). It is therefore tempting to view the two hormonal systems as somewhat independent regulators of intra-atrial (ANP) and ventricular (BNP) pressure, the secretion of both hormones being augmented when congestive heart failure supervenes.

ENDOTHELINS

The vascular endothelium, once considered to be an inert barrier between the blood and vascular wall, first gained recognition as a physiological regulator of vasomotor tone when prostacyclin, a potent vasodilator, was identified as a product of the endothelial cell.[171] Soon to follow were discoveries of other vasoactive compounds including an endothelium-derived relaxant factor (EDRF), now recognized as nitric oxide. In the course of bioassays for EDRF using medium from cultured aortic endothelial cells, a compound with potent coronary vasoconstrictor activity was identified.[172] Within three years,[173] the factor had been isolated, using recombinant DNA technology, and sequenced as a unique 21-amino acid peptide (endothelin) with highly potent and prolonged vasoconstrictor activity. Subsequently, diverse effects in other tissues have been

TABLE 154–1. COMPARISON OF ATRIAL NATRIURETIC PEPTIDE AND BRAIN NATRIURETIC PEPTIDE

	ANP	BNP
Sequence homology among species	Very strong	Weak
Major sites of gene expression	Cardiac atrium (brain)	Cardiac ventricle (brain)
Type of secretion	Regulated (atrium) Constitutive (ventricle)	Constitutive (ventricle)
Circulating form (humans)	Mostly small mol wt (28-amino-acid peptide)	Small (32-amino-acid peptide) and large mol wt
Receptors		
ANPR-A	++	+ (10% affinity of ANP)
ANPR-C	++	+ ? Other
Half-life (in plasma)	3 min	15–20 min
Arteriovenous ratio	Approx 2.0	Approx 1.3
Short-term actions	Negligible species-specificity	Species-specific
Natriuresis	+	+
Hemodynamic effects	+	+
Inhibition of R-A-A	+	+

confirmed, including a role in mitogenesis, cardiac contractility, and regulation of renin and aldosterone, as well as effects within the central nervous system.

Comparable in impact to the discovery of cardiac peptide hormones seven years earlier, the findings unleashed a major research effort culminating in the identity of at least three isoforms (each encoded by a distinct gene) and later the discovery of two unique receptors that mediate autocrine, paracrine, and possibly endocrine actions of these vasoactive peptides. Although the natriuretic peptide (vasorelaxant) family originating largely from the heart, and the endothelin (vasoconstrictor) family synthesized largely by local endothelial cells of blood vessels, could be viewed as counterbalancing hormone systems regulating cardiovascular homeostasis, it appears more likely that endothelins participate as *local* modulators of vascular tone rather than as circulating hormones. Nonetheless, as already shown for angiotensin II, endothelin and cardiac natriuretic peptides appear to be mutually opposing forces in many tissue and cellular pathways.

Structure, Synthesis, and Secretion

Endothelin (ET) was first identified in the supernatant of cultured porcine aortic endothelial cells. It is a 21-amino acid peptide (mol wt 2492) containing two intrachain disulfide bonds (Fig. 154–7) cross-linking the four cysteine residues.[174] Soon after the discovery of ET, two additional isoforms were identified from endothelial cell cultures derived from humans and other species. As shown in Figure 154–7, the three forms (ET-1, ET-2, and ET-3) in humans differ from each other only in respect to a few amino acid substitutions within the intrachain loop—sufficient, how-

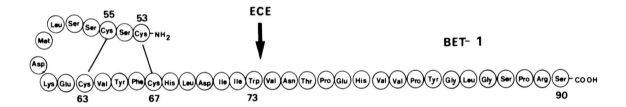

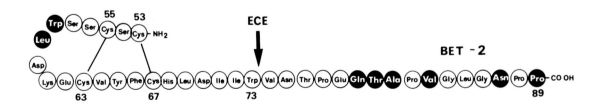

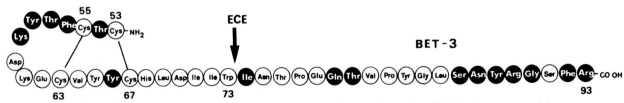

FIGURE 154–7. Amino-acid sequences of the three isoforms of the immediate biological precursor of human endothelin (BET). The *filled circles* represent amino-acid sequence changes compared with the big endothelin-1 sequence. The *arrow* indicates the proteolytic cleavage site (by endothelin-converting enzyme, ECE) responsible for the production of the biologically active mature endothelins. (Adapted from Rubanyi GM, Parker Botelho LH: Endothelins. FASEB J 5:2713–2720, 1991.)

ever, to confer quite different biological activities (see below). Although apparently unique among mammalian peptides, the structure of endothelins bears striking resemblance to sarafotoxin—a potent vasoconstrictor peptide isolated from venom of the Egyptian asp. Strong homology among ET's in mammals (porcine and human ET-1 are identical, as are rat and human ET-3) points to a common evolutionary origin and strong conservation of mature forms. The isolation of three distinct genes encoding the three isoforms in humans and other species has also confirmed close homology among the precursor peptides.

Transcription of the ET gene yields an mRNA species encoding a 203-amino acid precursor, prepro-ET, which (analogous to other peptide hormones) contains a 20-amino-acid residue signal (leader) sequence at the N-terminus. Processing occurs through the action of dibasic pair-specific endopetidases (recognition sites Lys 51-Arg 52 and Arg 91-Arg 92) to yield the 38-amino acid residue polypeptide pro-ET-1 (pro-ET$_{53-91}$, or "big" ET-1). As shown in the figure, there are small differences in the length and amino acid residues of the respective proforms of ET-1, ET-2, and ET-3. Further processing of pro-ET-1 occurs outside the endothelial cell by the action of a putative endothelin-converting enzyme (ECE), which in the instance of ET-1 cleaves the Trp$_{73}$-Val$_{74}$ bond to yield the mature form (ET-1, Cys$_{53}$-Trp$_{73}$). This step, which is important for the biological action of ET-1 (in vitro the proform has only 1 per cent of the vasoconstrictor effect of ET-1),[175] is yet to be fully clarified but appears to be mediated by a membrane-bond neutral metalloproteinase identified within both endothelial and vascular smooth muscle cells.[176] It appears likely that the form of this protease may vary in different tissues.

Evidence of ET gene expression has been confirmed in many studies using cultured endothelial cells together with studies of ET-1 mRNA distribution using in situ hybridization.[177] ET-1 mRNA (but not ET-2 or ET-3 gene transcripts) has been detected in cultured human epithelial, endothelial, and vascular smooth muscle cells[178] as well as within neurons of the paraventricular and supraoptic nucleus of the hypothalamus.[179] Recently prepro-ET-1 mRNA has been detected in human endometrium.[180]

Despite the widespread tissue distribution of ET-2 and ET-3, their precise source is currently unknown. Originally thought to be a product only of aortic endothelial cells,[173] subsequent studies of ET-1 mRNA distribution have shown gene expression in a wide variety of vascular tissue endothelial cells, including those of the small resistance blood vessels.[177] The process of peptide release is not well understood but appears to be constitutive—at least in cultured aortic endothelial cells[173]—which is consistent with the low levels of either pro or mature forms found inside the cell. Thus, production of ET appears to be regulated predominantly at the level of mRNA transcription, rather than release of preformed granules in response to stimuli. Induction of ET-1 mRNA (and/or increased peptide release) occurs in response to a variety of mechanical and chemical stimuli, including shear stress,[181] thrombin, transforming growth factor β (TGFβ), epinephrine, arginine vasopressin, angiotensin II, interleukin-1α, and hypoxia.[174, 182] Phorbol esters and calcium ionophores also stimulate gene expression. Some of the stimulatory effects of these factors are likely to be mediated by increase in intracellular ionic calcium and consequent protein kinase C activation.[183] Further, EDRF (NO) appears to inhibit the release of ET-1,[184] which suggests that an intracellular servomechanism (initiated by ET stimulation of EDRF; see below) may exist between the two vasoactive substances. It is obvious from this reasoning that a number of local factors such as pH, blood flow, and hormone levels could be important regulators of ET synthesis and release in vivo. Many tissue homogenates contain immunoreactive ET,[174] ET-1 being the predominant form in most studies.

Receptors and Intracellular Actions

In keeping with the diverse biological actions of ET (see later), specific cell surface binding of ET has been shown, using radioligand binding and autoradiography in vascular smooth muscle cells, adrenal glomerulosa cells, and renal glomeruli, as well as the inner medullary and papillary regions of the kidney.[185] ET receptors are also richly represented in coronary and intrasplenic arteries, pulmonary vessels, the heart, smooth muscle of the respiratory tract, and peripheral nerves, as well as within the central nervous system.[185] Binding of ET-1 in vascular smooth muscle cells is saturable, of high affinity (K_d 0.4 nM[186]), and characterized by slow (irreversible) dissociation. These features may explain in part the protracted nature of the vasoconstrictor action of ET. The range of dissociation constants (0.1–10 nM) of binding sites in various tissues is commensurate with a greater local concentration of ET than is found in plasma of normal human subjects. On these grounds (and in contrast to ANP), a physiological circulatory (hormone) role for ET appears unlikely.

Available evidence strongly supports the view that ET acts in a paracrine and autocrine manner to regulate vasomotor tone (Fig. 154–8). For example, release from the endothelial cell to the underlying vascular smooth muscle cell receptor for ET-1, initiating contraction and possibly facilitating cell growth/proliferation,[183] is consonant with the above findings. In addition, high-affinity ET binding sites are located on the endothelial cell itself and appear to mediate endothelial cell proliferation (mitogenesis).[187] Similarly, ET stimulates EDRF production from endothelial cells,[188] an action that may affect the nature and timing of the vasoconstrictor response. Other autocrine actions of ET (Fig. 154–8) include activation of angiotensin-converting enzyme and increased production of PGI$_2$.

The variation in potency of the three ET's in different tissues and the different structural requirements for EDRF release, as opposed to vasoconstriction, are consistent with the presence of multiple receptors for ET. Two distinct receptors, one highly selective for ET-1 (classified as ET$_A$ with K_d 0.18 nM) and likely to be the vascular smooth muscle ET receptor,[189] the other (ET$_B$) binding equally all three ET's and probably of endothelial cell origin,[190] have now been cloned and characterized. Both receptors are transmembrane proteins, similar to other G protein-coupled receptors, which when activated by ET lead to increased intracellular inositol phosphate production and elevation in free calcium. Both ET$_A$ and ET$_B$ receptors are widely distributed in many tissues, including the central nervous system. Taken together these findings suggest that ET$_A$ receptor mediates the paracrine (vasoconstrictor) action of ET-1, whereas the ET$_B$ receptor mediates the "non-selective" actions of endothelins, including autocrine func-

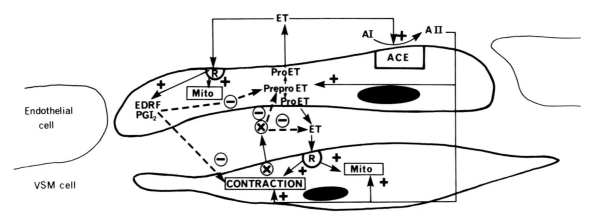

FIGURE 154–8. Autocrine and paracrine actions and modulation of biosynthesis and action of endothelin (ET) in the vascular wall. ET, formed from big ET outside the endothelial cell, can act in an autocrine fashion by stimulating production of endothelium-derived relaxing factors (PGI₂, EDRF), activating angiotensin-converting enzyme (ACE), and promoting gene expression and mitogenesis (Mito). In a paracrine fashion, ET binds to the underlying vascular smooth muscle (VSM) cell, triggers vasoconstriction, and may facilitate mitogenesis. The release of prostacyclin (PGI₂) and EDRF by ET from endothelial cells can mediate vasodilation. Facilitated production of angiotensin II (AII), on the other hand, acts synergistically with ET. The biosynthesis of ET is inhibited by EDRF and by unknown factors (X) released from VSM cells. Proteolytic enzymes at or near the VSM cell surface can degrade ET-1, reducing its bioactivity. *Continuous lines* and *arrows with positive* (+) *signs* indicate facilitation; *interrupted lines* with negative (−) *signs* indicate inhibition. (Adapted from Rubanyi GM, Parker Botelho LH: Endothelins. FASEB J 5:2713–2720, 1991.)

tions such as EDRF release and vasodilatation. Like other vasoactive hormones such as angiotensin II, norepinephrine, and arginine vasopressin, ET initiates vascular smooth muscle cell contraction by activating phospholipase C and associated "second messengers" of the phosphoinositol pathway, which in turn mobilizes intracellular calcium stores. Similar mechanisms of ET action have been found in cultured glomerular mesangial cells. In addition, ET stimulates incorporation of ³H thymidine into quiescent cultures of vascular smooth muscle cells, reflecting new DNA synthesis. These actions, along with enhancing expression of proto-oncogenes, presumably facilitate similar actions of angiotensin II.

Plasma Levels and Metabolism

ET immunoreactivity is present in normal human plasma but at levels less than 5 pmol/L or 12 pg/ml—well below those necessary to initiate biological effects in vitro[173] and much lower than the K_d of identified receptors (0.1–10 nM). Using HPLC techniques, Yamaji et al.[191] showed that pro-ET-1, ET-1, and small amounts of ET-3 were present in normal human plasma and cerebrospinal fluid. Surprisingly, the concentration of immunoreactive pro-ET-1 in plasma is reported to be higher than the mature peptide.[192] Pro-ET-1 is relatively inactive in vitro, but administration in vivo shows potency similar to the mature form, findings suggestive that there may be an important source of the converting enzyme outside the endothelium. Infusion of ET-1 in normal humans[193] shows that the hormone is rapidly cleared across the splanchnic (fractional extraction 75 per cent) and kidney (fractional extraction 60 per cent) tissues and disappears rapidly from arterial plasma (t½ 1.4 and 35 min for first and second phase disappearances curves respectively). Only one form of immunoreactive ET-1 was evident in plasma extracts subjected to reverse phase HPLC analysis. These findings are consistent with the rapid uptake of ET-1 by specific receptors, probably in a wide variety of vascular beds, including those of the lungs, heart,

liver, and kidney. ET is also rapidly cleared across the lung, explaining the reduced effects of intravenous compared to intra-arterial administration. Like ANP, ET-1 is hydrolyzed by endopeptidase EC 24.11 to several smaller (mostly inactive) metabolites,[194] but the importance of this pathway in ET-1 regulation and physiology in vivo is uncertain. Conceivably, EC 24.11 or other similar protease could participate in the degradation of ET adjacent to the vascular smooth muscle cell membrane.

Plasma immunoreactive (IR)-ET-1 is increased by orthostasis[195, 196] and decreased by volume expansion in normal subjects. Levels appear to be unaffected by cold stress or during short-term infusions of norepinephrine. A variety of disease states are associated with increased levels of plasma IR-ET-1, including myocardial infarction,[197] experimental heart failure,[198] septic shock, toxemia of pregnancy, systemic sclerosis, severe renal failure, and pulmonary hypertension.[199] Subjects with Raynaud's syndrome showed elevated values and augmented responses to local cooling[200] when compared to normal subjects. Some[201] but not all[202] studies report higher levels of IR-ET-1 in essential hypertension. Higher than normal levels have also been found in patients with advanced atherosclerosis.[203] In many of the above disorders the significance and source of the abnormal elevation in plasma hormone concentration are unclear. However, in at least one disorder—malignant hemangioendothelioma—a causal connection between hypertension and increased circulating level of ET-1 appears to have been established.[204]

As discussed later, the relevance of plasma ET-1 levels and the possible "hormonal" role of ET still remain in doubt. As indicated in Figure 154–8, the concentration of ET-1 released from endothelial/epithelial cells is presumably much higher at the interface with adjacent smooth muscle cell. Thus plasma (venous) levels may simply represent "spillover" analogous to plasma norepinephrine levels (which serve as markers of sympathetic nervous activity) and may have little physiological significance except perhaps in a few well-defined pathological states. It is to be noted that relatively high concentrations of IR-ET-1 are present in the cerebrospinal fluid,[191] seminal fluid plasma,[205] amniotic fluid, and urine,[206] presumably reflecting the activity of ET production in the relevant tissue of origin.

Biological Actions

Smooth muscle contraction, particularly of vascular smooth muscle of arteries and veins, is the best defined of the many biological actions of ET. In vitro studies indicate a vasoconstrictor potency some 5- to 10-fold that of angiotensin II. The vascular actions of ET-1, the most powerful vasoconstrictor yet isolated, exhibit several unique kinetic features, among them the slow onset of contraction that is sustained and difficult to reverse.[173] Similar effects are observed in vivo (despite the hormone's rapid disappearance rate) and are consistent with findings from kinetic studies of ^{125}I I-ET binding to high-affinity receptors.[207] This action of ET is presumably mediated by influx of extracellular calcium. ET vasoconstrictor actions are inhibited by ANP, possibly at steps subsequent to mobilization of intracellular calcium stores.[208] Interestingly, vasoconstriction is greater when ET is applied to the adventitia than following luminal application—the response of which is increased by removing the endothelium. These findings are consistent with an action of ET to increase EDRF and PGI_2 release (and other products of cyclooxygenase) from the endothelial cell[174]—events that are mediated presumably by the ET_B receptor and are also thought to account for the *initial* vasodilatation observed in vivo after large injections of ET. Vascular smooth muscle contraction induced by ET is critically dependent on the C-terminal tryptophan residue and the two intrachain bridges of which the outer (Cys_1–Cys_{15}) appears to be more important. All three isoforms of ET are qualitatively similar in their actions, although ET-1 is generally the most potent.[185] It now seems likely that these differences are due to different affinities for the ET_A and ET_B receptors and the variable distribution of these receptors in different tissues. Although the local concentration of pro-ET_1 in tissues is likely to be high, its biological activity in vitro is low (1 per cent of ET_1) and requires conversion (at sites still to be determined) to the mature peptide to be effective. ET stimulates DNA synthesis in cultured vascular smooth muscle cells and may be responsible for growth of vascular (intimal) smooth muscle cells that appear to initiate atherosclerosis. Since DNA synthesis is markedly inhibited by antiendothelin antibodies,[209] this mitogenic action of ET could be important in atherogenesis.

Other cardiovascular effects of ET include a dose-dependent positive inotropic effect (direct myocardial action) and an action to increase heart rate.[210] Many other effects, for instance, decrease in GFR, increase in renal vascular resistance, increased bronchial smooth muscle tone, are also likely consequences of endothelin's actions on intracellular calcium within smooth muscle cells. Similar intracellular mechanisms may underlie the inhibition of renin synthesis by ET[211] and the stimulatory effect of ET on the adrenal glomerulosa to increase synthesis and secretion of aldosterone.[212] ET-1 stimulates ANP production both in the heart[213] and in diencephalic neurons of the rat brain.[214] When infused intracerebroventricularly, ET-1 (like angiotensin II) increases arterial blood pressure and sympathetic

nervous activity. These findings strongly suggest a role (along with natriuretic peptides and angiotensin II) in the brain's regulation of cardiovascular function.[215]

The effects of infused ET in humans and experimental animals have confirmed many of the actions reported in vitro and ex vivo. However, it is important to note that effects of high plasma concentration contrived by infusion or injection of ET are likely to be quite different from those produced under physiological conditions by slow release from endothelial cells. Intravenous bolus injection of large doses of ET-1 induces transient hypotension followed by a sustained rise in blood pressure that continues well beyond the increase in plasma ET-1 concentration. The initial fall in blood pressure is likely to be due to ET-induced EDRF release and is more obvious after ET-3 injection. In anesthetized rats and dogs the pressor phase is associated with fall in cardiac output and reduction in heart rate. Systemic and coronary vascular resistance is markedly increased. In keeping with vasoconstriction, renal blood and GFR fall, sodium excretion is reduced, and renin secretion is increased after high doses (e.g., 50 ng/kg/min).[216] More revealing are the effects of small infusions. In anesthetized normal dogs,[217] infusion of ET-1 (2.5 ng/kg/min), sufficient to raise plasma IR-ET-1 twofold, increased renal and systemic vascular resistance without affecting mean arterial pressure or coronary blood flow. A sustained fall in heart rate and cardiac output also occurred. Even at these lower doses, hemodynamic responses continued well beyond the return of plasma ET-1 levels to basal levels. Although renin-aldosterone was unaffected in this study,[217] somewhat higher doses of ET (5 ng/kg/min) reduced renin activity but increased plasma aldosterone.[198]

In humans, step increases in plasma ET-1 (from 1.2 to 56 pmol/L, during exogenous infusion for 45 min) induced small increases in blood pressure (5 per cent), lowered heart rate, but in short-term studies did not affect plasma renin activity or aldosterone or ANP levels.[218] In another study of normal humans,[193] constant infusion of ET-1 (4 pmol/kg/min, achieving peak plasma ET-1 levels of 50 pmol/L at 20 min) induced a sustained fall in splanchnic and renal blood flow that was associated with increased splanchnic and renal vascular resistance and a 7 per cent rise in mean arterial pressure. These studies in normal humans suggest that large increments in ET-1 (as observed for instance in profound septic shock) may have hemodynamic effects, but do not address the likely effects of more physiological levels in plasma. Nonetheless, the studies of the Mayo group in dogs[217] clearly indicate that small increments (two-fold those of basal levels) may have hemodynamic actions particularly on renal vascular resistance and challenge deductions drawn from in vitro findings that predict that much higher concentrations (approximately 100 pmol/L) are required to induce vasoconstriction. Synergism of ET-1 with other vasoconstrictor peptides/factors (especially angiotensin II) could account for the different responses observed in vivo.

Interaction with Other Vasoactive Agents and Significance of Endothelin

Much remains to be learned about the role and significance of local ET, as opposed to circulating levels in blood.[219] Nonetheless it is clear that tissue concentration of ET has an important role in the long-term (hours) control of vasomotor tone and hence in the maintenance of peripheral vascular resistance and possibly therefore in regulating blood pressure in humans. Unlike ANP and BNP (which must circulate in blood from the heart to act peripherally) ET-1 is produced in a wide range of tissues in proximity to specific receptors. Just as ANP/BNP (and possibly CNP[51a]) appear to counterbalance the actions of circulating and tissue angiotensin II, a remarkable interplay among endothelins, angiotensin II, and ANP and BNP appears to dictate the local action of these hormones in many tissues.[114] In addition, ANP, CNP, and ET are good substrates for neutral endopeptidase, which may itself be subject to regulation in a variety of cell membranes. Although the importance of enzyme degradation at cellular level is still unclear, it should be noted that neutral endopeptidase 24.11 would reduce the activity of ANP and possibly reduce the action of angiotensin II. Neutral endopeptidase's action on ET production and degradation in vivo is unclear, but the enzyme has the potential to increase processing to the mature human, as well as to hydrolyze ET to inactive metabolites. Although likely to be important in controlling peripheral vascular resistance, the major role of tissue ET may be to counterbalance other endothelial factors (e.g., EDRF/NO, prostacyclin) contributing to the maintenance of blood fluidity and tissue perfusion.

REFERENCES

1. Guyton AC: Long-term arterial pressure control: An analysis from animal experiments and computer and graphic models. Am J Physiol 259:R865–R877, 1990.
2. de Bold AJ, Borenstein HB, Veress AT, Sonnenberg H: A rapid and potent natriuretic response to intravenous injection of atrial myocardial extract in rats. Life Sci 28:89–94, 1981.
3. Odar-Lederlof I, Theodorsson E, Ericsson F, Kjellstrand CM: Plasma concentrations of calcitonin gene-related peptide in fluid overload. Lancet 338:411–412, 1991.
4. Lundberg J, Torssell L, Sollevi A, et al: Neuropeptide Y and sympathetic vascular control in man. Regul Pept 13:41–52, 1985.
5. Said SI: Neuropeptides in blood pressure control. In Laragh JH, Brenner BM (eds): Hypertension, Pathophysiology, Diagnosis, and Management. New York, Raven Press, 1990, pp 791–804.
6. Ganten D, Paul M, Lang RE: The role of neuropeptides in cardiovascular regulation. Cardiovasc Drugs Ther 5:119–130, 1991.
7. de Bold AJ: Atrial natriuretic factor: A hormone produced by the heart. Science 230:767–770, 1985.
8. Kisch B: Electron microscopy of the atrium of the heart. Exp Med Surg 14:99–112, 1956.
9. Jamieson JD, Palade GE: Specific granules in atrial muscle cells. J Cell Biol 23:151–172, 1964.
10. Kangawa K, Matsuo H: Purification and complete amino acid sequence of alpha-human atrial natriuretic polypeptide (α HANP). Biochem Biophys Res Commun 118:131–139, 1984.
11. Sudoh T, Kangawa K, Minamino N, Matsuo H: A new natriuretic peptide in porcine brain. Nature 332:78–81, 1988.
12. Saito Y, Nakao K, Itoh H, et al: Brain natriuretic peptide is a novel cardiac hormone. Biochem Biophys Res Commun 158:360–368, 1989.
13. Sudoh T, Minamino N, Kangawa K, Matsuo H: C-type natriuretic peptide (CNP): A new member of natriuretic peptide family identified in porcine brain. Biochem Biophys Res Commun 168:863–870, 1990.
14. Tawaragi Y, Fuchimura K, Tanaka S, et al: Gene and precursor structures of human C-type natriuretic peptide. Biochem Biophys Res Commun 175:645–651, 1991.
15. Minamino N, Makino Y, Tateyama H, et al: Characterization of immunoreactive human C-type natriuretic peptide in brain and heart. Biochem Biophys Res Commun 179:535–542, 1991.
15a. Vollmar AM, Gerbes AL, Nemer M, Schulz R: Detection of C-type natriuretic peptide (CNP) transcript in the rat heart and immune organs. Endocrinology 132:1872–1874, 1993.
15b. Clavell AL, Sting AJ, Wei CM, et al: C-type natriuretic peptide: A selective cardiovascular peptide. Am J Physiol 264:R290–R295, 1993.
16. Koller KJ, Lowe DG, Bennett GL, et al: Selective activation of the B natriuretic peptide receptor by C-type natriuretic peptide (CNP). Science 252:120–123, 1991.
17. de Wardener HE: Kidney, salt intake, and Na+, K+-ATPase inhibitors in hypertension. Hypertension 17:830–836, 1991.
18. Hamlyn JM, Blaustein MP, Bova S, et al: Identification and characterization of a ouabain-like compound from human plasma. Proc Natl Acad Sci USA 88:6259–6263, 1991.
19. Matsuo H, Nakazato H: Molecular biology of atrial natriuretic peptides. Endocrinol Metab Clin North Am 16:43–61, 1987.
20. Rosenzweig A, Seidman CE: Atrial natriuretic factor and related peptide hormones. Annu Rev Biochem 60:229–255, 1991.
21. Gardner DG, Deschepper CF, Ganong WF, et al: Extra-atrial expression of the gene for atrial natriuretic factor. Proc Natl Acad Sci USA 83:6698–6701, 1986.
22. Chien KR, Knowlton KU, Zhu H, Chien S: Regulation of cardiac gene expression during myocardial growth and hypertrophy: Molecular studies of an adaptive physiologic response. FASEB J 5:3037–3046, 1991.
23. Brenner BM, Ballermann BJ, Gunning ME, Zeidel ML: Diverse biological actions of atrial natriuretic peptide. Physiol Rev 70:665–699, 1990.
24. Shiono S, Nakao K, Morii N, et al: Nature of atrial natriuretic polypeptide in rat brain. Biochem Biophys Res Commun 135:728–734, 1986.
25. Ritter D, Needleman P, Greenwald JE: Synthesis and secretion of an atriopeptin-like protein in rat kidney cell culture. J Clin Invest 87:208–212, 1990.
26. Schultz-Knappe P, Forssmann K, Herbst F, et al: Isolation and structural analysis of "urodilatin," a new peptide of the cardiodilatin (ANP) -family, extracted from human urine. Klin Wochenschr 66:752–759, 1988.
27. Goetz KL: Renal natriuretic peptide (urodilatin?) and atriopeptin: Evolving concepts. Am J Physiol 261:F921–F932, 1991.
28. Saper CB, Standaert DG, Currie MG, et al: Atriopeptin-immunoreactive neurons in the brain: Presence in cardiovascular regulatory areas. Science 227:1047–1049, 1985.
29. Itoh H, Pratt RE, Dzau VJ: Atrial natriuretic polypeptide inhibits hypertrophy of vascular smooth muscle cells. J Clin Invest 86:1690–1697, 1990.
30. Sundsfjord JA, Thibault G, Larochelle P, Cantin M: N-terminal fragment of proatrial natriuretic factors in the human circulation. J Clin Endocrinol Metab 66:605–610, 1988.
30a. Zeidel ML: Hormonal regulation of inner medullary collecting duct sodium transport. Am J Physiol 265:F159–F173, 1993.
31. Lim AT, Sheward WJ, Copolov D, et al: Atrial natriuretic factor is released into hypophysial portal blood: Direct evidence that atrial natriuretic factor may be a neurohormone involved in hypothalamic pituitary control. J Neuroendocrinol 2:15–18, 1990.
32. Lang RE, Tholken H, Ganten D, et al: Atrial natriuretic factor—a circulating hormone stimulated by volume loading. Nature 314:264–266, 1985.
33. Zimmerman RS, Edwards BS, Schwab TR, et al: Atrial natriuretic peptide during mineralocorticoid escape in the human. J Clin Endocrinol Metab 64:624–627, 1987.
34. Raine AE, Erne P, Burgisser E, et al: Atrial natriuretic peptide and atrial pressure in patients with congestive heart failure. N Engl J Med 315:533–537, 1986.
35. Webster MW, Sharpe DN, Coxon R, et al: Effect of reducing atrial pressure on atrial natriuretic factor and vasoactive hormones in congestive heart failure secondary to ischemic and nonischemic dilated cardiomyopathy. Am J Cardiol 63:217–221, 1989.
36. Nishida Y, Miyata A, Morita H: Lack of neural control of atrial natriuretic peptide release in conscious dogs. Am J Physiol 253:F1164–F1170, 1987.
37. Morris M, Alexander N: Baroreceptor influences on plasma atrial natriuretic peptide (ANP): Sinoaortic denervation reduces basal levels and the response to an osmotic challenge. Endocrinology 122:373–375, 1988.
38. Ruach AL, Callahan MF, Buckalew VM, Morris M: Regulation of plasma atrial natriuretic peptide by the central nervous system. Am J Physiol 258:R531–R535, 1990.
39. Charles CJ, Tang F, Cameron VA, et al: Intracerebroventricular atrial

natriuretic factor (ANF) antiserum inhibits volume-induced ANF in sheep: Evidence for the brain's regulation of ANF secretion. Endocrinology 129:2225–2230, 1991.

40. Itoh H, Nakao K, Yamada T, et al: Brain renin-angiotensin—central control of secretion of atrial natriuretic factor from the heart. Hypertension 11 (Suppl I):I-57–I-61, 1988.

41. Cuneo RC, Espiner EA, Crozier IG, et al: Chronic and acute volume expansion in normal man: Effect on atrial diameter and plasma atrial natriuretic peptide. Horm Metab Res 21:148–151, 1989.

42. Shin Y, Lohmeier TE, Hester RL, et al: Hormonal and circulatory responses to chronically controlled increments in right atrial pressure. Am J Physiol 261: R1176–R1187, 1991.

43. Volpe M, Pepino P, Lembo G, et al: Modulatory role of angiotensin-II in the secretion of atrial natriuretic factor in rabbits. Endocrinology 128:2427–2431, 1991.

44. Leitman DC, Murad F: Atrial natriuretic factor receptor heterogeneity and stimulation of particulate guanylate cyclase and cyclic GMP accumulation. Endocrinol Metab Clin North Am 16:79–105, 1987.

45. Maack T, Suzuki M, Almeida FA, et al: Physiological role of silent receptors of atrial natriuretic factor. Science 238:675–678, 1987.

46. Suga S, Nakao K, Hosoda K, et al: Receptor selectivity of natriuretic peptide family; atrial natriuretic peptide, brain natriuretic peptide, and C-type natriuretic peptide. Endocrinology 130:229–239, 1992.

47. Inagami T: Atrial natriuretic factor. J Biol Chem 264:3043–3046, 1989.

48. Anand-Srivastava MB, Sairam MR, Cantin M: Ring-deleted analogs of atrial natriuretic factor inhibit adenylate cyclase/cAMP system. J Biol Chem 265:8566–8572, 1990.

49. Hirata M, Chang C-H, Murad F: Stimulatory effects of atrial natriuretic factor on phosphoinositide hydrolysis in cultured bovine aortic smooth muscle cells. Biochim Biophys Acta 1010:346–351, 1989.

50. Cahill PA, Hassid A: Clearance receptor-binding atrial natriuretic peptides inhibit mitogenesis and proliferation of rat aortic smooth muscle cells. Biochem Biophys Res Commun 179:1606–1613, 1991.

50a. Levin ER: Natriuretic peptide C-receptor: More than a clearance receptor. Am J Physiol 264:E483–E489, 1993.

51. Wilcox JN, Augustine A, Goeddel DV, Lowe DG: Differential regional expression of three natriuretic peptide receptor genes within primate tissues. Mol Cell Biol 11:3454–3462, 1991.

51a. Suga S, Nakao K, Itoh H, et al: Endothelial production of C-type natriuretic peptide and its marked augmentation by transforming growth factor-β. Possible existence of "vascular natriuretic peptide system." J Clin Invest 90:1145–1149, 1992.

52. Smith JB, Lincoln TM: Angiotensin decreases cyclic GMP accumulation produced by atrial natriuretic factor. Am J Physiol 253:C147–C150, 1987.

53. Cahill PA, Redmond EM, Keenan AK: Vascular atrial natriuretic factor receptor subtypes are not independently regulated by atrial peptides. J Biol Chem 265:21896–21906, 1990.

54. Lanier-Smith KL, Currie MG: Glucocorticoid regulation of atrial natriuretic peptide receptors on cultured endothelial cells. Endocrinology 129:2311–2317, 1991.

55. Hirata Y, Ishii M, Matsuoka H, et al: Plasma concentrations of α-human atrial natriuretic polypeptide and cyclic GMP in patients with heart disease. Am Heart J 113:1463–1469, 1987.

56. Charles CJ, Espiner EA, Cameron VA, Richards AM: Hemodynamic, renal, and endocrine actions of ANF in sheep: Effect of 24-h, low dose infusions. Am J Physiol 258:R1279–R1285, 1990.

57. Bell GM, Atlas SA, Pecker M, et al: Diurnal and postural variations in plasma atrial natriuretic factor, plasma guanosine 3′:5′-cyclic monophosphate and sodium excretion. Clin Sci 79:371–376, 1990.

58. Sugawara A, Nakao K, Morii N, et al: α-Human atrial natriuretic polypeptide is released from the heart and circulates in the body. Biochem Biophys Res Commun 129:439–446, 1985.

59. Yandle TG, Espiner EA, Nicholls MG, Duff H: Radioimmunoassay and characterization of atrial natriuretic peptide in human plasma. J Clin Endocrinol Metab 63:72–79, 1986.

60. Ando K, Hirata Y, Emori T, et al: Circulating forms of human atrial natriuretic peptide in patients with congestive heart failure. J Clin Endocrinol Metab 70:1603–1607, 1990.

61. Yandle T, Crozier I, Nicholls G, et al: Amino acid sequence of atrial natriuretic peptides in human coronary sinus plasma. Biochem Biophys Res Commun 146:832–839, 1987.

62. Espiner EA, Nicholls MG: Human atrial natriuretic peptide. Clin Endocrinol 26:637–650, 1987.

63. Crozier IG, Nicholls MG, Ikram H, et al: Atrial natriuretic peptide in humans—Production and clearance by various tissues. Hypertension 8 (Suppl II):II-11–II-15, 1986.

64. Yandle TG, Richards AM, Nicholls MG, et al: Metabolic clearance rate and plasma half life of alpha-human atrial natriuretic peptide in man. Life Sci 38:1827–1833, 1986.

65. Richards AM, Wittert G, Espiner EA, et al: EC 24.11 inhibition in man alters clearance of atrial natriuretic peptide. J Clin Endocrinol Metab 72:1317–1322, 1991.

66. Richards M, Espiner E, Frampton C, et al: Inhibition of endopeptidase EC 24.11 in humans—renal and endocrine effects. Hypertension 16:269–276, 1990.

67. Schwartz J-C, Gros C, Lecomte J-M, Bralet J: Enkephalinase (EC 3.4.24.11) inhibitors: Protection of endogenous ANF against inactivation and potential therapeutic applications. Life Sci 47:1279–1297, 1990.

67a. Kenny AJ, Bourne A, Ingram J: Hydrolysis of human and pig brain natriuretic peptides, urodilatin, C-type natriuretic peptide and some C-receptor ligands by endopeptidase-24.11. Biochem J 291:83–88, 1993.

67b. Wei CM, Kao PC, Lin JT, et al: Circulating β-atrial natriuretic factor in congestive heart failure in humans. Circulation 88:1016–1020, 1993.

68. Yasue H, Obata K, Okumura K, et al: Increased secretion of atrial natriuretic polypeptide from the left ventricle in patients with dilated cardiomyopathy. J Clin Invest 83:46–51, 1989.

69. Nicklas JM, Benedict C, Johnstone DE, et al: Relationship between neurohumoral profile and one year mortality in patients with CHF and/or LV dysfunction. Circulation 84(Suppl II):II468, 1991.

70. Sugawara A, Nekar K, Sakamoto M, et al: Plasma concentration of atrial natriuretic polypeptide in essential hypertension. Lancet 2:1426–1427, 1985.

71. Atlas SA, Laragh JH: Atrial natriuretic factor and its involvement in hypertensive disorders. In Laragh JH, Brenner BM (eds): Hypertension: Pathophysiology, Diagnosis, and Management. New York, Raven Press, 1990, pp 861–883.

72. Sergev O, Racz K, Varga I, et al: Atrial natriuretic peptide in normal and low renin essential hypertension. Kidney Int 38:S107–S108, 1990.

73. Jin H, Chen Y-F, Yang R-H, et al: Impaired release of atrial natriuretic factor in NaCl-loaded spontaneously hypertensive rats. Hypertension 11:739–744, 1988.

74. Ferrari P, Weidmann P, Ferrier C, et al: Dysregulation of atrial natriuretic factor in hypertension-prone man. J Clin Endocrinol Metab 71:944–951, 1990.

75. Steinhelper ME, Cochrane KL, Field LJ: Hypotension in transgenic mice expressing atrial natriuretic factor fusion genes. Hypertension 16:301–307, 1990.

76. Gordon RD, Tunny TJ, Klemm SA, Hamlet SM: Elevated levels of plasma atrial natriuretic peptide in Bartter's syndrome fall to normal with indomethacin: Implications for atrial natriuretic peptide regulation in man. J Hypertension 4:S555–S558, 1986.

77. Shimizu K, Nakano S, Nakano Y, et al: Ectopic atrial natriuretic peptide production in small cell lung cancer with the syndrome of inappropriate antidiuretic hormone secretion. Cancer 68:2284–2288, 1991.

78. Maack T, Marion DN, Camargo MJ, et al: Effects of auriculin (atrial natriuretic factor) on blood pressure, renal function, and the renin-aldosterone system in dogs. Am J Med 77:1069–1075, 1984.

79. Atlas SA, Maack T: Effects of atrial natriuretic factor on the kidney and the renin-angiotensin-aldosterone system. Endocrinol Metab Clin North Am 16:107–143, 1987.

80. Lanese DM, Yuan BH, Falk SA, Conger JD: Effects of atriopeptin III on isolated rat afferent and efferent arterioles. Am J Physiol 261:F1102–F1109, 1991.

81. Sosa RE, Volpe M, Marion DN, et al: Relationship between renal hemodynamic and natriuretic effects of atrial natriuretic factor. Am J Physiol 250:F520–F524, 1986.

82. Janssen MT, de Zeeuw D, van der Hem GK, de Jong PE: Antihypertensive effect of a 5-day infusion of atrial natriuretic peptide in man. Hypertension 13:640–646, 1989.

83. Mizelle HL, Hildebrandt DA, Gaillard CA, et al: Atrial natriuretic peptide induces sustained natriuresis in conscious dogs. Am J Physiol 258:R1445–R1452, 1990.

84. Hildebrandt DA, Mizelle HL, Brands MW, et al: Intrarenal atrial natriuretic peptide infusion lowers arterial pressure chronically. Am J Physiol 259:R585–R592, 1990.

85. Field LJ, Veress AT, Steinhelper ME, et al: Kidney function in ANF-transgenic mice: Effect of blood volume expansion. Am J Physiol 260:R1–R5, 1991.

86. Cody RJ, Atlas SA, Laragh JH, et al: Atrial natriuretic factor in normal

subjects and heart failure patients—plasma levels and renal, hormonal, and hemodynamic responses to peptide infusion. J Clin Invest 78:1362–1374, 1986.

87. Crozier IG, Nicholls MG, Ikram H, et al: Haemodynamic effects of atrial peptide infusion in heart failure. Lancet 2:1242–1245, 1986.

88. Riegger GA, Elsner D, Kromer EP, et al: Atrial natriuretic peptide in congestive heart failure in the dog: Plasma levels, cyclic guanosine monophosphate, ultrastructure of atrial myoendocrine cells, and hemodynamic, hormonal, and renal effects. Circulation 77:398–406, 1988.

89. Abassi Z, Haramati A, Hoffman A, et al: Effect of converting-enzyme inhibition on renal response to ANF in rats with experimental heart failure. Am J Physiol 259:R84–R89, 1990.

90. Margulies KB, Perrella MA, McKinley LJ, et al: Angiotensin inhibition potentiates the renal responses to neutral endopeptidase inhibition in dogs with congestive heart failure. J Clin Invest 88:1636–1642, 1991.

91. Richards AM, Rao G, Espiner EA, Yandle T: Interaction of angiotensin converting enzyme inhibition and atrial natriuretic factor. Hypertension 13:193–199, 1989.

92. Margulies KB, Heublein DM, Perrella MA, Burnett JC: ANF-mediated renal cGMP generation in congestive heart failure. Am J Physiol 260:F562–F568, 1991.

93. Richards AM, Nicholls MG, Espiner EA, et al: Effects of α-human atrial natriuretic peptide in essential hypertension. Hypertension 7:812–817, 1985.

94. Richards AM, Espiner EA, Ikram H, Yandle TG: Atrial natriuretic factor in hypertension: Bioactivity at normal plasma levels. Hypertension 14:261–268, 1989.

95. Garcia R, Gutkowska J, Genest J, et al: Reduction of blood pressure and increased diuresis and natriuresis during chronic infusion of atrial natriuretic factor (ANF Arg 101-Tyr 126) in conscious one-kidney, one-clip hypertensive rats. Proc Soc Exp Biol Med 179:539–545, 1985.

96. Lappe RW, Smits JF, Todt JA, et al: Failure of atriopeptin II to cause arterial vasodilation in the conscious rat. Circ Res 56:606–612, 1985.

97. Shapiro JT, Deleonardis VM, Needleman P, Hintze TH: Integrated cardiac and peripheral vascular response to atriopeptin 24 in conscious dogs. Am J Physiol 251:H1292–H1297, 1986.

98. Valentin JP, Ribstein J, Mimran A: Effect of nicardipine and atriopeptin on transcapillary shift of fluid and proteins. Am J Physiol 257:R174–R179, 1989.

99. Huxley VH, Tucker VL, Verburg KM, Freeman RH: Increased capillary hydraulic conductivity induced by atrial natriuretic peptide. Circulation Res 60:304–307, 1987.

100. Villanueva MM, Nunes JP, Soares-da-Silva P: Relaxant effects of α-human atrial natriuretic peptide on venous smooth muscle. J Auton Pharmacol 11:139–145, 1991.

101. Bache RJ, Dai X-Z, Schwartz JS, Chen DG: Effects of atrial natriuretic peptide in the canine coronary circulation. Circ Res 62:178–183, 1988.

102. Thoren P, Mark AL, Morgan DA, et al: Activation of vagal depressor reflexes by atriopeptins inhibits renal sympathetic nerve activity. Am J Physiol 251:H1252–H1259, 1986.

103. Volpe M, Lembo G, Condorelli G, et al: Converting enzyme inhibition prevents the effects of atrial natriuretic factor on baroreflex responses in humans. Circulation 82:1214–1221, 1990.

104. Ferrari AU, Daffonchio A, Sala C, et al: Atrial natriuretic factor and arterial baroreceptor reflexes in unanesthetized rats. Hypertension 15:162–167, 1990.

105. Richards AM, Nicholls MG, Ikram H, et al: Renal, haemodynamic, and hormonal effects of human alpha atrial natriuretic peptide in healthy volunteers. Lancet 1:545–549, 1985.

106. Groban L, Cowley AW, Ebert TJ: Atrial natriuretic peptide augments forearm capillary filtration in humans. Am J Physiol 259:H258–H263, 1990.

107. Bruun NE, Skott P, Giese J: Renal and endocrine effects of physiological variations of atrial natriuretic factor in normal humans. Am J Physiol 260:R217–R224, 1991.

108. Parkes DG, Coghlan JP, McDougall JG, Scoggins BA: Long-term hemodynamic actions of atrial natriuretic factor (99–126) in conscious sheep. Am J Physiol 254:H811–H815, 1988.

109. Charles CJ, Espiner EA, Richards AM: Cardiovascular actions of ANF: Contributions of renal, neurohumoral and hemodynamic factors in sheep. Am J Physiol 264:R533–R538, 1993.

110. Garcia R, Thibault G, Gutkowska J, et al: Effect of chronic infusion of synthetic atrial natriuretic factor (ANF 8-33) in conscious two-kidney, one-clip hypertensive rats. Proc Soc Exp Biol Med 178:155–159, 1985.

111. Munzel T, Drexler H, Holtz J, et al: Mechanisms involved in the response to prolonged infusion of atrial natriuretic factor in patients with chronic heart failure. Circulation 83:191–201, 1991.

112. Baron DA, Lofton CE, Newman WH, Currie MG: Atriopeptin inhibition of thrombin-mediated changes in the morphology and permeability of endothelial monolayers. Proc Natl Acad Sci USA 86:3394–3398, 1989.

113. Lofton CE, Newman WH, Currie MG: Atrial natriuretic peptide regulation of endothelial permeability. Biochem Biophys Res Commun 172:793–799, 1990.

114. Kohno M, Yasunari K, Yokokawa K, et al: Inhibition by atrial and brain natriuretic peptides of endothelin-1 secretion after stimulation with angiotensin II and thrombin of cultured human endothelial cells. J Clin Invest 87:1999–2004, 1991.

115. Espiner EA, Richards AM: Atrial natriuretic peptide—an important factor in sodium and blood pressure regulation. Lancet 1:707–710, 1989.

116. Weidmann P, Hasler L, Gnadinger MP, et al: Blood levels and renal effects of atrial natriuretic peptide in normal man. J Clin Invest 77:734–742, 1986.

117. Garcia R, Thibault G, Gutkowska J, Cantin M: Effect of chronic infusion of atrial natriuretic factor on plasma and urinary aldosterone, plasma renin activity, blood pressure and sodium excretion in 2-K, 1-C hypertensive rats. Clin Exp Hypertens A8:1127–1147, 1986.

118. Nagano M, Bravo EL: Impaired aldosterone production by long-term infusion of atrial natriuretic factor. Am J Physiol 258:E51–E56, 1990.

119. Opgenorth TJ, Burnett JC, Granger JP, Scriven TA: Effects of atrial natriuretic peptide on renin secretion in nonfiltering kidney. Am J Physiol 250:F798–F801, 1986.

120. Goodfriend TL, Elliott ME, Atlas SA: Actions of synthetic atrial natriuretic factor on bovine adrenal glomerulosa. Life Sci 35:1675–1682, 1984.

121. Aguilera G: Differential effects of atrial natriuretic factor on angiotensin II and adrenocorticotropin-stimulated aldosterone secretion. Endocrinology 120:299–304, 1987.

122. Lotshaw DP, Franco-Saenz R, Mulrow PJ: Atrial natriuretic peptide inhibition of calcium ionophore A23187-stimulated aldosterone secretion in rat adrenal glomerulosa cells. Endocrinology 129:2305–2310, 1991.

123. Saito Y, Nakao K, Nishimura K, et al: Clinical application of atrial natriuretic polypeptide in patients with congestive heart failure: Beneficial effects on left ventricular function. Circulation 76:115–124, 1987.

124. Volpe M, Odell G, Kleinert HD, et al: Effect of atrial natriuretic factor on blood pressure, renin and aldosterone in Goldblatt hypertension. Hypertension 7(Suppl I):I43–I48, 1985.

125. Rabelink TJ, Koomans HA, van de Stolpe A, et al: Effects of atrial natriuretic peptide on distal tubule function in humans. Kidney Int 37:996–1001, 1990.

126. Samson WK: Atrial natriuretic factor and the central nervous system. Endocrinol Metab Clin North Am 16:145–161, 1987.

127. Burrell LM, Lambert HJ, Baylis PH: Effect of atrial natriuretic peptide on thirst and arginine vasopressin release in humans. Am J Physiol 260:R475–R479, 1991.

128. Ibanez-Santos J, Tsagarakis S, Rees LH, et al: Atrial natriuretic peptides inhibit the release of corticotrophin-releasing factor-41 from the rat hypothalamus in vitro. J Endocrinol 126:223–228, 1990.

129. King MS, Baertschi AJ: Physiological concentrations of atrial natriuretic factors with intact N-Terminal sequences inhibit corticotropin-releasing factor-stimulated adrenocorticotropin secretion from cultured anterior pituitary cells. Endocrinology 124:286–292, 1989.

130. Kovacs KJ, Antoni A: Atriopeptin inhibits stimulated secretion of adrenocorticotropin in rats: Evidence for a pituitary site of action. Endocrinology 127:3003–3008, 1990.

131. Fink G, Dow RC, Casley D, et al: Atrial natriuretic peptide is a physiological inhibitor of ACTH release: Evidence from immunoneutralization in vivo. J Endocrinol 131:R9–R12, 1991.

132. Wittert GA, Espiner EA, Richards AM, et al: Atrial natriuretic factor reduces vasopressin and angiotensin II but not the ACTH response to acute hypoglycaemia stress in normal men. Clin Endocrinol 38:183–189, 1993.

133. Unger T, Badoer E, Gareis C, et al: Atrial natriuretic peptide (ANP) as a neuropeptide: Interaction with angiotensin II on volume control and renal sodium handling. Br J Clin Pharmacol 30:83S–88S, 1990.

134. Standaert DG, Cechetto DF, Needleman P, Saper CB: Inhibition of the firing of vasopressin neurons by atriopeptin. Nature 329:151–153, 1987.

135. Badoer E, Unger T, Ganten D: Role of the endocrine brain in the

control of hypertension—angiotensin II and atrial natriuretic peptide in the brain. *In* Motta M (ed): Brain Endocrinology (ed 3). New York, Raven Press, 1991, pp 403–430.

136. Levin ER, Mills S, Weber MA: Central nervous system mediated vasodepressor action of atrial natriuretic factor. Life Sci 44:1617–1624, 1989.

137. Casto R, Hilbig J, Schroeder G, Stock G: Atrial natriuretic factor inhibits central angiotensin II pressor responses. Hypertension 9:473–477, 1987.

138. Ermirio R, Ruggeri P, Cogo CA, et al: Neuronal and cardiovascular responses to ANF microinjected into nucleus ambiguus. Am J Physiol 260:R1089–R1094, 1991.

139. Goetz KL: Evidence that atriopeptin is not a physiological regulator of sodium excretion. Hypertension 15:9–19, 1990.

140. Hirsch AT, Creager MA, Dzau VJ: Relation of atrial natriuretic factor to vasoconstrictor hormones and regional blood flow in congestive heart failure. Am J Cardiol 63:211–216, 1989.

141. Schrier RW, Howard RL: Unifying hypothesis of sodium and water regulation in health and disease. Hypertension 18 (Suppl III):III164–III168, 1991.

142. Westenfelder C, Birch FM, Baranowski RL, et al: Volume homeostasis in calves with artificial atria and ventricles. Am J Physiol 258:F1005–F1017, 1990.

143. Villarreal D, Freeman RH: ANF and the renin-angiotensin system in the regulation of sodium balance: Longitudinal studies in experimental heart failure. J Lab Clin Med 118:515–522, 1991.

144. Canton AD, Romano G, Conte G: Role of atrial natriuretic factor in renal adaptation to variation of salt intake in humans. Am J Physiol 258:F1579–F1583, 1990.

145. Stasch J-P, Hirth-Dietrich C, Kazda S, Neuser D: Role of endogenous ANP on endocrine function investigated with a monoclonal antibody. Peptides 11:577–582, 1990.

146. Cowley AW, Skelton MM: Dominance of colloid osmotic pressure in renal excretion after isotonic volume expansion. Am J Physiol 261:H1214–H1225, 1991.

147. Sudoh T, Maekawa K, Kojima M, et al: Cloning and sequence analysis of cDNA encoding a precursor for human brain natriuretic peptide. Biochem Biophys Res Commun 159:1427–1434, 1989.

148. Kojima M, Minamino N, Kangawa K, Matsuo H: Cloning and sequence analysis of cDNA encoding a precursor for rat brain natriuretic peptide. Biochem Biophys Res Commun 159:1420–1426, 1989.

149. Kambayashi Y, Nakao K, Kimura H, et al: Biological characterization of human brain natriuretic peptide (BNP) and rat BNP: Species-specific actions of BNP. Biochem Biophys Res Commun 173:599–605, 1990.

150. Sudoh T, Minamino N, Kangawa K, Matsuo H: Brain natriuretic peptide-32: N-terminal six amino acid extended form of brain natriuretic peptide identified in porcine brain. Biochem Biophys Res Commun 155:726–732, 1988.

151. Minamino N, Aburaya M, Ueda S, et al: The presence of brain natriuretic peptide of 12,000 daltons in porcine heart. Biochem Biophys Res Commun 155:740–746, 1988.

152. Mukoyama M, Nakao K, Hosoda K, et al: Brain natriuretic peptide as a novel cardiac hormone in humans—evidence for an exquisite dual natriuretic peptide system, atrial natriuretic peptide and brain natriuretic peptide. J Clin Invest 87:1402–1412, 1991.

153. Ogawa Y, Nakao K, Mukoyama M, et al: Natriuretic peptides as cardiac hormones in normotensive and spontaneously hypertensive rats—The ventricle is a major site of synthesis and secretion of brain natriuretic peptide. Circ Res 69:491–500, 1991.

154. Hosoda K, Nakao K, Mukoyama M, et al: Expression of brain natriuretic peptide gene in human heart—production in the ventricle. Hypertension 17:1152–1156, 1991.

155. Yokota N, Aburaya M, Yamamoto Y, et al: Increased plasma brain natriuretic peptide levels in DOCA–salt hypertensive rats: Relation to blood pressure and cardiac concentration. Biochem Biophys Res Commun 173:632–638, 1990.

156. Ueda S, Minamino N, Sudoh T, et al: Regional distribution of immunoreactive brain natriuretic peptide in porcine brain and spinal cord. Biochem Biophys Res Commun 155:733–739, 1988.

157. Yokota N, Aburaya M, Yamamoto Y, et al: Cardiac content of brain natriuretic peptide in DOCA–salt hypertensive rats. Life Sci 48:397–402, 1991.

158. Mukoyama M, Nakao K, Saito Y, et al: Human brain natriuretic peptide, a novel cardiac hormone. Lancet 335:801, 1990.

158a. Kinnunen P, Vuolteenaho O, Ruskoaho H: Mechanisms of atrial and brain natriuretic peptide release from rat ventricular myocardium: Effect of stretching. Endocrinology 132:1961–1970, 1993.

159. Shubeita HE, McDonough PM, Harris AN, et al: Endothelin induction of inositol phospholipid hydrolysis, sarcomere assembly, and cardiac gene expression in ventricular myocytes. A paracrine mechanism for myocardial cell hypertrophy. J Biol Chem 265:20555–20562, 1990.

160. Marumo F, Matsubara O, Masaki Y, et al: Degradation and distribution of brain natriuretic peptide in porcine tissues. J Endocrinol 132:101–106, 1992.

161. Yandle TG, Richards AM, Gilbert A, et al: Assay of brain natriuretic peptide (BNP) in human plasma: Evidence for high molecular weight BNP as a major plasma component in heart failure. J Clin Endocrinol Metab 76:832–838, 1993.

162. Togashi K, Kameya T, Ando K, et al: Brain natriuretic peptides in human plasma, spinal cord and cerebrospinal fluid. Clin Chim Acta 201:193–200, 1991.

163. Mukoyama M, Nakao K, Obata K, et al: Augmented secretion of brain natriuretic peptide in acute myocardial infarction. Biochem Biophys Res Commun 180:431–436, 1991.

164. Lang CC, Coutie WJ, Khong TK, et al: Dietary sodium loading increases plasma brain natriuretic peptide levels in man. J Hypertension 9:779–882, 1991.

164a. Mowani JG, McAlpine H, Kennedy N, Struthers AD: Plasma brain natriuretic peptide as an indicator for angiotensin-converting enzyme inhibin after myocardial infarction. Lancet 341:1109–1113, 1993.

164b. Nicholson S, Richards M, Espiner E, et al: Atrial and natriuretic peptide response to exercise in patients with ischemic heart disease. Clin Exp Pharm Physiol 20:535–540, 1993.

164c. Lang CC, Choy AJ, Turner K, et al: The effect of intravenous saline loading on plasma levels of brain natriuretic peptide in man. J Hypertension 11:737–741, 1993.

165. Norman JA, Little D, Bolgar M, Di Donato G: Degradation of brain natriuretic peptide by neutral endopeptidase: Species specific sites of proteolysis determined by mass spectrometry. Biochem Biophys Res Commun 175:22–30, 1991.

166. Lang CC, Motwani J, Coutie WJ, Struthers AD: Influence of candoxatril on plasma brain natriuretic peptide in heart failure. Lancet 338:255, 1991.

167. Song D-Li, Kohse KP, Murad F: Brain natriuretic factor—augmentation of cellular cyclic GMP, activation of particulate guanylate cyclase and receptor binding. FEBS Letters 232:125–129, 1988.

168. McGregor A, Richards M, Espiner E, et al: Brain natriuretic peptide administered to man: Actions and metabolism. J Clin Endocrinol Metab 70:1103–1107, 1990.

169. Holmes SJ, Espiner EA, Richards AM, et al: Renal, endocrine and hemodynamic effects of human brain natriuretic peptide in normal man. J Clin Endocrinol Metab 76:91–96, 1993.

170. Yoshimura M, Yasue H, Morita E, et al: Hemodynamic, renal, and hormonal responses to brain natriuretic peptide infusion in patients with congestive heart failure. Circulation 84:1581–1588, 1991.

171. Moncada S, Gryglewski R, Bunting S, Vane JR: An enzyme isolated from arteries transforms prostaglandin endoperoxides to an unstable substance that inhibits platelet aggregation. Nature 263:663–665, 1976.

172. Hickey KA, Rubanyi GM, Paul RJ, Highsmith RF: Characterization of a coronary vasoconstrictor produced by endothelial cells in culture. Am J Physiol 248:C550–C556, 1985.

173. Yanagisawa M, Kurihara H, Kimura S, et al: A novel potent vasoconstrictor peptide produced by vascular endothelial cells. Nature 332:411–415, 1988.

174. Rubanyi GM, Botelho LH: Endothelins. FASEB J 5:2713–415, 1988.

175. Kimura S, Kasuya Y, Sawamura T, et al: Conversion of big endothelin-1 to 21-residue endothelin-1 is essential for expression of full vasoconstrictor activity: Structure-activity relationships of big endothelin-1. J Cardiovasc Pharmacol 13:S5–S7, 1989.

176. Matsumura Y, Ikegawa R, Tsukahara Y, et al: Conversion of big endothelin-1 to endothelin-1 by two-types of metalloproteinases of cultured porcine vascular smooth muscle cells. Biochem Biophys Res Commun 178:899–905, 1991.

177. Nunez DJ, Brown MJ, Davenport AP, et al: Endothelin-1 mRNA is widely expressed in porcine and human tissues. J Clin Invest 85:1537–1541, 1990.

178. Resink TJ, Hahn AW, Scott-Burden T, et al: Inducible endothelin mRNA expression and peptide secretion in cultured human vascular smooth muscle cells. Biochem Biophys Res Commun 168:1303–1310, 1990.

179. Yoshizawa T, Shinmi O, Giaid A, et al: Endothelin: A novel peptide in the posterior pituitary system. Science 247:462–464, 1990.

180. Economos K, MacDonald PC, Casey ML: Endothelin-1 gene expression and protein biosynthesis in human endometrium: potential modulator of endometrial blood flow. J Clin Endocrinol Metab 74:14–19, 1992.

181. Yoshizumi M, Kurihara H, Sugiyama T, et al: Hemodynamic shear stress stimulates endothelin production by cultured endothelial cells. Biochem Biophys Res Commun 161:859–864, 1989.

182. Emori T, Hirata Y, Ohta K, et al: Secretory mechanism of immunoreactive endothelin in cultured bovine endothelial cells. Biochem Biophys Res Commun 160:93–100, 1989.

183. Simonson MS, Dunn MJ: Cellular signalling by peptides of the endothelin gene family. FASEB J 4:2989–3000, 1990.

184. Boulanger C, Luscher TF: Release of endothelin from the porcine aorta: Inhibition by endothelium-derived nitric oxide. J Clin Invest 85:587–590, 1990.

185. Brenner BM, Troy JL, Ballermann BJ: Endothelium-dependent vascular responses. J Clin Invest 84:1373–1378, 1989.

186. Hirata Y, Yoshimi H, Takata S, et al: Cellular mechanism of action by a novel vasoconstrictor endothelin in cultured rat vascular smooth muscle cells. Biochem Biophys Res Commun 154:868–875, 1988.

187. Vigne P, Marsault R, Breittmayer JP, Frelin C: Endothelin stimulates phosphatidylinositol hydrolysis and DNA synthesis in brain capillary endothelial cells. Biochemistry 266:415–420, 1990.

188. DeNucci G, Thomas R, D'Orleans-Juste P, et al: Pressor effects of circulating endothelin are limited by its removal in the pulmonary circulation and by the release of prostacyclin and endothelium-derived relaxing factor. Proc Natl Acad Sci USA 85:9797–9800, 1988.

189. Arai H, Hori S, Aramori I, et al: Cloning and expression of a cDNA encoding an endothelin receptor. Nature 348:730–732, 1990.

190. Sakurai T, Yanagisawa M, Takuwa Y, et al: Cloning of a cDNA encoding a non-isopeptide-selective subtype of the endothelin receptor. Nature 348:732–735, 1990.

191. Yamaji T, Johshita H, Ishibashi M, et al: Endothelin family in human plasma and cerebrospinal fluid. J Clin Endocrinol Metab 71:1611–1615, 1990.

192. Saito Y, Nakao K, Itoh H, et al: Endothelin in human plasma and culture medium of aortic endothelial cells: Detection and characterization with radioimmunoassay using monoclonal antibody. Biochem Biophys Res Commun 161:320–326, 1989.

193. Weitzberg E, Ahlborg G, Lundberg JM: Long-Lasting vasoconstriction and efficient regional extraction of endothelin-1 in human splanchnic and renal tissues. Biochem Biophys Res Commun 180:1298–1303, 1991.

194. Vijayaraghavan J, Scicli AG, Carretero OA, et al: The hydrolysis of endothelins by neutral endopeptidase 24.11 (enkephalinase). J Biol Chem 265:14150–14155, 1990.

195. Schichiri M, Hirata Y, Ando K, et al: Postural change and volume expansion affect plasma endothelin levels. JAMA 263:661, 1990.

196. Kaufmann H, Oribe E, Oliver JA: Plasma endothelin during upright tilt: Relevance for orthostatic hypotension? Lancet 338:1542–1545, 1991.

197. Miyauchi T, Yanagisawa M, Tomizawa T, et al: Increased plasma concentrations of endothelin-1 and big endothelin-1 in acute myocardial infarction. Lancet 2:53–54, 1989.

198. Cavero PG, Miller WL, Heublein DM, et al: Endothelin in experimental congestive heart failure in the anesthetized dog. Am J Physiol 259:F312–F317, 1990.

199. Yoshibayashi M, Nishioka K, Nakao K, et al: Plasma endothelin concentrations in patients with pulmonary hypertension associated with congenital heart defects—evidence for increased production of endothelin in pulmonary circulation. Circulation 84:2280–2285, 1991.

200. Zamora MR, O'Brien RF, Rutherford R, Weil JV: Serum endothelin-1 concentrations and cold provocation in primary Raynaud's phenomenon. Lancet 336:1144–1147, 1990.

201. Saito Y, Nakao K, Mukoyama M, Imura H: Increased plasma endothelin level in patients with essential hypertension. N Engl J Med 322:205, 1990.

202. Davenport AP, Ashby MJ, Easton P, et al: A sensitive radioimmunoassay measuring endothelin-like immunoreactivity in human plasma: Comparison of levels in patients with essential hypertension and normotensive control subjects. Clin Sci 78:261–264, 1990.

203. Lerman A, Edwards BS, Hallett JW, et al: Circulating and tissue endothelin immunoreactivity in advanced atherosclerosis. N Engl J Med 325:997–1001, 1991.

204. Yokokawa K, Tahara H, Kohno M, et al: Hypertension associated with endothelin-secreting malignant hemangioendothelioma. Ann Intern Med 114:213–215, 1991.

205. Casey ML, Byrd W, MacDonald PC: Massive amounts of immunoreactive endothelin in human seminal fluid. J Clin Endocrinol Metab 74:223–225, 1992.

206. Berbinschi A, Ketelslegers JM: Endothelin in urine. Lancet 2:46, 1989.

207. Martin ER, Marsden PA, Brenner BM, Ballermann BJ: Identification and characterization of endothelin binding sites in rat renal papillary and glomerular membranes. Biochem Biophys Res Commun 162:130–137, 1989.

208. Suzuki E, Hirata Y, Matsuoka H, et al: Effects of atrial natriuretic peptide on endothelin-induced vasoconstriction and intracellular calcium mobilization. J Hypertension 9:927–934, 1991.

209. Takagi Y, Fukase M, Takata S, et al: Autocrine effect of endothelin on DNA synthesis in human vascular endothelial cells. Biochem Biophys Res Commun 168:537–543, 1990.

210. Donckier JE, Hanet C, Berbinschi A, et al: Cardiovascular and endocrine effects of endothelin-1 at pathophysiological and pharmacological plasma concentrations in conscious dogs. Circulation 84:2476–2484, 1991.

211. Kurtz A, Kaissling B, Busse R, Baier W: Endothelial cells modulate renin secretion from isolated mouse juxtaglomerular cells. J Clin Invest 88:1147–1154, 1991.

212. Cozza EN, Gomez-Sanchez CE, Foecking MF, Chiou S: Endothelin binding to cultured calf adrenal zona glomerulosa cells and stimulation of aldosterone secretion. J Clin Invest 84:1032–1035, 1989.

213. Schiebinger RJ, Gomez-Sanchez CE: Endothelin: A potent stimulus of atrial natriuretic peptide secretion by superfused rat atria and its dependency on calcium. Endocrinology 127:119–125, 1990.

214. Levin ER, Isackson PJ, Hu RM: Endothelin increases atrial natriuretic peptide production in cultured rat diencephalic neurons. Endocrinology 128:2925–2930, 1991.

215. Lee M, de la Monte S, Ng S, Quertermous T: Expression of the potent vasoconstrictor endothelin in the human central nervous system. J Clin Invest 86:141–147, 1990.

216. Miller WL, Redfield MM, Burnett JC: Integrated cardiac, renal, and endocrine actions of endothelin. J Clin Invest 83:317–320, 1989.

217. Lerman A, Hildebrand FL, Aarhus LL, Burnett JC: Endothelin has biological actions at pathophysiological concentrations. Circulation 83:1808–1814, 1991.

218. Vierhapper H, Wagner O, Nowotny P, Waldhausl W: Effect of endothelin-1 in man. Circulation 81:1415–1418, 1990.

219. Battistini B, Chailler P, D'Orléans-Juste P, et al: Growth regulatory properties of endothelins. Peptides 14:385–399, 1993.

Hormonal Aspects of Hypertension

GORDON H. WILLIAMS
THOMAS J. MOORE

Hypertension has been estimated to be present in 40 to 50 million adults in the United States. A similar high percentage of adults in other developed countries has hypertension. Most of these individuals are assumed to have essential hypertension, with fewer than 10 per cent having secondary forms of hypertension. Traditional endocrine causes of hypertension include primary aldosteronism, Cushing's syndrome, pheochromocytoma, acromegaly, renal vascular disease, renin-secreting tumors, and hypercalcemia.[1] Of importance, nearly all secondary forms of hypertension have a hormonal basis (Table 155–1).

Understanding the pathophysiology of essential hypertension has progressed more slowly. In part, this has been because of the general assumption for many years that essential hypertension was a single entity. However, recent data strongly suggest that essential hypertension is a syndrome with several different causes.[2] Most of the reported pathophysiological mechanisms have an endocrine basis. Since over 60 per cent of the hypertensive population have a volume- or sodium-sensitive component to their arterial pressure, it is not surprising that abnormalities in the renin-angiotensin system have been most frequently described, particularly because of its relationship to aldosterone secretion and vascular responsiveness.

THE RENIN-ANGIOTENSIN SYSTEM

The juxtaglomerular apparatus of the kidney is made up of specialized cells that have the capacity to synthesize the enzyme *renin*. Renin is stored in granules in these cells, and its release is controlled by a variety of stimuli, including a change in renal perfusion pressure, potassium, angiotensin II, and the adrenergic nervous system. The substrate

for this enzyme is *angiotensinogen* (a circulating protein synthesized in the liver). The product of the interaction of the substrate with the enzyme is the decapeptide *angiotensin I*. A variety of tissues contain *angiotensin-converting enzyme*, which is capable of metabolizing the inactive angiotensin I to the active octapeptide, *angiotensin II*, by hydrolyzing the two C-terminal amino acids. The half-life of angiotensin II is short (seconds), while that of renin is much longer (10 to 20 min).[3]

Angiotensin II has two primary effects: it is a potent vasoconstrictor, and it increases aldosterone secretion. The renin-angiotensin system and aldosterone secretion are linked together in a negative-feedback loop. This feedback loop is designed primarily to regulate sodium homeostasis and only secondarily to modify arterial pressure.[4–6] Thus the critical elements of this feedback loop consist of its action on the renal vasculature to modify renal blood flow and its effect on aldosterone. These two effects work in concert: when sodium intake is restricted, angiotensin II levels increase, which reduces renal blood flow and increases aldosterone release. Both these effects increase sodium retention by the kidney. The opposite effect occurs when sodium intake is increased or plasma and extracellular volume are expanded.

Crucial for the function of this negative-feedback loop is the impact of dietary sodium intake on the responsiveness of the target tissues to angiotensin II[7, 8] (Fig. 155–1). In contrast to most other endocrine negative-feedback loops, the responses of the target tissues to angiotensin II vary depending on the level of sodium intake. Sodium restriction enhances the adrenal response to angiotensin II but reduces the vascular response. With sodium loading, the opposite effects occur. Thus sodium intake has a reciprocal influence on the vascular and adrenal responses to angio-

Table 155–1. Classification of Arterial Hypertension

I. Systolic hypertension with wide pulse pressure
  A. Decreased compliance of aorta (arteriosclerosis)
  B. Increased stroke volume
    1. Aortic regurgitation
    2. Thyrotoxicosis
    3. Hyperkinetic heart syndrome
    4. Fever
    5. Arteriovenous fistula
    6. Patent ductus arteriosus
II. Systolic and diastolic hypertension (increased peripheral vascular resistance)
  A. Renal
    1. Chronic pyelonephritis
    2. Acute and chronic glomerulonephritis
    3. Polycystic renal disease
    4. Renovascular stenosis or renal infarction
    5. Most other severe renal disease (arteriolar nephrosclerosis, diabetic nephropathy, etc.)
    6. Renin-producing tumors
  B. Endocrine
    1. Oral contraceptives
    2. Adrenocortical hyperfunction
      a. Cushing's disease and syndrome
      b. Primary hyperaldosteronism
        i. Adenoma
        ii. Bilateral hyperplasia
        iii. Glucocorticoid-remediable aldosteronism (GRA)
        iv. 11-hydroxysteroid dehydrogenase deficiency
      c. Congenital or hereditary adrenogenital syndromes (17α-hydroxylase and 11β-hydroxylase defects)
    3. Pheochromocytoma
    4. Myxedema
    5. Acromegaly
  C. Neurogenic
    1. Psychogenic
    2. "Diencephalic syndrome"
    3. Familial dysautonomia (Riley-Day)
    4. Polyneuritis (acute porphyria, lead poisoning)
    5. Increased intracranial pressure (acute)
    6. Spinal cord section (acute)
  D. Miscellaneous
    1. Coarctation of aorta
    2. Increased intravascular volume (excessive transfusion, polycythemia vera)
    3. Polyarteritis nodosa
    4. Hypercalcemia
  E. Unknown etiology
    1. Essential hypertension (>90 per cent of all cases of hypertension)
    2. Toxemia of pregnancy
    3. Acute intermittent porphyria

Reproduced with permission from Williams GH: Hypertensive vascular disease. *In* Isselbacher KJ, Braunwald E, Wilson JD, et al (eds): Harrison's Principles of Internal Medicine, 13th ed. New York, McGraw-Hill, 1994.

tensin II. This effect is likely to be of substantial relevance in allowing the renin-angiotensin-aldosterone feedback loop to make fine adjustments with chronic changes in sodium intake to more effectively maintain normal sodium and volume homeostasis.

The mechanisms responsible for the alteration in target tissue responsiveness to angiotensin II with changes in dietary sodium intake have been evaluated extensively. It is highly probable that the major factor modifying the vascular responses is the circulating levels of angiotensin II.[9–11] Thus, when the circulating levels are increased, there is classic down-regulation of the angiotensin II receptor and vice versa, thereby modifying the vascular responsiveness to angiotensin II in a predictable fashion.

How sodium intake modifies adrenal responses to angio-

tensin II is not as clearly established, although it is known that the final mechanism is a change in the level of aldosterone synthetase—the last step in aldosterone biosynthesis.[12–15] The mediator of this change is unclear, but it may be secondary to a change in the activity of a local adrenal renin-angiotensin system. In addition to the systemic or circulating renin-angiotensin system, several tissues, including the kidney, adrenal gland, vasculature, and brain, have local renin-angiotensin systems.[16–21] For example, all the components necessary to generate angiotensin II can be found within the glomerulosa cell of the adrenal gland.[22–24] It is this system which may, in part, mediate the change in adrenal sensitivity induced by changes in sodium intake (see Ch. 93).

RENIN CLASSIFICATION OF ESSENTIAL HYPERTENSION

Classifying patients according to their plasma renin activity became popular in the 1970's when it became evident that, compared with normotensive subjects, hypertensives displayed a broader range of plasma renin activity: low, normal, and elevated[25] (Fig. 155–2). Renin subgrouping provided the basis for the volume-vasoconstrictor model of hypertension.[26] Approximately 25 per cent of essential hypertensives had low renin levels in some studies. Low-renin subjects, in analogy with hyperaldosteronism, were thought of as volume-expanded. High-renin subjects were considered to have hypertension due to vasoconstriction. Since low-renin subjects responded well to diuretics and high-renin subjects to beta blockers (and other agents that blunt the renin-angiotensin system), it was thought that renin subgrouping would allow more precise antihypertensive therapy. It soon became evident, however, that therapeutic responses were not so specific. Subjects of all renin subgroups responded to diuretics, and many low-renin subjects responded well to converting enzyme inhibitors and other agents that block the renin-angiotensin system.[1] Because of this, renin subgrouping is no longer widely used clinically. However, a review of the topic is useful because renin subgrouping does provide a useful model for considering the pathophysiology of essential hypertension (volume-vasoconstrictor). In addition, recent studies of the "rare" syndrome of familial glucocorticoid-suppressible hyperaldosteronism suggest that documenting suppressed plasma renin levels in families with prevalent hypertension may provide an important clue to identifying this disorder.

Plasma Renin Activity Measurements

Early renin measurements were performed by bioassay, measuring the pressor response to human plasma infused into rats. Since 1970, however, the most commonly used assay measures *plasma renin activity*.[27] This consists of two steps. First, plasma is incubated at 37°C for a specific period of time, allowing the renin in the sample to cleave angiotensin I from angiotensinogen. The second step is to measure the angiotensin I thus formed by radioimmunoassay. Results of these assays are generally reported as nanograms of angiotensin I generated per milliliter of plasma per hour of incubation. Some laboratories prefer to add

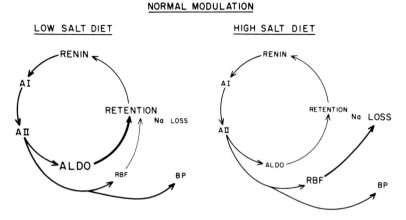

FIGURE 155–1. Impact of dietary sodium intake on responsiveness of angiotensin target tissues. Note that dietary sodium intake has a reciprocal influence on vascular and adrenal responses to angiotensin II. With sodium restriction, the adrenal response is enhanced but the vascular response is reduced. Sodium loading produces the opposite effect. (Reproduced with permission from Williams GH, Hollenberg NK: "Sodium-sensitive" essential hypertension: Emerging insights into pathogenesis and therapeutic implications. *In* Klahr S, Massry SG (eds): Contemporary Issues in Nephrology, 4th ed. New York, Plenum Press, 1985, p 303.)

an excess of angiotensinogen to the sample. This allows the renin activity measurement to be independent of the endogenous angiotensinogen concentration.

Several factors are known to affect the renin assay. Temperature and pH of the sample are particularly important.[28, 29] Plasma contains not only renin but also prorenin, a renin precursor with little renin-like activity. Prorenin can be activated during the assay unless pH and temperature are carefully controlled. Acidification of the sample to pH 3.3 was a common step in early assays to destroy angiotensinases in the plasma. However, when samples are acidified in this way and then restored back to a more neutral pH, prorenin in the sample can be activated. Similarly, if samples are thawed for assay and kept chilled (e.g., between 0 and +6°C), prorenin may be cryoactivated and again falsely elevate the renin activity assay.[29, 30]

Factors Affecting Plasma Renin Activity

As noted earlier, the amount of renin activity in plasma is dynamically regulated. Dietary sodium restriction, volume depletion with diuretics, and upright posture all increase plasma renin activity.[3] Not all studies of renin subgrouping have adequately controlled these factors. For example, one of the most widely used approaches to renin subgrouping utilized the relationship between plasma renin activity and 24-hour urinary sodium[26] (Fig. 155–3). The drawback of this so-called *renin-sodium nomogram* in defining low-renin hypertension is that, in subjects consuming more than 175 mEq sodium per day (i.e., 24-hour urinary sodium levels of 150 mEq or greater), plasma renin activity is suppressed even in normal subjects to near the lower limit of detectability of the assay. Thus this method

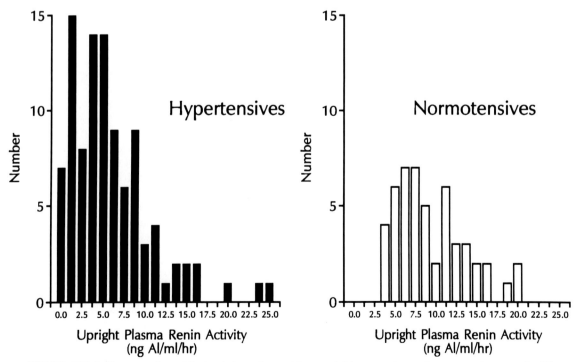

FIGURE 155–2. Plasma renin activity levels in patients with essential hypertension and normotensive controls. All patients were studied when in balance on a 10 mEq sodium/100 mEq potassium intake and after 2 h of ambulation in the morning. Note that the distribution in the hypertensive patients is more broad than in the normotensive subjects, but there is no clear bimodality of the levels in the hypertensive patients. (Adapted with permission from Tuck ML, Williams GH, Cain JP, et al: Relation of age, diastolic pressure and known duration of hypertension to presence of low renin essential hypertension. Am J Cardiol 32:637–642, 1973.)

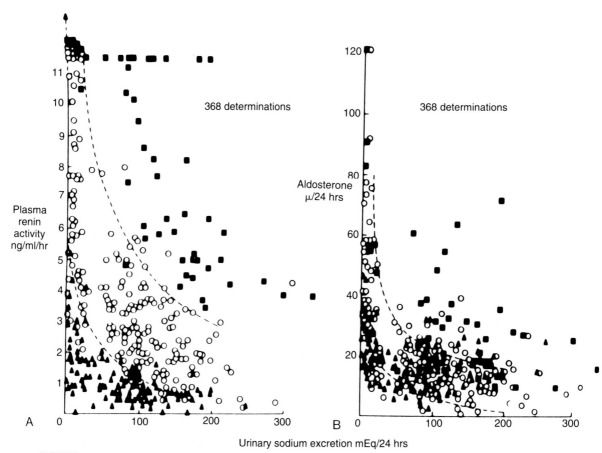

FIGURE 155–3. Relationship between sodium excretion and plasma renin activity, measured at noon, and aldosterone secretion in hypertension patients. The normal range is noted by the two dashed lines. Patients with low renin (▲), normal renin (○), and high renin (■) levels are separately noted. (Reproduced with permission from Sealey JE, Blumenfeld JP, Bell GM, et al: On the renal basis for essential hypertension: Nephron heterogeneity with discordant renin secretion and sodium excretion causing a hypertensive vasoconstriction–volume relationship. *In* Laragh JH, Brenner BM (eds): Hypertension: Pathophysiology, Diagnosis and Management. New York, Raven Press, 1990, p 1092.)

identifies low-renin hypertension best if dietary sodium is restricted before the sampling. Other investigators have attempted to standardize the conditions of posture and volume status of subjects before renin sampling.[25] These measures include a standardized sodium-restricted diet (e.g., 10 mEq sodium per day for 3 to 4 days) or volume depletion with furosemide in various dosage schedules. Assumption of the upright posture for 2 hours before sampling is also a commonly used stimulatory maneuver. Despite these attempts at standardization, it is clear that renin classification does not define discrete, distinct hypertensive subgroups. Mitchell and associates[31] reported a sizable experience from the National Institutes of Health (NIH).[31] Using the renin-sodium nomogram approach, they did duplicate determinations in 34 patients with normal- or low-renin hypertension. Thirty per cent of the subjects changed categories on retesting; 8 changed from the low- to the normal-renin group and 2 from the normal- to the low-renin group. Similarly, when 20 patients with low-renin hypertension by renin-sodium classification were recategorized according to their response to dietary sodium restriction, 55 per cent of the subjects changed from the low- to the normal-renin group. These results suggest that more vigorous attempts at renin stimulation (e.g., longer-term dietary sodium restriction, higher doses of furosemide,

etc.) result in a lower prevalence of low-renin hypertension in a given population.

Finally, the level of renin activity is affected by age (renin levels decline with aging) and by race.[25, 32, 33] Among hypertensive subjects, the prevalence of low-renin hypertension was 37 per cent in those over age 50 compared with 12 per cent in those younger than 40 years of age.[25] There is also a higher prevalence of low-renin hypertension among black patients. Channick and colleagues[34] studied 100 unselected hypertensives and found low renin levels in 26 per cent of the white subjects and 51 per cent of black subjects. These findings have been confirmed in other studies.[25, 35]

SECONDARY CAUSES OF HYPERTENSION: CONDITIONS IN WHICH THE ROLE OF HORMONAL FACTORS IS CLEAR

It is estimated that in less than 10 per cent of the hypertensive population is the cause of the elevated arterial pressure known. In these patients the cause is almost invariably hormonal, and appropriate treatment often leads to a cure. A detailed discussion of the pathophysiology, diagnosis, and treatment of these conditions has been given in other chapters of this text. It is important to note that because of the low probability a given patient with hypertension will have a correctable cause, mass screening for secondary causes is unwarranted. Factors that would increase the need for specific evaluation for a secondary form of hypertension include (1) hypertension resistant to treatment (i.e., requiring more than two antihypertensive agents), (2) hypertension first presenting in an individual either under age 30 or over age 55, or (3) signs or symptoms suggestive of a specific secondary form of hypertension.

Adrenal Causes of Hypertension

Hypertension can be caused by increased production of any of the three major adrenal secretory products: mineralocorticoids, glucocorticoids, or catecholamines.

Cushing's Syndrome (see Ch. 100)

The hypertension in Cushing's syndrome can be associated either with normal or low plasma renin activity levels.[3, 36] This is because glucocorticoids have two major effects related to their hypertensive potential. First, they increase production of the renin substrate angiotensinogen, which could lead to increased angiotensin levels. Second, they can increase sodium retention because the increased glucocorticoids can overwhelm the glucocorticoid-inactivating mechanisms in the kidney, i.e., 11-hydroxysteroid dehydrogenase activity[37, 38] (see Ch. 102). The former mechanism may predominate, since most patients with Cushing's syndrome do not have hypokalemia. While there is a loose correlation between the glucocorticoid level and the rise in arterial pressure, other factors also must be important in determining whether an individual with Cushing's syndrome develops hypertension. As might be anticipated, with the steroidogenic enzyme inefficiencies associated with adrenal carcinomas, there is an increased production of hypertensinogenic steroids (e.g., 11-deoxycorticosterone).[3] Patients with this condition are most likely to have hypertension and hypokalemia. Patients suspected of having Cushing's syndrome should be screened either with an overnight dexamethasone test or a 24-h urinary cortisol test, as noted in Chapter 100. After initial screening, definitive testing can then establish the specific cause of the Cushing's syndrome.

Mineralocorticoid Excess (see Ch. 102)

Because of the sodium retention induced by the relative or absolute increase in steroid production in patients in this group, all have low plasma renin activity.[3, 39] The most common form is primary aldosteronism due to a unilateral adrenal adenoma. Hypertension is clearly due to the excess mineralocorticoid activity. Nearly all patients also have hypokalemia unless they have been on a sodium-restricted diet or taking a potassium-sparing diuretic (e.g., spironolactone). Because there are no clinical clues to suggest this diagnosis, all patients with hypertension should have a serum potassium level measured prior to initiating therapy. While measurement of plasma renin activity was originally felt to be useful in screening for primary aldosteronism, it is no longer considered so because of the substantial number of patients with essential hypertension who have low

plasma renin activity levels (see below). Definitive diagnosis of primary aldosteronism is established by the presence of high, poorly suppressible plasma or urinary aldosterone levels following a sodium load. Because some patients with primary aldosteronism do not have an adrenal tumor, it is important to demonstrate anatomically the presence or absence of a tumor, because therapy for primary aldosteronism due to a tumor is quite different from that for the disease that results from bilateral hyperplasia.[3, 39] Rarely, patients with a tumor and mineralocorticoid excess fail to produce excess aldosterone but instead have excess production of 11-deoxycorticosterone. The definitive diagnosis in these patients is made by demonstrating a hypermineralocorticoid state with low aldosterone levels and elevated levels of 11-deoxycorticosterone. Finally, three other forms of mineralocorticoid excess are due to enzyme defects. In one form the defect is in the 11-hydroxysteroid dehydrogenase enzyme which is necessary to inactivate cortisol. These patients have normal glucocorticoid and low aldosterone levels, but the mineralocorticoid receptors in the kidney and potentially elsewhere are freely accessible to the glucocorticoids, thereby producing sodium retention and hypertension.[38] The second group of patients consists of those with classic congenital adrenal hyperplasia (see Ch. 104). Only the 11-hydroxylase and 17α-hydroxylase deficiency states have been associated with hypertension.[3, 40] Even in these cases, a substantial fraction of the patients do not have an elevated arterial pressure or other manifestations of mineralocorticoid excess (e.g., hypokalemia). Diagnosis is made by demonstrating elevated levels of precursor steroids behind the specific enzymatic defect. The last condition, discussed in greater detail below, is glucocorticoid-remediable aldosteronism. In these patients, aldosterone is inappropriately under the control of ACTH, thereby producing a relative hyperaldosterone state. Glucocorticoids are effective therapy.

The mineralocorticoid excess syndrome group of patients comprise fewer than 1 per cent of the total hypertensive population, with the majority of these patients having an aldosterone-producing tumor. Yet because this is a silent form of correctable hypertension, it is imperative that serum potassium levels be determined prior to initiating therapy in any patient with hypertension.

Pheochromocytoma

In contrast to patients with excess steroid secretion, patients with pheochromocytoma invariably have normal or high plasma renin activity and clearly have a vasoconstrictor form of hypertension. Definitive diagnosis is established by the measurement of excess production of epinephrine, norepinephrine, or their metabolites in the urine.[41, 42] A review of alternative procedures is given in Chapter 106. Pheochromocytoma should be ruled out in all cases of familial hypertension and in those patients with symptoms suggestive of episodic hypertension, even though the majority of patients with pheochromocytoma do not present in this way. Between 1 and 2 in 1000 patients with hypertension have a pheochromocytoma. Thus, even though it is an infrequent cause, the importance of being vigilant in searching for it in selected cases is critical, since, undetected, there is a high degree of morbidity and mortality. These patients may have traditional catecholamine-excess symptoms, including hypertension, tachycardia, cold, clammy skin, and/or paroxysms of headache, tachycardia, and a sense of impending doom. These symptoms can be controlled by α- or β-adrenergic blockers. The ultimate treatment is almost always resection of the tumor.

Renal Hypertension

Renal hypertension is one of the most common secondary forms of hypertension, being present in 3 to 5 per cent of the total hypertensive population. While the kidney produces a variety of hormones, the one whose excess production has been most clearly associated with a rise in arterial pressure is renin via its generation of angiotensin II, as described above, usually secondary to unilateral renal artery stenosis. It was initially assumed that these individuals would have consistently increased levels of plasma renin activity and angiotensin II. However, this has not proven to be correct primarily because of the substantial variation in plasma renin activity levels in normal subjects and in patients with essential hypertension, as noted above.[43] The classic form of renal hypertension is secondary to a stenosis in a main or segmental branch of one renal artery. With reduced perfusion to the affected kidney, excess production of renin occurs with increased generation of angiotensin II. This increased angiotensin II results in secondary aldosteronism and hypertension with suppression of renin from the contralateral kidney. The secondary aldosteronism also can produce hypokalemia.[3] Thus patients with renal artery stenosis and secondary aldosteronism can have many of the same clinical features associated with primary aldosteronism. The distinguishing feature is an elevated, rather than a low, plasma renin activity in the presence of hypokalemia. Unfortunately, fewer than one half of patients with renal artery stenosis actually have an increased level of renin activity. A far greater percentage of these individuals have evidence, however, of an activated renin-angiotensin system, as demonstrated by the fall in arterial pressure in response to administration of a competitive angiotensin antagonist (saralasin, 1-Sar 8-Ala, angiotensin II) or abnormalities in renal blood flow, as assessed by a renogram, in response to a converting-enzyme inhibitor. It is important to remember that renal vascular hypertension can occur even in the absence of a stenosis in the main renal artery. A segmental stenosis will produce the same clinical picture that occurs in individuals with a lesion in the main renal artery. Another rare form of renal hypertension occurs because of a renin-producing tumor, often located in the kidney but also seen in other tissues (e.g., ovary, pancreas).[45] Renin-producing tumors display all the features of renal artery stenosis except that a tumor is present rather than a lesion in the vascular supply to the kidney. Finally, renal parenchymal disease also may lead to an increased arterial pressure through activation of the renin-angiotensin system, particularly in individuals with accelerated hypertension.[43] In these cases, there is decreased segmental perfusion of the kidney due to inflammation or fibrosis in small intrarenal vessels. These patients also may have decreased ability to excrete a salt load. Therefore, confusion may exist in that plasma renin activity, particularly if the patient is on a normal- or high-salt diet, may actually be suppressed. Performing plasma renin activity measurements under carefully controlled conditions, as noted above, minimizes the confusion that can result from renal parenchymal disease.

The diagnosis of renal artery stenosis should be entertained in the following individuals: all patients with accelerated hypertension, hypertension beginning before age 30 or after age 55, hypertension and renal insufficiency, and difficult-to-control hypertension. The physical sign of an abdominal bruit also may warrant further evaluation for renal artery stenosis. Definitive diagnosis is usually established by documentation of a stenosis on a selective renal arteriogram and increased renin production from the side of the lesion with suppression of renin production from the contralateral kidney.[43] Care must be taken to interpret renin levels appropriately because of the impact of antihypertensive therapy and restricted dietary sodium intake (see above).

The treatment of renal artery stenosis has evolved substantially over the past several years. Three approaches are presently available: surgical repair, interluminal balloon dilatation (angioplasty), and medical therapy. Increasingly, angioplasty is the treatment of choice for most unilateral renal arterial lesions producing hypertension. However, for a substantial number of individuals, particularly those who are elderly, medical therapy with angiotensin-converting enzyme inhibitors may be effective. These agents, however, need to be used with caution in patients in whom bilateral renal disease may be present, since they may cause accelerated deterioration of renal function.

Oral Contraceptives

The most common secondary form of hypertension is due to the administration of oral contraceptives.[46] These agents are probably the cause of an elevated arterial pressure in 5 per cent of the total hypertensive population and in a substantial minority of women of reproductive age. The hypertensive effect appears to be limited to those patients taking estrogen-containing oral contraceptives. Estrogen increases the production of angiotensinogen, the renin substrate, thereby producing activation of the renin-angiotensin system. Because of the increased production of angiotensin II, both vasoconstriction and volume retention occur secondary to mild hyperaldosteronism and a reduction in renal blood flow. All women taking oral contraceptives have some increase in plasma renin activity, angiotensin II, and aldosterone levels. Yet only a small minority actually have a substantial rise in arterial pressure. Thus it is likely that those who develop hypertension have an additional factor which in combination with the increased production of angiotensinogen leads to the substantial rise in arterial pressure. This additional factor could be a genetically determined abnormality (similar to what occurs in essential hypertension), mild renal disease, obesity, or increased age (hypertension is significantly more frequent in women taking oral contraceptives over age 40).

Because there is no way of determining a priori which patient will develop hypertension with estrogen therapy, all patients should have their arterial pressure carefully monitored for the first 6 months of therapy. Patients with oral contraceptive–induced hypertension usually have these medications discontinued. While arterial pressure returns to normal in the majority of patients within 6 months, in a substantial minority the condition may persist. If oral contraceptives are required, then an antihypertensive agent which modifies angiotensin II production (converting enzyme inhibitors) would be most appropriate. Of interest is the relative lack of a hypertensinogenic effect of conjugated estrogens administered to postmenopausal women. This may be secondary to the lower dose of estrogen or to the absence of other hypertensinogenic factors produced by the normal ovary.

Hypercalcemia (see Chs. 63 to 65)

Calcium's role in modifying arterial pressure is controversial.[1, 47] Epidemiological studies suggest that an increase in dietary calcium intake can lower arterial pressure. On the other hand, an elevation in cytosolic calcium levels in circulating blood elements has been associated with hypertension. Finally, hypertension is commonly associated with hyperparathyroidism. Indeed, the frequency of hypertension in patients with hyperparathyroidism is approximately double that of the normal population. The mechanisms responsible for this hypertension are unclear. Since in some cases removal of the parathyroid adenoma does not correct the hypertension, it is likely that in some patients it is secondary to structural damage in the kidney (nephrocalcinosis). Recent studies have suggested that there may be an interrelationship between the renin-angiotensin-aldosterone system and the parathyroid-calcium system.[48] Administration of parathyroid hormone increases renin levels acutely. Likewise, administration of angiotensin II increases parathyroid hormone levels. Whether these effects are direct or indirect is still unclear. However, it is feasible that hyperparathyroidism with its chronically increased parathyroid hormone levels could induce a state of mild secondary hyperaldosteronism. While the level of activity of the renin-angiotensin-aldosterone system has been reported to be normal in hyperparathyroidism, studies that controlled dietary sodium intake, which may be necessary to distinguish a normal from a mildly hyperactive state, have not been reported.

Acromegaly

Patients with acromegaly have approximately a 40 per cent prevalence of hypertension.[49] In general, the hypertension appears to be of the low-renin type and therefore, presumably, secondary to volume expansion. Increased sodium retention can occur from one of two mechanisms. First, growth hormone can have a direct effect on the kidney, causing sodium retention, or second, growth hormone can modify adrenal responsiveness to angiotensin II, promoting a mild form of hyperaldosteronism. While some investigators have reported an increased frequency of primary aldosteronism itself in patients with acromegaly, other studies have not supported such a mechanism.[49] Finally, whether the acromegalic state produces some permanent change either in cardiac or renal function which contributes to the hypertension is unclear. There is only a poor correlation between the level of growth hormone and the level of arterial pressure in patients who have hypertension, although, in general, patients who are hypertensive have higher growth hormone levels than normotensive patients with acromegaly. The most effective treatments for the hypertension in patients with acromegaly are measures directed at lowering the growth hormone levels. Of the antihypertensive agents available, diuretics are the most appropriate first-line choice.

Diabetes Mellitus (see Ch. 90)

Hypertension is a common late sequela of diabetes mellitus.[49] Indeed, potentially more than half of diabetic patients also have hypertension. The mechanism underlying the elevated arterial pressure includes renal artery and renal parenchymal disease (see above), insulin resistance (see below), and volume overload associated with the hyperglycemic state. In general, the hypertension in diabetes appears to be volume-dependent. Yet converting enzyme inhibitors may be the treatment of choice because of their lack of adverse effects on glucose homeostasis, their ability to modify renal glomerular pressure (thereby reducing renal damage), and their beneficial effect on reducing proteinuria (probably secondary to their effect on glomerular hemodynamics, but tubular effects cannot be excluded).[50] Noteworthy is the presence of hyporeninemic hypoaldosteronism and hypertension in diabetic patients. This condition appears to be secondary to a juxtaglomerular derangement induced by atherosclerosis or to the metabolic derangements of diabetes. Also important to remember is the increased probability of bilateral renal artery stenosis in patients with diabetes. Both these conditions can lead to hyperkalemia and renal insufficiency, particularly if a converting enzyme inhibitor is given. Thus, in all patients with diabetes mellitus started on a converting enzyme inhibitor, renal function and serum potassium levels should be monitored over the first 2 to 3 weeks of therapy.

PRIMARY (ESSENTIAL) HYPERTENSION: A CONDITION IN WHICH HORMONES ARE PRESUMED TO BE INVOLVED

Pathophysiological Hypotheses of Low-Renin Essential Hypertension

Many investigators have suggested that low-renin hypertension is a volume-expanded form of hypertension. This conclusion is in part based on analogy with primary hyperaldosteronism. However, studies have not uniformly documented increases in plasma volume, extracellular fluid volume, or exchangeable sodium in low-renin subjects. This topic has been well summarized by Safar and associates.[51] Part of this discrepancy may be methodological. The precision of the volume measurements may not be adequate to detect the subtle changes in volume that might account for suppressed renin activity. In addition, not all studies carefully regulated sodium intake, and the age, gender, and race of the subjects in control groups versus hypertensive groups or low-renin versus normal-renin subjects were not always well matched.

Further evidence suggesting that low-renin hypertension

is a volume-expanded type of hypertension comes from the results of therapeutic trials. Low-renin subjects respond better to diuretic treatment than do normal-renin hypertensives.[52–54] Early reports that these subjects respond particularly well to spironolactone[52, 53] were not confirmed by later studies which showed an equally beneficial response to thiazide diuretics.[54, 55]

The cause of the presumed volume expansion in these subjects remains uncertain. The fact that arterial pressure responds well to spironolactone (a specific mineralocorticoid antagonist) and to aminoglutethimide (an inhibitor of adrenal steroid synthesis) has focused attention on the adrenal gland. Aldosterone levels are generally normal in low-renin hypertensives, although the aldosterone response to infused angiotensin II on a high-sodium diet is enhanced[56–58] (Fig. 155–4). Thus the potential exists that on a high-sodium diet a mild form of hyperaldosteronism may be present. Other studies have focused on the production of an unrecognized steroid as a potential cause of the volume expansion in low-renin hypertension.[59] Abnormalities of weak mineralocorticoids such as 18-hydroxydeoxycorticosterone or deoxycorticosterone have been reported in a minority of patients with low-renin hypertension.[60, 61] However, no consistent abnormality of steroid production has been identified to account for the majority of patients with low-renin hypertension.

Low-Renin Glucocorticoid-Remediable Hypertension

Glucocorticoid-remediable aldosteronism (GRA, also know as glucocorticoid-suppressible aldosteronism or dexamethasone-suppressible aldosteronism) was first described by Sutherland and colleagues in 1966.[62] These investigators described severe hypertension in a father and a son which was characterized by hypokalemia, excessive aldosterone production, and both the aldosterone excess and arterial pressure were ameliorated by dexamethasone administration. Subsequently, studies of other kindreds have demonstrated that this is an autosomal dominant defect characterized by early-onset hypertension, low plasma renin activity, excessive aldosterone production, and varying degrees of hypokalemia. In clinical practice, the family history and hypokalemia are usually the clinical clues that raise the possibility of this diagnosis. In addition to aldosterone excess, these subjects produce two abnormal hybrid steroids: 18-hydroxycortisol and 18-oxocortisol.[63] In normal individuals, the aldosterone synthase enzyme which converts corticosterone to aldosterone via oxidation of the 18 position of the steroid molecule is present only in the zona glomerulosa of the adrenal gland.[3] Conversely, 17-hydroxylase activity is limited to the zona fasciculata of the adrenal gland, where cortisol is produced. In patients with GRA, both enzymes appear to be working on the steroid nucleus, since the hybrid steroids are transformed in both the 17 and 18 positions. In normal subjects, cortisol is under the sole control of ACTH, while aldosterone production is mainly regulated by the renin-angiotensin system and potassium.[3] In GRA, both cortisol and aldosterone production are regulated by ACTH. This is evidenced by the facts that, in GRA, aldosterone follows the same circadian rhythm as cortisol, is suppressed by dexamethasone administration, and cannot be stimulated by administration of angiotensin II.[64, 65] Of interest, after the administration of dexamethasone and suppression of the hybrid steroid and aldosterone excess, the adrenal gland reacquires its aldosterone responsiveness to angiotensin II administration. This responsiveness is maintained as long as ACTH is suppressed with dexamethasone treatment.

A recent investigation of a large GRA kindred has allowed clarification of the pathophysiology of this disorder

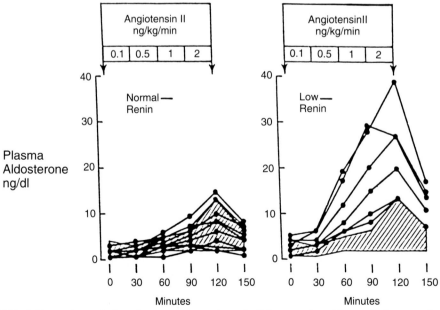

FIGURE 155–4. Comparison of adrenal responses to angiotensin II in normal- and low-renin hypertensive patients. Normal responses are shown in the shaded area. Note the hyperresponsiveness of the adrenal to angiotensin II in the low-renin essential hypertension patients. (Reproduced from Wisgerhof M, Brown, RD: Increased adrenal sensitivity to angiotensin II in low renin essential hypertension. J Clin Invest 61:1456–1462, 1978, by copyright permission of the American Society for Clinical Investigation.)

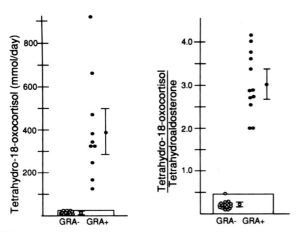

FIGURE 155–5. Urinary tetrahydro-18-oxocortisol levels and their ratio to tetrahydroaldosterone in a large glucocorticoid-remediable aldosteronism kindred. The normal range of these steroids is shown by the hatched area. (From Rich GM, Ulick S, Cook S, et al: Clinical characteristics of glucocorticoid-remediable aldosteronism in a large pedigree. Ann Intern Med 116:813–820, 1992.)

and of the genetic defect which causes it.[66, 67] Having identified a proband with GRA, all at-risk family members were investigated by screening 24-h urinary 18-hydroxycortisol and 18-oxocortisol to identify those members having the biochemical features of GRA (Fig. 155–5). Twelve positive family members were found. All 12 of these patients were either hypertensive or had high-normal arterial pressures compared with age-matched control subjects. Upright plasma renin activity on an unselected dietary sodium intake was suppressed in all 12 affected family members except 1 patient who was on a potassium-sparing diuretic (who had a normal PRA). Importantly, hypokalemia was not seen in this kindred, except in subjects who had developed hypokalemia on thiazide diuretic therapy. In fact, the serum potassium levels in affected family members were identical with those in unaffected members.

Because the abnormal hybrid steroids are 17- and 18-hydroxylated and regulated by ACTH, it was hypothesized that, in patients with GRA, both these genes were active in the zona fasciculata and regulated by ACTH. The gene encoding aldosterone synthase is structurally similar to the gene for steroid 11β-hydroxylase. These two genes have a 95 per cent identical nucleic acid sequence, and both reside on human chromosome 8. Using genetic markers for the 11β-hydroxylase gene, affected and unaffected family members were screened. One marker suggested the presence of a gene duplication in the affected family members of the pedigree. The structure of the abnormal duplicated gene was determined and found to contain the regulatory sequence allowing ACTH responsiveness at the 5′ region of the gene, the first portion of the 11β-hydroxylase coding region, fusion of the 11β-hydroxylase and aldosterone synthase sequences in the midportion of the gene, and exons 5 to 9 of aldosterone synthase at the end of the gene (Fig. 155–6). These findings confirm that in affected family members, the 11β-hydroxylase and aldosterone synthase genes have been fused by unequal crossing over, placing aldosterone synthase under ACTH regulation. Since 11β-hydroxylase is normally expressed in the zona fasciculata, affected family members can express both 11β-hydroxylase and aldosterone synthase in the zona fasciculata through

this genetic recombination, and this accounts for the hybrid steroid formation and aldosterone excess under ACTH control. Finally, 17 patients with GRA from 11 other pedigrees have been screened to determine whether this same gene duplication accounted for all cases of GRA.[68] Although the same type of unequal crossing over had occurred in all pedigrees, the specific cross-over break point varied, suggesting at least 8 independent mutations in these 11 kindreds. In all cases, however, the ACTH regulatory region, a portion of the 11β-hydroxylase gene and the aldosterone synthase gene were combined.

The clinical relevance of these findings lies in the fact that, heretofore, identification of GRA rested largely on clinical suspicion due to a positive family history of hypertension and *hypokalemia*. The New England kindred in which the genetic abnormality was first described did not have hypokalemia as a prominent feature. If hypokalemia is not a reliable index of GRA, then perhaps the clinical clues should rest on the family history and a *suppressed plasma renin activity*. Genetic testing of familial hypertension patients with low-renin hypertension will be needed to determine how common GRA is among low-renin subjects. Since patients with GRA respond not only to dexamethasone suppression but also to potassium-sparing diuretics (such as triameterene and spironolactone), there is an obvious similarity with the therapeutic success of these agents in low-renin hypertension. Screening for GRA in low-renin subjects might allow identification of unsuspected GRA, which would have implications both for specific therapy in individual patients and for family screening and early identification of affected family members.

Patients with GRA have traditionally been treated with glucocorticoids to suppress ACTH secretion, similar to what is done with individuals with congenital adrenal hyperplasia. However, often the dose of glucocorticoids necessary also induces cushingoid side effects. Thus the potential utility of aldosterone antagonists (i.e., spironolactone) is currently being explored as an alternative and/or adjunctive therapy to reduce the dose of glucocorticoids necessary to normalize blood pressure.

Nonmodulating Hypertension

In 1982, Shoback and colleagues[69] described a group of patients who belong to the normal- and high-renin subset

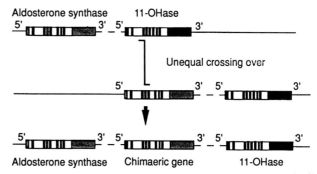

FIGURE 155–6. Schematic representation of the chimeric gene duplication found in patients with glucocorticoid-remediable aldosteronism. (Reprinted by permission from Lifton RP, Dluhy RG, Powers M, et al: A chimaeric 11β-hydroxylase/aldosterone synthase gene causes glucocorticoid-remediable aldosteronism and human hypertension. Nature 355:262, 1992. Copyright © 1992 Macmillan Journals Limited.)

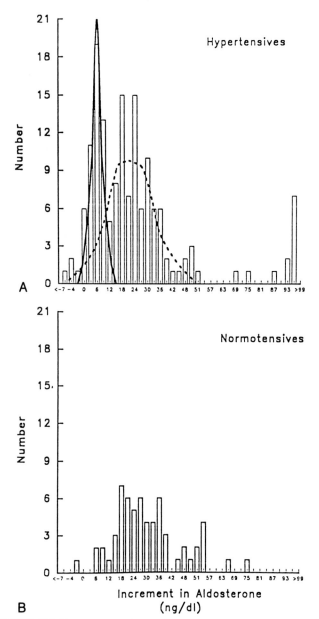

FIGURE 155–7. Increase in plasma aldosterone levels in response to a 3 ng/kg/min angiotensin II infusion in normotensive and hypertensive subjects. All subjects were in balance on a 10-mEq sodium intake. A, The response of 150 normal or high-renin essential hypertensive patients. Note the highly significant bimodal distribution ($p < 0.0009$). B, The response of 61 normotensive subjects free of known disease or family history of hypertension. (From Williams GH, et al: Non-modulation as an intermediate phenotype in essential hypertension. Hypertension 20:788–796, 1992. Reproduced with permission from the American Heart Association.)

of the hypertensive population. These individuals were distinguished from the rest of the hypertensive population by the failure of sodium intake to modify target tissue responsiveness to angiotensin II. Thus they were termed *nonmodulators.* Data dating back a decade before Shoback's report provide support for this hypothesis. For example, patients with hypertension who were placed on a low-sodium diet failed to increase their aldosterone secretion when challenged with a diuretic.[70, 71] Other reports documented that some patients with essential hypertension have a reduced renal arterial flow on a high-sodium diet when compared with normotensive subjects.[72, 73] Finally, one study reported

concurrent abnormalities in renal vascular responses to a high-salt diet and aldosterone responses to diuretic-induced volume depletion.[71] Even though patients with low-renin hypertension are excluded from the subset of patients termed *nonmodulators,* both low-renin and nonmodulating hypertensives have a salt-sensitive form of hypertension. The mechanisms underlying this salt sensitivity, however, are quite different.

Over the past decade, several reports have provided sufficient information that a determination of the presence or absence of nonmodulation can be made in the individual patient. These studies suggest that approximately 30 per cent of hypertensives are nonmodulators.[74] However, its frequency in a given population varies depending on the number of patients with low-renin hypertension.

Two techniques have been used to define nonmodulators. Both take advantage of the failure of sodium intake to modify tissue responses to angiotensin II in these patients.[2, 74] One is the adrenal response to angiotensin II. Nonmodulators are defined as those individuals who have an increment in aldosterone of less than 15 ng/dl in response to a 3 ng/kg/min angiotensin infusion when assessed on a 10-mEq sodium intake (Fig. 155–7). Alternatively, renal arterial flow responses, as determined by paraaminohippurate (PAH) clearance to the same dose of angiotensin II, can be measured on a high-sodium (200-mEq) diet. Under these conditions, a nonmodulator has a decrement in PAH clearance of less than 100 ml/min/1.73 m² when adjusted for age. While a clearer distinction between modulators and nonmodulators is possible using the adrenal criterion, it is more convenient to assess nonmodulators by the renal arterial flow criterion. When both ap-

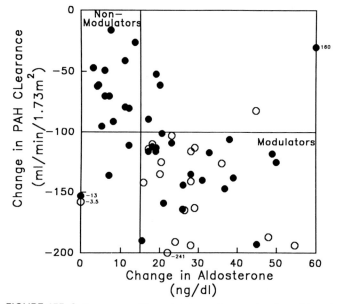

FIGURE 155–8. Responses of hypertensive and normotensive subjects to a 3 ng/kg/min angiotensin II infusion. Each subject was studied twice. Increments in plasma aldosterone were determined when the subjects were on a 10-mEq sodium diet, and decrements in PAH clearance were determined when they were in balance on a 200-mEq sodium diet. In 50 of the 59 subjects (85 per cent), the two indices agreed. (From Williams GH, et al: Non-modulation as an intermediate phenotype in essential hypertension. Hypertension 20:788–796, 1992. Reproduced with permission from the American Heart Association.)

NON-MODULATION

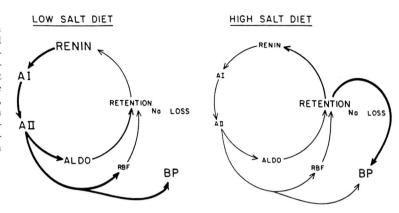

FIGURE 155–9. Diagrammatic representation of the defects in adrenal and renal vasculature responses to angiotensin II and their impact on arterial pressure and sodium handling in nonmodulation. Because of the failure of modulation, a greater activation of the renin-angiotensin system is observed on a low-salt diet. In contrast, on a high-sodium intake, because of the failure of an increase in renal blood flow, there will be sodium retention, which also can lead to an increase in arterial pressure. (From Williams GH, Hollenberg NK: "Sodium-sensitive" essential hypertension: Emerging insights into pathogenesis and therapeutic implications. *In* Klahr S, Massry SG (eds): Contemporary Issues in Nephrology, 4th ed. New York, Plenum Press, 1985, p 303.)

proaches have been used in individual patients, the concordance has been close to 85 per cent[74] (Fig. 155–8). Of critical importance is the need to perform the studies during precise sodium balance; as in normal subjects, both the adrenal and renal vascular responses to angiotensin II can be substantially different with only modest changes in sodium balance.[75, 76]

Pathophysiology of the Hypertension in Nonmodulators

While several mechanisms have been proposed to account for the increase in arterial pressure in nonmodulators, two are most likely. Each is related to the primary defect characteristic of nonmodulation, i.e., the failure of sodium intake to modify the adrenal and renal vascular responses to angiotensin II. First, it has been hypothesized that the renal blood flow defect may lead to abnormal sodium retention.[2] This is based on the assumption that the increase in renal blood flow observed when normal subjects are placed on a high-sodium diet would be absent in nonmodulators. This would limit their ability to excrete a salt load, resulting in an increase in arterial pressure (compare Figs. 155–2 and 155–9). Several lines of evidence support this hypothesis. First, in two separate studies, when the impact of sodium loading on renal blood flow was assessed, there was no increase in nonmodulators in contrast to the approximately 20 per cent increase observed in modulating hypertensive and normotensive subjects[69, 77] (Fig. 155–10). Second, when nonmodulators are given an acute salt challenge when in balance on a low-sodium diet, they excrete only half as much sodium as observed in normotensive and modulating hypertensive subjects.[78] Third, in response to a 5-day challenge of a high-sodium diet (200 mEq), nonmodulators retain approximately twice as much sodium as modulators.[79] Fourth, the half-time for achieving low-sodium balance when sodium is removed from the diet is approximately 24 h in normotensive subjects or modulating hypertensive patients. In contrast, the half-time in the nonmodulators is 50 per cent longer (36 h).[79] Finally, following 5 days of a high-salt diet, only nonmodulators increase their arterial pressure if low-renin hypertensive patients are excluded.[79] Thus nonmodulators have all the characteristics of a salt-sensitive form of hypertension. This is a feature shared by low-renin hypertensive patients, as described earlier. However, the mechanisms responsible for the increased salt retention are quite different.

A second mechanism proposed to increase arterial pressure in nonmodulators is likely to be less important because of the circumstances required to activate it.[2] As noted above, the renin-angiotensin system is linked to aldosterone secretion in a negative-feedback loop designed to maintain normal volume and sodium homeostasis. When nonmodulators are sodium-restricted, sensitivity of the adrenal gland to angiotensin II is not increased. Theoretically, to compensate for this lack of increased sensitivity, the renin-angiotensin system should be activated to a greater extent in nonmodulators. As a result, when sodium-restricted, nonmodulators should have the characteristics of an angiotensin-dependent hypertension. Two lines of evidence provide support for this hypothesis. First, renin and angiotensin levels tend to be higher in nonmodulators than in modulators.[74, 80] Second, when a competitive angio-

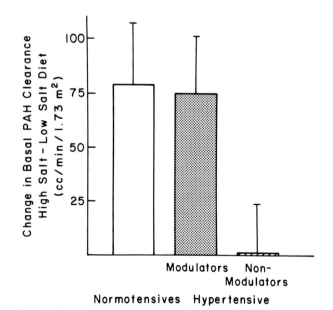

FIGURE 155–10. Impact of sodium intake on basal renal plasma flow. Renal plasma flow was estimated by PAH clearance, which was determined twice in each subject: once on a 10-mEq and once on a 200-mEq sodium intake. Sodium loading significantly increased PAH clearance in normotensive subjects and modulators, but not in nonmodulators. (Adapted from Redgrave J, Rabinowe S, Hollenberg NK, Williams GH: Correction of abnormal renal blood flow response by converting enzyme inhibition in essential hypertensives. J Clin Invest 75:1285–1290, 1985, by copyright permission of the American Society for Clinical Investigation.)

tensin II antagonist (saralasin) is given to sodium-restricted modulators and nonmodulators with similar plasma renin activity levels, the arterial pressure decline is nearly three-fold greater in the nonmodulators.[81]

Thus nonmodulators paradoxically have characteristics associated with both angiotensin II–dependent and sodium-sensitive hypertension, depending on the level of dietary sodium intake. Since in most circumstances patients are on a moderate- to high-sodium diet, the expression of their hypertension is commonly dominated by the renal vascular abnormality, i.e., sodium sensitivity.

Causes of the Nonmodulating Defect

Several lines of evidence suggest that the nonmodulating characteristic is secondary to a dysregulation of the local renin-angiotensin system in the adrenal and the kidney. First, in nonmodulators, renal blood flow is similar on a high- and low-salt diet.[69, 77] Since the major regulator of renal vascular resistance with changes in sodium intake is angiotensin II, this suggests that nonmodulators have increased angiotensin II levels on a high-salt diet. Yet the circulating levels of renin and angiotensin II, if anything, are lower on a high-salt diet in nonmodulators than in modulators.[74] Second, converting enzyme inhibitors, when administered for 2 days to nonmodulators on a high-salt diet, increase renal blood flow, thereby restoring it to the levels observed in modulating hypertensives and normotensive subjects on a high-salt diet[77] (Fig. 155–11). Third, the altered adrenal response to angiotensin II on a low-salt diet is also corrected by the administration of a converting

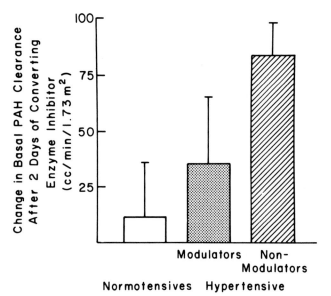

FIGURE 155–11. Renal blood flow as determined by PAH clearance in response to administration of a converting enzyme inhibitor. Each subject was maintained on a 200-mEq sodium intake, and PAH clearance was determined twice on each subject: once before and a second time 2 days after continuous administration of the converting enzyme inhibitor. No significant change in renal blood flow was observed in normotensive subjects, but a highly significant increase occurred in the nonmodulating patients. (From Redgrave JE, Rabinowe SL, Hollenberg NK, Williams GH: Correction of abnormal renal blood flow response to angiotensin II by converting enzyme inhibition in essential hypertensives. J Clin Invest 75:1285, 1985, by copyright permission of the American Society for Clinical Investigation.)

enzyme inhibitor, although it takes approximately 6 weeks before responses are restored to normal.[82, 83] Finally, converting enzyme inhibition also restores to normal the renal response to an acute sodium load.

Genetics of Nonmodulation

A considerable body of evidence has clearly established that arterial pressure is primarily determined by genetic factors, with a substantial impact by environmental forces.[84–88] Thus an intensive search has been conducted to determine if the nonmodulating characteristic is indeed an intermediate phenotype and, therefore, genetically determined. To establish this, it would be important to document the presence of several of the following findings: bimodality in the distribution of the nonmodulating characteristic in the hypertensive population, a strong family history of hypertension in nonmodulators, the presence of nonmodulating characteristics in normotensive subjects, and familial aggregation of the nonmodulating characteristic. At least three of the characteristics useful in defining nonmodulation show a bimodal distribution in the normal- and high-renin essential hypertensive population. The most dramatic of these is the bimodal distribution of the aldosterone secretory response to acute volume depletion when subjects are sodium-restricted[70, 71, 74] (Fig. 155–12). Nearly as dramatic is the change in the renal blood flow increment in response to a change in dietary sodium intake from low to high and the plasma aldosterone increment in response to a 3 ng/kg/min angiotensin II infusion in subjects studied on a low-sodium diet.[74] Thus, in contrast to other characteristics associated with hypertension, there is a clear bimodality in the nonmodulating trait. Second, nonmodulators have a much greater frequency of a positive family history for hypertensive relatives than do modulating hypertensive patients (85 versus 25 per cent).[79, 89] Third, at least three of the features of nonmodulation have been described in normotensive subjects, but only in those who have a positive family history for hypertension—a population which should be enriched with the gene(s) producing the nonmodulating trait.[89–92] Normotensive subjects with a positive family history for hypertension have a lower aldosterone response to acute administration of angiotensin II, particularly on a low-sodium diet, than do normotensive individuals with a negative family history for hypertension.[91] A Dutch study documents that normotensive individuals with a positive family history for hypertension have lower renal blood flow on a high-sodium diet than do subjects with a negative family history.[92] Finally, normotensive subjects with a positive family history for hypertension have an increase in renal blood flow on a high-sodium diet following the administration of a converting enzyme inhibitor, in contrast to the absence of such an effect in normotensive subjects with a negative family history.[90] Since these studies were drawn from quite distinct populations (Switzerland, the Netherlands, and Japan), it is likely that the nonmodulating phenotype is generally found throughout the world. A final study further supports the conclusion that nonmodulation is a genetically determined trait. When hypertensive siblings were evaluated for the presence or absence of the nonmodulating trait, there was substantial familial aggregation of nonmodulation.[93]

In summary, nonmodulators are a substantial subset of

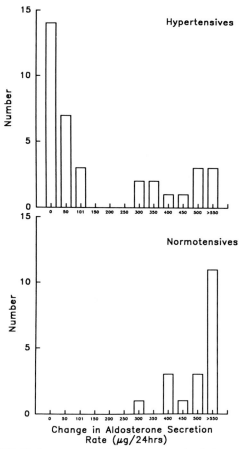

FIGURE 155–12. Increments in aldosterone secretion in hypertensive and normotensive subjects on a 10-mEq sodium intake. Subjects were given furosemide for 24 h to induce further volume depletion. The increment is the difference between the low-salt and the furosemide-stimulated aldosterone secretion. (From Williams GH, Dluhy RG, Lifton RP, et al: Nonmodulation as an intermediate phenotype in essential hypertension. Hypertension 20:788–796, 1992, with permission of the American Heart Association.)

the hypertensive population. Their arterial pressure is particularly sensitive to sodium intake, the trait appears to be inherited, and it is likely due to dysregulation of the local renin-angiotensin systems within the adrenal and kidney. Finally, therapeutically, converting enzyme inhibitors appear to be specific therapy for the hypertension in these patients, since they appear to correct the underlying defect(s) responsible for the elevated arterial pressure.

Insulin Resistance in Essential Hypertension

Essential hypertensive patients often have non-insulin-dependent diabetes mellitus (NIDDM) and/or obesity. Although these three conditions occur frequently, their degree of association is higher than one would assume, given the frequency of each in the general population.[94–98] This has led some to postulate that the cause for essential hypertension is insulin resistance. While substantial evidence supports this possibility,[95–102] some studies[103] have not observed an increased frequency of insulin resistance in essential hypertension. These discrepancies may be related in part to the observation that insulin resistance is associated with an increase in blood pressure only in some ethnic groups. For example, in one study, there appears to be little relationship between arterial pressure and insulin resistance in blacks or Pima Indians but a strong association in Caucasians[104] (Fig. 155–13). On the other hand, other studies examining hypertensive rather than normotensive subjects have suggested that there is a significant relationship between these two variables, even in blacks.[105, 106]

Part of the difficulty in interpreting many of the published studies is the variability of the definition of who is insulin-resistant. A variety of techniques have been used to assess insulin resistance in vivo.[107] One of the simplest measures for screening large populations has been the measurement of the fasting insulin and glucose levels or the performance of a glucose tolerance test with measurement of insulin levels. Although these techniques are not sufficiently precise to accurately quantitate the severity of the insulin resistance, the simultaneous presence of hyperinsulinemia with normal or elevated glucose levels strongly suggests that insulin resistance is present. However, often a more precise quantitation of the magnitude of insulin resistance is required. Three approaches have been used: the minimal model approach,[108] the insulin suppression test,[109] and the euglycemic insulin clamp technique.[110] The presumed "gold standard" of these is the euglycemic insulin clamp technique. It is not universally utilized because of the extensive personnel needs to complete the study safely and accurately.

Mechanisms Responsible for Insulin Resistance
(see Ch. 91)

There are several possible defects that could be responsible for the decrease in glucose metabolism observed in insulin-resistant states. These include alterations in binding to or signal transduction by the insulin receptor, defects in glucose transport, and metabolic abnormalities in glycolysis, glucagon synthesis, or glucose oxidation. Recent studies have suggested that one other mechanism possibly underlying insulin resistance is a raised cytosolic calcium level. Studying both rat and human tissue, Drazin and colleagues have reported that adipocyte sensitivity to insulin is reduced when cytosolic calcium levels are raised.[111–113] While this may be one mechanism inducing insulin sensitivity, other mechanisms also must exist, since Kelly and colleagues reported that insulin resistance was not always correlated with raised cytosolic calcium levels in adipocytes.[114] The cytosolic calcium theory is particularly intriguing for two reasons: First, insulin resistance per se may actually contribute to an increase in cytosolic calcium. This is based on the results of several studies suggesting that insulin can directly stimulate the calcium pump (calcium ATPase).[115, 116] Thus a cell that has a reduced insulin sensitivity would presumably have a reduced activity of the major transport process to pump calcium out of the cell. This would then result in an increase in cytosolic calcium levels. Second, both platelet and lymphocyte cytosolic calcium measurements have been performed in essential hypertensives as a potential reflection of vascular smooth-muscle cytosolic calcium. An elevation of cytosolic calcium has been demonstrated in the platelets in essential hypertensives by some[117–121] but not by others.[122] Platelet cytosolic calcium has been reported to correlate with arterial pres-

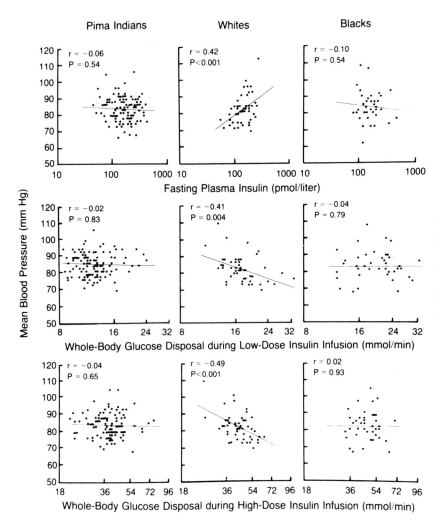

FIGURE 155–13. Glucose disposal rate determined by insulin clamp and fasting insulin levels in normotensive blacks, Caucasians, and Pima Indians. Note the significant correlation of arterial pressure with glucose disposal rates in the Caucasians but not in the other two subgroups. (From Saad MF, Lillioja S, Nyombab L, et al: Racial differences in the relationship between arterial pressure and insulin resistance. N Engl J Med 324:733–739, 1991, with permission of the Massachusetts Medical Society.)

sure by some[117, 123] but not by all[119, 121] investigators. It also has been reported to increase in response to dietary sodium loading in normotensive individuals with a positive family history for hypertension accompanied by an increase in arterial pressure.[124] An elevation in lymphocyte cytosolic calcium also has been demonstrated in hypertensive subjects.[125] In contrast to the platelet cytosolic calcium level, however, an increased lymphocyte cytosolic calcium level has not been correlated consistently with an increased arterial pressure.[123, 125] Interestingly, with weight reduction, a reduction in arterial pressure is accompanied by a reduction in platelet cytosolic calcium levels.[126] Weight reduction also reduces insulin resistance.

Relationship of Sodium Intake to Insulin Resistance

When sodium-restricted normotensive subjects are given a sodium load, there is an increase in insulin resistance, as determined by the euglycemic insulin clamp technique[127] (Fig. 155–14). This change (15 to 20 per cent) is similar (but opposite) to that observed when an individual loses weight. Thus the impact of dietary sodium intake on insulin sensitivity is substantial. Of interest, when patients with essential hypertension are assessed by similar techniques, there is minimal dietary sodium impact on insulin sensitivity. As a group, essential hypertensive patients, even when

adjusted for differences in weight, have glucose utilization rates considerably lower than normotensive subjects, whether they are on a high- or a low-sodium diet. Thus not only are patients with essential hypertension insulin-resistant, but they also have lost their sodium-mediated change in insulin sensitivity.

The mechanism underlying this sodium-mediated change in insulin sensitivity in normotensive subjects is unclear. However, of interest, when Sprague-Dawley rats are placed on a low-sodium diet, the number of renal insulin receptors and the mRNA levels for this receptor are substantially greater than when animals are placed on a high-sodium diet.[128] There is no change in the receptor's binding characteristics. Since insulin administered acutely produces renal sodium retention, the changes in the renal insulin receptor observed on a high-salt diet may assist the kidney to excrete a salt load. Since, in the human study, generalized insulin resistance was induced by sodium loading, it is likely that sodium intake modifies insulin receptors in a variety of tissues, specifically those which are involved in glucose homeostasis and the kidney.

Mechanisms Responsible for the Hypertension Associated with Insulin Resistance

Three major hypotheses have been developed to explain the role of insulin resistance in inducing an increase in

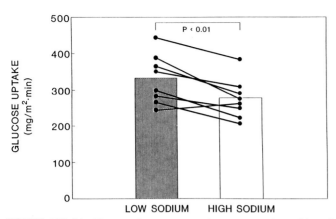

FIGURE 155–14. Glucose clearance rates in normotensive subjects in whom a euglycemic insulin clamp was performed. Each subject was studied twice: once on a 10-mEq sodium intake and a second time on a 200-mEq sodium intake. Note the 15 to 20 per cent decrease in glucose utilization when the subjects were studied on the high-sodium intake, suggestive of the induction of insulin resistance by salt loading. (From Donovan D, Solomon C, Williams GH, Simonson DC: Effect of dietary sodium intake on insulin sensitivity. Am J Physiol 264:E730–E734, 1993, with permission of the American Physiological Society.)

arterial pressure: (1) a defect in sodium handling by the kidney,[129] (2) an increased activation of the adrenergic nervous system,[95–101] and (3) increased vascular reactivity.[130] Both in human and animal studies, the acute administration of insulin induces sodium retention[129] (Fig. 155–15). Chronic studies have not been reported in humans, and in animals, chronic insulin administration does not seem to induce sodium retention.[131] However, because of the relationship between sodium intake, insulin sensitivity, and the number of renal insulin receptors, the chronic animal studies may be flawed. For example, insulin administration would acutely promote sodium retention in normal subjects or animals. This volume expansion would induce a state of insulin resistance, thereby reducing the efficacy of insulin in producing continued sodium reabsorption. However, patients with essential hypertension may already have down-regulated their insulin receptors. Therefore, the insulin-mediated sodium reabsorption may continue. Definite studies to test this possibility have not yet been reported.

Equally intriguing as the mediator of the hypertensive process with insulin resistance is insulin's effect on the adrenergic nervous system. It is quite clear that increases in insulin levels increase the activity of the adrenergic nervous system.[132] This leads to increased vasoconstriction, which under normal circumstances is counterbalanced by insulin's direct vasodilatory effect[133] (Fig. 155–16). However, in states where insulin resistance is already present as a primary defect and/or with chronic hyperinsulinemia, the relationship between insulin's vasoconstrictor effect, mediated through the adrenergic nervous system, and its direct vasodilatory effect may become unbalanced. A final possible mechanism which could increase arterial pressure is a change in vascular reactivity. Insulin could induce this by one of two mechanisms: (1) by increasing vascular smooth-muscle cytosolic calcium levels, as noted above, and (2) by inducing vascular hypertrophy and hyperplasia secondary to its mitogenic effect. Either or both of these mechanisms could lead to an increase in vascular resistance and reactivity.

In summary, insulin resistance is associated with an elevated arterial pressure in some patients with hypertension. This decrease in insulin sensitivity is observed even when differences in weight, age, lipid levels, or family history of diabetes are considered. There are theoretical reasons to suggest that insulin resistance and the hyperinsulinemia accompanying it could result in abnormalities in vascular and renal responses leading to increased vascular reactivity and sodium reabsorption. Furthermore, in patients with hypertension who have an underlying defect in the regulation of the insulin receptor, this defect will be magnified if obesity is present or diuretics and/or beta blockers are given. Both increase insulin resistance.[134]

Our understanding of how insulin resistance may increase arterial pressure is still limited. Indeed, it is unclear whether the insulin-resistant state is an actual cause of the elevated arterial pressure or an associated marker of some other defect which is the primary pathophysiological event.

CONCLUSION

Hormonal factors are clearly involved in the pathophysiology of most forms of secondary hypertension. Their role in the pathophysiology of the much more common group of patients with essential hypertension is less well-understood. Yet abnormalities in the renin-angiotensin-aldosterone system and insulin secretion have been associated with substantial subsets of the essential hypertensive population. Particularly intriguing are the mirror-image defects in some patients with low-renin essential hypertension (enhanced adrenal response on a high-sodium diet) and a sizeable fraction of the normal- and high-renin essential hypertensive group (nonmodulators with a decreased adrenal response to angiotensin II on a low-sodium diet). These reciprocal defects, because they are coupled to abnormalities in the regulation of the renin-angiotensin-aldosterone feedback loop and/or altered renal vascular responsiveness, lead to sodium-sensitive hypertension. In-

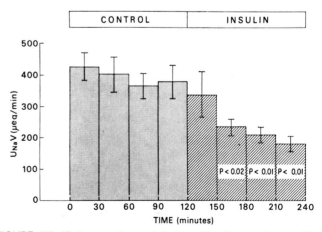

FIGURE 155–15. Impact of acute infusion of insulin on urinary sodium excretion in normal subjects. Patients were on an ad lib sodium diet and after four control urine collections, an insulin infusion was begun. Note the substantial fall in sodium excretion during the insulin infusion. (From Cooke CR, Andres R, Faloona GR, Davis PJ: The effect of insulin on renal handling of sodium, potassium, calcium and phosphate in man. J Clin Invest 55:845–855, 1975, with copyright permission of the American Society for Clinical Investigation.)

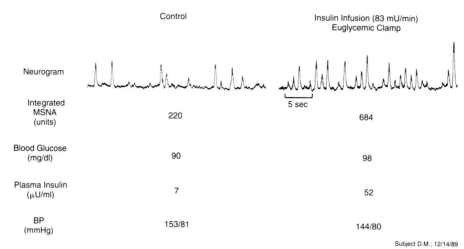

FIGURE 155–16. Forearm vascular and adrenergic nervous system responses to acute administration of insulin in a normal subject. Note the direct relationship between the activity of the adrenergic nervous system (as determined by direct nerve recording—integrated MSNA) and insulin levels and the inverse relationship between blood pressure and insulin. Additionally, forearm vascular resistance fell by 40 to 50 per cent when insulin was given. (From Anderson EA, Hoffman RP, Balon TW, et al: Hyperinsulinemia produces both sympathetic neural activation and vasodilation in normal humans. J Clin Invest 84:2246–2252, 1991, with copyright permission of the American Society for Clinical Investigation.)

deed, these subgroups may account for the vast majority of those individuals who have sodium-sensitive essential hypertension. Intriguing, but less well understood, is the potential role of hyperinsulinemia in inducing both increased vascular reactivity and sodium retention. Finally, the relationship among these three endocrine defects is uncertain. The potential that each of them is inherited provides entrée to a better understanding of these defects and the development of specific markers to identify patient subsets. The availability of such markers will have substantial implications for both prevention and specific therapy.

REFERENCES

1. Williams GH: Hypertensive vascular disease. *In* Isselbacher KJ, Braunwald E, Wilson JD, et al (eds): Harrison's Principles of Internal Medicine, 13th ed. New York, McGraw-Hill, 1994.
2. Williams GH, Hollenberg NK: Pathophysiology of essential hypertension. *In* Parmley WW, Chatterjee K (eds): Cardiology. Philadelphia, JB Lippincott Co, 1990, pp 1–18.
3. Williams GH, Dluhy RG: Diseases of the adrenal cortex. *In* Isselbacher KJ, Braunwald E, Wilson JD, et al (eds): Harrison's Principles of Internal Medicine, 13th ed. New York, McGraw-Hill, 1994.
4. Sokabe H: Physiology of the renal effects of angiotensin. Kidney Int 6:263–271, 1974.
5. Berne HA: Hormones and endocrine glands of fishes. Science 158:455–462, 1967.
6. Vinson GP, Whitehouse BJ, Goddard C, Sibley CP: Comparative and evolutionary aspects of aldosterone secretion and zona glomerulosa function. J Endocrinol 81:5P–24P, 1979.
7. Oelkers W, Brown JJ, Fraser R, et al: Sensitization of the adrenal cortex to angiotensin II in sodium-depleted man. Circ Res 34:69–77, 1974.
8. Hollenberg NK, Chenitz WR, Adams DF, Williams GH: Reciprocal influence of salt intake on adrenal glomerulosa and renal vascular responses to angiotensin II in normal man. J Clin Invest 54:34–42, 1974.
9. Strewler GJ, Hinrichs KJ, Guiod LR, Hollenberg NK: Sodium intake and vascular smooth muscle responsiveness to norepinephrine and angiotensin in the rabbit. Circ Res 31:758–766, 1972.
10. Devynck MA, Meyer P: Angiotensin receptors in vascular tissue. Am J Med 61:758–767, 1976.
11. Gunther S, Gimbrone MA Jr, Alexander RW: Regulation by angioten-
sin II of its receptors in resistant blood vessels. Nature 287:230–232, 1980.
12. Aguilera G, Catt K: Regulation of aldosterone secretion by the renin-angiotensin system during sodium restriction in rats. Proc Natl Acad Sci USA 75:4057–4061, 1978.
13. Platia MP, Catt KJ, Hodgen GD, Aguilera G: Angiotensin II receptor regulation during altered sodium intake in primates. Hypertension 8:1121–1126, 1986.
14. Williams GH, Hollenberg NK, Braley LM: Influence of sodium intake on vascular and adrenal angiotensin II receptors. Endocrinology 98:1343–1350, 1976.
15. Tremblay A, Parker KL, Lehoux JG: Dietary potassium supplementation and sodium restriction stimulate aldosterone synthase but not 11β-hydroxylase P450 messenger ribonucleic acid accumulation in rat adrenals and require angiotensin II production. Endocrinology 130:3152–3158, 1992.
16. Ganong WF: Angiotensin II in the brain and pituitary: Contrasting roles in the regulation of adrenohypophyseal secretion. Horm Res 31:24–31, 1989.
17. Grinstead WC, Young JB: The myocardial renin-angiotensin system: Existence, importance, and clinical significance. Am Heart J 123:1039–1045, 1992.
18. Rosenthal J, Thurnreiter M, Plaschke M, et al: Renin-like enzymes in human vasculature. Hypertension 15:848–853, 1990.
19. Printz MP: Regulation of the brain angiotensin system: A thesis of multicellular involvement. Clin Exp Hypertens 10:17–35, 1988.
20. Kifor I, Moore TJ, Fallo F, et al: Potassium-stimulated angiotensin release from superfused adrenal capsules and enzymatically-dispersed cells of the zona glomerulosa. Endocrinology 129:823–831, 1991.
21. Glorioso N, Atlas SA, Laragh JH, et al: Prorenin in high concentration in human follicular fluid. Science 233:1422–1424, 1986.
22. Kifor I, Moore TJ, Fallo F, et al: The effect of sodium intake on angiotensin content of the rat adrenal gland. Endocrinology 128:1277–1284, 1991.
23. Brecher AS, Shier DN, Dene H, et al: Regulation of adrenal renin messenger ribonucleic acid by dietary sodium chloride. Endocrinology 124:2907–2913, 1989.
24. Racz K, Pinet F, Gasc J-M, et al: Coexpression of renin, angiotensin and their messenger ribonucleic acids in adrenal tissues. J Clin Endocrinol Metab 75:730–737, 1992.
25. Tuck ML, Williams GH, Cain JP, et al: Relation of age, diastolic pressure and known duration of hypertension to presence of low renin essential hypertension. Am J Cardiol 32:637–642, 1973.
26. Laragh JH: Vasoconstriction-volume analysis for understanding and treating hypertension: The use of renin and aldosterone profiles. Am J Med 55:261–274, 1973.
27. Emanuel RL, Cain JP, Williams GH: Double antibody radioimmuno-

28. Hsueh WA, Carlson EJ, Israel-Hagman M: Mechanism of acid activation of renin: Role of kallikrein in renin activation. Hypertension 3:122–129, 1981.
29. Sealey JE, Moon C, Laragh J, Alderman M: Plasma prorenin: Cryoactivation and relationship to renin substrate in normal subjects. Am J Med 61:731, 1976.
30. Emanuel RL, Williams GH: Should blood samples for assay of plasma renin activity be chilled? Clin Chem 24:2042–2043, 1978.
31. Mitchell JR, Taylor AA, Pool JL, et al: Renin-aldosterone profiling in hypertension. Ann Intern Med 87:596–612, 1977.
32. Sambhi MP, Crane MG, Genest J: Essential hypertension: New concepts about mechanisms. Ann Intern Med 79:411–424, 1973.
33. James GD, Sealey JE, Mueller F, et al: Renin relationship dissects, race and age in a normotensive population. J Hypertens 4(suppl 5):S387–S389, 1986.
34. Channick BJ, Adlin EV, Marks AD: Suppressed plasma renin activity in hypertension. Arch Intern Med 123:131–140, 1969.
35. Mroczek WJ, Finnerty FA, Catt KJ: Lack of association between plasma renin and history of heart attack or stroke in patients with essential hypertension. Lancet 2:464–468, 1973.
36. Kaye TB, Crapo L: The Cushing syndrome: An update on diagnostic tests. Ann Intern Med 112:434–444, 1990.
37. Sudhir K, Jenning GL, Esler MD, et al: Hydrocortisone-induced hypertension in humans: Pressor responsiveness and sympathetic function. Hypertension 13:416–421, 1989.
38. Ulick S, Tedde R, Wang JZ: Defective ring A reduction of cortisol as the major metabolic error in the syndrome of apparent mineralocorticoid excess. J Clin Endocrinol Metab 74:593–599, 1992.
39. Melby JC: Diagnosis of hyperaldosteronism. Endocrinol Metab Clin North Am 20:247–255, 1991.
40. deSimone G, Tommaselli AP, Rossi R, et al: Partial deficiency of adrenal 11-hydroxylase: A possible cause primary hypertension. Hypertension 7:204–210, 1985.
41. Sheps SG, Jiang N-S, Klee GG, vanHeerdaen JA: Recent developments in the diagnosis and treatment of pheochromocytoma. Mayo Clin Proc 65:88–95, 1990.
42. Shapiro B, Fig LM: Management of pheochromocytoma. Endocrinol Metab Clin North Am 18:443–481, 1989.
43. Williams GH, Hollenberg NK: Renal vascular hypertension. In Klahr S, Massry SG (eds): Contemporary Nephrology, vol 2. New York, Plenum Press, 1983, pp 351–373.
44. Nally JV Jr, Chen C, Fine E, et al: Diagnostic criteria of renovascular hypertension with captopril renography: A consensus statement. Am J Hypertens 4:749S–752S, 1991.
45. Geddy PM, Main J: Renin-secreting retroperitoneal leiomyosarcoma: An unusual cause of hypertension. J Hum Hypertens 4:57–58, 1990.
46. Woods JW: Oral contraceptives and hypertension. Hypertension 11 (suppl II):II11–II15, 1988.
47. Criqui MH, Langer RD, Reed DM: Dietary alcohol, calcium and potassium. Circulation 80:609–614, 1989.
48. Grant FD, Mandel SJ, Brown EM, et al: Interrelationships between the renin-angiotensin-aldosterone and calcium homeostatic systems. J Clin Endocrinol Metab 75:988–992, 1992.
49. Williams GH, Braunwald E: Endocrine and nutritional disorders and heart disease. In Braunwald E (ed): Heart Disease, 4th ed. Philadelphia, WB Saunders Co, 1991, pp 1827–1855.
50. Keane WF, Anderson S, Aurell M, et al: Angiotensin converting enzyme inhibitor and progressive renal insufficiency: Current experience and future directions. Ann Intern Med 111:503–516, 1989.
51. Safar ME, London GM, Simon AC, Chau NP: Volume factors, total exchangeable sodium, and potassium in hypertensive disease. In Genest J, Kuchel O, Hamet P, Cantin M (eds): Hypertension: Physiopathology and Treatment. New York, McGraw-Hill, 1983, pp 42–53.
52. Cary RN, Douglas JG, Schwekert JR, Liddle GW: The syndrome of essentially hypertension and suppressed renin activity. Arch Intern Med 130:849–854, 1972.
53. Vaughn ED, Laragh JH, Gavras I, et al: Volume factor in low and normal renin essential hypertension: Treatment with either spironolactone or chlorathaladone. Am J Cardiol 32:522–532, 1973.
54. Adlin EV, Marks AD, Channick BJ: Spironolactone and hydrochlorothiazide in essential hypertension: blood pressure response and plasma renin activity. Arch Intern Med 130:855–858, 1972.
55. Douglas JG, Hollifield JW, Liddle GW: Treatment of low-renin essential hypertension: Comparison of spironolactone and a hydrochlorothiazide-treamterene combination. JAMA 227:518–521, 1974.
56. Kisch ES, Dluhy RG, Williams GH: Enhanced aldosterone response to angiotensin II in human hypertension. Circ Res 38:502–505, 1976.
57. Wisgerhof M, Brown RD: Increased adrenal sensitivity to angiotensin II in low-renin essential hypertension. J Clin Invest 63:1456–1462, 1979.
58. Marks AD, Marks DB, Kanefsky TM, et al: Enhanced adrenal responsiveness to angiotensin II in patients with low renin essential hypertension. J Clin Endocrinol Metab 48:266–270, 1980.
59. Woods JW, Liddle GW, Michelakis AM, Brill AB: Effect of an adrenal inhibitor in hypertensive patients with suppressed renin. Arch Intern Med 123:366–370, 1969.
60. Melby JC, Dale SL: Adrenal steroidogenesis in "low renin" or hyporeninemic hypertension. J Steroid Biochem 6:761–766, 1975.
61. Spark RF: Low renin hypertension and the adrenal cortex. N Engl J Med 287:343–349, 1972.
62. Sutherland DJ, Ruse JL, Laidlaw JC: Hypertension, increased aldosterone secretion and low plasma renin activity relieved by dexamethasone. Can Med Assoc J 95:1109–1119, 1966.
63. Ulick S, Chu MD: Hypersecretion of a new corticosteroid, 18-hydroxycortisol, in two types of adrenocortical hypertension. Clin Exp Hypertens [A] 4:1771–1777, 1982.
64. Connell JMC, Kenyon CJ, Corrie JET, et al: Dexamethasone-suppressible hyperaldosteronism. Hypertension 8:669–676, 1986.
65. Ganguly A: Glucocorticoid-suppressible hyperaldosteronism: An update. Am J Med 88:321–324, 1990.
66. Lifton RG, Dluhy RG, Powers M, et al: A chimaeric 11β-hydroxylase/aldosterone synthase gene causes glucocorticoid-remediable aldosteronism and human hypertension. Nature 355:262–265, 1992.
67. Rich GM, Ulick S, Cook S, et al: Clinical characteristics of glucocorticoid-remediable aldosteronism in a large pedigree. Ann Intern Med 116:813–820, 1992.
68. Lifton RP, Dluhy RG, Powers M, et al: The molecular basis of a hypertensive disease: Chimaeric gene duplications result in ectopic expression of aldosterone synthase and glucocorticoid-remediable aldosteronism. Nature Genet 2:66–74, 1992.
69. Shoback DM, Williams GH, Moore TJ, et al: Defect in the sodium-modulated tissue responsiveness to angiotensin II in essential hypertension. J Clin Invest 72:2115–2124, 1983.
70. Williams GH, Rose LI, Dluhy RG, et al: Abnormal responsiveness of the renin-aldosterone system to acute stimulation in patients with essential hypertension. Ann Intern Med 72:317–326, 1970.
71. Williams GH, Tuck ML, Sullivan JM, et al: Parallel adrenal and renal abnormalities in the young patients with essential hypertension. Am J Med 72:907–914, 1982.
72. Hollenberg NK, Merrill JP: Intrarenal perfusion in the young "essential" hypertensive: A subpopulation resistant to sodium restriction. Trans Assoc Am Physicians 83:93–101, 1970.
73. Hollenberg NK, Borucki LJ, Adams DF: The renal vasculature in early essential hypertension: Evidence for pathogenic role. Medicine 57:167–178, 1976.
74. Williams GH, Dluhy RG, Lifton RP, et al: Non-modulation as an intermediate phenotype in essential hypertension. Hypertension 20:788–796, 1992.
75. Adler GK, Moore TJ, Hollenberg NK, Williams GH: Changes in adrenal responsiveness and potassium balance with shifts in sodium intake. Endocr Res 13:439–445, 1987.
76. Rogacz S, Hollenberg NK, Williams GH: Role of angiotensin II in the hormonal, renal and electrolyte response to sodium restriction. Hypertension 9:289–294, 1987.
77. Redgrave JE, Rabinowe SL, Hollenberg NK, Williams GH: Correction of abnormal renal blood flow response to angiotensin II by converting enzyme inhibition in essential hypertensives. J Clin Invest 75:1285–1290, 1985.
78. Rystedt L, Williams GH, Hollenberg NK: The renal and endocrine response to saline infusion in essential hypertension. Hypertension 8:217–222, 1986.
79. Hollenberg NK, Moore TJ, Shoback D, et al: Abnormal renal sodium handling in essential hypertension: Relationship to failure of renal and adrenal modulation of responses to angiotensin II. Am J Med 81:412–418, 1986.
80. Moore TJ, Williams GH, Dluhy RG, et al: Altered renin-angiotensin-aldosterone relationships in normal renin essential hypertension. Circ Res 41:167–171, 1977.
81. Dluhy RG, Bavli SZ, Leung FK, et al: Abnormal adrenal responsiveness to angiotensin II dependency in high renin essential hypertension. J Clin Invest 64:1270–1276, 1979.
82. Taylor TT, Moore TJ, Hollenberg NK, Williams GH: Converting enzyme inhibition corrects the altered adrenal response to angiotensin II in essential hypertension. Hypertension 6:92–99, 1984.
83. Dluhy RG, Smith K, Taylor T, et al: Prolonged converting enzyme

inhibition in non-modulating hypertension. Hypertension 13:371–377, 1989.

84. Hayes CG, Tyroler HA, Cassel JC: Family aggregation of blood pressure in Evans County, Georgia. Arch Intern Med 128:965–975, 1971.

85. Annest JL, Sing CF, Biron P, Mongeau JG: Familial aggregation of blood pressure and weight in adoptive families: Estimation of the relative contributions of genetic and common environmental factors to blood pressure correlations between family members. Am J Epidemiol 110:492–503, 1979.

86. Morton NE, Guldbransen CL, Rao DC, et al: Determinants of blood pressure in Japanese-American families. Hum Genet 53:261–266, 1980.

87. Moll PP, Harburg E, Burns TL, et al: Heredity, stress, and blood pressure, a family set approach: The Detroit project revisited. J Chronic Dis 36:317–328, 1983.

88. Feinleib B, Garrison RJ, Fabsitz R, et al: The NHLBI twin study of cardiovascular disease risk factors: Methodology and summary of results. Am J Epidemiol 106:284–285, 1977.

89. Blackshear JL, Garnic D, Williams GH, et al: Exaggerated renal vasodilator response to calcium entry blockade in first-degree relatives of essential hypertensive subjects. Hypertension 9:384–389, 1987.

90. Uneda S, Fujshima S, Fujiki Y, et al: Renal hemodynamics and the renin-angiotensin system in adolescents genetically predisposed to essential hypertension. J Hypertens 2(3):S437–S439, 1984.

91. Baretta-Piccoli C, Pusterla C, Stadler P, Weidmann R: Blunted aldosterone responsiveness to angiotensin II in normotensive subjects with familial predisposition to essential hypertension. J Hypertens 6:57–61, 1988.

92. VanHooft IMS, Grobbee DE, Derkx FHM, et al: Renal hemodynamics and the renin-angiotensin-aldosterone system in normotensive subjects with hypertensive and normotensive parents. N Engl J Med 324:1305–1311, 1991.

93. Lifton RP, Hopkins PN, Williams RR, et al: Evidence for heritability of non-modulating essential hypertension. Hypertension 113:884–889, 1989.

94. Kahn CR: Insulin resistance: A common feature of diabetes mellitus (editorial). N Engl J Med 315:252–254, 1986.

95. Reaven GM, Hofman BB: Hypertension as a disease of carbohydrate and lipoprotein metabolism. Am J Med 8:2S–6S, 1989.

96. Pollare T, Lithell H, Selinus I, Berne C: Sensitivity to insulin during treatment with atenolol and metoprolol: A randomized, double-blind study of effects on carbohydrate and lipoprotein metabolism in hypertensive patients. Br Med J 298:1152–1157, 1989.

97. Laakso M, Sarlund H, Mykkanen L: Essential hypertension and insulin resistance in non-insulin-dependent diabetes. Eur J Clin Invest 19:518–526, 1989.

98. Halkin H, Modan M, Shefi M, Almog S: Altered erythrocyte and plasma sodium and potassium in hypertension: A facet of hyperinsulinemia. Hypertension 11:71–77, 1988.

99. DeFronzo RA, Ferrannini E: Insulin resistance: A multifaceted syndrome responsible for NIDDM, obesity, hypertension, dyslipidemia, and atherosclerotic cardiovascular disease. Diabetes Care 14:173–194, 1991.

100. Shen DC, Shieh SM, Fuh MM, et al: Resistance to insulin-stimulated-glucose uptake in patients with hypertension. J Clin Endocrinol Metab 66:580–583, 1988.

101. Pollare T, Lithell H, Berne C: Insulin resistance is a characteristic feature of primary hypertension independent of obesity. Metabolism 39:167–174, 1990.

102. Ferrannini E, Buzzigoli G, Bonadonna R, et al: Insulin resistance in essential hypertension. N Engl J Med 317:350–357, 1987.

103. Mbanya JC, Thomas TH, Wilkinson R, et al: Hypertension and hyperinsulinemia: A relation in diabetes but not essential hypertension. Lancet 1:733–734, 1988.

104. Saad MF, Lillioja S, Nyomba BL, et al: Racial differences in the relation between blood pressure and insulin resistance. N Engl J Med 324:733–739, 1991.

105. Falkner B, Hulman S, Tannenbaum J, Kushner H: Insulin resistance and blood pressure in young black men. Hypertension 16:707–711, 1990.

106. Manolio TA, Savage PJ, Burke GL, et al: Association of fasting insulin with blood pressure and lipids in young adults: The CARDIA study. Arteriosclerosis 10:430–436, 1990.

107. Bergman RN, Finegood DT, Ader M: Assessment of insulin sensitivity in vivo. Endocr Rev 6:45–86, 1985.

108. Bergman RN, Phillips LS, Cobelli C: Physiologic evaluation of factors controlling glucose tolerance in man: Measurement of insulin sensitivity and beta cell sensitivity from the response to intravenous glucose. J Clin Invest 68:1456–1466, 1981.

109. Harano Y, Hidaka H, Takatsuki K, et al: Glucose, insulin and somatostatin infusion for the determination of insulin sensitivity. Metabolism 27:1449, 1978.

110. DeFronzo RA, Tobin JD, Andres R: Glucose clamp technique: A method for quantifying insulin secretion and resistance. Am J Physiol 237:E214–E223, 1979.

111. Draznin B, Sussman KE, Eckel RH, et al: The existence of an optimal range of cytosolic free calcium for insulin-stimulated glucose transport in rat adipocytes. J Biol Chem 262:14385–14388, 1987.

112. Draznin B, Sussman KE, Eckel RH, et al: Possible role of cytosolic free calcium concentrations in mediating insulin resistance of obesity and hyperinsulinemia. J Clin Invest 28:1848–1852, 1988.

113. Draznin B, Lewis D, Houlder N, et al: Mechanism of insulin resistance induced by sustained levels of cytosolic free calcium in rat adipocytes. Endocrinology 125:2341–2349, 1989.

114. Kelly KL, Deeney JT, Corkey BE: Cytosolic free calcium in adipocytes: Distinct mechanisms of regulation and effect on insulin action. J Biol Chem 264:12754–12757, 1989.

115. Levy J, Gavin JR III, Hammerman MR, Avioli LV: Ca²⁺-Mg²⁺-ATPase activity in kidney vasolateral membrane in non-insulin-dependent diabetic rats: Effect of insulin. Diabetes 35:899–905, 1986.

116. Nagy K, Grunberger G, Levy J: Insulin antagonistic effects of insulin receptor antibodies on plasma membrane (Ca²⁺ + Mg²⁺) ATPase activity: A possible etiology of type B insulin resistance. Endocrinology 126:45–52, 1990.

117. Erne P, Bolli P, Burgisser E, Buhler FR: Correlation of platelet calcium with blood pressure: Effect of antihypertensive therapy. N Engl J Med 310:1084–1088, 1984.

118. Bruschi G, Bruschi ME, Caroppo M, et al: Cytoplasmic free [Ca²⁺] is increased in the platelets of spontaneously hypertensive rats and essential hypertensive patients. Clin Sci 68:179–184, 1985.

119. Cooper RS, Shamsi N, Katz S: Intracellular calcium and sodium in hypertensive patients. Hypertension 9:224–229, 1987.

120. Lechi A, Lechi C, Bonadonna G, et al: Increased basal and thrombin-induced free calcium in platelets of essential hypertensive patients. Hypertension 9:230–235, 1987.

121. Hvarfner A, Larsson R, Morlin C, et al: Cytosolic free calcium in platelets: Relationships to blood pressure and indices of systemic calcium metabolism. J Hypertens 6:71–77, 1988.

122. Dominiczak AF, Morton JJ, Murray G, Semple PF: Platelet cytosolic free calcium in essential hypertension: Responses to vasopressin. Clin Sci 77:183–188. 1989.

123. Pritchard K, Raine AEG, Ashley CC, et al: Correlation of blood pressure in normotensive and hypertensive individuals with platelet but not lymphocyte intracellular free calcium concentrations. Clin Sci 76:631–635, 1989.

124. Yamakawa H, Suzuki H, Nakamura M, et al: Role of platelet cytosolic calcium in the response to salt intake in normotensive subjects. Clin Exp Pharmacol Physiol 18:627–629, 1991.

125. Oshima T, Matsuura H, Kido K, et al: Intralymphocytic sodium and free calcium and plasma renin in essential hypertension. Hypertension 12:26–31, 1988.

126. Scherrer U, Nussberger J, Torriani S, et al: Effect of weight reduction in moderately overweight patients on recorded ambulatory blood pressure and free cytosolic platelet calcium. Circulation 83:552, 1991.

127. Donovan D, Solomon C, Seely EW, et al: Effect of dietary sodium intake on insulin sensitivity. Am J Physiol 264:E730–E734, 1993.

128. Sechi LA, Griffin CA, Grady EF, et al: Insulin receptor concentration and gene expression are modulated by sodium intake in the rat kidney. J Hypertens 9:S212–S213, 1991.

129. DeFronzo RA, Cooke CR, Adres R, et al: The effect of insulin on renal handling of sodium: Potassium, calcium and phosphate in man. J Clin Invest 55:845–855, 1975.

130. Weidmann P, Beretta-Piccoli C, Trost BN: Pressor factors and responsiveness in hypertension accompanying diabetes mellitus. Hypertension 7:II33–II42, 1985.

131. Hall JE, Coleman TG, Mizelle HL: Does chronic hyperinsulinemia cause hypertension? Am J Hypertens 26:171–173, 1989.

132. Anderson EA, Hoffman RP, Balon TW, et al: Hyperinsulinemia produces both sympathetic neural activation and vasodilation in normal humans. J Clin Invest 84:2246–2252, 1991.

133. Creager MA, Liang CS, Coffman JD: Beta-adrenergic–mediated vasodilator response to insulin in the human forearm. J Pharmacol Exp Ther 235:709–714, 1985.

134. Pollare T, Lithell H, Berne C: A comparison of the effects of hydrochlorothiazide and captopril on glucose and lipid metabolism in patients with hypertension. N Engl J Med 321:868–873, 1989.

Orthostatic (Postural) Hypotension

PHILIP E. CRYER

Orthostatic, or postural, hypotension is an abnormal fall in blood pressure when a person moves from the lying to the sitting or standing position. It is a common finding,[1] particularly in the elderly.[2] Although it can produce symptomatic cerebral hypoperfusion, including syncope, orthostatic hypotension is a clinical sign, not a diagnosis. It is the result of one or more of three fundamental mechanisms which can be produced by an array of disease processes, medications, or both. A supine to standing decrement in systolic blood pressure of 30 mmHg or more is often used to define orthostatic hypotension clinically.[1] However, decrements of 20 mmHg or more are a significant risk factor for falls and syncope and, in patients with diabetes mellitus, have been found to be associated with an increased 5-year mortality rate.[2]

The topic of orthostatic hypotension has been reviewed by the author in the broader context of disorders of the sympathochromaffin system[3] and by others in the context of autonomic failure,[4, 5] that of diabetic autonomic neuropathy,[6] and that of autonomic failure not due to diabetes mellitus.[7]

ORTHOSTATIC ADAPTATION

Physiology

Assumption of the upright position causes a sharp decrease in venous return (preload) to the heart because of pooling of an estimated 500 to 700 ml of blood in the distensible venous system, largely in the abdomen and lower extremities. In the absence of compensatory mechanisms, this would result in a corresponding decrease in cardiac output, arterial blood pressure, and tissue (including cerebral) perfusion. Syncope would result from the simple act of standing. Obviously, there are effective compensatory mechanisms.

The primary compensatory mechanism is activation of a baroreceptor-initiated, central nervous system–mediated sympathetic neural reflex. Activation of this reflex results in release of the neurotransmitter norepinephrine from axon terminals of sympathetic postganglionic neurons within the cardiovascular system. Through interaction with postjunctional alpha-adrenergic receptors, norepinephrine

causes arterial vasoconstriction in most of the extracerebral vasculature; the splanchnic vascular bed appears to play a particularly important role.[5] The resulting increase in systemic vascular resistance prevents a substantial fall in blood pressure; the pulse pressure normally narrows because of small decrements in systolic blood pressure, increments in diastolic blood pressure, or both. Although vasoconstriction is the predominant mechanism of maintenance of the blood pressure in the standing position, sympathetic norepinephrine release also limits the fall in venous return and in cardiac output through effects on the veins and the heart, respectively.

The majority of released norepinephrine is dissipated locally, either by reuptake into the axon terminal or uptake into cells adjacent to the synaptic cleft. Nonetheless, an estimated 10 per cent escapes into the circulation.[3] Therefore, as shown in Figure 156–1, assumption of the upright position normally causes a prompt, approximately two-fold increase in the plasma norepinephrine concentration.[3] Thus measurement of the plasma norepinephrine, along with the blood pressure and heart rate, response to standing can be used to assess the integrity of the sympathetic reflex arc in patients with orthostatic hypotension.[9–13]

While it is generally acknowledged that sympathetic neural norepinephrine plays a primary role in maintenance of the blood pressure in the standing position, other factors may be involved. For example, plasma vasopressin concentrations increase in the standing position, and administration of a vasopressin (V1) antagonist has been reported to cause orthostatic hypotension, albeit delayed, in some patients with diabetes mellitus and to worsen orthostatic hypotension in patients affected with this prior to drug administration.[14] However, orthostatic hypotension is not a feature of vasopressin deficiency (e.g., central diabetes insipidus). Similarly, plasma endothelin concentrations increase in the standing position, and reduced plasma endothelin responses have been reported in some patients with orthostatic hypotension.[15] Finally, the renin-angiotensin system is activated in the standing position, and a deficient response might theoretically contribute to development of orthostatic hypotension.[14] Again, however, orthostatic hypotension is not a feature of renin deficiency despite the resulting hypoaldosteronism. On the other hand, orthostatic hypotension is a consistent feature of autonomic (sympathetic) failure, as discussed later in this

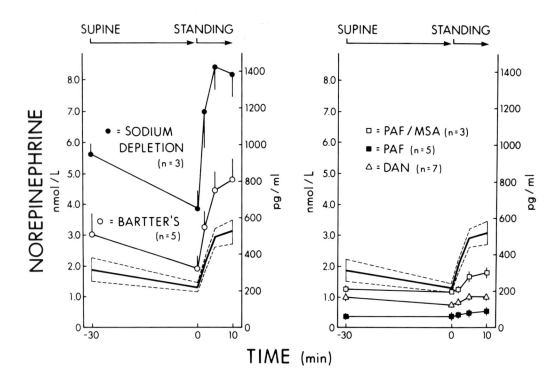

FIGURE 156-1. Mean *(heavy solid lines)* and 95 per cent confidence intervals *(interrupted lines)* of plasma norepinephrine concentrations measured in the supine and standing positions in 40 normal human subjects *(both panels)* and mean (±SE) plasma norepinephrine levels *(left)* in patients with sodium depletion *(closed circles)* and Bartter's syndrome *(open circles)* and *(right)* patients with progressive autonomic failure with multiple system atrophy (PAF/MSA, *open squares)*, progressive autonomic failure alone (PAF, *closed squares)*, and diabetic autonomic neuropathy (CDAN, *open triangles)*.

chapter. Thus, although it is conceivable that peptides such as vasopressin, endothelin, and angiotensin II play a supportive role in maintenance of the blood pressure in the standing position over time, it appears clear that the sympathetic nervous system plays the primary role in the short and probably the long term.

Additional factors are involved in maintenance of the blood pressure in the standing position. These include an adequate intravascular volume and a responsive cardiovascular system. Clearly, the integrity of the complex physiological regulation of these, discussion of which is beyond the scope of this chapter, is critical to the prevention of orthostatic hypotension.

Pathophysiology

Hyperadrenergic Orthostatic Hypotension

Clinically, orthostatic hypotension is most often the result of decreased intravascular volume or, less commonly, decreased vascular responsiveness to vasoconstrictors, particularly norepinephrine. The sympathetic reflex is, of course, intact. Indeed, the abnormal decrement in blood pressure causes an enhanced sympathetic response to standing, and the plasma norepinephrine increment is increased,[11, 12] as shown in Figure 156–1. Such patients have hyperadrenergic orthostatic hypotension.[3]

Hypoadrenergic Orthostatic Hypotension

Orthostatic hypotension also can be the result of a defect—afferent, central, or efferent—in the sympathetic reflex arc. This results in reduced norepinephrine release in response to standing. Thus, despite the resulting abnormal decrement in blood pressure, the plasma norepinephrine response to standing is reduced, as shown in Figure 156–1; indeed, it is often absent.[9, 10] Such patients have hypoadrenergic orthostatic hypotension.[3]

CLINICAL MANIFESTATIONS

Patients with orthostatic hypotension have normal (or elevated) blood pressures, and no symptoms referable to their blood pressure dysregulation per se, in the lying position. This is a key historical point. Symptoms that occur in both the lying and standing positions are not explicable on the basis of orthostatic hypotension. On the other hand, symptoms that occur only in the standing (or sitting) position strongly suggest abnormal orthostatic adaptation, which is easily confirmed by demonstration of an orthostatic drop in blood pressure, particularly if the symptoms are reproduced during that demonstration. Upon moving from the lying to the standing (or even the sitting) position, affected patients note a variety of symptoms such as lightheadedness, blurring or even loss of vision, and a profound sense of weakness. These may culminate in syncope. Nonetheless, patients typically have symptoms prior to syncope; syncope without premonitory symptoms is rarely if ever the result of orthostatic hypotension. Symptoms clear rapidly if the patient lies down. Postural symptoms are commonly worse on first arising in the morning (or on arising as to void during the night), after meals, and after exercise. Although often the case, symptoms need not occur immediately after arising. They can develop more gradually over time. Generally, standing quietly is particularly difficult for affected patients.

Despite the intensity of its symptoms, orthostatic hypotension per se is rarely fatal. It can be, however, if for some reason the patient cannot move to the lying position.

CAUSES

Hyperadrenergic Orthostatic Hypotension

As mentioned earlier, orthostatic hypotension is most commonly caused by intravascular volume contraction.

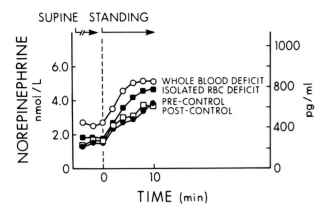

FIGURE 156–2. Plasma norepinephrine concentrations measured in the supine and standing positions in a normal subject in the basal state (pre-control, *closed circles*), after removal of 700 ml of whole blood (whole blood deficit, *open circles*), after reinfusion of the removed plasma (isolated red blood cell deficit, *closed squares*), and after subsequent reinfusion of the removed red blood cells (postcontrol, *open squares*). (Data from Tohmeh JF, Shah SD, Cryer PE: The pathogenesis of hyperadrenergic postural hypotension in patients with diabetes. Am J Med 67:772, 1979.)

Hemorrhage is a prominent example. As shown in Figure 156–2, a blood volume reduction of as little as 700 ml has been shown to cause a hyperadrenergic (increased plasma norepinephrine) response to standing[12]; hyperadrenergic orthostatic hypotension has been attributed to chronic reductions of red blood cell mass.[12] Sodium depletion is another common cause of intravascular volume contraction and orthostatic hypotension (see Fig. 156–1). This can be the result of excessive gastrointestinal or renal sodium losses with inadequate replacement. An example familiar to endocrinologists is sodium depletion resulting from hypoaldosteronism (see Chs. 99 and 103). In patients with Addison's disease (see Ch. 99), orthostatic hypotension attributable primarily to sodium depletion is compounded by reduced vascular responsiveness to norepinephrine.

Hyperadrenergic orthostatic hypotension caused by decreased responsiveness to norepinephrine is most commonly the result of the administration of vasodilator drugs. It is also part of the mechanism in Addison's disease, as mentioned, and the mechanism of orthostatic hypotension in Bartter's syndrome.[16] Thus the latter patients exhibit an enhanced plasma norepinephrine response to standing, as shown in Figure 156–1.

Clinically, abnormal postural adaptation represents a spectrum from normal maintenance of the standing blood pressure (resulting from an enhanced compensatory sympathetic response) with prominent tachycardia and sometimes disabling symptoms to frank orthostatic hypotension. The mechanisms of the former, the orthostatic tachycardia syndrome, are debated, but it clearly lies in the hyperadrenergic category.[17-19] It has been associated with unexplained reductions in blood volume and termed *idiopathic hypovolemia*,[18] and it is reported to improve following sodium loading.[17, 18] It also has been attributed to excessive gravitational pooling of blood, but defects in local autonomic innervation and vascular responsiveness to norepinephrine have not been found.[19, 20] Nonetheless, it has been reported to respond to octreotide and to ergot alkaloids.[20] On the other hand, evidence of postganglionic denervation of lower limb veins causing excessive gravitational blood pooling in patients further along the

spectrum, i.e., those with hyperadrenergic orthostatic hypotension, has been presented.[21]

These mechanisms—volume contraction and decreased vascular responsiveness—should be considered in all patients with orthostatic hypotension because they are often manageable. There can be multiple hypotensive mechanisms in a given patient, even a patient in whom autonomic failure, which is not treatable, is the primary mechanism. For example, otherwise trivial sodium depletion can result in symptomatic orthostatic hypotension, which can be treated with sodium repletion, in a patient with relatively mild autonomic failure.

Hypoadrenergic Orthostatic Hypotension

Hypoadrenergic orthostatic hypotension can result from afferent, central, or efferent lesions in the sympathetic reflex arc. Secondary causes of such lesions are listed in Table 156–1. In the absence of these, generalized autonomic failure is considered to be idiopathic or primary.

Primary Autonomic Failure

Despite some overlap, it is useful clinically to divide primary autonomic failure into two clinical and pathophysiological syndromes[1, 3, 5, 7, 22, 23]: progressive autonomic failure (idiopathic orthostatic hypotension, Bradbury-Eggleston syndrome) and progressive autonomic failure with parkinsonism or multiple system atrophy (Shy-Drager syndrome). These are abbreviated PAF and PAF/MSA, respectively, in this chapter. The etiology (or etiologies) of these disorders is unknown. It is not known whether they are two separate diseases or part of a spectrum of one disease. Pathological overlap, e.g., loss of neurons from the intermediolateral cell columns of the spinal cord, favors the latter interpretation and can be used as evidence against the simple designation of PAF as a disorder of the peripheral autonomic nervous system and PAF/MSA as a disorder of the central autonomic nervous system.[22, 23] Nonetheless, there are several clinical and pathophysiological differences between the syndromes.

PAF is characterized by hypofunction of the autonomic

TABLE 156–1. GENERALIZED AUTONOMIC FAILURE

A. Primary autonomic failure
  1. Progressive autonomic failure (idiopathic orthostatic hypotension, Bradbury-Eggleston syndrome)
  2. Progressive autonomic failure with parkinsonism or multiple system atrophy (Shy-Drager syndrome)
B. Secondary autonomic failure
  1. Metabolic disorders—diabetes mellitus, alcoholism, amyloidosis, others (porphyria, Tangier disease, Fabry's disease)
  2. Structural CNS disorders—trauma, tumors, or vascular lesions of the brain or spinal cord; syringomyelia
  3. Paraneoplastic autonomic failure
  4. Autoimmune disorders—acute and subacute dysautonomia, Guillain-Barré syndrome, pernicious anemia
  5. CNS infections—syphilis, Chagas' disease
  6. Others—hereditary sensory neuropathies, inflammatory neuropathies, familial dysautonomia (Riley-Day syndrome)

Modified, with permission, from Bannister R: Introduction and classification. *In* Bannister R (ed): Autonomic Failure. New York, Oxford University Press, 1983, p 1.

nervous system (both the sympathetic and the parasympathetic components) in the absence of other neurological dysfunction. Indeed, some physicians refer to this as "pure" autonomic failure. The defect in sympathetic function results in hypoadrenergic orthostatic hypotension. As shown in Figure 156–1, the plasma norepinephrine response to standing is reduced.[9, 10, 13, 23, 24, 25] The plasma norepinephrine response to stimulation of postganglionic neurons with edrophonium, an acetylcholinesterase inhibitor, has been found to be reduced in PAF but not in PAF/MSA.[13, 26] The urinary excretion of norepinephrine metabolites[27] and plasma norepinephrine levels[9, 10, 13, 23, 25, 28] are also lower in PAF compared with PAF/MSA. Taken together, these findings suggest more prominent damage to sympathetic postganglionic neurons in PAF than in PAF/MSA.

The defect in parasympathetic function can result in a variety of symptoms in PAF.[1, 3–7, 23, 29] These include genitourinary (urinary frequency, incontinence, or retention), gastrointestinal (diarrhea, fecal incontinence), and respiratory (sleep apnea, stridor) symptoms and hypohidrosis. Although it is typically slowly progressive and often produces substantial disability, PAF is consistent with survival for decades.

PAF/MSA is characterized by hypofunction of the autonomic nervous system clinically similar to that in PAF plus additional neurological disorders.[3–7, 22, 23, 29] The latter include striatonigral degeneration causing clinical Parkinson's disease. In addition, olivopontocerebellar atrophy (with gait disturbance and truncal ataxia) and pyramidal dysfunction (with hyperreflexia and extensor plantar reflexes) occur.[29] However, dementia is not a feature of PAF/MSA. PAF/MSA, in contrast to PAF, is typically rather rapidly progressive and debilitating. Death followed the onset of neurological manifestations by an average of 4 to 5 years in one series.[1]

Increased mononuclear leukocyte beta$_2$-adrenergic receptor and platelet alpha$_2$-adrenergic receptor densities, attributed to up-regulation in response to decreased norepinephrine levels, have been demonstrated in patients with primary autonomic failure.[30, 31] Given increased cardiovascular sensitivity to agonists in vivo,[31] adrenergic receptor up-regulation is thought to be a generalized phenomenon in such patients.

Hypoadrenergic orthostatic hypotension in the absence of parasympathetic hypofunction also occurs. It can result from dopamine β-hydroxylase deficiency[32–37] and has been attributed to an unexplained defect in norepinephrine release.[38] Patients with congenital dopamine β-hydroxylase deficiency can suffer hypothermia, hypotension, and hypoglycemia as neonates, but the disorder is characterized by severe orthostatic hypotension throughout later life. They have low plasma and urinary norepinephrine levels and elevated dopamine levels; the plasma norepinephrine-to-dopamine ratio is much less than 1.[35] Affected patients have been shown to have absent tissue dopamine β-hydroxylase immunoreactivity but normal tissue tyrosine hydroxylase and peptidergic immunoreactivity.[32, 34] Interestingly, treatment with 3,4-dihydroxyphenylserine, an unnatural catecholamine precursor that is converted to norepinephrine in the absence of dopamine β-hydroxylase, has been found to result in increased norepinephrine levels and marked improvement in orthostatic hypotension in patients with dopamine β-hydroxylase deficiency.[34–37]

Secondary Autonomic Failure

A number of causes of secondary autonomic failure are listed in Table 156–1. Of these, diabetic autonomic neuropathy is the most common. McLeod and Tuck[5] have emphasized that the peripheral neuropathies that most commonly include clinically important autonomic failure are those attributable to diabetes, amyloidosis, alcoholism (especially with Wernicke's encephalopathy), inflammatory neuropathy, and familial dysautonomia (Riley-Day syndrome). Although most of the disorders listed in Table 156–1 cause chronic autonomic failure, acute or subacute autonomic failure also occurs.[39] Typically, the latter develops in young, previously healthy individuals, evolves over 1 to 3 weeks, and resolves over months. Complete recovery is the rule, but there are sometimes residual defects. Initial symptoms are often gastrointestinal (vomiting, abdominal pain, diarrhea); syncope also can occur. An autoimmune mechanisms is often suspected. However, acute autonomic neuropathy can follow viral infections (including human immunodeficiency virus infection[40]), be associated with various autoimmune disorders or malignancies, or be secondary to porphyria, botulism, or various toxins.[39] The latter include the rodenticide Vacor and the chemotherapeutic agent vincristine. Orthostatic hypotension is the most common presenting feature in secondary autonomic failure, as it is in primary autonomic failure.[7]

DIAGNOSIS AND CLINICAL CLASSIFICATION

As mentioned earlier, orthostatic hypotension is suspected on the basis of symptoms that occur only in the upright position and resolve in the lying position. It is readily confirmed by measurement of the blood pressure in the lying and standing positions. The latter should be a routine part of the physical examination. Obviously, it is possible to diagnose asymptomatic orthostatic hypotension. While the latter does not require treatment, it represents a diagnostic clue.

A supine to standing decrement in systolic blood pressure of 30 mmHg or greater is generally considered diagnostic of orthostatic hypotension,[1] but decrements of 20 mm Hg are meaningful.[2] Indeed, the author considers any reproducible decrement in diastolic blood pressure abnormal and has used a 20 mmHg decrement in mean blood pressure as a diagnostic criterion.[11, 12] If the blood pressure does not decline promptly on arising in a patient with a suggestive history, the blood pressure should be measured repeatedly over 5 to 10 minutes of standing.

The heart rate should be recorded along with each blood pressure reading. A substantial increase in heart rate during orthostatic testing suggests that orthostatic hypotension is of the hyperadrenergic variety. On the other hand, the absence of an increase in heart rate suggests hypoadrenergic orthostatic hypotension. Intermediate heart rate increments, e.g., 10 to 20 beats/min, are, however, of little interpretive value. Measurement of the heart rate response also permits identification of bradycardic (vasovagal or vasodepressor) orthostatic hypotension, which can occur in apparently normal individuals and is generally not reproducible.

In patients with reproducible orthostatic hypotension

TABLE 156–2. CLINICAL TESTS FOR AUTONOMIC HYPOFUNCTION

TEST	NORMAL	BORDERLINE	ABNORMAL
Postural fall in blood pressure. Fall in systolic blood pressure (mmHg) after 2 min standing	<11	11–29	>29
Heart rate variation. Ratio of maximum to minimum heart rate (bpm) during deep breathing at 6 breaths/min	>15	11–14	<11
Heart rate response to standing. Ratio of the RR interval at approximately beat 30 to that at approximately beat 15 after initiation of standing (30:15 ratio)	>1.04	1.01–1.03	<1.01
Valsalva maneuver. Ratio of longest RR interval after to shortest RR interval during the Valsalva maneuver (40 mm Hg × 15 sec) with an aneroid manometer or modified sphygmomanometer (Valsalva ratio)	>1.20	1.11–1.120	<1.11
Sustained handgrip. Increase in diastolic blood pressure (mmHg) measured during 30 per cent of maximal handgrip for up to 5 min with a handgrip dynamometer	>15	11–15	<11

Used, with permission, from Ewing DJ: Practical bedside investigation of diabetic autonomic failure. *In* Bannister R (ed): Autonomic Failure. New York, Oxford University Press, 1983, p 371.

who are able to stand for at least 5 minutes, the plasma norepinephrine response to standing can be used to classify the disorder.[9–13] While the norepinephrine data illustrated in this chapter were determined with a single isotope derivative (radioenzymatic) method, high-pressure liquid chromatographic (HPLC) methods are available commercially and are adequate for plasma norepinephrine measurements. As shown in Figure 156–1, patients with hyperadrenergic orthostatic hypotension exhibit increased plasma norepinephrine responses, while those with hypoadrenergic orthostatic hypotension exhibit reduced plasma norepinephrine responses. Conservative criteria, based on the smallest and largest increments in plasma norepinephrine the author has observed in normal humans, are as follows: A supine to standing norepinephrine increment of less than 0.84 nmol/L (140 pg/ml) is low, while an absolute value of greater than 6.15 nmol/L (1040 pg/ml) is high. Interpretation of this maneuver sometimes requires judgment. For example, a low-normal norepinephrine response can be reasoned to be abnormally low in a patient with clear-cut orthostatic hypotension, since the lower blood pressure would be expected to stimulate an above-normal norepinephrine response if the sympathetic reflex were intact.

The use of orthostatic increments in plasma norepinephrine concentrations to assess patients with orthostatic hypotension has been criticized.[41] Esler and colleagues[41] have been pioneers in the development and application of isotopic techniques that independently quantitate the plasma norepinephrine appearance rate (or "spillover" rate to emphasize the fact that the plasma appearance rate is but a small fraction of the sympathetic neural norepinephrine release rate) and the plasma norepinephrine clearance rate. They have shown that patients with PAF can exhibit small orthostatic increments in plasma norepinephrine concentrations due to decreased norepinephrine clearance rather than increased norepinephrine spillover.[41] The plasma norepinephrine increments in their patients were smaller than those in their normal control subjects, even though the latter exhibited surprisingly small increments. Their point is, of course, well taken. However, its clinical relevance is debatable. Aside from the fact that isotopic measurements of norepinephrine kinetics are impractical in clinical practice, the clinical issue is to distinguish a hyperadrenergic (marked plasma norepinephrine incre-

ments) from a hypoadrenergic (minimal plasma norepinephrine increments) mechanism in a patient with orthostatic hypotension, not to distinguish either patient from persons with normal postural adaptation. As shown in Figure 156–1, the difference in the orthostatic plasma norepinephrine concentration responses between these two orthostatically hypotensive patient groups is substantially greater than that between those of either group and normal subjects.

The clinical utility of plasma norepinephrine measurements in the assessment of patients with orthostatic hypotension has not been evaluated critically. However, the author finds them useful in selected patients, typically those thought initially to have orthostatic hypotension due to a defect in the sympathetic reflex arc because of an associated disorder such as diabetes mellitus or parkinsonism or because of the absence of any other clinically apparent mechanism. Some such patients are found to have a hyperadrenergic pattern due to a treatable abnormality. Cardiovascular reflex tests, in addition to orthostatic blood pressure testing, of autonomic function also can be used to detect autonomic failure.[42–44] Some of these are listed in Table 156–2.

TREATMENT

General

The first principle of the management of a patient with orthostatic hypotension[1, 3, 4, 45–47] is careful consideration of potential remediable factors such as anemia, sodium depletion (including ill-advised dietary sodium restriction), or an offending medication. In the absence of such reversible factors, symptomatic therapy is often required. The objective of symptomatic therapy is to raise the standing blood pressure to a level that will prevent symptoms. It is not to raise the standing blood pressure to normal, since that would almost assuredly result in hypertension in the lying position. While the orthostatic blood pressure response should be followed during treatment, quantitation of standing time is often more useful in more severely affected patients.[46, 47]

Patients should be instructed to avoid rapid movement to sitting and standing position (with particular caution on first arising and after meals), activities that involve straining, unnecessary heat exposure, and prolonged bed rest. They also should avoid nonprescription medications that might worsen orthostatic hypotension. Physical maneuvers may raise the blood pressure.[47a]

Mechanical Measures

Most physicians recommend mechanical measures to patients with symptomatic chronic orthostatic hypotension.[1, 3, 4, 45–47] These include sleeping with the head of the bed elevated (to reduce natriuresis with fluid loss during sleep[48] and the use of elasticized support garments that extend from the feet to the costal margins (to reduce venous pooling during upright activity). To the author's knowledge, neither of these has been subjected to a rigorously controlled long-term clinical trial; clearly, they are impractical for some patients. Nonetheless, they are safe and are often recommended by clinicians with considerable experience who believe them to be effective.

Drug Therapy

The synthetic mineralocorticoid 9α-fluorohydrocortisone (Florinef), administered orally usually in doses of 0.1 to 0.3 mg or more daily, is the mainstay of drug treatment of chronic orthostatic hypotension.[1, 3, 4, 45–47] A potent sodium-retaining agent, if often relieves symptoms. The drug increases plasma volume transiently; over the long term it increases pressor sensitivity to norepinephrine and thus vascular resistance.[45, 49] Since the efficacy of 9α-fluorohydrocortisone is attributable to sodium retention, the physician should ensure a liberal sodium intake, with sodium chloride tablets if necessary. Indeed, in the author's experience, the most common cause of failure of 9α-fluorohydrocortisone therapy is the failure to provide a sufficiently high sodium intake. The latter can be documented with urinary sodium measurements. Although reluctance to recommend vigorous sodium loading for such often elderly patients is understandable because of the finite risk of precipitating cardiac failure, this is an unusual complication if cardiac function is adequate prior to therapy. On the other hand, hypokalemia is a common complication of 9α-fluorohydrocortisone and sodium chloride administration; potassium supplementation is often required. Another complication of effective therapy is hypertension in the lying position. Administration of a beta-adrenergic antagonist has been used to minimize this[1] but can precipitate cardiac failure. Although very large doses of 9α-fluorohydrocortisone (up to 2.0 mg daily!) have been used, side effects are generally proportional to the dose administered. It is useful to document positive sodium, and water, balance (an increase in body weight) and volume expansion (an increase in urinary sodium excretion) following initiation of a 9α-fluorohydrocortisone and sodium loading therapy. This, of course, requires several days.

If 9α-fluorohydrocortisone administration with sodium loading does not relieve orthostatic symptoms, most physicians continue these and add an additional drug.

The length of the list of other drugs that have been used to treat chronic orthostatic hypotension is in itself evidence of the lack of consistent efficacy of any one of these drugs. They include monoamine oxidase inhibitors (e.g., pargyline, tranylcypromine), cyclooxygenase inhibitors (e.g., indomethacin), dopaminergic agonists (e.g., metoclopramide, domperidone[50]), beta-adrenergic antagonists (e.g., propranolol, pindolol, xamoterol[51]), indirect-acting sympathomimetics (e.g., ephedrine, amphetamines, dietary tyramine), and direct-acting vasoconstrictors (e.g., the alpha-adrenergic agonists phenylephrine and phenylpropanolamine).

Drugs that produce venous as well as arterial constriction, such as midodrine, ergotamines, and clonidine, are conceptually appealing for the treatment of chronic orthostatic hypotension. Midodrine, an alpha-adrenergic agonist, appears effective in some patients, particularly those with less severe impairment of autonomic reflexes.[52, 53] With the exception of one report of efficacy of oral ergotamine tartrate,[54] oral, as opposed to parenteral, ergotamines have not been found to be effective, presumably because of their high first-pass hepatic extraction. Use of the combination of subcutaneous dihydroergotamine and oral caffeine has been reported.[55] Inhaled ergotamine tartrate has been shown to raise blood pressure and prolong standing time in patients with autonomic failure.[56] Clonidine, an alpha$_2$-adrenergic agonist, has been shown to raise the blood pressure in patients with severe autonomic failure and orthostatic hypotension but to lower blood pressure in less severely affected patients; the blood pressure response was inversely related to the plasma norepinephrine level.[57] Clonidine lowers blood pressure in normal individuals by suppressing central sympathetic outflow, but it also has a direct vasoconstrictive effect. Presumably the latter action predominates in patients with severe autonomic failure. Interestingly, in patients with less severe autonomic failure the alpha$_2$-adrenergic antagonist yohimbine has been shown to raise the blood pressure, presumably by enhancing endogenous norepinephrine release.[57, 58] Indeed, at this writing the author is inclined to try yohimbine when 9α-fluorohydrocortisone plus sodium loading is not sufficient to relieve symptoms of orthostatic hypotension.

Vasopressin analogues also have been tested in patients with autonomic failure.[59, 60] Desmopressin, given subcutaneously in the evening, was found to reduce nocturnal polyuria, diminish overnight weight loss, raise supine blood pressure, and reduce the orthostatic fall in blood pressure the following morning.[59] However, the drug can cause serious hyponatremia.[59]

Amezinium metilsulfate, a drug thought to increase endogenous norephinephrine release by inhibiting both monoamine oxidase and norepinephrine reuptake into sympathetic axon terminals, has been reported to increase sitting blood pressure and reduce orthostatic symptoms in patients with autonomic failure.[61] The norepinephrine precursor 3,4-dihydroxyphenylserine, used to treat patients with dopamine β-hydroxylase deficiency,[34–37] also has been used to treat generalized autonomic failure[62] and has been reported to be effective in PAF/MSA.[63]

Finally, with respect to drug treatment, the somatostatin analogue octreotide has been reported to prevent postprandial hypotension in patients with PAF/MSA, but not in those with PAF,[64] and to prevent glucose-induced hypotension in patients with autonomic failure.[65] The drug also has been reported to reduce orthostatic hypotension and prolong walking time in some patients with autonomic failure.[66, 67]

Other Approaches

Atrial pacing has been helpful in some patients with chronic orthostatic hypotension.[68, 69] Preliminary studies with a closed-loop computer-based system for blood pressure monitoring and controlled norepinephrine infusion were reported some years ago,[70] and an apparently successful example of this general approach has been reported.[71] Obviously, the safety and efficacy of these invasive approaches remains to be established. Nonetheless, further research into the treatment of chronic orthostatic hypotension is needed, since some patients are refractory to current treatment regimens and are disabled by their orthostatic hypotension.

ACKNOWLEDGMENTS: The author expresses gratitude to his several collaborators, to various research technicians, including particularly Mr. Suresh D. Shah, to the nursing staff of the Washington University General Clinical Research Center, headed by Ms. Carolyn E. Havlin, and to Ms. Mary Russo for preparation of this manuscript. The author's work cited was supported, in part, by U.S. Public Health Service Grants Mo1 RR00036, R01 DK 27085, and P60 DK 20579.

REFERENCES

1. Thomas JE, Schirger A, Fealey RD, Sheps SG: Orthostatic hypotension. Mayo Clin Proc 56:117–125, 1981.
2. Lipsitz LA: Orthostatic hypotension in the elderly. N Engl J Med 321:952–957, 1989.
3. Cryer PE: Diseases of the sympathochromaffin system. In Felig P, Baxter J, Frohman L (eds): Endocrinology and Metabolism (ed 3). New York, McGraw-Hill (in press).
4. Mathias CJ: Autonomic dysfunction. Br J Hosp Med 38:238–243, 1987.
5. McLeod JG, Tuck RR: Disorders of the autonomic nervous system. Ann Neurol 21:419–430, 1987.
6. Ewing DJ, Clarke BF: Diabetic autonomic neuropathy—Present insights and future prospects. Diabetes Care 9:648–665, 1986.
7. Ewing DJ: The clinical features of non-diabetic autonomic failure. Scott Med J 35:35–38, 1990.
8. Cryer PE, Santiago JV, Shah SD: Measurement of norephinephrine and epinephrine in small volumes of human plasma by a single isotope derivative method: Response to the upright posture. J Clin Endocrinol Metab 39:1025–1029, 1974.
9. Cryer PE, Weiss S: Reduced plasma norephinephrine response to standing in autonomic dysfunction. Arch Neurol 33:275–277, 1976.
10. Ziegler MG, Lake CR, Kopin IJ: The sympathetic nervous system defect in primary orthostatic hypotension. N Engl J Med 296:293–297, 1977.
11. Cryer PE, Silverberg AB, Santiago JV, Shah SD: Plasma catecholamines in diabetes: The syndromes of hypoadrenergic and hyperadrenergic postural hypotension. Am J Med 64:407–416, 1978.
12. Tohmeh JF, Shah SD, Cryer PE: The pathogenesis of hyperadrenergic postural hypotension in patients with diabetes. Am J Med 67:772–778, 1979.
13. Leveston SA, Shah SD, Cryer PE: Cholinergic stimulation of norepinephrine release in man: Evidence of a sympathetic postganglionic axonal lesion in diabetic adrenergic neuropathy. J Clin Invest 64:374–380, 1979.
14. Saad CI, Ribiero AB, Zanella MT, Mulinari RA, et al: The role of vasopressin in blood pressure maintenance in diabetic orthostatic hypotension. Hypertension 11(Suppl 1):I217–I221, 1988.
15. Kaufman H, Oribe E, Oliver JA: Plasma endothelin during upright tilt: Relevance for orthostatic hypotension. Lancet 338:1542–1545, 1992.
16. Silverberg AB, Mennes PA, Cryer PE: Resistance to endogenous norepinephrine in Bartter's syndrome: Reversion during indomethacin administration. Am J Med 64:231–235, 1978.
17. Rosen SG, Cryer PE: The postural tachycardia syndrome: Reversal of sympathetic hyperresponsiveness and clinical improvement during sodium loading. Am J Med 72:847–850, 1982.
18. Fouad FM, Tadena-Thoma L, Bravo EL, Tarazi RC: Idiopathic hypovolemia. Ann Intern Med 107:298–303, 1986.
19. Miller JW, Streeten DHP: Vascular responsiveness to norepinephrine in sympathicotonic orthostatic intolerance. J Lab Clin Med 115:549–558, 1990.
20. Hoeldtke RD, Davis KM: The orthostatic tachycardia syndrome: Evaluation of autonomic function and treatment with octreotide and ergot alkaloids. J Clin Endocrinol Metab 73:132–139, 1991.
21. Streeten DHP: Pathogenesis of hyperadrenergic orthostatic hypotension. J Clin Invest 86:1582–1588, 1990.
22. Bannister R: Introduction and classification. In Bannister R (ed): Autonomic Failure. New York, Oxford University Press, 1983, p 1-13.
23. Cohen J, Low P, Fealey R, et al: Somatic and autonomic function in progressive autonomic failure and multiple system atrophy. Ann Neurol 22:692–699, 1987.
24. Sever PS: Plasma noradrenaline in autonomic failure. In Bannister R (ed): Autonomic Failure. New York, Oxford University Press, 1983, p 155–173.
25. Goldstein DS, Polinsky RJ, Garty M, et al: Patterns of plasma levels of catechols in neurogenic orthostatic hypotension. Ann Neurol 26:558–563, 1989.
26. Gemmill JD, Venables GS, Ewing DJ: Noradrenaline response to edrophonium in primary autonomic failure: Distinction between central and peripheral damage. Lancet 1:1018–1021, 1988.
27. Kopin IJ, Polinsky RJ, Oliver JA, et al: Urinary catecholamine metabolites distinguish different types of sympathetic neuronal dysfunction in patients with orthostatic hypotension. J Clin Endocrinol Metab 57:632–637, 1983.
28. Goldstein DS, Polinsky RJ, Garty M, et al: Patterns of plasma levels of catechols in neurogenic orthostatic hypotension. Ann Neurol 26:558–563, 1989.
29. Bannister R: Clinical features of progressive autonomic failure. In Bannister R (ed): Autonomic Failure. New York, Oxford University Press, 1983, p 67–73.
30. Davies B: Adrenergic receptors in autonomic failure. In Bannister R (ed): Autonomic Failure. New York, Oxford University Press, 1983, p 174–200.
31. Senard JM, Vaet P, Durrieu G, et al: Adrenergic supersensitivity in parkinsonians with orthostatic hypotension. Eur J Clin Invest 20:613–619, 1990.
32. Robertson D, Goldberg MR, Onrot J, et al: Isolated failure of autonomic noradrenergic neurotransmission. N Engl J Med 314:1494–1497, 1986.
33. Man in't Veld AJ, Boomsma F, Moleman P, Schalekamp MA: Congential dopamine–beta-hydroxylase deficiency: A novel orthostatic syndrome. Lancet 1:183–187, 1987.
34. Mathias CJ, Bannister RB, Cortelli P, et al: Clinical, autonomic and therapeutic observations in two siblings with postural hypotension and sympathetic failure due to an inability to synthesize noradrenaline from dopamine because of a deficiency of dopamine beta hydroxylase. Q J Med 75:617–633, 1990.
35. Robertson D, Haile V, Perry SE, et al: Dopamine beta-hydroxylase deficiency: A genetic disorder of cardiovascular regulation. Hypertension 18:1–8, 1991.
36. Biaggioni I, Robertson D: Endogenous restoration of noradrenaline by precursor therapy in dopamine–beta-hydroxylase deficiency. Lancet 2:1170–1172, 1987.
37. Man in't Veld AJ, Boomsma F, van den Meiracker AH, Schalekamp MADH: Effect of an unnatural noradrenaline precursor on sympathetic control and orthostatic hypotension in dopamine–beta-hydroxylase deficiency. Lancet 2:1172–1175, 1987.
38. Nanda RN, Boyle FC, Gillespie JS, et al: Idiopathic orthostatic hypotension from failure of noradrenaline release in a patient with vasomotor innervation. J Neurol Neurosurg Psychiatry 40:11–19, 1977.
39. Hart RG, Kanter MC: Acute autonomic neuropathy. Arch Intern Med 150:2373–2376, 1990.
40. Cohen JA, Miller L, Polish L: Orthostatic hypotension in human immunodeficiency virus infection may be the result of generalize autonomic nervous system dysfunction. J Acquired Immune Deficiency Syndromes 4:31–33, 1991.
41. Esler MD, Meredith IT, Eisenhofer G, et al: Postural plasma noradrenaline responses are misleading as a test for autonomic failure in ortho-

static hypotension (Abstract). In Abstracts of the 7th International Catecholamine Symposium. Amsterdam, Excerpta Medica, 1992, p 87.

42. Hilsted J, Jensen SB: A simple test for autonomic neuropathy in juvenile diabetics. Acta Med Scand 205:385–387, 1979.

43. Ewing DJ: Practical bedside investigation of diabetic autonomic failure. *In* Bannister R (ed): Autonomic Failure. New York, Oxford University Press, 1983, p 371–405.

44. Johnson RH: Clinical assessment of sympathetic function in man. Methods Find Exp Clin Pharmacol 6:187–195, 1984.

45. Bannister R: Treatment of progressive autonomic failure. *In* Bannister R (ed): Autonomic Failure. New York, Oxford University Press, 1983, p 316–334.

46. Onrot J, Goldberg MR, Hollister AS, et al: Management of orthostatic hypotension. Am J Med 80:454–464, 1986.

47. Ahmad RAS, Watson RDS: Treatment of postural hypotension. Drugs 39:74–85, 1990.

47a. Wieling W, van Lieshout JJ, van Leeuwen AM: Physical manoeuvres that reduce postural hypotension in autonomic failure. Clin Autonom Res 3:57–65, 1993.

48. Kaufman H, Oribe E, Pierotti AR, et al: Atrial natriuretic factor in human autonomic failure. Neurology 40:1115–1119, 1990.

49. Chobanian AV, Volicer L, Tifft CCP, et al: Mineralocorticoid-induced hypertension in patients with orthostatic hypotension. N Engl J Med 301:68–73, 1979.

50. Sandra RGF, de Faria L, Zanella MT, et al: Peripheral dopaminergic blockade for the treatment of diabetic orthostatic hypotension. Clin Pharmacol Ther 44:670–674, 1988.

51. West JN, Stallard TJ, Dimmitt SB, et al: Xamoterol in the treatment of orthostatic hypotension associated with multiple system atrophy. Q J Med 74:209–213, 1990.

52. Kauffmann H, Brannan T, Krakoff L, et al: Treatment of orthostatic hypotension due to autonomic failure with a peripheral alpha-adrenergic agonist (midodrine). Neurology 38:951–956, 1988.

53. McTavish D, Goa KL: Midodrine: A review of its pharmacological properties and therapeutic use in orthostatic hypotension and secondary hypotensive disorders. Drugs 38:757–777, 1989.

54. Chobanian AV, Tifft CP, Faxon DP, et al: Treatment of chronic orthostatic hypotension with ergotamine. Circulation 67:602–608, 1983.

55. Hoeldtke RD, Cavanaugh ST, Hughes JD, Polansky M: Treatment of orthostatic hypotension with dihydroergotamine and caffeine. Ann Intern Med 105:168–173, 1986.

56. Biaggioni I, Zygmunt D, Haile V, Robertson D: Pressor effect of inhaled ergotamine in orthostatic hypotension. Am J Cardiol 65:89–92, 1990.

57. Robertson D, Goldberg MR, Tung C-S, et al: Use of alpha$_2$ adrenoceptor agonists and antagonists in the functional assessment of the sympathetic nervous system. J Clin Invest 78:576–581, 1986.

58. Onrot J, Goldberg MR, Biaggioni I, et al: Oral yohimbine in human autonomic failure. Neurology 37:215–220, 1987.

59. Mathias CJ, Fosbraey P, da Costa DF, et al: The effect of desmopressin on nocturnal polyuria, overnight weight loss, and morning postural hypotension in patients with autonomic failure. Br Med J 293:353–354, 1986.

60. Rittig S, Arentsen J, Sorenson K, et al: The hemodynamic effects of triglycyl-lysine-vasopressin (Glypressin) in patients with parkinsonism and orthostatic hypotension. Mov Disord 6:21–28, 1991.

61. Kita K, Hirayama K: Treatment of neurogenic orthostatic hypotension with amezinium metilsulfate, a new indirect sympathomimetic drug. Neurology 38:1095–1099, 1988.

62. Freeman R, Landsberg L: The treatment of orthostatic hypotension with dihydroxyphenylserine. Clin Neuropharmacol 14:296–304, 1991.

63. Kaufman H, Oribe E, Yahr MD: Differential effect of L-threo-3,4-dihydroxyphenylserine in pure autonomic failure and multiple system atrophy with autonomic failure. J Neural Transm 3:143–148, 1991.

64. Hoeldtke RD, Dworkin GE, Gaspar SR, et al: Effect of the somatostatin analogue SMS-201-995 on the adrenergic response to glucose ingestion in patients with postprandial hypotension. Am J Med 86:673–677, 1989.

65. Raimbach SJ, Cortelli P, Kooner JS, et al: Prevention of glucose-induced hypotension by the somatostatin analogue octreotide (SMS 210-995) in chronic autonomic failure: Hemodynamic and hormonal changes. Clin Sci 77:623–628, 1989.

66. Hoeldtke RD, O'Dorisio TM, Boden G: Treatment of autonomic neuropathy with a somatostatin analogue, SMS-201-995. Lancet 2:602–605, 1986.

67. Hoeldtke RD, Israel BC: Treatment of orthostatic hypotension with octreotide. J Clin Endocrinol Metab 68:1051–1059, 1989.

68. Kristinsson A: Programmed atrial pacing for orthostatic hypotension. Acta Med Scand 214:79–83, 1983.

69. Weissman P, Chin MT, Moss AJ: Cardiac tacypacing for severe refractory idiopathic orthostatic hypotension. Ann Intern Med 116:650–651, 1992.

70. Polinsky RJ, Samaras GM, Kopin IJ: Sympathetic neural prosthesis for managing orthostatic hypotension. Lancet 1:901–904, 1983.

71. Lehmann M, Peterson KG, Khalaf AN, et al: Improvement of the exercise capacity of a patient with primary orthostatic hypotension (primary sympathetic insufficiency) by programmed subcutaneous noradrenaline administration via microdosing pump. Klin Wochenschr 68:873, 1990.

Hormones and Blood Cell Production

DONALD METCALF
NICOS A. NICOLA
NICHOLAS M. GOUGH

The ambivalence of the title of this chapter reflects the difficulty endocrinologists have in coming to terms with the significance and implications of the numerous specific regulatory molecules that control crucial aspects of the biology of specific cell populations but have not yet been wholly embraced into the family of "hormones." This chapter will deal in detail only with the four colony-stimulating factors (CSF's), controlling granulocytic and macrophage production, and erythropoietin, controlling erythropoiesis.

REGULATORY CONTROL OF HEMOPOIETIC CELLS

Despite their apparently random admixture, hemopoietic populations are organized into a developmental sequence in which multipotential stem cells generate lineage-specific committed progenitor cells which, in turn, produce the dividing and maturing cells in that lineage.[1] Control of these processes is achieved by the use of a double control system: (1) local control by specialized stromal cells in the marrow and (2) control by a group of molecular regulators acting via specific membrane receptors on target cells (Fig. 157–1). No hemopoietic cells are capable of spontaneous proliferation, and all cell divisions require continuous stimulation by an appropriate regulator. Variation in the concentration of these regulators, whether circulating or locally produced, achieves the required level of mature cell production or functional activation.

Local Control Systems

Hemopoietic stromal cells are of special importance in controlling the formation and commitment of stem and progenitor cells. Early evidence for the probable importance of cell contact in the local control exerted by stromal

cells came from an analysis of the selective nature of hemopoietic colony formation initiated by stem cells seeding in the spleen and bone marrow of irradiated recipients.[2] This has been substantiated by the demonstration in tissue culture that adherent layers of stromal cells are particularly efficient in maintaining the numbers of stem and progenitor cells in contact with them in long-term cultured marrow cells.[3]

Marrow stromal cells can produce a number of hemopoietic regulatory factors, including interleukin 1 (IL-1),

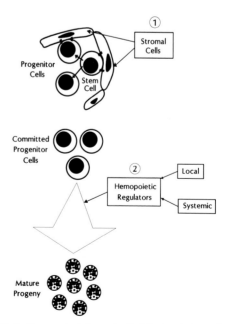

FIGURE 157–1. Hemopoiesis is controlled by local stromal cells and by hemopoietic regulators. Local control systems appear to have their most obvious impact on stem cell populations, whereas the hemopoietic regulators are prominent in controlling the production of maturing cells by progenitor cells.

granulocyte-macrophage colony-stimulating factor (GM-CSF), granulocyte colony-stimulating factor (G-CSF), macrophage colony-stimulating factor (M-CSF), IL-4, IL-6, IL-9, IL-11, stem cell factor (SCF), and leukemia inhibitory factor (LIF). In at least the cases of M-CSF and SCF, these regulators are able to be produced in both membrane-displayed and secreted forms, the membrane-displayed form being active in stimulating hemopoietic cells making effective cell contact.[4, 5] No regulator has yet been characterized that is only produced by stromal cells.

It remains unclear, therefore, whether the hemopoietic stromal cells are important because they produce unique molecules crucial for early events in hemopoiesis, whether the membrane display of regulators is a more effective method of presentation of regulators to early hemopoietic cells, or whether the stromal cells simply generate high local concentrations of soluble regulators within areas containing hemopoietic populations.

Regulatory Factors

Specific hemopoietic regulatory factors acting on hemopoietic populations can be produced locally, as noted above, or be produced elsewhere in the body and then act as conventional humoral regulators. To date, 19 hemopoietic regulators have been characterized, cloned, and produced recombinantly in an active form (Table 157–1). Almost all are glycoproteins with a relatively similar polypeptide molecular mass of 14 to 21 kDa.[6] Individual regulators vary widely in their range of responding target cells. At one extreme, erythropoietin action is restricted to erythroid and possibly megakaryocytic cells. At the other extreme, LIF has actions on hemopoietic cells of various types, osteoblasts, fibroblasts, neuronal cells, hepatocytes, myoblasts, and embryonic stem cells. There are no examples where the action of a hemopoietic regulator is absolutely confined to cells of a single hemopoietic lineage. As a consequence of this pattern, cells in any one lineage are potentially able to be influenced by multiple regulators, and the regulator design pattern is one of apparent redundancy (Fig. 157–2). There are some situations where regulator action tends to be sequential, but this sequential aspect of regulator control has been more emphasized than warranted by the actual data.

Regulator action is mediated by unique receptors on the

TABLE 157–1. THE HEMOPOIETIC REGULATORS

REGULATOR	ABBREVIATION	RESPONDING HEMOPOIETIC CELLS
Erythropoietin	Epo	E, Meg
Granulocyte-macrophage colony-stimulating factor	GM-CSF	G, M, Eo, Meg, E
Granulocyte colony-stimulating factor	G-CSF	G, M
Macrophage colony-stimulating factor	M-CSF	M, G
Multipotential colony-stimulating factor (interleukin 3)	Multi-CSF/IL-3	G, M, Eo, Meg, Mast, E, Stem
Interleukin 1	IL-1	T, Stem
Interleukin 2	IL-2	T, B
Interleukin 4	IL-4	B, T, G, M, Mast
Interleukin 5	IL-5	Eo, B
Interleukin 6	IL-6	B, G, Stem, Meg
Interleukin 7	IL-7	B, T
Interleukin 9	IL-9	T, Meg, Mast
Interleukin 10	IL-10	T
Interleukin 11	IL-11	Meg, B
Interleukin 12	IL-12	NK
Megakaryocyte colony-stimulating factor	Meg-CSF	Meg
Stem cell factor (Steel factor)	SCF	Stem, G, E, Meg, Mast
Leukemia inhibitory factor	LIF	Meg
Oncostatin M	OSM	?

G, granulocyte; M, macrophages; Eo, eosinophils; E, erythroid cells; Meg, megakaryocytes; Stem, stem cells; Mast, mast cells; T, T lymphocytes; B, B lymphocytes; NK, natural killer cells.

membranes of responding cells.[6] These are transmembrane glycoproteins and typically number a few hundred or, at most, a few thousand per cell. In some cases the ligand-activated receptor is comprised of a dimer of two receptor molecules, while in other cases high-affinity receptors are generated by complexing of a low-affinity receptor chain (α subunit) with a β subunit.[7]

In general, the amino acid sequences of the various hemopoietic regulators exhibit minimal evidence of homology that might suggest relatedness of the regulators. In contrast, there is clear evidence of the relatedness of many of the receptors which in fact comprise a superfamily of growth factor receptors, a family that includes those for some hormones such as prolactin and growth hormone[8] (Fig. 157–3). Two hemopoietic growth factors, SCF and M-

MULTIPLE REDUNDANT FACTORS CONTROL EACH HEMOPOIETIC LINEAGE

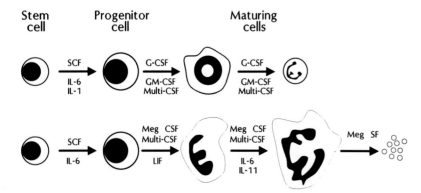

FIGURE 157–2. Hemopoietic cells, as exemplified by cells in the granulocytic and megakaryocytic lineages, are subject to control by multiple sets of hemopoietic regulators.

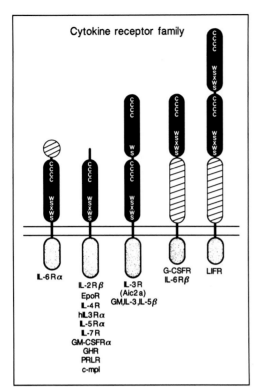

FIGURE 157–3. The membrane receptors for many of the hemopoietic regulators are members of the cytokine receptor superfamily in which receptors exhibit homologous regions in their extracellular domain.

CSF, have tyrosine kinase receptors that have domains of the immunoglobulin superfamily.

Stem cells appear to require stimulation by multiple regulators to respond by cell proliferation. Committed progenitor cells and their progeny can be stimulated to proliferate by single regulatory molecules. However, progenitor cells and their progeny characteristically co-express receptors for multiple regulators, and combinations of such regulators usually elicit additive or superadditive proliferative responses.

THE COLONY-STIMULATING FACTORS (CSF's)

There are six regulators with direct proliferative actions on granulocyte-macrophage precursors: the four colony-stimulating factors (CSF's), IL-6, and SCF. Of these, the major regulators are probably the CSF's. The CSF's were discovered and purified on the basis of their ability to stimulate granulocyte-macrophage progenitor cells to proliferate in semisolid cultures and form colonies of maturing granulocytes and/or macrophages.[9, 10]

The CSF's are glycoproteins, three of which have a single polypeptide chain, while the fourth, M-CSF, is a dimer of two apparently identical chains (Table 157–2). The size of the CSF polypeptide chains is similar (14,000 to 26,000 mol wt), but because of their widely varying carbohydrate content, the native CSF's can vary in their molecular weight from 18,000 to 140,000. The four CSF's share no significant sequence homology, but there are a number of reasons for regarding them as a related family of regulators. (1) Their actions on responding cells are comparable, and most of the cells simultaneously express receptors for all four CSF's, allowing subtle interactions between the CSF's. (2) The genes for GM-CSF and multipotential CSF (multi-CSF) lie adjacent on chromosome 5 in humans (11 in the mouse) and perhaps share common regulatory elements. (3) GM-CSF, multi-CSF, and G-CSF appear likely to have similar three-dimensional structures. (4) The receptors for G-CSF, GM-CSF, and multi-CSF exhibit obvious homology, and those for GM-CSF and multi-CSF share a common β subunit.

As their major action, all four CSF's stimulate the proliferation of granulocytic and macrophage cells, but G-CSF tends to be a selective stimulus for neutrophilic granulocyte formation while, conversely, M-CSF tends to be a selective stimulus for the formation of macrophages. GM-CSF and multi-CSF are stimuli for the formation of both granulocytic and macrophage cells.[11]

Each CSF has some ability to stimulate stem cells to proliferate and generate committed progenitor cells. This action requires collaboration with one or more additional

TABLE 157–2. MOLECULAR PROPERTIES OF HUMAN HEMOPOIETIC GROWTH FACTORS

	GM-CSF	G-CSF	M-CSF	MULTI-CSF (IL-3)	EPO
Leader sequence (aa)	17	30	31	19	27
Mature sequence (aa)	127	174; 177	158; 189	133	165
Predicted protein mol wt	14,465	18,600	26,000	15,400	18,398
Glycosylated mol wt (kDa)	15–35	20	45 + 60 (homodimer)	15–30	30–34
Cysteines (disulfides)	(54–96; 88–121)	17 (36–42; 64–74)	7, 31, 48, 90, 102, 139, 146	(16–84)	(7–161; 29–33)
Glycosylation sites					
N	Asn 19, 29	—	Asn 122, 140	Asn 15, 70	Asn 24, 38, 83
O	Ser 9, Thr 10	Thr 133	+	+	Ser 126
Alpha helix (%)	47	69		40	55
Predicted (actual) helix					
A	15–28 (13–28)	13–26, 49–57	15–38	19–27	3–20
B	34–41 (55–64)	70–97	46–61	56–68	55–77
C	55–75 (74–87)	106–130	73–93	71–85	90–113
D	97–117 (103–116)	155–175	110–130	103–121	129–151
Predicted active site	A21–31 C78–87	A20–46		Loop 29–50 D110–111	C99–100
Sequence identity (mouse/human)	56%	80%	75%	29%	79%

hemopoietic regulators, the most active of which are SCF (Steel factor), IL-1, and IL-6.[12]

Each CSF also has proliferative effects on hemopoietic cells outside the granulocyte-macrophage lineage and possibly on some nonhemopoietic cells. GM-CSF is a proliferative stimulus for eosinophils and at high concentrations for megakaryocytes and some erythroid precursors.[13] Multi-CSF is the most broadly acting of the CSF's, with the additional ability to stimulate the proliferation of eosinophils, megakaryocytes, erythroid cells, mast cells, and some stem cells.[14] Both G-CSF and GM-CSF have been reported to stimulate the proliferation of endothelial cells[15] and M-CSF the proliferation of placental trophoblast cells.[16] Small cell lung tumor cells and certain other types of cancer cells can express receptors for GM-CSF, but the data are conflicting whether GM-CSF has the ability to stimulate the proliferation of these cells.[17, 18]

Multiple Actions of the CSF's

Each CSF exhibits multiple actions on responding granulocytic and macrophage cells.

PROLIFERATIVE STIMULATION. Each CSF is a highly active proliferative stimulus, and the purified recombinant CSF's stimulate increasing colony formation at concentrations between 50 and 2000 pg/ml[11] (Fig. 157–4). Although some proliferation can be achieved by interrupted exposure to a CSF,[19] the long intracellular half-life of bound CSF receptors[6] makes it possible that sustained signaling could occur and be necessary throughout the cell cycle. If cells are not in cell cycle, then CSF stimulation forces the cells from G_1/G_0 into the S-phase of the cell cycle within 3 hours.[20] Thereafter, the concentration of CSF impinging on the responding cell determines the length of the cell cycle and the number of maturing progeny produced.[21] As CSF concentrations are increased, resulting cell production rises because of two mechanisms: the recruitment of extra (less responsive) progenitor cells into the pool of responding precursors and increased cell production by individual progenitor cells.

DIFFERENTIATION COMMITMENT. In the granulocyte-mac-rophage lineage, many progenitor cells are bipotential, with a capacity to form both granulocytic and macrophage progeny. The decision regarding which type of progeny to be produced appears able to be influenced by the action of a CSF such as M-CSF or G-CSF.[22]

More obvious examples of the ability of a CSF to initiate differentiation commitment have come from an analysis of CSF action on myeloid leukemic cells, where the CSF's can irreversibly suppress the self-generation of clonogenic cells and force the production of progeny that are committed to initiate differentiation into either the granulocytic or macrophage pathway.[23]

INDUCTION OF MATURATION. No single regulatory molecule could be expected to be able to intervene directly to control all the complex steps involved in granulocyte or macrophage maturation, but the data indicate that the CSF's can at least *initiate* maturation, even if the succeeding elements of the sequence are possibly programmed so as to be autoinducing.[22]

FUNCTIONAL ACTIVATION. The CSF's play a role in maintaining the integrity of membrane transport of ions and small metabolites. In the absence of adequate CSF concentrations, granulocyte-macrophage cells die prematurely by the process of apoptosis.[24] This action of the CSF's affects all cells in the sequence from progenitor cells to mature neutrophils and monocytes.

In addition, the CSF's have an important, if not exclusive, ability to stimulate many functions of mature granulocytic and macrophage cells. These actions range from enhancement of phagocytosis, intracellular killing of organisms, antibody-mediated cytotoxicity, and superoxide production to the production, particularly by monocytes and macrophages, of a wide range of biologically active molecules such as other hemopoietic factors (e.g., IL-1, CSF's or IL-6, and plasminogen-activator), interferon-γ, lysozyme, and tumor necrosis factor.[11, 25–28]

Interactions Between the CSF's and with Other Growth Factors

Most granulocyte-macrophage progenitor cells co-express receptors for all four CSF's and can potentially be

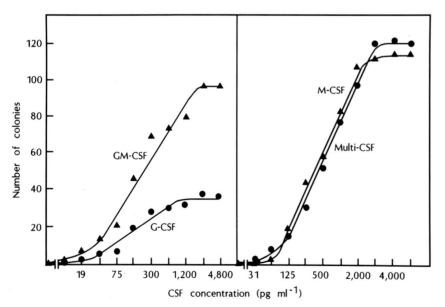

FIGURE 157–4. The formation of granulocyte and/or macrophage colonies by murine progenitor cells after stimulation by increasing concentrations of purified colony-stimulating factors. (From Metcalf D: The Florey Lecture 1991: The colony stimulating factors: Discovery to clinical use. Philos Trans R Soc Lond [Biol] 333:147–173, 1991.)

stimulated simultaneously by two or more CSF's. Co-stimulation leads to the formation of larger numbers of maturing granulocytes and macrophages by individual progenitor cells than does stimulation by twice the concentration of each CSF alone.[1, 29]

In a few exceptional situations, combinations of CSF's can result in antagonistic effects. With murine cells, the combination of GM-CSF with M-CSF is suppressive for the proliferation of some macrophage progenitor cells.[29] Similarly, when stimulating the functional activity of mature neutrophils, addition of GM-CSF can suppress the rise in alkaline phosphatase induced by stimulation using G-CSF.[30]

Combination of CSF's with regulators acting on stem cells, such as stem cell factor or IL-1, achieves a potentiation of granulocyte and macrophage formation that is much greater in magnitude than that observed following combinations of CSF's.[12, 31]

General Physiology of the CSF's

CSF's are products or potential products of a variety of cell types distributed widely throughout the body.[1, 32] They therefore display one of the characteristic features of hemopoietic regulators—the possibility of systemic action as a conventional humoral regulator or the possibility of exclusively local production and action. Only low levels of CSF's are detectible by bioassay or immunoassay in the tissues or serum. The production of CSF's is, however, highly labile, and following induction by, for example, endotoxin, IL-1, or foreign antigens, rates of transcription and/or stability of CSF mRNA can be altered dramatically within hours, resulting in major rises (up to 1000-fold) in CSF levels.

The half-life of CSF's in the circulation is relatively short (1 to 5 hours).[33] This, combined with the short half-life of CSF mRNA, means that following removal of an inductive signal, CSF levels can return to baseline values within 24 hours. The clearance and degradation systems for the CSF's are not well characterized, but major organs involved appear to be the liver and kidney.[32] In the case of M-CSF, it has been suggested that utilization by macrophages following internalization of occupied M-CSF receptors also might play a significant role.[34] Similarly, the half-life of G-CSF correlates inversely with the number of circulating neutrophils, suggesting that a similar mature cell consumption may play some role in determining the half-life of G-CSF.[35]

Effects of the CSF's in Vivo

Injections of CSF's into experimental animals, primates, or humans stimulate the production of the same hemopoietic subpopulations as are able to be stimulated by the particular CSF in vitro. Because of the relatively short half-life of CSF's in the circulation, injections of CSF's need to be given one to three times daily, and subcutaneous injection is the optimal route.[33]

CSF stimulation of white cell formation is achieved mainly by increased cell production in the bone marrow, but there is also an increase in the level of cell production in the spleen, causing some increase in spleen size. With high levels of stimulation, increased numbers of hemopoietic cells can appear in the liver, a normal site of hemopoiesis in fetal life and a potential hemopoietic organ in adult life.

The responses induced by each CSF differ in the types of cells responding and in the location of greatest rises in cell numbers. Thus G-CSF induces the largest rises in blood granulocytes, while GM-CSF induces the largest rises in macrophages locally, when injected into the peritoneal cavity.[11] CSF injections also enhance the functional activity of mature white cells, as observed by increased phagocytic or cytocidal activity—effects similar to those demonstrable in vitro.[11]

Where hemopoietic tissues have been damaged by irradiation or cytotoxic drugs, the injection of CSF's accelerates the rate of regeneration of the relevant hemopoietic population.[36, 37] The injection of CSF's also increases resistance in animals to challenge infection with microorganisms[38] and prevents death from infections in animals with marrow damage induced by irradiation.[39–42]

Effects of CSF Depletion

Proof of the role of the CSF's in maintaining basal hemopoiesis requires the demonstration that leukopenia results when antibodies to CSF are administered or that leukopenia is present if a CSF gene is abnormal and not expressed. To date, information of this type has been obtained only for M-CSF and G-CSF.

Mice with the genetic anomaly op/op develop an osteopetrotic state characterized by an absence of osteoclasts, grossly depleted macrophage numbers, and failure of teeth eruption. The gene responsible for this phenotype (op) is located on chromosome 3 in the same position as the gene encoding M-CSF. Analysis of the M-CSF gene in op/op mice has identified a debilitating frame-shift mutation in the M-CSF coding region and a consequent lack of production of biologically active M-CSF.[43] Administration of M-CSF to op/op mice corrects the osteoclast, macrophage, and teeth defects,[44] permitting the conclusion that, in normal health, M-CSF is mandatory for the development of major macrophage populations and their derivative osteoclasts.

When human G-CSF is injected into dogs, antibodies develop that are also able to neutralize canine G-CSF. In such dogs, the development of detectable antibody is paralleled by the development of neutropenia. Moreover, neutropenia can be induced in recipient dogs by injecting such antibody-containing serum.[45] These observations imply that G-CSF must be necessary to maintain the production of basal numbers of granulocytes.

Disease States Associated with Excess CSF Levels

The wide tissue distribution of potential CSF-producing cells makes it difficult to establish whether aberrant or excessive CSF production is a characteristic of, or is involved in, the pathogenesis of any disease state. In principle at least, elevated CSF production could occur in a local lesion without evidence of this being apparent from changes in CSF levels in the circulation.

Some information has been obtained on the consequences of sustained, extreme elevations of CSF's in mice resulting from the generation of transgenic animals[46] or the retroviral insertion of CSF cDNA into hemopoietic stem cells which are then used to repopulate irradiated recipients.[47–49] It was anticipated that sustained excessive growth factor stimulation might lead to leukemic transformation in the responding populations. While extreme hyperplasia of responding populations was achieved, in none of the model systems studied did myeloid leukemia develop. Perturbation of hemopoiesis by the selective stimulation of granulocyte and macrophage formation does not lead to significant depletion of stem cells or of progenitor cells in other lineages, presumably because of the substantial capacity of stem cells for self-renewal.

Chronic overstimulation of macrophages by grossly elevated GM-CSF levels leads to a wasting disease with ocular damage and chronic inflammatory lesions in muscle tissue[46, 50] that is possibly based on the induced overproduction by macrophages of tissue-damaging agents such as tumor necrosis factor (TNF), IL-1, interferon-γ, and plasminogen activator.[51] Comparable inflammatory diseases in humans might be based on local overproduction of CSF's active on macrophages.

Chronic overstimulation of neutrophils in mice by excess levels of G-CSF did not lead to overt disease,[48] while premature death occurred in association with excess numbers of tissue mast cells in mice with excess levels of multi-CSF.[49]

GRANULOCYTE-MACROPHAGE COLONY-STIMULATING FACTOR (GM-CSF)

The GM-CSF Protein

Human GM-CSF is a secreted monomeric glycoprotein containing 127 amino acids in the mature protein and 4 cysteine residues that form two internal disulfide bonds that are required for biological activity (see Table 157–2). GM-CSF can be heterogeneous in size and charge as a result of variable glycosylation. Glycosylation of GM-CSF appears to be only minimally involved in secretion and in-vivo clearance rates, but N-glycosylation reduces the biological activity of GM-CSF by reducing the receptor binding affinity through a slower kinetic association rate.[52]

GM-CSF was predicted to take up the conformational characteristics of a four α-helical bundle common to several cytokines and growth factors,[53] and this basic structure has been confirmed by x-ray crystallographic studies of the nonglycosylated form of human GM-CSF.[54] The face of the GM-CSF molecule containing the antiparallel C and A helices appears to be the region interacting with high-affinity cellular receptors.[55, 56]

The GM-CSF Gene

GM-CSF is encoded by a unique gene which comprises four exons spanning approximately 2.5 kilobase pairs of DNA in both mice and humans and which specifies a single mRNA of approximately 780 nucleotides.[57] The GM-CSF gene has been localized to 5q23–31 in humans and 11A5–B1 in the mouse. The GM-CSF gene is tightly linked structurally and possibly functionally to the gene encoding multi-CSF,[58, 59] with the two genes separated by only 9 kilobase pairs in humans and 14 kilobase pairs in the mouse. In both species, the multi-CSF gene lies 5′ of and in the same transcriptional orientation as the GM-CSF gene.[58]

Loss of a portion of the long arm of chromosome 5 is seen frequently in therapy-related myelodysplastic syndromes and acute leukemias.[60] A survey of a large number of cases of the 5q⁻ anomaly indicates that although the extent of the deletion is variable, there is a common region involved in all deletions, at or about 5q22–23. The close linkage of various hemopoietic regulator genes to this region of chromosome 5 has raised the suggestion that deletion of the gene(s) for various of these regulators may be a contributing factor in the genesis of leukemia,[61] but this seems unlikely.

Sources and Regulation of GM-CSF

A number of cell types have the capacity to synthesize GM-CSF: T lymphocytes, macrophages, endothelial cells, stromal cells, and fibroblasts.[57] In all cases, GM-CSF production requires inductive stimulation of the producer cell, for example, by other cytokines, antigens, or inflammatory agents. Injection of mice with bacterial endotoxin results in a rapid release of GM-CSF into the serum, probably from macrophages and endothelial cells. Almost all tissues and organs derived from endotoxin-primed mice, when cultured in vitro, release GM-CSF into the culture medium.[1]

GM-CSF–producing cells are thus widely dispersed in the body and in locations likely to make early contact with products of invading microorganisms. Although increased transcription of the GM-CSF gene is evident after inductive stimulation of most producer cell types,[62] quantitatively the more important mechanism may be posttranscriptional stabilization of the mRNA.[62, 63]

Receptors for GM-CSF and Multi-CSF (Interleukin 3)

Cellular receptors for GM-CSF and multi-CSF have a similar distribution on cells of the neutrophil, eosinophil, and macrophage lineages, with receptor numbers decreasing somewhat with cellular differentiation.[32] In humans, both receptors are also expressed on basophils, but in the mouse, mast cells express only multi-CSF receptors. Both receptors also can exist in two different states: a low-affinity state (K_D = 1 to 10 nM) with rapid dissociation kinetics and a high-affinity state (K_D = 30 to 100 pM) with slow dissociation kinetics[64, 65] (Table 157–3).

In humans, distinct low-affinity ligand-binding receptor subunits (α chains) have been cloned and shown to bind only the cognate ligand (K_D = 7 nM for GM-CSF, K_D = 100 nM for multi-CSF). Either of these two α chains can associate with a common β chain (which by itself can bind neither ligand) to form either a high-affinity GM-CSF or multi-CSF receptor complex.[66] Since there is some evidence that the β chain is responsible for cellular signaling, this arrangement may explain the common biological effects of these two CSF's and also the apparent cross-reactivity of GM-CSF and multi-CSF for receptor binding on hu-

TABLE 157–3. STRUCTURE OF HUMAN CSF RECEPTORS

		EC DOMAIN	NO OF AMINO ACIDS				CORE MOL WT (kDa)	GLYC MOL WT (kDa)	CHROMO-SOMAL LOCATION	K_D	NUMBERS PER CELL
			L	EC	TM	CYT					
GM-CSFR	α-chain	R-HD	22	297	27	54	44	85	X, Y, Par	7 nM, 50 pM	50–1000
Multi-CSFR	α-chain	R-HD	17	288	20	53	45	70	—	100 nM, 100 pM	50–1000
Multi-GMR	β-chain	(HD)$_2$	16	422	27	432	108	120	22q12	—	—
G-CSFR	α-chain	Ig-HD-(FBN-III)$_3$	25	601	24	187	91	150	1p34	100 pM	50–1000
EpoR	α-chain	R-HD	24	224	23	234	55	100, 85, 65	19p	100 pM, 1 nM	100–4000
M-CSF receptor		(Ig)5-TK		490	25	435	120	175	5q	100 pM	100–10,000

R, no identifiable domain structure; HD, hemopoietin domain; FBN-III, fibronectin III domain; Ig, immunoglobulin loop domain; L, leader; EC, extracellular; TM, transmembrane; CYT, cytoplasmic; PAR, pseudoautosomal region.

man cells. In the latter case, ligand-dependent association of one α chain with a common limiting β chain serves to deplete β chains and prevent the formation of the alternate αβ complex (Fig. 157–5). The same β chain is also utilized by a third α chain (the binding subunit of the IL-5 receptor) consistent with the common actions of GM-CSF, multi-CSF, and IL-5 on eosinophils and the capacity of each of these CSF's to compete for each other's receptor binding.[7, 66]

All the preceding α chains and the β chain are related in amino acid sequence and structure. They each contain a conserved 200 amino acid element in the extracellular ligand-binding domain of the receptor that is shared with the receptor for growth hormone, prolactin, IL-2 (β chain), IL-4, IL-6, IL-7, G-CSF, erythropoietin, LIF, and ciliary neurotrophic factor[8] (see Fig. 157–3). This structural element (the hemopoietin domain) is characterized by scattered amino acid conservation including 4 cysteine residues (that form two internal disulfide loops in the growth hormone receptor) and the sequence Trp-Ser-X-Trp-Ser. The structure of this domain has been determined by x-ray crystallography for the growth hormone–receptor complex and shown to form two antiparallel β barrel sheets that form the ligand-binding domain between them.[67] Growth factors with four α-helical bundles are predicted to interact with these β sheets, with the third or fourth helix interacting with one receptor subunit (α chain) and the first helix interacting with the other (β chain). This is consistent with the available data on the active sites of GM-CSF and multi-CSF which identify low-affinity binding sites on the third helix and high-affinity binding sites on the first helix.

The receptor subunits are much less conserved in their cytoplasmic domains and do not contain recognizable signal-transducing elements such as tyrosine kinase, phosphatase, or G-protein–binding domains so that the mechanisms by which they transduce signals remain unknown.

The GM-CSF Receptor Gene

In the human genome, the common β subunit of the GM-CSF, multi-CSF, and IL-5 receptors appears to be encoded by a unique gene located at 22q12–q13.[68] The gene encoding the α chain of the human GM-CSF receptor is located in the pseudoautosomal region (PAR), a region of approximately 2500 kilobase pairs of homologous sequence localized at the tip of the human sex chromosomes which recombines during male meiosis.[69] The GM-CSF receptor α chain gene has been localized to the middle of the PAR, approximately 1200 kilobase pairs from the telomere. There is a very high frequency of recombination within the PAR, and this region is rich in hypervariable repeat sequences. As a consequence, the GM-CSF receptor α chain gene is highly polymorphic.

The major GM-CSF receptor α chain mRNA is approximately 2.8 kilobases in length. Variant transcripts have been detected, one in particular lacking the region encoding the transmembrane region of the protein, but their significance is not yet known.

Biological Actions in Vitro

At concentrations of 20 to 2000 pg/ml, GM-CSF stimulates the in vitro proliferation of murine precursors of granulocytes, monocyte-macrophages, and eosinophils (see Fig. 157–4). At higher concentrations, GM-CSF also becomes a proliferative stimulus for megakaryocyte and some erythroid and multipotential precursors.[13] Macrophage precursors are stimulated to proliferate at lower concentrations than are granulocyte precursors. In cultures of human cells, the same range of responses is observed.[70]

Combination of GM-CSF with other CSF's leads to increased cell production[29, 71] and in cultures of human cells GM-CSF can greatly enhance their responsiveness to M-CSF.[72] When acting in collaboration with SCF, IL-1, or IL-

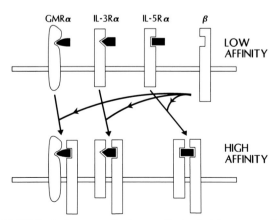

FIGURE 157–5. On human cells, the specific (α chain) receptors for GM-CSF, multi-CSF, and IL-5 share competitively a common β chain. Binding of the β chain confers high affinity on the receptor, with the β chain likely to initiate intracellular signaling.

6, GM-CSF can enhance the generation of committed progenitor cells from stem cells.[12, 31]

Because mature neutrophils, monocytes, and eosinophils express receptors for GM-CSF, these cells can have their viability prolonged by GM-CSF[73] and their functional activity increased.[27, 28, 74] Thus GM-CSF can be chemotactic for neutrophils, can enhance neutrophil adhesion to endothelial cells, and can prime neutrophils to produce superoxide in response to the polypeptide FMLP. Neutrophils also exhibit increased phagocytic activity and intracellular killing of microorganisms. Similarly, monocytes and macrophages can be stimulated to increase their phagocytic activity, cytoplasmic killing of microorganisms, and production of M-CSF, IL-1, G-CSF, interferon-γ, TNF, and plasminogen activator. Eosinophils are stimulated by GM-CSF to increase their production of superoxide and to exhibit increased antibody-dependent cytotoxicity for tumor cells.

Pharmacology

In the mouse, the second-phase half-life of injected GM-CSF is approximately 0.5 hour,[75] and in humans, it is 1 to 3 hours.[76] The subcutaneous or intraperitoneal injection of GM-CSF can produce more sustained rises in serum GM-CSF levels, presumably by providing a more slowly absorbed depot of GM-CSF.

After the intravenous injection of ^{125}I-labeled GM-CSF, the highest levels of labeling are observed in the liver and kidney, suggesting that these organs are the major location of degradation and clearance.[77]

Actions in Vivo

When injected in doses of 100 ng three times daily for 6 days into mice, GM-CSF elicits some elevation of granulocyte and monocyte levels in the peripheral blood.[75] In mice with much higher levels of GM-CSF, major elevations of granulocyte and monocyte levels develop.[47] Injection of GM-CSF into the peritoneal cavity of mice elicits enhanced mitotic activity in resident macrophages, with a 10- to 20-fold rise in macrophage, eosinophil, and neutrophil cell numbers and evidence of functional activation of the mature cells.[75] The data suggest that GM-CSF may have a stronger influence on cell proliferation and function in local tissues than on systemic granulocyte and monocyte levels.

In humans, the intravenous or subcutaneous administration of GM-CSF leads to an initial transient fall in circulating leukocytes, presumably due to increased margination of cells by adherence to endothelial cells.[78, 79] After a few hours, leukocyte levels commence rising due to an accelerated release of mature cells from the bone marrow. This process is progressively overridden by further rises resulting from the stimulation of increased granulocyte, monocyte, and eosinophil formation in the marrow.[28, 80, 81] The levels of granulocytes, monocytes, and eosinophils achieved in the circulation are dose-dependent, and elevated levels can be sustained for as long as GM-CSF injections are continued. Following cessation of administration of GM-CSF, white cell levels return to preinjection values within 1 to 2 days. In some patients, changes in platelet and hematocrit levels have been observed, but such responses are not typical.

GM-CSF also has the ability to elevate up to 10- to 30-fold the number of progenitor cells circulating in the peripheral blood without altering numbers in the bone marrow. This increase includes not only granulocyte-macrophage and eosinophil progenitors but also megakaryocyte and multipotential precursors.[82, 83]

The use of high doses of GM-CSF (>15 μg/kg/day) can produce certain adverse responses that may be the consequence of stimulation of heightened functional activity in monocytes and macrophages.[33] Use of lower doses of GM-CSF is effective in achieving adequate elevated white cell levels without most of these adverse responses.[28]

GRANULOCYTE COLONY-STIMULATING FACTOR (G-CSF)

The G-CSF Protein

G-CSF is a highly conserved glycoprotein with a molecular weight of 20,000 to 25,000 (see Table 157–2). In humans, G-CSF occurs predominantly as a 174 amino acid molecule, although an alternate form with three extra amino acids (Val-Ser-Glu) inserted after position 35 has been described. It contains two essential disulfide bonds and a single free cysteine at position 17. However, since murine G-CSF contains no free cysteine yet is active on human cells, this residue is not required for activity. G-CSF contains a single site of O-glycosylation with no N-glycosylation. The attached carbohydrate is not required for biological activity and receptor binding but does aid in the solubility and stability of G-CSF at neutral pH (especially in preventing aggregation).[84] G-CSF has been predicted to take up a four α-helical bundle topology similar to that of IL-2, GM-CSF, and growth hormone.[53]

The G-CSF Gene

G-CSF is encoded by an mRNA of approximately 1500 nucleotides transcribed from a unique gene comprising five exons and spanning approximately 2.3 kilobase pairs of DNA in both mice and humans.[85] While only one transcript of the murine G-CSF gene has been described, two transcripts of the human gene have been documented[86] which differ by the presence or absence of nine nucleotides in the coding region of the mRNA. The G-CSF gene is located at 17q11.2–21 in the human genome and 11D-E1 in the mouse.[85] Although the human gene is cytogenetically close to the chromosome 17 breakpoint of the t(15;17) translocation characteristic of acute promyelocytic leukemia, in functional terms the translocation breakpoint is distant and does not appear to involve the G-CSF gene.

Sources and Regulation of G-CSF Expression

G-CSF can be produced by a number of different cell types, including macrophages, vascular endothelial cells, fibroblasts, stromal cells, and mesothelial cells.[85] The T lymphocyte is not a major source of G-CSF, by contrast with GM-CSF. Levels of G-CSF production are normally low in cells, but increased production can be induced by exposure to agents such as lipopolysaccharide (endotoxin) and a range of cytokines.

A number of tumor cell lines have been observed to produce G-CSF constitutively, and certain patients with cancer exhibit a neutrophil leukocytosis that is based on tumor cell production of G-CSF. Resection of the tumor reduces circulating neutrophil levels.[87]

In most normal persons, G-CSF is not detectable in the circulation (i.e., its levels are below the detection limit of 30 pg/ml), or, if it is detectable, levels are below 100 pg/ml. During infections or following chemotherapy, G-CSF levels can be elevated and may exceed 2000 pg/ml.[88]

Both transcriptional[89, 90] and posttranscriptional[62, 91] mechanisms have been implicated as being responsible for the enhanced expression of G-CSF after cellular stimulation.

The G-CSF Receptor

In mice and humans, G-CSF receptors are located on blast cells, immature and mature neutrophilic granulocytes, and, to a lesser extent, monocytes and macrophages, with receptor numbers increasing with cellular maturation of murine cells but decreasing with maturation of human cells.[92, 93] On all cell types only a single class of high-affinity receptor has been detected ($K_D = 50$ to 200 pM)[64] (see Table 157–3).

The G-CSF receptor also belongs to the family of hemopoietin receptors, with the ligand-binding domain containing the 200 amino acid hemopoietin domain consensus[94] (see Fig. 157–3). It has a long cytoplasmic tail but no sequences characteristic of signal-transducing elements.

Unlike for many of the other hemopoietic receptors, no β chain has been described for the G-CSF receptor, and this receptor alone confers high-affinity binding and signaling when transfected into foreign cells. However, there is some evidence that the high-affinity signal-transducing form of the receptor is generated by homodimerization (as is the case for the growth hormone receptor) so that the G-CSF receptor might be considered a hybrid between α and β subunits.[95]

The G-CSF Receptor Gene

The human G-CSF receptor is encoded by a unique gene located on chromosome 1 at around band p34.[96] The gene spans approximately 16.5 kilobase pairs of DNA and comprises 17 exons.[97] In the murine genome, two unlinked G-CSF receptor loci have been identified. Although only a single predominant G-CSF receptor mRNA of 3.7 kilobases is detected by Northern blot analysis, multiple transcripts have been detected by cDNA cloning.[98, 99] The functional significance of the different forms of the G-CSF receptor potentially encoded by these different transcripts is unclear.

Biological Actions in Vitro

In cultures of mouse bone marrow cells, G-CSF in concentrations of 50 to 1000 pg/ml stimulates the formation of small, well-differentiated neutrophil-granulocyte colonies with an occasional granulocyte-macrophage or macrophage colony.[100] G-CSF has no ability to stimulate the proliferation of eosinophil, megakaryocyte, erythroid, or mast cells. The proliferative actions of G-CSF are enhanced by combination with other CSF's.[29]

The apparently selective action of G-CSF on cells of the neutrophil-granulocyte lineage is somewhat misleading. G-CSF can initiate cell division in many granulocyte-macrophage and macrophage progenitor cells but is unable to sustain their proliferation beyond a few days.[100] G-CSF also has proliferative effects on stem cells to form progenitor cells of a number of lineages when acting in combination with SCF and to a lesser degree with IL-6 or multi-CSF.[12, 31, 101]

In cultures of human marrow cells, G-CSF stimulates the formation of predominantly granulocytic colonies which reach their maximal numbers within 7 days of incubation.[19] The progenitors responding to G-CSF have the membrane phenotype of CD34+/CD33+, and, when acting alone, G-CSF has minimal proliferative effects on the more ancestral CD34+ cells but may hasten their transition to responsive CD33+ progenitor cells.[102]

G-CSF has the ability to induce commitment to granulocyte formation in bipotential granulocyte-macrophage progenitor cells[1] and to initiate the events leading to maturation in cells of the granulocytic lineage.[103] When acting on mature neutrophils, G-CSF can extend their lifespan in vitro, can stimulate enhanced superoxide production by them following priming by f-met-leu-phe, and can stimulate a respiratory burst in adherent neutrophils, enhanced phagocytic activity for microorganisms, and enhanced antibody-dependent cytotoxicity for tumor cells. G-CSF also can enhance membrane expression of the cell adhesion molecules CD11b and increase neutrophil binding to the endothelial receptor LAM-1.[26, 104]

Pharmacology

In hamsters, the second-phase half-life of intravenously injected G-CSF was 3.8 hours,[105] and in humans, it was 1 to 4 hours according to the dose administered.[33, 35] Injection intraperitoneally or subcutaneously allows more sustained elevations of serum G-CSF levels by providing a slowly absorbed depot of G-CSF.

Actions in Vivo

When injected into mice in doses of 0.1 to 10 μg/day, G-CSF elicits a dose-dependent elevation in neutrophil levels with no changes in other blood cells. According to the dose injected, neutrophil levels can be elevated up to and beyond 100,000/μl, and these can be sustained for as long as injections are continued.[106–108] G-CSF also elicits a rise in the percentage of granulocytic cells in the bone marrow and moderate spleen enlargement with, again, an increased percentage of granulocytic cells. In the mouse, the

G-CSF response is associated with a remarkable displacement of erythropoietic cells from the marrow to the spleen, where the percentage of erythroid cells rises from a normal level of 5 to 10 per cent to greater than 50 per cent, compensating for the reduced erythropoiesis in the marrow.[11, 107] Injection of G-CSF was observed to reduce the frequency of progenitor cells in the marrow but elevated their frequency 50-fold in the enlarged spleen. The frequency of stem cells also was elevated in the blood but 10-fold in the spleen.[107]

The unusually strong neutrophil response able to be elicited by G-CSF may depend on interaction with SCF in vivo. In Wᵛ mice whose hemopoietic cells lack receptors for SCF or in Steel mice whose production of SCF is abnormal, injections of G-CSF produce much lower elevations of neutrophil levels than in normal mice.[109]

In humans, injection of G-CSF in doses of 1 to 30 μg/kg/day induces a dose-dependent rise in neutrophil levels.[110, 111] In the first few hours following G-CSF injection, neutrophil levels fall transiently, probably due to induced adherence of neutrophils to capillary endothelium.[104] Levels then rise, probably initially due to an accelerated release of neutrophils from the bone marrow.[112, 113] After this phase, further rises in neutrophil levels are based on accelerated production of neutrophils in the marrow with elevations in the percentages of immature granulocytes in the marrow. When G-CSF–induced rises in neutrophil levels are occurring, some less mature granulocytes also can appear in the peripheral blood, and some of the mature neutrophils can exhibit prominent Döhle bodies or toxic granulation. Elevated neutrophil levels can be sustained for as long as injections are continued, but no fall occurs in the levels of other blood cells as a consequence of the increased production of neutrophils. Increased functional activity of neutrophils in G-CSF–injected subjects also has been documented.[114]

Some subjects injected with G-CSF exhibit slight spleen enlargement, and this may be due to increased spleen hemopoiesis comparable with that documented to occur in mice. G-CSF elicits an up to 100-fold rise in progenitor and repopulating cells in the peripheral blood in a response peaking 5 to 7 days after commencement of injections.[115]

The injection of G-CSF elicits remarkably few adverse responses, and no dose-limiting toxicity has been observed.[104]

MACROPHAGE COLONY-STIMULATING FACTOR (M-CSF OR CSF-I)

The M-CSF Protein

M-CSF differs from the other CSF's in that it is homodimeric and can exist in membrane-bound form. Moreover, it is translated from multiple transcripts, each of which encodes a transmembrane homodimer that can be cleaved proteolytically to generate soluble homodimers which can vary dramatically in their protein size and degree of glycosylation[116, 117] (see Table 157–2).

All the transcripts produce soluble M-CSF with full biological activity, indicating that only the most N-terminal 149 amino acids are required for activity. However, these molecules are only active as disulfide-bonded homodimers.

Cell surface–bound M-CSF and glycosaminoglycan-attached M-CSF also appear to be biologically active as disulfide-bonded homodimers, so these modifications may function primarily to localize M-CSF at specific cellular sites.

The M-CSF Gene

In contrast to the relatively simple structures and transcription patterns displayed by the GM-, multi-, and G-CSF genes, the M-CSF gene is far more complex.[118, 119] The M-CSF gene comprises 10 exons spanning approximately 20 kilobase pairs of DNA.[118] M-CSF mRNA's with a range of sizes from 1.6 to 4.5 kilobases have been observed. The relative functional importance of the different M-CSF proteins encoded by these mRNA's is unclear.

Although originally assigned to chromosomal location 5q33, it is now clear that the human M-CSF gene is in fact located at 1p13–p21.[120] The murine M-CSF gene is at 3F3 coincident with the op, or osteopetrosis, locus.[43]

Sources and Regulation of M-CSF Expression

M-CSF is detectable in moderate concentrations in the serum and tissues and in human urine.[121, 122] Levels of M-CSF are elevated in the serum and tissues during pregnancy in mice[121] and are also elevated in the serum during the acute phase of infections in mice and humans.[123]

M-CSF is the most readily detectable CSF produced in cultures of fibroblasts or of stromal cells from the bone marrow.[1, 25] It also can be produced by endothelial cells, monocytes, and a variety of tumor cells, but M-CSF appears not to be a product of mouse lymphocytes. The production of M-CSF by fibroblasts is inducible by IL-1, IL-6, GM-CSF, and endotoxin.

An unusual feature of M-CSF is its production in high levels by the pregnant mouse uterus.[121] In situ hybridization studies have localized the production mainly to the epithelium of the uterine wall. The close physical association resulting with M-CSF receptor–bearing cells in the placenta and the ability of M-CSF to stimulate the proliferation of trophoblast cells in vitro suggest that M-CSF may play an important role in the development or function of the placenta.[16]

A number of studies have indicated that, as for GM-CSF and G-CSF, both transcriptional and posttranscriptional mechanisms contribute to enhanced M-CSF mRNA expression, but the molecular dissection of sequences in the M-CSF promoter responsible for regulating gene expression is much less detailed than for the other CSF's.[62, 91, 119]

The M-CSF Receptor

The cellular receptor for M-CSF exists as a single high-affinity class ($K_D = 100$ pM) predominantly on cells of the monocyte-macrophage cell lineage and on placental trophoblasts and choriocarcinoma cell lines.[124] The M-CSF receptor is encoded by the c-fms proto-oncogene and is a single-chain integral transmembrane glycoprotein (see Table 157–3) with a cytoplasmic domain that contains residues characteristic of tyrosine kinases. The M-CSF receptor is most closely related to the receptors for platelet-derived growth factor (PDGF) and Steel factor, or stem cell factor, the latter receptor being encoded by the c-kit proto-oncogene.

Binding of M-CSF to its receptor results in receptor dimerization, activation of the tyrosine kinase activity of the receptor, and transphosphorylation on cytoplasmic tyrosines of the receptor subunits. Phosphorylation of Tyr 708 or Tyr 723 results in the interaction of the M-CSF receptor with the enzyme phosphatidyl inositol-3-kinase (PI3K) through a domain in the latter that is homologous to the src proto-oncogene (SH2 domain). Tyrosine 809 also appears to be required for the full mitogenic effects of the M-CSF receptor. Receptor mutants with phenylalanine at this position retain tyrosine kinase activity, bind PI3K, and induce expression of c-fos and junB, so additional interactions of the receptor with unknown effectors must be required for full mitogenicity.[125]

Several genes have been identified that are activated in macrophages by ligand-occupied M-CSF receptors. These include the immediate-early response genes c-fos, junB, and myc and the cell cycle progression genes (cyclins) CYL1 and CYL2. The induction of these latter genes in the G₁ phase of the cell cycle and the requirement for M-CSF to be present continuously through G₁ for mitogenesis suggest that these genes are crucial for entry into S-phase. They probably act as regulatory subunits of serine kinases related to p34-cdc-2, and their short half-lives and the requirement of new protein synthesis for their expression suggest that they may be directly involved in cell cycle progression.[126]

The M-CSF Receptor Gene (c-fms)

The M-CSF receptor is encoded by the cellular homologue (c-fms) of the transforming gene (v-fms) present in the Susan-McDonough strain of feline sarcoma virus.[125] The c-fms gene is located at 5q33.3 in the human genome,[61] within a chromosomal region frequently deleted in certain myelodysplastic syndromes and acute leukemias (see above). It is distant, however, from the critical region of 5q common to all 5q interstitial deletions. The c-fms gene spans a total of approximately 60 kilobase pairs of DNA and is composed of 21 or 22 exons depending on which promoter is used.[127] Interestingly, the c-fms exon 1 is located only 0.5 kilobase pairs downstream of the PDGF receptor gene.[127] The PDGF receptor gene has a similar genomic organization and encodes a tyrosine kinase receptor with clear sequence similarity to the M-CSF receptor, suggesting a common evolutionary origin.

Biological Actions in Vitro

In cultures of mouse bone marrow, M-CSF stimulates the formation of monocyte-macrophage colonies and a small number of granulocytic or granulocyte-macrophage colonies.[1, 29] M-CSF has no stimulating activity for eosinophils, megakaryocytes, erythroid, or mast cells.

In conventional cultures of human marrow cells in agar, M-CSF has virtually no proliferative effects, but if combined with low concentrations of GM-CSF, M-CSF exhibits a strong capacity to stimulate monocyte-macrophage colony formation.[72]

The proliferative actions of M-CSF are strongly enhanced by combination with IL-1 or IL-3 and possibly SCF. When used in such combinations, M-CSF may have the ability to stimulate some proliferation by stem cells and/or to stimulate the proliferation of more ancestral progenitor cells than the usual macrophage-committed progenitors, leading to the formation of giant macrophage-containing colonies.[128, 129]

M-CSF can act on bipotential granulocyte-macrophage progenitor cells to induce commitment to the macrophage lineage and presumably can initiate maturation events in such cells.[130]

In cultures deprived of M-CSF, the addition of M-CSF has an immediate effect of increasing protein synthesis in the cultured cells followed after an 8- to 12-hour interval by an increase in cells entering the S-phase of the cell cycle.[131] M-CSF has strong actions in stimulating the functional activity of mature macrophages. These include stimulation of phagocytosis with or without antibody, enhanced cytotoxicity for tumor cells, enhanced intracellular killing of microorganisms, and enhanced production of monocyte-macrophage products such as IL-1, interferon-γ, TNF, prostaglandin E (PGE), plasminogen activator, and other cytokines.[25, 132, 133]

Actions in Vivo

Intraperitoneal injection of recombinant M-CSF in doses of 100 ng three times daily to adult BALB/c mice had little effect on blood or marrow populations but did increase moderately the number of peritoneal macrophages.[11] Injection of M-CSF into M-CSF–deficient op/op mice enhanced the formation of osteoclasts, correcting pre-existing osteopetrosis and teeth eruption defects.[44] If injected locally into the peritoneal cavity, M-CSF also increased peritoneal macrophage numbers in these mice, but not when injected systemically. With subcutaneous injection, M-CSF increased peripheral blood monocyte numbers in such mice.[134]

When injected into primates, recombinant human M-CSF elevated blood levels of monocytes and promonocytes with some reduction in platelet levels. Such animals also exhibited decreases in plasma cholesterol.[133]

When injected into humans, native M-CSF has been reported to increase the regeneration of blood monocyte and neutrophil levels following chemotherapy and bone marrow transplantation.[135]

MULTIPOTENTIAL COLONY-STIMULATING FACTOR [MULTI-CSF (IL-3)]

The Multi-CSF Protein

Interleukin 3 (IL-3 or multi-CSF) is the least conserved of the colony-stimulating factors, with only 29 per cent sequence identity between the murine and human molecules. The mature murine molecule consists of 140 amino acids, although fully active N-terminally truncated (6 amino acids) forms also have been described (see Table 157–2). It contains 4 cysteine residues, and chemically synthesized derivatives of murine IL-3 have suggested that Cys 17 and 80 form a structurally essential disulfide bond, while the potential disulfide bond between Cys 79 and 140 is not essential.[136] Mature human IL-3 consists of 133 amino acids which include only 2 cysteine residues that form a homologous disulfide bond (Cys 16 and 84). Both human and murine IL-3 display considerable charge and size heterogeneity as a result of N- and O-glycosylation, but the attached carbohydrate is not required for biological activity and does not affect the specific biological activity or the clearance rate of IL-3.

Like other CSF's, IL-3 contains a considerable proportion of α helix (40 per cent) with some β structure (12 per cent) and is predicted to take up a four α-helical bundle configuration.[53]

The Multi-CSF Gene

Multi-CSF is encoded by a unique gene comprising five exons and spanning approximately 2.2 kilobase pairs of DNA in both mice and humans. Only one transcript of the multi-CSF gene has been documented, a mature mRNA of around 850 to 900 bases.[137]

The multi-CSF gene is tightly linked physically to the GM-CSF gene, at band 11A5–B1 in mice and 5q23–31 in humans.[137] As previously discussed for the GM-CSF gene, the multi-CSF gene is frequently deleted from 5q⁻ chromosomes but has not been implicated as anything more than coincidently deleted in this situation. Interestingly, however, the t(5;14) (q31;q32) translocation breakpoint, characteristic of a distinct subtype of acute B-lymphocytic leukemia with eosinophilia, has been shown to involve the juxtaposition of the multi-CSF and IgH genes, apparently resulting in excess multi-CSF production.[138]

Sources and Regulation of Multi-CSF Expression

In contrast to the other CSF's, multi-CSF is produced by a far more restricted set of cells: activated T lymphocytes and mast cells. Moreover, production of multi-CSF or expression of the multi-CSF gene have only been documented in such cell types in vitro, not in vivo, and it would appear that the expression of the multi-CSF gene is very tightly regulated. Certainly, expression of multi-CSF in T lymphocytes is secondary to, and possibly dependent on, expression of GM-CSF.[59] The rationale for such tight regulation may concern the potent mast cell–stimulating activity of multi-CSF. Interestingly, transcription of the multi-CSF gene appears to be dependent on the activity of an enhancer element located in the promoter region of the adjacent GM-CSF gene.[139]

Like GM-CSF, enhanced expression of the multi-CSF gene in T lymphocytes and mast cells appears to involve both transcriptional and post-transcriptional mechanisms, with enhanced stability of the mRNA appearing to play a major role.[140]

The Multi-CSF Receptor Gene

Currently, no details are available concerning the structure, arrangement, or location of either the murine or the human gene encoding the α chain of the multi-CSF receptor complex. As discussed above, the gene encoding the shared affinity converting, or β, subunit of the human GM-CSF/multi-CSF complex has been localized to 22q12–q13.[68]

Biological Actions in Vitro

In cultures of murine marrow cells, multi-CSF in concentrations of 50 to 2000 pg/ml stimulates the formation of colonies of granulocytes, macrophages, eosinophils, megakaryocytes, erythroid cells, and multipotential and blast cells.[14] Multi-CSF also can stimulate mast cell proliferation in appropriate cultures.[141] Stimulation by multi-CSF of the formation of megakaryocyte and blast cell colonies requires the use of relatively high concentrations.[14]

Multi-CSF has the most evident action on stem cells of all the CSF's, with a capacity, when acting alone, to stimulate some blast colony formation and some proliferation of purified stem cells.[29] When combined with other CSF's or IL-1, IL-6, and particularly SCF, multi-CSF has strong proliferative effects on stem cells to generate committed progenitor cell progeny.[12, 29]

In human cultures, multi-CSF has the capacity to stimulate colony formation by granulocyte, macrophage, eosinophil, megakaryocyte, blast, and mast cells.[142, 143] As is the case for murine cells, human multi-CSF is a particularly effective proliferative stimulus for early hemopoietic precursor cells in the stem cell compartment.

Like the other CSF's, multi-CSF has a capacity to stimulate the function of mature cells. Thus multi-CSF has been noted to stimulate the survival and functional activity of eosinophils[144] and monocyte cytotoxicity.[145] Because mature human neutrophils lack receptors for multi-CSF, their function is not influenced by multi-CSF.[146]

Actions in Vivo

When injected intraperitoneally in mice at doses of 200 ng three times daily for 6 days, multi-CSF induced moderate rises in blood eosinophil, neutrophil, and monocyte levels and some elevation of eosinophils and macrophages in the peritoneal cavity.[147] Bone marrow cellularity and composition were not altered substantially, but spleen size was increased slightly, with significant elevations in the percentage of nucleated erythroid cells. Major elevations were induced in megakaryocytes and progenitor cells in the spleen. The most striking response quantitatively was a 100-fold elevation of mast cells in the spleen, with smaller rises in the lymph nodes and skin.[14] Platelet responses in mice to the injection of multi-CSF have been equivocal.

Injection of multi-CSF into primates induced rises in the production of neutrophils, monocytes, platelets, and erythroid cells[148] and potentiated responses to subsequently administered GM-CSF.[149]

Injections of multi-CSF in humans have been reported to induce moderate elevations of neutrophils, monocytes, and eosinophils, with some rises in platelets and, less consistently, some rises in red cell numbers.[150, 151] In contrast to the effects of G-CSF and GM-CSF, the injection of multi-CSF induced only minor rises in progenitor cells in the peripheral blood.[152] Adverse responses included fever, headache, and flushing.

CLINICAL APPLICATIONS OF THE CSF'S

Three types of clinical situations permit a useful intervention with CSF treatment: (1) in cancer patients with reduced marrow populations and/or white cell levels following chemotherapy or marrow transplantation, (2) in patients with congenital neutropenia, cyclic neutropenia, or a myelodysplastic syndrome, and (3) in patients in whom inadequate resistance is being exhibited to severe infections.

Trials using GM-CSF demonstrated its ability to elevate neutrophil, monocyte, and eosinophil levels in patients with AIDS[153] and in cancer and lymphoma patients following chemotherapy.[80, 154] In further trials, GM-CSF was able to accelerate recovery of neutrophil and monocyte levels following bone marrow transplantation in patients with cancer and lymphoma and to reduce the frequency of marrow grafts that were followed by failure of adequate hemopoietic regeneration.[154, 155] In myelodysplastic patients with subnormal neutrophil and monocyte levels, GM-CSF increased levels of neutrophils, monocytes, eosinophils, and occasionally platelets and erythroid cells.[156–159]

G-CSF was able to elevate neutrophil levels in a dose-dependent manner in cancer patients prior to or following chemotherapy and to accelerate the regeneration of neutrophilic granulocytes in patients following marrow transplantation (Fig. 157–6) and in patients undergoing repeated cycles of chemotherapy.[110, 111, 160, 161] G-CSF also was able to elevate neutrophil levels in patients with myelodysplasia.[162, 163]

GM-CSF treatment appeared not to be effective in elevating neutrophil levels in patients with congenital neutropenia, but G-CSF treatment (5 to 10 μg/kg/day) was effective in elevating neutrophil levels to normal and in maintaining such levels.[164, 165] In patients with cyclic neutropenia, G-CSF treatment did not prevent the cyclic fluctuations in neutrophil levels of 18-day periodicity. Indeed, cycling in some patients persisted with a shorter periodicity of 12 to 14 days. However, the nadirs of such cycles were elevated and remained within the normal range for neutrophils.[166]

Administration of both types of CSF also has resulted in measurable increases in the functional activity of mature cells. GM-CSF has been reported to increase monocyte cytotoxicity[167] and superoxide production by granulocytes,[168] while G-CSF has been reported to increase neutrophil alkaline phosphatase, phagocytic activity, and superoxide production.[104]

The magnitude of the responses able to be elicited by the CSF's depends on the number of stem and progenitor cells available for stimulation, so, for example, responses are lower in patients who have undergone more intensive prior chemotherapy. Responses also have been limited in patients with severe aplastic anemia.

The CSF-induced rises in mature cell production can be

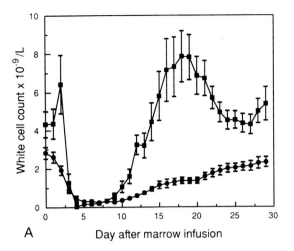

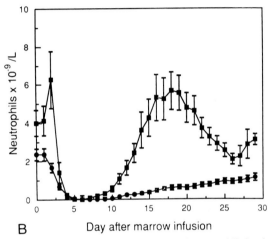

FIGURE 157–6. Acceleration of the recovery of neutrophils by the injection of G-CSF in patients with autologous bone marrow transplantation *(squares)* compared with recovery in control patients *(circles)*. (From Sheridan WP, Morstyn G, Wolf M, et al: Granulocyte colony stimulating factor and neutrophil recovery after high-dose chemotherapy and autologous bone marrow transplantation. Lancet 2:891–895, 1989.)

sustained without any depletion of cells in other lineages and without significant changes in the frequency of progenitor cells in the marrow. An unanticipated response to CSF injection has been a major increase of progenitor cells of all types in the peripheral blood. These numbers have risen up to 100-fold in G-CSF–injected patients[115] and 10- to 30-fold in GM-CSF–injected patients.[82, 83] Peripheral blood cells, harvested after CSF preinjection, have been used as a supplement to or in place of marrow in autologous transplantation in cancer patients. The regeneration of neutrophils and monocytes was not further accelerated, but a remarkable acceleration of platelet regeneration to normal levels was observed from the control delay of 39 days to 15 days.[169]

All clinical studies so far have documented some improvement in the frequency or severity of infections in these patient groups, a change most evident in patients with congenital or cyclic neutropenia. Available data on responses to recombinant multi-CSF are less extensive. However, in patients with myelodysplasia, multi-CSF treatment resulted in increased blood levels of neutrophils, monocytes, and eosinophils, with variable effects on platelet levels.[150] Comparable responses have been noted in cancer patients with marrow failure after chemotherapy.[151] No results of treatment with recombinant M-CSF have yet been reported, but in cancer patients following chemotherapy, the injection of purified urinary M-CSF was reported to accelerate the regeneration of both neutrophils and monocytes and was without significant adverse effects.[135]

Myeloid leukemia presents a potential problem with respect to CSF treatment because the leukemic populations in most patients with acute or chronic myeloid leukemia remain dependent on and responsive to proliferative stimulation by the CSF's.[23] Where chemotherapy, with or without marrow transplantation, is believed to have eliminated the leukemic clone, it appears reasonable to use the CSF's, as in other patients, to accelerate normal hemopoietic regeneration.

CSF treatment has proved useful in reducing hospitalization following chemotherapy or marrow transplantation and is likely to result in reduced morbidity and mortality from infections. It is clear, however, that the present method of administering single CSF's is not able to induce absolute protection against infections or a certain ability to resolve existing infections. It is likely that combinations of hemopoietic growth factors should improve existing results.

ERYTHROPOIETIN

The Erythropoietin (Epo) Protein

Erythropoietin is a secreted glycoprotein of molecular weight 34,000 (see Table 157–2). The mature protein consists of 165 amino acids (the C-terminal arginine is post-translationally cleaved in both natural and recombinant Epo), and this sequence is highly conserved between mice and humans (79 per cent identity). Human Epo contains two internal disulfide bonds that are essential for biological activity and three sites of N-glycosylation and O-glycosylation at Ser 126.[170, 171] N-glycosylation at Asn 38 and 83 is required for efficient secretion of Epo, and the added sugar increases the stability and solubility of Epo, although there is little effect on in vitro biological activity. Desialation of Epo exposes galactose residues that are recognized by the galactose receptor of the liver clearance system, thus resulting in increased serum clearance and severely reduced activity in vivo. Circular dichroism studies have revealed a high content of α-helix in Epo, and structural predictions have suggested that it has the conformation of a four α-helical bundle.[53]

The Erythropoietin Gene and Its Expression

Erythropoietin is encoded by a unique gene comprising five exons and spanning 3 to 3.5 kilobase pairs[172] located at 7q11–22 in the human genome[173] and 5G in the mouse.[174] The erythropoietin mRNA is 1.6 (human) to 1.8 (rat) kilobases long, with an unusually long 5′ untranslated region (approximately 230 nucleotides), the function of which is unknown.

The kidney is the major source of erythropoietin in the adult animal, and renal tissue hypoxia regulates erythro-

poietin production.[175, 176] Production of erythropoietin by the rat kidney under hypoxic conditions is the result of enhanced mRNA expression rather than release of pre-formed erythropoietin.[177, 178] In situ hybridization studies on kidneys of mice made profoundly anemic have shown erythropoietin mRNA expression in peritubular cells, tentatively identified as capillary endothelial cells, of the cortex and to a lesser extent the medulla.[179] In these studies, no specific hybridization was detected in glomerular or tubular cells. Not all the peritubular cells were erythropoietin mRNA–positive, and it is possible that the number induced to express erythropoietin is related to the severity of the anemia.

The molecular mechanisms by which hypoxia, or other stimuli such as cobalt, induce erythropoietin expression are uncertain, but it has been suggested that the oxygen sensor may be a heme protein. In the human hepatoma cell line Hep 3B, erythropoietin expression can be induced by hypoxia or cobalt, and both enhanced transcription and enhanced erythropoietin mRNA stability have been implicated.[180]

The Erythropoietin Receptor

The Epo receptor is displayed in low numbers (300 to 400/cell) on erythroid precursor cells and on megakaryocytes, but not on mature erythroid cells. Both high- ($K_D = 100$ pM) and low-affinity ($K_D = 1$ nM) states of the receptor have been described on erythroid cells[181] (see Table 157–3).

The cloned Epo receptor is also a member of the hemopoietin family of receptors (see Fig. 157–3). Like the G-CSF receptor, no β subunit has been described for the erythropoietin receptor, and when the receptor is transfected into foreign cells, both high-affinity binding and proliferative signaling are observed. Some evidence suggests that receptor homodimerization may be involved in high-affinity binding and cell signaling, and this is supported by receptor mutants where Arg 129 is altered to a cysteine residue. The mutation causes constitutive activation of the Epo receptor, presumably by the formation of covalent homodimers, and leads to oncogenic transformation of infected hemopoietic cells.[182] A second type of oncogenic activation of the Epo receptor occurs in erythroid precursor cells infected with the spleen focus–forming virus, where the envelope glycoprotein (gp55) of the retrovirus associates with and causes activation of the Epo receptor.[183]

The Erythropoietin Receptor Gene

The erythropoietin receptor is encoded by a unique gene comprising eight exons and spanning approximately 5 to 6 kilobase pairs of DNA.[184, 185] In the human genome, the erythropoietin receptor gene has been localized to 19p and in the mouse to chromosome 9.[186] Only one transcript of the erythropoietin receptor has thus far been defined. Although lacking a typical TATA box element, the genomic sequence spanning the region corresponding to the 5′ end of the erythropoietin receptor cDNA's has several hallmarks of a promoter region, including potential binding sites for the Sp1 and GATA-1 transcription factors.[184, 185] The latter is of particular interest because GATA-1 is a transcription factor implicated in erythroid differentiation and, moreover, has been shown to up-regulate the expression of the erythropoietin receptor promoter.[187]

Biological Actions in Vitro

In cultures of mouse bone marrow or fetal liver cells, erythropoietin stimulates proliferation of mature erythroid progenitors (CFU-E) to form small erythroid colonies.[188] Particularly when combined with SCF[189] or multi-CSF[190] and to a lesser degree GM-CSF,[191] erythropoietin is also able to stimulate the formation of large multicentric erythroid colonies by the most ancestral of the committed erythroid progenitor cells, the BFU-E. These combinations are also able to stimulate the formation of colonies derived from multipotential progenitor cells that contain erythroid and other hemopoietic lineage cells. With the exception of a relatively weak capacity of multi-CSF to stimulate some erythroid colony formation,[14] erythropoietin is the only known hemopoietic factor with the ability to stimulate the formation of maturing erythroid cells.

Erythropoiesis provides the clearest example of sequential regulatory control of blood cell formation. The generation of early erythroid cells requires stimulation by early-acting factors such as multi-CSF, SCF, or GM-CSF. On intermediate stages of erythropoiesis, erythropoietin acts in a synergistic manner with these factors, and for the later stages of erythropoiesis, erythropoietin becomes the dominant regulator of cell proliferation.

In cultures of human cells, erythropoietin is also a highly active proliferative stimulus for erythroid colony formation by CFU-E[192] and a subset of less mature erythroid precursors, the BFU-E.[193] As with murine cells, combination of erythropoietin with multi-CSF, SCF, or IL-3 is required to stimulate the proliferation of all available BFU-E.

The primacy of erythropoietin as the major regulator of the later stages of erythropoiesis is paralleled by an unusual degree of restriction in its range of action. Erythropoietin has no capacity to stimulate the formation of granulocytic, monocytic, eosinophil, or mast cells. Evidence has been conflicting on the apparent ability of erythropoietin to stimulate some megakaryocyte colony formation.[194, 195] Megakaryocytes do express receptors for erythropoietin,[196] allowing the possibility of a direct action, but its role as an important megakaryocyte-stimulating factor remains unproven.

Because the cells in erythroid colonies grown in serum-free cultures do mature to hemoglobinized and often enucleated cells, it is reasonable to conclude that erythropoietin, like the CSF's, may be capable of initiating maturation in erythroid precursor cells. Erythropoietin has been observed to increase globin mRNA transcription[197, 198] and to increase the concentration of hemoglobin in individual cells.[199] Erythropoietin receptors appear not to be expressed on mature red cells, reticulocytes, or the most mature nucleated erythroid cells, so no direct action of erythropoietin is possible on such cells.

Source, Distribution, and Production

In the adult, erythropoietin behaves as a classic hormone. It has a dominant single organ source, the kidney, and is detectable in the serum and urine.[181, 200, 201] However, there is also a component of local production and action in the biology of erythropoietin. In fetal life, the liver is the most important source of erythropoietin[202, 203] and is also the initial location of most erythropoietic cells.[204] Thus, since erythropoietin does not cross the placenta from the maternal circulation, the biology of erythropoietin in early fetal life is dominantly one of local production and action.

Even in adult life, the liver retains a capacity to produce erythropoietin,[205, 206] and because in unstimulated marrow cultures low levels of erythroid colony formation occur, it is likely that some cells in the marrow also exhibit a capacity for erythropoietin production. In the adult, approximately 95 per cent of the erythropoietin is produced in the kidney. While the use of antibodies to erythropoietin has documented the presence of erythropoietin in renal glomeruli,[207, 208] in situ hybridization studies have identified the interstitial cells adjacent to the renal tubules as the erythropoietin-producing cells.[179]

Extrarenal cellular sources of erythropoietin include Kupffer cells of the liver and possibly the macrophage-like nurse cells in the bone marrow at the center of small islands of erythropoietic cells.[209] In the early embryo, yolk sac cells also may be a source of erythropoietin.

A number of tumor cell types produce erythropoietin independently of the oxygen-carrying capacity of the blood.[210, 211] Outstanding among these in frequency are renal carcinomas, where perhaps 2 per cent produce erythropoietin, and Wilms' tumors in children, where two-thirds of patients exhibit increased erythropoietin production. In some instances, the raised levels of erythropoietin may not be produced by the tumor cells but rather by host cells in response to other tumor cell products, e.g., androgens or agents that induce a restricted or depleted blood volume.

Normal plasma levels of erythropoietin are 10 to 20 mU/ml,[212] and the second-phase plasma half-life of injected recombinant erythropoietin is 6 to 9 hours.[213] The plasma half-life of erythropoietin is more dependent on the glycoprotein moiety of the molecule than is the case for the CSF's, and as a consequence, only glycosylated erythropoietin is biologically effective when injected in vivo.[170]

Erythropoietin production is controlled mainly by renal tissue hypoxia,[175, 176] but it is unknown whether erythropoietin-producing cells sense levels of hypoxia or whether other cells in the kidney respond to hypoxia by releasing some signaling molecule. Since restriction of renal blood flow increases erythropoietin production markedly, it is less probable that such signals arise from anoxic tissues elsewhere to significantly influence the function of erythropoietin-producing cells in the kidney.

The relationship between erythropoietin and hemoglobin concentrations is log-linear,[212] except in situations where the anemia is secondary to renal disease or in states of chronic inflammation. Erythropoietin levels are reduced following transfusion[214] and can be almost completely suppressed in animals by hypertransfusion. In general, in disease states reducing oxygen demand, such as protein deprivation, hypophysectomy, or thyroidectomy, erythropoietin levels are also reduced.

Reduced oxygen availability at high altitudes results in elevated erythropoietin levels with consequent increased red cell production and secondary polycythemia. Following removal from hypoxic conditions, erythropoietin levels in humans return to normal within 24 hours.[215]

Because of the dominance of the renal sensing system, local anoxia in the kidney secondary to renal vascular disease can result in increased erythropoietin levels and abnormally elevated red cell production. A similar sequence can occur as a consequence of renal cysts or tumors that, by local pressure, induce local alterations in renal blood circulation.

Biological Actions of Erythropoietin in Vivo

In animals, the injection of erythropoietin increases iron incorporation into red cells, induces an elevated level of reticulocytes and mature red cells, and increases the number of erythroid precursors.[216, 217] This response is also seen in mice pretreated with cytotoxic drugs.

The injection of erythropoietin in humans elevated the frequency of both CFU-E and the less mature BFU-E in the marrow.[218] This implies, as was noted earlier in responses to injected CSF's, that the stem cell compartment is readily able to compensate for regulator-induced proliferation and depletion of progenitor cells.

The injection of erythropoietin has no influence on the levels of white cells or platelets, the observation of the latter casting some doubt on the significance of reported in vitro actions of erythropoietin in stimulating megakaryocyte proliferation in vitro.

Clinical Uses of Erythropoietin

The major current clinical use of erythropoietin is in the management of anemia developing as a consequence of chronic renal disease or bilateral nephrectomy.[219, 220] These situations involve a major loss of erythropoietin-producing cells, and erythropoietin treatment is essentially a replacement therapy comparable with the use of insulin in diabetes. Use of erythropoietin has almost entirely eliminated the requirement for blood transfusion for such patients, preventing the previous clinical problems of iron overload and the risks of hepatitis B or AIDS virus infection following repeated transfusions.

In initial studies, the injection of recombinant erythropoietin in doses of 15 to 150 U/kg intravenously two to three times weekly achieved target red cell and hemoglobin levels in virtually all patients within 2 to 3 months (Fig. 157–7), and the majority of such patients were able to be maintained indefinitely by the continuing use of recombinant erythropoietin. No example of acquired unresponsiveness or antibody formation to erythropoietin has been reported in such patients.[221] More recent studies indicate that the subcutaneous injection of erythropoietin is a more effective route of administration.

Enhanced erythropoiesis can only replace lost red cells at a speed dictated by the time required for erythroid precursor cell divisions and erythroid maturation. Because of this, erythropoietin treatment cannot substitute for blood transfusions in situations of acute blood loss. However, for scheduled surgery, prior administration of erythropoietin has permitted blood donation in sufficient volumes to per-

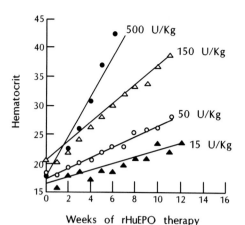

FIGURE 157–7. The hematocrit response to various doses of erythropoietin (rHuEPO) in patients with chronic renal disease. (Reproduced with permission from Eschbach JW, Egrie JC, Downing MR, et al: Correction of anemia of end-stage renal disease with recombinant human erythropoietin: Results of a phase I and II clinical trial. N Engl J Med 316:73–78, 1987.)

mit autologous transfusion during surgery and in many instances has eliminated the need for such transfusions.[222]

Erythropoietin has not been effective in the management of aplastic anemia, where severe intrinsic abnormalities exist in the hemopoietic precursor population that render the cells unresponsive to stimulation by erythropoietin.

Disease States Associated with Subnormal Erythropoietin Production

Subnormal erythropoietin production leads to the development of anemia with no other evident abnormalities in hemopoiesis. There are no known congenital anemias associated with subnormal erythropoietin production, and in adults, the most common disease state leading to failure of erythropoietin production is chronic renal disease.

Disease States Associated with Elevated Erythropoietin Production

Sustained elevations of erythropoietin levels result in the production of excess numbers of erythroid cells and in a state of induced or secondary polycythemia. In animal models, sustained elevation of erythropoietin levels has been achieved by generating transgenic mice with an inserted, abnormally regulated additional erythropoietin gene.[223] An alternative method is to repopulate irradiated mice with marrow cells containing a retrovirally inserted erythropoietin gene under strong independent promotion.[224] In these models, hematocrits in excess of 85 per cent can be generated, and such animals can die with the expected vascular complications of the induced high viscosity of the blood. These induced states of erythropoietin excess do not result in obvious abnormalities in the formation of other blood cells.

The most common disease state leading to excess erythropoietin is acute blood loss, a temporary situation which corrects itself when hemoglobin levels return to normal.

Extremely high levels of erythropoietin are present in patients with Diamond-Blackfan anemia, where the erythropoietin-producing cells are attempting unsuccessfully to stimulate an intrinsically abnormal set of progenitor cells to produce mature red cells.[212] More moderate elevations of erythropoietin are observed in polycythemia vera complicated by myelofibrosis, another situation in which the population of erythroid-forming cells is inadequate.

There are certain tumors—particularly renal tumors—where the tumor cells themselves produce erythropoietin which induces a secondary erythrocytosis not suppressible by the then elevated oxygen-carrying capacity of the blood.[210, 211]

REFERENCES

1. Metcalf D: The Hemopoietic Colony Stimulating Factors. Amsterdam, Elsevier, 1984.
2. Trentin JJ: Hemopoietic microenvironments. *In* Tavassoli M (ed): Handbook of the Hemopoietic Microenvironment, Princeton, NJ, Humana Press, 1989, pp 1–86.
3. Dexter TM, Spooncer E, Simmons P, Allen TD: Long-term marrow culture: An overview of techniques and experience. *In* Wright DG, Greenberger JS (eds): Long-Term Bone Marrow Cultures. New York, Alan R Liss, Kroc Foundation Series 18, 1984, pp 57–96.
4. Stein J, Borzillo GV, Rettenmier CW: Direct stimulation of cells expressing receptors for macrophage colony-stimulating factor (CSF-1) by a plasma membrane-bound precursor of human CSF-1. Blood 76:1308–1314, 1990.
5. Anderson DM, Lyman SD, Baird A, et al: Molecular cloning of mast cell growth factor, a hematopoietin that is active in both membrane bound and soluble forms. Cell 63:235–243, 1990.
6. Nicola NA: Hemopoietic cell growth factors and their receptors. Annu Rev Biochem 58:45–77, 1989.
7. Nicola NA, Metcalf D: Subunit promiscuity among hemopoietic growth factor receptors. Cell 67:1–4, 1991.
8. Bazan JF: Structural design and molecular evolution of a cytokine receptor superfamily. Proc Natl Acad Sci USA 87:6934–6938, 1990.
9. Bradley TR, Metcalf D: The growth of mouse bone marrow cells in vitro. Aust J Exp Biol Med Sci 44:287–300, 1966.
10. Ichikawa Y, Pluznik DH, Sachs L: In vitro control of the development of macrophage and granulocyte colonies. Proc Natl Acad Sci USA 56:488–495, 1966.
11. Metcalf D: The Florey Lecture 1991: The colony stimulating factors: Discovery to clinical use. Philos Trans R Soc Lond [Biol] 333:147–173, 1991.
12. Meunch MD, Schneider JG, Moore MAS: Interaction among colony stimulating factors, IL-1β, IL-6 and *kit* ligand in the regulation of primitive murine hematopoietic cells. Exp Hematol 20:339–349, 1992.
13. Metcalf D, Burgess AW, Johnson GR, et al: In vitro actions on hemopoietic cells of recombinant murine GM-CSF purified after production in *Escherichia coli*: comparison with purified native GM-CSF. J Cell Physiol 128:421–431, 1986.
14. Metcalf D, Begley CG, Nicola NA, Johnson GR: Quantitative responsiveness of murine hemopoietic populations in vitro and in vivo to recombinant multi-CSF (IL-3). Exp Hematol 15:288–295, 1987.
15. Bussolino F, Wang JM, Defilippi P, et al: Granulocyte- and granulocyte-macrophage colony stimulating factors induce endothelial cells to migrate and proliferate. Nature 337:471–473, 1989.
16. Arceci RJ, Shanahan F, Stanley ER, Pollard JW: Temporal expression and location of colony-stimulating factor (CSF-1) and its receptor in the female reproductive tract are consistent with CSF-1 regulated placental development. Proc Natl Acad Sci USA 86:8818–8822, 1989.
17. Dedhar S, Gaboury L, Galloway P, Eaves C: Human granulocyte-macrophage colony-stimulating factor is a growth factor active on a variety of cell types of nonhemopoietic origin. Proc Natl Acad Sci USA 85:9253–9257, 1988.
18. Miyagawa K, Chiba S, Shibuya K, et al: Frequent expression of receptors for granulocyte-macrophage colony-stimulating factor on human nonhematopoietic tumor cell lines. J Cell Physiol 143:483–487, 1990.
19. Begley CG, Nicola NA, Metcalf D: Proliferation of normal human promyelocytes and myelocytes after a single pulse stimulation by purified GM-CSF and G-CSF. Blood 71:640–645, 1988.
20. Moore MAS, Williams N: Functional, morphologic and kinetic analysis of the granulocyte-macrophage progenitor cell. *In* Robinson WA (ed): Hemopoiesis in Culture (DHEW Publication No 74–205) Washington, DHEW, 1973, pp 17–27.
21. Metcalf D: Clonal analysis of proliferation and differentiation of paired daughter cells: Action of granulocyte-macrophage colony-stimulating factor on granulocyte-macrophage precursors. Proc Natl Acad Sci USA 77:5327–5330, 1980.
22. Metcalf D: The molecular control of cell division, differentiation commitment and maturation in haemopoietic cells. Nature 339:27–30, 1989.
23. Metcalf D: The roles of stem cell self-renewal and autocrine growth factor production in the biology of myeloid leukemia. Cancer Res 49:2305–2311, 1989.
24. Williams GT, Smith CA, Spooncer E, et al: Haemopoietic colony stimulating factors promote cell survival by suppressing apoptosis. Nature 343:76–79, 1990.
25. Whetton AD, Dexter TM: Myeloid haemopoietic growth factors. Biochim Biophys Acta 989:111–132, 1989.
26. Demetri GD, Griffin JD: Granulocyte colony-stimulating factor and its receptor. Blood 78:2791–2808, 1991.
27. Gasson JC: Molecular physiology of granulocyte-macrophage colony-stimulating factor. Blood 77:1131–1145, 1991.
28. Grant SM, Heel RC: Recombinant granulocyte-macrophage colony-stimulating factor (rGM-CSF) Drugs 43:517–560, 1992.
29. Metcalf D, Nicola NA: The clonal proliferation of normal mouse hemopoietic cells: Enhancement and suppression of CSF combinations. Blood 79:2861–2866, 1992.
30. Teshima T, Shibaya T, Harada M, et al: Granulocyte-macrophage colony-stimulating factor suppresses induction of neutrophil alkaline phosphatase synthesis by granulocyte colony-stimulating factor. Exp Hematol 18:316–321, 1990.
31. Metcalf D: Lineage commitment of hemopoietic progenitor cells in developing blast cell colonies: Influence of colony stimulating factors. Proc Natl Acad Sci USA 88:11310–11314, 1991.
32. Metcalf D: The Molecular Control of Blood Cells. Cambridge, MA, Harvard University Press, 1988.
33. Leischke GJ, Burgess AW: Granulocyte colony-stimulating factor and granulocyte-macrophage colony-stimulating factor. N Engl J Med 327:28–35, 1992.
34. Tushinski RJ, Oliver IT, Guilbert LJ, et al: Survival of mononuclear phagocytes depends on a lineage-specific growth factor that the differentiated cells selectively destroy. Cell 28:71–81, 1982.
35. Layton JE, Hockman H, Sheridan WP, Morstyn G: Evidence for a novel in vivo control mechanism for granulopoiesis: Mature cell-related control of a regulatory growth factor. Blood 74:1303–1307, 1989.
36. Nienhuis AW, Donahue RE, Karlsson S, et al: Recombinant human granulocyte-macrophage colony-stimulating factor (GM-CSF) shortens the period of neutropenia after autologous bone marrow transplantation in a primate model. J Clin Invest 80:573–577, 1987.
37. Welte K, Bonilla MA, Gillio AT, et al: Recombinant human granulocyte colony-stimulating factor: Effects of hematopoiesis in normal and cyclophosphamide-treated primates. J Exp Med 165:941–948, 1987.
38. Matsumoto M, Matsubara S, Matsuno T, et al: Protective effect of human granulocyte colony-stimulating factor on microbial infection in neutropenic mice. Infect Immun 55:2715–2720, 1987.
39. Talmadge JF, Tribble H, Pennington R, et al: Protective, restorative and therapeutic properties of recombinant colony stimulating factors. Blood 78:2093–2103, 1989.
40. Tanikawa S, Nose M, Aoki Y, et al: Effect of recombinant human granulocyte colony-stimulating factor on the hematologic recovery and survival of irradiated mice. Blood 76:445–449, 1990.
41. Neta R, Oppenheim JJ, Douches SD: Interdependence of the radioprotective effects of human recombinant IL-1, TNF, G-CSF and murine recombinant GM-CSF. J Immunol 140:108–111, 1988.
42. Uckun FM, Souza L, Waddick KG, et al: In vivo protective effects of recombinant human granulocyte colony-stimulating factor in lethally irradiated mice. Blood 75:638–645, 1990.
43. Yoshida H, Hayashi S, Kunisada T, et al: The murine mutation osteopetrosis is in the coding region of the macrophage colony stimulating factor gene. Nature 345:442–444, 1990.
44. Wiktor-Jedrzejczak W, Urbanowska A, Aukerman SL, et al: Correction by CSF-1 of defects in the osteopetrotic op/op mouse suggests local, developmental and humoral requirements for this growth factor. Exp Hematol 19:1049–1054, 1991.

45. Hammond WP, Csiba E, Canin A, et al: Chronic neutropenia: A new canine model induced by human G-CSF. J Clin Invest 87:700–710, 1991.

46. Lang RA, Metcalf D, Cuthbertson RA, et al: Transgenic mice expressing a hemopoietic growth factor gene (GM-CSF) develop accumulation of macrophages, blindness and a fatal syndrome of tissue damage. Cell 51:675–686, 1987.

47. Johnson GR, Gonda TJ, Metcalf D, et al: A lethal myeloproliferative syndrome in mice transplanted with bone marrow cells infected with a retrovirus expressing granulocyte-macrophage colony-stimulating factor. EMBO J 8:441–448, 1989.

48. Chang JM, Metcalf D, Gonda TJ, Johnson GR: Long-term exposure to retrovirally expressed G-CSF induces a non-neoplastic granulocytic and progenitor cell hyperplasia without tissue damage in mice. J Lab Clin Invest 84:1488–1496, 1989.

49. Chang JM, Metcalf D, Lang RA, et al: Non-neoplastic hematopoietic myeloproliferative syndrome induced by dysregulated multi-CSF (IL-3) expression. Blood 73:1487–1497, 1989.

50. Metcalf D, Moore JG: Divergent disease patterns in granulocyte-macrophage colony-stimulating factor transgenic mice associated with different transgene insertion sites. Proc Natl Acad Sci USA 85:7767–7771, 1988.

51. Cuthbertson RA, Lang RA, Coghlan JP: Macrophage products IL-1α, TNFα and bFGF may mediate multiple cytopathic effects in the developing eyes of GM-CSF transgenic mice. Exp Eye Res 51:335–344, 1990.

52. Cebon J, Nicola NA, Ward M, et al: Granulocyte-macrophage colony-stimulating factor (rGM-CSF) from human lymphocytes: The effect of glycosylation on receptor binding and biological activity. J Biol Chem 265:4483–4491, 1990.

53. Parry DAD, Minasian E, Leach SJ: Cytokine conformations: Predictive studies. J Mol Recog 4:63–75, 1991.

54. Diederichs K, Boone T, Karplus PA: Novel fold and putative receptor binding site of granulocyte-macrophage colony-stimulating factor. Science 254:1779–1782, 1991.

55. Shanafelt AB, Miyajima A, Kitamura T, Kastelein RA: The amino terminal helix of GM-CSF and IL-5 governs high affinity binding to their receptors. EMBO J 10:4105–4112, 1991.

56. Lopez AF, Shannon MF, Hercus T, et al: Residue 21 of human granulocyte-macrophage colony-stimulating factor is critical for biological activity and for high but not low affinity binding. EMBO J 11:909–916, 1992.

57. Gough NM, Nicola NA: Granulocyte-macrophage colony stimulating factor. In Dexter T, Garland JM, Testa NG (eds): Colony-Stimulating Factors. New York, Marcel Dekker, 1990, pp 111–153.

58. Huebner K, Nagarajan L, Besa E, et al: Order of genes on human chromosome 5q with respect to 5q interstitial deletions. Am J Hum Genet 46:26–36, 1990.

59. Gough NM, Kelso A: GM-CSF expression is preferential to multi-CSF (IL-3) expression in murine T lymphocyte clones. Growth Factors 1:287–298, 1989.

60. Van den Berghe H, Vermaelen K, Mecucci C, et al: The 5q⁻ anomaly. Cancer Genet Cytogenet 17:189–255, 1985.

61. Le Beau MM, Westbrook CA, Diaz MO, et al: Evidence for the involvement of GM-CSF and FMS in the deletion (5q) in myeloid disorders. Science 231:984–987, 1986.

62. Falkenberg JHF, Harrington MA, Paus RA, et al: Differential transcriptional and post-transcriptional regulation of gene expression of the colony stimulating factors by interleukin 1 and fetal bovine serum in murine fibroblasts. Blood 78:658–665, 1991.

63. Thorens B, Mermod J-J, Vassalli P: Phagocytosis and inflammatory stimuli induce GM-CSF mRNA in macrophages through post-transcriptional regulation. Cell 48:671–679, 1987.

64. Nicola NA: Structural and functional characteristics of receptors for colony-stimulating factors. In Quesenberry PJ, Asano S, Saito K (eds): Hemopoietic Growth Factors. Amsterdam, Excerpta Medica, 1991, pp 101–120.

65. Nicola NA, Cary D: Affinity conversion of receptors for colony stimulating factors: Properties of solubilized receptors. Growth Factors 6:119–129, 1992.

66. Miyajima A: Molecular structure of the IL-3, GM-CSF and IL-5 receptors. Int J Cell Cloning 10:126–134, 1992.

67. De Vos AM, Ultsch M, Kossiakoff AA: Human growth hormone and extracellular domain of its receptor: Crystal structure of the complex. Science 255:306–312, 1992.

68. Shen Y, Baker G, Callen DF: Localization of the human GM-CSF receptor β chain gene to chromosome 22q12.2–22q13.1. Cytogenet Cell Genet (in press).

69. Gough NM, Gearing DP, Nicola NA, et al: Localization of the human GM-CSF receptor gene to the X-Y pseudoautosomal region. Nature 345:734–736, 1990.

70. Metcalf D, Begley CG, Johnson GR: Biologic properties in vitro of a recombinant human granulocyte-macrophage colony-stimulating factor. Blood 67:37–45, 1986.

71. Bot FJ, Van Ejik L, Schipper P, et al: Synergistic effects between GM-CSF and G-CSF or M-CSF on highly enriched human marrow progenitor cells. Leukemia 4:325–328, 1990.

72. Caracciolo D, Shirsat N, Wong GG, et al: Recombinant human macrophage colony-stimulating factor (M-CSF) requires subliminal concentrations of granulocyte/macrophage (GM)-CSF for optimal stimulation of human macrophage colony formation in vitro. J Exp Med 165:1851–1860, 1987.

73. Begley CG, Lopez AF, Metcalf D, et al: Purified colony stimulating factors enhance the survival of human neutrophils and eosinophils in vitro: A rapid and sensitive microassay for colony stimulating factors. Blood 68:162–166, 1986.

74. Lopez AF, Williamson DJ, Gamble JR, et al: Recombinant human granulocyte-macrophage colony-stimulating factor stimulates in vitro mature human neutrophil and eosinophil formation, surface receptor expression and survival. J Clin Invest 78:1220–1228, 1986.

75. Metcalf D, Begley CG, Williams D, et al: Hemopoietic responses in mice injected with purified recombinant murine GM-CSF. Exp Hematol 15:1–9, 1987.

76. Cebon JS, Bury RW, Lieschke GJ, Morstyn G: The effects of dose and route of administration on the pharmacokinetics of granulocyte-macrophage colony-stimulating factor. Eur J Cancer 26:1064–1069, 1990.

77. Burgess AW, Metcalf D: Serum half-life and organ distribution of radiolabeled colony stimulating factor in mice. Exp Hematol 5:456–464, 1977.

78. Arnout MA, Wang EA, Clark SC, Sieff CA: Human recombinant granulocyte-macrophage colony-stimulating factor increases cell-to-cell adhesion and surface expression of adhesion-promoting surface glycoproteins on mature granulocytes. J Clin Investig 78:597–601, 1986.

79. Griffin J, Sperfini O, Ernst TJ, et al: Granulocyte-macrophage colony-stimulating factor and other cytokines regulate surface expression of the leukocyte adhesion molecule-1 on human neutrophils, monocytes and their precursors. J Immunol 145:576–584, 1990.

80. Lieschke GJ, Maher D, Cebon J, et al: Effects of bacterially synthesized recombinant human granulocyte-macrophage colony-stimulating factor in patients with advanced malignancy. Ann Intern Med 110:357–364, 1989.

81. Herrmann F, Schulz G, Lindemann A, et al: Hematopoietic response in patients with advanced malignancy treated with recombinant human granulocyte-macrophage colony-stimulating factor. J Clin Oncol 7:159–167, 1989.

82. Socinski MA, Cannistra SA, Elias A, et al: Granulocyte-macrophage colony-stimulating factor expands the circulating haemopoietic progenitor cell compartment in man. Lancet 1:1194–1198, 1988.

83. Villeval J-L, Dührsen U, Morstyn G, Metcalf D: Effect of recombinant human granulocyte-macrophage colony-stimulating factor on progenitor cells in patients with advanced malignancies. Br J Haematol 74:36–44, 1990.

84. Oheda M, Hasegawa M, Hattori K, et al: O-linked sugar chain of human granulocyte colony-stimulating factor protects it against polymerization and denaturation allowing it to retain its biological activity. J Biol Chem 265:11432–11435, 1990.

85. Nicola NA: Granulocyte colony-stimulating factor. In Dexter TM, Garland JM, Testa NG (eds): Colony Stimulating Factors. New York, Marcel Dekker, 1990, pp 77–109.

86. Nagata S, Tsuchiya M, Asano S, et al: The chromosomal gene structure and two mRNAs for human granulocyte colony-stimulating factor. EMBO J 5:575–581, 1986.

87. Asano S, Urabe A, Okabe T, et al: Demonstration of granulopoietic factor(s) in the plasma of nude mice transplanted with a human lung cancer and in the tumor tissue. Blood 49:845–852, 1977.

88. Watari K, Asano S, Shirafuji N, et al: Serum granulocyte colony-stimulating factor levels in healthy volunteers and patients with various disorders as estimated by enzyme immunoassay. Blood 73:117–122, 1989.

89. Shannon MF, Pell LM, Lenardo MJ, et al: A novel tumor necrosis factor–responsive transcription factor which recognizes a regulatory element in hemopoietic growth factor genes. Mol Cell Biol 10:2950–2959, 1990.

90. Asano M, Nishizawa M, Nagata S: Three individual regulatory elements of the promoter positively activate the transcription of the

murine gene encoding granulocyte colony-stimulating factor. Gene 107:241–246, 1991.

91. Ernst TJ, Ritchie AR, Demetri GD, et al: Regulation of granulocyte- and monocyte-colony stimulating factor mRNA levels in human blood monocytes in mediated primarily at a posttranscriptional level. J Biol Chem 264:5700–5703, 1989.

92. Nicola NA, Metcalf D: Binding of ^{125}I-labeled granulocyte colony stimulating factor to normal murine hemopoietic cells. J Cell Physiol 124:313–321, 1985.

93. Nicola NA, Begley CG, Metcalf D: Identification of the human analogue of a regulator that induces differentiation in murine leukaemic cells. Nature 314:625–628, 1985.

94. Fukunaga R, Ishizaka-Ikeda E, Pan CX, et al: Functional domains of the granulocyte colony-stimulating (factor receptor). EMBO J 10:2855–2865, 1991.

95. Nagata S, Fukunaga R: Granulocyte colony-stimulating factor and its receptor. Prog Growth Factor Res 3:131–141, 1991.

96. Inazawa J, Fukunaga R, Seto Y, et al: Assignment of the human granulocyte colony-stimulating factor receptor gene (CSF3R) to chromosome 1 at region p35–p34.3. Genomics 10:1075–1078, 1991.

97. Seto Y, Fukunaga R, Nagata S: Chromosomal gene organization of the human granulocyte colony-stimulating factor receptor. J Immunol 148:259–266, 1992.

98. Fukunaga R, Seto Y, Mizushima S, et al: Three different mRNAs encoding human granulocyte colony-stimulating factor receptor. Proc Natl Acad Sci USA 87:8702–8706, 1990.

99. Larsen A, Davis T, Curtis BM, et al: Expression cloning of a human granulocyte colony-stimulating factor receptor: A structural mosaic of hematopoietic receptor, immunoglobulin, and fibronectin domains. J Exp Med 172:1559–1570, 1990.

100. Metcalf D, Nicola NA: Proliferative effects of purified granulocyte colony-stimulating factor (G-CSF) on normal mouse hemopoietic cells. J Cell Physiol 116:198–206, 1983.

101. Ikebuchi K, Ihle JN, Hirai Y, et al: Synergistic factors for stem cell proliferation: Further studies of the target stem cells and the mechanism of stimulation by interleukin-1, interleukin-6 and granulocyte colony-stimulating factor. Blood 72:2007–2014, 1988.

102. Ema H, Suda T, Miura Y, Nakauchi H: Colony formation of clone-sorted human hematopoietic progenitors. Blood 75:1941–1946, 1990.

103. Valtieri M, Tweardy DJ, Caracciolo D, et al: Cytokine-dependent granulocyte differentiation. Regulation of proliferative and differentiative responses in a murine progenitor cell-line. J Immunol 138:3829–3835, 1987.

104. Hollingshead LM, Goa KL: Recombinant granulocyte colony-stimulating factor. Drugs 42:300–330, 1991.

105. Cohen AM, Zsebo KM, Inoue H, et al: In vivo stimulation of granulopoiesis by recombinant human granulocyte colony-stimulating factor. Proc Natl Acad Sci USA 84:2484–2488, 1987.

106. Molineux G, Pojda Z, Dexter TM: A comparison of hematopoiesis in normal and splenectomised mice treated with granulocyte colony-stimulating factor. Blood 75:563–569, 1990.

107. Pojda Z, Molineux G, Dexter TM: Hemopoietic effects of short-term in vivo treatment of mice with various doses of rh-CSF. Exp Hematol 18:27–31, 1990.

108. Hattori K, Shimizu K, Takahashi M, et al: Quantitative in vivo assay of human granulocyte colony-stimulating factor using cyclophosphamide-induced neutropenic mice. Blood 75:1228–1233, 1990.

109. Cynshi O, Satoh K, Shimonaka Y, et al: Reduced response to granulocyte colony-stimulating factor in W/Wᵛ and Sl/Slᵈ mice. Leukemia 5:75–77, 1991.

110. Morstyn G, Campbell L, Souza LM, et al: Effect of granulocyte colony-stimulating factor on neutropenia induced by cytotoxic chemotherapy. Lancet 1:667–672, 1988.

111. Sekino H, Moriya K, Sugano T, et al: Recombinant human G-CSF (rG-CSF). Shinryo Shinrigaku 26:32–104, 1989.

112. Okada Y, Kawagishi M, Kusaka M: Neutrophil kinetics of recombinant human granulocyte colony-stimulating factor-induced neutropenia in rats. Life Sci 47:65–70, 1990.

113. Lord BI, Bronchud MH, Owens S, et al: The kinetics of human granulopoiesis following treatment with granulocyte colony-stimulating factor in vivo. Proc Natl Acad Sci USA 86:9499–9503, 1989.

114. Lindemann HA, Oster F, Haffner W, et al: Hematological effects of recombinant human granulocyte macrophage colony-stimulating factor in patients with malignancy. Blood 74:2644–2651, 1989.

115. Dührsen U, Villeval J-L, Boyd J, et al: Effects of recombinant human granulocyte-colony stimulating factor on hemopoietic progenitor cells in cancer patients. Blood 72:2074–2081, 1988.

116. Ceretti DP, Wignall J, Anderson D, et al: Human macrophage colony-stimulating factor: Alternative RNA and protein processing from a single gene. Mol Immunol 25:761–770, 1988.

117. Price LKH, Choi HU, Rosenberg L, Stanley ER: The predominant form of secreted colony-stimulating factor-1 is a proteoglycan. J Biol Chem 267:2190–2199, 1992.

118. Ladner MB, Martin GA, Noble JA, et al: Human CSF-1: Gene structure and alternative splicing of mRNA precursors. EMBO J 6:2693–2698, 1987.

119. Kawasaki ES, Ladner MB: Molecular biology of macrophage colony stimulating factor. In Dexter TM, Garland JM, Testa NG (eds): Colony Stimulating Factors. New York, Marcel Dekker, 1990, pp 155–176.

120. Morris SW, Valentine MB, Shapiro DN, et al: Reassignment of the human CSF1 gene to chromosome 1p13–p21. Blood 78:2013–2020, 1991.

121. Bartocci A, Pollard JW, Stanley ER: Regulation of colony-stimulating factor-1 during pregnancy. J Exp Med 164:956–961, 1986.

122. Stanley ER, Hansen G, Woodcock J, Metcalf D: Colony stimulating factor and the regulation of granulopoiesis and macrophage production. Fed Proc 34:2272–2278, 1975.

123. Cheers C, Haigh AM, Kelso A, et al: Production of colony stimulating factors (CSF's) during infection: Separate determinations of macrophage-, granulocyte-, granulocyte-macrophage- and multi-CSF's. Infect Immun 56:247–251, 1988.

124. Roberts WM, Shapiro LH, Ashmun RA, Look AT: Transcription of the human colony-stimulating factor-1 receptor gene is regulated by separate tissue-specific promoters. Blood 79:586–593, 1992.

125. Sherr CJ: Colony-stimulating factor-1 receptor. Blood 75:1–12, 1990.

126. Matsushimi H, Roussel MF, Ashmun RA, Sherr CJ: Colony-stimulating factor-1 regulates novel cyclins during the G1 phase of the cell cycle. Cell 65:701–713, 1991.

127. Roberts WM, Look AT, Roussel MF, et al: Tandem linkage of human CSF-1 receptor (c-fms) and PDGF receptor genes. Cell 55:655–661, 1988.

128. Bartelmez S, Stanley ER: Synergism between hemopoietic growth factors (HGF's) detected by their effects on cells bearing receptors for a lineage specific HGF: Assay for hemopoietin 1. J Cell Physiol 122:370–378, 1985.

129. McNiece IK, Kriegler AB, Bradley TR, Hodgson GS: Subpopulations of mouse bone marrow high-proliferative-potential colony-forming cells. Exp Hematol 14:856–862, 1986.

130. Metcalf D, Burgess AW: Clonal analysis of progenitor cell commitment to granulocyte or macrophage production. J Cell Physiol 111:275–283, 1982.

131. Tushinski RJ, Stanley ER: The regulation of mononuclear phagocyte entry into S phase by the colony stimulating factor, CSF-1. J Cell Physiol 122:362–369, 1985.

132. Lee MT, Warren MK: CSF-1 induced resistance to viral infection in murine macrophages. J Immunol 138:3019–3022, 1987.

133. Garnick MB, Stoudemire JB: Preclinical and clinical evaluation of recombinant human macrophage colony-stimulating factor (rhM-CSF). Int J Cell Cloning 8:(Suppl 1)356–373, 1990.

134. Kodama H, Yamasaki A, Nose M, et al: Congenital osteoclast deficiency in osteopetrotic (op/op) mice is cured by injections of macrophage colony-stimulating factor. J Exp Med 173:269–272, 1991.

135. Masaoka T, Motoyoshi K, Takaku F: Administration of the human urinary colony stimulating factor after bone marrow transplantation. Bone Marrow Transplant 3:121–127, 1988.

136. Clark-Lewis I, Hood LE, Kent SBH: Role of disulfide bridges in determining the biological activity of interleukin 3. Proc Natl Acad Sci USA 85:7897–7901, 1988.

137. Morris CF, Young IG, Hapel AJ: Molecular and cellular biology of interleukin-3. In Dexter TM, Garland JM, Testa NG (eds): Colony Stimulating Factors. New York, Marcel Dekker, 1990, pp 177–214.

138. Meeker TC, Hardy D, Willman C, et al: Activation of the interleukin-3 gene by chromosome translocation in acute lymphocytic leukemia with eosinophilia. Blood 76:285–289, 1990.

139. Nishida J, Yoshida M, Arai K, et al: Definition of a GC-rich motif as regulatory sequence of the human IL-3 gene: Coordinate regulation of the IL-3 gene by CLE2/GC box of the GM-CSF gene in T cell activation. Int Immunol 3:245–254, 1991.

140. Ryan GR, Milton SE, Lopez AF, et al: Human interleukin-3 mRNA accumulation is controlled at both the transcriptional and post-transcriptional level. Blood 77:1195–1202, 1991.

141. Yung Y-P, Eger R, Tertian G, Moore MAS: Long term in vitro culture of murine mast cells: II. Purification of a mast cell growth factor and its dissociation from TCGF. J Immunol 127:794–799, 1981.

142. Saeland S, Caux C, Favre C, et al: Effects of recombinant human interleukin-3 in CD34-enriched normal hematopoietic progenitors and on myeloblastic leukemia cells. Blood 72:1580–1588, 1988.

143. Sonoda Y, Yang YC, Wong GG, et al: Analysis in serum-free culture of the targets of recombinant human hemopoietic growth factors: Interleukin-3 and granulocyte-macrophage colony-stimulating factors are specific for early development stages. Proc Natl Acad Sci USA 85:4360–4364, 1988.

144. Rothenberg ME, Owen WF, Silberstein DS, et al: Human eosinophils have prolonged survival, enhanced functional properties and become hypodense when exposed to human interleukin-3. J Clin Invest 81:1986–1992, 1988.

145. Cannistra SA, Vellenga E, Groshek P, et al: Human granulocyte-monocyte colony-stimulating factor and interleukin 3 stimulate monocyte cytotoxicity through a tumor necrosis factor-dependent mechanism. Blood 71:672–676, 1988.

146. Lopez AF, Dyson PG, To LB, et al: Recombinant human interleukin-3 stimulation of hematopoiesis in humans: Loss of responsiveness in differentiation in the neutrophilic myeloid series. Blood 72:1797–1804, 1988.

147. Metcalf D, Begley CG, Johnson GR, et al: Effects of purified bacterially synthesized murine multi-CSF (IL-3) on hematopoiesis in normal adult mice. Blood 68:46–57, 1986.

148. Krumwich D, Seiler FR: In vivo effects of recombinant colony stimulating factors on hematopoiesis in cynomolgus monkeys. Transplant Proc 21:2964–2967, 1989.

149. Donahue RE, Seehra J, Metzger M, et al: Human IL-3 and GM-CSF act synergistically in stimulating hematopoiesis in primates. Science 241:1820–1823, 1988.

150. Ganser A, Seipelt G, Lindemann A, et al: Effects of recombinant human interleukin-3 in patients with myelodysplastic syndrome. Blood 76:455–462, 1990.

151. Ganser A, Lindemann A, Seipelt G, et al: Effects of recombinant human interleukin-3 patients with normal hematopoiesis and in patients with bone marrow failure. Blood 76:666–676, 1990.

152. Ottmann OG, Ganser A, Seipelt G, et al: Effects of recombinant human interleukin-3 on human hematopoietic progenitor and precursor cells in vivo. Blood 76:1494–1502, 1990.

153. Groopman JE, Mitsuyasu RT, DeLeo MJ, et al: Effects of recombinant human granulocyte-macrophage colony-stimulating factor on myelopoiesis in the acquired immunodeficiency syndrome. N Engl J Med 317:593–598, 1987.

154. Brandt SJ, Peters WP, Atwater SK, et al: Effect of recombinant granulocyte-macrophage colony-stimulating factor on hematopoietic reconstitution after high-dose chemotherapy and autologous bone marrow transplantation. N Engl J Med 318:869–876, 1988.

155. Neumanitis J, Singer JW, Buckner CD, et al: Use of recombinant human granulocyte-macrophage colony-stimulating factor in autologous marrow transplantation for lymphoid malignancies. Blood 72:834–836, 1988.

156. Antin JH, Smith BR, Holmes W, Rosenthal DS: Phase I/II study of recombinant human granulocyte-macrophage colony-stimulating factor in aplastic anemia and myelodysplastic syndrome. Blood 72:705–713, 1988.

157. Ganser A, Volkers B, Greher J, et al: Recombinant human granulocyte-macrophage colony-stimulating factor in patients with myelodysplastic syndromes: A phase I/II trial. Blood 73:31–37, 1989.

158. Thompson JA, Lee DJ, Kidd P, et al: Subcutaneous granulocyte-macrophage colony-stimulating factor in patients with myelodysplastic syndrome: Toxicity, pharmacokinetics and hematological effects. J Clin Oncol 7:629–637, 1989.

159. Vadhan-Raj S, Keating M, LeMaistre A, et al: Effects of recombinant human granulocyte-macrophage colony-stimulating factor in patients with myelodysplastic syndrome. N Engl J Med 317:1545–1552, 1987.

160. Gabrilove JL, Jakubowski A, Fain K, et al: Phase I study of granulocyte colony-stimulating factor in patients with transitional cell carcinoma of the urothelium. J Clin Invest 82:1454–1461, 1988.

161. Sheridan WP, Morstyn G, Wolf M, et al: Granulocyte colony stimulating factor and neutrophil recovery after high-dose chemotherapy and autologous bone marrow transplantation. Lancet 2:891–895, 1989.

162. Kobayashi Y, Okabe T, Ozawa K, et al: Treatment of myelodysplastic syndromes with recombinant human granulocyte colony-stimulating factor: A preliminary report. Am J Med 85:178–182, 1989.

163. Negrin RS, Haeuber DH, Nagler A, et al: Maintenance treatment of patients with myelodysplastic syndromes using human granulocyte colony-stimulating factor. Blood 76:36–43, 1990.

164. Welte K, Zeidler C, Reiter A, et al: Differential effects of granulocyte-macrophage colony-stimulating factor and granulocyte colony-stimulating factor in children with severe congenital neutropenia. Blood 75:1056–1063, 1990.

165. Bonilla MA, Gillio AP, Ruggeiro M, et al: Effects of recombinant human granulocyte colony stimulating factor on neutropenia in patients with congenital agranulocytosis. N Engl J Med 320:1574–1580, 1989.

166. Hammond WP, Price TH, Souza LM, et al: Treatment of cyclic neutropenia with granulocyte-colony-stimulating factor. N Engl J Med 320:1306–1311, 1989.

167. Wing EJ, Magee DM, Whiteside TL, et al: Recombinant human granulocyte/macrophage colony-stimulating factor enhances monocyte cytotoxicity and secretion of tumor necrosis factor α and interferon in cancer patients. Blood 73:643–646, 1989.

168. Kaplan SS, Basford RE, Wing EJ, Shadduck RK: The effect of recombinant human granulocyte-macrophage colony-stimulating factor on neutrophil activation in patients with refractory carcinoma. Blood 73:636–638, 1989.

169. Sheridan WP, Begley CG, Juttner CA, et al: Effect of peripheral-blood progenitor cells mobilised by filgrastim (G-CSF) on platelet recovery after high dose chemotherapy. Lancet 1:640–644, 1992.

170. Yamaguchi K, Akai K, Kawanishi G, et al: Effects of site-directed removal of N-glycosylation sites in human erythropoietin on its production and biological properties. J Biol Chem 266:20434–20439, 1991.

171. Wasley LC, Timony G, Murtha P, et al: The importance of N- and O-linked oligosaccharides for the biosynthesis and in vitro and in vivo biological activities of erythropoietin. Blood 77:2624–2632, 1991.

172. Jacobs K, Shoemaker C, Rudesdorf R, et al: Isolation and characterization of genomic and cDNA clones of human erythropoietin. Nature 313:806–810, 1985.

173. Watkins PC, Eddy R, Hoffman N, et al: Regional assignment of the erythropoietin gene to human chromosome region 7pter-q22. Cytogenet Cell Genet 42:214–218, 1986.

174. LaCombe C, Tambourin P, Mattei MG, et al: The murine erythropoietin gene is localized on chromosome 5. Blood 72:1440–1442, 1988.

175. Adamson JW, Eschbach JW, Finch CA: The kidney and erythropoiesis. Am J Med 44:725–733, 1968.

176. Jacobson L, Gurney C, Goldwasser E: The control of erythropoiesis. Adv Intern Med 10:297–327, 1960.

177. Bondurant MC, Koury MJ: Anemia induces accumulation of erythropoietin mRNA in the kidney and liver. Mol Cell Biol 6:2731–2733, 1986.

178. Schuster SJ, Wilson JH, Erslev AJ, et al: Physiologic regulation and tissue localization of renal erythropoietin messenger RNA. Blood 70:316–318, 1987.

179. Koury ST, Koury MJ, Bondurant MC, et al: Quantitation of erythropoietin-producing cells in kidneys of mice by in situ hybridization: Correlation with hematocrit, renal erythropoietin mRNA and serum erythropoietin concentration. Blood 74:645–651, 1989.

180. Goldberg MA, Gaut CC, Bunn HF: Erythropoietin mRNA levels are governed by both the rate of gene transcription and post-transcriptional events. Blood 77:271–277, 1991.

181. Krantz SB: Erythropoietin. Blood 77:419–434, 1991.

182. Longmore GD, Lodish HF: An activating mutation in the murine erythropoietin receptor induces erythroleukemia in mice: A cytokine receptor superfamily oncogene. Cell 67:1089–1102, 1991.

183. Li J-P, D'Andrea AD, Lodish HF, Baltimore D: Activation of cell growth by binding of Friend spleen focus-forming virus gp55 glycoprotein to the erythropoietin receptor. Nature 343:762–764, 1990.

184. Youssoufian H, Zon LI, Orkin SH, et al: Structure and transcription of the mouse erythropoietin receptor gene. Mol Cell Biol 10:3675–3682, 1990.

185. Penny LA, Forget BG: Genomic organization of the human erythropoietin receptor gene. Genomics 11:974–980, 1991.

186. Budarf M, Huebner K, Emanuel B, et al: Assignment of the erythropoietin receptor (EpoR) gene to mouse chromosome 9 and human chromosome 19. Genomics 8:575–578, 1990.

187. Zon LI, Youssoufian H, Lodish H, et al: Regulation of the erythropoietin receptor promoter by the cell-specific transcription factor GF-1 (ERYF-1, NF-E1) Blood 76(Suppl 1):174a, 1990.

188. Stephenson JR, Axelrad AA, McLeod DL, Shreeve MM: Induction of colonies of hemoglobin-synthesizing cells by erythropoietin in vitro. Proc Natl Acad Sci USA 68:1542–1546, 1971.

189. Broxmeyer HE, Hangoc G, Cooper S, et al: Influence of murine mast cell growth factor (c-kit ligand) on colony formation by mouse marrow hematopoietic progenitor cells. Exp Hematol 19:143–146, 1991.

190. Goldwasser E, Ihle JN, Prystowsky MB, et al: The effect of interleukin 3 on hemopoietic precursor cells. *In* Golde DW, Marks PA (eds): Normal and Neoplastic Hematopoiesis, vol 9. New York, Alan R Liss, 1983, pp 301–309.

191. Metcalf D, Johnson GR, Burgess AW: Direct stimulation by purified GM-CSF of the proliferation of multipotential and erythroid precursors. Blood 55:138–147, 1980.

192. Tepperman AD, Curtis JE, McCulloch EA: Erythropoietic colonies in cultures of human marrow. Blood 44:659–669, 1974.

193. Gregory CS, Eaves AC: Human marrow cells capable of erythropoietic differentiation in vitro: Definition of three erythroid colony responses. Blood 48:855–864, 1977.

194. Ishibashi T, Kaziol JA, Burstein SA: Human recombinant erythropoietin promotes differentiation of murine megakaryocytes in vitro. J Clin Invest 79:286–289, 1987.

195. Dessypris EN, Gleaton JH, Armstrong OL: Effect of human recombinant erythropoietin on human megakaryocyte formation in vitro. Br J Haematol 65:265–269, 1987.

196. Fraser JK, Tan AS, Lin F-K, Berridge MV: Expression of specific high affinity binding sites for erythropoietin on rat and mouse megakaryocytes. Exp Hematol 17:10–16, 1989.

197. Gross M, Goldwasser E: On the mechanism of erythropoietin-induced differentiation. Biochemistry 8:1795–1805, 1969.

198. Bottomley Ss, Smithee GA: Effect of erythropoietin on bone marrow delta aminolevulinic acid synthetase and heme synthetase. J Lab Clin Med 74:445–452, 1969.

199. Ganzoni A, Hillman RS, Finch CA: Maturation of the macroreticulocyte. Br J Haematol 16:119–135, 1969.

200. Jacobson LO, Goldwasser E, Fried W, Plzak L: Role of the kidney in erythropoiesis. Nature 179:633–634, 1957.

201. Sherwood JB, Robinson SH, Bassan LR, et al: Production of erythropoietin by organ cultures of rat kidney. Blood 40:189–197, 1972.

202. Fried W, Kilbridge R, Krantz S, et al: Studies on extrarenal erythropoietin. J Lab Clin Med 73:244–252, 1969.

203. Carmena AO, Lucarelli G, Carnevali C, Stohlman F: Effect of hypoxia on erythropoiesis in the newborn animal. Proc Soc Exp Biol Med 121:652–655, 1966.

204. Metcalf D, Moore MAS: Haemopoietic Cells. Amsterdam, North Holland, 1971.

205. Anagnostou A, Schade S, Barone J, Fried W: Effect of partial hepatectomy on extrarenal erythropoietin production in rats. Blood 50:457–462, 1977.

206. Brown S, Caro J, Erslev AJ, Murray TG: Spontaneous increase in erythropoietin and hematocrit value associated with transient liver enzyme abnormalities in an anephric patient undergoing hemodialysis. Am J Med 68:280–284, 1980.

207. Burlington H, Cronkite EP, Reincke U, Zanjani E: Erythropoietin production in cultures of goat renal glomeruli. Proc Natl Acad Sci USA 69:3547–3550, 1972.

208. Mori S, Saito T, Morishita Y, et al: Glomerular epithelium as the main locus of erythropoietin in human kidney. Jpn J Exp Med 55:69–70, 1985.

209. Vogt C, Pentz S, Rich IN: A role for the macrophage in normal hemopoiesis: III. In vitro and in vivo erythropoietin gene expression in macrophages detected by in situ hybridization. Exp Hematol 17:391–397, 1989.

210. Donati RM, McCarthy JM, Lange RD, Gallagher NI: Erythrocythemia and neoplastic tumors. Ann Intern Med 58:47–55, 1963.

211. Kazal LA, Erslev AJ: Erythropoietin production in renal tumors. Ann Clin Lab Sci 5:98–109, 1975.

212. Garcia JF, Ebbe S, Hollander L, et al: Radioimmunoassay of erythropoietin: Circulating levels in normal and polycythemic human beings. J Lab Clin Med 99:624–635, 1982.

213. MacDougal IC, Roberts DE, Neubert P, et al: Pharmacokinetics of recombinant human erythropoietin in patients on continuous ambulatory peritoneal dialysis. Lancet 1:425–427, 1989.

214. Adamson JW: The erythropoietin/hematocrit relationship in normal and polycythemic man: Implications for marrow regulation. Blood 32:597–609, 1968.

215. Finch CA, Lenfant C: Oxygen transport in man. N Engl J Med 286:407–415, 1972.

216. Spivak JL: The mechanism of action of erythropoietin. Int J Cell Cloning 4:139–166, 1986.

217. Papayannopoulou T, Finch CA: On the in vitro action of erythropoietin: a quantitative analysis. J Clin Invest 51:1179–1185, 1972.

218. Dessypris EN, Graber SE, Krantz SB, Stone WJ: Effects of recombinant erythropoietin on the concentration and cycling status of human marrow hematopoietic progenitor cells in vivo. Blood 72:2060–2062, 1988.

219. Eschbach JW, Egrie JC, Downing MR, et al: Correction of the anemia of end-stage renal disease with recombinant human erythropoietin: Results of a phase I and II clinical trial. N Engl J Med 316:73–78, 1987.

220. Bommer J, Kugel M, Schoeppe W, et al: Dose-related effects of recombinant human erythropoietin on erythropoiesis: Results of a multicenter trial in patients with end-stage renal disease. Contrib Nephrol 66:85–93, 1988.

221. Eschbach JW, Adamson JW: Correction of the anemia of hemodialysis (HD) patients with recombinant human erythropoietin (rHu Epo): Results of a multicenter study. Kidney Int 33:189(A), 1988.

222. Goodnough LT, Rudnick S, Price TH, et al: Increased preoperative collection of autologous blood with recombinant human erythropoietin therapy. N Engl J Med 321:1163–1168, 1989.

223. Gemenza GL, Traystman MD, Gearhart JD, Antonarakis SE: Polycythemia in transgenic mice expressing human erythropoietin gene. Proc Natl Acad Sci USA 86:2301–2305, 1989.

224. Villeval JL, Metcalf D, Johnson ER: Fatal polycythemia induced in mice by dysregulated erythropoietin (Epo) production by hematopoietic cells. Leukemia 6:107–115, 1992.

158

Endocrine-Immune Interaction

SEYMOUR REICHLIN

In higher forms of life, the major elements responsible for adaptation to perturbations in the environment and maintenance of homeostasis are the nervous, endocrine, and immune systems. Function of the endocrine and nervous systems is clearly linked, an insight that has come from discovery of the phenomenon of *neurosecretion* (recognition that neurons communicate by chemical messengers) and general acceptance of the view that most endocrine functions are regulated by hypothalamic hypophysiotropic hormones and that most hormones exert feedback effects on the brain.

Although endocrine effects on immune functions have long been known and documented by a voluminous literature, it is only in the past few years that the extent of the interactions between the immune and neuroendocrine systems has been recognized. Immune responses have been shown to alter brain and endocrine function, and in turn, neural and endocrine activity has been shown to modify immunological function. Molecular characterization of the lymphokines and thymokines (initially recognized as autocrine/paracrine regulators of immunocompetent cells) has revealed a complex secretory repertoire capable of influencing endocrine gland function both directly and indirectly through neuroendocrine control. Many of the regulatory peptides and their receptors previously thought to be specific to the brain or to the immune system are now known to be expressed by both and to influence endocrine function. These new insights have led to understanding of the way that the central nervous system can modify the capacity of the organism to cope with infection and toxins and to influence the course of autoimmune disease and possibly cancer through changes in immune surveillance.

These new lines of inquiry have led to a redefinition and expansion of some established disciplines and to the coining of several new terms. *Neuroimmunology* has traditionally referred to the study of immune reactions directly involving the central nervous system, for example, those involved in allergic encephalomyelitis, systemic lupus erythematosus, and multiple sclerosis. *Neuroimmunomodulation* refers to the influence of the nervous system on the immune response. *Neuroendocrinoimmunology* refers to the study of the way that the neuroendocrine system can regulate or modulate immunocompetent cells and the way these immune functional changes can, in turn, influence brain function and endocrine activity. *Psychoneuroimmunology* refers to the study of the effects of psychological status on immune function and the mechanisms of these effects. A number of recent monographs and reviews summarize current ideas in the field.[1-8]

Understanding of the *communicative* interactions between neuroendocrine and immune function has been gained at the same time that there has been an increasing understanding of the mechanisms underlying immune *diseases* of the endocrine glands. These mechanisms, which involve organ-specific antigens, stimulating and inhibitory antibodies, and the mobilization of tissue-destructive elements in the immune cascade, are responsible for a wide variety of common clinical disorders of the endocrine system, including type I diabetes, autoimmune thyroiditis, and Graves' disease. This aspect of the immune-endocrine interaction in the pathogenesis of endocrine disorders is reviewed in Chapter 159. The purpose of this chapter is to summarize what is known about the effects of the classical endocrine hormones on the immune response, about the role of immune cells and immunomodulators in the regulation of secretion of endocrine function, and about the way that neuroendocrine factors integrate these activities and to outline the more important ways in which these interactions are involved in pathogenesis of human disease.

LEVELS OF REGULATION IN THE IMMUNE SYSTEM

The immune system has evolved as a mechanism by which foreign organisms and molecules can be recognized and rendered harmless. To understand the way that the nervous system and classical endocrine hormones influence the immune response, it is essential to outline briefly the nature of the immune response, the chemical factors that regulate it, and the levels of control in the immune system which are accessible to hormonal and neural regulation.[9, 10] Put in the conceptual context familiar to endocrinologists, immune regulation is mediated by endocrine, paracrine, and autocrine factors. Endocrine factors secreted by immunocompetent cells are the circulating cytokines which influence proliferation and activation, paracrine factors are those in which cells are activated by direct contacts, and autocrine control is mediated by the cytokine secretion by activated cells themselves. Classical endocrine gland secretions may exert an influence at any of these levels.

Natural Immunity

Beyond the physical/anatomical barrier of the membranes that separate the internal and external environments such as skin and the linings of the hollow organs that communicate with the outside, *natural immunity* (which connotes the response to substances not previously experienced) is mediated by both cellular and humoral factors. The cellular factors include phagocytic cells of several types, macrophages (which sequestrate and destroy or inactivate invading toxins or organisms), polymorphonuclear leukocytes, and a population of lymphocytes designated *natural killer (NK) cells*, which can recognize foreign organisms or altered host cells (such as cancers) and destroy them by secreting toxic molecules and enzymes. Also included are fixed cells of the reticuloendothelial system, which, like their analogues, the circulating macrophages, ingest particles and release inflammatory mediators. Humoral factors include the cytokines and components of the complement cascade which interact with phagocytes to facilitate their ingestive and destructive capacity.

The ultimate purpose of both natural and acquired immunity is to sequester and destroy invading organisms and to inactivate toxic substances. These actions are mediated by pinocytosis and intracellular destruction (incorporation into lysosomes, proteolysis, oxidation) and by the production either directly or secondarily of small-molecular-weight inflammatory mediators such as prostaglandins, leukotrienes, and bradykinin[11] (Table 158–1). The production and release of these inflammatory mediators by activated lymphocytes are also targets for modulation by classical hormones.

Cytokines

Cytokines were initially called *lymphokines* because they were first discovered as secretory products of lymphocytes (see Ch. 157). The concept of lymphokines expanded with recognition that lymphocytes, monocytes, and macrophages secreted many different proteins and polypeptides

TABLE 158–1. INFLAMMATORY MEDIATORS SECRETED BY IMMUNOCOMPETENT CELLS THAT ARE SUPPRESSED BY GLUCOCORTICOIDS

Cytokines
    Interferon-γ
    Granulocyte-monocyte colony-stimulating factor
    Interleukin 1
    Interleukin 2
    Interleukin 3
    Interleukin 6
    Tumor necrosis factor
Inflammatory agents
    Eicosanoids
    Bradykinin
    Serotonin
    Histamine
    Plasminogen activator
    Collagenase
    Elastase

Data from Munck A, Guyre PM: Glucocorticoids and immune function. *In* Ader R, Felten DL, Cohen N (eds): Psychoneuroimmunology (ed 2). New York, Academic Press, 1991, pp 447–474.

which in addition to regulating proliferation and differentiation of the immune system possessed metabolic effects as well. With the discovery that identical molecules were expressed widely in many tissues and were involved in other functions not specifically immune, the more general term *cytokine* has now come into use. Cytokines are extremely powerful polypeptides that act at nanomolar and picomolar concentrations; it was not until the advent of molecular cloning methods that their structures were determined. The first lymphokine to be recognized was termed *endogenous pyrogen*, a fever-inducing factor that appeared in the blood following the injection of bacterial toxin (*exogenous pyrogen*[12]). This intermediary substance was postulated to be responsible for inducing fever; later it was found to induce metabolic effects termed the *acute-phase response* and to influence a variety of lymphocyte activities. The first endogenous pyrogen to be characterized by molecular cloning techniques was interleukin 1 (IL-1).[13] It has served as the archetypical cytokine, and numerous others have been similarly characterized.[9, 14–19] Within the immune system, cytokines regulate virtually every aspect of lymphocyte and macrophage function, determining, among other things, the expansion by proliferation of specific clones of lymphocytes, regulation of the presentation of signaling molecules on their surface, production of immune globulin, and enhancement of the killing activity of NK cells. Inflammatory cytokines are activated by many stimuli, including bacterial toxins, viruses, products of tissue injury, and foreign antigens. Some cytokines are inhibitory to immune functions.

Beyond the classical immune system, cytokines are secreted by endothelia, smooth-muscle cells, certain endocrine gland cells, keratinocytes, brain microglia and astrocytes, and pituitary folliculostellate cells. They are expressed as intrinsic cell regulators in most endocrine tissues and in the brain.

The list of recognized cytokines and their actions continues to grow.[9, 10, 14–19] Table 158–2 summarizes many of the better-established cytokines and their role in immuneregulation. One can distinguish cytokines released as part of natural immunity (unrelated to prior exposure to antigens) and cytokines involved in inducing a population of

TABLE 158–2. SEVERAL IMPORTANT CYTOKINES

CYTOKINE	NUMBER OF GENES	POLYPEPTIDE SIZE	PRIMARY EFFECTS
Mediators of natural immunity			
Interleukin 1	2 (IL-1a, 1b)	17 kDa	Activation, fever, acute-phase response
Interleukin 6	1	26 kDa	T-cell growth, acute-phase response
Tumor necrosis factor	1	17 kDa	Activation, acute-phase response, cachexia
Lower molecular weight inflammatory peptides	20 +		Leukocyte chemotaxis, activation
Mediators of lymphocyte activation, growth, and differentiation			
Interleukin 2	1	14–17 kDa	Growth, cytokine production, activation of NK cells, proliferation, B-cell stimulation
Interleukin 4	1	20 kDa	Growth of T and B cells
Transforming growth factor beta	2	14 kDa	Inhibits activation, proliferation, regulates growth

Modified from Abbas AK, Lichtman AH, Pober JS (eds): Cellular and Molecular Immunology. Philadelphia, WB Saunders Co, 1991.

specific antigens recognizing lymphocytes responsible for sensitization (see below). All the cytokines are polypeptides, ranging in size from 8 to 26 kDa. Unlike classical neuropeptides, most genes controlling their synthesis do not code for leader sequences, they are not packaged into secretory vesicles, and they are secreted constitutively. Regulation of cytokine synthesis and secretion is mediated through control elements encoded in the genome, which are activated following binding of cytokines, toxins, or hormones to specific cell membrane receptors.

Sequence analysis of receptors for cytokines and a number of other known tissue growth-regulating peptides shows a high degree of homology, leading to the speculation that all are evolved from a common ancestral gene.[18] Included in this immunoglobulin superfamily are receptors for IL-1, IL-6, IL-2β, IL-3, IL-4, IL-5, IL-7, erythropoietin (EPO), granulocyte colony-stimulating factor (G-CSF), granulocyte-macrophage colony-stimulating factor (GM-CSF), and leukemia inhibitory factor (LIF). In a sense, all autocrine and paracrine tissue growth factors such as epidermoid growth factor (EGF), nerve growth factor, (NGF), transforming growth factor beta (TGF-β), and the somatomedins[19] are cytokines, but common usage has restricted the term to those factors initially isolated from lymphocytes, mononuclear cells, or macrophages and which regulate lymphocyte proliferation and function.

Activated lymphocytes and mononuclear cells also can secrete polypeptides that are antagonists. One such, interleukin 1 receptor antagonist (IL-1RA), has been structurally characterized, shown to be homologous with IL-1α, and binds competitively to the IL-1 receptor.[14, 17] Synthesis and secretion of IL-1RA are regulated by many of the same stimuli that regulate synthesis of IL-1. Discovery of the IL-1RA shows that cytokines can act as an autocrine/paracrine control system.[18] Of the inhibitory cytokines, transforming growth factor beta (TGF-β) is of particular clinical interest. It may be responsible for the anergy observed in some patients with glioblastoma multiforme (where it is a paraneoplastic secretion),[20] is an important local suppressor in the uterus of maternal immune rejection of the fetus,[21, 22] and is an important mediator of immune suppression after immunization by the oral route.[23] Neuroendocrine and endocrine functions of the cytokines are reviewed in later sections.

Nitric Oxide

Nitric oxide (NO) has recently been recognized as an important communicating link among immune, endocrine, and neural systems.[24] This simple inorganic substance, formed enzymatically from arginine by at least two different NO synthases, can be induced in peripheral monocytes and macrophages,[25] in endothelial cells,[26] in neurons,[24] and in brain glia[28, 29] by exposure to several cytokines and bacterial toxins. NO acts like a neurotransmitter in brain, and its synthesizing enzymes are localized in anatomically selective areas.[24, 27] In isolated pancreatic islet β cells and in islet cell tumor lines (free of macrophages and endothelial cells), NO can be induced by IL-1β.[30] Following exposure to NO, glucose-stimulated release of insulin is inhibited.[31] It is likely that NO plays an important pathophysiological role. In the brain, the toxicity of glutamate receptor activation is greater in the presence of NO,[32] and in pancreatic islets, NO appears to kill cells by binding to mitochondrial iron-containing enzymes and inhibiting cAMP synthesis.[31]

Although not considered as classical cytokines, a number of well-characterized pituitary hormones and neuropeptides are secreted by immunocompetent cells (Tables 158–3 and 158–4). They may have some paracrine role (as yet not fully established) in mediating inflammation or in immunomodulation.[33–35] These are considered under individual pituitary hormones in a separate section below.

Locally derived secretory products of the lymphocyte/monocyte/macrophage population, classical endocrine gland secretions, circulating cytokines, thymic hormones (see below), and neuronal secretions (see below) influence virtually all aspects of natural immunity. These effects include modifications of the total immunocompetent cell mass in both the circulating cellular pool and those localized to lymphoid organs (spleen, lymph nodes, gut lymphocytes, Peyer's patches, and thymus). Classical endocrine hormones can modify cellular responsivity to foreign antigens, phagocytic function, complement levels, and the inflammatory cascade which follows activation of macrophages, monocytes, and polymorphonuclear leukocytes. Hormonal factors also can determine and regulate the adherence and selective sequestration of circulating immunocompetent cells (thus modifying the population of cells in the circulation) and can modify the traffic of lymphocytes between blood and lymphatic organs such as intestinal Peyer's patches.

Acute-Phase Response

In vertebrates, exposure to toxic antigens and products of damaged tissue, tumors, and viruses and bacteria in-

TABLE 158–3. PITUITARY HORMONES AND NEUROPEPTIDES
SECRETED BY IMMUNOCOMPETENT CELLS

NAME	STIMULI
Pituitary hormones	
ACTH	Lymphotropic viruses, bacterial toxin, CRH, arginine vasopressin, interleukin 1
Thyrotropin	TRH
LH	GnRH
FSH	Concanavalin A
GH	GH
PRL	Not known
Placental hormones	
Chorionic gonadotropin	Mixed lymphocyte reaction
Peptides	
CRH	Interleukin 1
GHRH	Unknown
Met-enkephalin	Concanavalin A
Arginine vasopressin	Unknown
Oxytocin	Unknown
NPY	Unknown
VIP	Histamine liberators
Somatostatin	
Substance P	
PTH-related peptide	
Calcitonin gene-related peptide	
Insulin-like GF (somatomedin C)	GH

From Blalock JE: Production of peptide hormones and neurotransmitters by the immune system. *In* Blalock JE (ed): Neuroimmunoendocrinology. Basel, Karger, 1992, pp 1–24.

duces a complex but stereotyped pattern of immunological, endocrine, and metabolic events termed the *acute-phase response* that affects virtually every organ in the body.[9, 14, 17, 36] A number of cytokines appear in the blood, including IL-1, IL-1RA, IL-6, and tumor necrosis factor alpha (TNF-α) (Fig. 158–1). Some are activated directly by the toxic factor or indirectly through the mediation of IL-1. The initial tissue source of circulating cytokines appears to be the vascular endothelium, reticuloendothelial cells, monocytes, macrophages, and lymphocytes. Within the brain, astroglia and microglia,[5] the choroid plexus,[37] and blood vessels secrete cytokines into the cerebrospinal fluid and contribute to the circulating pool.

Each of the three major acute-phase cytokines is capable of inducing a patterned neuroendocrine response which includes release of ACTH, cortisol, vasopressin, prolactin (PRL), and growth hormone (GH) and inhibition of thyroid-stimulating hormone (TSH), thyroxine secretion, gonadal steroids, and gonadotropins. Exposure to cytokines activates the sympathetic nervous system with release of epinephrine and norepinephrine.

Metabolic changes are dramatic. Tissue breakdown leads to striking negative nitrogen balance and inhibition of muscle protein synthesis. Liver function is dramatically altered, among the changes being inhibition of synthesis of albumin, thyroxine-binding prealbumin, thyroxine-binding protein, and iron- and copper-binding proteins and stimulation of synthesis of a family of acute-phase proteins which includes globulins, serum amyloid antecedant, C-reactive protein, and components of both the classical and alternative complement pathways.[36] The changes in liver function are mediated mainly by IL-6, whose secretion is induced by IL-1 and TNF. Adipose tissue is also affected, especially by TNF-α (first termed *cachectin* because it induced fat wasting

in rodents suffering from inflammation). Lipolysis is activated, and synthesis of fat from precursors is inhibited.[38]

Cardiovascular responses include decreased cardiac contractility and vasodilation leading to impaired perfusion and shock. Cytokine-induced production of NO by endothelia plays an important role in the circulatory response.[26, 39]

Brain function can be markedly influenced during the acute phase response.[3, 5, 8, 14, 17, 40] Fever (secondary to central prostaglandin secretion in the thermoregulatory areas of the brain), increased slow-wave sleep, drowsiness, disorientation, delerium, and coma can occur if sufficient antigen or cytokine is injected. It has been proposed that IL-1 may pass the blood-brain barrier to influence thermosensi-

TABLE 158–4. IMMUNOREGULATORY EFFECTS OF SEVERAL HORMONES AND NEUROPEPTIDES

HORMONE/ NEUROPEPTIDE	EFFECT
ACTH	Suppression of Ig and IFN-γ synthesis
	Augmentation of B-cell proliferation
	Suppression of IFN-γ–mediated macrophage activation
Glucocorticoids	Inhibition of all aspects of lymphokine synthesis and effects
Estrogens	Stimulation of a number of lymphocyte functions
GH	Enhancement of generation of T cells
PRL	Stimulation of thymulin secretion
	Stimulation of lymphocyte proliferation
TSH	Enhancement of Ig synthesis
hCG	Suppression of T_c and NK cell activity
	Suppression of T-cell proliferation
	Suppression of mixed lymphocyte reactions
	Generation of T_s cells
α-Endorphin	Suppression of Ig synthesis and secretion
	Suppression of antigen-specific helper T cell
β-Endorphin	Enhancement of Ig and IFN-γ synthesis
	Modulation of T-cell proliferation
	Enhancement of generation of T_c cells
	Enhancement of NK cell activity
	Chemotactic for monocytes and neutrophils
Leu- or met- enkephalin	Suppression of Ig synthesis
	Enhancement of IFN-γ synthesis
	Enhancement of NK cell activity
	Chemotactic for monocytes
Substance P	Augmentation of T-cell proliferation
	Degranulation of mast cells and basophils
	Enhancement of macrophage phagocytosis
	Elicitation of O_2, H_2O_2, and thromboxane B_2 production
AVP and oxytocin	Replacement of IL-2 requirement for IFN-γ synthesis
Somatostatin	Suppression of histamine and leukotriene D_4 release from basophils
	Suppression of T cell proliferation
VIP	Inhibition of mitogen-stimulated T cells through cAMP link
	Inhibition of release of T-lymphocytes from popliteal nodes
	Inhibition of migration of T-lymphocytes into mesenteric nodes
α-MSH	Suppression of IL-1 stimulated fever
	Suppression of monocyte secretion of IL-2
	Suppression of fibroblast production of prostaglandins
	Suppression of neutrophil migration

*Ig, immunoglobulin; IFN-γ, interferon-γ; NK cells, natural killer T cells; T_s cells, T suppressor cells; T_c cells, cytotoxic T cells.

Adapted from Blalock JE: A molecular basis for bidirectional communication between the immune and neuroendocrine systems. Physiol Rev 69:1–32, 1989.

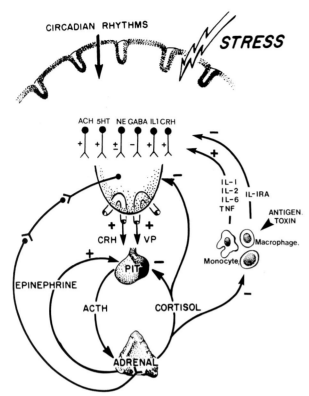

FIGURE 158–1. Hypothalamic-pituitary-adrenal-lymphocyte axis. This diagram illustrates the hypothalamic-pituitary control system of adrenal cortical secretion and its interaction with the peripheral immunocompetent cells. This relationship is an example of the "bidirectional communication" between the immune system and the brain. Superimposed on the normal negative-feedback relationship between circulating cortisol and ACTH are elements that override the system. These include environmentally and internally driven circadian rhythms, emotional and physical stress, and several different cytokines secreted by toxin-activated immunocompetent cells. These include IL-1, IL-2, IL-6, and TNF-α. IL-1 released from toxin-activated T cells in response to bacterial endotoxin in turn induces hypothalamic release of CRH and vasopressin, which stimulates ACTH secretion. The central CRH neuronal network also activates the peripheral autonomic nervous system to release epinephrine from the adrenal medulla, which synergizes with vasopressin and CRH. In turn, the circulating cortisol acts on peripheral immunocompetent cells to inhibit their activation and their secretion of bioactive cytokines, peptides, and other mediators of inflammation. Sympathetic nervous system activation inhibits NK activity. (Adapted, with permission, from Reichlin S: Neuroendocrinology. In Wilson JD, Foster DW (eds): Williams' Textbook of Endocrinology (ed 8). Philadelphia, WB Saunders Co, 1992, pp 135–221.)

tive neurons in the preoptic hypothalamus by way of the organum vasculosum of the lamina terminalis (OVLT), one of the periventricular organs that surround the third ventricle.[40] Alternatively, IL-1 (and some toxins) may act by stimulating cytokine secretion by brain vascular endothelia and/or choroid plexus.[37] Cytokine secretion by activated glia also may mediate the response.[40–43]

Acquired (Specific) Immunity

In addition to the capacity possessed by higher forms to exhibit cellular and humoral responses to first exposure to toxic substances, the immune system has the capacity to recognize foreign molecules (nonself) and differentiate them from endogenous molecules (self), to magnify the population of specifically responding cells, and to imprint

the capacity for highly specific recognition and "memory" of foreign substances. These activities include stimulation of populations of antibody-producing lymphocytes/plasma cells and specifically sensitized cytolytic T-lymphocytes (CTL).[9, 10]

Immunization, the process by which a foreign antigen (or bacterial/viral product) is recognized and then proceeds to activate the immune cascade, is initiated by the binding of the antigen to a membrane-bound protein in at least one clone of lymphocytes preprogrammed by chance arrangement of its structure to recognize that antigen (*clonal selection theory*). As outlined by Abbas et al.,[9] the "lymphocyte repertoire is extremely large. It is estimated that the mammalian immune system can discriminate at least 10^9 distinct antigenic determinants." Recognition molecules which belong to the immune globulin superfamily are localized only to B-lymphocytes, so named because they are analogous (in mammals) to lymphocytes in chickens whose direction of differentiation has been imprinted during their sojourn in a lymphatic gland of the gut termed the *bursa of Fabricius*. Internalized into the B-lymphocyte, the antigen or a fragment of it associates with an intrinsic B-cell protein termed the *major histocompatibility complex* (MHC type II). The MHC type II complex, translocated to the surface of the B-lymphocyte, is now capable of binding (in association with other interactive molecules) to a specific receptor on a T-lymphocyte. These membrane-bound protein-protein interactions lead to physical adherence of the two cells for a period long enough to activate the T cell. MHC–antigen complex activation of the T cell leads to enhanced gene transcription and expression, induction of several proto-oncogenes, the appearance of new proteins within the cell, expression of new receptors on the cell, induction of cytokine secretion, and expansion of a highly specific T-cell clone complementary to the specific activated B-cell clone. Cytokines produced during this interaction further stimulate T- and B-cell activity and enhance their immune cell–specific biological functions: expansion of the B-cell clone, stimulation of secretion of immune globulins, and expansion and activation of the T cells.

During the course of immunization, a host of regulatory cytokines is thus activated. Beyond their effects in modifying lymphocyte function, these regulatory cytokines acting singly and synergistically enter the blood and influence brain and endocrine activity. Steps of the immune cascade are susceptible to control by classical endocrine secretions. Each of the known pituitary hormones has either a direct effect on elements of the immune response or can act indirectly on immunocytes through the secretions of its respective target gland.

The Thymus and Thymic Hormones

An additional level of paracrine and endocrine control of the immune process is imposed by the thymus. Paracrine control is mediated by local cell-cell interactions within the thymus; endocrine control is mediated by the secretions of various cellular elements comprising intrinsic thymocytes (of various types), transient and resident lymphocytes, and macrophages. The thymus in microcosm illustrates the interactions among classical hormones, cytokines, intrinsic secretory cells, and the autonomic nervous system. To quote Jankovic,[44] "the immune microenvironment is composed of (a) T- and B-lymphocytes; (b) accessory nonlymphoid cells, such as epithelial cells, dendritic cells, macrophages; (c) hormones, which are released at remote sites and enter the immune micromilieu via blood capillaries; (d) cholinergic, adrenergic, peptidergic, and other neurons, which are involved in neuroimmune circuits; . . . (g) biologically active substances such as lymphokines, monokines, interleukins, immunoglobulins, complement, regulatory monoamines, neurotransmitters, and neuropeptides, produced by lymphoid and nonlymphoid cells, in situ or elsewhere."

A unique function of the thymus is the "imprinting" of lymphocytes to be either T or B type. Lymphocytes arising from primitive precursor cells in the bone marrow circulate to the thymus. Within the sinusoids of the thymus, a selective subpopulation of the lymphocytes is sequestered (presumably by adherence between specific membrane-bound proteins) for a period of time during which specific cell-cell interactions take place. These interactions ordain the function of that class of lymphocyte to be T cells (for *thymus*). T cells lack the ability to recognize foreign antigens as such but, when appropriately stimulated, are capable of inducing cytokine production and activating (helper T cells) or inhibiting immune responses (suppressor T cells). T cells bear membrane markers of their status—for example, the CD4 cell, so conspicuously involved in AIDS, is a helper T cell.

In addition to its role in defining the ultimate destiny of the lymphocyte, the thymus also secretes a family of regulatory proteins, some of which are unique to the thymus and others of which are expressed elsewhere as well.[45, 46] Many were first isolated from the thymus and as a group are designated *thymulins* (Table 158–5). In addition, most of the cytokines associated with lymphocytes and macrophages are secreted within the thymus, either by thymus epithelial cells or by the resident lymphocyte and mononuclear population. The thymus is innervated by both the cholinergic and sympathetic nervous systems, which, in addition to cholinergic and adrenergic secretions, deliver to the interstitial space a wide range of neuropeptides[47] (see Table 158–5). Receptors for neurotransmitters and neuropeptides are selectively present on thymus epithelial cells and/or lymphocytes. Many of the thymic peptides are secreted into the circulation and, as hormones, can modulate the immune process elsewhere.

Several thymic peptides have been reported to influence anterior pituitary secretion either through actions on the pituitary directly or indirectly through the hypothalamus.[45–48] Thymosin β4 stimulates release of luteinizing hormone by way of gonadotropin-releasing hormone (GnRH); thymosin fraction 5 stimulates GH and PRL secretion through a direct action on the anterior pituitary. Thymic factors that can stimulate the hypothalamic-pituitary-adrenal axis include thymosin fraction 5, thymopoietin, and thymosin α1. Reasons set forth by Hall et al.[47] for believing that thymosin α1 may play a physiological role in ACTH regulation are that circulating levels of this peptide fluctuate in parallel with plasma corticosterone (in the mouse) and that thymosin α1 immunoreactivity is demonstrable in the hypothalamus, where it may be part of an intrinsic neuropeptidergic system analogous to the central interleukinergic pathways.[49, 50] These provocative data notwithstanding, the way in which thymic hormones may interact in the regulation of reproduction and the adrenal stress response is incompletely understood.

The thymus is a conspicuous target of classical hormones. For example, glucocorticoids, estrogens, and testosterone induce thymus involution; development and maintenance of the thymus is GH- and PRL-dependent. These phenomena are discussed below.

The Autonomic Nervous System: Adrenal Medulla, Catecholamines, and Neural Innervation of Immune Organs

The nervous system exerts another level of immunomodulatory control through the sympathetic nervous system, acting systemically by release of epinephrine from the adrenal medulla and locally by release of norepinephrine and neuropeptides from sympathetic nerve endings.[51–56] Activation of the sympathetic nervous system or injection of epinephrine (in experimental animals and humans) causes leukocytosis, lymphopenia, lymphocytic margination (endothelial sequestration), and changes in the ratios of various types of lymphocytes. The principal immunoregulatory organs (lymph nodes, thymus, spleen, and intestinal Peyer's patches) are abundantly supplied by autonomic nerve fibers.[52, 54] The sympathetic nervous system is importantly involved in centrally induced immunosuppression. For example, it has been shown that intracerebroventricular injection of corticotropin-releasing hormone (CRH) inhibits the NK cell activity in peripheral blood; suppression is markedly attenuated in these animals and is reversed by pharmacological blockade of the autonomic nervous system.[53]

Sympathetic and sensory neurons also secrete a variety of neurotransmitters and neuropeptides, including substance P, vasoactive intestinal polypeptide (VIP), angiotensin II, calcitonin gene–related peptide (CGRP), and somatostatin.[3, 52, 54, 56] Neurosecretions known to influence lymphocyte function are contained in sympathetic nerves that innervate lymphoid tissues[54] (Table 158–6).

Neuroimmodulatory actions of VIP and substance P are the best characterized of the immunoregulatory peptides released from neurons and are considered here.

Vasoactive Intestinal Polypeptide

VIP, a 28 amino acid–containing peptide, is widely distributed in neurons of the brain, lung, and gastrointestinal tract. The peptide is derived by processing of a prohormone, the sequence of which also codes for a homologue, PHI (in pig), PHM in the human, which has biological properties similar to that of VIP and is co-secreted with VIP.[55, 57] VIP belongs to a peptide superfamily which includes glucagon, secretin, and corticotropin-releasing hormone (CRH). Its location both in neurosecretory neurons of the hypothalamus and within a population of pituitary cells and its capacity to induce PRL secretion indicate that it may serve as both a hypophysiotrophic factor and a paracrine/autocrine PRL-releasing factor.[58]

VIP also plays a role in neuroimmunomodulation. VIP-ergic neurons innervate major immunoregulatory tissues—lymph glands, thymus, intestinal Peyer's patches, and dif-

TABLE 158–5. THYMIC HORMONES

NAME	CHEMICAL PROPERTIES	BIOLOGICAL PROPERTIES
Thymic factors initially isolated from the thymus		
Thymosin fraction 5	Family of heat-stable acidic polypeptides, MW 1000–15,000	Induces T-cell differentiation, stimulates MIF, IL-2, interferons, other cytokines
Thymosin α1	28 AA, MW 3108, sequenced	Induces MIF, interferons, lymphokines, T cells
Thymosin α7	MW 2500	Enhances suppressor T cells
Thymosin α11	35 AA, sequenced	Similar to thymosin α1
Thymosin β4	43 AA	Induced TdT in bone marrow
Thymosin β8	39 AA	Not known
Thymosin β9	41 AA	Not known
Thymosin β10	42 AA	Not known
Thymic humoral factor	MW 3200	Restores T-cell reactivity
Thymopoietin	49 AA, MW 5562	Induces intrathymic lymphocytes; terminal pentapeptide, biologically active
Thymulin (FTS)	Nonapeptide, contains zinc	Enhances cytotoxic T cells, inhibits delayed immunity
Thymic factor X	MW 4200, sequenced	Restores delayed hypersensitivity
Thyrostimulin	Mixture of peptides	Induces T-lymphocyte function

Classical lymphokines
  Interleukins 1, 2, 4, 6, 7, TNF, and others.
Neuropeptides
  Neurotensin
  Somatostatin
  Oxytocin
  Vasopressin
  Neurophysins
  Substance P
  VIP
  Calcitonin gene-related peptide (CGRP)
  Metenkephalin
  ACTH
  Cholecystokinin
  Atrial natriuretic peptide
  Neurokinin A
Neural markers
  Neuron-specific enolase
  Chromogranin A
  A2B5
  HISL-5, -9, -14
  ID4

TABLE 158–6. NEUROTRANSMITTERS AND NEUROPEPTIDES FOUND IN NERVES INNERVATING LYMPHOID ORGANS

Bone marrow
  Norepinephrine
Thymus
  Norepinephrine
  Substance P, tachykinin
  Calcitonin gene-related peptide (CGRP)
  VIP
  NPY
Spleen
  Norepinephrine
  Substance P
  NPY
  CGRP
  VIP
  Somatostatin
  Interleukin 1
Lymph nodes
  Norepinephrine
  Substance P
  NPY
  VIP
  PHI
  CGRP

Data from Felton SY, Feldon DL: Innervation of lymphoid tissue. *In* Ader R, Feldon DL, Cohen N (eds): Psychoneuroendocrinology (ed 2). San Diego, Academic Press, 1991, pp 27–61.

increase in cAMP levels. Effective concentrations of peptide for most reactions are between 10^{-7} and 10^{-10} M and occasionally as low as 10^{-12} M. In view of the close association of nerves with lymphocytes, it is likely that levels in this range could be achieved in situ.

When studied in vitro, most experiments show that VIP is inhibitory to lymphocyte activity, including changes in response to lectin mitogens, immunoglobulin synthesis, and NK activity[59, 60] (Table 158–7). In the whole animal, the most striking effects of VIP appear to be on migration and recirculation of lymphocytes. The important observations supporting this contention are that output of lymphocytes from lymph nodes is markedly suppressed by VIP infusion (as determined by direct cannulation in sheep) and uptake increased into Peyer's patches of the gastrointestinal tract. There is definite selectivity in the type of T

TABLE 158–7. EVIDENCE FOR PROLACTIN-MEDIATED IMMUNOMODULATION

Prolactin receptors are expressed on lymphocytes (B and T) and monocytes.

Prolactin receptors bind cyclosporine, an immune suppressant.

Prolactin excess (in some systems) stimulates splenocyte and thymocyte proliferation, enhances NK cell activity, increases IL-1 production, and IL-2 receptor expression.

Prolactin deficiency inhibits delayed hypersensitivity, antibody production, mixed lymphocyte responses of splenocytes, T-cell proliferation, spleen and thymus growth, and production of cytokines.

Prolactin treatment restores immune function in hypophysectomized rat.

Paracrine/autocrine production of prolactin by lymphocytes. Prolactin is synthesized and secreted by human peripheral blood mononuclear cells. Incubation of lymphocytes with antiprolactin antibody prevents proliferative effects of concanavalin A, phytohemagglutinin, bacterial endotoxin, IL-2, and IL-4.

Mechanism of prolactin action: Prolactin must be internalized to nucleus.

fuse interstitial macrophages. As summarized by Ottaway,[59] high-affinity, high-specificity membrane receptors for VIP have been demonstrated in lymphocytes and other immunocompetent cells, as well as a class of low-affinity receptors. Many different types of human lymphocytes can bind VIP but with differences among cell types and in different states of activation. It has been estimated that the rich innervation of the gastrointestinal tract brings VIP-secreting neurons within 9.5 μm of 50 per cent of the volume of tissue and within 13 μm of 100 per cent of the gastrointestinal mucosa.[59]

Following occupancy of the VIP receptor, lymphocytes, in common with other VIP-sensitive cells, display a marked cell which is modulated with regard to both release from lymph nodes and uptake mechanisms. Further, the presence or absence of the VIP receptor on the lymphocyte appears to determine its uptake in gastrointestinal lymphatic tissue and/or depletion of receptor-inhibiting uptake. As a model of potential mechanisms of neuroimmunomodulation, redistribution of lymphocytes among various lymphoid structures is conceivably important, since it exposes lymphocytes to different imprinting and regulatory milieus. An example of how regulation of lymphocyte traffic from the gut may be important is the phenomenon of cell-mediated systemic immunomodulation generated by oral antigen immunization.[61]

The clinical relevance of VIP-immune interaction remains to be determined. One can speculate that VIP contributes to regulation of local immunity and is involved in pathogenesis of inflammatory bowel disease.

Substance P and Other Tachykinins

Substance P, an archetypical brain-gut peptide, was independently discovered in extracts of the intestine by Von Euler and Gaddum on the basis of its ability to contract guinea pig ileum and by Leeman and associates on the basis of its ability to stimulate secretion of saliva. It was not until the peptide was sequenced and assayed that it was shown to be the same substance.[62] It is an 11 amino acid peptide that belongs to a family of analogous peptides termed the *tachykinins* which have similar biological properties, react with substance P receptors, and have a similar carboxy-terminal sequence. Substance P and substance K are synthesized as part of the same prohormone, while the third tachykinin, neuromedin K, is a product of a different gene. Based on binding studies using native and synthetic modifications of the tachykinin structure, at least three different receptors have been identified which are relatively selective for each of the three tachykinins. Other members of the tachykinin family are found in amphibians, dogfish, and mollusks,[63] providing evidence for an ancient biological conservation of structure.

Substance P and substance K are found in a population of sensory neurons which mediate painful stimuli through multisynaptic pathways originating in the dorsal root entry zone of the spinal cord. When stimulated, substances P and K are released at sensory nerve endings activated by retrograde neurotransmission. Thus any structure with sensory innervation has the potential to be exposed to these tachykinins. Substance P also can be secreted by activated eosinophils.

In addition to their central nervous system (CNS) distribution, tachykinin receptors are found on a number of types of circulating and fixed cells, including monocytes, macrophages, lymphocytes, mast cells, and endothelia.[63–65]

Among the effects exerted by substance P (and other tachykinins) are release of histamine from mast cells, stimulation of monocyte chemotaxis, stimulation of production by monocytes of the acute-phase cytokines IL-1, IL-2, IL-6, interferon-γ, and TNF, proliferation of lymphocytes (most likely mediated by locally induced cytokines), and proliferation of connective-tissue elements including fibroblasts.[66, 67] Substance P enhances cellular chemotaxis and phagocytosis. Tachykinins reverse stress-induced thymic involution and alter lymph node release of lymphocytes.

Neurokinin type 2 receptors are the main tachykinin receptors involved in immune cell response.[65–67]

A number of studies suggest that substance P released from nerve endings may play a role in the course of inflammatory disease. For example, obliteration of the substance P (and presumably substance K) component of sensory inervation of the joint markedly reduces the severity of acute adjuvant-induced arthritis in the rat[68, 69] and can influence the course of skin delayed hypersensitivity.[63]

Neuropeptides Secreted by Immunocompetent Cells and Their Function

Still another level of potential control of the immune process is the secretion by immunocompetent cells of hormones, polypeptides, and receptors classically associated with neuronal tissue or endocrine cells[3, 6, 7, 33, 34] (see Tables 158–3 and 158–4). Proopiomelanocortin (POMC)–related peptides (ACTH, α-MSH, enkephalins, endorphins) and corticotropin-releasing hormone (CRH) are discussed in this section because most data suggest that autocrine/paracrine and neurosecretory factors are the most important aspect of their immunoregulatory function. GH and PRL will be discussed below in relation to the effects of pituitary hormones on immune function.

ACTH

The report by Smith and colleagues[70] that ACTH was detectable by immunohistochemical staining in mouse lymphocytes and that Newcastle virus stimulated lymphocyte ACTH secretion sufficiently to increase corticosterone in infected hypophysectomized mice was a landmark in the development of the concept of an endocrine-signaling function of immunocompetent cells. Some aspects of these original claims have been challenged seriously, but other aspects have been confirmed. In a highly critical study, Dunn et al.[71] attempted to repeat the original study and found that mice that were completely hypophysectomized did not secrete increased corticosterone levels when infected. The finding of adrenal cortical activation was attributed by these workers to incompleteness of the hypophysectomy. In the rat, Newcastle virus infection also was found to be ineffective in stimulating corticosterone secretion.[72]

Nevertheless, certain aspects of the initial assertion that lymphocytes secrete ACTH have been established. Messenger RNA isolated from murine lymphocytes displayed a coding sequence for ACTH which was identical with that of the pituitary, and ACTH isolated from lipopolysaccharide (LPS)-stimulated lymphocytes was shown to have the same amino acid sequence as that of the pituitary.[73, 74] Human lymphocytes also were shown to express POMC mRNA, but infection with Epstein-Barr virus (EBV) had no effect on gene expression.[75] ACTH exerts direct effects on lymphocytes. ACTH receptors were demonstrated on several lymphocyte lines by competitive displacement and by immunofluorescence using antisera directed against the adrenal ACTH receptor, and ACTH stimulated the accumulation of cAMP, a response similar to that observed in the adrenal cortex after ACTH stimulation.[76] ACTH stimulates B-cell growth in the mouse[77] and NK activity when administered intravenously.[78]

The relevance of either intrinsic or exogenous ACTH to lymphocyte function in the human has not been established. Treatment of normal volunteers with the glucocorticoid antagonist RU 486 (which produced a compensatory elevated ACTH) had no effect on a number of measures of lymphocyte activity.[79] In one report, lymphocytes isolated from the blood of a child with a genetically determined adrenal ACTH receptor defect was reported to show no ACTH binding, a finding interpreted to mean that ACTH deficiency was defective in all tissues,[80] but in a large pedigree of patients with ACTH insensitivity (Allgrove syndrome), no differences in ACTH binding to lymphocytes were observed; ACTH activation of lymphocyte cAMP was not demonstrable in either affected or normal individuals.[81] On the other hand, a case of Cushing's syndrome attributed to ectopic production of ACTH by an inflammatory mass has been reported.[82]

Other POMC-Derived Peptides

The POMC gene is expressed in monocytes and other lymphatic cells; the synthesis of ACTH, alpha melanocyte-stimulating hormone (α-MSH), β-lipotropin, endorphin, and enkephalins has been claimed, but disputed vigorously.[82a, b] These secretory products are generally inhibitory to a number of lymphocyte functions. As in the case of the pituitary corticotrope cell, exposure of lymphocytes to CRH enhances and treatment with glucocorticoids inhibits POMC gene expression. CRH, synthesized by activated mononuclear cells at sites of inflammation, has proinflammatory actions. Since receptors for ACTH, α-MSH, endorphins, and CRH are expressed in immunocompetent cells, the potential for paracrine and autocrine neuropeptide control of inflammation at the tissue level exists (see below).

ENDORPHINS. Several endorphins (and ACTH 1–39) bind to specific membrane receptors and exert a number of effects on immunocompetent cells, some stimulatory and some inhibitory. These effects include reduction in antibody production[83, 84] and stimulation of T-lymphocyte migration.[85] Immunosuppressive effects on Peyer's patch immunoglobulin secretion apparently are mediated by the delta class of opioid receptors. Delta opioid receptors are also involved in the inhibition of T-cell locomotion, as inferred from studies using a number of opioid peptides, including β-endorphin, met-enkephalin, leu-enkephalin, and other analogues.[85] Mu opiate receptors also may be involved. On the other hand, modulation of proliferation in response to lectin stimulation is highly variable, responses apparently dependent on the prior functional state of the lymphocyte population.[86]

MELANOCYTE-STIMULATING HORMONE (MSH). α-MSH exerts effects on the immune response and on cytokine-mediated CNS reactions. However, the physiological importance of the peripheral actions of this peptide has not been established, in part because α-MSH circulates as such only in those species such as the rat which have an intermediate pituitary lobe (where selective processing of the POMC peptide takes place); in the human, MSH can be detected in the circulation only during pregnancy, when intermediate lobe–type cells become activated. By contrast,

ACTH is secreted into the blood, but even under stress, levels present may be too low to influence immune function directly, as inferred from concentrations which are effective in vitro. Nevertheless, there are special locations in which biologically significant concentrations of α-MSH (and ACTH) may occur. Within the brain, specific melanotropinergic[87] and corticotropinergic[88] neuronal pathways have been documented; their distribution generally corresponds to the distribution of α-MSH and ACTH receptors.[89] Since monocytes and macrophages express the POMC gene, a marker that is enhanced following exposure to IL-1 and IL-6,[90] it is possible that MSH and ACTH may exert paracrine/autocrine effects on immune function or modulate central cytokine action.

Central melanotropinergic neuronal pathways are involved in regulation of core temperature. α-MSH is a powerful antipyretic, inhibiting fever induced by pyrogens with a molar potency compared with acetaminophen of 25,000:1 when administered directly into the brain or 20,000:1 when administered intravenously.[91] Like other antipyretic drugs, it does not lower body temperature except when fever has been induced by pyrogen administration. α-MSH receptors have been localized to several regions of the brain, including the preoptic hypothalamus, in which are localized temperature-regulating neurons.[89] It is likely that α-MSH acts by inhibiting local release of prostaglandins, since it does not block prostaglandin-induced fever. α-MSH is not the only temperature-lowering peptide. Vasopressin, ACTH 1–24, and α-MSH 11–13 are also active in this regard.[91]

Other reported peripheral anti-inflammatory actions of α-MSH in intact animals are inhibition of delayed hypersensitivity and reduction in the acute-phase response to IL-1 and TNF-α.[92] Effects of α-MSH on inflammatory responses in vitro have not been observed consistently. α-MSH was shown to inhibit mouse thymocyte proliferation and human fibroblast prostaglandin synthesis, the peculiar finding being a U-shaped dose-response curve.[93] This finding, though compatible with responses in the whole animal, was not confirmed by another group.[94] The mechanism of α-MSH response has not been determined. There are two or more types of α-MSH receptors in brain.[89, 95] It is possible that only one of the types is involved in regulation of inflammatory responses. For example, α-MSH is antipyretic when administered either intraventricularly or systemically, while the highly potent analogue Nle4-D-Phe7 (MSH) is effective only when administered intraventricularly. In contrast to the native compound, this analogue does not block thymocyte proliferation or fibroblast prostaglandin synthesis when tested in vitro (Tatro, personal communication).

An unusual MSH-related mechanism for immunosuppression of host response to infection with the parasitic trematode Schistosoma mansoni has been proposed by Duvaux-Miret et al.[96] The trematode worm secretes the POMC-related peptides ACTH and β-endorphin throughout its life history; host polymorphonuclear leukocytes and trematode macrophages secrete an endopeptidase which converts these peptides to α-MSH. These workers suggest that immunocytes from the snail-infected hosts are inactivated by the high concentrations of α-MSH so generated.

CORTICOTROPIN-RELEASING HORMONE (CRH). Immunoreactive CRH and mRNA coding for this peptide have been identified in lymphocytes,[97] and CRH receptors in the mouse spleen have been well characterized.[98] They are localized in the red pulp and marginal zone regions, which are known to be rich in macrophages. Absence of receptors in periarterial and peripheral follicular white pulp suggests that neither T- nor B-lymphocytes have specific CRF binding sites; rather, the receptors appear to be localized to macrophages.[98] The radioautographic data fit well with cell culture studies which show that CRH stimulation of β-endorphin secretion by lymphocytes can be induced only in the presence of monocytes.[99] Kavelaars et al.[99] conclude that CRH induces IL-1, and this, in turn, stimulates the lymphocytes. CRH also can be detected in the joint fluid of rats suffering from experimental inflammatory arthritis.[100] Since CRH stimulates lymphocyte secretion of inflammatory cytokines,[97] and since cytokines stimulate the expression of CRH, a mechanism exists for autocrine/paracrine interaction in local inflammation which may be of pathogenetic importance in autoimmune disease.[97, 100]

CRH thus plays several contradictory roles in modulating inflammation. At the peripheral level, it stimulates inflammatory cell response. As the principal activator of pituitary-adrenal secretion, it stimulates release of immunosuppressant glucocorticoids. And acting centrally, it activates the sympathetic nervous system, leading to suppression of NK activity.

EFFECT OF PITUITARY AND TARGET GLAND HORMONES ON IMMUNE FUNCTION

Anterior Pituitary

Prolactin

The role of prolactin (PRL) as an immunoregulator has come into sharp focus only recently [101–104] (see Table 158–7). Although stimulation of lactation (in mammals) has always been considered by mammocentric physiologists to be its principal function, PRL is an ancient and pleiotropic hormone which exerts a wide range of biological effects throughout the vertebrate kingdom, including modifications of fat metabolism, water balance, and behavior.[105] Its function as an immunoregulator in rodents first became apparent when it was shown to reverse the involution of the rat thymus following hypophysectomy, as well as in pituitary-deficient dwarf Snell mice. Efforts to document a direct stimulatory effect of PRL on lymphocyte function were initially relatively unsuccessful until Friesen and colleagues[106] showed that a T-cell line, the Nb2 cells, was dependent on PRL for growth and proliferation. Indeed, this cell line has been used successfully as the basis of a highly selective and sensitive bioassay for PRL.

Prolactin has been shown to modulate normal lymphocyte, thymocyte, splenocyte, and NK cell functions after binding to specific PRL receptors.[107, 108] With the finding that activated lymphocytes contain PRL mRNA and secrete PRL-like peptides[101, 109] and that PRL immunoneutralization inhibits lymphocyte function in vitro,[104, 110, 111] paracrine and autocrine secretion of PRL has emerged as a potential additional control loop. Effects of PRL include immunoneutralization of mixed lymphocyte cultures and

blockade of the proliferative response to nonspecific activators (concavalin A, phytohemagglutinin, bacterial toxin) and to IL-2 and IL-4.[111] Additional evidence supporting the paracrine/autocrine model is the finding that PRL induces expression of IL-2 and IL-2 receptor in lymphocytes[103] and receptors for PRL as well.[112] Stimulation of proliferation by IL-2 in a cloned mouse T-cell line required the presence of PRL (as well as of other peptides) and was therefore considered to be a "progression factor necessary but not sufficient for T-cell proliferation."[103] The combined presence of IL-2 and PRL led to full expression of such factors as interferon regulatory factor 1, c-myc, proliferating cell nuclear antigen, thymidine kinase, cyclin B, and histone H3. PRL alone induced only the expression of interferon regulatory factor 1. In the absence of PRL, IL-2 induced only expression of cyclin B and histone H3. These findings are used to support the hypothesis that PRL may enhance the expression of some genes necessary for entry into S-phase.[113] That PRL may act at a nuclear site is given further credence by the finding that PRL (after binding to its receptor) is translocated to a nuclear site,[113] where it activates a nuclear protein kinase C.[102] G-proteins also may mediate PRL responses.[114]

The relevance of PRL to immunomodulation has been tested in autoimmune disease. In rodent models, PRL restores the susceptibility to adjuvant arthritis after hypophysectomy[115] and advances the time of emergence and enhances the severity of spontaneous lupus syndrome in the B/W mouse.[116] Conversely, suppression of PRL secretion with the dopamine analogue bromocriptine diminishes the severity of several induced autoimmune disorders in rats, including allergic encephalomyelitis[117] and uveitis.[118]

Evidence linking PRL secretion to *human* autoimmune disease is still sketchy. That elevated PRL levels may be a pathogenetic factor in some disorders is suggested by the finding in some[119, 120] but not all[121] studies that the prevalence of antithyroid autoantibodies is greater than expected in patients with hyperprolactinemia. As in models of rodent autoimmune disease, a limited number of reports have documented that suppression of PRL by bromocriptine may benefit the course of several established or putative autoimmune diseases, including psoriasis,[122] iridocyclitis,[123] and iritis.[124]

The immunosuppressant drug cyclosporine may act in part by interfering with PRL-stimulated immunoreactivity. Cyclosporine binds to the PRL receptor and is displaced from the receptor by PRL.[125–127] Cyclosporine also acts through its binding to a nuclear element,[128] as has been claimed for PRL (see above).

In one limited study of a group of patients being evaluated after cardiac transplantation, serum PRL values in the week preceding biopsy were found to be significantly higher in the graft-rejecting group than in those whose cardiac biopsies showed no evidence of rejection.[129] If secondary to the rejection episode, elevated PRL might produce adverse effects, either by stimulating the immune system or by displacing cyclosporine from its receptors. Bromocriptine treatment reduced episodes of cardiac rejection (in cyclosporine-treated patients) over the initial 2 months,[130] a finding that parallels experiments in rats showing that rejection of cardiac[131] and kidney[132] transplants in animals receiving subtherapeutic doses of cyclosporine was reduced by bromocriptine.

Growth Hormone

Effects of growth hormone (GH) on many aspects of immune function have been recognized for nearly three decades. Current interest in the subject has been stimulated by the observations that several classes of immune-competent cells express surface GH receptors and that thymus involution induced by hypophysectomy or aging can be reversed by treatment with GH (as by PRL) and by demonstration that certain cytokines acting at the level of the hypothalamus or the pituitary influence GH secretion. These observations suggest that GH regulation of lymphocyte function may be part of feedback loops including the pituitary and hypothalamus and that regression of immunoreactivity seen in elderly individuals may be secondary to age-related changes in GH secretion. Several comprehensive reviews summarize this extensive literature.[104, 133–135]

GROWTH HORMONE DEFICIENCY. Among the early clues suggesting that immune function was influenced by GH was the finding in laboratory animals that hypophysectomy brought about a decrease in the size of the spleen and thymus[136] and reduced immune globulin response to immunization. More recently, it has been shown that these organs have a marked decrease in spontaneous splenic DNA synthesis.[106] The changes observed in animals are restored to or toward normal by administration of GH. Thymus regression after hypophysectomy also can be reversed by treatment with PRL.[106] It is possible that GH and PRL react with a common receptor.

The importance of GH immunomodulation in the human has not been established definitively. Its role is possibly important in hypopituitary children and adults and in the "physiological" GH deficiency of aging. Changes in GH-deficient children have not been consistent in all studies, some showing no differences in a number of immunological measures such as normal circulating immunoglobulins and normal lymphocyte responsiveness in vitro[137] and others showing reduced lymphocyte reactivity. For example, in one study of hypopituitary children, treatment with recombinant human GH brought about transient reduction in the percentage of B and T cells and decreases in lymphocyte mitogen responses and IL-2 receptor levels.[138] Children with hypopituitarism show a reduced secretion of the thymic hormone thymulin, which is restored by GH treatment.[139] The concentration of GH used may be critical; in mononuclear cells obtained from healthy adults, low concentrations of recombinant human GH stimulated lymphoproliferative responses to phytohemagglutinin, while high concentrations were inhibitory.[140]

In the hypopituitary adult, mitogenic responses of peripheral blood monocytes are normal but are further activated by GH treatment. Tumor cytotoxic activity of NK cells in the normal human also was enhanced by GH injections.[141]

GH REGULATION OF IMMUNOCOMPETENT CELLS. GH receptors identical with those of the liver have been demonstrated to be present in human lymphocytes and in thymus; in keeping with the idea that GH can act as a lymphokine is the demonstration of a homologous binding domain in receptors for GH, PRL, erythropoietin, IL-6, and IL-2.[108] Internalization of the GH receptor in lymphocytes is regulated by phorbol esters.[142] The extracellular domain of the lymphocyte receptor can be released following treatment with reducing substances which expose the peptide chain to proteolytic enzymes.[143]

GH binding to these receptors can activate a number of lymphocyte and macrophage functions. As summarized by Kelly[135] (Table 158–8), injections of GH enhance antibody synthesis and the rejection of skin grafts and increase the severity of adjuvant-induced arthritis. GH stimulates the expression of c-*myc* proto-oncogene in thymus and spleen[143] and the secretion of insulin-like growth factor I (IGF-I).[144, 145] In turn, IGF-I is stimulatory to a number of lymphocyte functions, including increase in thymidine incorporation into T cells and pro-B cell differentiation.[144, 146]

In macrophages obtained from hypophysectomized rats, exposure to GH increased the production of superoxide anion after exposure to zymosan. The intensity of the response was similar to that induced by interferon-γ.[147] This is an important function for killing of phagocytosed microorganisms. Exposure of lymphocytes to media conditioned by GH-treated lymphocytes enhances their proliferation. The factor may be one of the well-characterized cytokines, since both IL-1 and IL-2 secretion by lymphocytes was enhanced by exposure to GH.[148]

SECRETION OF GH AND GHRH BY LYMPHOCYTES. GH also may be a paracrine/autocrine regulatory factor in lymphocytes.[149] Two GH-immunoreactive species are secreted by lymphocytes—one of molecular weight 22,000 corresponding to pituitary GH and the other of molecular weight 100,000 which could be converted to the lower-molecular-weight form by incubation with reducing substances.[149] Confirmation that the cells synthesize GH was

TABLE 158–8. GROWTH HORMONE REGULATION OF ACTIVITIES OF CELLS OF THE IMMUNE SYSTEM

Growth hormone deficiencies and immunoregulation
  Thymic atrophy and wasting in mice and dogs
  Reduced antibody synthesis in mice
  Delayed skin-graft rejection in mice
  Normal lymphoid cell subsets and thymic histology with reduction in peripheral T and B cells
  Association of pituitary hypoplasia and thymic atrophy in humans
  X-linked GH deficiency and complete inability to synthesize antibodies
  Reduction in activity of NK cells in humans
  Defective allogeneic mixed-lymphocyte reaction
  Reduction in plasma thymulin in humans and mice
  Normal immunoglobulin concentrations and lymphoid cell subsets in humans
Growth hormone and the thymus gland
  Increases thymic size and DNA synthesis in young rodents
  Improves thymic size and morphology in aged animals
  Increases plasma thymulin in humans and dogs
Growth hormone and lymphoid cells
  Lymphocytes have receptors for growth hormone
  Augments antibody synthesis and reduces skin-graft survival in vivo
  Increases lectin-induced T-cell proliferation and IL-2 synthesis in vivo
  Stimulated proliferation of human lymphoblastoid cells
  Augments basal lymphocyte proliferation in vivo
  Increases activity of cytotoxic T-lymphocytes in vitro
  Augments activity of NK cells in vivo
  Synthesized by lymphoid cells
Growth hormone and phagocytic cells
  Primes macrophages for superoxide anion release in vitro and in vivo
  Augments respiratory burst in neutrophils from GH-deficient patients in vivo
  Increases basal respiratory burst of human neutrophils and inhibits activated burst in vitro
Growth hormone and hemopoiesis
  Augments neutrophil differentiation in vitro
  Augments erythropoiesis

Adapted from Kelly KW: Growth hormone, lymphocytes and macrophages. Biochem Pharmacol 38:705–713, 1989.

the demonstration of GH mRNA in cellular extracts. Release of lymphocyte GH is enhanced by phytohemagglutinin, a lectin that activates many different monocyte/lymphocyte functions, and is further enhanced by exogenous GH.[148] In contrast to control of the pituitary, neither growth hormone–releasing hormone (GHRH) nor somatostatin influenced GH secretion by lymphocytes.[150]

The most important finding supporting the view that GH is an autocrine/paracrine regulator of immune function is the demonstration that introduction of a GH antisense oligodeoxynucleotide in lymphocytes reduced responses to concanavalin A stimulation.[151]

Lymphocytes also have been shown to contain immunoreactive GHRH,[152] which is possibly an autocrine/paracrine factor as well, since GHRH added to lymphocytes in vitro stimulates proliferation and inhibits NK function.[153, 154]

ROLE OF GH IN THYMIC INVOLUTION IN AGING ANIMALS. In both rodents and humans, the thymus gland involutes progressively with age. Since GH secretion (and somatomedin C levels) decline with age[155] and GH is known to stimulate thymus growth, it has been postulated that thymus atrophy is due to an age-related decrease in GH secretion and, by inference, with the decline in lymphocyte reactivity seen in normal aging humans. GH injections or implantation of GH-secreting pituitary tumors in the rat reversed the thymic involution in aging[133, 134] and in the human stimulated production of the thymic hormone thymulin.[139] The extent to which reduced lymphocyte reactivity in normal older humans is due to the functional GH deficiency of aging and its relevance for immune surveillance of neoplasia and response to infection have not been determined.

Target Gland Hormones

Adrenal Steroids

GLUCOCORTICOIDS. Of the known effects of hormones on the immune system, those of the adrenal were the earliest to be recognized. As outlined by Munck and Guyre,[156] an excessive number of circulating white blood cells was described by Addison in 1855 in patients with adrenal tuberculosis; thymic hypertrophy following adrenalectomy was described in 1924. Selye's classic work (1936) showed that a wide variety of stresses brought about adrenal enlargement and thymus atrophy.[157] Since either adrenalectomy or hypophysectomy prevented stress-induced thymus atrophy, Selye concluded that thymus regression was secondary to pituitary-adrenal activation. The crucial findings that confirmed an anti-inflammatory action of the adrenal cortical secretions were the demonstration by White and colleagues[158] that injections of ACTH caused lymphopenia and thymus involution and the revolutionary demonstration by Hench and colleagues[159] that cortisone brought about remissions in patients with rheumatoid arthritis, a finding that earned these workers a Nobel Prize.

Although the anti-inflammatory effects of glucocorticoids became well known[11, 156, 160] and a cornerstone of clinical therapy, these actions were thought for many years to be "pharmacological" side effects and not relevant to physiological function. The prevailing view was that the physiological function of the adrenal cortical stress response was to provide increased amounts of glucocorticoids needed to increase the capacity of the organism to resist stress. This concept arose as a logical extension of Claude Bernard's theory of the constancy of the internal milieu and on W. B. Cannon's interpretation of the homeostatic function of the sympathetic nervous system response to stress. Hans Selye expanded the concepts of Bernard and Cannon to include the adrenal cortical response, bolstering his argument with the well-established facts that adrenalectomized animals and humans are more vulnerable to stress of any kind and that this vulnerability is reversed by glucocorticoid administration.

Within the last two decades, however, there has been a radical reinterpretation of the physiological function of the pituitary adrenal response to stress specifically induced by infection or bacterial toxins. Several groups of workers, including Besedovsky and colleagues[161, 162] and Munck and colleagues,[11, 156] have proposed that the major physiological function of glucocorticoid response in inflammatory stress is to modulate and suppress activation of the immune system and the tissue-damaging effect of inflammatory mediators arising during the expression of natural and acquired immunity. Viewed from an evolutionary standpoint, it can be postulated that the pituitary-adrenal response to stress has evolved as a means to control the defensive response that follows invasion by toxins, antigens, and microorganisms. Having so evolved, the system is now available to cope with other forms of stress, both physical and symbolic.

In support of the view that the immune-suppressive actions of the glucocortiocoids are manifestations of their *physiological* function is the impressive catalog of their actions on lymphocytes and macrophages.[11, 156, 160] These include inhibition of cytokine secretion by immunocompetent cells and the consequent loss of lymphocyte reactions which are secondary to cytokine actions. Among the factors inhibited are interferon-γ, granulocyte-monocyte colony-stimulating factor, interleukins 1, 2, 3, and 6, and tumor necrosis factor. The secretion of a variety of inflammatory mediators by activated lymphocytes and macrophages is also inhibited. These include bradykinin, serotonin, histamine, and the tissue destructive enzymes collagenase, elastase, plasminogen activators, and prostaglandins. Although it is likely that the major immunosuppressive actions of glucocorticoids are mediated through changes in cytokines, certain aspects of glucocorticoid action on macrophages may separately regulated. NK activity is suppressed by glucocorticoids,[163] as is lymphocyte viability (see below under "Apoptosis").

Apoptosis. Exposure of lymphocytes and related cell types to glucocorticoids induces "programmed cell death" in a process termed by Wyllie *apoptosis*.[164] Apoptosis can be defined as "a physiological process by which selected cells are deleted from a population in response to specific regulatory signals."[165] Apoptosis in lymphocytes and thymocytes is a response at the level of gene expression by activation of the glucocorticoid receptor.

Binding of the glucocorticoid receptor to glucocorticoid regulatory sites (GRE's) in target genes leads to the synthesis of one or more specific nonlysosomal endonucleases which degrade nucleosomal DNA. In turn, this leads to lysis of the cells. Essential to the induction of apoptosis in lymphocytes is an increase in calmodulin[166, 167] and an increase in intracytoplasmic Ca^{2+}. The destructive effect of glucocorticoids can be blocked by exposure to phorbol esters[168] or to IL-2.[169] Glucocorticoid induction of apoptosis is not confined to the lymphatic system. Activation of glucocorticoid receptors has been shown to induce cell death in hippocampal neurons and to potentiate cell death caused by other factors such as anoxia and excitation of the glutamate receptor. In contrast to the situation in lymphocytes, glucocorticoid-induced apoptosis in hippocampal neurons does not result from activation of endonucleases. The mechanism of neuronal damage is unknown.[170]

Although the major overall effect of glucocorticoids on lymphatic cells is to reduce activity and induce cell death, a number of proteins and genes are *activated*. In addition to increased calmodulin and endonuclease(s), glucocorticoids can induce IL-1 receptors.[171] Gene expression of mitochondrial phosphate carrier protein, immunoglobulin (Ig)–related glycocoprotein, and autoantigens for systemic lupus erythematosus and Graves' disease[167] has been demonstrated, and a number of other less well characterized mRNA sequences also appear, including a novel sequence corresponding to an as yet uncharacterized G-protein–coupled receptor.[168]

Inhibitory Nuclear Glucocorticoid Response Elements. Most biological effects of the glucocorticoids result in activation of genes and consequent *increased* protein expression brought about by binding to defined specific DNA response elements. The question as to whether glucocorticoid-receptor complexes inhibit gene expression by binding to specific *inhibitory* DNA response elements (negative glucocorticoid response elements) is an important one. Using site-directed mutagenesis in the IL-2 gene (whose expression is inhibited by glucocorticoids), Northrop and colleagues[172] have found a sequence which is required for glucocorticoid-induced inhibition of transfected Jurkat cells, a sequence distinct from previously established enhancer sequences. A somewhat more sophisticated mechanism of glucocorticoid inhibition has been proposed by Vacca et al.[173] These workers showed that two sequences in the IL-2 gene are synergistic for stimulation of gene expression: AP-1 motif and the NFAT (nuclear factor of activated T cells protein) motif. These authors postulate that glucocorticoids act by preventing the interaction of these regulatory sites.

Still another mechanism by which glucocorticoids inhibit cellular function is by interactions between the glucocorticoid receptor and AP-1. AP-1 is a protein complex of the c-*jun* and c-*fos* proto-oncogenes which is capable of binding (through c-*jun*) to the glucocorticoid receptor. One example of this mechanism is the finding that in the presence of high concentrations of c-*jun*, binding of the glucocorticoid receptor to the glucocorticoid response element is reduced, leading to transcriptional repression.[174] Thus glucocorticoid interaction with the AP-1 (nucleoprotein) pathway is influenced by the relative concentrations of proto-oncogenes of the *jun/fos* family.

Brain Versus Lymphocyte Glucocorticoid Receptor. One of the questions of great interest to those who have utilized the dexamethasone suppression test to characterize patients with depressive disorder is whether peripheral lymphocyte glucocorticoid receptors can be used as a measure of CNS glucocorticoid receptor. Type II glucocorticoid receptors are distributed widely in a number of brain sites as well as in peripheral lymphocytes; binding affinities are identical. In contrast, type I receptors (mineralocorticoid receptor) were found in the hippocampus but not in other brain regions or in lymphocytes.[175] Following adrenalectomy, type II receptors increase in hippocampus, frontal cortex, and hypothalamus but not in the pituitary nor in lymphoid tissues (lymphocytes, spleen, thymus). Large doses of corticosterone suppress receptors in all sites. These findings indicate that peripheral lymphocyte receptors can reflect changes in brain receptors but only under conditions which would have to be defined for each manipulation.

DEHYDROEPIANDROSTERONE (DHEA). DHEA and its sulfate (DHEAS) are present in blood in concentrations far in excess of that of any other steroid hormone. Generally considered to be an intermediate precursor to androgens, DHEA exerts immunomodulatory activities which are of unknown significance. The steroid binds specifically to a cytosolic and nuclear receptor in murine T cells which is slightly cross-reactive with cortisol and dihydrotestosterone. DHEA binding is not displaced by progesterone, dexamethasone, estradiol, androsterone, DHEAS (the sulfated form of DHEA) and β-etiocholanolone.[176] Both enhancing and inhibitory actions of DHEA on immune function have been described. DHEA increased IL-2 synthesis by helper T cells,[177] antagonized the suppressive effects of dexamethasone on lymphocyte, thymus, and splenic activity,[178, 179] and enhanced natural immunity to systemic viral infection[180] and acquired immunity in aged mice.[181] On the other hand, DHEA inhibits NK differentiation,[182] release of superoxide radical by alveolar macrophages,[183] lymphopoiesis,[184] and T-cell production of IL-4.[185] DHEA reduces antibody synthesis and is clinically beneficial in a mouse strain that develops spontaneous systemic lupus erythematosus.[186] The relevance of these findings to human immunoregulation is not known.

Gonadal Steroids

ESTROGENS AND PROGESTINS. Several striking observations indicate that females have more reactive immune systems than do males,[187–189] the best examples being the much higher incidence in women of autoimmune diseases such as systemic lupus erythematosus, Hashimoto's thyroiditis, rheumatoid arthritis, and Graves' disease.[189] Rodent models of autoimmune disease (e.g., genetically determined lupus in the NZB mouse) demonstrate the same striking sex differences, which can be modified by castration and estrogen replacement.[187–189] On the other hand, during pregnancy, the female immune system is inhibited, as shown by the appearance of immune tolerance to the fetus, to autoantigens, and to extrinsic antigens. The role of sex steroids in determination of these marked changes in immunoreactivity has received much attention, with data indicating effects at virtually all levels in immunoregulation, but the results of numerous studies have not as yet provided a clear understanding of the way in which estrogens exert their many effects and how they are integrated.[188, 189] There are unexplained discrepancies between studies of immunoreactivity in the intact animal and studies of isolated elements of the immune system.

Soluble cytoplasmic estrogen and progesterone receptors have been identified in T-lymphocytes, in thymic epithelial cells, and in the bursa of Fabricius (in chickens). These findings indicate that the sex steroids have the potential to exert their effects directly on immunocompetent cells and on thymus- and bursal-regulatory function.[189]

In virtually all rodent models, female animals show more intense responsivity to antigenic stimulation than do males. For example, antibody response to immunization, as measured by serum titers, and the number of antibody-producing splenic B cells is greater and skin-graft rejection is more consistent in female mice. The paradoxical finding that makes for difficulty in interpretation is that in virtually all studies, removal of estrogens by castration leads to *increased* humoral and cellular immunoreactivity; in keeping with the effects of castration, estrogen added in vitro to a variety of immune cell preparations is inhibitory. Among the immunosuppressive effects of estrogens are inhibition of mitogen-induced T-lymphocyte mitosis following exposure in vitro (an effect which may be concentration dependent) and reduced mitogen responsiveness of cells removed from animals or humans who have received estrogen therapy. Although virtually all published work on estrogen control of immunity has dealt with acquired immunity, depressed NK activity also has been demonstrated (in mice) following treatment with estrogen.[190]

If the direct effect of estrogens on immune function are inhibitory, it would have been expected that treatment with the antiestrogen tamoxifen would have stimulated immune function. On the contrary, lymphocytes from women being treated for breast cancer with tamoxifen showed reduced DNA synthesis after exposure to pokeweed mitogen[191] and, when added in vitro, inhibited splenocyte response to pokeweed mitogen.[192]

There are several possible explanations for the seemingly paradoxical effects of gender, ovarian function, and estrogens on immunoreactivity. In the whole animal, estrogen may act by reversing the immune-suppressive effects of androgens. This possibility is well supported by work on spontaneous lupus in the NZB mouse.[188, 189] Another possibility, proposed by Grossman,[189] is that sex steroids exert effects on the immune system at crucial stages in development to modify its subsequent reactivity. There are precedents for this type of mechanism; for example, sexual dimorphism of liver enzymes in the rat is determined by sexually dimorphic patterns of GH regulation at a critical stage of development.[193] An alternative (or complementary) explanation is that immune-regulatory elements are genetically linked to sex-determining chromosomes.[194] Still another explanation is that estrogens (and other sex steroids) may modify synthesis of other regulatory substances. For example, CD8[+] lymphocytes exposed to progesterone in vitro secrete a factor that inhibits mixed lymphocyte reactivity.[195]

Most of the work on estrogen effects on lymphocyte function has been done in rodents; studies of *human* lymphocyte reactivity have given somewhat ambiguous results. Addition of estradiol to human lymphocytes in vitro has been reported to either increase[196] or decrease[197] responsivity to phytohemagglutinin. Measurements of reactivity of lymphocytes removed during various stages of the menstrual cycle (and therefore exposed to physiological levels of hormones) showed no significant variations throughout the cycle in one study,[198] but in another study, T-cell number was reportedly reduced in the first half of the menstrual cycle.[199]

The most convincing evidence for an immunoregulatory action of estrogens (and progesterone) has come from studies of IL-1 secretion by monocytes isolated from women at different stages of the menstrual cycle or in menopause and by changes in IL-1 mRNA content. The

crucial findings, summarized by Polan et al.,[200] are that monocytes from postmenopausal (estrogen-deficient) women secrete more IL-1 than those from menstruating women, an effect that can be reversed by ovarian steroid treatment. Release of IL-1β from monocytes isolated during the luteal phase is much greater than that from monocytes isolated during the follicular phase. These data suggest that estrogens are inhibitory to lymphocyte reactivity, while progesterone may be stimulatory. Detailed study of dose-response curves indicates a biphasic response to progesterone, low levels being stimulatory and high levels (similar to those of pregnancy) being inhibitory to IL-1β secretion and IL-1β mRNA concentration. Polan et al.[200] associate these changes with temperature regulation—they propose that the postovulatory and early-pregnancy rise in body temperature may be due to progesterone-induced IL-1 production and that the late-pregnancy return to normal temperature may be due to the IL-1 inhibitory actions of high levels of progesterone.

The concentration of IL-1β in the blood of women at the time of ovulation is higher than at any other time during the cycle.[201] This effect is due either to hormonal changes, exerted directly or indirectly on the circulating monocyte/lymphocyte pool, or to activation of gonadotropin-dependent ovarian and/or uterine cytokine release (see below). The severity of angioneurotic edema may vary during phases of the menstrual cycle[202] and may benefit from antiestrogen administration or inhibition of gonadotropin secretion.

There seems little doubt that ovarian steroid hormone status is a determinant of lymphatic reactivity. Whether the effect is exerted directly on the circulating lymphocytes and monocytes or indirectly on effector tissues such as the thymus remains for study.

TESTOSTERONE. In contrast to the somewhat contradictory data documenting estrogen modulation of the immune process, most studies show that androgens are immunosuppressive. This is shown most dramatically by studies of spontaneous lupus in mice subjected to gonadectomy and testosterone therapy[188, 189, 203] and by the relatively low prevalence of autoimmune disease in males, both human and rodent.[187] A number of lines of evidence suggest that testosterone effects on lymphocytes are mediated indirectly. Lymphocytes apparently do not express androgen receptors, but thymus epithelial cells do.[203] Castration in males leads to thymic hypertrophy, and this is reversed by testosterone administration. The bursa of Fabricius in the chicken has androgen receptors and, like the thymus in mammals, is reduced in size following testosterone administration. Little is known about the molecular mechanisms of testosterone action on immunoregulatory tissue. One unique action of testosterone is to suppress the lymphocyte substance P receptor, an effect not shared with either estradiol or progesterone.[204]

Clinical advantage has been taken of the capacity of testosterone and other androgens to inhibit immune function. Thrombocytopenic purpura, an autoimmune disease characterized by the appearance of antiplatelet antibodies, is more common in women than in men. Testosterone and other androgen analogues such as danazol have been used clinically in the treatment of autoimmune hematological disease.[205]

IMMUNOMODULATION IN PREGNANCY. Suppression of fetal rejection by the mother, remission of autoimmune diseases such as rheumatoid arthritis, Hashimoto's thyroiditis, and Graves' disease, and anergy are examples of the striking reduction in cellular and humoral immunity that occurs in pregnancy. The mechanism of immunosuppression involves both circulating factors and those acting locally in the uterus; these complex interactions and the relative importance of each component have not been fully characterized. Each of the placental hormones secreted in high amounts during pregnancy has direct immunosuppressive properties. In addition to estrogens and progestins, human chorionic gonadotropin (hCG) is immunosuppressive. Further, factors arising in the uterus and/or placenta may act locally or systemically to suppress the immune system. These are summarized by Sargent and Redman.[206] Uterine prostaglandins are important in initiation and maintainance of normal implantation; uterine epithelial cells have been shown to secrete IL-1α, which regulates PGE_2 and PGE_{2a} secretion by uterine stromal cells.[207]

Humoral and cellular immunity to paternal antigens usually does not develop in normal pregnancies. NK activity during pregnancy is depressed from the first trimester to term, as is the proportion of T-helper cells, but antibody-dependent cellular cytotoxicity is unchanged. Trophoblast tissue secretes an immune suppressant factor or factors within 24 hours of fertilization. One candidate substance is transforming growth factor beta (TGF-β), which has been isolated from both mouse uterus and human placenta.[21, 22, 206] In the pregnant uterus, biologically active immune-suppressant factors as yet uncharacterized are induced by exposure to high levels of progesterone. Other circulating immunosuppressant factors also may be important; some may arise from the uterus itself. "They include α-fetoprotein, SP1, pregnancy-associated β$_2$-macroglobulin, early pregnancy factor, and products of the interaction between polyamine oxidase and polyamines."[206] The placenta is also a source of IL-1, IL-6, and TNF-α. Additionally, blocking antibodies of various types that can interfere with various stages of immune function have been identified in pregnancy serum.

Thyroid Hormones

Although much information is available about immune function in states of thyroid excess and deficiency, most of the data relate to the role of the immune system in the pathogenesis of the two most common autoimmune disorders of the thyroid, Graves' disease and Hashimoto's thyroiditis, and hence largely deal with sensitized or abnormal cells. Based on the finding that neither the spleen nor the thymus shows a significantly increased oxygen consumption after thyroxine or triiodothyronine administration,[208] lymphatic tissue was long thought to be unaffected by thyroid hormone. However, the presence of typical T_3 receptors in lymphocytes is clear evidence that thyroid hormone is potentially capable of exciting responses.[209] More recent studies report that lymphocytes from hyperthyroid individuals, studied by microcalorimetry, show increased metabolic rate.[210] Early literature summarized in 1976[211] concluded that thyroid deficiency caused a decrease in lymph node and splenic size and that thyroid hormone excess caused hypertrophy of these organs. But data relating thyroid hormone and thymus function were contradictory, both inhibitory and stimulatory effects having been de-

scribed. Similarly, both inhibitory and stimulatory effects on delayed hypersensitivity and on resistance to infection were reported.[211, 212]

Subsequent work using more modern methods for assessing lymphocyte function showed that thyroid-deficient rats had a decreased proportion of suppressor to helper T cells in the spleen and an opposite ratio in peripheral blood. Replacement T_3 corrected the abnormality, but high-dose T_3 did not alter the balance of suppressor/helper cells as compared with euthyroid animals.[213] Further evidence that thyroid hormone influences thyroid function is the finding by Fabris et al.[214] that blood levels of the thymic hormone thymulin (see section under "Thymus," above) are increased in hyperthyroidism and decreased in hypothyroidism,[214] findings that could be duplicated by treatment of mouse thymus in vitro.[215] One of the strengths of the Fabris et al. studies in humans is that altered thyroid activity in many of their patients was not due to autoimmune disease. The decline in NK activity with age (in the mouse) is parallel with the age-related decline in serum T_3 and T_4; return to youthful levels of thyroid hormone leads to restoration of NK activity.[216]

The issue of thyroid hormone modulation of the immune process is clinically relevant to the well-documented decrease in B-lymphocyte production of thyroid-stimulating immunoglobulin (TSI) that occurs during the course of antithyroid treatment of Graves' disease. In a carefully considered review of this issue, Cooper[217] concluded that reduction in thyroid hormone levels may inhibit TSI, but there is an important independent immunosuppressant effect of propylthiouracil unrelated to control of thyroid overactivity per se. Perhaps the most convincing data indicating that thyroid hormone is immunomodulatory come from the report that circulating blood levels of soluble IL-2 receptor (a marker of T-cell activation) are elevated in thyrotoxic patients suffering from either Graves' disease or toxic nodular goiter. Serum IL-2 receptor levels correlated significantly with free T_3 or free T_4 levels irrespective of the underlying autoimmune or nonautoimmune nature of the disease.[218] A similar correlation between IL-2 receptor and T_3 was observed in thyrotoxic patients treated with carbamazole, a thionamide that is not thought to have a direct effect on immune cells.[219]

EFFECT OF CYTOKINES ON NEUROENDOCRINE FUNCTION

Cytokines arising from peripheral immune activation or within the gland itself have many effects on endocrine gland function (Table 158–9). The best understood clinical neuroimmunomodulatory responses important in clinical neuroendocrinology are the pituitary-adrenal response to inflammation, the sick euthyroid syndrome, and inflammation-induced hypogonadism, "sick hypogonad syndrome." Of these, the pituitary-adrenal response is the best characterized and its clinical significance most clearly demonstrated.

One of the important concepts emerging from current research is that cells of the immune system can influence the brain and endocrine function. Besedovsky and Del Rey first proposed the view that the immune system has the capacity to sense the presence of foreign molecules and

TABLE 158–9. INFLUENCE OF CYTOKINES ON NEUROENDOCRINE FUNCTION

HYPOTHALAMIC-PITUITARY-ADRENOCORTICAL FUNCTION

Activates corticotropin-releasing hormone and vasopressin-containing hypophysiotropic pathways to stimulate corticotropin release and glucocorticoid release.

Activates downstream fibers projecting to sympathetic outflow neurons to stimulate peripheral autonomic and adrenal medullary secretion.

In some studies stimulates corticotropin and adrenal cortex directly.

HYPOTHALAMIC-PITUITARY-THYROID FUNCTION

Hypothalamus

LPS and IL-1 inhibit TRH synthesis.

LPS and IL-1 stimulate somatostatin secretion.

Glucorticoid excess inhibits TRH secretion.

TNF-α lowers hypothalamic TRH mRNA.

Anterior Pituitary

LPS stimulates pituitary production of IL-1 (mainly by the thyrotroph cells).

LPS stimulates IL-6 production by folliculostellate cells.

TNF-α reduces glycosylation of TSH, decreasing its biological potency.

Thyroid Gland

IL-1 decreases iodide uptake, cAMP accumulation, thyroglobulin synthesis and secretion, peroxidase gene expression.

TNF-α inhibits iodide uptake, inhibits response to TSH.

IFN increases expression of HLA Class I and Class II molecules, increases iodide uptake and cAMP accumulation but reduces thyroid peroxidase and blocks stimulation of T_3 release induced by thyrotropin.

Growth is stimulated by IL-1, and inhibited by IFN.

HYPOTHALAMIC-PITUITARY-GONADAL AXIS FUNCTION

Hypothalamus

Inhibits pulsatile GnRH secretion via activation of central CRH and VP pathways.

Ovary

Cytokines normally present are IL-1, IL-6, TNF-α.

IL-1 stimulates granulosa cell growth, inhibits luteinization.

IL-6 inhibits FSH-stimulated progesterone secretion.

TNF-α inhibits granulosa cell differentiation, inhibits estrogen synthesis and progesterone synthesis.

Testis

Intratesticular macrophages secrete IL-1, IL-6, and others.

Leydig cells secrete IL-1; Sertoli cells secrete IL-1 and IL-6.

IL-1 and TNF-α inhibit gonadotropin-stimulated Leydig cell secretion of testosterone.

Abbreviations: LPS, *E. coli* endotoxin, lipopolysaccharide; IL-1, interleukin-1; TRH, thyrotropin releasing hormone; CRH, corticotropin-releasing hormone; TNF-α, tumor necrosis factor-alpha; IL-6, interleukin-6; TSH, thyrotropin; cAMP, cyclic $3',5'$ adenosine monophosphate; IFN, interferon-gamma; VP, vasopressin.

Note that many manifestations of autoimmune thyroid disease are attributable to local cytokine release from various classes of activated lymphocytes and macrophages.

foreign organisms and to communicate this information to the brain and neuroendocrine systems.[161, 162] This interaction was described by Blalock as the "bidirectional communication" between the immune and neuroendocrine systems.[33, 34] Infection remote from the brain, systemic inflammation, bacterial and viral infections, and bacterial toxins can exert profound effects on brain function, effects that can be mimicked by systemic injection of IL-1, IL-2, IL-6, and TNF-α. Important manifestations of IL-1–mediated brain effects are fever, anorexia, drowsiness, increased slow-wave sleep, malaise, delirium, and coma. Con-

fusion, delirium, and other manifestations of moderate to severe acute brain syndrome were observed in the majority of patients treated with IL-2 and lymphokine-activated NK (LAK) cells[220] and in patients treated with IL-6 (Atkins et al., personal communication). Bacterial toxins, acting peripherally, initiate a cascade of production of lymphokines, including formation of IL-1, IL-2, IL-6, and TNF-α, which induce marked changes in liver function and in protein and fat metabolism (the "Acute-Phase Response," above). An important component of the acute-phase response is activation of pituitary-adrenal function.

Pituitary-Adrenal Regulation

Toxins and inflammatory cytokines stimulate the synthesis and secretion of CRH and vasopressin by direct actions at the level of the hypothalamus (see Fig. 158–1). Findings that support this contention include increased mRNA coding for CRH after systemic[221] or intracerebroventricular injection of IL-1,[222] increased release of CRH and vasopressin into the hypophyseal-portal blood,[223] increased CRH release from hypothalamic fragments in vitro following addition of IL-1,[224] and blockade of the response to systemic injections of IL-1 by use of anti-CRH antibody.[225, 226] Although IL-1 has been reported by some authors to stimulate the release of ACTH from pituitary cells in vitro[227] and from the mouse At-20 ACTH-secreting cell line,[228] others have been unable to show this.[229] In any case, the finding that immunoneutralization of CRH (and to a lesser extent of vasopressin) can block ACTH release in the whole animal[230, 231] is strong evidence that the most important locus of IL-1 effect is the hypothalamus.

The pituitary-adrenal response also can be mobilized by injections of IL-2,[232] IL-6,[233] TNF-α,[234] and other cytokines, indicating considerable redundancy in the immune limb of the activating system. In part, this is due to the capacity of cytokines to induce other cytokines and to be synergistic with one another.

These cytokines (and IL-1) may reach the hypothalamus from the periphery[40] but also can be generated within the hypothalamus in response to toxin exposure. Responsive cellular elements capable of transducing the toxin signal include astrocytes, microglia,[5, 41] and mast cells,[236] which make up an important component of the interstitial space, where they come into intimate contact with neurons. Each of these cell types is capable of secretion of one or more cytokines in response to toxin and other stimuli.

Further contributing to the IL-1 pool in the hypothalamus are a class of "interleukinergic" neurons containing IL-1β.[49, 50] These are distributed within the classic tuberoinfundibular pathway but are also found elsewhere in the brain, including (in the rat) the olfactory tubercle and the hippocampus.[50]

The neural distribution of IL-1 to the hippocampus may be important for brain functions unrelated to immune regulation. Receptors for IL-1 and several other cytokines are distributed in this region.[237] The hippocampus is importantly involved in memory consolidation and is a prominent site of lesions in Alzheimer's disease; IL-1 stimulates the production of Alzheimer precursor peptide in brain endothelial cells[238] and stimulates the synthesis of nerve growth factor.[239] The consequent release of glucocorticoids, in turn, modulates the intensity of the immune response, virtually all of whose components are inhibited by glucocorticoids, as summarized above.

An excellent example of the validity of this hypothesis has come from the study of immune responses in a strain of rats with a genetic defect in hypothalamic CRH synthesis. As demonstrated by Sternberg and collaborators,[240] rats of the Lewis strain develop acute arthritis when injected with streptococcal cell wall suspensions, whereas rats of the Fischer strain do not. Lewis rats differ from Fischer rats in that they do not show increased adrenal glucocorticoid release when challenged with antigen and do not increase their hypothalamic content of mRNA coding for CRH, as do Fischer rats. Measures that inhibit pituitary-adrenal function in Fischer rats convert their immune responses to those resembling the Lewis (susceptible) strain. Lewis rats are susceptible to many other forms of induced autoimmune disease.

Attempts have been made to extend this hypothesis to humans. A recent report suggests that patients suffering from rheumatoid arthritis have blunted or absent circadian rhythms of cortisol and fail to release ACTH normally after the trauma of surgery.[241]

Stimulation of release of ACTH is not the sole consequence (for immune regulation) of cytokine-induced activation of central CRH pathways. Neuropeptidergic CRH pathways form a widespread network outside the classic tuberoinfundibular (hypophysiotropic) system.[242] Hypothalamic CRH neurons project into the spinal cord by multisynaptic pathways that innervate cell bodies of origin of the autonomic nervous system. Following stimulation by toxins, IL-1, and other cytokines, a massive discharge of norepinephrine from peripheral sympathetic neurons and of epinephrine, from the adrenal medulla occurs.[51-56] This response has a number of consequences for immunity, including inhibition of NK activity and widespread changes in function of both circulating lymphocytes (which possess catecholamine receptors) and lymphoid organs (spleen, thymus, lymph nodes, Peyer's patches), which are abundantly supplied with sympathetic nerve endings (see above).

A peculiarity of the central CRH system is that it is associated with a specific binding protein. CRH binding protein, first discovered as a "carrier protein" responsible for the high circulating levels of CRH in pregnancy, is distributed within neurons of the brain.[243] How this binding interaction influences central responses to cytokines and its functional significance remain to be determined.

Pituitary-Thyroid Regulation

The bidirectional control of neuroendocrine function by inflammatory cytokines is also illustrated in humans in the *sick euthyroid syndrome*. This disorder, the most common thyroid disorder encountered in hospitalized patients, is characterized by low serum levels of T_3, normal or reduced levels of T_4, and inappropriately normal or low serum levels of thyroid-stimulating hormone (TSH).[244, 245] Altered metabolism of circulating thyroid hormones and intrathyroidal abnormalities are responsible for many of the manifestations (see below),[246] but the paradoxically low levels of TSH in these patients suggest, in addition, that the hypo-

thalamic-TSH feedback response to low thyroid hormone levels is inhibited. Inflammation and sepsis suppress TSH secretion through the action of inflammatory cytokines on both pituitary thyrotrope responsiveness to TRH[247] and hypothalamic function (see Table 158–9).

Injections of bacterial pyrogens, IL-1, and/or tumor necrosis factor reduce thyroid hormone and TSH levels in the rat,[248, 249] a finding that can be induced in the human as well.[250] Hypothalamic changes include decreased levels of mRNA coding for thyrotropin-releasing factor[251] and increased somatostatin secretion. In a brain cell culture system, IL-1 increased the concentration of somatostatin in the medium and the concentration of mRNA coding for somatostatin in the cells.[252] Increased somatostatin secretion has implications for GH regulation as well (see below). Bacterial endotoxins induce the synthesis within the pituitary itself of both IL-1 and IL-6 (see above), which may exert suppressive effects through a paracrine mechanism. The absence of clinical findings of hypothyroidism and the inappropriately low TSH also have been attributed to upregulation of the thyroid hormone receptor in peripheral tissues and the CNS.[253]

In contrast to the relatively well-documented teleological importance of the pituitary-adrenal counterregulatory response in inflammation outlined above, the homeostatic value of suppression of pituitary-thyroid function in the sick euthyroid state is less well established. Early literature that described the effects of thyroid state on resistance to infection indicated that with few exceptions, the hypothyroid state was protective of infected animals, fewer animals dying or with delayed death as compared with thyroid hormone–treated animals.[211, 212] In humans, restoration of the low T_3 levels of starved individuals to normal increases the severity of negative nitrogen balance[254]; the administration of T_4 to sick euthyroid patients had, in one limited study, no beneficial (or adverse) effect on disease outcome.[255]

Pituitary-Gonadal Regulation

Severe inflammatory illness also induces a reduction in gonadal function. In women, anovulation may result. In men, sepsis, burns, and trauma lower serum testosterone levels. Cytokine suppression of pituitary-gonadal function is exerted at many levels. IL-1 reaching the gonad by way of the circulation or released within the gonad as an autocrine/paracrine secretion inhibits steroidogenesis (see below). At the hypothalamic level, IL-1 inhibits pulsatile secretion of GnRH.[256] Inhibition of GnRH is most likely secondary to cytokine-induced activation of CRH and vasopressinergic neurons.[256]

Little is known about the functional significance of the gonadal suppression, its role in the negative nitrogen balance in severe stress, and its homeostatic function. One could argue on the basis of teleology that inflammation-induced gonadal dysfunction prevents reproduction in sick individuals.

GH Regulation

In humans, GH secretion is stimulated by injections of bacterial endotoxin or of cytokines released in response to endotoxin challenge. These include IL-1, IL-2, IL-6, and tumor necrosis factor alpha (TNF-α).[133, 135] In rats, the initial response to pyrogen exposure is inhibition of GH release.[257] The effect is dose-related, i.e., low doses stimulating and high doses inhibiting GH secretion.[257a] The locus of effect of the individual cytokines on the hypothalamus and pituitary and the pathways involved have not been fully worked out, in part because of limitations imposed by species differences in the way that GH is regulated. In humans, stress induces GH release, while in rats, GH secretion is both increased and decreased by cytokines. In isolated rat pituitary cells, IL-1, IL-6, and thymosin fraction 5 all stimulate the release of GH, and several cytokines are inhibitory. These include interferon-γ and TNF-α.[133, 135] In contrast, intraventricular injection of IL-1 stimulates GH release in the rat. Increases in somatostatin secretion are demonstrable in vitro (see above). The report that somatostatin secretion is the product of glial activation[258] suggests that cytokine effects on hypothalamic hypophysiotropic function may be mediated by changes in glial rather than neuronal activity. Enhanced hypothalamic somatostatin secretion could inhibit GH secretion.

GH released during inflammation (in humans) may serve a homeostatic function.[134, 135] GH released in response to inflammatory stress increases phagocytic activity of macrophages, stimulates production of IGF-I and TNF-α, and counteracts the deleterious metabolic effects of glucocorticoids secreted during inflammatory stimulation.

INTRINSIC CYTOKINES IN ENDOCRINE GLAND FUNCTION

Among the numerous tissue growth factors involved in differentiation and regulation of endocrine gland growth and function, the cytokines have a special place because they are involved in responses to local and remote inflammation as well as in physiological regulation. In addition to the participation of resident immunocompetent cells in local endocrine regulation, many endocrine cells themselves secrete one or more cytokines. These will be considered in relation to specific glands.

Pituitary

A role for the interleukins in the regulation of pituitary function was suggested by the finding that in some but not all experiments IL-1 could stimulate secretion of ACTH, PRL, and GH, a property shared with IL-6 (see above).[259] That these effects could be part of an intrinsic control system was first suggested by Denef and colleagues,[260, 261] who showed that pituitary cells grown in culture secreted IL-6 in response to exposure to IL-1, a finding confirmed by others.[262–264] Cell fractionation techniques appear to localize the source of secretion to the folliculostellate cell. This cell is a likely candidate for this function. It is embryologically related to brain astroglia, known to be sources of intracerebral IL-6, and displays a number of marker proteins that confirm its origin as part of the primordial brain tissue.[265] It does not secrete any of the classical anterior pituitary hormones but is the principal source of vascular endothelial growth factor and follistatin in the pituitary.[266]

The IL-6 secretory function of the pituitary has been studied extensively. IL-6 secretion is stimulated by IL-1, by bacterial endotoxin (*E. coli* lipopolysaccharide, LPS), by analogues of cAMP, by phorbol esters, by prostaglandin E_2, and by VIP.[259, 267]

Studies of toxin effect on the folliculostellate cell are important because they show how inflammation elsewhere in the body can exert an effect on intrapituitary cell regulation. IL-1 receptor has been demonstrated in a mouse ACTH-secreting pituitary cell line[268] and has been characterized as a type 1 receptor. Exposure of rat pituitary cells to human IL-1 receptor antagonist (IL-1RA) blocks the IL-6 response to both human and rat IL-1.[264] The effects of LPS, on the other hand, may not be mediated solely through IL-6 generation. In contrast to its effects in blocking LPS-induced IL-6 in brain, IL-1a does not block the effects of LPS in the pituitary, thus indicating that other mechanisms are involved. LPS may act on an LPS receptor[269] or via another cytokine such as TNF-α which has been demonstrated to release IL-6[270] or IL-2 and its receptor, which has been demonstrated in pituitary cells and has been shown to stimulate growth of the GH3 pituitary tumor cell line and to inhibit growth in primary pituitary cultures.[271]

IL-1 itself is also expressed in pituitary cells. Immunoreactive IL-1 was detected in a subpopulation of cells but only following challenge with bacterial lipopolysaccharide.[272] IL-1 is colocalized mainly with thyrotrope cells. Since TNF and IL-1 inhibit TRH-induced TSH release, these findings suggest that IL-1 exerts a paracrine inhibitory effect during systemic inflammation.

The mouse pituitary also secretes large amounts of macrophage inhibitory factor (MIF). Activated by toxins, it synergizes with TNF-α in causing shock.[272a]

Ovary

The importance of cytokines arising from within the ovary in the regulation of folliculogenesis, ovulation, and steroid secretion has become evident through a series of recent observations (reviewed in refs. 273 and 274). It has been pointed out that "unlike some gonadal compartments (e.g., the testicular seminiferous tubule), the ovary does not constitute an immunologically privileged site. Thus, resident ovarian (i.e., extravascular) mononuclear phagocytes (macrophages), lymphocytes, and polymorphonuclear granulocytes can be observed at various stages of the ovarian life cycle."[273] In addition to an invading population of macrophages and lymphocytes, cytokines may arise from nonimmune elements in the ovary, including the granulosa cell. Although macrophages found in the ovary may arise by invasion from the circulating blood, the major cells responsible for ovarian cytokine production are not "common" macrophages because they do not adhere to glass or plastic surfaces, as is typical of macrophages isolated from blood.[273]

Intraovarian cytokines play an important role in the development of the ovary, the process of ovulation and atresia, and the regulation of steroidogenesis of both estrogens and progestins. Intraovarian cytokine synthesis is regulated by gonadotropins and glucocorticoids and is also responsive to such stimuli as bacterial toxin (LPS) and circulating

IL-1—means by which systemic inflammation could influence ovarian activity.

Cytokines found in the ovary include IL-1, TNF-α, and IL-6. Evidence that they are secreted by ovarian cells is clear[274–276]; IL-1 arises from ovarian theca interstitial cells[276] and probably from invading macrophages and lymphocytes. Other macrophage secretory products, not classically defined as "cytokines," also influence ovarian function. These include basic fibroblast growth factor and transforming growth factors alpha and beta.

IL-1 stimulates granulosa cell growth and inhibits luteinization of granulosa cells, down-regulates FSH-stimulated granulosal LH receptors, and augments FSH-stimulated synthesis of 20α-dihydroprogesterone and progesterone. IL-6 inhibits FSH-stimulated progesterone production and promotes FSH-induced granulosa cell apoptosis.[277] Indeed, Hughes et al.[277] propose that cytokine-induced granulosa cell apoptosis is the triggering event that culminates in follicular atresia. TNF-α inhibits FSH-induced granulosa cell differentiation at the level of cAMP generation and attenuates estrogen and progestin synthesis through inhibition of specifically defined steroidogenic enzymes.[278]

Factors that regulate secretion of IL-6 and TNF-α from ovarian cells are summarized by Judd and Macleod,[274] who argue convincingly that factors that increase intracellular cAMP stimulate IL-6 and inhibit TNF-α secretion, while factors that activate intracellular protein kinase C or calcium stimulate secretion of both cytokines. Corresponding to their mode of action at the cellular level, LH and FSH stimulate IL-6 release and inhibit TNF-α release, while LPS, IL-1α, and IL-1β (which do not increase intracellular cAMP content) stimulate release of both IL-6 and TNF-α. Glucocorticoids suppress secretion of both cytokines, a finding that led Judd and MacLeod to propose that stress-induced adrenal cortical activation may serve to overcome the effects of inflammatory cytokines in the ovary. IL-1 gene expression in the ovary is stimulated by preovulatory secretion of gonadotropins.[276] In the human, IL-1 appears in the serum in the luteal phase of the cycle.[201] Intrinsic ovarian cytokines may interact in a complex autocrine/paracrine control loop: "In this system, IL-1 produced by the theca-interstitial cells stimulates the granulosa cells to produce IL-6 and TNF. The IL-6 and TNF released from the granulosa cells then serve as an autocrine and/or paracrine factor to regulate ovarian function."[274] At least one way in which the IL-1 effect is mediated is through stimulation of prostaglandin biosynthesis.[279]

Testis

It has long been known that acute illness leads to temporary infertility and suppression of gonadotropin secretion. Studies of the effects of inflammatory cytokines on elements of the testicle and the demonstration of intrinsic cytokine production in the testis have provided insights as to how systemic illness can affect gonadal function and raise the possibility that abnormalities in testicular cytokine secretion may be involved in some disorders of testicular function.

The testicle functionally consists of two compartments, a tubular space occupied by Sertoli cells and developing spermatocytes which are in contact with the lumen of the spermatic ducts and an interstitial space occupied by androgen-secreting Leydig cells.[280] In addition to the Leydig cells, the interstitial space contains macrophages. In the rat, there is one macrophage present for every four Leydig cells.[281] As summarized by Sun et al.,[281] "macrophages are often observed in intimate association with Leydig cells in the testis, with Leydig cell processes inserted into specialized invaginations on the macrophage surface. Highly specific Leydig cell–macrophage binding interactions have also been observed in vitro." Macrophage synthesis of a wide variety of cytokines within the testis is therefore possible and can be induced by any of the factors known to influence macrophage cytokine synthesis elsewhere, such as bacterial toxin, viral infection, IL-1, IL-2, and TNF-α. In addition to the activity of resident and invasive macrophages, new evidence indicates that specific cells of the testis are also capable of cytokine synthesis. Primary cultures of Leydig cells express IL-1α mRNA,[282] and Sertoli cells secrete both IL-1 and IL-6.[283] Both cytokines are activated by several stimuli, including bacterial toxin, IL-1, and stage-specific components of the spermatocyte.[283] Sertoli cells are also stimulated by particle-induced phagocytosis. In this regard, they resemble typical circulating macrophages and brain astrocytes and glia. Thus an extensive system for cytokine synthesis exists within the testis.

IL-1 inhibits gonadotropin-stimulated Leydig cell secretion of testosterone.[284–286] TNF-α also inhibits testosterone secretion,[287] and its effect is synergistic with that of IL-1. On other hand, under particular circumstances, IL-1 and TNF-α can stimulate testosterone secretion.[288] It is possible that cytokines other than IL-1 are involved in intratesticular androgen regulation. In the studies of Sun et al.,[281] media conditioned by macrophages in culture were potent inhibitors of Leydig cell secretion in an assay system that showed no effect from addition of purified IL-1α and IL-1β.

Pancreatic Islets

The intrinsic cytokine system of the pancreatic islets has been the focus of intense activity. Inhibition of insulin secretion has long been known to contribute to the impaired carbohydrate tolerance observed during bacterial infection in the human. Further, the recognition that Type I diabetes is due to an autoimmune invasion of islets by sensitized cytotoxic T cells has raised important questions about the role of inflammatory cytokines in B-cell dysfunction. These questions have been considered in detail by Argiles et al.[289] and Corbett et al.,[290] whose conclusions are summarized here. Most work has dealt with IL-1, receptors for which have been identified on pancreatic B cells. IL-1 generated by invading lymphocytes and macrophages or entering islets from peripheral blood may cause a transient stimulation of insulin, followed by inhibition of both basal and glucose-stimulated secretion. The suppressive phase is sustained and leads to impaired insulin biosynthesis, decreased insulin mRNA, decreased rate of mitochondrial glucose oxidation, decreased uptake of Ca^{2+}, and decreased cAMP and ATP production. Many of these inhibitory effects are also induced by TNF-α, with which IL-1 is synergistic. Over the long term, exposure to IL-1 leads to B-cell death.

A number of pathogenic mechanisms may be involved; generation of free oxygen radicals and production of nitric oxide (NO) are the most important. NO has been shown to be synthesized by induction of a specific synthase by IL-1, a phenomenon recognized in a variety of cell types in addition to macrophages. Working with islet cells isolated from rat pancreas and from a pancreatic tumor cell line, Corbett and colleagues[290] have shown that the B cell itself generates NO in response to IL-1β. These workers propose that NO can cause cell death by inactivating iron-sulfur clusters of mitochondrial iron-containing enzymes such as aconitase, leading to decreased levels of cellular ATP and inhibiting DNA synthesis. Incubation with the IL-1 receptor antagonist prevents B-cell damage.[291]

Thyroid

Thyroid dysfunction in systemic inflammatory disease results in the sick euthyroid state or low T_3 syndrome, also termed *nonthyroidal illness*, and involves abnormalities in peripheral thyroid hormone metabolism, thyroid gland activity, pituitary TSH secretion, and hypothalamic control. Mechanisms operative in the pituitary and hypothalamus were considered earlier. In this section, the effects of cytokines on the thyroid itself are considered.

Thyroidal effects of cytokines have been reviewed by Kennedy and Jones[246] (see Table 158–9). IL-1 can reach the gland either from the peripheral circulation or by secretion from invasive activated lymphocytes and macrophages, as occurs in autoimmune thyroiditis and Graves' disease. Virtually all steps in thyroid hormonogenesis and secretion are impaired. These include inorganic iodide uptake, thyroglobulin production, and peroxidase gene expression. Several responses to TSH are also impaired, including cAMP accumulation and endocytic mobilization of thyroglobulin. Paradoxically, IL-1 acts as a growth factor and may be responsible in part for the thyroid enlargement that sometimes occurs in autoimmune thyroiditis.[292] TNF-α exerts similar inhibitory effects on TSH-activated thyroid functions (see above). Interferon-γ also exerts effects on both antigen presentation and thyroid function. It stimulates the expression of class II antigens (a necessary part of antigen presentation for autosensitization) and stimulates iodide uptake and cAMP accumulation. On the other hand, interferon-γ inhibits thyroid peroxidase, blocks the increase induced by thyrotropin, and inhibits growth.

At the level of the pituitary, both IL-1 and TNF reduce TSH responsiveness to TRH, and TNF-α reduces glycosylation of TSH (hence reducing its biological potency). At the hypothalamic level (considered above), TRH secretion is reduced and somatostatin secretion is enhanced, changes that reduce the hypothalamic component of negative-feedback control, thus leading to inadequate compensatory TSH secretory response to low thyroid hormone levels.

PSYCHONEUROENDOCRINOIMMUNOLOGY

One of the areas of immunoendocrine interaction that has aroused considerable interest recently is that of psychoneuroendocrinoimmunology. A growing, albeit controversial, literature suggests that psychological factors can influence the onset and course of autoimmune disease and cancer. Since neuroimmunomodulation may be mediated by classical pituitary–target gland secretions and by neurotransmitters and neuropeptides, they are considered in this chapter.

An important basis for suspecting that emotional state determines immune function is the evidence from studies in experimental animals indicating that the immune response can be conditioned[293] and that stress such as crowding in rodents impairs natural immunity and increases the vulnerability of animals to certain infections and carcinomas.[1, 2, 8] Certain forms of stress and depression reportedly influence health, immune function, and the incidence and course of cancer in humans. These studies and their implications have been reviewed extensively.[1, 2, 8, 294] The data derived from the study of patients, though extensive and provocative, have been difficult to interpret and remain controversial.

REFERENCES

1. Ader R (ed): Psychoneuroimmunology. New York, Academic Press, 1981.
2. Ader R, Felton DL, Cohen N (eds): Psychoneuroimmunology (ed 2). New York, Academic Press, 1991.
3. Reichlin S: Neuroendocrinology. *In* Wilson JD, Foster DW (eds): Williams' Textbook of Endocrinology (ed 8). Philadelphia, WB Saunders Co, 1992, pp 135–221.
4. Kemeny ME, Solomon GF, Morley JE, Herbert TL: Psychoneuroimmunology. *In* Nemeroff CB (ed): Neuroendocrinology. Boca Raton, FL, CRC Press, 1992, pp 563–591.
5. Plata-Salaman CR: Immunoregulators in the nervous system. Neurosci Biobehav Rev 15:185–215, 1991.
6. Blalock JE (ed): Neuroimmunoendocrinology. Basel, Karger, 1992.
7. Janković BD: Opening remarks. Ann NY Acad Sci 496:1–2, 1987.
8. Reichlin S: Neuroendocrine-immune interactions. N Engl J Med 329:1246–1253, 1993.
9. Abbas AK, Lichtman AH, Pober JS (eds): Cellular and Molecular Immunology. Philadelphia, WB Saunders Co, 1991.
10. Paul WE (ed): Fundamental Immunology. New York, Raven Press, 1989.
11. Munck A, Guyre PM, Holbrook NJ: Physiological functions of glucocorticoids in stress and their relation to pharmacological actions. Endocr Rev 5:25–44, 1984.
12. Atkins E: Pathogenesis of fever. Physiol Rev 40:580–646, 1960.
13. Auron PE, Webb AC, Rosenwasser LJ, et al: Nucleotide sequence of human monocyte interleukin 1 precursor cDNA. Proc Natl Acad Sci USA 81:7907–7911, 1984.
14. Dinarello CA: Interleukin-1 and interleukin-1 antagonism. Blood 77:1627–1652, 1991.
15. Akira S, Hirano T, Taga T, Kishimoto T: Biology of multifunctional cytokines: IL-6 and related molecules (IL-1 and TNF). FASEB J 4:2860–2867, 1990.
16. Henderson B, Blake S: Therapeutic potential of cytokine manipulation. Trends Pharmacol Sci 13:145–152, 1992.
17. Dinarello CA, Wolff SM: The role of interleukin-1 in disease. N Engl J Med 328:106–113, 1993.
18. Kishimoto T, Akira S, Taga T: Interleukin-6 and its receptor: A paradigm for cytokines. Science 258:593–596, 1992.
19. Sporn MB, Roberts AB: Autocrine secretion—10 years later. Ann Intern Med 117:408–414, 1992.
20. Bodmer S, Strommer K, Frei K, et al: Immunosuppression and transforming growth factor beta in glioblastoma: Preferential production of transforming growth factor-beta2. J Immunol 143:3222–3229, 1989.
21. Das SK, Flanders KC, Andrews GK, Dey SK: Expression of transforming growth factor beta isoforms (beta 2 and beta 3) in the mouse uterus: Analysis of the perimplantation period and effects of ovarian steroids. Endocrinology 130:3459–3466, 1992.
22. Altman DJ, Schneider SL, Thompson DA, et al: A transforming growth factor beta 2 (TGF-beta 2)–like immunosuppressive factor in

amniotic fluid and localization of TGF-beta 2 mRNA in the pregnant uterus. J Exp Med 172:1391–1340, 1990.

23. Miller A, Lider O, al-Sabbagh A, Weiner HL: Suppression of experimental autoimmune encephalomyelitis by oral administration of myelin basic protein: V. Hierarchy of suppression by myelin basic protein from different species. J Neuroimmunol 39:243–250, 1992.

24. Snyder SH: Nitric oxide: First in a new class of neurotransmitters. Science 257:494–496, 1992.

25. Lowenstein CJ, Glatt CS, Bredt DS, Snyder SH: Cloned and expressed macrophage nitric oxide synthase contrasts with the brain enzyme. Proc Natl Acad Sci USA 89:6711–6715, 1992.

26. Beasley D, Schwartz JH, Brenner BM: Interleukin 1 induces prolonged L-arginine–dependent cyclic guanosine monophosphate and nitrite production in rat vascular smooth muscle. J Clin Invest 87:602–608, 1991.

27. Garthwaite J: Glutamate, nitric oxide and cell-cell signalling in the nervous system. Trends Neurosci 14:60–67, 1991.

28. Schmidt HH, Gagne GD, Nakane M, et al: Mapping of neural nitric oxide synthase in the rat suggests frequent co-localization with NADPH diaphorase but not with soluble quanylyl cyclase, and novel paraneural functions for nitrinergic signal transduction. J Histochem Cytochem 40:1439–1456, 1992.

29. Habicht GS, Katona LI, Benach JL: Cytokines and the pathogenesis of neuroborreliosis: Borrelia burgdorferi induces glioma cells to secrete interleukin-6. J Infect Dis 164:568–574, 1991.

30. Eizirik DL, Cagliero E, Bjorklund A, Welsh N: Interleukin-1 beta induces the expression of an isoform of nitric oxide synthase in insulin-producing cells, which is similar to that observed in activated macrophages. FEBS Lett. 308:249–252, 1992.

31. Corbett JA, Wang JL, Hughes JH, et al: Nitric oxide and cyclic GMP formation induced by interleukin 1 beta in islets of Langerhans: Evidence for an effector role of nitric oxide in islet dysfunction. Biochem J 287:229–235, 1992.

32. Dawson VL, Dawson TM, London ED, et al: Nitric oxide mediates glutamate neurotoxicity in primary cortical cultures. Proc Natl Acad Sci USA 88:6368–6371, 1991.

33. Blalock JE: A molecular basis for bidirectional communication between the immune and neuroendocrine systems. Physiol Rev 69:1–32, 1989.

34. Carr DJ, Blalock JE: Neuropeptide hormones and receptors common to the immune and neuroendocrine systems: Bidirectional pathway of intersystem communication. In Ader R, Felten DL, Cohen N (eds): Psychoneuroimmunology (ed 2). San Diego, Academic Press, 1991, pp 573–588.

35. Payan DG, McGillis JP, Goetz EJ: Neuroimmunology. Adv Immunol 39:299–323, 1986.

36. Casey LC, Balk RA, Bone RC: Plasma cytokine and endotoxin levels correlate with survival in patients with the sepsis syndrome. Ann Intern Med 119:771–778, 1993.

37. Nathanson JA: The blood-cerebrospinal fluid barrier as an immune surveillance system: Functions of the choroid plexus. Prog Neuroendocrinimmunol 2:96–101, 1989.

38. Beutler B: The tumor necrosis factors: Cachectin and lymphotoxin. Hosp Pract 28:45–56, 1990.

39. Nava E, Palmer RM, Moncada S: Inhibition of nitric acid synthesis in septic shock: How much is beneficial? Lancet 338:1555–1557, 1991.

40. Blatteis CM: Neuromodulative actions of cytokines. Yale J Biol Med 63:133–146, 1990.

41. Benveniste EN: Cytokines: Influence on glial cell gene expression and function. In Blalock JE (ed): Neuroimmunoendocrinology. Basel, Karger, 1992, pp 106–153.

42. Tatro JB, Romero L, Steere AM, Reichlin S: Induction of mitric oxide synthase and IL-6 in rat brain cells in culture by Borrelia burgdorferei cell walls. Submitted.

43. Romero LI, Schettini G, Lechan RM, et al: Bacterial lipopolysaccharide (LPS) induction of IL-6 in rat telencephalic cells is mediated in part by IL-1. Neuroendocrinology 57:892–897, 1993.

44. Jancovic BD: Opening remarks. Ann NY Acad Sci 496:1–2, 1987.

45. Oates KK, Goldstein AL: Thymosins: Hormones of the thymus gland. Trends Pharmacol Sci 5:347–352, 1984.

46. Hall NR, McGillis JP, Spangelo BL, Goldstein AL: Evidence that thymosine and other biological response modifiers can function as neuroactive immunotransmitters. J Immunol 135(Suppl 2):806S–811S, 1985.

47. Hall RS, O'Grady MP, Farah J Jr: Thymic hormones and immune function: Mediation via neuroendocrine circuits. In Ader R, Felten DL, Cohen N (eds): Psychoneuroimmunology (ed 2). San Diego, Academic Press, 1991, pp 515–528.

48. Milenkovic L, McCann SM: Effects of thymosin alpha-1 on pituitary hormone release. Neuroendocrinology 55:14–19, 1992.

49. Breder CD, Dinarello CD, Saper CB: Interleukin-1 immunoreactive innervation of the human hypothalamus. Science 240:321–324, 1988.

50. Lechan RM, Toni R, Clark BD, et al: Immunoreactive interleukin-1 beta localization in the rat forebrain. Brain Res 514:135–140, 1990.

51. Weiss JM, Sundar S: Effects of stress on cellular immune responses. Annu Rev Psychiatry 11:145–180, 1992.

52. Felton DL, Felton SY, Carlson SL, et al: Noradrenergic and peptidergic innervation of lymphoid tissue. J Immunol 135:755s–765s, 1985.

53. Irwin MR, Hauger RL, Jones L, et al: Sympathetic nervous system mediates central corticotropin-releasing factor induced suppression of natural killer cytotoxicity. J Pharmacol Exp Ther 255:101–197, 1990.

54. Felten SY, Felten DL: Innervation of lymphoid tissue. In Ader R, Felten DL, Cohen N (eds): Psychoneuroendocrinology (ed 2). San Diego, Academic Press, 1991, pp 27–61.

55. Madden KS, Livnat S: Catecholamine action and immunologic reactivity. In Ader R, Felten DL, Cohen N (eds): Psychoneuroendocrinology (ed 2). San Diego, Academic Press, 1991, pp 283–310.

56. Roszman TL, Carlson SL: Neurotransmitters and molecular signalling in the immune response. In Ader R, Felten DL, Cohen N (eds): Psychoneuroendocrinology (ed 2). San Diego, Academic Press, 1991, pp 311–335.

57. Said S, Mutt V (eds): Vasoactive intestinal peptide and related peptides. Ann NY Acad Sci 527: 1988.

58. Reichlin S: Neuroendocrine significance of vasoactive intestinal polypeptide. Ann NY Acad Sci 527:431–449, 1988.

59. Ottoway CA: Vasoactive intestinal peptide and immune function. In Ader R, Felten DL, Cohen N (eds): Psychoneuroimmunology (ed 2). San Diego, Academic Press, 1991, pp 225–262.

60. O'Dorisio MS: Neuropeptide modulation of the immune response in gut associated lymphoid tissue. Int J Neurosci 38:189–198, 1988.

61. Sayegh MH, Khoury SJ, Hancock WW, et al: Induction of immunity and oral tolerance with polymorphic class II major histocompatibility complex allopeptides in the rat. Proc Natl Acad Sci USA 89:7762–7766, 1992.

62. Eglezos A, Andrews PV, Boyd RL, Helme RD: Modulation of the immune response by tachykinins. Immunol Cell Biol 69:285–294, 1991.

63. Payan DG, McGillis JP, Goetzl EJ: Neuroimmunology. Adv Immunol 39:299–323, 1986.

64. Payan DG: Neuropeptides and inflammation: The role of substance P. Annu Rev Med 40:341–352, 1989.

65. Scicchitano R, Biennenstock J, Stanisz AM: In vivo immunomodulation by the neuropeptide substance P. Immunology 63:735–735, 1988.

66. Rameshwar P, Gascon P, Ganea D: Immunoregulatory effects of neuropeptides: Stimulation of interleukin-2 production by substance P. J Neuroimmunol 37:65–74, 1992.

67. Eglezos A, Andrews PV, Boyd RL, Helme RD: Modulation of the immune response by tachykinins. Immunol Cell Biol 69:285–294, 1991.

68. Kidds BL, Mapp PI, Gibson SJ, et al: A neurogenic mechanism for symmetrical arthritis. Lancet 2:1128–1130, 1989.

69. Lotz M, Carson DA, Vaughan JH: Substance P activation of rheumatoid synoviocytes: Neural pathway in pathogenesis of arthritis. Science 235:893–895, 1987.

70. Smith EM, Meyer WJ, Blalock JED: Virus-induced corticosterone in hypophysectomized mice: A possible lymphoid adrenal axis. Science 218:1311–1312, 1982.

71. Dunn AJ, Powell ML, Moreshead WV, et al: Effects of Newcastle disease virus administration to mice on the metabolism of cerebral biogenic amines, plasma corticosterone and lymphocyte proliferation. Brain Behav Immun 1:216–230, 1987.

72. Olsen NJ, Nicholson WE, DeBold CR, Orth DN: Lymphocyte-derived adrenocorticotropin is insufficient to stimulate adrenal steroidogenesis in hypophysectomized rats. Endocrinology 130:2113–2119, 1992.

73. Smith EM, Galin FS, LeBoef RD, et al: Nucleotide and amino acid sequence of lymphocyte-derived corticotropin: Endotoxin induction of a truncated peptide. Proc Natl Acad Sci USA 87:1057–1060, 1990.

74. Galin FS, LeBoeuf RD, Blalock JE: Corticotropin-releasing factor upregulates expression of two truncated pro-opiomelanocortin transcripts in murine lymphocytes. J Neuroimmunol 31:51–58, 1991.

75. Oates EL, Allaway GP, Armstrong GR, et al: Human lymphocytes produce pro-opiomelanocortin gene-related transcripts: Effects of lymphotropic viruses. J Biol Chem 263:10041–10044, 1988.

76. Johnson EW, Blalock JE, Smith EM: ACTH receptor-mediated induction of leukocyte cyclic AMP. Biochem Biophys Res Commun 157:1205–1211, 1988.
77. Brooks KH: Adrenocorticotropin (ACTH) functions as a late-acting B cell growth factor and synergizes with interleukin 5. J Mol Cell Immunol 4:327–325, 1990.
78. McGlone JJ, Lumpkin EA, Normal RL: Adrenocorticotropin stimulates natural killer cell activity. Endocrinology 129:1653–1658, 1991.
79. Laue L, Lotze MT, Chrousos GP, et al: Effect of chronic treatment with the glucocorticoid antagonist RU 486 in man: Toxicity, immunological, and hormonal aspects. J Clin Endocrinol Metab 71:1474–1480, 1990.
80. Smith EM, Brosnan P, Meyer WJ, et al: An ACTH receptor on human mononuclear leukocytes: Relation to adrenal ACTH-receptor activity. N Engl J Med 317:1266–1269, 1987.
81. Moore PS, Couch RM, Perry YS, et al: Allgrove syndrome: An autosomal recessive syndrome of ACTH insensitivity, achalasia and alacrima. Clin Endocrinol 34:107–114, 1991.
82. Dupont AGG, Somers AC, Van Steviteghem AC, et al: Ectopic adrenocorticotropin production: Disappearance after removal of inflammatory tissue. J Clin Endocrinol Metab 58:654–658, 1984.
82a. Sharp B, Linner K: Editorial: What do we know about the expression of proopiomelanocortin transcripts and related peptides in lymphoid tissue? Endocrinology 133:1921A–1921B, 1993.
82b. van Woudenberg AD, Metzelaar MJ, van der Kleij AAM, et al: Analysis of proopiomelanocortin (POMC) messenger ribonucleic acid and POMC-derived peptides in human peripheral blood mononuclear cells: No evidence for a lymphocyte-derived POMC system. Endocrinology 133:1922–1933, 1993.
83. Johnson HM, Smith EM, Torres BA, Blalock JE: Regulation of the in vitro antibody response by neuroendocrine hormones. Proc Natl Acad Sci USA 79:4171–4174, 1982.
84. Carr DJ, Radulescu RT, deCosta BR, et al: Differential effect of opioids on immunoglobulin production by lymphocytes isolated from Peyer's patches and spleen. Life Sci 47:1059–1069, 1990.
85. Heagy W, Laurance M, Cohen E, Finberg R: Neurohormones regulate T cell function. J Exp Med 171:1625–1633, 1990.
86. Heijnen CJ, Kavelaars A, Ballieux RE: Beta-endorphins: Cytokine and neuropeptide. Immunol Rev 119:41–63, 1991.
87. O'Donohue TL, Dorsa DM: The opiomelanotropinergic neuronal and endocrine systems. Peptides 3:353–395, 1982.
88. Joseph SA: Immunoreactive adrenocorticotropin in rat brain: A neuroanatomical study using antiserum generated against synthetic ACTH. Am J Anat 158:533–548, 1980.
89. Tatro JB: Melanotropin receptors in the brain are differentially distributed and recognize both corticotropin and alpha-melanocyte stimulating hormone. Brain Res 536:124–132, 1990.
90. Fukata J, Usui T, Naitoh Y, et al: Effects of recombinant human interleukin-1a, 1b, 2, and 6 on ACTH synthesis and release in the mouse pituitary tumour line AtT-20. J Endocrinol 122:33–39, 1988.
91. Lipton JM: Modulation of host defense by neuropeptide alpha-MSH. Yale J Biol Med 63:173–182, 1990.
92. Hiltz ME, Catania A, Lipton JM: Alpha-MSH peptides inhibit acute inflammation induced in mice by rIL-1 beta, rIL-6, rTNF-alpha and endogenous pyrogen but not that caused by LTB4, PAF and rIL-8. Cytokine 4:320–328, 1992.
93. Cannon JG, Tatro JB, Reichlin S, Dinarello CA: Melanocyte stimulating hormone inhibits immunostimulatory and inflammatory actions of interleukin 1. J Immunol 137:2232–2236, 1986.
94. Johansson O, Sandberg G: Effect of the neuropeptides beta-MSH, neurotensin, NPY, PHI, somatostatin and substance P on proliferation of lymphocytes in vitro. Acta Physiol Scand 137:107–111, 1989.
95. Mountjoy KG, Robbins LS, Mortrud MT, Cone RD: The cloning of a family of genes that encode the melanocortin receptors. Science 257:1248–1251, 1992.
96. Duvaux-Miret O, Stefano GB, Smith EM, et al: Immunosuppression in the definitive and intermediate hosts of the human parasite Schistosoma mansoni by release of immunoreactive neuropeptides Proc Natl Acad Sci USA 89:778–781, 1992.
97. Karalis K, Sano H, Redwine J, et al: Autocrine or paracrine inflammatory actions of corticotropin-releasing hormone in vivo. Science 18:421–422, 1991.
98. Webster EL, De Souza EB: Corticotropin-releasing factor receptors in mouse spleen: Identification, autoradiographic localization, and regulation by divalent cations and guanine nucleotides. Endocrinology 122:609–617, 1988.
99. Kavelaars A, Ballieux RE, Heijnen CJ: The role of interleukin-1 in the CRF- and AVP-induced secretion of ir-β-endorphin by human peripheral blood mononuclear cells. J Immunol 142:2338–2342, 1989.
100. Crofford LJ, Sano H, Karalis K, et al: Local secretion of corticotropin-releasing hormone in the joints of Lewis rats with inflammatory arthritis. J Clin Invest 90:2555–2564, 1992.
101. Pellegrini I, Lebrun J-J, Ali S, Kelly PA: Expression of prolactin and its receptor in human lymphoid cells. Mol Endocrinol 6:1023–1031, 1992.
102. Russell DH: New aspects of prolactin and immunity: A lymphocyte-derived prolactin-like product and nuclear protein kinase C activation. Trends Pharmacol Sci 10:40–44, 1989.
103. Clevenger CV, Sillman AL, Hanley-Hyde J, Prystowsky MB: Requirement for prolactin during cell cycle regulated gene expression in cloned T-lymphocytes. Endocrinology 130:3216–3222, 1992.
104. Kelley KW, Arkins S, Li YM: Growth hormone, prolactin, and insulin-like growth factors: New jobs for old players. Brain Behav Immun 6:317–326, 1992.
105. Nicoll CS. Prolactin. In Greep RO, Astwood EB (eds): The Pituitary. Philadelphia, American Physiological Society, 1978.
106. Berczi I, Nagy E, de Toledo SM, et al: Pituitary hormones regulate c-myc and DNA synthesis in lymphoid tissue. J Immunol 146:2201–2206, 1991.
107. Russell DH, Kibler R, Martrisian L, et al: Prolactin receptors in human T and B lymphocytes: Antagonism of prolactin binding by cyclosporin. J Immunol 134:3027–3031, 1985.
108. Kelly PA, Djiane J, Postel-Vinay M-C, Edery M: The prolactin/growth hormone receptor family. Endocr Rev 12:235–251, 1991.
109. Sabharwal P, Glaser R, Lafusae W, et al: Prolactin synthesized and secreted by human peripheral blood mononuclear cells: An autocrine growth factor for lymphoproliferation. Proc Natl Acad Sci USA 89:7713–7716, 1992.
110. Hartmann DP, Holaday JW, Bernton EW: Inhibition of lymphocyte proliferation by antibodies to prolactin. FASEB J 3:2194–2202, 1989.
111. Bernton EW, Bryant HU, Holaday JW: Prolactin and immune function. In Ader R, Felten DL, Cohen N (eds): Psychoneuroimmunology. San Diego, Academic Press, 1991, pp 403–428.
112. O'Neal KD, Schwarz LA, Yu-Lee L: Prolactin receptor gene expression in lymphoid cells. Mol Cell Endocrinol 82:127–135, 1991.
113. Clevenger CV, Altmann SW, Prystowsky MB: Requirement of nuclear prolactin for interleukin-2–stimulated proliferation of T lymphocytes. Science 253:77–79, 1991.
114. Too CK, Murphy PR, Friesen HG: G-proteins modulate prolactin- and interleukin-2–stimulated mitogenesis in rat NB2 lymphoma cells. Endocrinology 124:2185–2192, 1989.
115. Berczi I, Nagy E, Asa SL, Kovacs K: The influence of pituitary hormones on adjuvant arthritis. Arthritis Rheum 20:18–22, 1977.
116. McMurray R, Keisler D, Kanuckel K, et al: Prolactin influences autoimmune disease activity in the female B/W mouse. J Immunol 147:3780–3787, 1991.
117. Riskind PN, Massacesi L, Doolittle TH, Hauser SL: The role of prolactin in autoimmune demyelination: Depression of experimental allergic encephalomyelitis by bromocriptine. Ann Neurol 29:542–547, 1991.
118. Palestine AG, Muellenberg-Coulombre CG, Kim MK, et al: Bromocriptine and low dose cyclosporine in the treatment of experimental autoimmune uveitis in the rat. J Clin Invest 79:1078–1081, 1987.
119. Ferrari C, Boghen M, Paracchi A, et al: Thyroid autoimmunity in hyperprolactinaemic disorders. Acta Endocrinol 104:35–41, 1983.
120. Ishibashi M, Yamaji T: Immunological abnormalities associated with hyperprolactinemia. Program, The Endocrine Society, 71st Ann Meeting, June 21–24, 1989, p 407.
121. Thorner MO: Prolactin: Clinical physiology and the significance and management of hyperprolactinaemia. In Martini L, Besser GM (eds): Clinical Neuroendocrinology. London, Academic Press, 1977, pp 319–361.
122. Weber G, Frey H: Zur behandlung der Psoriasis arthropathica mit Bromocriptin. Z Hautkr 61:1456–1466, 1986.
123. Hedner LP, Bynke G: Endogenous iridocyclitis relieved during treatment with bromocriptine. Am J Ophthalmol 100:618–619, 1985.
124. Palestine AG, Nussenblatt RB, Gelato M: Therapy for human autoimmune uveitis with low-dose cyclosporine plus bromocriptine. Transplant Proc 20(Suppl 4):131–135, 1988.
125. Russell DH, Martrisian L, Kibler R, et al: Prolactin receptors in human lymphocytes and their modulation by cyclosporine. Biochem Biophys Res Commun 121:899–906, 1984.
126. Russell DH, Larson DF, Cardon SB, Copeland JG: Cyclosporine inhibits prolactin induction of ornithine decarboxylase in rat tissues. Mol Cell Endocrinol 35:159–166, 1984.

127. Russell DH, Kibler R, Martrisian L, et al: Prolactin receptors in human T and B lymphocytes: Antagonism of prolactin binding by cyclosporine. J Immunol 134:3027–3031, 1985.

128. Flanagan WM, Corthesy B, Bram RJ, Crabtree GR: Nuclear association of a T-cell transcription factor blocked by FK-506 and cyclosporin A. Nature 352:803–807, 1991.

129. Larson DF, Copeland JG, Russell DH: Prolactin predicts cardiac allograft rejection in cyclosporine immunosuppressed patients (Letter). Lancet 2(8445):53, 1985

130. Carrier M, Emery RW, Wild-Mobley J, et al: Prolactin as a marker of rejection in human heart transplantation. Transplant Proc 19:3442–3443, 1987.

131. Carrier M, Wild J, Pelletier LC, Copeland JG: Bromocriptine as an adjuvant to cyclosporine immunosuppression after heart transplantation. Ann Thorac Surg 49:129–132, 1990.

132. Wilner ML, Ettenger RB, Koyle MA, Rosenthal JT: The effect of hypoprolactinemia alone and in combination with cyclosporine on allograft rejection. Transplantation 49:264–267, 1990.

133. Weigent DA, Blalock JE: Growth hormone and the immune system. Prog Neuroendocrinimmunol 3:231–241, 1990.

134. Kelly KW: Growth hormone, lymphocytes and macrophages. Biochem Pharmacol 38:705–713, 1989.

135. Kelly KW: Growth hormone in immunobiology. In Ader R, Felten DL, Cohen N (eds): Psychoneuroimmunology (ed 2). New York, Academic Press, 1991, pp 377–402.

136. Nagy E, Berczi I: Immunedeficiency in hypophysectomized rats. Acta Endocrinol (Copenh) 89:530–537, 1978.

137. Spadoni GL, Cianfarani S, Baldini AA, et al: Laron dwarfism: Cellular unresponsiveness to GH demonstrated on cultured lymphocytes by a cytochemical method. Horm Metab Res 20:450–452, 1988.

138. Rapaport R, Peterson B, Skuza KA, et al: Immune functions during treatment of growth hormone-deficient children with biosynthetic human growth hormone. Clin Pediatr 30:22–27, 1991.

139. Mocchegiani E, Paolucci P, Balsamo A, et al: Influence of growth hormone on thymic endocrine activity in humans. Horm Res 33:248–255, 1990.

140. Bozzola M, Valtorta A, Moretta A, et al: Modulating effect of growth hormone (GH) on PHA-induced lymphocyte proliferation. Thymus 123:157–165, 1988–89.

141. Crist DM, Kraner JC: Supplemental growth hormone increases the tumor cytotoxic activity of natural killer cells in healthy adults with normal growth hormone secretion. Metab Clin Exp 39:1320–1324, 1990.

142. Suzuki K, Suzuki S, Saito Y, et al: Human growth hormone–stimulated growth of human cultured lymphocytes (Im-9) and its inhibition by phorbol diesters through down-regulation of the hormone receptors: Possible involvement of phosphorylation of a 55,000 molecular weight protein associated with the receptor in the down-regulation. J Biol Chem 265:11320–11327, 1990.

143. Trivedi B, Daughaday WH: Release of growth hormone binding protein from IM-9 lymphocytes by endopeptidase is dependent on sulfhydryl group inactivation. Endocrinology 123:2201–2206, 1988.

144. Merchav S, Tatarsky I, Hochberg Z: Enhancement of erythropoiesis in vitro by human growth hormone is mediated by insulin-like growth factor I. Br J Haematol 70:267–271, 1988.

145. Rom WN, Basset P, Fells GA, et al: Alveolar macrophages release an insulin-like growth factor I-type molecule. J Clin Invest 82:1685–1693, 1988.

146. Landreth KS, Narayanan R, Dorshkind K: Insulin-like growth factor-I regulates pro-B cell differentiation. Blood 80:1207–1212, 1992.

147. Edwards III CK, Ghiasuddin SM, Schepper JM, et al: A newly defined property of somatotropin: Priming of macrophages for production of superoxide anion. Science 239:769–771, 1988.

148. Schimpff RM, Repellin AM: In vitro effect of human growth hormone on lymphocyte transformation and lymphocyte growth factors secretion. Acta Endocrinol (Copenh) 120:745–752, 1989.

149. Weigent DA, Baxter JB, Wear WE, et al: Production of immunoreactive growth hormone by mononuclear leukocytes. FASEB J 2:2812–2818, 1988.

150. Hattori N, Shimatsu A, Sugita M, et al: Immunoreactive growth hormone (GH) secretion by human lymphocytes: Augmented release by exogenous GH. Biochem Biophys Res Commun 168:386–401, 1990.

151. Weigent DA, Blalock JE, LeBoeuf RD: An antisense oligonucleotide to growth hormone messenger ribonucleic acid inhibits lymphocyte proliferation. Endocrinology 128:2053–2057, 1991.

152. Stephanou A, Knight RA, Lightman SL: Production of a growth hormone–releasing hormone-like peptide and its mRNA by human lymphocytes. Neuroendocrinology 53:628–633, 1991.

153. Pawlikowski M, Zelazowski P, Dohler KD, Stepien H: Effects of two neuropeptides: Somatoliberin (GHRH) and corticoliberin (CRF) on human lymphocyte natural killer activity. Brain Behav Immun 2:50, 1988.

154. Zelazowski P, Dohler KD, Stepien H, Pawlikowski M: Effect of growth hormone–releasing hormone on human peripheral blood leukocyte chemotaxis and migration in normal subjects. Neuroendocrinology 50:236–239, 1989.

155. Hammerman MR: Insulin-like growth factors and aging. Endocrinol. Metab Clin North Am 16:995–1011, 1987.

156. Munck A, Guyre PM: Glucocorticoids and immune function. In Ader R, Felten DL, Cohen N (eds): Psychoneuroimmunology (ed 2). New York, Academic Press, 1991, pp 447–474.

157. Selye H: Thymus and adrenals in the response of the organism to injuries and intoxications. Br J Exp Pathol 17:234–248, 1936.

158. White A, Dougherty TF: The pituitary adrenotrophic hormone control of the rate of release of serum globulins from lymphoid tissue. Endocrinology 36:207–217, 1945.

159. Hench PS, Kendall EC, Slocumb CH, Polley HF: The effect of a hormone of the adrenal cortex (17-hydroxycorticosterone: compound E) and of pituitary adrenocorticotropic hormone on rheumatoid arthritis. Mayo Clinic Proc 24:181–197, 1945.

160. Bateman A, Singh A, Kral T, Solomon S: The immune-hypothalamic-pituitary-adrenal axis. Endocr Rev 10:92–112, 1989.

161. Besedovsky HO, Del Rey A: Physiological implications of the immune-neuro-endocrine network. In Ader R, Felten DL, Cohen N (eds): Psychoneuroimmunology (ed 2). San Diego, Academic Press, 1991, pp 589–608.

162. Besedovsky J, Del Rey A, Sorkin E, et al: Immunoregulatory feedback between interleukin-1 and glucocorticoid hormones. Science 233:652–654, 1986.

163. Callewaert DM, Moudgil VK, Radcliff G, Waite R: Hormone-specific regulation of natural killer cells by cortisol: Direct inactivation of the cytotoxic function of cloned human NK cells without an effect on cellular proliferation. FEBS Lett 285:108–110, 1991.

164. Wyllie AH: Glucocorticoid-induced thymocyte apoptosis is associated with endogenous endonuclease activation. Nature 284:555–556, 1980.

165. Caron-Leslie LM, Schwartzman RA, Gaido ML, et al: Identification and characterization of glucocorticoid-regulated nuclease(s) in lymphoid cells undergoing apoptosis. J Steroid Biochem Mol Biol 640:676–671, 1991.

166. Dowd DR, MacDonald PN, Komm BS, et al: Evidence for early induction of calmodulin gene expression in lymphocytes undergoing glucocorticoid-mediated apoptosis. J Biol Chem 266:18423–18426, 1991.

167. Baughman G, Harrington MT, Campbell NF, et al: Genes newly identified as regulated by glucocorticoids in murine thymocytes. Mol Endocrinol 5:637–644, 1991.

168. Forbes IJ, Zalewski PD, Giannakis C, Cowled PA: Induction of apoptosis in chronic lymphocytic leukemia cells and its prevention by phorbol ester. Exp Cell Res 198:367–372, 1992.

169. Nieto MA, Lopez-Rivas A: IL-2 protects T lymphocytes from glucocorticoid-induced DNA fragmentation and cell death. J Immunol 143:4166–4170, 1989.

170. Masters JN, Finch CE, Sapolsky RM: Glucocorticoid endangerment does not involve deoxyribonucleic acid cleavage. Endocrinology 124:3083–3088, 1989.

171. Fernandez-Ruiz E, Rebolla N, Nieto MA, et al: IL-2 protects T cell hybrids from the cytolytic effect of glucocorticoids: Synergistic effect of IL-2 and dexamethasone in the induction of high-affinity IL-2 receptors. J Immunol 143:4146–4151, 1989.

172. Northrup JP, Crabtree GR, Mattila PS: Negative regulation of interleukin 2 transcription by the glucocorticoid receptor. J Exp Med 175:1235–1245, 1992.

173. Vacca A, Felli MP, Farina AR, et al: Glucocorticoid receptor-mediated suppression of the interleukin 2 gene expression through impairment of the cooperativity between nuclear factor of activated T cells and AP-1 enhancer elements. J Exp Med 175:637–646, 1992.

174. Yang-Yen, H-F, Chambard J-C, Sun Y-L, et al: Transcriptional interference between c-Jun and the glucocorticoid receptor: Mutual inhibition of DNA binding due to direct protein-protein interaction. Cell 62:1205–1215, 1990.

175. Lowy MT: Quantification of type I and II adrenal steroid receptors in neuronal, lymphoid and pituitary tissues. Brain Res 503:191–197, 1989.

176. Meikle AW, Dorchuck RW, Araneo BA, et al: The presence of a dehydroepiandrosterone-specific receptor binding complex in murine T cells. J Steroid Biochem Mol Biol 42:293–304, 1992.

177. Daynes RA, Dudley DJ, Araneo BA: Regulation of murine lymphokine production in vivo: II. Dehydroepiandrosterone is a natural enhancer of interleukin 2 synthesis by helper T cells. Eur J Immunol 20:793–802, 1990.
178. Blauer KL, Poth M, Rogers WM, Bernton EW: Dehydroepiandrosterone antagonizes the suppressive effects of dexamethasone on lymphocyte proliferation. Endocrinology 129:3174–3179, 1991.
179. May M, Holmes E, Rogers W, Poth M: Protection from glucocorticoid induced thymic involution by dehydroepiandrosterone. Life Sci 46:1627–1631, 1990.
180. Loria RM, Padgett DA: Mobilization of cutaneous immunity for systemic protection against infections. Ann NY Acad Sci 650:363–366, 1992.
181. Ben-Nathan D, Lachmi B, Lustig S, Feuerstein G: Protection by dehydroepiandrosterone in mice infected with viral encephalitis. Arch Virol 120:263–271, 1991.
182. Risdon G, Moore TA, Kumar V, Bennett M: Inhibition of murine natural killer cell differentiation by dehydroepiandrosterone. Blood 78:2387–2391, 1991.
183. Rom WN, Harkin T: Dehydroepiandrosterone inhibits the spontaneous release of superoxide radical by alveolar macrophages in vitro in asbestosis. Environ Res 55:145–156, 1991.
184. Risdon G, Kumar V, Bennett M: Differential effects of dehydroepiandrosterone (DHEA) on murine lymphopoiesis and myelopoiesis. Exp Hematol 19:128–131, 1991.
185. Daynes RA, Araneo BA: Contrasting effects of glucocorticoids on the capacity of T cells to produce the growth factors interleukin 2 and interleukin 4. Eur J Immunol 19:2319–2325, 1989.
186. Matsunaga A, Miller BC, Cottam GL: Dehydroepiandrosterone prevention of autoimmune disease in NZB/W F1 mice: Lack of an effect on associated immunological abnormalities. Biochim Biophys Acta 992:265–271, 1989.
187. Schwartz R, Datta SK: Autoimmunity and autoimmune disease. In Paul WE (ed): Fundamental Immunology. New York, Raven Press, 1989, pp 819–866.
188. Grossman CJ: Regulation of the immune system by sex steroids. Endocr Rev 5:435–455, 1984.
189. Grossman C: Possible underlying mechanisms of sexual dimorphism in the immune response, fact and hypothesis. J Steroid Biochem 34:241–251, 1989.
190. Styrt B, Sugarman R: Estrogens and infection. Rev Infect Dis 13:1139–1150, 1991.
191. Paavonen T, Aronen H, Pyrhonen S, et al: The effects of antiestrogen therapy on lymphocyte functions in breast cancer patients. Acta Pathol Microbiol Immunol Scand 99:163–170, 1991.
192. Baral E, Kwok S, Berczi I: Suppression of lymphocyte mitogenesis by tamoxifen. Immunopharmacology 18:57–62, 1987.
193. Legraverend C, Mode A, Wells T, et al: Hepatic steroid hydroxylating enzymes are controlled by the sexually dimorphic pattern of growth hormone secretion in normal and dwarf rats. FASEB J 6:711–718, 1992.
194. Montgomery IN, Rauch HC: Experimental allergic encephalomyelitis (EAE) in mice: Primary control of EAE susceptibility is outside the H-2 complex. J Immunol 128:421, 1982.
195. Szekeres-Bartho J, Autran B, Debre P, et al: Immunoregulatory effects of a suppressor factor from healthy pregnant women's lymphocytes after progesterone induction. Cell Immunol 122:281–294, 1989.
196. Kalman B, Olsson O, Link H, Kam-Hansen S: Estradiol potentiates poke-weed mitogen-induced B cell stimulation in multiple sclerosis and healthy subjects. Acta Neurol Scand 79:340–346, 1989.
197. Bellini T, Degani D, Matteuzzi M, Dallocchio F: Effect of beta-estradiol on calcium response to phytohaemagglutinin in human lymphocytes. Biosci Rep 10:73–78, 1990.
198. Caggiula AR, Stoney CM, Matthews KA, et al: T-lymphocyte reactivity during the menstrual cycle in women. Clin Immunol Immunopathol 56:130–134, 1990.
199. Ressel M, Kohler G, Straube W: Behavior of T-lymphocytes during the normal menstrual cycle. Zentralbl Gynakol 110:619–622, 1988.
200. Polan ML, Kuo A, Loukides J, Bottomly K: Cultured human luteal peripheral monocytes secrete increased levels of interleukin-1. J Clin Endocrinol Metab 70:480–484, 1990.
201. Cannon JG, Dinarello CA: Increased plasma interleukin-1 activity in women after ovulation. Science 227:1247–1249, 1985.
202. Muhlemann MF, MacRae KD, Smith AM, et al: Hereditary angioedema and thyroid autoimmunity. J Clin Pathol 40:518–523, 1987.
203. McCruden AB, Stimson WH: Sex hormones and immune function. In Ader R, Felten DL, Cohen N (eds): Psychoneuroimmunology (ed 2). San Diego, Academic Press, 1991, pp 475–493.
204. Parnet P, Payan DG, Kerdelhue B, Mitsuhashi M: Neuroendocrine interaction on lymphocytes: Testosterone-induced modulation of the lymphocyte substance P receptor. J Neuroimmunol 28:185–198, 1990.
205. Donaldson VH: Danazol. Am J Med 87:49N–55N, 1989.
206. Sargent IL, Redman CWG: Immunobiologic adaptations of pregnancy. In Reece EA, Hobbins JC, Mahoney MJ, Petrie RH (eds): Medicine of the Fetus and Mother. Philadelphia, JB Lippincott, 1992, pp 25–40.
207. Jacobs AL, Carson DD: Uterine epithelial cell secretion of interleukin-1a induces prostaglandin E_2 (PGE$_2$) and PGF$_{2a}$ secretion by uterine stromal cells in vitro. Endocrinology 132:300–308, 1993.
208. Barker SB: Effect of triiodothyronine on oxygen consumption of tissues not responsive to thyroxine. Proc Soc Exp Biol Med 90:109–111, 1955.
209. Tsai JS, Samuels HH: Thyroid hormone action: Demonstration of putative nuclear receptors in human lymphocytes. J Clin Endocrinol Metab 38:919–922, 1974.
210. Valdermarsson S, Ikomi-Kumm J, Monti M: Thyroid hormones and thermogenesis: A microcalorimetric study of overall cell metabolism in lymphocytes from patients with different degrees of thyroid dysfunction. Acta Endocrinol (Copenh) 123:155–160, 1990.
211. Ahlqvist J: Endocrine influences on lymphatic organs, immune responses, inflammation and autoimmunity. Acta Endocrinol (Copenh) (Suppl 206):3–136, 1976.
212. Reichlin S, Glaser RJ: Thyroid function in experimental streptococcal pneumonia in the rat. J Exp Med 107:219–236, 1958.
213. Pacini F, Nakamura H, DeGroot LJ: Effect of hypo- and hyperthyroidism on the balance between helper and suppressor T cells in rats. Acta Endocrinol (Copenh) 103:528–534, 1983.
214. Fabris N, Mocchegiani E, Mariotti S, et al: Thyroid function modulates thymic endocrine activity. J Clin Endocrinol Metab 62:474–478, 1986.
215. Mocchegiani E, Amadio L, Fabris N: Neuroendocrine-thymus interactions: I. In vitro modulation of thymic factor secretion by thyroid hormones. J Endocrinol Invest 13:139–147, 1990.
216. Provinciali M, Muzzioli M, Di Stefano G, Fabris N: Recovery of spleen cell natural killer activity by thyroid hormone treatment in old mice. Natural Immunity and Cell Growth Regulation 10:226–236, 1991.
217. Cooper DS: Treatment of thyrotoxicosis. In Braverman LE, Utiger RD (eds): Werner and Ingbar's The Thyroid (ed 6). Philadelphia, JB Lippincott, 1991, pp 887–918.
218. Mariotti S, Caturegli P, Barbesino G, et al: Circulating soluble interleukin 2 receptor concentration is increased in both immunogenic and nonimmunogenic hyperthyroidism. J Endocrinol Invest 14:777–781, 1991.
219. Weryha G, Gobert B, Leclerc J, et al: Dynamic changes in soluble interleukin-2 receptor levels during treatment of Graves' disease. Horm Res 35:8–12, 1991.
220. Kennedy RL, Jones TH: Cytokines in endocrinology: Their roles in health and disease. J Endocrinol 129:167–178, 1991.
221. Denicoff KD, Rubinow DR, Papa MZ, et al: The neuropsychiatric effects of treatment with interleukin-2 and lymphokine-activated killer cells. Ann Intern Med 107:293–300, 1987.
222. Sternberg EM, Young WS III, Bernardini R, et al: A central nervous system defect in biosynthesis of corticotropin-releasing hormone is associated with susceptibility to cell wall-induced arthritis in Lewis rats. Proc Natl Acad Sci USA 86:4771–4775, 1989.
223. Kakucska I, Qi Y, Clark BD, Lechan RM: Endotoxin induced corticotropin-releasing hormone (CRH) gene expression in the hypothalamic paraventricular nucleus is mediated by central interleukin-1. Endocrinology 133:815–821, 1993.
224. Sapolsky R, Rivier C, Yamamoto G, et al: Interleukin-1 stimulates the secretion of hypothalamic corticotropin-releasing factor. Science 238:522–524, 1987.
225. Tsagarakis S, Gillies G, Rees L, et al: Interleukin-1 directly stimulates the release of corticotrophin-releasing factor from rat hypothalamus. Neuroendocrinology 49:98–101, 1989.
226. Berkenbosch F, Van Oers J, Del Rey A, et al: Corticotropin-releasing factor–producing neurons in the rat activated by interleukin-1. Science 238:524–526, 1987.
227. Bernton EW, Beach JE, Holaday JW, et al: Release of multiple hormones by a direct action of interleukin-1 on pituitary cells. Science 238:522–524, 1987.
228. Fukata J, Isui T, Naitoh Y, et al: Effect of recombinant human interleukin 1a, b, 2 and 6 on ACTH synthesis and release in the mouse pituitary tumor cell line AtT-20. J Endocrinol 122:33–39, 1989.
229. Navarra P, Tsagarikis S, Faria MS, et al: Interleukins-1 and -6 stimu-

late the release of corticotropin-releasing hormone-41 from rat hypothalamus in vitro via the eiconanoid cyclooxygenase pathway. Endocrinology 128:37–44, 1990.

230. Rivier C: Role of endotoxin and interleukin-1 in modulating ACTH, LH and sex steroid secretion. *In* Porter JC, Jezov A (eds): Circulating Regulatory Factors and Neuroendocrine Function. New York, Plenum Press, 1990, pp 295–301.

231. Smith EM: Hormonal activities of cytokines. *In* Blalock JE (ed): Neuroimmunoendocrinology. Basel, Karger, 1992, pp 154–169.

232. Cambronero JC, Rivas FJ, Borrell J, Guaza C: Interleukin-2 induces corticotropin-releasing hormone release from superfused rat hypothalami: Influence of glucocorticoids. Endocrinology 131:677–683, 1992.

233. Naitoh Y, Fukata J, Tominga T, et al: Interleukin-6 stimulates the secretion of adrenocorticotropic hormone in conscious, freely moving rats. Biochem Biophys Res Commun 155:1459–1463, 1988.

234. Sharp BM, Matta SG, Peterson PK, et al: Tumor necrosis factor-alpha is a potent ACTH secretogogue: Comparison to interleukin-1 beta. Endocrinology 124:3131–3133, 1989.

235. Loppnow H, Libby P: Proliferating or interleukin-1 activated human vascular smooth muscle cells secrete copious interleukin 6. J Clin Invest 85:731–738, 1990.

236. Theoharides TC: Mast cells: The immune gate to the brain. Life Sci 46:607–617, 1990.

237. Farrar WL, Kilian PL, Ruff MR, et al: Visualization and characterization of interleukin-1 receptors in brain. J Immunol 139:459–463, 1987.

238. Buxbaum JD, Oishi M, Chen HI, et al: Cholinergic agonists and interleukin-1 regulate processing and secretion of the Alzheimer beta/A4 amyloid protein precursor. Proc Natl Acad Sci USA 89:10075–10078, 1992.

239. Carman-Krzan M, Vige X, Wise BC: Regulation by interleukin-1 of nerve growth factor secretion and nerve growth factor mRNA expression in rat primary astroglial cultures. J Neurochem 56:636–643, 1991.

240. Sternberg EM: The stress response and the regulation of inflammatory disease. Ann Intern Med 117:854–866, 1992.

241. Chikanza IC, Petrou P, Kingsley G, et al: Defective hypothalamic response to immune and inflammatory stimuli in patients with rheumatoid arthritis. Arthritis Rheum 35:1281–1288, 1992.

242. Swanson LW, Sawchenko PE, Rivier J, et al: Organization of ovine corticotropin-releasing factor immunoreactive cells and fibers in the rat brain: An immunohistochemical study. Neuroendocrinology 36:165–186, 1983.

243. Potter E, Behan DP, Linton EA, et al: The central distribution of a corticotropin-releasing factor (CRF)–binding protein predicts multiple sites and modes of interaction with CRF. Proc Natl Acad Sci USA 89:4192–4196, 1992.

244. Wartofsky L, Burman KD: Alterations in thyroid function in patients with systemic illness: The ''sick euthyroid syndrome.'' Endocr Rev 3:167–217, 1982.

245. Arem R, Wiener GJ, Kaplan SG, et al: Reduced tissue thyroid hormone in fatal illness. Metabolism 42:1102–1108, 1993.

246. Kennedy RL, Jones TH: Cytokines in endocrinology: Their roles in health and disease. J Endocrinol 129:167–178, 1991.

247. Dubois J-M, Dayer J-M, Siegrist-Kaiser CA, Burger AG: Human recombinant interleukin-1b decreases plasma thyroid hormone and thyroid-stimulating hormone levels in rats. Endocrinology 123:2175–2181, 1988.

248. Pang XP, Hershman JM, Mirell CJ, Pekary AF: Impairment of hypothalamic-pituitary-thyroid function in rats treated with human recombinant tumor necrosis factor-alpha (cachectin). Endocrinology 125:76–84, 1989.

249. Hermus RM, Sweep CGJ, van der Meer MJM, et al: Continuous infusion of interleukin-1b induces a nonthyroidal illness syndrome in the rat. Endocrinology 131:2139–2146, 1992.

250. Van der Poll T, Romijn JA, Wiersinga WM, Saujerwein HP: Tumor necrosis factor: A putative mediator of the sick euthyroid syndrome in man. J Clin Endocrinol Metab 71:1567–1572, 1990.

251. Kakucska I, Romero LI, Clark BD, et al: Suppression of thyrotropin-releasing hormone gene expression by interleukin-1 beta (IL-1b) in the rat: Implications for nonthyroidal illness. Neuroendocrinology, in press.

252. Scarborough DE, Lee SL, Dinarello CA, Reichlin S: Interleukin-1 stimulates somatostatin biosynthesis in primary cultures of fetal rat brain. Endocrinology 124:549–551, 1989; erratum 124:2022, 1989.

253. Williams GR, Franklyn JA, Neuberger JM, Sheppard MC: Thyroid hormone receptor expression in the ''sick euthyroid'' syndrome. Lancet 2:1477–1481, 1989.

254. Gardner DF, Kaplan MM, Stanley CA, Utiger RD: Effect of tri-iodothyronine replacement on the metabolic and pituitary responses to starvation. N Engl J Med 300:579–584, 1979.

255. Brent GA, Hershman JM: Thyroxine therapy in patients with severe nonthyroidal illnesses and low serum thyroxine concentration. J Clin Endocrinol Metab 63:1–8, 1986.

256. Shalts E, Feng Y-J, Ferin M: Vasopressin mediates the interleukin-1a–induced decrease in luteinizing hormone secretion in the ovariectomized rhesus monkey. Endocrinology 131:153–158, 1991.

257. Kasting NW, Martin JB: Altered release of growth hormone and thyrotropin-induced by endotoxin in the rat. Am J Physiol 243:E332–E337, 1982.

257a. Payne LC, Obal F Jr, Opp MR, Krueger JM: Stimulation and inhibition of growth hormone secretion by Interleukin-1b: The involvement of growth hormone-releasing hormone. Neuroendocrinology 56:119–123, 1992.

258. Scarborough D, Simar MR, Lee SL: Interleukin-1b stimulates somatostatin synthesis in astrocyte subcultures derived from neonatal brain. Program, 73rd Annual Meeting of the Endocrine Society, Washington, DC, June 19–22, 1991, p 350.

259. Schwartz K, Cherny R: Intercellular communication within the anterior pituitary influencing the secretion of hypophysial hormones. Endocr Rev 13:453–475, 1992.

260. Vankelecom H, Carmeliet P, Van Damme J, et al: Production of interleukin-6 by folliculostellate cells of the anterior pituitary gland in a histiotypic cell aggregate culture system. Neuroendocrinology 49:102–106, 1989.

261. Allaerts W, Carmeliet P, Denef C: New perspectives in the function of pituitary folliculostellate cells. Mol Cell Endocrinol 71:73–81, 1990.

262. Spangelo BL, MacLeod RM, Isakson PC: Production of interleukin-6 by anterior pituitary cells in vitro. Endocrinology 126:582–586, 1990.

263. Spangelo BL, Judd AM, Isakson PC, MacLeod RM: Interleukin-1 stimulates interleukin-6 release from rat anterior pituitary cells in vitro. Endocrinology 128:2685–2692, 1991.

264. Romero LI, Lechan RM, Clark BD, et al: IL-1 receptor antagonist inhibits hIL-1 beta but not bacterial lipopolysaccharide (LPS) stimulated IL-6 secretion by rat anterior pituitary cells. Program, 73rd Annual Meeting of the Endocrine Society, Washington, DC, 1991, p 150.

265. Ishikawa H, Nogami H, Shirasawa N: Novel clonal strains from rat anterior pituitary producing S-100 protein. Nature 303:711–713, 1983.

266. Gospodarowicz D, Lau K: Pituitary follicular cells secrete both vascular endothelial growth factor and follistatin. Biochem Biophys Res Commun 165:292–298, 1989.

267. Schettini G: Interleukin 1 in the neuroendocrine system: From gene to function. Prog Neuroendocrinimmunol 3:157–166, 1990.

268. Koibayashi H, Fukata J, Tominaga T, et al: Regulation of interleukin-1 receptors on AtT-20 mouse pituitary tumour cells. FEBS Lett 298:100–104, 1992.

269. Romero LI, Lechan RM, Mancilla-Ramirez J, et al: Effect of human interleukin-1 receptor antagonist (IL-1Ra) on interleukin-1 and bacterial endotoxin-induced IL-6 secretion by rat anterior pituitary cells. Endocrinology (submitted).

270. Nash AD, Brandon MR, Bello PA: Effects of tumor necrosis factor-alpha on growth hormone and interleukin-6 mRNA in ovine pituitary cells. Mol Cell Endocrinol 84:1231–1237, 1992.

271. Arzt E, Buric R, Stelzer G, et al: Interleukin involvement in anterior pituitary cell growth regulation: Effects of IL-2 and IL-6. Endocrinology 132:459–467, 1993.

272. Koenig JI, Snow K, Clark BD, et al: Intrinsic pituitary interleukin 1b is induced by bacterial lipopolysaccharide. Endocrinology 126:3053–3058, 1990.

272a. Bernhagen J, Calandra T, Mitchell RA, et al: MIF is a pituitary-derived cytokine that potentiates lethal endotoxaemia. Nature 365:756–759, 1993.

273. Adashi EY: The potential relevance of cytokines to ovarian physiology: The emerging role of resident ovarian cells of the white blood series. Endocr Rev 11:454–464, 1990.

274. Judd AM, MacLeod RM: The regulation of interleukin 6 and tumor necrosis factor release from primary cultures of ovarian cells. Prog Neuroendocrinimmunol 5:245–255, 1992.

275. Sancho-Tello M, Perez-Roger I, Imakawa K, et al: Expression of tumor necrosis factor-a in the rat ovary. Endocrinology 130:1359, 1992.

276. Hurwitz A, Ricciarelli E, Botero L, et al: Endocrine and autocrine-mediated regulation of rat ovarian (theca-interstitial) interleukin-1b gene expression: Gonadotropin-dependent preovulatory acquisition. Endocrinology 129:3427–3429, 1991.

277. Hughes FM Jr, Fong Y-Y, Gorospe WC: Interleukin-6 stimulates apoptosis in rat granulosa cells: Development and utilization of an in vitro model. Program, 74th Annual Meeting of the Endocrine Society, Washington, DC, 1992, p 28.

278. Adashi EY: Cytokine-mediated regulation of ovarian functions: Encounters of a third kind. Endocrinology 124:2043–2045, 1989.

279. Kokia E, Hurwitz A, Ricciarelli E, et al: Interleukin-1 stimulates ovarian prostaglandin biosynthesis: Evidence for heterologous contact-independent cell-cell interaction. Endocrinology 130:3095–3097, 1992.

280. Griffin JE, Wilson JD: Disorders of the testes and the male reproductive tract. *In* Wilson JD, Foster DW (eds): Williams' Textbook of Endocrinology (ed 8). Philadelphia, WB Saunders Co, 1992, pp 799–852.

281. Sun X-R, Hedger MP, Risbridger GP: The effect of testicular macrophages and interleukin-1 on testosterone production by purified adult rat Leydig cells cultured under in vitro maintenance conditions. Endocrinology 132:186–192, 1993.

282. Wang D, Nagpal ML, Calkins JH, et al: Interleukin-1b induces interleukin-1a messenger ribonucleic acid expression in primary cultures of Leydig cells. Endocrinology 129:2862–2866, 1991.

283. Syed V, Gerard N, Kaipia A, et al: Identification, ontogeny, and regulation of an interleukin-6–like factor in the rat seminiferous tubule. Endocrinology 132:293–299, 1993.

284. Calkins JH, Sigel MM, Nankin HR, Lin T: Interleukin-1 inhibits Leydig cell steroidogenesis in primary culture. Endocrinology 123:1605–1610, 1988.

285. Calkins JH, Guo H, Sigel MM, Lin T: Differential effects of recombinant IL-1a and b on Leydig cell function. Biochem Biophys Res Commun 167:548–553, 1990.

286. Fauser BCJM, Galway AB, Hsueh AJW: Inhibitory actions of interleukin-1b on steroidogenesis in primary cultures of neonatal rat testicular cells. Acta Endocrinol (Copenh) 120:401–408, 1989.

287. Mauduit C, Hartmann DJ, Chauvin MA, et al: Tumor necrosis factor-α inhibits gonadotropin action in cultured porcine Leydig cells: Site(s) of action. Endocrinology 129:2933–2940, 1991.

288. Warren DW, Pasupuleti V, Lu Y, et al: Tumor necrosis factor and interleukin-1 stimulate testosterone secretion in adult male rat Leydig cells in vitro. J Androl 11:353–360, 1990.

289. Argiles JM, Lopez-Soriano J, Ortiz MA, et al: Interleukin-1 and beta-cell function: More than one second messenger? Endocr Rev 13:515–524, 1992.

290. Corbett JA, Lancaster JR Jr, Sweetland MA, McDaniel ML: Interleukin-1 beta–induced formation of EPR-detectable iron-nitrosyl complexes in islets of Langerhans: Role of nitric oxide in interleukin-1 beta–induced inhibition of insulin secretion. J Biol Chem 266:21351–21354, 1991.

291. Eizirik DL, Tracey DE, Bendtzen K, Sandler S: An interleukin-1 receptor antagonist protein protects insulin-producing beta cells against suppressive effects of interleukin-1b. Diabetologia 34:445–448, 1991.

292. Mine M, Tramontano D, Chinn WW, Ingbar SH: Interleukin-1 stimulates thyroid cell growth and increases the concentration of the c-*myc* protooncogene mRNA in thyroid follicular cells in culture. Endocrinology 120:1212–1214, 1987.

293. Ader R, Cohen NA: The influence of conditioning on immune responses. *In* Ader R, Felten DL, Cohen N (eds): Psychoneuroimmunology (ed 2). San Diego, Academic Press, 1991, pp 611–646.

294. Kiecolt-Glaser JK, Glaser R: Stress and function in humans. *In* Ader R, Felten DL, Cohen N (eds): Psychoneuroimmunology (ed 2). San Diego, Academic Press, 1991, pp 847–868.

159

Immunological Mechanisms Causing Autoimmune Endocrine Disease

KEVAN C. HEROLD
JOSÉ QUINTANS

Diseases of the endocrine organs are frequently caused by immune mechanisms. Any of the endocrine glands can be the focus of an autoimmune attack. The clinical manifestations of these ailments are diverse, ranging from the destruction of an endocrine organ (e.g., Hashimoto's disease or insulin-dependent diabetes mellitus) to overstimulation of the endocrine gland and hypersecretion of hormones (e.g., Graves' disease) (Table 159–1).

The development of endocrine disease by immunological mechanisms represents a failure to develop or maintain tolerance to self antigens. In most instances, the initiators of the immune response that results in disease have not been identified. Of those antigens which have been described as targets of autoimmunity, most are cellular components that are constitutively expressed (e.g., thyroid peroxidase,[1] glutamic acid decarboxylase,[2, 3] insulin[4]). Thus recent interest has focused on understanding how tolerance toward self proteins is established and maintained by the immune system and what kinds of breakdowns lead to endocrine diseases. In this chapter we will discuss antigen presentation, the acquisition and maintenance of tolerance toward self proteins in T and B lymphocytes, and what events may result in the breakdown in self tolerance and autoimmune disease.

To understand the pathophysiology of autoimmune disease requires an appreciation of how the immune system makes the operational distinction between self and nonself. Immune recognition is carried out by clonally distributed receptors of high specificity with a level of discrimination that precludes any fundamental distinctions between self and nonself on the basis of receptor design. As a result, the immune repertoire cannot predict the structure of either self or nonself and is generated randomly to anticipate all possible antigenic contingencies by including receptors for both self and nonself.[5] Self/nonself discrimina-

TABLE 159–1. ENDOCRINE DISEASES MOST LIKELY DUE TO AUTOIMMUNE MECHANISMS

Chronic lymphocytic thyroiditis (Hashimoto's disease)
Graves' disease
Postpartum thyroiditis
Insulin-dependent diabetes mellitus
Type B insulin resistance
Autoimmune hypoglycemia (Insulin antoantibodies)
Autoimmune oophoritis
Autoimmune orchitis
Addison's disease
Autoimmune hypophysitis
Autoimmune hypoparathyroidism
Type I polyendocrine autoimmunity
  Chronic mucocutaneous candidiasis
  Hypoparathyroidism
  Addison's disease
Adrenal medullary autoantibodies
Primary (adrenal) pigmented and nodular form of Cushing's syndrome

tion is imposed on lymphocytes after they express their clonal receptors through negative selection.[6] Tolerance, like immunity, is specific and clonal. Because it is not generally possible to follow the fate of individual cells, it has until recently been difficult to track the fate of autoreactive cells. A major experimental breakthrough for studies of tolerance was the introduction of transgenic mouse models. Transgenic mice expressing genes for T- and B-cell antigen receptors of known specificity contain large numbers of lymphocytes expressing the transgene receptors. When genes for foreign antigens targeted by the receptor transgenic products are also introduced, an ideal experimental model is created to follow the fate of transgenic lymphocytes after they encounter the transgenic antigen. Because molecular biology makes it possible to control the expression of the foreign antigens in selected tissues or organs, transgenic models are invaluable to study tolerance to antigens expressed in primary lymphoid organs as well as in the periphery.[7] Obviously, there are important differences between transgenic models and humans, and the extent to which they apply to lymphocyte development in normal mice or humans remains to be established. Because it is the authors' expectation that transgenic models will prove to be highly relevant, we will discuss them in some detail.

GENERAL MECHANISMS FOR ACQUISITION OF SELF TOLERANCE

Three major mechanisms are responsible for tolerance to self: clonal deletion,[8, 9] clonal anergy,[10–12] and clonal ignorance.[13, 14] In addition to the three primary mechanisms just mentioned, models based on the secondary suppression of self reactivity have been proposed and will be briefly mentioned below. Although, in the past, immunologists have been fond of regulatory models for the maintenance of tolerance,[15] the experimental evidence that links them to the pathogenesis of autoimmunity is scanty.

The most important and efficacious mechanism for tolerance involves clonal deletion, or abortion, of self-reactive clones.[6, 8, 9, 16–24] Clonal deletion occurs predominantly in immature lymphocytes, since they first express their clonal receptors in the primary lymphoid organs and operate concomitantly with lymphopoiesis throughout life.[16, 19, 23, 24] The engagement of the antigen-specific receptors with self antigens delivers a signal that leads to programmed cell death, or apoptosis. The success of clonal deletion is dependent on the availability of self antigens at tolerogenic concentrations and the correct functioning of the lymphocyte's apoptotic machinery. Apoptosis is developmentally regulated in lymphocytes to ensure their timely death following encounters with self antigens. In general, self-reactive clones with high-affinity receptors are more likely to be clonally deleted than those expressing low affinity for self.[14, 24, 25] In practice, this means that the process of clonal deletion is leaky and does not achieve complete removal of all self-reactive clones, particularly those of low affinity. As a consequence, self-reactive lymphocyte clones exist in normal individuals, and whether they ever cause autoimmunity depends on a variety of secondary circumstances (such as availability of co-stimulatory signals, concurrent inflamma-

tory processes, cross-reactivity with infectious agents) that will be discussed below. According to this developmental scenario, it is to be expected that a fraction of individuals will display autoimmunity. Given the tremendous diversity of the immune repertoire and the frequency of encounters with infectious agents, the amazing finding is that only 10 to 15 per cent of humans suffer from autoimmune disorders.

The second major mechanism that ensures self tolerance is clonal anergy, a state of specific functional unresponsiveness.[10–12, 26–28] In contrast to clonal deletion, anergy does not lead to apoptosis but rather results in a temporary dysfunction of lymphocyte reactivity to antigens. Because of this, anergy is potentially reversible[11, 29] and a less complete method for dealing with autoreactive cells. It is also less wasteful, since it gives the immune system another chance to reinterpret antigenic signals. In general, anergy results from the delivery of antigenic signals devoid of co-stimulation (see below), resulting in the functional uncoupling of one or more of the lymphocyte activation pathways.[11, 27, 28] Anergy is essential to maintain tolerance to peripheral antigens that are not present in the primary lymphoid organs at the time of lymphocyte development.

The third mechanism, called *clonal ignorance,* has been discovered in the last decade with the introduction of transgenic mice (see below).[13, 26, 30–32] Certain self antigens appear to be displayed in ways that escape detection by the immune system under normal circumstances. Because of this, neither clonal abortion nor anergy occur, and both self-reactive lymphocytes with the functional capacity to respond and their target antigens co-exist in a state of chancy ignorance. This is a precarious state, since self-reactive lymphocyte clones operationally ignore self antigens only as long as local conditions permit (e.g., absence of co-stimulation, cytokines).

An interesting aspect of the problem of self/nonself discrimination is the issue of tolerance to the clonal receptors themselves, particularly their unique antigenic features or idiotypes (see below). Because clonal receptors are so diverse and the relative concentrations of any of them too low, the idiotopic components of clonal receptors do not induce tolerance; that is, the immune system is not tolerant of its own clonally distributed receptors, and receptor/antireceptor immunity can, in principle, be a component of immune responses.[33] This is the conceptual basis for the idiotype network discussed below. The absence of tolerance to the idiotypical components of clonal receptors also provides the theoretical framework for proposals to prevent autoimmunity via anti-idiotypic vaccines,[34] i.e., by inducing immunity against the idiotypes expressed by the clonal receptors on self-reactive lymphocytes.

OVERVIEW OF HUMAN LYMPHOCYTE SUBSETS

Humans contain a rather impressive number of immunocompetent cells, approximately 2×10^{12} lymphocytes,[35] of which there are two major types, called T and B cells because of their origin, the thymus and the bone marrow, respectively. (Actually, B lymphocytes were originally named after the bursa of Fabricius, the avian organ responsible for their differentiation.)

Most lymphocytes are found in the primary and secondary lymphoid organs. A small fraction are present in the tissues, including 2 per cent found in the blood. Approximately 35 per cent of white blood cells are small lymphocytes, amounting to 2.5×10^3 cells per microliter in adult white and black Americans. T cells constitute 70 per cent of blood lymphocytes and B cells 10 to 15 per cent.[35, 36] The remaining 10 to 15 per cent of blood lymphocytes are large cells, approximately 15 μm in diameter with a cytoplasm rich in granules. Because of these physical attributes, the cells are called large granular lymphocytes (LGL's).

The most distinctive lymphoctye markers are the antigen-specific receptors, a molecular family of cell surface receptors exclusively made by lymphocytes.[37] T cells express a receptor complex consisting of antigen-specific receptors (T-cell receptors, TCR's) associated with a multi-molecular complex called CD3, responsible for signal transduction.[38] The part of the TCR complex that binds to foreign antigen includes a heterodimer consisting of alpha/beta or gamma/delta chains (Fig. 159–1). In humans, 95 per cent of circulating T cells are alpha/beta, and the remainder express gamma/delta chains.[39]

There are two major subsets of alpha/beta T cells characterized by the expression of either CD4 or CD8 on their surfaces. CD4 and CD8 are members of the immunoglobulin superfamily of cell surface molecules.[40, 41] Their NH2 domains bind class II and class I molecules, respectively, while their intracytoplasmic tails transduce activation signals. CD4+ T cells are called *helper cells* because they help B and T cells to proliferate and differentiate into effector cells. CD4+ T cells are functionally heterogeneous, comprising subsets with characteristic patterns of lymphokine secretion and function. The most distinctive subsets are referred to as Th0, Th1, and Th2.[42–45] Th0 cells represent the less differentiated subset of helper cell that can be driven by antigen and the appropriate antigen-presenting cell (APC) to differentiate into Th1 cells, which secrete interleukin 2 (IL-2) and interferon-γ (IFN-γ), or Th2 cells, which secrete IL-4, IL-5, and IL-10.[42, 43] Th1 cells mediate classical delayed hypersensitivity reactions, whereas Th2 cells provide help for B-cell responses. CD8+ T cells are called *cytolytic* or *killer cells* in recognition of their main functional trait, the ability to kill or lyse target cells, usually cells infected with virus or in grafts of foreign tissues. They also secrete cytokines, particularly IFN-γ.[43] Unlike LGL's with natural killer cell function, many of which also express CD8 (30 to 40 per cent of LGL's are CD8+), T cells require antigenic stimulation to become cytotoxic; i.e., T-cell–mediated killing is inducible and antigen-specific, whereas natural killer cell function is constitutive and nonspecific.[46, 47]

Because gamma/delta T cells do not express either CD4 or CD8, they are also called *double-negative T cells* or *CD3+/CD4−/CD8−/TCR gamma/delta cells* as opposed to the CD3+/CD4−/CD8+ or CD3+/CD4+/CD8− subsets of T cells with alpha/beta TCR's. Gamma/delta T cells are predominantly found in the subepithelial regions of the skin, respiratory, gastrointestinal, and genitourinary organs,[48] but their function is unclear. Because of their unique localization outside the conventional lymphoid organs, it is suspected that they carry out specialized defense reactions in the tissues directly exposed to the outside environment.

It is important to note that our description of T-cell subsets does not include "suppressor cells." Although much work has been done on suppressor cells, their existence as a discrete T-cell subset is questionable today.[49, 50] Nonetheless, suppressive phenomena clearly do occur. Studies with human cells have ascribed the ability of CD8+ T cells to inhibit the response of stimulated T and B cells to suppressor cells.[50] However, it has been difficult to isolate antigen-specific suppressor T cells and scrutinize them with the molecular probes currently available. Furthermore, recent work with transgenic mice has failed to provide any evidence for the operation of suppressor cells in tolerant mice. Much of the phenomena of the past can be reinterpreted on the basis of more recent findings: Many of the inhibitory effects of suppressor T cells are due to T-cell–derived cytokines with inhibitory properties. For example, Th1 and Th2 cells are reciprocally suppressive; i.e., IFN-γ inhibits many of the effects of IL-4, and IL-10 suppresses Th1 function.[43, 51] Imbalances in the Th1/Th2 ratios are thought to play a role in the pathogenesis of asthma and chronic infections such as leprosy[52] and also may be involved in autoimmune phenomena. It has been reported that in rats Th2 cells inhibit autoimmune encephalomyelitis caused by self-reactive Th1 cells.[51] In addition to the mutually antagonistic (suppressive) effects of cytokines, it is likely that certain kinds of direct cell-cell interactions between conventional lymphocytes generate "suppressive" signals as part of a physiological feedback between activated cells. Since co-stimulation is necessary for the induction of immunity, it is to be expected that the down-regulation of co-stimulatory signals (see below) will

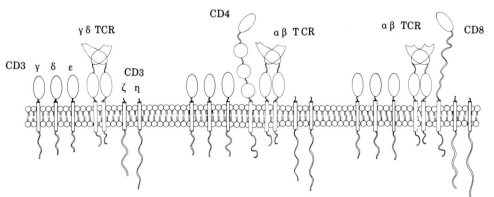

FIGURE 159–1. Structure of the T-cell receptor complex. The T-cell receptor complex is a molecular conglomerate containing the clonally distributed TCR heterodimers (α/β or γ/δ) and the nonclonal CD3 components responsible for transmitting activation signals following the engagement of the TCR with antigen plus MHC. The CD3 complex includes gamma, delta (both of which are unrelated to the gamma/delta chains of the TCR), epsilon, zeta, and eta chains. See text for further details.

become an important element in suppressor cell phenomenology.

B cells utilize a membrane version of the antibody molecule called *surface immunoglobulin,* (sIg) as antigen-specific receptors. As in T cells, sIg is part of a larger B-cell receptor complex containing transduction components related to CD3 but not yet placed within the CD charts.[53] B cells perform a dual function in immune responses as specialized APC's and antibody producers. They rely on sIg to bind unprocessed antigen. Cross-linking of sIg by multivalent antigenic determinants delivers the antigen-specific signal (often referred to as signal 1) required for clonal responses.[54] This essential signal prepares the B cell to receive additional signals and become fully activated. These additional signals (signal 2) are not antigen-specific and include cell-cell interactions with CD4+ T cells, cytokines, or bacterial products with mitogenic properties such as lipopolysaccharide. sIg cross-linking by antigen leads to the internalization of the antigen-receptor complexes and their subsequent degradation in the endosomal compartment. Proteolytic fragments of both the antigen and the sIg become associated with class II MHC molecules and are then transported to the B-cell surface for presentation to CD4+ T cells.[55] The interaction of an antigen-specific CD4+ T cell with antigen plus major histocompatibility complex (MHC) class II on the surface of the B cell results in T-cell help. "Help" is a complex and dynamic process that requires direct T–B-cell contact as well as cytokine-mediated effects. The cell-cell contacts are initiated by the clonally restricted interaction between the TCR, the CD4 complex, and its ligand, the MHC-bound peptide on the B-cell surface. This initial contact probably involves a small fraction (1 per cent or possibly less) of TCR and MHC molecules and needs to be followed by additional and stronger contacts mediated by other cell surface molecules (see "Co-stimulatory Molecules," below). Among the multiple pairs of cell adhesion molecules involved, one appears to have special significance for the delivery of help to B cells. In response to the direct contact with the B cell, T helper cells express a new ligand, a 39-kDa protein that interacts with CD40 on B cells.[56] The interaction between CD40 and its counter-receptor generates the signals required for T-cell–dependent B-cell activation. It should be noted that the T–B-cell engagement is not unidirectional, with the B cells acting as passive recipients of T-cell help. During T–B-cell interactions, B cells deliver differentiation signals to the T cells and modulate the quality and quantity of help generated. For example, it is thought that the B cell drives the differentiation of Th0 cells along the Th2 pathway.[42, 45]

In contrast to T cells, B lymphocytes cannot be unequivocally grouped into subsets with unique surface markers. All B cells make and secrete antibodies, although two major subpopulations of B cells display sufficient functional diversity to justify their classification as distinct subsets. CD5+ B cells (B1) differentiate in the omentum[57–59] and constitute the predominant B-cell type during fetal life. They tend to produce IgM antibodies with broad specificity for bacterial and self antigens. Although rheumatoid factor activity and anti-DNA antibodies are most frequently produced by B1 cells, their participation in autoimmune endocrine diseases remains to be demonstrated. An interesting example of B1 cell involvement in experimental autoimmunity is discussed below in the section dealing with B-cell tolerance.[60] B2 cells represent the conventional B cells that secrete all Ig classes based on their dependence on T-cell help.

From an operational standpoint it is helpful to classify B cells into two subsets: the B-cell subset that responds to polysaccharide antigens without T-cell help and the B-cell subset that responds to protein antigens in a T helper cell–dependent manner.[61] The B-cell responses to thymus-independent (TI) antigens are probably mediated by B1 or B1-like cells and provide a first line of defense against common bacterial pathogens. These TI responses consist mainly of IgM antibodies and do not lead to the generation of immunological memory. Their role in autoimmunity remains to be fully explored. The most relevant B-cell subset represents the conventional B2 cells that mount antibody responses against thymus-dependent protein antigens. The basic mechanism of T-cell help was outlined earlier. The B cell relies on its sIg clonal receptors to bind and internalize antigen that is then processed and presented on class II MHC molecules to helper T cells.[55] Following engagement of the TCR's with the MHC + peptide complex, a large number of pairs of cell adhesion molecules participate actively in the T–B-cell interaction. Several of these pairs deliver co-stimulatory signals to the B cell to promote its clonal expansion and differentiation. In addition, the activated T cells secrete cytokines such as IL-4, IL-5, and others that stimulate B-cell differentiation. The process of T-cell–dependent B-cell differentiation is complex and highly regulated with several possible outcomes: generation of memory cells, generation of highly differentiated effector cells that secrete all classes of Ig's, and selection of cellular mutants that have undergone a somatic hypermutation in their immunoglobulin genes.

PRESENTATION OF ANTIGENS TO T CELLS; RECOGNITION OF SELF PEPTIDES BY IMMUNE RESPONSE CELLS

The immune responses that cause autoimmune endocrine diseases are antigen-specific. That is, they are focused toward certain target peptides rather than involving generalized immune activation in a nonspecific manner. The specificity of this response is conferred by the ability of immune cells to respond exclusively to organ-specific antigens. However, antigen recognition by T and B lymphocytes differs: The antigen receptor on T cells recognizes protein sequences of 8 to 20 amino acids in length trapped in an MHC basket,[62, 63] whereas immunoglobulins, which are the antigen receptors (sIg) on B cells recognize three-dimensional structures present on unprocessed antigens.[57] The processing of proteins and the presentation of their peptide components to T cells requires a complex series of interrelated events that take place in specialized APC's, which include cells such as macrophages, dendritic cells, and, in certain situations, B cells. APC's perform two essential functions required for the initiation of immune responses: They display antigenic fragments associated with specialized antigen-presenting molecules, and they deliver co-stimulatory signals required for lymphocyte activation and differentiation.

The specialized antigen-presenting molecules are the cell surface glycoproteins encoded in the highly polymorphic major histocompatibility complex genes (MHC)

MHC Class I

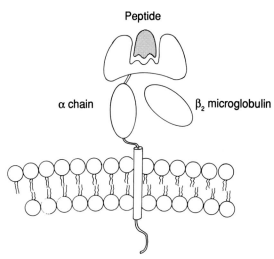

FIGURE 159–2. Structure of class I MHC molecules. Class I molecules are comprised of α_1, α_2, and the membrane-spanning α_3 domains and β_2-microglobulin. A peptide-binding basket is formed with a floor formed by four β-pleated sheets and sides by α helices. The peptide antigen, generally 8 to 10 amino acids in length, has both amino and carboxy ends as anchor points which are buried in the basket. Antigen (peptide) is required for surface expression of class I MHC molecules (see text).

called class I and II. MHC molecules are peptide-binding molecules that present intracellular peptides for recognition by T cells. Because T cells only recognize the complex MHC + peptide, T-cell recognition is said to be MHC restricted. In this manner, only peptides that can bind to MHC molecules can be "seen" by T cells.

MHC Class II

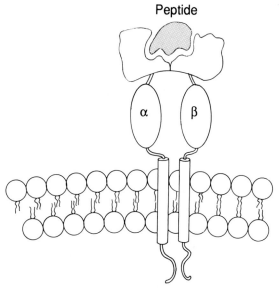

FIGURE 159–3. Structure of class II MHC molecules. The class II MHC molecules are heterodimers of α and β chains. A peptide basket is formed by β-pleated sheets on the floor and α helices on the sides. The peptides bound to class II molecules are larger than class I MHC molecules and range from 16 to 20 amino acids.

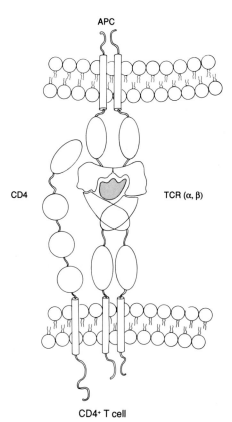

FIGURE 159–4. Interaction of TCR and CD8 with class I MHC molecules and peptide antigens. CD4 and CD8 are cell surface glycoproteins found on T cells. They are members of the Ig superfamily that bind Ig domains found in class II and class I molecules. They both consist of NH_2 terminal extracellular domains, a transmembrane component, and an intracellular tail linked to protein kinases involved in T-cell activation. CD4 contains four extracellular domains. The NH_2 terminal domain contains the site for binding the second domain of class II β chains and is nearby the receptor sites for gp120 from HIV. CD8 consists of two identical (homodimer) or similar (heterodimer) S—S linked chains configured as extended and glycosylated rods with a terminal Ig domain that contains the binding site for the α_3 domain of class I molecules.

MHC molecules sample the contents of the intracellular compartments and bring representative peptides to the cell surface for T-cell scrutiny.[64, 65] There are two major and separate intracellular sources of peptides, the biosynthetic and the catabolic pools, serviced by the class I and II MHC molecules, respectively (Figs. 159–2 and 159–3). MHC class I molecules specialize in the binding of endogenous peptides in the endoplasmic reticulum and in their subsequent transport to the cell surface for recognition by T cells expressing the MHC class I binding molecule CD8 (CD8 + T cells)[64] (Fig. 159–4). Class I MHC molecules are found on all cells, although the relative level of expression may differ considerably between organs, cell types, and even individual cells. MHC class II molecules (also referred to as Ia) bind exogenous peptides generated by proteolysis of extracellular material in the endosomal compartment and present them on the surface for recognition by T cells expressing the MHC class II binding molecule CD4 (CD4 + T cells)[65] (Fig. 159–5). The expression of class II MHC molecules is more restricted than that of class I. They are found on APC's such as macrophages and dendritic cells, B-lymphocytes, thymic epithelial cells, and, in humans, activated T lymphocytes.

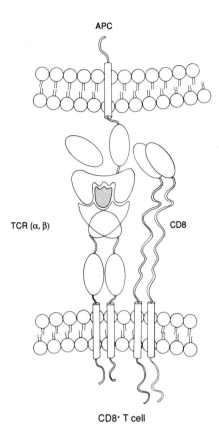

APC

TCR (α, β) CD8

CD8⁺ T cell

FIGURE 159–5. Interaction of TCR and CD4 with class II MHC molecules and peptide antigens.

The structures of MHC class I and II molecules reflect their specialized functions. Class I and II molecules both contain NH₂ terminal peptide binding baskets sitting on a structural platform made up of two immunoglobulin domains. MHC class I consists of an α chain with three extracellular domains associated noncovalently with the non-MHC peptide β₂-microglobulin[62] (see Fig. 159–2). The MHC class I basket is made up of the α₁ and β₂ domains supported by the Ig α₃- and β₂-microglobulin domains. MHC class II is a heterodimer of α and β chains, both of which are integral membrane proteins with two extracellular domains[63] (see Fig. 159–3). The α₁ and β₁ domains create the MHC class II basket that sits on top of the immunoglobulin α₂ and β₂ domains. For both classes of MHC molecules, the peptide-binding basket is made up of two domains each contributing four β-pleated sheets and one α helix. The β sheets form the bottom of the basket and the α helix the sides. Most of the polymorphic residues in MHC molecules reside in the sites involved in peptide; i.e., the different MHC alleles encode MHC molecules with different peptide-binding properties.

The complete amino acid sequences of many class I molecules are known, the three-dimensional structures of several class I molecules have been determined by x-ray crystallography, and the peptides trapped in the grooves of selected class I molecules have been isolated and sequenced.[62, 66] The MHC class I basket is a characteristic structure that accommodates peptides 8 to 10 amino acids long. Peptides lie extended in the cleft with their *N* and *C* terminals bonded to conserved residues of class I. A deep and highly polymorphic pocket (i.e., characteristic of each MHC allele) in the middle of the groove traps the peptide backbone, and several shallow pockets accommodate side chains. This arrangement permits class I molecules to trap and present a large number of peptides with different amino acid compositions. The peptides are buried in the groove, and only a few residues (three or four) stick out of the cleft to engage the TCR.

Peptide loading occurs in the endoplasmic reticulum as the MHC class I chains are being synthesized.[64] Peptide occupancy of the MHC class I basket confers the structural stability required for association with β₂-microglobulin and the subsequent transport and expression on the cell surface of the MHC heterodimer plus peptide. The peptide dependence of MHC class I molecules is an essential aspect of their biology, since, in general, in the absence of peptide, class I molecules are unstable and are not expressed on the cell surface.[67] MHC class I molecules are molecular filters that sample the endogenous pool of cellular peptides. As a consequence, class I MHC molecules cannot engage in peptide exchanges that could misrepresent the contents of the intracellular pool and cause bystander T-cell damage (see below). The peptides for class I MHC are produced predominantly in the cytosol in specialized proteolytic units called *proteasomes* and transported into the endoplasmic reticulum across membrane by ATP-dependent transporters.[68] Interestingly, the genes for the specialized components of the proteasomes and transporters are found within the MHC class II region.[68–71] Culture of cells with cytokines such as IFN-γ results in enhanced expression of proteasomes and peptide transporter genes as well as enhanced expression of class I MHC molecules on the cell surface.

Proteasomes function as intracellular peptide shredders that generate minipeptides suitable for MHC class I baskets.[68–71] Normally, the baskets are occupied by self components. Tolerance for these peptides is acquired either during thymic ontogeny[5, 6, 9, 72] or maintained through mechanisms in the periphery, as discussed below.[5, 7, 73–75] In general, the same peptides predominate on the surfaces of most cell types. However, tissue-specific components may fail to induce tolerance because they are not present during T-cell development in the thymus and are therefore a potential target of autoimmunity. This may occur particularly if their expression in the periphery is abnormally enhanced by concomitant pathological processes such as inflammation, infection, or other circumstances that may, for example, cause production of cytokines which increase MHC expression. The biological relevance of the MHC filter becomes obvious when considering what happens in infected cells. Cells harboring intracellular microbes (viruses in particular) will generate microbial peptides that compete with self peptides for MHC baskets and cell surface exhibition. The presence of these foreign components in MHC class I molecules triggers a T-cell reaction that by definition is focused on the cell surface. Peptides on class I MHC molecules are derived from within the cell and, under physiological conditions, do not freely exchange with exogenous peptides. This prevents noninfected cells from being erroneously targeted by cytotoxic cells.

Recently the three-dimensional structure of a class II MHC molecule has been determined.[75a] The MHC class II basket accommodates peptides 16 to 20 amino acids in length produced in the acidic endosomal compartment[76–78] (Fig. 159–3). The class II site appears to be open at one

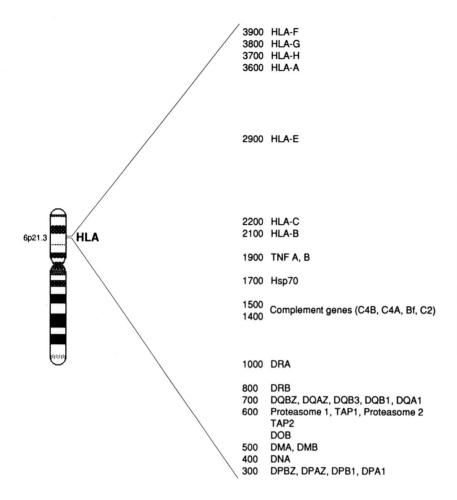

3900 HLA-F
3800 HLA-G
3700 HLA-H
3600 HLA-A

2900 HLA-E

6p21.3 HLA

2200 HLA-C
2100 HLA-B

1900 TNF A, B

1700 Hsp70

1500
1400 Complement genes (C4B, C4A, Bf, C2)

1000 DRA

800 DRB
700 DQBZ, DQAZ, DQB3, DQB1, DQA1
600 Proteasome 1, TAP1, Proteasome 2
TAP2
DOB
500 DMA, DMB
400 DNA
300 DPBZ, DPAZ, DPB1, DPA1

FIGURE 159–6. Organization of human MHC genes on chromosome 6. The diagram depicts the genetic organization of the MHC at 6p21.3. Numbers indicate base pairs ($\times 10^3$) from its origin. The region spans more than 3 million base pairs and contains over 70 functional genes. The class II region is proximal to the centromere and includes the class II regions DP, DN, DM, DO, DQ, and DR. The functional significance of many class II genes has not yet been established. In addition, the class II region contains four linked genes for proteasome components and peptide transporters (TAPs). The class I region is distal to the centromere and contains class 1a genes A, B, and C and 1b genes E to G. Other genes of immunological relevance are listed: TNF (tumor necrosis factor) A and B and the gene for Hsp70 (heat shock protein 70). (Adapted from Trowsdale J, et al: Map of the human MHC. Immunol Today 12:443, 1991.)

end so that the C end of the peptide can extend outside the groove. Another distinguishing feature of the class II peptides is the absence of conserved backbone motifs characteristic of the peptides bound by class I. This suggests that the class II configuration tolerates greater structural freedom in its ligands and probably can handle a larger repertoire of peptides than class I molecules. Unlike class I MHC molecules that must be loaded with a peptide in order to leave the endoplasmic reticulum and successfully reach the cell surface, class II MHC molecules co-migrate with chaperon proteins that prevent the occupancy of their baskets until they reach the endosomes. This molecular plug is the invariant chain, a highly glycosylated chaperon that helps to deliver MHC class II molecules to the endosomal compartment.[79, 80] There, dissociation of the invariant chain from class II MHC molecules renders the MHC molecule available for receipt of peptide. In the endosomal compartment, the invariant chain is removed by proteolysis, and the class II molecules expose their baskets to sample the peptide contents of the endosomes. In this manner, exogenous material that has been internalized and processed, as well as cell surface self components internalized during membrane turnover, competes for binding to MHC class II molecules. Successful binding leads to cell surface expression and eventual recognition by CD4+ T cells (see Fig. 159–4).

The human MHC is called HLA (for human leukocyte antigen), a region spanning over 3 million base pairs on the short arm of chromosome 6 where the genes for class I α chains, class II α and β chains, TAP's (transporters

associated with antigen processing), and proteasome subunits are found[81] (Fig. 159–6). The gene for β_2-microglobulin lies outside the HLA region on chromosome 15. The genetic organization of the region is complex and includes other genes in addition to the MHC genes just mentioned: genes for certain complement components, tumor necrosis factor α (TNF-α) and TNF-β, heat shock protein 70, and others. The genes encoding class I α chains are found in several loci called HLA-A, -B, -C, -E, -F, -G, and -H. Of these, A to C encode the classical transplantation antigen (also called type 1a MHC), and E to H represent recently described and less polymorphic MHC genes of unknown function. It is thought that most of the nonclassical or 1b type antigens represent mutated and nonfunctional genes. The genes encoding the class II α and β chains are located at several loci: HLA-DR, -DQ, -DP, -DO, and -DZ.

IMPLICATIONS FOR CONTROL OF IMMUNE RESPONSIVENESS BY THE MHC

The binding ability of MHC molecules is a key determinant of immune responsiveness; only those antigens which are able to bind to particular class I or class II MHC molecules have the ability to stimulate T cells and cause autoimmune disease. A peptide that does not have affinity for any of the allelic products of MHC genes present in an individual is invisible to T cells of individuals with that particular MHC haplotype and therefore cannot cause autoimmunity. This key function of the MHC is illustrated by the association of MHC alleles with autoimmune endocrine diseases. For example, 95 per cent of Caucasian individuals with insulin-dependent diabetes mellitus (IDDM) express either DR3 or 4 antigens, and the risk appears to be even stronger with HLA-DQ genes that are in linkage disequilibrium with these DR alleles.[82] In most of the HLA-DQ genes associated with IDDM, aspartic acid has been found to be absent at position 57 of the β chain, whereas in alleles associated with reduced risk of IDDM, aspartic acid is generally present at that position.[83–85] It is thought that this change in the sequence of the DQ β chain may alter the binding groove of the MHC basket and allow or prevent certain antigens from binding to the class II MHC molecule. This notion is supported by the observation that other HLA-DQ alleles associated with IDDM have in common a change in the same binding region of the molecule.[86] In addition, expression of diabetes in the NOD mouse, an animal model of IDDM, is closely linked to genes in the class II MHC.[87] Autoimmune thyroid disease is also strongly associated with class II MHC alleles (DR3).[88] While these examples clearly illustrate the relationship of the MHC to autoimmune phenomena, it is not immediately obvious how the MHC does it. In principle, any of three mechanisms discussed more fully below could account for the MHC effects: during ontogeny as a result of either positive or negative selection and in the periphery while fulfilling their roles as peptide-presenting molecules. Although it is not known, the most likely combination of MHC effects leading to autoimmunity would result from a failure to tolerize to certain tissue-specific peptides during lymphocyte development coupled with an abnormal ability to present peptides cross-reactive with self in the periphery.

The association of particular MHC alleles with autoimmune disease raises new possibilities for specific immunotherapy. If, in fact, the disease-associated alleles are uniquely able to bind disease-associated antigens, it should be possible to produce peptides that can specifically bind to the MHC molecules and inhibit the binding of the antigens responsible for disease. These peptides would therefore prevent initiation of an immune response restricted by specific class II MHC alleles. These so-called blocking peptides have been used successfully to prevent presentation of antigens by class II molecules in mice.[89, 90]

CO-STIMULATORY MOLECULES AND THEIR ABILITY TO REGULATE IMMUNE RESPONSES

Recognition of antigen/peptide in the antigen-binding basket of class I or class II MHC molecules alone is not sufficient for activation of T lymphocytes. It has been shown in transgenic mouse models, for example, that expression of foreign antigens on the surfaces of peripheral tissues does not result in autoimmunity.[7, 13, 30, 32] On the contrary, when foreign antigens are expressed on cell surfaces in the absence of co-stimulation, T-cell tolerance rather than immune responsiveness may occur (Fig. 159–7). It has been shown in vitro that interaction of T-cell receptor with antigen plus MHC molecule may render cells unresponsive to stimulation by antigen on modified APC's.[91, 92] This nonresponsive state may be prevented by addition of either IL-2 or third-party APC's which can pro-

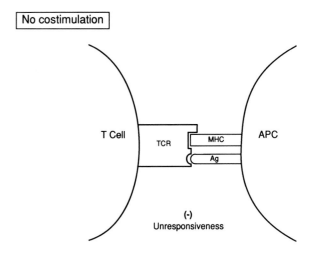

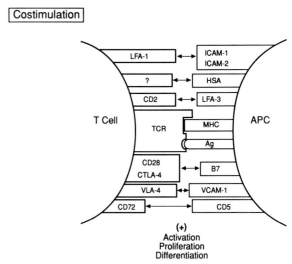

FIGURE 159–7. Co-stimulatory molecules in T-cell activation. Activation of T-lymphocytes involves two signals. The first is the cognate interaction of TCR with antigen plus MHC molecule (signal 1). However, this signal alone does not result in activation and may even cause nonresponsiveness of the T cell. When co-stimulatory signals (signal 2) are delivered together with signal 1, T-cell activation takes place. The minimal requirements for co-stimulation are not precisely defined, and several interactions have been postulated to be important. Co-stimulatory signals can be provided by antigen-presenting cells such as dendritic cells, macrophages, and B cells but are not antigen-specific. However, most endocrine cells do not express these molecules under normal conditions. The significance of these interactions on immune recognition of antigens on endocrine cells is discussed in the text.

vide the necessary co-stimulation. Co-stimulatory signals are generated through the interaction between molecules on the surfaces of T cells and ligands on the surfaces of APC's. The interactions between these molecules are not antigen-specific. The signal that is transduced following interaction of co-stimulatory molecule and its ligand may synergize or modulate signals resulting from the interaction of the TCR with the complex of antigen plus MHC molecule (see Fig. 159–7).

The co-stimulatory molecules initially identified are involved in cell-mediated lysis assays in vitro (Table 159–2). These molecules include lymphocyte function–related an-

TABLE 159–2. CO-SIMULATORS OF T-CELL ACTIVATION

MOLECULE	LOCATION	T-CELL LIGAND	COMMENT
ICAM-1 ICAM-2	Wide variety of tissues	LFA-1	ICAM is induced during inflammation ICAM-2 is constitutively expressed on endothelial cells; ICAM-1/LFA-1 interaction enhances T-cell activation. ICAM-1 also binds CD43.
B7	Activated B cells, macrophages, dendritic cells.	CD28	Both CD 28 and CTLA4 are T-cell co-receptors for B7. CD28 is expressed constitutively but has a lower avidity for B7 than CTLA4, which has increased expression after T-cell activation.
LFA-3	Widely distributed	CD2	Responsible for T-cell rosetting with erythrocytes. Interaction of CD2 and LFA-3 may function primarily to augment specific signaling through TCR.
VCAM (vascular adhesion molecule)	Vascular endothelial	VLA-4	VCAM is inducible. Interaction augments TCR-mediated T-cell proliferation.
?		HSA	HSA is present on B-cell blasts and at low levels on dendritic cells.

tigens 1, 2, and 3 (LFA-1, LFA-2, LFA-3).[93–95] LFA-1 (CD11a/CD18) and LFA-2 (CD2) are members of the integrin and immunoglobulin families, respectively, and their ligands on APC's are intercellular adhesion molecule 1 or 2 (ICAM-1 or -2) and LFA-3, respectively. Although the expression of LFA-1 is restricted to leukocytes, ICAM-1 is expressed on a wide variety of cells during inflammation, but only in limited cell types under normal conditions.[95] The importance of the ICAM-1/LFA-1 interaction has been shown recently in a model of allograft transplantation. Rejection of cardiac allografts was prevented when recipients were treated with monoclonal antibodies against ICAM-1 and LFA-1.[96] Activated T cells express CD2 (LFA-2), which accounts for their ability to form rosettes with erythrocytes that express LFA-3.[95, 97] The effect of the interaction of CD2 and LFA-3 may be to augment signals delivered following interaction of the TCR with antigen and MHC molecule. Other co-stimulatory molecule interactions serve to enhance adhesion between lymphocyte and APC.[98] Examples include the interaction between VCAM (vascular cell adhesion molecule) and VLA-4 or CD44 and Mel-14/LAM-1. The latter helps to direct lymphocyte circulation through lymph nodes.

B7 is a member of the immunoglobulin gene family, and its ligand on T cells is CD28.[99] B7 is found on the surfaces of B cells as well as other APC's, including dendritic cells and macrophages. Blocking the interaction between B7 and CD28 can prevent responses to alloantigens in vitro and can inhibit humoral immune responses in vivo.[100] Lenschow et al.[102] have shown recently that treatment with a fusion protein, CTLA4Ig, that consists of a CD28 homologue, CTLA4,[101] fused to human gamma globulin heavy chain, can prevent rejection of islet xenografts in mice. Interestingly, treatment of xenograft recipients with CTLA4 led to tolerance specific for xenoantigens. The authors of this study suggest that interaction of TCR with xenoantigen in the absence of a co-stimulatory signal leads to nonresponsiveness. This is supported by the observation that expression of class II MHC as an alloantigen on islets that do not express co-stimulatory molecules (in transgenic mice) and use of these cells as APC's can result in antigen-specific tolerance.[103] Tolerance in this setting may be similar to clonal anergy observed in vitro following stimulation of TCR without co-stimulation (see Fig. 159–7).

Most peripheral tissues do not constitutively express co-stimulatory molecules. This ensures that immune reactivity will not develop against antigens expressed on their cell's surfaces. This point is supported by the observation that endocrine cells, such as islet cells, function poorly as APC's.[103] With inflammation and production of cytokines, however, certain co-stimulatory molecules are induced[104] and may meet the requirements for antigen presentation. The importance of co-stimulatory molecules for recognition of autoantigens on endocrine tissues and autoimmunity has been shown in an adoptive transfer model of IDDM. In these studies (in NOD mice), blockade of an adhesion-promoting receptor on macrophages (CD11b/CD18) prevented adoptive transfer of disease by splenocytes from a diabetic animal to a nondiabetic mouse.[107] Furthermore, treatment of NOD mice with anti–ICAM-1 and anti–LFA-1 mAbs has been found to prevent development of diabetes in NOD mice or in multidose streptozotocin-induced diabetes mellitus.[106]

DEVELOPMENT OF TOLERANCE DURING T-CELL ONTOGENY IN THE THYMUS

The specificity of individual T cells is imparted during their development in the thymus during a complex and not completely understood process called *thymic education.*[107] Thymic lymphopoiesis is intense during development and declines after birth. A staggering 95 to 98 per cent of thymic lymphocytes die in situ, presumably because of the rigors of thymic education. The unique problem faced by T cells is how to express a diverse repertoire for foreign antigens that is both tolerant of self and MHC-restricted.

There are two separate lineages of T-cell differentiation, leading to alpha/beta or gamma/delta T cells. The gamma/delta T cells differentiate in waves with characteristic V gene expression and colonize mucosal sites where they may undergo additional steps of extrathymic differentiation.[48] As noted earlier, the function of gamma/delta T cells is unknown. We will focus our discussion on the development of the conventional or classical T cells. Alpha/beta T cells originate from blood-borne CD4−/CD8−/CD3−/TCR− precursor cells (Fig. 159–8). In the thymic cortex, the precursors become CD4+/CD8+ (double-positive) thymocytes expressing low levels of CD3 and TCR. TCR expression follows the productive rearrangements of β- and α-chain genes. TCR gene rearrangements are random and generate a huge repertoire of specificities (>10[9]).[108] The random rearrangement of TCR genes implies that each individual (even identical twins) possesses a unique T-cell repertoire, although reactivity against most antigens is conserved within a population. The random generation of the repertoire coupled with the stochastic nature of positive and negative selection may explain the discordance of certain autoimmune endocrine diseases among identical twins. The next well-defined step(s) in T-cell development is the differentiation of single-positive CD4+/CD8− or CD4−/CD8+ T cells. This requires the co-engagement of the TCR with either CD4 or CD8 on thymic MHC molecules.[109–112] Depending on the specificity of the TCR for class I or class II MHC molecules loaded with self peptides, the double-positive T cells will engage either CD4 or CD8 with appropriate MHC ligands and generate single-positive cells. It is likely that TCR binding in the absence of CD4/CD8 engagement causes apoptosis to ensure MHC restriction in the developing T cells.

Classical studies of bone marrow chimeric mice in which bone marrow progenitor cells were transferred to a host with a different MHC have shown that the developing cells become restricted to antigen in the context of the MHC of the host rather than the bone marrow source.[111, 113] These studies have shown that the radioresistant thymic epithelium is responsible for imprinting MHC restriction on developing thymocytes. Thus, from a developmental point of view, self refers to the MHC of the thymic epithelial cells in the context of which the capacity to recognize foreign antigens by T cells is imparted. The initial process of learning occurs through positive selection and indicates that thymocytes bearing receptors capable of interaction with self MHC on the thymic epithelium receive a positive signal that triggers their developmental progression.[5] More recent studies of this process, including those in transgenic mice that express a single T-cell receptor, have shown that positive selection requires direct interaction among the TCR, MHC, and accessory molecules and can be strongly influenced by the MHC haplotype expressed on the thymic epithelium.[110–113] The end result of this process is a repertoire dramatically skewed toward recognition of antigens bound to self MHC. In fact, selection for antigen reactivity can be induced if the antigen is appropriately presented in the thymus at the time of T-cell maturation.[114] Once this has been achieved, developing T cells face their next major hurdle, negative selection of self-reactive clones.

Several experimental systems have shown that cells with high avidity for self antigens and self MHC molecules undergo clonal deletion. For example, in mice, T cells that express the TCR β chain, Vβ6, are reactive with the murine minor lymphocyte stimulatory antigen (Mls[a]).[115] In mice that are Mls[a] autoreactive, CD4+ T cells expressing Vβ6 can be found in the cortex of the thymus, where immature cells reside, but are not found among the more mature thymocytes in the medulla and do not appear in the periphery. In addition to this example, studies with transgenic mice expressing TCR specific for the male (H-Y) antigens, other class II or class I MHC molecules, or peptides also have shown that clonal deletion is responsible for elimination of potentially autoreactive T cells from the repertoire of mature peripheral T cells.[23, 25] Transplantation studies have indicated that the cells responsible for clonal deletion are bone marrow–derived and migrate to the thymus.[113, 116] However, the precise identity of these APC's is not known. Some evidence suggests that extrathymic APC's migrating through the thymus may be able to mediate clonal deletion of immature CD4+/CD8+ thymocytes.[16]

Several important issues regarding selective events in the thymus remain unresolved. For example, it is not known how MHC recognition by developing thymocytes can mediate both positive and negative selection. It has been suggested that the MHC molecules on the cells that induce positive and negative selection express different peptides.[117–119] Present work with transgenic mice has suggested, for example, that the level of CD8 expression on developing T cells can determine the outcome of thymic

T Lymphocyte Ontogeny

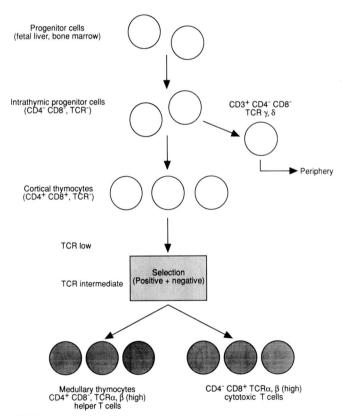

FIGURE 159–8. T-cell ontogeny. Bone marrow precursors which lack the phenotype of mature T cells migrate to the thymus during fetal life. They acquire expression of the T-cell receptor complex and both CD4 and CD8. However, most T cells do not mature further through events termed *positive* and *negative selection*; those cells which are able to react with foreign peptide plus MHC but are not reactive with self peptides expressed in the thymus at the time of ontogeny are selected for maturation. As the cells mature through these stages, they first express TCR with both CD4 and CD8 and then lose expression of either CD4 or CD8 and acquire the phenotype of mature T cells.

selection (in a class I–restricted response).[120] This indicates that quantitative differences in TCR-MHC recognition are a critical determinant of T-cell fate. The precise cellular and molecular events that result in apoptosis and the death of the developing thymocyte are largely unknown. Recent evidence suggests that expression of the proto-oncogene *bcl-2* may correlate with the mechanism whereby selected lymphocytes are saved from programmed cell death.[121–124] The *bcl-2* gene was identified in B-cell lymphomas and exhibits a novel localization—to the inner mitochondrial membrane—suggesting an important role in metabolic processes. The *bcl-2* protein is found in tissues characterized by apoptosis and is expressed in areas of surviving cells such as in the thymic medulla and germinal centers of lymph nodes. These and other observations suggest that *bcl-2* is expressed during T-cell maturation in T cells that survive cell death by apoptosis. Regulation of this or other developmental proteins may play an important role in prevention of autoimmune disease, as illustrated by the finding that *bcl-2* transgenic mice develop an autoimmune disease similar to systemic lupus erythematosus.[124] Thus, in one model system, autoimmunity may occur because autoreactive cells fail to die during development.

MECHANISMS OF TOLERANCE BY T CELLS FOR ANTIGENS NOT EXPRESSED IN THE THYMUS AT THE TIME OF T-CELL ONTOGENY

A number of different mechanisms are thought to be responsible for maintenance of tolerance to (self) antigens expressed on peripheral tissues.[26] Not all peptides bound to MHC molecules on peripheral tissues may be appropriately presented to the immune system, and not all peripheral tissues are capable of presenting antigens to the immune system. T cells, therefore, may not "see" antigens on the surfaces of these tissues because the density of MHC antigen complex is below a threshold needed to cause stimulation. In certain areas, T cells may not be able to gain access to antigens on the peripheral tissues. Receptors that direct T cells into the area of inflammation are not highly expressed under basal conditions, so the tissues may elude immune surveillance because T cells do not come in contact with the antigen. Local production of cytokines and inflammation can enhance expression of MHC molecules and co-receptors with the potential for recruitment of T cells to those sites.[104, 125]

Clonal anergy may be another mechanism for tolerance to peripheral tissues.[7, 26, 130–133] Even if antigen is available at sufficient levels, engagement of the TCR in the absence of the appropriate co-stimulatory signals may fail to induce activation (and may induce clonal anergy; see above). Under normal condition, peripheral tissues do not express the co-stimulatory molecules needed for T-cell activation. Thus interaction of a TCR with autoantigens on these peripheral tissues would be expected to result in antigen-specific nonresponsiveness. As discussed earlier, this is postulated to be the mechanism underlying the development of tolerance to xenoantigens when islet xenografts are transplanted followed by treatment with CTLA4Ig, which blocks co-stimulatory signals delivered via CD28.[102] If, however, sufficient APC's gain access to these antigens and present them to T cells, activation may occur.

In other systems, *clonal deletion* also has been shown to contribute to maintenance of tolerance to peripheral antigens.[8, 11, 21] This has been found in systems using the minor lymphocyte stimulatory antigen (Mls^a) discussed above. For example, when Mls^a-bearing cells are transferred into an Mls^b recipient, deletion of Vβ6+/CD4+ T cells occurs (see above).[11] The clonal elimination of these antigen-reactive cells is preceded by marked expansion of the cells. Thus, in this system, clonal deletion and tolerance are the end result of a powerful immune response. In other Mls-reactive systems (using V8.1+/CD4+ T cells which are also Mls^a-reactive), both clonal deletion and clonal anergy occur.[11] On the anergized cell in this system, TCR engagement does not result in IL-2 receptor expression or calcium mobilization, two early events in the activation of T cells. A defect in antigen-induced transcription of the IL-2 gene has been identified and ascribed to down-regulation of the transcription factor AP-1 in these cells.[28] T-cell anergy in these systems has been shown to depend on continuous exposure to antigen. When anergic T cells were removed from self antigen by adoptive transfer to a mouse strain without the antigen or by in vitro culture, nonresponsiveness was reversed, and the cells returned to normal functional status.[11] Anergic alloreactive T cells also have been found in the periphery of mice exposed to alloantigen (K^b) expressed on islet cells. In these mice, co-expression of IL-2 in the islet (as a transgenic) can reverse the T-cell anergy.[128]

The results from other model systems indicate that T cells may not undergo deletion or become anergized but may fail to respond to peripheral antigens in a manner best described as *clonal ignorance*.[7, 13, 76] In one example, expression of the alloantigen IA^d on the β cells of H-2^b mice failed to result in insulitis even though cells reactive with the alloantigen were present in the animal and responded to the alloantigen in vitro.[13] Results from doubly transgenic mice, expressing viral antigens in the periphery and autoreactive TCR, are also consistent with this mechanism.[30, 32] In mice expressing, in the pancreatic β cells, a transgene encoding glycoprotein from the lymphocytic choriomeningitis virus and TCR that recognizes the glycoprotein plus MHC, tolerance for both the glycoprotein and the β cells is seen. The tolerance is broken if the mouse is infected with live lymphocytic choriomeningitis virus. These results indicate, first, that T cells capable of reacting with the foreign protein are present in the animal despite the presence of tolerance to the foreign antigen. Furthermore, if the appropriate co-stimulatory signals are delivered, tolerance is reversed. In other transgenic model systems, variable amounts of organ inquiry have been found in tissues that express foreign antigens on peripheral tissues as transgenes. For example, in a different study, the expression of influenza virus hemagglutinin in the pancreatic β cells of transgenic mice did result in autoimmune diabetes that involves both a cellular and humoral islet-specific immune response.[130] In doubly transgenic mice that express the class I MHC alloantigen L^d on pancreatic exocrine tissue and TCR specific for L^d on T cells, an inflammatory response against the exocrine tissue is seen.[131] Together, these results suggest that when the frequency of antigen-reactive T cells is high when foreign antigen is present in abundance on peripheral tissues and/or when co-activation signals are delivered, immune reactivity may occur. If such requirements are not met, clonal ignorance for antigens on peripheral tissues prevails, and tissue damage does not occur.

MECHANISMS OF TOLERANCE IN THE B-CELL COMPARTMENT

Like T-cell ontogeny, B-lymphocyte development requires sequential gene rearrangements to create a diverse repertoire and selective steps that abrogate self-reactivity and adjust the repertoire to the environment. The basic points to consider about B-cell ontogeny are that DNA rearrangements of Ig genes occur in an antigen-independent fashion and create a huge repertoire of random Ig specificities ($>10^{10}$), including reactivity with self antigens. Autoreactive B cells are eliminated by clonal deletion at the immature B-cell stage, with other mechanisms operating later.[133] It is thought that positive selection by environmental antigens plays a crucial role in maintaining and shaping the B-cell repertoire. It is likely that most B cells are destined to die after a short life unless they receive a positive signal from environmental antigens and are recruited into a long-lived cellular pool. This mechanism guarantees that the randomly generated repertoire is shaped by the internal and external environments to remove both self-reactive and irrelevant specificities.

Precursor cells committed to the B-cell lineage first undergo DJ rearrangement to become pro-B cells.[54, 132] This is followed by the allelic exclusion of rearranged VH genes to generate functional heavy-chain genes in pre-B cells. Although it had been thought that pre-B cells contained only cytoplasmic μ chains, it is now known that these heavy chains pair up with surrogate light chains and are expressed on the pre-B cell surface. Whether surface expression is important for the selection of the B-cell repertoire or is simply required to foster light-chain gene rearrangements is not known. The κ locus rearranges first and, if it fails to produce functional genes, is followed by rearrangements in the λ locus. A successful rearrangement of either κ or λ genes leads to the production of conventional Ig molecules that are expressed as sIgM on immature B cells. This stage of B-cell differentiation is characterized by the susceptibility to apoptosis following receptor cross-linking. It is thought that tolerance to most self antigens occurs at this stage,[14, 17–22] before the immature B cell undergoes additional differentiation to become an antigen-reactive mature B cell expressing sIgM and sIgD.

As shown in Figure 159–9, there are two separate developmental pathways for B cells, one in the omentum and the other in the bone marrow.[57–59] The B1 pathway generates a self-renewing population of B cells that express several antiself specificities. Relatively little is known about self/nonself discrimination in the B1 subset. It has even been proposed that it comprises a separate immune system where self-reactivity is a physiological trait to maintain lymphocyte connectivity. Murakami et al.[60] have shown in a transgenic model that mature B1 cells may be susceptible to clonal deletion (apoptosis) if they encounter antigen. In this model, B1 cells express a transgene encoding anti-erythrocyte specificity. Approximately 50 per cent of transgenic mice suffered from autoimmune disease due to the presence of a small proportion of B cells that have escaped tolerance in the bone marrow and the spleen. These cells find a sanctuary in the peritoneal cavity and selectively expand as B1 cells in the absence of exposure to self antigen. The critical role of self antigen in the induction and maintenance of self tolerance was clearly documented using this model; injection of red blood cells into the peritoneal cavity of autoimmune transgenic mice caused apoptosis of the self-reactive B cells, and the mice recovered from anemia.

When antigens are present in low concentrations, e.g., albumin (such that fewer than 5 per cent of B-cell antigen receptors are occupied), there appears to be little effect of the autoantigen on the development or function of self-reactive B cells.[14, 133] For example, in double transgenic mice which express antilysozyme genes and very low concentrations of secreted lysozyme, B cells can be stimulated to secrete antilysozyme antibody in a normal fashion and actually secreted antibodies spontaneously. Thus clonal ig-

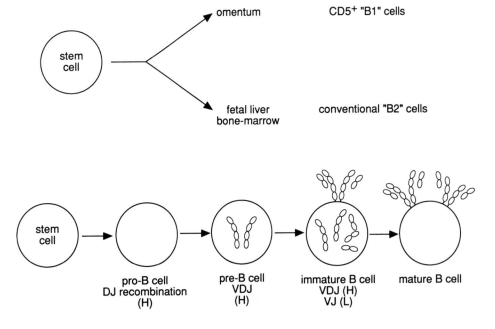

FIGURE 159–9. B-lymphocyte ontogeny. Two lineages of B cells have been described. B1 cells, which express the surface marker CD5, develop in the omentum and produce IgM antibodies with broad specificities, including self antigens. ''Conventional'' B2 cells comprise the B cells found elsewhere and can secrete all antibody isotypes. B-cell developmental stages involve rearrangement of heavy and light chains and surface expression of IgM. Finally, on mature B cells, IgM and IgD are expressed on the cells' surfaces.

norance may be operative for antigens that circulate in low concentrations such as thyroglobulin, insulin, or growth hormone and may explain the relatively common finding of autoantibodies against these proteins in normal individuals.

When antigen is present at higher concentrations (sufficient to occupy 45 per cent of antigen receptors on B cells), the outcome for autoantibody-producing B cells is different.[14, 132, 134] B-cell inactivation occurs in vivo in antilysozyme double-transgenic mice expressing soluble lysozyme. Although the B cells continue to reside as mature cells in the follicular mantle zones of spleen, lymph nodes, and Peyer's patches and express high-affinity antigen receptors, their ability to proliferate in response to stimulation is markedly impaired, and they do not make antibody. On these anergized cells there are changes in the antigen receptor function (there is a 20-fold decrease in membrane IgM) and changes in the B cell's potential to differentiate. Other models such as transgenic mice with anti–single-stranded DNA antibody genes or antierythrocyte autoantibody genes from NZB mice support the notion that clonal anergy may be a general mechanism for mediating B-cell tolerance to self antigens.[135] Of note, in the latter mice, tolerance may spontaneously break down in some of the animals, resulting in anemia.

In a process analogous to clonal deletion of T cells, B cells producing antibody against autoantigens with high affinity for B-cell receptors may undergo clonal deletion. In transgenic mice of the H-2K^k or H-2K^b haplotype, in which the majority of the B cells express a single antibody with specificity for these MHC molecules, most of B-lymphocytes die within the bone marrow and do not appear in the spleen or lymph nodes.[14, 17–20, 136] An identical process is seen in double transgenic mice bearing antilysozyme Ig and a membrane-bound form of lysozyme. In contrast to the anergized B cells seen with secreted lysozyme, mature lysozyme-binding B cells are not detected in mice expressing lysozyme in the cell-bound form.

In these examples using transgenic mice, the fate of a B cell producing an antiself specificity is determined by a number of factors[14] (Table 159–3). These include the concentration of self antigen with which the developing B cell has an encounter, the affinity of the B-cell antigen receptor for the ligand, the valency of the epitope, the stage of B-cell development when this encounter occurs, and other signals. As discussed earlier, data from the antilysozyme/lysozyme transgenic model have shown that although functional unresponsiveness and IgM modulation occur in the presence of lysozyme at a concentration of 10^{-10} M, this does not occur when the concentration of antigen is reduced tenfold and fewer than 5 per cent of the surface Ig receptors are occupied. Thus there appears

to be a threshold concentration of antigen necessary to cause down-modulation of B-cell receptors and anergy. Like developing T cells, immature B cells are more susceptible to deletion than mature cells. The threshold requirements for antigen and differences in susceptibility with stages of development suggest the possibility that other signals may in part determine the fate of encounter of the developing B cell with self antigen, but these signals are poorly understood.

T-cell help may be a key factor in the maintenance of B-cell tolerance. In mature B cells in which stimulation is dependent on T-cell help, tolerance is maintained by the CD4 helper T cells. For example, Karvelas and Nossal[137] have shown that immunological tolerance for antibody production against soluble human serum albumin resides in both T- and B-cell compartments. Using mixtures of cells adoptively transferred to irradiated recipients, these authors have shown that there is a major T-cell component in the process whereby soluble protein antigens ablate affinity maturation and memory cell generation by B cells.

The tolerance-inducing processes described so far are, despite significant differences in detail, basically similar in T and B cells. There is one situation that is unique to B cells because their immunoglobulin genes are subject to a somatic diversification process that does not occur in T cells, namely, somatic hypermutation.[138] Hypermutation of the V-gene segments is an antigen-driven and helper T cell–dependent process that occurs in the specialized environment of the germinal centers. It evolved as a means to diversify and improve the antibody repertoire by introducing a high rate of mutations in the gene segments encoding the antibody-binding sites. Its success requires the positive selection of mutants making "better" antibodies and the negative selection of mutants with antiself specificities. Positive selection is driven by antigen presented by follicular dendritic cells and is the basis for the improvements in the quality of antibody responses (often called *affinity maturation*) that occur late in the course of primary responses or after repeated antigenic challenges. Negative selection requires apoptosis of self-reactive mutants and is thought to be related to lack of expression of *bcl*-2. Obviously, any failure of the apoptotic machinery in B cells poses the risk of autoimmunity. The implications of this potential pathogenetic mechanism for endocrine autoimmune disease remains to be fully explored. In principle, mutant antibody genes could give rise to antibodies reactive with endocrine components that have not been represented in the selection process. Also, it is conceivable that mutated antibodies express internal images of endocrine components and mimic their biological effects (see Fig. 159–9 and the next section).

TABLE 159–3. B-CELL TOLERANCE IN TRANSGENIC MICE

OUTCOME	AUTO ANTIGEN	EXAMPLES
Clonal ignorance	Less than 10^{-10} M, occupying less than 5% of antigen receptors, low-affinity interaction	Insulin, thyroglobulin, albumin, soluble form of lysozyme
Clonal anergy	10^{-9} M, occupying about 45% of antigen receptors	Soluble form of lysozyme
Clonal deletion	Membrane-bound, high-affinity interaction	Membrane-bound lysozyme, anti-DNA antibodies, anti–class I MHC antibodies, treatment of mice from birth with antibodies to IgM

IDIOTYPE NETWORKS

Jerne[138] proposed in 1974 that the immune system is a functional network resulting from paratope-idiotope interactions. Idiotopes are self-epitopes of V domains located both within and outside the paratopes of Ig's and TCR's.[33, 139, 140] They are operationally defined by anti-idiotypic reagents (see Fig. 159–10). The typical anti-idiotypic probes are antibodies because relatively little is known about idiotype-specific (anti-idiotypic) TCR's or how to use them to define idiotypic markers. Internal image anti-idiotypic antibodies are those which can be used successfully as immunogens to generate antiantigen immunity. It has been suspected that autoantibodies with internal images of hormones or their receptor sites play a role in autoimmune disease, but the structural data documenting such a relationship has not been produced.

Initially postulated for B-cell idiotypes, the network theory is applicable to T cells and their receptors; TCR idiotypes have been used successfully to stimulate the production of anti-idiotypic T cells, and various types of idiotype-specific helper and cytotoxic effects have been reported in experimental models.[139] Jerne's theory has been a strong stimulant of immunological research and has generated much enthusiasm as well as some controversy. The idiotype network is perceived as a closed system of self-recognizing V domains found in lymphocytes. It is thought that the large repertoire of V domains contains representations of the antigenic universe in its internal images and has the intrinsic capacity to autoregulate itself through complementary anti-idiotypic interactions. It is clear that anti-idiotypes with powerful immunoregulatory properties can be produced with relative ease in experimental animals. A separate issue is whether or not the network operates physiologically in the course of immune responses. Notwithstanding the abundant literature on network dysfunction, the role of the idiotype network in autoimmunity and immunopathology is poorly defined. As noted in the introduction, the occurrence of idiotypic/anti-idiotypic reactions is to be expected, although it remains to be firmly established whether they are incidental or essential components of either immune function or dysfunction. There are descriptions of autoanti-idiotypic antibodies in various clinical settings, but there is no conclusive evidence to suggest that dysfunctions of the idiotype network are primarily responsible for disease states.[140]

MECHANISMS IN THE PATHOGENESIS OF AUTOIMMUNE ENDOCRINE DISEASE

Autoimmune Phenomena May Occur in Normal Individuals

The most frequent type of autoimmunity is asymptomatic. Signs of immune reactivity directed against endocrine tissues are a common finding among otherwise normal populations. In one cross-sectional study,[141] 10.3 per cent of women and 2.7 per cent of men without thyroid dysfunction were found to have thyroid autoantibodies. Only 5 to 10 per cent of individuals with thyroid autoantibodies will progress to overt disease. Similarly, 3.1 per cent of first-degree relatives of patients with IDDM have been found to have islet cell antibodies.[142] However, only 1 per cent of relatives progress to diabetes over a 7-year period, and only 68 per cent of these patients can be identified by the presence of autoantibodies. The prevalence of cell-mediated responses against endocrine tissues are not known, since assays to detect such responses are not available. It is likely, however, that the cell-mediated responses against endocrine tissues in the general population are greater than suspected. For example, focal thyroiditis can be found at autopsy in as many as 6 per cent of men and 22 per cent of women without known thyroid disease.[143] Thus low levels of hormonal and possibly cellular autoimmunity are tolerated in many normal individuals without progression to endocrine disease. Clearly, additional triggering events are needed to cause endocrine pathology.

Possible Triggers of Autoimmune Endocrine Disease

GENERAL STATEMENTS. The current paradigms of antigen presentation and MHC-restricted T-cell recognition have important implications for our understanding of autoimmunity. The MHC controls what T cells "learn" during ontogeny and what they recognize later in life. Co-stimulation largely determines how T cells react to what they see. Since infectious agents and their products are the most potent inducers of co-stimulatory signals, the potential association between infection and autoimmunity should not come as a surprise. For their function, MHC molecules are dependent on the production and availability of peptides generated by the proteasomes and endosomes; i.e., MHC function is primarily dependent on cel-

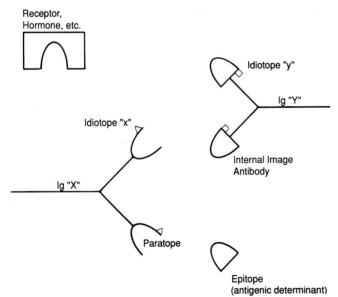

FIGURE 159–10. Idiotypic networks. A hormone receptor or other peptides may serve as an antigenic determinant for an immunoglobulin (IgX). The antigen-binding site of that immunoglobulin may in turn serve as an antigen (idiotope X) for a second antibody (idiotope Y). By virtue of its ability to bind the antigen-binding site of idiotope X, idiotope Y's antigen-binding site will form an internal image of the original antigenic determinant of idiotope X. Idiotope Y may therefore be capable of interacting with similar binding sites as the antigenic determinant such as the hormone receptor.

lular rather than immunological mechanisms. In practice, this means that much of autoimmunity may have to do with abnormal cell biology rather than with abnormal immunity, at least initially. For example, T-cell "education" (both positive and negative selection during ontogeny) is dependent on the intrathymic display of MHC antigens with peptides. It is not known how much of "self" is actually visible to T cells during ontogeny. It was noted earlier that a rigorous exposure to a diverse self leads to extensive clonal deletions and potential holes in the repertoire. Probably evolution tried to get away with T cells ignoring as much of self as practical (defined as risk of self-reactivity). There is general agreement that T cells do not become tolerized to all potential self antigens. Work on transgenic mice has clearly shown that tissue-specific antigens are invisible to T cells, a situation that emphasized the importance of mechanisms for peripheral tolerance and the critical role played by co-stimulatory signals. It is also not known whether endogenous class I–restricted self is more or less available than exogenous class II–restricted self. In principle, one could assume that CD8+ T cells have more opportunities to be tolerized than CD4+ T cells, since it is not clear how cytosolic components become exposed to the exogenous class II pathway. This is a crucial issue in autoimmunity, since CD8+ effector T cells and B cells are dependent on CD4+ helper T cells. Lack of tolerance in CD4+ T cells to intracellular self components may well be at the root of many autoimmune phenomena, since any number of nonspecific changes in the biology of cells could lead to abnormal exposure of previously hidden self components. Under these hypothetical circumstances, one would expect to find nontolerized B cells that are capable of presenting the previously hidden self antigen to helper cells. There are two possible outcomes of such a presentation event: induction of tolerance (if the APC's lack co-stimulatory properties, i.e., as is the case with nonactivated resting B cells) or a self-propagating process of autoimmunity. While in the past the contribution of self-reactive B cells to autoimmunity has been viewed exclusively from the perspective of autoantibody production, it is likely that their APC role may be more important during the inductive phases of autoimmunity. A good example of how this may happen was recently provided by Day et al.[144] These authors showed that targeting a self antigen to B cells prevented the induction of a cell-mediated autoimmune disease in rats.

FAILURE TO DEVELOP TOLERANCE TO ORGAN-SPECIFIC ANTIGENS DURING LYMPHOCYTE ONTOGENY. When lymphocyte development has been manipulated in experimental systems such that deletion of autoreactive T cells has not occurred in the thymus, autoimmune disease has been found to occur in the peripheral organs. If clonal deletion is interrupted in neonatal mice by administering the immunosuppressive agent cyclosporin A, the adult animals develop manifestations of autoimmune disease, including orchitis, pancreatitis, and isletitis.[145–147] The overexpression of *bcl*-2 discussed earlier is another example of this mechanism.[124] In these models, cells reactive with peripheral antigens are not removed from the repertoire during ontogeny and can be activated by the antigens on the peripheral organs. In this model of autoimmunity, the repertoire from normal individuals and individuals with disease would differ, in that the latter individuals would have cells that are reactive with peripheral antigens. In support of this notion,

T-cell reactivity against particular thyroid antigens has been found to differ in individuals with autoimmune thyroid disease compared with controls.[148] However, since, in general, phenotypic markers of endocrine antigen–reactive T cells (e.g., Vβ chain usage) are unknown for the T cells involved in endocrine diseases, it has not been possible to identify T cells reactive with endocrine antigens and study their presence in normal individuals. Placement of peripheral antigens in the thymus at the time of T-cell ontogeny can result in loss of susceptibility to autoimmune endocrine disease. For example, if antigen-bearing islets are placed into the thymus of neonatal prediabetic BB rats, the incidence of diabetes as adults is reduced.[149, 150] If antigen-bearing islets are placed into the thymus of adult mice followed by depletion of mature peripheral T cells and T-cell regeneration, mice previously susceptible to streptozotocin-induced autoimmune diabetes become resistant.[151] This tolerance, which is specific for islet antigens, can be broken by adoptive transfer of spleen cells from a normal syngeneic mouse. These findings are most consistent with deletion of those cells which cause diabetes by placement of islet antigens in the thymus during T-cell ontogeny.

A failure to delete autoreactive lymphocytes from the repertoire may be tightly linked to the MHC genes. As discussed earlier, the binding characteristics of the MHC gene products determine which antigens are presented to developing cells so that allelic variations in the gene sequences may dramatically alter the T-cell repertoire. Therefore, depending on the relative avidity for the antigen-MHC complex, autoreactive T cells may not be removed during negative selection and could cause autoimmunity when in the periphery. Faustman et al.[152] have found that expression of MHC class I gene products is lower on cells from humans and mice with diabetes compared with normal mice and humans. They ascribe their observations to a defect in processing of peptides for binding to class I MHC molecules. They postulate that in these patients and mice, the lower level of expression of class I products has resulted in a failure to delete islet antigen–reactive T cells during development. In their experiments, APC's from the diabetic twin discordant for diabetes showed reduced ability to stimulate automixed lymphocyte reactions to T cells taken from the nondiabetic twin.

This concept implies that autoimmunity may be oligoclonal (i.e., a limited number of lymphocyte clones are self reactive, making it possible to remove them and prevent disease without inducing global immunosuppression). For example, in an animal model of multiple sclerosis, experimental allergic encephalomyelitis (EAE), cellular responses against myelin basic protein (MBP) involve predominantly Vβ8.2+ T cells.[153] Removal of these cells in vivo with mAb can prevent the development of the disease.[154] It has even been possible to generate idiotopic responses against the TCR that can prevent autoimmune disease.[155–157] The experimental data thus far concerning the heterogeneity of T-cell responses in autoimmune endocrine diseases show evidence for both heterogeneous and more limited responses. For example, analysis of T cells infiltrating thyroid glands from patients with autoimmune thyroid disease show limited heterogeneity of the T-cell response.[158] However, a similar analysis of T cells infiltrating islets of Langerhans in NOD mice shows heterogeneity.[159–161] One of the important issues in studying these phenomena is the difficulty in identifying when the T-cell response begins because cells recruited later in the process may not respond to the primary antigen and the response may be more heterogeneous. Lehmann et al.[162] have found that during the inductive phase of EAE, immune tolerance toward a single determinant of MBP is impaired. In mice with chronic EAE, several additional determinants of MBP recall proliferative responses that had not stimulated responses during earlier phases of the disease. These determinants of MBP, which are cryptic during primary immunization, can become immunogenic later in the course of EAE. Therefore, the phenotypes of T cells that are found at the time of clinical presentation may not accurately reflect those of the cells which initiated the process or caused the earliest lesions.

EXPRESSION OF FOREIGN ANTIGENS ON THE SURFACES OF ENDOCRINE TISSUES. Foreign proteins, possibly even viral antigens, expressed on endocrine tissues through mechanisms described below may be recognized by the immune cells, and endocrine cells may be destroyed by virtue of their expression of these antigens. It should be noted, however, that expression of antigens (including alloantigens and viral peptides) on the surfaces of β cells as transgenes has often not resulted in immunological responses against those antigens despite the presence of antigen-reactive T cells in the circulation. Therefore, although immunological responses may be directed against foreign peptides on the surfaces of endocrine tissue, additional factors involving antigen processing and presentation and participation of co-stimulatory molecules are needed for the response to occur. In animal models, infection with a virus appears sufficient to trigger the immune response. Epidemiological data such as the seasonal occurrence of IDDM[163] or the finding of endogenous retroviral sequences in animal models[164] and patients with autoimmune endocrine disease suggest a pathogenic role for viruses in autoimmune endocrine disease. Recently, an association between human spumaretro virus, an endogenous retrovirus, and Graves' disease has been described.[165] Similar findings have been repeated in animal models of IDDM.[164] There are several examples in animal models of autoimmune endocrine diseases induced by viruses. The m variant of encephalomyocarditis virus can cause, in certain strains of mice, diabetes that is dependent on CD4+ T cells for its occurrence.[166] However, to date, a virus or other pathogenic organism that directly leads to autoimmune endocrine disease in humans has not been clearly identified. In one report, a strain of Coxsackie virus was isolated from a patient dying shortly after the onset of IDDM.[167] This virus showed tropism for pancreatic islets and could cause diabetes in laboratory animals. Guberski et al.[168] have identified a virus (Kilham's rat virus) that can cause diabetes in diabetes-resistant BB rats. In the latter, virus particles could be identified in spleen and liver but not in pancreatic islet cells. This raises the possibility that the pathogenesis of diabetes involves viral effects on immune regulation rather than direct effects on target tissues. In this regard, Oldstone et al.[169] have identified a strain of lymphocytic choriomeningitis virus that can infect CD4+ T cells in NOD mice and eliminate susceptibility to diabetes.

Several lines of evidence support the notion that mimicry between foreign peptides and autoantigens may result in autoreactivity. For example, a 64-kDa islet membrane protein that is recognized by autoantibodies in IDDM has been found recently to be glutamic acid decarboxylase.[2, 3]

Glutamate decarboxylase has molecular homology with the Coxsackie viral protein P2-C. Thus Coxsackie viral infection could precipitate anti–islet cell autoreactivity in genetically predisposed persons by inducing the formation of antibodies that, because of shared epitopes, react with islet cell glutamate decarboxylase.[170] A similar mechanism also may account for the high rate of development of IDDM in offspring of women who have had congenital rubella. Karjalainen et al.[171] have reported that patients with IDDM have antibodies that react with a discrete segment of bovine serum albumin (BSA), suggesting the possibility that mimicry between the BSA antigen and an islet antigen may trigger an anti-islet immune response. Although the relationship between dietary factors and development of autoimmune endocrine disease is still unresolved, a clear effect of dietary protein on the incidence of autoimmune diabetes has been demonstrated in experimental animals.[172, 173]

ACCESS OF THE IMMUNE SYSTEM TO ANTIGENS EXPRESSED ON PERIPHERAL ORGANS. The most well-characterized antigens of autoimmune endocrine disease, such as glutamic acid decarboxylase, insulin, microsomal antigen, thyroglobulin, and others, are constitutively expressed cellular proteins. Injury to endocrine tissue may cause shedding and presentation of antigens that are not normally available to the immune system. (Inflammation itself may lead to increased expression of homing receptors and co-stimulatory molecules.) If T-cell precursors reactive with these peripheral antigens are present in the circulation (presumably because the peripheral antigens were not expressed in the thymus at the time of T-cell ontogeny) and appropriate costimulatory signals are delivered, immune reactivity against these self proteins may occur.

Tissue injury may initiate this chain of events. An experimental model of autoimmunity that is believed to occur through this mechanism is diabetes induced with low doses of streptozocin in mice.[174–177] Streptozocin is an islet toxin that can induce diabetes when given in high dose because of its toxic effects on β cells. However, when given as five subdiabetogenic doses to certain strains of male mice, insulitis and hypoglycemia develop gradually. In this model, a T-cell–dependent immune response that occurs after injury to β cells is responsible for β cell destruction. Diabetes may be prevented by depletion of T cells and adoptively transferred with splenocytes.[176, 177]

It has been proposed that CD4+ T cells may gain access to self antigens as a result of heterotopic expression of class II MHC molecules.[178] Under normal condition, class II MHC molecules are not expressed on endocrine cells, and therefore, antigens that bind to these molecules are not presented to the immune system. However, the identification of class II MHC gene products by immunohistochemistry of thyroid cells has lead to the hypothesis that aberrant expression of class II MHC gene products may stimulate an immune response.[179] This hypothesis has been called into question on a number of accounts. First, it has been difficult to firmly establish that class II MHC expression does in fact occur on the surfaces of endocrine tissues in vivo and that the heterotopic expression of these molecules can initiate immune responses. Although treatment in vitro of certain endocrine cell lines with interferon-γ increases expression of MHC molecules, and thyrocytes do appear to express class II MHC gene products when stimulated with interferon-γ,[180] it is likely that the enhanced

MHC expression observed in endocrine tissues in vivo is secondary to exposure to cytokines rather than the primary event initiating autoimmunity. More recent studies of cells in the islets of Langerhans have shown that class II MHC expression is limited to immune cells (such as infiltrating macrophages) and is not seen on endocrine cells.[181] Data from transgenic models have indicated that it is unlikely that class II MHC expression alone on islet cells could initiate an immune response, since expression of even foreign class II MHC antigens on endocrine tissues as a transgene does not result in autoimmunity.[129] Finally, other data suggest that endocrine tissues that express class II MHC antigens as transgenes function poorly in antigen presentation. Islet cells that express class II MHC molecules may even induce anergy of antigen-reactive T cells.[103] Thus, although heterotopic expression of class II MHC molecules on endocrine tissues remains a plausible mechanism for breakdown of tolerance of CD4+ T cells, direct experimental evidence for this hypothesis is lacking.

DEFECTIVE IMMUNE REGULATION. The literature is replete with experimental findings that have been interpreted as defective immune regulation. These data include suggestions that antigen-specific and/or idiotype-specific suppressor cells may be responsible for maintenance of nonreactivity to self antigens. The argument has been that loss of inhibitory circuits leads to autoimmunity. Unfortunately, conclusions in these studies about lymphocyte function are often based on analysis of the phenotype of cells. This approach does not provide insight into mechanisms, since cells with the same cell surface markers may differ in their functional capabilities. However, certain specific examples do exist in experimental autoimmune endocrine diseases to indicate that regulatory networks may be involved in avoidance of autoimmunity.

Diabetes can be induced in a diabetes-resistant strain of BB/W rats by depletion of a subset of T cells that express RT-6 together with additional exogenous stimulation provided by mitogens.[182] RT-6+ T cells are present in normal rats but are not found in the peripheral T cells of diabetes-prone BB/W rats. Depletion of these cells with monoclonal antibodies leads to the development of diabetes in an MHC-identical, diabetes-resistant strain of rat. The functions of this subset of T cells as immune regulators may explain the ability of adoptive transfer of lymphocytes from diabetes-resistant BB rats to prevent diabetes in the diabetes-prone animals.[183] In NOD mice, the ability to adoptively transfer diabetes with spleen cells varies with the age of the recipient.[184] Before 6 weeks of age, pretreatment of the recipient is not needed, but after that age, adoptive transfer cannot be performed without irradiation. It has been suggested that cells capable of inhibiting the islet-reactive lymphocytes develop after 6 weeks, but in addition, cells capable of inhibiting diabetes may be present in the transferred cells. Islet-reactive T-cell clones have been isolated from NOD mice that are able to prevent IDDM,[185] as well as T-cell clones that can transfer IDDM.[186] The mechanisms for these "suppressor" effects are unknown. One possibility is that upon activation, these cells elaborate cytokines that are able to inhibit activation or cytokine production by other cells. Examples of cytokines that have these capabilities include interferon-γ and IL-10.

ROLE OF CYTOKINES. High local concentrations of cytokines appear capable of breaking tolerance to endocrine tissues. Those which are able to enhance antigen presentation or T-cell activation are most likely to do this. In doubly transgenic mice expressing alloantigen on the pancreatic β cells and TCR-reactive with the alloantigen, immune reactivity against the alloantigen and the β cells does not occur. However, T-cell responses can be stimulated if a third transgene, encoding IL-2 production by the β cells, is added.[128] Thus IL-2 may provide the signal to allow the alloantigen-reactive T cells to respond. Sarvetnick et al.[187, 188] have found that loss of tolerance, tissue destruction, and diabetes will occur with expression of IFN-γ in the β cells in the islets of Langerhans as a transgene. Both CD4+ and CD8+ T cells infiltrate the islets, and CD8+ T cells from these mice can lyse β cells in vitro. The mechanism of this effect is uncertain but is likely to involve the enhancement of antigen presentation and T-cell stimulatory signals.

EFFECTORS OF AUTOIMMUNE ENDOCRINE DISEASES

Most autoimmune endocrine diseases develop over a prolonged period of time, on the order of months to years. Although some diseases, such as IDDM, have an acute dramatic clinical presentation, evidence from studies of tissue-specific immunoglobulins indicates that signs of autoimmunity can be found years before clinical presentation of the disease.[189, 190] Over this period of time, the immune response against endocrine tissues may diversify as new epitopes are exposed with progressive cellular damage. Those cells recruited to the inflammatory reaction need not be reactive with the antigen that initiated the autoimmune response. Because of the increasing complexities of the response with time, animal models are most helpful in understanding the initiating events of disease and effector cells that are responsible for cellular damage. The chronic nature of the disease also implies that to be most effective, immunotherapies need to be administered at a preclinical stage of the disease, since by the time clinical presentation occurs, tissue damage is extensive and long-standing.

Immunoglobulins

Tissue-specific immunoglobulins have been described in most autoimmune endocrine diseases. The role of these immunoglobulins in the pathogenesis of autoimmune endocrine diseases, in general, is uncertain, but they have been very useful in prediction and diagnosis. In certain situations, such as measurement of islet cell antibodies and insulin-binding autoantibodies, together with loss of first-phase response to intravenous glucose, these tests can accurately predict future clinical IDDM in first-degree relatives of patients with IDDM.[189] In other situations, however, such as detection of thyroid autoantibodies, the serological markers indicate the presence of autoimmunity but are less accurate alone in predicting future disease.[141] In particular cases, clinical disease itself is due to the presence of immunoglobulins. Examples of such disease states are given below.

Autoantibodies that can stimulate the thyroid-stimulating hormone (TSH) receptor are responsible for the development of hyperthyroidism in Graves' disease.[191] There is some evidence that these IgG autoantibodies may be pauciclonal or even monoclonal in origin and may arise from one or a few B cells.[192] However, this issue is unresolved, and it is most likely that multiple TSH receptor autoantibodies, some blocking, some stimulating, and some even with anti-idiotypic activity, may occur.[193]

An analogous syndrome, type B insulin resistance, is due to the production of autoantibodies that bind to the insulin receptor and inhibit insulin action.[194] This usually results in diabetes without ketoacidosis but with severe insulin resistance. The levels of insulin in the serum in excess of 1000 μU/ml and massive doses of insulin (more than 10,000 units/day) are required for treatment, which is often ineffective. These antibodies are polyclonal and can be shown to impair insulin binding in vitro. Other autoantibodies, however, can directly stimulate the insulin receptor, resulting in hypoglycemia. These antibodies may occur spontaneously but also may evolve in patients with anti–insulin receptor antibodies. Many of these patients have other autoimmune features such as elevated levels of circulating IgG, including antinuclear antibodies, leukopenia, systemic lupus erythematosus, and others.

In IDDM, some serological factors are thought to cause functional impairments. Serum from patients with IDDM has been shown to cause impaired insulin release by cultured rat islets in response to glucose. More recently, Johnson et al.[195, 196] have suggested that immunoglobulins in IDDM may block glucose entry into β cells and thereby cause a reversible inhibition of insulin release by these cells. Their data suggest that these immunoglobulins are reactive with a glucose transporter found on islets (GLUT-2).

Autoantibodies that bind hormones may cause clinical disease by creating a repository of bound hormone that can release free hormone in an unpredictable manner and cause symptoms or by reducing the amount of free hormone available for binding to receptors. A well-described syndrome of hypoglycemia is caused by autoantibodies against insulin in patients who have never received exogenous insulin.[197-200] These polyclonal, low-affinity, high-capacity antibodies may periodically release bound insulin, causing hypoglycemia. Very little is known about the epitopes on human insulin that are recognized by the antibodies or the precipitating events in the pathogenesis of the disease. Most often patients are over 40 years age and have other manifestations of autoimmune disease such as antinuclear antibodies. Similar types of antibodies have been described in patients with multiple myeloma in which a monoclonal antibody that binds insulin has resulted in hypoglycemia.[201] An analogous syndrome has been described in which autoantibodies bind thyroid hormone.[202] This syndrome, however, is less commonly a cause of clinical disease because of the longer half-life of thyroid hormone.

Lymphocytes

In most experimental models of autoimmune endocrine diseases, T cells play a central role in the pathogenesis of the disease. For example, spontaneous thyroiditis in OS chickens is dependent on T cells because their complete removal within a day of hatching prevents disease later in life.[203] Experimental autoimmune thyroid disease also has been shown to be dependent on Lyt-1+ (T) cells; both Lyt-2+ (CD8+) and L3T4+ (CD4+) T cells are required for adoptive transfer of the murine disease.[204] Roep et al.[205] have isolated a T-cell clone from a patient with newly diagnosed IDDM that proliferates specifically to insulin secretory granule proteins (MW 35 to 41 kDa).[205] In all experimental models of IDDM, T-cell depletion prevents disease, and diabetes can be adoptively transferred with T cells or splenocytes.[166, 175, 177, 186, 206-210] Diabetes can be adoptively transferred to young BB rats with spleen cells cultured with Con A from diabetic BB rats.[211, 212] Transfer of diabetes is restricted to rats of the RT1u haplotype, but insulitis can occur in other haplotypes. In the case of IDDM in the NOD mouse, T-cell clones and bulk populations of T cells have been isolated that can adoptively transfer the disease.[186, 206-208] Both CD4+ and CD8+ splenocytes or T-cell clones are needed to transfer the disease. As found in other models of autoimmune endocrine disease, T-cell clones have been isolated that can proliferate specifically to islet antigens.[186, 206] Transgenic NOD mice have been prepared in which more than 95 per cent of the peripheral T cells express a TCR from a CD4+ islet–reactive T-cell clone.[206] In these mice, insulitis and diabetes occurred in a manner similar to spontaneous disease. The observations with this model indicate that in the NOD mice a single TCR is sufficient for pathogenesis of diabetes and that T cells can recognize islet antigens and gain access to the tissue, unlike other transgenic models discussed above. Experiments with bone marrow chimeras of (NOD × B10.D2)F1 mice have shown that the cells required for disease in NOD mice are bone marrow–derived and not affected by a nonsusceptible thymus.[207] Interestingly, when NOD mice were treated with anti–T-cell monoclonal antibodies to prevent diabetes, treatment was successful even when it commenced after the age at which T cells begin to infiltrate the islets of Langerhans.[212] Furthermore, when the treatment was then discontinued, tolerance to the development of the disease was seen. Although the mechanism of this phenomenon is still unresolved, it raises the possibility that autoimmune endocrine diseases may be prevented by treatment with T-cell–directed immunosuppressive therapy if the process can be indentified at an early, preclinical stage. The development of autoimmune diabetes in NOD mice correlates closely with T-cell responses to GAD. Kaufman et al. and Tisch et al. have shown that T-cell proliferative responses and immunoglobulin responses to recombinant GAD appear as insulitis develops.[212a, b] Intrathymic injection of GAD into young mice prevents diabetes, presumably because of loss of T-cell response to this protein. Interestingly, immunoglobulin responses are not eliminated by intrathymic injection of GAD (i.e., split tolerance).

Much less is known about the role of NK cells as effectors in endocrine diseases. These cytotoxic cells are neither MHC- nor antigen-restricted and do not express CD3 on their surfaces. It is noteworthy that in one biopsy from a patient with IDDM who died within 24 hours of diagnosis, NK cells could be identified in the islets together with T and B cells.[167] NK-cell abnormalities also have been identified in patients with autoimmune thyroid disease.[213]

Cytokines

Some experimental data have suggested that soluble mediators can directly damage endocrine tissues. For example, Bendetzen et al.[214] have shown that IL-1 has direct toxic effects on cultured cells and have postulated that its release in vivo may cause damage to insulin-producing cells.[214] Others have suggested that TNF with interferon-γ also may cause β cell damage.[215] IL-6 is produced by several types of cells, including mononuclear cells, vascular endothelial cells, and fibroblasts, and has diverse effects such as a growth factor for differentiated B cells. Diabetes may be prevented in NOD mice with antibodies that bind IL-6.[216] These observations raise the possibility that by virtue of their exquisite sensitivity to the toxic effects of these mediators, endocrine cells may fall prey to inflammatory responses that may occur in their vicinity. In this model, the antigen specificity is limited to the affector limb of the response. This notion is supported by the observation that frequent administration of conditioned media from splenocytes from diabetic BB rats cultured with Con A can induce diabetes at an early age in BB rats.[164] Autoimmune thyroid disease may appear in patients receiving high doses of rIL-2 as part of a therapy for malignant disease.[217] This is most likely due to the ability of IL-2 to stimulate thyroid-reactive T cells or even NK cells which express IL-2 receptors on their surfaces, but a clear understanding of this mechanism is not available.

Nonlymphoid Mononuclear Cells

Cells generally considered to function primarily as APC's also have been shown to be essential for the development of experimental autoimmune endocrine diseases. Macrophages produce IL-1 when activated, and administration to mice of silica particles, which impair macrophage function, can prevent development of autoimmune diabetes.[218] In a manner similar to the effects of IL-1, nitric oxide (NO) secreted in high concentrations by activated macrophages has been postulated to mediate destruction of islet cells in autoimmune diabetes.[219, 220] NO has been identified recently as an important mediator in the defense against tumor cells, fungi, protozoa, and mycobacteria and may have a role in immune regulation. Macrophages have been identified as the earliest cells infiltrating islets in experimental diabetes. Undoubtedly, these cells play an essential role because of their ability to present antigens and stimulate T cells, but the recent studies suggest that their soluble products have direct cytotoxic effects on endocrine cells.

CONCLUSION

By the time of clinical presentation, patients with autoimmune endocrine diseases manifest humoral and cellular immunity against self antigens, indicating that tolerance for these antigens has been lost. In this review we have provided a background for understanding how tolerance develops for antigens expressed by endocrine tissues under normal conditions and how this process may go awry, resulting in autoimmune endocrine disease. Tolerance for self antigens occurs through a series of developmental steps that remove or silence autoreactive B- and T-lymphocytes while fostering the development of cells reactive with foreign peptides. In this regard, the linkage between MHC genes and autoimmune endocrine diseases is not surprising, since MHC molecules control the gamut of antigens that can be presented to the immune system and hence determine how tolerance or immune reactivity develops. Additional mechanisms such as the co-stimulatory requirements for T-cell activation, inaccessibility of peptides to APC's and clonal deletion of antigen-reactive T cells operate in the peripheral tissues to limit autoreactivity of cells not removed during lymphocyte ontogeny. T-cell immune responses against even foreign antigens on peripheral tissue may not occur in the absence of appropriate APC's and co-stimulatory signals, indicating that factors other than the antigen itself are responsible for the initiation of autoreactivity. The initiation of T- and B-cell responses is critically dependent on activities of T helper cells, which therefore are the focus of mechanisms of pathogenesis.

Data from experimental models and most human data would support the notion that autoimmune endocrine diseases occur after chronic autoimmune responses that involve T-lymphocytes. Candidate antigens have been identified in the different disease states, but the involvement of these antigens in the initiation of disease has not been proven. Most of these antigens have been cellular proteins that are constitutively expressed by the endocrine tissues. However, the initiating factors in the diseases and key cellular structures involved in the immune responses remain unknown. Humoral responses against the target tissues have been demonstrated in all the human diseases as well as animal models, and in certain instances, autoreactive immunoglobulins can explain the pathogenesis of the disease. The immunoglobulin responses are important indicators of ongoing autoimmunity and, with appropriate supporting data, predict future disease.

Our understanding in the areas of antigen presentation and T- and B-cell activation suggests several new approaches to immunotherapy to prevent the development of autoimmune endocrine diseases. Most currently available immunosuppressive therapies are not specific in their sites of action. However, further understanding of the lymphocytes involved in the pathogenesis of these diseases and the mechanism of antigen presentation may afford more specific reagents that can be given safely to subjects before disease onset or to treat complications of the illnesses caused by immune mechanisms.

ACKNOWLEDGMENT: This work was supported by Grants K08 DK-01938 and R01 DK-44905 (to K.H.) and P01 CA-19266 from the National Institutes of Health.

REFERENCES

1. Weetman AP, McGregor AM: Autoimmune thyroid disease: Developments in our understanding. Endocr Rev 5:309–355, 1984.
2. Baekkeskov S, Nielsen J, Masner B, et al: Autoantibodies in newly diagnosed diabetic children immunoprecipitate human pancreatic islet cell proteins. Nature 298:167–170, 1982.
3. Baekkeskov S, Aanstoot HJ, Cristgau S, et al: Identification of the 64K autoantigen in insulin-dependent diabetes as the GABA-synthesizing enzyme glutamic acid decarboxylase. Nature 347:151–156, 1990.

4. Palmer JP, Asplin CM, Clemons P, et al: Insulin antibodies in insulin-dependent diabetics before insulin treatment. Science 222:1337–1339, 1983.

5. Schwartz RH: Acquisition of immunologic self-tolerance. Cell 57:1073–1081, 1989.

6. Hengartner H, Odermatt B, Schneider R, et al: Deletion of self-reactive T cells before entry into the thymus medulla. Nature 336:388–390, 1988.

7. Miller JFAP, Morahan G, Allison J, Hoffmann M: A transgenic approach to the study of peripheral T cell tolerance. Immunol Rev 122:103–116, 1991.

8. Jones LA, Chin LT, Longo DL, Kruisbeek AM: Peripheral clonal elimination of functional T cells. Science 250:1726–1729, 1990.

9. Kappler JW, Roehm N, Marrack P: T cell tolerance by clonal elimination in the thymus. Cell 49:273–280, 1987.

10. Hammerling G, Schonrich G, Momburg R, et al: Non-deletional mechanisms of peripheral and central tolerance: Studies with transgenic mice with tissue specific expression of a foreign MHC class I antigen. Immunol Rev 122:47–67, 1991.

11. Ramsdell F, Fowlkes BJ: Maintenance of in vivo tolerance by persistence of antigen. Science 257:1130–1133, 1992.

12. Nossal GJV, Pike BL: Clonal anergy: Persistence in tolerant mice of antigen-binding B lymphocytes incapable of responding to antigens or mitogen. Proc Natl Acad Sci (USA) 77:1602–1606, 1980.

13. Miller J, Daitch L, Rath S, Selsing E: Tissue-specific expression of allogeneic class II MHC molecules induces neither tissue rejection nor clonal inactivation of alloreactive T cells. J Immunol 144:334–341, 1990.

14. Goodnow CC: Transgenic mice and analysis of B cell tolerance. Annu Rev Immunol 10:489–518, 1992.

15. Asherson GL, Colizzi V, Zembalen M: An overview of T-suppressor cell circuits. Annu Rev Immunol 4:37–68, 1986.

16. Swat W, Ignatowicz L, von Boehmer H, Kisielow P: Clonal deletion of immature CD4+8+ thymocytes in suspension culture by extra-thymic antigen-presenting cells. Nature 351:150–153, 1991.

17. Nemazee D, Russell D, Dembic Z, Buerki K: Peripheral deletion of self-reactive B cells. Nature 354:308–311, 1991.

18. Nemazee D, Russell D, Arnold B, et al: Clonal deletion of autospecific B lymphocytes. Immunol Rev 122:117–132, 1991.

19. Nemazee DA, Buerki K: Clonal deletion of B lymphocytes in a transgenic mouse bearing anti-MHC class I antibody genes. Nature 337:562–566, 1989.

20. Nemazee DA, Buerki K: Clonal deletion of autoreactive B lymphocytes in bone marrow chimeras. Proc Natl Acad Sci (USA) 86:8039–8043, 1989.

21. Webb S, Morris C, Sprent J: Extrathymic tolerance of mature T cells: Clonal elimination as a consequence of immunity. Cell 63:1249–1256, 1990.

22. Hartley SB, Crosbie J, Brink R, et al: Elimination from peripheral lymphoid tissues of self-reactive B lymphocytes recognizing membrane-bound antigens. Nature 353:765–769, 1991.

23. Rocha B, von Boehmer H: Peripheral selection of the T cell repertoire. Science 251:1225–1228, 1991.

24. Murphy KM, Heimberger AB, Loh DY: Induction by antigen of intrathymic apoptosis of CD4+CD8+TCR^lo thymocytes in vivo. Science 250:1720–1722, 1990.

25. Teh H-S, Kishi H, Scott B, von Boehmer H: Deletion of autospecific T cells in T cell receptor (TCR) transgenic mice spares cells with normal TCR levels and low levels of CD8 molecules. J Exp Med 169:795–806, 1989.

26. Miller JFAP, Morahan G: Peripheral T cell tolerance. Annu Rev Immunol 10:51–70, 1992.

27. Blackman MA, Finkel TH, Kappler J, et al: Altered antigen receptor signaling in anergic T cells from self-tolerant T-cell receptor β-chain transgenic mice. Proc Natl Acad Sci USA 88:6682–6686, 1991.

28. Kang S-M, Beverly B, Tran A-C, et al: Transactivation by AP-1 is a molecular target of T cell clonal anergy. Science 257:1134–1138, 1992.

29. Goodnow CC, Brink R, Adams E: Breakdown of self-tolerance in anergic B lymphocytes. Nature 352:532–536, 1991.

30. Ohashi PS, Oehen S, Buerki K, et al: Ablation of ''tolerance'' and induction of diabetes by virus infection in viral antigen transgenic mice. Cell 65:305–317, 1991.

31. Bohme J, Haskins K, Stecha P, et al: Transgenic mice with I-A on islet cells are normoglycemic but immunologically intolerant. Science 246:1179–1183, 1989.

32. Oldstone MBA, Nerenberg M, Southern P, et al: Virus infection triggers insulin-dependent diabetes mellitus in a transgenic model: Role of anti-self (virus) immune response. Cell 65:319–331, 1991.

33. Quintans J, Zuckerman L: Idiotypes and immune networks. In Encyclopedia of Human Biology, Vol 4. San Diego, Academic Press, 1991, pp 313–317.

34. Cohen IR: Physiological bases of T-cell vaccination against autoimmune disease. Cold Spring Harbor Symp Quant Biol 54:879–886, 1989.

35. Hannet I, Erkeller-Yuksel F, Lydyard P, et al: Developmental and maturational changes in human blood lymphocyte subpopulations. Immunol Today 13:215–220, 1992.

36. Hsu S-M, Cossman J, Jaffe ES: Lymphocyte subsets in normal human lymphoid tissues. Am J Clin Pathol 80:21–30, 1983.

37. Malissen M, Minard K, Mjolsness S, et al: Mouse T cell antigen receptor: Structure and organization of constant and joining gene segments encoding the β polypeptide. Cell 37:1101–1110, 1984.

38. Jorgensen JL, Reay PA, Ehrich EW, Davis M: Molecular components of T cell recognition. Annu Rev Immunol 10:835–873, 1992.

39. Davis M: T cell receptor gene diversity and selection. Annu Rev Biochem 59:475–496, 1990.

40. Janeway CA: The T cell receptor as a multicomponent signaling machine: CD4/CD8 co-receptors and CD45 in T cell activation. Annu Rev Immunol 10:645–674, 1992.

41. Fleury SG, Crouteau G, Sekaly R-P: CD4 and CD8 recognition of class II and class I molecules of the major histocompatibility complex. Semin Immunol 3:177–186, 1991.

42. Abbas AK, Williams ME, Burstein HJ, et al: Activation and functions of CD4+ T-cell subsets. Immunol Rev 123:5–22, 1991.

43. Kelso A, Troutt AB, Maraskovsky E, et al: Heterogeneity in lymphokine profiles of CD4+ and CD8+ T cells and clones activated in vivo and in vitro. Immunol Rev 123:85–114, 1991.

44. Swain SL, Bradley LM, Croft M, et al: Helper T-cell subsets: Phenotype, function and the role of lymphokines in regulating their development. Immunol Rev 123:115–144, 1991.

45. Romagnani S: Human Th1 and Th2 subsets: Doubt no more. Immunol Today 12:256–261, 1991.

46. Young JD-E: Killing of target cells by lymphocytes: A mechanistic view. Physiol Rev 69:250–314, 1989.

47. Karlhofer FM, Ribaudo RK, Yokoyama WM. MHC class I alloantigen specificity of Ly-49+ IL-2–activated killer cells. Nature 358:66–70, 1992.

48. Allison JP, Havran WL: The immunobiology of T cells with invariant γΓ antigen receptors. Annu Rev Immunol 9:679–705, 1991.

49. Dorf ME, Bennacerraf B: Suppressor cells and immunoregulation. Annu Rev Immun 2:127–158, 1984.

50. Bloom BR, Salgame P, Diamond B: Revisiting and revising suppressor T cells. Immunol Today 13:131, 1992.

51. Powrie F, Mason D: OX-22^high CD4+ T cells induced wasting disease with multiple organ pathology: Prevention by the OX-22^low subset. J Exp Med 172:1701–1708, 1990.

52. Peltz G: A role for CD4+ T-cell subsets producing a selective pattern of lymphokines in the pathogenesis of human chronic inflammatory and allergic diseases. Immunol Rev 123:23–36, 1991.

53. Rolnick A, Melchers F: Molecular and cellular origins of B lymphocyte diversity. Cell 66:1081–1094, 1991.

54. Clark EA, Lane PJL: Regulation of human B-cell activation and adhesion. Annu Rev Immunol 9:97–127, 1991.

55. Finkelman FD, Lees A, Morris SC: Antigen presentation by B lymphocytes to CD4+ T lymphocytes in vivo: Importance for B lymphocyte and T lymphocyte activation. Semin Immunol 4:247–256, 1992.

56. Noelle RJ, Meenakshi R, Shepherd DM, et al: A 39-kDa protein on activated helper T cells binds CD40 and transduces the signal for cognate activation of B cells. Proc Natl Acad Sci USA 89:6550–6554, 1992.

57. Casali P, Notkins AL: CD5+ B lymphocytes, polyreactive antibodies and the human B-cell repertoire. Immunol Today 10:364–369, 1989.

58. Solvason N, Kearney JF: The human fetal omentum: A site of B cell generation. J Exp Med 175:397–404, 1992.

59. Hardy RR: Variable gene usage, physiology and development of Ly-1+ (CD5+) B cells. Curr Opin Immunol 4:181–185, 1992.

60. Murakami M, Tsubata T, Okamoto M, et al: Antigen-induced apoptotic death of Ly-1 B cells responsible for autoimmune disease in transgenic mice. Nature 357:77–80, 1992.

61. Fitch FW, Lancki DW, Gajewski TF: T-cell mediated immune regulation: Help and suppression. In Paul W (ed): Fundamental Immunology. New York, Raven Press, 1993.

62. Bjorkman PH, Saper MA, Samraoui B, et al: The foreign antigen binding site and T cell recognition regions of class I histocompatibility antigens. Nature 329:512–518, 1987.

63. Brown JH, Jardetzky T, Saper MA, et al: A hypothetical model of the

foreign antigen binding site of class II histocompatibility molecules. Nature 332:845–850, 1988.

64. Van Bleek GM, Nathensen SG: Presentation of antigenic peptides by MHC class I molecules. Trends Cell Biol 2:202–207, 1992.

65. Germain RN, Hendrix LR: MHC class II structure, occupancy and surface expression determined by post-endoplasmic reticulum antigen binding. Nature 353:134–139, 1991.

66. Rothbard JB, Gefter MC: Interactions between immunogenic peptides and MHC proteins. Annu Rev Immunol 9:527–565, 1991.

67. Townsend A, Ohlen C, Bastin J, et al: Association of class I major histocompatibility heavy and light chains induced by viral peptides. Nature 340:443–448, 1989.

68. Monaco JJ, Cho S, Attaya M: Transport protein genes in the murine MHC: Possible implications for antigen processing. Science 250:1723–1726, 1990.

69. Glynne R, Powis SH, Beck S, et al: A proteasome-related gene between the two ABC transporter loci in the class II region of the human MHC. Nature 353:357–358, 1991.

70. Brown MG, Driscoll J, Monaco JJ: Structural and serological similarity of MHC-linked LMP and proteasome (multicatalytic proteinase) complexes. Nature 353:355–357, 1991.

71. Cho S, Attaya M, Monaco JJ: New class II-like genes in the murine MHC. Nature 353:573–576, 1991.

72. Sambhara SR, Miller RG: Programmed cell death of T cells signaled by the T cell receptor and the α$_{3}$ domain of class I MHC. Science 252:1424–1427, 1991.

73. Allison J, Campbell IL, Morahan G, et al: Diabetes in transgenic mice resulting from over-expression of class I histocompatibility molecules in pancreatic β cells. Nature 333:529–533, 1988.

74. Morahan G, Allison J, Miller JFAP: Tolerance of class I histocompatibility antigens expressed extrathymically. Nature 339:622–624, 1989.

75. Morahan G, Hoffmann M, Miller JFAP: A non-deletional mechanism of peripheral tolerance in T cell receptor transgenic mice. Proc Natl Acad Sci USA 88:11421–11425, 1991.

75a. Brown JH, Jardetkz TS, Gorga JC, et al: Three-dimensional structure of the human class II histocompatibility antigen HLA-DR1. Nature 364:33–39, 1993.

76. Chicz RM, Urban RG, Lane WS, et al: Predominant naturally processed peptides bound to HLA-DR1 are derived from MHC-related molecules and are heterogeneous in size. Nature 358:764–768, 1992.

77. Hunt DF, Michel H, Dickinson TA, et al: Peptides presented to the immune system by the murine class II major histocompatibility complex molecule I-A^{d}. Science 256:1817–1820, 1992.

78. Sadegh-Nasseri S, Germain RN: A role for peptide in determining MHC class II structure. Nature 353:167–169, 1991.

79. Doyle C, Ford PJ, Ponath PD, et al: Regulation of the class II-associated invariant chain gene in normal and mutant B lymphocytes. Proc Natl Acad Sci USA 87:4590–4594, 1990.

80. Neefjes JJ, Ploegh HL: Intracellular transport of MHC class II molecules. Immunol Today 13:179, 1992.

81. Trowsdale J, Regousis J, Campbell RD, et al: Map of the human MHC. Immunol Today 12:443, 1991.

82. Bach FH, Rich SS, Barbosa RS, Segall M: Insulin-dependent diabetes-associated HLA-D region encoded determinants. Hum Immunol 12:59–64, 1985.

83. Todd JA, Acha-Orbea H, Bell JI, et al: A molecular basis for MHC class II–associated autoimmunity. Science 24:1003–1009, 1988.

84. Baish JM, Weeks T, Giles R, et al: Analysis of HLA-DQ genotypes and susceptibility in insulin-dependent diabetes mellitus. N Engl J Med 322:1836–1841, 1990.

85. Todd JA, Bell JI, McDevitt HO: HLA-DQβ gene contributes to susceptibility and resistance to insulin-dependent diabetes mellitus. Nature 329:599–604, 1987.

86. Nepom GT: Immunogenetics of HLA-associated diseases Concepts Immunopathol S:80–105, 1988.

87. Wicker L, Miller BJ, Coker LZ, et al: Genetic control of diabetes and insulitis in the nonobese diabetic (NOD) mouse. J Exp Med 165:1639–1654, 1987.

88. Moens H, Farid NR: Hashimoto's thyroiditis is associated with HLA-DRw3. N Engl J Med 299:133–134, 1978.

89. Guery JC, Sette A, Leighton J, et al: Selective immunosuppression by administration of major histocompatibility complex (MHC) class II-binding peptides: I. Evidence for in vivo MHC blockade preventing T cell activation. J Exp Med 175:1345–1352, 1992.

90. Adorini L, Barnaba V, Bona C, et al: New perspectives to immunointervention in autoimmune diseases. Immunol Today 11:383–387, 1990.

91. Jenkins MK, Schwartz RH: Antigen presentation by chemically modified splenocytes induces antigen-specific T cell unresponsiveness in vitro and in vivo. J Exp Med 165:302–319, 1987.

92. Mueller CL, Jenkins MK, Schwartz RH: Clonal expansion versus functional clonal inactivation: A co-stimulatory signalling pathway determines the outcome of T cell antigen receptor occupancy. Annu Rev Immunol 7:445–480, 1989.

93. Golde WT, Gay D, Kappler J, Marrack: The role of LFA-1 in class II restricted, antigen specific T cell responses. Cell Immunol 103:73–79, 1986.

94. Makgoba WW, Sanders ME, Luce GEG, et al: Functional evidence that ICAM-1 is a ligand for LFA-1 dependent adhesion in T cell-mediated cytotoxicity. Eur J Immunol 18:637–641, 1988.

95. Springer TA, Dustin ML, Kishimoto TK, Marlin SD: The lymphocyte function associated LFA-1, CD2 and LFA-3 molecules: Cell adhesion receptors of the immune system. Annu Rev Immunol 5:223–252, 1987.

96. Isobe M, Yagita H, Okumura K, Ihara A: Specific acceptance of cardiac allograft after treatment with antibodies to ICAM-1 and LFA-1. Science 255:1125–1227, 1992.

97. Brietmeyer JB, Daley JF, Leuine HB, Schlossman SF: The CD2 molecule is functionally linked to T3/Ti cell receptor in the majority of T cells. J Immunol 139:2899–2905, 1987.

98. Dustin ML, Springer TA: Role of lymphocyte adhesion receptors in transient interactions and cell locomotion. Annu Rev Immunol 9:27–66, 1991.

99. Liu Y, Linsley PS: Costimulation of T-cell growth. Curr Opin Immunol 4:265–270, 1992.

100. Linsley PS, Wallace PM, Johnson J, et al: Immunosuppression in vivo by a soluble form of the CTLA-4 T cell activation molecule. Science 257:792–795, 1992.

101. Brunet JF, Denizot F, Luciani MF, et al: A new member of the immunoglobulin superfamily CTLA-4. Nature 328:267–270, 1987.

102. Lenschow DJ, Zeng Y, Thistlethwaite JR, et al: Long-term survival of xenogenic pancreatic islet grafts induced by CTLA4Ig. Science 257:789–792, 1992.

103. Markmann J, Lo D, Naji A, et al: Antigen presenting function of class II MHC expressing pancreatic beta cells. Nature 336:476–479, 1988.

104. Campbell IL, Cutri A, Wilkinson D, et al: Intercellular adhesion molecule 1 is induced on isolated endocrine islet cells by cytokines but not by reovirus infection. Proc Natl Acad Sci USA 86:4282–4286, 1989.

105. Hutchings P, Rosen H, O'Reilly L, et al: Transfer of diabetes in mice prevented by blockade of adhesion-promoting receptor on macrophages. Nature 348:639–642, 1990.

106. Amano K, Yoneda R, Tominaga Y, et al: Association of ICAM-1 and LFA-1 molecules in the development of diabetes in NOD mice. Diabetes 41:38A, 1992.

107. Von Boehmer H: The developmental biology of T lymphocytes. Annu Rev Immunol 6:309–326, 1988.

108. Adkins B, Mueller C, Okada CY, et al: Early events in T cell maturation. Annu Rev Immunol 5:325–365, 1987.

109. MacDonald HR, Hengartner H, Pedrazzini T: Intrathymic deletion of self-reactive cells prevented by neonatal anti-CD4 antibody treatment. Nature 335:174–176, 1988.

110. Kisielow P, Teh HS, Bluthmann H, von Boehmer H: Positive selection of antigen-specific T cells in thymus by restricting MHC molecules. Nature 355:730–733, 1988.

111. Blackman M, Kappler J, Marrack P: The role of the T cell receptor in positive and negative selection of developing T cells. Science 248:1335–1337, 1990.

112. Aldrich CJ, Hammer RE, Jones-Youngblood S, et al: Negative and positive selection of antigen-specific cytotoxic T lymphocytes affected by the α3 domain of MHC I molecules. Nature 352:718–721, 1991.

113. Marrack P, Lo D, Brinster R, et al: The effect of thymus environment on development and tolerance. Cell 53:627–634, 1988.

114. Vukmanovic S, Grandea AG III, Faas SJ, et al: Positive selection of T-lymphocytes induced by intrathymic injection of a thymic epithelial cell line. Nature 359:729–732, 1992.

115. McDonald HR, Schreider R, Lees RK, et al: T cell receptor Vβ use predicts reactivity and tolerance to MIs^{a} encoded antigens. Nature 332:40–45, 1988.

116. Roberts JL, Sharrow SO, Singer A: Clonal deletion and clonal anergy in the thymus induced by cellular elements with different radiation sensitivities. J Exp Med 171:935–940, 1990.

117. Murphy DB, Lo D, Roth S, Brinster RL: A novel MHC class II epitope expressed in the thymic medulla but not cortex. Nature 338:765–768, 1989.

118. Lorenz RG, Allen PM: Thymic epithelial cells lack the capacity for antigen presentation. Nature 340:557–591, 1989.

119. Mizuochi T, Kasai M, Kokuho T, et al: Medullary but not cortical thymic epithelial cells present soluble antigens to helper T cells. J Exp Med 175:1601–1605, 1992.

120. Ingold AL, Landel C, Knall C, et al: Co-engagement of CD8 with the T cell receptor is required for negative selection. Nature 352:721–724, 1991.

121. Sentman CL, Shutter JR, Hockenbery D, et al: bcl-2 inhibits multiple forms of apoptosis but not negative selection in thymocytes. Cell 67:879–888, 1991.

122. DeFranco AL: bcl-2 to the rescue. Curr Biol 2:95–97, 1992.

123. Strasser A, Harris AW, Cory S: bcl-2 transgene inhibits T cell death and perturbs thymic self-censorship. Cell 67:889–899, 1991.

124. Strasser A, Whittingham S, Vaux DL, et al: Enforced Bcl-2 expression in B-lymphoid cells prolongs antibody responses and elicits autoimmune disease. Proc Natl Acad Sci USA 88:8661–8665, 1991.

125. Campbell IL, Wong GHW, Schrader JW, Harrison LC: Interferon-γ enhances the expression of the major histocompatibility class I antigens on mouse pancreatic beta cells. Diabetes 34:1205–1209, 1985.

126. Lo D, Burkly LC, Widera G, et al: Diabetes and tolerance in transgenic mice expressing class II MHC molecules in pancreatic beta cells. Cell 53:159–168, 1988.

127. Burkly LC, Lo D, Kanagawa O, et al: T cell tolerance by clonal anergy in transgenic mice with non-lymphoid expression of MHC class II I-E. Nature 342:564–566, 1988.

128. Heath WR, Allison J, Hoffmann MW, et al: Autoimmune diabetes as a consequence of locally produced interleukin-2. Nature 359:547–549, 1992.

129. Lo D, Freedman J, Hesse S, et al: Peripheral tolerance in transgenic mice: Tolerance to class II MHC and non-MHC transgene antigens. Immunol Rev 122:87–102, 1991.

130. Roman LM, Simons LF, Hammer RE, et al: The expression of influenza virus hemagglutinin in the pancreatic β cells of transgenic mice results in autoimmune diabetes. Cell 61:383–396, 1990.

131. Fields LI, Loh D: Organ injury associated with extrathymic induction of immune tolerance in doubly transgenic mice. Proc Natl Acad Sci USA 89:5730–5734, 1992.

132. Mason DY, Jones M, Goodnow CC: Development and follicular localization of tolerant B lymphocytes in lysozyme/anti-lysozyme IgM/IgD-transgenic mice. Int Immunol 4:163–175, 1992.

133. Goodnow CC, Crosbie J, Jorgensen H, et al: Induction of self-tolerance in mature peripheral B lymphocytes. Nature 342:385–391, 1989.

134. Goodnow CC, Crosbie J, Adelstein S, et al: Altered immunoglobulin expression and functional silencing of self-reactive B lymphocytes in transgenic mice. Nature 334:676–682, 1988.

135. Erikson J, Radic MZ, Camper S, et al: Expression of anti-DNA immunoglobulin transgenes in non-autoimmune mice. Nature 349:331–334, 1991.

136. Hartley SB, Crosbie J, Brink R, et al: Elimination from peripheral lymphoid tissues of self-reactive B lymphocytes recognizing membrane bound antigens. Nature 353:765–769, 1991.

137. Karvelas M, Nossal GJV: Memory cell generation ablated by soluble protein antigen by means of effects on T- and B-lymphocyte compartments. Proc Natl Acad Sci USA 89:3150–3154, 1992.

138. Jerne NK: Idiotypic networks and other preconceived ideas. Immunol Rev 79:5–35, 1984.

139. Gaulton GN, Greene MI: Idiotypic mimicry of biological receptors. Annu Rev Immunol 4:253–280, 1986.

140. Burdette S, Schwartz RS: Idiotypes and idiotypic networks. N Engl J Med 317:219–223, 1987.

141. Turnbridge WMG, Evered DC, Hall R, et al: The spectrum of thyroid disease in the community: The Whickham survey. Clin Endocrinol 7:481–492, 1977.

142. Riley WJ, Maclaren NK, Krisher J, et al: A prospective study of the development of diabetes in relatives of patients with insulin-dependent diabetes. N Engl J Med 323:1167–1172, 1990.

143. Williams ED, Doniach I: The post-mortem incidence of focal thyroiditis. J Pathol 83:255–264, 1962.

144. Day MJ, Tse AGD, Puklavec M, et al: Targeting autoantigen to B cells prevents the induction of a cell-mediated autoimmune disease in rats. J Exp Med 175:655–659, 1992.

145. Jenkins MK, Schwartz RH, Pardoll DM: Effects of cyclosporin A on T cell development and clonal deletion. Science 241:1655–1658, 1988.

146. Kosaka H, Matsubara H, Sogoh S, et al: An in vitro model for cyclosporin A–induced interference of intrathymic clonal elimination. J Exp Med 172:395–398, 1990.

147. Gao E-K, Lo D, Cheney R, et al: Abnormal differentiation of thymocytes in mice treated with cyclosporin A. Nature 336:176–179, 1988.

148. DeGroot LJ: Personal communication, 1992.

149. Posselt AM, Barker CF, Friedman AL, Naji A: Prevention of autoimmune diabetes in the BB rat by intrathymic islet transplantation at birth. Science 256:1321–1324, 1992.

150. Koevary SB, Blomberg M: Prevention of diabetes in BB/Wor rats by intrathymic islet injection. J Clin Invest 89:512–520, 1992.

151. Herold KC, Montag AG, Buckingham F: Induction of tolerance to autoimmune diabetes with islet antigens. J Exp Med 176:1107–1114, 1992.

152. Faustman D, Li XP, Lin HY, et al: Linkage of faulty major histocompatibility complex class I to autoimmune diabetes. Science 254:1756–1761, 1991.

153. Acha-Orbea H, Steinman L, McDevitt HO: T-cell receptors in autoimmune diseases. Annu Rev Immunol 7:371–405, 1989.

154. Acha-Orbea H, Mitchell DJ, Timmermann L, et al: Limited heterogeneity of T-cell receptors from lymphocytes mediating autoimmune encephalomyelitis allows specific immune interventions. Cell 54:263–273, 1988.

155. Vandenbark AA, Hashim G, Offner H: Immunization with a synthetic T-cell receptor V-region peptide protects against experimental autoimmune encephalomyelitis. Nature 341:541–544, 1989.

156. Howell MD, Winters ST, Olee T, et al: Vaccination against experimental allergic encephalomyelitis with T cell receptor peptides. Science 246:668–670, 1989.

157. Offner H, Hasshim GA, Vandenbark AA: T cell receptor peptide therapy triggers autoregulation of experimental encephalomyelitis. Science 251:430–432, 1991.

158. Davies TF, Martin A, Concepcion ES, et al: Evidence of limited variability of antigen-receptors on intrathyroidal T cells in autoimmune thyroid disease. N Engl J Med 325:238–244, 1991.

159. Waters SH, O'Neil JJ, Melican DT, Appel MC: Multiple TCR Vβ usage by infiltrates of young NOD mouse islets of Langerhans. Diabetes 41:308–312, 1992.

160. Candelias S, Katz J, Benoist C, et al: Islet-specific T-cell clones from nonobese diabetic mice express heterogeneous T-cell receptors. Proc Natl Acad Sci USA 88:6167–6170, 1991.

161. Nakano N, Kikutani H, Nishimoto H, Kishimoto T: T cell receptor V gene usage of islet β cell–reactive T cells is not restricted in nonobese diabetic mice. J Exp Med 173:1091–1097, 1991.

162. Lehmann PV, Forsthumer T, Miller A, Sercarz EE: Spreading of T-cell autoimmunity to cryptic determinants of an autoantigen. Nature 358:155–157, 1992.

163. Ludvigsson J, Afoke AO: Seasonality of type 1 (insulin-dependent) diabetes mellitus: Values of C-peptide, insulin antibodies and haemoglobin A1c show evidence of a more rapid loss of insulin secretion in epidemic patients. Diabetologia 32:84–91, 1989.

164. Rossini AA, Mordes JP, Like AA: Immunology of insulin-dependent diabetes mellitus. Annu Rev Immunol 3:289–320, 1985.

165. Lagaye S, Vexiau P, Morozov V, et al: Human spumaretrovirus-related sequences in the DNA of leukocytes from patients with Graves disease. Proc Natl Acad Sci USA 89:10070–10074, 1992.

166. Haynes MK, Huber SA, Craighead JE: Helper-inducer T-lymphocytes mediate diabetes in EMC-infected BALB/c ByJ mice. Diabetes 36:877–881, 1987.

167. Yoon J-W, Austin M, Onodera T, Notkins AL: Virus-induced diabetes mellitus: Isolation of a virus from the pancreas of a child with diabetic ketoacidosis. N Engl J Med 300:1173–1179, 1979.

168. Guberski DL, Thomas VA, Shek WR, et al: Induction of type 1 diabetes by Kilham's rat virus in diabetes-resistant BB/Wor rats. Science 254:1010–1013, 1991.

169. Oldstone MBA: Prevention of type 1 diabetes in nonobese diabetic mice by virus infection. Science 239:500–502, 1988.

170. Kaufman DL, Erlander MG, Clare-Salzler M, et al: Autoimmunity to two forms of glutamate decarboxylase in insulin-dependent diabetes mellitus. J Clin Invest 89:283–292, 1992.

171. Karjalainen J, Martin JM, Knip M, et al: A bovine albumin peptide as a possible trigger of insulin-dependent diabetes mellitus. N Engl J Med 327:302–307, 1992.

172. Elliott RB, Martin JM: Dietary protein: A trigger of insulin-dependent diabetes in the BB rat? Diabetologia 26:297–299, 1984.

173. Coleman DL, Kuzava JE, Leiter EH: Effect of diet on incidence of diabetes in nonobese diabetic mice. Diabetes 39:432–436, 1990.

174. Rossini AA, Like AA, Chick WL, et al: Studies of streptozotocin-induced diabetes. Proc Natl Acad Sci USA 74:2485–2490, 1977.

175. Herold KC, Bluestone JA, Montag AG, et al: Prevention of autoimmune diabetes with nonactivating anti-CD3 monoclonal antibody. Diabetes 41:385–391, 1992.

176. Herold KC, Montag AG, Fitch FW: Treatment with anti-T-lymphocyte

antibodies prevents induction of insulitis in mice given multiple doses of streptozotocin. Diabetes 36:796–801, 1987.

177. Kim YT, Steinberg C: Immunologic studies on the induction of diabetes in experimental animals, cellular basis for the induction of diabetes by streptozotocin. Diabetes 33:771–777, 1984.

178. Hanafusa T, Pujol-Borrell R, Chiovato L, et al: Aberrant expression of HLA-DR antigen on thyrocytes in Graves' disease: Relevance for autoimmunity. Lancet 2:1111–1115, 1983.

179. Pujol-Borrell R, Hanafusa T, Chiovato L, Bottazzo GF: Lectin-induced expression of DR antigen on human cultured follicular thyroid cells. Nature 304:71–73, 1983.

180. Weetman AP, Rees AJ: Synergistic effects of recombinant tumor necrosis factor (TNF) and gamma interferon on rat thyroid cell growth and Ia antigen expression. Immunology 63:285–289, 1988.

181. McInerney MF, Rath S, Janeway CA: Exclusive expression of MHC class II proteins on CD45+ cells in pancreatic islets of NOD mice. Diabetes 40:648–651, 199.

182. Like AA: Depletion of RT6.1+ T lymphocytes alone is insufficient to induce diabetes in diabetes-resistant BB/Wor rats. Am J Pathol 136:565–574, 1990.

183. Rossini AA, Faustman D, Woda B, Like AA: Lymphocyte transfusions prevent diabetes in the Biobreeding/Worcester (BB/W) rat. J Clin Invest 74:39–45, 1984.

184. Boitard C, Yasunami R, Dardenne M, Bach JF: T cell-mediated inhibition of the transfer of autoimmune diabetes in NOD mice. J Exp Med 169:1669–1680, 1989.

185. Pankewycz O, Strom TB, Rubin-Kelley VE: Islet-infiltrating T cell clones from non-obese diabetic mice that promote or prevent accelerated onset diabetes. Eur J Immunol 21:873–879, 1991.

186. Reich EP, Sherwin RS, Kanagawa O, Janeway CA: An explanation for the protective effect of the MHC class II I-E molecule in murine diabetes. Nature 341:326–328, 1989.

187. Sarvetnick N, Shizuru J, Liggitt D, et al: Loss of pancreatic islet tolerance induced by β-cell expression of interferon-γ. Nature 346:844–847, 1990.

188. Sarvetnick N, Liggitt D, Pitts SL, et al: Insulin-dependent diabetes mellitus induced in transgenic mice by ectopic expression of class II MHC and interferon-gamma. Cell 52:773–782, 1988.

189. Ziegler AG, Ziegler R, Vardi P, et al: Life-table analysis of progression to diabetes of anti-insulin autoantibody-positive relatives of individuals with type 1 diabetes. Diabetes 38:1320–1325, 1989.

190. Srikanta S, Ganda OP, Eisenbarth GS, Soeldner JS: Islet-cell antibodies and beta-cell function in monozygotic triplets and twins initially discordant for type 1 diabetes mellitus. N Engl J Med 308:322–327, 1983.

191. Kriss JP, Pleshakov V, Chien JR: Isolation and identification of the long-acting thyroid stimulator and its relation to hyperthyroidism and circumscribed pretibial myxedema. J Clin Endocrinol Metab 24:1005–1028, 1964.

192. Zakarija M: Immunochemical characterization of the thyroid-stimulating antibody (T Sab) of Grave's disease: Evidence for restricted heterogeneity. J Clin Lab Immunol 10:77–85, 1983.

193. Zakarija M, McKenzie JM, Banovac K: Clinical significance of assay of thyroid-stimulating antibody in Graves' disease. Ann Intern Med 93:28–32, 1980.

194. Moller DE, Flier JS: Insulin resistance: Mechanisms, syndromes, and implications. N Engl J Med 325:938–948, 1991.

195. Johnson JJ, Crider BP, McCorkle K, et al: Inhibition of glucose transport into rat islet cells by immunoglobulin from patients with insulin-dependent diabetes mellitus. N Engl J Med 322:653, 1990.

196. Unger RH: Diabetic hyperglycemia: Link to impaired glucose transport in pancreatic β cells. Science 251:1200–1205, 1991.

197. Goldman J, Baldwin D, Rubenstein AH, et al: Characterization of circulating insulin and proinsulin binding antibodies in autoimmune hypoglycemia. J Clin Invest 63:1050–1059, 1979.

198. Folling I, Norman N: Hyperglycemia, hypoglycemic attacks and production of anti-insulin antibodies without previous known immunization: Immunological and function studies in a patient. Diabetes 21:814–826, 1972.

199. Anderson JH Jr, Blackard WE, Goldman J, Rubenstein AH: Diabetes and hypoglycemia due to insulin antibodies. Am J Med 64:868–873, 1978.

200. Blackshear PJ, Rotner HE, Kriauciunas KAM, Kahn CR: Reactive hypoglycemia and insulin antibodies in drug-induced lupus erythematosus. Ann Intern Med 99:182–184, 1983.

201. Redmon B, Pyzdrowski KL, Elson MK, et al: Hypoglycemia due to a monoclonal insulin-binding antibody in multiple myeloma. N Engl J Med 326:994–998, 1992.

202. Sakata S, Nakamura S, Miura K: Autoantibodies against thyroid hormone of idiothyronine. Ann Intern Med 103:579–589, 1985.

203. Pontes de Carvalho LP, Templeman J, Wick G, Roitt IM: The role of self-antigen in the development of autoimmunity in obese strain chickens with spontaneous autoallergic thyroiditis. J Exp Med 155:1255–1266, 1982.

204. Sakaguchi S, Sakaguchi N: Organ-specific disease induced in mice by elimination of T cell subsets. J Immunol 142:471–480, 1989.

205. Roep BO, Arden SD, deVries RRP, Hutton JC: T-cell clones from a type-1 diabetes patient respond to insulin secretory granule proteins. Nature 345:632–634, 1990.

206. Haskins K, McDuffie M: Acceleration of diabetes in young NOD mice with a CD4+ islet-specific T cell clone. Science 249:1433–1436, 1990.

206a. Katz JD, Wang B, Haskins K, Beroist C, Mathis D: Following a diabetogenic T cell from genesis through pathogenesis. Cell 74:1089–1100, 1993.

207. Wicker LS, Miller BJ, Chai A, et al: Expression of genetically determined diabetes and insulitis in the nonobese diabetic (NOD) mouse at the level of bone marrow-derived cells. J Exp Med 167:1801–1810, 1988.

208. Miller BJ, Appel MC, O'Neil JJ, Wicker LS: Both the Lyt-2+ and L3T4+ T cell subsets are required for the transfer of diabetes in nonobese diabetic mice. J Immunol 140:52–58, 1988.

209. Koevary S, Rossini AA, Stoller W, et al: Passive transfer of diabetes in the BB/W rat. Science 220:727–729, 1983.

210. Like AA, Rossini AA, Appel M, et al: Spontaneous diabetes mellitus: Reversal and prevention in the BB/W rat with antiserum to rat lymphocytes. Science 206:1421–1423, 1979.

211. Nakano K, Mordes JP, Rossini AA: Host immunity in the Bio-Breeding/Worcester (BB/W) rat. Diabetologia 27:314A, 1984.

212. Shizuru JA, Taylor-Edwards C, Banks BA, et al: Immunotherapy of the nonobese diabetic mouse: Treatment with an antibody to T-helper lymphocytes. Science 240:659–662, 1988.

212a. Kaufman DL, Clare-Salzter M, Tion J, et al: Spontaneous loss of T-cell tolerance to glutamic acid decarboxylase in murine insulin-dependent diabetes. Nature 366:69–72, 1993.

212b. Tisch R, Yang X-D, Singer SM, et al: Immune response to glutamic acid decarboxylase correlates with insulitis in non-obese diabetic mice. Nature 366:72–75, 1993.

213. Amino N, Mori H, Iwatani Y, et al: Peripheral K lymphocytes in autoimmune thyroid disease: Decrease in Graves' disease and increase in Hashimoto's disease. J Clin Endocrinol Metab 54:587–591, 1982.

214. Bendtzen K, Mandrup-Poulsen T, Nerup J, et al: Cytotoxicity of human pl 7 interleukin-1 for pancreatic islets of Langerhans. Science 232:1545–1547, 1986.

215. Rabinovitch A, Sumoski W, Rajotte RV, Warnock GL: Cytotoxic effects of cytokines on human pancreatic islet cells in monolayer culture. J Clin Endocrinol Metab 71:152–156, 1990.

216. Campbell IL, Kay TWH, Oxbrow L, Harrison LC: Essential role for interferon-γ and interleukin 6 in autoimmune insulin-dependent diabetes in NOD/Wehi mice. J Clin Invest 87:739–742, 1991.

217. Atkins MH, Mier JW, Parkinson DR, et al: Hypothyroidism after treatment with interleukin-2 and lymphokine-activated killer cells. N Engl J Med 318:1557–1563, 1988.

218. Charlton B, Bacelj A, Mandel TE: Administration of silica particles or anti-Lyt2 antibody prevents β-cell destruction in NOD mice given cyclophosphamide. Diabetes 37:930–935, 1988.

219. Corbett JA, McDaniel ML: Does nitric oxide mediate autoimmune destruction of β-cells? Possible therapeutic interventions in IDDM. Diabetes 41:897–903, 1992.

220. Kolb H, Kolb-Bachofen V: Nitric oxide: A pathogenetic factor in autoimmunity. Immunol Today 13:157–159, 1992.

Polyglandular Failure Syndromes

ANDREW MUIR
DESMOND A. SCHATZ
NOEL K. MACLAREN

BACKGROUND

Constellations of multiple endocrine gland insufficiencies often associated with diseases of nonendocrine organs occur in individual patients and their families. Recognition of such "polyglandular" syndromes has evolved over the last century, as summarized in Table 160–1. In 1849, Thomas Addison first described the clinical and pathological features of adrenocortical failure in patients who also appeared to have pernicious anemia.[1] In their 1908 review of polyglandular insufficiencies (islet, thyroid, gonad, adrenal, anterior hypophysis), Claude and Gourgerot[2] suggested a common pathogenesis for these conditions. Mononuclear leukocyte infiltrates of goitrous thyroid glands were first noted by Hashimoto[3] in 1912, and a similar lesion of pancreatic islets, termed *insulitis*, was described by von Meyenburg[4] in 1940. It was Schmidt[5] in 1926 who documented the association between adrenocortical failure and thyroiditis, while Carpenter et al.[6] in 1964 expanded Schmidt's syndrome to include insulin-dependent diabetes mellitus (IDDM). A second association between mucocutaneous candidiasis and hypoparathyroidism was first described in 1929 by Thorpe and Handley.[7] Whitaker et al.[8] expanded this to a triad including adrenocortical insufficiency in 1956. The autoimmune pathogenesis of these disorders began to emerge that same year when Roitt et al.[9] discovered circulating precipitating autoantibodies to thyroglobulin in patients with Hashimoto's thyroiditis. Finally, in 1980, Neufeld et al.,[10] from our own group, distinguished the two major autoimmune polyglandular syndromes (APS's), as summarized in Table 160–2.

Type I APS is diagnosed when a patient manifests at least two of three key features: hypoparathyroidism, hypoadrenocorticism, and recurrent mucocutaneous candidiasis. This is a rare syndrome that usually presents with persistent candidiasis during the first decade of life and often beginning during infancy. It has been reported to affect males and females almost equally in a large American series,[11] but a modest female bias was observed in another collection of smaller reports.[12] The more common type II APS is characterized by adrenocortical insufficiency in conjunction with thyroiditis and/or IDDM. Its prevalence has not been formally established, but it has been estimated to be near 14 to 20 affected patients per million of the population.[13] The diagnosis of type II APS is frequently made during early adulthood through midlife and is three to four times more common in females. Distinctions between types I and II APS can occasionally become blurred in individual patients who may show features that are too incomplete to be defined as either type I or type II APS or that overlap between the two syndromes.

PATHOPHYSIOLOGY/BIOCHEMISTRY

The evidence supporting the autoimmune nature of the component diseases of the APS is compelling: (1) affected organs demonstrate a chronic inflammatory infiltrate composed mainly of lymphocytes, (2) some of the component diseases are associated with immune-response genes encoded by class II loci of the HLA complex, and (3) the syndromes are replete with autoantibodies reacting to target tissue–specific antigens. These autoantibodies may arise in a primary fashion through a breakdown in normal immunological tolerogenesis or by immunization with an environmental agent that is a molecular mimic of a self antigen (see below for discussion). Other autoantibodies appear to arise during a secondary immune response, stimulated by the release from damaged glands of intracellular antigens which are normally sequestered from the immune system. There are three main classes of organ-specific self antigens to which autoantibodies are directed in APS (Table 160–3). These are surface receptor molecules, intracellular enzymes which have a central role in a vital and unique cellular function of the target cell, and secreted proteins such as hormones produced by the affected organ. Examples of surface receptor molecules affected by autoimmunity include the thyrotropin receptor, as involved in Graves' disease as well as in atrophic thyroiditis, and a component of the glucose transport system of the pancreatic beta cell, as has been implicated to be a target in IDDM. Important enzymes that act as autoantigens include thyroid peroxidase (the so-called thyroid "microsomal" antigen) in Hashimoto's thyroiditis and the 21α-hydroxylase enzyme, essential to steroid hormone synthesis, in nontuberculous Addison's disease. Thyroglobulin, as tar-

TABLE 160–1. THE EMERGENCE OF THE POLYGLANDULAR SYNDROMES

EVENT	YEAR	REFERENCE
Description of adrenocortical atrophy in patients with pernicious anemia	1849	1
Hypothesis that polyglandular disease arises from a single process	1908	2
Description of mononuclear leukocyte infiltrate in goitrous thyroid glands	1912	3
Schmidt's syndrome described (thyroiditis and adrenalitis)	1926	5
Description of association between hypoparathyroidism and candidiasis	1929	7
Description of mononuclear leukocyte infiltrate in islets of Langerhans of diabetic patients	1940	4
Triad of hypoadrenocorticism, hypoparathyroidism, and candidiasis described	1956	8
Thyroid autoantibodies observed	1956	9
Thyroiditis induced in rabbits by immunizing with gland extract	1956	109
Indirect immunofluorescence labeling technique described	1959	110
Carpenter et al. expand Schmidt's syndrome to include insulin-dependent diabetes mellitus	1964	6
Clinical classification of distinct polyglandular autoimmune syndromes	1980	10,11

geted in Hashimoto's thyroiditis, or insulin and proinsulin, as involved in IDDM, are examples of autoantigenic endocrine cell products important to their respective autoimmune disease.

It is perplexing as to why the component diseases of APS co-exist, but one explanation may be that the affected glands share target antigenic epitopes. Experimental evidence for this possibility is lacking, with the exception of the "steroidal cell" autoimmunity syndromes, where the 17α-hydroxylase enzyme present in the testes, ovary, placenta, and adrenal cortex can readily explain the common involvement of these organs in affected patients. The authors submit that the explanation must lie in a poorly understood breakdown of peripheral (thymus-independent) self tolerance. In support of this possibility is the seemingly paradoxical defects in T-cell function which are profound in type I APS and more occult, but present nevertheless, in diseases such as IDDM. In the following we will discuss these manifestations in some detail.

Humoral Autoimmunity

The identification of circulating organ-specific autoantibodies provided the earliest and strongest evidence for the autoimmune pathogenesis of the APS's. Whereas patients with collagen-vascular diseases synthesize immunoglobulins that recognize non–organ-specific cellular targets such as nucleic acids or nucleoproteins, the endocrine autoimmunities are associated with autoantibodies that react to organ-specific antigens. While their pathogenic relevance remains unclear, their importance as diagnostic indicators and predictive markers of future disease is well established.[14–18] Most autoantibodies are detected by indirect immunofluorescent labeling of target organs. Procedures for procurement and processing of fresh frozen substrate tissues for such testing must be meticulously followed in order to obtain consistent and reliable results.[19] Attempts to simplify testing by introducing more sensitive and quantitative techniques have had variable successes.

Adrenal autoantibodies (AA) detected by indirect immunofluorescent labeling have been reported in at least two of every three patients with nontuberculous Addison's disease when tested at the time of their diagnoses.[20] All layers of the adrenal cortex bind AA with striking sparing of the adrenal medulla. Fluorescence of the zona glomerulosa in particular gives a distinctive pattern. Occasionally, AA-positive individuals who do not have overt adrenocortical failure can be identified by screening patients with au-

TABLE 160–2. THE AUTOIMMUNE POLYGLANDULAR SYNDROMES

TYPE I APS	TYPE II APS	FREQUENCY
Hypoparathyroidism Mucocutaneous candidiasis Adrenocortical insufficiency Ungual dystrophy, enamel hypoplasia, hypogonadism (♀ > ♂)	Adrenocortical insufficiency Thyroiditis Insulin-dependent diabetes mellitus	>40%
Malabsorption Alopecia (totalis or universalis) Pernicious anemia (juvenile onset) Thyroiditis Chronic active hepatitis		10–40%
Vitiligo Sjögren's syndrome Anterior hypophysitis Insulin-dependent diabetes mellitus	Hypogonadism (♀ > ♂) Vitiligo Alopecia Pernicious anemia (adult onset) Myasthenia gravis Celiac disease Rheumatoid arthritis Sjögren's syndrome	<10%

"Incomplete" autoimmune syndromes:
Thyroiditis and atrophic gastritis
Thyroiditis and insulin-dependent diabetes mellitus
Insulin-dependent diabetes mellitus and atrophic gastritis

TABLE 160–3. TYPES OF AUTOANTIGENS IN APS

TARGET ORGAN	ENZYMES	RECEPTORS	SECRETED CELL PRODUCTS
Islet	Glutamic acid decarboxylase$_{65}$	Insulin Glucose transporter (GLUT-2)	Insulin Proinsulin
Thyroid	Thyroid peroxidase	Thyrotropin	Thyroglobulin
Adrenal	21α-Hydroxylase 17α-Hydroxylase	ACTH	
Gonad	17α-Hydroxylase	Gonadotropin	
Gastric parietal cell	H⁺, K⁺-ATPase		Intrinsic factor

toimmune endocrine diseases or their family members. Up to 40 per cent of such apparently healthy individuals were reported to subsequently develop Addison's disease over a follow-up period of 6 months to 10 years.[16, 17] This risk was observed to be especially high if the autoantibodies fixed complement in vitro or were present in high titers. Another 20 per cent of asymptomatic AA-positive relatives were reported to have elevated basal serum levels of ACTH or renin or blunted adrenocortical responses to an intravenous infusion of ACTH, features that are indicative of subclinical glandular dysfunction (Fig. 160–1).

Some 15 per cent of AA-positive patients with Addison's disease also have an autoantibody that cross-reacts with other steroid-producing cells, i.e., placental syncytiotrophoblasts, ovarian luteal cells, and/or testicular Leydig cells. These "steroidal cell" autoantibodies (SCA) are distinguished from AA by their ability to be adsorbed from serum by preincubation with adrenal, gonadal (ovarian or testicular), or placental homogenates, whereas AA are removed from positive sera by prior exposure to adrenal homogenates exclusively. When detected, SCA indicate a high risk for future gonadal failure, especially in females.[15, 21]

Whereas cellular immune mechanisms are thought to cause glandular destruction, a pathogenic role for humoral autoreactivity in autoimmune oophoritis has been suggested by studies showing complement-mediated cytotoxicity of cultured granulosa cells in the presence of sera from affected patients but not in the presence of sera from control patients.[22] Binding of SCA to granulosa cells by indirect immunofluorescence, however, can only be demonstrated when autoantibodies are present in high titers.

Screening of a fetal adrenal expression library revealed that 17α-hydroxylase, a 55-kDa gonadal and adrenal steroid biosynthetic P$_{450}$ microsomal enzyme, was an autoantibody target in 21 of 35 type I APS patients but in neither of 2 patients with isolated Addison's disease.[23] Thus this hydroxylase appears to be an important target antigen of SCA, and its identification should lead to the development of specific and readily available diagnostic tests for gonadal/adrenal autoimmunities. At variance with this study were immunoprecipitation experiments identifying a 55-kDa autoantigen in normal adrenocortical tissue but not in placenta using sera from patients with AA-positive but SCA-negative Addison's disease.[24] Most recently, sera of addisonian patients without gonadal insufficiency have been found to Western blot the cytochrome P$_{450}$ 21α-hydroxylase enzyme, suggesting that this protein is an adrenocortical-specific autoantigen in the disease.[25] The syndrome of deficient adrenocorticoid action in the face of normal serum hormone levels among patients with the acquired immune

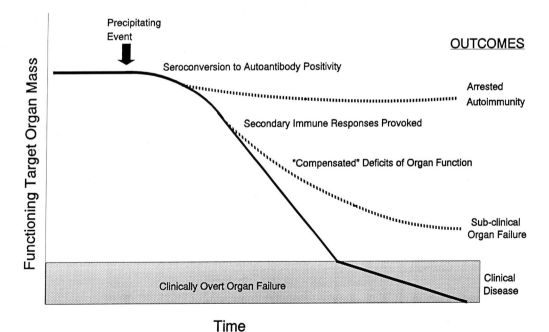

FIGURE 160–1. The proposed natural history of endocrine autoimmunity. Autoimmune attack of target organs often begins in people who have a genetic predisposition after an unknown precipitating event (*arrow*). The early process manifests itself by provoking autoantibody production, and it may arrest at that stage (*top broken line*). Progressive disease, associated with secondary responses against antigens released by damaged tissue, is initially detectable by minimal biochemical abnormalities, such as elevations of trophic hormones. Organ function loss may plateau before the threshold of critical organ mass is reached (*lower broken line*), or it may progress to clinically overt disease (*solid line*). Hormone replacement therapy may decelerate the destruction of surviving tissue, but at this late stage, complete organ atrophy is inevitable.

deficiency syndrome (AIDS) has been attributed to auto-immunity to cortisol itself,[26] a claim that awaits independent confirmation. Undoubtedly, current molecular biological techniques will permit the rapid characterization of many more organ-specific autoantigens in these diseases.

The existence of parathyroid gland–specific autoantibodies in patients with hypoparathyroidism is debated. While they were reported by indirect immunofluorescent labeling in 38 per cent of 74 affected patients, parathyroid autoantibodies also were identified in 6 per cent of 245 healthy control subjects in the same study.[27] Subsequent investigations have found that antiparathyroid serological immunoreactivity is rare in patients with failed glands[28] and usually is not parathyroid-specific.[29] Indeed, antibodies considered to be against parathyroid antigens have been confused with mitochondrial autoantibodies in previous reports. Recent studies of humoral sensitivity to parathyroid tissue may have delineated a tissue-specific response to antigens within the endothelial component of the gland.[30]

The intensive studies of humoral autoimmunities against antigens expressed by the pancreatic beta cell (e.g., islet gangliosides, insulin, proinsulin, glutamic acid decarboxylase [GAD_{65}]) and the thyroid gland (e.g., thyroid peroxidase, thyroglobulin, thyrotropin receptors) highlight the complexity of disease-autoantibody relationships. While immunoglobulins against the thyrotropin receptor may stimulate or inhibit both thyroid gland activity and growth, no consistently discernible effect on thyroid function has yet been attributed to autoantibodies that recognize thyroid peroxidase or thyroglobulin (see Table 160–3). Nevertheless, immunization of susceptible strains of mice with thyroglobulin in complete Freund's adjuvant induces a thyroid-specific immune infiltrate in experimental allergic thyroiditis (EAT).[31] Islet cell autoantibodies (ICA) are important predictors of future disease in patients at high risk for IDDM, yet ICA also occur in many patients with type I APS, a syndrome with only a low likelihood of progression to clinically overt IDDM. Direct evidence of ICA heterogeneity has emerged, suggesting that GAD_{65} represents but one of the islet cell autoantigens detected by indirect immunofluorescent labeling.[32] Type I APS patients appear to have ICA directed predominantly against GAD_{65} but presumably lack other components of the pathogenic process (e.g., antigen-specific cytotoxic T lymphocytes) that are necessary to produce beta-cell damage and thus overt hyperglycemia.

Achlorhydria and pernicious anemia occurring as part of the APS are associated with the presence of circulating autoantibodies against gastric parietal cells (PCA) and, less frequently, intrinsic factor (IFA). Approximately 10 per cent of patients with IDDM have co-existing circulating PCA, of whom many only develop achlorhydria.[33] The pathogenic importance of these immunoglobulins is suggested by their toxic effects on the gastric mucosa of frogs and guinea pigs.[34, 35] The parietal cell proton pump (H^+,K^+-ATPase) represents at least one target of PCA.[36] Thus PCA appear to be primarily associated with achlorhydria, while IFA may arise secondarily as a consequence of gastric cell damage and are associated with increasing likelihood of clinical pernicious anemia.

Antimelanocyte autoantibodies have been demonstrated in a small number of individuals with type I APS and vitiligo, but a similar association has not been made in patients with isolated vitiligo.[37] The antigen involved in this reaction has not been identified. Antibodies detected by indirect immunofluorescent labeling of hypothalamic vasopressin-producing cells also have been reported in a small number of patients with central diabetes insipidus who had other autoimmune endocrinopathies.[19] In a report of 19 patients with a variety of endocrine autoimmunities, autoantibodies against anterior pituitary lactotrophs were detected,[38] and scattered reports of humoral responses against somatotrophs and perhaps even gonadotrophs also have been published but not independently confirmed. Rarely, if ever, have these patients had symptomatic disease of the hypothalamic-pituitary axis, however. In contrast, among 30 reported patients with proven or presumed symptomatic lymphocytic hypophysitis, autoantibodies directed against the pituitary gland have been described only once.[39] Using transformed rodent pituitary cell lines as a substrate in an indirect immunofluorescence assay, immunoglobulins that specifically bound the hypophyseal cells in culture were observed in the serum of humans with the empty sella syndrome.[40] The authors believe that pituitary autoimmunity is an area of potential research that needs more attention.

The antibodies described above that react with cellular enzymes or hormones generally have unknown pathogenic significance. The functional role of autoantibodies that alter organ function by binding to their hormone receptors is, however, readily understandable. Whereas autoantibodies that bind thyrotropin and acetylcholine receptors have been long recognized to have pathogenic importance in Graves' disease and myasthenia gravis, respectively, a similar mechanism has only recently emerged as a potential pathogenic process in other endocrine autoimmunities. Thus immunoglobulins that recognize receptors for gonadotropins, insulin, or ACTH receptors may inhibit the action of their respective hormone ligands[41] (see Table 160–3).

Among those type I APS patients with chronic active hepatitis, autoantibodies against mitochondrial, nuclear, or smooth-muscle antigens are frequently found, albeit their clinical significances are also unclear. Abnormal B-lymphocyte function has been variably described in patients with APS. Deficiency of IgA is the most common feature, and high levels of IgG and IgE also have been observed in some patients.[42, 43] Age-specific expansions of activated CD5+ B lymphocytes were observed in patients with IDDM,[44] and if so studied, a similar phenomenon may be found in other endocrine autoimmunities.

Cellular Autoimmunity

The pathologic observations and experimental investigations of cellular immunity in multiorgan autoimmunity have yielded results that are similar to those found in the more intensive studies of isolated thyroid and pancreatic islet disease. In this section, therefore, information derived from research into APS and other autoimmune disorders will be combined to review the principles of autoimmunity that are important in APS pathogenesis.

The gross and microscopic pathological changes in types

I and II APS are similar to those of the component-isolated endocrinopathy. Histological examinations of affected adrenal, thyroid, and parathyroid glands, ovaries, pancreatic islets, and gastric mucosa have all yielded similar results.[20, 45-53] A mononuclear leukocyte infiltrate that is comprised mainly of lymphocytes with some macrophages, natural killer (NK) cells, and plasma cells is typically seen. The infiltrating lymphocytes are of both B and T lineages, while the T-cell population includes both the CD4+ and CD8+ subsets and often displays activation markers.[45, 49] Sparing of adjacent nontarget tissue is striking in all organs. As the disease approaches its final stages, atrophy predominates within the gland. Fibrosis eventually becomes a prominent finding in most affected glands and may highlight islands of surviving endocrine tissue that are both hyperplastic and hypertrophied, as illustrated by "regenerative nodules" in the adrenalitis lesions of Addison's disease. Such attempts at regeneration are invariably accompanied by continued inflammation.

Effector Functions

The presence of circulating tissue-specific autoreactive leukocytes in APS patients was first demonstrated by the elaboration of migration inhibitory factors (MIF's) after incubation of target-organ homogenates with peripheral blood mononuclear cells (PBMC's) from affected individuals. Subsequently, increased levels of PBMC's expressing activation markers such as HLA class II antigens have been observed in patients with early but not end-stage IDDM, Graves' disease, thyroiditis, Addison's disease, and oophoritis.[45, 54] Since surface antigen phenotyping does not reliably distinguish lymphocytes with different functions, cytokine production profiles of PBMC's are coming under scrutiny. Diminished production of interleukin 2 (IL-2) and interferon-γ in response to mitogen has been observed in patients at high risk for IDDM.[55] In contrast, autologous thyroid cells elicited interferon-γ production by PBMC's harvested from patients with autoimmune thyroid disease but not from those with nontoxic goiters or thyroid cancer.[56] Examinations of affected end organs obtained early in the disease process will ultimately be more informative than those of circulating lymphocytes. Unfortunately, tissue specimens obtained at or after the time disease becomes clinically apparent contain infiltrates that represent a complex response against a multitude of antigens. They are thus unsuitable for studies of autoimmune initiators. As programs of disease prediction expand, improved availability of more appropriate organ specimens with early autoimmune infiltrates is expected. Animal models of disease are now being used to follow the kinetics of leukocyte infiltration of autoimmune targets. In NOD mice (described below), descriptions of early insulitis have described initial infiltration by macrophages and CD8+ T lymphocytes, followed by CD4+ T lymphocytes and B lymphocytes.[57]

It appears unlikely that the action of a single T-lymphocyte clone can result in clinically important organ failure, since adoptive transfer of either IDDM or thyroiditis requires transfusion of both CD4+ and CD8+ lymphocytes. Nonetheless, it is likely that autoimmunity against a single antigen initiates disease. Target-organ invasion by restricted T-cell families, identified by their expression of T-cell receptor genes that contain uniquely rearranged variable (V) or complementarity-determining regions (e.g., CDR3), or monoclonal expansion of B lymphocytes has not been demonstrated convincingly in either APS. Preferential use of certain TCR families may occur, however, in an antigen-specific fashion during the inductive events.[58]

Despite the multitude of investigations, the sequence of effector events leading to eventual cell destruction has not been resolved with any certainty. It has been difficult to determine how the local effects of cytokines (released from either leukocytes, damaged endothelium, or possibly endocrine epithelium[20, 59]), aberrant expression of major histocompatibility antigens (class I and/or class II),[45, 50, 60] and adhesion molecules (ICAM-1)[61, 62] on the endocrine epithelium surface contribute to the pathological process. In diabetic rodents, beta-cell expression of class I MHC is observed early in the pathogenic sequence, perhaps enhancing the ability of CD8+ T cells to lyse these cellular targets. Later, there may be enhanced class II reactivity due to the invasion of macrophages and perhaps some patchy aberrant expression of these antigens on pancreatic beta cells. Some have suggested that T-cell elaboration of interferon-γ may have an important role in cell destruction, since it can be cytotoxic either alone or in combination with tumor necrosis factor.[63] These two cytokines also have been reported to increase aberrant class II MHC expression on thyroid,[64] islet,[65] and ovarian granulosa cells.[66] The beta cells are especially sensitive to cytotoxic effects of IL-1, an effect that may operate through cytokine-mediated accumulation of local nitric oxide (NO).[67] Recently, it has been suggested that cellular lysis through inflammation is often perpetuated by generation of NO,[67, 68] but it remains to be shown whether this mechanism will prove to be the principal mode of glandular cell destruction in the APS.

Recurrent mucocutaneous candidal infections in type I APS which are often resistant to treatment most certainly reflect an abnormality of T-lymphocyte function. No specific T-cell defect to account for these findings has been consistently identified, albeit one must exist.[54] The possible role of the elusive transfer factor remains unclear.[69] Again, this is an area where further investigation is needed.

Immunoregulatory Functions

The classical concept of autoimmune disease arising from a "forbidden" lymphocyte clone that has escaped intrathymic deletion is incomplete, since some potentially autoreactive T lymphocytes are regularly found circulating in healthy individuals. Autoimmunity caused by such cells is normally prevented through the active induction of clone-specific anergy by a process that remains poorly defined. Deficiencies of this immunoregulation may allow potentially autoreactive lymphocyte clones to become activated and thus pathogenic. Diminished suppressor activity has been demonstrated in patients with both IDDM and thyroiditis, while functional defects of both CD4+CD45RO+ (helper-inducer) and CD4+CD45RA+ (suppressor-inducer) T cells have been related to IDDM.[55, 70, 71] Such defects may result, at least in part, from deficiencies of cytokines such as IL-2 or interferon-γ.

Animal Models

Experimental animal models of spontaneous autoimmune IDDM (BioBreeding [BB] rat and nonobese diabetic [NOD] mouse) and thyroiditis (obese strain [OS] chicken, Buffalo and BB rats, NOD mouse) have provided much of the current insights into the humoral and cellular mechanisms of organ-specific autoimmunity. Models of induced immune-mediated disease against other endocrine organs also have been devised using immunizations with purified antigens (e.g., thyroglobulin,[31] zona pellucida peptide[72]) or tissue homogenates (e.g., adrenal,[20, 73] ovary,[74] and hypophysis[73]) suspended in an immune adjuvant. How well these induced disease states mimic their spontaneously occurring human counterparts remains problematic.

The most convincing evidence that endocrine autoimmunities are T lymphocyte–mediated has come from demonstrations that their courses can be altered by a variety of immunomodulating treatments, including corticosteroids, azathioprine, cyclosporin A, γ-irradiation, cyclophosphamide, antilymphocyte antibodies, immune adjuvants, and neonatal thymectomy. Adoptive transfer of IDDM, oophoritis, orchitis, and atrophic gastritis has been achieved by passing splenocytes from affected rodent donors to unaffected recipients.[54]

Polyglandular autoimmunity, including oophoritis, orchitis, gastritis, and thyroiditis, was induced in genetically susceptible mice by depleting T lymphocytes permanently (through thymectomy between the second and fourth day of life)[75] or transiently (through neonatal administration of cyclosporin A).[76] Such interventions may interfere with the normal negative selection against the release of potentially autoreactive T lymphocytes by the healthy thymus. Neonatal thymectomy has been a particularly important model for delineating mechanisms of immune regulation in APS. Using this model, it has been demonstrated that early interactions between the lymphoid system and the target organ are important in the pathogenesis of autoimmunity[77] and that CD4+ splenocytes from adult but not neonatal mice contain regulatory populations that are able to prevent the transfer of autoimmune endocrinopathies.[75]

Microinjection of genetic material into mouse embryos to create transgenic animals has been an important technique for the study of autoimmune disease. This method has created an entire literature on the importance of prenatal antigen exposure in tolerogenesis.[78] Selective mating of transgenic mice also permits the creation of animals with specific gene deletions. The microinjection of a structural gene coupled to an insulin promotor into mouse zygotes has allowed the β-cell–specific expression of a transgene product to be induced. Thus β-cell production of interferon-γ has led to diabetes.[79] Substitutions of NOD mice I-A genes or promotion of expression of I-E genes into the mouse major histocompatibility (MHC) complex have powerfully prevented IDDM in these mice.[80] It is expected that this technique will eventually allow direct assessment of the pathogenic importance of target-organ autoantigen production, but to date, experiments have been confounded by transgene-induced cytotoxicity.

Environmental Factors

If environmental precipitators of autoimmunity exist, they continue to be elusive. While the links between con-genital rubella infection, IDDM, and hypothyroidism are well known, the associations between IDDM and other viruses such as Coxsackie B, mumps, and cytomegalovirus[81] are poorly documented, as is the putative link between thyroiditis and *Yersinia enterocolitica*.[45] A retroviral protein found in islets of diabetic patients was reported to be recognized by insulin autoantibodies, probably by molecular mimicry.[82] An infectious trigger of polyglandular autoimmunity has not been reported in human epidemiological studies; nonetheless, reovirus type I infection in susceptible mice causes IDDM and growth failure. In addition, the synthesis of autoantibodies against the pancreas, anterior hypophysis, and gastric mucosa was reported.[83]

Immune stimulation by dietary antigens has been proposed as a primary pathogenic event in IDDM. While nitrosamines in smoked meats have been implicated,[84] dietary proteins have received more attention. Diabetes-susceptible BB rats are protected from disease when bovine protein sources are removed from their diets.[85] In humans, prolonged breast feeding and delayed introduction of cow's milk have been reported to reduce the risk of future IDDM,[86] while international comparisons show a positive correlation between IDDM prevalence and cow's milk ingestion ($r = 0.96$).[87] Circulating antibodies against a peptide with homology to both bovine serum albumin and a human islet surface protein have been observed in IDDM patients.[88] The importance of these observations will be addressed in a controlled clinical trial aimed at preventing IDDM by removing cow's milk from infant diets. The role of dietary triggers of APS has not been examined.

Genetics

While the pathogenic processes of type I and type II APS appear to be similar, their genetics are distinct. Type I is usually reported to be a sporadic disease but has been observed among siblings, suggesting that an autosomal recessive mode of inheritance also can occur.[12] While isolated Addison's disease has a strong association with the class II HLA alleles DR3 and DR4, no such relationships are apparent in addisonian patients with type I APS.[89] One Finnish report, however, suggested that HLA-A28 occurred more frequently in type I APS patients,[90] but these observations have not been reported by others.

Type II APS is commonly inherited as an autosomal dominant trait with incomplete penetrance and is related to the HLA-DR3 and -DR4 phenotypes.[89] However, thyroid autoimmunity in pedigrees with IDDM may segregate independently from the HLA complex.[33] The molecular genetics of the α and β chains of the HLA-DQ protein so intensively investigated in IDDM have not yet been closely examined in APS patients. As discussed elsewhere, unique amino acid sequences in the DQα and DQβ chains that probably relate to the antigen-binding cleft of the class II molecule are important to the inherited susceptibility to IDDM. Multiple genes are likely to be involved in the APS's, and those outside the HLA complex have yet to be identified.

THE CLINICAL SPECTRUM OF APS

An important responsibility for the clinician managing patients with endocrine gland deficiencies is to consider whether an individual having a single endocrine autoimmunity is at risk for the occurrence of polyglandular disorders. Clues uncovered by a thorough history and physical examination may reveal the true multifocal nature of a patient's condition. Subclinical or "compensated" deficiencies, identified by elevations of tropic hormones (e.g., normal thyroxine but elevated thyrotropin in Hashimoto's disease), reflect early gland destruction which may be detected during the evaluation of more progressive and symptomatic disease in other glands. Once recognized, each individual hormone deficiency should be treated and monitored using the same therapeutic replacement regimens as those used for patients who have isolated gland dysfunction. The authors urge the use of full diagnostic autoantibody panels followed by monitoring of the function of any targeted organ for all Addison's disease probands and their immediate relatives and in patients with IDDM complicated by the presence of circulating thyroid gland autoantibodies.

Type I APS

Type I APS is diagnosed when two of the three defining diseases are present (i.e., mucocutaneous candidiasis, hypoparathyroidism, adrenocortical insufficiency). The first sign is invariably mucocutaneous candidiasis. Any young person afflicted by troublesome moniliasis should be assessed for a possible T-lymphocyte deficiency state as well as for type I APS. In one study, nearly 45 per cent of pediatric patients with refractory monilial infections but no overt underlying T-cell defect had an autoimmune endocrinopathy.[91] Of the 50 to 100 per cent of type I APS patients who develop recurrent monilial infection, most have lesions that are restricted to the skin, nails, and oral and perianal mucosa. Whereas remissions of varying length occur, progressive courses are common, and gastrointestinal involvement can become severe, especially when complicated by bacterial overgrowth, chronic diarrhea, or gastrointestinal hemorrhages. More than 75 per cent of type I APS patients develop hypoparathyroidism, usually presenting before age 10 years. Severe hypocalcemia manifested by carpopedal spasms, seizures, or laryngospasm can be the presenting feature of type I APS, especially in young children. Adrenocortical failure typically develops between the ages of 10 and 30 years. Deficiencies of mineralocorticoids and glucocorticoids usually arise simultaneously, but their onsets can be dissociated by up to 5 years.[92]

Females suffer from gonadal insufficiency more often than males and usually present with maturational arrest after the onset of a normal pubarche and menarche. Autoimmune oophoritis also may present with failed pubertal development or with menstrual irregularities and polycystic ovaries.[93]

Fat malabsorption, which may be episodic, has been linked by some to hypoparathyroidism. More likely causes include IgA deficiency, gluten sensitivity, and bacterial overgrowth of the upper small bowel. Deficiencies of iron or vitamin B_{12} result from parietal cell autoimmunity with subsequent early appearance of achlorhydria followed by intrinsic factor deficiency and pernicious anemia. Typical atrophic gastritis arises in 15 per cent of type I APS cases with a mean age at onset of 16 years.[92] Studies of Finnish patients have particularly emphasized manifestations of type I APS in the teeth and integument. In decreasing order of frequency, enamel hypoplasia, ungual dystrophy (pitting), keratopathy, and tympanic membrane sclerosis have all been reported at rates from 33 to 77 per cent.[92] Vitiligo may be missed if not specifically sought using ultraviolet light. Alopecia totalis or universalis is frequent, but all types occur. It has been suggested that hair loss may diminish after treatment of hypoparathyroidism is started,[12] but this does not reflect the authors' experience. The appearance of hepatomegaly or jaundice with dark urine and clay-colored stools often heralds the onset of chronic active hepatitis. It occurs in up to 10 per cent of patients and is not associated with persistent immunological hypersensitivity to hepatitis viruses. Sjögren's syndrome (parotitis, arthritis, and sicca syndrome) is not infrequent, while IDDM, chronic thyroiditis, and hypophysitis are distinctly uncommon.

Type II APS

Type II APS is far more common than type I and is diagnosed when a patient has adrenocortical deficiency with IDDM, chronic lymphocytic thyroiditis, or Graves' disease. Unlike type I APS, this syndrome can be more difficult to recognize before the onset of clinically significant multigland disease. The disease commonly manifests in the third or fourth decade, but it is not uncommon before or after these ages. It is heralded by adrenocortical failure in almost half the cases, although this estimate may be skewed by a selection bias in the literature. As many as 20 years can elapse before polyglandular involvement becomes evident. Furthermore, isolated thyroiditis and IDDM are common enough in these age groups that routine adrenal autoantibody screening of such affected patients is not justified unless adrenocortical insufficiency is clinically suspected. The authors recommend routine thyroid autoantibody screening of all IDDM patients and full endocrine autoantibody testing in those found to be positive. However, physicians should routinely elicit historical and physical features relevant to the diagnostic triad in all patients with IDDM and/or autoimmune thyroiditis. A family history of polyglandular failure is often present in past generations that can serve as a flag for those patients who need extra monitoring. The presence of extraendocrinological manifestations such as alopecia or vitiligo is less common than in type I APS, but when such manifestations are present, they are important clinical indicators, especially if they are profound. The mortality risk of untreated adrenocortical failure in the 2 per cent of patients with myasthenia gravis who develop associated endocrinopathies requires that all these patients under 40 years should be assessed closely for endocrinological disorders during their initial investigations.

Other Associations with APS

Rare diagnoses have on occasion been reported in association with an APS. The authors and others have followed patients with type I APS who developed severe, idiopathic, noninflammatory myopathy with eventual respiratory failure. Separate reports suggested that pure red cell hypoplasia and male infertility in patients with type I APS responded well to glucocorticoid therapy.[94, 95] In rare cases, neo-osseous porosis and sarcoidosis have been linked to type I and type II APS, respectively.[96, 97]

Differential Diagnosis

The differential diagnosis of APS at the time of initial presentation varies according to the disease manifested. When evidence of a second autoimmunity is present, consideration should be given to whether the patient has type I or type II APS, since future monitoring and prognosis are different for these two syndromes. Other diagnostic considerations are summarized in Table 160–4. Chromosomal disorders such as trisomy 21 and Turner's syndrome (45X,O and its genetic variants) are associated with an increased risk for endocrine autoimmunities, especially Hashimoto's thyroiditis (up to 30 per cent) and IDDM (some 5 per cent).[98, 99] The primary hypogonadism of Turner syndrome, however, is not of autoimmune origin, and apparent growth hormone deficiencies in some of these females may resolve after estrogen priming. DiGeorge syndrome is a developmental disorder of the branchial arches that results in facial deformities, aortic arch anomalies, and thymic and parathyroid gland agenesis. These patients develop hypoparathyroidism and mucocutaneous candidiasis, which are usually diagnosed in infancy, but have few to no circulating T-lymphocytes and produce no autoantibodies. Kearns-Sayre syndrome is a myopathic disease that is associated with hypoparathyroidism, primary hypogonadism, IDDM, and hypopituitarism. Cardiac conduction defects are common, and muscle biopsies are usually diagnostic. Wolfram's syndrome or DIDMOAD (diabetes insipidus, diabetes mellitus, optic atrophy, nerve deafness) is an uncommon congenital condition that presents in young children. Congenital rubella is associated with the later onset of IDDM and hypothyroidism. The POEMS syndrome (plasma cell dyscrasia with polyneuropathy, organomegaly, endocrinopathy, M protein, and skin changes) occurs mainly in Japanese patients. It is associated with IDDM and primary hypogonadism. Thymomas (malignant more so than benign) are associated with myasthenia gravis in up to 50 per cent of cases. They arise most commonly after 40 years of age in myasthenic patients and may be seen in association with Cush-

ing's syndrome, Graves' disease, or Addison's disease.[100] Hemochromatosis usually presents with lethargy, malaise, abdominal pain, and hypermelanotic skin lesions. The similarity to Addison's disease can become confusing in patients with either IDDM or secondary hypogonadism induced by pancreatic or hypophyseal iron deposition. Rarely, thyroid, parathyroid, or adrenocortical insufficiencies have been reported in hemochromatosis. Myotonic dystrophy is associated with primary testicular atrophy, alopecia, and less frequently, diabetes mellitus (usually related to insulin resistance).

Diagnostic Protocols

Two major laboratory approaches are used to diagnose an APS. First, serum screening for autoantibodies is used to (1) verify the autoimmune nature of disease in patients with polyglandular insufficiencies, (2) identify patients affected by an isolated endocrinopathy who are likely to develop multiorgan autoimmunities, and (3) screen family members of APS patients, even if those relatives are currently asymptomatic. A complete screening panel includes assessments of adrenal (21-hydroxylase), steroidal cell (17-hydroxylase), thyroid (peroxidase and thyroglobulin), islet cell (GAD_{65} and nonGAD), and parietal cell (H^+, K^+-ATPase) autoantibodies (see Table 160–3). Thyroid-stimulating immunoglobulins may be required in selected patients. A single negative examination does not rule out the possibility of future disease, and annual follow-up tests are optimal. The predictive value of a positive result has already been outlined above.

Second, assessments of end-organ function in autoantibody-positive individuals are required. Serum levels of thyrotropin, calcium, phosphorus, and fasting glucose performed annually can effectively assess thyroid, parathyroid, and pancreatic islet function of asymptomatic patients. Suspicion of subclinical gland dysfunction should prompt a complete functional evaluation of the suspect gland before determining a final diagnosis. Gonadal dysfunction is diagnosed when random serum gonadotropin levels are elevated in the face of low sex steroid levels.

While depression of early morning serum cortisol levels and electrolyte disturbances represent changes which occur at or just before the clinical onset of adrenocortical failure, it is best to follow individuals at high risk for hypoadrenocorticism (those with AA or SCA) annually by seeking inappropriate elevations of basal serum ACTH levels (midafternoon or later) and supine (>1 hour) plasma renin activity (PRA). To date, the authors have determined no clinically relevant advantage to screening for adrenal gland dysfunction by formal ACTH testing or preceding PRA assessments by salt deprivation. In our studies, serum ACTH levels above 75 and 55 pg/ml at 6:00 and 20:00 hours, respectively, indicated that the anterior hypophysis was responding to adrenocortical insufficiency and thus warranted follow-up with a complete adrenocortical function assessment.[16]

Annual hemoglobin or hematocrit determinations are essential, with accompanying examinations of the blood film for erythrocyte and polymorph morphology. When nutritional deficiencies are suspected, serum levels of ferritin and/or vitamin B_{12} and red cell folate determinations are indicated.

Fat malabsorption in APS may occur for many reasons,

TABLE 160–4. DIFFERENTIAL DIAGNOSIS OF APS

Type I APS
Type II APS
Thyrogastric autoimmunity
Chromosomal disorder (45X,O; trisomy 21)
Kearns-Sayre syndrome
Congenital rubella
DiGeorge syndrome
Wolfram's syndrome (DIDMOAD)
POEMS
Thymoma
Hemochromatosis
Myotonic dystrophy

some of which are reversed with proper treatment. It is therefore mandatory that it be completely investigated. Stool examinations for ova and parasites are helpful for diagnosing *Giardia lamblia* infections, but it may be necessary to obtain duodenal fluid or a jejunal biopsy for direct examination and culture. Bacterial overgrowth can be diagnosed with duodenal aspirate, and a small bowel biopsy is required to diagnose villous morphology. Serum IgA levels also should be assessed.

Patients with suspected recurrent mucocutaneous candidal infections which have been refractory to topical medication should have the diagnosis confirmed at least initially by culturing scrapings from the periphery of an affected area.

Therapy

It has already been suggested that the key to successfully managing patients with an APS is to identify and treat their autoimmunities before they cause significant morbidity and mortality. The treatment of organ insufficiencies is identical whether it occurs in isolation or as part of an APS. Replacement therapy remains the cornerstone. Patient education about the nature of the disease is often critical to the early recognition of new autoimmunities, and as with any chronic disease, individualized needs for psychosocial support must be assessed. Genetic counseling is also warranted, and additional affected family members should be sought by specific tests. Emergency identification should be worn at all times by APS patients, and the use of increased corticosteroid doses at times of acute stress usually averts adrenal crises in those with Addison's disease. The authors believe that exogenous glucocorticoid supplements given at times of acute stress are well advised in those asymptomatic individuals who have biochemical evidence of asymptomatic adrenocortical disease.

Of all the endocrine components of an APS, only IDDM does not carry a satisfactory prognosis when managed with well-monitored hormone replacement therapies. The long-term vascular complications have thus made IDDM a candidate for aggressive experimental approaches. Results of controlled trials using cyclosporin A and azathioprine for treating newly diagnosed IDDM have indicated that some metabolic benefits are provided, albeit they are not often long-lived, even with continued immunotherapy.[101, 102] Anecdotal reports of improved orchitis,[95] oophoritis,[103] and hypophysitis[104] after immunosuppressive corticosteroid treatments are provocative but require systematic evaluation. For now, all immunomodulating therapies must be considered experimental and should be prescribed only in the setting of a controlled clinical trial. As more autoantigens are identified and the disease pathogenesis becomes better understood, selective therapies that do not cause generalized immunosuppression may be developed. Still further in the future lies the prospect of curative organ transplantation. Pancreatic and, to a lesser extent, islet transplants are currently used in kidney graft recipients with IDDM.[105] Adrenal gland transplants have been successful in experimental rodents[106] and humans.[107]

The introduction of ketoconazole has helped greatly with the treatment of chronic mucocutaneous candidiasis, which is commonly resistant to topical antimicrobials. The drug frequently causes gastrointestinal upset and can interfere with glucocorticoid and sex steroid biosynthesis. Elevations of hepatic transaminases are usually transient, but fatal hepatic necrosis can rarely be caused by ketoconazole.

The management of fat malabsorption should be first aimed at diagnosing and treating reversible causes. Bacterial overgrowth often responds to broad-spectrum oral antibiotics. *Giardia lamblia* is best treated with quinacrine hydrochloride or metronidazole, and villous atrophy, seen especially in type II APS, typically responds to dietary gluten withdrawal. If no specific cause for fat malabsorption is found, then nutritional support with fat-soluble vitamin and medium-chain fatty acid supplements may be required. This is best done in consultation with a nutrition or gastroenterology specialist.

Improved survival for patients with chronic active hepatitis has been achieved with new regimens of immunomodulating agents such as prednisone, cyclosporin A, and azathioprine.[108] Tertiary hepatic care is indicated for patients who develop this illness.

Prognosis

The impact of an APS on a given patient's lifestyle varies considerably owing to differences in a host of disease-dependent, patient-dependent, family-dependent, and physician-dependent factors. All patients with either type I or type II APS are committed to a regimen of lifelong hormone, mineral, and/or vitamin replacement. While it is usually best to counsel patients to continue participating in all their regular activities, health care providers must be mindful that an APS disease can dramatically alter a patient's life (e.g., an airline pilot who develops IDDM).

Systematic studies of the long-term prognosis in APS patients are lacking, but clinical impressions are that the type II APS patients have rates of morbidity and mortality that are identical to those of the component diseases when they occur in isolation. Adrenal crises are still a significant cause of preventable mortality, and uncontrolled thyroid hormone imbalances can rarely present as emergencies, especially in the elderly. The complications of IDDM, both acute and chronic, are as important in the APS setting as in isolated pancreatic disease.

While many patients diagnosed with type I APS lead a full and vigorous life,[92] poorer outcomes are common. Some develop a course of recurrent illnesses starting in their second decade of life. Problems include asthenia which is often of uncertain etiology, recurrent opportunistic infections which presumably arise because of a T-lymphocyte deficiency, and chronic active hepatitis which continues to be one of the most common causes of mortality in type I APS. Mortality near the end of the second or during the third decade is not uncommon.

CONCLUSION

Syndromes of multiorgan failure induced by autoimmunity occur in well-recognized patterns and can be detected at an asymptomatic stage by screening high-risk individuals for circulating autoantibodies. Such antibodies are of diagnostic importance also in symptomatic patients. Optimal management includes close anticipatory monitoring so that early treatment of organ failure can be instituted, thereby preventing irreversible morbidity or even death. Currently, treatment is limited to pharmacological replacements and psychosocial support; however, increases in our understanding of the pathogenesis of these conditions should lead to treatments that will prevent progression to complete end-organ destruction. Over recent years, dramatic progress has been made in the identification of target antigens and epitopes involved in the autoimmune organ-specific diseases which are components of the APS. Clearly, more needs to be learned about the defective peripheral immune tolerance that these patients must have toward their own glands.

REFERENCES

1. Addison T: Anaemia—Disease of the suprarenal capsules. Lond Med Gaz 8:517–518, 1849.
2. Claude H, Gourgerot H: Insuffisance pluriglandulaire endocrinienne. J Physiol Pathol Gen 10:469–480, 1908.
3. Hashimoto H: Zur kenntnis der lymphomatosen veranderung der schilddruse (struma lymphomatosa). Acta Klin Chir 97:219–248, 1912.
4. von Meyenburg H: Uber "Insulitis" bei diabetes. Schweitz Med Wochenschr 71:554–557, 1940.
5. Schmidt MB: Eine biglandulare erkrankung (Nebennieren und Schilddrusse) bei Morbus Addisonii. Verh Dtsch Pathol Ges 21:212–221, 1926.
6. Carpenter CCJ, Solomon N, Silverberg SG, et al: Schmidt's syndrome (thyroid and adrenal insufficiencey): A review of the literature and a report of fifteen new cases including ten instances of coexistent diabetes mellitus. Medicine 43:153–180, 1964.
7. Thorpe ES, Handley HE: Chronic tetany and chronic mycelial stomatitis in a child aged four-and-one-half years. Am J Dis Child 38:328–338, 1929.
8. Whitaker J, Landing BH, Esselborn VM, Williams RR: The syndrome of familial juvenile hypoadrenocorticism, hypoparathyroidism and superficial moniliasis. J Clin Endocrinol 16:1374–1387, 1956.
9. Roitt IM, Doniach D, Campbell PN, Hudson RV: Autoantibodies in Hashimoto's disease (lymphadenoid goitre). Lancet 2:820–821, 1956.
10. Neufeld M, Maclaren N, Blizzard R: Autoimmune polyglandular syndromes. Pediatr Ann 9:154–162, 1980.
11. Neufeld M, Maclaren NK, Blizzard RM: Two types of autoimmune Addison's disease associated with different polyglandular autoimmune (PGA) syndromes. Medicine 60:355–362, 1981.
12. Brun JM: Juvenile autoimmune polyendocrinopathy. Horm Res 16:308–316, 1982.
13. Maclaren NK, Riley WJ: Autoimmune endocrinopathies. In Samter M, Talmage DW, Frank MM, et al (eds): Immunological Diseases of the Endocrine System. Boston, Little, Brown, 1988, pp 1737–1764.
14. Riley WJ, Maclaren NK, Krischer J, et al: A prospective study of the development of diabetes in relatives of patients with insulin-dependent diabetes. N Engl J Med 323:1167–1172, 1990.
15. Elder M, Maclaren N, Riley W: Gonadal autoantibodies in patients with hypogonadism and/or Addison's disease. J Clin Endocrinol Metab 52:1137–1142, 1981.
16. Ketchum CH, Riley WJ, Maclaren NK: Adrenal dysfunction in asymptomatic patients with adrenocortical autoantibodies. J Clin Endocrinol Metab 58:1166–1170, 1984.
17. Betterle C, Scalici C, Presotto F, et al: The natural history of adrenal function in autoimmune patients with adrenal autoantibodies. J Endocrinol 117:467–475, 1988.
18. Leisti S, Ahonen P, Perheentupa J: The diagnosis and staging of hypocortisolism in progressing autoimmune adrenalitis. Pediatr Res 17:861–867, 1983.
19. Scherbaum WA: Autoimmune hypothalamic diabetes insipidus. Prog Brain Res 93:283–292, 1992.
20. Bigazzi PE: Autoimmunity of the adrenals. In Volpe R (ed): Autoimmunity and Endocrine Disease. New York, Marcel Dekker, 1985, pp 345–373.
21. Ahonen P, Miettinen A, Perheentupa J: Adrenal and steroidal cell antibodies in patients with autoimmune polyglandular disease type I and risk of adrenocortical and ovarian failure. J Clin Endocrinol Metab 64:494–500, 1987.
22. McNatty KP, Short RV, Barnes EW, Irvine WJ: The cytotoxic effect of serum from patients with Addison's disease and autoimmune ovarian failure on human granulosa cells in culture. Clin Exp Immunol 22:378–384, 1975.
23. Krohn K, Uibo R, Aavik E, et al: Identification by molecular cloning of an autoantigen associated with Addison's disease as steroid 17α-hydroxylase. Lancet 339:770–773, 1992.
24. Furmaniak J, Talbot D, Reinwein D, et al: Immunoprecipitation of human adrenal microsomal antigen. FEBS Lett 231:25–28, 1988.
25. Winquist O, Karlsson F, Kämpe O: 21-Hydroxylase, a major autoantigen in idiopathic Addison's disease. Lancet 339:1559–1562, 1992.
26. Salim YS, Faber V, Wiik A, et al: Anti-corticosteroid antibodies in AIDS patients. APMIS 96:889–894, 1988.
27. Blizzard RM, Chee D, Davis W: The incidence of parathyroid and other antibodies in the sera of patients with idiopathic hypoparathyroidism. Clin Exp Immunol 1:119–128, 1966.
28. Chapman CK, Bradwell AR, Dykks PW: Do parathyroid and adrenal autoantibodies coexist? J Clin Pathol 39:813–814, 1986.
29. Betterle C, Caretto A, Zeviani M, et al: Demonstration and characterization of anti-human mitochondria autoantibodies in idiopathic hypoparathyroidism and in other conditions. Clin Exp Immunol 62:353–360, 1985.
30. Fattorossi A, Aurbach GD, Sakaguchi K, et al: Anti-endothelial cell antibodies: Detection and characterization in sera from patients with autoimmune hypoparathyroidism. Proc Natl Acad Sci USA 85:4015–4019, 1988.
31. Elrehewy M, Kong YM, Giraldo AA, Rose NR: Syngeneic thyroglobulin is immunogenic in good responder mice. Eur J Immunol 11:146–151, 1981.
32. Atkinson MA, Kaufman DL, Newman D, et al: Islet cell cytoplasmic autoantibody reactivity in insulin-dependent diabetes. J Clin Invest 91:350–356, 1993.
33. Maclaren NK, Riley WJ: Thyroid, gastric, and adrenal autoimmunities associated with insulin-dependent diabetes mellitus. Diabetes Care 8(Suppl 1):34–38, 1985.
34. Loveridge N, Bitensky L, Chayen J, et al: Inhibition of parietal cell function by human gammaglobulin containing gastric parietal cell antibodies. Clin Exp Immunol 41:264–270, 1980.
35. Tanaka N, Glass GBJ: Effect of prolonged administration of parietal cell antibodies from patients with atrophic gastritis and pernicious anemia on the parietal cell mass and hydrochloric acid output in rats. Gastroenterology 58:482–494, 1970.
36. Burman P, Mardh S, Norberg L, Karlsson FA: Parietal cell antibodies in pernicious anemia inhibit H^+, K^+-adenosine triphosphatase, the proton pump of the stomach. Gastroenterology 96:1434–1438, 1989.
37. Betterle C, Mirakian R, Doniach D, et al: Antibodies to melanocytes in vitiligo. Lancet 1:159, 1984.
38. Bottazzo GF, Pouplard A, Florin-Christensen A, Doniach D: Autoantibodies to prolactin-secreting cells of human pituitary. Lancet 2:97–101, 1975.
39. Cosman F, Kalmon DP, Holub DA, Wardlaw SL: Lymphocytic hypophysitis: Report of 3 new cases and review of the literature. Medicine 68:240–256, 1989.
40. Komatsu M, Kondo T, Yamauchi K, et al: Antipituitary antibodies in patients with the primary empty sella syndrome. J Clin Endocrinol Metab 67:633–638, 1988.
41. Wilkin TJ: Receptor autoimmunity in endocrine disorders. N Engl J Med 323:1318–1324, 1990.
42. Arulanantham K, Dwyer JM, Genel, M: Evidence for defective immunoregulation in the syndrome of familial candidiasis endocrinopathy. N Engl J Med 300:164–168, 1979.
43. Eisenbarth GS, Wilson PN, Ward F, et al: The polyglandular failure syndrome: Disease inheritance, HLA-type, and immune function studies in patients and families. Ann Intern Med 91:528–533, 1979.
44. Schatz DA, Lang F, Cantor AB, et al: CD5+ B lymphocytes in high-risk islet cell antibody-positive and newly diagnosed IDDM patients. Diabetes 40:1314–1318, 1991.
45. Volpé R: Immunology of human thyroid disease. In Volpé R (ed): Autoimmune Diseases of the Endocrine System. Boca Raton, Fla, CRC Press, 1990, pp 73–239.
46. Brenner O: Addison's disease with atrophy of the cortex of the suprarenals. Q J Med 22:121–144, 1928.
47. Gloor E, Hurlimann J: Autoimmune oophoritis. Am J Clin Pathol 81:105–109, 1984.

48. Sedmak DD, Hart WR, Tubbs RR: Autoimmune oophoritis: A histopathologic study of involved ovaries with immunologic characterization of the mononuclear cell infiltrate. Int J Gynecol Pathol 6:73–81, 1987.
49. Bottazzo GF, Dean BM, McNally JM, et al: In situ characterization of autoimmune phenomena and expression of HLA molecules in the pancreas in diabetic insulitis. N Engl J Med 313:353–360, 1985.
50. Foulis AK, Liddle CN, Farquharson MA, et al: The histopathology of the pancreas in type I (insulin-dependent) diabetes mellitus: A 25-year review of deaths in patients under 20 years of age in the United Kingdom. Diabetalogia 29:267–274, 1986.
51. Muir A, Schatz DA, Maclaren NK: Autoimmune Addison's disease. In Bach JF (ed): Immunoendocrinology: Seminars in Immunopathology. New York, Springer-Verlag, 1993, 14, pp 275–284.
52. Craig JM, Schiff LH, Boone JE: Chronic moniliasis associated with Addison's disease. Am J Dis Child 89:669–684, 1955.
53. Roitt IM, Doniach D: Gastric autoimmunity. In Miescher PA, Müller-Eberhard HJ (eds): Textbook of Immunopathology. New York, Grune & Stratton, 1976, pp 737–749.
54. Muir A, Maclaren NK: Autoimmune diseases of the adrenal glands, parathyroid glands, gonads, and hypothalamic-pituitary axis. Endocrinol Metab Clin North Am 20:619–644, 1991.
55. Schatz DA, Riley WJ, Maclaren NK, Barrett DJ: Defective inducer T-cell function before the onset of insulin-dependent diabetes mellitus. J Autoimmunity 4:125–136, 1991.
56. Aguayo J, Sakatsume Y, Jamieson C, et al: Nontoxic nodular goiter and papillary carcinoma of the thyroid gland are not associated with peripheral blood lymphocyte sensitization to thyroid cells. J Clin Endocrinol Metab 68:145–149, 1989.
57. Jarpe AJ, Hickman MR, Anderson JT, et al: Flow cytometric enumeration of mononuclear cell populations infiltrating the islets of Langerhans in prediabetic NOD mice: Development of a model of autoimmune insulitis for type I diabetes. Reg Immunol 3:305–307, 1991.
58. Davies TF, Martin A, Concepcion ES, et al: Evidence of limited variability of antigen receptors on intrathyroidal T cells in autoimmune thyroid disease. N Engl J Med 325:238–244, 1991.
59. Campbell IL, Harrison LC: Molecular pathology of type I diabetes. Mol Biol Med 7:299–309, 1990.
60. Bottazzo GF, Todd I, Rirakian R, et al: Organ-specific autoimmunity: A 1986 overview. Immunol Rev 94:137–169, 1986.
61. Bagnasco M, Caretto A, Olive D, et al: Expression of intercellular adhesion molecule-1 (ICAM-1) on thyroid epithelial cells in Hashimoto's thyroiditis but not in Graves' disease or papillary thyroid cancer. Clin Exp Immunol 83:309–313, 1991.
62. Campbell IL, Cutri A, Wilkinson D, et al: Intercellular adhesion molecule-1 is induced on endocrine islet cells by cytokines but not by reovirus infection. Proc Natl Acad Sci USA 86:4282–4286, 1989.
63. Rabinovitch A, Sumoski W, Rajotte R, Warnock GL: Cytotoxic effects of cytokines on human pancreatic islet cells in monolayer culture. J Clin Endocrinol Metab 71:152–156, 1990.
64. Hamilton F, Black M, Farquharson MA, et al: Spatial correlation between thyroid epithelial cells expressing class II MHC and interferon-gamma–containing lymphocytes in human thyroid autoimmune disease. Clin Exp Immunol 83:64–68, 1991.
65. Pujol-Borrell R, Todd I, Doshi M, et al: HLA class II induction in human islet cells by interferon-gamma plus tumour necrosis factor or lymphotoxin. Nature 326:304–306, 1987.
66. Hill JA, Welch WR, Heidi MP, et al: Induction of class II major histocompatibility complex antigen expression in human granulosa cells by interferon gamma: A potential mechanism contributing to autoimmune failure. Am J Obstet Gynecol 162:534–540, 1990.
67. Corbett JA, McDaniel ML: Does nitric oxide mediate autoimmune destruction of β-cells? Possible therapeutic interventions in IDDM. Diabetes 41:897–903, 1992.
68. Kolb H, Kolb-Bachofen V: Nitric oxide: A pathogenic factor in autoimmunity. Immunol Today 13:157–160, 1992.
69. Kirkpatrick CH: Transfer factor. CRC Crit Rev Clin Lab Sci 12:87–122, 1980.
70. Serreze DV, Leiter EH: Defective activation of T suppressor cell function in nonobese diabetic mice. J Immunol 140:3801–3807, 1988.
71. Faustman D, Schoenfeld D, Ziegler R: T-lymphocyte changes linked to autoantibodies: Association of insulin autoantibodies with CD4+CD45R+ lymphocyte subpopulation in prediabetic subjects. Diabetes 40:590–597, 1991.
72. Rhim SH, Millar SE, Robey F, et al: Autoimmune disease of the ovary induced by ZP3 peptide from the mouse zona pellucida. J Clin Invest 89:28–35, 1992.
73. Levine S: Allergic adrenalitis and adenohypophysitis: Further observations on induction and passive transfer. Endocrinology 84:469–475, 1969.
74. Damjanović M: Experimental autoimmune oophoritis: II. Both lymphoid cells and antibodies are successful in adoptive transfer. Autoimmunity 9:217–223, 1991.
75. Smith H, Lou Y-H, Lacy P, Tung KSK: Tolerance mechanism in experimental ovarian and gastric autoimmune diseases. J Immunol 149:2210–2218, 1992.
76. Sakaguchi S, Sakaguchi N: Organ-specific autoimmune disease induced in mice by elimination of T cell subsets: V. Neonatal administration of cyclosporin A causes autoimmune disease. J Immunol 142:471–480, 1989.
77. Taguchi O, Nishizuka Y: Autoimmune oophoritis in the thymectomized mouse: T cell requirement in the adoptive cell transfer. Clin Exp Immunol 42:324–331, 1980.
78. Ferrick DA, Ohashi PS, Wallace VA, et al: Transgenic mice as an in vivo model for self-reactivity. Immunol Rev 118:257–283, 1990.
79. Sarvetnick N, Shizuru J, Liggitt D, et al: Loss of pancreatic islet tolerance induced by β-cell expression of interferon-γ. Nature 346:844–847, 1990.
80. Lund T, O'Reilly L, Hutchings P, et al: Prevention of insulin-dependent diabetes mellitus in nonobese diabetic mice by transgenes encoding modified I-A β-chain or normal I-E α-chain. Nature 345:727–729, 1990.
81. Schatz D, Winter W, Maclaren N: Immunology of insulin-dependent diabetes. In Volpé R (ed): Autoimmune Diseases of the Endocrine System. Boca Raton, Fla, CRC Press, 1990, pp 241–296.
82. Hao W, Serreze DV, Leiter EH, et al: Insulin (auto)antibodies from human IDDM cross-react with retroviral antigen p73. Diabetes 43(Suppl. 1):37A, 1992.
83. Haspel MV, Onodera T, Prabhakar BS, et al: Virus-induced autoimmunity: Monoclonal antibodies that react with endocrine tissues. Science 220:304–306, 1983.
84. Helgason T, Jonasson MR: Evidence for a food additive as a cause of ketosis-prone diabetes. Lancet 2:716–720, 1981.
85. Daneman D, Fishman L, Clarson C, Martin JM: Dietary triggers of insulin-dependent diabetes in the BB rat. Diabetes Res 5:93–97, 1987.
86. Virtanen SM, Rasanen L, Aro A, et al: Infant feeding in Finnish children less than 7 years of age with newly diagnosed IDDM: Childhood Diabetes in Finland Study Group. Diabetes Care 14:415–417, 1991.
87. Dahl-Jørgenesen K, Joner G, Hanssen KF: Relationship between cow's milk consumption and incidence of IDDM in childhood. Diabetes Care 14:1081–1083, 1991.
88. Karjalainen J, Martin JM, Knip M, et al: Evidence for a BSA peptide as a candidate trigger of type I diabetes. N Engl J Med 327:302–307, 1992.
89. Maclaren NK, Riley WJ: Inherited susceptibility to autoimmune Addison's disease is linked to human leukocyte antigens-DR3 and/or DR4, except when associated with type I autoimmune polyglandular syndrome. J Clin Endocrinol Metab 62:455–459, 1986.
90. Ahonen P, Koskimies S, Lokki ML, et al: The expression of autoimmune polyglandular disease type I appears associated with several HLA-A antigens but not with HLA-DR. J Clin Endocrinol Metab 66:1152–1157, 1988.
91. Herrod HG: Chronic mucocutaneous candidiasis in childhood and complications of non-Candida infection: A report of the pediatric immunodeficiency collaborative study group. Pediatrics 116:377–382, 1990.
92. Ahonen P, Myllärniemi S, Sipilä I, Perheentupa J: Clinical variation of autoimmune polyendocrinopathy-candidiasis-ectodermal dystrophy (APECED) in a series of 68 patients. N Engl J Med 322:1829–1836, 1990.
93. Lonsdale RN, Roberts PF, Trowell JE: Autoimmune oophoritis associated with polycystic ovaries. Histopathology 19:77–81, 1991.
94. Mandel M, Etzioni A, Theodor R, Passwell JH: Pure red cell hypoplasia associated with polyglandular autoimmune syndrome type I. Isr J Med Sci 25:138–141, 1989.
95. Tsatsoulis A, Shalet SM: Antisperm autoantibodies in the polyglandular autoimmunity (PGA) syndrome type I: Response to cyclical steroid therapy. Clin Endocrinol 35:299–303, 1991.
96. Vela BS, Dorin RI, Hartshorne MF: Case report 631: Neo-osseous porosis (metaphyseal osteopenia) in polyglandular autoimmune (Schmidt) syndrome. Skeletal Radiol 19:468–471, 1990.
97. Walz B, From GL: Addison's disease and sarcoidosis: Unusual frequency of co-existing hypothyroidism (Schmidt's syndrome). Am J Med 89:692–693, 1990.

98. Jones KL: Smith's Recognizable Patterns of Human Malformation (ed 4). Philadelphia, WB Saunders Co, 1988, pp 74–79.

99. Hall JG, Gilchrist DM: Turner syndrome and its variants. Pediatr Clin North Am 37:1421–1440, 1990.

100. Engel EG: Myasthenia gravis and other disorders of neuromuscular transmission. *In* Braunwald E, Isselbacher KJ, Petersdorf RG, et al (eds): Harrison's Principles of Internal Medicine. New York, McGraw-Hill, 1987, pp 2079–2082.

101. Silverstein J, Maclaren N, Riley W, et al: Immunosuppression with azathioprine and prednisone in recent onset insulin dependent diabetes mellitus. N Engl J Med 319:599–604, 1988.

102. Martin S, Schernthaner G, Nerup J, et al: Follow up of cyclosporin A treatment in type I (insulin dependent) diabetes mellitus: Lack of long-term effects. Diabetalogia 34:429–434, 1991.

103. Rabinowe SL, Berger M, Welch WR, Dluhy RG: Lymphocyte dysfunction in autoimmune oophoritis. Resumption of menses with corticosteroids. Am J Med 81:347–350, 1986.

104. Mayfield RK, Levine JH, Gordon C, et al: Lymphoid adenohypophysitis presenting as a pituitary tumour. Am J Med 69:619–623, 1980.

105. Sutherland DER: Current status of pancreas transplantation. J Clin Endocrinol Metab 73:461–463, 1991.

106. Ricordi C, Lacy PE, Santiago JV, et al: Transplantation of parathyroid, adrenal cortex and adrenal medulla using procedures which successfully prolonged islet allograft survival. Horm Metab Res Suppl 25:132–135, 1990.

107. Yu XC, Yu TL, Zhang SZ, Liu DF, Jia JH: Homotransplantation of adrenal gland. Chin Med J Engl 104:487–490, 1991.

108. Stravinoha MW, Soloway RD: Current therapy of chronic liver disease. Drugs 39:814–840, 1990.

109. Rose NR, Witebsky E: Studies on organ specificity: V. Changes in the thyroid gland of rabbits following active immunization with rabbit thyroid extracts. J Immunol 76:417–427, 1956.

110. Holborow EJ, Brown PC, Roitt IM, Doniach D: Cytoplasmic locaton of "complement-fixing" auto-antigen in human thyroid epithelium. Br J Pathol 40:583–588, 1959.

Index

Note: Page numbers in *italics* refer to illustrations; page numbers followed by t refer to tables.

Adipose tissue *(Continued)*
  aromatase activity in, 2475
  at menarche, 2556–2557, *2558*, 2561
  atrophy of, in insulin therapy, 1498
  brown, 2267
    in thermogenesis, 2252
  cell enlargement in, 2631–2632
  chorionic somatomammotropin effects on, 2185
  deficiency of, in insulin resistance, *1598*, 1599–1600
  distribution of, aging and, 2719–2720
    criteria for, 2628, *2629*
    disorders associated with, 2720, 2722
    in Cushing's syndrome, 1741–1743, 1742t, *1742–1744*
    in obesity classification, 2644
    measurement of, 2626
    mortality and, 2638–2639, *2639*, 2648
  energy storage in, 1389–1390, 1390t, 2631, *2632*, 2664
  excessive. See *Obesity.*
  fatty acid transport from, in ketogenesis, *1509*, 1509–1510
  fetal, 2267, *2268*
  glucocorticoid receptors in, 1662
  glucose metabolism in, 1396t, 1396–1397, 1401, *1401*
  glucose transport in, insulin and, 1381
  hypertrophy of, in insulin therapy, 1498
  insulin metabolism in, 1359
  lipid synthesis in, 1406
  lipolysis in, 2664, *2665*
  measurement of, 2625t, 2625–2628, *2626–2627*
  natural history of, 2634–2635
  ontogeny of, 2631
  proliferation of, 2631
  regional mobilization of, 2654–2655
  suction-assisted removal of, 2655
  upper body, disorders associated with, 2722
  visceral, measurement of, 2626, 2628
    mortality risk from, 2648
  white, 2267
Adiposogenital dystrophy, 151
Adipsic hypernatremia, 417, 417t
Adipsin, 2667
Adolescents, bone mass in, 1234–1235
  hyperthyroidism in, 794–795
  hypothyroidism in, 793–794, 793t–794t, *794*
  oral contraceptives for, 2152
  puberty in. See *Puberty.*
  sexual behavior in, 1982–1984
  thyroid function in, 792–793, *793*
Adrenal androgens. See *Androgen(s), adrenal;* specific hormone.
Adrenal cortex, adenoma of, aldosterone-producing. See *Conn's syndrome.*
  aldosteronism in, 1778, *1778*
  angiotensin II-responsive, 1783t, 1789
  Cushing's syndrome in, 1747, 1748
  hypercortisolemia in, 1716–1717, *1716–1717*
  imaging of, 1716–1717, *1716–1717*, 1726
  vs. ectopic ACTH syndrome, 2773
  vs. idiopathic aldosteronism, 1787
  angiotensin II synthesis in, 1672
  carcinoma of, aldosteronism in, 1778, 1789
    Cushing's syndrome in, 1748
    imaging of, *1713*, 1726, *1726*
  cells of, in ovarian tumors, 2118–2119
  diseases of. See also specific disease, e.g., *Cushing's syndrome.*
    historical overview of, 1628

Adrenal cortex *(Continued)*
  failure of, hypoaldosteronism in, 1805
  fetal, 2193–2195, *2194*
  function of, in aging, 2712–2713
    in hypothyroidism, 761
    in pregnancy, *2295*, 2295–2298, *2297*
    testing of, *1735–1736*, 1735–1738
      in aldosteronism, 1779–1788, *1780–1781*, 1782t–1783t, *1784–1787*
      in Cushing's syndrome, 1750–1756, 1751t–1752t, *1753–1756*
      in pregnancy, *2295*, 2295–2298, *2297*
  historical overview of, 1627–1629
  hormones of. See also *Cortisol; Glucocorticoid(s);* specific hormone, e.g., *Aldosterone.*
    historical background of, 1627–1629, 1642–1644
    in hypertension, 2921–2922
    secretion of, in aging, 2712–2713
      in obesity, 2642–2643, 2643t
      rhythms of, 2525–2526, *2526–2527*
  hyperplasia of, macronodular, 1717–1718, *1717–1718*, 1748
  imaging of, in Cushing's syndrome, 1716–1719, *1716–1719*, 1719t
  intracellular transduction mechanisms in, 1673–1674, *1674*
  renin-angiotensin system of, 1673
  scintigraphy of, *1715*, 1715–1716, *1786–1787*, 1787
  tumors of. See also *Adrenal cortex, adenoma of.*
    hyperandrogenism in, 2103
    in multiple endocrine neoplasia, 2818
Adrenal gland. See also *Hypothalamic-pituitary-adrenal axis.*
  anatomy of, 1711–1712, *1712*
  androgen secretion from, 2093–2094, *2094*
  atrophy of, imaging of, 1720, *1721*
    in fungal infections, 1732
  autoantibodies to, 3014–3015, 3015t
  blood supply of, 1711
  cortex of. See *Adrenal cortex.*
  corticotropin-releasing hormone in, 349
  disease of, menstrual cycle disorders in, 2072
  embryology of, 2244–2245
  enzymes of, in fetus, 2245
  failure of, primary, 347
  fetal, 1841–1842, *1841–1842*, 2190, 2193–2195, 2244–2245
  function of, testing of, 1926–1927
    tests for, *1735–1736*, 1735–1738
      in Cushing's syndrome, 1750–1756, 1751t–1752t, *1753–1756*
  granulomatous disease of, 1720–1721, *1722*
  hemochromatosis of, imaging of, 1721, *1722*
  hemorrhage of, adrenal insufficiency in, 1732
    imaging of, 1721, *1722*
  hormones of. See *Cortisol; Glucocorticoid(s);* specific hormone, e.g., *Aldosterone.*
  hyperplasia of. See *Adrenal hyperplasia.*
  hypoplasia of, congenital, delayed puberty in, 1961
    with hypogonadism, genetic defect in, 130t, 139
  imaging of, 1711–1730
    anatomic considerations in, 1711–1712, *1712*
    arteriography in, 1714, 1869
    computed tomography in, 1712, *1712–1713*, 1787–1788, 1868
    for venous sampling, 1714–1715
    in aldosteronism, 1719–1720, *1720–1721*

Adrenal gland *(Continued)*
  in Cushing's syndrome, 1716–1719, *1716–1719*, 1719t
  in insufficiency, 1720–1723, *1721–1723*, 1723t
  in pheochromocytoma, 1723–1724, *1723–1725*
  in tumors, 1724, 1726–1727, *1726–1727*
  magnetic resonance imaging in, 1712–1714, *1713–1714*, 1787–1788, 1869
  scintigraphy in, *1715*, 1715–1716, *1786–1787*, 1787, 1869
  ultrasonography in, 1715
  injury of, adrenal insufficiency in, 1732–1733
  insufficiency of. See *Adrenal insufficiency.*
  medulla of. See *Adrenal medulla.*
  metastasis to, adrenal insufficiency in, 1733
  pigmented nodular disease of, 1717, *1718*, 1748
  "puberty" of. See *Adrenarche.*
  removal of. See *Adrenalectomy.*
  sex steroid secretion by, postmenopausal, 2130–2131, *2131*
  tumors of. See *Adrenal tumors.*
  venography of, in aldosteronism, 1786–1787, *1786–1787*
Adrenal hyperplasia, congenital, 1813–1835, 1843, 2098–2099
  definition of, 1813
  delayed puberty in, 1960
  enzyme defects in, 130t, 139–140
  forms of, 1813–1815, 1814t
  from prenatal exogenous hormones, 1980–1981
  historical background of, 1815
  hypogonadism in, 2381, 2383
  imaging in, 1721, 1723, *1723*, 1723t
  in cholesterol desmolase deficiency, 1814t, 1814–1815, 1825, 1827
  in corticosterone methyloxidase II deficiency, 1814t, 1822–1823, *1823*
  in dexamethasone-suppressible hyperaldosteronism, 1823
  in 11β-hydroxylase deficiency, 1813, 1814t, 1821–1822, *1821–1822*
    prenatal diagnosis of, 1830
  in 21-hydroxylase deficiency, 1813, 1814t, 1815–1821
    classic type, 1815–1818, *1816–1817*
    diagnosis of, 1819–1821, *1820*
    epidemiology of, 1815
    molecular genetics of, 1819, *1819–1820*
    nonclassic type, *1817*, 1818t, 1818–1819
    prenatal diagnosis of, 1829–1830
  in 17α-hydroxylase/17,20-lyase deficiency, 1814, 1814t, 1825, *1827*
  in 3β-hydroxysteroid dehydrogenase deficiency, 1813–1814, 1814t, 1823–1825, *1824*, *1826*
  precocious puberty in, 1967–1968, 1969–1970
  prenatal diagnosis of, 1829–1830
  prenatal treatment of, 1830–1831, *1830–1831*
  pseudohermaphroditism in, 1913t, 1913–1917, 1923–1924, *1924*
  sexual behavior in, 1980, 1981
  testicular tumors in, 2445
  transmission of, 1813
  treatment of, 1827–1829, *1828*, 2105
  vs. premature adrenarche, 2097–2098
  lipoid, 1827, 1913–1914
  massive macronodular, Cushing's syndrome in, 1748

Agonadism, 1905t, 1905–1906

Ahistrom syndrome, obesity in, 2646t

AIDS. See *Human immunodeficiency virus infection.*

Airway tone, in diabetes mellitus, 1552

Akee fruit, ingestion of, hypoglycemia from, 1611

Alanine, formation of, in fasting, 1393, *1393*
  in gluconeogenesis, *1606*, 1607
  levels of, in hypoglycemia, 2270, *2270*

Alanine cycle, in starvation, 2665, *2665–2666*

Albright's hereditary osteodystrophy, 1136, 1141–1143, *1143–1144*
  diagnosis of, 1146t, 1146–1147
  G protein mutation in, 130t, 142
  genetics of, 1145–1146

Albumin, abnormalities of, thyroid hormone disorders in, 570
  absence of, 881
    thyroid hormone disorders in, 570
  deficiency of, calcium levels in, 1130
    growth attenuation in, 2578
  gene of, mutation in, 130t, 136
  measurement of, in nutritional assessment, 2671
    in urine, 1573
  steroid binding to, 2025
  thyroid hormone binding to, 560
    changes in, 570
    mechanism of action of, 560–561
    metabolism of, 561t
    properties of, 561t, 563
  urinary, in diabetic nephropathy, 1573–1575

Alcohol use and abuse, hepatitis in, anabolic steroids in, 2368
  testicular function in, 2395–2396, 2396t
  hypoglycemia in, 1611–1612
  hypoparathyroidism in, 1126
  hypophosphatemia in, 1215–1216
  in diabetic diet, 1491
  ketoacidosis in, vs. diabetic ketoacidosis, 1512t
  maternal, fetal alcohol syndrome from, 2465t
  thyroid-stimulating hormone deficiency in, 213

Aldose reductase, in diabetic neuropathy, 1539–1540, 1540t
  inhibitors of, in diabetic neuropathy therapy, 1558

Aldosterone, actions of, 1668–1669, *1669*
  sites of, 1668
    specificity-conferring enzymes in, 1678
  androgen receptor binding affinity of, 2341t
  biochemistry of, 1677–1681
  deficiency of. See *Hypoaldosteronism.*
  in adrenal insufficiency, 1738
  in fetus, 2245
  in hydrogen ion transport, 1681
  in hypertension, 2924, *2924*
  in ketoacidosis, 1511t
  in potassium excretion, 1694–1695, *1695*
  in potassium homeostasis, 1672–1673
  in potassium transport, 1681
  in pregnancy, 1703, *2297*, 2297–2298
  in sodium homeostasis, 1669–1672, *1671, 1689*, 1689–1690, *1691*
  in sodium transport, 1679–1681
  in sodium/hydrogen antiporter activity, 1681
  levels of, in ACTH stimulation test, 1737
  measurement of, in aldosteronism diagnosis, 1780–1781
  placental transport of, 2240
  receptors for, 1677–1678
    classic, 1677–1678

Aldosterone *(Continued)*
  defects in, pseudohypoaldosteronism in, 1807–1808
  membrane, 1678
  secretion of, ACTH effects on, 362
    atrial natriuretic peptide inhibition of, 2903, *2903*
    deficient, *1804*, 1804–1807
    feedback regulation of, 1668–1669, *1669*
    inhibitors of, 1670
    intracellular transduction mechanisms in, 1673–1674, *1674*
    potassium intake and, 1672–1673
    regulation of, 1695–1698, *1696*, 2917–2918, *2919*
    renin-angiotensin systems in, 1670, 1670t, 1672–1673
    sodium intake and, 1670–1672, *1671*
    stress hormones in, 1673, 1673t
  structure of, *94*, 1792, *1793*
  synthesis of, 1632, *1698*, 1699, 1804, *1804, 1814, 1837, 2094*
  urinary, measurement of, 1780–1781

Aldosterone oxidase. See *Aldosterone synthase (corticosterone methyl oxidase II).*

Aldosterone synthase (corticosterone methyl oxidase II), 1822
  activity of, potassium effects on, 1673
    sodium restriction effects on, 1671
  deficiency of, adrenal hyperplasia in, 1822–1823, *1823*
    hypoaldosteronism in, *1804*, 1804–1805
  gene of, duplication of, 2925, *2925*
    11β-hydroxylase gene hybridization with, 1776, *1777*, 2925, *2925*
    mutation of, 130t, 140
  in aldosterone synthesis, 1699

Aldosterone-induced proteins, 1679–1680

Aldosterone-renin ratio, in aldosteronism, 1776t, 1781–1782

Aldosteronism, definition of, 1702
  hypertension in, 2921
  in 18-hydroxycortisol excess, 1699
  in oral contraceptive use, 2922–2923
  in ovarian tumor, 2123
  primary, 1775–1789
    clinical features of, 1779
    definition of, 1775
    dexamethasone (glucocorticoid)-suppressible, 1776, *1777*, 1783t, 1789–1790, 1821, 1823, 2924–2925, *2925*
    diagnosis of, 1779–1788, *1780–1781*, 1782t–1783t, *1784–1787*
    differential diagnosis of, 1779
    etiology of, 1776t, 1776–1778, *1777*
    familial type II, 1778
    glucocorticoid-suppressible, 1776, *1777*, 1783t, 1789–1790, 1821, 1823, 2924–2925, *2925*
    idiopathic, 1776–1778, 1783t
      vs. adenoma, 1787
    imaging of, 1719–1720, *1720–1721*
    in adrenal carcinoma, 1778, 1789
    in adrenal hyperplasia, 1789
    in adrenocortical adenoma, 1778, *1778*
    in angiotensin II-responsive aldosterone-producing adenoma, 1783t, 1789
    in children, 1779
    in ovarian carcinoma, 1778–1779
    in pregnancy, 1779, 2298
    incidence of, 1779
    normokalemic, 1779
    pathology of, *1778*, 1778–1779
    prevalence of, 1775–1776, 1776t

Aldosteronism *(Continued)*
    treatment of, 1788–1789
    vs. pseudoaldosteronism, 1798
  secondary, 1702–1705
    causes of, 1702
    compensatory aldosterone secretion in, 1702–1704
    definition of, 1702
    edematous disorders in, 1704–1705

Aldosteronoma, imaging of, 1719–1720, *1720–1721*

Alimentary hypoglycemia, 1611

Alkali ingestion, hypercalcemia in, 1087–1088

Alkaline phosphatase, deficiency of, hypophosphatasia in, 1220
  in bone formation, 1194
  in malignancy-associated hypercalcemia, 1071–1072
  in renal osteodystrophy, 1160–1161
  in vitamin D-dependent rickets, 1174t
  measurement of, in bone metabolism evaluation, 1233
    in Paget's disease, 1266–1267
  placental, 2197
  secretion of, in malignancy, 2783

Alkalosis, in milk-alkali syndrome, 1088
  metabolic, calcium reabsorption in, 1023
    in Cushing's syndrome, 1745
    in malignancy-associated hypercalcemia, 1071
    in mineralocorticoid excess, 1700–1701
  respiratory, phosphate reabsorption in, 1032

Allantois, 1888, *1889*

Allergy, to insulin therapy, 1498

Allgrove syndrome, 2972

Allopurinol, in nephrolithiasis, 1185

Alloxan, pancreatic islet damage from, 1427

Alopecia, in hypocalcemia, 1124
  in vitamin D resistance, 1007
  in vitamin D-dependent rickets, 1176
  male-pattern, androgens in, 2096, *2096*

Alpha cells. See *A cells, pancreatic.*

Alpha-adrenergic activity, in growth hormone regulation, 306

Alpha-chlorhydrin, as contraceptive, 2451

Alpreolol, action of, on adrenergic receptors, 1856

Altitude, erythropoietin production and, 2957–2958
  puberty timing and, 1956

Alton giant, 320, *320–321*

Aluminum, absorption of, 1155, 1163, *1163*
  accumulation of, in renal failure, *1154*, 1154–1155
  determination of, in bone, 1161
  in parathyroid hormone secretion regulation, 940
  in phosphate-binding agents, safe use of, 1162–1163, *1163*
  in renal osteodystrophy, 1161–1162
  intoxication with, bone disease in, 1222–1223
    hypercalcemia in, 1087
    prevention of, 1162–1163, *1163*
    treatment of, 1166–1167
  osteomalacia caused by, *1154*, 1154–1155, 1159, *1160*, 1222–1223

Alytesin, physiology of, 2879

Alzheimer's disease, interleukin-1 in, 2979–2980
  somatostatin levels in, 272
  thyrotropin-releasing hormone in, 200

Amenorrhea, alternating with dysfunctional uterine bleeding, 2074, *2074*
  bone density measurement in, 1229

Biological rhythms (Continued)
 of gonadotropic axis, 2530–2532, 2531
 of insulin secretion, 2533–2536, 2534–2535
 of lactotropic axis, 2529–2530
 of pineal gland, 2536–2538
 of somatotropic axis, 2527–2529, 2528
 of thyrotropic axis, 2532–2533, 2533
 seasonal, 2518–2519, 2519
 ultradian, 2512–2517, 2513, 2515, 2517–2518
Biophysical profile, in diabetic pregnancy, 1470
Biopsy, bone, 1206, 1207
 endometrial, in ovulation documentation, 2081
 fine needle, of parathyroid glands, 1111
  of thyroid, 640–641, 838, 838–839, 905, 906
 gonadal, in sexual differentiation disorders, 1927
 muscle, in diabetic neuropathy, 1557
 nerve, in diabetic neuropathy, 1557
 parathyroid glands, 1111, 1114
 pituitary tumor, 499
 testis, 2415–2416, 2415–2416
 thyroid, 640–641, 838, 838–839, 905, 906
Bisalbuminemia, 570
Bisphosphonates, in hypercalcemia, 1095–1096, 1096–1097, 1099t
 in osteoporosis, 1238, 1244, 1245
 in Paget's disease, 1269–1270
Bladder, dysfunction of, in diabetes mellitus, 1550, 1560
Blastocyst, implantation of, 2172, 2172
Bleeding. See Hemorrhage.
Blindness, circadian rhythms in, 2508, 2509
 sleep disorders in, 440
Blood cells, production of. See Hematopoiesis.
Blood disorders, in Graves' disease, 688–689
Blood pressure. See also Hypertension; Hypotension.
 atrial natriuretic peptide effects on, 2902, 2903
 control of, dietary, 1489
 glucocorticoid effects on, 1648–1649
 in vasopressin regulation, 410, 410
 maintenance of, in postural change, 2935–2936, 2936
 sodium excretion and, 1694, 1694
Blood urea nitrogen, in hyperosmolar coma, 1517, 1517t
 in hyperparathyroidism, 1049
 in ketoacidosis, 1511t–1512t, 1512–1513
Blood vessels, calcification of, in renal failure, 1158, 1158
Blood volume, anabolic steroid effects on, 2369
 in vasopressin regulation, 410, 410
Blood-brain barrier, 153–154
Blood-testis barrier, 2312, 2312, 2322
Bloom's syndrome, 2565t, 2565–2566
Body compartments, measurement of, 2625–2626, 2626
Body fat. See Adipose tissue.
Body mass index, aging and, 2719–2720, 2720t
 health, 2627–2628
 in obesity measurement, 1490
 measurement of, 2627, 2627
 vs. mortality, 2638, 2639, 2647–2648, 2648
Body surface area, in resting metabolic rate calculation, 2635–2636
Body temperature. See Temperature, body.
Body weight. See Weight.
Boldenone, structure of, 2364
Bombesin (gastrin-releasing peptide), 2612
 in ACTH regulation, 364

Bombesin (gastrin-releasing peptide) (Continued)
 in corticotropin-releasing hormone potentiation, 347
 in pituitary hormone regulation, 187t
 physiology of, 2879
 secretion of, in thyroid carcinoma, 861
Bone, basic multicellular units of, 1196
 biopsy of, 1206, 1207
 calcitonin gene-related peptide effects on, 985, 986
 calcium in, 1016, 1016
 cells of, 1191–1193, 1191–1193. See also Osteoblast(s); Osteoclast(s).
 cysts of, in dialysis-related amyloidosis, 1158
 deformities of, in rickets, 1207–1208
 density of, in osteomalacia, 1209, 1210
  in pseudohypoparathyroidism, 1142
  measurement of, 1229–1233, 1230, 1231
 differentiation of, 2549–2550
 disorders of, after renal transplantation, 1167
  aluminum-related, 1154, 1154–1155
  in renal failure. See Renal osteodystrophy.
  metabolic. See also Osteomalacia; Osteoporosis; specific disease, e.g., Osteitis fibrosa/osteitis fibrosa cystica.
   classification of, 1200–1201
   concept of, 1200
  Paget's. See Paget's disease (bone).
 formation of, endochondral, 1194–1195, 1195
  evaluation of, 1233–1234
  in Paget's disease, 1266–1267
  intramembranous, 1194–1195, 1195
  measurement of, 1266–1267
 growth of, 1190–1198, 1191–1197, 2549–2550, 2557, 2558t–2560t, 2559–2560
  in adolescents, 1234–1235
  in growth hormone excess, 320t, 320–322, 320–322
  in hypothyroidism, 794
  in thyroid hormone resistance, 883, 883–884
  radiation therapy effects on, 2582
  rickets and, 1207–1208
 histology of, in malignancy-associated hypercalcemia, 1061–1062, 1062
  in vitamin D-dependent rickets, 1174t
 in hyperparathyroidism, 1050–1051, 1051
 in hyperthyroidism effects, 690
 lamellar, 1193–1195, 1194–1196
 late, 1208
 loss of. See also Bone, resorption of; Osteoporosis.
  in hyperprolactinemia, 395–396
 mass of, factors affecting, 1234–1235
  in acromegaly, 1242
  peak, 1234–1235
 metabolism of, in hypothyroidism, 761
  phosphate in, 1026
 metastasis to, bone resorption in, 1063
  hypercalcemia in, 2785
 mineralization of, 1194
  aluminum effects on, 1154, 1154–1155, 1222
  at puberty, 1235
  defects of, 1204t, 1204–1207, 1205–1207. See also Osteomalacia; Rickets.
   etiology of, 1204t
   in renal failure, 1156, 1156
   in vitamin D deficiency, 1248
  inhibition of, 1198
  mechanisms of, 1198, 1198–1199
  pH requirements for, 1214
  phosphate in, 1026
  requirements for, 1204

Bone (Continued)
 vitamin D in, 1004–1005, 1212–1213
 modeling of, 1195
 organic components of, 1190–1191
 organization of, 1190–1198, 1191–1197
 ossification of, endochondral, 1194–1195, 1195
  intramembranous, 1194–1195, 1195
  vs. age, 2557, 2559–2560
 Paget's disease of. See Paget's disease (bone).
 pain in, in fibrogenesis imperfecta ossium, 1221
  in osteomalacia, 1208
  in Paget's disease, 1263
  in renal failure, 1157
 parathyroid hormone-related protein effects on, 970–971
 properties of, 1190
 proteins of, 1190–1191
 remodeling of, 1195–1197, 1196–1197, 1233
  in pseudohypoparathyroidism, 1137
 resorption of. See also Osteoclast(s).
  bisphosphonates in, 1095–1096
  calcitonin in, 981–982, 981–983
  estrogen replacement in, 2133–2135, 2134–2135
  evaluation of, 1233–1234
  factors affecting, 2134
  glucocorticoids in, 1243
  hypercalcemia in, 1085–1086
  in acidosis, 1214–1215, 1215
  in androgen deficiency, 1240–1241
  in estrogen deficiency, 1236–1237, 1237
  in hypophosphatemia, 1026
  in malignancy-associated hypercalcemia, 1061–1062, 1062
  in Paget's disease, 1260–1263, 1260–1263, 1266
  in remodeling, 1195–1197, 1196–1197
  measurement of, 1266
  mechanisms of, 1198, 1198–1199
  parathyroid hormone in, 931–932, 932t
  thyroid hormone effects on, 1245–1247, 1247
  vitamin D action on, 1004, 1005
 structure of, 1190–1198, 1191–1197
 vitamin D action on, 1004–1005, 1005
 woven, 1193, 1193–1195
Bone acidic protein, 1190
Bone age, adult height prediction from, 2557, 2558t–2560t, 2559–2560
 definition of, 2557
 determination of, in delayed puberty evaluation, 1964
 growth disorders classified by, 2562–2563, 2562–2563, 2564t
Bone GLA protein, 1190
 measurement of, in Paget's disease, 1267
Bone marrow, failure of, anabolic steroids in, 2366–2367
 colony-stimulating factor treatment in, 2955, 2955
 Paget's disease of, 1261, 1261
Bone morphogenetic protein, 1199, 2604
Bone scan, in malignancy-associated hypercalcemia, 1072
 in Paget's disease, 1263, 1263
 in renal osteodystrophy, 1159–1160, 1160
Bone sialoprotein, 1190
Boucher-Neuhäser syndrome, delayed puberty in, 1962
Brachydactyly, in Albright's hereditary osteodystrophy, 1142–1143, 1143–1144
Bradbury-Eggleston syndrome, 2937, 2937t

β-Endorphin *(Continued)*
  synthesis of, 13, *13, 359,* 359–360
    in placenta, 2242
Endorphin(s), in immunoregulation, 2967t, 2972
  measurement of, in pheochromocytoma, 1867
  neuronal pathways for, *182*
  secretion of, in paraneoplastic syndromes, 2757t
  synthesis of, 2755, *2755*
Endosomes, in insulin degradation, 1383
  in receptor-mediated endocytosis, 32–33, *33*
  in thyroglobulin transport, *509,* 513, 533
Endostyle, in thyroid development, 518
Endothelial growth factor, 2592
Endothelins, 2907–2912
  actions of, 2911–2912
    intracellular, 2909–2910, *2910*
  distribution of, 2909
  gene of, 2909
  in aldosterone secretion, 1673
  in parturition, 2214
  isoforms of, *2908,* 2908–2909
  levels of, 2910–2911
  metabolism of, 2910
  physiology of, 2882
  precursors of, *2908,* 2908–2909
  receptors for, 2909–2910
  secretion of, 2909
    in postural change, 2935
    inhibition of, 2902
  structure of, *2908,* 2908–2909
  synthesis of, *2908,* 2908–2909, *2910*
Endothelium-derived relaxing factor, 2907, 2909–2910, *2910*
  osteoclast activity and, 982, *982*
Endotoxemia, hypothalamic-pituitary-adrenal axis response in, *345*
Endotoxin. See *Lipopolysaccharide.*
End-stage renal disease, in diabetes mellitus, 1574
  prevalence of, 1570
  treatment of, 1580–1586, *1580–1586,* 1581t–1583t
  in diabetic nephropathy, 1574
Endurance training, adaptation to, *2698,* 2698–2699
Energy/fuel. See also *Carbohydrates; Glucose; Lipid(s); Protein.*
  distribution of, 1390–1391
  expenditure of, 1397, 1397t
    components of, *2636*
    in hypothyroidism, 760
    in obesity, 2637
    in starvation, 2667
    individual variation in, 2648
    measurement of, 2634–2637, *2636*
  intake of, determination of, 2637
  metabolism of, 1389–1390, 1390t
  requirements of, in nutritional therapy planning, *2672,* 2672–2673, 2673t
    in weight loss diet, 2649, 2649t
  sources of, 1389–1390, 1390t
  storage of, 1389–1390
    in adipose tissue, 2631, *2632*
  transport of, placental, 2258–2261, *2259*
Engorgement, breast, in lactation, 2234
Enhancer(s), in gene expression, *8,* 8–9, *10*
Enhancer-binding proteins, as transcription factors, 126, *126*
Enkephalin(s), in ACTH regulation, 364
  in gonadotropin-releasing hormone secretion, 2000

Enkephalin(s) *(Continued)*
  in immunoregulation, 2967t, 2972
  in reproductive behavior, 453–455, *455*
  neuronal pathways for, *182*
  physiology of, 2880–2881
  secretion of, ectopic, 2775
    in obesity, 2642
    in paraneoplastic syndromes, 2757t
  vs. endorphins, 362
Enkephalinase, in atrial natriuretic peptide metabolism, 2900
Enteral nutrition, 2675–2676
  complications of, 2673–2674
Enteric hyperoxaluria, 1187
Enteritis, regional, growth attenuation in, 2578, *2578*
Enterochromaffin cells, in carcinoid tumor, 2804
Enterogastrone, 2873
Enteroglucagon, physiology of, 2875
Enteroglucagonoma, 2886
Enteroinsular axis, 1278, 1344
Enteropathy, gluten (celiac disease), gastrointestinal hormone action in, 2883
Enterostatin, in appetite control, 2632–2633
Entrainment, of circadian rhythms, *2490–2491,* 2490–2492, 2495, 2497
Entrapment neuropathy, in diabetes mellitus, 1555
Environmental factors, in diabetes mellitus, 1426t, 1426–1427
  in polyglandular failure syndromes, 3018
  in spermatogenesis, 2409
Enzyme(s). See also specific enzyme.
  genes of, mutations in, detection of, 134–135
    diseases caused by, 130t, 139–140
  inhibitors of, in obesity treatment, 2654
  placental, 2197
Enzyme-linked immunosorbent assay, for thyroid hormones, 623
Enzyme-multiplied immunoassay technique, for thyroid hormones, 623
Eosinophil granule major basic protein, placental, 2197t
Eosinophilic granuloma, delayed puberty in, 1961
  of hypothalamus, 486
Ependymal zone, of median eminence, 153
Ependymoma, precocious puberty in, 1969
Ephedrine, in obesity, 2654
Epidermal growth factor, 2600–2603
  actions of, 2602–2603
    intra-ovarian, 2024
  gene of, 2601, *2601*
  heparin-binding, 2600, *2601*
  in adrenal androgen control, 1841
  in benign prostatic hyperplasia, 2466t, 2466–2467, *2467*
  in fetus, 2251
  in lactation, 2230
  in mammary growth, 2226
  in ovary, 2024
  in parathyroid hormone-related protein/peptide gene expression, 970
  in placental growth, 2176
  in prolactin gene regulation, 375
  in Sertoli cells, 2325
  in steroid synthesis, 2095
  in thyroid hormone mediation, 787
  in thyroid regulation, 543t, 544
    of cell growth and differentiation, *553,* 553–554, *555*
  nomenclature of, 2600
  placental transport of, 2240, 2240t

Epidermal growth factor *(Continued)*
  precursors of, 2601, *2601*
  receptor for, 2602
    activation of, 41–42
    in fetus, 2251
    oncogenes and, 59, 59t
    serine phosphorylation of, 45
    structure of, 28, *28, 2597*
  secretion of, ectopic, 2792
  structure of, 2600–2601, *2601*
Epidermoid cyst, parasellar, 462, 482, *485*
Epididymis, examination of, 2410, *2410*
  obstruction of, infertility in, 2418–2419
  surgery on, 2419
Epinephrine, actions of, 1854, 1858, 1859t
  drug effects on, 180t
    on adrenergic receptors, 1856t
  deficiency of, in diabetes mellitus, 1554
  distribution of, 157
  in ACTH regulation, 363
  in aging, 2714
  in corticotropin-releasing hormone regulation, 343
  in exercise, *2695, 2698*
  in fetus, 2248, *2248,* 2267
  in gluconeogenesis, 2267
  in glucose metabolism, 1394, 1409, 1607–1608, *1608*
  in glycogen metabolism, 47
  in gonadotropin secretion, 1993, *1994*
  in gonadotropin-releasing hormone secretion, *1999,* 1999–2000
  in hypoglycemia, 1607–1608, *1608*
  in ketoacidosis, 1511, 1511t
  in lipolysis, 2667
  in parathyroid hormone secretion, 940
  in prolactin secretion, 185
  insulin response to, 1356
  localization of, 157
  measurement of, in plasma, 1866–1867
    in urine, 1865–1866, 1866t
  placental transport of, 2240–2241
  secretion of, from pheochromocytoma, 1853, 2834, *2835*
  thyroid hormone effects on, *194*
  structure of, *1855*
  synthesis of, *179,* 1854, *1855*
Epiphysis, growth abnormalities of, in hypothyroidism, 794
Epiphysis cerebri. See *Pineal gland.*
Epithelial cells, thyroid, abnormal replication of, 773
Epostane, in progesterone synthesis inhibition, 2210
Equilibrium dialysis, isotopic, in free thyroid hormone measurement, 626–627
Ergocalciferol. See *Vitamin D₂.*
Ergolines. See also *Bromocriptine.*
  in acromegaly, 324–325, *325*
Ergosterol. See *Provitamin D₂ (ergosterol).*
Ergot derivatives, in orthostatic hypotension, 2940
  in prolactinoma, 189
ERK. See *Mitogen-activated protein kinase.*
Erythema, in glucagonoma, 2885–2886
Erythema gyratum repens, as paraneoplastic syndrome, 2761
Erythroblastosis fetalis, growth disorders in, 2567
  hypoglycemia in, 2273
Erythrocytes, glucose levels in, 1390–1391
  glucose metabolism in, 1395–1396, 1396t
  Graves' disease effects on, 688

Hypotension *(Continued)*
    classification of, 2938–2939, 2939t
    clinical manifestations of, 2936
    definition of, 2935
    diagnosis of, 2938–2939, 2939t
    hyperadrenergic, 2936–2937, *2936–2937*
    hypoadrenergic, *2936*, 2936–2938, 2937t
    in diabetes mellitus, 1551, 1560
    in pheochromocytoma, 1862
    pathophysiology of, 2936, *2936*
    treatment of, 2939–2941
    vs. normal orthostatic adaptation, 2935–
        2936, *2936*
Hypothalamic amenorrhea. See under
    Amenorrhea.
Hypothalamic diabetes insipidus, 413t, 413–
    414, *414*
Hypothalamic hypothyroidism, 757, *757*
    neonatal, 790
Hypothalamic-pituitary axis, anatomy of, 152–
    154
    defects of, in Turner's syndrome, 1909, *1909*
    historical aspects of, 151–152
    hormones of, 154–156, *155*
    in B cell development, 1283
    in childhood, 245, 794
    in fetus, 783–784, *784*, 784t
    in hypothyroidism, in children, 794
    in puberty regulation, 1945t, 1946, 1948
    neurotransmitters of, 156–157
    regulation of, neurotransmitters in, 182t
Hypothalamic-pituitary-adrenal axis,
        abnormalities in, amenorrhea in, 2053
    corticotropin-releasing hormone in. See *Corticotropin-releasing hormone.*
    evaluation of, in sexual differentiation disorders, 1926–1927
    hormones of, immunoregulatory, 1648
    in obesity, 2642–2643, 2643t
    of fetus, 2244–2245
    regulation of, acetylcholine in, 183
        catecholamines in, 181, 183
        cytokines in, 1645, 2979t, 2979–2980
        serotonin in, 183
    resetting of, in glucocorticoid resistance,
        1770, 1770–1771
    response of, in endotoxemia, *345*
        in stress, 343
    suppression of, adrenal insufficiency in, 1733,
        1733t
Hypothalamic-pituitary-adrenal-lymphocytic
    axis, 2967, *2968*
Hypothalamic-pituitary-adrenal-ovarian axis,
    postmenopausal, *2131*
Hypothalamic-pituitary-gonadal axis, 242, 242–
    243
    disorders of, 347–349, *348*
    evaluation of, 490–491
        in sexual differentiation disorders, 1926–
            1927
    of fetus, 2245–2246
    regulation of, cytokines in, 2979t, 2980
Hypothalamic-pituitary-ovarian axis, disorders
        of, 2062–2071, *2063*. See also *Ovarian
        failure.*
    hypothalamic failure in, 2064t, 2064–2065,
        2065
    pituitary failure in, 2064t, 2064–2065, *2065*
    gonadotropin secretion and, 1993–1994,
        1994
Hypothalamic-pituitary-thyroid axis, drugs
        affecting, 648–652, 652t
    evaluation of, 641–646, 642t–643t, *642–643*,
        645

Hypothalamic-pituitary-thyroid axis *(Continued)*
    in pregnancy, 803, *805*
    in thyroid regulation, 575–576, 602. See also
        Thyrotropin-releasing hormone.
    of fetus, 2246–2247
    regulation of, cytokines in, 2979t, 2980
    thyrotropin-releasing hormone in, 196–197,
        197
Hypothalamus. See also entries beginning with
    Hypothalamic.
    anatomy of, 152–154
    astrocytoma of, 463
    blood supply of, 153
    blood-brain barrier permeability at, 154
    circadian rhythm pacemaker in, 2493–2497,
        2496
    computed tomography of, 468
    disorders of, adrenal androgen levels in, 1844
        amenorrhea in, 253, *253*, 2064t, 2064–
            2065, *2065*
        appetite disorders in, 2632–2633, *2633*,
            2634t
        growth hormone deficiency in, 2574
        hyperprolactinemia in, 394, 394t
        hypogonadotropic disorders in, *251*, 253,
            253, 255
        hypothyroidism in, 212
        in aging, 2703–2704
        in anorexia nervosa, *2683*, 2683t, 2683–
            2685
        obesity in, 2581, 2632–2633, *2633*, 2645
        thyroid-stimulating hormone response to
            TRH in, 199t, 199–200
    embryology of, 2244
    function of, aging and, 2703–2704
        atrial natriuretic peptide effects on, 2904
        cytokine effects on, 2979t, 2979–2981
        in food intake, 2634, *2635*
    gangliocytoma of, 463
    germ cell tumors of, 463
    glioma of, imaging of, 479, *482*
    gomitoli of, 161
    granulomatous disease of, *485*, 486
    hamartoblastoma of, 463
    hamartoma of, 463
        imaging of, 482, *484*
        precocious puberty in, 1969, *1972–1973*
    hormones of, 151–152, 154–156. See also
        specific hormone.
        in pituitary function testing, 292, 292t–293t
        regulation of, 1645
    infundibulum of. See *Infundibulum; Median
        eminence.*
    injury of, obesity in, 2646
    ''mechanical,'' in ovulation induction, 2043,
        2043
    metastasis to, imaging of, 477, 479, *479*
    neurotransmitters of, 156–157, *182*. See also
        specific neurotransmitter.
    nuclei of, 152, 152t
        hypophyseotropic hormones in, 154–156,
            155
        neurotransmitters in, *155*, 156–157
    reproductive behavior and, 445–457
        cell groups responsible for, 445–447, *446*,
            448
        control of, 449–451
        coordination of, 456
        gene products in, 455–456
        molecular mechanisms of, 451–454, *453–
            455*
        neural circuits for, 448–449, *449*
    sarcoidosis of, testicular function in, 2397

Hypothalamus *(Continued)*
    sex differentiation of, 1893–1894, *1894*,
        1978–1979
    thyroid hormone resistance in, 214
    tumors of, amenorrhea in, 253
        astrocytoma as, 463
        delayed puberty in, 1960
        diabetes insipidus in, 413
        germ cell, 463
        glioma as, 479, *482*
        growth hormone deficiency in, 331
        hamartoma as, 463, 482, *484*
        infundibular, 482
        lipoatrophy in, 1599
        mass effects of, 459t, 459–460
        metabolic sequelae of, 460t–461t, 460–462
        metastatic, 477, 479, *479*
        neurological effects of, 459t
        types of, 463
Hypothermia, in hypothalamic lesions, 460
    in myxedema coma, 765–766
    neonatal, hypoglycemia in, 2273
Hypothyroidism, 752–768
    adrenal function in, 761
    after parathyroidectomy, 1119
    after radiation therapy, 755
    after radioactive iodine treatment, 681
    after thyroidectomy, 755
    autoimmune, in pregnancy, 810
    biochemical changes in, 635t
    bone metabolism in, 1245
    calcium reabsorption in, 1023
    cardiovascular effects of, 759–760
    causes of, 753t–754t, 753–758, *754*, *757*
        differential diagnosis of, 793, 793t
        in neonates, 792
        in pregnancy, 809
    central (secondary), 212, 757, *757*
    clinical features of, *758*, 758t, 758–762
        in children, 793–794, *794*
    congenital, 789t, 789–792, *791*, 871–872
        vs. cretinism, 829
    cretinism in. See *Cretinism.*
    definition of, 752
    diagnosis of, 2090
        in neonates, 790–791, *791*
        in pregnancy, 809–810
    differential diagnosis of, in children, 793,
        793t
    endocrine function in, 761–762
    familial, TSH gene mutation in, 209–210, *210*
    fertility effects of, 799–800, 2090
    fluid and electrolyte metabolism in, 760
    free thyroid hormones in, 626
    frequency of, 752
    gastrointestinal effects of, 760
    goiter in. See *Goiter.*
    gonadal function in, 761
    growth disorders in, 2577
    gynecomastia in, 2478
    hematopoietic effects of, 760
    hyperprolactinemia in, 2066
    hypothalamic, 757, *757*, 790
    idiopathic (atrophic thyroiditis), 753
    immune function in, 2978
    in aging, 2711
    in anorexia nervosa, 2683
    in antithyroid agent ingestion, 756–757
    in congenital defects, 755–756
    in fetus, 789–790, 804–805
    in iodide abnormalities, 756, 873–874
    in iodotyrosine dehalogenase deficiency,
        880–881

Metyrapone test, for adrenal function, 1736–1737
 in Cushing's syndrome, 1754–1755
Metyrosine, in pheochromocytoma, preoperative, 1870
Mevalonate, in cholesterol synthesis, 2020, *2020*
Mexiletine, in neuropathic pain, 1559, *1559*
Mibolerone, structure of, *2364*
Mice. See *Mouse.*
Microadenoma, pituitary. See under *Pituitary adenoma.*
Microalbuminuria, in diabetic nephropathy, 1573–1575
β_2-Microglobulin, accumulation of, in dialysis, 1158
Micronodular adrenal disease, Cushing's syndrome in, 1748
Micropenis, sexual differentiation disorders with, 1923
Micropinocytosis, of thyroglobulin, *512*, 512–513, 532, 550
Microprolactinoma, treatment of, 189
Microsomal proteins, thyroid, antibodies to, 634
Microsomes, antibodies to, in thyroid disease, 729t, 729–730
Midgets, 2563
Midline defects, congenital, delayed puberty in, 1960
Midrodrine, in orthostatic hypotension, 2940
Mifepristone. See *RU 486.*
Miglitol, in diabetes mellitus, 1495
Migration inhibitory factors, in polyglandular failure syndromes, 3017
Milk. See also *Lactation.*
 composition of, 2232–2233
 lipids of, synthesis of, 2227, *2227*
 oral contraceptives in, 2153
 prolactin in, 378
 synthesis of, 2226–2227, *2227*
 thyroid hormone measurement in, 632–633
 vitamin D-fortified, 995
 witch's, 2225, 2474
 yield of, vs. prolactin concentration, 2228–2229
Milk-alkali syndrome, hypercalcemia in, 1087–1088
Milk-ejection reflex, 424–425, 2231
Milkman's syndrome, 1209
Miller and Moses water deprivation test, 494
Millet, as goitrogen, 823
Mineralization, bone. See under *Bone.*
Mineralocorticoids. See also *Aldosterone.*
 deficiency of, clinical features of, 1732
 in adrenal insufficiency, 1732
 excess of. See also *Aldosteronism; Conn's syndrome.*
 apparent, 1678
 acquired, 1795t, 1795–1798
 clinical spectrum of, 1792, 1794t
 congenital, 1791–1795, *1793–1794,* 1794t
 diagnosis of, 1792, 1794, *1794*
 ectopic ACTH syndrome as, 1796–1797
 essential hypertension as, 1797–1798
 from exogenous mineralocorticoids, 1798
 glucocorticoid resistance as, 1797
 pathophysiology of, 1792, *1793,* 1795–1796
 prevalence of, 1792
 treatment of, 1794–1795
 corticosterone in, 1791
 deoxycorticosterone in, 1791

Mineralocorticoids (Continued)
 electrolyte metabolism in, 1699t, 1699–1701, *1700*
 hypertension in, 2921
 in adrenal carcinoma, 1789
 in adrenal hyperplasia, 1789
 in angiotensin II-responsive aldosterone-producing adenoma, 1789
 in ectopic ACTH syndrome, 1796–1797
 in essential hypertension, 1797–1798
 in glucocorticoid resistance. See *Glucocorticoid(s), resistance to.*
 in 11β-hydroxylase deficiency, 1790–1791
 in 17α-hydroxylase deficiency, 1790
 in Liddle's syndrome, 1798
 in mineralocorticoid therapy, 1798
 in pseudoaldosteronism, 1798
 exogenous, apparent mineralocorticoid excess syndrome from, 1798
 receptors for, 1644
 affinity of, 1698
 classic, 1677–1678
 dysfunction of, in apparent mineralocorticoid excess, 1792, *1793–1794,* 1794
 pseudohypoaldosteronism in, 1807–1808
 feedback via, 1645–1646
 functions of, 1677–1678
 in brain, 1649–1650
 membrane, 1678
 sites of, 1668, 1689–1690
 structure of, 1677
 resistance to, 1807–1809
 type I (classic form), 1807–1808
 type II (Gordon's syndrome), 1808–1809
 secretion of, *1698,* 1698–1699, 2713
Minerals, in diabetic diet, 1491
MIT. See *Monoiodotyrosine (MIT).*
Mithramycin. See *Plicamycin (mithramycin).*
Mitochondria, gigantism of, in acidophil stem-cell adenoma, 169, *170*
 glucose oxidation in, in glucose metabolism, 1332
 in calcium regulation, 70–71, *71*
 steroid synthesis in, *1633,* 1633–1635, *1635*
Mitochondrial phosphoprotein pp30, as labile protein factor, 1634–1635
Mitogen-activated protein kinase, 44, *44*
 actions of, 47–48
 in insulin action, 1373, *1374,* 1380
Mitogen-activated protein kinase-kinase, 44, *44,* 47–48
 in insulin action, 1380
Mitogenesis, bombesin in, 2612
 growth factors in, 2592
 insulin-like growth factor in, 317
 of thyroid cells, 552–554, *553*
Mitosis, in growth, 2549
Mitotane, in Cushing's disease, 1757
Mixed antiglobulin test, for sperm antibodies, 2412
Möbius syndrome, delayed puberty in, 1962
 hypogonadism in, 2381
Model-based methods, for hormone secretion analysis, 2523
MODY (maturity-onset diabetes of youth), 1412t, 1413–1415, 1457
Molar disease. See *Trophoblastic disease.*
Molar thyrotropin, measurement of, 637
Molecular biology techniques, blotting procedures as, 123–124, *124,* 124t
 cloned cDNAs in, 123
 functional assays as, 133–135, *135*
 in clonality determination, 141–142
 in disease, 120–140, 130t

Molecular biology techniques (Continued)
 endocrine syndromes as, 139
 from binding protein mutations, 136–137
 from gene deletions and mutations, 131t, 131–135, *132–135,* 134t
 from hormone mutations, 135–136, *136*
 from receptor mutations, 137, 137–138
 from signaling system mutations, 142–143, *143*
 from somatic mutations, 140–143, *143*
 from steroidogenic enzyme mutations, 139–140
 from transcription factor mutations, 138–139
 in DNA library preparation and screening, 121–122, *123*
 in DNA sequencing, 122–123, *123*
 in gene expression analysis, 123–124, *124,* 124t
 in gene regulation evaluation, 124–125, *125*
 in gene structure analysis, 119–123, *120–123*
 in post-transcriptional regulation assessment, 124–125
 in protein expression studies, 127–128
 in subcloning DNA into plasmids, 122, *123*
 in transcription factor-DNA interaction analysis, 126–127, *126–127*
 in transient gene expression studies, 125, *125*
 nuclear run-on assays as, 124
 polymerase chain reaction as. See *Polymerase chain reaction.*
 restriction fragment length polymorphisms as. See *Restriction fragment length polymorphisms.*
 Southern blot as, 131, *132*
 transgenic models in, 128–129, *129*
Moloney murine leukemia virus, gene of, thyroid response element sequences in, *588*
Mondini's cochlea, in Pendred's syndrome, 877
Monoacylglycerol, in arachidonic acid cascade, 2215, *2215*
Monoamine oxidase, in catecholamine metabolism, 1855, *1855*
Monocytes, insulin binding to, 1446, *1447*
 prolactin in, 387, *387*
 vitamin D action on, 1006
Monoiodothyronine (T_1), measurement of, 630
 normal levels of, *622,* 630
 structure of, *622*
Monoiodotyrosine (MIT), 522, *522–523*
 defective coupling of, 872t, 877–878, *878*
 deiodination of, 534
 levels of, in iodine deficiency, 825
 normal, *622,* 631
 measurement of, 631
 proportion of, 608
 radioiodide labeled, in deiodinase activity measurement, 646
 secretion of, 534
 structure of, *622*
 synthesis of, 524, 529, *530–531*
Mononeuropathy, in diabetes mellitus, 1547–1548
Mononuclear cells, vitamin D action in, *1005,* 1005–1006
Mood, oral contraceptive effects on, 2146
Moon facies, in Cushing's syndrome, 1741, *1743*
Moore-Federman, 2571t
"Morning-after pill," 2159, 2159t
Morphine, in corticotropin-releasing hormone regulation, 344

Morris, syndrome of (androgen resistance), *1920*, 1920–1921

Mortality, in breast cancer, 2847
  in Cushing's syndrome, 1763
  in diabetes mellitus, with autonomic neuropathy, 1556
    with nephropathy, 1586, *1586*
  in hyperparathyroidism, 1048
  in nonthyroidal illnesses, prediction of, 666, *666*
  in oral contraceptive use, 2152
  in thyroid carcinoma, 840, *840*, 842–844, *844*

Morula, blastocyst formation from, 2172

mos oncogene, in receptor regulation, 113

Motilin, in pituitary hormone regulation, 187t
  physiology of, 2875–2876

Motor neuropathy, in diabetes mellitus, 1546–1547

Mouse, *little*, receptor defects in, 56
  transgenic, applications of, 128–129, *129*
    in multiple endocrine neoplasia, 2827

Movement disorders, thyrotropin-releasing hormone in, 200

mRNA. See *RNA, messenger.*

MSHs. See *Melanocyte-stimulating hormones.*

Mucopolysaccharide storage diseases, growth disorders in, 2569

Mucormycosis, in ketoacidosis, 1515

Mucosa, neuromas of, in multiple endocrine neoplasia, *2836*, 2836–2837

Mucus, cervical. See under *Cervix.*

Müllerian ducts, 1891–1892, *1892–1893*

Müllerian inhibiting substance/factor. See *Antimüllerian hormone.*

Müllerian tubercle, 1891, *1892*

Multinodular goiter. See under *Goiter.*

Multiple autoimmune endocrinopathy. See *Polyglandular failure syndromes.*

Multiple endocrine insufficiency. See *Polyglandular failure syndromes.*

Multiple endocrine neoplasia, clinical features of, 2816–2819
  diagnosis of, 867
  growth hormone-releasing hormone and, 284–285
  overlap syndrome in, 2815
  paraneoplastic syndromes and, 2766
  parathyroid pathology in, 1107
  prognosis for, 863
  type 1, 2815–2831
    adenomas in, 319
    adrenal cortical tumors in, 2818
    age of onset of, 2822, *2822*
    animal models for, 2817
    asymptomatic, 2823–2825, *2824–2825*
    carcinoid tumors in, 2818
    carriers of, 2825, *2825*
    circulating growth factor in, 2826–2827
    genetics of, 130t, 133, *134*, 140–141, 863, *2819–2825*, 2819–2826
    historical aspects of, 2815–2816
    insulinoma in, 1612
    lipomas in, 2818
    pancreatic tumors in, 2817–2818
    parathyroid tumors in, 1045–1046, 2816–2817
    pheochromocytoma in, 1863–1864
    pituitary tumors in, 2818
    screening for, 2823–2825, *2824–2825*
    thyroid tumors in, 2819
    treatment of, 2816–2819
    tumors characteristic of, 2815, 2816t
    vs. type 2, 2815, 2816t
  type 2, classification of, 863

Multiple endocrine neoplasia *(Continued)*
  diseases in, 910t, 910–911, *911*
  epidemiology of, 2832
  genetics of, 130t, 140–141, 863, 2839–2841, *2840–2841*
  historical aspects of, 2832
  incidence of, 2832
  pathophysiology of, 2823, *2823*
  treatment of, 911
  vs. type 1, 2815, 2816t
  type 2A, 864, 2580
    clinical features of, 2832–2837, *2833–2836*
    cutaneous amyloidosis variant of, *2836*, 2935
    definition of, 2832
    genetics of, 2840–2841, *2841*
    hyperparathyroidism in, 2835, 2839, 2842
    overlap with type 2B, 2837
    parathyroid carcinoma in, 1045
    pheochromocytoma in, 1863t, 1863–1864, 2834–2835, *2835*, 2838–2839, 2842
    screening for, 2837–2839, *2838*
    thyroid carcinoma in, *2833–2834*, 2833–2835, 2837–2838, *2838*, 2841–2842
    treatment of, 2841–2842
    tumors characteristic of, 2815, 2816t
  type 2B, 864, *865–866*, 867
    clinical features of, 2835–2837, *2836*
    definition of, 2832
    gene of, 130t
    hyperparathyroidism in, 2842
    mucosal neuromas in, *2836*, 2836–2837
    overlap with type 2A, 2837
    pheochromocytoma in, 1863t, 1863–1864, 2835–2836, 2842
    screening for, 2839
    treatment of, 2841–2842
    tumors characteristic of, 2815, 2816t
  type 3, nerve growth factors in, 2611
    pheochromocytoma in, 1863t, 1863–1864

Multiple hormone resistance, in pseudohypoparathyroidism, 1144–1145

Multiple lentigenes syndrome, hypogonadism in, 2381

Multiple myeloma, hypercalcemia in, 1062–1063
  osteomalacia in, 1219–1220

Multiple organ failure syndrome, nutritional therapy in, 2674–2675

Multiple sclerosis, somatostatin levels in, 273

Multipotential colony-stimulating factor. See under *Colony-stimulating factor(s).*

Multisubunit receptors family, 23t, 25t, *29*, 29–30

Mumps, orchitis in, 2391–2392

Munchausen's syndrome, factitious Cushing's syndrome in, 1749–1750

Muscle, adrenergic receptors in, 1857t
  androgen receptors in, 2369
  atrophy of, in hyperparathyroidism, 1051–1052
    testicular function in, 2396
  biopsy of, in diabetic neuropathy, 1557
  disorders of, as paraneoplastic syndromes, 2760
  glucose metabolism in, *1395*, 1395–1397, 1396t, 1401–1402, *1401–1402*
    in exercise, 2694
  glucose transport in, insulin and, 1381
  glycogenolysis in, 1390
  hypertrophy of, in anabolic steroid use, 2369
  hypothyroidism effects on, 759
  insulin metabolism in, 1359
  insulin resistance in, 1446

Muscle *(Continued)*
  proteolysis of, in fasting, 1393, *1393*
  smooth, parathyroid hormone-related protein effects on, 971–972
  weakness of, in Cushing's syndrome, 1744
    in diabetic neuropathy, 1546–1547
    in hyperparathyroidism, 1051–1052
    in hypoaldosteronism, 1804
    in osteomalacia, 1208
    in phosphate deficiency, 1025–1026
    in renal failure, 1157
    in rickets, 1208

Muscular dystrophy, myotonic, testicular failure in, 2392

Mutagenesis, in receptor structure studies, 22–23

Mutation, detection of, methods for, 131t, 131–135, *132–135*, 134t
  diseases caused by, 129–131, 130t
    binding protein disorders as, 130t, 136–137
    endocrine syndromes as, 130t, 139
    identification of, 131t, 131–135, *132–135*, 134t
    signal pathway disorders as, 130t, 142–143, *143*
    transcription factor disorders as, 130t, 138–139
  in multiple endocrine neoplasia, 133, *134*
  in thyroid medullary carcinoma, 864
  knockout gene approaches in, 129, *129*
  of aldosterone synthase gene, 1776, *1777*
  of androgen receptor genes, 2339–2340, 2340t–2341t
  of chorionic somatomammotropin gene, 2186
  of cyclin D1 gene, 130t, 143
  of enzyme genes, 130t, 139–140
  of G protein genes, 1140–1141, *1141*, 1145–1146
  of glucocorticoid receptor genes, 108, *1770*, 1770–1774, *1772–1773*
  of hormone genes, 130t, 135–136, *136*
  of 11β-hydroxylase gene, gene of, 1822, *1822*
  of 3β-hydroxysteroid dehydrogenase gene, 1824, *1824*
  of hypoxanthine phosphoribosyltransferase gene, 259, *260*, 319
  of insulin gene, 1601t–1602t, 1601–1602
  of insulin receptor gene, 1375, *1376*, 1597, 1597t, 1597–1598
  of parathyroid hormone precursor genes, *1129*, 1129–1130
  of pit-1 gene, 210, *210*, 374
  of progesterone receptor gene, 108
  of protein genes, site-directed, 128
  of receptor genes, 54–56, *55*, 55t
    nuclear, 130t, *137*, 137–138
  of thyroglobulin gene, 878–880, *879*
  of thyroid hormone receptor genes, 595, *595*, 881–884, *882–883*
  of thyroid-stimulating hormone genes, 209–210, *210*
  site-directed, 125, *125*, 128
  somatic, endocrine neoplasia in, 140–143, *143*

Myasthenia, as paraneoplastic syndrome, 2760

Myasthenia gravis, Graves' disease with, 719, *719*
  thyroid antibodies in, 738t

Mycoplasmal infections, infertility in, 2089

Myelin, abnormal composition of, diabetic neuropathy and, 1541
  glycation of, diabetic neuropathy and, 1540

Pituitary adenoma *(Continued)*
  treatment of, 324, 500–502, 501t. See also *Transsphenoidal surgery.*
  types of, 166
  vs. aneurysm, 464
  vs. craniopharyngioma, 462–463
  vs. metastatic tumor, 464
  vs. Rathke's cyst, 462
Pituitary adenylate cyclase-activating peptide, 2878–2879
Pituitary apoplexy, 165, 472, *474*
Pituitary gland. See *Pituitary.*
Pituitary hormones. See also specific hormone.
  deficiency of, after radiation therapy, 501
    combined, 210, *210*
    in craniopharyngioma, 462–463
  excess of. See also *Acromegaly;* specific hormone.
    pituitary function testing in, 494t–495t, 494–495
  in immunoregulation, 2973–2975, 2974t
  of fetus, 2244t–2245t, 2244–2247
  replacement therapy with, 502–503
  secretion of. See also entries beginning with *Hypothalamic-pituitary.*
    cytokine effects on, 2981
    from immunocompetent cells, 2966, 2967t
    in aging, 2704–2709
    pulsatile, 2513–2514
    regulation of, neuropeptides in, 186–188, 187t
      neurotransmitters in, 181–186, 182t
      somatostatin in, 272
      therapeutic interventions for, 188–189
    rhythms of, 2487–2488, *2488*
    tests for. See *Pituitary, function of, testing of.*
  thymic hormone effects on, 2969
Pituitary hypothyroidism, 757
  neonatal, 790
Pituitary stalk, compression of, 459
Pituitary transcription factor, 374
Pituitary tumors. See also *Pituitary adenoma.*
  ACTH-secreting, localization of, 1756
  angiography of, 469
  biopsy of, 499
  carcinoma as, 166
  cavernous sinus venography in, 467
  complications of, 458t, 458–459
  computed tomography of, 467–469, *468, 470–471,* 472
  corticotropinoma as, 1758–1759
  craniopharyngioma, 166
  Cushing's disease in. See *Cushing's disease (pituitary-dependent Cushing's syndrome).*
  delayed puberty in, 1960
  differential diagnosis of, 459
  granular cell, 462
  growth hormone deficiency in, 331
  growth hormone secretion from, 318–319
  hyperprolactinemia in, 2066
  hypothalamic involvement of, metabolic sequelae of, 460t–461t, 460–462
  in multiple endocrine neoplasia, 2818
  magnetic resonance imaging of, 469, *470–473,* 472
  mass effects of, 459t, 459–460
  metastatic, 463–464, 464t
  natural history of, 458t, 458–459
  neurological effects of, 459t
  oncocytoma as, 174–175, *175*
  prolactin cell hyperplasia in, 163
  prolactinoma as. See *Prolactinoma.*
  radiation therapy for, 500–502, 501t
  radiography of, 467

Pituitary tumors *(Continued)*
  recurrent, after surgery, 500
  secondary, 166
  thyroid-stimulating hormone response to TRH in, 199t, 199–200
  tomography of, 467
  transsphenoidal surgery in. See *Transsphenoidal surgery.*
  treatment of, 2066–2067
    hormone replacement therapy after, 502–503
  vs. ectopic growth hormone-releasing hormone syndrome, 2776
Pituitary-adrenal axis. See *Hypothalamic-pituitary-adrenal axis.*
Placenta, ACTH processing in, 360
  amino acid transport in, 2259, 2261
  aromatase activity in, 2194–2195
  blood supply of, 2175
  calcium transport in, 972, *972*
  carbohydrate transport in, 2260–2261
  catecholamine transport in, 2240–2241
  cholesterol receptors on, 2190–2191
  chorion frondosum of, 2173, *2173, 2175*
  chorion laeve of, *2173,* 2175, *2175,* 2196
  deiodinases in, 783
  development of, 2239–2240
  enzymes of, 2197, 2197t
    secretion of, in malignancy, 2783
  formation of, *2172–2176,* 2172–2177
  fuel transport in, 2258–2261, *2259*
  functions of, 2258–2259
    DHAS loading test for, 1844
  glucose transport in, 1465
  glycogen synthesis in, 2261
  growth of, 2175–2177, *2176,* 2551
  hormone transport in, 2240t, 2240–2241
  hormones of, 2171–2172, 2241–2243, 2287–2288, *2288.* See also *Chorionic gonadotropin.*
    activins as, 2190
    amniotic, 2196
    chorionic proopiomelanocortin peptides as, 2189, *2189*
    chorionic somatomammotropin as, 2183–2187, *2184–2185*
    corticotropin-releasing hormone as, 350, *2187–2188,* 2187–2189, 2295
    estrogens as, 2193–2196, *2194–2195,* 2241, *2241*
    gene expression of, 2178
    growth hormone as. See *Growth hormone, placental.*
    inhibins as, 2010, 2190, *2191*
    neuropeptide, 2189–2190, *2190,* 2242–2243
    polypeptide, 2242
    progesterone as, 2241
    progestins as, 2190–2193, *2192–2193*
    steroid, 1841, *1841*
  insulin metabolism in, 1359, 1464
  iodide transport by, 804
  lactate transport in, 2261
  lipid transport in, 2259, 2259–2260
  permeability of, 2240t, 2240–2241
  polypeptide transport in, 2240, 2240t, 2259
  pregnancy-associated plasma protein A in, 2197, 2197t
  pregnancy-specific β_1-glycoproteins in, 2197, 2197t
  protein transport in, 2259
  proteins in, 2196–2197, 2197t
  species variation in, 2239–2240
  steroid hormone transport in, 2240, 2240t

Placenta *(Continued)*
  structure of, *2172–2176,* 2172–2177, 2239
  thyroid hormone transport in, 803–804, 2240, 2240t
  thyrotropic activity in, 676–677
  thyrotropin-releasing hormone in, 199
  trophoblast of. See *Trophoblast; Trophoblastic disease.*
  villi of, 2172–2174, *2172–2174*
Placental lactogens. See *Chorionic somatomammotropin (placental lactogen).*
Plasma, somatostatin in, 270t
  volume of, in pregnancy, 2287
Plasma membrane, thyroid hormone action in, 585, 585t
  turnover of, in thyroglobulin transport, 514
Plasma protein receptor family, 25t, 30–31
Plasma renin activity, factors affecting, 2919–2920, *2920*
  in aging, 2713
  in hypertension classification, 2918–2920, *2919–2920*
    inhibition of, atrial natriuretic peptide in, 2903, *2903*
  measurement of, 2918–2920
  in aldosteronism, 1781, 1783t
Plasmacytoma, of pituitary, 464
Plasmids, DNA subcloning into, 122, *123*
Plasminogen activator, in Sertoli cells, 2325
Platelet(s), function of, phosphate in, 1026
Platelet-activating factor, in parturition, 2213, 2216
Platelet-derived growth factor, 2592
  actions of, 2607–2608, *2608*
  gene of, 2607
  historical aspects of, 2606
  in benign prostatic hyperplasia, 2466t, 2466–2467
  in bone resorption regulation, 1199
  in placental growth, 2176
  nomenclature of, 2606
  precursors of, 2607
  processing of, 2607
  receptor for, 28, *28,* 2607, *2607*
    activation of, 41–42
    oncogenes and, 59, 59t
  signaling of, 2607
Plicamycin (mithramycin), in hypercalcemia, 1097, 1100t
  in Paget's disease, 1270
Plummer's disease, 777, *777*
Plurihormonal adenoma, 175
P-Mod-S protein, in Sertoli cells, 2316–2317, 2324
Pneumothorax, in parenteral nutrition, 2674
POEMS syndrome, vs. polyglandular failure syndrome, 3020
Poikiloderma congenita, growth disorders in, 2571t
Poikilothermia, in hypothalamic lesions, 460
Poisoning, aluminum. See *Aluminum, intoxication with.*
  heavy metal, osteomalacia in, 1220
  organic, vs. diabetic ketoacidosis, 1512t
Poland syndrome, hypogonadism in, 2381
Poly-A tail, of RNA, 121
Polyadenylation, in gene expression, *10,* 10–11
  of RNA, 121
Polycystic ovarian syndrome, 2124
  amenorrhea in, 2068–2069
  anovulation in, 2055–2056, *2055–2056,* 2073, 2100
  clinical characteristics of, 2100
  diagnosis of, 2099–2100

Pregnancy (Continued)
follicle cyst in, 2125
glomerular filtration rate in, 2287
glucagon secretion in, 1466
glucocorticoid levels in, 2295, 2295
glucose screening in, 1420
goiter in, 800t, 805
Graves' disease in, 705–706
growth hormone secretion in, 318
human chorionic gonadotropin in. See *Chorionic gonadotropin, human.*
hyperandrogenism in, 2103
hypercalcemia in, 2299–2300
hyperemesis gravidarum in, 2294, 2294–2295
hyperparathyroidism in, 1054–1055
hyperprolactinemia and, 398–399
hyperreactio luteinalis in, 2125
hyperthyroidism in, 705–706, 800t, 806t, 806–808, 2293–2295, 2294
neonatal Graves' disease in, 792
hypothalamic-pituitary-thyroid axis in, 803, 805
hypothyroidism in, 762, 800t, 808–810, 2295
immunomodulation in, 2977–2978
in vitamin D-dependent rickets, 1177
inhibin in, 2014
insulin dynamics in, 1355, 1464–1465
insulin-like growth factor-I levels in, 2290
iodide in, deficiency of, 2292
levels of, 611
metabolism of, 801, 801t
ketoacidosis in, vs. diabetic ketoacidosis, 1512t
luteoma in, 2125
maintenance of, after ovarian removal, 2036
menstruation after, 2152–2153
metabolism in, 1464–1466
monitoring of, chorionic gonadotropin measurement in, 2181–2182, 2182t
progesterone assay in, 2193
obesity in, 2640–2641
oral contraceptive ingestion during, 2150
oral contraceptives after, 2152–2153
ovarian tumors in, 2120–2121
ovulation after, 2152–2153
oxytocin receptor in, 426
parathyroid gland function in, 2298–2299, 2299
pheochromocytoma in, 1872–1873, 2298, 2842
pituitary tumor enlargement in, 2066–2067
placental growth hormone levels in, 2185
plasma volume in, 2287
prevention of. See *Contraceptives.*
prolactin cell hyperplasia in, 162–163, 163
prolactin in, 2227
secretion of, 378
synthesis of, 376–377
prolactinoma in, 2289, 2289, 2289t
prolonged, 2207, 2207t
rates of, 2405
renin levels in, 2297, 2297–2298
tests for, chorionic gonadotropin measurement in, 2181–2182, 2182t
thyroid disorders in, carcinoma as, 812–813
goiter as, 800t, 805
hyperthyroidism as, 705–706, 800t, 806t, 806–808, 2293–2295, 2294
hypothyroidism as, 800t, 808–810, 2295
nodules as, 800t, 812
types of, 799, 800t
wastage in, 800

Pregnancy (Continued)
thyroid function in, 609–612, 612, 649, 801t, 801–805, 802–805, 2292–2293, 2293–2294
thyroid hormone levels in, 611, 672, 801–802, 802–803
thyroiditis after. See *Thyroiditis, autoimmune (Hashimoto's disease), postpartum.*
thyroxine-binding globulin levels in, 565, 611, 612
virilization in, 2103
vitamin D-binding proteins in, 1001
wastage in, thyroid disorders and, 800
weight gain in, 2640–2641, 2644
with diabetes, 1469
with intrauterine device in place, 2163–2164
Pregnancy protein 19, 2177t
Pregnancy-associated plasma protein A, 2197, 2197t
Pregnancy-specific β₁-glycoproteins, 2197, 2197t
Pregnenediol, formation of, in pregnancy, 2192
urinary, monitoring of, for fertile period determination, 2144
Pregnenolone, androgen synthesis from, 1836, 1837
corticosteroid synthesis from, 1631, 1631–1632
excess of, in 3β-hydroxysteroid dehydrogenase deficiency, 1824, 1914
in benign prostatic hyperplasia, 2463t
steroid synthesis from, 2020, 2020–2021, 2315, 2315
androgenic, 2093, 2094
synthesis of, 1631, 1631, 1634, 2020, 2020–2021, 2093, 2094, 2314–2316, 2315
defects in, pseudohermaphroditism in, 1913t, 1913–1914
testosterone synthesis from, 2351, 2352
Pregnenolone sulfate, synthesis of, in fetal adrenal cortex, 2194, 2194
Prelysosomes, in endocytosis, 32–33, 33
in thyroglobulin transport, 509, 513, 533
Premature infants. See *Neonates, premature.*
Premature ovarian failure. See under *Ovarian failure.*
Premenstrual syndrome, 1985
luteinizing hormone secretion in, 2532
thyroid function and, 800
Prenatal diagnosis, of sexual differentiation disorders, 1930, 1930t
Prenatal genetic screening, chorionic gonadotropin assay in, 2182
Preoptic region, reproductive behavior and, 445–447, 446, 448
Preproenkephalins, genes of, 356–357
in reproductive behavior, 455
Preproglucagon, 1337, 1338, 1339
Prepro-gonadotropin-releasing hormone, 220, 220–221
Preproinsulin, 1300–1301, 1301
gene of, mutation of, 136
Preproopiomelanocortin, 359
endopeptidase cleavage of, 359, 359
Prepropancreatic polypeptide, 1318, 1319
Preproparathyroid hormone, 933–934, 934–935, 936
gene of, mutation of, 1129, 1129–1130
Prepropeptides, processing of, 360–361
Preprosomatostatin, 271, 1317, 1318
Preprotachykinin, 2881
Pressure-natriuresis-diuresis response, 1694, 1694, 1700
Preterm labor, endocrinology of, 2218
Pretibial myxedema. See *Myxedema, pretibial.*

Previtamin D₃, synthesis of, 992, 992–994, 994
Priapism, in impotence treatment, 2438–2439
Principal cell, in electrolyte transport, 1689
Proatrial natriuretic peptide, 2896–2897
Probucol, in dyslipoproteinemia, 2749t–2750t
Procollagen, measurement of, in bone metabolism evaluation, 1233
Production rate, of ovarian hormones, 2025, 2025t
Proenkephalin, in reproductive behavior, 453–455, 455
Progeria, 2571t
Progesterone, actions of, intra-ovarian, 2024
after embryo transfer, 2091
androgen receptor binding affinity of, 2341t
antagonists to, 110
binding proteins for, 2025–2026
in androgen synthesis, 2022
in androstenedione synthesis, 2093, 2094
in benign prostatic hyperplasia, 2463t
in chorionic gonadotropin synthesis, 2180
in corticosteroid synthesis, 1631, 1631–1632
in follicular fluid, 2035, 2035, 2095, 2095
oocyte maturity and, 2041
in gonadotropin secretion, 248–249, 1997
in gonadotropin-releasing hormone regulation, 1997, 2001, 2001, 2003, 2004
in hypothalamic amenorrhea, 2052, 2052
in intrauterine devices, 2161, 2161
in lactation, 2230
in luteal phase defects, 2090
in mammary growth, 2226
in polycystic ovarian syndrome, 2055–2056, 2056
in pregnancy, 2190–2193, 2192–2193, 2210t, 2210–2211
species dependent on, 2208, 2208t
in reproductive behavior, actions of, 449, 449
hypothalamic control of, 450
molecular mechanisms of, 451
in testosterone synthesis, 2352
in vitamin D metabolism, 1002
levels of, normal, 2025t
vs. inhibin levels, 2013, 2013
maternal ingestion of, fetal effects of, 1923
measurement of, in ovulation documentation, 2081
in pregnancy, 2193
metabolism of, 2020–2021, 2021, 2025t
in pregnancy, 2192, 2193
placental, 2190–2193, 2192–2193
placental transport of, 2240
receptor for, content of, factors affecting, 2027–2028
DNA binding of, 105
in breast cancer, 2851
in endometrium, 2857–2858
mutations in, 108
on lymphocytes, 2976–2977
phosphorylation of, 111
purification of, 96–97, 96–98
regulation of, 112
reproductive behavior and, 451–453, 453
thyroid hormone receptor homology to, 593
transcription activation functions of, 106–107
transformation of, 95, 95–96
transport of, 110
resistance to, receptor gene mutation in, 108
secretion of, 2022
from corpus luteum, 2035–2036
from ovarian tumor, 2115
from placenta, 2191–2192, 2192

Quetelet index, 2627, *2627*
Quingolide. See *CV205–502 (mesulergine, quingolide).*

R 1881, structure of, *94*
R5020 (progestin), actions of, 2028
Rabson-Mendenhall syndrome, insulin resistance in, 1599
Rachitic disease. See *Rickets.*
Radial neuropathy, in diabetes mellitus, 1547
Radiation, testicular failure in, 2392
Radiation therapy, bone growth disorders in, 2582
 cranial, amenorrhea in, 253
  delayed puberty from, 1960
  short stature in, 290
 for acromegaly, 324
 for carcinoid tumor, 2810
 for craniopharyngioma, 463
 for Cushing's disease, 1759
 for gonadotrophic adenoma, 264, 264t
 for Graves' ophthalmopathy, 720–721
 for hyperprolactinemia, 399–400, 402
 for pituitary tumor, 500–502, 501t
 for prostate cancer, 2859–2860
 for subacute thyroiditis, 746
 for testicular tumor, germ cell, 2442
 for thyroid carcinoma, 851, 851t
 for thyroid nodule, 905
 hypothyroidism after, 755
 ovarian failure in, delayed puberty in, 1962
 parathyroid adenoma in, 1045
 semen cryopreservation before, 2429
 side effects of, 501–502
 testicular injury in, 1963, 2408–2409
 thyroid carcinoma caused by, 840–841, *841*, 905, 908
Radiculopathy, abdominal, in diabetes mellitus, 1548
Radioactive iodide. See *Iodine and iodide, radioactive.*
Radioactive iodide uptake test, of thyroid function, 618–620, 619t–620t, *619–620*
 in iodide deficiency, 827
 in subacute thyroiditis, 745, *745*
Radiography, in delayed puberty evaluation, 1964
 of sellar region, 467
 of thyroid, 639–640
Radioimmunoassay, for cyclic adenosine monophosphate, 1112
 for follistatin, 2012
 for gonadotropins, 237
 for growth hormone-releasing hormone, 284
 for inhibin, 2011
 for parathyroid hormone, 1075–1080, *1078–1079*
 for prolactin, 375
 for somatostatin, 269–270, 270t
 for thyroglobulin antibodies, 728, *729*, 729t
 for thyroid hormones, 622–623
 for thyroid-stimulating hormone, 641
 vs. radioreceptor assay, 19
Radioisotope tests, of bone metabolism, 1233
 of glucose metabolism, 1391–1392
 of thyroid function, 618–621, 619t–620t, *619–620*, 638t, 638–639
Radioligand assays, for gonadotropins, 237
 for thyroid hormones, 622–623
Radioreceptor assay, 19, *19*
 for prolactin, 375
Radioreceptor-to-radioimmunoassay ratios, in ovarian failure, 252, *252*

Radiosurgery, of pituitary, in Cushing's disease, 1759
Raf protein kinase, 44, *44*
 actions of, 48
 activation of, *46, 47*
RAIU test. See *Radioactive iodide uptake test.*
Ranatensins, physiology of, 2879
Randle cycle, 1393, *1404*, 1404–1405
Ranitidine, in Zollinger-Ellison syndrome, 2817
ras genes and proteins, growth factors and, 2614
 in insulin signal transmission, 1380
 in protein kinase activation, *46*
 in receptor regulation, 113
 in signal transduction, 43–44, *44*
 in thyroid carcinoma, 842
 mutation of, 130t, 142, *143*
  detection of, 133, *133*
Ras guanine nucleotide-releasing factor, 43, *44*
Receptor(s), acetylcholine, 26, 31
 adrenergic. See *Adrenergic receptors.*
 affinity labeling of, 96, *96*
 affinity of, 19–20, 56
 androgen. See *Androgen(s), receptor for.*
 angiotensin, 1673–1674, *1674*
 antibodies to, 19
 antigen-specific, *2992*, 2992–2993
 atrial natriuretic peptide, 1691
 benzodiazepine, as labile protein factor, 1634–1635
 binding to, in cAMP-dependent signaling, 79, *79*
 calcitonin, 24t, 26, 982–983, *983*
 calcium, 941
 catecholamine, vs. gonadotropin receptors, 238
 cellular content of, regulation of, 112–113
 cholecystokinin, 2872, *2873*
 cholesterol, 2190–2191
 chorionic gonadotropin, 231, 237–238
 cloning of, 21–23, 98–99, 2991
 colony-stimulating factor. See under *Colony-stimulating factor(s).*
 complexes of, with antagonists, 109–110, 110t
 consensus, *100*, 102, 104t
 corticotropin-releasing hormone, 342
 cross-reactivity of, 58, *58*, 58t
 cytokine, 308, *309*, 382–383, *383*
 degradation of, 32–34, *33*, 33t
 dehydroepiandrosterone, 1838
 dephosphorylation of, 111
 desensitization of, 51–54, *52–54*, 53t, 75
  adrenergic, 27, 84–86, *85*
  endocytosis in, 32–34
 dihydropyridine, *40*
 dioxin, 99
 disorders of, 54–60, *55*, 55t, *57–59*, 58t–59t
  in pseudohypoparathyroidism, *1139*, 1139–1141
 DNA-binding domains of, 99, *100–102*, 104–105
 dopamine, 380, 1856, 1858
 down-regulation of, 52–53
 ectopic, 2792–2793
 endothelin, 2909–2910
 epidermal growth factor. See under *Epidermal growth factor.*
 erythropoietin, 382, *383*, 2956–2957
 estrogen. See under *Estrogen(s).*
 fibroblast growth factor, 28, 41–42, 2609
 follicle-stimulating hormone, 231–232, 237–238, 2022, *2022*, 2316
 functions of, 17–18. See also *Nuclear receptor(s), structural-functional relationships of.*

Receptor(s) *(Continued)*
 G protein, 2022
 gamma-aminobutyric acid. See under *Gamma-aminobutyric acid.*
 genes of, 99, *101*
  mutation of, 130t, *137*, 137–138
 glucagon, 24t, 26, *1344*, 1344–1345
 glucocorticoid. See under *Glucocorticoid(s).*
 glucose, 1329
 glutamate, 26
  metabotropic, 23t–24t, 26
 glycine, 31
 gonadotropin, 237–238
 gonadotropin-releasing hormone, 218, 225–227, *226*, 1996, *1996*
 granulocyte colony-stimulating factor, 382, *383*, 2611
 granulocyte-macrophage colony-stimulating factor, 382, *383*
 growth hormone. See under *Growth hormone.*
 growth hormone-releasing hormone, *281*, 281–282
 guanylate cyclase, 23t, 25t, 29
 hematopoietic growth factor, 30
 hepatocyte growth factor, 29, 42, 2613
 historical studies of, 93–99, *94–98*
 hybrid, insulin-like growth factor-insulin, 315, 1377, 1593–1594
 immunochemistry of, 97, *97*
 in calcium regulation, 72–73, *73*
 in endocytosis, 32–34, *33*, 33t
 in phosphoinositide-specific phospholipase C activation, 67t, 67–69
 in Sertoli cells, 2323
 insulin. See under *Insulin.*
 insulin receptor-related, 1376–1377
 insulin-like growth factors. See under *Insulin-like growth factor(s).*
 interferon, 30, 382, *383*
 interleukin. See under *Interleukin(s).*
 Janus kinase family, 29, *29*
 leukemia inhibitory factor, 2611
 ligand-binding domains of, 99, *100–101*, 105, 108
 lipoprotein, high-density, 2735
  low-density, 30, 2732–2734, *2733*, 2739
 localization of, 98, *98*
 luteinizing hormone. See under *Luteinizing hormone.*
 mannose-6-phosphate, 31, 2596, *2597*
 melanocyte-stimulating hormone, 56
 melatonin, 433, 441–442
 membrane. See *Membrane receptors.*
 mineralocorticoid. See under *Mineralocorticoids.*
 multiple ligands reacting with, 26
 multisubunit, 23t, 25t, *29*, 29–30
 mutations of, 54–56, *55*, 55t
 natriuretic peptide, *2898*, 2898–2899
 nerve growth factor, 25t, 28–30, 2611
 neuromedin B, 2880
 neuropeptide Y, 2881
 nuclear. See *Nuclear receptor(s).*
 numbers of, disorders of, 56
 odorant (rhodopsin-type), 23t–24t, 26, *27*
 on target vs. nontarget cells, 20
 oncostatin M, *2611*
 opioid, 2880–2881
 orphan, 22, 96, 99, 591
 oxytocin. See under *Oxytocin.*
 parathyroid hormone, 942–945, *943*, 948–949, 1141
 parathyroid hormone-related peptide, 942–945, *943*

ISBN 0-7216-4265-9

90038

9 780721 642659